SPECIAL FEATURES—cont'd

Client Education Guides

Continued on inside back cover

ELSEVIER

evolve

The Latest *Evolution* in Learning.

Evolve provides online access to free learning resources and activities designed specifically for the textbook you are using in your class. The resources will provide you with information that enhances the material covered in the book and much more.

Visit the Web address listed below to start your learning evolution today!

▶▶ **LOGIN:** *http://evolve.elsevier.com/Black/medsurg/*

Evolve Student Learning Resources for Black and Hawks: *Medical-Surgical Nursing: Clinical Management for Positive Outcomes,* 7th edition, offers the following features:

- **Open-Book Quizzes:** Each chapter includes interactive self-assessment tools such as multiple choice, fill-in-the-blank, and matching with instant scoring and feedback at the click of a button. Crossword puzzles provide a fun and effective way to reinforce chapter key terms.
- **WebLinks:** An exciting resource that lets you link to hundreds of websites carefully chosen to supplement the content of the textbook. The WebLinks are regularly updated, with new ones added as they develop.
- **Concept Map Creator:** An exciting tool that walks you through the thinking process of creating individualized Concept Maps, from initial diagnoses to interventions to outcomes to a completed plan of care.
- **Additional Resources:** Content comes alive with health assessment animations and videos, a glossary of audio pronunciations, a Fluid & Electrolyte self-study module, and more!
- **Enhanced Web Content:** Discussions of Case Management, Diversity in Health Care, and Ethical Issues in Nursing enhance the wealth of content included in the text. Appendixes, Clinical Pathways, Spanish Assessment phrases and Spanish Client Education Guides provide useful tools for clinical practice. Care Plans, Bridges to Home Health Care, Complementary and Alternative Therapies, Case Studies, and Thinking Critically discussions all serve to reinforce the text content.

Think outside the book... *evolve.*

The CD-ROM included with every copy of *Medical-Surgical Nursing: Clinical Management for Positive Outcomes,* 7th edition, features:

- **Open-Book Quizzes** to test your knowledge with interactive exercises and crossword puzzles
- **Additional Resources** to bring the content alive with health assessment animations and videos and a Fluid & Electrolyte self-study module
- **Case Studies** followed by interactive learning activities and a care plan
- **Discussions for Thinking Critically Questions**

Medical-Surgical Nursing

Clinical Management for Positive Outcomes

Medical-Surgical Nursing

Clinical Management for Positive Outcomes

7th edition

Joyce M. Black, PhD, RN, CPSN, CWCN
Associate Professor
College of Nursing
University of Nebraska Medical Center
Omaha, Nebraska

Jane Hokanson Hawks, DNSc, RN, BC
Professor of Nursing
Midland Lutheran College
Fremont, Nebraska

ELSEVIER
SAUNDERS

Volume 1

ELSEVIER
SAUNDERS

11830 Westline Industrial Drive
St. Louis, Missouri 63146

MEDICAL-SURGICAL NURSING: CLINICAL
MANAGEMENT FOR POSITIVE OUTCOMES
Copyright © 2005 by Elsevier Inc. All rights reserved.

Single Volume 0-7216-0220-7
2-Volume Set 0-7216-0221-5

NOTICE

Nursing is an ever-changing field. Standard safety precautions must be followed, but as new research and clinical experience broaden our knowledge, changes in treatment and drug therapy may become necessary or appropriate. Readers are advised to check the most current product information provided by the manufacturer of each drug to be administered to verify the recommended dose, the method and duration of administration, and contraindications. It is the responsibility of the licensed prescriber, relying on experience and knowledge of the patient, to determine dosages and the best treatment for each individual patient. Neither the publisher nor the author assumes any liability for any injury and/or damage to persons or property arising from this publication.

Previous editions copyrighted 2001, 1997, 1993, 1987, 1980, 1974.

International Standard Book Number 0-7216-0220-7 (Single Volume)
0-7216-0221-5 (2-Volume Set)

Executive Publisher: Barbara Cullen
Senior Developmental Editor: Victoria Bruno
Developmental Editor: Adrienne Simon
Publishing Services Manager: Deborah L. Vogel
Senior Project Manager: Jodi M. Willard
Senior Designer: Kathi Gosche

Printed in United States of America

Last digit is the print number: 9 8 7 6 5 4 3 2 1

When I walked into the hospital, I used to see a sign that said,
"Enter in to learn, go forth to serve." Therefore this book
is dedicated to those students and patients who taught me the
value of caring and teaching, and I hope they can serve others
through my efforts here. I appreciate the quiet contributions of
my colleagues. And I thank my family—Steve, Jon, Katy,
and Tricia—for their ongoing understanding of the
considerable strain on my time and energy.
J.M.B.

To the patients, nurses, students, and faculty I learn from;
to my parents, Esther and the late Charles Hokanson, who
helped me become the person I am; and to my husband,
Edward, and my daughter, Jennifer, whose support
and understanding remain constant.
J.H.H.

Joyce M. Black, PhD, RN, CPSN, CWCN, is an Associate Professor at the University of Nebraska Medical Center College of Nursing in the Adult Health and Illness Department. She teaches junior-level nursing students in medical-surgical nursing and supervises the research activities of several graduate students. Dr. Black received her Doctorate from the University of Nebraska Medical Center College of Nursing in Omaha, Nebraska, in 1999; her Master of Science in Nursing degree from the University of Nebraska Medical Center College of Nursing in 1981; her Bachelor of Science in Nursing degree from Winona State University in Winona, Minnesota; and her Associate's degree in Nursing from Rochester Community College in Rochester, Minnesota.

Dr. Black has had several years of clinical experience as a medical-surgical nurse at Saint Mary's Hospital in Rochester, Minnesota, which is affiliated with the Mayo Clinic. Her clinical practice has been in orthopedics, critical care, burn care, respiratory diseases, wound care, and plastic surgery. She is certified by the American Society of Plastic Surgical Nurses and by the Wound, Ostomy and Continence Nurses Society. Dr. Black also serves as the editor of *Plastic Surgical Nursing* and as a member of the Board of Directors for the National Pressure Ulcer Advisory Panel. Her area of research is in deep tissue injury, pressure ulcers, and wound healing.

Jane Hokanson Hawks, DNSc, RN, BC, is a Professor of Nursing at Midland Lutheran College, Fremont, Nebraska. She teaches sophomore students in medical-surgical nursing and senior students in advanced medical-surgical nursing and nursing management. Dr. Hawks received her Doctorate of Nursing Science in collegiate nursing education from Widener University in Chester, Pennsylvania; her Master of Science in Nursing degree in medical-surgical nursing and nursing administration from the University of Nebraska Medical Center College of Nursing in Omaha, Nebraska; and her Bachelor of Science in Nursing degree from St. Olaf College in Northfield, Minnesota.

Dr. Hawks has worked in and has taught medical-surgical nursing for more than 26 years. She has practiced in a variety of areas, including critical care, renal transplantation, orthopedics, general surgery, and urology. She serves as the editor of *Urologic Nursing*. Her areas of research include empowerment, mentoring, nursing education, active teaching strategies, and alcoholism. She and her colleagues developed the NANDA nursing diagnosis Altered Family Process: Alcoholism (now known as Dysfunctional Family Processes: Alcoholism). Dr. Hawks co-authored *Mentoring for Mission: Nurturing New Faculty at Church-Related Colleges*, which was published in 2003 and funded through a grant from the Lilly Fellows Foundation.

Section Editors

Robert G. Carroll, PhD
Professor,
Department of Physiology,
Brody School of Medicine,
East Carolina University,
Greenville, North Carolina

Annabelle M. Keene, MSN, RN, BC
School Nurse,
Bellevue Public Schools,
Bellevue, Nebraska;
Formerly, Associate Professor,
College of Saint Mary,
Omaha, Nebraska

Sheila Melander, DSN, RN, ACNP-C, FCCM
Professor,
School of Nursing,
University of Tennessee at Memphis,
Memphis, Tennessee;
Cardiovascular Acute Care Nurse Practitioner,
Owensboro, Kentucky

Contributors

Mary A. Allen, MS, RN
Medical Officer/Nurse Consultant,
National Institute of Allergy and Infectious Diseases,
National Institutes of Health,
Bethesda, Maryland

Donna M. Barker, MS, APN/CNS, ONC
Clinical Nurse Specialist, Orthopedics,
Barrington, Illinois

Francie Bernier, MSN, BSN, RNC
Doctoral Student,
University of Virginia,
School of Nursing,
Charlottesville, Virginia;
Clinical Education Specialist,
Hollister, Inc.,
Libertyville, Illinois

Meg Blair, MSN, RN, CEN
Assistant Professor,
Nebraska Methodist College;
Staff Nurse,
Emergency Department,
Creighton University Medical Center,
Omaha, Nebraska

Lisa Bowman, MSN, RN, CRNP, CNRN
Nurse Practitioner,
Clinical Research Coordinator,
Thomas Jefferson University Hospital,
Philadelphia, Pennsylvania

Patricia C. Buchsel, MSN, BSN, FAAN
Chief Operating Officer,
Creative Cancer Concepts, Inc.,
Rockwall, Texas;
Clinical Faculty,
School of Nursing,
University of Washington,
Seattle, Washington

Andrea R. Cain, BSN, RN
Registered Nurse,
Gupta & Mills Cardiology,
Owensboro, Kentucky

Candace Cantwell, RD, RN, CNSD
Clinical Nurse,
Medical Intensive Care Unit,
University of Pennsylvania Medical Center,
Philadelphia, Pennsylvania

Robert G. Carroll, PhD
Professor,
Department of Physiology,
Brody School of Medicine,
East Carolina University,
Greenville, North Carolina

Verna Benner Carson, PhD, MS, APRN/PMH
National Director of RESTORE Behavioral Health,
Tender Loving Care Home Health Care,
Lake Success, New York;
Formerly, Associate Professor,
School of Nursing,
University of Maryland,
Baltimore, Maryland

Linda K. Clarke, MS, RN, CORLN
Head and Neck Nurse Specialist,
Greater Baltimore Medical Center,
Baltimore, Maryland

Charlene Compher, PhD, RD, FAAN
Assistant Professor in Nutrition Science,
School of Nursing,
University of Pennsylvania,
Philadelphia, Pennsylvania

Linda Carman Copel, PhD, RN, CS, DAPA
Associate Professor,
College of Nursing,
Villanova University,
Villanova, Pennsylvania

Tricia C. Corbett, MSPH
Clinical Instructor,
School of Nursing,
University of Washington,
Seattle, Washington

Pamela Cornwell, MA, RN
Assistant Director of Patient Care Services,
Shriners Hospitals for Children,
Sacramento, California

Melissa Craft, MS, RN, AOCN
Assistant Clinical Professor,
University of Oklahoma,
Oklahoma City, Oklahoma;
Oncology Clinical Nurse Specialist,
Breast Imaging of Oklahoma,
Edmund, Oklahoma

Sherill Nones Cronin, PhD, RN, C
Professor of Nursing,
Director, MSN Program,
Bellarmine University;
Nurse Researcher,
Jewish Hospital,
Louisville, Kentucky

Susan L. Dean-Baar, PhD, RN, CRRN, FAAN
Associate Professor,
Associate Dean for Academic Affairs,
School of Nursing,
University of Wisconsin at Milwaukee,
Milwaukee, Wisconsin

Jean Elizabeth DeMartinis, PhD, APRN (FNP-C)
Associate Clinical Professor,
Creighton University,
Omaha, Nebraska;
Cardiology and Prevention Specialist,
Nurse Practitioner,
MidAmerica Cardiovascular Institute,
Omaha, Nebraska

Peggy Doheny, PhD, RN, ONC
Professor,
College of Nursing,
Kent State University,
Kent, Ohio

Charlotte Eliopoulos, PhD, RNC, MPH, ND
President,
Health Education Network,
Glen Arm, Maryland

James A. Fain, PhD, RN, BC-ADM, FAAN
Associate Professor,
Associate Dean for Academic Programs,
Graduate School of Nursing,
University of Massachusetts at Worcester,
Worcester, Massachusetts

Kathryn Fiandt, DNS, MSN, BSN, FNP, BC
Associate Professor,
University of Nebraska Medical Center;
Clinical Director,
University of Nebraska Medical Center,
Family Health Care Center,
Omaha, Nebraska

Mary L. Fisher, PhD, RN, CNAA, BC
Associate Professor,
School of Nursing,
University of Indiana;
PRN Staff Nurse,
St. Vincent Health Services,
Indianapolis, Indiana

Nancy J. Girard, PhD, MSN, RN, FAAN
Associate Professor,
Chair,
Acute Nursing Care Department,
School of Nursing,
University of Texas Health Sciences Center at San
    Antonio,
San Antonio, Texas

Mikel Gray, PhD, CUNP, CCCN, FAAN
Nurse Practitioner,
Department of Urology;
Professor,
School of Nursing,
University of Virginia,
Charlottesville, Virginia

Catherine Gregory, MSN, BSN, PNP, PALS, ABLS
Pediatric Nurse Practitioner,
Burn Surgery,
Shriners Hospital for Children,
Sacramento, California

Sheila A. Haas, PhD, RN
Dean and Professor,
Marcella Niehoff School of Nursing,
Loyola University at Chicago,
Chicago, Illinois

Diana P. Hackbarth, PhD, RN
Professor,
Marcella Niehoff School of Nursing,
Loyola University at Chicago,
Chicago, Illinois

Margie J. Hansen, PhD, MSN, BSN, RN
Clinical Associate Professor of Nursing,
University of North Dakota,
Grand Forks, North Dakota

Karen A. Hanson, MS, RN, CNP
Nurse Practitioner,
Division of Gastroenterology and Hepatology,
Mayo Clinic,
Rochester, Minnesota

Debra E. Heidrich, MSN, RN, AOCN, CHPN
Guest Lecturer,
Wright State University,
Dayton, Ohio

Esther A. Hellman, PhD, MS, BSN
Assistant Professor,
Creighton University School of Nursing,
Omaha, Nebraska

Beverly E. Holland, MSN, RN, RhD, ARNP
Adult Nurse Practitioner,
Tabler Group, Mental Health Services,
Louisville, Kentucky

Rhonda Holloway, MBA, RN, NP
Private Practice,
Denver, Colorado

Roberta A. Jorgensen, MS, BSN
Gastrointestinal Nurse Coordinator,
Mayo Clinic,
Rochester, Minnesota

Esperanza Villanueva Joyce, EdD, CNS, RN
Nursing Dean and Professor,
Our Lady of the Lake College,
Baton Rouge, Louisiana

Annabelle M. Keene, MSN, RN, BC
School Nurse,
Bellevue Public Schools,
Bellevue, Nebraska;
Formerly, Associate Professor,
College of Saint Mary,
Omaha, Nebraska

Patricia A. Keresztes, PhD, CCRN
Assistant Professor of Nursing,
Purdue University Calumet,
Hammond, Indiana

Helene J. Krouse, PhD, APRN, BC, CORLN, FAAN
Professor,
Assistant Dean for Adult Health,
College of Nursing,
Wayne State University,
Detroit, Michigan

Kim K. Kuebler, MN, RN, ANP-CS
Clinical Coordinator, Oncology,
Emory University Hospital,
Atlanta, Georgia

Judi L. Kuric, PhD, MSN, RN, APRN-BC, CRRN-A, CNRN
Assistant Professor,
University of Southern Indiana;
Acute Care Nurse Practitioner,
Neuro Rehab Solutions,
Evansville, Indiana

Louise Nelson LaFramboise, PhD, RN
Assistant Professor,
College of Nursing,
University of Nebraska Medical Center,
Omaha, Nebraska

Joan M. Lappe, PhD, RN
Professor,
Creighton University School of Nursing,
Omaha, Nebraska

Anne M. Larson, PhD, MS, BA, BC-ANA
Professor of Nursing,
Midland Lutheran College,
Fremont, Nebraska;
Registered Nurse on call, Intensive Care Unit,
Alegent Health,
Immanuel Medical Center,
Omaha, Nebraska

Mira Lessick, PhD, MSN, BSN, RN
Associate Professor,
University of Toledo,
Toledo, Ohio

Patricia A. MacDonald, BSN, RN, NP
Consultant, Rheumatology,
University of Chicago,
Chicago, Illinois

Donna W. Markey, MSN, RN, ACNP-CS
Instructor,
School of Nursing;
Nurse Practitioner,
Digestive Health Center,
Oregon Health and Sciences University,
Portland, Oregon

Karen S. Martin, MSN, RN, FAAN
Health Care Consultant,
Martin Associates,
Omaha, Nebraska

Cynthia McCurren, PhD, MSN, BSN, RN
Associate Professor,
Associate Dean,
School of Nursing,
University of Louisville,
Louisville, Kentucky

Norma D. McNair, MSN, RN, CCRN, CNRN, APRN-BC
Assistant Clinical Professor,
School of Nursing,
University of California at Los Angeles;
Clinical Nurse Specialist,
Neuroscience/Orthopedics,
University of California at Los Angeles Medical Center,
Los Angeles, California

Patricia Meier, MA, BSN, AOCN
Staff Nurse,
Mercy General Health Partners,
Muskegon, Michigan

Sheila Melander, DSN, RN, ACNP-C, FCCM
Professor,
School of Nursing,
University of Tennessee at Memphis,
Memphis, Tennessee;
Cardiovascular Acute Care Nurse Practitioner,
Owensboro, Kentucky

Lindsay Ann Middelton, BSN, RN, CGC
Genetic Counselor,
Clinical Research Nurse,
National Institutes of Health,
National Cancer Institute,
Urology Oncology Branch,
Bethesda, Maryland

*Melanie S. Minton, MBA, BSN, RN, CNRN
Lead Business Faculty,
LeTourneau University,
Houston, Texas;
Director and Educator,
Neuroscience Nursing,
Memorial Hermann Memorial City Hospital,
Houston, Texas

Kim Miracle, MSN, RN, C
Clinical Nurse Specialist,
Outcomes Manager,
Jewish Hospital,
Louisville, Kentucky

Anita E. Molzahn, PhD, MN, BScN, RN
Professor,
School of Nursing,
University of Victoria,
Victoria, British Columbia,
Canada

---

*Deceased.

Mark Moyad, MD, MPH
Phil F. Jenkins Director of Complementary Medicine,
Urologic Oncology,
Clinical Cancer Researcher/Consultant,
University of Michigan,
Ann Arbor, Michigan

Elizabeth A. Murphy-Blake, MSEd, MSN, APRN-C, FNP-C
Nurse Practitioner,
Veterans Administration Medical Center,
Omaha, Nebraska

Susan Newton, MS, BSN, RN, AOCN
Field Manager,
Oncology Nursing,
Ortho Biotech Oncology,
Bridgewater, New Jersey

Noreen Heer Nicol, MS, BS, RN, FNP
Clinical Senior Instructor,
School of Nursing,
University of Colorado,
Denver, Colorado;
Affiliate Assistant Professor,
School of Nursing,
University of Northern Colorado,
Greeley, Colorado;
Chief Clinical Officer,
National Jewish Medical and Research Center,
Denver, Colorado

Cheryl M. Noetscher, RN, BSN, MS
Manager,
Care Management,
St. Joseph's Hospital Health Center,
Syracuse, New York

Barbara B. Ott, PhD, RN
Associate Professor,
Villanova University,
Villanova, Pennsylvania

Jeannine M. Petit, MSN, BSN, CNRN, GNP-C
Nurse Practitioner,
Neurology Department,
Medical College of Wisconsin,
Milwaukee, Wisconsin

Mary Ellen Pike, MSN, BSN, RN
Assistant Professor,
Bellarmine University,
Louisville, Kentucky

Kathleen A. Popelka, DNSc, CFNP
Nurse Practitioner,
Women Veteran Manager,
Veterans Administration Medical Center,
Omaha, Nebraska

Sharon R. Redding, MN, RN
Associate Professor of Nursing,
College of Saint Mary;
Staff Nurse,
Alegent Bergan Mercy Medical Center,
Omaha, Nebraska

Marlene Reimer, PhD, RN, CNN(C)
Professor,
Faculty of Nursing,
University of Calgary,
Calgary, Alberta,
Canada

Dottie Roberts, MSN, MACI, CMSRN, RN, BC, ONC
Clinical Nurse Specialist,
Rehabilitative/Medical Services,
Palmetto Baptist Medical Center,
Columbia, South Carolina

M. Lynn Rodgers, MSN, RNC, CCRN, CNRN, ACNP-BC
Acute Care Nurse Practitioner,
Deaconess Hospital,
Evansville, Indiana

Helen Murdock Rogers, DNSc, RN
Associate Professor,
Chairperson,
Nursing Department,
Worcester State College,
Worcester, Massachusetts

Vicki M. Ross, PhD(C), RN
Doctoral Candidate,
University of Kansas,
Kansas City, Kansas

Linda M. Scott, MS, CRNP
Nurse Practitioner,
The National Institutes of Health,
Bethesda, Maryland

Carol A. Sedlak, PhD, RN, ONC
Associate Professor,
College of Nursing,
Kent State University,
Kent, Ohio

Judy Selfridge-Thomas, MSN, RN, CEN, FNP
Nurse Practitioner,
Department of Emergency Medicine,
St. Mary Medical Center,
Long Beach, California;
San Pedro Peninsula Hospital,
San Pedro, California

Nancy Shoemaker, MS, APRN/PMH
Preceptor, Graduate Nursing Students,
School of Nursing,
University of Maryland;
Nurse Psychotherapist,
University of Maryland Fayette Street Clinic,
Baltimore, Maryland

Mary Sieggreen, MSN, APN, NP, CUN
Associate Professor,
Clinical Nursing,
Wayne State University;
Vascular Nurse Practitioner,
Harpen University Hospital,
Detroit Medical Center,
Detroit, Michigan

Karen A. Sikorksi, MS, BSN, APN
Clinical Nurse Specialist, Pain,
OSF Saint Anthony Medical Center,
Rockford, Illinois

Sarah C. Smith, MA, BS, RN, CRNO
Advanced Practice Nurse,
Educational Associate,
Department of Ophthalmology and Visual Sciences,
University of Iowa Health Care,
Oxford, Iowa

Dianne M. Smolen, PhD, RN, C, CNS
Professor and Director, Continuing Nursing Education,
School of Nursing,
Medical College of Ohio,
Toledo, Ohio

Christine Stewart-Amidei, MSN, RN, CNRN, CCRN, CS
Advanced Practice Nurse,
Neurosurgery,
University of Chicago,
Chicago, Illinois

Nancy Evans Stoner, MSN, RN, CNSN
Clinical Nurse Specialist,
Nutrition Support,
University of Pennsylvania Medical Center,
Philadelphia, Pennsylvania

Janice Tazbir, MS, CCRN
Associate Professor of Nursing,
Purdue University Calumet,
Hammond, Indiana;
Staff RN, Intensive Care Unit,
University of Chicago,
Chicago, Illinois

Amy Verst, MSN, RN, CPNP, ATC
Assistant Professor,
Bellarmine University,
Louisville, Kentucky

Carol Weber, PhD, MSN, BSN, RN
Professor of Nursing,
Regis University,
Denver, Colorado

Ann H. White, PhD, RN
Associate Professor of Nursing,
University of Southern Indiana,
Evansville, Indiana

Bernadette White, MSN, RN, APRNc, HTP
Assistant Professor,
Creighton University School of Nursing,
Omaha, Nebraska

Connie White-Williams, MSN, RN, FNP
Affiliate Faculty,
Cardiothoracic Transplant Coordinator,
University of Alabama at Birmingham,
Birmingham, Alabama

Nancy L. York, MSN, RN
Assistant Professor,
Lansing School of Nursing and Health Sciences,
Bellarmine University,
Louisville, Kentucky

Reviewers

Mike Aldridge, BSN, RN, CCRN
Children's Hospital of Austin,
Austin, Texas

Gwen Anderson, PhD, RN
San Diego State University,
San Diego, California

Carol Pappas Appel, MSN, RN, CNP, AOCN
Barbara Ann Karmanos Cancer Institute,
Detroit, Michigan

Rebecca S. Appleton, PhD, RN
Marshall University,
Huntington, West Virginia

Susan B. Battistoni, PhD, RN
Salisbury University,
Salisbury, Maryland

Susan Birkhead, BSN, MPH
Samaritan Hospital,
Troy, New York

Jonathan S. Black, BS
University of Nebraska Medical Center,
Omaha, Nebraska

Terry Butkus, MSN, RN, FNP
University of Nebraska Medical Center,
Omaha, Nebraska

Elizabeth M. Carson, EdD, MS, RN
Saint Anthony College of Nursing,
Rockford, Illinois

Janet E. Cuddigan, PhD, RN
University of Nebraska Medical Center,
Omaha, Nebraska

R. Eric Doerfler, MSN, NP
Nightingale Health Centers, Inc.,
Harrisburg, Pennsylvania

Diane K. Dressler, MSN, RN, CCRN
Marquette University,
Milwaukee, Wisconsin

Rebecca Ann Fountain, MSN, RN
University of Texas at Tyler,
Tyler, Texas

Joy L. Haagsma, MSN, RN
Cape Cod Community College,
West Barnstable, Massachusetts

Linda E. Hein, MSN, RN, CNS, HNC, CHTP,
  Reiki Master
Veterans Administration Medical Center,
Portland, Oregon;
Private Practice,
Vancouver, Washington

Robbie Helmich Henson, PhD, RN
Oklahoma Baptist University,
Shawnee, Oklahoma

Karen L. Heys, MN, RN
Everett Community College,
Everett, Washington

Sadie Pauline Hutson, MSN, RN, CRNP
University of Pennsylvania,
Philadelphia, Pennsylvania

Molly Ann Hoffman Jalufka, BSN, RNC, TNCC
The Victoria College,
Gonzales, Texas

Jennifer Kane, BSN, RN
Massachusetts General Hospital,
Boston, Massachusetts

Joan A. Masters, PhD, RN, GNP
Northeastern University,
Boston, Massachusetts

Sharon J. Olsen, MS, RN, AOCN
Johns Hopkins University,
Baltimore, Maryland

Debra L. Schutte, PhD, RN
University of Iowa,
Iowa City, Iowa

Lynda Shand, PhD, MA, RN
College of New Rochelle,
New Rochelle, New York

Julie A. Slack, MSN, RN
Mohave Community College,
Kingman, Arizona

Judith Blanche Sweet, MS, RN, FNP
University of California at San Francisco,
San Francisco, California

Scott Carter Thigpen, MSN, RN, CCRN, CEN
South Georgia College,
Douglas, Georgia

Peggy Tidikis-Menck, PhD, RN
University of Nebraska Medical Center,
Omaha, Nebraska

Susan C. Vaughn, MSN(C), BSN, RN
Gentiva Health Services,
Charlotte, North Carolina

Rosalee C. Yeaworth, PhD, RN, FAAN
University of Nebraska Medical Center,
Omaha, Nebraska

Preface

It is our conviction that a book is not a static document. Certainly, a book—bound and printed—portrays health care at a given moment in time. By making the seventh edition of *Medical-Surgical Nursing* a web-enhanced textbook, we are able to provide instructors and students with a guide to delivering safe and appropriate nursing care as well as with enhanced resources from the web that are constantly changing and reflective of day-to-day changes in health care. To that end, we see this book as a "work in progress." Future editions will continue to improve, and we appreciate your comments, questions, and corrections to guide our ongoing work. We can improve only with your input. We also realize that educators and students must share in the task of bringing the book to life.

PHILOSOPHY AND APPROACH

This textbook grows out of the belief that nurses and physicians do not compete with each other but instead collaborate to reach certain outcomes in cooperation with the client and family. Nonetheless, nursing and medicine are separate disciplines. Consequently, nursing and medical content are not intermingled in this text. However, because nursing and medicine are collaborative efforts, it is often difficult for nursing students to understand one without having an understanding of the other. We therefore present thorough coverage of both nursing management and medical management.

With the increased emphasis on outcomes in health care, we have organized client care under the heading of Outcome Management. Several headings appear under this heading, including Medical Management, Nursing Management of the Medical Client, Surgical Management, and Nursing Management of the Surgical Client, as appropriate.

In this text, we use the nursing process to describe nursing management, but we do not apply the nursing process to every disorder. Instead, we have designated the nursing process for major or prototypical disorders. Within the presentation of the nursing process for those disorders, we have developed nursing diagnoses and collaborative problems, as appropriate, with their own outcomes and interventions. Collaborative problems define those client problems that cannot be resolved through independent nursing actions; they are potential complications that may develop because of a disorder, surgical procedure, or nonsurgical treatment. Collaborative problems complete the picture of nursing care and eliminate the need to force-fit every client problem into the framework of a nursing diagnosis. We have written Outcomes and Interventions sections for *each* identified nursing diagnosis and collaborative problem because we have found from our teaching experience that students cannot easily pull apart lists of diagnoses followed by lists of outcomes and interventions and then rebuild them into care plans.

ORGANIZATION

This edition is organized from simple to complex and from common to uncommon disorders. The early portion of the text focuses on the care of clients usually assigned to beginning students. The book then progresses to address the care of clients with more complex disorders, which are more commonly taught in upper division classes.

The format of the text has remained the same but is now divided into 18 units. The first five units are devoted to content that is applicable to all medical-surgical clients. The material in this first portion of the book will guide the student in learning to provide comprehensive care regardless of the specific diagnosis or problem. Concepts that span medical-surgical practice, such as health promotion, care delivery settings, physical assessment, complementary and alternative therapies, fluid and electrolyte balance, genetics, infectious diseases, pain, palliative care, perioperative care, and oncology, are found in this portion of the book. The remainder of the text is divided into common responses to health disorders. These units begin with a review of anatomy and physiology, followed by a chapter on health and diagnostic assessment; one or more "nursing care" chapters then present the nursing care of clients with specific disorders. We have added two new Anatomy and Physiology Reviews to address physiologic genomics and arousal, pain, and conscious awareness. A brief description of each unit is described below.

Unit 1 discusses health promotion and self-care and includes chapters related to health promotion in both middle-aged and older adults. Chapter 4 discusses history taking, physical assessment, and diagnostic testing. Chapter 5 is a new chapter that provides an overview of complementary and alternative therapies.

Unit 2 presents an overview of nursing and health care today. Chapter 6 describes the "stakeholders" in health care delivery, because medical-surgical nurses (not just managers) in all areas of practice must become increasingly aware of how health care is financed. Because the practice of medical-surgical nursing is not confined to certain areas, this edition contains more material on nursing care and philosophy in various care settings. Chapters 7 through 12 address nursing care in ambulatory, acute, intensive care, home health, long-term care, and rehabilitation settings. A new chapter on intensive care and rehabilitation nursing can be used to orient new students to these care settings.

Unit 3 looks at concepts that provide the foundations of care for medical-surgical clients, including separate chapters on fluid and electrolyte disorders. Other chapters address acid-base disorders and the surgical experience.

Unit 4 discusses physiologic concepts basic to medical-surgical nursing care. The unit begins with a new genetics chapter (Chapter 17) and continues with chapters related to cancer, infectious disorders, and wound healing.

Unit 5 covers psychosocial concepts basic to medical-surgical nursing care. The unit begins with a chapter on pain management and continues with chapters on palliative care, sleep and rest disorders, psychosocial and mental health concerns, and substance abuse.

Units 6 through 17 focus on the management of clients with specific disorders. Each unit begins with a structure and function overview of the pertinent body systems, followed by a nursing assessment chapter. The structure and function overview has been shortened and redesigned, and more artwork has been added for each body system.

In general, the discussion of specific disorders includes headings for Etiology, Pathophysiology, Clinical Manifestations, and Outcome Management. Because increasingly more nursing care is being directed toward health promotion, in this edition we have added content that focuses on health promotion, health maintenance, and health restoration to the Etiology topics in the disorders chapters. To emphasize the importance of understanding pathophysiology and its relationship to the treatment of a disorder, we have incorporated headings in the management sections that will help the student see the relationship between the pathophysiologic changes and specific strategies to promote positive outcomes in nursing management. The term *clinical manifestations* has been selected to encompass signs and symptoms along with diagnostic findings. The term *manifestations* replaces "signs and symptoms" in all chapters except one; in Chapter 23 on palliative care, *symptom management* is the preferred term.

Unit 18 presents the care of clients with multisystem disorders. Chapter 82 looks at organ donation issues, the transplantation process, quality-of-life issues, and specific interventions for clients requiring organ transplantation. Shock and multisystem disorders are discussed in Chapter 83. Chapter 84 examines the basic concepts of triage, ethical issues, and maintaining the chain of custody of medicolegal evidence. Chapter 84 also organizes emergency conditions by various nursing diagnoses identified and treated.

Hallmark Features

A completely new design focuses on guiding the reader to the Evolve website, where a wealth of supplemental content resides. Each chapter opens with a listing of web enhancements, which introduces the reader to that chapter's features on the Evolve website. All of the web features—including features that begin in the text and continue on the Evolve website with interactive exercises and bonus material—contain a reference within the text and are designated with an `evolve` icon in the margin. The following is a list of our hallmark features, including a description and the location of the feature:

- **Concept Maps** are flowcharts linking pathophysiological processes, clinical manifestations, and medical and nursing interventions. This feature appears throughout the text.
- **Case Studies** present complex client scenarios with in-depth detail—most with multiple clinical problems. This feature contains an introduction in the text; the Evolve website contains the body of the case study and the discussions, multiple-choice questions, and a nursing care plan.
- **Client Education Guides** act as examples to help students teach clients how to collaborate in their own care; these guides are worded in client-centered language. Some guides appear on the Evolve website, and others remain in the text for this edition. All Client Education Guides are translated into Spanish and appear on the Evolve website.
- **Care Plans** present nursing care using the nursing process format and highlight both nursing diagnoses and collaborative problems, expected outcomes, interventions with rationales, and evaluations. Some care plans appear on the Evolve website, but the majority remain in the text for this edition.
- **Bridge to Home Health Care** boxes describe specific applications and strategies for medical-surgical care in the home. Some bridges appear on the Evolve website, and others remain in the text for this edition.
- **Management and Delegation** boxes present the primary concerns nurses need to address when delegating care activities to unlicensed assistive personnel. This feature appears in the text and includes new topics such as Delegation in Health Care Delivery, Postoperative Care: Vital Signs, and Management of Clients with Vascular Disorders.
- **Bridge to Critical Care** boxes are an integrated feature to highlight major critical care concerns. This feature appears in the text and now includes a new bridge on defibrillation.
- **Critical Monitoring** boxes highlight those clinical manifestations that must be reported to the physi-

cian without delay. This feature appears throughout the text. New Critical Monitoring features for this edition include Ruptured Abdominal Aortic Aneurysm, Acute Pulmonary Edema, Digoxin Toxicity, Angina from Impending Myocardial Infarction, Headache, and Myasthenic and Cholinergic Crises in Clients with Myasthenia Gravis.

- **Physical Assessment Findings in the Healthy Adult** serve both to remind students of the relevant normal findings for each body system and to demonstrate how to chart those findings with clinical precision. This feature appears in the text.
- **Diversity in Health Care** boxes are focused discussions of health and illness related to particular populations. This feature appears on the Evolve website.
- **Ethical Issues in Nursing** boxes feature an ethical dilemma in the form of a question, with the discussion immediately following. This feature remains on the Evolve website for this edition.
- **Case Management** boxes, written by a practicing case manager, present key coordination and anticipatory issues under consistent headings of Assess, Advocate, and Prevent Readmission, thus linking nursing care with client-focused case management. This feature appears on the Evolve website.
- **Clinical Pathways** are excerpted from actual pathways used in specific hospitals. They are accompanied by a guide to show what should occur during specific times in the pathway and how to stay on track when caring for the client. This feature appears on the Evolve website.
- **Thinking Critically Questions** conclude each nursing care chapter. This feature presents short, typical client scenarios and pose questions about what actions to take. Discussions for all the questions are provided on the Evolve website.
- **NOC boxes** appear in chapters that contain nursing diagnoses content. The chapter opens with the appropriate suggested NOC outcome labels for the nursing diagnoses presented in the body of the text, thus emphasizing the importance of outcomes at the outset of the chapter.
- **Anatomy and Physiology Reviews** introduce each body system unit and provide a brief review of the relevant anatomy and physiology of the body system.
- **Appendixes** on Religious Beliefs and Practices Affecting Health Care, A Health History Format That Integrates the Assessment of Functional Health Patterns, and Laboratory Values of Clinical Importance in Medical-Surgical Nursing appear on the Evolve website.

NEW CONTENT AND FEATURES

In addition to the hallmark features listed in the previous section, the seventh edition includes six new boxed features, as well as a new and unique icon. This edition also features four new chapters and two new Anatomy and Physiology Reviews.

Four New Chapters

- Complementary and Alternative Therapies (Chapter 5) discusses why people choose alternative therapies and issues related to discussing complementary and alternative therapies with clients. The chapter provides students with the necessary understanding of complementary and alternative therapy.
- Critical Care (Chapter 9) provides a basic understanding of the topic of critical care, an area in which medical-surgical nurses are exposed.
- Rehabilitation (Chapter 12) provides a basic understanding of the topic of rehabilitation, an area in which medical-surgical nurses are exposed.
- Genetics (Chapter 17) discusses basic concepts of genes, chromosomes, and DNA, as well as the nursing role in genetic care. The chapter provides a basic understanding of molecular genetics and principles of human genetics in order to function effectively in today's health care arena.

Two New Anatomy and Physiology Reviews

Physiologic Genomics (Unit 4) is the unit opener for chapters on genetics, perspectives in oncology, cancer, wounds, and infectious disorders. It prepares the student for the chapters in the unit.

Arousal, Pain, and Conscious Awareness (Unit 5) is the unit opener for chapters on pain, palliative care, sleep, psychosocial, and substance abuse. It prepares the student for the chapters in the unit.

New Features

- **Web enhancements boxes** appear on each chapter opener and list the chapter features that appear on the Evolve website.
- **Integrating Pharmacology** boxes explain and explore common classifications of medications that are routinely used to treat a specific condition. These features help students understand how medications can be synergistically used for disease management. This feature appears throughout the text.
- **Genetic Links** boxes "link" a disease with its corresponding genetics. This feature provides the student with the description, genetics, diagnosis/testing, and management of a specific disease and appears throughout the text.
- **Terrorism Alert** boxes provide cutting-edge material on bioterrorism. They aid the student in recognizing the clinical manifestations and diseases associated with bioterrorism. This feature appears throughout the text.
- **Evidence-Based Practice in Action** boxes have been revamped for this edition. Applicable management chapters will feature these boxes in the text and

present a synopsis of the research with 4 to 5 supporting article summaries.

- **Evidence-based** content is noted in the margin by an **EB** icon. This icon introduces the concept of evidence-based (research-based) practice and provides numerous practical examples of how it relates to nursing practice.
- **Complementary and Alternative Therapy** boxes have been completely rewritten for this edition and present nontraditional therapies used by clients and health care providers to treat various conditions. They discuss alternative and complimentary therapies related to specific diseases or body systems. Some boxes are featured in the text, and others appear on the Evolve website.
- **Spanish Assessment Phrases** are listed on the Evolve website.
- **NIC, NOC, NANDA** appendixes located on the Evolve website list all of the labels for NIC and NOC as well as NANDA diagnoses.

ANCILLARY PACKAGE

Student Ancillaries

The **Evolve website** is available at http://evolve.elsevier.com/Black/medsurg/ and features a wealth of assets:

- New **Evolve Learning Resources,** which provide students with open-book quizzes that consist of crossword puzzles, multiple-choice questions, matching questions, and fill-in-the-blank questions for each chapter. Students are prompted at both the beginning and end of each chapter to take advantage of these resources.
- **Special Features,** which include Web-Only Features that appear on the Evolve website (Appendixes, Case Management, Clinical Pathways, Diversity in Health Care, Ethical Issues in Nursing, and Spanish Assessment Phrases); Web-Partial Features, with some features appearing in the text and others appearing on the Evolve website (Bridge to Home Health Care, Care Plans, Client Education Guides, Complementary and Alternative Therapy); and Web-Enhanced Features that start in the text and continue on the Evolve website (Case Studies, Concept Maps, and Thinking Critically).
- **Case Studies** and their accompanying discussions, multiple-choice questions, and a nursing care plan.
- Discussions for the **Thinking Critically** questions.
- Online **Concept Map Creator,** which is a one-of-a-kind program that allows students to create customized concept maps. Students are prompted to enter the following client data: medical diagnosis, pathophysiology, risk factors, clinical manifestations, nursing diagnoses, collaborative problems, expected outcomes, and nursing interventions. The program then generates a concept map in two for-

mats: (1) a graphic "map" that clearly illustrates the relationships among various client data and components of the nursing process, and (2) a tabular word processing file that students may print and use to record client responses/evaluation data, thereby completing the nursing process.

- **Fluid and Electrolyte Module,** which is a user-friendly tutorial that helps students master the difficult concepts of fluid and electrolyte balance and imbalance. This self-paced program includes animations to help illustrate important concepts, and an accessible and inviting user interface helps make the program easy to navigate. The program is divided into five sections: an introduction, three sections on fluid and electrolyte balance and imbalance, and a quiz section with approximately 75 questions to test students on information learned throughout the program.
- Seventy-five **Animations, Video Clips, and Audio Clips** from *Health Assessment Online,* which feature a cutting-edge collection of supplemental online materials. This library of electronic assets provides a wealth of online resources to draw from this highly visual topic.
- More than 45 **bonus Health Assessment Full-Color Images** covering all body systems.
- **Audio Pronunciations** for more than 250 words from Dorland's Dictionary.
- **Content Updates** from the authors.
- **WebLinks** for each chapter.

The **new Student CD-ROM** packaged with the text contains the following:

- **Open book quizzes** consisting of crossword puzzles, multiple-choice questions, matching questions, and fill-in-the blank questions for each chapter give students the chance to assess their understanding of the chapter.
- The **Fluid and Electrolyte Learning Module** gives the student a self-guided opportunity to learn and master this complex content.
- **Case Studies** with discussions, multiple-choice questions, and a nursing care plan provide real-life examples of clients with complex problems.
- **Physiologic Animations** from *Health Assessment Online* demonstrate complex processes to help students grasp underlying concepts.
- Discussions for the **Thinking Critically** questions give students an opportunity to compare their responses to those of the authors.

The **Virtual Clinical Excursion** workbook/CD-ROM guides students through a multi-floor virtual hospital to care for highly complex and diverse clients. Students will be able to collect client data from various sources (reports, charts, medication administration record, and short video clips and audio clips of nurse-client interactions); work with data entry and retrieval screens; record client data; analyze and interpret data to reach conclusions about complex problems; listen to a report and itemize a client's problems and high-priority concerns; administer medications; and more.

The **Study Guide** is in the traditional print format text but is completely rewritten for this edition. It contains exercises such as compare and contrast similar disorders or clinical manifestations, short answer, reflective (why instead of what), diagram of treatment (e.g., ask where drugs should be placed), best practices, application questions (specific client, not a case study), drug dosages (from IV to oral), decipher what's wrong with sample documentation, sample interventions, keeping skills sharp (safety, drug dosage/math, communication/assessment), and concept map exercises.

Instructor Ancillaries

The **Instructor's Resource** is available both online and on CD-ROM! Instructors also have access to the student resources. The Instructor's Resource includes the following helpful aids:

- **Instructor's Manual (IM)** consists of critical points to emphasize and facilitate student learning for both the classroom and the clinical setting. The classroom activities include Review Activity, Class Assignments, Lecture/Discussion, Guest Speakers, Group Activities, and Concept Map Activity (if applicable). The clinical activities include Skills Laboratory, Clinical Site Activities, and Clinical Conference Activities.
- The **PowerPoint Presentation** consists of approximately 1500 lecture slides, providing instructors with text lecture slides for each unit.
- The computerized **Test Bank** has approximately 2500 questions, including more than 400 questions in the new NCLEX alternate item format. Each test question includes a rationale, Nursing Process step, Cognitive Level, NCLEX category of client needs, and text reference.
- The **Image Collection** consists of more than 800 full-color images from the text and other sources.
- This resource will also contain **WebLinks** to various related websites.

The **Evolve Course Management System** is an interactive learning environment that works in coordination with **Medical-Surgical Nursing, 7th Edition,** to provide Internet-based course management tools you can use to reinforce and expand on the concepts you deliver in class. You can use Evolve to:

- Publish your class syllabus, outline, and lecture notes.
- Set up "virtual office hours" and e-mail communication.
- Share important dates and information through the online class *Calendar.*
- Encourage student participation through *Chat Rooms* and *Discussion Boards.*

ACKNOWLEDGMENTS

We have been asked several times, "Isn't a revision a lot less work than a new book?" You would think so, but it's amazing—a revision is no less work than a new book.

A project of this size certainly could not be accomplished without the collaboration of many people. First and foremost, we recognize the importance of the clinical expertise of our many contributing authors, which enables us to present a new edition that continues to be the "gold standard" for textbooks of medical-surgical nursing. We would also like to thank the special feature contributors.

There are also many people at Elsevier who have made this monumental task a "do-able" task. Thank you, Barbara Nelson Cullen, Executive Publisher, for your ongoing encouragement, help, and support. Thank you, Victoria Bruno, Senior Developmental Editor and Adrienne Simon, Developmental Editor, for your help and day-to-day management, keeping us on track to meet the production schedule. Your organization made this project move well. Thanks also to Victoria for hiring the ancillary writers and developing all the ancillaries, including the Evolve website. Thank you, Catherine Ott, Senior Editorial Assistant, for handling the countless administrative tasks associated with the publication of the book and ancillaries, as well as for coordinating the peer reviews of the book. Thank you, Graphic World, for providing wonderful full-color illustrations. Thank you, Jodi Willard, Senior Project Manager, for keeping the book on schedule and for making this aspect of the book publication go smoothly. Finally, we want to thank *you*—educators and students—for allowing us to join you in the teaching and learning of medical-surgical nursing. We trust that you will find the seventh edition of *Medical-Surgical Nursing: Clinical Management for Positive Outcomes* a valuable asset.

Joyce M. Black and Jane Hokanson Hawks

Contents

Promotion of Self-Care

Health Promotion

Esther A. Hellman

As a result of the growing prevalence of chronic conditions and the related cost burden, health promotion and illness prevention are increasingly important.[8] This chapter describes epidemiologic concepts and health promotion theories and shows how these concepts and theories are used in managing chronic conditions, which can occur across the life span. Health promotion concepts in two groups of the adult population are described in Chapters 2 and 3.

CONCEPT OF HEALTH

Nursing practice is directed and guided by an understanding of the definition of health and the factors that impact a client's health framework. The definition of health is broad and incorporates concepts of physical, mental, and social well-being. In 1947 the World Health Organization (WHO) definition of health emphasized several holistic qualities: "Health is a state of complete physical, mental, and social well-being and not merely the absence of disease or infirmity."[37] Since 1947 alternate definitions of health have been proposed. Some definitions portray health and illness on an interactive continuum, with multiple configurations ranging from depletion of health (death) to high-level wellness.[24] High-level wellness is further conceptualized as self-actualization and maximization of a person's potential.

Other definitions describe health as a unidirectional developmental process consisting of a unitary patterning of person and environment. When each person is viewed as being part of a complex, interconnected social, biologic, and environmental system, health can be better understood. Table 1-1 lists various definitions of health.

In general, today's definitions of health reflect a multidimensional, holistic, and subjective view. Individual definitions and perceptions of health are taken into account. The meaning of health can be viewed in many contexts, such as historical, social, personal, scientific, philosophical, and spiritual. These meanings will always exist in the various contexts of individual human experience, are sometimes contradictory, and often overlap. Cultural ideologies and tradition also influence one's image of health.

In the nurse-client relationship, nurses respect the clients' unique psychosocial, spiritual, and cultural needs and advocate for their health choices and decisions. Nurses support client participation in the process of actualizing a defined image of health and do not negate the ability of clients to form their own image of health. They include clients' perceptions when assessing their health to understand fully the priority of their values and perceptions of these complex interactions.[19] During the course of the client's lifetime and experiences, the client's definition of health may change.

evolve *Be sure to check out the bonus material on the Evolve website and the CD-ROM, including free self-assessment exercises.*
http://evolve.elsevier.com/Black/medsurg/

TABLE 1-1	*Definitions of Health*
Nursing Model	**Definition**
King's goal attainment theory	Health is a dynamic life experience. "Dynamic" implies a continuous adjustment to stressors in internal and external environments and the use of one's resources to achieve maximum potential.
Leininger's transcultural model	Health refers to "beliefs, values, and action patterns that are culturally known and used to preserve and maintain personal or group well-being, and to perform daily role activities."[23a]
Levine's conservation principles	Health is defined in terms of an Anglo-Saxon word meaning "whole." Patterns of wholeness change with growth and development. Health and disease patterns reflect adaptive change.
Neuman's systems model	Health is a condition in which the parts and subparts of the whole person are in harmony.
Orem's self-care model	Health is a state of wholeness, including a person's parts and modes of functioning.
Pender's health promotion model	"Health is a manifestation of evolving patterns of person-environment interaction throughout the life span."[25]
Rogers' unitary person model	Health and illness are seen as expressions of the interaction of a person and the environment in the process of unfolding consciousness.
Roy's adaptation model	Health is a process or state of being and a process of becoming an integrated whole.
Watson's model of human caring	Health is more than the absence of disease. It is a harmony within the mind, body, and soul.
World Health Organization	Health is a "state of complete physical, mental, and social well-being and not merely the absence of disease or infirmity."[37]

Concept of Wellness

Dunn was the first to define and describe *wellness,* a term and an idea that was the precursor to the health promotion movement.[5] His now-classic definition of what he termed *high-level wellness* is "an integrated method of functioning which is oriented toward maximizing the potential of which the individual is capable within the environment where he is functioning." Dunn stressed that wellness is an ongoing process directed toward higher potential, not a static goal, and that high-level wellness is a feeling of being "alive to the tips of the fingers, with energy to burn, tingling with vitality."[5] He postulated that health professionals tend to focus on disease rather than on wellness because their training is disease focused rather than wellness or prevention oriented. It is easier to fight against disease than to fight for a condition of greater wellness.

Travis popularized the theoretical concept of wellness through development and teaching of the wellness model (Figure 1-1). The effect of this model resulted in the recognition that wellness requires attention; it does not happen automatically. The left side of the figure represents the biomedical model. The client exhibits manifestations of a disease, is treated, and is brought back to a neutral point where disease manifestations have been alleviated. In the case of chronic illness, disease manifestations are controlled and minimized. The right side represents the wellness model and the potential for high-level health and wellness. The biomedical and wellness models can work in harmony. The nurse can use the wellness model anywhere on the health-illness continuum by encouraging clients to move past the neutral point, as far

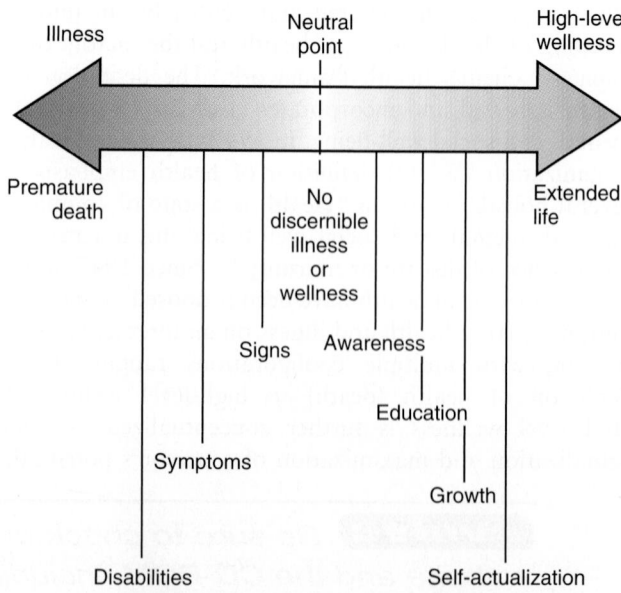

FIGURE 1-1 Travis' wellness model.

toward high-level wellness as possible. For example, if clients are ill, treatment is important, but clients should not stop there. After recovery, clients should practice healthy behaviors (such as regular exercise, stress management, and eating a low-fat, balanced diet) to minimize future illnesses and progress to a higher level of wellness.

Wellness is the quality or condition of being well, even among people with chronic illness, especially of being robust, healthy, and fit. Wellness is not simply the absence of clinical manifestations; it incorporates positive mental, physical, and spiritual well-being. High-level wellness is a method of functioning oriented toward maximizing individual potential within the environment. High-level wellness involves (1) progression toward a higher level of functioning, (2) integration of the whole being, and (3) an open-ended future with the challenge of fuller potential.

Relationships Among Disease, Illness, Health, and Wellness

In the biomedical model, disease is identified by clinical manifestations and explained by the presence of an organic cause of a disorder. A person who has a disease has a medically defined condition similar to that suffered by others (e.g., diabetes mellitus or hepatitis).[3] In contrast, when using a multicausal perspective to define disease, both biological and psychological influences are important; and the interrelationship of environmental, physical, and social factors is relevant. Disease results from interacting systems at the cellular, tissue, organismal, interpersonal, and environmental levels. Disease may be defined as "the failure of a person's adaptive mechanisms to adequately counteract stimuli and stresses, resulting in functional or structural disturbances."[6]

As mentioned earlier, multicausal and biopsychosocial theories of disease causation more closely approximate reality and increase the chances of discovering factors that are amenable to intervention. See the Diversity in Health Care feature on Health and Illness Beliefs and Practices on the website.

In contrast to the concept of disease, illness has a broader meaning and includes the perception and the response of clients to the disease. Illness is a state of being with social and psychological as well as biomedical components. Illness is a disenabling response, a mismatch between a person's needs and the resources available to meet those needs; it signals that the present balance is not working.[5] A person can have a disease without feeling ill. A seemingly healthy person may have an early form of disease without clinical manifestations. For example, young adults in their teens or twenties may already have heart disease, such as atherosclerosis, without manifestations of disease.[28] Although such people appear healthy, if they continue unhealthy habits such as smoking, eating a high-fat diet, and not exercising, the heart disease will progress until clinical manifestations appear. Similarly, injury changes the balance on the wellness continuum (see Figure 1-1). Injuries usually require treatment; after recovery or rehabilitation, people can achieve higher levels of wellness by practicing healthy behaviors.

In summary, disease, illness, health, and wellness are related concepts. Disease and health must be considered together because without disease there is no need to discuss health.[6] Disease is a state of disequilibrium, whereas health is a state of equilibrium, or balance.[5] Health and illness are dynamic patterns that change with time and social circumstances; they are not mutually exclusive. There are degrees of health and illness; clients with cancer and others with chronic diseases can achieve personal levels of wellness. Health is a resource for everyday living. High-level wellness maximizes one's potential capacity and is a component of the highest level of health.

CONCEPT OF HEALTH PROMOTION

Health promotion is the process of fostering awareness, influencing attitudes, and identifying alternatives so that people can make informed choices and change behavior to achieve an optimal level of physical and mental health and improve their physical and social environments. According to WHO, health promotion includes activities that encourage healthy lifestyles, create supportive environments for health, strengthen community action, reorient health service, and build healthy public policy. Health promotion has to do with acquiring mental, physical, and spiritual assets to protect and buffer people from disease as well as to move them along a continuum toward high-level wellness.

Health promotion programs are designed to improve the health and well-being of BOTH individuals and communities through empowerment. Clients are empowered through the provision of information, skills, services, and support needed to undertake and maintain positive lifestyle changes. Health promotion activities are geared toward individuals, families, and communities. WHO defines *community* as a social group determined by geographical boundaries or common values and interests. Community members know and interact with one another. The community within a particular social structure creates norms, values, and social institutions.

Health is affected by the extent of control or mastery people have over their lives or by the amount of power or powerlessness felt. Health promotion involves empowering the client. *Empowerment* gives the client power by transferring from the nurse knowledge, skills, resources, access, and language. The nurse can empower the client by teaching about self-care so that the client can progress toward a self-determined and self-fulfilling life.

Evolution of the Concept of Health Promotion

During the 1970s and 1980s, the field of health promotion grew alongside the emerging ideology and practice of wellness. Initially, it found expression in Canada with the Lalonde Report[14] and in the United States in the Surgeon General's Report, *Healthy People*.[29] Both documents discuss the significance of environmental factors in influencing health and are not limited to mention of individual lifestyle or personal behavior issues, which are hallmarks of the wellness movement. The Lalonde Report made recommendations in four equally weighted areas: (1) human biology, (2) environment, (3) lifestyle, and (4) health care organization. The Surgeon General's Report noted that lifestyle influenced health more than the other categories did. It argued that Americans are killing themselves, not only by careless habits but also by polluting the environment and permitting harmful social conditions to exist. For the first time, attention was directed toward environmental issues such as control of toxic agents and occupational health and safety. In addition, the nation's health strategy was reformulated to emphasize the prevention of disease and the promotion of health. This strategy was to be accomplished over the next decade by the development and implementation of 15 targeted preventive health services, health protection activities, and health promotion activities.

In 1991 *Healthy People 2000* was published with an updated set of measurable goals and priority areas for improving the health of the nation by the year 2000.[30] Three broad goals were identified: (1) increasing the span of healthy life for Americans, (2) reducing health disparities among Americans, and (3) achieving access to preventive services for all Americans. Specific goals, objectives, and strategies were delineated for achieving 22 priorities in health promotion, health protection, and preventive services.

Healthy People 2010 is the current working document for the improvement of health and prevention of disease for this decade.[33] *Healthy People 2010* is grounded in research and science, built through public consensus, and designed to measure progress toward achieving the goals. The two overarching goals for this decade are (1) to increase quality and years of healthy life and (2) to eliminate health disparities. Ten leading health indicators that reflect the major public health concerns facing Americans in the 21st century have been identified: (1) physical activity, (2) overweight and obesity, (3) tobacco use, (4) substance abuse, (5) responsible sexual behavior, (6) mental health, (7) injury and violence, (8) environmental quality, (9) immunization, and (10) access to health care. The health indicators support the goals for the health of the nation and serve as a link to 467 objectives that are organized into 28 focus areas.

Nurses have long conducted health promotion activities, and the definition and scope of professional nursing practice include health promotion activities. In its social policy statement, the American Nurses' Association (ANA) defined nursing as having four essential features[1]: (1) attention to the full range of human experiences and responses to health and illness without restriction to a problem-focused orientation; (2) integration of objective data with knowledge gained from an understanding of the client's or group's subjective experience; (3) application of scientific knowledge to the processes of diagnosis and treatment; and (4) provision of a caring relationship that facilitates health and healing.

To promote health, nurses must understand the complex social, political, and economic forces that shape the lives of individuals, families, and communities. A nurse who is active socially and politically models the ANA social policy statement that delineates involvement in social reform as being a part of nursing practice. The policy states, among other concerns, the "provision for the public health through use of preventive and environmental measures and increased assumption of responsibility by individuals, families, and other groups."[1] Labonte, a health educator, believed that the ultimate challenge is to create social and health conditions that allow all the world's citizens to achieve a state of good health.[13]

Epidemiologic Concepts

Epidemiology is the study of patterns of health, disease, disability, death, and other problems in a population. Epidemiology focuses on how diseases originate and spread.[16] A major epidemiologic goal is identifying aggregates, or subpopulations, at high risk for acquiring a disease and then modifying or reducing those risks. For example, smokers have a three-fold higher risk for development of cardiac disease compared with nonsmokers. Nurses can modify or reduce a smoker's risk of cardiac disease by counseling about how to accomplish smoking cessation. Risk factors and levels of prevention are epidemiologic concepts.

Risk Factors

Risk factors are factors whose presence is associated with increased probability of the occurrence of an illness or disease. A health risk factor can be the client's age, gender, lifestyle, personal health history, or family health history. When clients have certain risk factors that indicate they are "at high risk" of developing a disease, it does not mean that they are sure to develop this disease, just as being "not at high risk" does not guarantee the clients will not develop this disease. Health risk factors can be categorized (Table 1-2):

- *Genetic* or *biologic* (age, race, family history)
- *Behavioral* (health habits, such as eating a high-fat diet, not exercising, smoking, ineffective stress management)

Text continued on p. 15

TABLE 1-2	*Health Promotion and Risk Management*		

		Screening and Preventive Measures	
Risk Factor	**Potential Health Problem**	**Self-Care**	**Professional Level**

Race

Black	Hypertension	Self-monitor BP Avoid salt in diet Maintain ideal body weight Seek professional care if systolic BP >140 or diastolic BP >90	Monitor if BP is elevated or client is taking antihypertensive medications
White (fair skin tones)	Skin cancer	Limit exposure to sun Wear protective clothing Use sunscreen with SPF 15 or above Perform monthly head-to-toe skin inspection Seek professional care if change noted in any moles or birthmarks, or if new growths or patches do not heal	Monitor skin lesions Skin biopsy or excision and follow-up treatment
	Osteoporosis	See self-care and professional level measures listed under "Personal Habits—Inadequate calcium intake"	
Japanese	Stomach cancer	Know suspicious GI symptoms: pain, hematemesis, melena, weight loss, nausea, and so on*	Follow-up for laboratory tests and special diagnostic procedures
Hispanic	Diabetes mellitus	Regular exercise and weight control Consume balanced diet of no more than 30% fats with complex carbohydrates Know symptoms of hyperglycemia: polydipsia, polyuria, polyphagia, and delayed wound healing*	Diet counseling Follow-up for laboratory tests, diagnostic procedures, and blood glucose monitoring and control
Native American	Alcohol abuse and related diseases	Abstinence Limit alcohol intake to 1 oz/day or less if personal tendency (e.g., 1 to 2 mixed drinks or cans of beer) Know symptoms of alcoholism* Join self-help support group such a Alcoholics Anonymous (AA)	Assessment of history and physical condition Referral to a detoxification program Counseling for client and family

Genetic or Family-Related

Overweight	Obesity-related disease Cancer	Monitor weight once per week Perform regular, sustained exercise Consume balanced diet (no more than 30% fats, and calories should not exceed metabolic needs) Join self-help group such as Weight Watchers	Diet counseling Follow-up for morbid obesity (>100% of ideal body weight)
Diabetes mellitus	Diabetes mellitus or glucose intolerance	Regular exercise and weight control Consume balanced diet Know symptoms of hyperglycemia: polydipsia, polyuria, polyphagia, and delayed wound healing*	Follow-up for laboratory tests, special diagnostic procedures, and blood glucose monitoring and control

BP, Blood pressure; *BSE,* breast self-examination; *ECG,* electrocardiogram; *GI,* gastrointestinal; *HIV,* human immunodeficiency virus; *IU,* international units; *SPF,* sun protection factor; *STDs,* sexually transmitted diseases; *TSE,* testicular self-examination.

*Seek professional care if symptoms are present.

Continued

TABLE 1-2	*Health Promotion and Risk Management—cont'd*		
		Screening and Preventive Measures	
Risk Factor	**Potential Health Problem**	**Self-Care**	**Professional Level**
Genetic or Family-Related—cont'd			
Hypertension	Cardiovascular disease Renal disease Retinopathy Stroke	Regular, sustained exercise Consume balanced diet Avoid excess salt intake Maintain ideal body weight Regular BP checks (self or professional) Take BP medication daily	Regular follow-up for diagnostic studies and laboratory work Monitor compliance
Heart disease (onset before age 50)	Cardiovascular disease	See "Hypertension" Know symptoms of heart disease: chest pain, dyspnea, cyanosis* Stop smoking Monitor resting pulse rate Low saturated fat diet Regular exercise	Annual physical examination, including ECG and laboratory tests Refer to smoking cessation clinics Diet counseling
Breast cancer (in mother or sister)	Breast cancer	Learn to perform BSE Perform BSE monthly	Regular professional breast examination as indicated for age and personal history Regular mammography as indicated for age
Age-Related			
Vision changes	Strabismus	Monitor for difficulty focusing, especially on near objects See ophthalmologist if symptoms occur Schedule regular eye examinations as indicated for age	Follow-up for complete eye examination and possible neurologic examination
	Visual acuity changes, cataracts, glaucoma, or macular degeneration	Monitor visual acuity See ophthalmologist if vision is "fuzzy," or if seeing halos around lights Schedule regular eye examinations	Complete eye examination to screen for cataracts, glaucoma, and macular degeneration as indicated for age
	Injury or trauma	Wear protective eye gear when engaging in activity likely to result in projectiles or blunt trauma See ophthalmologist if injury should occur	Provide prompt diagnosis and treatment if injury occurs
Falls	Injury or trauma	Keep environment illuminated Remove loose scatter rugs Use a night-light Install handrails and grab bars Wipe up spills immediately	Provide prompt diagnosis and treatment if injury occurs
Self-medication errors	Overmedicating or undermedicating	Request and use prepackaged unit dose medications Prepare medicines in a well-lit area Wear corrective lenses when preparing medicines	Careful assessment of medication history; monitor for toxic response

BP, Blood pressure; *BSE*, breast self-examination; *ECG*, electrocardiogram; *GI*, gastrointestinal; *HIV*, human immunodeficiency virus; *IU*, international units; *SPF*, sun protection factor; *STDs*, sexually transmitted diseases; *TSE*, testicular self-examination.
*Seek professional care if symptoms are present.

TABLE 1-2	*Health Promotion and Risk Management—cont'd*		
		Screening and Preventive Measures	
Risk Factor	**Potential Health Problem**	**Self-Care**	**Professional Level**

Age-Related—cont'd

Risk Factor	Potential Health Problem	Self-Care	Professional Level
Hearing problem	Presbycusis	Avoid exposure to loud noises Wear earplugs when exposed to loud noise levels, and limit lengths of exposure	Complete audiometric screening as appropriate for age and personal history
	Injury or trauma	Avoid putting sharp objects into ear canals Know symptoms of ear infections: pain, discharge from ear canal, vertigo, and fever*	Follow-up for prompt diagnosis and treatment if injury or infection occurs
Inadequate dental hygiene	Dental caries Periodontal disease Premature loss of teeth	Brush teeth regularly after meals and at bedtime Floss teeth daily Have damaged teeth repaired or replaced promptly Follow recommendations for fluoride treatments; use fluoridated toothpaste Schedule regular dental checkups	Complete dental checkups, with yearly follow-up Fluoride treatments as indicated for age and locale
Impaired immune system integrity	Community-acquired infections	Keep immunizations current as recommended for age Receive vaccinations for influenza yearly and pneumococcal infection as indicated Seek professional care if symptoms of infection occur	Prompt diagnosis and treatment if a contagious disease or infection is suspected
Impaired mobility	Falls	See self-care measures listed for falls related to vision changes under "Age-Related" Use mobility-assistance devices (e.g., cane or walker) Avoid hazardous surfaces, such as wet floors and icy pavements	Prompt diagnosis and treatment if injury occurs

Biologic

Risk Factor	Potential Health Problem	Self-Care	Professional Level
Hyperlipidemia, hypercholesterolemia	Cardiovascular disease	Consume balanced diet low in saturated fats Exercise regularly Avoid or stop smoking Have blood lipid and cholesterol levels monitored periodically as recommended	Regular follow-up for monitoring serum levels
Hyperglycemia	Diabetes mellitus	Consume diet low in fats and simple carbohydrates Include complex carbohydrates Exercise regularly Have blood glucose levels monitored periodically as recommended Self-monitor blood glucose levels if diabetic and following a prescribed medical regimen	Regular follow-up for monitoring control of blood glucose levels Adjustment of medical treatment as indicated by laboratory results

Continued

TABLE 1-2	*Health Promotion and Risk Management—cont'd*		
		Screening and Preventive Measures	
Risk Factor	**Potential Health Problem**	**Self-Care**	**Professional Level**
Biologic—cont'd			
Hypersensitivity reactions	Allergic reactions, including rhinitis, bronchospasm, asthma, eczema, and atopic dermatitis	Avoid known allergens Seek prompt medical treatment if self-care measures are ineffective Discuss with physician whether allergen sensitivity testing and treatment for desensitization is indicated Wear a MedicAlert tag Learn to use and carry an emergency kit (e.g., epinephrine [Adrenalin] if indicated)	Prompt diagnosis and treatment if severe reactions or complications occur Initiation of desensitization therapy if indicated
Personal Habits			
Inadequate rest and sleep	Fatigue Lowered resistance to illness	Obtain sufficient sleep to feel rested on awakening (amount varies with individual need) Avoid sedatives, caffeine, alcohol Seek professional care if chronic fatigue interferes with activities of daily living	Complete history and physical examination Evaluation in a sleep laboratory
Irregular diet habits	Obesity, diabetes, hypertension, cardiovascular disease, irritability, depression, and hyperactivity or hypoactivity	Consume meals at regular times each day Eat three balanced meals per day Limit intake of salt, caffeine, refined sugar, and fats Perform regular exercise Monitor weight weekly See self-care measures listed under obesity, diabetes, hypertension, and cardiovascular disease	Regular follow-up to monitor existing health problems Prompt diagnosis and treatment if a health problem arises
Inadequate calcium intake	Osteoporosis	Consume elemental calcium in recommended amount per day for age and gender. Recommended amounts range from 1000 to 1500 mg/day Limit milk products as source of calcium; include other sources of dietary calcium, such as broccoli, carrots, green beans, spinach, collard greens, and rhubarb Consume 400-800 international units/day of vitamin D Engage in daily weight-bearing activity such as walking	Follow-up for periodic physical examination Possible estrogen hormone replacement therapy, when indicated Diet counseling
Excess fat intake	Colon cancer Possible breast cancer	Consume diet low in saturated fats, such as that found in beef; substitute with fish, poultry, and beans Limit milk products and eggs Include fiber in diet, such as from grains and cereals Know symptoms of colon cancer (blood in stool, change in bowel habits) and breast cancer (lump, discharge, pain)* Have stool specimen tested for occult blood Perform BSE monthly	Follow-up for laboratory tests and possible diagnostic procedures Diet counseling

BP, Blood pressure; *BSE,* breast self-examination; *ECG,* electrocardiogram; *GI,* gastrointestinal; *HIV,* human immunodeficiency virus; *IU,* international units; *SPF,* sun protection factor; *STDs,* sexually transmitted diseases; *TSE,* testicular self-examination.
*Seek professional care if symptoms are present.

TABLE 1-2	*Health Promotion and Risk Management—cont'd*		
		Screening and Preventive Measures	
Risk Factor	**Potential Health Problem**	**Self-Care**	**Professional Level**

Personal Habits—cont'd

Risk Factor	Potential Health Problem	Self-Care	Professional Level
Low fiber intake	Colon cancer	Consume diet high in fiber, including cereals and grains, especially bran Know symptoms of colon cancer (see earlier)* Have stool specimen tested for occult blood	Follow-up for laboratory tests and diagnostic procedures Supplemental fiber to include in diet
Alcohol abuse	Alcoholism Cancer of mouth, throat, esophagus, larynx, and liver Accidents, including those that result in death Cirrhosis Esophageal varices Pancreatitis Dementia	Abstinence, if high risk for alcoholism Limit alcohol intake to 1 oz or less per day if no personal tendency (e.g., 1 to 2 mixed drinks or cans of beer) Know the symptoms of alcoholism* Join self-help support group, such as Alcoholics Anonymous, if alcohol consumption interferes with performance of job or interpersonal relationships	Careful assessment of history and physical condition Referral to a detoxification program, if indicated Counseling Family counseling and support are often necessary (e.g., Al-Anon, Ala-Teen)
Drug abuse	Harmful side effects Drug interactions Allergic reactions Hepatitis HIV	Use prescribed medications only as directed Discard outdated medications Limit use of over-the-counter drugs to only those necessary Avoid recreational drug use Know symptoms of substance abuse* If using intravenous drugs, do not share needles or syringes	Careful assessment of history and physical condition Referral to a detoxification program, if indicated Counseling Family counseling and support are often necessary Screening for HIV infection
Tobacco use	Cancer of mouth or lung Cardiovascular disease Respiratory disease	Avoid tobacco use in any form Limit use, if unable to quit Know symptoms of tobacco-related health problems: persistent cough, oral sore that does not heal, hoarseness that persists, blood in sputum* Have regular health checkups Avoid exposing others to sidestream smoke Attend support group to help stop smoking, such as Smokers Anonymous	Follow-up for laboratory tests and special diagnostic procedures Counseling for help to stop smoking Referral of family members (if indicated) for health assessment if exposed to sidestream smoke
Safety	Unintentional injury or death	Use safety equipment as indicated (seat belts, helmet, eye shield, life vest) Learn how to swim Never drink and drive; appoint a designated driver Do not operate equipment or engage in hazardous activity if taking medication that causes drowsiness Develop safety awareness (e.g., learn to identify unsafe situations and avoid them or take corrective action)	Thorough teaching about medications and their side effects Prompt diagnosis and treatment if an injury occurs

Continued

TABLE 1-2	*Health Promotion and Risk Management—cont'd*		
		Screening and Preventive Measures	
Risk Factor	**Potential Health Problem**	**Self-Care**	**Professional Level**
Personal Habits—cont'd			
Sun exposure	Sunburn Skin cancer	See self-care measures listed under skin cancer related to race	See measures listed under skin cancer related to race
Lifestyle			
Lack of regular exercise	Obesity Cardiovascular disease	Engage in regular aerobic exercise (brisk walking, biking, jogging, swimming) at least 3 times/week for 30 to 40 minutes each Warm up prior to exercising to increase flexibility and reduce chance of injury Do not begin an exercise program until evaluated by health care professional for a baseline health assessment Follow professional advice regarding type of exercise program and intensity of training Wear appropriate gear for activity as protection Consume a balanced diet Know warning signals of when to stop exercising (e.g., dizziness, chest pain)*	Baseline health assessment prior to beginning exercise program Prompt diagnosis and treatment if complications or injury occurs Periodic assessment of cardiovascular status and endurance
Stress and coping ability	Many health problems are related to high stress levels and inadequate coping	Decrease level of stress whenever possible Develop a variety of coping skills Practice relaxation techniques (e.g., biofeedback, imagery, meditation, self-hypnosis) Recognize effects of stress on self Develop a support network* Modify lifestyle to reduce stress	Counseling for stress management Referral to appropriate support system as indicated by the individual circumstances Teaching regarding relaxation techniques Careful assessment and treatment if psychosomatic health problems develop
Lack of self-care activities to promote health	Cancer of breast, testis, or prostate	Monthly practice of BSE or TSE Regular professional examination as indicated for age	Periodic, regular examination
	Cancer of the cervix	Obtain regular pelvic examination and Papanicolaou (Pap) smear as indicated for age and sexual activity status	Periodic, regular examination with follow-up as necessary
	Vision and hearing problems	See self-care measures under age-related health problems	See measures listed under age-related health problems for vision and hearing
	Dental and gum disease	See self-care measures under age-related health problems	See measures listed under age-related health problems for dental hygiene
	Tetanus Influenza Pneumonia	Keep immunizations current*	Prompt diagnosis and treatment if an infectious disease occurs

BP, Blood pressure; *BSE*, breast self-examination; *ECG*, electrocardiogram; *GI*, gastrointestinal; *HIV*, human immunodeficiency virus; *IU*, international units; *SPF*, sun protection factor; *STDs*, sexually transmitted diseases; *TSE*, testicular self-examination.
*Seek professional care if symptoms are present.

TABLE 1-2	*Health Promotion and Risk Management—cont'd*		
		Screening and Preventive Measures	
Risk Factor	**Potential Health Problem**	**Self-Care**	**Professional Level**
Lifestyle—cont'd			
	Cancer	Know the seven warning signs: change in bowel or bladder habits, a nonhealing sore, unusual bleeding or discharge, lump or thickening in breast or other area, difficulty swallowing or indigestion, change in mole or wart, and persistent cough or hoarseness* Know and follow current recommendations for prevention and early entry into the health care system	Follow-up for laboratory tests and special diagnostic procedures Prompt diagnosis and treatment
High-risk sexual activity	Unplanned pregnancy	Use contraceptive method acceptable to self and partner Prenatal care	Counseling regarding options for contraceptives Counseling regarding pregnancy outcome options
	Cervical cancer	Abstain from early, frequent sexual activity Limit number of sexual partners Limit number of childbirths Schedule regular Pap smear as recommended for age	Regular professional pelvic examinations and Pap smears as indicated by health behavior profile
	STDs, such as HIV infection and herpes	Limit number of sexual partners Avoid anal intercourse Use condoms Avoid oral-genital intercourse Avoid oral contact with body fluids (semen, blood, feces, urine) Seek professional care for regular, periodic assessment if engaging in high-risk sexual activity Know symptoms of STDs (e.g., sore on genitals or mucous membranes, discharge from penis or vagina, abnormal bleeding, dyspareunia) Refrain from sexual activity if symptoms of STDs develop	Follow-up for prompt diagnosis and treatment should STD be suspected Counseling regarding safe sex practices Referral to public health for contact and follow-up for possible infected partners
Travel	Diseases prevalent in locale	Obtain necessary vaccinations before departure Seek prompt treatment if illness develops while traveling or after return	Prompt diagnosis and treatment if illness occurs
Environmental and Occupational			
Sports	Fractures, sprains, and strains	Have a baseline health assessment prior to beginning a sport Wear protective gear to avoid injury (e.g., eye shield, helmet, padding)* Follow recommendations for warm-up and cool-down exercises Limit mobility of injured body part until rehabilitation begins	Prompt diagnosis and treatment of injuries Rehabilitation

Continued

TABLE 1-2	Health Promotion and Risk Management—cont'd		
		Screening and Preventive Measures	
Risk Factor	**Potential Health Problem**	**Self-Care**	**Professional Level**
Environmental and Occupational—cont'd			
Outdoor activity	Sunburn Skin cancer Frostbite Hypothermia or hyper- thermia	Wear protective gear appropriate for the weather Use sunscreen with an SPF of 15 or above Limit exposure to extremes of heat or cold Learn survival tactics relative to activity Know early signs of hypothermia (disorientation) and hyperthermia (dry, hot skin) Attempt to seek medical treatment as soon as possible if a problem arises Avoid future exposure to extremes of heat or cold because of increased vulnerability	Prompt diagnosis and treatment if a problem occurs See measures listed under skin cancer related to race
Loud noise	Hearing loss	Limit exposure to loud music and machinery Wear protective earplugs Have regular screening of hearing and seek professional care if hearing loss is evident	Regular, complete audiometric screening, as appropriate
Chemical fumes, airborne particle exposure	Respiratory diseases Cancer	Provide adequate ventilation Wear protective gear (goggles, respirators) Limit exposure when possible (chemicals, dry cleaning fluid, film processing, mining, asbestos exposure, household cleaners) Evaluate occupational risks Reduce exposure by changing jobs, if necessary Know symptoms of possible disease, such as hoarseness, persistent cough, hemoptysis, chronic dyspnea* Avoid smoking	Prompt diagnosis and treatment if disease should occur
Stress-provoking activity	Many stress-related health problems may occur	See "Stress and coping ability" under Lifestyle	Counseling regarding stress management
High–accident-risk activity (also see "Safety" under Personal Habits)	Unintentional injury or death	Avoid high–accident-risk activities Learn safety measures Practice safety measures so they become habitual Use safety equipment such as goggles, helmets Get sufficient rest Avoid alcohol, drugs, or medications known to cause drowsiness when engaging in high-risk activity Obtain treatment if injury occurs	Prompt diagnosis and treatment if an accidental injury occurs
Low-level electromagnetic radiation exposure	Cancer of brain or eye Leukemia Sarcoma Possible birth defects	Limit exposure Monitor immediate environment for radiation levels Promptly seek health assessment and treatment for possible problems	Prompt diagnosis and treatment if a health problem occurs

BP, Blood pressure; *BSE,* breast self-examination; *ECG,* electrocardiogram; *GI,* gastrointestinal; *HIV,* human immunodeficiency virus; *IU,* international units; *SPF,* sun protection factor; *STDs,* sexually transmitted diseases; *TSE,* testicular self-examination.
*Seek professional care if symptoms are present.

TABLE 1-2	*Health Promotion and Risk Management—cont'd*		
		Screening and Preventive Measures	
Risk Factor	**Potential Health Problem**	**Self-Care**	**Professional Level**
Socioeconomic			
Recent immigration	Diseases common to locale of origin or where traveled	Obtain necessary immunizations before departure Seek professional care if symptoms of disease occur, especially during or after recent travel	Careful assessment of history and physical examination Prompt diagnosis and treatment if a health problem occurs
Lack of adequate health insurance coverage	Delayed or postponed treatment of health problems Undetected health problems	Use free walk-in health care facilities	Referral to social services or welfare agency for assistance with applying for available health care, such as Medicaid or Medicare

- *Environmental* (for example, living in an area with frequent smog warnings)

The risk level for disease or illness may be assessed through a health-risk appraisal that identifies potential health threats before illness or disease development and provides clients with a way to evaluate their vulnerability to identified potential health threats (see Chapter 4). The Health Risk Appraisal questionnaire covers such areas as personal and family history of illnesses and medical conditions, lifestyle habits, general health status, and satisfaction with life. This information helps the nurse to identify high-risk clients and to individualize health promotion interventions.

Risk factors are a key to health promotion interventions. Numerous risk factors, when left unattended or unacknowledged, can become life threatening. Once identified, risk factors can be addressed, and a primary prevention program can be initiated. It is important to distinguish between *modifiable* risk factors (those capable of being changed) and *nonmodifiable* risk factors (those that are unchangeable, e.g., genetic or biologic factors). Common modifiable risk factors include (1) tobacco use; (2) dietary indiscretion, deficiencies, and overconsumption (obesity); (3) sedentary lifestyle; (4) alcohol and drug abuse; (5) fatigue and lack of sleep; (6) pollution, such as noise, air, and environment; (7) unsafe sexual behavior; and (8) misuse of motor vehicles and or firearms.

Levels of Prevention

Prevention means averting the development and progression of disease.[15] Preventing disease can be grouped into three levels, which are named for the stage of disease they target. The levels of prevention are primary, secondary, and tertiary. Table 1-3 identifies selected behaviors associated with these levels.

Primary Prevention. *Primary prevention* involves health promotion activities that provide protection against the occurrence of a specific illness or disease.[15] Primary prevention interventions are done before the client develops a disease and do not include therapeutic treatment or identification of manifestations. It does include health promotion (e.g., teaching clients about healthy lifestyle behaviors) and specific protection interventions (e.g., immunizations) to decrease vulnerability to illness or dysfunction. A health promotion program can be developed to increase immunity and strengthen the body and mind. Everyday behavior can be examined to guide primary prevention. For example, impaired mobility is usually preventable. If a client is at risk for impaired mobility, nursing intervention can prevent impairment. For the client who has arthritis and currently does not have mobility problems, encouraging the client to eat a well-balanced diet and to engage in specific exercises may help prevent or delay the development of mobility problems.

Secondary Prevention. *Secondary prevention* refers to health behavior that promotes the early detection (case finding or screenings) and treatment of disease and the limitation of disability.[15] Screening primarily identifies cases in an early stage of disease, when treatment is more effective. (See the table on the Recommendations for Common Screening Procedures and Health Management Behaviors Across the Life Span on the website.) *evolve*

Using the immobility example to examine secondary prevention, the nurse monitors clients for early manifestations of immobility in clients with risk factors. Causes of physical immobility may be (1) decreased energy from ischemia, hypoxia, malnutrition, and electrolyte imbalance; (2) lack of innervation, as in central nervous system or peripheral nerve impairment; (3) decreased musculoskeletal strength, as in endocrine diseases, disuse syndrome, and scar tissue formation; and (4) pain, which in-

TABLE 1-3	*Behaviors Associated with Each Level of Prevention*	
Level of Prevention	**Type of Behavior***	
Primary	Stop smoking, or do not start smoking	
	Avoid overexposure to the sun	
	Support antipollution legislation	
	Practice safe sex, monogamy, or abstinence	
	Obtain genetic counseling for family-linked disorders	
	Design and follow a regular exercise plan	
	Maintain ideal body weight	
	Maintain a low-cholesterol, low-fat, high-fiber nutritious diet	
	Wear a seat belt and helmet	
	Identify and eliminate stressors	
	Limit alcohol intake, and never drink and drive	
	Have regular dental care	
Secondary	Obtain genetic counseling for family-linked disorders	
	Undergo screening for tuberculosis	
	Obtain tonometry yearly after age 40 for glaucoma screening	
	Have yearly Pap smears and mammograms per recommended guidelines	
	Have eye examinations every 2 years	
	Practice monthly self-breast, self-testicular, self-skin, and self-oral examinations	
	Undergo a physical examination yearly after age 40	
	Self-monitor blood pressure for hypertension	
Tertiary	Have a complete blood count before chemotherapy	
	Have speech therapy after a stroke	
	Participate in cardiac rehabilitation	
	Have breast reconstruction	
	Participate in stroke or coma rehabilitation	

*Preventive behaviors identified are representative and are not intended to be inclusive.

hibits movement and the desire to move. The nurse monitors for changes in individual norms and for manifestations of early sequela. If manifestations of immobility can be detected early, before even the client is aware of them, many immobility complications can be avoided. Nursing actions, such as thorough assessments and early interventions (applying heat, balancing exercise and rest, and administering prescribed anti-inflammatory drugs), can help prevent a serious mobility problem.

Tertiary Prevention. *Tertiary prevention* is directed toward rehabilitation after a disease or condition already exists to minimize disability and help the client learn to live productively with limitations. Tertiary prevention is used to prevent damage, pain, and other complications when the disability is permanent and irreversible. It minimizes the effects of disease and disability by surveillance and maintenance aimed at preventing complications and deterioration and maximizing the optimal level of functioning. It incorporates creative problem-solving approaches in the design, implementation, and evaluation of nursing intervention to support the client's achievement of successful adaptation to known risks, optimal reconstitution, or establishment of high-level wellness.

Continuing the immobility example, muscle and joint degeneration and metabolic and circulatory disturbances occur when a client is immobile for any length of time. After the client has definite manifestations of immobility, the nurse develops a rehabilitation plan. The plan implements (1) active exercise, (2) passive mobilization, (3) frequent position changes, and (4) balanced diet. Tertiary preventive outcome goals are optimal rehabilitation to higher level of wellness within parameters that the client can achieve.

Models of Health Promotion
Social scientists have worked on models of health-related behavior change or health promotion behavior. The models look at factors that affect individual readiness to take health action.[4] Nurses use health promotion models to motivate clients to make health behavior changes.

Social Cognitive Theory
Bandura developed the Social Cognitive Theory to explain human behavior. The model is based on the premise that human behavior is influenced by "reciprocal determinism" between cognition, behavior, and environment.[2] According to this theory, both efficacy and outcome expectations are crucial for behavioral change. The central concept is self-efficacy. Perceived self-efficacy or efficacy expectation is a judgment of one's ability to execute a specific behavior.

People with high self-efficacy are more confident of their abilities to maintain behavioral change (e.g., exercise adherence, smoking cessation, or achievement of ideal weight). They will attempt to execute the behavior more readily, with greater intensity, and with greater perseverance in response to initial failure than people with comparatively weaker self-efficacy. Interventions to increase self-efficacy include (1) *performance attainment*—having clients successfully execute the behavior; (2) *vicarious experiences*—watching others successfully enact the behavior; (3) *verbal persuasion*—convincing clients of their capability to execute the behavior; and (4) *physiologic states*—helping clients to expect and interpret various physiologic states (e.g., stress, anxiety, fatigue, pain) that may occur when the behavior is executed.

Interventions to increase perceived self-efficacy may be beneficial when the nurse is encouraging health-protecting and health-promoting behaviors. Social Cognitive Theory affects behavior change through the following phases:

1. Promoting and motivating clients to change a target behavior
2. Providing skills training and behavior modeling so that clients can acquire the specific behavioral change skills
3. Developing support networks to help maintain the new behavior
4. Maintaining the behavior through reinforcement
5. Generalizing to other levels of interaction, from the family to the community

Health Belief Model

The Health Belief Model attempts to explain why some people who are illness free take actions to avoid illness, whereas others do not. This model is based on the idea that people want to avoid negatively valued outcomes or personal threats, such as illness, disability, nonproductivity, discomfort, and death. The Health Belief Model includes five factors, identified and illustrated in Box 1-1. Cognitive and emotional beliefs identify individuals' readiness to change behavior.[12] Before people take action to change a behavior (whether it is smoking, not being immunized, or engaging in unprotected sexual activity), they must first feel personally threatened by the disease.

> ### BOX 1-1 The Health Belief Model: Client Characteristics and Starting an Exercise Program
>
> 1. *Perceived susceptibility to a problem.* Negative effects of not exercising (identified as threatening) include difficulty managing weight, lack of energy, and increased risk of coronary artery disease.
> 2. *Perceived seriousness of a problem.* The client feels that the identified negative effects of not exercising are serious problems.
> 3. *Perceived benefits and barriers to taking action.* If an exercise program is started, the benefits (weight loss and maintenance, more energy, better health) will be greater than any barriers (lack of time, cost of equipment, lack of an exercise partner).
> 4. *Cues to action.* The client has been exposed to action cues. An exercise room is available to employees at work, and the company's nurse practitioner has advised the client to begin an exercise program.
> 5. *Self-efficacy* (the behavior is doable). The client is confident that he or she will be able to begin and continue a regular exercise program.

Thus, they must feel personally susceptible to a disease (perceived susceptibility) with serious or severe consequences (perceived seriousness).[12] Once they perceive a threat to their health and their perceived benefits outweigh their perceived barriers, these clients are most likely to undertake the recommended preventive health action.

Health Promotion Model

Pender's Health Promotion Model emphasizes developing individual resources to enhance well-being.[25] This model demonstrates complex biopsychosocial processes that motivate people to engage in behaviors directed toward health enhancement.[25] The model links individual characteristics and experiences and behavior-specific cognitions and affects (including benefits of and barriers to action and interpersonal and situational influences) to a commitment to a health-promoting behavior. The final behavioral outcome is also influenced by the immediate competing demands and preferences, which can derail an intended health-promoting action (e.g., selecting a meal with a high-fat rather than a low-fat content because of taste preferences).

Transtheoretical Model and Stages of Change

The Transtheoretical Model, developed by Prochaska and DiClemente,[26] identifies stages of change: The individual moves from (1) not thinking about change in the near future *(precontemplation)*, (2) to thinking seriously about making a change *(contemplation)*, (3) to planning actively and starting a behavior change *(preparation)*, (4) to making overt changes *(action)*, and (5) to taking steps to maintain changes and avoid relapse *(maintenance)*. This model stages the client's readiness to change and incorporates (1) the pros and cons of a behavior change, (2) self-efficacy, and (3) change processes. For example, a client who states no intention of beginning an exercise program would be in the precontemplation stage for exercise. The model is a guide for assessing a client's readiness to change and for developing stage-specific health interventions.[3]

Teaching and Motivating Clients

Nurses encounter clients during times of major health changes and are in key positions to help them make decisions and adopt behaviors that greatly alter health. To assist others effectively in making healthy decisions and changes, nurses must teach about healthy behaviors, function as role models, and understand the concepts of motivation.[9] The previously described health promotion models can be used as client teaching guides to identify areas for client assessment and crucial teaching content to facilitate the desired behavioral changes. An example of client teaching using the Transtheoretical Model follows.[26] This example can be applied to any change in health behavior, such as quitting smoking, starting a regular exercise program, or eating a low-fat, balanced diet.

According to the Transtheoretical Model, the client's readiness to change must be assessed before any instruction about changes in health behavior can be initiated. The nurse determines the stage of change by assessing the client's intention to make the desired healthy behavior change and by assessing the client's progress toward making the change. Then an intervention is used that is specific to and appropriate for the client's stage of change.

Both practice and research have demonstrated that giving information to clients does not in itself bring about healthy behaviors. Nurses frequently give up trying to teach because of a lack of client motivation. When this occurs, the client may be labeled as "noncompliant" or "difficult." Instead, it may be that the client cannot relate to the intervention because it is not directed at the client's specific stage of behavioral change, situation, or cultural perspective. It is important to ask clients about their perceived benefits of changing the behavior as well as about barriers to changing the behavior.

Motivating others to change health behaviors involves the following:

- Clients must believe that the problem is solvable.
- Clients must view the solution as something they want to do.
- Clients must feel competent to carry out the behavior successfully.
- Clients must feel able to overcome barriers to change.
- Clients must experience positive feedback and consequences.

The nurse's role is to use multiple skills to empower clients to engage in healthy behaviors. Approaches include helping clients to identify their values and to explore feelings about themselves, with emphasis on identifying strengths. Helping clients set goals (developing intrinsic motivation) greatly enhances the likelihood of achieving the desired behavioral changes. Nurses assist clients in differentiating perceived from actual barriers and in promoting behaviors to overcome the actual barriers. Whenever possible, nurses should act as models of health with a joyful zest for living, thus providing a living example.

Multifactorial Aspects of Chronic Disease

A century ago our ancestors fought infectious and communicable diseases. Although serious infectious diseases are still a public health threat, most life-threatening diseases today are those that become chronic as a result of metabolic abnormalities induced by health risk factors such as genetic or biologic (aging), behavioral (nutri-

tion), and environmental influences. Figure 1-2 shows the association between multiple risk factors and chronic diseases. Health risk factors reflect a multicausal theory of disease causation. The relationships among health risk factors and disease are examined in the following text.

Genetic or Biologic Health Risk Factors

Heredity and Disease. Genetic aspects of disease have been recognized for many years. Over the past 10 years, a great deal of effort has been put into creating a physical map of the human genome, that is, discovering the order of genes within the genome and placing navigational landmarks on these genes.[17] The genome contains the master blueprint for all cellular structures and activities for the lifetime of the cell or organism. Working toward the assembly of the complete sequencing of the genome's physical map has assisted in identifying more disease-causing genes. Currently, more than 4000 diseases, for example, sickle cell anemia and cystic fibrosis, are known to be genetic and inherited from the individual's mother or father. Moreover, it is now known that alterations in our genes play a role in common conditions such as heart disease, diabetes, and many types of cancer. Recent technology has allowed researchers to develop therapy to treat altered gene structures and to clone a new being.

More than one fifth of the human genes differ in form from one person to another. This remarkable degree of genetic variation among normal people is what accounts for natural variations in attributes such as height, hair color, intelligence, personality, and blood pressure. Through the proteins that genes encode, genes determine how efficiently individuals process foods, how effectively they detoxify poisons, and how vigorously they respond to infections. These genetic differences affect each person's ability to handle environmental challenges, including those that produce disease. In every disease, there is some degree of genetic interaction with the environment. Common disorders, such as heart disease and most cancers, arise from a complex interaction among multiple genes and between genes and factors in the environment. Because of the rapidly advancing science in genetics, features throughout this text discuss the genetic basis of disease.

Many diseases have their roots in our genes. In the case of a recessive disease, if one abnormal gene is inherited, the child does not show manifestations of clinical disease, but they pass the abnormal gene to 50% (on average) of their offspring. In the case of a dominant disorder, if one abnormal gene is inherited, the child will likely show the disease. Such diseases are termed *genetic disorders;* an example is Huntington's chorea, which is a progressive neurologic disease caused by an inherited dominant gene mutation.

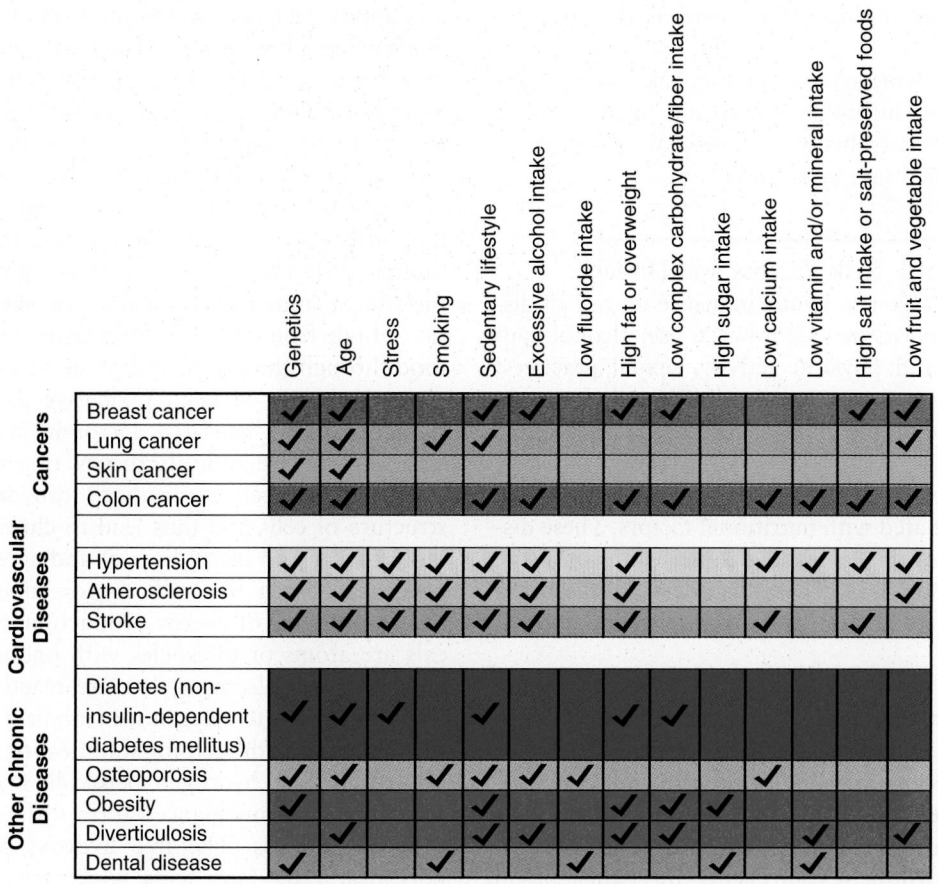

FIGURE 1-2 Multiple risk factors have been linked to many chronic diseases. It is theorized that exposure to lifestyle risk factors may interact with genetic predisposition to cause the disease. (Modified from Whitney, E.N., & Rolfes, S.R. (2002). *Understanding nutrition*, [9th ed.]. Belmont CA: Wadsworth Publishing.)

New approaches to the treatment of genetic disease include gene therapy. Once the disease-causing defective gene has been identified, gene therapy makes it possible to correct such defects in the function of cells. *Gene therapy* involves the injection of a normal copy of deoxyribonucleic acid (DNA) fragments into cells of clients with the disease. The fragments find their way to the nucleus and repair enzymes to restore normal function to the cell. Today research is being conducted on the use of gene therapy in the treatment of Alzheimer's disease, muscular dystrophy, cystic fibrosis, and some forms of primary and secondary epilepsy. Gene therapy is a rapidly evolving form of treatment, and other new approaches include the promotion of new blood vessel growth *(angiogenesis)* for clients who have impaired circulation associated with disorders such as cancer, macular degeneration, coronary heart disease, and diabetes.

Aging and Disease. There is an increased risk for all diseases with aging, especially cancer. Older clients tend to attribute aches and pains to aging itself and often are less likely to have routine preventive screenings. Older clients are more prone to injury and acute infections (especially respiratory) than younger clients. Contributing to this are the increased occurrence of chronic illness, decreased reserves of energy, and decreased ability to respond physiologically to stress. It is common to see an older client who is mentally competent become confused during the stress of acute illness, often resulting from renal and hepatic changes.[34] Recovery from acute illness takes longer than in a younger client, and it is possible that the previous level of functioning will not be regained.

Even though the risk of disease and disability clearly increases as the individual ages, poor health is not an inevitable consequence. Much of the illness, disability, and death associated with chronic disease are avoidable through known early detection and prevention interventions. Common nursing interventions in the care of the older client include promotion of physical safety, prevention of alterations in skin integrity, promotion of social interactions, promotion of adequate nutrition, and cancer screenings. It should never be presumed that all older clients are weak and debilitated. The nurse's role in health promotion among older clients is described in Chapter 3.

Historically, a wide array of factors has been thought to cause diseases, including spirits and imbalances. A history of health care historical overview of causes of disease is presented on the website.

Behavioral Health Risk Factors and Disease

Several behaviors exert a strong influence on risk of disease. These behaviors include tobacco use, alcohol consumption, diet and physical activity, sexual practices, and inadequate stress management.[10] The following sections concentrate on the influence of diet on disease.

Diet and Disease. Heart disease, cancer, stroke, and liver disease are associated with nutritional factors. These disorders are four of the 10 leading causes of death in the United States (Box 1-2). These disorders are discussed in Chapters 47 (diabetes), 54 (hypertension), and 72 (stroke).

Diet and Heart Disease. A diet that is high in saturated fats and cholesterol is linked to increased blood cholesterol levels and a greater risk for heart disease. Saturated fat raises blood cholesterol more than other forms of fat. Reducing saturated fat to less than 10% of dietary calories will help your clients lower their blood cholesterol level. Atherosclerosis and heart disease are discussed in Unit 13.

Diet and Cancer. Cancer is a disease of multiple origins, such as heredity, smoking, and environmental exposure. Some cancers have dietary links. Many people fear that food additives are *carcinogens* (cancer-causing substances). In fact, food additives have little to do with cancer; however, contaminants of food, entities that get into foods by accident, may be powerful carcinogens, such as pesticides and bacteria. Consuming a high-fat diet has also been implicated in cancer. Animals that have been exposed to a carcinogen and given a high-fat

diet appear to have greater numbers of tumors than animals given a low-fat diet. Thus fat appears to be a cancer promoter, perhaps by (1) causing the body to secrete more hormones, such as estrogen; (2) promoting the secretion of bile into the intestine, where organisms can convert the bile into compounds that cause cancer; or (3) incorporating into cell membranes and changing them so they offer less resistance to carcinogenic invaders. It is thought that fiber and vegetables might help to reduce the risk of some forms of cancer by speeding the excretion of bile from the body, decreasing the transit time of food through the colon, and reducing exposure.

Antioxidants in Diet. Oxidative damage to cells is thought to be a causative factor in disease and aging. The oxygen free radicals theory of aging and disease states that oxygen free radicals can damage the basic structure of cells and thus lead to chronic diseases (notably cancer and heart disease) and accelerate the aging process. Oxygen free radicals, or superoxide radicals, are by-products of energy production. Superoxide radicals are atoms or molecules with one or more pairs of unpaired, free electrons that are reactive. The radicals commonly bind to oxygen for stabilization. The oxygen then binds to hydrogen for stabilization. The product of this reaction is hydrogen peroxide, which is toxic to cells. The most unbalanced form of free radicals is free hydroxy radicals. The free hydroxy radicals bind to polyunsaturated fatty acids, which are commonly found in cell membranes and membranes of organelles within the cell. If the free radical binds to the lysosome, the cell is destroyed.

The body's defense mechanisms against these free radicals are referred to as *antioxidants*. Antioxidants help deactivate *free radicals*. The antioxidants include vitamins C and E and beta-carotene (vitamin A). Vitamin E and selenium in cell membranes are oxidized by the free radicals, much as fatty acid is. Vitamin E neutralizes the free radical and prevents it from attaching to a fatty acid. In the process, vitamin E is damaged. The damaged vitamin E is restored by vitamin C. The role of beta-carotene in free radical antioxidation is not clear. Vitamins A and E are carried by the low-density lipoproteins (LDLs). Plants are vital sources of antioxidants for humans and other animals. In addition, hundreds of dietary supplements now trumpet the antioxidants they contain; however, it is better to get beta-carotene from food (e.g., carrots, spinach, cantaloupe) than from pills.

Beta-carotene (vitamin A) regulates *cellular differentiation,* a process that goes awry in cancer. Some people think that if they take vitamin A supplements, their risk of cancer will be reduced. This area is still being studied, but it appears that the fiber in foods containing vitamin A is more important than the vitamin itself. Other antipromoters of cancer include vitamin B_6, folate, pantothenic acid, vitamin B_{12}, iron, zinc, selenium, and antioxidants, such as vitamins C and E. Some non-nutrient

---

BOX 1-2   *Ten Leading Causes of Death*

1. Heart disease
2. Cancer
3. Stroke
4. Chronic lower respiratory disease
5. Accidents
6. Diabetes
7. Pneumonia and influenza
8. Alzheimer's disease
9. Nephritis, nephritic syndrome, and nephrosis
10. Septicemia

compounds are found in foods from the cabbage family. These foods produce chemicals that activate enzymes that destroy carcinogens. The research base for the synthetic form of antioxidants and other cancer-preventing vitamin supplements is less conclusive. Dietitians recommend eating vegetables and consuming various foods to dilute the effects of harmful cancer promoters but may or may not recommend taking vitamin supplements.

Alcohol Consumption and Disease. Moderate alcohol intake plays several roles in health. Some of the beneficial effects of components in red wine include flavonoids and other antioxidants. Research indicates that moderate alcohol intake (one glass of red wine per day) may raise high-density lipoprotein (HDL) levels, anticlotting properties, and reduces the risk of heart disease.[36] Alcohol is addictive, however, and a high intake of alcohol is associated with hypertension, stroke, liver disease, and several types of cancer, including some found in the head, neck, and reproductive system.

Inadequate Stress Management and Disease. The perceived stresses associated with behavioral and environmental causes contribute to illness and disease.[18] When an individual perceives a stressful situation, the stress response is initiated, releasing catecholamines. Repeated activation of the stress response and the resulting deterioration that the body experiences are called *allostatic load*. Allostatic load is influenced by the way individuals manage and perceive stress. It is also influenced by diet, alcohol, exercise, tobacco, and sleep. This stress response triggers disease causing physiologic events, including modulation of the immune system. An abnormal response to the allostatic load is *autoimmunity*, which literally means immunity against oneself. In addition, asthma, diabetes, various gastrointestinal disorders, heart disease, and viral infections are negatively influenced by stress.

Environmental Health Risk Factors

Studies in cancer causation have revealed that chemicals in the workplace, for example, asbestos, diesel fumes, and radiation, are responsible for specific cancers. Such discoveries have left the impression that most human cancers are associated with environmental chemical contamination. This opinion has led to public pressure on government to control chemical contamination as a key means of cancer prevention. Careful analysis of the causative elements in each type of cancer, however, has shown that prevailing lifestyles in a given population (especially tobacco use, nutritional variations, and physical activity) account for most of the incidence of cancer.

Sun exposure increases the risk of skin cancers. The populations most sensitive to the sun's effects are those with fair skin, such as people of Celtic descent. The chief cause of skin cancer is damage to DNA from ultraviolet light. An allegedly "healthy" look (tanned skin) can have unhealthy consequences. The belief that sun exposure is needed for vitamin D absorption is obsolete in most countries because milk is supplemented with vitamin D. Children who have no sun exposure and do not drink milk can be at risk for rickets from low vitamin D levels. Adults who do not consume adequate vitamin D develop osteomalacia. Veiled Arabic women constitute a high-risk group because they shield their skin from the sun and may have a low intake of milk and other sources of vitamin D.[7]

Air and water pollution can lead to disease. Air pollution, smog, and haze contain a mixture of industry and automotive chemicals, such as solvents, metals, and unburned fuel. Air pollution increases the risk of asthma and lung cancer. Water pollution has caused endemic infections with various microorganisms. In many parts of the world, the greatest problem is a shortage of clean nonpolluted water.

Interrelationship of Health Risk Factors

A person's body, mind, and the environment all function together to determine whether illness develops. The brain helps to maintain an internal milieu and assists the body in adapting to the external environment. The response can affect the body's functioning. The way the brain defines a situation can evoke chemical and nervous system reactions. When people habitually respond to every frustration, disappointment, or loss as if it is a matter of life and death, then the endocrine, musculoskeletal, and autonomic nervous systems overrespond. If people view life as requiring constant domination of things and people, they can have excessive production of cholesterol, triglycerides, norepinephrine, adrenocorticotropic hormone, and insulin. This attitude may contribute to deficient levels of pituitary growth hormone.

The function and balance of neurotransmitters (chemical messengers, such as enkephalins and endorphins) can be influenced by drugs, viruses, bacteria, poor nutrition, defective genes, aging, or the perception of stress. Tissue damage can result from normal bodily processes that go awry or are disrupted; these processes include (1) neurotransmitter activity in the brain, (2) the stress hormones of the adrenal glands and nervous system, and (3) the helper and suppressor cells of the immune system. For example, excessive stress hormones (corticosteroids, catecholamines) can lead to artery damage or may suppress the action of antibodies and natural killer cells, which protect the body from foreign invaders and tumor development. Deficient suppressor cells may permit overaction of the immune system to the point at which the body starts attacking itself, such as in rheumatoid arthritis. Autoimmune disorders are discussed in Chapter 79.

The brain is central to any change in health because it is the mediator between the external and internal environments. Through the brain's interpretation, we can change an environment, leave it, or engage in it; or we can decide to rest, exercise, or diet. Ultimately, illness involves a combination of mind-body factors. These factors interact to produce symptoms. It is not uncommon to experience depression with physical illness or to have physical manifestations of mental or emotional illness.

Increasingly, scientific study is directed toward the mind-body interactions. The increase in chronic conditions and the disillusion with medical care have led to increased use of alternative or complementary practices, which are often based on mind-body connection theory, are wellness oriented, are less intrusive, and have fewer side effects. The Office of Alternative Medicine within the National Institutes of Health funds research to evaluate the effectiveness of alternative medical treatment.

HEALTH PROMOTION AND ILLNESS PREVENTION INTERVENTIONS

Health promotion and illness prevention interventions are essential for everyone, including people who have chronic conditions.[27] Chronic conditions account for about 80% of all medical expenses.[7] Chronic conditions usually cannot be cured, but health promotion and illness prevention interventions can improve the quality of life for those with chronic conditions and have the potential to reduce medical expenses. A health risk appraisal should be done, with risk-reduction interventions tailored to each individual's need. A general discussion of health promotion follows. Health promotion for young and middle-aged adults is described in Chapter 2; for older clients, see Chapter 3.

Modifying Behavioral Health Risk Factors

Nutrition and exercise are addressed together because they work synergistically to promote high-level wellness. Sedentary living and the lack of sound nutrition contribute to major risk factors, such as obesity, hypercholesterolemia, and muscular atrophy. When people begin to modify one of these two areas, the other area often receives attention at the same time.

Nutrition

Nutrition has moved into the forefront as a prominent component of health promotion and disease prevention. A correlation exists between what we eat and how we feel; the potential for development of disease is also correlated with nutritional status and habits. Cardiovascular disease (CVD), cancer, type 2 diabetes, and osteoporosis are three common afflictions that are directly related to nutrition to some degree. Scores of other conditions related to poor nutrition may be less crippling, but they clearly affect how we feel (e.g., dental caries, constipation, and acne). The U.S. Department of Agriculture (USDA) has revised its dietary recommendations and has created the "food pyramid" (see Chapter 2), which includes food groupings and provides suggested servings from each group.[11,32]

Nutritional Deficits. Deficits in nutritional intake can result in stunted growth, reduced metabolic function, delayed or premature cessation of reproductive function, and increased risk for less serious illnesses. Mechanisms of homeostasis protect the body from temporary deficits, but chronic nutritional deprivation creates a susceptible host for the diseases of malnutrition. Three classic deficiency diseases are *scurvy* (vitamin C deficiency), *beriberi* (thiamin deficiency), and *pellagra* (niacin deficiency). Malnutrition also increases susceptibility to infection (see Chapter 21) and decreases wound-healing ability (see Chapter 20).

Nutritional Excesses. Overeating or eating too many of the wrong foods can also cause illness and disease. In the United States, an epidemic increase in the incidence of obesity has occurred over the past 20 years in all sociodemographic groups. About 20% of Americans are obese, and 11 million Americans are severely obese, meaning they are more than 100 pounds overweight or weigh twice their ideal body weight.[33] Many people eat foods that are high in fat, sugar, protein, simple carbohydrates, caffeine, and alcohol. Being overweight or obese increases the risk of diabetes, abnormal cholesterol levels, high blood pressure, and cancer (see Chapter 2). Researchers estimate that being overweight or obese led to an additional $22.17 billion in direct medical costs for the treatment of CVD in 1996 ($31 billion in 2001 dollars, 17% of the total direct medical cost of treating CVD).[35]

Balanced Nutrition. Healthy nutrition is defined as a balance of nutrients, fiber, fluids, vitamins, and minerals. Whenever possible, foods should be free of chemicals, additives, preservatives, and toxins. Clients should eat fresh foods, fruits, vegetables, legumes, and lean meats and should avoid high-fat, overprocessed, and fried foods. The U.S. government recommends a diet with less fat and more complex carbohydrates (see Chapter 2). Clients can use a food diary (see Chapter 30) to assess their food intake.

Exercise

A new way of thinking about fitness is depicted in Chapter 2. Exercise, like nutrition, should be balanced and performed on a regular basis. Currently, the U.S. Surgeon General recommends adults exercise for about 30 minutes each day, and recently the Institute of Medicine recommended at least 1 hour of exercise per day.[11,31] This exercise can be done in a series of "brisk" 10-minute activity periods and has the same beneficial results as a continuous workout.[22] Exercise tones and strengthens internal organs and the circulatory, respiratory, and musculoskeletal systems. The components of fitness are multiple (warm-up, aerobic exercise, cooldown, resistance training, and stretching), and all aspects should be part of a routine.

Exercise does not reverse pathophysiologic changes but conditions muscles to work more efficiently. Exercise also stimulates the production of endorphins (which promote the feelings of well-being), increases production of HDLs, assists in weight control, decreases risk of some cancers, and increases activity tolerance.

According to recent data from the National Health and Nutrition Examination Survey, most individuals' estimated caloric and fat intake has actually gone down; however, their amount of physical activity has also gone down.[35] A physical exercise program coupled with a balanced nutritional diet is the most effective way to actualize promotion of physical health and combat weight gain. Eating and exercising wisely develop strength and endurance, a more youthful appearance, increased vitality, appropriate posture, and general physical stamina (see Chapters 2 and 3).

Empowerment

Empowerment involves helping clients assume control and mastery over all aspects of their lives. This involves health care as well as social and political environments. It is crucial to accept clients as the experts in their own experience and definition of health. At the basic level, *empowerment* means a transfer of skills, resources, access, and language so that the client with a chronic condition can be as independent as possible. Empowerment can occur only in a supportive environment. The nurse must learn how to establish and maintain an empowering environment in which the client sees the potential and value in seizing power and being independent.

In the United States, changing social beliefs about individual rights and normality have influenced state and federal laws. This legislation has contributed to a decrease in attitudinal and architectural barriers to social integration as well as to increased availability of health care, housing, employment, recreation, and transportation for ill people. Nurses can encourage clients to be politically active and can also be active themselves in advocating for the health care rights of those with chronic conditions.

Developing Human Potential

Current definitions of *health* refer to the achievement of maximum potential, or *self-actualization* (see Table 1-1). In the domain of health promotion, people develop and maintain life potentials, becoming the best and healthiest they can. The more time and energy devoted to developing strengths, the less likely problems are to develop. The physical potentials of nutrition and exercise were discussed earlier.

Each physical body is unique. Through the senses of sight, hearing, touch, taste, and smell, we gather experience of the world. When the body is nurtured, it increases in strength, vitality, energy, sexuality, and the capacity to communicate and connect with other potentials. Our picture of the world is created uniquely from mental stimuli. It is through logical processes that we learn to understand fully, enjoy, and appreciate many of life's greatest pleasures. Growth is possible when we are receptive to information, suggestions, and help.

Emotions are feelings, the inner and outer responses to the events encountered in life. One of the greatest challenges is to acknowledge, own, express, and understand one's emotions. Increasing attention to the development and balancing of this potential allows spontaneity and positive zest for living to emerge.

Spirit comes from one's roots and inner core of being. It is related to the universal need to understand the human experience of life on earth. Where did we come from? Where are we going? What is our purpose? Why do good and evil exist? What occurs after death? Who or what put this life form together? Development of the spiritual potential allows for the transcendence of the experience of oneness, peace, harmony, and connection with the universe.

We cannot live purposeful lives without meaningful relationships. We may not share a house with anyone, but many of us live in neighborhoods and all of us are part of communities, cities, and states. Our relationships extend to our nation and to the whole of planet earth. The challenge in relationships is to extend ourselves and to learn how to exchange feelings of honesty, trust, intimacy, compassion, openness, and harmony. When we share our feelings and experiences, true interchange occurs. It is through our attitude and orientation that we affect the outcome of all our encounters.

People have enormous capacity for making choices either consciously or unconsciously. Health and balance occur when we use the skill of effective choice making. Each of us is responsible for assessing our values and desires. No one else can make decisions for us.

Milio[21] contends that the focus on choice is paramount in shaping the overall health for the person as well as for the society as a whole. Our range of choices is affected by personal resources, which include awareness, knowledge, our own beliefs, and our family's beliefs. Time, money, support of family and friends, and the urgency of other priorities influence what choices are made. Milio notes that "most human beings, professional or nonprofessional, provider or consumer, make the easiest choices available to them most of the time."[20] The nurse needs to try to recognize this tendency when working with clients. Lifestyle behavioral patterns are not isolated choices unrelated to social, personal, or economic circumstances.

Stress Management

All of us have experienced stress, but each of us has different perceptions and thoughts about it. What are your perceptions? Think of a recent stressful event at home or at work that involved you and someone else. How did you react? How did the other person react? Was there a different reaction to the same event? Stress is an individual matter. No two people respond in completely the same manner. In a given situation, one person may perceive a challenge, whereas the other perceives a serious stressor. The way in which each situation is perceived affects health both directly and indirectly.

One factor that can alter a stress response is the environment, such as social supports, physical setting, and organizational factors. Social supports can buffer individuals from the potentially negative effects of stressors, and people who have strong social supports may live longer and have a lower incidence of physical illness. Other factors are internal, such as personality, personal resources, temperament, history, and genetic variables. (Within the personal aspect of the stress response is how the stressor is appraised and how the person copes with the stressor.)

The expression of emotion, especially anger, is one coping style. One might think that the expression of anger would have a negative effect on illness outcome; surprisingly, however, the outcome after expression of negative emotions depends on the disease. Frequently, expressing hostility and anger increased survival in people with cancer, but in people who had lung disease, the expression of anger and other negative emotions increased their manifestations and adverse physiologic changes (e.g., hypoxia) occurred.

Social Support. Scientists have long noted a link between social relationships and health. Socially isolated people are less healthy, both psychologically and physically, and are more likely to die than people who are more socially integrated; however, the actual cause and effect are not clear. Are unhealthy people less likely to have and maintain social relationships, or does the lack of social relationships cause people to become ill and die? Do people in a social network provide a basis of health?

As we learn more about chronic illnesses, the role of social support seems even stronger. Physiologic studies have shown a link between the amygdala and the hypothalamus in the brain and positive social relationships. Social contact decreases levels of hormones such as cortisol, epinephrine, and norepinephrine. From a psychological standpoint, social relationships provide a sense of meaning or coherence that promotes a healthy lifestyle. Social support may help a client adhere to medical treatment and seek medical care. Marriage, a widely studied area of social support, may be simultaneously a source of stress and support, but regardless of the quality of the interaction, marriage is a form of support. Frequently, a quick deterioration in the health of a survivor is seen after the death of a spouse. Health care providers must make use of a client's social support network, including the network in the treatment regimen and assessing the impact of illness on the partner.

Self-Help Groups. Self-help groups are growing in industrialized nations. It is estimated that there are at least 500,000 to 750,000 self-help groups in the United States, with at least 10 to 15 million members. Some groups are approved by various organizations. Reach for Recovery, an organization for women who have had a mastectomy, is approved by the American Cancer Society. Informal groups also exist, such as people caring for older, infirm parents in their homes, who meet to discuss common problems. Self-help groups are recognized and accepted as a form of assistance to meet people's needs. The largest groups help people with mental illnesses, and the second largest groups help people with acquired immunodeficiency syndrome (AIDS).

There are two types of self-help groups. One is the Twelve-Step program, of which Alcoholics Anonymous is the prototype. The other is a group whose members share common experiences. Characteristics of both types of groups include (1) helping with cognitive restructuring of an event or experience; (2) instructing in adaptive skills; and (3) fostering emotional support, personal disclosure, socialization, taking actions together, empowerment, self-reliance, and self-esteem.

Developing Coping Skills. Many practical methods exist to cope with stress. Planning is one effective way to reduce adverse effects. For example, we prepare for predictable life changes, such as marriage, job change, or retirement. We plan by establishing goals. Through planning, we develop a belief system that allows us to dictate our life and our experience. Setting goals facilitates this belief system because it serves as a reminder that we have the power to create new experiences in our lives. Goals should include areas such as meaning and purpose, fun and play, exercise, nutrition, work, and relaxation.

The most widely practiced and possibly the most effective exercise for immediate stress reduction is to evoke the *relaxation response:*

1. When first learning to do this, remove yourself from the source of stress, assume a relaxed posture, and begin taking deep breaths through your nose.
2. Consciously and progressively relax all of your muscles.

3. Begin thinking of your strengths and imagining a successful outcome.

4. Realize that, in the great scheme of things, this event, whatever its nature, is only a minor event. Evoking the relaxation response induces a decrease in sympathetic nervous system activity and produces an altered, quieted state of consciousness.

5. As you begin to appreciate the effects of the simple progressive relaxation technique, you may want to explore and develop more long-term stress management techniques, such as biofeedback training, yoga, *Tai Chi*, meditation, and guided imagery.

Mind-Body Views and Alternative Therapies

Various mind-body therapies have been introduced to Western medicine. Biofeedback, autogenic training, therapeutic touch, guided imagery, and focused thought are examples. Mind-body therapies can influence the immune system, help manage pain, and reduce stress and anxiety. An example of the positive influences of a mind-body therapy is teaching a client to slow down, simplify, and fully relax so that the client might experience enhanced life satisfaction and beneficial immune system changes.

The Office of Alternative Medicine recently reviewed the use of acupuncture for treatment of chronic conditions. Acupuncture was found to be effective for addictions and psychiatric disorders; allergy and immunology; general pain; headaches; and nausea, vomiting, and postoperative problems.[23] Another effective therapy was the integration of behavioral and relaxation approaches into the treatment of chronic pain and insomnia (see also Chapters 22 and 24 and the Complementary and Alternative Therapy feature on Spirituality and Health at right).[23] Various forms of complementary and alternative therapies are presented throughout this textbook.

Modifying Environmental Health Risk Factors

Environment is one of the four primary determinants of health. It is not enough to think solely in terms of self or of our immediate surroundings when we think of health promotion. We are not just members of families, communities, states, or regions; we are intertwined with one another and linked as a global family. What affects one of us now has a ripple effect and affects us all. Because of the population explosion and congested urban living conditions, it is easy to affect another person's living environment. For example, it is possible to pollute the air by driving a car with a defective exhaust pipe, to impinge on auditory air space by playing loud music, or to create an eyesore by littering. Collectively, we can pollute the environment to such a great degree that life itself is threatened.

COMPLEMENTARY AND ALTERNATIVE THERAPY

Spirituality and Health

A growing body of research is showing that spiritual or spiritually related activities may in fact be protective of health.[5] For many people, spirituality may mean their particular religious practice; for others, it may be their own personal views and beliefs or the way they feel connection to something beyond themselves. In fact, connectedness may be an important component of spirituality and its positive health benefits. The social and communal aspects of many religions and spiritual practices may be a common denominator in the health benefits seen. Conversely, social isolation is considered a factor in poor health.[3]

Levin has researched the epidemiology of religion and has found that people who were more religious or spiritual also had better health, greater well-being, and less depression.[2] Research into the effects of intercessory prayer (prayers said on someone else's behalf), sometimes without their being aware of it consciously, is both intriguing and controversial. Preliminary data from a pilot study of a number of interventions, including intercessory prayer, in a group of clients with unstable angina and infarction showed the least adverse outcomes when they were mentioned in the prayers of others.[1] Such studies are difficult to conduct and to evaluate. Yet other research has shown that when a certain percentage of a population is engaged in Transcendental Meditation, the incidence of violence decreases in surrounding populations.[4] Such research leads some to speculate that there is a field of consciousness of which we are all a part.

Some studies have shown that clients with cancer who participate in support groups show improvement in quality of life and in survival time.[3] Perhaps this is because "all relationships are spiritual." The more intimate and loving one's relationships, the better this is for one's health.[3]

References
1. Horrigan, B. (1999). Mitchell W. Krucoff, MD, The Mantra Project. *Alternative therapies in health and medicine. 5*(3):75-82.
2. Horrigan B. (1999). Jeff Levin, MPH, PhD, The Power of Love. *Alternative Therapies in Health and Medicine, 5*(4):78-86.
3. Ornish D. (1998). *Love and survival.* New York: Harper-Collins.
4. Sharma, H. & Clark, C. (1998). *Contemporary ayurveda.* Philadelphia: Churchill Livingstone.
5. Ziegler, J. (1998). Spirituality returns to the fold in medical practice. *Journal of the National Cancer Institute, 90,* 1255-1257.

Health promotion, because it addresses the whole self and the whole human family, must also address protection of the environment. It is not within the scope of this chapter to delineate ways to do this; its purpose is to stimulate an awareness that each of us can play a role in cleaning, maintaining, and striving to improve environmental conditions to the best of our ability.

CONCLUSIONS

Health promotion is a key watch phrase for the 21st century. Nurses are encouraged to develop a consciousness that includes attention to the social, political, and economic aspects of the environment. Once we recognize that establishing health-promoting behaviors can alter the presence or absence of good health, specific interventions must be delineated and disseminated to the subsets of the population that can benefit. All clients, including those with chronic conditions, have the potential to achieve improvements in quality of life and health care savings with interventions of health promotion and illness prevention. Appraisal of health risk can reveal which risk-reduction interventions would be helpful. Models of health promotion serve as a guide for motivating clients to make health behavioral changes. A broad understanding of chronic conditions will widen the nurse's role and will assist the nurse in providing holistic nursing care to facilitate client and family adaptation and ameliorate the course of a chronic condition.

BIBLIOGRAPHY

1. American Nurses' Association. (1995). *Nursing's social policy statement*. Washington, DC: Author.
 2. Bandura, A. (1986). *Social foundations of thought and action: A social cognitive theory* (p. 22). Englewood Cliffs, NJ: Prentice-Hall.
3. Cassidy, C. (1999). Using the Transtheoretical Model to facilitate behavior change in patients with chronic illness. *Journal of the American Academy of Nurse Practitioners, 11,* 281-287.
4. Downie, R., Tannahill, C., & Tannahill, A. (1996). *Health promotion models and values* (2nd ed.). New York: Oxford University Press.
5. Dunn, H. (1961). *High-level wellness*. Arlington, VA: R.W. Beatty.
6. Edelman, C., & Mandle, C. (Eds.). (2001). *Health promotion throughout the life span* (5th ed.). St. Louis: Mosby.
7. el-Sonbaty, M., & Abdul-Ghaffar, N. (1996). Vitamin D deficiency in veiled Kuwaiti women. *European Journal of Clinical Nutrition, 50,* 315-318.
8. Fox, P., & Fama, T. (1996). *Managed care and chronic illness: Challenges and opportunities*. Gaithersburg, MD: Aspen.
9. Gochman, D. (Ed.). (1997). *Handbook of health behavior research: I: Personal and social determinants*. New York: Plenum Press.
 10. Institute of Medicine. (2001). *Health & behavior: The interplay of biological, behavioral, & societal influences*. Washington, DC: National Academy Press.
 11. Institute of Medicine. (2002). *Dietary reference intakes for energy, carbohydrates, fiber, fat, protein and amino acids (macronutrients)*. Washington, DC: National Academy Press.

12. Janz, N., Champion, V., & Strecher, V. (2002). The Health Belief Model. In K. Glanz, B. Rimer, & F. Lewis (Eds.), *Health behavior and health education: Theory, research, and practice* (3rd ed). San Francisco: Jossey-Bass.
13. Labonte, R., et al. (2002). Community capacity building: a parallel track for health promotion programs. *Canadian Journal of Public Health, 93,* 181-182
14. Lalonde, M. (1974). *A new perspective on the health of Canadians*. Ottawa: Government of Canada.
15. Leavell, H., & Clark, E. (1965). *Preventative medicine for the doctor in his community: An epidemiologic approach*. New York: McGraw-Hill.
15a. Leininger, M. (1978). *Transcultural nursing: Concepts, theories, and practices*. New York: John Wiley and Sons.
16. Lilienfeld, A. (1976). *Foundations of epidemiology*. New York: Oxford University Press.
17. Little, J., et al. (2002). Reporting, appraising, and integrating data on genotype prevalence and gene-disease associations. *American Journal of Epidemiology, 156,* 300-310.
18. McEwen, B. (2002). The neurobiology and neuroendocrinology of stress implications for post-traumatic stress disorder from a basic science perspective. *Psychiatric Clinics of North America, 25,* 469-494, ix.
19. Mendelson, C. (2002). Health perceptions of Mexican American women. *Journal of Transcultural Nursing, 13,* 210-217.
20. Milio, N. (1976). A framework for prevention: Changing health damaging to health-generating life patterns. *American Journal of Public Health, 66,* 435-439.
21. Milio, N. (2001). Evaluation of health promotion policies: Tracking a moving target. *World Health Organization Regional Publications. European Series, 92,* 365-385.
22. Murphy, M., et al. (2002). Accumulating brisk walking for fitness, cardiovascular risk, and psychological health. *Medicine & Science in Sports & Exercise, 34,* 1468-1474.
23. National Institutes of Health, Office of Alternative Medicine. (2002). Grant award and research data. Bethesda, MD: Office of Alternative Medicine. Available at http://nccam.nih.gov/health/acupuncture.
24. Newman, M. (1987). Health conceptualizations: Nursing emergency paradigm: The diagnosis of pattern. In McLean J., (Ed.), *Classification of nursing diagnosis*. St. Louis: Proceedings of the Seventh Conference.
25. Pender, N. (1996). *Health promotion in nursing practice* (3rd ed.). Stamford, CT: Appleton & Lange.
26. Prochaska, J., Redding, C., & Evers, K. (2002). The Transtheoretical Model and stages of change. In K. Glanz, B. Rimer, & F. Lewis (Eds.), *Health behavior and health education: Theory, research, and practice* (3rd ed). San Francisco: Jossey-Bass.
27. Smedley, B., & Syme, S. (Eds.). (2001). *Promoting health: intervention strategies from social and behavioral research*. Washington, DC: National Academy Press.
28. Tuzcu, E., et al. (2001). High prevalence of coronary atheroscle- rosis in asymptomatic teenagers and young adults: evidence from intravascular ultrasound. *Circulation, 103,* 2705-2710.
29. U.S. Department of Health and Human Services. (1979). *Healthy* *people: The Surgeon General's report on health promotion and disease prevention*. Washington, DC: U.S. Government Printing Office.
30. U.S. Department of Health and Human Services. (1991). *Healthy* *people 2000: National health promotion and disease prevention objectives*. (PHS No. 91-50213.) Washington, DC: U.S. Government Printing Office.

EB 31. U.S. Department of Health and Human Services. (1996). *Physical activity and health: A report of the Surgeon General.* Atlanta: National Center for Chronic Disease Prevention and Health Promotion.

EB 32. U.S. Department of Health and Human Services. (2000). *Nutrition and your health. Dietary guidelines for Americans.* (5th ed.) Washington, DC: U.S. Department of Agriculture.

EB 33. U.S. Department of Health and Human Services. (2000). *Healthy People 2010.* (2nd ed.) 2 vols. Washington, DC: U.S. Government Printing Office.

EB 34. Wakefield, B. (2002). Risk for acute confusion on hospital admission. *Clinical Nursing Research, 11,* 153-172.

35. Wang, G., et al. (2002). Economic burden of cardiovascular disease associated with excess body weight in U.S. adults. *American Journal of Preventive Medicine, 23,* 1-6. EB

36. Wannamethee, S., & Shaper, A. (1999). Type of alcoholic drink and risk of major coronary heart disease events and all-cause mortality. *American Journal of Public Health, 89,* 685-690. EB

37. World Health Organization. (1947). Constitution of the World Health Organization. *Chronicle of the World Health Organization, 1*(1-2), 29-43.

Health Promotion in Middle-Aged Adults

Kathryn Fiandt

evolve

Web Enhancements

Ethical Issues in Nursing
What Values are Represented in the Nurse-Client Relationship?

http://evolve.elsevier.com/Black/medsurg/

Appendix A
Religious Beliefs and Practices Affecting Health Care

It is essential that nurses be knowledgeable regarding health promotion and disease prevention. When providing holistic care, think beyond current health problems to the client's general well-being and future risks for illness or injury. This can be particularly important when working with young and middle-aged adults who rarely visit health care providers except for family planning, childbearing needs, acute illness, or injury episodes. It is not uncommon for young and middle-aged adults to go 10 years between health care visits. Because of the rarity of contacts with this population, take every opportunity to address health risks and risk management in these age groups.

HEALTH RISKS

The leading causes of death in young adults are motor-vehicle and other unintentional injuries, homicide, suicide, malignant neoplasms, and heart disease. In middle-aged adults, the risk of premature death from cancer or heart disease increases.[45] In both age groups, death from human immunodeficiency virus (HIV) infection has increased; of the more than one million persons with acquired immunodeficiency syndrome (AIDS) in the United States, most are 20 to 40 years of age.[15]

Healthy People 2010,[43] the federal population-based health objectives, identified the leading indicators of health that apply to young and middle-aged adults (Table 2-1). Nurses can assist in achieving these goals by assessing the client's lifestyle and risk status and by intervening to modify poor habits and reduce risk. This chapter describes the components of a healthy lifestyle, including health promotion (primary prevention), risk assessment, and risk management, specifically disease prevention (*primary* prevention) and early detection (*secondary* prevention) in the young and middle-aged populations.

HEALTH PROMOTION

Health promotion involves activities that promote general well-being. These activities are categorized as patterns of healthy eating, healthy activity, and effective coping with stress. The concept of health promotion is described in Chapter 1. The following topics describe specific health promotion activities.

Healthy Eating

Healthy eating is a cornerstone of a healthy lifestyle. In a recent report of the Institute of Medicine,[24] the first major revisions in the recommendations for healthy eating and activity in more than a decade were presented. These recommendations were based on a comprehensive review of the research in the area of diet and exercise. The Institute of Medicine recommendations regarding a healthy diet for young and middle-aged adults are summarized in Table 2-2. An important addition to dietary recommendations is that the total number of calories

evolve Be sure to check out the bonus material on the Evolve website and the CD-ROM, including free self-assessment exercises.

http://evolve.elsevier.com/Black/medsurg/

TABLE 2-1	Healthy People 2010 *Leading Health Indicators for Young and Middle-Aged Adults*

1. Increase the proportion of adults who engage regularly, preferable daily, in moderate physical activity for at least 30 minutes per day.
2. Reduce the proportion of adults who are obese.
3. Reduce cigarette smoking by adults.
4. Reduce the proportion of adults using any illicit drug during the past 30 days.
5. Reduce the proportion of adults engaging in binge drinking of alcoholic beverages during the past month.
6. Increase the proportion of sexually active persons who use condoms.
7. Increase the proportion of adults with recognized depression who receive treatment.
8. Reduce deaths caused by motor-vehicle accidents.
9. Reduce homicides.
10. Reduce the proportion of nonsmokers exposed to environmental tobacco smoke.

Data from U.S. Department of Health and Human Services. (January 2000). *Healthy People 2010.* (Conference Edition, in Two Volumes). Washington, DC: Author.

TABLE 2-2	Summary of Institute of Medicine Dietary Recommendations

1. The total recommended number of calories consumed should be based on age, gender, height, weight, and one of four activity levels. (See Institute of Medicine, p. 5.1 for formula.)
2. Dietary Reference Intakes are recommended intakes of some nutrients (i.e., carbohydrate, fiber, fatty acids, cholesterol, protein, amino acids) for both good health and prevention of chronic disease. In addition to recommended intakes, tolerable upper intake levels of these nutrients are provided.
3. Recommended ranges of dietary sources of calories are carbohydrates 45% to 65%, protein 10% to 35%, and fat 20% to 35%. It is recommended that these be considered together to ensure that total calories per day do not exceed expenditure.
4. Fewer than 25% of total calories should be from added sugars. Added sugars are those incorporated into food and beverages during production and are distinguished from natural sugars such as those found in milk (lactose) and fruit (fructose).
5. Because saturated fat, cholesterol, and trans fatty acids serve no health benefit, it is recommended that intake be reduced to the lowest level possible needed to maintain a nutritionally adequate diet.
6. Whenever possible, monounsaturated and polyunsaturated fats should be substituted for saturated fat, cholesterol, and trans fatty acid.
7. Two polyunsaturated fats are essential and available only from food sources. These are alpha-linolenic acid (an omega-3 fatty acid) and linoleic acid (an omega-6 fatty acid).
8. The recommended intake of alpha-linolenic acid is 17 g for adult men and 12 g for adult women. Good dietary sources include vegetable oils such as safflower oil or corn oil.
9. The recommended intake of linoleic acid is 1.6 g for adult men and 1.1 g for adult women. Good dietary sources of this fat include milk and some vegetable oils, such as soybean oil and flaxseed oil.
10. Recommended daily intake of total* fiber for young and middle-aged adults is 38 g for men and 25 g for women.
11. Recommended levels of dietary protein for adults are 0.8 g per kilogram of body weight.

Data from Institute of Medicine. (2002). *Dietary reference intakes for energy, carbohydrate, fiber, fat, fatty acids, cholesterol, protein, and amino acids.* Washington, DC: National Academy Press.
*Total fiber includes both *dietary* fiber, the edible, nondigestible component of carbohydrates, and lignin, and *functional* or supplemental fiber sources such as psyllium or pectin.

recommended should be based on the client's age, gender, height, weight, and one of four activity levels. The activity levels are sedentary, low active, active, and very active. Following this guideline ensures that calorie recommendations for a client take into account all the factors that determine the energy they expend, and thus their caloric needs. Too often, as will be discussed later, our clients consume more calories than needed for energy and health; this results in overweight and chronic health problems.

To use the guidelines effectively for achieving healthy eating patterns, clients must be able to read nutrition labels. The food labeling system mandated by the U.S. Food and Drug Administration (FDA) is designed to assist consumers in making informed decisions regarding the foods they purchase. The Nutrition Facts label (Figure 2-1) is a tool to identify both serving size and the nutritional components of the food item.

Nurses who are knowledgeable about the composition of a healthy diet and the Nutrition Facts label can assist clients to adopt healthy eating patterns. Young and middle-aged adults are often in excellent health but may have poor eating patterns that lay the foundation for future health problems. In addition, these clients may already have health problems as a result of poor eating patterns. Health patterns of concern include obesity, cancer risk, osteoporosis, and cardiovascular disease. Obesity and cancer risks are discussed here. Chapter 28 covers osteoporosis, Chapters 57 and 58 cover heart disease, and Chapter 54 covers hypertension.

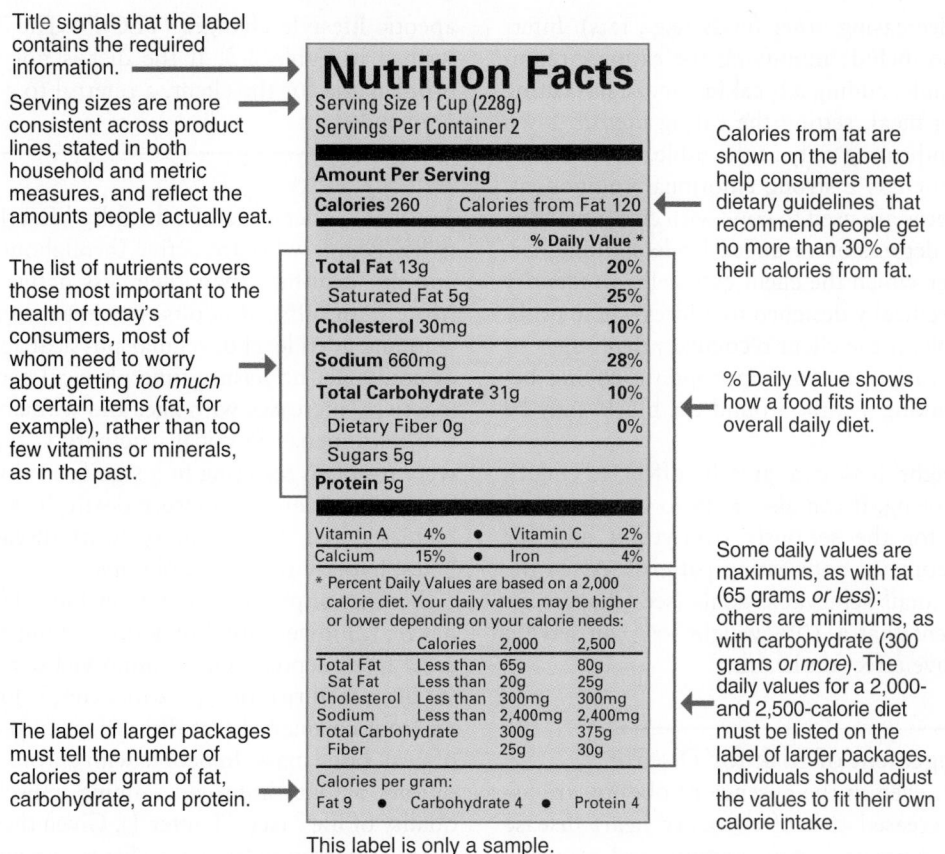

Nutrition Facts
Serving Size 1 Cup (228g)
Servings Per Container 2

Amount Per Serving

Calories 260   Calories from Fat 120

% Daily Value *

Total Fat 13g   20%
  Saturated Fat 5g   25%
Cholesterol 30mg   10%
Sodium 660mg   28%
Total Carbohydrate 31g   10%
  Dietary Fiber 0g   0%
  Sugars 5g
Protein 5g

Vitamin A   4%   •   Vitamin C   2%
Calcium   15%   •   Iron   4%

* Percent Daily Values are based on a 2,000 calorie diet. Your daily values may be higher or lower depending on your calorie needs:

	Calories	2,000	2,500
Total Fat	Less than	65g	80g
Sat Fat	Less than	20g	25g
Cholesterol	Less than	300mg	300mg
Sodium	Less than	2,400mg	2,400mg
Total Carbohydrate		300g	375g
Fiber		25g	30g

Calories per gram:
Fat 9   •   Carbohydrate 4   •   Protein 4

This label is only a sample.

FIGURE 2-1 Guide to using a food label. (Modified from U.S. Food and Drug Administration. [December 10, 1992]. The new food label. *FDA Backgrounder,* 1-9.)

Obesity

Current estimates are that 23% of the U.S. population are obese (body mass index [BMI] ≥30 kg/m²). The *Healthy People 2010*[43] goals include reducing the number of obese Americans to 15%; however, in the last 20 years the percent of people who are obese has increased by 50%. In addition, the percentage of the adult U.S. population who are overweight (BMI 25 to 29.9 kg/m²) is estimated to be 55%. Both obesity and overweight pose serious health risks. Overweight persons (this includes all obese people) have an increased risk for heart disease, hypertension, type 2 diabetes, degenerative joint disease, sleep apnea, and gallbladder disease.[37] When overweight is associated with a high-fat diet, the risk of breast, colon, rectum, and prostate cancer increases. Take every opportunity to measure height and weight and to calculate BMI (see Chapter 30) and also to advise clients when they fall outside the range of healthy weight.

Management of the Overweight Client. The basic therapeutic approach to overweight is to modify eating patterns through improving the *quality* (versus *quantity*) of foods eaten. The focus is on making positive changes in eating patterns. Specific modifications include (1) de-

creasing portion size, (2) modifying the composition of the diet through substitution and modification of foods consumed, and (3) changing eating behaviors. The second therapeutic component of obesity management is improving activity patterns (see later discussion).

Assessment. Before recommending diet modifications, assess the client's current eating patterns. Simple dietary assessment tools include a 24-hour diet recall and use of a 3-day dietary log in which the client records all food and drink for 3 days, one of which should be a weekend day. The 24-hour diet recall is ideal for obtaining information at the time of the nurse–client encounter. The 3-day dietary log includes not only what food was eaten but when, why, and how the client ate. This tool assists both the nurse and the client in recognizing eating patterns and problematic eating behavior. Chapter 30 discusses nutritional assessment.

Intervention. Once eating patterns have been assessed, collaboratively develop a list of problems and a mutually agreed-on, realistic plan for addressing these problems with the client. Focus interventions on changing foods eaten through substitution (e.g., carrots for candy), increasing certain foods (e.g., fruits and vegetables), or decreasing other foods (e.g., fats). Interventions can also include modifying the eating circumstances, for example, adding a breakfast meal, not eating after the evening meal, setting the eating utensil down between bites, and eating only at the table.

Eating behavior has a strong emotional component. Poor eating patterns are used to cope with emotional discomfort such as depression or anger. Understanding circumstances under which the client eats helps to identify interventions specifically designed to address these problems. For example, if the client recognizes that anger or fatigue leads to eating, a more appropriate coping behavior, such as taking a walk around the block, may be identified.

Although weight loss can greatly affect a client's health and well-being, it can also seem to be a hopeless task, especially for the seriously overweight and for adults with a lifetime of poor eating patterns. Assist the client in setting small achievable goals (see Chapter 1). Reassure the client that a 10% weight loss can have a substantial positive effect on health.[17]

Diet and Management of Risk for Disease

Diets high in fat, even in the absence of obesity, are associated with increased risk of coronary heart disease and cancer of the breast, colon, rectum, and prostate. The American Cancer Society (ACS)[2] recommends decreasing the risk for cancer by eating a variety of healthful foods with an emphasis on plan sources, eating five or more servings of a variety of fruit and vegetables daily, choosing whole grains, limiting consumption of red meats, and choosing foods that help maintain a healthy weight. For clients who are at increased risk for coronary heart disease, as determined by borderline or elevated serum cholesterol levels and identified risks, the National Cholesterol Education Panel recommends therapeutic lifestyle changes (TLC).[30] The TLC diet is described in Table 2-3. If the diet is not successful or is problematic for the client, a referral to a dietitian is recommended.

Healthy Activity

Another cornerstone of a healthy lifestyle is healthy activity. People who are active throughout life live longer and are healthier than their less active counterparts.[35] More than 60% of adults, however, do not achieve the recommended level of regular physical activity, and 40% of adults get no leisure-time physical activity.[43] Physical inactivity increases with age, and women are more inactive than men.[44] Physical inactivity is a serious, nationwide problem resulting in a significant burden of unnecessary illness and premature death. It is associated with increased risk for coronary heart disease, type 2 diabetes, hypertension, and obesity.

Benefits of physical activity include (1) weight maintenance, (2) lower blood pressure, (3) improved mood, (4) relief from depression, (5) improved sense of well-being, (6) decreased risk of type 2 diabetes, (7) reduced mortality from coronary heart disease, and (8) increased levels of peak bone mass. In people with chronic, disabling conditions, activity improves stamina, muscle strength, and quality of life[19] (see Chapter 1). Given these benefits, take every opportunity to assess clients' activity patterns, and work with them to improve activity levels.

Management of the Inactive Client. Current activity recommendations are that every adult in the United States should accumulate an hour of moderately intense activity every day.[24] This recommendation is based on extensive research on what the average person needs to do to maintain a healthy weight. Activity can be accumulated, but it should occur in blocks of at least 8 minutes and should be perceived as moderate or high intensity.[4,23] In

TABLE 2-3	*Nutrient Composition of the TLC Diet*
Nutrient	**Recommended Intake**
Saturated fat*	Less than 7% of total calories
Polyunsaturated fat	Up to 10% of total calories
Monounsaturated fat	Up to 20% of total calories
Total fat	25-35% of total calories
Carbohydrate†	50-60% of total calories
Fiber	20-30 g/day
Protein	Approximately 15% of total calories
Cholesterol	Less than 200 mg/day
Total calories (energy)‡	Balance energy intake and expenditure to maintain desirable body weight/prevent weight gain

From Third Report of the Expert Panel on Detection, Evaluation, and Treatment of High Blood Cholesterol in Adults (Adult Treatment Panel III). Retrieved September 2, 2002, from http://nhlbi.nih.gov/guidelines/cholesterol.
*Trans fatty acids are another LDL-raising fat that should be kept at a low intake.
†Carbohydrate should be derived predominantly from foods rich in complex carbohydrates, including grains, especially whole grains, fruits, and vegetables.
‡Daily energy expenditure should include at least moderate physical activity (contributing approximately 200 Kcal per day).

addition, people who are very fit and engage in high-intensity activity can achieve similar health benefits in 30 minutes of high-intensity activity on most days. Simple walking is an excellent initial activity that requires no special equipment and can be done anywhere. Although this level of activity is ideal, you can advise your clients that important benefits can be obtained through modest amounts of daily physical activity[36] as they begin an exercise program.

Most research indicates that counseling clients to increase their physical activity is rarely effective in initiating behavioral change.[49] A trial of the effect of brief counseling suggests, however, that highly structured and specific programs might, with minimal expense or time, be effective in promoting healthy patterns of physical activity in clients (see Chapter 1).[7]

Assessment. Intervention to improve activity patterns begins with assessment of the client's current activity pattern. Two effective tools are the 24-hour recall and a 3-day activity log. In the 24-hour recall, help the client identify all forms of activity during that day. Focus on activity that was sustained for at least 8 minutes and perceived as moderate to heavy exertion. Encourage the client to be thorough by giving examples, such as time spent doing housework. Then sum the total number of minutes spent in moderate or heavy activity per day.[6]

During assessment, begin developing ideas for new activity opportunities. This information will be useful later for developing an intervention plan.

Benefits outweigh the risks with the current recommendation for moderate physical activity. Before beginning an activity program, however, all clients should be screened for risks that contraindicate unsupervised activity. People with known health problems, especially those involving cardiac risk, including hypertension, elevated serum cholesterol, cigarette smoking, diabetes, and a family history of early heart disease, should be evaluated by their health care provider before increasing physical activity levels.[42]

Intervention. Once the activity pattern has been assessed and there are no evident risks requiring further evaluation, work with the client to identify problem areas and develop a plan to increase physical activity. The *Activity Pyramid* is an excellent tool for beginning instruction (Figure 2-2). The Activity Pyramid is a pictorial representation of the principles of healthy activity and can be used during nurse–client encounters to provide basic information.

The Exercise Prescription. A written exercise prescription[16] specifies recommended activity. The exercise prescription has four major components:
- *Mode,* or the type of activity engaged in
- *Intensity* with which the activity is performed

FIGURE 2-2 The Activity Pyramid. (Copyright ©1999, Park Nicollet *HealthSource* ® Institute for Research and Education, Minneapolis, MN.)

TABLE 2-4	*Examples of Moderate Levels of Activity*

Around the House

Washing windows or floors
Washing and waxing the car
Walking and running with children
Climbing stairs
Pushing a stroller
Raking leaves
Shoveling snow
Digging and weeding in the garden

Sports and Leisure Activities

Volleyball or basketball
Bicycling
Social dancing (fast)
Walking (briskly)
Skiing
Swimming

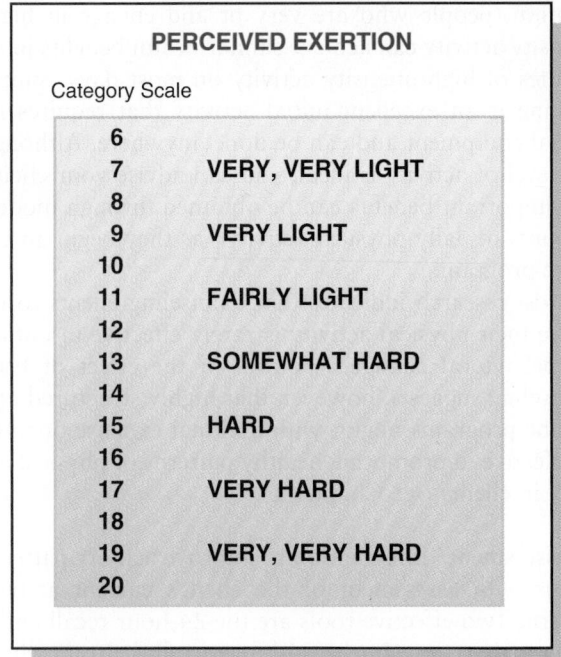

FIGURE 2-3 The Borg perceived exertion scale. (From Strauss, R.H. [Ed.]. [1991]. *Sports medicine* [2nd ed.] Philadelphia: W.B. Saunders.)

- *Duration* of time
- *Frequency*

As noted earlier, the minimum goal for an exercise program is a moderate-intensity *(intensity)* physical activity performed for a total of at least 60 minutes *(duration)* most days of the week *(frequency)*. Many activities that are a part of most people's daily routine can serve as the mode of a physical activity program, including walking, housework, child care, and gardening (Table 2-4).

Intensity is an essential component of an activity. The recommendations are based on moderate intensity. Instruct clients how to assess exertion level. One simple means of measuring perceived exertion is the *talk test;* clients should be able to talk but only a few words at a time when engaged in the activity. If they can carry on a normal conversation, they are not working hard enough; if they cannot talk at all, they are working too hard. Another measure of intensity is the *Borg rating* of perceived exertion (Figure 2-3).

Overcoming Barriers. Research indicates that people who successfully incorporate physical activity into their daily lives are confident in their ability to perform the activity, find it pleasurable, and have social support.[4,6] Activities should also be convenient and realistic.

Simple strategies can increase the likelihood of success in implementing an activity program. On the basis of the assessment of the client's activity level, (1) advise the client to increase time spent in current moderate-intensity activities, (2) help the client identify pleasurable activities to incorporate into the current routine, and (3) encourage the client to identify friends or family members who can serve as a support system and, ideally, who can join in the planned activity.

Activity plans should include a monitoring method, such as a log, and a reward system. Help clients identify

potential barriers and assist them in developing a plan to overcome them. Although the primary goal of a regular activity plan is to improve physical health, many benefits relate to feelings of well-being. When working with a client to improve activity patterns, use interventions that increase self-efficacy by choosing realistic activities and goals.

One successful strategy for increasing physical activity is to increase social support within the community as well as within the client's social circle. Use every opportunity to support community projects that promote physical activity, such as developing hiking, walking, and biking trails or opening schools for community recreation. If security is a concern, support efforts to organize a community watch unit or to develop a walking club to take advantage of safety in numbers. Occupational health nurses can encourage employers to develop on-site programs to support employee health. Nurses who regularly work with clients to develop activity programs can maintain a comprehensive listing of community resources available to support activity plans. Community nursing organizations can develop a volunteer pool to work with walking clubs in area malls, perform blood pressure screenings, and provide health education classes.

Tools for Assisting Clients with Healthy Eating and Activity

A variety of programs is available to nurses who regularly work with clients to improve their eating and activity behaviors. An excellent resource for working with overweight clients is the report of the Expert Panel on the Identification, Evaluation, and Treatment of Overweight and Obese Adults.[31] This document is a detailed guide for the treatment of overweight and obesity. Materials include information on nutrition and exercise, Weekly Food and Activity Diaries, Guides to Behavior Change and Physical Activity, and tools to help the clinician evaluate the client's risks and motivation and to set goals. The entire document is available online at www.nhlbi.nih.gov.

Another source of tools for counseling clients regarding physical activity and nutrition is the PACE Project (Patient-centered Assessment and Counseling for Exercise and Nutrition).[7,26] The PACE Project provides a system of materials designed to assess a client's readiness to modify physical activity and eating, to screen for activity contraindications, and to develop and implement an individualized activity and nutrition program. PACE Project materials can be accessed online at www.paceproject.org.

Whichever tools are used, the intervention program chosen by the nurse should include a personalized eating program and exercise prescription and a plan for identifying and overcoming probable barriers to implementation and maintenance of the plan (see Chapter 1).

Stress

Stress, the body's response to demands, seems to be increasing in today's world. Physical demands for adaptation are compounded by the adaptive responses required by the volume of information and the decisions required for existence in today's society. Stress is usually the result of an imbalance between the demands placed on a person and one's ability to adapt. *Stress management,* the final cornerstone of a healthy lifestyle, is the ability to cope with these adaptive demands effectively.

Dysfunction in one's ability to adapt and manage stress has a negative effect on health[10]:

1. *Behavioral* responses to stress include decreased ability to think clearly and function, increased tobacco and alcohol use, overeating, and disrupted sleep patterns.
2. *Emotional* responses include depression, anger, decreased self-esteem, apathy, and impatience.
3. *Physical* responses to stress can include tight, sore neck and shoulder muscles, increased blood pressure and heart rate, palpitations, chest discomfort, headaches, gastrointestinal upset, and fatigue.

Management of Stress

Assessment. Today it seems that people are always "stressed," often blaming stress for their physical and mental problems. As a result, clients may request help in coping with stress. Assessment of the problem is the first step in intervention. Include a thorough history of the cognitive, emotional, and physical manifestations that lead clients to conclude that they are stressed. Assess the problems or situations that seem to precipitate stress and the behavioral and emotional responses to it (i.e., how clients feel and act when the problem is present). Also evaluate how clients currently cope with the problem (see discussion of coping in Chapters 1 and 25). Help the person recognize ineffective coping and develop a plan to cope effectively with the stress.

Intervention. Stress management has three components: stress resistance, cognitive reappraisal, and effective coping skills.

Stress Resistance. Stress resistance involves decreasing the body's response to stress, healthy eating and activity, and relaxation techniques. Physical activity can be a *positive* stressor; that is, activity requires an adaptive response, and, when performed properly, it results in physical changes that counter the normally negative effects of stress. Physical activity improves mental function, decreases depression, and increases physical endurance.

Healthy eating can increase resistance to stress, and unhealthy eating adds to stress. Healthy eating aids stress resistance; however, some foods are associated with effective or ineffective coping. Complex carbohydrates (e.g., breads, beans, grains) provide a sustained source of energy and have a relaxing effect, whereas fruits, vegetables, and protein provide energy and increased physiologic ability to cope. Intake of simple carbohydrates (e.g., sugar) can temporarily increase energy, but this rise is then quickly followed by weakness and lethargy as the blood glucose level drops. Overeating, an ineffective means of coping, can result in decreased energy and lowered self-esteem. The stimulant caffeine induces the fight-or-flight biologic response and can exacerbate the physical damage that results from stress when it is consumed in excess.

Sleep and rest are natural forms of relaxation that are essential for healing and repairing the physiologic consequences to stress. Inadequate rest worsens stress, especially through impaired mental functioning. Chapter 24 discusses promoting positive outcomes in clients with sleep and rest disorders. In addition to sleep and rest, people can practice techniques to facilitate physical and mental relaxation. *Progressive relaxation* is a technique of slowly focusing on each muscle group, tensing the muscles for 5 to 7 seconds, and then relaxing them. This process promotes learning how to relax the entire body and particularly benefits people with muscle tension or spasm, insomnia, and neck or back pain. Many forms of relaxation involve *breathing techniques,* such as breath awareness, deep breathing, and the purifying breath.[12]

Meditation, once considered an alternative practice, is an established form of relaxation therapy. Research has shown that physiologic changes, such as lowering blood pressure and decreasing heart disease risk, occur as a result of meditation. There are several active or passive forms of meditation, including focusing on breath awareness or a *mantra,* meditative movement such as *yoga* or *Tai Chi,* mindfulness, and prayer.

Cognitive Reappraisal. The goal of cognitive reappraisals or restructuring is to change the perception or interpretation of events as stressors. Cognitive reappraisal is based on the assumption that a major factor in stress is the individual's perception of the event or experience as a stressor.[27] Three common techniques are presented.

Thought stopping is an ideal intervention for "worriers" (i.e., people who obsessively maintain ongoing inner dialogues of "what if" or "I can't"). Clients identify the obsessive thought and allow the self to imagine a situation involving the thought. As the obsessive dialogue begins, the person interrupts the dialogue with a loud "STOP!" and substitutes a positive thought. The goal of this process is to learn to disrupt obsessive and nonproductive thoughts automatically with a positive message.

Refuting irrational ideas, like thought stopping, involves interventions designed to disrupt obsessive, nonproductive thoughts. The intervention derives from rational emotive therapy, which is based on the belief that much stress is related to common irrational beliefs such as "I must be perfect in everything I do" and "It's absolutely necessary that I have love and approval from my peers and family at all times." To overcome these stressful beliefs, the client first identifies the irrational idea and then identifies the facts, such as "no one is perfect all the time." Clients also need to explore their emotional response to stressful thoughts. The client then substitutes rational self-talk for the previous irrational self-talk. This particular intervention is very effective for self-directed, empowered people.

Guided imagery, a form of relaxation, is an excellent method of cognitive reappraisal. Guided imagery is usually practiced under the direction of a trained therapist. The therapist assists the client to visualize a stressful event, become worried, and then to switch to a relaxing event or to rework the situation so that it is less stressful. Alternatively, the therapist may help the client into a guided dialogue with his or her inner self or may act as a guide to help with problem solving.

Effective Coping. Effective coping involves recognition of the problem causing stress and, through problem-solving skills, development and implementation of an effective strategy to cope with or solve the problem. Effective coping skills include time management, assertiveness, solution-oriented therapy, and development of a support system.[12,27] Often clients use ineffective coping strategies, usually designed to avoid the problem, resulting in repression of associated unpleasant emotions. Addictive behaviors, such as alcohol abuse and overeating, often begin as ineffective coping strategies.

Effective coping starts with identifying the problem. Help the client to differentiate the problem from the emotional response to the problem. Once the problem is identified, several issues must be addressed before one can work on problem-solving skills.

First, does the problem really exist, or is it imagined? People often worry about imagined problems. Help the client assess validity of the problem before working on a solution.

Second, is the problem really important or just a nuisance? If the problem is not important, use cognitive reappraisal techniques to put the problem in perspective.

Third, does the problem have feasible solutions? Some problems (an untimely death or catastrophic illness) are beyond control. In these cases, the goal is not problem resolution but acceptance. The individual will need support to learn from the problem and to develop an ongoing support system for assistance through the crisis.

Important, controllable problems are amenable to intervention or action responses using standard problem-solving, assertiveness, and time management skills. Nurses often assist people in distress. Mastering effective coping skills can be an asset in clinical practice; however, nurses often work with people experiencing crises in which basic coping strategies are not enough. Develop a network of counseling and support resources to which clients can be referred.

PREVENTION OF INJURY AND ILLNESS

The greatest causes of injury and premature death in young and middle-aged adults include accidents, particularly motor-vehicle accidents, and violence, particularly suicide and homicide.[43,45] Risk identification and risk management counseling can prevent illness and injury in these populations. Place particular emphasis on preventable causes of accidents, specifically the use of drugs and alcohol, and preventable causes of cancer, specifically smoking. In addition, always be aware of the risk for domestic or spousal abuse.

Accidents

Because motor-vehicle accidents are the leading cause of death in young adults, prevention counseling should focus on the regular use of lap and shoulder belts and refraining from drug or alcohol use while driving. Because of the significant impact of drugs, alcohol, and tobacco on health, most prevention measures are devoted to screening and intervening in alcohol, drug, and tobacco abuse. The following discussion focuses on screening and primary prevention measures. Chapter 26 describes secondary intervention for clients who have abuse problems.

Alcohol Abuse

Alcohol abuse results in specific health problems, including withdrawal syndrome; hepatitis, cirrhosis, and pancreatitis; and cancers of the liver, oropharynx (especially in smokers), and esophagus as well as an increased risk of breast cancer. In addition to diseases clearly associated with alcohol abuse, "problem drinkers" have increased mortality from all causes, beginning with four drinks per day for men and two drinks per day for women. Alcohol is associated with more than 50% of all injuries (44% of all traffic accidents), fires, drownings, homicides, and suicides.[45]

Problem drinkers are more likely to be seen in primary care clinics and hospitals. They often do not present with manifestations of dependence that would immediately result in identification of the problem. All clients, not just those with obvious problems, should be screened for problem drinking. Nurses are in a position to identify problem drinking because their role includes obtaining a comprehensive psychosocial history (see Chapter 4).

Various tools are available to screen for problem drinking. The mnemonic CAGE is a useful popular four-item tool[45]:

- C = Have you ever felt you ought to *Cut* down on drinking?
- A = Have people *Annoyed* you by criticizing your drinking?
- G = Have you ever felt bad or *Guilty* about your drinking?
- E = Have you ever had a drink first thing in the morning to steady your nerves or get rid of a hangover *(Eye-opener)*?

If problem drinking is suspected or if the client answers "yes" to any item, the Alcohol Use Disorders Identification Test (AUDIT) may be administered. The AUDIT is a 10-item tool developed by a six-nation team in conjunction with the World Health Organization (WHO). The AUDIT is highly sensitive and specific[25,39] and can easily be included in a social history format. Score the AUDIT tool (Table 2-5) by summing the total points for all answers. Drinking is considered problematic if the score is 8 points or more.

Do not hesitate to screen for problem drinking. If you suspect that a client has a drinking problem (based on screening), briefly state so to the client. Be sure to have an established support and referral network of clinical specialists to assist the client and family with acceptance and management of problem drinking.[45] Chapter 26 details interventions for clients who have substance abuse problems.

Drug Abuse

Unfortunately since 1992, after years of decline in drug use, abuse of illicit and legal drugs has been on the increase. More than 5.5 million Americans are affected by drug abuse, and 50% of these people are in the criminal justice system. Drug abuse is more common among men, the unemployed, and people without a high school education. Although drug abuse is more prevalent in urban communities, rural communities are not immune. Drug abusers are at increased risk for HIV infection and other communicable diseases. Drug abuse is a significant factor in homicides, suicides, and motor-vehicle accidents.[45]

Be aware of the hazards of drug abuse and of the possibility of drug abuse in clients. Several standardized tools can be used to screen for drug abuse, but none has well-established validity or reliability.[45] Take every opportunity to assess for drug abuse.[5] Following your questions regarding tobacco and alcohol use, ask the client about drug use as a routine part of lifestyle assessment, (see Chapter 4). State questions directly ("Do you currently use any other drugs such as marijuana ['pot,' 'weed'] or cocaine ['crack']?"). If the answer is "no," one can follow with "Have you ever used any other drugs?" If the client indicates current or past use of illicit drugs, further explore the patterns of use.

Advise abusing and high-risk clients (adolescents, males, people exposed to users of drugs) of the hazards of substance abuse. Advise users to stop or cut down, and offer help through referral (see Chapter 26 for interventions for substance abuse problems).

Smoking Cessation

More than 25% of Americans smoke, and thousands of children begin smoking every day.[32] Smoking is directly linked to many forms of cancer, heart disease, and hypertension. It is a risk factor in health problems as diverse as osteoporosis, ulcer disease, and low birth weight in babies. Smoking accounts for one of every five deaths in the United States,[45] making tobacco the single greatest cause of disease and premature death in the United States. All nurses should have the skills necessary to help people who are ready to stop smoking and to help motivate people who are not at a point where they can stop. In 2000 the *Treating Tobacco Use and Dependence Guidelines*[50] were published. These guidelines were sponsored by the U.S. Public Health Service and were the result of the collaboration of several public and private agencies to develop evidence-based guidelines on tobacco abuse. These guidelines are listed in Table 2-6. The core premise of the guidelines is that tobacco abuse is a chronic disease and as such puts responsibility on the nurse, along with other health care providers, to provide ongoing counseling, support, and treatment.[3]

Intervention. Smoking cessation intervention can be seen as a stepped process. The first step is to ask all clients if they smoke. When a person who smokes is identified, the nurse then asks whether he or she is willing to quit now. The treatment algorithm then guides the nurse on means to support smoking cessation through brief support interventions or provides strategies to enhance motivation to quit. The nurse can personalize the need to stop smoking, for example, by reminding parents of young children of the increased risk for ear

TABLE 2-5	*The Alcohol Use Disorders Identification Test (AUDIT) Structured Interview*				
	Score*				
Question	**0**	**1**	**2**	**3**	**4**
How often do you have a drink containing alcohol?	Never	Monthly or less	2-4 times/mo	2-3 times/wk	4 or more times/wk
How many drinks do you have on a typical day when you are drinking?	None	1 or 2	3 or 4	5 or 6	7-9†
How often do you have 6 or more drinks on one occasion?	Never	Less than monthly	Monthly	Weekly	Daily or almost daily
How often during the last year have you found that you were unable to stop drinking once you had started?	Never	Less than monthly	Monthly	Weekly	Daily or almost daily
How often last year have you failed to do what was normally expected from you because of drinking?	Never	Less than monthly	Monthly	Weekly	Daily or almost daily
How often during the last year have you needed a first drink in the morning to get yourself going after a heavy drinking session?	Never	Less than monthly	Monthly	Weekly	Daily or almost daily
How often during the last year have you had a feeling of guilt or remorse after drinking?	Never	Less than monthly	Monthly	Weekly	Daily or almost daily
How often during the last year have you been unable to re-member what happened the night before because you had been drinking?	Never	Less than monthly	Monthly	Weekly	Daily or almost daily
Have you or has someone else been injured as a result of your drinking?	Never	Yes, but not in last year (2 points)		Yes, during the last year (4 points)	
Has a relative, doctor, or other health worker been concerned about your drinking or sug-gested you cut down?	Never	Yes, but not in last year (2 points)		Yes, during the last year (4 points)	

From U.S. Preventive Services Task Force. (1996). *Guide to clinical preventive services* (2nd ed.). Baltimore: Williams & Wilkins.
*Score of greater than 8 (out of 41) suggests problem drinking and indicates the need for more in-depth assessment. Cut-off of 10 points recommended by some to pro-vide greater specificity.
†Five points if response is 10 or more drinks on a typical day.

infections and asthma the child may have or the type of role model the parent is presenting. Women should be reminded that smoking increases the risk of osteoporosis and premature aging of the skin, and asymptomatic men should be reminded of the increased risk for emphysema, heart disease, and lung cancer.

Once the client is identified as a smoker and is advised of the need to stop smoking, assessment of the motiva-tion to change is next (see Chapter 1). If a client ex-presses any interest in changing the smoking behavior, from cutting down to stopping, ask what can be done to help assure the client that the nurse is supportive of his or her efforts. Success is more likely if people spend thoughtful time planning the behavior change[16] in prepa-ration to quit. Help the client evaluate his or her smok-ing patterns to personalize the plan. Suggestions include

TABLE 2-6	*Guidelines for Tobacco Use and Dependence*

1. Tobacco dependence is a chronic condition that often requires repeated intervention; however, effective treatments exist that can produce long-term or even permanent abstinence.
2. Because effective tobacco dependence treatments are available, every patient who uses tobacco should be offered at least one of these treatments.
   Patients willing to try to quit tobacco use should be provided treatments identified as effective.
   Patients who are unwilling to try to quit tobacco use should be provided a brief intervention designed to increase their motivation to quit.
3. It is essential that clinicians and health care delivery systems institutionalize the consistent identification, documentation, and treatment of every tobacco user seen in a health care setting.
4. Brief tobacco dependence treatment is effective, and every patient who uses tobacco should be offered at least brief treatment.
5. There is a strong dose-response relation between the intensity of tobacco dependence counseling and its effectiveness. Treatments involving person-to-person contact are consistently effective, and their effectiveness increases with the treatment intensity (e.g., minutes of contact).
6. Three types of counseling and behavioral therapies are especially effective and should be used with all patients attempting tobacco cessation:
   a. Provision of practical counseling (problem solving/skills training)
   b. Provision of social support as a part of treatment (intra-treatment social support)
   c. Help in securing social support outside of treatment (extratreatment social support)
7. Numerous effective pharmacotherapies for smoking cessation now exist. Patients attempting smoking cessation should be advised to seek pharmacologic treatment.
8. Tobacco dependence treatments are both clinically effective and cost-effective relative to other medical and disease prevention interventions. As a result, insurers and purchasers of health care should ensure that tobacco dependence treatment be a reimbursable health care service.

Modified from U.S. Public Health Service. (2000). *Treating tobacco use and dependence: Clinical Practice Guideline.* Retrieved September 2, 2002, from http://www.surgeongeneral.gov/tobacco.

(1) cleaning the house just before stopping to rid it of tobacco odor, (2) getting rid of all cigarettes, and (3) setting up a support network. Advise the client to inform friends who smoke that he or she is trying to quit and that they should respect this by not smoking around the client or not offering cigarettes. If the client's history in-

TABLE 2-7	*Things to Do Instead of Smoking*

- Take a slow, deep breath of fresh air.
- Take a walk.
- Chew on a piece of gum or a carrot or hard candy.
- Drink a glass of water.
- Think about your children.
- Brush your teeth.
- Play with worry beads.
- Pray or meditate.
- Think about the money you are saving.
- Smile.

dicates a high degree of nicotine addiction, offer advice about or referral for nicotine replacement.

Finally, assist the client in problem-solving strategies and skills to assist them in their effort. This might include addressing how the client will manage "triggers" to smoking (e.g., alcohol or anxiety-producing situations) and alternatives to smoking. When the urge to smoke strikes, advise the client to walk and learn deep breathing to work through the urge. Table 2-7 lists suggested activities to substitute instead of smoking.

In addition to explaining smoking cessation, be aware of community resources to which clients can be referred for assistance. Provide a variety of motivational literature to clients, such as the excellent materials by the ACS and the American Lung Association. Support community-based smoking cessation interventions, including a smoke-free work environment and participation in such community programs as the National Smoke-Off day.

The *Treating Tobacco Use and Dependence*[50] guidelines offers many resources to assist the nurse in smoking cessation efforts. These resources include suggestions for system-based changes as well as evidence-based strategies for increasing the likelihood of success. The guidelines are available online or can be ordered at the U.S. Public Health Service website.

Passive Smoking

Passive smoking, or exposure to second-hand smoke, also places people at increased risk for heart disease and cancer. The Atherosclerosis Risk in the Community (ARIC) study in 1994 indicated that nonsmokers who are regularly exposed to environmental tobacco smoke have a 20% increase in progression of atherosclerosis compared with nonsmokers who are not exposed to tobacco smoke.[22] Identify persons who are exposed to environmental tobacco smoke, and help them devise ways to modify their risk. Ideally, risk modification involves smoking cessation on the part of a family member; however, people are often exposed to tobacco smoke in their work environment (e.g., bars, casinos), and the client may have to make difficult decisions regarding risk management versus livelihood and family. In these cases, the nurse's role as a client advocate can be to support social efforts to limits unwanted exposure to passive smoke, such as laws to limit smoking in public places.

Domestic Abuse

The Surgeon General's report in the mid-1980s identified domestic violence as a public health issue. Estimates are that from one million[45] to four million[20] women are victims of assault, robbery, or rape by a spouse, ex-spouse, or intimate partner each year. Too often, this violence escalates to murder; 50% of murders are committed by an intimate partner.[20] An estimated 35% of women are seen in emergency departments for abuse and that 30% of women seen in primary care are abuse victims.[38] One study of inpatient female psychiatric clients found that 64% reported abuse as adults.[38] Although men are not immune from domestic abuse, most victims are women; therefore, this discussion focuses on the abuse of women.

Nurses in all clinical settings see women who are abused; they must, therefore, be aware of the risk of violence and must be comfortable addressing abuse risk issues in client encounters. The American Nurses' Association position paper, *Physical Violence Against Women*,[11] supports the need to (1) increase nurses' awareness of and sensitivity to the problem of physical violence against women; (2) work to reduce injuries, psychological trauma, and cost that are a result of such violence; and (3) increase nurses' awareness of their role in assessing, intervening for, and preventing physical violence against women.[38]

Assessment. Although nurses often work with women who are victims of abuse, this text emphasizes (1) the identification of risk for abuse and (2) interventions to prevent abuse before it starts. Identification begins with recognizing characteristics common to abused women. Characteristics of women at increased risk for violence include living in households with high degrees of stress, being abused as a child, and marrying young.[38, 45] Abused women often display low self-esteem and experience helplessness.[20,38] In addition, certain characteristics in the woman's partner can increase her risk, such as having been abused or observed abuse as a child, abusing drugs or alcohol, having controlling behaviors, and pathologic jealousy. In addition, men who repetitively abuse women verbally often escalate to physical violence over time, during periods of high stress, or when a woman is pregnant.[38] Remember, any woman can be a victim of abuse, and any man can be an abuser. Routine screening for a history of abuse or current abuse in all women is an appropriate component of a psychosocial history (see Chapter 4).

The Partner Violence Screen (PVS)[14] is brief, easy to use, and accurate in identifying abuse. The tool consists of three questions:
1. Have you been hit, kicked, punched, or otherwise hurt by someone within the past year? If so, by whom?
2. Do you feel safe in your current relationship?
3. Does a partner from a previous relationship make you feel unsafe now?

Intervention. Once a woman is identified as being at risk for violence either through having established risk factors or having been abused in the past, work with her to develop an individualized plan designed to prevent future violence. The plan may include assertiveness training, participation in a woman's empowerment or support group, self-esteem work, and social services assistance to improve her educational and economic status.[21,28] Additional prevention strategies include community health nurse visits to high-risk families and community-wide media campaigns to enhance public awareness of the problem.[38] Explain stress management strategies, especially effective coping (see earlier discussion), to help the client to avoid violence.

If a woman is identified as being in a currently violent relationship, intervention needs to be focused on safety. This woman is at high risk for sustaining significant injury or death. Therefore, nurses who screen for domestic violence must have a clearly established protocol for ensuring that every effort has been made to protect the woman. This protocol should be developed in collaboration with local law enforcement agencies and women's safety groups (e.g., YWCAs or other agencies).[13]

Infectious Diseases

With the exception of HIV disease, infectious diseases are not a major cause of illness or premature death in young and middle-aged adults; however, these groups are not immune to problems related to infectious diseases. Two activities are essential for protection from infectious diseases in these populations: (1) maintaining up-to-date immunizations and (2) practicing safe sex.

Immunization

The U.S. Preventive Services Task Force (USPSTF)[45] recommends that all young and middle-aged adults have a tetanus-diphtheria booster vaccination every 10 years and that women of childbearing age who do not have proven immunity to rubella have a rubella vaccination.

Hepatitis B. People at risk for hepatitis B should receive the hepatitis B vaccination series. These risk factors[45] include frequent occupational exposure to blood and blood products, men who have sex with men, injection drug users and their partners, people with multiple (>6 lifetime) sexual partners, people who have had a sexually transmitted disease (STD), and people who travel to countries where hepatitis B is endemic.

Meningococcal Meningitis. Recently a resurgence of concern about meningococcal meningitis in college students and discussion of the value of immunizing college students has occurred. Although the risk is low, the Centers for Disease Control and Prevention (CDC) Advisory Committee on Immunization Practices[9] (ACIP) currently recommends that clinicians inform incoming college freshman who will be living in dormitories and their families about the risk of meningococcal disease and the availability of vaccine. If the student wishes to decrease the risk, he or she should be offered the vaccine or directed to a source for vaccination. The risk for all other groups of college students is the same as that for the general population and does not justify consideration of vaccination.

Varicella (Chickenpox). In addition, the ACIP[8] recommends varicella (chickenpox) vaccine for susceptible (i.e., nonimmune) adults in the following high-risk groups: (1) persons who live or work in environments where transmission of varicella is likely (e.g., teachers of young children, day care employees, and residents and staff members in institutional settings); (2) persons who live and work in environments where transmission can occur (e.g., college students, inmates and staff members of correctional institutions, and military personnel); (3) nonpregnant women of childbearing age; (4) adults living in households with children; and (5) international travelers.

Safe Sex

There are dozens of infectious STDs. Of these, HIV infection and hepatitis B and C can result in significant morbidity and premature death; others result in permanent infection (e.g., herpes simplex) or infertility (e.g., gonorrhea). Risk factors for contracting a STD include the following:

1. Having a high number of sex partners
2. Having sex with a person who engages in high-risk behavior (e.g., multiple partners)
3. Having sex for money
4. Having sex with an intravenous (IV) drug user

People who abuse drugs and alcohol are at increased risk, even if they do not abuse IV drugs, because they are more likely to engage in high-risk sexual behaviors while in an impaired state. Do not hesitate to screen for high-risk sexual behavior, and advise clients about the risks and behaviors to protect from infection. Safe sex behavior includes the following:

1. Abstaining from sex
2. Maintaining a mutually monogamous relationship with a noninfected partner

3. Avoiding sexual contact with casual or high-risk partners
4. Using male or female condoms consistently and appropriately

Present information regarding referral sources in the community to assist clients with free or low-cost screening and treatment for STDs and information regarding sources of low-cost condoms. If you work in an ambulatory clinic or a community-based practice, consider finding a source of low-cost condoms and making them available at little or no cost to persons at high risk.[45] Chapters 43 and 80 cover working with clients who have STDs, including AIDS.

SCREENING FOR DISEASE

Secondary prevention includes early detection of illness. Early identification is key to preventing premature death from many catastrophic illnesses, including coronary heart disease, cancer, and type 2 diabetes mellitus. Be aware of the risks for diseases and the current recommendations regarding screening and take every opportunity to advise clients of the need for regular screening (see Chapter 4). Facilitating early detection of disease saves lives.

Recommendations for Screening

The U.S. Preventive Services Task Force[45] (USPSTF) issued its landmark report regarding the effectiveness of preventive services in 1989 and updated its recommendations in 1996; these recommendations are currently under a third revision. These recommendations are the "gold standard" of screening services, and nurses should be familiar with them. In addition to screening, the USPSTF recommends many of the counseling, immunization, and chemoprophylaxis measures discussed earlier in this chapter. The recommendations are specific to age groups (except for pregnant women) and differentiate screenings recommended for all people in the group from screenings recommended for those with high-risk characteristics.

Screening recommendations are based on several factors that apply to populations rather than to individuals. The screening test must be reasonably priced, sensitive, and specific to the problem. In addition, there is generally no value to screening for diseases for which there is no treatment or when treatment does not improve either the quality of life or longevity. As a result, many tests do not meet requirements for an effective screening program.

Screenings recommended for the general population 11 to 24 years of age are listed in Table 2-8. Screenings recommended for the general population between the ages of 25 and 64 years are listed in Table 2-9.

Depression

More than 19 million people in the United States suffer from depression. Major depression is a significant cause of disability and accounts for two thirds of all deaths

TABLE 2-8	Recommended Screenings for the General Population Ages 11 to 24 Years		
Screening	**Frequency**	**For**	
Height and weight	Periodic*	Obesity	
Blood pressure	Periodic*	Hypertension	
Pap smear (females)	At least every 3 years	Cervical cancer	
Chlamydia screen (females)	With Pap smear	*Chlamydia trachomatis*	
Rubella serology (females)†	Once	Non-immune status	
Assess for problem drinking	Periodic	Problem drinking	
Depression	Periodic	Depression	

Modified from U.S. Preventive Services Task Force. (1996). *Guide to clinical preventive services* (2nd ed.). Baltimore: Williams & Wilkins; and U.S. Preventive Services Task Force (2002). *Screening: Depression.* Update, 2002 Release. Retrieved August 27, 2002, from http://www.ahcpr.gov/clinic/uspstfdepr.
*Clinician discretion.
†In women with childbearing potential with incomplete vaccination history.

TABLE 2-9	Recommended Screenings for the General Population Ages 25 to 64 Years		
Screening	**Frequency**	**For**	
Blood pressure	Periodic*	Hypertension	
Height and weight	Periodic*	Obesity	
Total blood cholesterol†	Every 5 years	Coronary heart disease risk	
Pap smear (females)	At least every 3 years	Cervical cancer	
Fecal occult blood test‡	Annually	Colorectal cancer	
Mammogram and clinical breast exam§	Annually	Breast cancer	
Rubella serologic testing (females)‖	Once	Non-immune status	
Assessment for problem drinking	Periodic*	Problem drinking	

From U.S. Preventive Services Task Force. (1996). *Guide to clinical preventive services* (2nd ed.). Baltimore: Williams & Wilkins; and U.S. Preventive Services Task Force (2002). *Screening: Depression.* Update, 2002 Release. Retrieved August 27, 2002, from http://www.ahcpr.gov/clinic/uspstfdepr.
*Clinician discretion.
†Males age 35-64; females age 45-64.
‡Over age 50, or sigmoidoscopy less often.
§Females ≥ 50 years.
‖In women of childbearing age with an inaccurate vaccination history.

from suicide annually.[43] In addition, depression is associated with many other medical problems,[43] including heart disease, diabetes and chronic obstructive pulmonary disease (COPD). Despite the significant impact of depression on the health of the population, it is estimated that fewer than 25% of people suffering from depression receive treatment.[43] As a result, the recommendation of the USPSTF is for routine screening of adults for depression in clinical practices.[46] A variety of depression screening tools is available (see Chapter 25). Nurses who screen for depression should have a clearly established protocol in place to ensure that the client is referred for accurate diagnosis and effective treatment.

Breast Cancer

Breast cancer is the most common cause of cancer among women in the United States. More than 175,000 women are diagnosed with breast cancer annually, and more than 40,000 women die of breast cancer annually. Breast cancer death can be significantly reduced by early diagnosis. Women are screened for breast cancer in three ways: mammography, clinical breast examination, and breast self-examination. Of these, mammography is the most sensitive.[43]

The USPSTF[47] and the ACS[1] recommend that women 40 years of age and older have regular (every 1 to 2 years) mammograms. Although the USPSTF[47] states that there is insufficient evidence to support the value of clinical breast examination, the ACS[1] also recommends that women 20 to 39 years of age have clinical breast examinations every 3 years.

In addition, the USPSTF indicates that there is insufficient evidence to recommend for or against breast self-examination (BSE); however, the ACS[1] recommends that all women 20 years of age and older perform BSE on a monthly basis. Nurses can teach women how to do these self-examinations.

Women can use BSE to assess their breasts. When women perform BSE properly and regularly, they can note early changes in their breasts and seek further evaluation. A major barrier to BSE is lack of confidence. Take time when working with women to ensure that they are confident of their skill and have had all their questions addressed. The BSE technique is described in Figure 2-4.

When teaching, emphasize that the examination should be done every month and at the end of menses in all menstruating women. Advise nonmenstruating women to pick one day a month (e.g., the first day of the month) to do BSE. Inform women that most breast lumps are benign but it is essential that they seek professional evaluation if they find anything that concerns them. Chapter 39 discusses physical assessment of the breast, including the clinical breast examination.

FIGURE 2-4 Self-examination of female breasts and axillae. Accomplished by observation and palpation. The client assumes various positions for observation while standing in front of a mirror. **A,** Arms are relaxed at the sides. Next, lean forward. **B,** Raise arms high overhead. Press arms behind head. **C,** Rest palms on hips, and firmly press inward to flex chest muscles. **D,** In shower, examine the breast contours. **E,** Method of palpating breast. With fingers flat, gently press with small circular motions around an imaginary clock face; begin at 12 o'clock. Move an inch at a time toward the nipple. **F,** As a final step, squeeze the nipple gently between the thumb and index finger. Palpation of the breast is accomplished while lying down. **G,** Position to examine inner breast. **H,** Position to examine axilla. **I,** Position to examine outer breast. **J,** Repeat the entire process for opposite breast and axilla. (See text and Chapters 39 and 42 for discussion of technique and observations.)

Prostate Cancer

Nearly 40,000 men die annually of prostate cancer. Men at increased risk include those who have a first-degree relative (e.g., father, brother, son) with prostate cancer and African Americans. Despite the prevalence of the disease, neither the USPSTF[45] nor the American Academy of Family Physicians[29] recommends *routine* screening for prostate cancer because early screening and treatment have not proved beneficial. They do recommend, however, counseling clients about known risks for prostate cancer and the uncertain benefits of screening. The ACS[1] and the American Urological Association[29] suggest that men should be offered screening for prostate cancer using a prostate-specific antigen test and a digital rectal examination starting at age 50 (at age 45 for African-American men) (see Chapter 39).

When advising men about screening, keep in mind the man's prostate cancer risk factors, his general health, and his desires. Generally, prostate cancer screening should not be done in men older than 70 years of age or who have significant underlying illness that would result in a life expectancy of less than 10 years.[29]

Colorectal Cancer

Colorectal cancer is the second most common form of cancer in the United States, and it accounts for more than 55,000 deaths per year. If the disease is found while still localized, survival rates are at 91%. If the disease is found when it has spread, the survival rate is much lower.[45] Therefore, early detection of the disease is essential. Risk factors include uncommon hereditary familial polyposis syndromes and ulcerative colitis of more than 10 years' duration. More common risk factors include a family history of colorectal cancer, especially in young and middle-aged adults, and possibly high-fat and low-fiber diets.[45]

Current recommendations are for annual screening of adults over 50 years of age for colorectal cancer using fecal occult blood testing (FOBT).[48] People who are at increased risk might benefit from beginning screening at 40 years of age. FOBT is easily done at home, but the client should be instructed on dietary restrictions, specifically, no raw meat; no aspirin or nonsteroidal anti-inflammatory agents, and no vitamin C in doses greater than 250 mg for 48 hours before and during specimen collection. Specimens should be kept away from heat and should be tested within 2 weeks of collection. Both the USPSTF[48] and the American Cancer Society[1] recognize the potential value of either a sigmoidoscopy every 5 years in combination with annual FOBT testing or a colonoscopy every 10 years, but there are insufficient data to support either of these options for routine screening.

CONCLUSIONS

Health promotion and disease prevention activities are at the core of health care for young and middle-aged adults. Be familiar with current recommendations regarding healthy eating and activity patterns and with strategies for coping with daily stressors. Take every opportunity to work with clients to assist them to implement healthy lifestyles. Include risk assessment, risk management, and appropriate screening for diseases when working with these populations. Based on assessment results, provide education and appropriate referral.

BIBLIOGRAPHY

1. American Cancer Society. (2002). *Guidelines for the early detection of cancer.*
2. American Cancer Society. (2002). *The complete guide—nutrition and physical activity.* Retrieved August 27, 2002.
3. Anderson, J.E., et al. (2002). Treating tobacco use and dependence: An evidence-based clinical practice guideline for tobacco cessation. *Chest, 121* (3), 932-941.
4. Bonheur, B., & Young, S. (1991). Exercise as a health-promoting life-style choice. *Applied Nursing Research, 4*(1), 2-6.
5. Burns, C.M. (1993). Assessment and screening for substance abuse: Guidelines for the primary care nurse practitioner. *Nurse Practitioner Forum, 4*(4), 199-206.
6. Burns, K. (1996). A new recommendation for physical activity as a means of health promotion. *Nurse Practitioner, 21*(9), 18, 21-22, 26, 27.
7. Calfas, K., et al. (1996). A controlled trial of physician counseling to promote the adoption of physical activity. *Preventive Medicine, 25,* 225-233.
8. Centers for Disease Control. (May 28, 1999). Prevention of Varicella updated recommendation of the Advisory Committee on Immunization Practice (ACIP). *Morbidity and Mortality Weekly Report, RR06,* 1-5.
9. Centers for Disease Control. (June 30, 2000). Meningococcal disease and college students. *Morbidity and Mortality Weekly Report, 49* (RR07), 11-20.
10. Chrousos, G., & Gold, P. (1992). The concepts of stress and stress system disorders. *Journal of the American Medical Association, 267*(9), 1244-1252.
11. Council of Community Health Nurses. (1991). *Physical violence against women: ANA position statement.* Kansas City, MO: American Nurses' Association.
12. Davis, M., Eshelman, E., & McKay, M. (1995). *The relaxation and stress reduction workbook* (4th ed.). Oakland, CA: New Harbinger Publications.
13. Domestic violence: Ending the cycle of abuse. (1998). *Clinician Reviews, 8*(1), 55-57, 61-62, 67-68, 71.
14. Feldhaus, K., et al. (1997). Accuracy of three brief questions for detecting partner violence in the emergency department. *Journal of the American Medical Association, 277,* 1357-1361.
15. Ferri, R. (June 25, 1988). Treating HIV infection. *The Clinical Advisor,* 30-36.
16. Franklin, B., Buchal, M., & Hollingsworth, V. (1991). Exercise prescription. In R. Strauss (Ed), *Sports medicine* (2nd ed.). Philadelphia: W. B. Saunders.

EB 17. Goldstein, D. J. (1992). Beneficial effects of modest weight loss. *International Journal of Obesity, 16*, 397-415.

18. Gorin, S. S. (1998). Smoking cessation. In S. S. Gorin & J. Arnold (Eds.), *Health promotion handbook.* St. Louis: Mosby.

19. Grubbs, L. (1993). The critical role of exercise in weight control. *Nurse Practitioner, 18*(4), 20, 22, 25-26, 29.

20. Hoff, L. A. (1992). Battered women: Understanding, identification, and assessment. *Journal of the American Academy of Nurse Practitioners, 4*(4), 148-155.

21. Hoff, L. A. (1993). Battered women: Intervention and prevention. *Journal of the American Academy of Nurse Practitioners, 5*(1), 34-39.

EB 22. Howard, G., et al. (1998). Cigarette smoking and progression of atherosclerosis: The Atherosclerosis Risk in Communities (ARIC) study. *Journal of the American Medical Association, 279*(2), 119-124.

23. Jones, K. D., & Jones, J. M. (1997). Physical activity and exercise. *Clinician Reviews, 7*(3), 81-83, 86-88, 93-94, 97-98, 101-102, 104.

EB 24. Institute of Medicine. (2002). *Dietary reference intakes for energy, carbohydrate, fiber, fat, fatty acids, cholesterol, protein, and amino acids.* Washington, DC: National Academy Press.

25. Isaacson, J., Butler, R., & Zackarek, M. (1994). Screening with the Alcohol Use Disorders Identification Test (AUDIT) in an inner-city population. *Journal of General Internal Medicine, 9,* 550-553.

EB 26. Long, B. J., et al. (1996). A multisite field test of the acceptability of physical counseling in primary care: Project PACE. *American Journal of Preventive Medicine, 12*(2), 73-81.

27. McCloskey, J. C., & Bulechek, G. M. (1996). *Nursing intervention classification* (2nd ed.). St. Louis: Mosby.

28. McWhirter, E. H. (1994). *Counseling for empowerment.* Alexandria, VA: American Counseling Association.

29. Naitoh, J., Zeiner, R. L., & Dekernion, J. B. (1998). Diagnosis and treatment of prostate cancer. *American Family Physician, 57*(7), 1531-1539.

EB 30. Third Report of the National Cholesterol Education Program (NCEP) Expert Panel on Detection, Evaluation, and Treatment of High Blood Cholesterol in Adults (Adult Treatment Panel III). (2001). Bethesda, MD: U.S. Department of Health and Human Services, Public Health Service, National Institutes of Health, National Heart, Lung, and Blood Institute.

EB 31. National Heart, Lung, and Blood Institute (NHLBI), NHLBI Obesity Education Initiative Expert Panel. (June 1998). *Clinical guidelines on the identification, evaluation, and treatment of overweight and obesity in adults: The evidence report.* Bethesda, MD: National Institutes of Health, National Heart, Lung, and Blood Institute.

32. Novak, J. C. (1998). Effective smoking cessation strategies. *Clinical Letter for Nurse Practitioners, 2*(1), 1-6.

33. Reference deleted in proofs.

34. Padden, D.L. (2002). The role of the advanced practice nurse in the promotion of exercise and physical activity. *Topics in Advanced Practice Nursing Journal, 2*(1).

35. Paffenbarger, R. S., et al. (1986). Physical activity, all-cause mortality, and longevity in college alumni. *New England Journal of Medicine, 314*(10), 605-613.

36. Pate, R. R., et al. (1995). Physical activity and public health. *Journal of the American Medical Association, 273*(5), 402-407.

37. Pi-Sunyer, F. X. (1993). Medical hazards of obesity. *Annals of Internal Medicine, 119*(7), 655-660.

38. Quillian, J. P. (1995). Domestic violence. *Journal of American Academy of Nurse Practitioners, 7*(7), 351-358.

39. Saunders, J., et al. (1993). Development of the Alcohol Use Disorders Identification Test (AUDIT): WHO collaboration project on early detection of persons with harmful alcohol consumption. II. *Addiction, 88,* 791. EB

40. Strauss, R. H. (1991). *Sports medicine* (2nd ed.). Philadelphia: W.B. Saunders.

41. Sugg, N. K., & Inui, T. (1992). Primary care physicians' response to domestic violence. *Journal of the American Medical Association, 267*(23), 3157-3160.

42. U.S. Department of Health and Human Services. (1998). *Clinician's handbook of preventive services* (3rd ed.). Washington, DC: U.S. Government Printing Office.

43. U.S. Department of Health and Human Services. (2000). *Healthy* EB *people 2010.* (Conference Edition, in Two Volumes). Washington, DC: Author.

44. U.S. Department of Health and Human Services. (1996). *Physical* EB *activity and health,* S/N 017-023-00196-5. Washington, DC: U.S. Government Printing Office.

45. U.S. Preventive Services Task Force. (1996). *Guide to clinical pre-* EB *ventive services* (2nd ed.). Baltimore: Williams & Wilkins.

46. U.S. Preventive Services Task Force. (2002). Screening for depres- EB sion: Recommendations and rationale. *Annals of Internal Medicine, 136*(10), 760-764.

47. U.S. Preventive Services Task Force. (2002). Screening for breast EB cancer: Recommendations and rationale. *Annals of Internal Medicine,137*(5 pt 1), 344-346.

48. U.S. Preventive Services Task Force. (2002). Screening for colorec- EB tal cancer: Recommendations and rationale. *Annals of Internal Medicine, 137*(2), 129-131.

49. U.S. Preventive Services Task Force. (2002). Behavioral counseling EB in primary care to promote physical activity: Recommendations and rationale. *Annals of Internal Medicine, 137*(3), 205-207.

50. Fiore, M.C., et al. (2000). Treating tobacco use and dependence: EB Clinical practice guidelines. Rockville, MD: U.S. Department of Health and Human Services, Public Health Service.

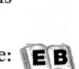

evolve *Did you remember to check out the bonus material on the Evolve website and the CD-ROM, including free self-assessment exercises?*

http://evolve.elsevier.com/Black/medsurg/

Health Promotion in Older Adults

Beverly E. Holland
Cynthia McCurren

evolve

Web Enhancements

Bridge to Home Health Care
  Detecting Elder Abuse
Care Plan
  The Older Client at Risk for Relocation Stress Syndrome

http://evolve.elsevier.com/Black/medsurg/

Ethical Issues in Nursing
  What Values Are Represented in the Nurse-Client Relationship?
  How Can You Be a Client Advocate to Older Adults?
Appendix A
  Religious Beliefs and Practices Affecting Health Care

The population of the United States is aging, producing a number of health care issues. Therefore, health promotion in older adults merits special attention. According to the Administration of Aging,[1] persons 65 years of age or older numbered 35 million in 2000. They represented 12.4% of the U.S. population: about one in every eight Americans. The number of older Americans increased by 3.7 million (12%) since 1990. In 2000 the group of adults 75 to 84 years of age (12.4 million) was 16 times larger than in 1900, and the 85+ group (4.2 million) was 34 times larger. There were 50,545 centenarians (100+ years) in 2000, representing a 35% increase from 1990.[1]

The older population will continue to grow (Figure 3-1). The most rapid increase is expected between the years 2010 and 2030, when the "baby boom" generation (those born between 1946 and 1964) reaches 65 years of age. By 2030 there will be about 70 million older persons, more than twice their number in 2000, and they will represent 20% of the population.[1] The older adult population is currently the fastest growing segment in the nation. Concern for rapidly increasing aging populations is an international dilemma.

The aging of America has profound implications for nursing practice across all settings, including acute care, the community, and long-term care. More than 48% of hospital patients, 80% of home-care patients, and 85% of all residents of nursing homes are older adults.[21] The overwhelming majority of nurses practicing in the United States today are, by default, geriatric nurses. Nurse experts on aging agree that nurses need information to provide appropriate care to older people. Nurses who care for older clients must be aware of the unique physical, psychosocial, legal, ethical, and economic issues surrounding the aging process. Knowing what resources, services, and options are available at the federal, state, and local levels is essential.

Nurses must understand the normal aging process and be prepared to care for clients who have chronic disorders and complex acute conditions. Normal aging changes the structure and function of various organ systems. Pathologic processes often present and progress differently in older adults, necessitating adaptation of interventions. Selected effects of aging as they relate to assessment, disease presentation, and nursing intervention appear throughout this book in discussions of the different body systems and their disorders.

This chapter examines late adulthood and the implications for nursing practice from a holistic perspective. The focus is on health promotion, disease prevention, and content unique to elder care to ensure overall well-being in older adults.

evolve Be sure to check out the bonus material on the Evolve website and the CD-ROM, including free self-assessment exercises.

http://evolve.elsevier.com/Black/medsurg/

Nursing Outcomes Classification (NOC)
for Nursing Diagnoses—Clients at Risk for Relocation Stress Syndrome

Relocation Stress Syndrome	Depression Control	Psychosocial Adjustment: Life Change
Anxiety Control	Depression Level	Quality of Life
Caregiver Adaptation to Patient Institu-	Grief Resolution	Sleep
tionalization	Loneliness	Social Support
Coping	Mood Equilibrium	

NURSING AND THE STUDY OF AGING

The American Nurses' Association (ANA)[2] has identified standards of *gerontological nursing* practice. *Gerontological nursing* is the ANA's term for nursing specializing in the care of older adults. These standards include practice guidelines for health promotion, health maintenance, disease prevention, and self-care, with a goal of restoring and maintaining optimal physical, psychological, and social functioning. Organizational standards for nursing service, research, ethics, and professional development are also included. *Standards of Gerontological Nursing Practice* defines what gerontological nurses can do and outlines their unique contributions by describing and prescribing professional nursing practice related to care of older adults.

The ANA provides three levels of gerontological nursing certification:

- Gerontological nurse
- Gerontological clinical nurse specialist (GCNS)
- Gerontological nurse practitioner (GNP)

Advanced-practice nurses (GNPs and GCNSs) have diverse opportunities for practice. They can manage many health problems that occur among residents in skilled nursing facilities, retirement communities, day care settings, ambulatory care settings, hospitals, and private practice. Gerontological nurse specialists can also assume roles in education, counseling, case management, and long-term care administration.

Emerging Profile of the Older Population

Ethnicity

In 2000, 16.4% of persons 65 years of age and older in the United States were minorities: 5.6% Hispanics, 8% African Americans, 2.4% Asians and Pacific Islanders, and fewer than 1% Native Americans or Native Alaskan. By 2030 this percentage is expected to increase to 25.4%.[1] Caregivers who work with diverse older Americans must consider ethnic origin in relation to health and illness issues, family and social support, and interaction within the health care system.

Aging, Gender, and Marital Status

In 2000 there were 20.6 million women over age 65 years and 14.49 million older men. Life expectancy for men is 81 years and for women 84 years. Among people 65 years and older, 74% of men live with their spouses, compared with only 43% of women. Almost half of all older women in 2000 were widows.[1] Traditionally, women have assumed dependent roles, letting others make their decisions, including treatment choices. In general, these women are vulnerable; nurses need to ensure that they receive their share of medical resources and quality health care.

Economic Forces

The largest single income source for an older adult is the Social Security benefit, accounting for 38% of the income of the older population. Other contributing sources include income from assets, pensions, and earnings. In 2000 the median yearly income for older men was $19,168; for older women, it was $10,899. The poverty rate was 10.2% among all older adults in 2000, and another 6.7% of older adults were classified as "near-poor."[1]

Educational Issues

In 2000, 70% of older adults had completed high school, a significant increase from 1970, when only 28% had done so. Bachelor's degrees had been earned by 16% in

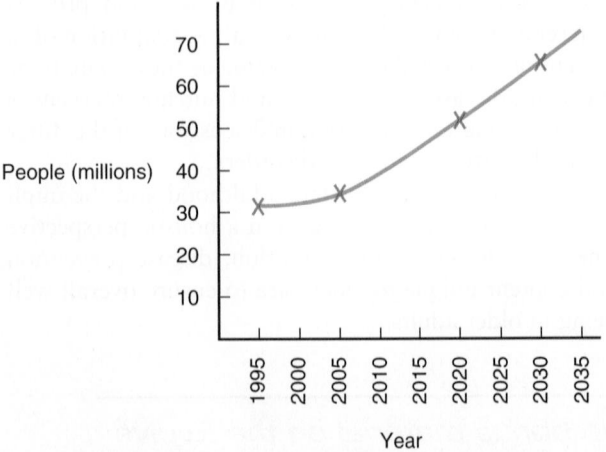

FIGURE 3-1 Projected rise in U.S. population 65 years of age and older.

2000. There is great disparity in educational levels among various ethnic groups, most markedly among African-American and Hispanic older adults, in whom the rate of finishing high school is 46% and 37%, respectively.[1]

Cultural Aspects

The United States has many ethnocultural groups interacting within one society. Culture defines who is old, establishes rituals for identifying older adults, sets socially acceptable roles and expectations for behavior of older adults, and influences attitudes toward older adult members.

The definitions of functional and chronological aging indicate that there are no arbitrary or widely accepted markers for old age. The prevailing definition of old age in the United States is considered age 65; there are diverse perceptions of old age in various cultures. People may be recognized as older adults as early as age 40 among Southeast Asian and Native American groups. Social changes, such as becoming grandparents and retirement, or changes in functional status rather than chronological age, mark entrance into old age in different cultures. Clients may be chronologically old but, in functional terms, are active and productive.

When working with older people, nurses should use a holistic approach. Holistic care encompasses understanding the interaction of culture, socioeconomic background, and spirituality as well as the physiologic and psychological processes of the person. Chapter 4 discusses psychosocial and cultural assessment. A holistic approach takes into account the complexities of the interactions and delivers individualized care to meet each client's needs.[19]

Nurses who care for older clients and families from different cultural backgrounds notice that family relationships vary within a cultural context. The availability of physical and personal support from family members can facilitate the older person's ability to maintain independence, cope effectively with acute and chronic illnesses, remain functional and productive despite disability, and experience a peaceful death.

Older adults who have made major lifestyle adjustments from their homelands to the United States and from rural to urban settings may be unaware of health care alternatives (e.g., preventive programs, benefits, and screening programs) for which they are eligible. The nurse can help clients in evaluating their social networks, seeking assistance for health care needs, activating social contacts for support, and developing culturally competent care plans.

Health Promotion, Maintenance, and Restoration in Older Clients

Older adults are more likely to suffer from multiple chronic and disabling illnesses than are younger adults (see Chapter 2). Approximately 80% of older adults in the United States have one or more chronic diseases.[25] Chronic conditions result in limitations in the *activities of daily living* (ADL). In 1998, among those 65 to 74 years of age, 28.8% reported a limitation caused by a chronic condition. In those over 75 years of age, more than half (50.6%) reported limitations from chronic disorders.[1] Heart disease, cancer, and strokes account for 66% of deaths in persons older than 65 years of age. Clients with hypertension, arthritis, pulmonary disorders, diabetes, visual and hearing problems, dementia, and depression require ongoing care and rehabilitation.[10]

A traditional perception of *health* as the absence of disease or disability is clearly not applicable to most older people. A more appropriate focus is on health as a state of mind and on the ability to live and function effectively in society. Health encompasses an interaction of physical, functional, and psychosocial factors. Health promotion goals, therefore, must include individual and group efforts related to spiritual, emotional, psychosocial, and physical concerns (see Chapter 1). Desired outcomes of health promotion programs should include the following:

1. Maximizing functional independence, thereby reducing dependency
2. Decreasing mortality
3. Decreasing morbidity, including impairment
4. Maintaining or improving quality of life (QOL)
5. Promoting behavioral change when necessary
6. Increasing productivity

Older adults can make efforts to control aspects of their health and move toward wellness (Table 3-1). Nursing has a prominent role in helping older adults practice health promotion, including self-care, physical activity, nutritional awareness, and stress management.

Quality of Life

The concept of QOL is difficult to define. It is recognized that QOL contains factors internal to the individual and external factors affecting that person. Researchers attempt to measure QOL using scales, interviews, and questions. What is generally agreed on is that QOL is subjective and varies with the individual's perception of health and his or her capabilities. A definition by Rene Dubos[7] addresses the subjective and multidimensionality of QOL by saying, "Men naturally desire health and happiness. . . . The kind of health that men desire . . . is not necessarily a state in which they experience physical vigor and a sense of well-being, not even one giving them a long life. It is, instead, the condition best suited to reach goals that each individual formulates for himself" (p. 228). Normal physiologic aging changes and chronic health conditions have a large impact on a person's perceived QOL. Some other factors that affect perceived QOL include autonomy, stress, and feeling lack of control or powerlessness.

TABLE 3-1	*Health Promotion, Maintenance, and Restoration Activities for Older Adults*	
Promotion*	**Maintenance†**	**Restoration‡**
Primary Prevention (prevents occurrence of specific disease and provides specific protection)	*Secondary Prevention* (early detection and treatment and limitation of disability)	*Tertiary Prevention* (rehabilitation after disease)

Use of seat belt
Smoking cessation programs
Diet low in fat, high in fiber
Regular weight-bearing exercise
Weight control
Education in osteoporosis: calcium and vitamin D intake
Limiting alcohol ingestion
Dental care
 	
Vaccinations
  Tetanus-diphtheria toxoid
  Pneumococcus
  Influenza
	Self-Examination
	  Testicular self-examination
	  Breast self-examination
	Complete Physical Examination
	  Blood pressure
	  Electrocardiogram
	  Total cholesterol with high-density lipoprotein
	  Mammography with clinical breast examination
	  Digital rectal examination
	  Fecal occult blood testing
	  Thyroid-stimulating hormone test
	  Pelvic examination with Pap smear
	  Prostate examination
	  Sigmoidoscopy
	
	Counseling **Counseling and Referral**
	  Sexuality Hearing examination
	  Urinary incontinence Visual examination with
	  Depression/life glaucoma test
	    satisfaction Dental examination and
	                cleaning
		Rehabilitation
		  Post-stroke rehabilitation
		  Cardiac rehabilitation
		  Pulmonary rehabilitation
		  Orthopedic rehabilitation
		  Reminiscence therapy

*Health promotion activities for older adults are similar to recommendations for all adults.

†Recommendations on frequency of examinations vary depending on the recommending organization (American College of Physicians, American Cancer Society, U.S. Preventive Services Task Force, and American Geriatrics Society) and the risk factors and presenting manifestations of the individual.

‡Rehabilitation programs are interdisciplinary and are developed to meet the specific needs and deficits of the person.

Self-Care and Self-Responsibility

As older adults become better informed and increasingly aware of the self-help movement, health care expectations also rise. The desire to be in control of one's body, mind, and spirit and to assume responsibility for one's own wellness increases. This does not mean that traditional health care providers are ignored. Instead, strategies are taught that enable people to respond to their body signals and to take action accordingly. The nurse can help the aging person understand this shared role (between the individual and health care professionals) for maintaining wellness, counsel older adults about factors that can alter wellness, and provide information about available alternatives (see Chapter 1). Given adequate information, older adults can practice effective self-care through a process of examining choices and making informed, meaningful decisions.

Most older persons want to have as much control as possible over their body, mind, and spirit. Assessment should include an evaluation of self-care, with an emphasis on abilities rather than disabilities. Suggested preventive practices are discussed in Chapters 1, 2, and 4.

Physical activity, nutrition, and stress management are also factors in geriatric wellness.

Physical Activity

Exercise and activity are essential for health promotion and maintenance and for achieving an optimal level of functioning (see Chapters 1 and 2). Approximately half of the physical deterioration in the older adult population is caused by disuse rather than by the aging process or disease. Positive effects of exercise on health include (1) increased energy, (2) improved eating and sleeping, (3) decreased discomfort and stress, and (4) decreased smoking and alcohol use.[8]

Physiologically, benefits to the cardiopulmonary, vascular, and musculoskeletal systems result in (1) improved oxygen transport, (2) decreased blood pressure and pulse rate, (3) increased vital lung capacity, (4) decreased body fat and increased lean body mass, (5) reduced osteoporosis, and (6) increased muscle strength and joint flexibility. Positive psychological changes occur as well, including improved cognitive functioning and a heightened sense of well-being.

FIGURE 3-2 Today's older adult is interested in maintaining strength and endurance.

BOX 3-1   *Risk Factors for Malnutrition in the Older Adult Population*

*D*isease
*E*ating poorly
*T*ooth decay or oral pain
*E*conomic hardship
*R*educed social contact
*M*ultiple medications
*I*nvoluntary weight loss or gain
*N*eeds assistance with self-care
*E*lder older than 80 years

From the Nutrition Screening Initiative in conjunction with the American Academy of Family Physicians, the American Dietetic Association, and the National Council on the Aging (1993).

Before beginning an exercise program, older clients should have a physical examination, which may include an exercise stress test. One of the best exercises for an older adult is walking, with progression to 30-minute sessions three to five times each week. Swimming and dancing are also beneficial. Age alone does not preclude older people from pursuing a range of physical activities; the issue is simply one of physical tolerance. Older adults confined to a chair or with limited mobility can perform adapted exercises. At many senior centers, wellness programs, and fitness clubs, consultants, instructors, or physical therapists can help the client establish an individualized exercise program (Figure 3-2).

Nutrition

Nutritional status is important to an older person's ability to remain healthy, to maintain structural integrity, to think clearly, and to possess the necessary energy to engage in social and fitness activities. Several physiologic changes related to aging can affect nutritional status.

Socioeconomic factors can contribute to malnutrition. With reduced income, some older adults may restrict food intake to near-starvation levels because they may choose to pay rent and buy medicine over spending for food. Diets may be unbalanced because of the expense of fresh fruits, vegetables, and meats. Lack of transportation and the inability to carry heavy quantities of groceries can prohibit some people from obtaining food. Living alone can also be associated with poor nutrition because many older adults lose the motivation to prepare a balanced diet for just themselves.

Psychologically, depression and stress can affect nutritional status. Both conditions can lead to overeating or undereating. Medications can influence nutrition, producing side effects of increased or decreased appetite, constipation, nausea, or decreased absorption. Additionally, drugs such as diuretics can affect fluid and electrolyte balance, leading to problems with dehydration and constipation.

Physiologically, energy requirements lessen with age because of a decline in basal metabolic rate and often a reduction in physical activity. The need for vitamin D, vitamin B_6, and calcium to protect against osteoporosis increases, and increased fiber intake is recommended to reduce the apparent risk of some forms of cancer and to promote bowel function. Unexplained weight loss of more than 5% in 1 month or more than 10% in 6 months is cause for concern. Clients at risk for nutritional problems should be identified (Box 3-1; see also Chapter 30). When no physical cause can be identified, older adults with altered nutrition should be referred to community resources for assessment and assistance related to food, finances, and dental care.

Stress Management

Any real or perceived threat to one's physical, emotional, and social well-being can create stress (see Chapters 1 and 2). Life's later years can include changes such as acute or chronic illness, retirement, death of significant others, financial hardship, or relocation, resulting in stress that can be overwhelming. Although the sources of stress may vary, the physiologic outcomes are similar. Stimulation of the sympathetic nervous system results in the release of epinephrine, norepinephrine, and adrenal glucocorticoids. Prolonged stress can result in serious consequences, including heart disease, hypertension, stroke, cancer, gastric ulcers, skin problems, complications of underlying disorders, and numerous social and emotional problems.

The way in which an older person adapts to change and stress is influenced by personality traits, past coping strategies, and spirituality. Spirituality extends beyond religion to include contemplation, experiential learning, recognition through growth, discovery and acceptance, new connections, and letting go. Growth, self-discovery, and connecting with others support older people in times of stress, reinforce a sense of self-worth, and provide confidence to overcome obstacles.

Encourage the client to respond to stress in a healthy manner. Balancing nutrition, rest, and exercise; remaining connected with others; and having a sense of inner peace can help with stress management. Explain methods of relaxation, including biofeedback, meditation, progressive relaxation, breathing-control exercises, physical activity, and involvement in pastimes that provide respite from stressful demands (see Chapters 1 and 2).

Teaching

Encouraging health promotion and disease prevention among older adults requires effective teaching. Teaching older adults is similar to teaching members of any age group in that individual characteristics and learning needs must be considered. General guidelines for teaching older adults are listed in Box 3-2.

NORMAL AGING AND COMMONLY OCCURRING PATHOLOGIC PROCESSES

Aging has been defined as a universal, internally predictable biologic process following maturity. It is characterized by changes accumulated over time that increase susceptibility to disease and ultimately lead to death. Physiologically, aging in the absence of disease involves a steady decline in the functional reserve of organ systems and homeostatic controls, especially when a person is under stress. In addition to disease, nutritional status and other extrinsic factors (i.e., environment, activity, medication, depression) are superimposed on the basic process of aging and create individual differences in how one experiences aging.

PRESENTATION OF ILLNESS

With advanced age, the body does not respond as vigorously to illness or disease because of diminished physiologic reserve. People often attribute discomforts to "old age" and accept the changes as inevitable, thus failing or refusing to seek help for potentially treatable conditions. A frequent complicating factor in identifying and treating disease in older people is the presence of multiple ailments. The number of pathologic conditions that a person has at one time is strongly correlated with age.[30] The presenting picture may be further complicated by atypical or altered presentation of disease (i.e., weakness, weight loss, confusion, or failure to thrive). Each of these factors presents a challenge; conduct careful and thorough assessments and analyses of manifestations to promote appropriate treatment.

> **BOX 3-2**   *Guidelines for Effectively Teaching Older Adults*
>
> **Vision**
> 1. Provide large, easy-to-read typeface
> 2. Emphasize contrasting colors: black and white
> 3. Avoid blues and greens
> 4. Use nonglare paper
> 5. Write short, simple paragraphs
> 6. Make sure eyeglasses are in place and clean
>
> **Hearing**
> 1. Speak slowly
> 2. Enunciate clearly
> 3. Lower the pitch of your voice
> 4. Eliminate background noise
> 5. Face the learner
> 6. Use nonverbal cues
> 7. Make sure client's hearing aid is in place and is working properly
>
> **Energy Level/Attention**
> 1. Use short teaching sessions
> 2. Offer liquid refreshment and bathroom breaks
> 3. Promote comfort
>
> **Information Processing and Memory**
> 1. Present most important information first
> 2. Clarify information with use of examples that the client can relate to
> 3. Motor skills: Teach one step at a time, demonstrate, allow for return demonstration
> 4. Encourage association between items
> 5. Be concrete and specific
> 6. Eliminate distractions
> 7. Encourage verbal interactions
> 8. Correct wrong answers and reinforce correct answers
> 9. Offer praise and encouragement

Atypical or altered presentation of disease can be displayed in various ways. For example, an older adult with pneumonia may exhibit confusion and may have an increased respiratory rate and generalized weakness instead of the classic manifestations of productive cough, fever, and chest pain. Frequently, manifestations in one organ system may cause abnormality in another system, resulting in manifestations unrelated to the actual problem, such as confusion accompanying a urinary tract infection. Chronic conditions can mask the presence of acute illness, as can be seen in new-onset heart failure, in which orthopnea might be hidden if a person regularly uses multiple pillows because of gastroesophageal reflux, arthritis, or obesity.

Finally, expected manifestations may not be present at all, as in the case of a myocardial infarction unaccompanied by chest pain. Table 3-2 summarizes common

TABLE 3-2	Structural and Functional Changes and Common Health Problems in Older Adults	
System	**Normal Changes Associated with Aging**	**Common Health Problems**
Cardiovascular	Decreased contractility, impaired coronary artery blood flow, altered preload and afterload, increased atherosclerotic plaques	Hypertension, ischemic heart disease, heart failure, cardiac dysrhythmia, valvular heart disease, peripheral vascular disease, varicose veins, dehydration, stroke/transient ischemic attack
Neurologic/behavioral	Decreased speed of neural conduction, decreased number of brain cells, decreased neurotransmitters, decreased rapid eye movement sleep, decreased cerebral circulation	Parkinsonism, essential tremor, Alzheimer's disease or dementia, depression, anxiety, psychosis or paranoid state, sleep disturbance, subdural hematoma, trigeminal neuralgia
Respiratory	Increased rigidity of thoracic cage, decreased elasticity, decreased vital capacity, increased residual volume, decreased cough efficiency, decreased ciliary action	Pneumonia, chronic obstructive pulmonary disease, dyspnea
Gastrointestinal	Decreased secretion of gastric acid, delayed gastric emptying, decreased gastrointestinal motility, altered nutrient digestion, altered bowel function, weakening of lower esophageal sphincter	Diverticula or diverticulitis, constipation, diarrhea, gastroesophageal reflux or hiatus hernia, fecal incontinence, colorectal cancer, rectal prolapse, dysphagia, anorexia, gallbladder disease
Genitourinary	Decreased bladder capacity, decreased concentrating and diluting abilities, decreased creatinine clearance, increased prostate size	Renal insufficiency, urinary incontinence, urinary tract infection, enlarged prostate or prostate cancer, sexual dysfunction
Endocrine/metabolic	Decreased basal metabolism, altered pancreatic function, decreased testosterone, estrogen, progesterone	Diabetes mellitus, hyperthyroidism or hypothyroidism, thyroid cancer, hypercalcemia or hypocalcemia, hyperlipidemia, hypokalemia, hyponatremia, gout
Musculoskeletal	Decreased bone density, decreased muscle size and strength, degenerated joint cartilage	Paget's disease, osteoporosis, osteomalacia, rheumatoid arthritis, osteoarthritis, polymyalgia rheumatica, spondylosis, fractures, foot pathology, gait disturbance, falls
Autonomic nervous system	Decreased reaction time and coordination, decreased temperature regulation, decreased sensitivity of baroreceptors	Falls, accidental injuries, orthostatic hypotension, impaired body temperature regulation
Hematologic and immune	Decreased erythropoietin production, decreased intrinsic factor, decreased functioning T and B cells and monocytes	Iron deficiency anemia, pernicious anemia, anemia of chronic disease, cancer, autoimmune disorders
Oral	Decreased salivary secretion, decreased oral motor apparatus, loss of teeth	Periodontal disease; problems with speech, chewing, and swallowing
Sensory	Decreased accommodation, decreased visual acuity, decreased hearing of high-pitched frequencies	Visual impairment, hearing impairment, diminished smell or taste
Dermatologic	Decreased elasticity, decreased secretion of natural oil and perspiration, thinning of skin, decreased heat regulation, decreased epidermal renewal, decreased inflammatory response	Pressure sores, basal cell and squamous carcinoma, herpes zoster, seborrheic and actinic keratosis, stasis dermatitis, pruritus, hypothermia or hyperthermia
Reproductive	Female: vaginal mucosal thinning, atrophy, decreased breast tissue, sexual dysfunction Male: decreased sexual desire	Female: Cervical cancer, breast cancer Male: prostate cancer, impotence

structural and functional changes associated with normal aging and presents common diseases, disorders, and injuries frequently seen in older adults. Risk factors for many chronic diseases in old age are manifested in early to middle adulthood (see Chapters 47, 54, 63, and 72). Increasing age and chronic disease, functional disabilities, and hospitalization intensify the demand and need for health care services, which has implications in any health care setting.

FUNCTIONAL STATUS

Functional ability is the result of the combined effect of disease and disability on the person's ability to carry out the tasks associated with everyday living. Maintaining optimal function allows the older adult to remain as independent as possible. With a goal of assisting the older adult to live independently as long as possible and to prevent hospitalization and institutionalization, the functional assessment can detect problem areas and make recommendations that could allow changes to be made that would allow them to remain independent. For example, many older adults fear the loss of the ability to drive. A functional assessment may determine that the cause of the problem (i.e., vision, hearing) can be corrected and the person would not have to give up driving or the independence it provides.[8]

A *functional assessment* is a systematic measure of objective performance in areas of daily living. It measures ADL and instrumental ADL (IADL). Basic self-care skills or ADL are the essential activities and tasks performed to get through the day: dressing, eating, ambulating, toileting, and hygiene. ADL assessment helps to determine the need for daily personal care and to plan long-term care.[15] A corresponding rise in functional dependence related to ADL occurs with increasing age.[1]

The IADL are more complex and are essential to community living situations. IADL include ADL and shopping, housework, managing money, food preparation, and transportation.[17] Evaluation of IADL is used to determine what type of assistance people in an independent or semi-independent setting may need. The ability to perform IADL is less important in institutional settings than in community settings, although the assessment can prove important for discharge planning when the client is returning to the home environment.

Assessment of functional status of the older adult is important when detecting disease and dysfunction, selecting appropriate interventions, and evaluating the results of those interventions. A comprehensive functional assessment would include ADL and IADL, balance and mobility, cognitive abilities, vision and hearing, bowel and bladder function, nutritional status, and environmental factors. Research has found that functional impairments (both physical and psychosocial) are reliable early indicators of active illness in older people.[5,8]

On completion of a functional assessment, a management plan can be developed. This plan may include coordination of environmental changes, facilitation for the use of assistive devices, and arrangements for community referrals for services that would allow the person to remain in the chosen environment.

Functional assessment instruments generally include scales for measuring ADL[15] and IADL.[17,18] Observation, interview, mental status,[11,26] and depression screening[29] can assess psychosocial functioning and provide information about cognitive functioning, perceptual-motor skills, insight, reasoning, and contact with reality. Chapters 4 and 69 describe mental status assessment.

Physiologic Factors That Influence Functional Status

Sleep
Older adults fall asleep with more difficulty, awaken more readily and more frequently, spend more time in the drowsiness stage, and spend less time in deep sleep than do younger adults.[30] Functionally, these changes have little impact on the daily life of the older adult; however, adverse reactions can occur when these changes coincide with illness, stress, daily demands, or certain medications, such as hypnotic, antidepressant, diuretic, and some antihypertensive medications. Sleep disorders and their treatments are discussed in Chapter 24.

Sensory Impairments
Normal aging results in some sensory impairment (see Table 3-2). Vision and hearing are senses that individuals rely on to communicate and to function in the environment. Sensory impairments can affect safety, communication with others, performance of daily activities, and quality of life. Assessment suggests that limitations in ADL are more likely to occur in older people with sensory impairments than in those without sensory loss. Vision changes can affect the performance of a variety of daily activities: driving a vehicle; shopping for groceries; negotiating stairs; maneuvering safely in dark or unfamiliar environments; seeing markings on clocks, radios, thermostats, appliances, and televisions; and reading newspapers, signs, directories, and labels on food items and medication containers. Besides influencing daily activities, impaired vision increases the risk of falling. Impairments and treatment for vision and hearing disorders are discussed in Chapters 67 and 68.

Mobility and Balance
Mobility is essential for maintaining independence. Serious consequences occur when mobility declines. Older people use mobility and balance to assess whether they

are in relatively good or poor health. At least half of older adults have some limitation in function that prevents them from being fully independent.

Mobility depends on the ability to maintain balance and strength. Decreased functioning of various body systems can affect balance and strength and may place the person at risk. Decreases in functional status can be caused by impaired sensory ability (vision and hearing), cardiopulmonary disorders (dysrhythmia, postural hypotension, chronic obstructive pulmonary disease), neurologic disorders (parkinsonism and problems that affect gait, balance, sway, and reaction time), and depression. Side effects from medications also increase risk. The side effects of hypovolemia, postural hypotension, excessive sedation, decreased cognitive functioning, and loss of postural control can negatively affect mobility and balance.[32] Chronic disorders that increase with age and that affect functional ability include osteoporosis, osteoarthritis, and rheumatoid arthritis (see Chapters 28 and 79).

Unstable balance is of concern because the risk of falling increases with age. Each year, 25% to 35% of healthy community-dwelling adults between 65 and 75 years of age report a significant fall. This rate rises to 32% to 42% for those over 75 years of age.[12] In hospitals, falls constitute the largest category of reported incidents.

The effect of falls in older adults is far reaching. Falls contribute to significant morbidity and mortality.[32] Consequences of falls consume a large portion of health care dollars in the United States, and fear of subsequent falls contributes to restricted activity and mobility and to reduced independence. This self-restriction contributes to functional decreases and social isolation, thus setting up a spiral of downward decline. Up to 40% of all nursing home admissions are related to falls and instability.[32]

Psychosocial Factors That Influence Functional Status

Although physiologic changes and chronic illnesses associated with aging may affect functional abilities, psychosocial changes are often the most challenging and demanding. Some challenges arise from physical changes, but many are caused by changes in roles, relationships, and living environments. These changes tax coping abilities and energies.

Ageism

Ageism refers to the prejudices and stereotypes applied to older people purely because of their age. Ageism, like racism and sexism, is a way of labeling a group of people and not allowing them to be individuals with unique ways of living. Prejudice toward older adults is often an attempt by younger generations to shield themselves from their own eventual aging and death. Such stereotyping allows younger individuals to see older people as different from themselves, and they ultimately cease to identify with older people as human beings. An awakening comes when these younger people age and find themselves the victims of the same stereotypes and attitudes.

The significance of ageism is considerable. Ageism can affect a person's self-confidence, disempower by limiting potential, and cause early or excessive dependency. It can also affect well-being by influencing the attitudes of health care providers and political powers. Typically, the diagnosis and treatment of disease in older adults is less aggressive; programs are generally underfunded; and the ability of older adults to remain a contributing force, as perceived by society, is reduced simply because of chronologic age.[8]

Negativism can have a devastating effect and can cause older adults to adopt modes of dependency, helplessness, and a negative self-image, leading to increased vulnerability to biopsychosocial stressors.[10] Images of older persons as being dependent, deteriorating beyond rehabilitative efforts, and being physically and mentally unappealing can lead to reluctance among professionals to care for them. This can result in carelessness about the quality of care delivered; however, each older adult has the potential for rehabilitation, treatment, self-actualization, or improvement in QOL and well-being, regardless of how small that potential may be.

Multiple Losses

Many losses inevitably occur in later life. Assessing the impact of the losses and supporting older adults are major goals. Aging persons experience personal, social, and economic losses. Among the most devastating are "people" losses—parents, friends, spouse, or children (Figure 3-3). Other typical losses may include loss of one's

FIGURE 3-3 Loss of loved ones may result in an emotional burden accompanied by mental and physical effects.

home, possessions, pets, employment, social position, or financial security. An "overload" state can result when losses become multiple; the emotional upheaval becomes a catalyst, and the result is mental confusion, withdrawal, helplessness, and depression.

Relocation is one type of loss that can produce psychosocial changes and changes in mortality and morbidity.[6] Armer[4] examined the personal perceptions of the relocation event to rural relocating older adults. Central to the reaction and adjustment to relocation was whether the move was one of choice. Other influencing factors included social support and interaction, prior life satisfaction, and recency of loss. Individuals at high risk for poor relocation adjustment have low self-esteem, no friends or support, many worries, high levels of alienation, poor self-perception of health, and depression. Interventions to help with relocation include assessing for risk factors, empathizing with the difficulties of the move, and suggesting positive resources to effectively cope. See the Care Plan feature on The Older Client at Risk for Relocation Stress Syndrome on the website. Adjustment to loss is a challenge at any age. For older adults, resolution of grief over loss may not always be achieved but can be integrated into their lives without causing dysfunction.

Neglect and Abuse

Neglect and abuse are complex, serious issues affecting older adults in all settings. It is estimated that 10% of adults over 65 years of age have been victims of abuse or neglect, and it is also believed that about four times as many incidents occur but are never reported.[34] Elder abuse encompasses emotional, sexual, and physical neglect as well as physical and sexual violence and financial abuse. It is not uncommon for adults to experience several types of abuse simultaneously. Without intervention, abuse tends to escalate. See the Bridge to Home Health Care feature on Detecting Elder Abuse on the website.

Elder abuse has emerged as a significant aspect of family violence for several reasons. One is the increased number of older adults. As more people live to an advanced age, more adult children are assuming the caregiver role. If the adult child is unprepared for this responsibility, abuse and neglect may occur. Because an older person's dependency needs increase with time, the stress and burden of caregiving also increase, thus raising the risk of abuse. It is the responsibility of the health care provider, both ethically and legally, to be aware of the obvious and subtle signs of abuse and neglect and, as a client advocate, to encourage and coordinate assistance for victims and abusers. The passage of elder abuse and adult protective services laws has led to increased reporting of mistreatment and self-neglect, which has resulted in greater recognition of the problem.

MENTAL HEALTH DISORDERS IN OLDER ADULTS

Dementia, Delirium, and Depression

Dementia (specifically Alzheimer's disease) and delirium (also known as "confusion") are discussed in Chapter 74 along with their pathophysiology, clinical manifestations, assessment, and management. The focus here is on three important conditions in older adults: dementia, delirium, and depression. Clinically, the presenting manifestations of these conditions in older clients can be similar. A differential diagnosis is essential.

Disorders associated with cognitive decline are among the most common and frightening problems faced by older adults. A common myth is that older adults inevitably experience cognitive decline as a consequence of aging. Serious difficulties with thinking clearly and remembering are abnormal consequences at any age and are manifestations of medical illness or altered psychosocial well-being.[10]

The stereotypical view that cognitive decline is a normal part of aging prevails. For this reason, an acute deterioration in cognition is frequently overlooked; undetected cases of cognitive disorders have ranged from 30% to 84%.[9] Because many older adults believe that cognitive decline is part of aging, they do not seek medical attention when they notice changes in processing stimuli or in responding to stressful life events. Family members may react to acute cognitive changes as the "beginning of the end" and may prematurely plan for alternative living arrangements and entertain other actions and thoughts that may be unnecessary.

Dementia

Dementia is a clinical syndrome characterized by severe intellectual deterioration that interferes with one's ability to cope with daily life. It is gradually progressive and *irreversible*. Deficits occur in memory, language, perception, praxis, learning, problem-solving, abstract thinking, and judgment. Approximately 10% of people 65 to 74 years of age have dementia; the prevalence increases to 47% for those older than 85 years.[16] Dementia can be *primary*, as with Alzheimer's disease, multi-infarct dementia, alcoholism, and Pick's disease, or *secondary* to other causes, as with Parkinson's disease and trauma. Causes of dementia can vary, but the clinical presentation is similar regardless of cause. Therefore, the descriptive term *dementia of Alzheimer's type* is generally used.

Before a diagnosis of dementia is made, all potential physical and psychosocial causes of cognitive decline should be ruled out. The onset and progressive nature of the cognitive decline should be documented, and serial neuropsychological testing should be performed. The diagnosis can be complicated when delirium, depression, or both are superimposed on dementia.

Delirium

Delirium is a syndrome characterized by global cognitive impairment of abrupt onset that is *reversible*. This condition becomes irreversible only if underlying causes are undetected or treated unsuccessfully. Delirium is also known as acute confusion, reversible dementia, pseudosenility, acute brain failure, and clouded mental state. Attention deficits are the most significant feature of delirium. Other diagnostic criteria include disorganized thinking, reduced level of consciousness, perceptual disturbances, disturbances of the sleep-wake cycle, increased or decreased psychomotor activity, disorientation, and memory impairment.

Delirium is one of the most prevalent cognitive disorders among hospitalized older clients. It is associated with higher mortality, prolonged hospital stays, longer nursing time than necessary for the admitting diagnosis, and a higher rate of nursing home placement.[27] Delirium is often the presenting manifestation of physical illness in an older person, exceeding the indicators of fever, pain, and tachycardia. It has been associated with a variety of conditions, especially adverse drug reactions, metabolic disorders (e.g., electrolyte disorders, renal failure, respiratory failure, and endocrinopathies), cardiac failure, cerebrovascular disorders, infection (especially pulmonary, renal, or neurologic), anemia, and surgery. Psychosocial factors can also cause or contribute to a delirious state; these include bereavement, relocation, and sensory deprivation or overstimulation.

The key to differentiating delirium from dementia is assessment of the onset of the cognitive manifestations. Onset of delirium is rapid, occurring within hours to days; dementia onset is slower and more gradual. It is imperative that reversible delirium not be classified as dementia. A comprehensive investigation of all possible physical and psychosocial factors that might cause altered cognition must be conducted.

Depression

Research suggests that significant manifestations of depression occur in approximately 10% to 15% of all community-dwelling older adults over 65 years of age; among institutionalized older adults, the prevalence rate increases to 50% to 75%.[10] Depression is a complex syndrome that manifests itself in a variety of ways in older people. The most common manifestations are *vegetative*, which include insomnia, fatigue, weight loss, constipation, preoccupation with physical health, and thoughts of death. Older adults who are suffering from depression may also exhibit sadness, crying, anxiety, irritability, or paranoia.

Depression can also lead to cognitive impairment. It is estimated that depression-associated cognitive disorders occur in 10% to 29% of depressed older adults.[26] Therefore, differentiation between depression-related cognitive alteration and dementia may be difficult. Depressed clients often look and act demented, and they perform poorly on mental status tests; however, the vegetative signs of depression are not usually seen in demented people. Features supporting a diagnosis of depression versus dementia include recent onset of depressive symptoms and inconsistencies with actual functional performance and cognitive testing. Table 3-3 contrasts the primary clinical features of delirium, dementia, and depression.

Elderly Suicide

Suicide is a real and serious risk among older persons. The suicide rates increase with age and are highest among older widowed white men who live alone.[31] Intentional self-starvation or engaging in activities that oppose therapeutic need or threaten a medical problem (e.g., noncompliance with dietary restrictions, intentional medication misuse) may be suicidal gestures. Asking the individual about recent losses, lifestyle changes, new or worsening health problem, depression and changes in support system may indicate suicidal ideation. Often the individual may present with diffuse, nonspecific complaints that are not properly diagnosed or treated as depression. The suicidal older adult needs close observation, treatment of underlying depression, and a safe environment to prevent self-harm.

Treatment Strategies

Several strategies are used to help older clients who have dementia, delirium, or depression. Gerontological nurses commonly use four strategies: (1) reality orientation, (2) validation therapy, (3) remotivation therapy, and (4) reminiscence therapy. Treatment modalities and their specific application are described in gerontological nursing and psychiatric literature.[8]

Substance Use Disorders

Substance use disorders refer to ingestion of any compound in quantities that may be harmful to health or well being,[3] including overindulgence in legal drugs, alcohol, nicotine, caffeine, nonprescription over-the-counter drugs and preparations, prescription drugs, controlled drugs (e.g., meperidine or codeine), and illegal drugs (see Chapter 26).

As many as 31% of community-dwelling older adults and 18% to 49% of institutionalized older adults have serious problems related to alcohol use.[20] Alcohol abusers can be divided into two types: (1) long-term abusers and (2) recent-onset abusers.[20] Long-term drinkers show abusive alcohol use throughout their

TABLE 3-3	*Common Mental Health Disorders in Older Adults: Clinical Features*		
	Delirium	**Dementia**	**Depression**
Description	A reversible, acute confusional state	A gradually progressive, irreversible cognitive decline	A reversible affective feeling associated with sadness, which may vary from mild downheartedness or a feeling of indifference to a feeling of great despair beyond hope
Onset	Rapid, acute, often at night	Slow, gradual	Gradual or sudden
Duration	Days to weeks, but usually less than 1 month	Continuous, ongoing, months to years	Varies from weeks to years
Disorientation	Present, especially for time; tendency to mistake unfamiliar for familiar persons, places	May be absent in mild states of dementia	May seem disoriented to place or time
Thinking	Slow or accelerated; may be dream-like, impoverished	Impoverished; poor abstracting ability	Slowed thinking, indecisiveness
Memory	Short-term memory impaired; long-term memory intact	Short-term memory impaired; long-term memory may be affected	May seem impaired for recent and remote events
Attention	Consistently impaired; easily distracted; fluctuates	Typically intact	Complaints or evidence of diminished ability to concentrate
Alertness	Reduced or increased, but awareness always affected	Typically normal; may be reduced	Psychomotor agitation or retardation
Perception	Invariably affected, especially at night; often have hallucinations	May be intact; usually no hallucinations	May have auditory hallucinations
Sleep	Sleep-wake cycle altered	Usually normal for age	Insomnia or hypersomnia
Course	Typically fluctuates with lucid intervals and exacerbations	Relatively stable over course of a day	Usually rapid progression
Affect	Intermittent fear, perplexity, bewilderment	Flat or indifferent	Sad, worried, anxious, hopeless; may slow agitation or apathy
Cause	Multiple potential causes (e.g., surgery, infection, drugs)	Unknown, possible environmental, hereditary, chemical	Secondary to other mental illness; related to loss, physical illness, medications, loneliness

Data from American Psychiatric Association. (2000). *Diagnostic and statistical manual of mental disorders* (4th ed.). Washington, DC: Author.

lives; they are at risk for serious medical problems and generally have alienated their families and social support systems.

Recent-onset drinkers may be reacting to some event, such as loss of a loved one, or they may have general negative feelings, such as helplessness or depression stemming from role losses in later life.[20] The recent-onset alcohol abuser is more successful in substance abuse treatment than the long-term abuser. Learning new coping skills and increasing socialization often help the recent-onset drinker to overcome problems.

Non-alcohol substance disorders in older adults are divided into illicit drug abuse and prescription drug abuse. Cross-sectional data indicate a low prevalence of illicit drug use among older adults, but longitudinal data suggest that health care professionals can anticipate much larger numbers of drug users as the baby boomers age. Many of these baby boomers will bring their drug-using habits into old age with them. Studies indicate that cannabis (hashish) abuse may become a major problem.[20]

It is difficult to determine the extent of prescription drug abuse by older people. Researchers contend that thousands of older Americans are "hooked" on their prescription drugs in an "inadvertent addiction."[20] The cycle of addiction usually begins benignly with a medication or

BRIDGE TO HOME HEALTH CARE
Managing Multiple Medications

Clients who take several medications often need help to understand the best procedures and to follow instructions as closely as possible. Failure to take the right drug at the right time and in the proper way often results in relapses, rehospitalizations, or nursing home placement.

Review all prescription and nonprescription medications, and carefully explain the administration schedule to the client and family members. Tailoring the schedule to the client's lifestyle increases the likelihood that the instructions will be followed. For example, if the client goes to bed at 7:00 PM, be sure that the last dose is scheduled at that hour.

Some people need minimal help with organizing their drugs and dosages. They may benefit from any number of compliance aids that can be purchased at pharmacies, such as containers with separate compartments for each day of the week. The challenge is greater when the client has a complex medication program; reduced strength and dexterity; or a visual, hearing, cognitive, or other impairment in functional status. These clients may need to purchase an automated medication dispenser that emits visual cues, such as flashing strobe lights, or audible cues, such as beeps.

Although units vary, an automated dispenser must be simple to use. One such dispenser can be programmed easily to provide a reminder at the right time for up to four times a day for a week.

This dispenser helps the client manage complex schedules, is tamper proof, and dispenses only the pills needed from a supply cassette in a removable drawer. Other automated dispensers have light-emitting diode (LED) screens on which preprogrammed messages, such as "Take with food" or "Take 30 minutes before food," serve as additional reminders.

Determine how and when the client will obtain refills. If the client has no transportation, a pharmacy may have a delivery service or a family member can obtain them. A social service referral is needed if the client cannot pay for prescriptions.

Monitor the client for side effects. Many people stop taking essential medications because of unpleasant side effects. Sometimes the client can manage this problem effectively by changing the times of doses or by taking the medication with food.

Instruct the client on drug storage. Some drugs are sensitive to light; others must be secured to decrease the risk of overdoses. All medications must be safely kept away from any children who visit or live in the household.

Simplicity is the key to successful medication management. Regularly evaluate the client's regimen and household routines, and discuss any changes that would make things easier with the client, family members, and physician.

---

a drink for pain or anxiety. Physicians often are unaware of the problem, and they may also be unaware of the number of medications a client is taking because several different physicians may issue the prescriptions.

MEDICATION USE IN OLDER ADULTS

Appropriate drug use is one of the most important determinants of quality of life in the geriatric population. Medications are the most common therapeutic intervention for diseases in older adults and are increasingly common as a component of health promotion and disease prevention. Drugs have the capacity for great benefit as well as significant harm for older adults. Older adults consume nearly 30% of all prescription drugs and spend more than $15 billion annually on medication.[20,24] The average number of prescribed medications increases with age, with older adults filling an average of 7.5 to 17.9 prescriptions per year.[24] Older adults who live in long-term care facilities typically receive eight or more medications a day.[20] In addition to prescription drug use, 70% to 80% of older adults self-medicate with over-the-counter drugs without consulting a health care professional.[24]

See the Bridge to Home Health Care feature on Managing Multiple Medications, above.

The most commonly used drugs by the older population include cardiovascular agents, antihypertensives, analgesics, antiarthritic agents, sedatives, tranquilizers, laxatives, and antacids.[24] The most commonly used over-the-counter drugs include analgesics, antacids, cold remedies and decongestants, diuretics, laxatives, and sleep aids.[24] Older adults are increasingly using herbal remedies, which are often considered safe by consumers but can be an overlooked source of adverse effects and drug interactions. Drug use will continue to rise as the number of adults age 65 and older grows and new pharmacologic therapies for chronic conditions and disorders are brought to market. When used properly, drugs can be beneficial; when used inappropriately, they threaten one's functional abilities and health.

The effects of drugs can be beneficial or harmful. A confounding factor in the effectiveness of drug therapy is related to age-related body system changes (Table 3-4). Drug interactions increase with age and the number of drugs taken. Nearly one third of older adults report

TABLE 3-4	*Medication Effects in the Older Adults*

Pharmacokinetics refers to how the body handles the drug; this includes absorption, distribution, metabolism, and elimination of the drug. **Pharmacodynamics** or drug activity refers to the actual effects of the drug in the body; this includes additive, synergistic, antagonistic and potentiation effects.

Drug Dynamics	Impact on Older Person
Absorption: Movement of the drug into the circulation	Absorption is affected by age-related changes in stomach emptying, changes in gastric pH, gastrointestinal motility, and nutritional status (especially low serum albumin levels). Therefore, the medication stays in the stomach or intestine longer and takes longer for effect to be obtained.
Distribution: Movement of the drug throughout the body	The adequacy of the circulatory system and ability of the drug to enter the cell impact distribution. It is altered by reduced cardiac output, decrease in total body water, and increase of adipose tissue. These changes may result in higher than usual blood levels of water-soluble drugs and storage of lipid soluble drugs in fatty tissue, resulting in toxicity and less drug reaching the site of action due to storage.
Metabolism: Breakdown of the drug in the body, primarily the liver	Breakdown altered by size of liver and portal circulation; therefore, the drug stays in the body longer and may show prolonged responses.
Elimination: Removal of the drug from the body, primarily the renal system	Age-related changes in renal function, renal blood flow, glomerular filtration, and tubular secretion may affect duration and intensity of drug responses in the body.
Additive Effects: Two drugs with similar pharmacologic actions produces increased effect (e.g., 1 + 1 = 2), which can be positive or negative	Negative additive effects can occur with the use of a diuretic (e.g., furosemide) for a cardiovascular disorder and aminoglycoside antibiotic (e.g., tobramycin) for an infection, the result can be increased damage to hearing and balance (ototoxicity) and to the kidneys (nephrotoxicity).
Synergistic Effect: Two drugs whose combined effects are greater than the sum of each drug acting alone (e.g., 1 + 1 = 3)	Positive synergistic interaction occurs when hypertension is treated with a diuretic (e.g., hydrochlorothiazide) and a beta-adrenergic blocker (e.g., atenolol). This combination lowers blood pressure than either drug alone.
Antagonistic Effect: Effect of two drugs is less than the sum of the effects of the drugs acting separately, causes a diminished therapeutic effect (e.g., 2 + 2 = 3)	Reduced anticoagulation occurs when warfarin is given with phenytoin.
Potentiation Effect: One drug increases the effect of a second drug	Acetaminophen is given with codeine with the result being increased analgesia.

Data from Gutierrez, K. (1999). *Pharmacotherapeutics: Clinical decision-making in nursing.* Philadelphia: W.B. Saunders.

adverse reactions to medications, accounting for as many as 10% of their hospitalizations.[22]

Polypharmacy is described as the use of excessive or unnecessary medications that increase the risk of drug interactions and other adverse drug reactions. Ironically, drug reactions that mimic medical-physical complaints are often treated with another drug. Polypharmacy has many consequences, including adverse drug effects, adverse interactions with other drugs and food, duplication of therapy, decreased quality of life, and unnecessary financial and societal costs.[22,24] Polypharmacy is consid-

ered by *Healthy People 2010*[14] to be one of the principal drug safety problems in the United States.

CONTINUUM: HEALTH CARE AND LIVING ARRANGEMENTS

Aging adults have complex needs that often require care from multiple care settings, including hospitals, day treatment services, home care, hospice and long-term care (Chapters 7 to 12). The services provide acute care, diagnostic, preventive, therapeutic, rehabilitative, maintenance, and palliative care. Today's economy is promoting change in health care institutions that affect the continuum of health care. Many institutions, facilities, and services are merging into integrated systems. An *integrated* system provides a seamless delivery of services and encompasses the entire range of health, community-based, and in-home services. Advantages of an integrated system include a single point of access and entry, assessment and coordination of appropriate care services, and assured quality of care in a cost-effective, time-efficient system.

In the United States, approximately 32 million people over 65 years of age have a current or potential need for more assistance and support in their living environment.[8] These individuals frequently choose alternative living arrangements. The continuum of housing, or alternative living arrangements, offers choices to individuals that can maximize independence, safety, counteract dependency, and preserve health and QOL. As a person's physical and medical capabilities change, they often find they can no longer live in their home but want to remain independent as long as possible. The continuum of housing provides all levels of living arrangements so that older adults can move from one living arrangement level to another as needed without having to leave their community and friends and includes retirement homes/apartments, adult day care, assisted living and long-term nursing facilities (see Chapter 11).

Health Care for Older Adults

Provision of care to older adults has recently become more challenging and expensive because of advances in technology, legal interpretations of needed health care, more complex health care, and control of costs implemented by changed health care delivery systems (managed care).[10] Technology and medical advances in health care now allow people to live longer even when they have a variety of health care problems. These advances may sustain life even when an older person's quality of life becomes limited.

Older adults are the largest consumers of health care and have more interactions with health care providers than any other age group.[28] The largest third-party payer for older adult health care is the government (Medicare, Medicaid, state and local programs).[28]

Medicare (Title 18 of the Social Security Act) is a federal program available to those 65 years of age and older who have paid into social security, are disabled, or have end-stage renal disease. Special circumstances allow disabled and those with endstage renal disease to qualify for Medicare before the age of 65 years. Although most older adults receive Medicare benefits, Medicare does not provide comprehensive coverage of health care expenses. Medicare has two parts. Part A is available to all who qualify and provides hospital services and some home health and skilled nursing home services. Part B is optional and the individual must pay a monthly premium. It covers physician services, outpatient hospital care, occupational therapy, physical therapy, some home health, laboratory services, ambulance transportation, prosthesis and some equipment and supplies. Medicare does not cover prescriptions, nor does it cover most preventive care, including vision, hearing, or dental examinations. Currently legislators are looking at new programs or revisions to Medicare that would allow older adults coverage for needed prescription drugs.

Medicaid (Title 19 of the Social Security Act) is a federal and state program that provides medical services to the aged poor, the blind, the disabled, and families with dependent children. Because Medicaid is a federal-state program, criteria for acceptance vary from state to state. Medicaid covers costs of physicians, inpatient and outpatient hospital care, prescription drugs, and skilled nursing facilities. Medicaid provides coverage of nursing home care for a large percentage of older adults in nursing homes.[28]

Currently many older adults have problems accessing adequate health care. Some of the primary problems include transportation to health care providers for those who no longer drive, the cost of outpatient prescription drugs, health care providers who are unaware of specialized care older adults may need, and paying for health care not covered by Medicare. Multiple chronic problems often necessitate multiple providers of care and many prescription medications.

Many more older adults are in the health care system each year, and the cost of goods and services is constantly rising. It is projected that by the year 2040, Medicare and Medicaid will account for 45% of health care expenditures.[33] The astronomic costs of health care are fueling national debates on what services should be provided and how to reduce or control these costs. To reduce total costs may require extensive cuts in services to older adults. Government health insurance (Medicare) and health assistance (Medicaid) programs will change, and these changes will have ramifications for all Americans. Several agencies, including aging associations, societies, and institutes, have websites that can be found on the WebLinks icon on the website. *evolve*

Managed Care

Health care delivery is changing. Among the major shifts taking place is the rapid growth of managed care. *Managed care* is a system that provides structure and focus for overseeing the use, cost, quality, and effectiveness of health care services. The basic concept of managed care revolves around accountability and standardization of care for a given disorder or for a specific population. The development of DRGs (diagnostic related groups) and critical paths or care paths for nursing care of specific health problems seen in the hospital has increased standardization and accountability. These measures have decreased lengths of stay and care costs. The increasing number of frail older persons with chronic disorders has resulted in pressure to move Medicare into a managed care system. As this occurs, the thrust of managed care services will be to coordinate and integrate health services and resources to improve quality, to provide service flexibility, to contain cost, and to help the older person maintain function and independence as long as possible.

Acute Care

Most nurses who care for older adults provide care in an inpatient hospital setting. Clients 65 years of age and older account for almost half of all inpatient hospitalization days.[16] This setting can be for an emergency or acute illness, such as a stroke or hip fracture (see Chapters 8 and 9) or exacerbation of a chronic condition, such as diabetes mellitus or chronic obstructive lung disease (see Chapters 47 and 63).

Hospitals are developing new ways of delivering care to older adults to improve both quality and efficiency. Some hospitals are establishing geriatric units with specially trained staff who work together as a *multidisciplinary team*. The core team typically includes a geriatrician (physician with specialized training in caring for older adults), nurses, a pharmacist, a social worker, various rehabilitation therapists (e.g., speech, physical, and occupational), dietetics, and mental health professionals (e.g., psychologists or psychiatrists). These programs focus on helping older adults with complex problems to remain at their highest possible level of functioning. They can lead to improved assessment and diagnosis, more appropriate placements, fewer prescribed medications, and reduced health care costs.

Long-Term Care

Long-term care refers to care services that range from informal assistance provided by family and friends, to formal medical and supportive services provided in the home, to specialty facilities for rehabilitation, to care in a nursing facility (see Chapter 11). Long-term care services assist those with chronic disabilities and decreasing health status to maintain their physical, social, and psychological functioning. Traditionally, nursing home care has been synonymous with long-term care, but this is misleading. Many older persons with disabilities are as likely to receive long-term care at home as in a nursing home. Long-term care accounts for 25% of all health care expenditures for older persons.[8]

Home Health Care

Home health care is skilled care received in the home for persons who meet specific criteria. Home health care can provide a wide variety of services, such as skilled nursing care, rehabilitation services, mental health nursing, social services, nutritional counseling, provision of some medical supplies and equipment, and personal care as-

sistance (see Chapter 10). Medicare may cover some of these services for a limited time for clients who meet specific criteria.

Case Management

Older clients and their families often have difficulty negotiating the health care delivery system. The older client may require specialized care in a variety of settings over long periods. The nursing case manager understands the physical and psychosocial needs involved as well as the best community resources to meet those needs and can be a valuable asset to the client and the family. The case manager works closely with a variety of other health care providers in a multidisciplinary manner to obtain services and resources for the older client, in the best setting, with the highest quality of care, and at an affordable cost. The case manager may work with adult children who have primary caregiver responsibilities but live in another area. Nursing case management provides comprehensive, individualized, and economic care for older clients with complex chronic health needs. The goal is to meet the needs of the client and support the caregiver while coordinating access to cost-effective services.

ETHICAL ISSUES THAT AFFECT OLDER ADULTS

Whatever the setting, daily challenges occur for the older client that require an advocate. An advocate represents the interests of others by acting in their behalf, educating them and their family, or influencing policies that affect them.[8] Issues of autonomy, competency, and self-determination arise frequently when working with older adults. It is important to know and understand the issues to serve as a client advocate and to ensure that both the client and family are informed.

Autonomy

Autonomy is the personal freedom and independence to direct one's own life and make choices for and about oneself. Autonomous people are capable of rational thought and problem solving. They can identify problems, understand the situation, search for alternatives, and select solutions that allow continued personal freedom.

Loss of autonomy, and therefore independence, is a real fear among older adults. No autonomous adult wishes to give up the right to decide when to get up, when to go to bed, what to eat, or what interests and activities to pursue. In many institutional settings, autonomy becomes restricted when schedules must be met and the older person moves slowly; when decreases in hearing and processing slow decision making; and when the person's decision does not coincide with the family's or health care provider's ideas.

A nurse has the responsibility to encourage the older person's autonomy in any way possible. This can be done by supervision and education of staff to listen and allow the person time to make choices and discussions with family members about what is occurring and how they can enhance the older person's autonomy.

Competence or Capacity

The term *competence* is a legal term used in regard to a client's actions. Health care professionals use the term *capacity* to describe a person's ability to make decisions, to make rational choices, to understand the consequences of their choices, to fulfill one's role adequately, and to handle one's affairs.[23] Capacity is a basic assumption on which the actions of autonomy are based. Increasingly, nurses encounter clients who are confused or mentally impaired. Do these individuals have the capacity to give consent for tests and procedures? Can they decide whether to proceed with, stop, or refuse treatment? Can they make end-of-life decisions?

Competence usually describes a status—the ability to make all or no decisions for oneself. Competence is a legal determination made by a judge. Adults are presumed to be legally competent unless there is evidence of an inability to care for oneself or to manage affairs or both. The court generally appoints a guardian for the individual judged to be incompetent.

Capacity is not absolute; it recognizes that a person may be able to make some decisions and not others, may have decisional capacity only at certain times, or or and that some decisions require a higher level of capacity than others. Health care professionals must be sensitive to the fact that some residents are lucid during certain hours of the day and disoriented or confused at other times, requiring consideration of appropriate timing for the discussion of treatment options and matters that require a decision.

Self-Determination

The Patient Self-Determination Act (PSDA) legislation was passed in 1990. This act required every health care institution that received federal funds to inform individuals receiving services of their right to plan for their future care through the use of advance directives. Advance directives encourage individuals to be active partners in guiding their medical treatment and to claim their rights in treatment decisions. Self-determination, capacity, and autonomy are closely related in decision making associated with future treatment and end-of-life decisions.

Advance Directives

Advance directive is an umbrella term for any document used to protect the individual's wishes for and interests in decisions about life-sustaining measures.[13] If available, advance directives can minimize potential conflict within a family once the person loses decision-making capacity and alleviate the burden of guilt that family members may feel about decisions to withdraw or withhold treatment. These documents include the *living will* and the *durable power of attorney for health care.*

Living Will

A *living will* affirms a person's right and desire to refuse a life-prolonging intervention and becomes effective when the person is determined to be terminally ill or near death. A living will, sometimes called a *treatment directive,* is typically a series of instructions regarding the withholding, withdrawing, or implementing of life-sustaining medical care in the event of terminal illness. It is limited to the instructions in the document and only applicable for terminal illness or when death is imminent.[13] Relatives who disagree with the stated terms have been known to override the individual's wishes and not honor the living will.

Durable Power of Attorney for Health Care

Durable power of attorney for health care is a private legal relationship created in which one person grants another person (called the *proxy*) the authority to make decisions regarding health care for the person if he or she is mentally unable to make decisions as the result of an accident, illness, or mental incapacity.[13] This document is not limited to life-sustaining measures but can apply to nursing facility placement, surgery, or other forms of non-emergency treatment. The proxy can guide the overall course of the individual's treatment by consenting to treatment as well as by refusing care. The proxy can clarify a living will or make decisions independently according to the client's values in situations that a living will might not address. Use of a proxy is a recommended procedure for clients with dementia and other disorders in which capacity is anticipated to decline. Older people generally name a spouse or an adult child as proxy. The proxy designee must be able to seek and understand medical information, communicate with health care professionals, and advocate effectively on behalf of the older adult. The proxy must be faithful to the older adult's wishes and well-being and must be willing to assume the burden of difficult decisions to honor the client's wishes.

An advance directive, although a legal document, can be disregarded or overridden. Situations in which advance directives have been disregarded include (1) family opposition, (2) caregiver's disregard for or lack of knowledge about an advance directive, and (3) state laws that mandate responding emergency medical technicians (EMTs) and paramedics to resuscitate before transporting to a hospital. To guard against these occurrences, nurses should encourage families to discuss end-of-life decisions before their occurrence, especially if the condition is one of terminal illness. Nurses should be knowledgeable of and share with the family the state laws directing emergency medical services (EMS), and if there are forms declining EMS resuscitation with transport.

To educate the public about advance directives, nurses must know the different types and encourage families to discuss and be knowledgeable of their loved one's wishes. Once an advance directive is available and placed on the client's chart, all caregivers should be made aware of its existence and every effort should be made to honor the individual's wishes (see Chapter 23).

CONCLUSIONS

Opportunities to care for older adults exist in all settings. The number of older adults requiring health care is considerable. For too long, nurses working with older adults have been preoccupied with loss, disability, chronic disease, long-term care, and medication use. As nurses, we need to look at the positive aspects of aging, the factors that allow older people to continue to function well despite the changes of aging. We need to teach older adults about things that are modifiable. It is never too late to change behaviors and to improve health status and quality of life.

Many of the hospitalized clients we work with will be discharged to their homes with continued care needs. The role of the nurse in acute care and community settings—to act as an advocate and to promote the physical and mental well-being of older people—will be extremely important.

Given that older adults are the fastest growing segment of the population in the United States, every nurse involved with adult health care undoubtedly will at some point be challenged to meet the unique needs of these clients. A holistic perspective is necessary to meet the physiologic, psychological, sociologic, and spiritual needs of older adult client.

BIBLIOGRAPHY

1. Administration on Aging. (2001). A profile of older Americans: 2001. Available: http://www.aoa.gov/aoa/STATS/profile/2001/highlights.html.
2. American Nurses' Association. (1995). *Scope and standards of gerontological nursing practice.* Washington, DC: Author.
3. American Psychiatric Association. (1994). *Diagnostic and statistical manual of mental disorders* (4th ed.). Washington, DC: Author.
4. Armer, J. (1996). An exploration of factors influencing adjustment among relocating rural elders. *Image, 28*(1), 35-38.
5. Besdine, R.W. (1983). The educational utility of comprehensive functional assessment in the elderly. *Journal of the American Geriatrics Society, 31,* 651-656.
6. Castle, N.G., (2001). Relocation of the elderly. *Medical Care Research and Review, 59* (3), 291-333.
7. Dubos, R. (1959). Mirage of health: Utopias, progress and biological change. Garden City, NJ: Doubleday.
8. Ebersole, P., & Hess, P. (Eds.). (1998). *Toward healthy aging* (5th ed., pp. 1-29). St. Louis: Mosby.
9. Eden, B., & Foreman, M.D. (1996). Problems associated with under recognition of delirium in critical care: A case study. *Heart Lung,* 25 (5), 388-400.
10. Eliopoulos, C. (2001). *Gerontological nursing* (5th ed). Philadelphia: Lippincott–Williams & Wilkins.
11. Folstein, M.F., Folstein, S., & McHugh, P.R. (1975). Mini mental state: A practical method for grading the cognitive states of patients for the clinician. *Journal of Psychiatric Research, 12,* 189-198.
12. Girardi, M., et al. (2001). Predicting fall risk in an elderly population: A computer dynamic posturography versus electronystagmongraphy test results. Incidence, onset, and associated factors. *Laryngoscope 111*(9), 1528-1532.
13. Gunter-Hunt, G., Mahoney, J.E., & Sieger, C.E. (2002). A comparison of state advance directive documents. *The Gerontologist 42*(1), 51-60.
14. Healthy People 2010. Leading health indicators. Available: http://www.healthypeople.gov/LHI/lhiwhat.htm.
15. Katz, S., et al. (1963). Studies of illness in the aged. The index of ADL: A standardized measure of biological and psychosocial functions. *Journal of the American Medical Association, 185,* 915-919.
16. Kennedy-Malone, L., Fletcher, K.R., Plank, L.M. (2000). *Management guidelines for gerontological nurse practitioners.* Philadelphia: F.A. Davis.
17. Lawton, M.P., and Brody, E.M. (1969). Assessment of older people: self-maintaining and instrumental activities of daily living. *The Gerontologist, 9*(3), 179-186.
18. Mahoney, F.I., & Barthel, D.W. (1965). Functional evaluation: The Barthel index. *Maryland State Medical Journal, 14,* 61-65.
19. McKenna, W.A. (1995). Transcultural perspectives in nursing care of the elderly. In M.M. Andrews & J.S. Bole (Eds.), *Transculture concepts in nursing care* (pp. 203-234). Philadelphia: Lippincott-Raven.
20. Menninger, J.A. (2002). Assessment and treatment of alcoholism and substance-related disorders in the elderly. *Bulletin of the Menninger Clinic 66*(2), 166-183.
21. Mezey, M. (1996). Challenges in providing care for persons with complex chronic illness. In R.H. Binstock, L.E. Cluff, & O. Von Merix (Eds), *The Future of Long-Term Care* (119-142). Baltimore, MD: John Hopkins University Press.
22. Michocki, R.J. (2001). Polypharmacy and principles of drug therapy. In A.M. Adelman and M.P. Daly, *20 Common problems in geriatrics* (pp 69-81). New York: McGraw-Hill.
23. Miller, C.A. (1995). *Nursing care of older adults: Theory and practice* (2nd ed.). Philadelphia: Lippincott-Raven.
24. Pepper, G.A. (1999). Drug use and misuse. In J.T. Stone, J.F. Wyman, & S.A. Salisbury (Eds.), *Clinical gerontology nursing: A guide to advanced practice* (2nd ed.). Philadelphia: W.B. Saunders.
25. Program Resource Development, American Association of Retired Persons. (1998). *A profile of older Americans (1997)* [brochure]. Washington, DC: Author.
26. Ramsdell, J., et al. (1990). Evaluation of cognitive impairment in the elderly. *Journal of General Internal Medicine, 5,* 55-64.
27. Rapp, C.G., (2001). Acute confusion/delirium protocol. *Journal of Gerontological Nursing, 27*(4), 21-23.
28. Rowland, D., & Garfield, R. (2002). Health care for the poor: Medicaid at 35. *Health Care Financing Review 22*(1), 23-35.
29. Sheikh, J. J., and Yesavage, J.A. (1986). Geriatric depression scale (GDS): Recent evidence and development of a shorter version. *Clinical Gerontologist, 5*(1/2), 165-173.
30. Stone, J. K., Wyman, J. F., & Salisbury, S. A. (1999). *Clinical gerontological nursing: A guide to advanced practice* (2nd ed.). Philadelphia: W. B. Saunders.

31. Szanto, K., et al. (2002). Identification of suicidal ideation and prevention of suicidal behavior in the elderly. *Drugs & Aging* *19*(1), 11-24.

32. Tideiksaar, R. (1997). *Falling in old age* (2nd ed.). New York: Springer.

33. U.S. Senate Special Committee on Aging. (1989). *Developments in aging: 1988* (Committee Publication No. 101-4). Washington, DC: U.S. Government Printing Office.

34. Wieland, D. (2000). Abuse of older persons: An overview. *Holistic Nursing Practice, 14*(4), 40-50.

Health Assessment

Annabelle M. Keene

evolve

Web Enhancements

Assessment of the client provides baseline data for the nursing process. Assessment enhances identification of physical and psychosocial needs. The nurse's knowledge and expertise affect the level of assessment. Some assessment skills are basic, such as taking a temperature. Advanced assessment skills are learned and practiced in order to provide interventions and to evaluate health maintenance and promotion practices.

Become familiar with the parameters of human behavior and physiology in order to recognize abnormal situations. Normal ranges for psychosocial behavior may vary, whereas many physiologic manifestations have narrowly defined limits. For example, cell death occurs if body temperature is either too high or too low; the defined parameters are a matter of a few degrees. In contrast, depression in survivors following the death of a loved one is expected, but prolonged depression may signal mental illness. Skillful assessment requires careful observation and the ability to decide whether an observation is normal. Consider unique circumstances when comparing assessment findings to standardized norms.

Evaluate the client's reaction to the assessment process as well as the possible implications of the findings. Nursing diagnoses associated with health assessment include Anxiety, Fear, Deficient Knowledge, Powerlessness, and Situational Low Self-Esteem. Include in each nursing diagnosis the specific cause leading to the problem. For example, a woman having a breast examination may be anxious because she never has had such an examination before or she may fear that a lump will be found.

Assessment requires skill and judgment. This chapter provides information for developing expertise in health assessment. Proficiency requires extensive practice. Seek guidance from a skilled, competent practitioner. A broad knowledge base, repeated practice, and access to a mentor foster the ability to discriminate among findings.

Health assessment focuses on the client and has several parts. The health history contains subjective information, whereas the physical examination is objective information. Diagnostic tests provide objective data about a client's health status. Each client is unique with complex physical and psychosocial interactions. Conduct health assessment free from bias, prejudice, and

evolve *Be sure to check out the bonus material on the Evolve website and the CD-ROM, including free self-assessment exercises.*
http://evolve.elsevier.com/Black/medsurg/

stereotyping. For example, an older client with several chronic health problems may not have immediate health care needs, yet the potential for complex health problems exists. Conversely, a young adult may appear "healthy" when, in fact, overwhelming psychosocial problems or needs affect both current and future health status. An individualized approach to health assessment provides a valid database for nursing care.

HEALTH HISTORY

Health assessment begins with the health history interview. The purpose of the interview is to collect the client's subjective data. Observe the client throughout the interaction. Your observations will become part of the objective data of the physical examination that follows.

THE HEALTH HISTORY INTERVIEW

Accuracy

Assess the accuracy and completeness of the data throughout the health history interview. Validation allows formulation of accurate nursing diagnoses. Determine whether the client is a reliable historian, able and willing to provide information. The client may be (1) unconscious or disoriented and unable to cooperate; (2) willing to cooperate but hindered by circumstances, such as a language barrier or anxiety; or (3) unwilling and mistrustful about cooperating because of anger or depression.

If the client cannot provide information, seek secondary sources, such as significant others or an interpreter. Information content and accuracy may be influenced by the perceptions and biases of the secondary sources as well as by their knowledge of the problem and recall ability.

Stereotyping jeopardizes collection of accurate data. False assumptions and generalizations may alienate the client and interfere with development of trust. A mistrustful client is reluctant to divulge sensitive information, perhaps fearing rejection or ridicule, resulting in inaccurate or missed nursing diagnoses.

Similarities among people result in their being grouped according to age, gender, ethnic background, common occupation, recreational activity, health risk behavior, or type of health problem. Each person is also unique. Reliable research findings concerning group characteristics or similarities may be applied to a specific client who belongs to that group. For example, the incidence of hypertension is higher in blacks than in whites, and regular blood pressure screening should be included at every health care visit. Generalizations, particularly those grounded in assumptions or prejudice or based on limited experience, are potentially harmful.

Physical appearance or presenting manifestations may bias one's perception of a client. Similar manifestations may have different origins. For example, a client with an uneven, lurching gait and garbled speech may appear to be intoxicated or under influence of a controlled substance. In fact, the client might have residual neurologic deficits from a head injury. Initial inaccurate judgment may be costly in wasted time and effort and may result in a strained nurse-client relationship. Box 4-1 includes guidelines that may reduce stereotyping during health assessment.

Computerized health history assessment is available in clinical settings, particularly ambulatory care settings. Computer programs for history taking result in accurate, legible databases when data are entered correctly. Either the client or the nurse, using interactive programs, records the data directly. Data also may be entered from a client-completed questionnaire, which is reviewed and validated by a nurse skilled in health assessment. Computerized health histories tend to be complete because pertinent assessment areas are included in the programs. Branching programs direct collection of additional data when the client responds with significant information.

Depth

Many factors influence the level of assessment. Ideally, data are collected at one time and in sufficient depth to allow problem identification; however, this may not always be practical. The interview setting may be less than ideal (the scene of a motor vehicle accident). The client's reason for seeking health care may preclude in-depth interviewing (a ruptured appendix). The client's attention span, energy, and comfort level may affect ability to participate (acute pain).

In an acute situation:
1. Collect data pertinent to the immediate problem and assess the client's present health status.
2. Tailor the health history interview to include pertinent data while striving to be thorough.
3. Update and enlarge the database as indicated by the client's condition.

In clinical practice, many agencies provide specific health history formats. These formats are designed to meet agency purposes and may vary considerably in depth and level. Tailor the health history interview to the needs of the client and the agency. For example, you might arrange to meet several brief times with clients who have limited abilities or special needs (impaired

BOX 4-1	*Reducing Stereotyping During the Health Assessment*

- Do not manipulate a client's information to make it fit a cultural image.
- Do not assume that all of a client's manifestations stem from the identified medical diagnosis.
- Do not categorize a client by appearance or behavior.
- Do not ignore any aspect of the client's presentation.

hearing or limited intellectual capacity), or an interpreter may be required when a language barrier exists.

Long Format

The health history model presented in this chapter is an *exhaustive,* or long format (see the website for an example). This holistic approach, although time-consuming, elicits a wealth of data and allows thorough assessment of how the client functions within multiple aspects. The exhaustive approach may be impractical in an acute care setting, especially in one sitting. However, to make accurate nursing diagnoses and to identify etiology, you must know each component of the history and should learn how to collect a complete database, over time if necessary. Students often learn history-taking skills in a laboratory setting using the exhaustive model. They must also learn to modify the technique to an actual setting and to a client's ability.

Short Format

An *episodic* health history assessment often suffices when a client presents with an uncomplicated, short-term health problem, such as an earache. Use a systematic approach to collect data significant to the problem (Box 4-2). Proficiency in all areas of health history assessment, which are discussed in this chapter, is necessary to conduct an accurate episodic assessment.

GUIDELINES FOR THE HEALTH HISTORY INTERVIEW

External (environmental and interpersonal) and internal (intrapersonal and physiologic) factors affect the health history interview. Data quality and quantity are enhanced by sensitivity to the client and by one's skill level with the interview process.

Preparation of the Environment

The following guidelines apply:
1. When possible, conduct the interview in a comfortable setting. Using a quiet room with a closed door decreases interruptions. If the client cannot leave a setting (a multibed room or an emergency department cubicle), screen the area by drawing the privacy drapes.
2. Reduce or eliminate distractions (turn off the television) and inform colleagues to avoid interruptions.
3. Use facing comfortable chairs to help establish rapport. Adjust the distance between chairs to the client's preference and sense of personal space.
4. Ensure a moderate room temperature to promote comfort.
5. Provide indirect lighting to prevent glare and strong shadows that may distort observation of nonverbal cues.

Preparation of the Client

The following guidelines apply:
1. After introductions, explain the nature and purpose of the health history interview.
2. Speak in a moderate tone of voice, calmly and patiently.
3. Ask nonprobing, client-centered questions, which help put the client at ease. As the interview progresses, focused questions and therapeutic communication techniques help identify problem areas.
4. Alternate between open-ended and closed questions, depending on the data being elicited.
5. Throughout the interview, observe nonverbal communication for signs of discomfort with topics under discussion. These areas may need gentle, further exploration (with client permission), either during the interview or at a later time.
6. Respect the client's wish to decline discussing a topic.
7. Be aware of your interview style and skills. Nonverbal behavior can either facilitate or inhibit client responses and affect the quality of the historical data.

Preparation of the Interviewer

The following guidelines apply:
1. Reduce repetitious questioning and proceed in a structured yet flexible manner. Until you are comfortable with the format, use a pocket-sized outline of the health history as an aid.
2. Take *brief* notes and inform the client in advance that you will be taking notes so as not to disrupt the flow of the interview. Avoid extensive note taking, because it suggests that you are not listening attentively.
3. Compile the written history after the interview. The data may be recorded on a laptop computer during the interview.
4. Terminate the interview by summarizing highlights and allowing the client to add or clarify information.
5. Inform the client about how the physical examination will proceed.

BOX 4-2	*An Episodic Health History Format*

Include these elements in an episodic (short) health history:
- Client's statement of the problem (chief complaint)
- Symptom analysis
- Review the body system to which the symptom belongs
- Explore the symptom's relationship to other body systems (include a review of associated body systems)
- Investigate the current problem's relationship to the client's past health and health maintenance and promotion practices

COMPONENTS OF THE HEALTH HISTORY

The health history includes subjective data regarding the following:

- Biographical and demographic information
- Health history including review of systems (ROS)
- Family health history
- Psychosocial assessment
- Appraisal of the client's health maintenance and health promotion behaviors to assess health risks

Health history assessment may be organized according to a nursing theory (Orem's theory of self-care) or by health behavior patterns (Gordon's functional health patterns). A *format* is a tool for collecting comprehensive data. In this chapter, the health history format is an *evolve* extended health database model (see the website). Another type of health history format integrates the assessment of functional health patterns.

If data are available in other forms, compile them, thereby enhancing and expediting the interview. A single complete database is preferable for reference and retrieval of information.

Biographical and Demographic Information

The extent and type of biographical and demographic information may vary, depending on agency protocol. Include the date of the interview because the information gathered constitutes the baseline assessment. If the client's health status changes, the health history and physical examination reflect the extent of the change over time.

Biographical and demographic data provide clues about personal health risk. For example, some health risk may be ascribed to age, gender, family history, and location of residence. Various health screening procedures or recommendations are made based on age, gender, or other background data. Examples of recommended procedures include periodic pelvic examinations and monthly breast self-examinations for women, periodic prostate examinations and monthly testicular self-examinations for men, and regular screening of visual acuity and testing for glaucoma as a person ages.

Current Health

Current health status describes the reason for the health care visit.

Chief Complaint

Begin with the client's subjective statement of the reason for seeking health care (the *chief complaint*). The response may indicate concerns or anxiety on the part of the client or significant others and reveals the client's perception of the health problem. The client may talk about what the problem means and how he or she is coping. Al-lowing the client to elaborate can assist in avoiding generalizations. When the client reports a past or current health problem, proceed with a *symptom analysis*.

Symptom Analysis

Symptom analysis is a detailed description of the health problem. In this book, the term *manifestations* is used synonymously with *symptoms*. In addition to assessing the following characteristics, ask the client to provide an opinion about the cause of the manifestation or problem. Clients often have insight as to the nature and the cause of their problems and sometimes express fears and concerns while discussing them. Explore fears and concerns to identify and treat client responses to health problems.

Timing. Timing includes onset, duration, and frequency. *Onset* refers to when a manifestation was first noticed (hours, days, months ago). *Duration* is how long the manifestation lasts (minutes, hours, days, weeks). The manifestation may occur continuously, intermittently, regularly, or irregularly. *Frequency* is how often a manifestation occurs (daily, weekly, monthly).

Quality. Ask the client to discriminate manifestation quality with adjectives such as sharp, stabbing, dull, aching, cramping, cold, searing, burning, numb, tingling, loose, solid, soft, hard, tight, or crushing.

Quantity. Assist the client in describing the size, amount, number, or extent of manifestations as well as the severity or intensity. Quantify pain severity by asking the client to rate it on a scale (1 to 10). Assess the manifestation's effect by asking how usual daily activities have been affected, for example, "Describe how the pain has interfered with what you usually do. Does it keep you awake at night? Has it affected your appetite?"

Location. Ask where a manifestation, such as pain, is located on the body and whether it moves or is stationary, for example, "Does the pain stay in one place, or does it move around?" Asking the client to point helps define the location.

Precipitating Factors. Ask what the client was doing at the time the manifestation was first noticed. Does the client know what may have led to the manifestation's occurrence?

Aggravating and Relieving Factors. Ask the client to recall whether any factors alleviate the manifestation or make it worse, for example, "Is there anything that makes the manifestation go away or become less uncomfortable?" "Is there anything that makes the manifestation become worse?"

Associated Manifestations. Inquire whether the client has noticed anything in conjunction with the manifestation. For example, "Does the manifestation ever occur at other times or only when _____?"

When a manifestation is reported, assess all associated physiologic areas; for example, for epigastric pain, review gastrointestinal (GI), endocrine, and psychological systems. The epigastric pain may be related to problems in any of these body systems. If the reported manifestation is urinary incontinence, include the following:

1. Timing (when did the urine leakage start?)
2. Quality (are incontinent episodes accompanied by dysuria?)
3. Quantity (amount of urine leakage per occurrence, effect of episodes on daily activities)
4. Precipitating factors (obesity, pregnancy, vaginal delivery)
5. Aggravating factors (coughing, sneezing, straining, lifting, caffeine intake)
6. Relieving factors (frequent toileting, medication, pelvic muscle toning exercises)
7. Associated manifestations (urgency, urinary retention, constipation)

Location does not apply in this example.

The review of body systems (described later in this chapter) should include the urinary (renal), reproductive, and GI systems as well as a careful diet history.

Past Health History

The past health history may be important for determining both current and future health risk status. For example, the client who has not had chickenpox may be at risk when a community outbreak occurs or when exposed to herpes zoster (shingles). Further assess risk status and provide information about the varicella vaccination. Throughout this part of the health history interview, note areas to explore, such as use of alternative or complementary therapies (see Chapter 5).

Past health history data include information about the client's growth and development, immunization status, past illnesses (usual childhood diseases as well as those occurring in adulthood), presence of serious or chronic illnesses, hospitalizations, surgeries, serious injuries or accidents, obstetric history (if applicable), last visits to health care providers, allergies, and medications.

Family Health History

The family health history helps to identify family-linked (familial) diseases that affect health status and risk for potential health problems. The nurse should do the following:

1. Inquire about relationships of family members, their ages (if living), the age at which they died, the cause of death (if known), and the presence of significant illness or health problems.

2. Diagram the data as a visual display to track health risk status (Figure 4-1).
3. Include a statement summarizing health problems in the family.

Health problems of interest include heart disease, hypertension (high blood pressure), stroke, epilepsy (seizures), migraines or headaches, mental illness, Alzheimer's disease, Huntington's chorea, alcoholism, tuberculosis, asthma, allergies, diabetes mellitus, thyroid problems, eating disorders, obesity, kidney disease, arthritis, cancer (type), sickle cell anemia, anemia, hemophilia, human immunodeficiency virus infection, and developmental delay.

Psychosocial History

Psychosocial assessment is an important part of the health history. A complete psychosocial assessment, although lengthy, is essential to a client-centered approach. Integrate psychosocial assessment throughout the history interview. In-depth assessment is done after the physical health history, once you have established rapport. Psychosocial assessment also may be done earlier, after the family health history.

Psychological status affects many areas of human development and behavior, such as intellectual development and capability, motivation, perception and insight, decision-making, speech and communication, motor ability, sleep and rest patterns, and nutrition and elimination patterns. It is impossible to separate a human into discrete components. Different dimensions (psychological, sociologic, physiologic) interact and affect each person's behavior and responses to the environment. Interrelationships among the dimensions are neither static nor predictable. Physiologic responses to health problems are more predictable and objectively observed, whereas two people who are faced with identical problems may not react the same way emotionally. For this reason, psychosocial assessment may be less reliable than objective assessment of physical findings. However, one may be able to develop skill and expertise in psychosocial assessment by collecting both subjective and objective data.

Psychosocial assessment assists the nurse in understanding a client's response to circumstances and events, which, in turn, influence the client's ability to function. This understanding enables comprehensive care based on accurate nursing diagnoses. Approximately two thirds of the disorders that nurses independently identify and treat are psychosocial. Accurate assessment of responses to health problems enables the client to return to optimal levels of both physiologic and psychological functioning.

Performing the psychosocial assessment requires sensitivity and interpersonal skills. Ability to establish a therapeutic relationship directly affects the quality of the

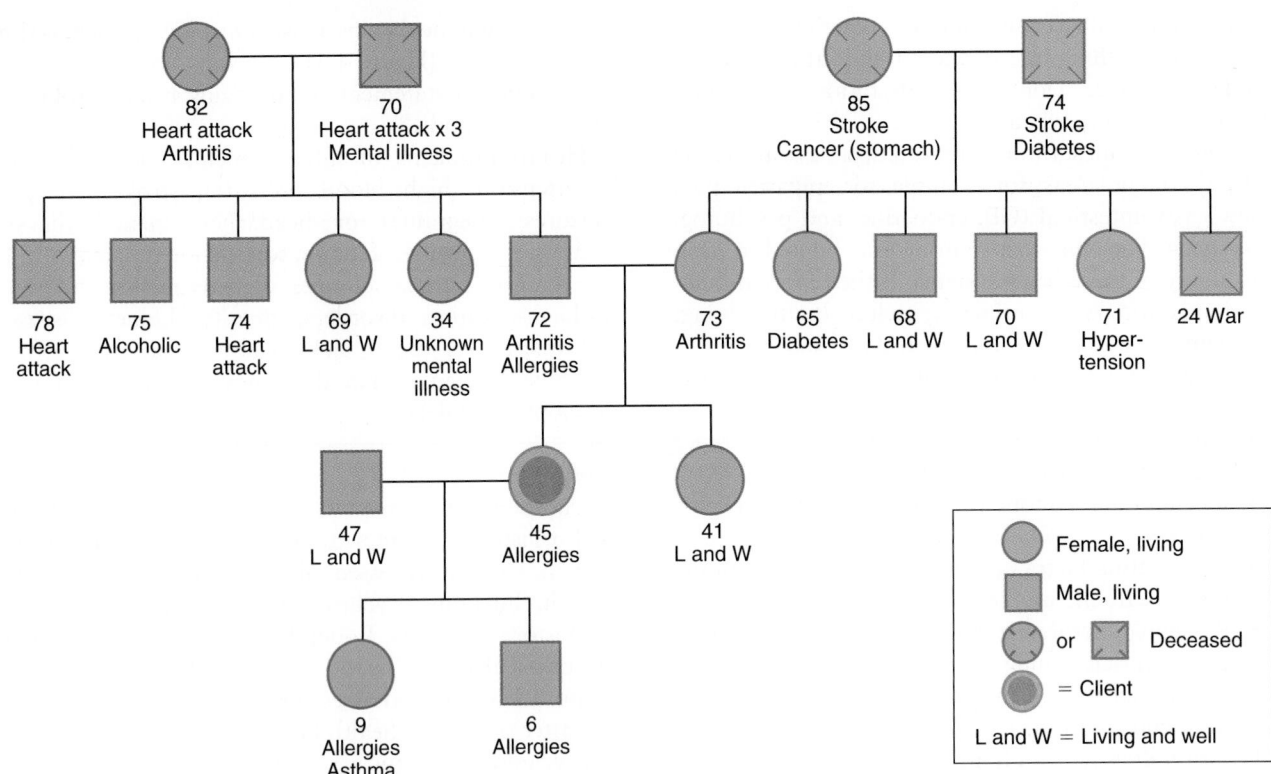

FIGURE 4-1 Family history diagram. A diagram such as this one assists in determining a client's risk for various disorders. In this case, the diagram indicates a woman with an increased inherited risk of cardiovascular disease (heart attack and stroke) and arthritis.

data. Because many topics are highly personal, it is imperative to be tactful and nonjudgmental and to handle confidential information professionally. An atmosphere of trust encourages the client to divulge sensitive information. Convey interest by listening attentively, making eye contact, and using skillful interview techniques. Your personal value system may influence or bias perception of a client's behavior and experiences. Self-awareness helps one to remain nonjudgmental. Free from bias, a trusting relationship promotes sharing of relevant information. Making accurate observations and sharing them allow the client opportunity to validate the nurse's perceptions and inferences.

Nature of Psychosocial Assessment

Psychosocial assessment encompasses gathering information about *psychological patterns* (nonphysical components, such as thoughts, feelings, motivations, mental status, personal strengths, and weaknesses) and *social experiences* (parts of life that are affected by or dependent on others). The term *psychosocial* denotes the melding of the two dimensions; it is impossible to separate the effects of psychological factors from those of social factors. Similarly, the psychosocial dimension intertwines with the physiologic dimension. All dimensions interact to produce a unique individual.

Psychosocial Risk Factors

During the health history interview, assess factors indicating risk for or an actual psychosocial problem. Box 4-3 lists guidelines for identifying psychosocial risk factors. If risk factors are present, proceed with a detailed assessment. An interview guide for in-depth assessment of selected areas of psychosocial status appears on the website. The guide includes questions that may be asked *evolve* during a cultural assessment.

Psychological Assessment

The psychological dimension includes perceptions about mood, thoughts, feelings, motivations, stressors, personal strengths and weaknesses, values and beliefs, and spirituality. Responses and interpretations are reflected in thought processes and in what is said and done. Observe the client's appearance and behavior throughout the interview. Observations, when validated, assist in understanding psychological status. Record subjective data in the health history and objective data in the physical examination report.

General Appearance. Appearance and behavior reflect the client's mental status and comfort level with the interview. Observe the client's posture, nonverbal behav-

---

BOX 4-3 *Identifying Psychosocial Risk Factors*

Social History
Social history includes information about the client's family members, social network, and lifestyle. Ask if others are available to provide emotional support to the client during stressful times. This support system may include pets.

Personal and Family History
A personal or family history of psychosocial problems increases a client's risk of having problems. A client may fear recurrence of an emotional or mental health problem or worry that he or she has inherited a family-linked illness, such as schizophrenia.

Level of Stress
Change and loss are two major influences that produce stress in individuals. Clients who have experienced stressful events within the past year are at risk for development of health problems. Assess the client's present stress level compared to the response to previous stressful events.

Usual Coping Pattern
The usual coping pattern refers to how the client copes with a serious problem or manages high levels of stress. Ask the client to describe a particularly stressful situation and how it was managed. Assess whether the client's usual coping style is adequate and appropriate for the current situation. Other coping strategies may be necessary. Psychosocial reactions to health problems are highly individual and usually occur as the client and significant others cope with the effects of illness.

Changes in Neurophysiologic Function
Neurophysiologic changes include physical manifestations of psychological stress. The stress response, regardless of its cause, results in altered levels of neurotransmitters, such as norepinephrine and serotonin, which then affect the sympathetic and parasympathetic nervous systems. The client's usual body functions, such as sleep and rest patterns, appetite, energy level, sexual function, and elimination patterns, can be affected.

Level of Understanding About Health Problem
Explore the client's level of understanding. The client may not comprehend what has happened or could happen as a result of a health problem. The client may have unrealistic expectations of the health care team. Determine how threatening a particular health problem is and whether the client has been able to prepare psychologically for its effects.

Mental Status
Mental status refers to the client's current emotional, intellectual, and perceptual functioning. If a dysfunction is evident, describe the problem.

Personality Style
Personality style is the way a client usually interacts with others. Examples include dependent, independent, controlled, relaxed, dramatic, suspicious, accepting, self-sacrificing, superior, inferior, uninvolved, involved, mixed (a combination of two predominant styles), or no predominant style.

Major Psychosocial Reactions
Reactions include disruption in the ability to trust, maintain self-esteem, retain feelings of control, cope with loss and guilt, and maintain intimacy.

---

ior, facial expression, manner of dress with regard to the climate and occasion, grooming and hygiene, and attitude toward the assessment interview (cooperative, hostile, withdrawn). For example, "The client is dressed neatly, sits back in the chair, and answers questions without hesitation."

Motor Activity. Note motor ability, gait, coordination, reaction time, and unusual body movements (gestures, tics, tremors, foot tapping, hand wringing, grimacing, or other repetitive movements). For example, "The client drummed his fingers on the table before answering."

Behavior. Activities observed by others constitute behavior. *Verbal* behavior is what is said and includes voice tone; *nonverbal* behavior concerns observable behavior, such as posture, movement, and facial expression. Observe and record both verbal and nonverbal behaviors.

Behavior is central to psychological assessment. Accurate assessment dictates that observed behavior be de-scribed rather than interpreted. "The client is crying" is an observed behavior, whereas "The client is depressed" is a judgmental statement. Without further assessment, the nurse does not know why the client is crying. If the client states, "I feel depressed," record "States she feels depressed."

Mental Status. Mental status assessment consists of evaluating behavior (verbal and nonverbal) and asking a series of questions. The purpose is to discover problems that may require further assessment and intervention. The level and depth of questioning vary, depending on individual circumstances. Assess a client who is alert and cooperative by listening and observing carefully during the interview. The client's responses provide information about orientation, mood, memory, attention span, general knowledge, language abilities, thought processes, judgment, and insight.

If a client demonstrates impaired cognitive function, perform an abbreviated mental status examination (see

Chapter 69). Disturbances in mood or thought processes (such as suicidal ideation) warrant a complete, detailed mental status examination. Even though mental status data are collected during the health history, record this information with the physical examination data. The following areas are included.

Level of Consciousness. Level of consciousness is the state of awareness. The client must be alert, not just awake, for a mental status assessment (see Chapter 69). Cue the client that the questions may seem "silly" but are to be answered anyway.

Orientation to Person, Place, Time, and Circumstances. Ask the client to explain the reason for seeking health care. If the reply is unclear or if the client digresses, ask the client to state his or her name, to identify the present location, and to specify the date and time.

Mood and Affect. *Mood* is the subjective description of a personal emotion that is pervasive and sustained. Record whether the described mood matches the present situation. For example, "The client stated she was 'happy and going to celebrate' when informed that the results of her tests were normal."

Affect is the observable, outward demeanor that depicts the current emotional state, such as fear, anger, resentment, depression, anxiety, or elation. A *flat affect* is a lack of any facial expression or emotional response and is accompanied by a monotonous voice. A *blunted affect* is greatly reduced in intensity but still appropriate to the situation. Note whether the observed affect matches the immediate circumstances. For example, "When informed that discharge from the hospital was postponed because of an infection, the client first cried, then shouted at the nurse to leave the room." This indicates the client first was upset and then became angry that the discharge was delayed because of a complication. Both reactions are understandable, given the situation.

Speech and Communication (Language). Evaluate the physical ability to speak and communicate by focusing on *how* the client talks, not the topic of speech. Observe tone of voice, pitch, rate of speech, articulation, length of responses, pauses, and pauses before the client replies to questions (latency).

Thought Processes and Content. Assess whether speech progresses logically and whether the stream of thought is spontaneous, natural, organized, logical, relevant, coherent, and goal-directed. What the client says should be consistent.

Attention Span. Assess the client's ability to focus or concentrate on a task or activity over time, such as com-

pleting history forms or answering questions. If results are uncertain, further evaluate the attention span using the following tests:
1. *Digit span,* a test in which the nurse identifies a series of five to seven numbers forward and up to five numbers backward and the series is repeated by the client.
2. *Serial 7s and 3s,* a test in which the client's attention span as well as calculation ability are tested. The client subtracts 7 (or 3) from 100 and continues to subtract 7 (or 3) until unable to go any further.

Memory: Immediate, Recent, and Remote. Assessment of memory usually begins with recall of the past health history. Ask the client to recall information: (1) within seconds (repeat a series of numbers), (2) within several minutes to hours (recall specific words later during the interview or recall what was eaten yesterday), and (3) within hours, months, or years (identify where the client grew up). Be able to verify the client's answers.

General Fund of Knowledge. Ask the client to identify commonly known places, events, and people. This can be done casually during conversation.

Calculations. Ask the client to perform simple arithmetic functions (addition, subtraction, multiplication, division) without using pencil or paper (see Serial 7s, above).

Abstract Reasoning and Thinking. Answers to general questions ("Why did you come to the hospital?") are usually sufficient to assess abstract reasoning. If reasoning is impaired, ask the client to think beyond the concrete dimension by explaining a common proverb or by explaining similarities or differences between selected concepts, such as "A bird in the hand is worth two in the bush" or "What is the difference between a tree and a bush?"

Perceptual Distortion. The client should be able to discriminate reality from misperceptions. Ask the client to describe any illusions or hallucinations by asking about each of the senses. For example, "Do you ever feel that you are hearing sounds that other people do not?"

Judgment. Assess judgment (decision-making ability) within the context of the health history interview as the client discusses actions and decisions made in daily living. To assess further, ask about a realistic rather than a hypothetical situation. For example, "What would you do when a prescribed medication has run out?"

Insight. Assess insight throughout the interview as the client explains the nature of the current health problem and his or her expectations of the health care team.

Evaluate whether the client demonstrates ability to perceive the self realistically and accurately.

When assessing mental status, individualize questions to the client's circumstances. Variables affecting one's ability to respond to specific questions include the following:

- Level of education
- Cultural background
- Degree of exposure to knowledge and information
- Familiarity with the language and vocabulary
- Perceived acceptance by the nurse

For example, it may be revealing to ask a teenager the name of a current popular singer but inappropriate to ask the same question of an older person. A client who has not progressed beyond a third grade level of education may be incapable of performing complicated arithmetic calculations. A proverb widely known in one culture may be meaningless to someone from a different cultural background. Finally, you must have access to correct answers for the questions asked, particularly those relating to personal circumstances, such as the location of the client's home, date and place of birth, and names of family members.

Other Psychological Factors. Assess additional psychological factors, such as personality style (see Box 4-3), motivation, and personal strengths, while interacting with the client and significant others. Although nurses do not usually participate in formal psychological testing, data from formal testing can be used to supplement psychosocial data collected in nurse-client interactions and in the health history.

Motivation. Motivation is highly individual and is influenced by personal needs and desires, goals, hopes, and aspirations. Attempt to determine motivation for seeking health care. If the client is ill, ascertain the motivation for returning to an optimal level of wellness.

Personal Strengths. Use the client's strengths to plan care. *Resources* are personal elements that determine an individual's capability to adapt to challenges and threatening stressors. *Internal* resources are *physiologic* (immune system, nutritional state, physiologic defense systems, genetic predisposition to health, current state of each body system) and *psychological* (defense mechanisms, interpersonal style, usual coping ability, current coping ability, and spiritual state, such as the will to live). *External* resources include the social environment (usual coping style of the family, availability of social support, and the assessment skills of the health care providers) and the physical, economic, and cultural environments.

Values and Beliefs. The value system and beliefs determine whether the client views health care as worth-

while. The client's values and beliefs may differ from yours. Accept them as valid because they help provide insight into behavior.

Spirituality. Spiritual beliefs have implications for well-being, such as sustaining hope or assisting with coping during periods of stress. Include spirituality assessment as part of the health history and explain the purpose for asking about it. This portion of the history is usually addressed at the end of the interview after a trusting nurse-client relationship is established. Because spirituality is personal, respect a client's wishes not to discuss this topic. Ask whether the client prefers to consult someone else when spiritual support is needed.

Sociologic Assessment

The *sociologic dimension* includes information about social roles and functions. Assess psychosocial development, social network, socioeconomic status, lifestyle, and sexuality. View the client both as an individual and as a member of a social network.

Psychosocial Development. *Psychosocial development* refers to a person's level of growth and development, including the life developmental processes and phases of growth and maturation. Psychosocial development occurs across the life span and includes physical, emotional, psychological, social, and cognitive components. Components are not distinct from one another, and progress through life's stages and phases is neither predictable nor inflexible. An understanding of human growth and development provides a foundation from which to assess the client.

Social Network. A *social network* is the group of people that surrounds, interacts with, and sustains a person with intimacy, social integration, nurturing, reassurance, and assistance. The nurse becomes part of a client's social network when the client enters the health care system; however, the client continues to receive support from the established social network.

Collect social network data by observing the client during interactions with family and visitors; ask questions about interpersonal relationships and determine whether there are certain individuals with whom the client prefers to maintain contact. Do not assume that only family members are the most important people. When planning care, include the significant others who may be experiencing stress along with the client.

Socioeconomic Status. An individual's economic position within society is referred to as *socioeconomic status*. Ask about factors that affect financial and social well-being because they have implications for planning individualized health care, such as (1) occupation, (2) current employment status, (3) work-related concerns, (4) financial concerns, (5) effect of the client's health status on the ability to work and on finances, (6) perceived effect that the client's socioeconomic status has on access to the health care system, (7) educational background, and (8) hopes and goals.

Lifestyle. Usual daily patterns of living are referred to as *lifestyle*. Lifestyle is closely associated with socioeconomic status but also includes relationships with others. Assess the following as they apply to the client's health:

- Usual roles and functions
- Work and study habits
- Leisure and relaxation activities
- Type and location of residence
- Living arrangements
- Usual manner of transportation
- Proximity of close friends
- Importance and influence of cultural beliefs on diet and health-seeking behavior or treatment
- Health habits (use of alcohol, medications, nicotine, recreational drugs)
- Stress level
- Coping methods used to relieve stress and their effectiveness
- Usual sleep pattern
- Degree of satisfaction with current status

Sexuality. *Sexuality* is the behavioral expression of one's sexual identity. It involves sexual relationships between people as well as the perception of one's maleness or femaleness (gender identification). Many aspects of sexuality affect health status and are significant to nursing care and client outcomes. Aspects include (1) physical health problems that affect sexual behavior (mastectomy, colostomy, skin lesions, venereal diseases, paralysis, physical deformities), (2) concerns with sexual performance (impotence, premature ejaculation, inability to achieve orgasm, infertility), (3) issues of sex role function (homosexuality, bisexuality, sexual ambiguity, transsexual surgery), and (4) effects of environmental restrictions on sexual performance (residency in a long-term care facility).

Sexuality and sexual behavior are sensitive topics. Clients may want to discuss sexuality issues and may look for permission to do so. Become comfortable with sexuality issues and do not allow personal beliefs and values to interfere with professional care. Accept and interact with clients without judging them or their behavior.

Cultural Assessment

Cultural assessment is a systematic examination of the cultural beliefs, values, and practices as they apply to determining health care needs. These needs, and any culture-based interventions, must be viewed from the client's cultural context. Cultural assessment tends to be broad because it seeks information about group values, beliefs, and behaviors. Also assess what the larger group's tenets mean to the individual.

Assess the following cultural components and their implications for health status:

- Identification with a cultural group
- Communication (language spoken, need for interpreter)
- Values, beliefs, and attitudes
- Cultural sanctions and restrictions
- Health-related beliefs and practices (special rituals or foods, sick role behavior, use of a "healer")
- Nutritional beliefs and practices (special foods, fasting)
- Socioeconomic issues (support system, social network, financial concerns)
- Educational background (primary language, learning style)
- Religious beliefs and practices (implications when ill, special healing rituals)

Further information about cultural assessment is available on the website, which includes Diversity in Health Care boxes on Introduction to Cultural Aspects of Health Care and on Communicating with Culturally Diverse Clients.

Guide to Psychosocial Assessment

Although discussed separately, psychological and sociologic assessments are often combined. You may collect psychosocial data that indicate a psychiatric disorder. If this situation occurs, consult with other health care professionals, such as a psychiatric clinical nurse specialist and the client's physician.

Review of Systems

The ROS is a head-to-toe review of the physical health history for each body system. This review provides a focus for the physical examination. Data may be collected when the client completes a checklist form that is reviewed and expanded as necessary by a health care professional. In an episodic (short-format) health history, focus on those systems pertinent to the problem.

Examples of ROS data are included in the health assessment chapters in this book. A more complete listing may be found on the website.

HEALTH PROMOTION AND HEALTH RISK APPRAISAL

Health risk appraisal examines factors that affect potential for developing a particular health problem. Risk factors are (1) *genetic* or *biologic* (race, family history, personal history), (2) *behavioral* (health habits such as smoking), or (3) *environmental* (living in a locale with smog). Determining health risk status identifies high-risk clients who may benefit from timely intervention. Explain the difference between being *at increased risk for development* of a health problem and the inevitability of *actual development of* a health problem. In health risk appraisal, assess the client's willingness and motivation to modify or reduce risk factors. For example, a client who smokes is at higher risk for pulmonary disease than a nonsmoker. You may believe that the client *should* stop smoking; however, without a desire to stop, teaching is ineffective. This client may be labeled "noncompliant" by the health care team when the client is only following a personal decision to keep smoking. Conversely, a female client at risk for osteoporosis may say that she is concerned and desires to reduce her risk. This client is receptive to teaching about increasing dietary calcium intake and engaging in regular weight-bearing activity.

Health risk factors are categorized for assessment purposes. Some risk factors are potentially hazardous for many people (ground water pollution in a community dependent on wells for its water supply). Other risk factors may adversely affect a limited group of individuals (particle inhalation in insulation installers). Still other risk factors are significant for a family group (genetic diseases, such as Huntington's chorea). Risk categories include the following:

- Race and genetic or family-related factors
- Age-related factors
- Biologic factors
- Personal habits
- Lifestyle factors
- Environmental and occupational factors
- Socioeconomic factors

A summary of health risk factors, their commonly associated health problems, and suggested health promotion behaviors or screening procedures that may reduce potential risk or facilitate early detection are listed in Chapters 1 and 2. Awareness of health risk factors may motivate a client to seek screening procedures and to practice health promotion behaviors, particularly for health problems that are treatable or manageable through timely intervention. Environmental and occupational risk factors are linked with specific health problems and may be susceptible to change. Socioeconomic risk factors are less easily eliminated; however, their effects may be modified through skillful case finding and risk management.

Assess the client's risk profile throughout the health history interview. A client with multiple risk factors linked to specific health problems is at greater risk for development of those problems than the client with fewer or no risk factors. People in hazardous occupations include firefighters, police, miners, heavy equipment operators, lumber and construction workers, factory and textile workers, musicians, and workers who use chemicals or pesticides, such as farmers, landscapers, gardeners, painters, and artists. Risk for *accidental injury* or *trauma* has been linked to multiple stressors, inadequate coping ability, mental and physical fatigue, decreased reaction time, and substance abuse. Stressors include strained interpersonal relationships, physical or psychological abuse, inadequate financial resources, a recent change in lifestyle, sensory stimulation overload, nutritional deficits, and hazardous environments. Lifestyle and personal habits greatly affect health status, and many are modifiable.

After assessing the risk profile, evaluate the client's health risk status. Examine each identified risk factor with the client to determine whether its effects can be modified. If the client is interested in reducing health risks (stopping smoking or wearing seat belts), intervene either directly or indirectly. Discuss approaches to behavior changes. *Direct* interventions include teaching to provide information and counseling to reinforce behavior. *Indirect* interventions include referral to an appropriate community resource or other health care professional (nutritionist, smoking-cessation program, counselor, support group for substance abusers, dieters' support programs).

The goals for the client are (1) to take responsibility for modifying factors that can affect health and (2) to strive for optimal health. Box 4-4 illustrates how to integrate health risk appraisal into the history interview.

Health Promotion Across the Life Span

Health promotion needs change with age and gender. For example, the risk for development of cancer of the bowel or breast is greater in people older than age 50 years than in younger people.

Specific screening procedures are performed during health assessment to determine potential and actual health problems. For example, after age 40 years, glaucoma screening is recommended every 2 years. For health maintenance and prevention, specific health management behaviors are recommended based on age. For example, routine childhood vaccinations for immunization against contagious diseases are administered according to a schedule that correlates with the development of the immune system as well as with periods when exposure is most likely to occur. Adults may be deficient in routine vaccinations or may not have been exposed to childhood contagious diseases. These clients should have screening antibody assays and immunizations if indicated.

Recommendations for common screening procedures and health management behaviors across the life span are listed in Chapters 1 and 2. Recommendations change periodically as research and epidemiologic studies reveal information about occurrence and as newer, more easily applied or sensitive screening methods are developed. Become familiar with the most current recommendations.

Chapter 19 discusses risk factors for the common types of cancer as well as primary risk factors and secondary type of cancer prevention. The American Cancer Society guidelines are given for early detection in asymptomatic populations.

BOX 4-4   *Example of Integrating Health Risk Appraisal into the History Interview*

Biographical and Demographic Data
S.W. is a 28-year-old single white female. Self-employed as a clothing designer. Self-insured. Admitted to nursing unit after surgical repair of the right knee.

Health Maintenance Activities
Annual checkups for teeth, vision, Pap smear. No breast self-examination. Last physical examination 18 months ago.

Personal Habits
Denies smoking. Consumes one to two alcoholic drinks or glasses of wine most days. Uses own automobile frequently; wears seat belts "when [she] remembers to put them on." Tans twice a week for 30 minutes.

Diet
No restrictions; likes most foods. Limits sugar and salt intake. Typical 24-hour diet includes Food Guide Pyramid groups. Usually eats breakfast and dinner; lunch consumed "on the run." Dines out often with clients.

Exercise
Jogs 2 to 3 miles per week and performs step aerobics once per week. Fell while jogging 3 weeks ago; injured right knee.

Stress Management
Feels "moderate" pressure to succeed in business. Life becomes "hectic" when new fashion lines shown. Uses imagery for relax- ation (usually effective). Denies current problems with stress management.

Sleep and Rest
Gets 6 to 7 hours of sleep per night and feels rested.

Sexuality
Sexually active since age 18. Reports five or six partners in past 10 years, with one partner for past 2 years. Prescribed oral contraceptive for 6 years. Partner does not use condoms.

Past Health History
No previous illness, injury, or surgery. No allergies.

Family Health History
Mother had breast cancer at age 42; treated with surgery and is currently healthy. No other known family-linked health problems.

Health Risk Appraisal
S.W. is at risk for (1) breast cancer, (2) possible skin cancer, (3) automobile-related injury or death, (4) possible sexually transmitted diseases, including human immunodeficiency virus infection, and (5) recurrent injury to the right knee. She also is at risk for health problems related to alcohol consumption, inadequate nutrition, inadequate exercise patterns, and a stress-producing lifestyle. There may be concerns about financial security that can be explored with S.W. during further questioning.

Screening Tests and Procedures
Screening tests and procedures help to assess for a health problem (a skin test for tuberculosis) or for risk of future health problems (serum cholesterol screening for the risk of atherosclerosis). When inquiring whether the client has had a specific screening test or procedure, such as an eye examination or mammogram, ask when the test was last performed and what the results were. Use this information to assess health risk status and to recommend further follow-up or screening procedures.

ORGANIZING THE HEALTH HISTORY INTERVIEW
Organize the data collected during the health history interview by topical areas. Use a comprehensive, flexible approach while allowing for in-depth focus assessment in areas of concern. Include a head-to-toe assessment. Various formats are helpful for conducting a health history interview. Gordon's functional health patterns (FHPs) are an example.

FHPs may be used to collect health history data. This approach assists in identifying health patterns, devia- tions from these patterns, and actual or potential nursing diagnoses. Each of the 11 patterns has its own as- sessment criteria (see the example on the website).

RECORDING THE HEALTH HISTORY INTERVIEW
Record interview data in the health record according to agency protocol. The format is organized and may be a narrative, an outline, or a checklist with written supplementary comments. Record all pertinent data (both positive and negative findings). Data are clear, concise, comprehensive, and consistent, with no gaps or areas of ambiguity. Use approved agency abbreviations and terminology, when possible, to promote communication among health care team members.

APPLYING THE NURSING PROCESS TO HEALTH ASSESSMENT
In health assessment, seek to gather as much data about the client as possible, both subjective and objective. Analyze the data to determine the client's needs and responses to potential and actual health problems. Con-

BOX 4-5	*Applying the Nursing Process to Health Assessment: Case Example*

Introduction

Mrs. L. is a 58-year-old, healthy-looking woman who visits a glaucoma screening booth at a health fair. The nurse integrates health assessment data and the nursing process while talking to Mrs. L. and testing her visual acuity.

Biographical Data

Married. Full time legal secretary. One married child out of state.

Physical Health History

No significant health problems. Postmenopausal. Sees rings around lights. Decreased side vision when reading.

Health Risk Appraisal

Mother had cataracts. Family history positive for hypertension. Nearsighted since age 10 and wears corrective lenses. Last eye examination 5 years ago. Has smoked one pack of cigarettes per day for 40 years.

Physical Examination

Snellen chart results (with corrective lenses) are O.D. (right eye) = 20/40, O.S. (left eye) = 20/30, O.U. (both eyes) = 20/30. Visual fields to confrontation reveal superior fields less than those of the examiner. Pupils react sluggishly to accommodation. Further physical examination limited because of setting.

Nursing Diagnosis

High risk for ineffective health maintenance related to visual changes (decreased visual acuity and peripheral vision), family history of hypertension, and smoking history.

Expected Outcomes

Long Term

Mrs. L. will maintain present visual acuity and prevent further loss of vision.

Short Term

1. Mrs. L. will verbalize an understanding of the need for an immediate, complete ophthalmologic examination.
2. Mrs. L. will identify an ophthalmologist whom she will contact no later than tomorrow for an appointment.

Interventions

1. Discuss results of visual screening and their significance with Mrs. L.
2. Explain risk factors for glaucoma and Mrs. L.'s risk profile.
3. Assist Mrs. L. in choosing an ophthalmologist.
4. Provide Mrs. L. with pamphlets about glaucoma from the National Society to prevent Blindness.
5. Give Mrs. L. an addressed postcard that is to be returned by the ophthalmologist after the first visit.

Evaluation

Long Term

Ask Mrs. L. to restate her understanding of the need to have regular visual checkups by an ophthalmologist and to follow the recommended medical regimen for eye care.

Short Term

Ask Mrs. L. whom she plans to contact for an eye appointment and when she intends to do this.

---

sider the client's preferences when formulating nursing diagnoses that are amenable to intervention. Establishing realistic goals and outcome criteria and planning interventions follow in logical order (Box 4-5).

PHYSICAL EXAMINATION

The physical examination is performed after the health history interview. Physical examination skills require use of the ears, eyes, and senses of touch and smell. Repeated practice reinforces integration of these skills. Learn the techniques and correct use of equipment as well as how to discriminate "normal" from "abnormal" findings.

Collect objective data systematically during the examination to supplement and validate subjective data. Evaluate both types of data to enhance holistic perception of the client. Ask about abnormal physical findings. For example, if a mass is found during palpation, ask whether the area is tender to touch. Record the client's reply in the physical examination portion of the data-

base ("nontender") even though the data are subjective. If you palpate a lump or mass not reported initially during the history interview, ask whether the client is aware of the mass's existence. If the client knows that the mass is present or reports related manifestations, proceed with a symptom analysis (see Symptom Analysis earlier in this chapter). Record these subjective data in the health history.

Physical examination is used in many settings. Health fairs, screening clinics, physicians' offices, independent practice clinics, home health care, and hospitals are some examples. Client health needs determine the extent and depth of examination. For example, a home health nurse visits a client who has had total hip replacement surgery. During the initial visit, the nurse performs a baseline assessment. During subsequent visits, the initial assessment findings guide evaluation of the client's progress (increased mobility and strength in the operative leg). Similarly, a coronary care nurse conducts periodic examinations of a client after a myocardial infarction to assess for life-threatening complications.

PURPOSE OF THE EXAMINATION

The purpose of physical examination is to differentiate normal from abnormal physical findings. A foundation of basic anatomy (structure) and physiology (function) is key to developing skill, expertise, and an appreciation for the wide range of findings that are considered normal. In addition to collecting baseline data, use assessment skills to make clinical judgments about health status and to evaluate the effectiveness of health care interventions (see the home health and coronary care examples mentioned on p. 79).

LEVELS OF PHYSICAL EXAMINATION

The level of physical examination depends on client needs:

1. A *screening* physical examination is an organized, superficial check of major body systems to detect abnormalities or possible problems.
2. If a problem is detected, the examination focuses on a *regional* or *branching* examination, which is an in-depth assessment of a specific body system. This chapter describes the screening adult physical examination; regional examinations are discussed in the assessment chapters for each body system. A table illustrating a complete head-to-toe examination is on the website.
3. A *complete* physical examination includes ancillary procedures such as x-ray studies and clinical laboratory tests.

In the clinical setting, *periodic head-to-toe assessment* updates baseline data and assesses changes in health status. Individualize the depth of body system examinations according to client needs. For example, assess a client with a neurologic problem using a Mini-Mental State assessment tool such as the Glasgow Coma Scale in addition to the head-to-toe evaluation (see Chapter 69). A client with intact neurologic function would not require this depth of assessment. An example of a head-to-toe periodic assessment guide appears in Box 4-6.

ACCURACY OF THE PHYSICAL EXAMINATION

The physical examination validates data collected during the health history interview. As with the health history, strive to collect accurate, thorough data. If you encounter difficulty with an assessment technique or question the accuracy of a finding, consult with colleagues. A second opinion or evaluation may be needed.

PHYSICAL EXAMINATION AND THE NURSING PROCESS

An accurate database is essential for formulating individualized nursing diagnoses. It may be misleading to diagnose a problem on the basis of one assessment find-

---

> **BOX 4-6** *Head-to-Toe Periodic Assessment Guide*
>
> 1. *Vital signs:* Temperature, pulse, respirations, blood pressure
> 2. *Pain:* Location, type, quality, intensity
> 3. *Neurologic:* Orientation (person, place, time, situation), level of consciousness, gait, extremity color/movement/sensation (CMS), pupillary responses to light
> 4. *Pulmonary:* Respiratory pattern and effort; breath sounds; cough quality; sputum production, color, and quantity
> 5. *Cardiovascular:* Heart sounds and rhythm, pulses (radial, dorsalis pedis, and posterior tibial), capillary refill, edema (location and amount), skin color and temperature
> 6. *Gastrointestinal:* Oral assessment, abdominal appearance, bowel sounds, bowel elimination pattern
> 7. *Genitourinary:* Bladder distention, voiding pattern
> 8. *Integumentary:* Skin integrity, wounds, dressings, drainage
> 9. *Psychosocial:* Sociability, affect, anxiety, attitude
>
> Note: Perform additional assessments according to the client's specific health status and needs.

---

ing. *Significant* findings (data that are either abnormal or indicate a potential risk) cue the collection of additional information. A complete assessment is necessary before data can be grouped and a cause determined. The initial physical assessment is the baseline for the client's functional ability. Physical assessment is also used as intervention (monitoring lung sounds) to evaluate changes in the client's physical condition and to determine whether expected outcomes have been achieved.

TECHNIQUES OF THE PHYSICAL EXAMINATION

Four primary techniques are used in physical assessment: *inspection, palpation, percussion,* and *auscultation.* These techniques enhance the data collected by observation of the ears, eyes, and senses of touch and smell and are used during the examination of each body region (Figure 4-2).

Inspection

Inspection is the systematic, deliberate visual examination of the entire client or a body region. Inspection yields information about size, shape, color, texture, symmetry, position, and deformities. It is the first examination technique and begins at the outset of the client-nurse interaction. For example, inspect facial skin while collecting the history. Complete inspection before progressing to the hands-on techniques of palpation, percussion, and auscultation.

Conduct inspection in a well-lighted setting. Uncover the body region or part to permit complete visualization while draping the rest of the body to preserve modesty

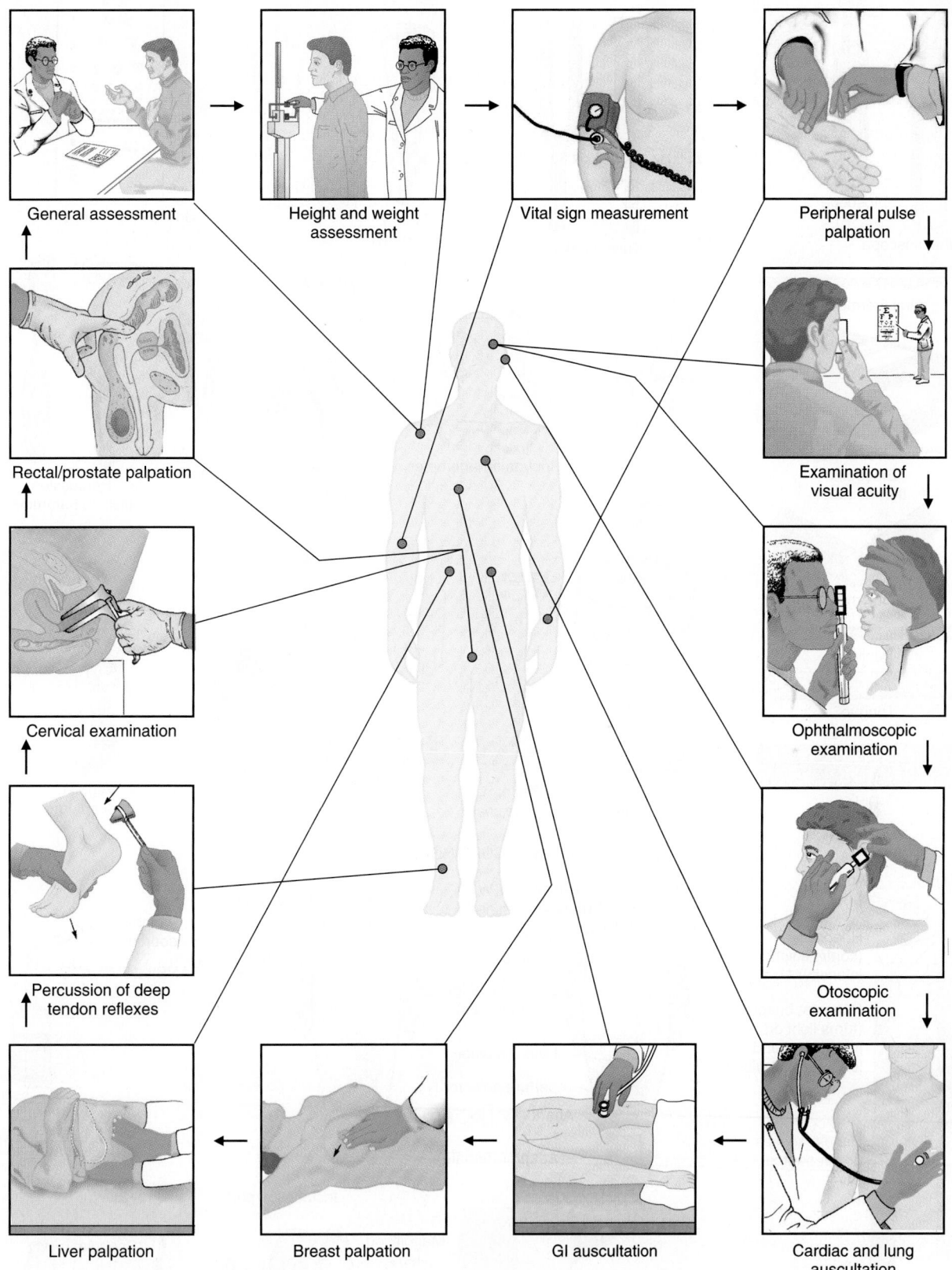

FIGURE 4-2 Common techniques of physical assessment used in a head-to-toe screening examination. The examiner wears gloves for the pelvic, rectal, and prostate examinations.

FIGURE 4-3 Instruments used in a physical examination.

and comfort. During inspection, compare observations with the known parameters of normal findings in clients of similar age, gender, race, and ethnicity.

Inspection is enhanced with special instruments such as a penlight, oto-ophthalmoscope, and various specula (nasal and vaginal) that permit visual access to body cavities and orifices (Figure 4-3). Other equipment includes tongue blades, a marking pen, a ruler, a tape measure, skinfold calipers, a goniometer, and eye charts.

Palpation

Palpation, generally the second physical assessment technique, is the use of touch. During palpation, exert varying amounts of pressure to determine information about masses, pulsation, organ size, tenderness or pain, swelling, tissue firmness and elasticity, vibration, crepitation, temperature, texture variation, and moisture. Also use palpation to assess masses for position, size, shape, consistency, and mobility.

Technique. Use the most sensitive parts of your hands and fingers to palpate specific characteristics. For example, the *fingertips* or *pads* are the most sensitive for fine touch and are used to palpate pulses, lymph nodes, and breast tissue. Use the *dorsum,* or back of the hand and fingers, to discriminate changes in skin temperature (see Chapter 50). Use the *palmar surface* of the hand over the metacarpophalangeal joints and the *ulnar aspect* to assess vibration of the lung with vocalization (tactile fremitus). Assess position, consistency, mobility, size, shape, and skin turgor by lightly grasping tissue between the *thumb* and *index finger.*

Facilitate palpation by positioning the client comfortably. This minimizes muscle tension and lessens the possibility of mistaking such tension for muscle rigidity. Improve relaxation by having warm hands and short fingernails and by using a gentle approach. Encourage the client to take slow, deep breaths. Apply tactile pressure, and increase pressure gradually. Prolonged pressure decreases sensitivity in the palpating hand.

Before palpating, ask the client to indicate tender areas. Palpate tender areas last while you observe for nonverbal signs of discomfort or pain. Examine these areas, but note that this may result in discomfort and reluctance to continue.

Levels of Palpation. Palpation proceeds from light to deep (Figure 4-4).

For *light* palpation, depress the underlying tissue approximately 1 to 2 cm (½ to ¾ inch). After light palpation, use deep palpation to determine the size and condition of underlying structures, such as abdominal organs.

For *deep* palpation, depress the underlying tissue approximately 4 to 5 cm (1½ to 2 inches), proceeding cautiously, because prolonged pressure can potentially in-

FIGURE 4-4 Palpation techniques. **A,** Light palpation employs the lightest possible pressure to assess structures under the surface of the skin, such as lymph nodes. **B,** Deep palpation is used to assess the condition of underlying organs, such as in the abdomen, using one or both hands. **C,** Bimanual palpation is used to trap and assess hard-to-palpate organs, such as the kidneys, or to stabilize an organ with one hand while the other hand palpates, as in liver palpation.

jure internal organs. Use one or both hands (bimanual palpation).

For *bimanual* palpation, place one hand lightly on the client's skin (the sensing hand). Place the other hand (active hand) over the sensing hand to apply pressure. The sensing hand does not apply direct pressure and remains sensitive to underlying organ characteristics.

In one variation of bimanual palpation, one hand positions or stabilizes an organ while the other hand palpates (liver, spleen, kidney, or breast or uterus and adnexa during gynecologic examination). Another variation involves trapping structures that move between the two hands, such as the kidney with respiration. (See also gynecologic assessment, Chapter 39.)

Precautions. Take precautions during palpation. For example, palpate an artery so that blood flow is not obstructed. Do not palpate the carotid arteries simultaneously because of the possibility of restricting blood flow to the brain.

Percussion

Percussion is used to assess tissue density with sound produced from striking the skin. Usually the third technique in physical assessment, percussion allows examination of 3 to 5 cm of tissue depth. Evaluate the sounds and tissue vibrations that result from percussion in relation to the underlying body structures. Percussion of body structures containing air, fluid, and solids produces various sounds, depending on density. Percussion helps confirm suspected abnormal findings from palpation and auscultation, such as a mass or consolidation in the lungs.

The two primary methods of percussion are direct and indirect (Figure 4-5).

Direct Percussion

Direct percussion involves striking the body surface either with one or two fingers or with the fist (*blunt* percussion). Use it primarily to assess the sinuses and over the thin chest wall of a small adult or a child. Perform blunt percussion to elicit tenderness from an underlying structure, such as the kidney, not to produce a sound. Use of a reflex hammer is another example of blunt percussion.

Indirect Percussion

Technique. *Indirect* percussion involves striking an intermediary finger or hand that is placed firmly on the body's surface. Dexterity and practice are required to attain proficiency in this technique. Place the distal phalanx of the middle finger *(pleximeter)* (see Figure 4-5) firmly on the skin surface over soft tissue. Hyperextend the remaining fingers so that only the single digit is in contact with the skin. The *plexor* must strike the pleximeter sharply and quickly; do this by relaxing the wrist, keeping the forearm stationary, and striking with the fingertip (not the pad). Errors in technique diminish (damp) the sound produced. Common errors include (1) placing the pleximeter over bone, (2) resting the palm or other fingers of the nondominant hand on the body surface, (3) losing contact between pleximeter and skin surface, (4) delivering a weak blow with the plexor, and (5) striking the pleximeter at a point other than the distal joint.

For an accurate comparison of sounds, deliver the same amount of force with each blow. A light, quick blow produces the clearest sound. The blows may be repeated rapidly two or three times to assess the sound.

Types of Sounds. Indirect percussion results in five characteristic sounds:

1. *Flatness,* a soft, high-pitched, short sound produced by very dense tissue such as muscle. Percussion of the thigh reproduces a characteristic flat sound.
2. *Dullness,* a soft to moderately loud sound of moderate pitch and duration. It is produced by less dense, mostly fluid-filled tissue, such as the liver and spleen, and has a thudding quality.
3. *Resonance,* a moderate to loud sound of low pitch and long duration. It results from the air-filled tissue of the normal lung and has a hollow quality.
4. *Hyperresonance,* a very loud, low-pitched sound lasting longer than resonance. It is produced by the overinflated, air-filled lungs of a person with pulmonary emphysema, or it may be heard in a child's lung because of a thin chest wall. Hyperresonance has a booming quality.
5. *Tympany,* a loud, high-pitched, moderately long sound with a drum-like, musical quality. It results from enclosed, air-containing structures, such as the stomach (gastric bubble) and bowel. It can be reproduced by percussion over a puffed cheek.

Auscultation

Auscultation is listening to internal body sounds to assess normal sounds and detect abnormal sounds. It is the final step in the physical examination. Use a stethoscope to enhance sounds. The sounds commonly assessed by auscultation include those produced by the heart, lungs, abdomen, and vascular system. Become proficient at auscultation by knowing which sounds are produced by each body structure and the location at which they are most readily heard. Recognizing abnormal sounds is easier once the normal sounds have been mastered.

Acute hearing ability, a reliable stethoscope, and knowing how to use the stethoscope are essential. Stethoscopes that amplify sounds are available for those who have difficulty hearing. The basic stethoscope has a chest piece with a bell and diaphragm and single or double tubing connected to double ear tubes (binaurals). A tension bar between the binaurals holds the ear pieces firmly in place and reduces kinking of the tubing.

Technique. Hold the *diaphragm* between the index and middle fingers firmly against the skin surface; use it to hear high-pitched sounds, such as lung sounds, heart sounds, and blood pressure. Place the *bell* lightly in contact with the skin to hear low-pitched sounds, such as murmurs and bruits. Place the *chest piece* on the skin so

DIRECT PERCUSSION

INDIRECT PERCUSSION

FIGURE 4-5 Techniques for the two primary types of percussion, direct and indirect. **A** and **B**, *Direct percussion.* **A,** Use one or two fingers to percuss directly against a body surface, such as over the sinuses, to elicit tenderness. **B,** Use the ulnar surface of your fist to gently strike the surface of the body over an underlying organ, such as at the costovertebral junction to assess for kidney tenderness. **C-E,** *Indirect percussion.* **C,** Place the distal phalanx of the middle finger of your nondominant hand (the pleximeter) on the skin over soft tissue. Bend the middle finger of your dominant hand at its distal interphalangeal joint to create a "hammer" (or plexor). **D,** Pivot the plexor down quickly in an arc to strike the pleximeter. **E,** Place the palm of your left hand over the area to be percussed. Gently strike the left hand with the ulnar surface of your right fist.

that it is between bones and not over them, because bone does not transmit sound. Clothing and excessive chest hair interfere with sound transmission and may introduce artifacts. Snug-fitting *earpieces* occlude the external ear canal to enhance sound transmission from the chest piece. Keep the *tubing,* no longer than 12 to 15 inches

for the best sound transmission, free of contact with all surfaces to prevent extraneous noises.

A quiet environment is essential for auscultation. Close the door, and draw the cubicle curtains. If necessary, turn down the television or radio volume after informing the client about the importance of decreasing external sounds. Concentrate on the part being auscultated to determine what is causing the sounds you hear. Once you understand the source and characteristics of normal body sounds, it is easier to recognize abnormal sounds and their origin.

Types of Sounds. There are four characteristic auscultation sounds:

1. *Pitch,* the number or frequency of sound wave cycles per second. Varying the frequency alters the pitch. For example, a high frequency results in a high-pitched sound, whereas a low frequency produces a low-pitched sound. Heart murmurs can be either high-pitched or low-pitched, depending on the structural cause. Pitch is a diagnostic clue.
2. *Intensity,* the amplitude of a sound wave. The greater the amplitude, the louder the sound; the lower the amplitude, the softer the sound.
3. *Duration,* the length of time a sound endures; it may be long, medium, or short.
4. *Quality,* a description of a sound's character, such as "gurgling," "blowing," "whistling," or "snapping."

Olfaction

Olfaction is the use of the sense of smell to detect body odors. The sense of smell helps detect abnormalities not readily recognized by other means, such as inspection. For example, the smell of ammonia in urine suggests a urinary tract infection; a strong, musty odor from a casted body part suggests a wound infection under the cast; a strong, fruity breath odor indicates enhanced production of ketone by-products. Consider olfactory findings with other assessments to determine the nature of the client's health problem.

GUIDELINES FOR PHYSICAL EXAMINATION

Physical examination proceeds in a logical, orderly fashion. The approach commonly follows a head-to-toe organization so that findings are complete. This is not an absolute rule, and the nurse who is beginning to use physical assessment skills must practice and develop a system that is comfortable to use. Once a system is developed, use it routinely to avoid inadvertently omitting portions of the examination. For a successful physical assessment, you must know both the techniques and the parameters of normal findings. Consult the following guidelines to plan and conduct a physical examination.

Preparation of the Environment

To prepare for physical examination, ensure that the environment is private, quiet, comfortable (neither too warm nor too cool), and well lighted. An examination may be conducted in a special room in an office or clinic, in a client's bedroom in the home, or in the area enclosed by drawn curtains around a client's bed in a hospital room. Eliminate or control extraneous noises to enhance concentration and to encourage the client to feel free to discuss problems or concerns.

Preparation of Equipment

Assemble all necessary equipment before beginning. Arrange equipment in order of use to facilitate examination. Practice picking up equipment, holding it in the position of use, making adjustments, assembling, and disassembling. Check equipment for adequate functioning. It is embarrassing as well as time-consuming to hunt for a replacement bulb for the oto-ophthalmoscope or to discover that the battery needs recharging in the middle of an examination.

Equipment commonly used in physical examination is shown in Figure 4-3. Additional equipment may include cotton balls, gauze sponges, a watch with a second hand, supplies for specimens, and substances to test the senses of taste and smell.

Preparation of the Client

Prepare the client physically and psychologically for the physical examination. Before beginning, instruct the client to empty the bladder. If a urine specimen is needed, instruct the client in the technique for collection. An empty bladder facilitates examination of the abdomen, genitalia, and rectum.

Draping

Physical preparation also includes instructing the client to dress according to the type and extent of examination to be conducted. A gown and drapes provide privacy (Figure 4-6).

Positioning

During the examination, assist the client in assuming different positions to facilitate assessment and minimize position changes. Figure 4-6 illustrates common positions for examination and the areas of the body that are assessed. Consider client limitations that may prevent optimal positioning, such as arthritis, back injury, joint deformities, or weakness. The client may have to assume an alternative position to complete the examination. Some positions may be uncomfortable or embarrassing. Keep the client in these positions only as long as required and drape to prevent unnecessary exposure.

Psychological Preparation

Approach the client professionally and calmly. An organized, efficient approach and a relaxed tone of voice and facial expression put the client at ease and promote trust. The client may be anxious about the examination

POSITION	AREAS EXAMINED	RATIONALE	CONTRAINDICATIONS
Sitting	Vital signs, head and neck, back, posterior and anterior thorax and lungs, breasts, axillae, heart, upper and lower extremities, reflexes	Sitting upright allows for full lung expansion and better visualization of upper body symmetry.	Older and weak clients may be unable to sit without support. An alternate position is supine with the head of the bed elevated.
Supine	Vital signs, head and neck, anterior thorax and lungs, breasts, axillae, heart, abdomen, extremities, peripheral pulses	This is a relaxed position for most clients. It provides access to pulse sites and prevents contracture of abdominal muscles, especially if a small pillow is placed under the knees.	Clients with cardiovascular and respiratory problems may be unable to lie flat without becoming short of breath. An alternate position is to raise the head of the bed. Clients with lower back pain may be unable to lie flat without flexing the knees.
Dorsal recumbent	Abdomen and external genitalia	Flexed knees reduce tension on lower back and abdominal muscles and increase client comfort.	Same as for supine. The client should not raise the arms over the head or clasp the hands behind the head because this increases contraction of the abdominal muscles.
Lithotomy	Female genitalia, reproductive tract, and rectum	This position maximally exposes the genitalia and facilitates the insertion of a vaginal speculum.	This position is assumed immediately before it is needed because it is embarrassing and uncomfortable. The client is kept draped. Clients with arthritis or joint deformity may be unable to assume this position. Alternate positions are dorsal recumbent and Sims'.
Sims' (posterior view)	Rectum, vagina	Flexion of the upper hip and knee improves exposure of the rectal area.	Clients with deformities of the hip or knee may be unable to assume this position. Older and obese clients may be uncomfortable.
Prone	Posterior thorax, hip movement, popliteal pulses	This position is used to assess hip extension. Sometimes popliteal pulse palpation is facilitated in this position.	This position is not well tolerated by older clients or clients with cardiovascular or respiratory problems.
Knee-chest	Rectum, prostate	This position provides maximal exposure of the anal and rectal areas and facilitates insertion of instruments into the rectum.	Poorly tolerated by clients with cardiovascular or respiratory problems. Clients with difficulty flexing hips or knees may be unable to assume this position.
Standing, bent over examining table	Rectum, prostate	This is a more comfortable position than knee-chest and allows for palpation of the prostate gland.	This position is assumed immediately before it is needed because it is embarrassing. Clients with back problems may need assistance.

FIGURE 4-6 Draping and positioning the client to facilitate assessment and protect privacy.

and about the possibility of finding something abnormal. Some agencies require the presence of a second staff person of the same gender as the client for examination of breasts and genitalia when the examiner is of the opposite gender. Explain what will be done before proceeding so that the client knows what to expect and cooperates fully.

Explain the examination in general terms, then provide a detailed explanation as you examine each body system. Simple terms are less confusing and less threatening than complicated explanations. Encourage the client to verbalize discomfort as the examination proceeds.

Be sensitive to the client who is uncomfortable with exposing body parts to anyone other than those who are culturally sanctioned. For example, in some cultures, a woman is restricted from revealing most of her body to a male other than her husband or immediate family. In other cultures, women are restricted from touching men other than their immediate male relatives.

Watch facial expressions and body language throughout the examination. Nonverbal communication may convey anxiety, fear, or concern. For example, the client may pull the drape closely around the body, or muscles may be tight and tense. In extreme instances, the client may wish to stop the examination and you should comply. Never coerce the client to continue. Attempt to explain the purpose of the examination and to clarify misconceptions.

Preparation of the Examiner
On meeting the client, begin the physical examination by focusing on appearance, movements, position, and reaction to the assessment process. Have a mental plan (assisted by an outline or checklist) so that you cover the major portions of the examination. The outline may include the general sequence, methods, equipment, and techniques needed to examine each body system.

Organization
Organization and efficiency provide a framework for a thorough physical assessment without wasting time or energy. Minimize position changes to reduce client fatigue. Use a piece of equipment to examine an entire region or body system. For example, use the reflex hammer to test deep tendon reflexes in quick succession, proceeding from upper to lower extremities, while the client is either seated or supine.

Sequence of Examination
The importance of organizing the physical examination systematically has already been discussed. A suggested format for sequencing the adult general screening physi-

cal examination that integrates a head-to-toe approach incorporating regional assessments as well as each body system may be found on the website. Develop an individual style and approach to obtain the data necessary to diagnose the client's responses to physical problems, yet be flexible enough to accommodate individual needs.

Knowledge of Structure and Function
Anatomic landmarks are reference points for locating areas to examine and for recording findings. Reference to an anatomy book is recommended for the beginning practitioner in physical examination. Descriptive terms and anatomic reference points are discussed further as examination of each body system is discussed.

ADULT GENERAL SCREENING PHYSICAL EXAMINATION

General Survey
The general survey begins the physical examination and includes observing the overall appearance and behavior, obtaining vital signs, and measuring height and weight.

General Appearance and Behavior
Evaluate observations regarding general appearance and behavior in relation to the client's background (culture, educational level, socioeconomic status, current health, and illness status). Manifestations of problems or abnormalities direct attention to specific body areas as the examination proceeds. For example, the client who is unkempt and has obvious body odor needs thorough examination of the hair, skin, and nails for assessment of hygiene. General appearance and behavior assessments include the following.

Apparent Age, Gender, and Race. Because a client's appearance may or may not match chronologic age, direct assessment to each body system for potential problems related to aging. Other assessments are gender-specific and affect the type of procedures performed. Interpret data and make recommendations for health teaching and further screening based on the client's health risk profile (see Health Promotion and Health Risk Appraisal earlier in this chapter).

Apparent State of Health. Assess whether the client looks "healthy," frail, or ill. Note deformities or absent body parts.

Manifestations of Distress or Discomfort. The client may display obvious manifestations of pain (wincing), anxiety (eyes darting around room), difficulty breathing (gasping), or other problems. Adapt the examination by including only the necessary assessments. The ideal situation is one in which the client is comfortable and in no acute distress.

Body Build. Assess body build for proportionate distribution of weight for height. Body build may be thin, obese, trim, or muscular, and it may reflect the level of wellness, age, and lifestyle.

Posture. Posture may reflect mood or the presence of a physical problem. Observe posture throughout the assessment process. Normal findings are an erect posture while standing, with the shoulders and hips aligned over the knees and ankles. Sitting posture is with a straight back and slight rounding of the shoulders. Deviations from normal include stooping, slouching, and a curved posture. An ethnic variation may include an increased forward lumbar spine curvature (lordosis) accompanied by a forward tilt of the pelvis and abdominal protrusion.

Gait. Observe gait as the client enters the examination room or ambulates. Gait should be smooth and coordinated with arms swinging freely at the sides, opposite to leg movements. The head and face should orient in the direction of movement. Shuffling steps and hesitancy are abnormal findings. Note devices to assist ambulation.

Movements. Observe body movements as the examination proceeds. They are usually purposeful and controlled without tremors, tics, muscle fasciculations, spasticity, or decreased muscle tone. Note immobile body parts.

Dress. The manner of dress should be appropriate to the time of year, temperature, age, socioeconomic status, and current circumstances. A depressed client may wear clothing that is dull, unkempt, or mismatched. A client with a thyroid disorder may be dressed more warmly than others (hypothyroid) or may wear lightweight clothing despite a cool or cold environment (hyperthyroid).

Hygiene and Grooming. Note the cleanliness of hair, nails, skin, and clothes. Does the client present a pleasant image? Consider what activity the client engaged in before the examination and whether it affects appearance.

Body and Breath Odor. Note odors in relationship to activity level, such as strenuous exercise. Deficient hygiene may result in body and breath odors that are considered unpleasant or offensive. Odors include cigarette smoke, perfume, perspiration, alcohol, acetone, blood, decaying tissue, or an associated disease process.

Mental Status. Mental status includes level of consciousness, orientation, affect, speech, and thought processes. If abnormalities are noted in these areas, proceed with a full mental status assessment (see Mental Status under Psychological Assessment earlier in this chapter and Chapter 69).

Level of Cooperation. Assess the client's cooperation with the examination. Is the client interested, concerned, and willing to discuss information, or is the client silent, withdrawn, hostile, angry, or suspicious? Is the client relaxed and able to engage in eye contact, or is the client tense and avoid eye contact? Consider cultural influences when assessing eye contact and body language. In some cultures, direct eye contact is perceived as being hostile or as dominant behavior and averted eyes are the norm when talking to another person. Similarly, members of some cultural groups do not directly face a person while talking if that person is perceived as an authority figure.

Height and Weight

Measure height and weight while the client is standing. This often is done immediately after the health history interview, before the client sits on the examination table. Use a balance scale (see Figure 4-3), which is usually accurate. (Alternatives to the standing platform scale include bed and chair scales.) The standing scale has a telescoping ruler to measure height.

Compare height and weight with published reference ranges. Weight should fall within range for gender, height, and body frame. (Determining body frame, ideal body weight, and body mass index is discussed in Chapter 30.) Adjust weight for clients who are missing all or part of an extremity (amputation) to account for the absent body mass using a chart or table for segmental weights.

Balance (Romberg's Test)

After measuring height and weight and before the client sits down, assess balance. Romberg's test and the test for pronation assess cerebellar function and may be done later during the neurologic examination. Instruct the client to stand quietly with hands at the sides and feet together. Once equilibrium is attained, instruct the client to close the eyes. The client should be able to stand upright with minimal swaying and no loss of balance. Stand close by and intervene in case the client begins to lose balance and fall. While the client is standing, ask the client to raise and extend arms to shoulder height, then close the eyes. The client should be able to maintain the arms in extension with no downward drifting or pronation (pronation sign). (See other cerebellar assessments in Chapter 69.)

Once Romberg's test is completed, you may assess visual acuity if the eye chart is located at the correct distance from the examination table. Otherwise, test visual acuity when the eyes are examined. Instruct the client to sit on the edge of the examination table for assessment of vital signs.

Vital Signs

Once the client is comfortably seated, measure vital signs after a brief stabilization period. Measure body temperature and blood pressure during the general survey. You may measure specific vital signs during examination of the upper extremities or heart (peripheral pulse) and thorax (respirations). A nursing fundamentals textbook would describe the techniques of vital signs measurement and equipment selection. (See the Management and Delegation feature on Measuring and Recording Vital Signs and Other Client Data, below.)

Temperature. Oral body temperature ranges from 96.8° to 99.5° F (36° to 37.5° C), with an average of 98.6° F (37° C). Body temperatures greater than the normal range are *hyperthermic*; those less than the normal are *hypothermic*.

Pulse. Resting pulse rate ranges from 60 to 100 beats/min. A rate greater than 100 beats/min is *tachycardia*; a rate less than 60 beats/min is *bradycardia*. Note general characteristics of the pulse, such as rhythm (regular or irregular), amplitude (weak or bounding), and pattern. Rhythm is regular, with pulsations occurring at equal intervals and of similar amplitude. A slight variation in rhythm occurs with respiration and is normal. Describe *pulse amplitude* (Box 4-7) and any irregular patterns. See also Chapter 53.

Respiration. Respirations range from 12 to 20 breaths/min. They have a regular, smooth pattern and consistent

---

BOX 4-7	*Recording Pulse Amplitude*

Absent: Indiscernible to palpation
Weak, thready: Difficult to palpate and easily obliterated by slight pressure
Normal: Easily palpable and can be obliterated only with strong pressure
Bounding: Easily palpable, forceful, and not easily obliterated by pressure

---

MANAGEMENT AND DELEGATION

Measuring and Recording Vital Signs and Other Client Data

The measurement and recording of routine vital signs may be delegated to unlicensed assistive personnel. Delegate collection of data only when you are caring for a stable client. Emphasize the following when delegating these tasks to assistive personnel:

1. *Blood pressure.* Place the blood pressure cuff 1 to 2 inches above the antecubital fossa, with the cuff bladder overlying the brachial artery. For the leg, place the blood pressure cuff 1 to 2 inches above the popliteal space, with the cuff bladder overlying the popliteal artery. The size of the cuff should accommodate the circumference of the client's arm or leg. If the client has contraindications to blood pressure measurement on the arm or leg, inform the assistive personnel.
2. *Pulse.* Count the radial pulse for 30 seconds and multiply by 2. If the pulse seems irregular, count it for a full minute.
3. *Respiratory rate.* Count the rate of respiration without the client's being aware that it is being done. This prevents the client from consciously controlling the respiratory rate. If the respiratory rate is regular, count the rate for 30 seconds and multiply by 2. If the respiratory rate is irregular, count the rate for a full minute.
4. *Temperature.* Designate the route by which the temperature should be taken. Delay taking oral temperatures for 15 minutes if the client has just eaten, smoked, or consumed a hot or cold liquid. If the client has dry mucous membranes and cannot hold the thermometer under the tongue with the lips closed, use the axillary, rectal, or tympanic route. If the client has contraindications to rectal temperature measurement, inform the assistive personnel.
5. *Oxygen saturation.* Designate the type of pulse oximeter sensor to be used. If a finger or toe sensor is used, you may need to remove nail polish or artificial nails. The skin at the sensor site should be clean, dry, and intact.

Findings that are immediately reportable to you, the RN, should be described for the assistive personnel. These findings may include a blood pressure outside the range of 95/60 mm Hg to 120-139/80 mm Hg or may be defined by the client's baseline blood pressure. Pulse rates less than 60 or greater than 110 beats/min as well as any irregular pulse or inability to locate a pulse should be reported. Adult respiratory rates less than 10 or greater than 20 should be reported to you, as should any irregular respiratory pattern. Temperatures outside the normal range of 97.6° to 99.4° F should be reported. An oxygen saturation level below 96% should be brought to your attention.

Even though you have delegated the collection of this information, you remain responsible for the review and interpretation of the data as well as for the full health assessment of the client. Assess cardiovascular and respiratory status daily and more frequently as the client's clinical condition warrants.

Verify the competence of the assistive personnel in performing each of these tasks during orientation and annually thereafter. Include the proper recording of the vital signs and any other client data delegated for collection.

depth. They are quiet and effortless, without abnormal sounds such as wheezing. Respiratory depth reflects *tidal volume* (the amount of air taken in with each breath). Use the rise and fall of the chest to estimate whether respirations are shallow, moderate, or deep. Note the respiratory pattern and record its characteristics (see Figure 61-3). See also Chapters 61 and 69.

Blood Pressure. Blood pressure varies greatly among individuals. Normal systolic pressure ranges from 100 to 140 mm Hg, and diastolic pressure ranges from 60 to 90 mm Hg. It is more accurate to evaluate consecutive blood pressure readings over time rather than use an isolated measurement for determining blood pressure abnormalities. *Hypotension* is a systolic pressure less than 95 mm Hg or diastolic pressure less than 60 mm Hg. *Hypertension* is a systolic pressure greater than 140 mm Hg or diastolic pressure greater than 90 mm Hg. In 2003, the JNC 7 Report recommended that clients with systolic pressure levels of 120 to 139 mm Hg and/or diastolic pressure levels of 80 to 89 mm Hg be considered prehypertensive and practice health-promoting lifestyle modifications to prevent cardiovascular disease.[10a] Note the difference between the systolic and diastolic pressure readings *(pulse pressure)*. Report a difference of more than 40 mm Hg, which is abnormal. A slightly elevated blood pressure may be considered a normal finding in older people.

Assess blood pressure with the bell of the stethoscope initially. Assess both arms and compare the two readings. A pressure difference of 5 to 10 mm Hg between the two arms is insignificant. Report larger differences. Assess for an *auscultatory gap* the first time a client's blood pressure is measured. This phenomenon occurs as a period of silence between two levels of systolic pressures that may range as much as 40 mm Hg. See also Chapter 53.

Skin Color

Assess overall skin color during the health history interview, but conduct a more thorough assessment during the remainder of the examination. Observe the face and visible skin surfaces for color tones that should be congruent with the client's stated race. Abnormal findings include pallor (paleness), flushing or a ruddy complexion, cyanosis (blue cast), jaundice (yellow cast), and areas of irregular pigmentation. See also Chapter 50.

Processing the Data

Comparison of Findings

Use the client as a "control," or self-standard, for comparison during the physical examination. Compare findings from one side of the body with those from the opposite side *(bilateral comparison)*. Even though both sides of the human body are not exactly identical (symmetrical), similarities in structure and appearance are individualized and unique. Comparisons are useful and valid for findings such as a joint deformity or an extremity swelling. If a part of a limb is missing (such as from an amputation), a bilateral comparison is impractical; compare findings with a known standard.

Comparison with Known Standards

Compare physical examination findings with known parameters of "normal" for age, gender, and racial background. For example, decreased skin elasticity and loss of subcutaneous adipose tissue are expected findings for an older client but not for a 30-year-old.

Suspected Problem Areas

Examine known or suspected problem areas carefully. Include areas identified during the health history interview as well as those predicted to be at risk based on the client's history and reactions to the physical examination. For example, thoroughly assess mouth and neck structures of the client who reports difficulty swallowing (see Chapters 30 and 44). To allay anxiety, explain why a particular portion of the examination is more thorough.

Health Teaching

The physical examination process lends itself to health teaching and opportunities to provide accurate information and correct misconceptions. Examples include reinforcing techniques for self-examination and having the client perform a return demonstration.

TERMINATING THE HEALTH ASSESSMENT

After completing the examination, close the client's gown or allow the client to dress (assist if needed) and to assume a comfortable position. Summarize findings in understandable terms. If a serious abnormality is found, consult with the client's health care provider or refer the client to another health care professional for further assessment after explaining the general nature of the abnormality and the need for further examination.

Discard disposable, used equipment and supplies according to agency protocol. Clean or restock equipment for future use.

RECORDING THE FINDINGS

Document physical examination findings using accurate, descriptive terms. Avoid vague, subjective terminology, such as "normal," "slight," "moderate," "healthy," or "poor," because they are easily misinterpreted. Strive to be objective, concise, clear, and thorough. However, it is better to err on the side of verbosity than to describe a significant finding vaguely or inadequately. A detailed recording is the baseline for comparison with future physical findings.

During the examination, briefly note abnormal findings for later retrieval and detailed documentation. This avoids interrupting the flow of the examination to record detailed observations. After the examination, combine normal and abnormal findings in the final document.

HEALTH ASSESSMENT, NURSING DIAGNOSIS, AND NURSING PROCESS

After collecting baseline data (the results of both the health history and the physical examination), summarize the client's health problems. Assess the areas of strength and health risk profile. Formalize and prioritize nursing diagnoses. Reexamine and validate the tentative diagnoses formulated after the health history interview in light of the physical examination findings.

Determine which health problems are nursing diagnoses and which are collaborative problems. Make referrals when indicated to ensure continuity of care and either resolution or effective management of the health problems.

DIAGNOSTIC ASSESSMENT

Diagnostic assessment refers to the various tests used to detect disease and to evaluate the nature and extent of disease. During diagnostic assessment, nursing responsibilities range from preparing a client, to interpreting test results, to determining whether a client requires immediate medical intervention. This section discusses the general nursing management of clients undergoing a variety of common laboratory, imaging, endoscopic, and cytologic diagnostic tests. Specific information about individual tests is found throughout the book.

GENERAL NURSING MANAGEMENT

Assessment

If a client is scheduled for a diagnostic test, you need to assess the client's ability to participate. Limitations in physical condition, sensory ability, psychological condition, and functional status can affect the successful performance of a diagnostic test. For instance, disorders of the cardiovascular or respiratory system may severely limit tolerance for required position changes. Sensory limitations (impaired hearing or speech) or mental impairment may interfere with the client's ability to understand or accomplish the test.

Assessment of self-care ability, mobility, and nutritional status can also help you determine the client's ability to participate in diagnostic testing. Clients with impaired mobility, restricted self-care ability, or nutritional deficits may require extra assistance or interventions before or during testing. If agitated or unable to lie still, for example, the client may need a sedative before undergoing a lengthy imaging test. Many imaging tests require the client to lie motionless for 30 minutes or more. For many tests, the client must have fasted for 6 to 8 hours; if the client does not follow directions for fasting, then the test is usually postponed.

Nursing Interventions

Independent nursing interventions commonly needed by clients undergoing diagnostic tests include (1) preparation based in part on your assessment of the client's ability to participate, (2) collection of data, (3) collection and transport of specimens and clients, (4) monitoring during diagnostic testing, and (5) supportive teaching. It is crucial to obtain adequate specimens (Box 4-8).

Interdependent nursing interventions commonly include (1) transcribing orders, (2) consulting with laboratory and radiology technicians, (3) sedating the client, and (4) interpreting test results to determine whether immediate action is required. Consider the underlying pathophysiologic status, current medical treatment, and laboratory result when assessing the need for immediate attention from a physician. For example, if a serum potassium level increases from 2.5 to 2.8 mEq/L, cardiac rhythm is stable, and 80 mEq of potassium is infusing in 1 L of intravenous fluid, you may notify the physician about the potassium level during usual rounds. In contrast, if the potassium level decreases from 2.5 to 2.0 mEq/L and the client has a flattened T wave and ventricular dysrhythmia, immediately notify the physician about the change in the client's status.

| **BOX 4-8** | *Obtaining Adequate Specimens* |

- Ensure confidentiality and privacy for the client.
- If a culture is required, obtain it before initiating antibiotics, if possible.
- Avoid contamination of the specimen with secretions or excretions from uninvolved areas.
- Collect the correct amount of fluid or tissue for the sample.
- Use the proper instruments and collection tubes or bottles.
- To avoid contamination, do not open the collection bottle until you have the specimen.
- Label all containers accurately. Include the name of the client, source of the specimen, and date and time collected.
- Deliver the specimen to the laboratory immediately or keep it at the recommended temperature.

SPECIFICITY AND SENSITIVITY OF DIAGNOSTIC TESTS

It would be ideal if all diagnostic (or screening) tests were 100% accurate. They are not. False-positive and false-negative results occur. Test effectiveness is evaluated by specificity and sensitivity.

Specificity is the ability of a test to correctly identify a person who is disease free. It equals the number of true-negative results divided by the sum of true-negative and false-positive results. A *false-positive* result indicates that a client has the disease or disorder being tested when he or she does not have that disease or disorder.

Sensitivity is the ability of a test to correctly identify a disease. Sensitivity equals the number of true-positive results divided by the sum of true-positive and false-negative results. A *false-negative* result indicates that a client does not have the disease or disorder being tested, when he or she does have that disease or disorder.

No test is 100% specific and 100% sensitive because of (1) limitations inherent in the test and (2) various factors that can affect all tests. For example, the antinuclear antibody (ANA) test is highly sensitive for detecting systemic lupus erythematosus but is not specific because clients with rheumatoid arthritis may also have positive ANA results. The closer a test is to 100% on both counts, the more reliable its results.

MEASUREMENTS USED TO REPORT LABORATORY TEST RESULTS

Reference Values

The term *reference value* (rather than "normal value") is used for reporting laboratory studies because different laboratories may produce different values. In addition, some tests (serum calcium level) have more than one accepted reference value.

Laboratory results may be influenced by several factors. The time of day, temperature, altitude, stress felt by the client, medications taken, and underlying disorder may all have an effect. When analyzing laboratory test results, consider all influencing variables.

International System of Units

A comprehensive modern form of the metric system is the *International System of Units,* commonly called the *SI system* (from its French name, Système Internationale d' Unités). The SI system provides a common international language for units of measurement. Meter and kilogram are used for length and weight. Moles are used to express amounts per volume. A *mole* is the quantity of a substance in grams that is equal to its molecular weight.

Most Americans are more familiar with mass concentration units (such as milligrams) than with moles, and the United States has been slow to adopt the SI system.

The rationale for changing to SI units is that biologic components react in vivo on a molar basis. Thus, moles offer a better understanding of the relative amounts of components of body fluids and of biologic processes and their interrelationships.

LABORATORY DIAGNOSTIC TESTING

Nurses perform diagnostic tests in many practice settings. Some tests can be delegated to assistive personnel, as discussed in the Management and Delegation feature on Performing Specimen Collection and Testing on p. 94. No matter who performs a test, an accurate outcome depends on correctly collecting the right specimen in the proper container at the proper time. Anyone performing a diagnostic test should do the following:

1. Carefully follow the instructions on test kits, and maintain the integrity of all test materials.
2. When necessary, protect the test materials from light and moisture.
3. Always check the expiration dates.

In addition to performing tests, you may be responsible for ongoing care of portable testing equipment. Equipment requires routine maintenance, quality assurance checks, and recalibration, just as in a full-scale diagnostic laboratory. Standardized specimens should be analyzed on a routine schedule according to the agency's quality control standards and those mandated by the American Society of Pathologists and the Joint Commission on the Accreditation of Healthcare Organizations. The reliability of test results depends on the accuracy of procedures and equipment and the integrity of test materials.

Microbiology Studies

Many microbiology studies can be used to identify infection-causing organisms—bacteria, viruses, fungi, and protozoa—and to guide treatment. Several tests can be performed to identify a specific microorganism:

1. A *smear* is a specimen that has been spread across a glass slide. It is examined under a microscope, usually after being stained.
2. A *stain* is the application of dye or a combination of dyes to help identify microorganisms. Gram's stain is a quick, commonly used method to identify general strains of bacteria by their color. Gram-positive organisms stain purple-black. Gram-negative organisms stain pink. Knowing whether a bacterium is gram-positive or gram-negative can assist in choosing an initial treatment until the specific bacterium is identified by culture.
3. A *culture* is the placement of microorganisms on culture plates to facilitate their growth. Afterward, the microorganisms can be isolated and identified. The culture process may take a few hours to several weeks, depending on the organism.

Sensitivity studies determine the type of antibiotic that will impede the growth of the organism. Small disks

MANAGEMENT AND DELEGATION

Performing Specimen Collection and Testing

Collection of the following specimens may be delegated to unlicensed assistive personnel:

Specimen	Procedure
Sputum	Culture and sensitivity testing
Urine	Routine urinalysis
	Urine electrolyte measurements
	24-hour urine collection
	Culture and sensitivity testing for clean-catch and indwelling catheter specimens
Stool	Culture and sensitivity testing

Testing of the following specimens may be delegated to unlicensed assistive personnel:

Specimen	Procedure
Blood	Bedside blood glucose monitoring
Urine	Test-strip (dipstick) analysis
	Specific gravity determination
Stool	Occult blood test

Delegation of the tasks listed above requires that you give instructions on the following topics:

• Type of specimen to be collected and collection container in which it should be placed
• Client label with the appropriate information required by your laboratory
• Specimen request form to accompany the specimen
• Proper method of recording blood glucose, urine test-strip analysis, specific gravity, and stool occult blood results

After initial orientation, the assistive personnel should demonstrate competence in the performance of these tasks. Describe any findings that assistive personnel should report immediately to you, such as blood glucose levels outside the range of 70 to 180 mg/dl, urine that looks cloudy or seems to contain sediment, and obvious evidence of blood in urine, sputum, or stool. Inability to obtain the specimen should also be reported immediately.

Note: Delegating the collection of blood specimens may be permitted in some institutions, in states whose practice acts permit this. This very specialized skill requires venipuncture training and competence beyond the scope of most unlicensed assistive personnel.

several antibiotics to which a microorganism is susceptible. The physician then chooses a treatment based on cost, adverse drug effects, and so on.

Culture and sensitivity tests are commonly performed together to both identify an infecting microorganism and to determine appropriate drug treatment. On a physician's order, these tests may be abbreviated as *C & S*.

Specimen collection and handling are common procedures that can increase the risk of disease transmission if they are done incorrectly. To help prevent disease transmission, wash your hands thoroughly and frequently, and wear appropriate personal protective equipment—especially gloves—whenever you could be exposed to a client's body fluids. Properly label specimens and place in plastic containers to reduce the risk of transmission to other personnel.

Blood Cultures

Normally, blood is sterile. If bacteria enter the bloodstream (*bacteremia*), they can cause severe infections. *Septicemia* is systemic disease caused by bacteria and their toxins in the blood. Blood cultures are commonly obtained from clients who have unexplained fever, a high risk of sepsis, or appear to be in septic shock.

To collect blood for culture, thoroughly clean the skin at the selected puncture site. Draw samples at specific intervals (30 minutes apart, for example) or draw a second specimen from the other arm. Blood samples may be examined for anaerobic or aerobic microorganisms. Ideally, blood culture specimens should be collected before antibiotic therapy begins or other blood samples are collected (if ordered at the same time).

If the client has already received an antibiotic, laboratory personnel can add certain enzymes to the growth medium to eliminate the activity of the antibiotic. Note on the laboratory request slip that the client is receiving an antibiotic. Once the specimen is obtained, the client should receive prescribed antibiotics and antipyretics.

Wound Cultures

Infection delays wound healing. Therefore, material from inside a wound may be obtained for culture to detect and identify microorganisms. Ideally, the specimen is collected using aseptic technique before the client receives an antibiotic. Additional precautions (wearing a mask, gown, and gloves) may be needed to collect specimens from draining wounds.

Culturettes (sterile, cotton-tipped applicators in special containers) are commonly used for collecting wound culture specimens; they should be used as follows:

1. Place the cotton tip deep into the wound without touching the surrounding skin.
2. Swab the wound where the purulent drainage is most profuse.

saturated with antibiotics are placed on the culture plate. In time, the culture is examined again. If the antibiotic stopped the growth of the microorganism, the microorganism is *sensitive* to the antibiotic; if the antibiotic does not halt the growth of the microorganism, the microorganism is *resistant* to it. Sensitivity reports typically list

3. Return the applicator to the holder and break the bottom of it to release the culture medium.

A syringe and needle can also be used to aspirate and transfer infectious material from a wound.

Note on the request slip which antibiotics the client is taking and the specific site from which the specimen was obtained. After collecting the specimen, administer antibiotics prescribed.

Urine Cultures

Normally, urine is sterile. However, urinary tract infection (UTI) is a common disorder. Women are susceptible to UTIs because of their short urethras. In addition, nosocomial UTI is a common sequela (consequence) of indwelling catheterization. The test used most often to detect bacteria in urine uses a *clean-catch* (or midstream) specimen. Clean-catch collection minimizes contamination of the specimen by organisms on the perineal skin. To obtain the specimen correctly, the client (1) cleans the perineum, (2) starts voiding, (3) stops voiding, (4) resumes voiding, then (5) catches the specimen in a sterile container.

As an alternative, a specimen may be collected from an indwelling catheter. Urine standing in the collection bag undergoes chemical changes, may be contaminated with bacteria, and does not reflect the client's current urinary status; as a result, it should never be used as a specimen. Instead, obtain a specimen from the catheter or drainage tubing. Avoid opening the drainage system to air, which might introduce microorganisms. Most urinary drainage systems have a self-sealing, covered specimen collection port built into the top of the drainage tubing. Clean this area, then aspirate the specimen with a sterile needle and syringe. You may need to clamp the tubing below the port for 15 to 20 minutes to allow enough urine to accumulate.

If there is no collection port and the catheter is not rubber-like silicone (Silastic), use a small 25-gauge needle and syringe to aspirate urine from the catheter itself. Using aseptic technique, insert the needle into the catheter distal to the sleeve leading to the balloon, slant the needle toward the drainage tubing, and make sure it does not enter the balloon lumen. Puncture the catheter at an angle to allow it to reseal after you withdraw the needle. This procedure cannot be performed with a Silastic catheter because it will not reseal after being punctured.

At times you may need to perform a straight catheterization to obtain a urine specimen for culture. Select a straight catheter of the smallest size. Insert it into the bladder under aseptic conditions, allowing urine to flow directly from the end of the catheter into the sterile specimen container. Some agencies provide special kits that include a catheter attached to a test tube. Only rarely are urine specimens collected by catheterization because the catheter may introduce organisms into the urinary tract.

Blood Studies

Blood may be collected by venipuncture, microcapillary collection, serial port sampling, and arterial blood sampling. Check your facility's laboratory procedures to review collection procedures, available equipment, biohazard disposal procedures, and standard precautions.

Venipuncture

The procedure for venipuncture is described in Box 4-9. Table 4-1 explains the various tubes, called Vacutainer tubes, used for drawing blood. The vacuum tubes fill automatically with blood. Before drawing a specimen, make sure that (1) the proper tube is selected and (2) specimens from one type of tube are not mixed with those from another tube. When cells are damaged, potassium leaks and platelets migrate. A concern is that multiple venipuncture attempts or contamination with EDTA (ethylenediaminetetraacetic acid, an anticoagulant) may distort serum potassium test results. Therefore, draw specimens for potassium measurements early and consider that abnormal serum potassium readings may result from multiple punctures or contamination. Specimens for vacuum collection tubes without additives should be drawn first to prevent contamination by samples from additive-containing vacuum tubes.

A suggested sequence of tubes to use for blood specimen collection to prevent contamination is as follows:

1. Microbiology culture specimen tubes
2. Tubes without additives (red, speckled, or gold top)
3. Citrate-containing tubes (blue top)
4. Heparin-containing tubes (green or dark blue top)
5. EDTA-containing tubes (lavender top)
6. Oxalate/fluoride-containing tubes (gray top)

When obtaining blood from a superficial hand vein, use a butterfly needle. Insert the needle and, after blood flashback is noted in the tubing, use a syringe or Vacutainer tube to withdraw blood from the vein.

Microcapillary Collection

Microcapillary blood collections may be used for a variety of purposes, including peripheral testing in clinics, for very young or very old clients, and for clients with skin disorders. The procedure for microcapillary collection is similar to that for venipuncture. The site of the skin puncture is usually the finger tip. (An ear lobe may be used for clients with edema.) No tourniquet is used.

Use the following procedure for microcapillary blood collection:

1. Hold the finger firmly.
2. Clean the area with povidone-iodine or 70% alcohol.

BOX 4-9   *Procedure for Venipuncture*

1. Check physician's request to verify test and time requested, client's name, and client's identification number.
2. Select materials needed: alcohol swabs, cotton or gauze swab, adhesive bandage, gloves, labels, needle, sharps container, tube holders, tourniquets, and Vacutainer tube or syringe (if using a butterfly needle).
3. Label Vacutainer tube with client's name and identification number, collection date and time, specimen source, and test.
4. Greet client, check test requested and client's name and identification number, and determine client's preparation for test. Wash your hands.
5. Place the client's arm in a position comfortable for the client and convenient for you. Support it on a firm surface. The client should be sitting or lying down.
6. Assemble the needle, needle holder, Vacutainer tube, alcohol swabs, cotton or gauze swab, and bandage. Take care not to engage the Vacutainer tube. Place any additional Vacutainer tubes in a convenient location. Use a 20- or 21-gauge, 1- to 1½-inch needle for antecubital veins.
7. Apply the tourniquet tightly enough to distend the veins but not so tightly that it cuts off circulation. Tell the client to open and close his or her fist several times and to keep it closed while you locate a vein. If it is difficult to locate a vein, wrap the arm in a warm compress to promote venous distention. You may use a blood pressure cuff to distend the veins; obtain a pressure between the client's systolic and diastolic readings. Remember that a tourniquet or blood pressure cuff should never remain on the client's arm for more than 1 to 2 minutes.
8. Choose the site. Try to locate the median cubital vein. Other acceptable veins are the cephalic and basilic veins. If hand veins are selected, use a 23- or 25-gauge needle.
9. Put on gloves. Clean the venipuncture site with 70% isopropyl alcohol by making outward concentric circles. Allow the site to air-dry or wipe with sterile gauze.
10. Anchor the vein by stretching the skin below the site with your thumb. Reassure the client that any discomfort will be brief. Insert the needle bevel-up into the vein, and engage the Vacutainer tube. The needle should be at about a 15-degree angle to the client's arm and directly in line with the vein. If multiple samples are needed, remove the tube as soon as the blood flow stops and insert the next tube into the needle holder. Once good blood flow is established and before the final tube is filled, release the tourniquet.
11. Remove the last Vacutainer tube from the needle holder. Remove the needle with a swift motion, and quickly apply clean cotton or gauze over the puncture site. Apply pressure, or ask the client to apply pressure to the puncture site. Properly dispose of the needle in the sharps container. (Do not lay down or recap the needle.) Immediately label the specimen. Remove your gloves, and wash your hands. Record the client's name, the test performed, disposition of the specimen, and any condition not meeting specimen collection criteria.

TABLE 4-1   *Tubes Used for Venipuncture*

Stopper Color	Principal Anticoagulant or Additive and Mode of Action	Commonly Used for
Red	None. Clot activator and gel separator enhances clot formation.	Cell/blood typing Serum blood group antibody testing; alkaline phosphatase; amylase; blood urea nitrogen (BUN); Creatine phosphokinase (CPK); calcium; cholesterol
Speckled	None.	Compatibility testing; drug monitoring; glucose; high-density lipoprotein (HDL); human immunodeficiency virus (HIV); iron profile; low-density lipoprotein (LDL)
Gold (Hemoguard)	None.	Liver enzymes; potassium; protein; rapid plasma reagin (RPR); sodium; triglycerides
Lavender	Ethylenediaminetetraacetic acid (EDTA) binds calcium.	Complete blood count (CBC); erythrocyte sedimentation rate (ESR); hemoglobin electrophoresis; platelet count; reticulocyte count; sickle cell screen; white blood cell differential
Blue	Sodium citrate binds calcium.	Activated partial thromboplastin time (aPTT); individual coagulation factor studies; fibrin degradation products (FDPs); fibrinogen; prothrombin time (PT)
Green	Heparin inactivates thrombin and thromboplastin.	Ammonia; chromosome screening; lupus erythematosus cell, preparation; HLA typing
Gray	Sodium fluoride oxalate binds calcium. Sodium fluoride inhibits glycolysis.	Glucose
Dark or royal blue	Heparin inactivates thrombin and thromboplastin.	Trace metals (e.g., lead)

Modified from Flynn, J. C., Jr. (1999). *Procedures in phlebotomy* (2nd ed.). Philadelphia: W.B. Saunders.

3. Use a microlance (instead of a needle and Vacutainer tube) to puncture the finger pad off-center and perpendicular to the fingerprint lines.
4. Wipe away the first drop of blood with sterile gauze because it contains plasma, which may affect the accuracy of results.
5. Place the hand in a dependent position, and allow the next drops to flow without squeezing. Use a microtube or pipette to collect the specimen.
6. After blood collection, maintain pressure on the puncture site until bleeding has stopped.

Serial Port Sampling

Serial port sampling refers to collection of blood specimens from an indwelling venous catheter. This method reduces the discomfort caused by multiple venipunctures. Preparation for serial port sampling is similar to that for venipuncture:

1. Stop the intravenous fluid flow.
2. After opening the stopcock or choosing the lumen, use a 10-ml syringe to aspirate 10 ml of blood from the indwelling catheter.
3. Discard the first sample.
4. Use another 10-ml syringe (or 20-ml syringe, depending on the number of tests) to aspirate the specimen.
5. Flush the indwelling line with saline and heparin according to agency protocol.
6. Return the stopcock to the original position and adjust the intravenous fluid rate as needed.

Arterial Blood Sampling

Blood is collected from an artery for blood gas analysis and, rarely, for other studies. The technique of *arterial blood sampling* is discussed in Chapter 61. Because this method raises a risk of bleeding and nerve injury, arterial blood sampling is performed only by staff with special training. Blood gas analysis is discussed in Chapter 15.

Urine Studies

Urinalysis

Urinalysis is one of the oldest and most common laboratory tests. It is economical and noninvasive, the specimen is easily obtained, and results are available quickly. Urinalysis yields a large amount of information about possible disorders of the kidney and lower urinary tract, and systemic disorders that alter urine composition. Normal urinalysis results can help exclude a number of alternative diagnoses (Table 4-2).

Urinalysis data include color, specific gravity, pH, and the presence of protein, red blood cells (RBCs), white blood cells (WBCs), bacteria, leukocyte esterase, bilirubin, urobilinogen, glucose, ketones, casts, and crystals.

TABLE 4-2	*Normal Findings in a Routine Urinalysis*
Component	**Normal Values**
Color	Pale yellow to deep amber
Opacity	Clear
Specific gravity	1.002-1.035
Osmolality	275-295 mOsm/L
pH	4.5-8.0
Glucose	Negative
Ketones	Negative
Protein	Negative
Bilirubin	Negative
Red blood cells	None to 3
White blood cells	None to 4
Bacteria	None
Casts	None
Crystals	None

Normal urine does not contain protein, bilirubin, urobilirubin, glucose, ketones, bacteria, or leukocyte esterase. A few RBCs, WBCs, casts, and crystals are normal (see Chapter 34).

A *random-specimen urinalysis* can be collected at any time. In general, an early morning specimen gives more definitive results because the urine is concentrated and is not influenced by diet. Generally, no specific client preparation is needed. Collect the urine in a clean container. This type of specimen cannot be used for culture and sensitivity tests because neither the container nor the collection technique is sterile.

12- or 24-Hour Urine Collection

A *timed collection of urine* allows for quantitative analysis of specific substances and is more accurate than a random one-time specimen. A 12- or 24-hour specimen is usually collected in one large container. A chemical preservative in the container and refrigeration during the collection process may be needed. If refrigeration is not available, place the specimen container in ice or in insulated ice packs. Replace the cooling agent frequently to maintain the specimen at the necessary temperature. If the client has an indwelling catheter, the bag can be placed on ice during the timed collection period.

When specimen collection begins, the client voids (or the urine collection bag is emptied) and this urine is discarded. All urine voided over the next 12 or 24 hours, as indicated, is placed in the container. After 12 or 24 hours from the time of the first voiding, instruct the client to void again (or empty the urine collection bag) and add this urine to the specimen. A major requirement during the collection process is careful communication among all persons involved. If any single urine specimen is inadvertently discarded, the entire procedure must begin anew. The client should also be instructed to moderately limit the amount of fluids consumed and to avoid alcohol. Other specific instructions may be needed, such as avoiding certain foods or medications.

DIAGNOSTIC IMAGING

Imaging refers to representations produced by radiography (x-rays), nuclear magnetic resonance, tomograms, ultrasound, radioisotopes, and so forth. Methods range from simple x-ray studies to complex and expensive imaging using magnetic fields and radiowaves. Review your facility's protocol, especially the guidelines for preparation and follow-up care. You may need to consult with the imaging (radiology) department to obtain written guidelines for preparation and postimaging care, or to coordinate multiple studies. For example, barium studies may make visualization for other abdominal tests impossible for up to 2 days.

Explain the procedure and answer questions. Many procedures may take up to an hour (follow-up x-ray studies are sometimes obtained 30 minutes after an injection). Suggest that the client void before the procedure, unless the bladder must be full for the procedure.

Radiography

Procedure

Radiography is the most widely used diagnostic procedure for the study of soft tissues and bones. A radiograph, commonly called an "x-ray," is an image of a negative on photographic film made by exposing the film to x-rays that have passed through the body. The energy of the x-rays is adjusted by varying the voltage in the x-ray tube. Because each part of the body absorbs some of the x-rays, variable amounts of exposure are needed for optimal results, depending on the body part being examined.

Tissue is called *radiopaque* when transmission of x-rays is partially blocked, such as by bone. Bone appears white on x-ray film. Tissues are *radiolucent* when they allow x-rays to penetrate. Lung is translucent and therefore appears dark on x-ray film. The images on x-ray films are two-dimensional, so that multiple views are often needed, such as anteroposterior (AP, front to back), posteroanterior (PA, back to front), lateral (LAT, from the side), or oblique (OBL, at an angle). Note the position of the x-ray view for proper interpretation; this information is usually recorded by the x-ray technician.

X-ray examinations are used to (1) establish the presence of a mobility or structural problem, (2) follow progress, and (3) evaluate treatment. Features shown by an x-ray study can help diagnose a suspected problem. For example:

- A radiopaque (rather than radiolucent) area in the lung, which may mean pulmonary edema, pneumonia, or a tumor (Figure 4-7)

FIGURE 4-7 A chest radiograph showing right middle lobe pneumonia *(arrow)*. The consolidation of lung tissue makes the area appear radiopaque.

- Alterations in normal contour or density of bones, as in fractures or osteoporosis (Figure 4-8)
- Changes in fat lines around soft tissues (with tumor or inflammation present, fat tissue is replaced by soft tissues)
- Enlargement in shadows produced by organs (an enlarged heart shadow possibly meaning an enlarged heart from heart failure or athletic activity)

Two potential risks from repeated exposure to radiation are genetic and somatic. The *genetic risk* involves changes in chromosomes. If a developing (first trimester) fetus is exposed to radiation, the chromosomes can mutate and the baby can be born with deformities; the eggs and sperm can be damaged by radiation, which may lead to deformities in future offspring.

Somatic changes occur in body tissues that receive excessive or repeated doses of radiation. The risks from radiation exposure are cumulative and therefore are potentially more dangerous to health care personnel than to clients. Side effects of the use of radiation for cancer treatment are discussed in Chapter 19.

Several safety measures are used to avoid exposure to x-rays. The walls in rooms in which x-ray machines are located are lined with lead. Lead-lined protection, such as aprons, eyeglasses, and thyroid shields, are used by imaging personnel. Maintaining adequate distance is

FIGURE 4-8 X-ray showing a right hip (arrow) fracture.

also important, and x-ray rooms have a protective divider for the technician. When x-ray studies are obtained outside the radiology department, less protection may be available. If you must remain with a client during an x-ray exposure, wear a lead apron. Other personnel should step outside the room during the exposure. Clients are given lead aprons to shield their reproductive organs (gonads). Radiology personnel also wear a film badge to monitor accidental exposure.

Preprocedure Care

Before the x-ray procedure, ask the client to remove any radiopaque objects (jewelry, belts, or metal buttons) and to wear a gown. Additional preparation depends on the type of study. The client may be asked to assume various positions so that x-ray films can be obtained from the most useful angles.

Because various positions may be difficult or painful and x-ray tables are hard, the client may need analgesia and other pain-relieving interventions before and after the x-ray study. Nursing care for the client having diagnostic imaging studies focuses on client preparation and follow-up care.

You may be asked to monitor a physiologically unstable client during an imaging procedure, in which case you need an oximetry monitor, a sphygmomanometer, a stethoscope, extra intravenous fluids, and an emergency cart. Note pertinent findings—such as the presence of a pacemaker or an artificial joint—on the x-ray request.

Postprocedure Care

Although special care is not usually needed after an x-ray procedure, in some instances specific postprocedure care is needed. Postprocedure care, when indicated, is discussed in the following sections.

Chest X-Rays

Chest x-rays may be obtained to detect pulmonary disease and the status of respiratory problems or trauma and to confirm the placement of an endotracheal or tracheostomy tube. Complete details are presented in Chapter 61. There is no specific follow-up care.

Plain Abdominal Films

A plain abdominal film—*flat plate* or KUB, which stands for *k*idney, *u*reter, *b*ladder—can reveal such abnormalities as tumors, obstructions, abnormal gas collections, and strictures. No follow-up care is needed for this study.

Skeletal X-Rays

When fractures are suspected, x-ray studies are ordered for the bones in question. Generally, the procedure is not painful unless the extremity has to be moved for positioning. Examples of some x-ray projections are:

- Waters' projection, a PA view of the skull to show the orbits and maxillary sinuses. If a cervical spine fracture is suspected, the physician orders a lateral cervical spine x-ray study instead.
- Towne's projection, an AP view demonstrating the occipital bone and facial structures, such as the zygomatic arch.
- Panoramic (sometimes called Panorex, from the name of a machine), a 180-degree view of the teeth and jaw.

Fluoroscopy

Fluoroscopy is a radiographic technique that permits direct observation of the body. The body part under examination is positioned between an x-ray tube and a fluorescent screen. X-rays pass through the body and project the targeted organs or bones onto the fluoroscopic screen as visual images. The benefit of fluoroscopy is that joint actions, organs, and entire body systems can be observed directly and dynamically (as they move). Radiopaque and radiolucent media enhance visualization.

Fluoroscopy can be used to monitor the progress of other diagnostic studies. For example, the progress of a radiopaque catheter can be observed as it is threaded through an artery or vein; or the progress of radiopaque barium can be seen as it is swallowed and moves through the GI tract.

Tomography

Tomography is a radiographic technique that produces images of body tissues in a single plane or slice. Sequential images are obtained by moving the x-ray tube as it projects views at varying levels of tissue depth. Tomograms can be static body-section radiographs or can be combined with reconstruction tomography, as in computed tomography (CT) and positron emission tomography (PET), which are discussed later in this chapter.

Contrast X-Ray Studies

Contrast studies use radiopaque media to enhance visualization of an organ system or tissue under study. Contrast media include barium and various dyes.

Upper Gastrointestinal Series. An upper GI series, also known as a *barium swallow,* permits radiologic visualization of the esophagus, stomach, and duodenum using fluoroscopy. It can aid in the detection of strictures, ulcers, tumors, polyps, hiatal hernias, and motility problems. A detailed discussion of the upper GI series and related client care is found in Chapter 30.

Lower Gastrointestinal Series. A lower GI series, which requires a barium enema, is performed to visualize the position, movements, and filling of the colon. Barium is instilled rectally, and radiographs are obtained with or without fluoroscopy. This test can aid in detecting tumors, diverticula, stenoses, obstructions, inflammation, ulcerative colitis, and polyps. See Chapter 34 for a detailed discussion of this procedure and related care.

Computed Tomography

Procedure

Computed tomography scans highlight differences in bone and soft tissue. The images are generated by computerized synthesis of x-ray data obtained in many different directions in a cross-sectional plane or slice. The computed data are assembled as three-dimensional images. CT is used to identify space-occupying lesions (masses) and shifts of structures caused by neoplasms, cysts, focal inflammatory lesions, and abscesses of the head, chest, abdomen, pelvis, and extremities (Figure 4-9). To distinguish normal tissue from abnormal masses, a contrast medium (dye) may be administered. The CT scan can be performed quickly, within 20 minutes, not including analysis.

Preprocedure Care

Before a CT scan, make sure that the client has given informed consent and answer any questions about the procedure. Explain that fasting usually is not required for a CT scan of the head, but ask whether or not the client becomes nauseated easily; if so, adjust food and fluid intake accordingly. For example, some clients prefer a light breakfast to reduce nausea and others prefer an empty stomach. Fasting is usually required for a CT scan of the abdomen. Explain that a contrast agent is commonly given. Because the contrast material is

FIGURE 4-9 Computed tomography scans are obtained at various cross-sections of the brain. The image in **A** illustrates the cross-section used for the scan shown in **B.**

iodine-based, ask about allergies to iodine or contrast dyes (Box 4-10).

If the CT scan is of the client's head, remove any objects from the hair (wigs, barrettes, earrings, hair pins) before the test begins. The client's hair should be combed smooth.

Explain the client's role during the scan. The client is positioned supine, and the body part to be scanned is placed into the doughnut-shaped ring of the scanner. The technician moves the table from a control room to direct the study to different areas. The client can expect to hear mechanical noises coming from the scanner. Some clients may feel claustrophobic during the test, but assure them that it is possible to communicate with the technician.

Emphasize that the client must remain still during the scan. If unable to comply, sedation or even general anesthesia may be required. If sedation is needed, tell the client to (1) avoid alcohol and caffeine on the day of the scan, (2) avoid eating for 2 hours before the scan, (3) arrange for someone to drive home after the scan, and (4) avoid driving for at least 12 hours after the scan.

Postprocedure Care

After the test, assess the client for reactions to the contrast agent, hematoma at the injection site, and the quality of pulses in the limb used for injection of the contrast agent. The client may resume normal activities unless additional diagnostic tests are planned. Tell the client to expect diuresis from the dye, and encourage drinking plenty of fluids to flush the dye and prevent nephrotoxic injury.

Magnetic Resonance Imaging

Procedure

Magnetic resonance imaging (MRI) is a noninvasive test that uses powerful magnetic fields and radiofrequency pulses to produce the image; therefore, the client is not exposed to ionizing radiation. The magnet in the scanner is 30,000 times more powerful than the earth's magnetic field. Consequently, this test cannot be performed if clients have pacemakers, metal implants, some types of ventilators, or embedded metal fragments, such as shrapnel (Box 4-11). The powerful magnet may move

---

BOX 4-10   *Use of Contrast Agents*

Certain disorders, such as tumors, are better visualized with the use of a contrast agent. Other disorders, such as bleeding and edema, can be seen better without a contrast agent. The use of contrast agents is potentially dangerous. They may irritate blood vessels, and some clients may have allergic reactions to them that, if left untreated, may develop into anaphylactic shock.

Preprocedure Care

Before a test involving a contrast agent, ask the client whether he or she has ever had an allergic reaction to contrast dye or iodine. Note the type of allergic response on the record; for example, "Client states that he developed hives when a dye was injected for another test." Some clients report allergies, but when asked to explain the reaction, they state that they "feel warm" when given the dye. This is a normal reaction, not an allergic one.

Some clients are given contrast agents even though they report a contrast allergy. To reduce the severity of the reaction, these clients are pretreated with an antihistamine or corticosteroids. Therefore do not assure the client with a reported allergy to dye that a contrast agent will not be given. Even if the client says that he or she has no history of allergy, watch for symptoms of an allergic reaction after injection of a contrast agent. Some anaphylactic reactions have occurred with the first dose of dye. Tell the client that it is normal to feel a hot, flushed sensation and metallic taste in the mouth when the dye is injected. Tell the client to report any difficulty breathing or itching to staff in the radiology department.

Postprocedure Care

After the procedure, the client can usually resume normal activities. Diuresis will occur shortly after the use of a contrast agent. If the client is able to do so, encourage drinking at least one glass of water or other liquid an hour after the procedure. Replacement fluid may be needed, and the client should be assessed for fluid balance. The fluid balance in clients with renal or cardiac disease should be assessed carefully after a series of tests requiring intravenous contrast agents.

Complications

Complications rarely occur with the use of contrast agents but include local and systemic allergic reactions, spasm, occlusion of the vessel by a clot, and bleeding at the injection site. Assess the affected limb for color, warmth, pulses distal to the injection site, bleeding or hematoma formation, and mobility.

Assess the client for clinical manifestations of an allergic reaction, including pallor, tachycardia, restlessness, sneezing, coughing, erythema, tachypnea, respiratory distress, facial flushing, urticaria, pruritus, hypotension, nausea, vomiting, headache, convulsions, flank pain, hematuria, and oliguria. Assess for these reactions after the dye is injected, because clients have experienced respiratory or cardiac arrest while undergoing x-ray study. Emergency equipment should always be available.

| BOX 4-11 | *Contraindications to MRI: Implanted Metal Objects** |

- Bullets if ferromagnetic (steel shotgun pellets)
- Cardiac pacemaker
- Implanted cardioverter defibrillator (ICD)
- Implanted drug infusion pump
- Intracranial aneurysm clips
- Metal fragments visible in the eye
- Pulmonary artery catheter
- Shrapnel

*Consult with the radiologist if in doubt.

FIGURE 4-10 A normal magnetic resonance image. This sagittal section shows the cerebrum, ventricles, cerebellum, and medulla.

these objects inside the client's body or may interfere with their function. MRIs also are not performed for pregnant clients.

When looking at an MRI study, the image is opposite to that of a CT scan: Bone appears black on an MRI scan and white on a CT scan (Figure 4-10). A contrast agent may be used to augment the images.

Preprocedure Care

Explain the purpose of the MRI scan, the sounds and sensations that the client will hear and feel during the examination, and the client's role during the test. Obtain informed consent.

Before the test, the client should remove all metal-containing objects (brassiere, jewelry, watch, and so on). Note the presence of any internal metal objects, such as a prosthesis or pacemaker for the physician. Intravenous fluid pumps need to be removed during the test. Special MRI-compatible monitoring devices, such as pulse oximeters and electrocardiogram leads, can be used.

The client can eat normally and take prescribed medication before an MRI scan of the head. When the scan involves the GI system, the client must fast for 6 hours before the procedure. Tell the client to lie still during the procedure, which can take from 60 to 90 minutes. Clients who are agitated or unable to remain motionless may require sedation before the scan (see sedation instructions under Computed Tomography: Preprocedure Care). If a contrast agent is planned, ask whether the client tends to become nauseated easily, and adjust the intake of food and fluids accordingly.

The client lies supine on a narrow, padded table. Because the scanner makes loud clanging noises, the client should wear earplugs or headphones. Some clients may feel claustrophobic during the test; assure them it is possible to communicate with the technician.

Postprocedure Care

After the test, the client may resume previous activities and diet. Tell the client to expect to experience diuresis

if a contrast agent was used for the MRI study (see instructions for CT).

Positron Emission Tomography

Procedure

PET scanning produces images of metabolic and physiologic function. PET scans have diagnostic value because the function of diseased tissue commonly differs from that of normal tissues. The client is given doses of strong radioactive tracers *(radionuclides)*, which emit signals to show their uptake and distribution. The images are formed by computer analysis of photons detected by annihilation of positrons emitted by the radionuclides (Figure 4-11). PET has three primary uses:

- To determine the amount of blood flowing into specific body tissues
- To reveal how adequately tissues use blood receptors, such as medications and neurotransmitters
- To measure blood flow, glucose metabolism, and oxygen extraction

PET is used in the diagnosis of stroke, brain tumors, and epilepsy, and to chart the progress of Alzheimer's disease, Parkinson's disease, head injury, schizophrenia, bipolar disorder, and cardiac hypoxemia.

Preprocedure Care

Explain the purpose of the test, the sounds and sensations that the client will hear and feel during the examination, and the client's role during the test. Obtain informed consent. In contrast to CT and MRI machines, the PET scanner is quiet. The client should fast for 4 hours before the scan. If the client is diabetic, it is preferred that the blood

FIGURE 4-11 A positron emission tomographic scan showing decreased metabolic activity after a seizure (noted as green areas on the scan).

glucose be below 150 g/dl. The client must remain motionless for about 45 minutes. An agitated client may require sedation. (See instructions for sedation under Computed Tomography: Preprocedure Care.)

Postprocedure Care
No special care is required after a PET procedure.

Angiography
Procedure
Angiography is a radiographic technique that uses a contrast agent to assess blood vessels and the flow of blood through them. A common form of angiography is coronary angiography, which determines the degree of obstruction in myocardial circulation (Figure 4-12). Angiography can also be used to outline veins (venography) or lymphatic vessels (lymphography). The terms angiogram and arteriogram are used interchangeably in practice.

Preprocedure Care
Before angiography, make sure the client understands the procedure and has given informed consent. Note any known allergies to contrast agents or iodine. Collect baseline assessment data: vital signs, quality and symmetry of pulses in the limbs, level of consciousness, speech patterns, and estimates of limb strength. The same assessments are made after the procedure. *A detailed baseline is crucial to accurate assessment of postprocedure changes.*

FIGURE 4-12 Coronary angiography shows stenosis, or narrowing *(arrow),* of the left anterior descending coronary artery. (From Braunwald, E. [2001]. *Heart disease: A textbook of cardiovascular medicine* [6th ed.]. Philadelphia: W.B. Saunders.)

In most facilities, the client is given nothing by mouth for 6 to 8 hours before angiography. Some facilities allow fluids to reduce the risk of dehydration and clotting. Follow your facility's protocol. The planned puncture site may be shaved.

Postprocedure Care
Decreased perfusion of the distal limb from hemorrhage or hematoma at the puncture site and an allergic reaction to the contrast agent are the two major complications that can develop after angiography. Assessment is crucial to their early detection. Follow your facility's protocol for postprocedure care. Usually, it consists of the following steps:

1. If the femoral approach was used, keep the leg immobile; tell the client not to flex the hip or leg for 12 hours. If the brachial approach was used, release the pressure dressing and apply an elastic bandage to the client's arm; the arm must remain straight. Limb movement can dislodge the clot at the puncture site and result in bleeding.
2. Monitor vital signs every 15 minutes for 2 hours, then hourly until stable. Review the manifestations of an allergic reaction (see Box 4-10).
3. Keep a sandbag on a femoral puncture site to maintain pressure on the site. Check puncture sites every 15 minutes for 2 hours, then hourly.
4. Monitor distal pulses every 15 minutes for 2 hours, then hourly until stable. Assess quality of the pulses and note capillary filling time. Notify physician if the quality of the pulse changes.
5. Expect diuresis, provide ample fluids, and keep a urinal or bedpan nearby.
6. Resume prescribed medications and usual diet.

Ultrasonography

Procedure

Ultrasonography (also called *ultrasound* or *echography*) uses high-frequency sound waves to depict soft tissues. Ultrasonography works on the same principle as sonar and radar. When ultrasound waves are directed into the body, they spread through the tissues. Because tissues differ in density, the sound waves are reflected (bounced back) in various ways in different tissues. The reflected waves are processed, shown as an image, and recorded.

Ultrasound can be used to assess many structures in the body, including the heart, great vessels, liver, gallbladder, pancreas, breast, uterus and ovaries, scrotum, kidney, and thyroid gland (Figure 4-13). It is commonly used in obstetrics to determine gestational age. There is no exposure to ionizing radiation during this test, and it is noninvasive.

Preprocedure Care

No special care is required before ultrasonography. Explain the purpose of the test and what to expect. A gel is applied to the skin, and a transducer (a device that changes reflected high-frequency sound to electrical energy) is moved on the skin surface above the target organ. The procedure is painless and fairly quick.

Sometimes a bowel preparation with laxatives is used for viewing the abdominal organs. The bladder must be full to view the uterus. The room lighting may need to be dimmed for the technician to see the oscilloscope.

Postprocedure Care

No special care is required after an ultrasound study.

FIGURE 4-13 Normal ultrasound series of right breast.

Radionuclide Imaging

Procedure

Radionuclides are radioisotopes (radioactive forms of some elements) or tracers that are used to visualize organs or regions that cannot be seen on plain films. Radioisotopes are treated the same as normal elements by living cells. Their radiation can be detected by suitable counters. Radionuclide studies may be used to diagnose disorders of the heart, thyroid, liver, brain, bone, kidney, spleen, pancreas, lung, and gallbladder.

Various isotopes are used because they concentrate in a target organ or body fluid. For example, thallium concentrates in the heart, whereas iodine concentrates in the thyroid. An artificial radioactive element (technetium) is used extensively. Technetium emits gamma radiation only and therefore is safer than other isotopes that emit more damaging radiation. When combined with pyrophosphate given intravenously, technetium is taken up by bone and the entire skeleton can be surveyed. This technique is helpful in detecting bone tumors (Figure 4-14). When combined with albumin, technetium concentrates in the lung and can be used to estimate pulmonary blood flow. It can also be used to investigate lesions in other organs and has largely replaced radioactive iodine for thyroid assessment.

Depending on the intended diagnostic purpose, a blocking agent may be administered before the radionuclide to prevent uptake by certain tissues. The blocking agent is not radioactive. For example, iodine is normally concentrated in the thyroid gland. When iodine-tagged radionuclides are used other than in thyroid studies, Lugol's solution is given to block the uptake of iodine-tagged radionuclides by the thyroid.

The radionuclide is administered orally or intravenously about 1 to 3 hours before the test to allow time for distribution. During this time, have the client drink extra fluids to clear the portion not taken up by the tissues. After the waiting period, the client is placed on a table and an imaging device records the activity of the emitted radiation.

Radioactivity may be increased or decreased in comparison with normal activity in the organ. Areas of decreased activity, called *cold-spot imaging*, usually indicate tissues that are functioning improperly. This is common when normal tissues have been replaced by tumor. Increased activity, called *hot-spot imaging*, may occur in tissues that are metabolically more active. For example, a diseased thyroid gland or bone infection may be detected by hot-spot imaging.

Preprocedure Care

Tell the client that the radionuclide contains very little radioactivity. If an abdominal scan is scheduled, the client may need an enema first. Make sure that the radionuclide test is scheduled before any tests that use iodinated contrast agents or barium. These substances block the exit of protons from radionuclides. This is especially important with radioactive iodine thyroid scans. The use of contrast agents for other studies can block uptake of radioactive iodine for months. Obtain informed consent.

Obtain the following information from the client:

- Age, weight, and height to calculate the amount of radioactive substance to be used
- Menstrual history to rule out pregnancy (pregnancy is a contraindication to many radionuclide studies)
- Breast-feeding status (breast-feeding is a contraindication to many radionuclide studies)

FIGURE 4-14 A technetium scan of the skeleton shows an area of increased radionuclide density on the right tibia that is a bone tumor. (From Walter, J.B. [1992]. *An introduction to the principles of disease* [3rd ed.]. Philadelphia: W.B. Saunders.)

- History of allergy
- Recent exposure to radionuclides
- Presence of internal prostheses that could block the view of the organ
- Current treatments, such as the need for oxygen, telemetry, or timed specimen collections

Postprocedure Care

Tell the client to drink extra fluids; otherwise, no special care is required.

ENDOSCOPY

Endoscopy is direct visualization of a body system or part by means of a lighted, flexible tube. This method is more accurate than radiologic examination because the physician can directly observe sources of bleeding and surface lesions and can determine the status of healing tissues. Arthroscopy, bronchoscopy, and gastrointestinal endoscopy are examples of this type of diagnostic technique.

Endoscopic procedures require signed consent. Provide complete client education to enhance cooperation. Tell the client not to drive a motor vehicle for at least 12 hours after endoscopy if sedation was used during the procedure. (See instructions for sedation under Computed Tomography: Preprocedure Care.)

Arthroscopy

Arthroscopy is an endoscopic examination of a joint. An arthroscope is a thin fiberoptic instrument that allows examination of various joints without need for a large incision. Biopsy specimens can be obtained, articular cartilage abnormalities assessed, loose bodies removed, and cartilage trimmed. Further discussion of arthroscopy is found in Chapter 27.

Bronchoscopy

Bronchoscopy is the passage of a lighted bronchoscope, either rigid or flexible, into the bronchial tree for diagnostic or therapeutic purposes. This procedure is discussed in Chapter 61.

Endoscopy of the Gastrointestinal Tract

Endoscopy of the upper GI tract consists of esophagoscopy and esophagogastroduodenoscopy (Figure 4-15). These procedures are useful for assessing acute or chronic GI bleeding, pernicious anemia, esophageal injury, dysphagia, substernal pain, and epigastric discomfort (see Chapter 30). Endoscopy of the lower GI tract consists of proctosigmoidoscopy and colonoscopy (see Chapter 33).

CYTOLOGIC STUDIES

Cytology is the study of the anatomy, physiology, pathology, and chemistry of the cell. One of the most common cytologic studies is a staining technique devel-

A   B

FIGURE 4-15 Endoscopy showing normal gastric mucosa (**A**) and normal duodenal mucosa (**B**).

oped by George Papanicolaou—the *Pap test,* which is used to detect malignant cells. Usually, this test is used to study vaginal or cervical cells. Sometimes it may be used for other tissue cells obtained easily by smearing or scraping, as from the mouth, genital tract, or anus.

Tissues not available for scraping must be obtained by *biopsy,* which is the removal of tissue for diagnostic study. The tissue removed must be (1) representative of the tissue in question, (2) large enough to be examined, and (3) kept intact until studied. Many times a fixative or refrigeration is used to prevent tissue decomposition. Some tissues are not placed in fixative, such as breast tissue to be analyzed for hormones.

Biopsy procedures are either closed or open.

Closed Biopsy

In a *closed biopsy,* no surgical incision is used. Examples include the following:

- *Needle aspiration biopsy.* A trocar or needle is inserted into the tissue. The aspirated cells are then examined. This technique is common for the biopsy of breast masses.
- *Stereotactic needle aspiration biopsy.* A three-dimensional view of the abnormal tissue is created. On the basis of the imaging results, a needle is inserted into the mass. The client must be able to remain motionless for 20 to 60 minutes while the coordinates are determined. This technique is used for biopsy of certain lung lesions.
- *Core needle biopsy.* A special needle cuts a specimen from tissues not in view. This technique is common for biopsy of the kidney, prostate, liver, lung, and thyroid gland.
- *Punch biopsy.* A small specimen is removed by means of a special instrument that pierces the organ directly or through the skin. This technique is commonly used for biopsy of the skin or the cervix.
- *Brush biopsy.* Cells and tissue fragments are removed by a stiff bristle brush. The brush is advanced into the target area through an endoscope. Areas sampled in this way are the renal pelvis and bronchus.

Open Biopsy

A surgical incision is needed for an *open biopsy.* There are two types:

- *Excisional biopsy.* The entire lesion and a margin of surrounding normal tissue are removed. This is the procedure of choice in most cases.
- *Incisional biopsy.* A selected part of the lesion is removed. This form of biopsy is commonly completed during endoscopic examination.

Sections

Procedure

Two methods are used to assess for malignant cells from tissue samples:

1. *Frozen sections* are used for rapid microscopic diagnosis. A thin slice of tissue is cut from the frozen specimen and examined. The procedure requires about 10 to 15 minutes. The pathologist can determine whether malignancy is present and whether the entire tumor has been removed by looking for a margin of tumor-free tissue.
2. *Permanent sections* require about 48 hours. The tissue is placed in a fixative and then examined. It can be stained to facilitate pathologic study.

Preprocedure Care

Before a biopsy, explain the purpose of the procedure and obtain informed consent. The client may express concern or anxiety about the possible results of the biopsy; be empathetic with the client and family. Some clients sign a permit that allows surgical excision of the mass if it is found to be malignant on frozen section. In these situations, perform a complete baseline assessment for postoperative comparison. Certain types of biopsy require the client's cooperation. For example, to reduce the risk of laceration during biopsy of the liver, the client is instructed to hold his or her breath.

Postprocedure Care

Postprocedure care varies with the type of biopsy done. If organs such as the liver, lung, or kidney are sampled, the client has a risk of bleeding, peritonitis, and pneumothorax. Tailor the specific interventions to match the client's needs. Guidelines for care are offered in assessment chapters throughout this book.

CONCLUSIONS

The health history is the first component of health assessment. The history constitutes the subjective data and guides thorough assessment of specific concerns or areas identified through health risk appraisal. The history can be recorded in many ways, such as through computerized database assessments or on paper. Although a thorough history may seem time-consuming, the data provided are crucial to fully understanding the client's special needs.

The physical examination is the second part of health assessment, following the health history, in which objective data are collected through inspection, palpation, percussion, and auscultation. Once all data are collected, compare the findings with known standards and make appropriate referrals, intervene, or provide health teaching.

Diagnostic testing is common in both hospital and ambulatory care settings. A growing number of tests are performed, processed, or both at the point of care rather than in a laboratory. Become familiar with the various tests on urine, blood, and other body fluids. In many settings, nurses collect these specimens. Understanding how to collect the specimen and knowing the client care needed before and after the procedure are important aspects of nursing management. Diagnostic assessment of organs mandates an understanding of the test and the proper scheduling of multiple tests to avoid losing time. In addition, most laboratories call or Fax results to the nurse, who is then responsible for determining whether the results warrant notification of the physician.

BIBLIOGRAPHY

1. Ackley, B.J., & Ladwig, G.B. (2002). *Nursing diagnosis handbook: A guide to planning care* (5th ed.). St. Louis: Mosby.
2. Ainslie, G., et al. (1998). Psychosocial history by automated self-report. *Federal Practitioner, 15*(3), 33-40.
3. Andrews, M.M., & Boyle, J.S. (Eds.). (2002). *Transcultural concepts in nursing care* (4th ed.). Philadelphia: Lippincott Williams & Wilkins.
4. Barry, P.D. (1996). *Psychosocial nursing: Care of physically ill patients and their families.* Philadelphia: Lippincott Williams & Wilkins.
5. Bozzo, J. (1999). Databases and nursing outcomes. *American Journal of Nursing, 99*(4), 22.
6. Bickley, L.S., & Szilagyi, P.G. (2003). *Bates' guide to physical examination and history taking* (8th ed.). Philadelphia: Lippincott Williams & Wilkins.
7. Carr, M.W., & Grey, M.L. (2002). Magnetic resonance imaging: Overview, risks, and safety measures. *American Journal of Nursing, 102* (12), 26-33.
8. Carson, V.B. (1999). *Spiritual dimensions of nursing practice* (2nd ed.). Philadelphia: W. B. Saunders.
 9. Centers for Disease Control and Prevention (2002). Recommended childhood immunization schedule—United States, 2002. *Morbidity and Mortality Weekly Report, 51*(02), 31-33.
10. Chernecky, C.C., & Berger, B.J. (2001). *Laboratory tests and diagnostic procedures* (3rd ed.). Philadelphia: W. B. Saunders.
10a. Chobanian, A., et al. (2003). The seventh report of the Joint National Committee on Prevention, Detection, Evaluation, and Treatment of High Blood Pressure: The JNC 7 Report. *Journal of the American Medical Association, 289*(19), 2560-2572.
11. Clark, C.C. (2000). *Integrating complementary health procedures into practice.* New York: Springer.
12. Cook, L. (1999). The value of lab values. *American Journal of Nursing, 99*(5), 66-75.
13. D'Avanzo, C.E., & Geissler, E.M. (2003). *Pocket guide to cultural assessment* (3rd ed.). St. Louis: Mosby.
14. Edelman, C., & Mandle, C. (Eds.). (2002). *Health promotion throughout the life span* (5th ed.). St. Louis: Mosby.
15. Flynn, J.C. (1999). *Procedures in phlebotomy* (2nd ed.). Philadelphia: W. B. Saunders.
16. Fuster, V., et al. (Eds.). (2001). *Hurst's the heart* (10th ed.). Philadelphia: Lippincott Williams & Wilkins.
17. Giger, J., & Davidhizar, R. (Eds.). (1999). *Transcultural nursing: Assessment and intervention* (3rd ed.). St. Louis: Mosby.
18. Gordon, M. (1994). *Nursing diagnosis: Process and application* (3rd ed.). St. Louis: Mosby.
19. Halpern, N.A., & Brentjens, T. (1999). Point of care testing informatics: The critical care–hospital interface. *Critical Care Clinics, 15*(3), 577-591.
20. Huff, R.M., & Kline, M.V. (Eds.). (1999). *Promoting health in multicultural populations: A handbook for practitioners.* Thousand Oaks, CA: Sage.
21. Jarvis, C. (2000). *Physical examination and health assessment* (3rd ed.). Philadelphia: W. B. Saunders.
22. Jastremski, C.A. (1999). Nursing informatics: Issues for critical care medicine. *Critical Care Clinics, 15*(3), 563-576.
23. Leasia, M.S., & Monahan, F.D. (2002). *A practical guide to health assessment* (2nd ed.). Philadelphia: W. B. Saunders.
24. Malarky, L.M., & McMorrow, L.M. (2000). *Nurse's manual of laboratory tests and diagnostic procedures* (2nd ed.). Philadelphia: W. B. Saunders.
25. Norred, C.L., Zamudio, S., & Palmer, S.K. (2000). Use of complementary and alternative medicines by surgical patients. *AANA Journal, 68*(1), 13-18.
26. North American Nursing Diagnosis Association (NANDA). (2003). *Nursing diagnoses: Definitions and classification, 2003-2004.* Philadelphia: Author.
27. Pagana, K.D., & Pagana, T.J. (2002). *Mosby's manual of diagnostic and laboratory tests* (2nd ed.). St. Louis: Mosby.
28. Pender, N.J. (2002). *Health promotion in nursing practice* (4th ed.). Upper Saddle River, NJ: Prentice-Hall.
29. Purnell, L., & Paulanka, B. (1998). *Transcultural health care: A culturally competent approach.* Philadelphia: F.A. Davis.
30. Rahe, R.H. (1975). Life changes and near-future illness reports. In L. Levi (Ed.), *Emotions: Their parameters and measurement.* New York: Raven Press.
31. Rochman, R. (2000). Are computerized patient records for you? *Nursing, 30*(10), 61-62.

32. Rutenberg, C.O. (2000). Telephone triage. *American Journal of Nursing, 100*(3), 77-81.

33. Seidel, H.M., et al. (1999). *Mosby's guide to physical examination* (4th ed.). St. Louis: Mosby.

34. Society of Actuaries and Association of Life Insurance Medical Directors of America. (1983). *Metropolitan Life Insurance Co. build study.* New York: Author.

35. Spector, R.E. (2000). *Cultural diversity in health and illness* (5th ed.). Upper Saddle River, NJ: Prentice-Hall.

36. Staggers, N., Thompson, C.B., & Snyder-Halpern, R. (2001). History and trends in clinical information systems in the United States. *Journal of Nursing Scholarship, 33*(1), 75-81.

37. Strub, R.L., & Black, F.W. (2000). *The mental status examination in neurology* (4th ed.). Philadelphia: F.A. Davis.

38. Swartz, M.H. (2002). *Textbook of physical diagnosis: History and examination* (4th ed.). Philadelphia: W. B. Saunders.

39. U.S. Department of Health and Human Services. (1998). *Clinician's handbook of preventive services* (2nd ed.). Washington, DC: U.S. Government Printing Office.

40. Warner, P.H., Rowe, T., & Whipple, B. (1999). Shedding light on the sexual history. *American Journal of Nursing, 99*(6), 34-40.

41. Wilson, S.F., & Giddens, J.F. (2001). *Health assessment for nursing practice* (2nd ed.). St. Louis: Mosby.

42. Zoorob, R., & Morelli, V. (Eds.). (2002). Alternative therapies. *Primary care: Clinics in Office Practice, 29*(2).

Complementary and Alternative Therapies

Mark Moyad
Jane Hokanson Hawks

Complementary and alternative medicine (CAM) has received an enormous amount of attention around the world over the past decade. Nurses need to be well informed about various CAM modalities that clients might be using because of the increased interest in CAM as well as less restrictive regulation of many products. Many clients are afraid to disclose their use of herbs and other CAM therapies. In addition, many clients who use prescription drugs concurrently with CAM therapies could face possible health risks as a result of adverse reactions. A well-informed, nonjudgmental nurse is able to instill trust and gain an accurate picture of the client's CAM use as well as provide valuable information about safety issues.

This chapter begins with an overview of CAM. The second part of the chapter discusses a few issues and regulations that could aid the health professional in understanding CAM. A partial list of CAM therapies appears next and is followed by an explanation of the CAM boxes that appear throughout the book. CAM therapies to be assessed specifically related to disorders are identified in each assessment chapter of the book.

COMPLEMENTARY, ALTERNATIVE, AND INTEGRATIVE THERAPIES

Complementary and alternative medicine is defined by the National Center for Complementary and Alternative Medicine (NCCAM) as a group of diverse medical and health care systems, practices, and products that are not presently considered part of conventional medicine.[16] The NCCAM branch of the National Institutes of Health (NIH) was established in 1998 to ensure high-quality scientific research into CAM practices, to conduct and support basic and clinical research on CAM modalities, and to provide information about CAM to health care providers and consumers.[9,16,21]

According to the NCCAM,[21] complementary and alternative therapies are not the same. *Complementary* medicine is used *together with* conventional medicine. *Conventional medicine* is defined by NCCAM as medicine practiced by holders of M.D. (medical doctor) and D.O. (doctor of osteopathy) degrees and by allied health professionals, such as nurse-practitioners or advanced-practice nurses, registered nurses, physical therapists,

TABLE 5-1	*Five Types or Classifications of CAM Therapies*
Classification	**Description**
Alternative medical systems	Alternative medical systems are built on complete systems of theory and practice. Homeopathic and naturopathic medicine are examples that have developed in Western cultures. Examples of systems that have developed in non-Western cultures include traditional Chinese medicine and Ayurveda.
Mind-body interventions	Mind-body medicine uses a variety of techniques designed to enhance the mind's capacity to affect bodily function and manifestations. Some techniques that were considered CAM in the past have become mainstream (e.g., client support groups and cognitive-behavioral therapy). Other mind-body techniques are still considered CAM, including meditation, prayer, mental healing, and therapies that use creative outlets such as art, music, or dance.
Biologically based therapies	Biologically based therapies in CAM use substances found in nature, such as herbs, foods, and vitamins. Some examples include dietary supplements, herbal products, and the use of "natural" but scientifically unproved therapies such as shark cartilage to treat cancer.
Manipulative and body-based methods	Manipulative and body-based methods in CAM are based on manipulation or movement of one or more parts of the body. Some examples include chiropractic or osteopathic manipulation and massage.
Energy therapies	Energy therapies involve the use of energy fields. Biofield therapies are intended to affect energy fields that purportedly surround and penetrate the human body. The existence of such fields has not yet been scientifically proven. Some examples include qi gong, Reiki, and therapeutic touch. Bioelectromagnetic-based therapies involve the unconventional use of electromagnetic fields such as pulsed fields, magnetic fields, or alternating current or direct current fields.

Data from National Center for Complementary and Alternative Medicine (2003). *What is complementary and alternative medicine (CAM)?* Retrieved October 21, 2003, from http://nccam.nih.gov/health/whatiscam/index.htm; and Hawks, J., & Moyad, M. (2003). CAM: Definition and classification overview. *Urologic Nursing, 23*(3), 221-223.

and psychologists. Other terms for conventional medicine include allopathy; mainstream, Western, orthodox, and regular medicine; and biomedicine. Some conventional practitioners are also practitioners of CAM. An example of a complementary therapy is using aromatherapy to help lessen a client's discomfort following surgery.[9,21]

Alternative medicine is used *in place of* conventional medicine. An example of an alternative therapy is using a special diet to treat cancer instead of undergoing surgery, radiation, or chemotherapy that has been recommended by a practitioner of conventional medicine such as an oncologist.[9,21]

Integrative medicine *combines* mainstream medical therapies and CAM therapies for which there is some high-quality evidence of safety and effectiveness. Nurses often combine therapies when they use massage, touch, distraction, and relaxation techniques in addition to traditional use of analgesics for pain such as postoperative pain, cancer pain, and chronic pain control for clients.[9,21]

The major categories or domains of CAM therapies are described in Table 5-1.[9,21]

WHY DO PEOPLE CHOOSE ALTERNATIVE THERAPIES?

Several factors have contributed to the increasing interest in CAM modalities.[9] Lazar and O'Connor (1997) cite high personal involvement in decision-making and the hope for gaining therapeutic benefit as the two main reasons why clients choose CAM therapies. See Box 5-1 for other reasons.[9,13,21] All these factors contribute to the increased interest in CAM modalities.

Almost 50% of the population in the United States has used CAM at some point.[3,9] In fact, more visits to alternative-medicine practitioners have occurred recently compared with total visits to all primary care providers. Internationally, widespread prevalence of these therapies has been reported. For example, in parts of Europe and Australia, more than 50% of the population have used CAM.[3,9,15] The most rapidly growing area of CAM is the use of dietary supplements (herbs, vitamins, minerals, and other compounds).[3] Currently more than 20,000 herbal and related compounds or products are being sold or used in the United States alone.[26] Sales of dietary

BOX 5-1	*Factors Affecting the Use of Alternative Therapies*

- Desire for control over decision-making
- Hope to gain therapeutic benefit
- Desire to avoid toxicities, invasiveness, or other qualities of conventional treatments
- Need to control undesirable side effects of conventional therapies
- Preference for natural over synthetic medications
- Dissatisfaction with attitudes and practitioners of conventional medicine
- Failure to determine diagnosis
- Failure of conventional therapy
- Chronic illnesses with poor prognosis
- Acute or chronic conditions for which conventional treatments are lacking or disappointing
- Healing system that is part of a client's cultural or identity-group heritage
- Reduced insurance coverage
- Restraints on access to health care
- Increased costs of prescriptions and services
- Increased interest in preventive strategies and holistic approaches to health such as eating a more nutritionally sound diet, maintaining fitness, and reducing stress

BOX 5-2	*Methods to Facilitate Discussion of CAM Therapies*

- Give permission for clients to raise the topic and ask questions.
- Ask, in every history and physical examination, "What else are you doing to care for your health?"
- Listen for nondisclosing cues or references that may represent a client's efforts to "test the waters" without making full disclosure.
- Become familiar with local patterns of use.
- Be frank about what you do not know.
- Seek more information from clients and other sources such as the NCCAM website (http://nccam.nih.gov/health).
- When asking clients about medications, ask specifically about any supplements or herbs.

Data from Hawks, J., & Moyad, M. (2003). CAM: Definition and classification overview. *Urologic Nursing, 23*(3), 221-223; Lazar, J., & O'Connor, B. (1997). Talking with patients about their use of alternative therapies. In J. Randall, & J. Lazar (Eds.), *Primary Care: Complementary and Alternative Therapies in Primary Care, 24*(4), 669-714.

supplements have increased substantially, from $8.8 million in 1994 to almost $16 billion in 2002.[15]

ROLE OF THE NURSE

The nurse is often the health care provider who obtains a health history from the client and has the responsibility for initiating the discussion about the use of CAM modalities.[9] As the initiator, the nurse establishes a respectful and open communication environment in which the client feels safe and welcome to speak freely. Questions related to CAM use should be asked with each interaction because the client's interest in CAM might change over time or could vary with changes in the client's health status or that of other members of their family or social network.[9,13] Box 5-2 outlines guidelines for initiating a discussion about CAM with clients.[9,13] Nurses have a responsibility to educate clients about possible adverse reactions, to provide information from the NCCAM, and to teach lifestyle-modification behaviors (such as nutritionally sound diet, weight-loss strategies, stress-reduction strategies, exercise and fitness) that could prevent the development of acute or chronic problems.[9,24,25,28]

Issues related to regulation, quality, safety, and efficacy should be considered when discussing CAM with clients.[5,9] Many herbal products in the United States are considered dietary supplements and thus are not regulated as medicines and not required to meet the standards for drugs specified in the Federal Food, Drug, and Cosmetic Act. Quality of products from available product information should be screened and information gathered about the manufacturer, the composition and storage of the product, and its correct and safe use.[5,9]

Contrary to popular belief, herbal remedies and dietary supplements can pose health risks because of adverse reactions or interactions with prescribed drugs. Only a fraction of the thousands of medicinal plants used worldwide has been tested in randomized, controlled trials, many of which involved nurse researchers.[9] Further study is warranted for many commonly available products. Many of these issues are discussed in more detail in the next section.

It is important for the nurse to know that dietary supplement and herb manufacturers are not held to the same strict standards as are manufacturers of pharmaceuticals. Herb manufacturers are not required by law to demonstrate the safety, efficacy, or quality of their products. Therefore chemical analysis of samples labeled as the same product, but purchased from various suppliers, has revealed wide variations in quality and chemical content.[9,21] This lack of regulation is likely to continue.

As a result of the increased interest in CAM, nurses are encountering increasing numbers of clients who are using one or more of the "nontraditional" methods that constitute CAM.[9] Clients may self-medicate with a host of CAMs. Some clients will not realize that these products can interfere with prescribed medication, anesthesia, or surgery. Other clients may sense "feelings of disbelief" by practitioners about the effectiveness of CAM modalities and thus not disclose their use. Because of these differing perceptions, certain issues must be considered when discussing CAM therapies with clients.

ISSUES RELATED TO DISCUSSING COMPLEMENTARY AND ALTERNATIVE THERAPIES WITH CLIENTS

1. **Realize the impact of the U.S. 1994 Dietary Supplement Health and Education Act (DSHEA) and that some dietary interventions/supplements may gain U.S. Food and Drug Administration (FDA) approval to advertise a health benefit.** Both Houses of Congress and President Clinton easily approved the DSHEA in 1994, and it basically allowed manufacturers to regard almost any compound as a "supplement."[15,27] These rules apply specifically to the labels of dietary supplements and prevent manufacturers from making unsubstantiated claims that their supplement treats, cures, mitigates, diagnoses, or prevents a disease. Therefore manufacturers can only make a general claim and no specific claims on the supplement bottle. For example, a company could state "promotes circulation health" on a vitamin E bottle, but they cannot claim something specific such as "lowers low-density lipoproteins (LDL)." Some manufacturers, however, have been guilty of outrageous claims on Internet sites or in other promotional material because the ruling applies only to bottle labels. See the Complementary and Alternative Therapy feature on Internet Marketing of Herbal Products, below.

COMPLEMENTARY AND ALTERNATIVE THERAPY

Internet Marketing of Herbal Products

The largest review of websites advertising and selling nutritional supplements was recently analyzed by researchers. A total of 443 websites were evaluated in this study. Interestingly, a total of 81% of the retail websites made one or more health claims, and 55% of these sites claimed to treat, prevent, diagnose, or cure specific diseases. More than 50% of the websites with a health claim omitted the standard federal disclaimer. This is a big concern because consumers may be misled by vendors' claims that herbal supplements can affect diseases, despite regulations by the government prohibiting such claims. Health professionals need to be aware of the widespread and easily accessed information. Obviously, more regulation by the government is needed.

Reference

Data from Morris, C., & Avorn, J. (2003). Internet marketing of herbal products. *Journal of the American Medical Association, 290,* 1505-1509.

The main problem with the DSHEA ruling of 1994 is that it places the actual burden of proof on the U.S. federal government.[27] Hence, even when false claims are made without any medical research or evidence, the U.S. government must prove that the claim is actually false, which is contrary to the situation for pharmaceutical manufacturers, who must prove that their product is safe and effective. Reasons why Congress should pass such an act that virtually allows free reign to one group and tight restrictions to another include the following: (1) a large proportion of Congressional men and women or their spouses used dietary supplements; (2) the large lobby group of the supplement industry has enough clout to influence the rules; and, finally, (3) Congress took a "how can it hurt" approach.[15] Regardless of the reasons, the DHSEA ruling is one of many rulings that is partially responsible for the current situation.

Interestingly, a recent large-scale survey suggests that people in the United States do not believe that conventional health practitioners know much about supplements and are probably biased against them.[3] Most participants surveyed, however, also favored the following: (1) increasing government regulation of supplements to determine whether claims are accurate; (2) allowing the FDA to evaluate the safety of new dietary supplements before they are marketed; and (3) increasing the overall authority of the FDA to eliminate supplements found to be unsafe.

2. **Realize that the 1994 DSHEA did not apply to food manufacturers and what they may be able to claim or not claim.** In the past, food manufacturers were not given as free a reign as the dietary supplement manufacturers. It was difficult to get foods passed as potential sources of health unless clinical evidence existed to support the use of the food product for health. A new ruling directed by the FDA, however, should have a profound influence on what the public will see on future food labels.[15] Food companies now can make health claims on labels if most of the scientific evidence supports a benefit. The FDA claims that the new ruling may promote better education and guidance for a public that wants to eat healthier. Regardless, if a company exceeds the boundaries of a health claim, the FDA has a right to remove the health claim. A recent example is that companies that sell tomato products claim that these products may reduce the risk of prostate cancer.[15] The claim is allowed because some epidemiologic evidence supports a lowering of prostate cancer risk with tomato products.[8] The public can expect hundreds of these claims to appear on food labels in the next few years.

3. **Realize that other government rulings play a role in which of the dietary supplements are available for purchase.** Currently, numerous anabolic steroids are

available for over-the-counter (OTC) purchase. Hormone precursors such as dehydroepiandrosterone (DHEA) and androstenedione (Andro) are two popular supplements. These estrogen or testosterone precursors demonstrated an ability to change hormone levels dramatically in men and women of various age groups. DHEA and Andro have caused dramatic reductions in high-density lipoproteins (HDL, or "good cholesterol") in some studies. These supplements are available for purchase because of the passage in 1990 of Anabolic Steroid Control Act.[27] This act requires all four of the following criteria to be met for the removal of any anabolic dietary supplement: (1) the molecular structure is related to testosterone; (2) its pharmacology action is related to testosterone; (3) the substance cannot be an estrogen, progestin, or corticosteroid; and (4) it cannot promote muscle growth.

Andro and DHEA have a molecular structure and pharmacology related to testosterone and are not an estrogen, progestin, or corticosteroid. These supplements are still available for purchase because they have not been shown to promote muscle growth in past clinical trials using small dosages. It is possible that they promote this kind of muscle growth when greater dosages are used, but these trials have not been initiated. Therefore under federal law, companies are allowed to sell these types of supplements even though they may be harmful.

4. **Realize the importance of the placebo effect.** Randomized, controlled trials are generally considered the standard for determining causality.[4] Some studies use a placebo group when justified. Otherwise, studies use the standard treatment as the comparison group.

A placebo is a chemically inert substance that is administered in the same manner as the chemical or substance being studied. A placebo effect suggests that the persons being treated with the placebo experienced an improvement in their condition as the result of psychological or other factors rather than because of the inert substance administered. The results of drug studies that do not use placebos are always subject to doubt because the proportion of the effect that is attributable to psychological factors and the proportion that is caused by the drug cannot be determined.[6] The first article on the placebo effect was published by Pepper in 1945.[17] Ten years later Beecher proposed that about one third of clients in clinical trials experience a placebo effect.[2]

Although later studies demonstrated the placebo's dramatic effect when studying some conditions,[23] the one-third response may be an inadequate oversimplification for research studies today. Currently many conditions have demonstrated that objective evaluations (with serum and imaging tests) demonstrate little if any placebo response. For example, drugs that

use only objective evaluation (serum studies) for the assessment of benefits tend to have little to no placebo response. Statin drugs (HMG-CoA reductase inhibitors) have become the primary and standard prescription medications for the reduction of elevated cholesterol levels in men and women.[12] Because of the increasing number of FDA-approved statins, the drugs tend to be compared with each other in randomized trials.

Nevertheless, a few placebo comparisons with statin drugs have been completed. A study of more than 6500 men with a mean age of 45 to 64 years of age and an average cholesterol level of 272 mg/dl were assigned to take pravastatin (Pravachol) or placebo.[20] The average follow-up for this trial was almost 60 months. Pravastatin decreased plasma cholesterol by 20% and LDL by 26%; however, no change was observed in the placebo group. Another study of a variety of dosages of atorvastatin (Lipitor) was completed after only 6 weeks in 65 clients.[19] People receiving atorvastatin experienced mean decreases in LDL cholesterol of 37%, 42%, 50%, 52%, and 59% at dosages of 10, 20, 40, 60, or 80 mg once daily. The placebo group had an actual 0.3% increase in LDL after this same tested period. Finally, a study of atorvastatin (Lipitor), lovastatin (Mevacor), pravastatin (Pravachol), simvastatin (Zocor), and placebo was recently conducted for 24 weeks in type 2 diabetic clients with elevated cholesterol.[7] Reductions in LDL cholesterol of 21% to 37% were demonstrated with drug treatment compared with 1% with placebo. Reductions in total cholesterol of 18% to 29% were observed compared with 1% with placebo. Increases in HDL of 3.2% to 7.4% also were observed compared with an actual slight decrease (0.5%) in the placebo group. Therefore treating certain conditions and evaluating them objectively over a short or long period do not seem to demonstrate any benefit for some placebo groups; cholesterol-lowering trials with statin drugs are an example of this general observation.

Subjective improvements or self-evaluations tend to have greater placebo responses for conditions such as depression, hair loss, benign prostatic hyperplasia, and sexual dysfunction.[11,14,15] It is not unusual to observe a 25% to 50% placebo response rate in some studies. In other words, a fourth to half of clients taking a sugar pill claim a response that is equivalent to the drug itself, although these clients did not know they were taking a placebo. Some of the best-selling supplements in the United States today are for conditions that have enormous placebo response rates.[15]

Dietary supplements and herbal medications are enjoying an increasing amount of popularity and use, but more randomized trials are needed in this discipline before certain supplements can be recommended.[4] With more people seeking some relief from a specific condition with a CAM, it is important for nurses to explain to clients the need for further research before the effects of many CAM modalities are known.[15]

5. **Realize that at least 30% of all modern drugs are actually derived from plants.** A partial list of some common drugs that are derived from plants is found in Table 5-2.[26] Therefore the potential exists for numerous herbal medicines to have some role in our current health care system. The lack of randomized trials for most herbal products makes it difficult for health care professionals currently to recommend or not recommend many herbal products. Nurses need to emphasize this when discussing CAM modalities with clients.

6. **Be careful about using the word *antioxidant* to describe any dietary supplement.** Many people refer to dietary supplements as antioxidants; however, this is a myth because no supplement is actually a pure antioxidant.[10] Vitamins C, E, and beta-carotene are redox agents. This means that in some situations (food) they are antioxidants, but in other circumstances, when given in higher doses, they can act as pro-oxidants. Pro-oxidants can produce millions if not billions of harmful free radicals and can be harmful in some situations. In the Alpha Tocopherol, Beta-Carotene Cancer (ATBC) Prevention Trial published initially in 1994, researchers found that beta-carotene supplements were associated with 18% more lung cancer in smokers versus placebo.[22] This was a randomized, double-blind, placebo-controlled, primary prevention trial comparing daily supplementation with vitamin E, beta-carotene, both, or placebo in more than 29,000 Finnish male smokers. This trial demonstrated that neither vitamin supplement prevented lung cancer, but beta-carotene may have increased the risk. All-cause mortality was also not affected. This trial demonstrated the potential pro-oxidant effect of certain supplements in certain clients. Therefore a diet study is not necessarily tantamount to a dietary supplement study and vice-versa.

Antioxidant vitamins in food are balanced biochemistry. They are part of a mixture of redox agents, partly in reduced form and partly in oxidized form. In addition, these foods contain hundreds of other phytochemicals,[10] which is why a balanced, diverse, and moderate diet of healthy foods and beverages makes the most sense unless a clinical trial suggests otherwise. This important point should be discussed with clients who believe that if they consume a vitamin C pill it might be an adequate substitute for certain fruits and vegetables high in vitamin C.

7. **Realize that although numerous studies of alternative medicines have failed to demonstrate a benefit, numerous recent clinical trials suggest that in some qualifying people, an alternative medicine might provide a substantial benefit.** Randomized, controlled trials and other studies have demonstrated that certain people should be good candidates for some dietary supplements.[15] For example, one of the most recent and best

TABLE 5-2	*Common Plant-Derived Conventional Medicines*	
Drug	**Plant Name**	**Drug Classification**
Atropine	*Atropa belladonna*	Anticholinergic, antispasmodic, antidysrhythmic
Capsaicin	*Capsicum frutescens*	Topical analgesic
Cocaine	*Erythroxylon coca*	Topical anesthetic
Codeine	*Papaver somniferum*	Analgesic
Colchicine	*Colchicum autumnale*	Antigout
Digoxin	*Digitalis purpurea*	Antidysrhythmic
Ephedrine	*Ephedra sinica*	Appetite suppressant
Ipecac	*Caphaelis ipecacuanha*	Antidote, emetic
Physostigmine	*Physostigma venenosum*	Cholinergic
Quinine	*Cinchona officinalis*	Antimalarial, antimyotonic
Salicylin	*Salix purpurea*	Analgesic, antipyretic
Scopolamine	*Datura fastuosa*	Antiemetic, anticholinerigic
Senna	*Cassia acutifolia*	Laxative
Taxol	*Taxus brevifolia*	Antineoplastic
Vincristine	*Catharanthus roseus*	Antineoplastic

Data from Winslow, L.C., & Kroll, D.J. (1998). Herbs as medicines. *Archives of Internal Medicine, 158*(9), 2192-2199.

examples is derived from a randomized trial of more than 3500 people over 60 years of age.[1] Researchers found that people diagnosed with intermediate to advanced age-related macular degeneration (AMD) who took a specific daily combination supplement (500 mg of vitamin C, 400 international units of vitamin E, 15 mg of beta-carotene, and 80 mg of zinc) for 6 years versus placebo could reduce their risk of visual impairment. This same trial revealed, however, that people with an early diagnosis of AMD did not benefit from taking the supplement.

Another recent but shorter (6 month) randomized trial from Europe demonstrated that a combination B-vitamin supplement (1 mg of folic acid, 400 µg of B_{12}, and 10 mg of B_6) could be beneficial (versus placebo) specifically for clients after coronary angioplasty.[18] Clients receiving the supplement significantly reduced their homocysteine levels and decreased the need for another revascularization procedure and reduced the risk of early death from any cause compared with clients receiving a placebo.

Nurses should encourage a client to discuss specific supplements with their primary health care provider and realize that the final decision can be made only after an extensive medical evaluation. This method is applied when deciding on any conventional treatment for a specific medical condition. If the individual and provider agree, then a treatment or medication may be recommended. CAM overall should not be treated any differently.

COMMON COMPLEMENTARY AND ALTERNATIVE THERAPIES ACCORDING TO NCCAM CLASSIFICATIONS

Note: These therapies are not necessarily advocated by the authors but are provided as a simple introduction to some of the more common CAM modalities. This is only a partial list of CAM therapies. More specific clinical trials that suggest a benefit or harm with these therapies are found in boxes in many chapters of this textbook.

Table 5-3 provides examples of CAM alternative medical systems. Table 5-4 summarizes examples of CAM mind-body interventions. Table 5-5 describes examples of CAM biologically based therapies. Table 5-6 outlines examples of CAM manipulative and body-based methods. Table 5-7 provides examples of CAM energy therapies.

COMPLEMENTARY AND ALTERNATIVE THERAPY FEATURES THROUGHOUT THE TEXTBOOK

Effective or ineffective CAM clinical trials are included throughout this text in their appropriate setting. For example, trials of cholesterol-lowering supplements are boxed and placed in the section on cardiovascular disease. Hundreds of trials have been completed in the last decade. Many of the findings of these studies appear in

TABLE 5-3	*Examples of CAM Alternative Medical Systems*
CAM	**Description**
Acupuncture/traditional Chinese medicine	Practiced in China for more than 2500 years. Theory of acupuncture espouses belief that there are pathways of energy flow (Qi) throughout the body that are vital for health. A trained acupuncturist can correct inadequate Qi at various sites with the insertion of needles or applying heat or electrical stimulation at a number of acupuncture points.
Ayurevda (ah-yur-VAY-dah)	Practiced primarily in Indian subcontinent for 5000 years. Includes diet, herbal remedies and massage and emphasizes the use of body, mind, and spirit in disease prevention and treatment.
Curanderismo	This system of beliefs or folk medicine is especially popular in some Hispanic-American communities. It includes a variety of techniques such as healing rituals, spirituality, herbal medicines, and psychic healing.
Homeopathic medicine	Involves belief that "like cures like" meaning that small highly diluted quantities of medicinal substances are given to cure manifestations, when the same substances given at higher or more concentrated doses would actually cause those manifestations.
Naturopathic medicine	Practitioners work with natural healing forces within the body with a goal of helping the body heal from disease and attain better health. Practices may include dietary modifications, massage, exercise, acupuncture, minor surgery, and various other interventions.

TABLE 5-4	*Examples of CAM Mind-Body Interventions*
CAM	**Description**
Aromatherapy	Use of fragrant compounds or essential (volatile) oils extracted from plants. They are used to improve mood and overall health. They can be inhaled or applied during massage. Some of the popular compounds include chamomile, eucalyptus, jasmine, lavender, peppermint, and rosemary.
Art, music or dance therapy	Use of drawing or art, music, or dance to help individuals cope or express emotions.
Biofeedback	Treatment that utilizes monitoring devices to assist individuals to make them more aware of their physiology and to allow them better self-control over such things as blood pressure, muscle tension, temperature, and bladder control.
Hypnosis	In this state of restful alertness a practitioner makes the client more aware of his or her surroundings to change behavior or promote more healthful practices such as smoking cessation.
Imagery	In these mental exercises the client's mind and thoughts are supposed to impact or assist a certain outcome. For example, a client receiving chemotherapy has an image of the drug literally destroying cancer cells in the body. A variety of visualization techniques are used to promote mental and physical well-being.
Meditation	Uses reflection or mental concentration to create a higher sense of well-being and relaxation. The individual is supposed to eliminate extraneous and mundane thoughts with the overall goal of elevating the mind to a different level. Two broad categories of meditation exist. First, there are the techniques that place emphasis on concentration, or so-called transcendental meditation. Second are the techniques that place emphasis on mindfulness (Vipassana). These techniques can be acquired from experienced teachers during a series of sessions. The overall effects of meditation are derived from deep relaxation. For example, a relaxation response in the area of cardiovascular physiology may occur by reducing heart rate and blood pressure, or an endocrine response may occur by reducing the level of stress hormones.
Shamanism	This type of folk medicine uses spiritual healing and is actually performed by a shaman or an individual recognized by some people and tribes who believe he or she has special religious or magical powers of healing. There is no strong scientific evidence to support a beneficial effect of shamanism, but currently it is being rigorously tested at some academic medical centers. In addition, some current uses of this therapy (imagery) may reduce stress and anxiety; however, it should not be used in place of conventional treatment.
Spiritual healing	This is the direct interaction between the healer and a client with the intention of improving the client's overall or specific condition or potentially curing the disease. The treatment itself can occur through personal contact or from a distance. Several variations of this therapy exist, including Reiki, intercessory prayer, faith healing, and therapeutic touch. Therapists of one group see themselves as separate from other groups. The primary claim of healers seems to be the promotion or facilitation of self-healing and well-being.
Tai Chi	This is actually an ancient form of martial arts that uses slow, controlled movements, meditation, and breathing to improve overall health and well-being. This form of therapy needs to be taught and should be used in addition to conventional treatment.
Yoga	This type of exercise teaches specific postures and breathing exercises. This form of therapy has been shown at least to improve quality of life for some clients by leading to relaxation and reduced stress levels. Yoga should be taught by a certified instructor because some of the postures could result in injury without proper teaching techniques.

TABLE 5-5	Examples of CAM Biologically Based Therapies
CAM	**Description**
Alternative diets	More than 40 alternative diets claim to prevent or treat a variety of conditions including cancer. Some examples include macrobiotic diets (based on belief that disease is caused by an imbalance of yin and yang) and the Gerson diet (vegan diet).
Dietary supplements (e.g., herbs, vitamins, minerals)	More than 20,000 herbal and dietary supplements are sold in the United States.

TABLE 5-6	Examples of CAM Manipulative and Body-Based Methods
CAM	**Description**
Chiropractic medicine	System of health care, begun in 1895 by Daniel Palmer, based on the belief that the nervous system is the most critical part of an individual's state of health. According to the theory, diseases are a result of "nerve interference," caused by spinal subluxations, which respond to manipulation of the spine. Chiropractors use spinal manipulations, mobilizations, and other types of natural medicines.
Massage	Involves rubbing, manipulation, and kneading of the body's muscle and soft tissue. It may reduce stress, anxiety, pain, and depression. Many conventional medical practitioners use or recommend massage to relieve clinical manifestations along with standard treatment. For example, the use of massage to decrease lymphedema caused by some treatments of breast and other cancers may help to reduce swelling.

TABLE 5-7	Examples of CAM Energy Therapies
CAM	**Description**
Cymatic therapy	Sir Peter Manners, MD, developed this non-audible sound therapy, which uses hand-held devices to transmit sound energy or waves through the skin. When the waves reach the internal body they are to restore the body's basic rhythms and boost immune function.
Magnetic therapy	Involves the use of a variety of different sizes and shapes of individual magnets on the body to reduce pain and treat disease.
Qi gong (chee-GUNG)	A component of traditional Chinese medicine that combines movement, meditation, and regulation of breathing to enhance the flow of qi (energy) in the body, improve blood circulation, and enhance immune function.
Reiki (RAY-kee)	A Japanese word representing "Universal Life Energy." Reiki is based on the belief that when spiritual energy is channeled through a Reiki practitioner, the client's spirit is healed, which in turn heals the physical body.
Therapeutic touch	Derived from ancient technique called *laying-on of hands* and based on a premise that it is the healing force of the therapist that affects the client's recovery; healing is promoted when the body's energies are in balance; and by passing their hands over the client, healers can identify energy imbalances.

boxes within specific chapters of the book to facilitate nurses who work with clients who may want to discuss CAM therapies in conjunction with conventional medical treatments.

BIBLIOGRAPHY

 1. Age-Related Eye Disease Study Research Group. (2001). A randomized, placebo-controlled, clinical trial of high-dose supplementation with vitamins C and E, beta carotene, and zinc for age-related macular degeneration and vision loss: AREDS Report No. 8. *Archives of Ophthalmology, 119*(10), 1417-1436.

 2. Beecher, H.K. (1955). The powerful placebo. *Journal of the American Medical Association, 159,* 1602-1606.

 3. Blendon, R.J., et al. (2001). Americans' views on the use and regulation of dietary supplements. *Archives of Internal Medicine, 161*(6), 805-810.

 4. Byers, T. (1999). What can randomized controlled trials tell us about nutrition and cancer prevention? *Cancer: Cancer Journal for Clinicians, 49,* 353-361.

5. DeSmet, P. (2002). Herbal remedies. *The New England Journal of Medicine, 347*(25), 2046-2056.

6. Gall, M., Gall, J., & Borg, W. (2003). *Educational research: An introduction* (7th ed.). Boston: Allyn and Bacon.

 7. Gentile, S., et al. (2000). Comparative efficacy study of atorvastatin vs. simvastatin, pravastatin, lovastatin and placebo in type 2 diabetic patients with hypercholesterolaemia. *Diabetes Obesity and Metabolism, 2,* 355-362.

 8. Giovannucci, E. (1999). Tomatoes, tomato-based products, lycopene, and cancer: review of the epidemiologic literature. *Journal of the National Cancer Institute, 91,* 317-331.

9. Hawks, J., & Moyad, M. (2003). CAM: Definition and classification overview. *Urologic Nursing, 23*(3), 221-223.

10. Herbert, V. (1994). The antioxidant supplement myth. *American Journal of Clinical Nutrition, 60,* 157-158.

 11. Hrobjartsson, A., & Gotzsche, P.C. (2001). Is the placebo powerless? An analysis of clinical trials comparing placebo with no treatment. *New England Journal of Medicine, 344,* 1594-1602.

 12. Knopp, R.H. (1999). Drug treatment of lipid disorders. *New England Journal of Medicine, 341,* 498-511.

13. Lazar, J., & O'Connor, B. (1997). Talking with patients about their use of alternative therapies. *Primary Care: Complementary and Alternative Therapies in Primary Care, 24*(4), 699-714.

14. Lue, T.F. (2000). Erectile dysfunction. *New England Journal of Medicine, 342,* 1802-1813.

15. Moyad, M.A. (2003). *The ABCs of nutrition and supplements for prostate cancer.* Ann Arbor, MI: JW Edwards Publishing.

 16. National Center for Complementary and Alternative Medicine. (2003). What is complementary and alternative medicine (CAM)? Retrieved October 21, 2003, from the World Wide Web: http://nccam.nih.gov/health/whatiscam/index.htm.

 17. Pepper, O.H.P. (1945). A note on placebo. *Annals of the Journal of Pharmacology, 117,* 409-412.

 18. Schnyder, G., Roffi, M., Pin, R., et al. (2001). Decreased rate of coronary restenosis after lowering of plasma homocysteine levels. *New England Journal of Medicine, 345*(22), 1593-1600.

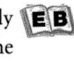 19. Schrott, H., et al. (1998). A multicenter, placebo-controlled, dose-ranging study of atorvastatin. *Journal of Cardiovascular and Pharmacologic Therapy, 3,* 119-124.

 20. Shepherd, I., et al. (1995). Prevention of coronary heart disease with pravastatin in men with hypercholesterolemia. West of Scotland Coronary Prevention Study Group. *New England Journal of Medicine, 333,* 1301-1307.

21. Skidmore-Roth, L. (2001). *Mosby's handbook of herbs & natural supplements.* St. Louis: Mosby.

22. The Alpha-Tocopherol, Beta Carotene Cancer Prevention Study Group. (1994). The effect of vitamin E and beta carotene on the incidence of lung cancer and other cancers in male smokers. *New England Journal of Medicine, 330,* 1029-1035.

23. Turner, J.A., et al. (1994). The importance of placebo effects in pain treatment and research. *Journal of the American Medical Association, 271,* 1609-1614.

24. Wender, R., & Nevin, J. (Eds.) (2002). *Primary Care: Preventive Medicine, 29*(3), 475-766.

25. Wierenga, M. (Ed.). (2002). *The Nursing Clinics of North America: Lifestyle Modification, 37*(2), 225-371.

26. Winslow, L.C., & Kroll, D.J. (1998). Herbs as medicines. *Archives of Internal Medicine, 158*(9), 2192-2199.

27. Yesalis, C.E. (1999). Medical, legal, and societal implications of androstenedione use. *Journal of the American Medical Association, 281*(21), 2043-2044.

28. Zoorob, R., & Morelli, V. (Eds.). (2002). *Primary Care: Alternative Therapies, 29*(2), 231-473.

Health Care
Delivery Systems

Overview of Health Care Delivery

Mary L. Fisher

evolve

Web Enhancements   http://evolve.elsevier.com/Black/medsurg/

Diversity in Health Care   How Can You Ensure the Ethical Use of Educational Materials
  Health Care Practitioners   for Clients?
Ethical Issues in Nursing   Appendix A
  Can the Underinsured Client Be Cared for Adequately?   Religious Beliefs and Practices Affecting Health Care

Nurses in the United States practice within a diverse and complex health care system. During the 1980s and 1990s, the system experienced a dramatic growth in scientific knowledge, coupled with an explosion of technology. This also was a period of increased competition and regulation. Additionally, the financing of health care was revolutionized in 1983, when prospective payment was introduced and later as managed care began to dominate the market. These events have had a profound impact on the practice of nursing. Understanding who the major stakeholders are within the field of health care and understanding recent health care history are crucial to the practice of professional nurses (see the Management and Delegation feature on Delegation in Health Care Delivery on p. 122). This chapter informs beginning practitioners of these changes and trends to prepare them for active roles in shaping the health care system in the new millennium.

MAJOR STAKEHOLDERS IN THE HEALTH CARE SYSTEM

Government

The role of government in the administration of health care in the United States cannot be overestimated. Many federal governmental health care efforts are headed by a cabinet-level officer, the Secretary for Health and Human Services, who runs the Department of Health and Human Services, founded in 1980. A complete listing of the governmental programs and entities under the Secretary are listed on the Health and Human Services website at http://hhs.gov/about/orgchart.html.[21]

Health care expenditures accounted for 20% of the federal government's budget in 1995; by 2001, expenditures were $647 billion,[11,12] with 45% of health care dollars being funded by government programs, especially Medicare (a federal program projected to be funded at $269.6 billion for 2003) and Medicaid (a joint federal-state initiative funded at $266 billion for 2003).[12] Other important sources of federal government funding are the Department of Veterans Affairs (VA), funded at $25.9 billion for 2003,[19] which oversees the VA health care system, and the Department of Defense, funded at 8 billion for 2002-2003, which funds health care for members of the armed forces and their dependents.[18] Workers' compensation, a joint federal and state program, was funded at $14.1 billion for 1997.[22] In addition, state and local governments support local indigent care through various mechanisms.

As the major payer, the federal government has been active in regulating the health care industry. Approximately 40% of hospital beds are occupied on any given day by Medicare recipients. Therefore, hospitals have great incentive to comply with regulations promulgated by the federal government, because they can be fined or "decertified" as a provider of care to Medicare clients if they do not. Noncompliance can result in the loss of millions of dollars of income for the hospital.

---

evolve *Be sure to check out the bonus material on the Evolve website and the CD-ROM, including free self-assessment exercises.*

http://evolve.elsevier.com/Black/medsurg/

MANAGEMENT AND DELEGATION

Delegation in Health Care Delivery

Delegation in health care has been evolving since the 1980s. The aging population, increasing health care costs, and shrinking workforce of registered nurses (RNs) has forced hospitals and other health care institutions to increase the use of unlicensed assistive personnel (UAP) in all settings. The National Council of State Boards of Nursing (NCSBN) and many national professional nursing organizations have formulated resources and position statements on the role of UAP in health care and more specifically on the role and responsibilities of licensed and unlicensed health care providers in delegating aspects of care for clients.

The NCSBN[1] concerns itself largely with the regulatory issues raised by the use of UAP as well as protection of the public's health, safety, and welfare. It provides guidance for individual state boards of nursing that are responsible for regulating nursing and the delegation process in their jurisdiction. Almost every state's nurse practice act and administrative rules address concepts of delegation. It is the nurse's responsibility to be aware of the nurse practice act and delegation regulations for the state in which he or she practices.

Professional nursing organizations offer position statements regarding nursing practice and the delegation of responsibilities to UAP. These aim to protect client rights and preserve the interests of professional nursing practice.

Delegation is transferring to a competent individual the authority to perform a selected nursing task in a selected situation. In doing so, the nurse retains accountability for the delegation. Accountability implies being responsible and answerable for actions or inactions of self or others in the context of delegation.

In general, the appropriate activities for consideration in delegation decision-making include tasks that do the following:

- Reoccur in daily care of a client or group of clients
- Do not require the unlicensed assistant to exercise nursing judgment
- Do not require complex application of the nursing process
- Have predictable results with minimal associated risks for the client
- Use a standard, unchanging procedure

The "Five Rights of Delegation"[2] are a valuable resource for clarifying the critical elements of the delegation decision-making process.

Right task	The activities and tasks you consider to delegate use standard, unchanging procedures and have a predictable outcome; the activities and tasks reoccur in the daily care of the client or population of clients and do not require nursing judgment.
Right circumstances	Delegation follows your individual client assessment and plan of care. The task complexity matches the UAP competency level and level of available supervision.
Right person	Your individual client assessment and UAP competency serves as the basis for your delegation decisions. Your own competency and skill level allows for your delegation of tasks and activities.
Right communication	You communicate delegation on a client- and UAP-specific basis, including specific data to be collected and reported, specific activity to be performed, expected results, potential complications and expectations, and communication of data and observations.
Right supervision	You supervise performance of activities, provide directions and clear expectations, and evaluate entire delegation process and the client's response.

Delegation considerations reflecting these Five Rights of Delegation are incorporated throughout this text. These considerations provide guidance as you prepare to assume responsibility for the care of your clients with accompanying accountability for your delegation practices.

References
1. National Council State Boards of Nursing. (1995). *Delegation: Concepts and decision-making process.* Position paper, Chicago, IL.
2. Available: *http://www.ncsbn.org/public/regulation/delegation* "Five Rights of Delegation."

Government regulation is frequently opposed by the health care industry because it often affects the health care practitioner's autonomy. In 1991, for example, the U.S. Supreme Court upheld the right of the federal government to restrict health care providers in family planning clinics that receive federal funds from informing pregnant women about abortion options (*Rust v. Sullivan*). Since the Supreme Court ruling, health care workers in the clinics had to alter their practice or be subject to penalty. Strong condemnation of this restriction was voiced by the American Nurses' Association (ANA) and the American Medical Association (AMA), among others. Legislation to modify the regulation was eventually passed.

The authors would like to thank Bonita Ann Pilon for her contribution to this chapter in the fifth edition of *Medical-Surgical Nursing.*

The federal government is the biggest source of funding for biomedical research. Established in 1989, the Agency for Health Care Policy and Research (AHCPR; now called the Agency for Healthcare Research and Quality, or AHRQ), conducts research on costs, quality, and medical effectiveness of health care. AHRQ received $306 billion in 2002, the majority of which was awarded in grants and contracts.[2] The National Institutes of Health (NIH), the principal biomedical research agency of the government through its 27 institutes and centers, received $23.4 billion for fiscal year 2002, 82% of which supports research and training.[25] The government also directs public health programs through the Centers for Disease Control and Prevention (CDC), which received $3.1 billion for fiscal year 2000.[8] The growth of scientific knowledge related to health care is highly dependent on government funding. Nurse researchers are recipients of research grants through various government agencies, most notably the National Institute for Nursing Research, established at NIH in 1993.[16] Its budget for 1999 was $70 million.[26] Research funds are an important source of revenue for major medical centers and university-affiliated hospitals.

Physicians

The role of physicians in the health care system in the United States is an important one. Physicians provide direct medical services to clients in a variety of settings, including offices, clinics, hospitals, and freestanding centers. In addition, physicians control 60% to 80% of hospital costs through their decisions regarding the use of resources. As gatekeepers to inpatient care, physicians decide which clients to admit, where to admit clients, the length of stay, the quantity of ancillary services, whether to perform surgery, when to initiate and to discontinue treatment regimens, and which medications to prescribe.

Because physicians strongly influence health care use, health care agencies and clients are often dependent on physicians. Agencies such as hospitals rely on their medical staffs to admit clients who generate income for the hospital. Therefore, physicians are customers of the hospital, just as clients are. As a result, physicians and their lobby groups, such as the AMA, usually have strong political influence within hospital organizations, the health care system, legislatures, and government-regulating agencies.

Many physicians perceived a decline in their dominance and control of health care during the 1980s and 1990s. These perceived and real losses have created anxiety and prompted defensive tactics among some members of the profession toward a restructured health care system. The traditions that define medical practice, such as autonomy, professional control, solo medical practice, and fee-for-service entrepreneurialism, are being ques-

tioned and reformed. Some contend that physicians will enjoy less control in a restructured health care environment than they have in the past. In keeping with this trend toward the loss of physician power, the AMA took the unprecedented step in 1999 of forming a collective bargaining arm to assist physicians in seeking input into practice changes.

Whereas Western practitioners are the main group sanctioned by American society to treat disease, traditional cultural and folk practitioners are a presence in the ethnic segments of society. Providers must recognize the place of traditional healers for an ethnically diverse population (see the Diversity in Health Care feature on Health Care Practitioners on the website). *evolve*

Hospital Administrators and Governing Boards

The chief executive, chief financial officer, chief nursing officer, and governing boards of hospitals strongly influence health care delivery in their institutions. In addition, most hospitals are members of the American Hospital Association (AHA), which represents the industry's efforts to influence legislation, regulation, judicial decisions, and health policy. The AHA filed a suit in the early 1990s to stop the National Labor Relations Board from implementing new collective bargaining rules. The suit went to the Supreme Court, where the rules were upheld, but they have had little impact in fostering collective bargaining as the AHA has feared.[6] The AHA also worked to block regulations from the Health Care Financing Administration, which effectively decreased reimbursement for capital costs to hospitals from Medicare.[20]

Business and Industry

By the year 2003, health care costs were projected to represent 15% of the gross domestic product, or $1.65 trillion.[9,10] These costs are the highest of any industrialized nation, making American products less competitive in the world economy. For example, health care costs for automobile workers add $1100 to the cost of every car made in the United States.[17] This continuing trend is best illustrated by comparing the cost of prescription drugs in the United States with that of other wealthy nations: Great Britain's cost is 33% less; Canada's, 37% less; France and Italy's, 47% less.[1]

American industries have a big stake in controlling these costs. As health care costs increased in the mid-1990s (~5% per year),[13] the influence of business and industry increased as well. Health insurance programs (e.g., Blue Cross/Blue Shield, commercial insurance) are purchased mainly through employee benefit programs. As the cost of health care increases, insurance costs increase as well, forcing businesses to assume greater financial burdens to insure employees and their dependents, as well as leading to salary stagnation as employers allocate dollars for insurance rather than salary increases. Costs for products increase accordingly.

One major reason for the increase is that the health care industry shifts costs by increasing charges to individuals and small payers to offset underpayment by Medicare, Medicaid, and other contracted payers. The result is that the private sector, insured clients, and employers pay more for care. During the past decade, business and industry leaders protested the increased costs and began to take collective action to drive costs down. Some strategies have included the following:

- Increased deductibles
- Larger and more frequent co-payments
- Reduced benefits and services
- Initiation of managed care programs
- Mandatory second opinions
- Precertification of admission
- Increased contracting of care to health maintenance organizations (HMOs) and preferred provider organizations (PPOs)

By 1997, 85% of the enrolled work force was in some type of managed care plan.[22]

In some areas of the United States, industry leaders have formed coalition groups that lobby their state government for laws to restrict health care spending, limit malpractice liability, and provide major reform for the health care system. Increasingly, large businesses have contracted for health care services directly with hospitals and physician groups, demanding—and receiving—significant discounts for care. The influence of large employers is expected to remain strong within the health care industry.

The Public

Despite decades of public policy designed to reduce health costs, U.S. health care spending was estimated to exceed $1.6 trillion or $5757 per capita annually by 2003.[9] The American public has a stake in health care from several perspectives. First, as consumers of health care services, the public is concerned with the quality, cost, and access to care. Many Americans believe that health care is a right and should be universally available to all citizens, regardless of the cost. Paradoxically, however, most do not want to pay these costs in the form of increased taxes.

People who are uninsured (~44 million, 86% of whom are employed workers and their families) or underinsured (Medicare recipients have no prescription medication coverage) do not have equal access to health care services that income and insurance provide.[20] This uninsured figure represents 16% of the non–older adult population.[13] Women and children are among those who suffer the most; 25% of the uninsured are children.[13] Because people have not agreed on the model for health care reform or the role of government, several ideas are being explored by various interest groups.

The public also is composed of voters who can elect representatives to enact laws protecting their health care interests. Often, citizens band together to influence the passage of health-related legislation. In 1990, activist groups concerned about acquired immunodeficiency syndrome (AIDS) strongly lobbied Congress to ensure passage of the Ryan White bill (Public Law 101-381), which provided funds for AIDS education, service, and research. The American Association of Retired Persons (AARP) is another prominent group that actively supports health care legislation targeted to older people. Although many other consumer groups are concerned with health care issues, AIDS and breast cancer activist groups and the AARP represent some of the larger and more vocal constituencies that currently influence the health care industry.

Overall, public values regarding health care are changing. People are interested in receiving quality health care at a reasonable cost. In addition, the public has a more positive view of health promotion and illness prevention than in the past. Health care resources remain focused on illness, however, with only 1% of health care expenditures going to public health.[20]

Nurses

Nurses outnumber physicians, dentists, pharmacists, and every other single group of health care providers in the United States. As of 2001, there were 1.99 million registered nurses (RNs) employed in nursing.[33] Among the 2.16 million RNs projected for 2005, about two thirds will work in hospitals, a distribution that has remained constant since the mid-1980s. The number of RNs has increased by 40% since 1980. From 1980 through the mid-1990s, the percentage of RNs employed in hospitals was stable at 67%. The percentage dipped to 60% in 1996, reflecting trends toward community and outpatient care and nurses' growing concern with health maintenance, health promotion, and health education. Hospital nurses are projected to account for 61% of the nursing work force in 2005.[33]

The average age of nurses has increased steadily since the 1980s. The median age for RNs neared 43 years in 2000. As health care demands continue to increase with an aging population, the demographics of an aging nursing work force project a 7% shortage in nursing supply versus demand by 2005.[33]

Racial and ethnic minorities, except Asians, are underrepresented in nursing.[27] The U.S. Bureau of Census in 1996 estimated that 72% of Americans were white, in contrast to 90% of nurses being white.[32]

Although the influence of such a large group of health care providers should be noticed, the greatest impact—and the most frequently discussed aspect of nursing—has been the recurring shortage of RNs. The voice of nursing has been heard lately, as thousands protest downsizing of hospitals, replacement of RNs by less skilled workers, and layoffs. However, the collective expertise and leadership of nurses has not yet been fully utilized to shape the reform era. Nursing's response to rapid market changes has been largely reactionary.

In 1991, the ANA, in collaboration with the National League for Nursing, the American Organization of Nurse Executives, the American Association of Colleges of Nursing, and other organized nursing groups, introduced *Nursing's Agenda for Health Care Reform.* The authors[3] stated that

> Nurses provide a unique perspective on the health care system. Our constant presence in a variety of settings places us in contact with individuals who reap the benefits of the system's most sophisticated services, as well as those individuals seriously compromised by the system's inefficiencies . . . . America's health care system is . . . very costly, its quality inconsistent, and its benefits unequally distributed. . . . In short, health care is neither fairly nor equitably delivered to all segments of the population.

Nursing's health care reform proposal attempted to address the cost, quality, and access dilemmas facing the nation. This endeavor was a proactive attempt by the nursing profession to significantly alter existing health policy. A 1999 publication by ANA, *Legislative and Regulatory Initiatives for the 106th Congress,* proposed mobilizing nurses politically to enact continuing influence on health care policy.[4]

FINANCING OF HEALTH CARE SERVICES

Funding Mechanisms

Health care is paid for in various ways. The major funding programs are defined in Box 6-1.

The health care industry has evolved through significant phases since the 1920s with regard to quality, cost, and access. To understand current issues, it is useful for nurses to understand the past, which was characterized by two major periods: (1) the *period of expansion* and (2) the *period of regulation and cost containment.* The current climate is known as the *period of reform.*

Period of Expansion

During the late 1920s, a congressional committee studied various facets of health care organization and financing. It was found that the cost of health care per illness had substantially increased with the emergence of hospitalization as the appropriate method of treating illness.[28] These increasing costs, coupled with the financial problems created by the Depression of 1929, led to financial difficulties for community general hospitals. Consequently, the need to spread financial risk across the community was recognized. Prepayment plans for hospital care spread slowly during the 1930s and evolved into the Blue Cross system.

Private Health Insurance

Blue Cross plans had two goals: (1) to provide a stronger financial base for community hospitals and (2) to move the risk of economic loss caused by hospitalization away from single individuals to larger groups of people. Because these objectives were considered socially desirable, Blue Cross, and later Blue Shield organizations, benefited from favorable legislation exempting them from some of the more stringent requirements for commercial insurance companies.

The evolution of Blue Cross/Blue Shield plans and their availability to the average worker signaled the beginning of an era in which the actual cost of health care became separated from the person who purchased the care (the insurance effect). Such a separation causes the cost of health care to appear artificially low to the client who, in turn, can afford to buy more services.

Demand for health care services, as a result of insurance, grew rapidly in the 1940s and 1950s. Because of economic wage and price controls during and after World War II, salary increases to workers were limited. Fringe benefits came into vogue as a means of attracting and retaining workers. Unions began bargaining for fringe benefits in lieu of unobtainable salary increases. As a consequence, health insurance became widely available to American workers and their families. The consumption of health care services, in turn, increased.

Another important event was the passage of the Social Security Act of 1935. This legislation established as social policy the right of older people to financial security. Although health care was not affected by this law at the time of its passage, the Social Security Act would later become the vehicle through which health care needs of older people and the poor would be addressed.[15]

Hill-Burton Act

After World War II, it was apparent that the nation's hospitals were obsolete and poorly distributed to meet the population's needs. There had been great shifts from rural to urban areas during the war. Immediately after the war, the baby boom began. The private sector had difficulty meeting the need for improved health care facilities. Congress responded by passing the Hospital Survey and Construction Act of 1946 (the Hill-Burton Act).[16]

The overt purpose of the Hill-Burton Act was to eliminate shortages of hospitals, especially in rural and economically depressed areas. Ratios of beds-to-population were used to measure shortage. Funds generated by the act were dispersed over 28 years (1946-1974). The act was amended during that time to include not only construction of new facilities but also modernization of existing facilities and, later, construction of emergency departments and neighborhood health centers.[14]

BOX 6-1 *Major Health Care Funding Programs in the United States*

Medicare

A federally funded and administered national health insurance program for citizens age 65 years and older and for certain other clients, such as those with end-stage renal disease, regardless of age. Medicare began in 1966 and is paid for through the payroll taxes of all workers (a portion of Social Security deductions) and through monthly premiums paid by recipients. The program covers both hospitalization and physician costs, but deductibles and restrictions apply. Medicare determines the maximum allowable fee for service. Health care providers receive 80% of this fee from Medicare and can bill only for the balance of the allowable fee. The maximum allowable fee is often much less than the true value of the service.

In 1983, the federal government instituted major changes in the way hospitals were reimbursed for Medicare clients. Previously, hospitals had been reimbursed costs plus an additional amount. Since 1983, hospitals have received compensation on a *prospective* basis. Hospitals are paid one predetermined sum for a given diagnosis. Similar types of diagnoses and conditions are grouped together, weighted for severity or intensity of illness, and assigned a dollar value for compensation; these are called diagnosis-related groups (DRGs). If the client's care (e.g., acute myocardial infarction) costs the hospital *more* than Medicare's payment, the hospital *loses* money. If the costs are less than the reimbursement amount, the hospital keeps the profit. This system has caused dramatic changes as hospitals struggle to survive financially. In 2004, Congress passed a bill to fund prescriptions for Medicare recipients.

Medicaid

A joint federal and state program administered by the state governments. This insurance program provides limited funding for hospital and medical care costs of low-income citizens. Each state sets the income levels that determine eligibility. As a result, some states provide more services than others can afford. The state must budget money from its own revenues for the program matched by the government. The federal portion is always larger than the state portion.

Blue Cross and Blue Shield

Private not-for-profit health insurance companies set up through special legislation in the 1930s. The "blues" are the largest single insurer outside the federal government from which businesses and industry can purchase health insurance for employees. Both hospital and medical care insurance are available.

Commercial Insurance Companies

For-profit businesses (e.g., Traveler's, Metropolitan Life). These agencies usually sell a host of insurance packages. Businesses or individuals may buy health insurance from a commercial carrier.

Self-Insurance

Businesses that develop their own insurance programs for employees. More companies are setting aside funds (which can be millions of dollars) to cover the risk of their self-insurance program. The company may hire Blue Cross and Blue Shield or a commercial insurer to administer the program, including receiving, reviewing, and paying claims.

HMO

A health maintenance organization representing a system of bundled services. Clients pay a monthly premium to the HMO, which entitles them to checkups and preventive care, medical care, prescriptions, and hospitalization if needed. The HMO employs its own physicians and other health care providers and may own or manage its own hospitals. Some HMOs charge the clients a co-payment for some services, such as prescriptions and office visits. Clients are restricted to using only HMO facilities and physicians. If clients go outside the system, they must pay for part or all of their expenses (except in emergencies or during travel).

PPO

A preferred provider organization is a group consisting of physicians, usually at least one hospital, and ancillary providers that coalesces to form a system of care. This system is marketed and sold, contractually, to employers. The physicians, hospital, and others remain independent agents who agree to treat certain clients (those who join the PPO) at discounted prices.

Workers' Compensation

A federally mandated, state-funded, and state-administered insurance program available to workers injured on the job. Each employer is assessed a payroll tax, which funds the plan. Clients file claims through the employer to secure funds for treatment.

Private Pay

A term used to describe clients who have no insurance and who must pay the entire health care bill.

Uncompensated Care

Health care delivered that is not paid for by an insurance program or by clients themselves. Many private pay clients contribute to the amount of uncompensated care when they cannot pay the high costs of health care. Other sources of uncompensated care include the differences between what the care costs and what Medicare or Medicaid pays the provider. By law, providers cannot bill anyone for the difference and must absorb the loss of revenue.

Capitation

A form of payment between the purchaser of health care and the provider. Capitation is often used when a large organization contracts for health services from a provider, such as a hospital or home health agency. The provider is paid in one of two ways: (1) a flat fee is paid per incident of care (no care, no payment) or (2) the provider receives a flat fee per person enrolled in the health plan for a defined level of care whether or not the enrollee seeks care. If few enrollees use the service, the provider does well financially. If not, the provider must care for every enrollee who seeks care regardless of whether the total money received covers the cost of the care provided.

Implicit within this legislation was the social policy of ensuring access to health care for all. The solution to the social problem of inadequate access was to construct more health care facilities. To ensure that people with limited ability to pay were actually served by the agencies receiving Hill-Burton Act money, the legislation stipulated a unique payback scheme. Each facility had to provide care to indigent clients, on an annual basis, that was equal in dollar value to the amount of money received by the hospital, prorated over a specified time period, usually 20 years. Much like a mortgage payment, the hospital provided free care each year equal to its annual repayment amount. These health services were provided, in lieu of payment, to people with limited access because of poverty.

The Hill-Burton Act's approach to indigent care was a noble one but did not succeed in providing access for all indigent clients. During the long payback period, the cost of health care increased dramatically as a result of new technology and inflation. Many hospitals began meeting their obligations for free care in a few weeks' time each year. After those obligations were met, hospitals were not legally bound to treat indigent clients. By the early 1970s, the bed shortage addressed by Hill-Burton legislation had reversed itself and an oversupply appeared to exist. In 1974, the act was allowed to expire.

Medicare/Medicaid Enacted

The early 1950s featured continued wage and price controls, growth of health insurance coverage among workers, and increased discussion of a national health insurance program. National health insurance was viewed as a means of insuring every American citizen against economic loss caused by the high cost of illness, regardless of employment status, age, or health status. This concern repeatedly asserted itself during President Truman's administration. The medical and hospital lobby successfully fought such legislation as late as 1952.[29]

By the mid-1960s, a new social problem was identified as the nation's priority: poverty. The War on Poverty during the Johnson Administration (1963-1968) provided the impetus for passage of the first national health insurance plans, for which the federal government was both the insurance carrier and the payer of a large portion of the premium. These insurance programs, known as Medicare and Medicaid, were passed as amendments to the Social Security Act in 1965.[16] The social problem of poverty was translated more specifically into limited access to health care services by the elderly and the non-elderly poor as the result of inability to pay. The social policy expressed by both pieces of legislation implied that access to health care for all citizens was a right. Government had an obligation to ensure that right.

Funding for the Medicare hospitalization plan (Part A) is provided by a payroll tax collected from every worker who pays Social Security taxes. The medical payment component (Part B) for physician care is paid by the enrollee through monthly premiums. The Medicare program is administered by the federal government through the Department of Health and Human Services (DHHS) Health Care Financing Administration.

Administration of Medicaid is delegated to the states, which must provide certain core services but are free to tailor other services to meet specific population needs. The states also determine eligibility requirements, which vary considerably from state to state. Funding for Medicaid is provided by a matching formula specific to each state. The federal funds are always the greatest portion of each Medicaid dollar spent. States receive differing amounts of federal money, thus providing different ranges of care, because some states can match more federal dollars than others through larger state tax revenues.

Implementation of Medicare and Medicaid substantially increased the federal government's (and, to a lesser extent, the state governments') role in the health care market. The federal government became the single largest purchaser of health care services. Subsequently, it played a growing role in regulating the health care industry in both cost and quality.

Period of Regulation and Cost Containment

In 1974, Congress passed the National Health Planning and Resources Act (Public Law 93-641), which required states to develop a statewide health plan for the use of resources. States were also required to review providers' requests to initiate or expand health services.[23] This review process, known as *certificate of need* (CON) review, required providers to demonstrate sufficient need for the service before the request was approved. This legislation represented the first federal government effort to combine health planning and regulation in one program. It was also the first significant attempt to control health care costs through the elimination of duplicate services and facilities. It was designed to curb the oversupply and increasing technology of facilities that arose during the period of expansion.

Because the CON regulation did nothing to change incentives to hospitals in the competitive health care market, it could not control costs and by the late 1970s was curtailed as a federal effort.[23] Results of CON studies support this evaluation. Steinwald and Sloan[30] suggested that "certificate-of-need controls, initiated by the states and mandated by PL 93-641, may be regarded as a classic example of regulatory failure."

During the 1970s, some state governments undertook their own regulatory programs. Rate controls were in place in at least eight states by the end of the decade. According to Steinwald and Sloan,[30] such programs "all respond to the evils of cost-based reimbursement—they seek to counteract the unrestrained nature of hospital reimbursement by superimposing constraints that the market cannot provide."

States with mandatory rate-setting programs represented the most stringent group of prospective reimbursement programs operating during the late 1970s. The rates of increase in total hospital expenses in the eight mandatory states were 9.7% and 8.6% for the years of 1976-1977 and 1977-1978, respectively, versus 15.8% and 14% for the other states and the District of Columbia.[30]

These data and other studies clearly indicated that prospective rate-setting was more effective in controlling health care costs than the CON controls were. Reimbursement for Medicaid clients also had moved to a prospective system in many states, whether or not the state had mandatory rate-setting.

Federal Prospective Payment Systems

The federal government, very aware of the increasing cost of health care and continuing as the nation's largest purchaser of care, began to look at methods of prospective reimbursement that could be used by the Medicare program. Research studies were underway at Yale University and other centers to develop a system of prospective payment. These studies were closely followed and sometimes funded by DHHS, previously called the Department of Health, Education, and Welfare.

The hospital industry adopted its own form of regulation in December 1977. Known as the Voluntary Effort (VE), it consisted of "joint activities at the state level by the American Hospital Association, the American Medical Association, and the Federation of American Hospitals (the for-profit hospitals' trade organization) to control the rate of growth of hospital costs."[30] Results of the VE were mixed. A study by the Congressional Budget Office indicated a small, nonsignificant negative effect on hospital expenditures. A second study found a significant negative effect on the cost per admission and cost per patient day. However, the second study indicated that the cost savings were not passed on to the consumers because hospital profits increased during the same period (1978-1980).[30]

The inability of various regulatory programs to control the increasing cost of health care (from 9% of the gross national product in 1978 to 13% by 1992) became a primary issue with Congress. The nation was trying to recover from economic recession, and inflation in all sectors of the economy was of grave concern. In addition, the population was aging and the ratio of workers (who paid Medicare taxes for hospitalization insurance) to older people (who spent the dollars paid in by using hospital services) was shrinking. Projections that the Medicare Trust Fund would be bankrupt began in the mid-1980s and continue, with Congress taking only intermediate steps to bail out the program instead of overhauling the entire health care system.

For example, the Tax Equity and Fiscal Responsibility Act, passed by Congress in July 1982, contained temporary limits on Medicare payments and directed the Secretary of DHHS to develop a *prospective payment system* (PPS) for Medicare.[16] The Secretary was instructed to report back to Congress by December 1982 on the status of such a system.

In December 1982, Secretary Richard Schweiker recommended to Congress that a PPS based on *diagnosis-related groups* (DRGs), developed by researchers at Yale University, be used for all Medicare clients. In March 1983, Congress passed amendments to the Social Security Act authorizing such a system. This system was to replace the *cost-based retrospective payment system* used to determine Medicare payments to hospitals. All hospitals serving Medicare clients were to switch to PPS except for certain sole community providers, specialty hospitals, and some psychiatric units within general hospitals.

The program became operational on October 1, 1983. Hospitals were phased into the system over the subsequent 11 months, when their fiscal year began. A formula was calculated for each hospital to determine its initial reimbursement rate under DRGs. Data were gathered from the hospital's own cost history (using a base year) and from a cost history by geographical region; a national rate was also established. These rates were weighted and blended to determine the exact rate of reimbursement per DRG. Since the PPS was initiated, several adjustments have been made in blending. The goal is still to move all hospitals toward one national rate.

Private Sector Response

Government was not the only entity involved with rising health care costs during the early 1980s; business and industry were also concerned because they paid the majority of the health insurance premium costs for employees. Local and regional business leaders come together to discuss and remedy the worsening situation. With the implementation of PPS for Medicare clients, these business coalitions were joined by Blue Cross organizations and other commercial insurers. These new groups held a common fear: hospitals would shift uncompensated costs generated by Medicare clients to clients who were still reimbursed retrospectively on a "cost-plus" basis. As a result of that fear, Blue Cross and other insurers have begun to restructure their payment systems to protect themselves from potential or actual cost shifting. These fears were warranted, because cost shifting became and remains a reality.

PPS has yielded other results as well. Hospitals and other health care providers increasingly compete for non-Medicare clients who are more favorably reimbursed. Hospitals also compete for certain Medicare clients whose DRG rate has been profitable for the hospital. Much traditional inpatient care has been shifted to the outpatient system or to the client's home, where the cost of care is less. Insurers and providers have teamed up in creative arrangements designed to hold down costs and yet remain competitive. Such arrangements have created alternative delivery systems based on greater efficiency and decreased costs. Among these are HMOs, PPOs, and independent practice associations. The number of outpatient surgical centers (freestanding and hospital-based) and freestanding emergency clinics has increased rapidly.

Providers have been marketing health services to businesses and the public. HMOs and PPOs, for example, seek to contract with employers to be the sole insurer for employee groups. *Capitation* has emerged as a popular form of PPS within these arrangements. Capitation is a per-member per-month fee paid in advance for a specified set of health care services. This money is given to providers up front, whether or not clients use services. The health care provider must provide care even if all of the up front fees have been used.

Medicare also is interested in capitation as a means of payment for its enrollees. In some regions, Medicare enrollees already receive care through an HMO that receives capitation payments from the federal government. The AHA projected that most Medicare clients would be covered by capitation by the early 1990s.[17] This prediction has yet to become a reality, with many HMO providers threatening to pull out of the Medicare sector because of reimbursement concerns.

Complex *oversight systems* within managed care limited the rate of cost growth through the 1990s, but this restraint did not come without costs. The public grew wary of roadblocks to receiving needed services and applied growing pressure on Congress to control HMO gatekeeping abuses. Perhaps heralding a new trend, United Health Care (UHC), the nation's second largest health insurer, began dismantling the costly oversight structure in late 1999.[5] Physicians in UHC plans no longer need permission for client tests and admissions. Citing studies indicating that the oversight cost more than it saved and disrupted coordination of care, the insurer led the way for the next phase of managed care reform.[5]

Period of Reform

By 1992, the United States began to reform its health care financing system. With the election of President Clinton, a Democrat, and with continued control of Congress by the same party, passage of national health care reform legislation seemed inevitable. President Clinton introduced the Health Security Act in early 1994, after almost a year of deliberation by economists, business

people, and health care providers. First Lady Hillary Rodham Clinton chaired the panel, which attempted to examine the current system's problems (access, cost, quality) to identify the national priorities, including a new emphasis on illness prevention.[27] Much controversy surrounded this ad hoc group. No representation was allowed from organized medicine or other provider organizations. Testimony was sought from these groups, but the actual crafting of the reform plan and ensuing legislation was carried out by the task force. The plan that emerged was so complex that it contained more than 100 pages in published form. The legislation that was sent to Congress was more than 1000 pages.

President Clinton's plan met opposition from within his own party as well as from outside. Everyone publicly agreed that the system needed to be reformed, but no one could agree about how much reform was needed or could be afforded. At one point in 1994, at least six different pieces of health care reform legislation were being considered by Congress. The main points of contention centered on (1) universal access and how to pay for it and (2) employer mandates, which require all employees to be covered by insurance provided by the employer. As a result of these issues and of a general lack of political support by Congress for the President, federal health care reform initiatives did not pass. In fact, no bill was moved out of committee for a vote.

The support for reform, however, did not die in Washington. A number of states passed legislation and policy directives to halt the escalation of costs and to provide increased access to services for citizens regardless of ability to pay. Tennessee led the way in 1994, when it moved all Medicaid recipients into a managed care plan, with capitation paid to managed care companies, which, in turn, provided a full range of health care services to recipients. Tennessee is still in the forefront of state managed care reform, with 1.3 million Medicaid eligible and uninsured and uninsurable people being covered.[31]

By 1996, more than one third of all Medicaid recipients nationwide were enrolled in some form of managed care. The Balanced Budget Act of 1997 enabled states to convert to managed care without the need for a federal Medicaid waiver.[9] The law established minimum standards for Medicaid managed care contracts, added qualifying conditions for companies to participate in the program, and ensured better access and coverage for recipients.[9]

The Health Insurance Portability and Accountability Act of 1996 created national standards for the availability and portability of individual health insurance coverage. This bill was, in part, an effort to reduce the ever increasing number of uninsured. It requires coverage for pre-existing conditions after 12 months and provides for continuation of group health insurance after COBRA (Consolidated Omnibus Budget Reconciliation Act) coverage ends for people who meet eligibility criteria.[24]

Reform also is being driven by the health care industry itself. During 1994, Columbia Health Care System, based in Dallas, acquired Hospital Corporation of America and Health Trust, both based in Nashville, to form the largest for-profit health care delivery system in the world. In addition to owning 220 hospitals, this corporation aggressively acquired primary care practices of physicians in both rural and urban areas. Using such a strategy, Columbia Health Care System is creating a network of integrated delivery systems that focuses on primary care as the most desirable and least costly level of care, with secondary and tertiary care available when needed. With such network in place in numerous markets across the United States, Columbia actively seeks managed care contracts from large employers, generally paid on a capitation basis, although discounted reimbursement mechanisms are still mixed with fee-for-service in most markets.

The response by the not-for-profit sector has varied. In some competitive markets, the not-for-profit hospitals have banded together to form their own integrated delivery systems to compete for managed care contracts. In other areas, some not-for-profits have entered into joint venture arrangements with the for-profit sector or have been purchased by large for-profit systems. This consolidation trend continued throughout the 1990s.

Since the early 1980s, the health care system has undergone rapid change. The system is still evolving, however, and the end product is difficult to foresee. Scarcity of and competition for human and financial resources are the dominant operating forces. This situation creates a dilemma with regard to social values of the past: health care as a right versus scarcity. Nurses must recognize and grapple with these forces and the dilemmas involved in shaping the nation's future health care system.

CONCLUSIONS

Our health care system is large and complex, with many stakeholders. It is also a system under considerable pressure to change as a direct result of increasing costs and lower accessibility to basic care for many citizens. This is the environment in which nursing practice takes place. Nurses are in the mainstream of service to both advantaged and disadvantaged clients. Nurses play a crucial role in delivering health care. Many believe that nurses may be the key to revamping the health care system to one that provides access to basic primary care for all citizens. The contribution of the nursing profession to the nation's health has never been more important.

BIBLIOGRAPHY

1. Abundis, J., & Rechin, K. (1999, November 18). Drug prices cheaper abroad. *USA Today*, p. 1.
2. Agency for Healthcare Research and Quality. (2002). *AHRQ fiscal year 2002 budget in brief*. U.S. Department of Health and Human Services (online). Available: *http://www.ahcpr.gov/about/cj2002/budbrf02.htm*.
3. American Nurses' Association. (2002). *Agenda for health care reform*. Kansas City, MO: (online). Available: *http://www.ana.org/readroom/rnagenda.htm*.
4. American Nurses' Association. (1999). *Legislative and regulatory initiatives for the 106th Congress*. Kansas City, MO: Author.
5. Appleby, J. (1999, November 9). Health plan eases doctor oversight. *USA Today*, p. 1.
6. Buerhaus, P.I., Staiger, D.O., & Averback, D.I. (2000). Implications of an aging registered nurse workforce. *Journal of the American Medical Association*. *283*(22), 2948-2954.
7. Campbell, P. W., & Healy, P. (1999, November 5). House approves 15% budget increase for the NIH—but with a hitch. *Chronicle of Higher Education, A36*, 38.
8. Centers for Disease Control and Prevention. (1999). *2000 budget*. Centers for Disease Control and Prevention, U.S. Department of Health and Human Services (online). Available: *http://www.cdc.gov/2000bdg/cdcbud.pdf*.
9. Centers for Medicare and Medicaid Services. (2003). Table 1: *National health expenditures and selected economic indicators, levels and average annual percent change: Selected calendar years 1980-2011*. Available: *http://cms.hhs.gov/statistics/nhe/projections-2001/t1.asp*.
10. Centers for Medicare and Medicaid Services. (2003). Table 2: National health expenditure amounts, and average annual percent change by type of expenditure: Selected calendar years 1980-2011. Available: *http://cms.hhs.gov/statistics/nhe/projections-2001/t2.asp*.
11. Centers for Medicare and Medicaid Services (2003). *Highlights: National health expenditures, 2001*. Centers for Medicare and Medicaid Services, U.S. Department of Health and Human Services (Online). Available: *http://cms.hhs.gov/statistics/nhe/historial/highlights.asp*.
12. Centers for Medicare and Medicaid Services. (2003). Table 3: National health expenditures aggregate and per capita amounts, percent distribution and average annual percent change by source of funds: Selected calendar years 1980-2011. Available: *http://cms.hhs.gov/statistics/nhe/projections-2001/t3.asp*.
13. Centers for Medicare and Medicaid Services (2003). Table 3: National health expenditures by source of funds and type of expenditure selected: Calendar years 1996-2001. Centers for Medicare and Medicaid Services (online). Available: *http://cms.gov/statistics/nhe/historical/t3.asp*.
14. Center for Public Service. (2002). *Government's 50 greatest endeavors: Enhance the nation's health care infrastructure*. The Brookings Institution. (online). Available: *http://www.brook.edu/dybdocroot/gs/cps/50ge/endeavors/healthcare.htm*.
15. Clark, M.J. (2002). The healthcare context. *Nursing in the Community: Dimensions of Community Health Nursing* (3rd ed.). Stamford, Conn: Appleton-Lange.
16. Clark, M.J. (2002). The historical context. *Nursing in the community: Dimensions of Community Health Nursing* (3rd ed.). Stamford, Conn: Appleton-Lange
17. Clemen-Stone, S., Eigsti, D.G., & McGuire, S.L. (1998). Occupational health nursing. In S. Clemon-Stone (Ed.), *Comprehensive community health nursing* (5th ed., pp. 537-566). St. Louis: Mosby.
18. Department of Defense. (2003). Defense budget materials, FY 2003 budget. Available: *http://www.dod.mil/comptroller/defbudget/fy2003/*.
19. Department of Veterans Affairs. (2003). VA Fact Sheets. Available: *http://www.va.gov.opa/fact/docs/vafacts.htm*.
20. Hassmiller, S.B. (2002). The public and primary healthcare systems. In M. Stanhope & J. Lancaster (Eds.), *Foundations of community health nursing: Community-oriented practice*. St. Louis: Mosby.

21. Health and Human Services. (2002). Organizational chart. (online). Available: *http://www.hhs.gov/about/orgchart/html*.

22. Health Care Financing Administration. (1999). *Expenditures for health services and supplies under public programs by type of expenditure and program: Calendar year 1997.* Health Care Financing Administration, U.S. Department of Health and Human Services (online). Available: *http://www.hcfa.gov/stats/nhe-oact/tables/t18.htm*.

23. Jacobs, P. (1995). Economics of healthcare. In G.L. Deloughery (Ed.), *Issues and trends in nursing* (pp. 97-128). St. Louis: Mosby.

24. McIntosh, M.A. (2002). The cost of healthcare to Americans. *JONA's Law, Ethics, and Regulations, 4*(3), 78-89.

25. National Institutes of Health. (2003). *An overview.* National Institutes of Health, U.S. Department of Health and Human Services (online). Available: *http://www.nih.gov/about/NIHoverview.html #mission.*.

26. National Institute for Nursing Research. (1999). Minutes of the National Advisory Council for Nursing Research (online). Available: *http://www.nih.gov/ninr/about/advcouncil/meetings/minutes/99.pdf*.

27. O'Neil, E., & Coffman, J. (Eds.). (1998). *Strategies for the future of nursing.* San Francisco: Jossey-Bass.

28. Pilon, B.A., & Davis, S. (1988). Healthcare delivery cost containment practices: History, current status, future directions. In N. Sanders (Director), *Cost management education for nurses* (Contact No. 240-86-0064). Washington, DC: Division of Nursing, Bureau of Health Professions, Health Resources and Services Administration, U.S. Department of Health and Human Services.

29. Poen, M. (1979). Politics, then health: The Medicare compromise. In *Harry S. Truman versus the medical lobby* (pp. 174-209). Columbia, MO: University of Missouri Press.

30. Steinwald, B., & Sloan, F. (1981). Regulatory approaches to hospital cost containment: A synthesis of the empirical evidence. In M. Olsen (Ed.), *A new approach to the economics of health care* (pp. 272-307). Washington, DC: American Enterprise Institute.

31. TennCare. (2003). *What is TennCare* (online). Available: *http://www.state.tn.us/tenncare/what.is.html*.

32. U.S. Bureau of Health Professions. (1996). *National sample survey of registered nurses.* Washington, DC: Government Printing Office.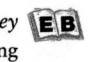

33. U.S. Department of Health and Human Services. (2002). RN statistics, projected supply, demand, and shortages of registered nurses: 2000-2020. National Center for Workforce Analysis. Available: *http://bhpr.hrsa.gov/healthworkforce/rnproject/report.htm*.

Ambulatory Health Care

Sheila A. Haas
Diana P. Hackbarth

In any given year, most Americans are not hospitalized, but the average person makes 3.3 ambulatory care visits per year.[7] This makes ambulatory settings the major site for health care delivery in the United States. Ambulatory care visits are increasing for several reasons:

1. The number of hours or days people stay in hospitals for illness, surgery, or complex treatments has decreased. More clients are seen in ambulatory settings for posthospital visits and follow-up care.
2. New technology has made ambulatory settings the site for people to undergo many surgical and complex procedures that previously required hospitalization.
3. Advances in the treatment of chronic health problems have made it possible to treat and monitor a client's progress in ambulatory care settings and avoid costly hospitalization. As a result, both the numbers and the acuity of people cared for in ambulatory settings have increased.

There are numerous advantages to providing health care in ambulatory settings. People prefer care close to home, with providers they know and with whom they have a relationship. Clients often feel less stress because they are not separated from their family, significant others, and community. Care in the community decreases exposure to nosocomial infections and other hazards of hospitalization. Ambulatory care is often less costly than hospitalization, saving money for clients, insurance companies, employers, and the government.

Socioeconomic factors have also encouraged the growth of ambulatory care. The growth of managed care organizations has increased the demand for primary care services and ambulatory facilities. Clients who are insured through a managed care plan often must see a primary care provider before obtaining referrals to specialty or hospital care. The variety of care modalities offered in ambulatory care has escalated, and the demand for professional nurses to work in ambulatory care has never been greater. The opportunities for professional nurses to work in ambulatory care settings are expected to increase in the years to come.

DEFINITION AND CHARACTERISTICS OF AMBULATORY CARE NURSING

Nurses have worked in ambulatory care settings for many years. Ambulatory care nurses take care of people in all age groups and with all diagnoses, both those who are healthy and those with acute, chronic, or life-threatening health problems. The definition of ambulatory nursing was developed by a panel of expert ambulatory care nurses who participated in focus groups of ambulatory care nurses across the United States.[5] The following factors have been identified as characteristics of ambulatory care nursing[5]:
- Nursing autonomy
- Client advocacy
- Skillful, rapid assessment

- Holistic nursing care
- Client teaching
- Wellness and health promotion
- Coordination and continuity of care
- Long-term relationships with clients and families
- Telephone triage, instruction, and advice
- Client and family control as major caregivers, users of the health care system, and decision makers regarding compliance with care regimen
- Collaboration with other health care providers
- Case management

Based on these characteristics, the American Academy of Ambulatory Care Nursing (AAACN)[1,5] defined ambulatory care nursing as follows:

Ambulatory care nursing includes those clinical, management, educational, and research activities provided by registered nurses for and with individuals who seek care and assistance with health maintenance and/or health promotion. These individuals engage predominantly in self-care and self-managed health activities or receive care from family and significant others outside an institutional setting.

Ambulatory care nursing takes place on an episodic basis, is less that 24 hours in duration, and occurs as a single encounter or a series of encounters over time. Ambulatory nurse-patient encounters take place in health care facilities as well as in community-based settings, including but not limited to schools, workplaces, or homes. The focus of ambulatory care services encompasses use of cost-effective ways to assist patients in promoting wellness, preventing illness, and managing acute and chronic diseases to effect the most attainable positive health status over the life span.

Characteristics of ambulatory care present the following challenges for nurses:

1. *Visit encounters are short,* the number of client visits per day is great, and the assessment time is compressed. In contrast to the hospital nurse, who can return to a client confined to bed to retrieve data that may have been missed, the ambulatory care nurse who misses collecting data may not be able to obtain it until the next visit. Because visits are short, the ambulatory care nurse cannot do an extensive assessment on every client but must do a focused assessment. This aspect is often a difficult transition for nurses who have worked in hospital settings.
2. Control of care and treatment modalities is in the hands of the client and family, *not* the health care provider. In the hospital, the nurse administers medications, administers the treatments, or supervises others providing care to the client. In ambulatory care, however, the client chooses to schedule a visit, keep an appointment, take prescribed medications, or undergo treatments as he or she sees fit. The nurse must become a teacher, coach, and ad-

vocate as well as a treatment provider because clients and families must follow through with the treatment plan on their own between visits.
3. In ambulatory care, many members of the health care team work together, and their roles often do not have clear boundaries. Nurses must be strong communicators and collaborators, often functioning as a team leader or team facilitator.
4. In ambulatory care, contacts with the nurse are frequently maintained through *communication devices* such as the telephone and computer. Ambulatory care nurses need highly developed assessment and communication skills, as well as critical thinking and judgment, in order to interpret data and to refer the client for appropriate follow-up.
5. Finally, there is *constant pressure* to increase efficiency and effectiveness of care. Nurses are working to standardize care so that health promotion, disease prevention, and early detection and treatment of health problems become integral to the ambulatory care client encounter.[5]

CONCEPTUAL MODELS THAT INFLUENCE AMBULATORY CARE NURSING PRACTICE

The Clinical Model

The organization of ambulatory care services in the United States is based on a complex mix of historical, philosophical, political, and economic factors. The way in which policy-makers, health care providers, and ordinary citizens conceptualize health and disease has a profound effect on how health care is delivered.[6]

Most health policy experts agree that the current health care system is based on the clinical or medical model.[6,9,28,29] In this model, health is conceptualized as the absence of the clinical manifestations of disease.[30] It is assumed that the body is a machine and that modern medical technology can use physical and chemical interventions to "fix the machine" whenever it is broken.[30] This has led to great emphasis on expensive, acute care with high-technology treatments and relatively little attention to prevention, public health, environmental measures, or personal responsibility for health.[6,29]

Most ambulatory care services, except for certain public health programs, are outgrowths of this clinical model. Services were traditionally organized around physicians' delivery of reimbursable clinical model care to people who sought care only when they were ill. The traditional nursing role in ambulatory care supported physician control and the clinical model of care delivery. Although the clinical model has led to great advances in scientific medicine and technology, the focus on body parts rather than the whole, and the lack of emphasis on prevention, have been problematic.

Many nurse theorists, primary care providers, and public health advocates look at health in a *holistic* way. Nurses are educated to (1) consider the whole person, family, and environment; (2) address both actual and potential health problems; and (3) emphasize health teaching, prevention, and self-care as well as care of the sick. Newer, more holistic conceptual models are becoming increasingly important in ambulatory care. These models have been delineated by health care scholars, national and international health advocacy organizations, and ambulatory care nurses themselves.

Levels of Prevention Model

The Levels of Prevention Model, advocated by Leavell and Clark in 1965,[23] has influenced both public health practice and ambulatory care delivery worldwide. This model suggests that the natural history of any disease exists on a continuum, with health at one end and advanced disease at the other. The model delineates three levels of the application of preventive measures that can be used to promote health and arrest the disease process at different points along the continuum.[23] The goal is to maintain a healthy state and to prevent disease or injury.

People experiencing acute or chronic disease, as well as healthy populations, are all candidates for primary prevention measures. The Levels of Prevention Model is appropriate in all health care settings and in any population group. The *Healthy People 2010 Objectives for the Nation* includes two overarching goals of reducing health disparities and increasing both the length and quality of life; it also includes leading health indicators and objectives to reduce mortality and morbidity at all three levels of prevention.[35] Most of these objectives can be implemented in ambulatory settings or through population-focused interventions in the community.

Primary Prevention

Primary prevention encompasses both health promotion and specific protection.[23] Health promotion includes interventions such as health education, information on growth and development, nutrition, and exercise as well as the provision of adequate housing, safe working conditions, and other services. For example, an ambulatory care nurse might provide telephone consultation and teaching to a new mother concerned about well baby care.

Specific protection interventions are targeted at specific health risks, injuries, and diseases. For example, immunizations protect against particular infectious diseases; seat belts reduce injuries in automobile crashes; smoking cessation reduces the risk of cancers and heart disease; reducing air pollution prevents exacerbations of asthma and bronchitis; a high-calcium diet with over-the-counter calcium supplements and weight-bearing exercise helps menopausal women prevent osteoporosis.

Primary prevention interventions may be targeted at individual clients, families, groups, communities, or populations.

Secondary Prevention

Secondary preventive measures include early diagnosis and prompt treatment as well as disability limitation.[23] Case finding, screening, and treatment of disease by medical or surgical interventions to arrest the disease process and prevent further complications are all part of secondary prevention. An ambulatory care nurse carrying out a multiphasic health screening for hypertension, diabetes, and hypercholesterolemia would be practicing secondary prevention. Other examples are administering chemotherapy to a client with cancer and positioning a client in the recovery room after outpatient surgery to ensure proper alignment of the extremities.

Tertiary Prevention

Tertiary prevention is the provision of measures to rehabilitate a person or group so they can maximize their remaining capacities.[23] Cardiac rehabilitation nurses, physical and occupational therapists, and many home care nurses focus on tertiary prevention. An example of tertiary prevention in the ambulatory surgery recovery room is teaching crutch walking to a client after foot surgery.

Primary Health Care, Primary Care, and Managed Care Models

Primary health care focuses on the universal right to basic health care. *Primary care* focuses on integrated care coordinated by one primary provider. *Managed care* approaches the use of health care services from a cost-containment perspective. *Primary prevention* is often confused with the concepts of primary health care and primary care.[17] In addition, many managed care organizations use primary care providers, such as family practice physicians and nurse practitioners, in a "gatekeeper" function, causing further confusion. Box 7-1 compares and contrasts these conceptual models. These models, as well as the clinical model and the ambulatory care nursing conceptual framework, have influenced the organization of practice in ambulatory care settings.

AMBULATORY CARE NURSING CONCEPTUAL FRAMEWORK

The Ambulatory Care Nursing Conceptual Framework was developed by a think tank of experts who are also members of the AAACN.[10] The AAACN member experts work in ambulatory care settings, perform

---

BOX 7-1   *Health Care Models*

Primary Health Care

- WHO definition (1978)[37]: "essential health care made universally accessible to individuals and families in the community through their full participation and at a cost the community and country can afford."
    Assumes community involvement
    Includes both personal health care services and population-based public health services
    Aimed at prevention as well as treatment of disease
    Aimed at improving health status of the population or community

Primary Care

- IOM definition (1994)[20]: "provision of integrated accessible health care services by clinicians who are accountable for addressing a large majority of personal health care needs, developing a sustained partnership with patients, and practicing in the context of family and community."
- IOM definition (1978)[21]: "personal health care services that are accessible, comprehensive, coordinated, and continuous. Care delivered by accountable providers of personal health services.
- Starfield definition (1992)[31]:
    First contact—source of care available in a timely manner

    Longitudinal—not episodic, focused on person, not episode of disease; client sees provider as regular source of care
    Comprehensive—includes services for common problems
    Coordinated—provider coordinates care when client is sent elsewhere for referrals, procedures, and therapies

Managed Care

- Enthoven definition (1993)[8]:
    Integrated financing and delivery systems with per capita prepayment and with providers placed at risk for cost and quality of care
    First contact—ensure access to basic services; restrict access to specialized services through "gatekeeper" function of primary provider
- Starfield definition (1992)[31]:
    Longitudinal—not addressed
    Comprehensive—not addressed
    Coordinated—gatekeeper as coordinator; goal is to eliminate unnecessary and inappropriate care; may also restrict access to appropriate care
    Reduction in cost; cost containment
    Health status of population—not addressed; in HMO organizations, goal is to keep enrolled population healthy in order to reduce utilization cost

IOM, Institute of Medicine; *WHO*, World Health Organization.

---

research, and write about ambulatory care nursing. A conceptual framework is a diagram that:

- Specifies major concepts, skills, and responsibilities in an area of practice
- Reflects values and beliefs as well as the experiential knowledge of a practice discipline
- Delineates the relationships between major concepts and skills
- Acts as a model to help organize practice, guide the development of educational materials, create test items for certification examinations, and develop orientation programs
- Forms the basis of performance appraisal instruments for ambulatory care nurses

The conceptual framework shown in Figure 7-1 delineates three roles for ambulatory care nurses: (1) the Clinical Nursing Role, (2) the Organizational/Systems Role, and (3) the Professional Role.[10] Each role has several dimensions that vary, depending on the size of the ambulatory care setting. For example, staff nurses working in large settings where there are multiple nurses and nurse managers do not need to do many of the more managerial dimensions under the Organizational/Systems Role. In smaller settings, they would likely practice in all three roles. The Ambulatory Care Nursing Conceptual Framework was used to structure the Ambulatory Care Nursing Core Curriculum written for nurses to use in preparation for certification in ambulatory care.

As seen in Figure 7-1, client populations may be healthy, acutely ill, chronically ill, or terminally ill. Role dimensions highly valued by nurses are all included in this conceptual framework:

- Primary, secondary, and tertiary prevention
- Teaching and client advocacy
- Care management, a feature of primary care
- Evidence-based practice

AMBULATORY CARE PRACTICE SETTINGS

Historically, health services in the United States were delivered to people in their homes by itinerant physicians, midwives, barbers, nurses, and "medicine men," who learned their trade through an unregulated apprentice system. In some urban areas, freestanding dispensaries were established as charity for the poor and a place for would-be physicians to learn their trade.[32] These dispensaries dissolved into outpatient departments once a system of voluntary hospitals was developed and nursing and medical education was upgraded and standardized in the beginning of the 20th century.[32]

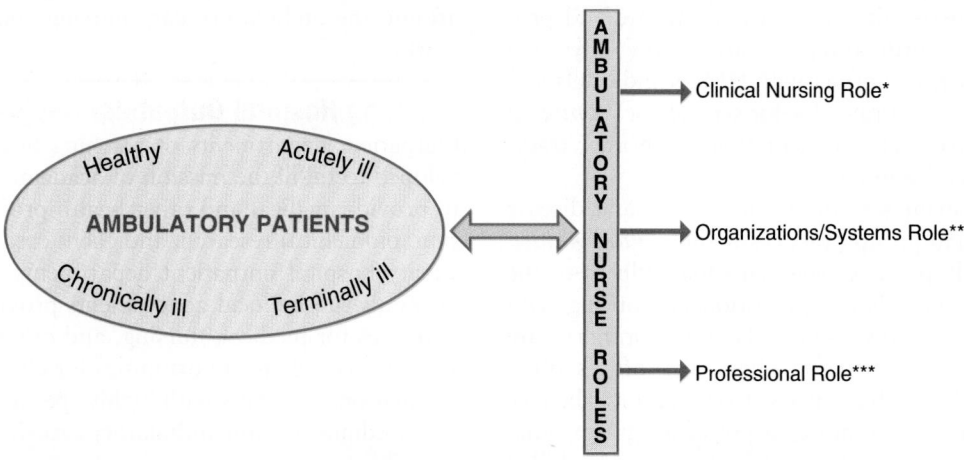

Clinical Nursing Role*
Patient Education
Advocacy (compassion, caring,
    emotional support)
Care Management
Assessment, Screening, Triage
Telephone Practice
Collaboration/Resource
    Identification and Referral
    Clinical Procedures,
    Independent/Interdependent/
    Dependent
Primary, Secondary, and
    Tertiary Prevention
Communication/Documentation
Outcome Management
Protocol Development/Usage

***Organizations/Systems
    Role*
Practice/Office Support
Healthcare Fiscal Management
    (reimbursement and coding)
Collaboration/Conflict
    Management
Informatics
Context of Care Delivery/
    Models
Care of the Caregiver
Priority Management/
    Delegation/Supervision
Ambulatory Culture/Cross-
    Cultural Competencies
Ongoing Political/
    Entrepreneurial Skills
Structuring Customer-Focused
    Systems
Workplace Regulatory
    Compliance (EEOC, OSHA)
Advocacy Inter-organizational
    and in Community
Legal Issues

***Professional Role
Evidence-Based Practice
Leadership Inquiry and
    Research Utilization
Clinical Quality Improvement
Staff Development
Regulatory Compliance (Risk
    Management)
Provider Self-Care

FIGURE 7-1 Ambulatory Care Nursing Conceptual Framework. (Modified from Haas, S. [1998]. Ambulatory care nursing conceptual framework. *AAACN Viewpoint, 20*[3], 16-17, with permission.)

For the purposes of data collection, the National Center for Health Statistics classifies ambulatory care settings into three main groups: physicians' offices, hospital outpatient departments, and hospital emergency departments (EDs).[7,24,27] Each of these may sponsor many types of ambulatory care programs, both on-site and geographically dispersed in communities. With the advent of managed care insurance plans, health maintenance organizations (HMOs) and preferred provider organizations (PPOs) have been developed as both sites and payment mechanisms for ambulatory care delivery.

Physician Offices

Almost 81% of the more than 1 billion annual ambulatory care visits in the United States occur in physicians' offices.[7] Increasingly, physicians are abandoning solo practice and aligning themselves in group practices to consolidate resources to meet the challenges of managed

care contracting. About two thirds of physicians practice in a group setting.[7] In the past, many group practices consisted of groups of specialists, such as cardiologists or oncologists. Today, larger group practices often include primary care physicians. About one fourth of physician office visits are to general and family practice physicians; 15.2% to internists; 12.6% to pediatricians; and 7.9% to obstetric and gynecology physicians,[7] all considered primary care providers. The remaining visits are to specialists.

Physician group practices usually operate on a for-profit basis and seek fee-for-service payment directly from clients or through third party payers such as insurance companies, Medicare, and Medicaid. In a *fee-for-service* system, providers get paid separately for each service they provide; the more services they provide, the more revenue they generate. In *integrated* delivery systems, hospitals align with several physician group practices to increase the hospital referral rate and provide increased coordination of care. Many physician group practices also contract with HMOs and PPOs and offer either reduced-rate fee-for-service or *capitated* (prepaid at a fixed rate) services along with their traditional fee-for-service practices.[6]

The predominant way of viewing health and disease in most physician group practices is the *clinical model*. However, family practice physicians may adhere to the *primary care model*. Nurse practitioners working with primary care physicians also ascribe to the primary care model. In the past, nurses in physicians' offices often served a clerical as well as an assistive function. The role of the ambulatory care nurse in physician group practices is evolving to meet the need for increasingly skilled technical services, especially in specialty practices such as oncology, freestanding birthing centers, and surgical centers.

Community Hospital Outpatient Departments

Community hospital clinic services began in the latter part of the 19th century and took over the functions of the freestanding dispensaries.[32] Clinic services were consistent with the mission of the religious and ethnic groups that organized voluntary community hospitals. This mission included both a charitable function for the community and a place for local physicians to practice.[9] Physicians were often assigned to staff hospital clinics as a duty, in return for the privilege of hospitalizing their clients.[22,29] Nurses trained in diploma schools staffed both the hospital and clinics.

Today, nonprofit community hospitals still provide varying amounts of uncompensated care in their outpatient departments as part of their obligation to provide "community benefits" as not-for-profit corporations. However, their goal is to maximize revenues by attracting individuals or employee groups who have insurance coverage. Thus, outpatient services constitute a key source of revenue for hospitals. Approximately 8.2% of all ambulatory care visits occur in hospital outpatient departments.[24]

Both primary care and specialized care in a clinical model may be offered. Ambulatory services may be housed adjacent to the hospital or be freestanding in the community. Services may include outpatient surgery, emergency centers, cardiac rehabilitation centers, drug and alcohol treatment programs, mobile vans, women's health or breast centers, work site health promotion, oncology centers, home care, hospice, and community health promotion.[29] Many integrated health care systems have freestanding satellite ambulatory care sites that offer primary care services for managed care enrollees. Specialized clinics and health promotion programs staffed by nurses also exist in community hospital outpatient settings. Some of these programs are organized around the ambulatory care nursing conceptual framework.

Teaching Hospital Outpatient Departments

Outpatient departments of teaching hospitals were developed to fulfill the mission of academic health centers: to provide medical and other health professional education, biomedical research, and client care services.[29] University hospital outpatient departments and most large hospitals run by local governments provide learning experiences for medical, nursing, and other health science students as well as opportunities for clinical research on populations of clients with highly specialized needs. Veterans Administration ambulatory care departments serve a similar function.

Clinical services are often organized around medical specialty areas for the convenience of providers. Some are regional referral centers, whereas others, especially those that are tax-supported, may provide a full range of services, including primary care for the poor.[29] Most teaching hospitals maintain a nonprofit status and provide care for those with public or private insurance as well as uncompensated care for uninsured clients (whose diseases may provide good learning experiences). Many hospitals have satellite ambulatory care centers. With the growth of managed care, increased competition, and decreased reimbursement from Medicaid, Medicare, and insurance companies, teaching hospitals are increasingly concerned with maximizing revenue from insured clients and ensuring a flow of paying clients to make up for empty inpatient beds or discounted client charges.

University hospital outpatient departments have traditionally espoused the clinical model and have been driven and controlled by physicians. There are, however, some nurse-managed hospital clinics that deal with specific client populations, such as clients with chronic leg ulcers or those who need monitoring of warfarin (Coumadin) therapy. Nurses play a major role in client and family teaching and as case managers for clients with catastrophic and chronic illnesses. For example, nurses case-manage the care of heart transplant clients, trauma victims, oncology clients, and high-risk mothers and infants.

Health Maintenance Organizations

HMOs began more than 50 years ago and proliferated during the 1990s in response to both federal enabling legislation and market forces. HMOs provide a defined population with a stated range of services through the prepayment of an annual or monthly capitation fee. With *capitation,* providers receive the same amount of money per client per month, no matter how many or how few services a client uses that month or year. Thus there is no incentive to provide expensive tests or treatments that the client may not need. HMOs are systems of care that integrate the insurance and payment mechanisms and the actual delivery of health care services.[6] About one fourth of ambulatory care visits are financed through an HMO mechanism.

HMOs began as nonprofit organizations but increasingly have been purchased by the for-profit sector. Philosophically, the concept of an HMO differs from traditional ambulatory services, in that value is placed on prevention and maintaining health in order to avoid more costly specialist or inpatient services. Care is coordinated by a primary care provider who acts as a gatekeeper. The goal is to lower costs through the provision of primary care, coordination of services, utilization management, and elimination of the "incentives" of the fee-for-service payment system.[6]

Many HMOs employ nurse practitioners, nurse-midwives, and physician assistants as primary care providers. In addition to the clinical model, HMOs espouse wellness, health maintenance, and primary care. Nursing, with its more holistic approach to client care, can play an influential role in managed care settings.

Emergency Departments

Almost 10.6% of ambulatory care visits are provided in EDs.[27] About three fourths of ED visits are made by persons who walk in, whereas 14% arrive by either ground or air ambulance. Triage staff in EDs classify clients in terms of the immediacy of their need to be seen in a timely manner. In 2000, ED staff classified 15.7% of visits as emergent, 31.2% as urgent, 16.9 as semiurgent, 10.7 as not urgent, and the remaining as unclassified.[27] The average waiting time for an emergent visit is 24 minutes nationally, whereas nonurgent clients must wait an hour or more, up to 24 hours, in many U.S. EDs.[27] Low-income families, the unemployed, and members of minority groups are most likely to be uninsured. Uninsured people and those whose health care is funded through Medicare and Medicaid use disproportionately more ED services for nonurgent care than those who have private insurance.[27] In the United States, there are 41.2 million uninsured and many more underinsured people who lack access to appropriate primary care services in their communities.[29] Because EDs are organized according to the clinical model and are set up to meet acute care needs, they are far from the ideal place to provide primary care services.

Other Ambulatory Care Settings

Many other settings provide a wide array of ambulatory care services. One unique type of ambulatory care organization is a Nurse-Managed Center or Nursing Center. These nurse-staffed community centers may provide primary health care services, home care, hospice, college health services, work site health promotion, school nursing, or wellness services. Many Nursing Centers were de-

veloped by schools of nursing as faculty practice sites and clinical sites for undergraduate and graduate students. Others were federally funded demonstration projects. Most Nurse-Managed Centers employ Advanced Practice Nurses (APNs) and are organized around a nursing or primary health care model.

Other settings in which ambulatory care nurses practice include government-funded public health clinics, migrant and community health centers, homeless shelters, school-based health centers, Native American Health Service clinics, and other community-based organizations that serve special population groups. These are either tax-supported or private nonprofit organizations. Many community-based organizations are organized around a primary health care or public health model. Most include population-based preventive services as well as personal health care.

CHARACTERISTICS OF AMBULATORY CARE CLIENT POPULATION

Each year in the United States, people make more than a billion ambulatory visits. Women make more visits than men, and older adults make an average 7.5 visits a year compared with about three visits a year for children.[7,24] The overall visit rate for whites is not significantly different than that for African Americans,[7] although African Americans are more likely to use hospital outpatient departments than whites.[7,24] Figure 7-2 shows the distribution of ambulatory care visits, categorized by clients' expressed reasons for the visit. Figure 7-3 depicts the distribution of ambulatory care visits by primary

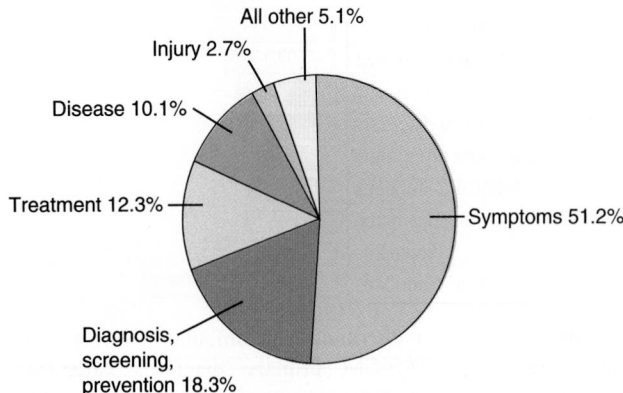

FIGURE 7-2 Percent distribution of physician's office and outpatient ambulatory care visits by client's principal reason for visit: United States, 2000. (From Cherry, D.K., & Woodwell, D.A. [2000]. *National ambulatory medical care survey: 2000 summary, no. 328.* Hyattsville, MD: National Center for Health Statistics; and Ly, N., & McCraig, L.F. [2000]. *National hospital ambulatory medical care survey: 2000 summary, no. 327.* Hyattsville, MD: National Center for Health Statistics.

diagnosis in the United States in 2000. Difficulty breathing, a manifestation of many problems including lung, heart, and allergic conditions, is a common reason for visits.

Ambulatory clients are often classified by their *health status*. A client may be essentially healthy but acutely ill at the time of the visit, such as a client with otitis media or appendicitis. The client can be expected to return to wellness once the acute problem is cured. Another client may be chronically ill but managing the chronic illness well. A young asthmatic person with peak flow readings within normal limits is an example. A client may be chronically ill and have an acute episode, such as an older diabetic client with influenza. Finally, a client may be terminally ill with end-stage renal disease or liver failure and require supportive care.

Ambulatory clients may also be classified by a major *illness*, body system, and typical *treatment* needed. For example, teaching hospital outpatient settings often have specific clinics for people with diabetes or heart failure; some have ear, nose, and throat clinics or urology clinics for people with maladies of certain body systems. Others have programs such as a "Coumadin clinic" and "cast clinic," which classify clients according to the type of treatment to be administered. Ambulatory clients may also be classified in terms of *age*, such as pediatric, adolescent, and geriatric.

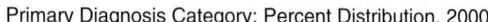

Primary Diagnosis Category: Percent Distribution, 2000

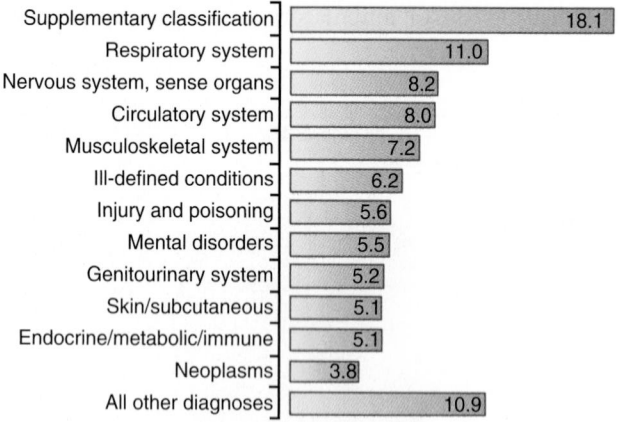

Category	Percent
Supplementary classification	18.1
Respiratory system	11.0
Nervous system, sense organs	8.2
Circulatory system	8.0
Musculoskeletal system	7.2
Ill-defined conditions	6.2
Injury and poisoning	5.6
Mental disorders	5.5
Genitourinary system	5.2
Skin/subcutaneous	5.1
Endocrine/metabolic/immune	5.1
Neoplasms	3.8
All other diagnoses	10.9

FIGURE 7-3 Percent distribution of ambulatory office visits categorized by ICD-9-CM primary diagnosis categories: United States, 2000. "Supplementary classification" is used for visits not related to illness or injury, such as general medical examinations, health supervision, and normal prenatal care. (From Cherry, D.K., & Woodwell, D.A. [2000]. *National ambulatory medical care survey: 2000 summary, no. 328.* Hyattsville, MD: National Center for Health Statistics; and Ly, N., & McCraig, L.F. [2000]. *National hospital ambulatory medical care survey: 2000 summary, no. 327.* Hyattsville, MD: National Center for Health Statistics.)

Another means of categorizing clients is by the type or source of *reimbursement* for the care provided; (e.g., private insurance, Medicare, Medicaid, worker's compensation, or self-pay). Because about 15% of the U.S. population lacks health insurance, payment for care is a problem for many individuals and families. Ambulatory care clients also may be defined by the type of *service*, such as primary care, which includes pediatrics, obstetrics and gynecology, family practice, and internal medicine.

As mentioned earlier, in ambulatory care it is the client, client's family, or significant other who initiates an encounter or visit, travels to and from the ambulatory care setting, and chooses to collaborate with the ambulatory interdisciplinary team regarding wellness behaviors and the treatment regimen. Thus, the ambulatory care team must know, understand, and respect the client's culture, traditions, and perspective on health and illness. Cultural competence is essential, because the client, family, or significant other manages and provides health care during visits and during the interval between visits and the client controls health care decisions. Respectful communication facilitates the long-term relationships that clients often have with ambulatory care nurses and other providers.

RESEARCH IN AMBULATORY CARE NURSING

Although nurses have been working in ambulatory settings for many years, little research on the work and role of ambulatory care nurses has been done. Such research is needed for many reasons[18]:

- To help develop new models of nursing care delivery
- To delineate position descriptions for nurses working in ambulatory care
- To develop standards of client care and professional nursing practice
- To create both performance improvement programs and nursing intensity systems to determine the number and types of nursing personnel needed

One of the earliest studies, done by Hooks and colleagues in 1980,[19] delineated barriers to ambulatory nursing practice. Verran, in 1981,[36] developed seven areas of nursing responsibility in ambulatory care using a Delphi method and the opinion of expert ambulatory care nurses. In 1985, Tighe and associates[34] further refined Verran's areas of responsibility by adding planning. In 1995, Hackbarth and co-workers[18] and Haas and colleagues[13-16] conducted a national survey of ambulatory care nurses working in many types of ambulatory care settings. An analysis of these data provided insight into the dimensions of the current staff nurse role and the dimensions of the future staff nurse role in ambulatory care.

In current practice, Hackbarth and co-workers[18] found that ambulatory care nurses spent much of their time performing activities in dimensions named Enabling Operations and Technical Procedures. These activities include locating records, ordering supplies, taking vital signs, setting up rooms, assisting with procedures, and administering oral or intramuscular (IM) medications. Some of these activities could have been done by clerks or nursing assistants. Relatively less of the staff nurse's time was spent on more professional activities in the dimensions named Telephone Communication, Advocacy, Teaching, and Care Coordination.

When nurses surveyed by Haas and Hackbarth[13] were asked what they would like to be doing in the future, they indicated that they would prefer to accomplish more activities in higher-level professional dimensions such as Teaching, Care Coordination, and Expert Practice. They even foresaw another dimension, labeled Technical Procedures (Figure 7-4). The implications of this research are clear. Nurses in many ambulatory settings need to have sufficient numbers of competent assistive personnel to whom they can delegate Enabling and Technical procedures if they are to have sufficient time to perform activities in higher-level dimensions such as Teaching, Advocacy, Care Coordination, High Tech Procedures, and Expert Practice.

Ambulatory care nurse researchers are involved in specifying ambulatory care nursing quality indicators[26,33] and ambulatory nursing outcomes.[25] Examples of ambulatory nursing quality indicators include appropriate services, client satisfaction, risk reduction, level of functioning, symptom severity protective factors in the client's environment, and strength of the therapeutic alliance.[33] Seven common Ambulatory Care Nursing Outcomes are (1) vital signs status, (2) knowledge: health promotion, (3) medication response, (4) physical aging status, (5) health-seeking behavior, (6) acceptance: health status, and (7) compliance behavior.[25] The Nursing Outcomes Classification is used to define and specify each of these outcomes.

DIMENSIONS UNIQUE TO NURSING PRACTICE IN AMBULATORY CARE

Telehealth Nursing Practice

One dimension of the professional nurse's role that is unique in ambulatory care settings is telephone communication, or Telehealth Nursing Practice. Telehealth Nursing Practice is defined as "nursing practice using the nursing process to provide care for individual patients or defined patient populations through telecommunications media."[2] Criteria for Telehealth Nursing Practice include the following[2]:

- Using protocols, algorithms, or guidelines to assess and address client needs systematically

Ambulatory Professional Nurse **Current Clinical Practice** Core Role Dimensions	Ambulatory Professional Nurse **Future Clinical Practice** Core Role Dimensions
Enabling operations Technical procedures Nursing process Telephone communication Advocacy Teaching Care coordination Expert practice within setting	Enabling operations Technical procedures Nursing process Telephone communication Advocacy Client teaching Care coordination Expert practice/community outreach
Ambulatory Professional Nurse **Current Quality Improvement and Research** Core Role Dimensions	Ambulatory Professional Nurse **Future Quality Improvement and Research** Core Role Dimensions
Quality improvement Research Continuing education	Quality improvement Research Continuing education

FIGURE 7-4 Current and future ambulatory professional nurse dimensions. (Data from Haas, S.A., & Hackbarth, D.P. [1995]. Dimensions of the staff nurse role in ambulatory care: Part III: Using research data to design new models of nursing care delivery. *Nursing Economics, 13*[4], 230-241; and Hackbarth, D.P., et al. [1995]. Dimensions of the staff nurse role in ambulatory care: Part I: Methodology and analysis of data on current staff nurse practice. *Nursing Economics, 13*[2], 89-98.)

- Prioritizing the urgency of client needs
- Developing a collaborative plan of care with clients and their support systems; the plan of care may include wellness promotion, prevention education, care counseling, disease state management, and care coordination
- Evaluating outcomes of practice and care

Telehealth Nursing Practice is not new and has been described in the literature since the 1960s. Communication by telephone for health guidance is common in pediatric practices, obstetrics and gynecology practices, primary care practices, and EDs. Clients often call ambulatory care settings to report manifestations of illness and to seek advice. A 1997 document published by the AAACN identifies standards that define the responsibilities of both clinical nurses and managers when providing care via the telephone.[4]

The *Nursing Intervention Classification* (NIC) lists four telephone nursing interventions:

- Telephone consultation
- Telephone follow-up
- Telephone triage
- Telephone surveillance

Each of these interventions was proposed by Haas and Androwich in 1999[11]:

EB

1. *Telephone consultation.* The nurse assesses the client's need and readiness to learn, teaches clients, and provides advice based on protocols approved for use with telephone nursing practice. Assessing a client by telephone is far more difficult for the nurse than a face-to-face meeting with a client. The nurse must have expert communication skills to elicit information when no visual or physical assessment cues are available. The nurse must listen for nuances in the client's communication, such as inflection, pitch, volume, and rate of speech. The telephone encounter time is limited. There is no time to reflect or have second thoughts. Although telephone assessment has some pitfalls, there are some benefits, too.

2. *Telephone follow-up* is used for clients who have had ambulatory surgery or complex treatments. The nurse calls the client within a specified period to assess how well the client is recovering and to provide guidance for any problems. Especially when the nurse is calling the client, the nurse must protect the confidentiality of the client and should speak with family members or significant others only if the client has given permission. Many clients appreciate telephone follow-up. It connotes caring and concern on the part of the nurse and the ambulatory care organization, and it gives the client ready access to a health professional.

3. With *telephone triage,* clients are sorted by telephone encounter based on the immediacy of the need and the type of problem. In ambulatory care, a nurse talks with a client calling from home and assesses the type of problem, how the problem should be resolved, whether the client should be seen in person and when, and who should resolve the problem.

4. Nurses use *telephone surveillance* to work with data coming into a central ambulatory site from monitoring equipment used by clients at home. For example, cardiac monitoring or high-risk obstetric monitoring can be accomplished by connecting the monitoring equipment to a computer or telephone in the client's home.

Telephone triage and telephone consultation by nurses has increased with the growth of managed care health insurance plans. Nurses use commercially available protocols or protocols that have been developed by physicians and nurses in their own ambulatory care organization to assess the client over the telephone and to recommend approved interventions. Nurse telephone consultation and telephone triage have some advantages. They make nurses and expert health advice readily available, they may save a trip to the ambulatory care site, and, for many clients, they provide a knowledgeable and caring person to ask about a problem.

Professional nurses have stated strongly that Telehealth Nursing Practice should be part of the professional nurse's role.[5] It should not be done by licensed practical nurses (LPNs) or assistive personnel such as receptionists or schedulers. It requires critical thinking and judgment as well as assessment and evaluation skills. Nurses need to attend educational programs designed to help them develop the knowledge and skills needed to practice these techniques effectively. Every telephone encounter should be documented on the client's medical record, including assessment data, analysis, recommendations made to the client, and the client's level of understanding of instructions, (e.g., when to come in or to call back).

Expert Practice Within the Setting

Another unique dimension of the current clinical nurse's role in ambulatory care is Expert Practice Within the Setting. Ambulatory care nurses who develop expertise with specific client populations often are in charge of nurse-run clinics such as incontinence clinics, Coumadin clinics, or wound care clinics. In a nurse-run clinic, a nurse with at least a bachelor's degree in nursing, plus experience and continuing education, works with physicians to develop protocols. Nurses monitor clients during ambulatory visits and suggest interventions for common problems that clients experience.

Nurses and clients express high levels of satisfaction with nurse-run ambulatory programs. Clients can call a nurse who knows them and their problems and who has insight into their problems. The nurse often acts as their advocate in the health care system. Nurses find this type of work rewarding because they have long-term relationships with clients and families and can see the results of their teaching, advocacy, and nursing interventions.

Ambulatory Care Interdisciplinary Team

Nurses working in ambulatory settings are members of an interdisciplinary team. They work collaboratively with physicians; midlevel providers, such as nurse practitioners (NPs), nurse midwives, and physician assistants (PAs); LPNs and licensed vocational nurses (LVN); medical assistants (MAs); nurse assistants (NAs); and clerks, receptionists, and schedulers.

The challenges in working with a large team are numerous. Roles often are blurred, especially when people have worked together in the same clinic for many years. Sometimes team members may be asked to perform beyond their legal scope of practice; at other times, nurses may do assistive or clerical work. Both situations can prevent clients from receiving care from the best prepared provider. Nurses must continually negotiate and advocate for clients within and beyond the team.

Nurses must also delegate appropriately to assistive workers. Nurses must be aware of the specifications of their state Nurse Practice Act and delegate to LPNs and LVNs only what is legally within their scope of practice. For example, MAs in some states may administer immunizations when they have the requisite training and when they are supervised by licensed professional nurses or physicians; in other states, this might be illegal. Supervision in ambulatory care is challenging.[12] State Nurse Practice Acts often legally define both the delegation and the supervision to be done by professional nurses.

Professional and Legal Considerations

Standards of Care

Standards are written authoritative statements developed and disseminated by a professional organizational or governmental or regulatory agency by which the quality of practice, services, research, or education can be judged.[1] In 1987, the AAACN developed *Ambulatory Care Nursing Administration and Practice Standards*. These are revised and updated periodically, most recently in 2000.[1] There are nine standards: Structure and Organization of Ambulatory Care Nursing, Staffing in Ambulatory Care, Competency, Ambulatory Nursing Practice, Continuity of Care, Ethics and Patient's Rights, Environment, Research, and Quality Management. AAACN also developed and published the *Telephone Nursing Practice Administration and Practice Standards* in 1997[4] and the revised update *AAACN Telehealth Nursing Practice Administration and Practice Standards*

in 2001.[2] The American Nurses' Association also published *Core Principles on Telehealth* in 1998.[3]

Ambulatory care nurses are also guided by other sets of standards. To provide services, an ambulatory care setting must be in compliance with its state's Department of Health rules and regulations and must operate in compliance with Occupational Safety and Health Administration standards. Evidence-based practice guidelines are available through the Agency for Health Care Research and Quality, which has guidelines for many common health problems such as chronic pain, incontinence care, depression, and sickle cell anemia. These are available at website http://www.ahrq.gov. Professional nursing organizations, such as the American Nurses' Association and Oncology Nurses Society, also have specific client population standards.

Competence

Competence is the "demonstrated knowledge, skills, and ability to effectively carry out the requirements of a given role. Nurse competence is circumscribed by the individual nurse's education, knowledge, certification, experience and abilities."[5] Ambulatory care nurses demonstrate competence in core clinical practice dimensions, such as client teaching. They also have competencies that reflect the unique clinical dimensions of ambulatory care nursing, such as telephone nursing, and that correspond to the needs of the particular client populations served and the nursing interventions commonly required by such populations. For example, ambulatory oncology clients are a specific population for whom competence with chemotherapy administration is a requisite nursing intervention competence. Ambulatory care nurses who work in smaller ambulatory settings may also be required to exhibit competencies in dimensions within the leadership role, such as regulatory compliance and risk management. Any nurse who works with assistive personnel must be competent in delegation and supervision.

Certification

Holding certification in a specialty practice area such as ambulatory care nursing is a way of demonstrating competence to consumers and colleagues. To obtain certification, practicing nurses prepare for and take an examination that is developed by a panel of experts and administered by a recognized certification agency. With increasing numbers of nurses practicing in ambulatory care and the evolution of the Ambulatory Care Nursing Conceptual Framework,[10] the AAACN and the American Nurses Credentialing Center service have developed a certification examination for nurses working in staff nursing positions in ambulatory care. The examination was administered for the first time in the fall of 1999.

To qualify for the examination, ambulatory care nurses must meet the requirement for hours of experience in ambulatory care nursing. To maintain certification, ambulatory nurses must continue to practice in the clinical area for the specified number of hours per year and accumulate a specified number of hours of sanctioned continuing education. Ambulatory care nurses are often certified in more than one area of specialty nursing practice. A nurse working with oncology clients might be certified in oncology nursing as well as ambulatory care nursing. AAACN has led the development of the Ambulatory Care Nursing Conceptual Framework, core curriculum, and ambulatory certification. AAACN website address is http://www.inurse.com and the e-mail address is aaacn@ajj.com.

Regulatory Compliance

Ambulatory settings must be licensed in the state in which they are located; they may earn and maintain credentials, such as accreditation by a national association like the Joint Commission on Accreditation of Healthcare Organizations (JCAHO). Accreditation offers the opportunity for an organization to be evaluated by an external group that assesses the quality of care provided. Accreditation demonstrates compliance with a uniform set of standards; it allows comparisons with other organizations and enhances the organization's competitive edge.

Three major accreditation agencies publish standards and offer external validation of quality of care for ambulatory care organizations:

1. JCAHO serves hospital-affiliated ambulatory care organizations as well as freestanding ambulatory care settings.
2. The National Committee for Quality Assurance serves managed care organizations and uses the Health Plan Employer Data and Information Set report cards.
3. The Accreditation Association for Ambulatory Health Care serves freestanding ambulatory surgery centers, medical group practices, student health centers, and office-based surgeons' practices.

All accreditation organizations use standards developed by the accreditation organization and on-site surveys done by teams of experts.

Multi-State Licensure

Multi-state licensure is an issue that has emerged because (1) there are increasing numbers of national health care systems, (2) Telehealth Nursing Practice is more common, and (3) people are more mobile in seeking care. The legal authority for practice is a concern for any professional nurse who provides care for people located in a state in which the nurse is not licensed. Nurses who must be concerned about multi-state licensure are (1) nurses working in integrated delivery systems and regional referral health care systems in which people come for care from other states, (2) flight nurses, and (3) Telehealth practice nurses. If a nurse cares for a client by telephone, computer, or monitoring device and the client is located in a state where the nurse is not licensed, the nurse faces the risk of being cited for practicing without a license in the client's home state.

The *Mutual Recognition Model,* implemented through an *Interstate Compact,* has been recognized as the preferred model of nurse licensure. The National Council of State Boards of Nursing has been working to educate nurses about the Interstate Compact. Information is available on their website at http://www.ncsbn.org. The Interstate Compact is a legal document that must be adopted by each state legislature. After adoption, nurses obtain a license in their home state but are able to communicate with clients in other states without violating the Nurse Practice Act in the client's home state if that state has also passed Interstate Compact legislation. The advantages of the Interstate Compact or "the one license concept" are reduced barriers to interstate practice, improved tracking for disciplinary purposes, cost-effectiveness, unduplicated counts of nurses, maintenance of a state-based system of licensure, and expanded consumer access to qualified nurses. Only a few states have adopted the Interstate Compact thus far. It may be several years before all states adopt the Interstate Compact. Until all states have adopted the Interstate Compact, nurses need to be aware of the implications of practicing across state lines.

TRENDS AND DIRECTIONS FOR THE FUTURE

Demographic and socioeconomic trends in the United States are expected to continue to challenge ambulatory care nurses. Among these challenges are (1) rapid changes in technology, (2) increased emphasis on demonstrated outcomes, (3) aging of the population, (4) reduced revenue to health care organizations from managed care contracts, (5) the large number of uninsured people, and (6) the growing shortage of nurses. A unified system ensuring access to health care for all Americans does not seem imminent.

Many believe, however, that the nation is experiencing a fundamental shift in emphasis on the concept of health itself, with the focus changing from the old clinical model to a wellness orientation. According to Shi and Singh,[29] health care is changing (1) from an *illness* orientation to a *wellness* orientation; (2) from an *acute* care emphasis to *primary* care; (3) from *inpatient* to *outpatient* services; (4) from *individual* health to *community* well-being; (5) from *fragmented* care to *managed* care; (6) from *independent* institutions to *integrated* systems; and (7) from service *duplication* to a *continuum* of services. If these predictions are correct, the well-educated ambulatory care nurse will be at the forefront of the health care delivery system in this new millennium.

CONCLUSIONS

Ambulatory care nursing is one of the fastest-growing areas of nursing specialty practice. Ambulatory care nurses are not only expert clinicians but also expert communicators. They play key roles in facilitating the client's successful progress through the integrated delivery systems. Ambulatory nurses make quality health care accessible.

BIBLIOGRAPHY

1. American Academy of Ambulatory Care Nursing. (2000). *Ambulatory care nursing administration and practice standards.* Pitman, NJ: Anthony J. Jannetti, Inc.
2. American Academy of Ambulatory Care Nursing. (2001). AAACN Telehealth nursing practice definition. *AAACN Viewpoint 24(4),* 10.
3. American Nurses' Association. (1998). *Core principles on telehealth.* Washington DC: American Nurses Publishing.
4. American Academy of Ambulatory Care Nursing. (1997). *Telephone nursing practice administration and practice standards.* Pitman, NJ: Anthony J. Jannetti, Inc.
5. American Academy of Ambulatory Care Nursing and American Nurses Association. (1997). *Nursing in ambulatory care: The future is here.* Washington, DC: American Nurses Publishing.
6. Bodenheimer, T., & Grumbach, K. (2002). *Understanding health policy: A clinical approach.* New York: Lange Medical Books/McGraw Hill.
7. Cherry, D.K., & Woodwell, D.A. (2002). *National ambulatory medical care survey: 2000 summary. Advanced data from vital and health statistics; No. 328.* Hyattsville, MD: National Center for Health Statistics.
8. Enthoven, A. (1993). The history and principles of managed competition. *Health Affairs* (suppl.), 24-28.
9. Ginzberg, E. (1994). *The road to reform.* New York: The Free Press.
10. Haas, S. (1998). Ambulatory care nursing conceptual framework. *AAACN Viewpoint, 20(3),* 16-17.
 11. Haas, S., & Androwich, I. (1999). Telephone consultation. In G. Bulecheck & J. McCloskey (Eds.), *Nursing interventions: Effective nursing treatments.* Philadelphia: W.B. Saunders.
12. Haas, S., & Gold, C. (1997). Perspectives in ambulatory care: Supervision of unlicensed assistive workers in ambulatory settings. *Nursing Economics, 15(1),* 57-59.
13. Haas, S.A., & Hackbarth, D.P. (1995). Dimensions of the staff nurse role in ambulatory care: Part III: Using research data to design new models of nursing care delivery. *Nursing Economics, 13(4),* 230-241.

14. Haas, S.A., & Hackbarth, D.P. (1995). Dimensions of the staff nurse role in ambulatory care: Part IV: Developing nursing intensity measures, standards, clinical ladders, and QI programs. *Nursing Economics, 13(5),* 285-294.
15. Haas, S.A., & Hackbarth, D.P. (1997). The role of the nurse manager in ambulatory care: Results of a national survey. *Nursing Economics, 15(4),* 191-203.
16. Haas, S.A., et al. (1995). Dimensions of the staff nurse role in ambulatory care: Part II: Comparison of role dimensions in four ambulatory settings. *Nursing Economics, 13(3),* 152-165.
17. Hackbarth, D. (1995). Institute of Medicine revised definition of ambulatory care. *Viewpoint, 17(4),* 1-4.
18. Hackbarth, D.P., et al. (1995). Dimensions of the staff nurse role in ambulatory care: Part I: Methodology and analysis of data on current staff nurse practice. *Nursing Economics, 13(2),* 89-98.
19. Hooks, M., Dewitz-Arnold, D., & Westbrook, L. (1980). The role of the professional nurse in the ambulatory care setting. *Nursing Administration Quarterly, 4(4),* 12-17.
20. Institute of Medicine. (1994). *Defining primary care: An interim report.* Committee on the future of primary care. Washington, DC: National Academy Press.
21. Institute of Medicine. (1978). Primary care medicine: A definition. In *A manpower policy for primary health care: Report of a study.* Washington, DC: National Academy Press.
22. Kovner, A. (1996). *Health care delivery in the United States* (6th ed.). New York: Springer.
23. Leavell, H.R, & Clark, E. (1965). *Preventive medicine for the doctor in his community: An epidemiologic approach.* New York: McGraw-Hill.
24. Ly, N., McCaig, L.F. (2002). National hospital ambulatory medical care survey: 2000 outpatient department summary. *Advanced data from vital and health statistics: No. 327.* Hyattsville, MD: National Center for Health Statistics.
25. Mastel, P. (2001). Ambulatory nursing outcomes. *AAACN Viewpoint, 23(4)* 6-7.
26. Mastel, P. (2000). Report cards: Proving the value of ambulatory care nursing. *AAACN Viewpoint 22(6),* 16-22.
27. McCaig, L.F., Ly, N. (2002). *National hospital ambulatory medical care survey: 2000 emergency department summary. Advance data from vital and health statistics; No. 326.* Hyattsville, MD: National Center for Health Statistics.
28. McKeown, T. (1978). Determinants of health. *Human Nature, 1(4),* 60-67.
29. Shi, L., & Singh, D. (2001). *Delivering health care in America* (2nd ed.). Gaithersburg, MD: Aspen.
30. Smith, J. (1983). *The idea of health: Implications for the nursing professional.* New York: Teachers College Press.
31. Starfield, B. (1992). *Primary care: Concept, evaluation and policy.* New York: Oxford University Press.

32. Starr, P. (1982). *The social transformation of American medicine.* Cambridge, MA: Basic Books.

 33. Swan, B.A. (2001). Ambulatory care nursing quality indicators: AAACN pilot survey. *AAACN Viewpoint 23*(2), 6-10.

34. Tighe, M.G., et al. (1985). A study of the oncology nurse role in ambulatory care. *Oncology Nursing Forum, 12*(6), 23-27.

35. U.S. Department of Health and Human Services. (2000). With understanding and improving health and objectives for improving health, 2 vols. In *Healthy people 2010* (2nd ed.). Washington DC: U.S. Government Printing Office.

36. Verran, J.A. (1981). Delineation of ambulatory care nursing practice. *Journal of Ambulatory Care Management, 4*(2), 1-13.

37. World Health Organization. (1978). *Primary health care: Report of the international conference on primary health care. Alma-Ata, USSR.* Geneva: Author.

Acute Health Care

Mary Ellen Pike

evolve

Web Enhancements

http://evolve.elsevier.com/Black/medsurg/

Ethical Issues in Nursing
  Is Whistle Blowing Ever the Right Thing to Do?

Appendix A
  Religious Beliefs and Practices Affecting Health Care

If you talk to a nurse who has worked in a hospital setting for the past 15 to 20 years, you are likely to hear about how much hospitals have changed. It is true. Today's hospitalized clients are sicker than they were years ago, in part because of advances in health care technology that have enabled them to survive disease and serious medical conditions longer. In the past, some of the nurse's caseload included clients who were nearly well. Today clients who are not acutely ill are discharged from the hospital and are treated in outpatient settings and by their families or significant others at home. Therefore the caseload for hospital nurses today consists of seriously ill clients. This chapter discusses the many reasons for this change and addresses what it is like to work in a hospital today.

HISTORY OF HOSPITAL NURSING

At the beginning of the twentieth century, most nurses were employed by affluent clients in the client's home. Nurses worked on a fee-for-service basis and were paid by the client or the client's family. A nurse worked with only one client all day long. This early form of nursing care was called *private duty nursing*. Private-duty nurses provided physical, psychological, and social care. Hospitals were for the poor and for those with communicable diseases. Clients were hospitalized to protect society from them. Hospitals were considered undesirable places to work.

During the Great Depression, many nurses could no longer find employment in the client's home. They were forced to work in hospitals, and in many instances they worked for room and board rather than for a salary. The Blue Cross plan, developed in 1929, offered a form of prepaid insurance to help people pay their hospital bills. During the 1930s and 1940s, more and more people purchased such insurance to protect themselves against hospital costs. The fact that hospitals could be more assured of payment put them on a sounder financial footing, and the demand for hospital-based nurses increased dramatically.

Until the early 1980s, the demand for hospital care continued to climb. Private insurance and government entitlement programs such as Medicare and Medicaid, established in 1965, allowed clients to be cared for without regard to cost. The need for nurses continued to rise, resulting in a cycle of nursing shortages every few years.

In the 1970s and 1980s, the cost of hospital care soared. Insurance companies and employers who covered health insurance premiums demanded government intervention to stem the rise in costs. In 1983 a new payment system, diagnosis-related groups (DRGs), a prospective payment system, was introduced. The hospital was paid a set amount of money based on the client's diagnosis. If the client required fewer days in the hospital than the DRG allowed, the hospital made money. If the client required more days, the hospital lost money. The incentive resulted in hospitals attempting to decrease every client's length of stay (LOS).

The 1990s was the decade of cost containment, with the Balanced Budget Acts of 1997 and 1999 greatly

---

evolve Be sure to check out the bonus material on the Evolve website and the CD-ROM, including free self-assessment exercises.

http://evolve.elsevier.com/Black/medsurg/

147

influencing hospital care. Hospitals changed from a client-driven, fee-for-service system to a payer-driven, capitated, managed care system. Physicians, who are subjected to utilization reviews, unhappily found third-party payers in control of hospital costs.

As a consequence of cost containment, hundreds of hospitals closed. Some hospitals merged with others to form a health care "system" in efforts to reduce costs, combine services, and attract third-party payment contracts. Some mergers were contested, such as "surprise" mergers, which fueled the uncertain climate in acute care.

ACUTE CARE HOSPITALS

The American Hospital Association defines a hospital as an institution with the primary function of providing diagnostic and therapeutic client services for a variety of medical conditions, both surgical and nonsurgical. Acute care hospitals are distinguished from long-term care facilities such as nursing homes, rehabilitation centers, and psychiatric hospitals by the fact that the average client stay is less than 30 days. Such hospitals are one of three types: government, voluntary/not-for-profit, and for-profit.

Types of Hospitals

Government-Sponsored Hospitals

These hospitals receive local, state, or federal government support. Examples include the Army, Navy, Veterans Affairs, Public Health Service, and Department of Justice prison hospitals. State-supported facilities include psychiatric hospitals, state university hospitals, and state prison hospitals. Locally supported institutions include county and city hospitals. Their services are often provided at no cost or at a reduced cost to the client. Many of the clients, even if employed, have no health care benefits.

Voluntary/Not-for-Profit Health Agencies

Voluntary health agencies are nonprofit, tax-exempt organizations designed to meet the health care needs of the general public. Despite their name, nonprofit organizations still need to be concerned with their financial status because the hospital must have adequate resources to meet its expenses, plan for expansion, and survive economic downturns. Examples include hospitals that are church affiliated, those owned by special-interest groups (such as the Shriners), and those treating specialties such as cancer or other chronic disorders.

For-Profit Hospitals

For-profit *(proprietary)* hospitals have the same goal as businesses: to generate profit. Like voluntary hospitals, they serve the general public. The hospitals are privately owned by large corporations, are parts of chains of hospitals, or are owned by single owners. These hospitals have stockholders. An advantage to the larger chains of hospitals is that they can purchase medical supplies in greater volume and therefore at less cost. They may have a slight advantage when contracting for third-party payment because of their ability to reduce costs.

Magnet Hospitals

Any of the preceding types of hospitals may also be designated a *magnet hospital*. Such a designation is given to hospitals that have a reputation for providing excellent nursing care and for having good medical outcomes. These hospitals often provide medical services for complex problems that require a team of health care providers, which would be too expensive to replicate in multiple sites. For example, clients who require organ transplantation or care after a serious injury are commonly cared for in these institutions. The hospitals have a high retention rate of their staff because of their high morale and good payment systems.

Client Admissions

Clients in acute care hospitals include those who are acutely ill; victims of trauma who have a potentially critical condition; those who need intensive monitoring, complex diagnostic studies, surgery, or complex treatments; and clients who have an exacerbation of a chronic disorder.

Clients can be admitted to a hospital in several ways (Box 8-1). Once the client is admitted, a primary physician (also called the *attending physician*) oversees the client's care. The clients may be referred to one or more physician specialists to diagnose and treat problems out-

---

BOX 8-1   *How Clients Are Admitted to a Hospital*

Direct
A client is seen in a physician's office, and it is determined that the client needs nursing care and specialized monitoring.

Emergency
A client is seen in the emergency department, and it is determined that the client needs surgery, nursing care, and/or specialized monitoring. The disease that has been diagnosed or is considered likely cannot be managed on an outpatient or self-care basis.

Scheduled
A client has elected to undergo surgery or special diagnostic testing that requires specialized monitoring or nursing care during recovery.

side the primary physician's practice area. Some hospitals are now using "hospitalists" to care for clients while they are in the acute care setting. *Hospitalists* are physicians who manage the care of hospitalized clients, allowing primary physicians and specialists to focus on clients outside the hospital setting.

Acute care is a costly service that relies on technology and the expertise of the health care team to arrive at a diagnosis, initiate treatment, stabilize the condition, and prepare for transition to a less costly level of health care.

Although nursing care is the primary reason for hospitalization, many other people are involved directly and indirectly in a client's care (Box 8-2).

Efficiency Measures

Hospitals continuously assess their outcomes and financial health by reviewing cost-benefit and clinical analysis data from their service lines. *Service lines* can be defined as care given to groups of clients with similar problems. For example, care of clients with heart disease or heart

---

BOX 8-2 *Personnel and Departments in a Hospital*

Professional Services

Medical Staff. Consists of private practice or group practice physicians who have their own offices and use the hospital services for care of specific problems. Also made up of physicians who may work for the hospital in departments such as surgery, laboratory, radiology, and emergency.

Nursing Service. Largest group of client care providers in the hospital. Nurses are employed by the nursing service department and provide client care in the hospital in areas where no direct client care is given (such as administration and hospital-based education programs).

Pharmacy. Consists of pharmacists and technicians who dispense medications prescribed by physicians. Pharmacy staff also monitor the use of regulated medications, such as narcotics. Many pharmacists also teach clients about their medications.

Rehabilitation Services. Physical therapists treat diseases and injuries by restoring, improving, or maintaining the client's functional ability or status to increase musculoskeletal strength to prevent further problems. Occupational therapists teach clients ways to overcome or reduce the problems in activities of daily living resulting from their disabilities.

Support Services

Administration. Hospital staff who are accountable for the operation of the entire hospital or institution. May include the hospital president, vice-presidents, and nurse-managers who supervise client care on a given nursing unit.

Biomedical Engineering Department. Maintains the elaborate equipment in the hospital to ensure safe and proper functioning and adherence to government regulations.

Business Departments. Several departments manage the business of the hospital based on both client income and outgoing expenses (salaries, purchasing, operation of the building). The admitting office collects information on insurance and assigns a room to the client. The business office lists all client charges, prepares the hospital bill, submits it to insurance companies, and records payments received. Payroll departments monitor hours worked, disperse salaries to the employees, and keep records. Purchasing departments disperse money for purchase of new supplies.

Cardiopulmonary. Includes the specialties of respiratory therapy and cardiac diagnostics.

Central Service/Material Management Department. Maintains supplies needed for client care. Provides stock supplies of routinely used items on the nursing units. Cleans and resterilizes reusable supplies.

Development/Community Relations. Volunteers and professional staff who often raise funds for various hospital projects (e.g., building projects). May be combined with the marketing department.

Dietary. Prepares food for client and staff daily. Dieticians assess and manage nutritional needs of hospitalized clients.

Environmental Services. Clean the hospital, including client rooms.

Information Technology. Computer support staff is growing in most hospitals because of the increasing use of computers. Staff members focus on design and support mechanisms for electronic data retrieval and storage.

Laboratory. Conducts diagnostic tests to help identify illness. Technicians commonly work in radiology and the various laboratories. Laboratory technicians usually collect blood samples from clients; nurses often collect all other specimens and may collect blood.

Laundry. Launders, sorts, and presses several hundred pounds of linen each day. New linen is delivered to each nursing unit daily. These services may be contracted out ("outsourced") to local providers.

Medical Records. Stores medical records for all clients. If a client is rehospitalized, former medical records are often important in diagnosis of new problems. Also compiles data for retrieval for reimbursement, service trending, and outcomes research.

Human Resources Department. Hires new employees and concentrates on employee relations. Human resources departments may serve in public relations roles to inform the hospital staff, clients, media, and public about the hospital and its operations. Public relations services may also be provided by the marketing department.

Volunteer Services. Operates coffee shops and gift shops, delivers mail to clients, and often raises funds for various hospital projects.

surgery would make up one service line. Many communities with two or more hospitals collaborate and then delineate service lines for each institution. For example, one hospital might provide all psychiatric services, another might have a stroke unit, and another could provide rehabilitation services. This is a cost-effective and a resource-effective method of providing care because duplication is eliminated. Clinical outcomes are generally improved when the volume of cases increases because the staff members become familiar with typical responses of clients and can detect complications earlier.

Post-Acute Care

Post-acute care is one of the fastest-growing segments of health care. It is designed to fill the gap between acute care and long-term or home care and is identified by a number of terms, including progressive, transitional, intermediate, telemetry, or step-down units. In some hospitals, nursing units or beds on a given unit can serve a dual purpose. These *swing beds* can be used either for acute care or for post-acute care, depending on the circumstances. Not all clients experience post-acute care. If the client can provide his or her own care at home, discharge to home is appropriate. Even if some nursing care is still required, home health care may be used to assist the client.

Examples of post-acute clients include those recovering from myocardial infarction (heart attack) or open heart surgery; those who must be weaned from a ventilator; those who need wound management after burn injury or for multiple pressure ulcers; those who require more rehabilitation after stroke or orthopedic surgery; or those who have complex medical conditions such as diabetes or digestive or renal problems. Care is delivered at a fraction of the cost or at about 30% of the cost of an acute care unit.

Post-acute units in a nursing home or rehabilitation facility include many clients who are Medicare beneficiaries, whose younger counterparts with the same level of disability would receive home care. Chronic post-acute units manage clients with little hope of ultimate recovery and functional independence. The goal of care for all clients in post-acute care is to send them home or to a less expensive level of care, such as to long-term care or assisted-living centers.

ROLES OF NURSES IN HOSPITALS

Nursing is a service provided both to individual clients and to aggregates of people (e.g., families, groups, communities, populations). To fulfill nursing's commitment to contribute to the health care of people, professional nurses assume multiple roles and responsibilities. Although these roles tend to overlap, they are important to distinguish. Nurses in the acute care hospital setting are providers of direct care, educators, researchers, and managers.

Provider of Direct Care

Most people are familiar with nurses as providers of *direct care*. Nurses assess, care for, educate, and comfort clients. Nurses provide direct care in all settings and along all dimensions of the health-illness continuum, from health promotion to critical care and death.

Indirect care consists of processes that support the actual bedside nursing care. Sometimes this level of care is labeled *interdependent*. The nurse interprets physicians' orders, administers medication, and provides treatment for the client when performing interdependent care.

Educator

Professional nurses provide formal and informal education to their clients, individually and in groups. Informal education goes on almost continually; clients are taught about medications while the medications are being administered, about the importance of assessment parameters when wound care is being done, and so on. The importance of informal education should not be underestimated.

Formal education is usually provided to groups of clients and their families. The nurse may use a classroom or bring videotapes, audiotapes, or a laptop computer into the client's room. Advantages of formal education are that the client is usually prepared for learning, significant others are included, and the material presented is consistent from client to client. Many hospitals have formal educators on their staff for clients with complex learning needs. Certified diabetes educators, certified lactation specialists, oncology nurse specialists, and enterostomal therapists are examples of nurses who teach clients in the hospital and often follow up with clients when they are back in the community.

Finally, some nurses specialize in education and rehabilitation. These nurses often work in cardiac and pulmonary rehabilitation and may have a subspecialty such as exercise physiology. Their role is to assist in the rehabilitation of clients after myocardial infarction, heart failure, chronic obstructive pulmonary disease, or transplantation.

Researcher

Most nurses would not identify themselves as *researchers*, and yet they are. Most acute care hospitals have research committees that select areas for study. Hospital nurses can identify topics to research, help develop and implement a study, collect data, and present and utilize the study's findings. Examples may include skin care or discharge teaching protocols. A master's or doctoral prepared nurse usually directs the study. Cost-containment and evidence-based practice have prompted research of many clinical practices.

Manager

The term *manager* in this discussion means the person who coordinates human and material resources in providing care to clients. *Human resources* include (1) the client, (2) the nurse, (3) the family or significant others, (4) professional colleagues, (5) support groups (e.g., the American Cancer Society), and (6) resource groups (e.g., Vocational Rehabilitation). *Material resources* include equipment and supplies. Time is also an important resource. Finally, outcome is an important consideration in health care management. Outcomes are detailed in the next section.

The first episode of client management that you encounter as a nurse is providing timely care to one client. Effective time management for one client is difficult at first because of interruptions and lack of familiarity with equipment and procedures. Even while caring for only one client, stay on time with assessments, medications, and treatments. Most of these aspects of nursing care are scheduled more than once every 24 hours; if late, the next treatment or medication may need to be delayed. As you gain experience, care of multiple clients becomes efficient.

NURSING CARE DELIVERY SYSTEMS

How client care is delivered on any nursing unit is very important. Several models are in use today, and each has its advantages and disadvantages.

Total Care Nursing

Total care nursing is the oldest of the care delivery systems. One nurse is assigned to one client and provides all care. The one-to-one pattern is common in critical care, with student nurses, and with private duty nurses. The advantage is that the client needs to work with only one nurse, and that one nurse can focus on meeting all needs of the client and family. The disadvantage is that any given nurse must be proficient in all nursing tasks and problem-solving areas.

Functional Nursing

Functional nursing is a system of care that concentrates on duties. It can be seen as an "assembly line" of care. Functional nursing began during World War II, when the demand for client care outstripped the supply of nurses. The registered nurse (RN) coordinates care for an entire unit or team. Other nurses are assigned to pass medications and perform treatments. Personnel with less training are assigned to provide more basic care (e.g., giving baths, making beds).

An advantage of this system is that care can be provided at a lower cost. Disadvantages are that the client interacts with several people, psychosocial needs are seldom met, and the RN seldom cares directly for the client and must rely on others' assessments of the client's prob-

lems. Each member of the working group is highly dependent on the other members. Functional nursing is still commonly used in skilled nursing and long-term care facilities. When there is a shortage of nurses, functional nursing is also considered in other settings.

Team Nursing

In *team nursing,* the RN works with one or more health care personnel to provide care for four or more clients. Team nursing was developed in the 1950s. World War II had drawn many nurses from hospitals, creating a nursing shortage and necessitating the increased use of unlicensed assistive personnel and licensed practical nurses (LPNs). Team nursing was considered one approach to using people's skills more effectively.

Advantages are that an RN is usually head of the team and generally knows the clients. In addition, the team leader can provide guidance to new or inexperienced nurses and other staff. As in functional nursing, the talents and abilities of each member of the health care team are used. Disadvantages are that (1) it is fairly expensive (because care is fragmented), (2) a lack of delegation skills by RNs may reduce efficiency, and (3) the "team" is often one RN and a nursing assistant (who may be working with more than one team).

Primary Nursing

Primary nursing is a model of care delivery that emerged during the 1980s to meet the increasingly complex needs of clients. The goal is for each client's care to be comprehensive and coordinated, from admission to discharge. Each client is assigned an RN as the primary nurse, and that nurse always provides care for that client when he or she is working. In addition, associate nurses provide care when the primary nurse is absent.

Advantages are obvious: (1) the client has the same nurse, (2) the client's psychosocial needs can be met, (3) communication with the physician is improved, and (4) the nurse feels autonomous. Disadvantages are (1) the increased cost in hiring a large RN staff and (2) possible role confusion between primary and associate nurses.

Case Management

Case management is a care delivery mode that incorporates concepts of continuity and efficiency in addressing long-term physical, psychological, and social needs of clients. The primary goals of case management are promoting self-care, upgrading the quality of life, and using resources efficiently. Case managers are nurses who coordinate care of a group of clients, monitor the implementation of interdisciplinary care plans, and maintain communication with third-party payers and referral sources.

A key distinction in the nurse's role in the case management system is that it transcends nursing unit and physician service (e.g., cardiology) boundaries. The nurse follows the client through the entire stay in the health care system and back into the community. Case managers must have a thorough knowledge of third-party reimbursement patterns and rules, community resources, and discharge planning techniques. Many hospitals have developed plans called *clinical pathways* or case management plans to direct client care and recovery from predictable problems. Several clinical pathways are presented on the Evolve website along with a discussion of how to use them.

In reality, most acute care hospital units use a combination of nursing care delivery models to provide care to clients. For instance, an oncology unit that has repeat clients may use primary nursing, whereas a large medical-surgical unit might use a team approach; when staffing is low, functional nursing might be used to accommodate the contributions of various care providers.

MANAGEMENT AND DELEGATION

Today, in an effort to control costs, almost all hospitals have hired *unlicensed assistive personnel* to provide care. Other than on-the-job training, these personnel receive little formal training. The use of less trained and educated personnel to perform nursing duties is changing the face of nurse staffing in hospitals. The use of unlicensed assistive personnel is increasing despite the inconclusive amount of research demonstrating their effectiveness on client outcomes.

Different terms are used for *nurse extenders* (which may include unlicensed assistive personnel), such as *unit assistants, primary practice partners,* and *patient care attendants*. Nurse extenders with more advanced skills might be called *clinical technicians*. Assistive personnel may help with clinical duties, nonclinical duties, or both. Some of the duties that may be delegated include giving baths, taking vital signs, serving food and collecting trays, performing unit-based laboratory tests (e.g., finger sticks for blood glucose assessment), 12-lead electrocardiograms (ECGs), and skin care.

Nurses need to learn when to delegate. For example, the nurse may delegate a bed bath and linen change for a client who is stable and may give the bath herself to an unstable or new client. This book offers many examples of appropriate delegation to unlicensed assistive personnel (see the list of Management and Delegation features on the inside back cover).

In planning the use of nurse extenders, nurse managers and their staff must consider many key questions (Box 8-3). Two issues that demand particular attention are (1) the functions that only an RN can perform (2) and the minimum level of RN staffing required to provide safe client care. Nurses may have been taught that only RNs can or should perform certain clinical duties, and they may therefore have difficulty delegating them to less qualified personnel. As the pressure mounts to delegate tasks to lower-paid workers, nurses will need to develop managerial skills, especially those of leadership, delegation, and supervision. Nurses will remain profes-

---

BOX 8-3 *Critical Considerations for Delegating Care to Unlicensed Assistive Personnel*

- What are the appropriate core duties of a registered nurse (RN)?
- Who should perform which tasks?
- What can be delegated?
- What is an appropriate and cost-effective staff mix?
- What is the risk management and liability at each level of caregiver?
- Who can substitute for whom?
- Who is the least expensive worker to do each task?
- How much management or supervision is needed?
- What is the philosophical commitment to the provision of total patient care by the RN here?
- Will lowering the qualification of staff add further stress and frustration to our staff?
- How will this affect recruitment?
- What is the impact on collective bargaining?

From Gardner, D.L. (1991). Issues related to the use of nurse extenders. *Journal of Nursing Administration, 21*(10), 40-45.

---

sionally accountable for client outcomes whether or not the specific tasks that contribute to those outcomes have been performed by nurses or by nurse extenders. Each nurse must clearly understand what the agency defines as the role and duties of the RN, LPN, LVN (licensed vocational nurse), and the various nurse extenders.

ENSURING QUALITY HEALTH CARE DELIVERY

Amid the fast-paced changes occurring in health care delivery, health care professionals remain responsible for ensuring quality client care. Quality client care is the outcome of the integrated health care team approach, which involves the corporate and hospital or agency administration, medical staff, board of trustees, employees, community, and client. Contract services, community resources, transfer agreements, and the expertise of social workers or case managers enable client transitions to alternate levels of care to occur in a continuous, coordinated, almost seamless fashion.

Through work-redesign and skill-mix reallocation, institutions are focusing goals on achieving efficient client outcomes. *Work redesign* involves studying a job over a fixed period to discover if and how a certain job function might be made more efficient. *Skill mix* is determined by studying the ratio of RNs to LPNs/LVNs and nurse assistants on a unit. The best skill mix delivers quality care while also controlling costs.

The "one-level-of-care" philosophy ensures that clients receive optimal care in all areas of an institution. For example, the same monitoring pertains when intravenous (IV) conscious sedation is administered in the endoscopy unit as when general anesthesia is administered in the operating room or emergency department.

Evidence-based practice is a concept used to improve care to achieve client outcomes. It uses research findings that are grounded in science along with client characteristics to guide clinical practice, thereby preventing practice being directed by tradition or personal preference and setting the stage for quality client care.

The Clients' Rights to Quality Care

Clients have an increased awareness of the quality-of-care issue. They are demanding and receiving more information before the initiation of treatments. Increasingly, clients' requests for information about costs, risks, benefits, and alternatives to suggested therapies are being honored. No longer automatically submissive to the suggested care, the client is becoming a participant and partner in health care, with the expectation of receiving quality care from all health care professionals.

Client rights have also reached a new level of importance for the health care consumer. Regulating agencies, insurance carriers, third-party payers, and providers are responding to ensure that these fundamental rights are maintained and that clients receive quality services.

Providing Quality Client Care

Any plan for providing client care involves the following aspects:

- Strategic planning to serve as a guideline for the continued or expanded services provided by the health care agency
- Budgeting process to assist the institution in studying, spending, and using the information to reduce costs or maintain them at the present rate
- Performance improvement plan to show the steps taken to improve performance based on monitoring and evaluation of staff performance
- Risk management input to identify and eliminate potential injuries to staff and clients
- Utilization review data to explore items such as acuity levels (a degree of severity of illness that affects the amount and complexity of care the client requires), outcomes, and costs and to discover what is and is not effective care
- Client satisfaction survey results, which gather data from clients at various stages of their stay in the agency (e.g., preprocedure, admission procedure, discharge)
- Physician input to incorporate professional input into client care planning
- Census data to plot current and future trends of health care in the organization

Changes in client population, diagnoses, programs, or staffing that would necessitate changes in the type, level, or amount of care are reviewed on an ongoing basis. Other factors contributing to quality care include (1) the adherence to, monitoring of, and evaluation of care given according to professional standards; (2) Joint Commission on the Accreditation of Healthcare Organizations (JCAHO) and Department of Health criteria; and (3) input from other regulatory agencies. In addition, clinical pathways, clinical practice guidelines, standards of practice and care, and competence standards serve as models for professional delivery of client care.

Staffing for Quality Care

Health care institutions use a combination of methods to ensure a staff of caregivers who can deliver quality care to clients. Two methods include (1) the daily collection of census data (a count of the number of clients occupying beds on any given day) and (2) determination of acuity levels.

Staff members are assigned or reassigned to units that have the greatest need for their expertise and experience. Staffing adjustments caused by the fluctuation of census data and acuity levels are accomplished by using per diem (daily) staff and other creative measures to ensure safe client care.

Today service-line leaders and empowered directors and managers are instrumental in adjusting strategies based on the many shifting variables that affect client care. Input from the employees who actually provide care is also helpful in redesigning and improving the quality of care. Because caregivers are directly involved with client care, they can contribute in important ways by reporting problems that can be addressed in a timely fashion. Such input, especially when acted on by management, helps staff members feel valued.

Unfortunately, adequate staffing is not always ensured. Today RNs are still in short supply. In an attempt to make the most effective use of available nursing staff, *cross-training* has evolved in hospitals. Whereas in the past nurses typically were assigned to one unit, where they could become familiar with the other personnel and the unit routine, today's hospital nurses may be cross-trained to work effectively in two or more units (e.g., a surgical unit and a cardiac intensive care unit). Nurses are assigned to the unit where they are most needed and may arrive for work not knowing in advance the work assignment for that day. Nurses may also be assigned to similar areas (e.g., orthopedics) but at different hospitals within the larger system as a result of mergers and acquisitions. This new scenario is often stressful for nurses and other staff members.

Nursing Intensity Classification

To ensure that staffing is adequate, one must understand how ill any given group of clients is and how much nursing care they will require. Hospitalized clients are classified according to several systems in an attempt to determine *nursing intensity,* a combination of the amount of care and the skill level at which care is provided (Table 8-1). Usually, physical care and psychosocial and

TABLE 8-1	Patient Care Classification Using Four Levels of Nursing Care Intensity			
Area of Care	**Category 1**	**Category 2**	**Category 3**	**Category 4**
Eating	Feeds self or needs little food	Needs some help in preparing; may need encouragement	Cannot feed self but is able to chew and swallow	Cannot feed self and may have difficulty swallowing
Grooming	Almost entirely self-sufficient	Needs some help in bathing, oral hygiene, hair combing, and so forth	Unable to do much for self	Completely dependent
Excretion	Up and to bathroom alone or almost alone	Needs some help in getting up to bathroom or using urinal	In bed, needs bedpan or urinal placed; may be able to partially turn or lift self	Completely dependent
Comfort	Self-sufficient	Needs some help with adjusting position or bed (e.g., tubes, IV lines)	Cannot turn without help, get drink, adjust position of extremities, and so forth	Completely dependent
General health	Good—in for diagnostic procedure, simple treatment, or surgical procedure (D & C, biopsy, minor fracture)	Mild symptoms—more than one mild illness, mild debility, mild emotional reaction, mild incontinence (not more than once per shift)	Acute symptoms—severe emotional reaction to illness or surgery, more than one acute illness, medical or surgical problem, severe or frequent incontinence	Critically ill—may have severe emotional reaction
Treatments	Simple—supervised ambulation, dangle, simple dressing, test procedure preparation not requiring medication, reinforcement of surgical dressing, change pad, vital signs once per shift	Any category 1 treatment more than once per shift, Foley catheter, care, I & O, bladder irrigations, sitz bath, compresses, test procedures requiring medications or follow-ups, simple enema for evacuation, vital signs q 4 hr	Any treatment more than twice per shift, medicated IV lines, complicated dressings, sterile procedures, care of tracheotomy, Harris flush, suctioning, tube feeding, vital signs more than q 4 hr	Any elaborate or delicate procedure requiring two nurses, vital signs more often than q 2 hr
Medications	Simple, routine, not needing preevaluation or postevaluation; medications no more than once per shift	Diabetic, cardiac, hypotensive, hypertensive, diuretic, anticoagulant medications, prn medications, more than once per shift, medications needing preevaluation or postevaluation	Unusual amount of category 2 medications; control of refractory diabetics (need to be monitored more than q 4 hr)	More intensive category 3 medications; IV lines with frequent, close observation and regulation
Teaching and emotional support	Routine follow-up teaching; clients with no unusual or adverse emotional reactions	Initial teaching of care of ostomies, new diabetics, tubes that will be in place for periods of time; conditions requiring major change in eating, living, or excretory practices; clients with mild adverse reactions to their illness (e.g., depression, being overly demanding)	More intensive category 2 items; teaching of apprehensive or mildly resistive clients; care of moderately upset or apprehensive clients; confused or disoriented clients	Teaching of resistive clients, care and support of clients with severe emotional reaction

Modified from Marquis, B. L., & Huston, C.J. (1996). *Leadership roles and management functions in nursing* (p. 266). Philadelphia: J. B. Lippincott.
D & C, Dilatation and curettage; *I & O,* input and output; *IV,* intravenous.

teaching skills are included. For example, a stable comatose client might require a large amount of low-complexity care that could be provided by unlicensed assistive personnel. In contrast, a newly diagnosed diabetic teenager with several personal and family problems may require less time for care, but the care should be provided by an RN. A wide variety of tools is used to measure client acuity and nursing care intensity.

Measurement of nursing intensity is often difficult. Tools designed by health consultants are frequently used to gather the necessary data to determine intensity. Some hospitals, however, develop their own instruments. Examples of tools used include a variety of client classification systems, Nursing Intervention Classification (NIC), Nursing Outcomes Classification (NOC), and the newer Oulu Patient Classification and the Professional Assessment of Optimal Nursing Care Intensity Level (PAONCIL). The data from the tools are used to provide a plan for staffing, reduce costs, improve care and heighten client satisfaction.

Client Satisfaction Surveys

As in business, health care providers have learned that it is easier to keep customers than to find new ones. Client satisfaction surveys are commonly given to the client on discharge or sent to the client's home shortly after discharge. Clients are often asked about their perception of medical care, nursing care, ancillary care, the environment, and follow-up care.

Sometimes client satisfaction surveys are discounted because of the fact that the client has limited knowledge of what would constitute "reasonable" care. To overcome this feeling of helplessness by the client, some hospitals inform clients of the services they can reasonably expect while hospitalized. For example, clients are told that they can reasonably expect adequate pain management. Then clients are asked to evaluate whether the outcome was met during the stay. This excellent change reminds all health care providers that the client's opinion should always be one indicator of quality of care.

REGULATORY REQUIREMENTS AND ISSUES

Regulatory agencies have the primary goal of enhancing the public's ability to secure adequate health care. Health care agencies are surveyed periodically to ensure that they comply with specific rules and regulations. A survey is an in-depth study of a health care institution (e.g., a hospital or a long-term care facility) according to specific criteria set forth by the regulating agencies involved. All aspects of the institution's services are inspected. Important performance areas include client assessment, medication administration, use of restraints, client and family education, staff training, information management, and organizational performance. After the

survey is completed, a report of findings is compiled and the institution is notified of its status. If a criterion is not met satisfactorily, the institution is notified, given time to correct the deficiency, and reevaluated at a later date. Sometimes the reevaluation is unannounced.

Public disclosure of survey findings has begun. Hospital surveys completed after 1994 are made available to the public, media sources, insurance companies, third-party payers, clients, and competing institutions. Other health care delivery services function under the same disclosure rules for compliance with regulations of the inspecting agencies.

Regulatory Agencies and Statutes

Several regulatory agencies have statutes that must be met by hospitals. These laws govern hiring and employment, quality controls, and conditions of the work site to reduce hazards. A full description of these laws is beyond the scope of this book; we will look at only a few of them. Employment laws include the equal employment opportunity laws that ensure equal rights in the workplace for racial and ethnic minorities, women, older adults, and the handicapped.

The *Civil Rights Act* of 1964 laid the foundation for equal employment in the United States. The thrust of Title VII of the Civil Rights Act is two-fold: (1) it prohibits discrimination based on factors unrelated to job qualifications, and (2) it promotes employment based on ability and merit. The areas of discrimination specifically mentioned are race, color, religion, gender, and national origin.

In 1967 Congress enacted the *Age Discrimination and Employment Act* (ADEA). Its purpose was to promote the employment of older people based on their ability rather than on their age. In early 1978 the ADEA was amended to increase the protected age to 70 years. Although people feared that this act would have serious consequences for labor-intensive occupations, such as nursing, many people are opting for earlier retirement and problems have not been reported.

The *Rehabilitation Act* of 1973 required all employers with government contracts of more than $25,000 to take affirmative action to recruit, hire, and advance handicapped people who are qualified. In 1990 Congress passed the *Americans with Disabilities Act* to eliminate discrimination against Americans with physical or mental disabilities in the workplace and in social life. Disability is defined as "any physical or mental impairment that limits any major life activity." This includes not only all people with obvious physical disabilities but also those with cancer, diabetes, human immunodeficiency virus (HIV) infection, acquired immunodeficiency syndrome (AIDS), and recovering alcoholics and drug users. The act not only prohibits discrimination but also delineates clear, enforceable standards.

The *Occupational Safety and Health Act* (OSHA) is broadly written legislation that requires a place of employment to be free from recognized hazards and to develop environmental safety laws for the safety of the employees. The Department of Labor enforces this act. Since the inception of OSHA, many companies have contended that the costs of meeting OSHA standards have excessively burdened American business; however, unions have asserted that the federal government has never adequately staffed or funded the Occupational and Health Administration. They have charged that OSHA has been negligent in setting standards for toxic substances, carcinogens, and other disease-producing agents.

Ethical Issues

Ethical issues in acute care commonly occur when the nurse is caught in the middle between clients, physicians, administrators, and other nurses and feels powerless to change the situation. Ethical distress can lead to negative consequences for everyone involved. Nurses are often called on to assist families in making informed decisions about client care, and they must be familiar with ethical, legal, economic, and emotional factors that affect the family's decision.

Legal Issues

Nurses have more responsibility today than in the past. Expanded roles open the doors to greater legal risk. The nurse's employer is obligated to carry malpractice insurance for its employees. You should know what is covered in the policy. In addition, you should consider carrying individual malpractice insurance.

Proper documentation is crucial to serve as evidence of the quality of nursing care provided. The court still assumes that if something was not noted in a chart, it was not done. Be specific, and document nursing actions taken and the client's response (e.g., pain reduction). If unusual events occur, complete an incident report. The benefit of incident reports is that they allow analysis of adverse client events. They should not be treated as a punitive activity but rather as a method of promoting quality care and risk management. Errors are examined to determine whether or not the error was due to a system problem (e.g., a faulty electrical outlet that leads to a fire or an improperly mounted side rail that allows a client to fall). If a lawsuit is filed, incident reports usually are not revealed; instead, the court system relies on the information in the medical record.

Cultural Issues

Nurses who practice in the 21st century will be interacting with an increasingly multicultural American society. Areas of the United States that had few immigrants now see people from all over the world. This diverse population requires that nurses be able to recognize differences and to be sensitive to those differences in perceptions of health and illness, in communication styles, and in nontraditional approaches to health care. Culturally competent care in its broadest sense is knowing, explaining, interpreting, and predicting nursing care within the knowledge of the client's cultural and ethnic beliefs and practices, whether the client is well or sick.

PERFORMANCE IMPROVEMENT AND GOALS

Hospitals and other health care organizations have been challenged by their goal of attaining a planned, systematic, multidisciplinary, nationwide approach to designing, measuring, assessing, and improving performance. These institutions generally seek to enhance their measurement activities as they relate to institutional quality indicators (Box 8-4). These indicators generally include the following:

- Results of basic clinical indicators
- Continuous quality improvement
- Access to care issues

BOX 8-4 | *Clinical Indicators with a Focus on High-Volume, High-Risk, and Problem-Prone Issues*

The community/clinic focus includes the following:
- Communicable diseases (e.g., TB, HIV)
- Low birth weight as a percentage of live births
- Births to mothers 10 to 17 years of age as a percentage of all live births
- Percentage of women receiving prenatal care during the first trimester
- Breast cancer rates and mammography statistics
- Immunization rates
- Return visits to the same level of care or visit within 72 hours to a higher level of care
- Accessibility, availability, and acceptability of care
- Appropriateness and relevance of care (e.g., based on diagnostic laboratory work, symptomatology)
- Appropriateness of treatment frequency
- Intake system
- Provision for information on an emergency or after-hours basis
- Client education
- Consultation
- Documentation including, for example, transfers and advance directives
- Availability of emergency carts/equipment
- Use of leasing for expensive/alternative resources
- Client record
- Client rights, including advance directives, informed consent, and special concern for abuse victims and for those with cultural diversity

- Consumer satisfaction and judgment input
- JCAHO indicators
- Human resource management
- Organization performance

Health care organizations are in the midst of a transition to performance improvement from traditional quality assurance.

RISK MANAGEMENT

Risk management is a planned program of loss prevention and liability control. Its purpose is to identify, analyze, and evaluate risks followed by a plan of reducing the frequency of accidents and injuries. The program requires a team of people from all departments in the institution. The risk manager or safety committee administers the program and serves as the liaison between the hospital administration, the risk management committee, and others as well as between insurance representatives, institution attorneys, and others. Risk managers have no typical profile and can be nurses, administrators, lawyers, or former insurance representatives.

Nursing personnel are crucial to a successful risk management program. The five areas of highest risk in the hospital are (1) medication errors, (2) complications from diagnostic or treatment procedures, (3) falls, (4) client or family dissatisfaction, and (5) refusal of treatment or refusal to sign consent for treatment. Medical records and incident reports serve as documents of accountability. Incident reports are used to analyze problems within the five categories and to plan for corrective actions.

THE FUTURE OF ACUTE CARE HOSPITAL NURSING

Acute care nursing will remain a challenging area in which to practice. Major changes will continue in health care delivery, and it will be essential that nurses take a primary position to help ensure that quality client care remains a priority. The following are a few of the trends that will influence the delivery of care in hospitals:

- As technology makes care in other settings more affordable, the acuity of clients in hospitals will increase, which will prompt the use of master's prepared, acute care nurse practitioners and clinical nurse specialists in the acute care setting.
- The 79 million baby boomers as well as their aging parents will present an unparalleled need for health care.

- Health care will be directed at populations rather than individuals. Examples include hospitals providing flu shots, community education programs, and screenings.
- Bioterrorism concerns will result in acute care hospitals taking the lead for disaster preparation. The skills of nurses working in acute care will be utilized in a variety of settings.
- A growing number of health care workers and clients will be immigrants and speak English as a second language.
- There will be continued emphasis on cost containment with projected cuts in entitlement programs.
- The hospital work force may be a virtual work force with a core of flexible workers and, based on acuity and census, other workers who contract for periods of time. Examples include employee health, accounting, computer personnel, and nursing staff.
- The length of a shift for nurses and rate of error will be examined.

CONCLUSIONS

Acute care hospital-based nursing has changed. Years ago, clients could stay in the hospital until they felt well enough to go home. Cost-containment issues have demanded that clients today spend as little time as possible in acute care and quickly move to less expensive areas for care. Professional nurses are the cornerstone of high-quality care during these shortened stays. All health care providers are trying to maintain excellence in health care during these changing times, and it is essential that nursing do so as well because excellence in health care is the primary reason the client is hospitalized.

BIBLIOGRAPHY

1. Baker, J. (2002). Medicare payment system for hospital inpatients: Diagnosis related groups. *Journal of Health Care Finance, 28*(3), 1-13.
2. Berke, W., & Ecklunc, M. (2002). Keep pace with step-down care. *Nursing Management, 33*(2), 26-29.
3. Buchan, J. (1999). Still attractive after all these years? Magnet hospitals in a changing health care environment. *Journal of Advanced Nursing, 30*(1), 100-108.
4. Coffman, S. (2001). Examining advocacy and case management in managed care. *Pediatric Nursing, 27*(3), 287.
5. Coile, R. (2001). A millennium mindset: The long boom. *Journal of Healthcare Management, 46*(2), 86-90.
6. Coile, R. (1999). Healthcare 2020: The new rules of society. *Health Management Technology, 20*(8), 44-48.

7. Costello, M.A. (2002). California seen as nurse-patient ratio testing ground. *AHA News, 38*(3), 2.

8. Cudney, A. (2002). Providing high-quality healthcare that is safe: Are we up to the task? *Journal of Healthcare Management, 47*(2), 77-80.

9. Deaton, C. (2001) Outcomes measurement and evidence-based nursing practice. *Journal of Cardiovascular Nursing, 15*(2), 83-86.

10. Driever, M.J. (2002). Issues in clinical nursing research: Are evidence-based practice and best practice the same? *Western Journal of Nursing Research, 24*(5), 591-597.

11. Driscoll, S.A. (2002). Guest editorial: The changing workforce. *Nursing Administration Quarterly, 26*(2), VII-VIII.

EB 11a. Fagerstrom, L., et al. (2000). Validation of a new method for patient classification, the Oulu patient classification. *Journal of Advanced Nursing, 31*(2), 481-490.

EB 11b. Fitzpatrick, J. (1999). Shift work and its impact upon nurse performance: Current knowledge and research issues. *Journal of Advanced Nursing, 29*(1), 18-27.

12. Geier, W. (1999). Caring side-by-side with acute care nurse practitioners. *Nursing Management, 30*(9), 32-34.

13. Kenny, P.A. (2001). Maintaining quality care during a nursing shortage using licensed practical nurses in acute care. *Journal of Nursing Care Quality, 15*(4), 60-69.

14. Lewis, P.S. & Latney, C. (2002). Achieve best practice with an evidence-based approach. *Nursing Management, 33*(12), 24-28.

15. McCloskey, D.J., et al. (2001). Determining cost of nursing interventions: A beginning. *Nursing Economics, 19*(4), 146-160.

16. McCullough, C.S. (Ed.). (2001). *Creating responsive solutions to healthcare change.* Indianapolis, IN: Center Nursing Press.

17. McDonald, M. (2001). The hospitalist movement: Wise or wishful thinking? *Nursing Management, 32*(3), 30-31.

18. Piotrawski, J. (2002). A post-acute turnaround. *Modern Healthcare, 32*(18).

19. Rosenfeld, P. (2001). Use of acute care nurse practitioners. *American Journal of Nursing, 101*(5), 61-63.

20. Shullanberger, G. (2000). Nurse staffing decisions: An integrative review of the literature. *Nursing Economics, 18*(3), 124-135.

21. Skuteris, L. (2002). A new approach to assessing staffing effectiveness. *Nursing Management, 33*(7), 12-13.

22. Sultz, H., & Young, K. (1999). *Health Care USA.* (2nd ed.). Gaithersburg, MD: Aspen.

23. Walsh, E. (2003). Get real with workload measurement. *Nursing Management, 34*(2), 38-42.

24. Washburn, E.R. (2001). Fast forward: A blueprint for the future from the institute of medicine. *Physician Executive, 27*(3), 8-14.

25. Wolf, E. (2001). Providing culturally appropriate care: A tale of two hospitals. *Healthcare Executive, 16*(2), 12-17.

Critical Care

M. Lynn Rodgers

The first step inside an intensive care unit, or ICU, can be overwhelming. The machinery is complex, medications are potent, stress and worry are visible on the faces of the families, and alarms seem to sound endlessly. The ICU can be intimidating and confusing. The reality is that the ICU is a place where skilled nurses, doctors, technologists, pharmacists, respiratory therapists, and others competently care for the sickest clients in the hospital. Their efforts are rewarding: More than 96% of clients admitted to the ICU are discharged alive.

Critical care is a term used to describe "the care of patients who are extremely ill and whose clinical condition is unstable or potentially unstable."[20] Although formally this specialty is less than 40 years old, clients with life-threatening illnesses have been organized into specific geographical areas for many years before designated critical care units were developed. Florence Nightingale in the 1880s detailed the benefits of grouping postoperative clients together to optimize their care and recovery. John Hopkins Hospital in Baltimore developed a three-bed postoperative neurosurgical unit in the early 1890s. In 1927 a unit specifically for premature infants was established in Chicago.[20]

HISTORY OF CRITICAL CARE

Nursing and technology continued to evolve in the 20th century to meet the ever-changing needs of society and its population. During World War II, "shock wards" were developed to meet the needs of injured solders. After the war, a nursing shortage spurred the development of post-anesthesia care units (PACUs) to ensure prompt attentive care for clients emerging from anesthesia. By 1960 almost every hospital in the United States could boast of such recovery rooms. During the late 1940s, the polio epidemic required the use of iron lungs as well as tracheotomy procedures and manual ventilation to support clients with respiratory paralysis. The physical needs were so great that intensive nursing care was required by these clients. In the 1950s, mechanical ventilation was developed. Again it was found that care of clients requiring ventilatory support was more efficient when clients were grouped together in a single unit.[1,20]

Soon general ICUs were developed for other very ill clients. By 1958, 25% of community hospitals in the United States with more than 300 beds reported having at least one ICU. By the end of the 1960s, almost every hospital in the United States had at least one ICU. Today more than 5000 ICUs exist in the United States, many of them very specialized, caring for highly specific groups of clients. Examples include cardiovascular, trauma, neurologic, surgical, cardiovascular surgical, pediatric, respiratory, transplantation, burn, neonatal, spinal cord injury, and medical ICUs to name a few.[1,20] Today stays in critical care units are common, and 80% of Americans will experience the critical care unit as a client or a family member.

REASONS FOR ADMISSION TO THE INTENSIVE CARE UNIT

The most common reasons for admission to ICU are for intensive monitoring and life-supportive care or for intensive nursing care that cannot be provided on a general medical surgical floor. Clients may be admitted following surgery, from the emergency room, or from the other floors within the hospital.

Common conditions necessitating admission to ICU include the following:

- Respiratory difficulties impairing the client's ability to ventilate or oxygenate: These problems often include disorders such as pneumonia, pulmonary embolism, drug overdose, and respiratory distress. Ventilators, also called *respirators,* may be required to assist with breathing. The use of these devices requires intense monitoring and skilled care providers to asssess both the equipment and the client's response.

- Circulatory problems such as hypotension (low blood pressure) or cardiac rhythm disorders: Clients may have had a myocardial infarction (heart attack), may be bleeding from internal or external wounds, or may have irregular heart rhythms that have become life threatening. The term *hemodynamically unstable* is used to describe these clients. Clients are routinely placed on cardiac rhythm monitors. They also may require sophisticated monitoring of cardiac output and pressures within the heart.

- Neurologic changes, such as loss of consciousness or changes in mental status: Intensive monitoring of the client's neurologic status provides needed data on the progress or deterioration of the brain's perfusion. Clients with head injuries, brain surgery, stroke, or spinal cord injury are admitted to the ICU for frequent reassessment.

- Life-threatening infection or the risk of infection, such as burn wounds or sepsis, requires intensive care to control the blood pressure and maintain perfusion of the heart, brain, lungs, and kidneys. Clients with sepsis or large open wounds require very intensive care for medication administration and fluid management.

- Metabolic problems, such as abnormal electrolytes from diabetes, renal failure, or acid-base imbalances require intensive monitoring and medication titration to control and treat complications.

- Clients who have had open heart surgery, thoracic surgery, brain surgery, extensive abdominal surgery, or orthopedic surgery are admitted postoperatively to the ICU for monitoring. Clients who have less invasive procedures, but have a personal history of cardiac or pulmonary disease, may also be admitted for observation and frequent assessment.

NEEDS OF THE CRITICALLY ILL CLIENT AND FAMILY

Clients in the ICU are at a most vulnerable stage. Not only do these clients have great physical needs, but their emotional, psychological, social, and environmental needs must be identified. Critically ill clients often experience pain, immobility, disorientation, and sleep deprivation. They can feel isolated, anxious, and depressed. Fears about their treatments, the unknown, and even death are not unusual. Everything in their environment is stress producing—unusual machines, loud noises, equipment alarms, constant light, and constant attention, staff conversations, physical restraints, lack of privacy, inadequate control of pain and anxiety, and separation from significant others.[4,6,7] Alteration of sleep quality and quantity in the critically ill client can have important adverse consequences, including impaired immunity and healing, an increase in oxygen consumption and carbon dioxide production, negative nitrogen balance, and stimulation of the "fight or flight" response of the sympathetic nervous system (Figure 9-1). An overwhelming sense of powerlessness is the overall recurrent theme verbalized by critically ill clients. Characteristics of hopelessness can actually impede recovery and lead to specific behavioral and physiologic changes (Box 9-1).[11] Because of airway devices, medications, or physical pathology, many critically ill clients cannot communicate their needs well, making their situation even more stressful. Even with the best of circumstances and nursing care, critically ill clients can experience delirium, often called *ICU psychosis*[7,9,11] (see also Chapter 24).

The critical care nurse has a great responsibility in controlling the environment to avoid or diminish the stressors that are specific to the critically ill client. Allowing open visitation as able, providing appropriate day and night cycles of activity and sleep, and controlling noise and conversation can allow the client a more restful and therapeutic recovery. Providing privacy and explaining all equipment, noise, and activities can be comforting measures for the critically ill client as well as his or her family. Designing some type of simple communication system to allow the client at least to answer "yes" or "no" questions is important. The nurse must adequately assess the client's analgesia and sedation needs. Often few overt clues are evident that the client requires such medications. Looking at subtle changes in vital signs or behavior and routinely providing sedation and analgesia are frequently required.[10] Lastly, the nurse may need to control open visitation to balance clients' needs for rest with families' needs to be close to their loved one.

Family Needs

Families and significant others of the critically ill client also have many stressors and important needs. The im-

FIGURE 9-1 Systems participating in the stress response. *ADH*, Antidiuretic hormone; *ACTH*, adrenocorticotropic hormone; *B-LPH*, beta-lipoprotein hormone blood pressure; *GH*, growth hormone; *HR*, heart rate; *PRL*, prolactin; *RR*, respiratory rate; *TSH*, thyroid-stimulating hormone. (Modified from Carrieri-Kohlman, V., West, C.M., & Lindsay, A.M. [2003]. *Pathophysiological phenomena in nursing* [3rd ed.]. Philadelphia: W.B. Saunders.)

BOX 9-1   *Characteristics of Hopelessness*

- Crying
- Decreased or flat affect
- Decreased response to stimuli
- Decreased verbalization
- Diminished interest in external objects
- Interference with learning
- Irritability
- Lack of involvement in care
- Lack of motivation or initiative
- Motionlessness
- Muteness
- Passivity
- Reduced activity
- Sad expression
- Sense of incompetence
- Sleep disorders
- Social withdrawal
- Tenseness
- Weakness
- Weight loss

From Gelling, L. (1999). The role of hope for relatives of critically ill patients: A review of the literature. *Nursing Standard, 14*(1), 33-38.

pact of critical illness is great. Despite efforts of the critical care nurse to defuse the critical care experience, family crises may develop. As the demands on the family increase, adaptation and coping mechanisms are depleted, anxiety levels are heightened, and maladaptation may occur. This maladaptation can manifest as fear, guilt, anger, and hostility as well as physiologic illnesses (Figure 9-2). Too often the critical care environment adds to the stress.[7,9,11] For more information on evaluating the needs of families of the critically ill, see the Critical Care Family Needs Inventory feature on the website.

Family members must have their physical and emotional needs met. Some ICUs assign a specific person to assist family and visitors of critical care clients. Such "visitor assistants" can concentrate on the family so that the nurse can spend more time with the client. Nationwide, many ICUs have adopted a password system to allow family members to obtain information from the nurse by phone. On admission to the ICU, the family establishes a password that they must give to the nurse whenever they call in to inquire about the client's condition. The family then shares this password only with those whom they want to have access to client information. Confidentiality must be protected by ensuring that only the proper persons receive the protected client in-

FIGURE 9-2 Hoff's crisis paradigm. (From Hoff, L.A. [2001]. *People in crisis: Clinical and public health perspectives* [5th ed.]. San Francisco: Jossey-Bass.)

formation. Family housing is also a top priority in today's hospitals. Some clients stay in the ICU for weeks at a time. Family members are frequently exhausted and welcome comfortable, private accommodations that are close to the ICU or hospital. Some hospitals even provide complimentary beverages or meals. Many times the stay in the ICU is harder on the family than on the client. Unfortunately, research indicates that most nurses and physicians underestimate critical care families' needs for information, proximity, and assurance, no matter how well they feel they are meeting these needs.[2,3,6] See the Evidence-Based Practice in Action feature on Family Needs in the Intensive Care Unit, below.

CRITICAL CARE NURSING

"Critical care nurses concentrate specifically on the care of clients with life-threatening problems."[1] Interventions for these clients must be adjusted continually based on constant monitoring of their response to treatment. Because of the multidisciplinary nature of critical care, coordination of care is essential. The critical care nurse is primarily responsible for such coordination. Continuous nursing vigilance is the key to this nursing specialty and can make a significant difference in client outcomes.[9,10] The critical care nurse does not just use the latest machines and technologies to provide highly technical nurs-

ing, although maintaining technological devices is crucial.[12] Creating an environment that promotes healing or an optimal health level in a nurturing, caring manner is especially essential for a critically ill client to ensure positive optimal outcomes.[7,9,11,21] Often complementary and alternative therapies, such as massage, prayer, music therapy, and therapeutic energy provision, assist the critical care nurse in providing such a healing environment.[7,21]

Providing such care must include not only the client but also his or her family members and significant others. Many times the critically ill client does not remember his or her ICU stay; however, the time in the critical care unit is often a significant emotional event and is traumatic for his or her loved ones. Often the only coping mechanism families have is hope. It is extremely essential that the critical care nurse foster this coping mechanism because hope can fortify a family's inner strength and helps the family members look beyond the present situation of pain and suffering.[11] Nurses have a fiduciary relationship with their clients and families; in other words, nurses have an ethical and legal obligation to act in their best interest.[5] The American Association of Critical-Care Nurses (AACN) defines this advocacy as "respecting and supporting the basic values, rights and beliefs of the critically ill client." Box 9-2 further delineates the advocacy role of the critical care nurse.[1]

EB EVIDENCE-BASED PRACTICE IN ACTION

Family Needs in the Intensive Care Unit

Meeting client and family needs has been a concern of nurses and managers for many years. The study of family needs in the intensive care unit (ICU) has been a research focus for many decades. Molter, a well-known critical care author and practitioner, developed a tool called the Critical Care Family Needs Inventory (CCFNI). This tool has been used by many staff nurses to ensure that nurses meet both the client's and the family's needs while their loved one is in the ICU.[4]

When the issue was first addressed, many thought that nurses' perceptions of family needs would be the same as the client's and the family's perceptions. This indeed was found to be true. In general, the three most important needs consistently identified by clients and families were proximity, assurance, and information. The top nine priorities of critical care families were as follows[1-4]:

- Assurance that the best care was being given to their family member by caring personnel
- To feel that there was hope
- To know the prognosis
- To understand how the client was being treated medically
- To be reassured that it is all right to leave for a while
- To feel accepted by hospital staff
- To feel someone is concerned for the family's health

- To feel the hospital personnel care about the client
- To have explanations given in terms that can be understood.

Implications

As shown by this list of priorities, nursing can do much to alleviate many of the stressors that face our critical care patients and family members. Much can be accomplished by listening to clients and their families and by taking time to meet their needs. Nurses have the knowledge base and the opportunities to address and meet almost all of the priorities listed here.

References
1. Azoulay, E., et al. (2001). Meeting the needs of the intensive care unit patient families. *American Journal of Respiratory Critical Care Medicine, 163*(1), 135-139.
2. Bijttebier, P., et al. (2001). Needs of the relatives of critical care patients: perceptions of relatives, physicians and nurses. *Intensive Care Medicine, 27*(1), 160-165.
3. Kosco, M., & Warren, N.A. (2000). Critical care nurses' perceptions of family needs as met. *Critical Care Nursing Quarterly, 23*(2), 60-72.
4. Molter, N.C. (1979). Needs of relatives of critically ill patients: A descriptive study. *Heart & Lung, 8*(2), 332-339.

The critical care nurse will do the following:

1. Respect and support the right of the patient or the patient's designated surrogate to autonomous informed decision-making.
2. Intervene when the best interest of the patient is in question.
3. Help the patient obtain necessary care.
4. Respect the values, beliefs, and rights of the patient.
5. Provide education and support to help the patient or the patient's designated surrogate make decisions.
6. Represent the patient in accordance with the patient's choices.
7. Support the decisions of the patient or the patient's designated surrogate, or transfer care to an equally qualified critical care nurse.
8. Intercede for patients who cannot speak for themselves in situations that require immediate action.
9. Monitor and safeguard the quality of care the patient receives.
10. Act as liaison between the patient, the patient's family, and health care professionals.

From American Association of Critical-Care Nurses. (2003). Retrieved December 2003: http://www.aacn.org.

Critical Care Practice Settings and Roles

Critical care nursing is not limited to designated critical care units. In 2000 the Department of Health and Human Services identified that about 31% of all hospital nurses work with critically ill clients in ICU, PACU, emergency room (ER) and in step-down units.[1] It is not the location of care that is important, however. Critical care nursing is not nursing in a specific place; rather, it is nursing with a specific mind-set that utilizes a specialized body of knowledge and skills. Critical thinking and clinical decision-making become more consistent the longer the critical care nurse practices in the critical care environment.[13] Debate is ongoing as to the appropriateness of novice nurses in the critical care setting. Many believe that because of the level of expertise required to care for these clients, novice nurses may not be best suited for this level of practice. On the other hand, if the time in orientation is designed especially to meet the needs of these clients, and the time in orientation is sufficient, many experts believe that this setting is appropriate for the novice nurse.[18]

The critical care nurse must constantly keep up with the latest information and become proficient with more complex new technologies and treatments.[1,12] The need for such nursing skills and knowledge will only increase as the population grows older and sicker. Today's changes in technology and health care will keep more of our population out of the hospital, but those who are admitted to critical care units will be more severely ill than ever before.

Critical care nurses are found in a variety of formal roles: bedside nurse, critical care educator, case management, unit or department manager, clinical nurse specialist, and nurse practitioner. Although all these roles are important, the bedside nurses are the backbone of critical care nursing. Only they are with the client on a 24 hours a day, 7 days a week. The critical care educator can educate clients; the case manager can promote appropriate and timely care; the manager can direct them; the clinical nurse specialist can help to plan client care; and the nurse practitioner can order treatments and medications. Ultimately, however, it is the bedside critical care nurse who coordinates the entire team's efforts to implement the plan of care and modify it as needed by the client's response.

Advanced Practice Nurses in Critical Care

Advance practice nurses in critical care are registered nurses with a master's degree who have a specialty in critical care. The critical care clinical nurse specialist (CNS) uses an advanced level of knowledge of critical care, pharmacology, and pathophysiology in completing the role of educator, consultant, manager, researcher, and practitioner.[8] The acute care nurse practitioner (ACNP) provides advanced nursing care to acutely and critically ill clients in a wide variety of settings, including the emergency department, ICUs, and step-down units. Making rounds, developing a plan of care, and performing specific advanced procedures are all tasks the ACNP may do. Some ACNPs serve as intensivists and may insert central lines or chest tubes, assist with surgery or intubation, or complete various functions once reserved for physicians.[14]

CRITICAL CARE PROFESSIONAL ORGANIZATIONS

Critical care practitioners are specifically supported by two national organizations, AACN and the Society of Critical Care Medicine. These organizations provide practice guidelines, opportunities for networking, educational programs, professional publications, scholarship and grant money, research opportunities, Internet resources, and practitioner support. In addition, both are considered as the "official" professional organizations that speak on behalf of critical care. Representatives from these organizations are often asked to testify or provide information for various national and state legislative organizations.

CONCLUSIONS

Critical care nursing occurs in a variety of settings. Health care will be pressed to provide efficient and cost-effective services. Government subsidies of health care may not be able to keep up with the demand. An impending shortage of nurses in the next 10 years will challenge our health care institutions. Aging nurses are retiring or leaving critical care. Young or new nurses must step up to meet the exciting challenges of critical care nursing. Despite all the challenges of the future, the center of all health care will still be the client, and the critical care nurse will be there at the client's side.

BIBLIOGRAPHY

1. American Association of Critical-Care Nurses. (2003). Retrieved December 2003: http://www.aacn.org.
2. Azoulay, E., Chevret, S., &, Leleu, G. (2000). Half the families of ICU patients experience inadequate communication with physicians. *Critical Care Medicine, 28*(8), 3044-3049.
3. Azoulay, E., et al (2002). Impact of a family information leaflet on effectiveness of information provided to family members of intensive care unit patients: A multicenter, prospective, randomized, controlled trial. *American Journal of Respiratory Critical Care Medicine, 165*(4), 438-442.
4. Azoulay, E., et al. (2001). Meeting the needs of the intensive care unit patient families. *American Journal of Respiratory Critical Care Medicine, 163*(1), 135-139.
5. Benner, P. (2003). Enhancing patient advocacy and social ethics. *American Journal of Critical Care, 12*(4), 374-375.
6. Bijttebier, P., et al. (2001). Needs of the relatives of critical care patients: perceptions of relatives, physicians and nurses. *Intensive Care Medicine, 27*(1), 160-165.
7. Chlan, L. (2002). Integrating nonpharmacological adjunctive interventions into critical care practice: a means to humanize care? *American Journal of Critical Care, 11*(1), 14-16.
8. Cohen, S.S., et al. (2002). The synergy model and the role of clinical nurse specialists in a multihospital system. *American Journal of Critical Care, 11*(5), 436-446.
9. Dang, D., et al. (2002). Postoperative complications: does intensive care unit staff nursing make a difference? *Heart & Lung, 31*(3), 219-228.
10. Frazier, S.K., et al. (2002). Critical care nurses' assessment of patients' anxiety: reliance on physiological and behavioral parameters. *American Journal of Critical Care, 11*(1), 57-64.
11. Gelling, L. (1999). The role of hope for relatives of critically ill patients: a review of the literature. *Nursing Standard, 14*(1), 33-38.
12. Happ, M.B. (2000). Preventing treatment interference: the nurse's role in maintaining technological devices. *Heart & Lung, 29*(1), 60-69.
13. Hicks, F.D., Merritt, S.L., and Elstein, A.S. (2003). Critical thinking and clinical decision making in critical care nursing. *Heart & Lung, 32*(3), 169-180.
14. Kleinpell, R.M. The nurse practitioner in the acute care setting: an expanding role. Session IV-Q. Program and abstracts of the American Academy of Nurse Practitioners 16th Annual National Conference; June 28-July 1, 2001; Orlando, FL.
15. Kosco, M., & Warren, N.A. (2000). Critical care nurses' perceptions of family needs as met. *Critical Care Nursing Quarterly, 23*(2), 60-72.
16. Medina, J., (2000). *Standards for acute and critical care nursing* (3rd ed.). Aliso Viejo, CA: American Association of Critical Care Nurses.
17. Molter, N.C. (1979). Needs of relatives of critically ill patients: A descriptive study. *Heart & Lung, 8*(2), 332-339.
18. Reisling, D.L. (2002). Early socialization of new critical care nurses. *American Journal of Critical Care, 11*(1), 11-26.
19. Rodgers, M.L. (2003). Retention and recruitment survey of ICU nurses. *Unpublished Manuscript.* Deaconess Hospital, Evansville, IN.
20. Society of Critical Care Medicine. (2003). Retrieved December 2003: http://www.sccm.org.
21. Tracy, R.F., et al. (2003). Nurses' attitudes towards the use of complementary and alternative therapies in critical care. *Heart & Lung, 32*(3), 197-209.

 evolve Did you remember to check out the bonus material on the Evolve website and the CD-ROM, including free self-assessment exercises?

http://evolve.elsevier.com/Black/medsurg/

Home Health Care

Karen S. Martin

evolve

Web Enhancements   **http://evolve.elsevier.com/Black/medsurg/**

Bridge to Home Health Care
  Finding Financial Help
  Medicare and Medicaid Coverage of Home Health Services

Ethical Issues in Nursing
  How Should Nurses Respond to Conflicts Between Clients and
  Family Members in the Home Health Care Setting?
Appendix A
  Religious Beliefs and Practices Affecting Health Care

This chapter is intended to serve as a bridge for nurses making the transition from inpatient or long-term care to home health care and community service settings. Included is a summary of the trends, general philosophy, risks, and practice of home health care. This chapter is designed for the student or practitioner whose primary or recent clinical experience has been in hospital, assisted living, nursing home, or other long-term care facilities. *Home health care nursing* is defined as the skilled services needed to treat individuals' disease and disability in collaboration with their families and designated caregivers.[23,33] *Community health nursing* is defined as a synthesis of nursing and public health practice that is comprehensive and is intended to promote and preserve the health of populations.[23,33] In this chapter, community health nursing is used as an umbrella term to encompass all the diverse types of home health care and community services, settings, and providers. Home health settings in which nurses commonly practice include hospital-based, visiting nurse, tax-supported, and privately or corporately owned agencies. Other community health nursing settings include tax-supported public health agencies, nursing centers, schools, wellness and occupational health programs, parish nursing programs, clinics for the homeless, case management programs, and other programs.

Features called *Bridge to Home Health Care*, written by nurses and other community professionals to describe their practice, are scattered throughout this book and are included on the website. These features address environmental, psychosocial, physiological, and health-related behavior concerns experienced by clients and their families. The Bridge to Home Health Care features help you gain insight into the roles and responsibilities of the nurse in home health care as it is practiced with clients and families every day. You can use this information as you consider and make referrals for follow-up care.

The bibliography in this chapter provides more extensive information about home care, public health, and related topics. After reading the chapter, you may discuss what community opportunities you will have as a nursing student. If you are a staff nurse, you may consider making an appointment to accompany a colleague who practices in a home care, public health, clinic, or school setting to learn more about the specialty. This chapter and the Bridge to Home Health Care features together provide a review of or an introduction to the world of home health care and community practice.

TRENDS

The need for home health care and community services has grown explosively as a result of consumer demand, the advent of Medicare reimbursement for home health services, the aging of the population, federal legislation that encouraged the expansion of home care, escalating

evolve *Be sure to check out the bonus material on the Evolve website and the CD-ROM, including free self-assessment exercises.*
http://evolve.elsevier.com/Black/medsurg/

health care costs, and the rise of managed care. Currently, more than 20,000 Medicare-certified and noncertified home health agencies provide service in the United States, a 1000% increase over 20 years. Between 1967 and 2001, Medicare home health expenditures grew from $50 million to $41 billion.[8,27]

These trends reflect a shift in the delivery of health care services from the hospital to the community. Ideally, this shift will decrease fragmentation and produce an improved health care system in which providers work together in the interest of their clients. The shift also has the potential to increase provider accountability and result in a more systematic delivery model that is driven by outcome data. A *seamless health care system* is the term used to describe this model, a system that includes a wide array of services and providers who collaborate as team members.

Although the recipients of home health care have diverse needs, circulatory disease is the primary medical diagnosis for more than half of clients admitted for service. Diabetes and cancer are the next most frequent diagnoses.[27] In general, the clients who receive home health care tend to be in the older adult population; this trend is likely to continue. Consider the following projections[1,34]:

- Since 1900, the percentage of people older than age 65 years has tripled; those 85 years and older increased by 34 times.
- More than 35 million people are older than age 65 years.
- People older than age 65 years account for one third of health care consumption; they may represent half of the total health care dollars spent by the year 2040.
- More than half of older adults have chronic illnesses that cause activity limitations.
- Up to 60% of older adults do not take their medications properly.
- The 4 million men and women older than age 85 years constitute the fastest-growing subset of older adults, with a growth rate nearly three times that of the overall older adult population.

Because the growth of home health care promises to continue, community health nurses face many challenges. The number of clients and complexity of their needs are increasing dramatically, as are the numbers and types of community health staff members and agency programs. At the same time, demands from consumers and payers for comprehensive, economical services are increasing, the availability of staff and reimbursement is decreasing, and regulatory demands are increasing.

Since 1997, dramatic legislative and regulatory changes occurred that reduced Medicare-Medicaid reimbursement to home health agencies. The stated purposes of the regulations were to introduce a prospective payment system that would standardize requests for payment from all home care agencies, initiate a per-client service limit, change billing procedures, and mandate the use of the Outcome and Assessment Information Set (OASIS). Nurses complete versions of the OASIS first after adult clients are admitted to service, then at interim periods, and finally at client dismissal.[8,21,37]

Reimbursement continues to be a challenge and responsibility that frequently confronts the nurse who practices in home health or community settings (see the Bridge to Home Health Care feature on Finding Financial Help on the website). A nurse in a hospital, nursing home, or other long-term care facility may not know the cost of service or supplies and may not need to discuss charges with clients and their families. In home health care agencies, however, it is usually nurses who collect financial data, either at intake or when providing the initial services. Data include:

- The source of payment
- Verification of eligibility for Medicare, Medicaid, or other programs providing payment
- Preauthorization approval from a managed care or other third-party payer
- Other details

Home health agencies bill third-party payers for most services; Medicare, Medicaid, and other public programs are common sources. Some clients pay for services themselves (private pay) or receive services that are paid for by private insurance, United Way, foundations, or grants. Often, reimbursement regulations are complex and require extensive paperwork for both nurses and clients.[21,37] Clients may ask their nurses for assistance as they try to deal with those regulations (see the Bridge to Home Health Care feature on Medicare and Medicaid Coverage of Home Health Services on the website for a summary of eligibility, requirement, and coverage information that home health nurses must know).

PERSPECTIVES

The specialty of home health care and community nursing has a long and distinguished history in the United States, even though it received little attention from the public or the nursing profession until the 1990s. In 1877, Francis Root was employed in New York City as the first home visit nurse. In 1893, Lillian Wald and Mary Brewster established the Henry Street Settlement in the same city. Their goal was to offer public health nursing and community programs to people of all ages who were at high risk of developing health problems and to those with acute and chronic health problems. Lillian Wald had the vision to[11]:

- Initiate programs and group activities at the settlement to meet the community's health-related, educational, social, and employment needs
- Send nurses from the settlement to make home visits and provide care to new mothers, infants, and the sick

• Forge alliances with business and political leaders to obtain support for her programs

This comprehensive approach can be called *community health nursing* and represents a true blend of public health and home care practice. Collaboration between the Henry Street staff and the New York City Mission home visit staff followed and led to the formation of the Visiting Nurse Service of New York, the largest single provider of home health care services in the United States. Soon, organized home visit programs were established in populated areas along the East Coast. Lillian Wald's vision of preventive, curative, and social services for the entire community spread throughout New York City and the rest of the nation. By 1912, as many as 2500 nurses were employed by 900 independent visiting nurse associations.[11]

By 1963, there were 1100 home health and home care aide organizations and hospices in the United States that employed professional registered nurses. The enactment of national Medicare legislation in 1965 accelerated the rate of agency growth. More than 20,000 Medicare and non-Medicare certified home care agencies now offer services to 7.6 million clients.[27] About 600,000 community health nurses are employed by home care and public health agencies, school systems, ambulatory care, and industry. That number is expected to escalate dramatically in the next 10 years.[16]

Agencies that provide Medicare- and Medicaid-certified services must meet minimum national standards; state standards also exist. Some agencies voluntarily participate in the Community Health Accreditation Program and the Joint Commission on Accreditation of Healthcare Organizations national accreditation programs. Nurses and other professional staff are required to meet licensure requirements but not consistent competence standards. Accreditation and competence are becoming important concerns to administrators, practitioners, and the public because of the increased use of technology and high-risk procedures and medications in the home. To be competent, practitioners need adequate orientation, equipment, and supervision; they also need to repeat high-risk procedures with sufficient frequency that they maintain their skills.

Collaboration and communication among members of all disciplines are necessary in home health care and community settings. Nurses make up the largest group of practitioners, although most home health agencies also employ or contract with home health aides and other paraprofessionals as well as other professionals. Physical therapists, occupational therapists, social workers, and speech pathologists are usually on staff. Registered dietitians, pharmacists, dentists, physicians, and clergy may be part of the team as well. Agency staff members also need to coordinate referrals and communicate about client services with various community providers.

Historically, Lillian Wald at Henry Street and other community nurses demonstrated collaboration and communication skills as part of their practice. During the 1990s, a new role, that of case manager, was developed. Nurse case managers are employed by home health agencies, hospice programs, health maintenance organizations, physician group practices, private insurance companies, public health departments, school systems, and managed care organizations. Although their responsibilities vary, they attempt to coordinate the delivery and payment of services that target clients' needs.

COMMUNITY-ORIENTED PHILOSOPHY

The client who receives services may be an individual, a family, a group, or a community.[3,23,33] As home health care and community practitioners have had the opportunity to work with clients over time, they have espoused a number of core values that influence their practice. Multidisciplinary collaboration and a seamless health care environment have already been mentioned. In addition, community health nurses have frequently conducted prevention and health promotion programs involving immunizations, smoking cessation, breast self-examination, and similar concerns.[33]

Nurses in home health care and community settings refer to those they serve as clients, patients, consumers, or customers. Regardless of the term used or whether terms are used interchangeably, nurses tend to base their practice on beliefs related to the consumer movement. Included are beliefs that people have both rights and responsibilities and that they must be knowledgeable about their own health care and be actively involved in decisions. These beliefs are linked to issues of access, cost, and quality as well as the concepts of primary health care applicable at a national and an international level. For international use, the World Health Organization[36] defined *health* as a state of complete physical, mental, and social well-being and not merely the absence of disease or infirmity; the definition further states that health is a fundamental human right and that attainment of the highest possible level of health is an important worldwide social goal.

The power of the client is an important core value for home health care and community providers.[31,33] When a practitioner enters a client's home, it is the client, not the practitioner, who is in charge. In the hospital or nursing home, the nurse gives the client medications and changes dressings. In the home, nurses assist clients in providing their own care or assist family members or informal caregivers in providing that care.[18,19,31] The family and other informal caregivers are critical members of the health care team. Their beliefs about health care practice and treatment, the extent of their skills, and their availability influence or even determine whether a client can remain at home and the outcome of the client's care.

Hospice programs provide some of the most dramatic examples of the power of clients. The agency's hospice team usually consists of nurses, home health aides, social workers, pharmacists, registered dietitians, chaplains, and volunteers. Team members also work with the client's physician and other social service agencies. The role of the team is to support end-of-life decisions made by clients and their families.

Staff members who provide services to clients, their families, and other informal caregivers in their homes are human bridges to home health care. This is true whether the staff member is a nurse, another professional, or a paraprofessional. To maximize outcomes of care, all members of the home health and community team should follow some basic principles as they practice their specialty:

- You are a guest in your client's home and neighborhood. Your behavior and your manners must convey that you recognize this role.
- Respect the client's cultural, religious, and ethnic heritage. Hesitate before contradicting that heritage. Clients are more likely to follow their heritage than your advice.
- The client may not respect *your* cultural, religious, and ethnic heritage. If you are a male nurse, the client may expect, and even request, a female nurse. Develop interpersonal skills—and a tough skin.
- Almost every home health client has family members or significant others who offer advice and can serve as either your advocate or your foe. Try to enlist them as your advocate.
- The client "owns" the health-related problem that initiated your services. That problem is just one portion of the client's past, present, and future. Thus, it is the client who experiences, learns to understand, and ultimately solves the problem. It is your goal to help clients and their families become independent as quickly as possible. Talk to your peers and supervisors if you sense that you may be losing that perspective.
- Enjoy the unique autonomy and challenges of providing highly complex care in the home and community setting. Home health practice requires integration of high-technology skills, teaching, case management, and monitoring. Remember the need for communication with other members of the health care team. The nurse is usually responsible for judging whether or not the client can safely remain at home, and other team members need to share the information the nurse has through oral and written means.
- Maintain your sense of humor. You will need it!

Risks

Home health care staff and students should consistently practice the Boy Scout motto, "Be prepared." Preparedness is essential regardless of your responsibilities, the size of your agency or organization, or its geographical location. If you work in a hospital or nursing home, colleagues, technology, supplies, and references are nearby. When you visit a home, school, clinic, or other community site, you are usually on your own. Help and information may be available via extra supplies in the trunk of your car, a cell phone, a computer, a pager, or a Fax machine, but help may not be available immediately.

Always consider your safety and that of your client. Plan carefully to minimize the risks of accidents or violence. Know your agency's emergency preparedness and response plan, especially since the advent of bioterrorism.[7] If an accident or violence occurs, you must know how to intervene immediately and appropriately. For example, when selecting individuals, families, or groups for a student assignment, it is necessary to evaluate the client's needs, the student's educational and life experiences, the faculty member's skills and availability, where the clients are located, the timing of the visit, the availability of other sources of help, and the student's method of transportation and familiarity with the neighborhood.

It is also important to establish an excellent working relationship among the students, faculty, and staff of the agency or institution to enhance safety and the quality of the experience for all. To improve communication and safety for both clients and students, strategies such as shared home visits, student learning centers, nursing centers, and homeless clinics are being used.[12,17,32] The Nightingale Tracker, a computerized communication system, and other tools and techniques are additional strategies to link faculty and students as described later in this chapter.

Resources

The home health care student and staff nurse have valuable resources that contribute to their ability to provide high-quality care: education, experience, and common sense. Use these resources consistently when making home visits.

Education

Regardless of the stage of your education or the length of time since graduation, faculty and materials provide valuable professional information. Formal and informal education beyond the professional program is important for practicing community health nurses; many educators are increasingly interested in partnerships with practitioners and agencies.[12,17] Consider courses in first aid, cardiopulmonary resuscitation, computers, the Internet, cultural awareness, community resources, current affairs, and political, legal, financial, and ethical issues. Read relevant publications and attend relevant conferences. Remember what you learned, and keep updating your knowledge.

Experience

Your professional and life experiences contribute to your technical and interpersonal skills. Know where you are and take action in the areas in which you need to improve.[4] Discuss your career goals and opportunities with a trusted friend. Take every opportunity to observe a colleague providing care or completing other responsibilities, such as completing documentation. Learn how to organize your practice and avail yourself of excellent practice pointers, including those on the website.

Common Sense

Some aspects of practice in community settings are not the same as practice in the acute care setting. Develop and use your intuition, and listen to it.[23] Expert home health care practitioners are known for their caring, flexibility, persistence, and ability to improvise. They use sound judgment to alter everything from their schedule to their interventions according to their circumstances and available resources. Expert practitioners have more than a plan A as they begin to work with a client; they can move to a plan B or plan C at a moment's notice.

PROVIDING CARE

The concepts and principles involved in home health care and other community practice settings are closely related to those of nursing practice in the hospital, outpatient departments, and long-term care. The assessment, problem identification (diagnosis), planning, intervention, and evaluation steps of the nursing process provide an important foundation for that practice. Specific systems that you may use in home health or community care include the Omaha System and the Nightingale Tracker.

The Omaha System

The Omaha System was developed and refined through three Visiting Nurse Association (VNA) of Omaha research projects funded by the Division of Nursing, U.S. Department of Health and Human Services, between 1975 and 1986. Research on reliability, validity, and usability was also completed.[23,30]

The Omaha System is designed to facilitate nursing practice, documentation, and information management. It is a series of cues or feedback loops that help remind the user about possible client problems and intervention options and about ways to evaluate the effect of the care provided. Structured language and codes enhance the precision of recording and ease of communication. Users can communicate their conclusions orally, through printed paper forms, or electronically.

The Omaha System provides a clinical data framework for agencies or programs that use manual or automated versions of client records. Establishing a clinical database that is reliable and valid enables a user to generate reports that contribute to program evaluation,

long-range planning, compliance with regulations required by accreditation organizations and third-party payers, and outcome statistics required by many governing board members and third-party payers. The public health nurses, managers, and administrators at Washington County Public Health and Environment, Stillwater, MN, use their outcome measurement data for just those purposes.[25,26] Many home health and community agencies are making dramatic progress in their efforts to improve their client records and to develop integrated clinical and financial management information systems.[15,34] However, agencies and software vendors must follow the complex and lengthy regulations of the Health Insurance Portability and Accountability Act of 1996, a challenge to practitioners, administrators, third-party payers, computer vendors, faculty members, and students who are involved in any health care delivery.[34]

Initial users of the Omaha System were community home care, public health, and school practice professionals in the United States. Both the number and type of Omaha System users are expanding dramatically to include nursing center staff, hospital-based and managed care case managers, nursing educators and students, acute care staff, researchers, and the international community. Such expansion reflects the trends already described in this chapter and the trend among all types of health care providers to automate the handling of clinical data.[5,6,9,13,20,24,35] The Omaha System includes one of the vocabularies recognized and disseminated by the American Nurses' Association.[2]

Figure 10-1 illustrates the concepts of the nursing process as they relate to the Omaha System. The circular

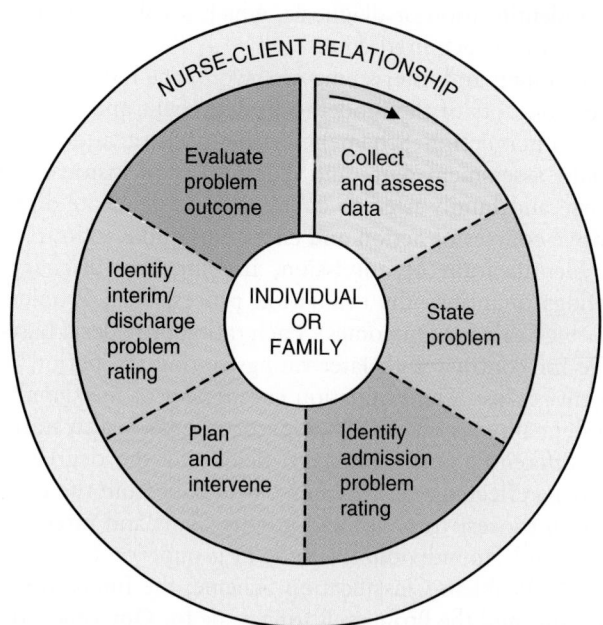

FIGURE 10-1 Steps of the nursing process as they relate to the Omaha System. (From Martin, K.S., & Scheet, N.J. [1992]. *The Omaha System: Applications for community health nursing* [p. 34]. Philadelphia: W.B. Saunders.)

model shown depicts the dynamic, interactive nature of the nursing process, the nurse-client relationship, and the related theories of diagnostic reasoning and clinical judgment, sometimes referred to as *analytic reasoning* or *expert knowledge*. The Omaha System is a research-based nursing diagnosis, intervention, and outcome measurement classification or taxonomy developed by practicing nurses.[22,23,30] The Problem Classification Scheme, the Intervention Scheme, and the Problem Rating Scale for Outcomes are components of the system. The relationships among the nursing process, the Omaha System, and home health care practice are described next.

A community health nurse begins service to a client after an intake or referral process. During the nurse's initial visit and all other visits, the vital importance of establishing and maintaining a positive nurse-client relationship must be recognized. Freeman and Heinrich[14] emphasized that a positive relationship is developed, not discovered. Such a relationship promotes quantity and quality of data and enhances the potential for success and client progress in relation to all components of the nursing process.

A nurse's initial activities include data collection, assessment, and analysis (i.e., Problem Classification Scheme). This process involves gathering, clustering, combining, summarizing, and validating diverse subjective and objective information about each family member, the family as an interacting unit, and the sociocultural and physical environment. A community health nurse uses principles of epidemiology to enhance systematic data collection and assessment and to identify patterns within client data. The conclusion and logical end product of the data collection and assessment process is problem identification or diagnosis, which involves interpretation of the acquired data.

Planning and intervening are two of the most important concepts of the model to both a client and a nurse (i.e., Intervention Scheme). Based on client and nurse goals, assessment data, and diagnostic conclusions, the nurse and family need to collaborate to delineate alternative courses of action and choose and take action.

Identification of admission, interim, and discharge ratings quantifies the evaluation process (i.e., Problem Rating Scale for Outcomes). Each rating provides a baseline for contrast with later ratings during the period of client service. The evaluation component of the Omaha System allows a nurse to compare a client's health status at different points in time to determine the degree of nursing effectiveness. The nurse uses data from the evaluation process to revise and modify plans and interventions with an individual, family, or group.[25,26]

The Problem Classification Scheme, the Intervention Scheme, and the Problem Rating Scale for Outcomes follow principles of taxonomy and consist of terms and codes arranged from general to specific. Terms are intended to be simple, clear, and concise.

The Problem Classification Scheme

The Problem Classification Scheme is a taxonomy of client problems or nursing diagnoses that has been developed from actual client data (Box 10-1). It consists of 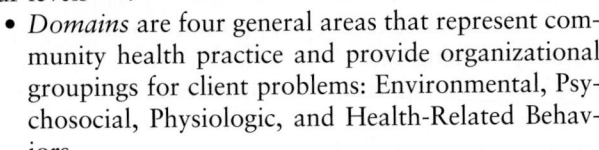 four levels[22,23]:

- *Domains* are four general areas that represent community health practice and provide organizational groupings for client problems: Environmental, Psychosocial, Physiologic, and Health-Related Behaviors.
- *Problems* are 40 nursing diagnoses that represent matters of difficulty and concern that adversely affect any aspect of the client's well-being. Examples include Caretaking/parenting, Integument, and Nutrition.
- *Modifiers* are the two sets of terms used to identify ownership of the problem and degree of severity in relation to client interest, risk factors, and signs and symptoms.
- *Manifestations* are the objective and subjective evidence of a client's problem.

The Problem Classification Scheme offers a view of the wide range of client concerns that the home health or community provider addresses. These include physical, emotional, social, spiritual, and economic concerns. Thus, this tool is used as a framework for assessment during a home or clinic visit and for documentation of the service provided. In that way, it constantly reminds the provider that the client needs to be viewed holistically and not as a "colostomy case" or a drug user, for example. The OASIS data set was not designed to be an assessment framework, but the OASIS items can be integrated into the agency's assessment form, such as a form based on the Problem Classification Scheme.[34,36]

Caretaking/parenting, a problem from the Psychosocial domain, appears in Box 10-2. It has nine manifestations, including difficulty providing physical care–safety as well as expectations incongruent with stage of growth and development. For example, you visit a 14-year-old mother and her newborn to provide information about infant growth, development, and care. You may record the following:

1. The problem: Caretaking/parenting.
2. Manifestations: Difficulty providing physical care–safety and expectations incongruent with stage of growth and development.
3. More specific descriptive and quantitative clinical data on the client's manual or automated record.

Integument, a problem from the Physiologic domain, also appears in Box 10-2. Integument has 10 manifestations, including lesion and drainage. If you care for a client whose infected wound requires cleaning and a dressing change, you may record the following[22]:

1. The problem: Integument.
2. Manifestations: Lesion and drainage.

BOX 10-1   *Domains and Problems of the Problem Classification Scheme*

Domain I. Environmental
The material resources, physical surroundings, and substances both internal and external to the client, home, neighborhood, and broader community.

1. Income
2. Sanitation
3. Residence
4. Neighborhood/workplace safety
5. Other

Domain II. Psychosocial
Patterns of behavior, communication, relationships, and development.

6. Communication with community resources
7. Social contact
8. Role change
9. Interpersonal relationship
10. Spirituality
11. Grief

12. Emotional stability
13. Human sexuality
14. Caretaking/parenting
15. Neglected child/adult
16. Abused child/adult
17. Growth and development
18. Other

Domain III. Physiologic
Functional status of processes that maintain life.

19. Hearing
20. Vision
21. Speech and language
22. Dentition
23. Cognition
24. Pain
25. Consciousness
26. Integument
27. Neuro-musculo-skeletal function
28. Respiration
29. Circulation

30. Digestion-hydration
31. Bowel function
32. Genito-urinary function
33. Antepartum/postpartum
34. Other

Domain IV. Health-Related Behaviors
Activities that maintain or promote wellness, promote recovery, or maximize rehabilitation potential.

35. Nutrition
36. Sleep and rest patterns
37. Physical activity
38. Personal hygiene
39. Substance use
40. Family planning
41. Health care supervision
42. Prescribed medication regimen
43. Technical procedure
44. Other

Data from Martin, K.S., & Scheet, N.J. (1992). *The Omaha System: Applications for community health nursing.* Philadelphia: W.B. Saunders.

BOX 10-2   *Problems, Modifiers, and Signs/Symptoms from the Problem Classification Scheme*

14. Caretaking/parenting:
    Health promotion
    Potential impairment
    Impairment
    01. difficulty providing physical care/safety
    02. difficulty providing emotional nurturance
    03. difficulty providing cognitive learning experiences and activities
    04. difficulty providing preventive and therapeutic health care
    05. expectations incongruent with stage of growth and development
    06. dissatisfaction/difficulty with responsibilities
    07. neglectful
    08. abusive

    09. other
26. Integument:
    Health promotion
    Potential impairment
    Impairment
    01. lesion
    02. rash
    03. excessively dry
    04. excessively oily
    05. inflammation
    06. pruritus
    07. drainage
    08. ecchymosis
    09. hypertrophy of nails
    10. other

Data from Martin, K.S., & Scheet, N.J. (1992). *The Omaha System: Applications for community health nursing.* Philadelphia: W.B. Saunders.

---

3. More specific descriptive and quantitative clinical data on the client's form or automated record.

Table 10-1 illustrates these two examples of assessment and nursing diagnosis documentation as well as terms and codes from the other two Omaha System schemes. Note that it depicts only part of the documentation for two nurse-client visits, not complete record entries.

The Intervention Scheme
The Intervention Scheme is a systematic arrangement of nursing actions or activities designed to help users identify and document plans and interventions in relation to specific client problems and other concepts of the nursing process (Box 10-3). It represents a research-based effort to link the effectiveness of interventions with diagnoses.[22]

TABLE 10-1	*Application of the Omaha System*				
Client Data	**Problems and Signs/Symptoms**	**Problem Rating Scale for Outcomes**	**Intervention Categories**	**Intervention Targets**	

Psychosocial Domain

Jane Doe: 14-year-old new mother with 2-day-old infant boy. Says she is "scared." Has not cared for infants; asking how to hold and feed. Wants son to sleep at least 6 hr. No family in area.	14. Caretaking/parenting: actual/family
	    01. difficulty providing physical care/safety
	    05. expectations incongruent with stage of growth and development
		Knowledge = 2
		Behavior = 3
		Status = 2
			I. Health Teaching, Guidance, and Counseling
			III. Case Management
				01. Anatomy/physiology
				04. Bonding
				08. Caretaking/parenting skills
				59. Support group	

Physiologic Domain

John Brown: 82-year-old just discharged after hemicolectomy. Has infected incision. Recalls some of discharge instructions.	26. Integument: actual/individual
	    01. lesion
	    07. drainage
		Knowledge = 4
		Behavior = 3
		Status = 3
			I. Health Teaching, Guidance, and Counseling
			II. Treatments and Procedures
				14. Dressing change/wound care
				50. Signs/symptoms—physical
				14. Dressing change/wound care
				50. Signs/symptoms—physical	

The first level consists of four categories:

1. Health Teaching, Guidance, and Counseling
2. Treatments and Procedures
3. Case Management
4. Surveillance

Categories are broad areas that provide a structure for describing actions or activities. One or more categories are used to develop a plan or document an intervention specific to a client problem.

The second level is an alphabetical listing of 62 targets. *Targets* are objects of nursing intervention or nursing activities that further describe problem-specific intervention categories. For the problem Integument and the category Treatments and Procedures, useful targets include dressing change/wound care and manifestations—physical. For Caretaking/parenting and the category Health Teaching, Guidance, and Counseling, possible targets are anatomy/physiology, bonding, and growth/development.

The third level is designed for client-specific information. Users generate pertinent, concise words or phrases as they develop plans or document care provided to a specific client. Although it was not part of the research projects, VNA of Omaha staff organized their suggestions into care planning guides.[22]

Table 10-1 presents the use of intervention categories, targets, and client-specific information to describe and document a plan or intervention category specific to

a client problem such as Integument or Caretaking/parenting. Again, note the definitions and diversity of community interventions. Nurses and other providers who practice in the community must be generalists and must develop competence in providing "hands-on" bedside care and technical skills as well as educational, referral, monitoring, and motivational skills. Recall that the client owns the health-related problem and is the only one who ultimately solves the problem.

The Problem Rating Scale for Outcomes

The Problem Rating Scale for Outcomes is a framework for measuring a client's problem-specific Knowledge, Behavior, and Status. The scale is intended to measure the client's progress and provide both a guide for practice and a method of documentation. The scale was designed for use throughout the time of client service. When establishing the initial ratings for client problems, the user creates an independent data baseline, capturing the condition and circumstances of the client at a given point in time. This admission baseline is used to compare and contrast the client's condition and circumstances with those ratings completed at later intervals and at client discharge. The comparison or change in ratings over time can be used to identify the client's progress in relation to interventions and the effectiveness of the plan of care.[25,26]

BOX 10-3 *Intervention Scheme*

Categories

I Health Teaching, Guidance, and Counseling
Health teaching, guidance, and counseling are nursing activities that range from giving information, anticipating client problems, encouraging client action and responsibility for self-care and coping, to assisting with decision making and problem solving. The overlapping concepts occur on a continuum with the variation due to the client's self-direction capabilities.

II Treatments and Procedures
Treatments and procedures are technical nursing activities directed toward preventing signs and symptoms, identifying risk factors and early signs and symptoms, and decreasing or alleviating signs and symptoms.

III Case Management
Case management includes nursing activities of coordination, advocacy, and referral. These activities involve facilitating service delivery on behalf of the client, communicating with health and human services providers, promoting assertive client communication, and guiding the client toward the use of appropriate community resources.

IV Surveillance
Surveillance includes nursing activities of detection, measurement, critical analysis, and monitoring to indicate client status in relation to a given condition or phenomenon.

Targets

1. Anatomy/physiology
2. Behavior modification
3. Bladder care
4. Bonding
5. Bowel care
6. Bronchial hygiene
7. Cardiac care
8. Caretaking/parenting skills
9. Cast care
10. Communication
11. Coping skills
12. Day care/respite care
13. Discipline
14. Dressing change/wound care
15. Durable medical equipment
16. Education
17. Employment
18. Environment
19. Exercises
20. Family planning
21. Feeding procedures
22. Finances
23. Food
24. Gait training
25. Growth/development
26. Homemaking
27. Housing
28. Interaction
29. Laboratory findings
30. Legal system
31. Medical/dental care
32. Medication action/side effects
33. Medication administration
34. Medication set-up
35. Mobility/transfers
36. Nursing care, supplementary
37. Nutrition
38. Nutritionist
39. Ostomy care
40. Other community resource
41. Personal care
42. Positioning
43. Rehabilitation
44. Relaxation/breathing techniques
45. Rest/sleep
46. Safety
47. Screening
48. Sickness/injury care
49. Signs/symptoms—mental/emotional
50. Signs/symptoms—physical
51. Skin care
52. Social work/counseling
53. Specimen collection
54. Spiritual care
55. Stimulation/nurturance
56. Stress management
57. Substance use
58. Supplies
59. Support group
60. Support system
61. Transportation
62. Wellness
63. Other

Data from Martin, K.S., & Scheet, N.J. (1992). *The Omaha System: Applications for community health nursing.* Philadelphia: W.B. Saunders.

The Problem Rating Scale for Outcomes is a five-point ordinal scale comprising three subscales, or concepts (Table 10-2). *Concepts* are three major areas that represent the basic client issues of knowing (Knowledge), doing (Behavior), and being (Status):

- *Knowledge* refers to the ability of the client to remember and interpret information.
- *Behavior* consists of the observable responses, actions, or activities of the client fitting the occasion or purpose.
- *Status* is the condition of the client in relation to objective and subjective defining characteristics.

The scale for each of the concepts has five categories or degrees for response. For example, for the problems Integument and Caretaking/parenting, the nurse identifies baseline Knowledge, Behavior, and Status ratings during the first home or clinic visit.

Automation and the Nightingale Tracker
The Omaha System has been described as a model for practice, documentation, and information management. The critical need to generate, store, analyze, and distribute clinical data with the help of automated information systems exists in all health care settings. For a few years early in the 1980s, the VNA developed and sold computer software. Soon other groups and agencies developed their own Omaha System software. Early in the 1990s, software companies started to develop commer-

TABLE 10-2	*Problem Rating Scale for Outcomes*				
Concept	1	2	3	4	5
Knowledge: the ability of the client to remember and interpret information	No knowledge	Minimal knowledge	Basic knowledge	Adequate knowledge	Superior knowledge
Behavior: the observable responses, actions, or activities of the client fitting the occasion or purpose	Not appropriate	Rarely appropriate	Inconsistently appropriate	Usually appropriate	Consistently appropriate
Status: the condition of the client in relation to objective and subjective defining characteristics	Extreme signs/symptoms	Severe signs/symptoms	Moderate signs/symptoms	Minimal signs/symptoms	No signs/symptoms

Data from Martin, K.S., & Scheet, N.J. (1992). *The Omaha System: Applications for community health nursing.* Philadelphia: W.B. Saunders.

cially available software for home health agencies, public health departments, nursing centers, and colleges of nursing.[10,13,15,28,29]

The presence of faculty and nursing students in service settings, especially students who are just beginning their nursing education, introduces additional challenges related to practice, documentation, and information management. Unlike hospital practice, community health practice may involve faculty remaining at the college or service setting while their eight or more students make independent visits and see clients at homes, clinics, schools, or other sites. These faculty and students, especially students in their early semesters of education, need to maintain communication while traveling and providing client care. Students may need to communicate with faculty quickly and often for the safety of both clients and students. These needs can be met by using reliable and efficient automated point-of-care information systems.

To help nursing students and faculty, the Helene Fuld Trust provided a research and development grant to FITNE to develop the Nightingale Tracker, a computerized communication system using portable hand-held computers. Students use the Nightingale Tracker to document the services they provide, send and receive Fax and e-mail messages, and browse the Internet. They can also use it as a speaker phone.[10,13]

The Omaha System terminology was selected as the clinical vocabulary for the Nightingale Tracker and is used by students as they complete clinical assignment activities. Such activities include assignment generation, preplanning, postclinical documentation, and evaluation follow-up. Since the Nightingale Tracker was released in 1998, students and faculty users have come to include associate degree, baccalaureate degree, registered nurse completion, and graduate nurse programs.[9,10,28,29] Some schools and colleges base their curriculum on the Omaha System.[24]

CONCLUSIONS

Home health care and community service settings are experiencing both unprecedented growth and financial constraints. Decreased agency revenue can lead to layoffs, decreased salary and benefits, increased workloads, and a sense of insecurity. Increases in client caseloads and services, staff, and budget can be exciting. At the same time, when the internal systems of agencies experience extra pressure and become overloaded, employees are more likely to become frustrated and stressed and to make errors. Teamwork, development, and improvement of systems are critical. Practitioners, administrators, students, and faculty need to use a variety of methods to communicate efficiently and work together to provide effective, high-quality services.

BIBLIOGRAPHY

1. Administration on Aging. (2002). *A profile of older Americans 2001: The older population* and *Health, health care, and disability.* Available: http://www.aoa.dhhs.gov/.
2. American Nurses' Association. *NIDSEC: Recognized languages for nursing.* Available: http://www.nursingworld.org/nidsec/classlst.htm.
3. Anderson, E.T., & McFarlane, J. (2000). *Community as partner* (3rd ed.). Philadelphia: Lippincott Williams & Wilkins.
4. Benner, P. (1984). *From novice to expert.* Menlo Park, CA: Addison-Wesley.
5. Bowles, K.H. (1999). The Omaha System: Bridging hospital and home care. *On-line Journal of Nursing Informatics* [On-line], *3*(1). Available: http://www.eaa-knowledge.com/ojni/ni/dm/ojni.html.
6. Button, P., et al. (1998). Challenges and issues related to implementation of nursing vocabularies in computer-based systems. *Journal of the American Medical Informatics Association, 5*(4), 332-334.
7. Centers for Disease Control and Prevention. (2002). *Anthrax and public health emergency preparedness and response.* Available: http://www.cdc.gov.

8. Centers for Medicare and Medicaid Services. (2002). *Conditions of participation: Home health agencies, national health expenditures: 1980-2010,* and *Health Insurance Portability and Accountability Act of 1996.* Available: http://www.cms.hhs.gov.

9. Connolly, P.M., Huynh, M.-P.T., & Gorney-Moreno, M.J. (1999). Cutting edge or over the edge? Implementing the Nightingale Tracker. *On-line Journal of Nursing Informatics* [On-line], *3*(1). Available: http://www.eaa-knowledge.com/ojni/ni/dm/ojni.html.

10. Connolly, P., & Elfrink, V.L. (2002). Using information technology in community-based psychiatric nursing education: The SJSU/NT project. *Home Health Care Management and Practice, 14*(5), 344-352.

11. Dolan, J.A., Fitzpatrick, M.L., & Herrmann, E.K. (1983). *Nursing in society: A historical perspective* (15th ed.). Philadelphia: W.B. Saunders.

12. Donovan, N. (2002). Providing a home care clinical experience that benefits, patients, students, and agencies. *Home Healthcare Nurse, 20*(7), 443-448.

13. Elfrink, V.L. (1999). The Omaha System: Bridging nursing education and information technology. *On-line Journal of Nursing Informatics* [On-line], *3*(1). Available: http://www.eaa-knowledge.com/ojni/ni/dm/ojni.html.

14. Freeman, R., & Heinrich, J. (1981). *Community health nursing practice* (2nd ed.). Philadelphia: W.B. Saunders.

15. Handly, M.J., et al. (2003). Essential activities for implementing a clinical information system in public health nursing. *Journal of Nursing Administration, 33*(1), 14-16.

16. Health Resources and Services Administration. (2002). *The registered nurse population: Findings from the National Sample Survey of Registered Nurses.* Washington, DC: Author.

17. Hamner, J.B., et al. (2002). Community-based service learning in the engaged university. *Nursing Outlook, 50*(2), 67-71.

18. Heineken, J., & McCoy, N. (2000). Establishing a bond with clients of different cultures. *Home Healthcare Nurse, 18*(1), 45-52.

19. Lester, N. (1998). Cultural competence: A nursing dialogue. *American Journal of Nursing, 98*(8), 26-33.

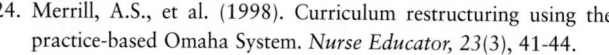 20. Martin, K.S. (1999). The Omaha System: Past, present, and future. *On-line Journal of Nursing Informatics* [On-line], *3*(1). Available: http://www.eaa-knowledge.com/ojni/ni/dm/ojni.html.

21. Martin, K.S. (2000). Home health care, outcomes management, and the Land of Oz. *Outcomes Management for Nursing Practice, 4*(1), 7-12.

22. Martin, K.S., & Scheet, N.J. (1992). *The Omaha System: A pocket guide for community health nursing.* Philadelphia: W.B. Saunders.

23. Martin, K.S., & Scheet, N.J. (1992). *The Omaha System: Applications for community health nursing.* Philadelphia: W.B. Saunders.

24. Merrill, A.S., et al. (1998). Curriculum restructuring using the practice-based Omaha System. *Nurse Educator, 23*(3), 41-44.

25. Monsen, K.A., & Martin, K.S. (2002). Developing an outcomes management program in a public health department. *Outcomes Management, 6*(2), 62-66.

26. Monsen, K.A., & Martin, K.S. (2002). Using an outcomes management program in a public health department. *Outcomes Management, 6*(3), 120-124.

27. National Association for Home Care. (2002). *Basic statistics about home care 2001.* Available: http://www.nahc.org.

28. Nightingale Tracker Field Test Nurse Team. (1999). Designing an information technology application for use in community-focused nursing curriculum. *Computers in Nursing, 17*(2), 73-81.

29. Nightingale Tracker Field Test Nurse Team. (2000). A comparison of teaching strategies for integrating technology into clinical nursing education. *Nurse Educator, 25*(3), 136-144.

30. Omaha System. (2002). Available: http://www.omahasystem.org.

31. Reif, L.J., & Martin, K.S. (1996). *Nurses and consumers: Partners in assuring quality in the home.* Washington, DC: American Nurses Publishing.

32. Schoneman, D. (2000). Surveillance as a nursing intervention: Use in community nursing centers. *Journal of Community Health Nursing, 19*(1), 33-47.

33. Stanhope, M., & Lancaster, J. (Eds.). (2004). *Community and public health nursing* (6th ed.). St. Louis: Mosby.

34. U.S. Department of Health and Human Services, National Center for Health Statistics. (2002). Health, United States, 2002. Available: http://www.cdc.gov/nchs/hus.htm.

35. Westra, B.L., & Solomon, D.A. (1999). The Omaha System: Bridging home care and technology. *On-line Journal of Nursing Informatics* [On-line], *3*(1). Available: http://www.eaa-knowledge.com/ojni/ni/dm/ojni.html.

36. World Health Organization/UNICEF. (1978). *Primary health care: Alma-Ata Conference.* Geneva: Author.

37. Zuber, R.F. (2002). Assessing Medicare eligibility. *Home Healthcare Nurse, 20*(7), 425-430.

Long-Term Care

Charlotte Eliopoulos

evolve

Web Enhancements

http://evolve.elsevier.com/Black/medsurg/

Appendix A
Religious Beliefs and Practices Affecting Health Care

Of all the types of health care settings, long-term care facilities (LTCFs) are perhaps the most misunderstood and criticized. The media give prime coverage to the small minority of facilities that have substandard conditions while ignoring the majority that provide compassionate, competent care on a daily basis. Some professionals who have never worked in an LTCF believe that this setting is a simple, nonchallenging environment in which to work. Many families assume that nursing home staff are untrustworthy, uncaring, and lazy.

In reality, residents of LTCFs receive competent care and enjoy a good quality of life. Despite significantly fewer resources available to them, compared with those found in hospitals and other care settings, LTCFs provide adequate care for highly dependent residents. The wide range of physical and mental conditions of residents, combined with the high prevalence of individuals of advanced age, make them a complex population for whom to care. Because physicians typically are not on the premises at all times, nurses must be highly competent in assessing residents, recognizing changes in status, and communicating needs to physicians. It is not unusual to find special relationships between residents and their caregivers, who often assume a family surrogate role. Why is there such a discrepancy between the reality and perception of LTCFs? Much of this is the result of the manner in which these facilities have developed. A brief review of the growth of LTCFs may offer some insight into the current challenges confronting this care setting.

GROWTH OF LONG-TERM CARE FACILITIES

By the end of the 17th century, most European countries had created institutions to care for the mentally ill, aged, developmentally disabled, orphaned, poor, criminals, and people with contagious diseases. It was not unusual for a single institution to house all of these various types of people together. The interest was not to provide highly specialized and individualized care but rather to segregate these people from the rest of society. Not surprisingly, low public interest and limited funds caused conditions to become inhumane in these institutions.

Until the 19th century, the United States had few institutions. People who were sick, old, or disabled were expected to receive care at home, from private help or family. As the population grew, however, so did the number of people without the financial or family resources to provide care, and hospitals and other forms of inpatient care were needed. Hospitals, staffed by physicians who at that time were from society's elite, were less than enthusiastic about having poor people with long-term care needs remaining in their beds for extended periods. Pressure grew to create facilities that could house and care for persons over the long term. In response, communities developed institutions that were given names such as *almshouse hospital, asylum, homes for the incurable,* and *chronic disease hospital.* Most often, these institutions were located on the outskirts of

evolve Be sure to check out the bonus material on the Evolve website and the CD-ROM, including free self-assessment exercises.

http://evolve.elsevier.com/Black/medsurg/

town where the average citizen would not have to have contact with the residents.

These early facilities relied on charities and meager public funds for their existence, and conditions were poor. A physician from that era, writing about those early institutions, described conditions such as grossly inadequate supplies, food so insufficient that many residents experienced recurrent incidents of scurvy, and residents forced to sleep on the floor because of overcrowding, rampant theft, open drunkenness, and sexual relations between residents and their caregivers.[8] Residents were expected to work for their keep, and recovered residents who had no family or home in the community, remained in the institution and cooked, cleaned, or cared for other residents in exchange for room, board, and a small salary. In this environment, high quality of life, rehabilitation, residents' rights, and individuality were foreign concepts. With these conditions, most people did not view institutions that provided long-term care as highly desirable options.

The enactment of the Social Security Act in 1935 afforded older adults the means to purchase care privately and not rely on charitable or public institutions. An informal long-term care system began to grow as people rented rooms of their homes to older adults who needed room, board, and perhaps some basic personal care assistance. Many of these homes were operated by nurses, or women who called themselves nurses, thus, the term *nursing home* began to be more widely used. Small nursing homes began to appear, often developed by religious or public agencies (e.g., Jewish homes for the aged, county rest homes) and sometimes by private individuals. At this time, the government had little involvement in nursing home operations; there were no government regulations pertaining to nursing home care and no government reimbursement for long-term care services.

In 1946, the federal government took a noticeable step in promoting nursing home growth through the Hill-Burton Hospital Survey and Construction Act. This Act provided funds for hospital construction, but other institutions, such as nursing homes, could also obtain funds if they met certain conditions. Because the construction requirements were developed for hospitals, the nursing homes that obtained these funds constructed facilities that were similar to hospitals. Rather than creating an environment designed for the unique needs of chronically ill individuals who would reside in the setting for an extended period of time, nursing homes resembled acute hospitals in appearance and style of operation (e.g., white uniforms, rigid schedules, limited visitation schedules, subservient role of residents).

By the 1960s, the "graying of the population" was being realized. As the numbers of older adults grew, so did their need for health services. During the Kennedy-Johnson era, federal programs proliferated to assist the disabled, aged, and other special groups. In 1965, Medicare and Medicaid were developed to ensure a minimum level of health care for the aged and poor. There was considerable interest in the existing health care system in providing nursing home reimbursement through Medicare and Medicaid. The American Medical Association lobbied to have reimbursement for extended care facilities to ease the problems that acute hospitals were experiencing, that is, clients were staying in hospitals and often no longer needed acute care services, but remained in the hospital because they lacked the means to pay for nursing home care. The owners of LTCFs also lobbied Congress to provide government funding for care in their facilities. Congress responded by including provisions for reimbursement for nursing home care in Medicare and Medicaid.

Along with funding came regulations—the standards or conditions that facilities had to meet in order to qualify for funds. Initially, the regulations included requirements for 24-hour licensed nursing coverage, individualized care plans, provisions for special diets, and other good standards of practice. However, only a small minority of the existing LTCFs could meet the standards at the time and protested that it would not be possible for them to participate in the Medicare and Medicaid programs. Again, with strong lobbying efforts, these conditions were waived, and facilities were able to take advantage of government reimbursement for long-term care without having to meet what were good, basic standards. (It is interesting that there was no noticeable voice from nurses, even though these facilities were called *nursing* homes.)

With eased standards and an influx of government reimbursement, the number of nursing homes grew (Table 11-1). This rapid and unregulated growth led to problems, some of which made front page headlines. Short

TABLE 11-1	Growth of Nursing Homes and Nursing Home Residents in the 20th Century	
Year	No. of Nursing Homes	Residents (in Thousands)
1940	1,200	25
1960	9,582	290
1970	22,004	1,076
1980	30,111	1,396
1990	14,744	1,558
1999	18,000	1,965

From U.S. Department of Commerce, Table 175. (2001). Nursing homes: Selected characteristics: 1985 to 1999. *Statistical Abstract of the United States.* (121st ed, p. 116) Washington, DC: Bureau of the Census.

staffing, substandard care, and abuse were among the conditions that the media exposed and that helped to generate the negative image of LTCFs that continues to shadow this care setting. The public was outraged and demanded action. In response, the Department of Health and Human Services commissioned the Institute of Medicine (IOM) to study these facilities and recommend changes. The IOM study confirmed the widespread poor quality of care that existed in LTCFs and emphasized the need to develop stricter regulations.[6] In response, highly stringent regulations were enacted under legislation called the *Omnibus Budget Reconciliation Act of 1987 (OBRA)* which produced profound reforms in nursing home care. Some of the conditions that LTCFs must meet are described in Box 11-1. Both the conditions and enforcement provisions are more stringent. Facilities that do not meet the conditions described in regulations can receive sanctions that include termination of Medicare and Medicaid reimbursement. As a result of the new regulations and strict enforcement of them, conditions in LTCFs have improved.

This history can help you to understand some of the reasons for the persistent negative image of LTCFs. Furthermore, it demonstrates that the importance of an active role for nursing in developing new health services and clearly defining nursing services that contribute to high-quality care. Nursing leadership was sorely lacking as nursing homes grew and as non-nurses determined nursing's function, role, and staffing requirements. The results speak for themselves.

RESIDENTS OF LONG-TERM CARE FACILITIES

Residents of LTCFs can be of any age, although most are older adults. The risk of being in an LTCF increases with each decade of life; the average age of residents is 82 years.

Women outnumber men by a ratio of 3 to 1, and 90% are single or widowed. A majority of residents are white; less than 10% are black and less than 3% Hispanic.

Most residents have conditions that impair their self-care capacity or require interventions that they cannot perform independently. About one half have a progressive cognitive impairment, such as Alzheimer's disease, arthritis, cardiovascular disease, or a combination of illnesses. Nearly 3 of every 10 residents have impaired vision, and about one fourth have impaired hearing. Most residents need assistance with at least several activities of daily living (ADL). Although most residents spend the remainder of their lives in the facility, an increasing number do recover, have restored function, and return to the community. In the past, some who might have remained in the hospital during recovery are now convalescing in nursing homes as a result of changes in reimbursement policies. The quality and quantity of caregiver support, rather than the medical diagnosis, determine one's risk of being admitted to an LTCF. For every resident in a nursing home, at least two equally disabled people are living in the community, receiving care from family or paid caregivers.[7] Often it is a change in status of the caregiver that precipitates the dependent person's admission to an LTCF. This reinforces the importance of assessing the family and assisting these caregivers in using interventions and resources that promote and maintain their health and well-being.

STAFF OF LONG-TERM CARE FACILITIES

Nearly 1 million nursing employees work in LTCFs in the United States and most of these are unlicensed personnel.[17] Regulatory standards are basic, and the only specific staffing requirements in federal regulations are that (1) a registered nurse (RN) must be on duty at least

---

BOX 11-1   *Protections Afforded to Residents of Long-Term Care Facilities as Described in Regulations**

Resident Rights
- To have rights as citizen and resident protected
- To be informed of rights, rules, regulations, and responsibilities
- To inspect and obtain copies of records
- To be informed of health status
- To refuse treatment or participation in research
- To be informed of charges
- To be informed of eligibility for Medicaid
- To be informed of process for filing a complaint with the state agency

- To choose and know physician and method of contacting physician
- To be informed of changes in status, room, roommate, or rights
- To proper management of personal funds
- To have privacy respected
- To voice grievances
- To examine survey results
- To perform or refuse to perform services for the facility, and to be compensated for services performed
- To send and receive mail

*This represents a brief outline of regulations included in the Omnibus Budget Reconciliation Act (OBRA). Please consult the full set of OBRA and state regulations for a complete description of regulatory requirements.

Continued

BOX 11-1 *Protections Afforded to Residents of Long-Term Care Facilities as Described in Regulations—cont'd*

Resident Rights—cont'd
- To have access to stationery, postage, and writing implements
- To receive visitors
- To use telephone privately
- To retain and use personal possessions
- To share a room with a spouse
- To self-administer drugs unless determined to be unsafe

Admission, Transfer, Discharge
- To have legitimate reason for discharge
- To be free from solicitation of gifts or money as condition for admission
- To have written policies regarding services provided by facility

Resident Behavior and Facility Practices
- To be free from restraints used for purpose of discipline or staff convenience
- To be free from verbal, physical, or mental abuse, punishment, or seclusion
- To have alleged and known abuse incidents investigated and reported according to state law

Quality of Life
- To have dignity maintained and promoted
- To choose activities and care
- To organize and participate in resident groups
- To participate in social, religious, and community activities
- To have program of activities directed by qualified personnel
- To have social services provided by qualified personnel
- To have clean, safe, home-like environment
- To have private closet space, adequate lighting, and comfortable room temperatures

Resident Assessment
- To have a comprehensive assessment conducted within the first 14 days of admission and at least annually thereafter
- To be reassessed whenever there is a change in status
- To have a comprehensive care plan developed within 7 days after completion of assessment
- To have a discharge plan and summary as needed

Quality of Care
- To receive necessary services and treatments to maintain or improve condition
- To be free from developing pressure ulcers, incontinence, contractures, or dehydration unnecessarily
- To be adequately nourished and hydrated
- To not receive unnecessary drugs
- To be free from significant medication errors

Nursing Services
- To have nursing personnel provided consistent with level of care and needs of residents

Dietary Services
- To have at least 3 well-balanced meals provided daily, including special diets
- To have department employ qualified personnel and follow standards for safe food procurement, preparation, and storage

Physician Services
- To be under the care of a physician
- To have the physician adhere to standards of practice

Specialized Rehabilitative Services
- To have physical therapy, occupational therapy, or speech-language therapy arranged for or provided as needed

Dental Services
- To be assisted in obtaining dental services

Pharmacy Services
- To have the facility adhere to standards for prescribing, pouring, administering, and monitoring medications

Infection Control
- To have the facility establish and maintain an infection control program

Physical Environment
- To have the facility follow standards of Life Safety Code

Administration
- To have facility be licensed by state
- To have qualified administrator
- To have nursing assistants complete training program and competency evaluation
- To have a designated medical director
- To provide or arrange for laboratory and diagnostic services
- To have clinical records safeguarded and maintained as required by state law
- To have facility emergency and disaster plans
- To have facility make transfer agreements with hospitals
- To have a utilization review committee in effect
- To have facility maintain a quality assessment and assurance committee that meets at least quarterly and develops and implements corrective actions for deficiencies

8 consecutive hours per day, 7 days a week and (2) a full-time director of nursing must be on staff if the facility has more than 60 beds. The proportion of other nursing staff is not stated, although it is required that "the facility provide 24-hour nursing services which are sufficient to meet total nursing care needs."[4] The fact that most direct nursing care is provided by nursing assistants presents special challenges to nurses who must supervise these caregivers.[5]

NURSING RESPONSIBILITIES

Assessment

The facility is required to assess residents within the first 14 days of admission and at least annually thereafter; residents are to be reassessed whenever there is a change in their status. The Minimum Data Set (MDS) is the tool on which the assessment is to be documented, and an RN coordinates its completion (Figure 11-1). Problems in need of care planning are generated from the information on the MDS.

As numerous as the items are on the MDS, it is not a *comprehensive* assessment; it is a *minimum* assessment. Important pieces of information are not captured, such as the client's self-concept, spirituality, sense of power, knowledge of health condition and self-care practices, sexuality, patterns of solitude, sense of purpose, immunity, stress management, use of alternative therapies, and attitudes regarding health status and death. Because these are important areas for consideration in the long-term care of residents, you may want to supplement the MDS with these additional assessment data. Although the MDS assessment tool may be formally completed periodically, high-quality care relies on the nurse's assessment of residents with every nurse-resident contact. For example, when administering a medication, you can observe the resident's coloring and respirations, note any change in mood, and ask about the status of a previous manifestation. Often residents do not have the ability to identify and report changes in their own health status, and astute nursing assessment is thus crucial. The need to be alert to changes in status is reinforced by the reality that physicians typically do not see residents on a daily basis and must rely on nurses to detect and report manifestations.

The advanced age of the residents can create challenges in assessment. Age-related changes can cause atypical manifestations in older adults. For example, instead of high fever and coughing, clinical manifestations of pneumonia in older adults may include confusion, loss of appetite, and fatigue with activities that caused no difficulties in the past. This challenges nurses to know the norms for individual residents and to identify subtle clues of illnesses so that problems can be identified early. Timely recognition and communication of manifestations to the physician can help prevent complications.

Care Planning

Regulations require that a care plan be written for each resident within 7 days after completion of the assessment. The care plan is an *interdisciplinary* one; nurses coordinate the input offered by each discipline and ensure that the plan is written in a correct, timely manner (Box 11-2). To the extent possible, the resident and the family should actively participate in the development of the care plan.

A care plan is not merely a paperwork requirement but a working tool to guide nursing actions; it is a blueprint for nursing actions. Goals and actions that are no longer relevant need to be revised. All members of the team, particularly nursing assistants who perform most direct care activities, must be familiar with the care plan. Typically, it is the nurse's responsibility to review the care plan with unlicensed caregivers to ensure they understand the actions that must be implemented and the observations that must be reported.

Caregiving

The direct caregiving role of nurses varies from facility to facility. In some LTCFs, nurses perform selected roles, such as administering medications and treatments; in others, they may be involved in total care activities. During the pre-employment interview, nurses should review the job descriptions for their specific positions to ensure that they have a realistic view of their role.

In addition to caregiving activities that might be performed in any setting (e.g., medication administration, treatments), special nursing support is required by residents and their families as they adjust to the LTCF. Few individuals have had experiences that prepared them for living in or having a loved one in a nursing home. Residents face many adjustments.

Environment

Many people have lived in the same home for several decades before admission and could probably locate objects in their homes blindfolded. When moved into an LTCF, they are faced with adapting to the layout of a new setting and other new components of their environment, such as paging systems, odors, and sounds. They no longer have ready access to their own refrigerator if they are hungry or a spare bedroom where a grandchild can spend the night. Their personal space has shrunk to a bed, a few chairs, a closet, and several drawers. People can enter their space and invade their privacy at any hour of the day or night.

Routines

New residents soon learn that they must adjust to facility routines and schedules. They may have to take a morning shower, although they may have taken a bed-

Resident _____ Numeric Identifier _____

MINIMUM DATA SET (MDS) — *VERSION 2.0*
FOR NURSING HOME RESIDENT ASSESSMENT AND CARE SCREENING
FULL ASSESSMENT FORM
(Status in last 7 days, unless other time frame indicated)

SECTION A. IDENTIFICATION AND BACKGROUND INFORMATION

1. RESIDENT NAME
a. (First)   b. (Middle Initial)   c. (Last)   d. (Jr./Sr.)

2. ROOM NUMBER

3. ASSESSMENT REFERENCE DATE
a. *Last day of MDS observation period*
Month — Day — Year
b. Original (0) or corrected copy of form (enter number of correction)

4a. DATE OF REENTRY
Date of reentry from most recent temporary discharge to a hospital in last 90 days (or since last assessment or admission if less than 90 days)
Month — Day — Year

5. MARITAL STATUS
1. Never married   3. Widowed   5. Divorced
2. Married   4. Separated

6. MEDICAL RECORD NO.

7. CURRENT PAYMENT SOURCES FOR N.H. STAY
(Billing Office to indicate; check all that apply in last 30 days)
Medicaid per diem   a.
Medicare per diem   b.
Medicare ancillary part A   c.
Medicare ancillary part B   d.
CHAMPUS per diem   e.
VA per diem   f.
Self or family pays for full per diem   g.
Medicaid resident liability or Medicare co-payment   h.
Private insurance per diem (including co-payment)   i.
Other per diem   j.

8. REASONS FOR ASSESSMENT
[Note—If this is a discharge or reentry assessment, only a limited subset of MDS items need be completed]
a. Primary reason for assessment
1. Admission assessment (required by day 14)
2. Annual assessment
3. Significant change in status assessment
4. Significant correction of prior full assessment
5. Quarterly review assessment
6. Discharged—return not anticipated
7. Discharged—return anticipated
8. Discharged prior to completing initial assessment
9. Reentry
10. Significant correction of prior quarterly assessment
0. NONE OF ABOVE
b. Codes for assessments required for Medicare PPS or the State
1. Medicare 5 day assessment
2. Medicare 30 day assessment
3. Medicare 60 day assessment
4. Medicare 90 day assessment
5. Medicare readmission/return assessment
6. Other state required assessment
7. Medicare 14 day assessment
8. Other Medicare required assessment

9. RESPONSIBILITY/ LEGAL GUARDIAN
(Check all that apply)
Legal guardian   a.
Other legal oversight   b.
Durable power of attorney/health care   c.
Durable power of attorney/financial   d.
Family member responsible   e.
Patient responsible for self   f.
NONE OF ABOVE   g.

10. ADVANCED DIRECTIVES
(For those items with supporting documentation in the medical record, check all that apply)
Living will   a.
Do not resuscitate   b.
Do not hospitalize   c.
Organ donation   d.
Autopsy request   e.
Feeding restrictions   f.
Medication restrictions   g.
Other treatment restrictions   h.
NONE OF ABOVE   i.

SECTION B. COGNITIVE PATTERNS

1. COMATOSE
(Persistent vegetative state/no discernible consciousness)
0. No   1. Yes *(If yes, skip to Section G)*

2. MEMORY
(Recall of what was learned or known)
a. Short-term memory OK—seems/appears to recall after 5 minutes
0. Memory OK   1. Memory problem **2**
b. Long-term memory OK—seems/appears to recall long past
0. Memory OK   1. Memory problem **2**

⬜ = When box blank, must enter number or letter.

🄰 = When letter in box, check if condition applies

Code "—" if information unavailable or unknown

Form 1728RHH   © 1997 Briggs Corporation, Des Moines, IA 50306 (800) 247-2343 PRINTED IN U.S.A.
Copyright limited to addition of trigger system.

3. MEMORY/ RECALL ABILITY
(Check all that resident was normally able to recall during last 7 days)
Current season   a.
Location of own room   b.
Staff names/faces   c.
That he/she is in a nursing home   d.
NONE OF ABOVE are recalled   e.

4. COGNITIVE SKILLS FOR DAILY DECISION-MAKING
(Made decisions regarding tasks of daily life)
0. INDEPENDENT—decisions consistent/reasonable
1. MODIFIED INDEPENDENCE—some difficulty in new situations only **2**
2. MODERATELY IMPAIRED—decisions poor; cues/supervision required **2**
3. SEVERELY IMPAIRED—never/rarely made decisions **2, 5B**

5. INDICATORS OF DELIRIUM— PERIODIC DISORDERED THINKING/ AWARENESS
(Code for behavior in the last 7 days.) [Note: Accurate assessment requires conversations with staff and family who have direct knowledge of resident's behavior over this time.]
0. Behavior not present
1. Behavior present, not of recent onset
2. Behavior present, over last 7 days appears different from resident's usual functioning (e.g., new onset or worsening)
a. EASILY DISTRACTED—(e.g., difficulty paying attention; gets sidetracked) 2 = **1, 17***
b. PERIODS OF ALTERED PERCEPTION OR AWARENESS OF SURROUNDINGS—(e.g., moves lips or talks to someone not present; believes he/she is somewhere else; confuses night and day) 2 = **1, 17***
c. EPISODES OF DISORGANIZED SPEECH—(e.g., speech is incoherent, nonsensical, irrelevant, or rambling from subject to subject; loses train of thought) 2 = **1, 17***
d. PERIODS OF RESTLESSNESS—(e.g., fidgeting or picking at skin, clothing, napkins, etc.; frequent position changes; repetitive physical movements or calling out) 2 = **1, 17***
e. PERIODS OF LETHARGY—(e.g., sluggishness; staring into space; difficult to arouse; little body movement) 2 = **1, 17***
f. MENTAL FUNCTION VARIES OVER THE COURSE OF THE DAY—(e.g., sometimes better, sometimes worse; behaviors sometimes present, sometimes not) 2 = **1, 17***

6. CHANGE IN COGNITIVE STATUS
Resident's cognitive status, skills, or abilities have changed as compared to status of **90 days ago** (or since assessment if less than 90 days)
0. No change   1. Improved   2. Deteriorated **1, 17***

SECTION C. COMMUNICATION/HEARING PATTERNS

1. HEARING
(With hearing appliance, if used)
0. HEARS ADEQUATELY—normal talk, TV, phone
1. MINIMAL DIFFICULTY when not in quiet setting **4**
2. HEARS IN SPECIAL SITUATIONS ONLY—speaker has to adjust tonal quality and speak distinctly **4**
3. HIGHLY IMPAIRED/absence of useful hearing **4**

2. COMMUNICATION DEVICES/ TECHNIQUES
(Check all that apply during last 7 days)
Hearing aid, present and used   a.
Hearing aid, present and not used regularly   b.
Other receptive comm. techniques used (e.g., lip reading)   c.
NONE OF ABOVE   d.

3. MODES OF EXPRESSION
(Check all used by resident to make needs known)
Speech   a.
Writing messages to express or clarify needs   b.
American sign language or Braille   c.
Signs/gestures/sounds   d.
Communication board   e.
Other   f.
NONE OF ABOVE   g.

4. MAKING SELF UNDERSTOOD
(Expressing information content—however able)
0. UNDERSTOOD
1. USUALLY UNDERSTOOD—difficulty finding words or finishing thoughts **4**
2. SOMETIMES UNDERSTOOD—ability is limited to making concrete requests **4**
3. RARELY/NEVER UNDERSTOOD **4**

5. SPEECH CLARITY
(Code for speech in the last 7 days)
0. CLEAR SPEECH—distinct, intelligible words
1. UNCLEAR SPEECH—slurred, mumbled words
2. NO SPEECH—absence of spoken words

6. ABILITY TO UNDERSTAND OTHERS
(Understanding verbal information content—however able)
0. UNDERSTANDS
1. USUALLY UNDERSTANDS—may miss some part/intent of message **2, 4**
2. SOMETIMES UNDERSTANDS—responds adequately to simple, direct communication **2, 4**
3. RARELY/NEVER UNDERSTANDS **2, 4**

7. CHANGE IN COMMUNICATION/ HEARING
Resident's ability to express, understand, or hear information has changed as compared to status of **90 days ago** (or since last assessment if less than 90 days)
0. No change   1. Improved   2. Deteriorated **17***

TRIGGER LEGEND
1 - Delirium
2 - Cognitive Loss/Dementia
4 - Communication
5B - ADL Maintenance
17* - Psychotropic Drugs
(For this to trigger, O4a, b, or c must = 1-7)

MDS 2.0   1/30/98

FIGURE 11-1 Sample section of the Minimum Data Set (MDS) assessment tool for nursing home resident assessment and care screening. Other sections would include Vision Patterns, Mood and Behavior Patterns, Psychosocial Well-Being, Physical Functioning and Structural Problems, and Continence in Last 14 Days. (© 1997, Briggs Corporation, West Des Moines, IA.)

BOX 11-2 *Characteristics of an Effective Care Plan*

- Is based on needs as identified in the Minimum Data Set assessment tool
- Contains goals and actions to address current needs and to prevent new problems
- States goals that are realistic, clear, specific, and measurable
- Lists actions that are related to each goal that include discipline responsible for implementation and specific directions
- Is accessible and utilized by all caregivers
- Is evaluated at least quarterly and revised as necessary, especially when a significant change in condition occurs

---

time bath for more than 70 years. They may have a full breakfast placed before them at 8:00 AM when they seldom ate a bite of food before noon. After decades of staying awake and listening to the radio until 2:00 AM, they are told that "lights out" is 9:00 PM.

People

After years of being on a first-name basis with neighbors, store clerks, the mail carrier, and the auto repairman, residents must learn a cast of new players. In addition to meeting other residents, they may meet at least three nurses and three nursing assistants who will care for them over a 24-hour period, the facility's medical director, administrator, social worker, housekeeper, dietitian, activities therapist, clergy, and several therapists. They must learn not only the names but also the roles of these people and how to communicate with them.

Independence

Despite a staff's best efforts to afford residents the right to make decisions, there is a loss of independence when people become residents of a nursing home. They cannot scramble an egg in the middle of the night, have a friend stay over for a few days, or paint the walls the color of their choice. They must report their whereabouts and needs to staff, and they depend on others for the basics of bringing them food and taking them to the toilet.

These adjustments also affect family members at the same time that they are facing their own changing roles and responsibilities in regard to their relationship with the resident. Both residents and their families can experience such reactions as anxiety, depression, anger, helplessness, withdrawal, grief, and inattention to self-care practices. You can protect the health of residents and their families and facilitate a positive adjustment to the LTCF by taking some of the actions described in Box 11-3.

During caregiving activities, make sure that *holistic care* is provided; such care implies that every aspect—body, mind, spirit—is being addressed. This integration of body, mind, and spirit results in more powerful and meaningful care than if each aspect is addressed separately. Some ways in which holistic nursing is demonstrated are listed in Box 11-4.

Communication

As mentioned earlier, the LTCF nurse carries significant responsibility for identifying and obtaining timely treatment of complications and new health problems. Because of their regular and close contact with residents, nursing assistants may be the first and only caregivers to detect changes in health status (e.g., a developing pressure ulcer or a change in eating pattern); therefore, effective channels of communication are crucial in reporting these findings. Conducting rounds, reading what has been documented, and asking specific questions are among the measures you can use to learn about a resident's condition.

You also must make sure that physicians learn of changes in a resident's condition in a timely manner. Documenting in a resident's record is not necessarily sufficient, particularly because most attending physicians do not visit LTCF residents on a daily basis and seldom have the time to scan all notations when they do visit. You must promptly communicate any changes and relevant information (e.g., abnormal laboratory results, family complaints) to physicians.

Between their scheduled visits to the facility, physicians may generate new orders, which often are communicated by telephone. Facilities may differ in regard to the personnel who can accept telephone orders; therefore, it is best to check with the individual facility's policy. The following should be done to promote safety in telephone orders:

1. Provide the physician with complete information that can aid in medical decision-making (e.g., clinical manifestations, current and usual vital signs, prescribed medications, unusual incidents, and other relevant facts).
2. Avoid making a medical diagnosis. Report clinical manifestations and allow the physician to make a medical judgment.
3. Take the order directly from the prescribing physician, not through office staff.
4. Repeat the order; if possible, have the physician Fax a copy of the written order.
5. Have the order signed within 24 hours.
6. If there is anything that seems inappropriate about the order, question the physician. If the response from the attending physician still leaves doubt, consult with the facility's medical director and director of nursing.

BOX 11-3 Helping New Residents and Families

1. *Learn about the unique characteristics of each resident.*
   a. Find out not only about the health conditions residents have but also who they are as people and the lives they have lived.
   b. Engage residents and families in conversations about residents' histories.
   c. Complete a *Profile Poster* similar to the one shown below to help staff and other residents learn about the unique backgrounds of residents and who they are as individuals.

Profile Poster

Name: *Mary Auchmeyer Luggi*
Recent home: *New York City*
Childhood home: *Frankfurt, Germany*
Schools attended: *New York City College*
Spouse's name: *Gus Luggi (deceased)*
Occupation: *High school home economics teacher*
Children: *Son: Gus Luggi Jr, Daughter: Emily Smythe*
Grandchildren: *Tom 21, Amelia 19, Gus 15, Ginny 14, Sammie 13*
Hobbies, interests: *Quilting, baseball, singing*
Other tidbits: *Travelled on several missionary trips to India, speaks German, Italian, and French*

Photos of resident and family can be added

---

2. *Identify residents' needs, preferences, and level of physical and mental function.*
   a. Assess how well residents can meet their activities of daily living and the assistance they need.
   b. Ask about their preferences in regard to food likes and dislikes, sleep and nap habits, bathing, and other activities.
   c. Incorporate findings into their plan of care.
3. *Explain and educate.*
   a. Orient residents and families to the layout of the facility, staff, routines, and activities.
   b. Explain procedures before doing them.
   c. Be available to discuss residents' and families' concerns and to answer questions.
4. *Promote maximum independence.*
   a. Encourage residents to do as much for themselves as possible.
   b. Explain to residents and families the value of residents being independent.
   c. Give residents opportunities to make decisions regarding their care and activities.
5. *Make residents and families feel comfortable.*
   a. Be courteous and patient; understand that the stress associated with admission can cause residents and family members to make demands, complain, ask many questions, and forget what has been told to them.
   b. Provide privacy during visitation.
   c. Inform families of the location of visitor lounges, cafeteria, and vending machines.
6. *Be holistic.*
   a. Being holistic means that we are concerned with the whole person: body, mind, and spirit.
   b. Try to help residents meet physical, emotional, social, and spiritual needs to promote their physical, emotional, social, and spiritual health.

From Eliopoulos, C. (1997). Helping new residents and families. *Long-Term Care Educator, 8*(12), 6.

BOX 11-4 Holistic Nursing in Long-Term Care Facilities

Nurses can promote holistic care in long-term care facilities by:

- Assisting residents to achieve a higher potential of functioning
- Supporting residents in their efforts to promote health and prevent complications
- Learning about the unique life stories of residents
- Ensuring that residents receive care that is consistent with their values and beliefs and respecting cultural differences
- Aiding residents and families in discovering meaning in health status and in life and death
- Strengthening residents' abilities to live in harmony with their health condition
- Assisting residents in maintaining their connections with family, friends, and the community within and outside the facility
- Helping residents boost their natural healing abilities
- Facilitating hope and a sense of purpose in residents' lives
- Supporting residents as they respond to their spiritual identity or relate to a higher power
- Providing a nurturing and healing caregiving environment
- Offering opportunities for residents to experience joy and satisfaction
- Protecting residents from threats to their health or well-being, and promoting highest quality of life
- Adhering to accepted standards of nursing practice

From Eliopoulos, C. (1999). *Nursing administration of long-term care facilities* (3rd ed.). Glen Arm, MD: Health Education Network.

Management

Nurses hold a variety of administrative and managerial positions in LTCFs, such as director of nursing, assistant director of nursing, supervisor, unit manager or head nurse, charge nurse, and staffing coordinator. Even if they do not hold these formal titles, most LTCF nurses must perform some management functions, such as the following:

- Delegating assignments
- Supervising other staff
- Evaluating performance
- Implementing disciplinary actions
- Completing reports
- Reviewing and auditing records
- Communicating needs to other departments
- Investigating, reporting, and recording incidents and accidents
- Handling complaints
- Ordering supplies
- Communicating with insurers, regulatory agencies, and other parties

To manage effectively, your knowledge and skills must exceed those used in clinical nursing activities. You must be knowledgeable of regulations, reimbursement programs, and legal aspects of nursing practice and employee-employer relations. You must also be skillful in assertiveness, coaching, counseling, accurate documentation, organization, time management, and communication.

OTHER FORMS OF LONG-TERM CARE

This chapter has focused on the role of nurses in the LTCF. However, the LTCF is only one part of the long-term care system, and other forms of long-term care are available, such as those in the following list. Other forms of long-term care and the resources to find them are presented on the website with this text:

1. *Subacute or transitional care.* For people who require ongoing care or recovery for an acute condition but do not need to receive the services on an acute hospital unit. The subacute care unit can be separate parts of a hospital or nursing home, or it can be an entire facility dedicated to this purpose.
2. *Assisted living facility.* A form of housing that provides 24-hour staffing, meals, supervision of medications, and personal care assistance.
3. *Adult day care.* A daytime program for people who typically have the same level of impairments as nursing home residents but who receive care in the community, usually by family members. The client

is transported to the center and receives structured activities, meals, personal care assistance, and health care supervision.

4. *Home care.* For community-based people who are homebound and who need caregiving assistance or special treatments.
5. *Hospice.* For people who are terminally ill and in need of care. This care can be provided in the home or in a day hospital setting. Care of the dying is a common experience in long-term care. Caring behaviors of the staff at the time of death, allowing the family to be involved with the resident, and providing spiritual support are important and valued nursing functions.[18]

Each of these types of care has unique regulations and conditions for reimbursement.

CONCLUSIONS

The roles and responsibilities of nurses in LTCFs are varied and complex. Residents possess a wide range of physical and mental conditions that require expert assessment, interventions, and monitoring. The inability of many residents to accurately express their needs and age-related alterations in the presentation of clinical manifestations presents special challenges in detecting changes in status. The absence of physicians in the facility on a daily basis places a greater burden on nurses to identify and seek treatment of residents' problems. The high proportion of unlicensed staff demands that nurses be effective managers. An abundance of regulatory and reimbursement requirements demand that nurses be knowledgeable of these topics.

The reality that most residents will not only receive care, but will *live* in the facility for the remainder of their lives causes nurses often to serve as surrogate family. Very few practice settings offer nurses the opportunity to fill such a wide and varied range of roles. Rather than a simple, nonchallenging practice setting, LTCFs challenge nurses to use a wide range of knowledge and skills as they establish meaningful long-term relationships with residents and their families. To fill the roles and responsibilities competently, LTCF nurses must be among their profession's best.

BIBLIOGRAPHY

1. Eliopoulos, C. (1999). *Integrating alternative and conventional therapies: Holistic care for chronic conditions.* St. Louis: Mosby.
2. Eliopoulos, C. (2002). *Nursing administration of long-term care facilities* (6th ed.). Glen Arm, MD: Health Education Network.

3. Eliopoulos, C. (1998). *Transforming nursing homes into healing centers: A holistic model for long-term care* (p. 48). Glen Arm, MD: Health Education Network.

4. *Federal Register.* (1989). Rules and Regulations (Vol. 54, No. 21). Section 483.26(c), February 2, 1989.

 5. Hall, L.M., & O'Brien-Pallas, L. (2000). Redesigning nursing work in long-term-care environments. *Nursing Economics, 18*(2), 79-87.

6. Institute of Medicine, Committee on Implications of For-Profit Enterprise in Health Care. (1986). Profits and health care: An introduction to the issues. In B.H. Gray (Ed.), *For-profit enterprise in health care* (pp. 3-18). Washington, DC: National Academy Press.

7. Kane, R.L., & Kane, R.A. (1997). Long-term care. In C.K. Cassel, et al. (Eds.), *Geriatric medicine* (3rd ed., pp. 81-96). New York: Springer.

8. Lawrence, C. (1905). *History of the Philadelphia almshouses and hospitals* (pp. 52, 123). Privately printed.

9. Mezey, M.D. (2001). *The encyclopedia of elder care.* New York: Springer.

10. National Committee to Preserve Social Security and Medicare. (1997). *Nurse staffing in nursing homes: Viewpoint.* Legislative Agenda for the 105th Congress, April 1997.

 11. Nay, R. (1998). Contradictions between perceptions and practices of caring in long-term care of elderly people. *Journal of Clinical Nursing, 7*(5), 401-408.

12. Rice, V.H. (1997). Ethical issues relative to autonomy and personal control in independent and cognitively impaired elders. *Nursing Outlook, 45*, 27-34.

13. Rosenberg, C.E. (1987). *The care of strangers: The rise of America's hospital system.* New York: Basic Books.

14. Ross, M.M., et al. (2001). Family caregiving in long-term-care facilities. *Clinical Nursing Research, 10*(4), 347-368.

15. Thomas, W.H. (1996). *Life worth living. How someone you love can still enjoy life in a nursing home.* The Eden Alternative in action. Acton, MA: VanderWyk & Burnham.

16. Thurmond, J.A. (1999). Nurses' perceptions of chemical restraint use in long-term care. *Applied Nursing Research, 12*(3), 159-162.

17. U.S. Department of Commerce. (2001). Table 175: Nursing homes—Selected characteristics: 1985 to 1999. *Statistical Abstract of the United States: 2001* (121st ed., p. 116). Washington, DC: Bureau of the Census.

18. Wilson, S.A., & Daley, B.J. (1999). Family perspectives on dying in long-term-care settings. *Journal of Gerontological Nursing, 25*(11), 19-25.

Rehabilitation

Susan L. Dean-Baar

Advances in sciences and technology are having a dramatic impact on health care as the population continues to live longer but with an increasing number of chronic conditions. Concurrent changes in health policy and the financing of health care delivery are decreasing the length of stays in acute care settings. The cumulative effect of these changes is resulting in an increasing number of clients requiring rehabilitation services after an episode of acute care. These rehabilitation services can be provided in a variety of settings. Today's nurse who is caring for clients on a medical-surgical unit needs to be familiar with the rehabilitation component of the continuum of care so that he or she can make appropriate referrals and prepare clients for the rehabilitation experience.

On the surface, rehabilitation settings can look much the same as acute care settings. The philosophy of these settings, however, differs significantly. In today's health care environment it is important to prepare clients and families for this change so that they can interpret provider behaviors correctly. In acute care settings clients are viewed as individuals with an illness that needs to be either cured or controlled through symptom management, and the focus is predominately on the current episode of care. In contrast, the focus of health care providers in rehabilitation settings is to support individuals and family members in learning skills that will assist them to live with a chronic illness or disability. This difference in approach is not always easy for clients and families to see, especially when a client receives both acute care and rehabilitation care in the same hospital. When a client is transferred from one care unit to another and both units have similar physical characteristics and room layouts, it becomes critical that the client be orientated as to what to expect and the differences in routine that he or she may experience. This chapter provides an overview of important rehabilitation principles and concepts that can assist clients and their families in making a successful transition from the acute care phase of the health care continuum to the rehabilitation phase.

Rehabilitation is an interdisciplinary specialty that supports a dynamic process of helping an individual to achieve a life that is as independent and self-fulfilling as desired in the physical, emotional, psychological, social, or vocational areas of functioning. *Rehabilitation nursing* is defined as "the diagnosis and treatment of human responses of individuals and groups to actual or potential health problems relative to altered functional ability and lifestyle."[1]

WORLD HEALTH ORGANIZATION FRAMEWORK

The World Health Organization's International Classification of Functioning, Disability, and Health (ICF)[11] provides a framework for the description of health and health-related states that benefit from rehabilitation services. The ICF framework describes the relationship between body functions and structures, activities and participation, environmental factors, and personal factors (Figure 12-1). A review of the definitions of each of these components is important because these terms may be used differently in other areas. The ICF defines *body functions* as the physiologic functions of body systems and includes psychological functions. *Body structures* are the anatomic parts of the body, such as organs and limbs and their components. *Impairments* are problems in body function or structure that deviate significantly from the expected norm. Impairments can have different characteristics and may be slight or severe; temporary or permanent; intermittent or continuous; and progressive, regressive, or static. *Activities* are the execution of a task or action by an individual, and *participation* is involvement in a life situation. In the ICF model environmental and personal components are contextual factors that can impact an individual's health status. *Environmental factors* are the external physical, social, and attitudinal factors that can positively or negatively influence an individual's capacity to perform functions. The impacted functions may be at the body function or structure level, the individual level, or a societal level. Personal factors are the non-health condition features of an individual's life, such as gender, race, age, lifestyle habits, education, behavior, and character style.

The ICF provides a framework that shows the importance of a comprehensive assessment to determine the impact that a health condition or disease may have on an individual. A wide variation in impairment may occur as a result of changes to body function or structure. The degree to which activities and participation are affected can be influenced significantly by contextual environmental and personal factors. When impairments lead to a decreased ability to engage in activities and participa-

tion, the individual may benefit from rehabilitation services. The results of a comprehensive assessment would assist in determining the level of rehabilitation services required and the setting in which the services would be best provided.

REHABILITATION SETTINGS

Rehabilitation services are provided in a variety of settings, depending on the array and intensity of services that are required. Individuals with an impairment that minimally impacts functional ability may be able to receive rehabilitation services in an outpatient setting. More complex impairments may require services that can be provided in the home setting or in a day treatment program. Individuals with impairments that affect multiple functional abilities may require a period of inpatient rehabilitation services in either a subacute or acute rehabilitation setting. Acute rehabilitation may be provided in free-standing rehabilitation hospitals or on dedicated units within hospitals. Subacute rehabilitation may be provided in long-term care facilities or on dedicated units within hospitals. Each type of setting has clear admission and discharge criteria to assist with determining the most appropriate placement for a client. As in other areas of health care, the trend has been toward shorter lengths of inpatient rehabilitation stays and the use of more community-based rehabilitation services.[2]

Current Medicare regulations require that at least 75% of clients on an acute Medicare-certified rehabilitation unit have a discharge diagnosis from the following:

- Stroke
- Spinal cord injury
- Congenital deformity
- Amputation
- Major multiple trauma
- Fracture of femur (hip fracture)
- Brain injury
- Polyarthritis, including rheumatoid arthritis
- Neurologic disorders, including multiple sclerosis, motor neuron disease, polyneuropathy, muscular dystrophy, and Parkinson's disease
- Burns

This list is currently being reconsidered and might change. In addition to the diagnosis requirement, Medicare requires that a client be able to participate actively in at least 3 hours of therapy a day and need at least two therapeutic modalities in addition to rehabilitation nursing and medicine.

REHABILITATION GOALS

The Association of Rehabilitation Nurses defines the goal of rehabilitation nursing as "to assist the individual who has a disability and/or chronic illness in restoring, maintaining, and promoting his or her maximal health."[1] Achievement of this goal requires nurses to practice with the following foci. Rehabilitation is a

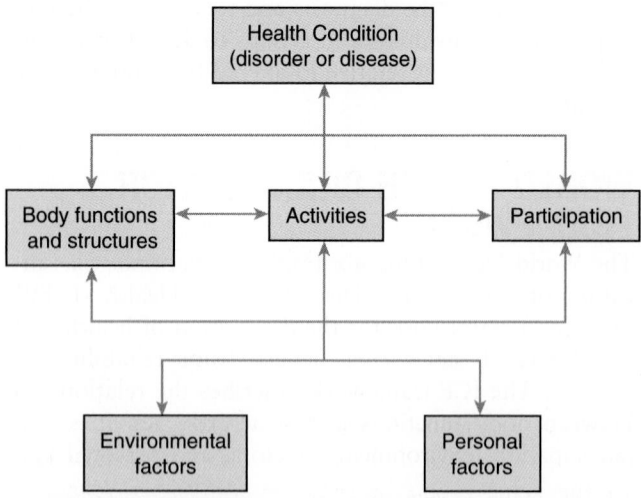

FIGURE 12-1 Interactions between the components of the International Classification of Functioning, Disability, and Health. (From World Health Organization [2001]. *International classification of functioning, disability, and health [ICF].* Geneva, Switzerland: Author.)

client-centered approach to achieving a maximum level of functioning and self-sufficiency in all spheres of life: physical, mental, social, emotional, educational, vocational, and economic. The emphasis is on abilities and developing methods for functional substitution where appropriate. Rehabilitation is not time specific but rather an ongoing process that may include periods of intense focus. Inherent within rehabilitation is a great deal of learning or relearning of a variety of life activities to support participation in life situations. Achieving the goal of rehabilitation requires nurses to focus on an optimal level of wellness and prevention of complications, which requires early intervention in the illness stage to limit disabling effects and conditions. In all phases of health care, it is crucial to assist the client and family in understanding the health condition that has led to functional impairments and the relationship of wellness-focused interventions (e.g., nutrition, exercise, physical activity) to learning how to manage the chronic illness or disability. An additional focus important to achieving the goal of rehabilitation is a return to and successful functioning within the community. This focus must include a realistic appraisal of the client's potential functional ability and interdependence with family, the environment, and social institutions. Identifying options and alternatives available for participation in activities that are important to the individual may play a large role in returning the client to the community. A final major focus to include in determining how to fulfill the goal of rehabilitation is the need to understand what an acceptable quality of life is for each client. Each individual brings a personal perspective to defining an acceptable quality of life, and the rehabilitation process is facilitated when nurses and the health care team understand the meaning and important aspects of quality of life for a specific client. Several key principles emerge from the goal and foci of rehabilitation.

KEY PRINCIPLES IN REHABILITATION

Rehabilitation is *client centered* and de-emphasizes the medical diagnosis and the disciplines that may be involved in the treatment of the client. The client and his or her unique needs are the focus; the rehabilitation plan is built on that focus. Health professionals provide expertise to the client and family and respect the client's ultimate right to make decisions regarding outcomes and the interventions to support his or her achievement. Families and significant others are an integral part of achieving client-centered care. Early assessment to identify the role family members will play in the post-acute and rehabilitation life of the client will allow the health care team to ensure that family members are prepared with the skills and knowledge that will be needed.

Rehabilitation is also a *goal-oriented approach* to care. Individual goals are determined in conjunction with the client and the rehabilitation teams professional

expertise. Pre-admission assessments are completed to ascertain the existence of reasonable goals that could be accomplished through participation in rehabilitation.

Goals are established to support the individual's improvement in *functional ability.* The rehabilitation process focuses on the functional presentation of the individual and on developing an individualized approach to maximize functional abilities by training, retraining, and the use of adaptive equipment. The focus on functional ability extends beyond physical functioning and also addresses functioning in areas such as social, emotional, and vocational issues. Assessment of functional ability and the potential for improvement are essential components in determining an individual's potential for rehabilitation.

A common assessment tool used in clinical practice to determine an individual's level of functional ability is the Functional Independence Measures (FIM).[4] The FIM includes an assessment of 18 areas of functioning related to self-care, sphincter management, transfers, locomotion, communication, and social cognition. Each area is assessed using a seven-point scale ranging from total dependence (1) to total independence (7). A maximum score of 126 would indicate total independence in all areas. The conceptual basis of the FIM has been incorporated into the Inpatient Rehabilitation Facility-Patient Assessment Instrument (IRF-PAI), which is the required uniform assessment tool completed for all Medicare clients admitted to acute rehabilitation settings.

Rehabilitation is provided using a *team approach.* The team comprises health care professionals who assist the client in developing and maintaining progress toward realistic goals. Box 12-1 identifies the members of the rehabilitation team. The only constant on any rehabilitation team is the client. All other members of the team vary depending on the needs of the client. The team approach to rehabilitation requires the coordination and cooperation of a variety of professionals with different areas of expertise. Teams can be described as having multidisciplinary, interdisciplinary, or transdisciplinary characteristics.[5] All three types of teams include members that are relevant to the care of the client. In a multidisciplinary team the members complete discipline specific evaluations of and goals for the client. There is little cross-disciplinary planning, and communication between team members focuses on sharing of information about the activities of each discipline. Interdisciplinary teams include collaboration among the members on the team. The entire team sets client goals, and then each discipline develops a plan for how each will contribute to the achievement of those goals. Transdisciplinary teams identify a primary therapist who is responsible for implementing the plan of care for a client. Transdisciplinary team members show evidence of several unique attributes, including role extension, role enrichment, role expansion, and role release.[7] Other team members provide information to the primary therapist, whose role it is to provide many of the therapies that the client requires. The boundaries of specific disciplines are blurred in a transdisciplinary team. Flexibility, cross-training, and good communication are essential to the effective use of a transdisciplinary team model. This model of care can be very effective for clients who require longer-term rehabilitation and a smaller number of health care providers with whom to interact, for example, clients with significant cognitive sequelae following a traumatic brain injury.

A successful rehabilitation experience requires attention to how the client and his or her family define an acceptable *quality of life.* Quality of life is influenced by numerous personal factors that must be identified and discussed to establish a rehabilitation plan of care. This plan should facilitate the maintenance or restoration of an acceptable quality of life that recognizes the uniqueness and wholeness of each individual. Research in quality of life for individuals with chronic illness has identified numerous factors that must be taken into consideration.[8] Health and functional issues include perception of the intrusive nature of manifestations, psychological and spiritual issues, social and economic issues (e.g., emotional support, cultural life, employment, and financial factors), and family issues. These aspects of living with a chronic illness or disability must be considered when discussing quality of life with clients and families.

Rehabilitation also includes a *wellness* focus. For many clients engaged in rehabilitation, it is not realistic to plan for a return to perfect health and an absence of illness. The focus becomes one of achieving the highest level of wellness possible. This is accomplished through

maintaining, restoring, and promoting healthy lifestyles in a manner that recognizes all aspects of the client's health: physical, emotional, psychological, and spiritual. Wellness is facilitated when interventions are included in the acute care setting to prevent and minimize complications such as pressure sores, decreased range of motion, and deconditioning.

The trajectory of many chronic illnesses and disabilities is one of continuous *change.* Coping with change is an innate characteristic of living with a chronic illness or disability. Acknowledgment of this phenomenon can be helpful to clients and families when coupled with assurance that one benefit of rehabilitation is the development of skills and knowledge that will assist with managing the many changes experienced over the trajectory of most chronic illnesses and disabilities. Most nurses and health care providers interact with clients and families at only one point of the health care delivery system. Providing care at each point in the system that acknowledges an awareness of the total trajectory and includes interventions to assist clients and their families in developing the skills needed to manage changes in their health conditions will enhance a client's and his or her family's ability to cope with changes successfully.

All persons diagnosed with a chronic illness or disability will experience a psychological reaction to this change in their lives. Nurses play an important role in supporting clients and families through the *coping and adjustment* process. Each client will have a unique response that will be influenced by many personal and contextual factors. Winterhalter[10] describes the advantages of using a stage model as a theoretical base for understanding the reactions that may be observed and the interventions that are most appropriate for each stage. Each client and family member will travel through this experience differently. The various responses and stages that are commonly described may or may not be present for each individual, and the intensity or length of each response can vary widely from one client to another. An individual's response may be influenced by the meaning of the event to him or her, past coping experiences, and others' reactions to the event. Common responses include denial, grieving, uncertainty, hopelessness, hopefulness, and eventual adaptation to the condition.

An understanding of the role that *culture* plays in the rehabilitation experience for clients is also needed. Cultural competence in rehabilitation nursing includes cultural awareness, cultural knowledge, cultural encounters, cultural skills, and cultural desire.[3] The provision of culturally sensitive care will enhance the ability of the rehabilitation process to achieve the predetermined rehabilitation goals.

A pivotal concept in rehabilitation is *client and family education.* In rehabilitation, this is a collaborative process among all members of the team that must be accomplished in partnership with the client and family.

BOX 12-1 *Rehabilitation Team Members*

- Client
- Family
- Registered nurse
- Physicians (physiatrists and others)
- Physical therapist
- Occupational therapist
- Speech/language pathologist
- Audiologist
- Psychologist
- Social worker
- Recreational therapist
- Vocational rehabilitation counselor
- Respiratory therapist
- Dietitian
- Chaplain
- Orthotist/prosthetist
- Insurance case manager

Several recent studies found a discrepancy in the perception of health care providers and clients and families in the effectiveness of current efforts in client education. Smith and Testani-Dufour[9] identified the need to individualize the teaching methods used to accommodate personal factors of the learner even when standardized materials have been developed. Paterson, Kieloch, and Gmiterek[6] report that families have limited recollection of teaching that has occurred by members of the rehabilitation team. They suggest that there are many reasons that such a discrepancy exists between what providers have documented has been taught and what family members recall being taught. These reasons include the manner in which the content was taught, the relevance of the content to the learner, and the family's emotional state at the time the teaching occurred. These are very real constraints that providers face in today's health care systems.

To optimize the effectiveness of client and family teaching, education must be designed, delivered, and reinforced in ways that are accessible and meaningful. Education needs to be present in appropriate levels and formats at all levels of the health care system so that it is available whenever the learner is ready to learn.

REHABILITATION PROCESS

The rehabilitation process can be affected by many factors, including the attitudes of the client, his or her family, and members of the rehabilitation team; financial resources; environmental barriers; the availability of community resources; and educational and occupational barriers. The rehabilitation process involves the creative talents of various disciplines to develop a planned sequence of services designed to meet the unique needs of each client in a manner that maximizes the contributions of each member of the team.

The assessment phase of the rehabilitation process requires an initial focused assessment to determine whether a client would benefit from rehabilitation services and, if so, what would be the most appropriate setting for provision of those services. The decision about the most appropriate setting to provide rehabilitation will be determined by analyzing the client's needs and medical stability, the client's therapy needs, the services offered in that setting, the intensity and skill level of the needed nursing services, the gap between the client's current functional level and the level realistically thought to be achievable as a result of rehabilitation, and the location of the setting. Once a determination has been made

that rehabilitation services are appropriate, an in-depth assessment is completed by each member of the rehabilitation team who will be involved in the provision of services to that client. The areas commonly included in this assessment are physical, functional ability, psychological, emotional, cognitive, mental status, social support, behavioral, communication, financial, previous patterns of coping, and family. Factors that may influence discharge and transition planning are identified early in the rehabilitation process.

On completion of the assessment, a set of goals and anticipated outcomes are established for the client and family and a plan is established for the achievement of those goals. Within the plan will be interventions directed at restoring lost functional abilities, promoting client and family adjustment and adaptation to the new health status and level of functioning, preventing secondary complications, and adapting the discharge environment to support the client's level of functional ability. Throughout implementation of the rehabilitation plan of care, ongoing evaluation of progress toward goals will occur. Team conferences are a standard part of comprehensive rehabilitation programs. The frequency at which team conferences occur is dictated by the setting where the client is receiving care and the requirements of the insurance or payer.

Transitions from one level of care to another can be stressful for clients and families. Without anticipatory guidance before the transfer to a rehabilitation setting, a client making the transition from an acute care setting to a rehabilitation setting might view the differences in routine in the rehabilitation setting as disturbing. The client or family might perceive encouragement from a nurse or a therapist in the rehabilitation setting to be independent with some aspect of daily care as poor quality of care if adequate orientation has not occurred to explain the differences in philosophy between the acute care and the rehabilitation setting. Another stressful transition can be the discharge from the rehabilitation setting to home or other community setting. Clients and families are often not secure in their ability to use the new skills and knowledge that they have gained as a result of rehabilitation. Clients and caregivers may feel overwhelmed by the amount of information they have been given and fearful of their ability to manage all the aspects of care still needed after discharge. It is critical for clients and families to have appropriate resources and referrals in place to ensure the most successful possible transition to the community.

CONCLUSIONS

Rehabilitation is needed by an increasing number of individuals because the ability to live a longer, productive life with multiple chronic conditions. Nurses in acute care settings have an important role in identifying clients who will benefit from rehabilitation services. Nurses and other health care providers who understanding the rehabilitation process can help to minimize the fragmentation in care that clients sometimes feel in today's health care delivery system. Preparation for and discussion about rehabilitation and incorporation of basic rehabilitation principles in acute care will assist with a smooth transition for clients and families.

BIBLIOGRAPHY

1. Association of Rehabilitation Nurses. (2000). *Standards and scope of rehabilitation nursing practice.* Glenview, IL: Author.
2. Buchanan, L.C., & Neal, L.J. (2002). Community-based rehabilitation. In S. Hoeman (Ed.), *Rehabilitation nursing: process, application, & outcomes* (3rd ed.). St. Louis: Mosby.
3. Campinha-Bacote, J. (2001). A model of practice to address cultural competence in rehabilitation nursing. *Rehabilitation Nursing, 26,* 8-11.
4. Deutsch, A., Braun, S., & Granger, C. (1997). The functional independence measure (FIM instrument). *Journal of Rehabilitation Outcomes Measurement, 1,* 67-71.
5. Mumma, C.M., & Nelson, A. (2002). Theory and practice models for rehabilitation nursing. In S. Hoeman (Ed.), *Rehabilitation nursing: Process, application, & outcomes* (3rd ed.). St. Louis: Mosby.
6. Paterson, B., Kieloch, B., & Gmiterek, J. (2001). 'They never told us anything': Postdischarge instruction for families of persons with brain injuries. *Rehabilitation Nursing, 26,* 48-53.
7. Reilly, C. (2001). Transdisciplinary approach: An atypical strategy for improving outcomes in rehabilitative and long-term acute care settings. *Rehabilitation Nursing, 26,* 216-220, 244.
8. Schirm, V. (2002). Quality of life. In I.M. Lubkin & P.D. Larsen (Eds.), *Chronic illness: Impact and interventions* (5th ed.). Boston: Jones & Bartlett.
9. Smith, M.S., & Testani-Dufour, L. (2002). Who's teaching whom? A study of family education in brain injury. *Rehabilitation Nursing, 27,* 209-214.
10. Winterhalter, J. (2001). Psychosocial issues for the person with chronic illness or disability. In J. Derstine & S.D. Hargrove (Eds.), *Comprehensive rehabilitation nursing.* Philadelphia: W.B. Saunders.
11. World Health Organization (2001*). International classification of functioning, disability, and health (ICF).* Geneva, Switzerland: Author.

Unit 3

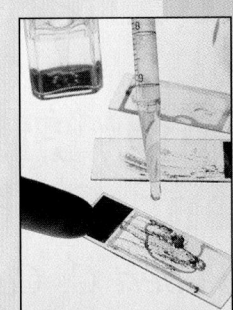

Foundations of Medical-Surgical Nursing

Anatomy and Physiology Review

Body Fluid Compartments and Cellular Function

Robert G. Carroll

Life requires a barrier between the organism and the environment. For animals, this barrier is the epithelium of the skin. At the microscopic level, this barrier is the cell membrane. Consequently, the anatomy and physiology review chapters focus both on (1) the external environment and the internal environment, and (2) the extracellular composition and the intracellular composition. *Anatomy* is the study of structure, including those barriers. *Physiology* is the study of movement across those barriers.

BODY FLUID COMPARTMENTS AND EXCHANGE

Water is the major body component, accounting for approximately 60% of adult body weight. The body gains water primarily from eating and drinking, and a small amount is generated from metabolism. Water is lost from the body as urine, feces, sweat, and insensibly from respiration and the skin surface. Sweat and saliva are dilute, hypotonic fluids. Most other fluids lost from the body are isotonic and have an osmolarity close to that of plasma. In all cases, water must cross an epithelial cell barrier (skin or gastrointestinal tract) to enter or exit the body.

Within the body, water is in one of two compartments. Two thirds of the body water is within the cells (intracellular fluid), and one third of body water is outside of the cells (extracellular fluid). Water can freely cross the cell membrane and move from one compartment to the other. In contrast, ions cannot easily cross the cell membrane, and intracellular ion composition is dramatically different from extracellular fluid ion composition (Table U3-1). Because ions cannot cross the cell membrane, they exert an ionic pressure that determines water movement into and out of the cell. For example, if extracellular fluid osmolarity increases, water exits the cell and moves into the extracellular space.

The extracellular fluid compartment is more complex. Most of the extracellular fluid is in the space between the cells, the interstitial fluid. Some of the fluid is the plasma of the vascular space. Exchange between the interstitial and plasma spaces is determined by the balance of the hydrostatic pressure and the osmotic pressure generated by the plasma proteins (see the Unit 12 Anatomy and Physiology Review for more details). The plasma is a key extracellular space, because compounds and fluid entering and exiting the body must first pass through the plasma before entering the cells. The most common extracellular ions are sodium, chloride, and bicarbonate.

TABLE U3-1	Chemical Compositions of Extracellular and Intracellular Fluids	
	Extracellular Fluid	**Intracellular Fluid**
Na^+	142 mEq/L	10 mEq/L
K^+	4 mEq/L	140 mEq/L
Ca^{2+}	2.4 mEq/L	0.0001 mEq/L
Mg^{2+}	1.2 mEq/L	58 mEq/L
Cl^-	103 mEq/L	4 mEq/L
HCO_3^-	28 mEq/L	10 mEq/L
Phosphates	4 mEq/L	75 mEq/L
SO_4^{2-}	1 mEq/L	2 mEq/L
Glucose	90 mg/dl	0 to 20 mg/dl
Amino acids	30 mg/dl	200 mg/dl ?
Cholesterol Phospholipids Neutral fat	0.5 g/dl	2 to 95 g/dl
Po_2	35 mm Hg	20 mm Hg ?
Pco_2	46 mm Hg	50 mm Hg ?
pH	7.4	7.0
Proteins	2 g/dl (5 mEq/L)	16 g/dl (40 mEq/L)

From Guyton, A.C., & Hall, J.E. (2000). *Textbook of medical physiology* (10th ed.). Philadelphia: W.B. Saunders.

CELL STRUCTURE AND FUNCTION

The cell is the basic unit of structure and function in biologic systems. Two fundamental types of cells are recognized on the basis of composition and organization: *prokaryotic* and *eukaryotic*. Cells found in the human body and in higher plants and animals are eukaryotic, having a defined nucleus containing deoxyribonucleic acid (DNA). A less complex bacterial cell is prokaryotic, because it has DNA but lacks a nucleus. The differences between these two cell types allow clinicians to attack a prokaryotic pathogen selectively *in vivo* and to use drugs that do not damage eukaryotic cells. Viruses are not true cells because they cannot replicate independently. Antiviral medications are directed against the unique aspects of the viral replication process. In this chapter, the term *cell* is synonymous with eukaryotic cell.

All cells, regardless of type, have the same basic structural pattern: a cytoplasmic matrix surrounded by a plasma membrane (Figure U3-1). Numerous *organelles* (membrane-limited structures with a complex infrastructure and unique functions) are scattered within the cytoplasm. Their compartmentalization allows multistage metabolic and physiologic events to occur simultaneously while keeping one function separate from another.

Cells perform the basic functions of life. Cells transfer energy, take up and assimilate materials from outside the cell, synthesize macromolecules, maintain a homeostatic environment, and reproduce (Table U3-2).

Most of the mass of a cell is water (70% to 85%), which aids in thermal regulation and serves as a solvent for (1) electrolytes, (2) organic molecules, and (3) chemical reactions. *Electrolytes* in the cytoplasm help maintain stable electrical and pH environments and assist with various metabolic and physiologic activities. The most common intracellular electrolytes are potassium, phosphate, and magnesium. *Molecules* within the cell consist mostly of sugars, fatty acids, amino acids, and nucleotides. These are metabolized for energy or used to synthesize macromolecules (lipids, proteins, nucleic acids, and their conjugates).

Cell Membrane Regulates Transport

The cell membrane is an organized layer of phospholipids and proteins (Figure U3-2). This dynamic structure serves a number of functions: (1) to separate the intracellular fluid from the extracellular fluid, (2) to regulate exchange and communication across the cell membrane, and (3) to provide structural support for the cell. Membranes also surround intracellular organelles,

FIGURE U3-1 A "typical" cell showing the internal organelles in the cytoplasm and the nucleus.

TABLE U3-2	*Cell Structures and Their Functions*	
Structure	**Description**	**Function**
Cell Nucleus		
Nucleus	Large structure surrounded by double membrane; contains nucleolus and chromosomes	DNA is transcribed using RNA to make proteins
Nucleolus	Granular body; consists of RNA and protein	Ribosomal RNA synthesis; ribosome subunit assembly
Chromosomes	Complexes of DNA and protein known as chromatin become visible as rod-like structures when cell divides	Contain genes that transmit hereditary information and govern cell structure and activity
Cytoplasmic Organelles		
Cell membrane	Boundary of cell	Encloses cell contents; regulates movement of materials into and out of the cell; maintains cell structure; communicates with other cells
Endoplasmic reticulum (ER)	Network of internal membranes extending throughout the cytoplasm; two types: smooth and rough; smooth lacks ribosomes on the outer surface; rough has ribosomes on the outer surface	Site of membrane lipids and proteins; origin of intracellular transport vesicles carrying proteins to be secreted; smooth ER is used for lipid biosynthesis and drug detoxification; rough ER is site of protein manufacturing
Ribosomes	Granules composed of RNA and protein, some attached to ER, some free in cytoplasm	Synthesize polypeptides
Golgi complex	Stacks of flattened membrane sacs	Modifies proteins; packages secreted proteins; sorts other proteins to vacuoles and other organelles
Lysosomes	Membranous sacs	Contain enzymes to break down ingested materials, secretions, and waste
Vacuoles	Membranous sacs	Transport and store materials, waste, and water
Mitochondria	Sacs consisting of two membranes; inner membrane is folded to form cristae and encloses matrix	Site of most reactions of cellular respiration; transformation of energy originating from glucose or lipids into ATP
Microbodies (e.g., peroxisomes)	Membranous sacs containing a variety of enzymes	Sites of many diverse metabolic reactions
Cytoskeleton		
Microtubules	Hollow tubes made of tubulin protein	Provide structural support; provide for cell movement and cell division
Microfilaments	Solid, rodlike structures consisting of actin protein	Provide structural support; provide for cell movement and cell division
Centrioles	Pairs of hollow cylinders located near the center of the cell	Spindles form between centrioles during mitosis; may anchor or organize microtubule formation
Cilia	Short projections extending from the surface of the cell, covered by plasma membrane	Regulate movement of material on surface of cell and some tissues
Flagella	Long projections made of microtubules; extend from surface of the cell; covered with plasma membrane	Provide for cellular locomotion by sperm cells

ATP, Adenosine triphosphate; *DNA,* deoxyribonucleic acid; *RNA,* ribonucleic acid.

EXTERIOR OF CELL

INTERIOR OF CELL

FIGURE U3-2 The cell membrane is composed of a bimolecular layer of lipids, primarily phospholipid and cholesterol. Proteins can be attached or embedded in the membrane. Peripheral proteins are attached to the surface; integral proteins are embedded in the cell membrane.

TABLE U3-3	*Mechanisms of Membrane Transport*
Mechanism	**Common Examples**
Passive (High to Low, No ATP)	
Osmosis	Movement of water through a lipid portion of the membrane
Diffusion	Movement of gasses and small hydrophilic molecules (oxygen, carbon dioxide, nitrogen, glycerol, urea) through the lipid portion of a membrane
Facilitated diffusion	Movement of glucose, some ions, and amino acids via specific carrier proteins
Active (Low to High, Uses ATP)	
Pumps	Hydrogen, sodium, and potassium ions moved by protein pumps
Endocytosis	Intake of substance by creating a vesicle
Pinocytosis	Random uptake of small amounts of extracellular fluid and solutes
Phagocytosis	Large-scale uptake of particles and cells; especially important in defense
Receptor-mediated	Specific uptake of molecules after binding to a ligand
Exocytosis	Secretion of products and wastes via secretory vesicles

ATP, Adenosine triphosphate.

such as vacuoles, mitochondria, Golgi apparatus, and the nucleus, where they perform an equivalent role.

Proteins in the cell membrane selectively regulate the cellular entry and exit of water soluble materials. Movement across the membrane can be passive down a concentration gradient (from high to low concentration) or active against gradient (from low to high). Active transport processes require energy. The basic transport mechanisms are summarized in Table U3-3 and illustrated in Figure U3-3.

Cell membrane channels regulate ion movement and consequently membrane electrical charge. Some of the channels leak continuously, and some are gated (opened by stimuli). A *ligand-gated* channel changes shape when a signaling molecule (e.g., protein, hormones, nitric oxide) binds to it, then opens and closes. These channels are seen in cells that respond to hormones, drugs, or neurotransmitters. A *voltage-gated* channel opens or closes when there are changes in the electrical voltage across the membrane. A *mechanically gated* channel opens in response to deforming forces, such as pressure or friction.

Some cell surface glycoproteins serve as mammalian blood group antigens (e.g., ABO, Rh). Others act as histocompatibility antigens, which detect self and non-self in immune function, important in tissue matching for tissue and organ transplants.

Nucleus Contains the Genetic Material

The nucleus is the most prominent organelle in the eukaryotic cell. It is surrounded by a porous double membrane (the *nuclear envelope*). Within the nucleus are one or more nucleoli, visible among a mass of chromosomes. The nucleus contains the genetic material of the cell in the form of chromatin threads composed of DNA. Each cell, except the reproductive cells, contains a person's full genetic complement of DNA (46 chromosomes).

The DNA contains the blueprint for all the proteins in the body. The DNA in the nucleus is unable to pass through the nuclear envelope into the cytoplasm; yet it is in the cytoplasm that polypeptides and proteins are synthesized. These proteins are used for structure or control of all metabolic and physiologic activities of the cell. Therefore DNA must transfer its instructions for synthesizing proteins to ribonucleic acid (RNA) molecules that can carry the information from the nucleus to the cytoplasm. It does this through a two-step process: transcription and translation.

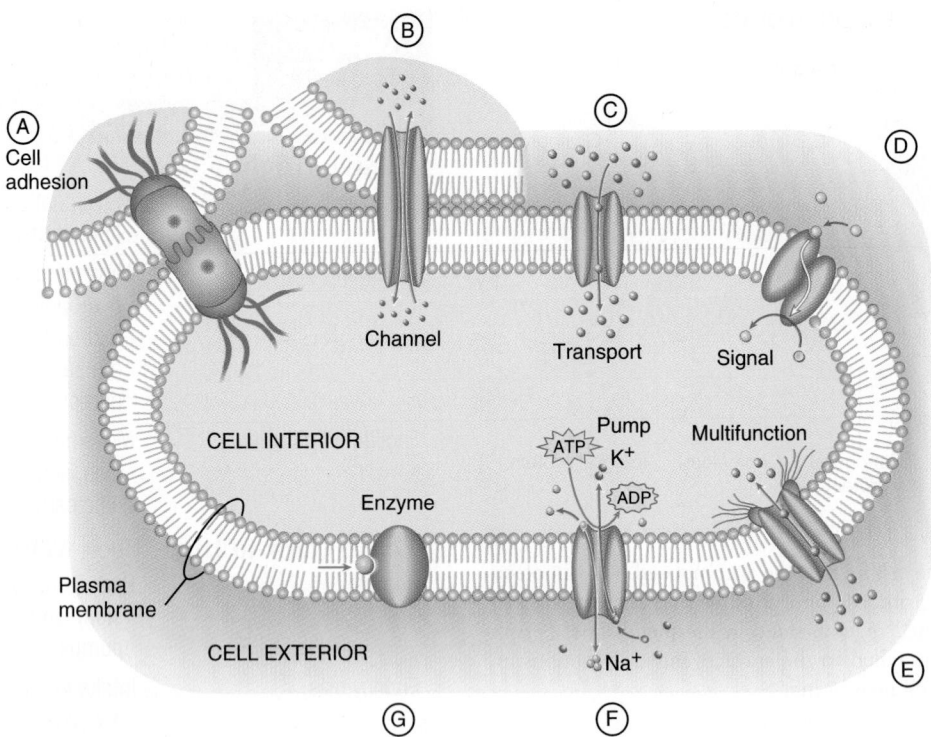

FIGURE U3-3 The cell membrane is responsible for adhesion to adjacent cells (**A**) and movement of substances in and out of the cell. Several mechanisms are required: gap junctions allow communication between neighboring cells by transfer of small molecules (**B**); passive transport of molecules (**C**); signal receptor proteins that bind to surface signal molecules and transfer a message to the cell interior (**D**); use of integral proteins to transport specific molecules (**E**); ATP-driven pumps to actively transport ions from one compartment to another (**F**); and use of membrane-bound enzymes, which have active sites on either side of the cell membrane (**G**). *ADP,* Adenosine diphosphate; *ATP,* adenosine triphosphate.

Transcription

DNA serves as a template for the assembly of molecules of RNA. The two linked chains of DNA separate from one another, exposing part of the base sequence. RNA links to the DNA template and then serves as the messenger (mRNA) and moves from the nucleus to the cytoplasm for protein synthesis.

Translation

At the ribosome, mRNA is used to assemble proteins in specific order. This step (translation) requires that the mRNA bind to the ribosome and that the ribosome "read" the RNA. Transfer RNA (tRNA) transports the amino acids in the cytoplasm to the ribosome, and the protein is assembled. In a human body, roughly 100,000 genes produce about 60,000 essential proteins. A single cell can synthesize about 20,000 different proteins. Because the entire genetic code is contained in each cell, abnormal genetic control, such as cancer, often results in cells producing proteins that they normally do not produce.

CELL REPLICATION

Besides producing proteins, most body cells also must reproduce themselves. In the healthy adult body, somatic cells replicate at varying rates. The cells of the skin and mucous membranes, the blood-forming cells in the bone marrow, and some cells in the reproductive system are replaced at a high constant rate. A second group of cells, such as hepatocytes and differentiated lymphocytes, undergoes replication only in response to a stimulus. A third group of cells has limited or no replicative capabilities. Individual smooth muscle cells may reproduce only once or twice in a lifetime; striated muscle cells (heart and skeleton) and neurons (except for olfactory cells) do not normally replicate, and therefore any loss is permanent. Research efforts seek to restore replicative function to neurons, providing a mechanism to treat the irreversible paralysis of clients with spinal cord injury.

Stages of Replication

The process of cell replication begins with replication of the genetic information. The DNA divides and serves as a template for its own replication. Once the DNA has

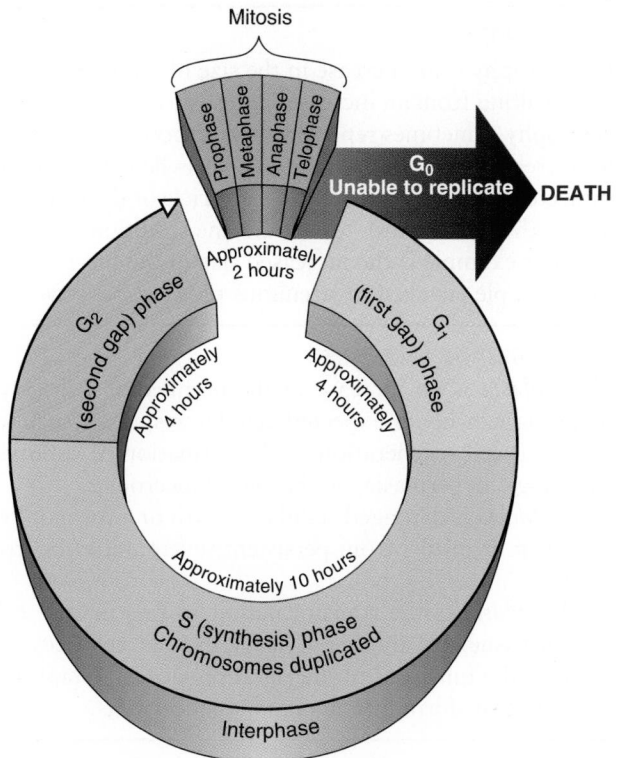

FIGURE U3-4 Phases in the life cycle of a cell. Actual times vary, depending on the type of cell.

duplicated, eukaryotic cells may divide by *mitosis* or *meiosis.* Somatic cells divide exclusively by mitosis, which produces two daughter cells with genetic content identical to that of the parent cell (unless altered by mutation). A cell undergoing mitosis follows a cyclic sequence that is driven by a combination of signals from inside and outside the cell (Figure U3-4).

Mitosis involves several steps:

1. In *prophase,* two centrioles move toward opposite poles of the cell, fibers become visible, and the nucleolus disappears. The chromatin threads of DNA become visible as structures called *chromosomes.*
2. During *metaphase,* the nuclear envelope has completely disappeared and the chromosomes are attached to their centromeres. At the end of this stage, the chromatin divides into separate strands of chromosomes.
3. *Anaphase* further divides the cell with evidence of pinching of the cell membrane.
4. In the last phase *(telophase),* the cell divides into two identical daughter cells having the same genetic content as the parent cell.

Replicating reproductive eukaryotic cells divide by *mitosis* and *meiosis.* Gametogenesis produces four progeny cells, each having one half of the genetic content of the starting cell (23 rather than 46 chromosomes).

Replication Errors (Mutations)

A major genetic problem is maintaining the integrity of the message contained in the nuclear DNA. Errors that occur in the replication process are called *mutations.* Mutation in a somatic cell may be beneficial or inconsequential at one extreme; at the other, it may result in cell death or malignancy. Mutation occurring during gametogenesis is passed on to the offspring. Thousands of abnormal changes are likely to occur on a daily basis during replication of human DNA because of thermal effects and inappropriate metabolic events. In nearly all cases, however, the DNA is restored to normal configurations by a variety of repair mechanisms. Abnormal genes that escape repair may result in diseases such as phenylketonuria or sickle cell disease.

Biotechnologists are applying recent advances in genetic engineering to the prevention and therapy of diseases. Using restriction *endonuclease* (which hydrolyzes or cuts DNA at specific sequences) and *DNA ligase* (which recombines the cut ends of DNA fragments), biotechnologists can cut selected genes out of sections of human DNA molecules, insert them into bacterial *plasmids* (extrachromosomal genetic elements in bacteria that can incorporate segments of human DNA), and produce large quantities of the gene product. Many benefits are being realized and anticipated from the use of this technology:

- Increased yields and improved antimicrobial action of antibiotics
- More effective and safer virus vaccines (prepared from gene components)
- Ability to produce mammalian proteins, including clotting factors, insulin, human growth hormone, and interferons
- Development of "magic bullets" for treating many conditions, including tumors, through precise modification of reactive sites in antibodies
- Development of transgenic plants and animals for increasing and improving nutritional sources for humans

CELL DEVELOPMENT

Human life begins as an undifferentiated single cell, derived from the fusion of a male gamete (sperm) with a female gamete (ovum). By about the seventh day after fertilization, the original cell (or zygote) has already undergone several cycles of replication. The progeny cells begin to develop into distinctive tissues. In the embryo and fetus, these fully differentiated cells can be distinguished on the basis of both form and function.

When tissues in the developing organism reach genetically programmed size limits, the rate of cell reproduction begins to slow and finally stops or attains a steady-state replacement level. This form of growth regulation (called *contact* or *density-dependent inhibition*) is initiated by physical (contact) and chemical (nutrient and cytokine) levels. Cell replication is described later in this review.

CELLS IN TISSUES AND ORGANS

Cells working together as a unit are called *tissues*. Tissues unite to form individual *organs*. The four major specialized types of cells that unite into larger tissue units are the following:

1. *Epithelial cells* are arranged in sheets. They cover the outside of the body (epidermis) and form the absorptive linings of the body's cavities and tubular structures (such as mucosa and glands).
2. *Nerve cells* form the highly specialized, irritable, and conductive nerve tissue.
3. *Muscle cells* allow mobility of body parts as well as mobility of substances (such as air, blood, and waste) within the body by contracting and relaxing.
4. *Connective tissue cells* support other cells and tissues. They include blood cells and structural cells found in bones, tendons, and ligaments. Blood cells carry oxygen to the tissues and carbon dioxide and wastes from the tissues. They also defend the body against foreign substances. Structural cells build the bony scaffolding and form the critical intercellular proteins that bind together the cells of the body. Collagen is an important extracellular connective tissue protein.

ALTERATIONS IN CELL STRUCTURE AND FUNCTION

The major causes of cellular alterations include changes in gene structure and function (either newly acquired or hereditary) and degeneration of normal tissue due to aging, excessive use, or infiltration by foreign substances (including fat, water, glycogen, and proteins).

Atrophy

Atrophy is the wasting or decrease in size of a normally developed organ. This condition results from a decrease either in the number of cells or in the size of the cells composing it. Atrophy may follow disuse of an organ. For example, muscle atrophy may develop following denervation or prolonged immobilization. Muscular atrophy caused by aging can be greatly minimized by physical activity. Because the adrenal glands normally secrete corticosteroids, atrophy of these glands can occur when large doses of corticosteroids are administered over a prolonged period. Atrophy also accompanies the normal physiologic aging process. The thymus gland increases in size during childhood and gradually atrophies during adolescence. The ovaries atrophy after menopause.

Hypertrophy

Hypertrophy is an increase in the size of an organ or tissue resulting from an increase in the size of the cells. Hypertrophy sometimes represents the response of an organ to a greater workload. For example, when the heart is subjected to great strain, the left ventricle of the heart enlarges (hypertrophies) to handle the additional stress. Another example is the increased size of the biceps muscle in people engaged in strenuous physical activity.

Precancerous Changes

Hyperplasia is an increase in the number of cells. Hyperplasia can be an expected cellular response, such as increased cell regeneration in the formation of calluses. Pathologic hyperplasia can become cancerous.

Dysplasia is deranged cellular growth or a form of hyperplasia. It results from persistent severe injury or irritation.

Metaplasia is the transformation of one mature cell type or tissue into another. Usually, the new cell does not perform the functions of the cell it replaced. Metaplastic cells can transform into malignant cancer cells.

Neoplastic (Cancerous) Changes

Neoplastic change is characterized by disturbances in cell differentiation and growth. When normal cells undergo transformation into cancerous cells, they fail to respond to normal regulatory forces and instead show unrestrained growth. These unregulated replicating cells *(neoplasms)* may then invade contiguous healthy tissues or become detached from the primary tumor and spread *(metastasize)* to other parts of the body where they continue to divide. This alteration in normal cell reproduction is discussed in greater detail in Chapter 18.

Aging

In a young healthy person, cells are biochemically active, have a high turnover rate (in some tissues), and have a high rate of metabolic and physiologic efficiency. In older adults, cells are less active, have a slower turnover rate, and begin to decline in efficiency. Aging cells shrink in size, protein synthesis slows, the Golgi apparatus shows signs of disintegration, and the mitochondria may undergo fragmentation. Aging affects every system of the body (Table U3-4).

Numerous theories exist regarding the aging process, but little is certain about how age-related changes occur. The age range of a cell is great. In the mature adult, an epithelial cell lining the intestinal tract lives only about 1½ days; a red blood cell can survive for 120 days. At the other extreme, nerve cells have a potential life expectancy of 100 years or more. In the immune system, immunocompetent cells appear to remain constant in numbers as people age but lose some of their interactive and regulatory properties. The resulting alteration in immune func-

TABLE U3-4	*Physiologic Changes of Aging: An Overview*
System	**Physiologic Changes**
Cardiovascular	Decreased vessel elasticity due to calcification and connective tissue (increased pulmonary vascular resistance) Decreased number of heart muscle fibers, with increased size of individual fibers (hypertrophy) Decreased filling capacity Decreased stroke volume Decreased sensitivity of baroreceptors Degeneration of vein valves
Respiratory	Decreased chest wall compliance due to calcification of the costal cartilage Decreased alveolar ventilation Decreased respiratory muscle strength Air trapping and decreased ventilation due to degeneration of lung tissue (decreased elasticity)
Renal and urinary	Decreased glomerular filtration rate due to nephron degeneration (decreased 33% to 50% by age 70) Decreased ability to concentrate urine Decreased ability to regulate hydrogen (H^+)

Gastrointestinal	Decreased muscular contractions
	    Decreased esophageal emptying
	    Decreased bowel motility
	Decreased production of hydrochloric acid (HCl), enzymes, and intrinsic factor
	Decreased hepatic enzyme production and metabolic capacity
	Thinning of stomach mucosa

Neurologic and sensory	Degeneration and atrophy of nerve cells
	    Decrease of 25% to 45% in neurons
	    Decrease in neurotransmitters
	    Decreased rate of conduction of nerve impulses
	    Loss of taste buds
	Loss of auditory hair cells and sclerosis of the eardrum

Musculoskeletal	Decreased muscle mass Bone demineralization Joint degeneration, erosion, and calcification
Immune	Decreased inflammatory response Decrease in T-cell function due to involution of the thymus gland
Integumentary	Decreased subcutaneous fat Decreased elastin Atrophy of the sweat glands Atrophy of the epidermal arterioles, causing altered temperature regulation

From Copstead, L.C., & Banasik, J. (2000). *Pathophysiology.* Philadelphia: W.B. Saunders.

tion is responsible for the increased incidence of autoimmune disease, the appearance of tumors, and the greater susceptibility to infection seen in the older population.

One theory of aging is that unrepaired mutations accumulate on DNA, causing changes that lead to aging. For example, highly specialized cells (such as nerve cells) do not reproduce. When these cells die from injury or disease and are not replaced, the remaining cells must assume their functions. The greater workload may stress these cells, cause them to age faster, and hasten their dying.

Another hypothesis is that all people are born with a genetic clock that governs their life span. This theory is based on the observation that each cell type has a finite number of divisions. This concept is supported in part by similarities in life spans seen in various family groups.

Mechanisms of Cell Damage

When cells are injured, the injured organelles no longer carry out their specific functions (e.g., mitochondria stop producing ATP). The extent of the damage depends on (1) the nature, intensity, and duration of the stressor; (2) whether the blood supply to the cells is affected; and (3) the state of differentiation or metabolic activity of the cells. Indeed, two clients exposed to the same injurious substance may not sustain the same degree of injury because of the influence of modifying factors. For example, a person's nutritional and emotional state can have a profound impact on the extent and consequences of a slight to moderate level of injury. However, there is a point after which cell death inevitably occurs. The mechanisms responsible for the transition from reversible to irreversible cellular damage are not completely understood.

Hypoxia

Hypoxia (inadequate tissue oxygenation) is a leading cause of cell injury and death. Hypoxia can occur as a result of the following:

- Vascular disease or injury, which impedes blood flow to tissues
- Insufficient oxygenation of blood caused by conditions such as carbon monoxide poisoning

Depending on the severity of the hypoxic state, cells compensate and recover or are killed. (For example, if the femoral artery becomes stenotic, the skeletal muscles of the legs eventually atrophy as a result of the inadequate blood flow and the consequent reduced oxygen supply. Severe or chronic hypoxia results in cell injury or death.)

The most common cause of hypoxia is *ischemia,* or reduced blood supply. Progressive hypoxia caused by gradual narrowing of arteries *(atherosclerosis)* is better tolerated than sudden anoxia caused by an obstruction in the blood supply.

Viral Injury

Viruses have been described as mobile genetic elements protected by outer layers of protein and lipoprotein. Viruses attach to specific receptors on host cell surfaces and are taken up by endocytosis. The nucleic acid core of the virus passes through the vesicular membrane into the interior of the host cell. The viral genome then subverts the metabolic machinery of the host cell and begins to make viral components. While inside the host cell, the virus is protected from the host's reactive cells and solutes. The assembled *virions* may then exit the cell either by lysing the cell remnant or by permitting the host cell to remain viable while continuously secreting virions across the cell membrane. Viruses damage host cells by killing them, depriving them of nutrients, or causing cells to transform into a tumor state.

Nutritional Imbalance

Inadequate protein intake decreases the function of the intestinal mucosa and pancreas, which in turn reduces nutrient absorption. Plasma proteins, especially albumin, help retain fluid in blood vessels. When levels of plasma proteins decline, fluid tends to move into interstitial spaces, causing edema. Antibodies or immunoglobulins are protein; therefore the lack of proteins adversely affects immune system function and increases the risk of infection.

Inadequate carbohydrate intake forces the body to use fats for energy. The liver becomes overwhelmed and ketone bodies are formed that accumulate in the blood, a condition known as *ketosis.* Ketosis develops because of the rapid breakdown of fatty acids stored in adipose tissue. Fatty acids are used for energy when the daily intake of carbohydrates is less than 50 g. Clients at high risk for ketosis include those with diabetes, those on starvation diets, and those on low-carbohydrate diets.

Increased fat intake often causes fat deposition in heart, liver, and muscle and may lead to obesity, coronary heart disease, stroke, or breast and colon cancer.

Growth factors include amino acids, purines and pyrimidines, and vitamins. These nutrients are required but cannot be synthesized. Insufficient quantities of these substances can seriously impair the ability of the cell to take up and metabolize nutrients or to synthesize macromolecules for structural building and reproduction.

CELL DEATH

Cells die as a result of being traumatized, through alteration by disease, from failure caused by genetic alterations, or through a programmed process called *apoptosis.* Apoptosis usually does not disturb the steady-state nature of the tissue and thus gives no sign of its occurrence.

CONCLUSIONS

Cells are the basic units of life, and they serve many functions. The integrity and existence of the organism is dependent on the individual and collective ability of body cells to digest and assimilate substances, protect themselves by reacting to stimuli, replicate, metabolize, and produce energy. When cells lose their ability to function normally because of injury or attack by pathogens, the organism becomes distressed and disease develops.

Recent advances in molecular biology are providing the means for great improvements in the diagnosis and treatment of many human diseases. Professionals should keep current in the field in order to comprehend the nature and consequences of the pathologic changes associated with disease processes and to enhance their ability to make and evaluate therapeutic decisions.

BIBLIOGRAPHY

1. Berne, R., et al. (2004). *Physiology* (5th ed.). St. Louis: Mosby.
2. Kierszenbaum, A.L. (2002). *Histology and cell biology: An introduction to pathology.* St. Louis: Mosby.
3. Guyton, A., & Hall, J. (2001). *Textbook of medical physiology* (10th ed.). Philadelphia: W. B. Saunders.
4. Silverthorn, D. (2001). *Human physiology* (2nd ed.). Saddle River, NJ: Prentice Hall.
5. Yeh, E. (1998). Life and death of the cell. *Hospital Practice,* August 15, 85-92.

Clients with Fluid Imbalances

Bernadette White

evolve

Web Enhancements

http://evolve.elsevier.com/Black/medsurg/

Appendix A
Religious Beliefs and Practices Affecting Health Care

Appendix C
Laboratory Values of Clinical Importance in Medical-Surgical Nursing

Dehydration is the most common fluid and electrolyte imbalance in the United States. The Centers for Medicare and Medicaid Management have identified dehydration as one of the most frequent diagnoses upon hospital admission, present in more than 1 million admissions per year. Dehydration is especially common among older adults and, therefore, is expected to increase as the population ages. Dehydration carries a 17% to 45% morbidity and mortality rate.[17] The cost to society includes not only the cost of hospital care for diagnosis and treatment of the dehydration and its secondary complications, but also for the financial and psychological loss to the family and society of a productive contributor.

This chapter provides the basic knowledge necessary to promote positive health outcomes for clients at risk for fluid and electrolyte imbalances. Positive health outcomes are achieved through health promotion, health maintenance, and health restoration strategies. Clearly, water is not only responsible for the body's structure and function, it is also necessary for the maintenance of equilibrium and of life itself. The introductory chapter to this unit reviews fluid compartments and the regulation of fluid movement between compartments.

EXTRACELLULAR FLUID VOLUME DEFICIT

Extracellular fluid volume deficit (ECFVD), commonly called *dehydration,* is a decrease in intravascular and interstitial fluids. ECFVD is a common and serious fluid imbalance that results in vascular fluid volume loss *(hypovolemia)*. Losses can be *mild,* with a loss of 1 to 2 L of water (2% of body weight); *moderate,* with a loss of 3 to 5 L of water (5% of body weight); or *severe,* when 5 to 10 L of water (8% of body weight) is lost.

Etiology

Average daily fluid intake for adults is about 1500 to 2000 ml. In addition, about 800 ml of fluid is consumed through solid foods. Fluid balance is maintained in the body because the intake of fluids equals the excretion of fluids. This simple concept can be used to explain common causes of fluid imbalances. A lack of fluid intake, excessive fluid output, or both can lead to dehydration. Conversely, excessive fluid intake and a lack of fluid excretion can lead to overhydration. Furthermore, alteration in any of the regulators of fluid balance—thirst, hormones, lymphatic system, kidneys—increases the risk for or can cause an actual fluid imbalance (Figure 13-1).

Lack of Fluid Intake

Cognitive and physical impairments can quickly reduce water intake. For example, clients who are hospitalized, chairbound, or bedbound may not be able to reach their water or may be too confused to realize they are thirsty. People with dysphagia or at risk for aspiration may not be able to swallow fluids safely. Tube-fed people who are not given adequate free water or who are fed hypertonic formulas are also at risk. Community-dwelling older

evolve Be sure to check out the bonus material on the Evolve website and the CD-ROM, including free self-assessment exercises.
http://evolve.elsevier.com/Black/medsurg/

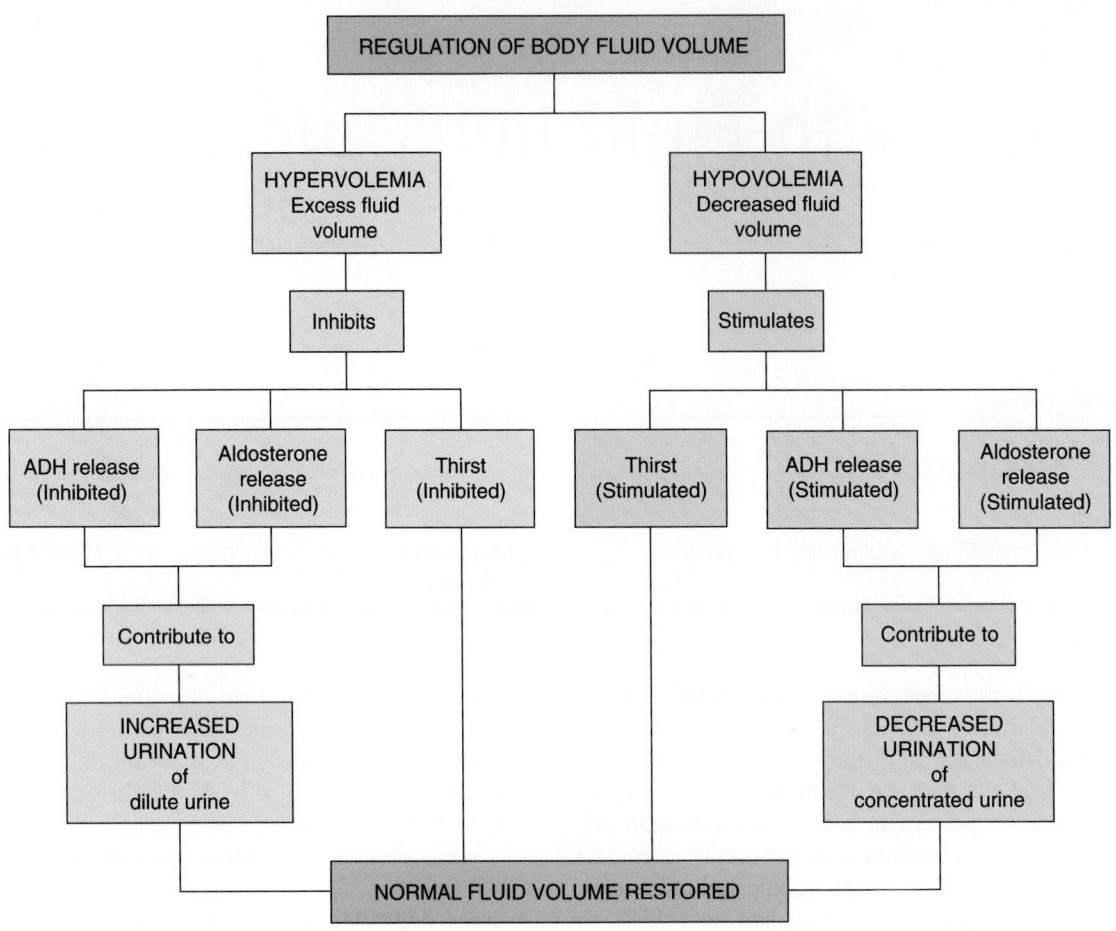

FIGURE 13-1 Regulation of body fluid volume depends on antidiuretic hormone (ADH), aldosterone, and thirst and fluid dynamics. (From White, B. [1994]. Maintaining fluid and electrolyte balance. In V.B. Bolander [Ed.], *Sorensen and Luckmann's basic nursing: A psychophysiologic approach* [3rd ed.]. Philadelphia: W.B. Saunders.)

adults may have decreased access to fluids because of financial or transportation barriers or debilitation. For many of these reasons, nursing home residents older than 85 years of age appear to be at greatest risk for dehydration.[2,7,15]

Impaired thirst mechanisms can also decrease fluid intake. The thirst mechanism is usually triggered by low blood pressure or a fluid volume depletion as small as 0.5%. The sensation of a dry mouth also stimulates thirst. Clients may experience dry mouth from salivary gland dysfunction, head or neck radiation, smoking, mouth breathing, oxygen therapy, hyperventilation, and anticholinergic medications (such as atropine).

Most healthy people respond to decreased fluid levels by drinking fluids and thus maintain balance. However, the thirst mechanism is depressed in people with debilitating illnesses and in older adults, even healthy older adults.[5] Several disorders also lead to inappropriate thirst mechanisms. People with excess fluids in the interstitial space but depleted fluids in the vascular space are commonly thirsty. Any stimulant that results in an increased renin-angiotensin-aldosterone response causes sodium retention that, in turn, also stimulates the thirst response. Clients with heart failure commonly experience this problem.

Osmolality also influences thirst. Hypo-osmolality inhibits the thirst response; conversely, hyperosmolality leads to thirst. It is common to find comatose and confused people with high plasma osmolality, but they are unable to recognize the urge to drink.

Excess Fluid Losses

Unmonitored use of potent diuretics (e.g., furosemide), severe vomiting, and diarrhea are common causes of dehydration. These conditions are commonly associated with other clinical manifestations as well, such as changes in electrolytes. Potential causes of fluid loss include fever, diaphoresis, hyperglycemia, gastrointestinal suction, ileostomy, fistulae, burns, blood loss, hyperventilation, hyperthyroidism, decreased antidiuretic hormone (ADH) secretion, diabetes insipidus (nephrogenic and neurogenic), Addison's disease or adrenal crisis, and the diuretic phase of acute renal failure.

Again, older adults are at risk for excessive fluid losses for several reasons: (1) decreased renal concentration of urine, (2) an altered ADH response, and (3) an increase in body fat and thus a decrease in total quantity of body water in proportion to body weight.[5] Increased drug-drug interactions and multiple chronic diseases potentiate the risk for fluid imbalances.

Third-space fluid shifts (shifting of fluid from the vascular space to interstitial space where fluid cannot be easily exchanged) can result in a fluid deficit in the vascular compartment. Spaces that are susceptible to third-spacing include the peritoneal, pericardial, pleural, and joint cavities. Abdominal third-spacing is called *ascites*.

Pathophysiology

Fluids are normally found in three spaces: inside the cells (intracellular), around the cells (interstitial), and in the bloodstream (intravascular). The pathophysiology of dehydration is seen when the normal compensation for fluid loss in the bloodstream cannot be corrected by stored fluid elsewhere. When fluids are lost from the intravascular spaces due to lack of intake or excess loss, interstitial fluids move in to restore vascular volume. Because the actual volume of fluid in the interstitial space is limited, other compensation systems are initiated to restore fluid volume. ADH and aldosterone secretion increase to reabsorb water and sodium in the kidney. Fluids are also reabsorbed from the ileum and large colon. The *baroreceptors* sense low blood pressure, and the sympathetic nervous system is stimulated to increase peripheral vasoconstriction and the heart rate. Vasoconstriction moves fluids from the periphery (legs, gastrointestinal tract) into circulation. Increasing sodium levels in the blood is also sensed by the osmoreceptors in the hypothalamus, which signals the thirst mechanism. These compensatory processes occur repeatedly in normal healthy people. When fluid loss continues or when the compensation fails to restore blood volume, the person becomes dehydrated.

If the dehydration is not corrected through the aforementioned mechanisms, fluid is shifted from the cells into the vascular system. The loss of cellular fluid is dangerous because the cells need fluid for cellular function. Less fluid is available for temperature regulation via sweating, and a lowered blood volume decreases the body's ability to transport core heat to the periphery for conductive loss. There is less cerebrospinal fluid and less fluid in the fat pads around the eyes. If cerebral cells become dehydrated, the vessels may be stretched and bleed or go into spasm, and thought processes may be impaired. If sodium is lost, the muscle and nerve functions that depend on this electrolyte are slowed. A full discussion of sodium imbalances is provided in Chapter 14.

There are three types of extracellular fluid (ECF) volume deficits:

- *Hyperosmolar (hypertonic)* fluid volume deficit: water loss is greater than electrolyte (sodium) loss
- *Iso-osmolar (isotonic)* fluid volume deficit: water and electrolyte (sodium) losses are equal
- *Hypotonic* fluid volume deficit: electrolyte loss is greater than fluid loss (rare)

Clinical Manifestations

Loss of Body Weight

Fairly rapid weight loss is an early and common result of fluid loss, because water is a major portion of body weight. A mild ECFVD exists when weight loss equals 2% of body weight. For example, in a client who weighs 150 pounds (68 kg), a 2% loss equals 1.4 L of water. Weight is the most accurate measure of fluid status, because it is less likely to be inaccurate if the client is weighed on the same scale, with the same clothes and at the same time each day.

Changes in Intake and Output

Intake and output (I & O) measurements provide another means of assessing fluid balance. These data provide insight into the cause of the imbalance (such as decreased fluid intake or increased fluid loss). These measurements are not as accurate as body weight, however, because of relative risk of errors in recording.

Thirst is an early clinical manifestation of ECFVD in a conscious person; however, thirst is diminished in older adults, so it is not an accurate indicator. Clients often request plain, cold water rather than carbonated or caffeinated beverages. This is advantageous because caffeine is a diuretic and sweet fluids may not quench thirst.

Urine output usually decreases with ECFVD because of the effects of ADH and aldosterone. Urine is usually concentrated, with specific gravity greater than 1.030 and urine osmolality greater than 1000 mOsm/kg. For many years, it was thought that the kidneys had to excrete at least 30 ml of urine per hour as a mechanism for waste removal. Currently, a urine output of 400 to 500 ml/day (16 to 20 ml/hr) is considered *oliguria* and indicates a marked compromise in kidney function. In most people (perhaps not the critically ill), urine output varies throughout the day. Normally, urine output is low and concentration is higher during the night. Thus, the view that urine should flow constantly at 30 to 40 ml/hr appears to lack justification.

People who are at risk for becoming dehydrated because they do not have the ability to concentrate urine are those who produce inadequate amounts of ADH (e.g., clients with diabetes insipidus) and those who do not respond normally to ADH (e.g., older adults) and those with inability to concentrate urine (e.g., clients with kidney failure).

Changes in Vital Signs

Inadequate fluid volume also leads to a decrease in systolic blood pressure, a weak pulse, and a decrease in central venous pressure (CVP) and pulmonary capillary wedge pressure (PCWP). For every liter of fluid lost, the cardiac output decreases by 1 L/min, the heart rate increases 8 beats/min, and the core temperature increases by 0.3° C (0.6° F).[6] Postural hypotension is a classic sign of decreased fluid volume. It is defined as a decrease in systolic blood pressure of more than 25 mm Hg, a decrease in diastolic pressure of more than 20 mm Hg, and a pulse increase of 30 beats/min or more when the client stands up.

Sympathetic nervous system stimulation leads to vasoconstriction and increases the heart rate to compensate for the altered tissue perfusion. Without restoring fluids, the vasoconstrictive and tachycardic (rate >100 beats/min) responses provide only a minimal and temporary compensation. If these responses continue, tissue perfusion is further compromised. Serious fluid loss can lead to systolic blood pressures less than 70 mm Hg. Low systolic pressure impairs tissue perfusion to vital organs that have high metabolic demands, such as cerebral, cardiac, and kidney tissues.

Flat jugular veins in a supine position and a prolonged peripheral venous filling time of more than 5 seconds are also noted. Because of the inability to cool the body core, an elevated temperature is common and can reach 105° F.

Manifestations of Cellular Dehydration

The mucous membranes of the mouth and eyes become dry even though fluid is recruited from the interstitial spaces. The lips can crack, and furrows may be seen on the tongue. Swallowing can become difficult.

Tenting of the skin (decreased turgor) occurs when the skin tissues tend to stick together because of the decreased interstitial fluid. Tenting is not diagnostic of fluid deficit in older adults because tenting commonly results from loss of elastin in the skin in this population. Soft and sunken eyes may be noted. Muscle weakness from an imbalance of sodium and potassium occurs early and becomes worse as the deficit progresses. Feces become hard and decreased in number because of compensatory reabsorption of fluid from the colon.

Cerebral signs are always considered serious because it means that intracellular fluid (ICF) compartmental shifting has occurred. Early signs include apprehension, restlessness, and headache. As the deficit progresses, hallucinations, maniacal behavior, and confusion occur, followed by coma.

Diagnostic Findings

In hyperosmolar fluid deficit, more solvent is lost than solutes, which creates hemoconcentration. Plasma sodium concentration is also increased *(hypernatremia)*. The following elevations are typical findings secondary to a hemoconcentrated state:

- Osmolality greater than 295 mOsm/kg
- Plasma sodium level greater than 145 mEq/L
- Blood urea nitrogen (BUN) greater than 25 mg/dl
- Plasma glucose greater than 120 mg/dl
- Hematocrit greater than 55%
- Urine specific gravity greater than 1.030

Specific gravity is a numeric value of urine concentration using solute-solvent relationships. Very concentrated urine has a high specific gravity. High specific gravity readings indicate dehydration or increased ADH. Glucose, protein, and dyes falsely elevate specific gravity. Urine specific gravity can be measured by using a urinometer or by sending a urine sample to the laboratory for testing.

Hypernatremia usually indicates hyperosmolality, and hyponatremia usually indicates hypo-osmolality. Box 13-1 shows how to calculate plasma osmolality. Urine specific gravity may also be used as an indirect measurement of osmolality.

Outcome Management

The seriousness of a client's manifestations and the aggressiveness of treatment are related to both the *amount* and *acuteness* of the fluid loss, and the client's state of health at the time of loss. Sudden loss of fluid does not give the compensatory mechanisms time to adapt; severe loss is often beyond the potential of compensatory mechanisms to adapt, resulting in vascular collapse or shock. A thorough history and physical examination, including collection of such demographic variables as age, gender, culture, presence of chronic diseases, and socioeconomic status, are critical to identifying realistic and measurable outcomes. Dehydration can occur volitionally (by choice) in terminally ill clients, and for those clients treatment may be withheld to meet their desires. There is increasing evidence that dehydration in the terminally ill

---

BOX 13-1   *How to Calculate Plasma Osmolality*

To calculate plasma osmolality, you must know the plasma sodium (Na) level. Additionally, you should know the glucose level and urea/nitrogen (BUN). The first formula may be used as a rough estimate of the plasma osmolality; the second formula gives a more exact plasma osmolality value.

$2 \times$ Plasma Na = Plasma osmolality

$2 \times$ Plasma Na + (BUN/3) + (Glucose/18) = Plasma osmolality is not painful because perception and level of consciousness are decreased by the ketone and other metabolic accumulation and increased production in endorphins is increased.[14,19]

Medical treatment of fluid volume deficit depends on the acuteness and severity of the fluid deficit. The goals of treatment are to restore normal fluid volumes by using fluids similar in composition to those lost, to replace ongoing losses, and to correct the underlying problem (such as vomiting or diarrhea).

Fluid Restoration

Oral Rehydration. If the fluid loss is mild, the thirst mechanism is intact and the client can drink fluid, replace the fluids orally. Oral glucose replacement solutions are palatable, inexpensive, and a good source of fluid, glucose, and electrolytes. These solutions are quickly absorbed even when the client has diarrhea or is vomiting. Cola drinks should be avoided because they do not contain adequate electrolyte replacement, the sugar content may lead to osmotic diuresis, and the caffeine may lead to diuresis.

Intravenous Rehydration. When the fluid loss is severe or life-threatening, intravenous (IV) fluids are used for replacement. The volume of fluid is calculated on the basis of the client's weight and the presence of any other comorbidities, such as, cardiac, renal, liver, or pulmonary disorders that would decrease the ability of the body to rid excess fluids. The type of solution used is based on the type of fluid lost from the body. Generally, isotonic ECFVD is treated with isotonic solutions, hypertonic ECFVD is treated with hypotonic solutions, and hypotonic ECFVD is treated with hypertonic solutions. Common IV fluids are listed in Table 13-1. Sodium solutions should be infused at a rate of 0.5 to 1 mEq/L/hr. If fluid is given too rapidly, cerebral edema may result.

Monitoring for Complications of Fluid Restoration. Fluid administration is based on the client's overall condition. A client with severe ECFVD accompanied by severe heart, pulmonary, liver, or kidney disease cannot tolerate large volumes of fluid or sodium without the risk for development of heart failure. For unstable clients, monitors are used to detect increasing pressures from fluids (e.g., measurement of right atrial and pulmonary artery pressure). If the deficit has existed for more than 24 hours, it is dangerous to correct this deficit too rapidly. Urine output, body weight, and laboratory values of sodium, osmolality, urea/nitrogen (BUN), and potassium are monitored closely.

Correction of the Underlying Problem. Antiemetic and antidiarrheal drugs may be prescribed to correct problems with nausea and vomiting or diarrhea. Antibiotics

may be used in clients with infectious diarrhea. Antipyretic agents may be used to reduce body temperature. Clients who are taking diuretics should have the benefits versus the risks examined of continuing the medication.

■ Nursing Management of the Medical Client Assessment

Obtain the client's history of fluid losses. If the cause is infectious, isolation may be warranted.

Assess the client's vital signs every 2 to 4 hours, depending on the severity of the fluid loss; compare them with baseline vital signs and report marked differences. Assess for postural (orthostatic) blood pressure and pulse changes by taking blood pressure and pulse with the client lying down. Then have the client stand up; repeat the blood pressure and pulse measurements after 1 minute. Report a drop in standing systolic blood pressure of 25 mm Hg or more from the supine blood pressure; report pulse increases of more than 30 beats/min. Autonomic neuropathy seen in diabetes, dysrhythmias, and some medications (e.g., antihypertensive agents) can also cause postural hypotension.

Assess the peripheral vein filling time daily. Veins with normal fluid volume should fill in 3 to 5 seconds when the arm is lowered below the level of the heart.

Monitor intake, output, and daily weights accurately in high-risk clients. Be certain that all sources of intake (including liquids with meals and between meals, with medications, in IV lines, in tube-feedings, and in IV or tube flushes) and all sources of output (including urine, diarrhea, diaphoresis, and hyperventilation) be recorded accurately. If the ECFVD is mild, assess urine output every 8 hours and compare daily outputs. Absence of adequate renal perfusion for several hours may result in permanent renal damage. Whenever the output decreases to less than 0.5 ml/kg/hr for 2 consecutive hours, urine output must be assessed hourly.

Teach unlicensed assistive personnel to report urine outputs of less than 0.5 ml/kg/hr for 2 consecutive hours or less than 240 ml for an 8-hour period. Provide other instructions as well (see the Management and Delegation feature on Care of Clients with Fluid Volume Deficit on p. 211). Instruct the client to report fluids consumed in addition to the fluids on food trays and urine output not measured.

Monitor plasma sodium, urea/nitrogen (BUN), glucose, and hematocrit levels to determine plasma osmolality. Assess for confusion, an early manifestation of ICF involvement.

Determine a history of chronic illnesses that may impair the ability to tolerate fluids at rapid speeds. Lung, renal, and heart disease reduce the body's ability to move fluids through the vascular system. Record the client's lung sounds on admission to serve as a baseline for later comparison.

TABLE 13-1 *Intravenous Water and Electrolyte Solutions*

Solution (Abbreviation)	Contents	Uses	Comments
Hypotonic			
5% dextrose in water (D₅W)	50 g dextrose No electrolytes	Replaces deficits of total body water Not used alone to expand ECF volume because dilution of electrolytes can occur	Supplies 170 kcal/L and free water Distilled water cannot be given IV because it would cause hemolysis of RBCs Dextrose is metabolized on first pass through the liver, leaving a solution of water but without the hemolytic problems
Isotonic			
0.9% NaCl (normal saline solution, NS, 0.9% NS)	154 mEq/L of Na and Cl	ECF deficits in patients with low serum levels of Na or Cl and metabolic alkalosis Before and after the infusion of blood products	Not used for routine administration of IV fluids because it contains more sodium than ECF (140 mEq of NaCl and 103 mEq of Cl) Expands plasma and interstitial volume and does not enter cells
Lactated Ringer's solution (LR)	130 mEq/L Na 4 mEq/L K 3 mEq/L Ca 109 mEq/L Cl 28 mEq/L lactate	ECF deficits, such as fluid loss with burns and bleeding and dehydration from loss of bile or diarrhea	Solution is roughly isotonic to plasma but does not contain magnesium or phosphate Lactate is equivalent to bicarbonate, and solution can be used to treat many forms of acidosis Cannot be used in people with alkalosis; solutions of acetate Ringer's are better for these clients
Hypertonic			
Lactated Ringer's solution with 5% dextrose (D₅/LR)	50 g dextrose 130 mEq/L Na 4 mEq/L K 3 mEq/L Ca 109 mEq/L Cl 28 mEq/L lactate	ECF deficits, such as fluid loss with burns and bleeding and dehydration from loss of bile or diarrhea Provides modest calories (170 kcal)	This solution is hypertonic because it is the combination of two solutions (D₅W and LR) See other comments on individual solutions
5% dextrose and normal saline (D₅/0.9 NS)	50 g dextrose 154 mEq/L Na and Cl	ECF deficits in patients with low serum levels of Na or Cl and metabolic alkalosis Before and after the infusion of blood products Provides modest calories (170 kcal)	This solution is hypertonic because it is the combination of two solutions (D₅W and NS) See other comments on individual solutions
5% dextrose and 0.45% normal saline (D₅/0.45 NS; D₅/½ NS)	50 g dextrose 77 mEq/L Na and Cl	Can be used as an initial fluid for hydration because it provides more water than sodium Provides modest calories (170 kcal)	Commonly used as a maintenance fluid
5% dextrose and 0.225% normal saline (D₅/0.2 NS; D₅/¼ NS)	50 g dextrose 34 mEq/L Na and Cl	Can be used as an initial fluid for hydration because it provides more water than sodium Provides modest calories (170 kcal)	Commonly used as a maintenance fluid

Na, Sodium; *Cl,* chloride; *K,* potassium; *Ca,* calcium; *ECF,* extracellular fluid; *NS,* normal saline; *RBC,* red blood cells; *IV,* intravenously; *kcal,* kilocalories.

MANAGEMENT AND DELEGATION
Care of Clients with Fluid Volume Deficit

When working with unlicensed assistive personnel in the care of clients with fluid volume deficit, remind them to do the following:

- Keep fresh water or other fluids in an easily accessible location. Remind older clients to drink fluids hourly because their thirst mechanism is diminished.
- Try to provide fluids of choice every 1 to 2 hours.
- Encourage family members to assist with fluid intake.
- Provide oral care every 2 hours to help decrease discomfort from dry mucous membranes.
- Record intake accurately. Remember, a cup of ice chips provides one-half cup of water.
- Assist clients as necessary to the bathroom, commode, or bedpan every 2 hours. If the client is wearing disposable briefs, assess for incontinence and the need for perineal care at least every 2 hours.
- Record all output accurately. Include the amount of urine, the number of episodes of incontinence, and the measured amount of any diarrhea.
- Report diarrhea, excessive sweating, or rapid breathing.
- Report urine that is dark, produced at less than 0.5 ml/kg/hr over 2 consecutive hours, or produced at more than 150 ml/hr.
- Report weight changes of 2 pounds or more from the previous day.

FIGURE 13-2 Skin turgor assessment. This assessment can be done on the forearm. Skin that does not flatten immediately after release is called "tenting," an example of fluid volume deficit in a young to middle-aged adult. Assessment for tenting is not appropriate for older adults.

years of age. A slower response may indicate loss of interstitial fluids. Generalized weakness may develop because of changes in sodium levels.

Diagnosis, Outcomes, Interventions

Diagnosis: Deficient Fluid Volume. Deficient fluid volume is the state in which a person has vascular, interstitial, or intracellular dehydration. The nursing diagnosis is *Deficient Fluid Volume related to insufficient fluid intake, vomiting, diarrhea, hemorrhage, or third-space fluid loss such as ascites or burns.*

Outcomes. The desired outcome is return of normal levels of body fluids. The goal statement may be that the client will have restoration of normal fluid volume, improvement in fluid volume, or no further fluid losses depending on the clinical situation. Indicators of adequate fluid volumes include the following:

- Oral intake between 1500 and 2500 ml or more in 24 hours
- Urine output greater than 0.5 ml/kg/hr
- Stable blood pressure and pulse in the supine and standing positions
- Increasing body weight of about 0.5 to 1 pound per day
- Absence of crackles (fluid in alveoli), an indicator of fluid overload from overcompensation
- Moist tongue and mucous membranes
- Urea/nitrogen (BUN), plasma sodium, hematocrit, and osmolality levels approaching normal ranges over the first 48 to 72 hours

Assess the client's weight and height, do not rely on the client's stated weight on admission. Weigh the client daily on the same scale, at the same time of day, with the client wearing clothing of similar weight. Orthostatic hypotension may be present, so help the client onto the scale. Analyze changes in daily weights. A loss of 2.2 pounds is equivalent to 1 L of fluid. Therefore, an 8-pound weight loss equals about 3.5 L of fluid, or a moderate fluid volume deficit.

Assess the oral cavity between the gums and cheek for dryness of the mucous membranes and the tongue for dryness and longitudinal furrows.[7,16] Use an oral assessment guide (see Chapter 4 for an example of how to derive a numerical rating of oral health). Another reliable method of testing for dryness of the mouth is to place your finger on the mucous membranes where the gums and cheek meet. When ECFVD is present, your finger will not glide easily because of dryness. Note any speech and swallowing difficulty. Assess closely for dried and adherent mucus on the soft palate.

Check skin turgor by gently pinching and lifting the skin (Figure 13-2). Usually, skin returns to a normal position within 1 or 2 seconds in people younger than 65

Interventions

Restore Oral Fluid Intake. Give small amounts of fluids "of choice" hourly to older, confused, or debilitated clients and to those who require restraints. Keep fluids fresh and within reach. Use orthotic devices as appropriate for those who can assist in their own fluid intake. If a client's lips are dry, he or she may be unable to suck on a straw. Wet the lips and mouth first to facilitate sucking. Give antiemetics as needed to control nausea before drinking. When appropriate, begin with clear liquids, such as oral replacement fluids, broth, or gelatin. Progress to full liquids and then solid foods, if tolerated without vomiting or aspiration. Encourage family members to participate in feeding.

If dysphagia (difficulty in swallowing) is present, consult the physician regarding swallowing studies. Once the problem has been identified, a speech pathologist can provide exercises to help the client. Reinforce the speech therapist's prescription during each feeding. You may need to give thickened fluids, elevate the headrest to 90 degrees before meals and for 1 hour after feeding, and flex the client's head slightly forward at the start of a swallow. Decrease the risk of aspiration by placing small amounts of food on the side of the mouth that has the best sensation and muscle strength. Teaching the client to chew slowly and to swallow two or three times with each mouthful and inspecting the mouth for food pocketing can also decrease the risk of aspiration. Assessing the fit of dentures is also important.

Restore Fluids by Intravenous Routes. Administer IV fluids cautiously to clients with ECFVD. Ideally, a large IV gauge (e.g., 18- to 20-gauge) should be used; however, most clients have venous collapse, and it is difficult to find a vein. A small IV site may be used initially; once fluids are reestablished, a larger needle can be inserted if fluids or an IV access is still needed. Use an IV pump to regulate IV infusion and to decrease the risk of too rapid an infusion. Monitor IV solutions, IV sites, and client outcomes hourly.

Rapid fluid replacement often results in overflow diuresis without cellular replacement. Diuresis compounds dehydration and may result in hypernatremia. In older adults or in those with renal or cardiac disease, rapid fluid administration may also result in pulmonary overload.

Reduce the Risk of Deficient Fluid Volume. If your assessment indicates no fluid deficit but a risk of fluid deficit, the format for writing the problem statement is *Risk for Deficient Fluid Volume related to (risk factor).* Interventions are focused on health promotion and maintenance strategies that decrease the likelihood of a deficit. The goal of oral fluid promotion and maintenance is to maintain the level of fluid intake at 1500 ml for 24 hours.

If the client is fed by tube, give water boluses with hypertonic tube-feedings. Recommended dilution is 1 ml of water per 1 kilocalorie (kcal) of feeding formula. For example, if a can of formula has 380 kcal in 240 ml of formula, give an additional 140 ml of water, for a total of 380 ml of fluid.

Control the Underlying Problems. Diarrhea has several causes. Examine the client's prescription and nonprescription (over-the-counter, herbal) medication list. If the onset of the diarrhea was at the same time as the new elixir drug with sorbitol, a common cause of osmotic diarrhea, consult the pharmacist regarding pills rather than the elixir form. Consider viral infections because many have been known to result in lactose intolerance. If this is the cause, encourage the client to avoid milk-based products. Avoiding fatty or fried foods also decreases diarrhea and enhances digestion.

Give prescribed antiemetics for nausea, antipyretics for fever, and antibiotics for infection.

Monitor for Complications. When fluid balance is compromised, a person is at risk for tissue breakdown. Apply a moisturizer or skin barrier to protect the skin from the irritants, enzymes, and microorganisms found in urine and feces. Continue to assess lung sounds for manifestations of fluid overload (crackles) from overcorrection.

Diagnosis: Impaired Oral Mucous Membrane. The nursing diagnosis of *Impaired Oral Mucous Membrane related to lack of oral intake or other causes* is a common problem in clients with dehydration.

Outcomes. The desired outcome is that the mucous membranes are restored with expected outcomes of having an improvement in oral score. In addition, the client's tongue, gums, and lips should become moist and the mouth, gums, and teeth should be clean and free of accumulations of dried mucus.

Interventions. Give oral care with a regular toothbrush or a foam toothbrush every 2 to 4 hours, and apply lip moisturizer. Rinse the client's mouth every 1 to 2 hours. Examine the client's mouth with a penlight to make sure that it remains free of debris. Avoid mouthwashes with an alcohol base, which can dry the mucous membranes. The frequency of oral care should be increased to hourly if there is no improvement. Artificial saliva can also be used for the client with a very dry and fissured mouth.

Diagnosis: Risk for Injury. If orthostatic hypotension is present, *Risk for Injury* is another problem that needs to be addressed.

Outcomes. The desired outcome is that the client will remain free of injury as evidenced by no manifestations of falls (bruises, bumps, abrasions) or reported episodes of falls.

Interventions. Provide safety through step-progression position changes. Step-progression gives the client's body time to adapt to changes in position. First, raise the head of the bed. Next, assist the client to sit at the edge of the bed in a "dangling" position until the dizziness has subsided. Have the client stand, and assist the client to a chair. Do not progress to the next position until the client tolerates the current one (i.e., without dizziness or marked hypotension). Place alarm monitors on clients who are confused and tend to get out of bed without assistance. Restraints may be needed if all other measures to control behavior do not work.

Evaluation

Mild to moderate fluid deficits should be corrected in 8 to 24 hours. More severe fluid losses may take several days, especially when they occur in older adults.

■ Self-Care

Client teaching is one of the primary interventions for promoting and maintaining fluid balance. Teach clients with mild fluid deficit to replace fluid with clear liquids, 30 to 60 ml or more hourly, as tolerated, to decrease nausea and replace electrolytes. Teach the importance of consulting a physician if an illness lasts longer than 24 hours or if the person is older or has a chronic illness, such as diabetes mellitus or liver, kidney, or heart disease.

Health promotion teaching is critical for those who actively exercise.[6] Teach people who exercise to do the following:

* Understand the importance of exercise and heat acclimatization
* Avoid exercise during high heat and humidity
* Wear appropriate clothing (excess clothing decreases evaporation)
* Use more caution to prevent heat exhaustion if the client is obese, because obesity impairs the sweating mechanism
* Drink cool water before exercise, 150 to 200 ml every 15 minutes during exercise, and after finishing exercise, and add 500 to 700 kcal of carbohydrates (for energy and sodium) if exercise is prolonged; do not wait for thirst to appear before drinking
* Avoid rapid fluid replacement, because this fluid only overflows to the kidneys
* Use caution when taking medications that interfere with thermoregulation, such as thyroid replacement, amphetamines, beta-blockers, haloperidol, antihistamines, anticholinergic drugs, and phenothiazines

Encourage diabetic clients who exercise to wear or carry Medic-Alert identification, to increase their protein intake, to decrease refined sugar intake, and to reduce insulin to half the usual dosage or to an amount recommended by the physician. Teach people taking cortisone the importance of not missing doses, of carrying Medic-Alert identification, and of consulting a physician about increased dosage during physical or emotional stress to prevent adrenal crisis.

Reducing fluid intake as a way of decreasing urinary incontinence in older adults is inappropriate.[15] Limited fluid intake increases bladder irritability, leading to uninhibited contractions, and alters the neurologic stimulus that controls normal bladder emptying. Emphasizing the importance of drinking even in the absence of thirst, teaching pelvic muscle exercises, and instituting a toilet schedule may help an older person overcome the problem of incontinence.

INTRACELLULAR FLUID VOLUME DEFICIT

Dehydration can become so severe that the cells become dehydrated. This condition is relatively rare in a healthy adult, but it occurs often in older people and in those with conditions that result in acute water loss. Compensatory attempts to combat the fluid deficit have the same physiologic basis as in ECFVD. Thirst and oliguria are the most common compensatory signs. Cellular manifestations are due to the dysfunction in the cerebral cells and include fever and central nervous system (CNS) changes, such as confusion, and if not corrected can lead to cerebral hemorrhage and coma.

The desired outcome is restoration of fluid volume, which is initially addressed through IV replacement. Once the client becomes stable, the focus of medical management is correction or control of the underlying cause. The focus of nursing management is on prevention or early detection of complications secondary to the pathology or the treatment. Interdisciplinary communication is critical to the achievement of positive outcomes.

EXTRACELLULAR FLUID VOLUME EXCESS

ECF volume excess (ECFVE) is fluid overload or overhydration. Excess fluids can be found in the vascular system, a problem called *hypervolemia,* or in the interstitial spaces, a problem usually called *third-spacing* (see later discussion). The water and sodium retained is in the same proportions as it exists in other ECF, and therefore is referred to as *iso-osmolar (isotonic) fluid volume excess.*

Etiology

ECFVE can develop from two processes: (1) simple overloading with fluids and (2) failure to excrete fluids. ECFVE often results from an increase in the total body sodium. Causes of ECFVE are listed in Table 13-2.

Fluid overload also results from renal disorders that impair glomerular filtration of sodium and water. As

TABLE 13-2	Etiology of Extracellular Fluid Volume Excess
Etiologic Factor	**Examples**
Compromised regulation of fluid movement and excretion	Cirrhosis of the liver Decreased plasma protein Heart failure Hypothyroidism Lymphatic or venous obstruction Renal disorders
Excessive ingestion of fluids or foods containing sodium	Excessive amounts of saline intravenous fluids Ingestion of high-sodium foods Excessive use of enemas with sodium (e.g., Fleet's) or medications with sodium (e.g., Alka-Seltzer)
Increased antidiuretic hormone (ADH) and aldosterone	Certain barbiturates and narcotics (e.g., morphine) Cushing's syndrome General anesthesia Glucocorticoid use Hyperaldosteronism Syndrome of inappropriate antidiuretic hormone (secretion)

fluid volume increases, the heart attempts to compensate through tachycardia and hypertrophy. When compensatory mechanisms fail, heart failure results. Uncontrolled heart failure can lead to multiple organ failure and death from massive water retention, also known as *anasarca.*

Conditions that cause a decrease in plasma protein (mainly albumin), such as liver or renal, disease, burns, or protein malnutrition, result in a decreased oncotic pressure in the blood. The loss of oncotic pressure from low albumin decreases reabsorption from the tissue spaces at the venous end and peripheral edema. Ascites may also result (Figure 13-3, *B*).

When lymphatic channels are obstructed or have been removed or damaged, tissue oncotic pressure increases and leads to edema (Figure 13-3, *C*). Edema can also develop from any condition that triggers the inflammatory response and thus results in increased capillary permeability, such as tissue trauma (Figure 13-3, *D*).

Pathophysiology

With a fluid volume excess, the hydrostatic pressure of the fluid is higher than usual at the arterial end of the capillary, pushing excess fluids into the interstitial spaces. The fluid is not reabsorbed at the venous end of the capillary because the oncotic pressure is too low to

pull the fluids back across the capillary membrane. Usually the residual fluids are removed by the lymphatics, but in the case of edema, the fluid volume overloads the lymph system and stays in the interstitial space, leading to peripheral edema (Figure 13-3, *A*).

The process of edema can be progressive. As the fluid pressure increases in the interstitial area and tissues, it creates a resistance to forward blood flow and increases resistance throughout the circulatory system. This process is called *increased peripheral vascular resistance* and eventually it creates a gradient that resists left ventricular output. Blood is unable to be propelled forward and it backs up across the alveolocapillary membrane of the lungs, resulting in pulmonary edema. Because the lungs are low-pressure organs, they also offer little resistance to fluid accumulation. Pulmonary edema develops quickly in clients with distention of the left side of the heart muscle in those persons who have an impaired myocardial pump. If the right side of the heart fails, peripheral edema occurs through the same retrograde process. Left-sided heart failure may lead to right-sided failure and vice versa. Therefore pulmonary and peripheral edema may exist simultaneously.

Clinical Manifestations

Fluid volume excess in the lungs leads to coughing, dyspnea, and crackles that can be auscultated over the involved lung area. The alveolar fluid accumulation also leads to impaired oxygen (O_2) and carbon dioxide (CO_2) transport between the capillaries and alveoli, resulting in pallor, cyanosis, decreased tissue perfusion (measured by pulse oximetry), and increased CO_2 blood gas abnormalities. Manifestations are from increasing hydrostatic pressure in the pulmonary capillaries, which results in shifting of fluid to the alveolar sacs. If hydrostatic pressure continues to rise, fluid shifts into the pleural spaces as well; this is known as *pleural effusion.*

Cardiovascular manifestations are numerous. Delayed emptying and filling of the right ventricle leads to systemic venous engorgement, including signs of jugular venous distention, peripheral vein filling time greater than 5 seconds, a bounding pulse and elevated blood pressure, and increased right atrial (CVP) and pulmonary capillary wedge pressure (PCWP). If the delayed ventricular filling overdistends the ventricles, an extra heart sound (S_3) can often be auscultated with the bell of the stethoscope.

Fluid accumulates in the interstitial compartments, especially in the gravity-dependent tissues of the legs and sacrum. Edema may develop in the feet in ambulatory people and in the sacrum of bedridden clients. The continued increase in fluid pressure also causes fluid shifting into the visceral tissues. Thus, the client may exhibit signs of organ dysfunction specific to the tissues involved (e.g., anorexia and bloating from stomach in-

FIGURE 13-3 Mechanisms of edema formation. **A,** Fluid overload. **B,** Decreased plasma and albumin. **C,** Altered lymphatic function. **D,** Tissue injury.

volvement). Rapid weight gain is a classic sign of fluid overload regardless of the system responsible for the overload.

If any early changes in cerebral function develop, such as confusion and headache, suspect ICF shifting. As the fluid excess increases in the cerebral cells, lethargy occurs, followed by seizures and then coma.

With fluid overload, the excess fluid volume dilutes the concentration of solutes. Typical findings include the following:

- Plasma osmolality less than 275 mOsm/kg
- Plasma sodium less than 135 mEq/L, depending on the type of fluid excess
- Hematocrit less than 45%
- Specific gravity less than 1.010
- BUN less than 8 mg/dl

These results must be evaluated in the context of the client's manifestations and the possibility of other pathologic processes. For example, blood loss would also cause a decreased hematocrit; a decreased protein intake would result in decreased urea nitrogen levels. The volume of water may mask electrolyte and other solute levels. For example, the plasma sodium level may appear to be within the normal range because of excess water retention, even though the actual sodium level is increased.

Outcome Management

A thorough clinical history of contributing and causative factors, medication history, manifestations of fluid overload, and laboratory findings are essential to identifying appropriate interventions. Reduction of dietary sodium, restriction of fluids, and pharmacologic interventions are the major treatments for ECFVE.

Restriction of Sodium and Fluids

Because sodium retains water, sodium intake is commonly restricted especially in those clients with renal or heart dis-ease. According to the usual definitions, a *mildly* restricted sodium diet contains 4 to 5 g of sodium, a *moderately* restricted diet contains 2 g of sodium, and a *severely* restricted diet contains 0.5 g of sodium (see Chapter 14, Box 14-1, for a list of high- and low-sodium foods).

Promoting Urine Output

Mild diuretics and digitalis promote fluid loss and improve myocardial contractility. Many diuretics cause potassium and magnesium to be excreted along with the sodium and water. To counteract this, a combination of potassium-wasting and potassium-sparing diuretics may be prescribed.

Several studies have found improved myocardial contractility and decreased morbidity and mortality in clients with heart failure who, in addition to digitalis, have received angiotensin-converting enzyme (ACE) inhibitors and low-dose beta-blockers. Many of these clients showed such an improvement in their overall cardiac function that they did not need diuretics. When ACE inhibitors are used, clients should be monitored for hyperkalemia because of the potassium-sparing effect of the ACE inhibitor.

■ Nursing Management of the Medical Client
Assessment

Monitor the client's vital signs for a bounding pulse, elevated blood pressure, or both every 4 to 8 hours. Assess the apical pulse if the radial pulse is irregular or if the client is taking cardiac medication. Assess breath sounds every 4 to 8 hours for crackles especially in the bases of the lung, rhonchi, or wheezes. Assess for changes in respiratory effort with activity or rest. Note the position of comfort that the client prefers. Most dyspneic clients sit erect to ease the effort of breathing. If clients remain upright for continued periods of time, assess the skin of the sacrum for signs of pressure ulcers. Use caution before lowering the client's head if a supine position worsens breathing.

Each morning, palpate the sacrum and legs for pitting edema and observe the client for hand and bilateral neck vein engorgement. Jugular vein distention at or above a 45-degree headrest suggests ECFVE. Hand veins that do not flatten within 3 to 5 seconds when the hand is raised above the heart level suggest fluid overload. Assess the condition of skin on the legs. Edematous skin is fragile and is at risk for injury (e.g., tearing) and decreased perfusion, which may lead to pressure sores.

Compare I & O every 4 to 8 hours. Weigh the client daily; do not rely on stated weights. Determine whether the client has had expected weight loss or unexpected weight gain. Edema does not usually occur until 3 L or more of excess fluid has accumulated. If edema seems pronounced in the extremities or abdomen, measure the area in the same site each shift and compare the data.

Monitor plasma osmolality, sodium level, hematocrit, and urine specific gravity. Observe for changes in level of consciousness, which may indicate the more serious complication of ICF shifting.

Diagnosis, Outcomes, Interventions

Diagnosis: Excess Fluid Volume. The diagnostic statement is written *Excess Fluid Volume* related to (specific cause, such as heart, renal, or liver failure). Be certain to specify the cause in your client's case. If your client has heart failure, also consider using the nursing diagnosis *Decreased Cardiac Output.*

Outcomes. The desired outcome is return of normal levels of body fluids. Indicators of adequate fluid volumes include:
- Stable blood pressure and pulse
- Decreasing body weight of about 0.5 to 1 pound per day
- Absence of manifestations of ICFVE, such as confusion
- Absence of manifestations of ECFVE, such as coughing, crackles, dyspnea, jugular venous distention, peripheral edema, S_3 gallop rhythm
- Urea/nitrogen, plasma sodium, hematocrit, and osmolality approaching normal levels in 48 to 72 hours
- Absence of manifestations of overcorrection, such as hypotension, dry mucous membranes

Interventions

Reduce Sodium and Fluid Intake. Fluid management becomes extremely important in clients with ECFVE. Strict I & O may be crucial. Include fluids on meal trays and those given with medications as part of the total fluid intake. Collaborate with the dietitian in planning fluid restrictions. Schedule oral medications at meal times, if possible, to limit fluid intake. Use minimal amounts of water (5 to 10 ml) to dissolve crushed medications that need to be given by feeding tube. Cold fluids decrease the sensation of thirst more than warm or hot fluids. Give the client ice chips, if allowed, and provide frequent oral care to decrease the thirst sensation (1 cup of ice equals ½ cup of water). Teach clients to hold the water in their mouth for a while to rehydrate the tongue, rather than swallowing it quickly. Instruct clients about the rationale for fluid and sodium restrictions.

Use IV pumps to control IV fluid intake. Use only isotonic saline for bladder and nasogastric tube irrigations. Monitor clients who have received intraoperative irrigations with hypotonic solutions (e.g., bladder, prostate, hysteroscopic surgeries) for fluid overload and consult the physician about changing postoperative irrigations to normal saline.

Sodium is a common ingredient in foods, and to many clients the low-sodium diet is bland. Suggest alternatives for seasoning, such as lemon, garlic, or pepper, to enhance the taste of foods and increase dietary compliance. Salt substitutes are available but clients should be cautioned regarding the use of potassium salt substitutes if they are on ACE inhibitors or have renal disease (both cause potassium retention). Potassium salt substitutes are also "saltier" than sodium chloride, so the client should use them sparingly to avoid creating a metallic taste with the food.

Mobilize Fluid. Instruct the client who has dependent leg edema to avoid long periods of standing and to sit with legs elevated. Bedrest alone promotes diuresis, particularly in clients with heart failure. Mobilization of edema in the supine position is probably due to diminished pooling of venous blood, a resultant increase in effective circulating blood volume and thus renal perfusion. Do not elevate the legs in severe edema. Although elevation may help reduce swelling, the rapid return of pooled blood from the swollen legs can overwhelm the heart.

Reduce Complications. Elevate the head of the bed 30 to 45 degrees to decrease venous return, which decreases cardiac workload and allows for improved diaphragmatic excursion, both of which improve oxygenation. This position also promotes jugular venous drainage, which improves cerebral perfusion. If dyspnea or orthopnea is present, position the client in semi-Fowler's or Fowler's position. Consult with the physician for an order to adjust oxygen to keep oxygen saturation greater than 90%.

If the client is taking diuretics and digitalis, monitor plasma electrolytes and anticipate digitalis toxic effects resulting from hypokalemia. Report the abnormal levels of plasma electrolytes, especially potassium levels.

When peripheral tissue perfusion is altered because of edema or vascular disease, provide frequent skin care, turn the client often, control moisture, and prevent friction and shear. The heel is especially at risk for decreased capillary blood flow. Therefore, it is important to keep the client's heels elevated off the mattress and to remove elastic stockings when nonblanchable erythema is noted. Lubricate the skin on the legs to prevent cracks and fissures.

Modifications for Older Clients

In general, these interventions are the same for the older client; however, response time is usually slower and the risk for side effects is higher because of poorer renal and liver function and problems with drug interactions.[43] For instance, digitalis toxicity is much more common in older adults. Some diagnostic studies may not be as accurate in this population. For example, a person with protein malnutrition, which is more common in older adults, may have renal insufficiency but may have a normal urea/nitrogen level (BUN) because of the lack of protein. Thus, it is very important to monitor creatinine levels; this provides a more precise reflection of renal function.

Evaluation

Correcting ECFVE is a slow process, especially when it results from an organ disorder. Most clients are discharged without complete resolution of peripheral edema but with improvement in pulmonary edema and breathing. Self-care instructions are critical.

■ Self-Care

If the client is going home on a low-sodium diet, review allowed and restricted foods with the client and the person who prepares the meals. Many canned foods, pre-prepared foods, and seasonings are high in sodium and should be avoided; fresh and frozen foods are usually lower in sodium. Buying these items in season and freezing them for later use saves money and provides more nutrients. Encourage the food purchaser to read food labels and to avoid products with high levels of sodium or salt and food whose labels contain the word "sodium" or the symbol "Na" as a prefix. Avoid drinking or cooking with softened water, which is high in sodium. Water may need to be obtained from another source, or a water distiller may be needed.

Suggest alternatives for seasoning to enhance the taste of foods and to increase dietary compliance. Adding fresh lemon to vegetables and main dishes, condiments that come in powder form (such as garlic), or other low-sodium seasonings that can be found at food stores can improve taste. *People taking ACE inhibitors cannot use potassium salt substitutes.*

If fluids are restricted, help the client and family plan for how fluids can be spaced. Recognize the cultural variations in fluid consumption. In Western society, offering a guest something to drink is a common practice and may influence total fluid consumption.

The client should be weighed daily. Instruct the client and family to notify the physician if weight gain of more than 3 pounds per week is noted, a marked reduction in urine output occurs, or if increased shortness of breath with exertion or especially at rest is seen. Other reasons to call the physician include new-onset headaches, confusion, seizures, or a deterioration in level of consciousness.

INTRACELLULAR FLUID VOLUME EXCESS: WATER INTOXICATION

Although the cells are usually resistant to fluid shifts, certain conditions can lead to an intracellular fluid volume excess (ICFVE). Conditions that cause acute or severe fluid volume excesses have a higher incidence of ICF overload. This is because the adaptive mechanisms may be unable to compensate for large or sudden fluid excesses.

ICFVE results from either water excess or solute deficit, primarily sodium. In water excess, the number of solutes is normal but they are diluted by excessive water. In solute deficit, the amount of water is normal but there are too few particles per liter of water.

The most common cause of ICFVE is the administration of excessive amounts of hypo-osmolar IV fluids, such as 0.45% (half-strength) saline solution or 5% dextrose in water (D_5W). ICFVE may occur in clients who receive continuous IV D_5W or in older clients who consume excessive amounts of tap water without adequate nutrient intake. Syndrome of inappropriate antidiuretic hormone (SIADH) also leads to ICFVE regardless of whether the SIADH is caused by CNS trauma, the stress of surgery, pain, or opioid use.

People with certain psychiatric disorders, such as schizophrenia, often have compulsive water consumption behaviors, which can lead to water intoxication. Monitor for compulsive water consumption in people with a history or current manifestations of an organic psychiatric illness.

Hypo-osmolar fluids in the vessels move by osmosis to the region of higher concentration of sodium in the cells in an attempt to maintain equilibrium. Too much fluid accumulating in the cells causes cellular edema. Cerebral cells absorb hypo-osmolar fluid more quickly than do other cells. Thus, these cell changes often present the earliest warning signs of intracellular shifting.

All neurologic manifestations are secondary to the increasing intracranial pressure (ICP). Most ICP syndromes progress in a cephalocaudal order. Thus, the early signs, such as changes in mental status, are seen in the brain and, as pressure increases to below the cortex, pupillary changes occur. Vital sign changes begin when the pressure is at the level of the hypothalamus and brain stem (late stages of ICP increase).

Because ICF excess is often associated with ECF excess, it is common to see a plasma sodium level of less than 125 mEq/L and a decreased hematocrit. However, there is no plasma test to reflect the cell fluid volume. Diagnostic tests, such as computed tomography and mag-

netic resonance imaging, are more helpful in identifying causes underlying the syndrome of ICFVE.

Neurologic cells are vulnerable to fluid excess or deficit. The first priority is to reduce ICP with steroids and osmotic diuretics. Equally as important is identifying and addressing the cause of the fluid volume excess. Immediate surgical intervention may be critical.

If SIADH is an impending risk, early administration of IV fluids containing some sodium chloride (NaCl) may prevent it. Saline solutions, such as $D_5/0.45\%$ NaCl, increase the osmolality of vascular fluid and prevent or help correct hypo-osmolality.

Because brain tissue has a narrow margin in which life is sustained, frequent monitoring and early intervention are critical. Perform neurologic checks, including level of consciousness, vital signs, reflexes, and pupillary responses, every hour if cranial changes are present. Cerebral perfusion is altered if systolic blood pressure drops too low or rises too high. Notify the provider if the client's sensorium changes from the baseline assessment, if systolic blood pressure is less than 100 mm Hg or greater than 160 mm Hg, or if other signs persist or worsen.

Monitor IV fluids and I & O hourly, and monitor weight daily. Polyuria is a good sign and indicates that fluid has shifted to the vascular space and to the renal tubules, where it can be excreted. Administer antiemetics prophylactically, as appropriate, to promote food and fluid ingestion and retention and to decrease the risk of vomiting, which worsens the increased ICP.

Provide safety measures when the client displays behavioral changes, such as confusion or disorientation. Keep the bed in a low position with bedside rails raised. Keep suction equipment at the bedside in anticipation of seizures. If a client has a seizure, protect the client from injury and maintain airway patency by turning the client to one side to displace the tongue. Remain at the bedside until the client is safe and document all phases of the seizure.

If the manifestations of increased ICP are improving, then the client is at less risk for complications. *Time equals brain cell survival.* The longer the manifestations of increased ICP persist and the more serious they are, the graver the prognosis.

EXTRACELLULAR FLUID VOLUME SHIFT: THIRD-SPACING

An extracellular fluid volume shift is basically a change in the location of ECF between the intravascular and the interstitial spaces. Fluid shifts are of two types: (1) *vascular* fluid shifts to interstitial spaces and (2) *interstitial* fluid shifts to vascular spaces. Fluid that shifts into the interstitial spaces and remains there is referred to as *third-space fluid.* This abnormal fluid accumulation not only results from pathologic conditions but also reflects an inability of the lymphatic system to compensate. Common sites of third-spacing include the pleural cavity, peritoneal cavity, and pericardial sac. Third-space fluid is physiologically useless because it does not circulate to provide nutrients for cells.

Etiology

Fluids can move into interstitial spaces because of increased hydrostatic pressure, increased capillary permeability, decreased serum protein levels, obstruction of the venous portion of the capillary, or nonfunctional lymphatic drainage systems.

Any pathologic process that triggers the inflammatory or ischemic processes can lead to fluid shifting. For example, massive fluid shifts from the vascular to the interstitial spaces can be seen in crush injuries, major tissue trauma, major surgery, extensive burns, acid-base imbalance, bowel obstruction, and sepsis.

Decreased protein intake, production, or storage, or increased loss as seen in protein-calorie malnutrition and in liver and kidney disease can lead to hypoalbuminemia. Bowel disorders that reduce protein absorption can reduce serum levels. Other conditions that cause a loss of protein, such as large draining wounds or burns, also deplete protein stores. Increased protein anabolism can occur in the healing phase of fractures or wounds; increased protein catabolism can occur with fever, infection or sepsis, and malignancy.

Altered lymphatic function and venous thrombosis impair fluid return to the right atrium, thus promoting third-spacing. The decreased colloidal osmotic pressures from the impaired protein synthesis, as noted earlier, is only compounded by the portal hypertension that accompanies end-stage liver disease, leading to third-spacing in the peritoneal cavity (ascites).

Pathophysiology

Tissue injury causes the release of histamine and bradykinin, resulting in increased capillary permeability, which allows more fluid, protein, and other solutes to move into the interstitial spaces than normal. This form of fluid shift may be time-limited. The early stages of inflammation last about 24 to 48 hours; the capillary membrane heals and the fluid returns to the venous system. It may take longer in conditions with prolonged inflammatory responses or severe tissue injury.

Protein malnutrition leads to fluid shifts because protein is not present to pull fluid back into the capillary at the venous end. This form of fluid shifting is usually long term and can be seen in children who are malnourished and have large protruding abdomens and pencil-thin legs.

Two phases of fluid shift are associated with tissue injury:

1. Fluid shifts from vascular to interstitial spaces, which leads to a risk for fluid volume deficit *(hypovolemia)* (see Figure 13-3, *D*). Severe hypo-

volemia may lead to vascular collapse and death. If cellular damage is severe, a toxic response may occur from intracellular ions, such as potassium, which leak into the vascular spaces.

2. As the capillary membrane heals, fluid shifts back from the interstitial to the vascular space, which leads to a risk for fluid volume excess *(hypervolemia)*. If the hypervolemia is severe, it may lead to heart failure. Intracellular potassium ions shift back into the cell during this phase, which increases the risk for hypokalemia.

Clinical Manifestations

Clinical manifestations of a fluid shift from the vascular to the interstitial spaces are similar to the manifestations of hypovolemia because the fluid is not in the vascular system. Typical clinical manifestations include pallor, cold limbs, weak and rapid pulse, hypotension, oliguria, and decreased levels of consciousness. Body weight does not change because fluid has not been lost; it has been redistributed. Severe losses can result in hypovolemic shock.

If fluid collects and obstructs an organ, nerve, or vessel, other clinical manifestations may arise. For example, bowel sounds may change throughout the abdomen. Extremities may become pale, cool, and pulseless if fluid obstructs blood vessels or nerves. Laboratory results may indicate an elevated hematocrit, sodium, BUN, and urine specific gravity.

When fluid returns to the blood vessels, the clinical manifestations are similar to those of fluid overload. Signs may include a bounding pulse, crackles, engorgement of peripheral and jugular veins, and an increase in blood pressure. Laboratory results may indicate a decrease in hematocrit and BUN. Other abnormal findings depend on the area of the body affected.

Outcome Management

As with fluid volume deficit and fluid volume excess, third-spacing is only a manifestation. It is crucial that the underlying cause be identified through a thorough history and physical examination so that interventions can be targeted to the desired outcomes.

Medical treatment begins with determining the cause of the fluid volume shift. If the third-spacing of fluid has occurred around the heart (pericardial effusion), lung (pleural effusion), or in the peritoneal cavity (ascites), the physician removes the excess fluid by tapping the space with a large-bore needle); these procedures are known as pericardiocentesis, thoracentesis, and paracentesis, respectively.

Replace Fluids

When hypovolemia results from tissue injury, such as burns or crush injuries, a large volume of isotonic IV fluid administration is required to replace intravascular volume. When there is evidence of capillary healing (increase in urine output without additional fluids), albumin may be given to replace the protein lost from the trauma and to promote restoration of capillary oncotic pressures. Because third-spacing is a common occurrence after major surgery, maintaining IV fluid intake is essential to maintaining kidney perfusion. The amount of fluid infusion may be three times greater than urine output. Generally, fluids are titrated to maintain an adequate blood pressure, CVP, PCWP, and urine output. During the first 24 to 72 hours when there is an increase in ADH and the healing phase is beginning with fluid moving back into the vessels, the client is at risk for fluid overload if the fluid replacement is too rapid.

Stabilize Other Problems

Some etiologies of fluid shifting are life-threatening and must be treated aggressively. For example, sepsis causes major increases in capillary permeability and must be treated with IV antibiotics and, usually, vasoactive medications to maintain blood pressure. Bowel obstructions can cause major third-spacing and lead to gangrene; surgical repair is critical. Serious inflammatory disorders require massive doses of steroids to stabilize the mast cell membrane.

■ Nursing Management of the Medical Client

If shock-like symptoms are present, assess vital signs every hour until the blood pressure is greater than 90 mm Hg; progress up to every 8 hours as the client's condition stabilizes. If fluid loss is a result of ascites or peripheral edema, the fluid shift is slower and changes in vital signs are usually subtle.

Monitor IV fluid replacement needs. If fluids are administered too rapidly, fluid overload or hypervolemia may occur. Assess for early signs of fluid overload, such as crackles, difficulty in breathing, and neck vein engorgement. Notify the physician if these signs are present. Anticipate a reduction in IV fluid needs as the third-space fluid shifts back into the plasma during the capillary repair stage.

If the third-spacing is in the abdomen, as with ascites, measure the client's abdominal girth every 8 hours. If a limb is involved, measure the circumference of the limb and assess peripheral pulses every 8 hours. Use preventive measures to prevent skin breakdown of edematous areas.

Monitor urine output every hour, and report an output of less than 0.5 ml/kg/hr if it persists for more than 2 hours. The client may need more fluids, not diuretics. Urine output is usually reduced after tissue injury because of decreased renal circulation and a fluid shift into the injured tissue spaces. One to 3 days after tissue injury, fluid returns to the circulation and the kidneys excrete excess fluid unless renal function is impaired, the injury was massive, or the client has impaired adaptive mechanisms. Monitor plasma levels of BUN and creatinine.

CONCLUSIONS

Fluid imbalances are common problems, especially in high-risk populations, such as older adults and clients with acute illnesses or multiple pathologic processes. Many health care disciplines work collaboratively toward maintaining or restoring fluid balance. The role of nursing in this collaborative effort is focused on health promotion activities, including teaching positive health behaviors, health maintenance activities (including early detection and consultation with other disciplines), and prevention and early detection of complications from the underlying diseases, coexisting conditions, or treatment. Through these interventions, the nurse plays a critical role in assisting clients and their families achieve positive health outcomes.

THINKING CRITICALLY *evolve*

1. The admitting department has just called your floor to secure a room for a 59-year-old woman with a history of 2 days of vomiting and diarrhea and a temperature of 103° F secondary to suspected influenza virus. The client has a past medical history of hypertension and heart failure. Home prescriptions include digoxin, 0.125 mg/day; furosemide (Lasix), 40 mg bid; and potassium chloride, 40 mEq/day. The client has also been advised to consume a low-sodium diet. An IV line of D_5/NS with 30 mEq of potassium chloride was started.
Factors to Consider. What is the priority risk/problem for this client? What are the desired outcomes? What are the critical assessments? What medical management and nursing strategies do you anticipate?

2. A middle-aged client is admitted to your unit with shock-like symptoms from a massive burn wound. He has pale skin, cold limbs, hypotension, and a weak, rapid pulse. Urine output via the indwelling catheter is decreased. His level of consciousness varies from an

adequate response to little or no response to external stimuli.

Factors to Consider. What is the priority risk or problem in this scenario? What are the desired outcomes? What are the critical assessments? What medical management and nursing strategies do you anticipate during this phase of fluid shifting from the vascular spaces to the interstitial spaces? How will they change when the fluid shifts back into the vascular spaces?

Discussions for these questions can be found on the website and the CD-ROM.

BIBLIOGRAPHY

1. Arief, I. (1999). Fatal postoperative pulmonary edema: Pathogenesis and literature review. *Chest, 115*(5), 1371-1377.
2. Bennett, J. (2000). Dehydration: Hazards and benefits. *Geriatric Nursing, 21*(2), 84-88.
3. Casa, D.J. (1999). Exercise in heat: I. Fundamentals of thermal physiology, performance implications, and dehydration. *Journal of Athletic Training, 34*(3), 246-252.
4. Cooper, A., & Moore, M. (1999). IV fluid therapy. *Australian Nursing Journal, 7*(5), 2-4.
5. Edwards, S. (2001). Regulation of water, sodium and potassium: Implications for practice. *Nursing Standard, 15*(22), 36-42.
 6. Galloway, S.D. (1999). Dehydration, rehydration, and exercise in the heat: Rehydration strategies for the athletic competition. *Canadian Journal of Applied Physiology, 24*(2), 188-200.
7. Hamilton, S. (2001). Detecting dehydration malnutrition in the elderly. *Nursing, 31*(12), 56-57.
8. Huether, S., & McCance, K. (2000). *Understanding pathophysiology* (2nd ed.) St. Louis: Mosby.
9. Iggulden, H. (1999). Dehydration and electrolyte disturbance. *Elderly Care, 11*(3), 17-23.
10. Innis, J. (2002). Treating nephrogenic diabetes insipidus. *Dimensions of Critical Care Nursing, 21*(3), 98-99.
11. Kayser-Jones, J., et al. (1999). Factors contributing to dehydration in nursing homes: Inadequate staffing and lack of professional supervision. *Journal of the American Geriatric Society, 47*(10), 1187-1194.
12. Maughan, R.J. (1999). Exercise in the heat: Limitations to performance and the impact of fluid replacement strategies. *Canadian Journal of Applied Physiology, 24*(2), 149-151.
13. May D.L. (1998). The relationship between self-induced water intoxication and severity of psychiatric symptoms. *Archives of Psychiatric Nursing, 12*(6), 335-343.
14. McAulay, D. (2001). Dehydration in the terminally ill patient. *Nursing Standard, 16*(4), 33-37.
15. Mentes, J. (2000). Hydration management protocol. *Journal of Gerontological Nursing, 26*(10), 6-15.
16. Primrose, W.R., et al. (1999). Indices of dehydration in elderly people. *Age Ageing 28*(4), 411-412.
17. Sansevero, A. (1997). Dehydration in the elderly: Strategies for prevention and management. *Nurse Practitioner, 22*(4), 41-70.
18. Schmidt, T. (2000). Assessing a sodium and fluid imbalance. *Nursing, 30*(1), 18.
19. Smith, S., & Andrews, M. (2000). Artificial nutrition and hydration at the end of life. *Medical Surgical Nursing, 9*(5), 233-247.
20. Zembrzuski, C. (2000). Nutrition and hydration. *Journal of Gerontological Nursing, 26*(12), 6-7.

Clients with Electrolyte Imbalances

Bernadette White

evolve

Web Enhancements

Bridge to Home Health Care
  Managing Intravenous Therapy
Appendix A
  Religious Beliefs and Practices Affecting Health Care

http://evolve.elsevier.com/Black/medsurg/

Appendix C
  Laboratory Values of Clinical Importance in Medical-Surgical Nursing

ELECTROLYTE IMBALANCES

Electrolytes are various chemicals that can carry positive or negative electrical charges. Electrolytes exist in the blood as acids, bases, and salts (such as sodium, calcium, potassium, chlorine, magnesium, and bicarbonate) and can be measured by laboratory studies of the plasma. Electrolytes are important because they are what cells (especially nerve, heart, muscle) use to maintain voltages across their cell membranes and to carry electrical impulses (nerve impulses, muscle contractions) across themselves and to other cells. The kidneys work to keep the electrolyte concentrations in the blood constant despite changes in the body. For example, when a person exercises heavily, electrolytes are lost in the sweat, particularly sodium and potassium. These electrolytes must be replaced to keep the electrolyte concentrations of body fluids constant.

An electrolyte imbalance is present whenever there is an excess or deficit in the plasma level of a specific ion. Terms used to describe the imbalance contain the prefix *hyper-* for increased or *hypo-* for decreased, followed by the name of the electrolyte (in its Latin form for sodium and potassium) and then the suffix *-emia* to indicate presence in the blood, as measured in the plasma. For example, *hyponatremia* means low plasma sodium, and *hyperkalemia* means elevated plasma potassium. *Hyper-*

calcemia and *hypermagnesemia* indicate elevated calcium and magnesium levels, respectively.

Electrolyte imbalances are common, so to help clients achieve the most positive health outcomes, you must understand the underlying causative disorders and conditions as well as the risk factors for electrolyte imbalance and become an active participant in health promotion, health maintenance, and health restoration interventions.

Etiology and Risk Factors

Anyone who has decreased intake, decreased availability, or increased loss of electrolytes is at risk for electrolyte deficit. When body fluids are lost, the electrolytes in them are also lost. For example, the loss of gastric juice through vomiting may lead to the loss of several electrolytes. Conversely, increased intake or increased retention of an electrolyte or decreased ability to excrete certain electrolytes may increase the risk for electrolyte excess. For example, ingestion of excess sodium bicarbonate for indigestion can alter both sodium level and acid-base balance.

Pathophysiology

Before you can fully understand the pathophysiology of electrolyte imbalances, you need to first understand the physiology of the action potential. Conduction of electrical current depends on normal membrane

evolve *Be sure to check out the bonus material on the Evolve website and the CD-ROM, including free self-assessment exercises.*

http://evolve.elsevier.com/Black/medsurg/

permeability, transportation of electrolytes, and ion concentrations. Common problems that alter the conduction of electrical current include problems with membrane permeability, ionic gradients, and concentrations.

Cells are quickly damaged by lack of blood flow or oxygen. Cardiac, nerve, and muscle cells can be damaged by lack of blood flow (as during periods of ischemia), altered by toxins (as from various medications), or directly injured (as in crush or stab injuries). Such damage typically increases the permeability of the cell membrane and increases its tendency to "fire." This phenomenon can be seen in cardiac cells after ischemia. Cardiac cells that normally do not generate action potentials begin to do so, causing abnormal heart rhythms. This same phenomenon can be the cause of seizures following brain injury.

Potassium levels can significantly influence the resting membrane potential (Figure 14-1). When potassium levels are lower than normal, the resting membrane potential becomes more positive. It requires less stimulus to make it fire. Cells so affected are called *hypopolarized* and respond to a weaker stimulus. Conversely, when potassium levels are higher, the resting membrane potential decreases and the cell is less excitable. Such cells are called *hyperpolarized* and require a stronger-than-normal stimulus to reach threshold potential and to generate an action potential. Sodium and calcium also alter resting membrane potential.

Diagnosis

A wide range of clinical manifestations should raise suspicion about a possible electrolyte imbalance (see the Critical Monitoring feature on Fluid and Electrolyte Imbalance Secondary to Any Disorder/Condition on p. 225). The diagnosis of electrolyte imbalance is made through clinical assessment and measurement of plasma levels in laboratory studies. Currently, measurement of intracellular levels of electrolytes is too costly; thus, plasma levels are used for diagnostic evaluation.

Plasma values for electrolytes can be expressed as milliequivalents per liter (mEq/L), or milligrams per deciliter (mg/dl). Values reported as mEq/L can be converted to mg/dl by multiplying by 1.2.

Using a "Collaborative Problem" Format

Currently there are no NANDA diagnoses for electrolyte imbalances. The Iowa Interventions Project approached these disorders as collaborative problems and developed a research-based list of critical and supporting activities for management of 15 fluid and electrolyte disorders. Because the nursing role primarily involves collaborating with the physician, the goal statements are also phrased differently. Note that each expected outcome is preceded by the phrase "The nurse will monitor the client for." Nursing diagnoses that may apply to clients with electrolyte imbalances include *Risk for Injury, Risk for Ac-*

tivity Intolerance, Risk for Decreased Cardiac Output, Impaired Oral Mucous Membranes, and *Risk for Impaired Skin Integrity.* Or you may use the appropriate collaborative problem taxonomy to identify the problem—*hyponatremia* or *hypernatremia, hypokalemia* or *hyperkalemia, hypocalcemia* or *hypercalcemia, hypomagnesemia* or *hypermagnesemia,* and *hypophosphatemia* or *hyperphosphatemia.*

SODIUM IMBALANCES

Sodium deficit is known as *hyponatremia;* sodium excess is known as *hypernatremia.* Chloride is the anion that usually accompanies sodium; therefore levels of chloride decrease or increase along with levels of sodium. Mani-

FIGURE 14-1 Electrocardiographic changes seen in potassium imbalances. (From Huether, S., & McCance, K. [2000]. *Understanding pathophysiology* [2nd ed.]. St. Louis: Mosby.)

festations of chloride imbalance are usually associated with the cation imbalance. Any condition that alters the renin-angiotensin-aldosterone system, kinin system, or atrial natriuretic or antidiuretic hormonal response places a person at risk for sodium imbalances.

HYPONATREMIA

Natrium is the Latin word for sodium. Hyponatremia is defined as a plasma sodium level less than 135 mEq/L. It is one of the most common electrolyte disorders in adults, especially older adults. Hyponatremia is usually associated with changes in fluid volume status. The four types of hyponatremic states are as follows:

- Hypovolemic hyponatremia
- Euvolemic hyponatremia
- Hypervolemic hyponatremia
- Redistributive hyponatremia

When sodium loss is greater than water loss, *hypovolemic hyponatremia* occurs. *Euvolemic hyponatremia* results when the total body water (TBW) is moderately increased and the total body sodium remains at a normal level. *Hypervolemic hyponatremia* results when a greater increase occurs in TBW than in total body sodium. In *redistributive hyponatremia,* no change occurs in TBW or total body sodium; water merely shifts between the intracellular and extracellular compartments relative to the sodium concentration.

Etiology and Risk Factors

Table 14-1 lists the most common pathophysiologic causes of hyponatremia. Hyponatremia can also occur in persons who are considered healthy. For example, athletes and outdoor laborers are at risk for hyponatremia from excessive perspiration. Any person with an altered thirst mechanism or without access to fluids, or one who attempts to rehydrate too rapidly after excessive fluid loss, is at risk for hyponatremia. Older adults are at increased risk because of their relatively lower percentage of TBW. The preoperative use of laxatives, multiple pathologic conditions, spinal anesthesia, and noninfectious postoperative complications increase risk factors for death from hyponatremia in older adults after surgery.

With cardiac, renal, and liver disease, the total body sodium is usually high, although the plasma sodium level may appear normal or low because of dilution from water retention. In such instances, the increase in TBW is generally greater than the sodium level indicates. Renal causes of hyponatremia stem from the inability to excrete sufficiently dilute urine. Normally, when hyponatremia and hypo-osmolality occur, diuresis follows to promote the return of sodium and water levels to homeostasis.

Pathophysiology

Most pathophysiologic changes caused by hyponatremia result from the decreased excitability of the membranes

TABLE 14-1	*Clinical Conditions and Disorders That May Cause Hyponatremia*
Type of Hyponatremia	**Clinical Conditions and Disorders**
Hypovolemic hyponatremia	Renal loss of sodium from diuretic use, diabetic glycosuria, aldosterone deficiency, intrinsic renal disease
	Extrarenal loss of sodium from vomiting, diarrhea, increased sweating, burns, high-volume ileostomy
Euvolemic hyponatremia	Sodium deficit resulting from SIADH or the increased secretion of ADH due to pain, emotion, medications; some cancers and CNS disorders
Hypervolemic hyponatremia	Edematous disorders resulting in sodium deficits; congestive heart failure, cirrhosis of the liver, nephrotic syndrome, acute and chronic renal failure
Redistributive hyponatremia	Pseudohyponatremia, hyperglycemia, hyperlipidemia

ADH, Antidiuretic hormone; *CNS,* central nervous system; *SIADH,* syndrome of inappropriate (secretion of) antidiuretic hormone.

from a loss of sodium and changes in water volume. Recall that most sodium is outside the cell. Less sodium is available to move across the excitable membrane, resulting in delayed membrane depolarization. Excitable tissues vary in their response to decreased sodium. The cells most sensitive to change are the central nervous system (CNS) cells.

As the concentration of sodium decreases in the extracellular fluid (ECF), the difference in gradient between the ECF and intracellular fluid (ICF) compartments also decreases. When the extracellular sodium level decreases, the ECF becomes hypo-osmolar. This osmotic shift can lead to intracellular edema. Water moves into the cell to the area of greater concentration to rebalance the water concentration. An increase in brain cell volume as small as 5% can cause brain herniation. Brain cells attempt to compensate by reducing cerebral blood flow, shifting cerebral spinal fluid, and decreasing the brain's intracellular osmolality. Intracellular osmolality is reduced through decreasing the amount of intracellular ions, such as sodium and potassium, and amino acids.

Clinical Manifestations

Clinical manifestations of hyponatremia vary with the cause, type, and rate of onset of sodium or fluid imbalance. A person with a plasma sodium level of 120 mEq/L that developed slowly may be asymptomatic. The same plasma sodium level resulting from an acute loss may be life-threatening.

EB When plasma sodium concentration is greater than 125 mEq/L, clinical manifestations may not be apparent. Early neurologic manifestations of headache and apprehension are from increased fluid shift into the cerebral cells. As intracranial pressure increases and plasma sodium level decreases to 115 mEq/L, severe neurologic changes such as confusion, hallucinations, behavioral changes, and seizures occur. Continued shifting of water into the intracellular compartment leads to brain herniation, resulting in coma and death.

Cardiovascular manifestations—such as a decrease in systolic and diastolic blood pressures, orthostatic hypotension, and a weak, thready pulse—are due to a decrease in vascular volume secondary to sodium and water loss. Tachycardia is a compensatory response that is the direct result of triggering of the release of sympathetic catecholamines by the baroreceptor reflex. Chemoreceptors in the aortic arch and carotid bodies also trigger sympathetic responses if the oxygen, carbon dioxide, or hydrogen levels become affected. In severe hypovolemic hyponatremia, a shock-like state occurs, with blood pressures of 60 mm Hg and below. An exception is hypervolemic hyponatremia, in which the excess volume causes elevated blood pressure and a full, rapid pulse.

Crackles in the lungs are from fluid shifting into the pulmonary alveoli secondary to increasing fluid pressures in the pulmonary capillaries. The increasing left ventricular fluid pressure leads to a retrograde increase in pressure in the left atrium and pulmonary vasculature. The changes in respiratory rate and difficulty breathing—such as tachypnea, dyspnea, orthopnea, and feeling short of breath—are from presence of fluid in the alveoli, which alters oxygen and carbon dioxide exchange. Alterations in respiratory pattern, such as with Cheyne-Stokes respirations, neurogenic hyperventilation, apneustic breathing, or ataxic breathing, are from progressive increases in intracranial pressure.

Hyponatremia causes gastrointestinal (GI) manifestations, such as nausea, vomiting, hyperactive bowel sounds, abdominal cramping, and diarrhea, because sodium is a crucial component of normal neuromuscular activity of smooth muscle. A decrease in sodium causes increased excitability of the neurons that innervate the smooth muscle.

Although not life-threatening, the dryness of the skin, tongue, and mucous membranes that results from the decreased interstitial volume caused by a sodium deficit has other, more serious implications. There is a higher risk for altered integrity of the skin and oral mucous membranes, which increases the risk of infection and results in increased health care needs and costs.

A laboratory finding of a plasma sodium level less than 135 mEq/L is diagnostic of hyponatremia. However, as noted previously, most clients are not symptomatic until levels reach 125 mEq/L or less. Because chloride is the main anion associated with sodium, a chloride level less than 98 mEq/L is a common finding. A decreased concentration of sodium is also reflected in a plasma osmolality of less than 275 mOsm/kg. The kidney attempts to compensate for the body's loss of sodium by decreasing urinary losses; thus, a typical urine sodium level is less than 40 mEq/L. If the hyponatremic state and body fluid volume disorders are not corrected, potassium, calcium, chloride, and bicarbonate electrolyte imbalances may also occur.

Outcome Management
■ Medical Management

Medical management is determined by the cause of the hyponatremia, the type of hyponatremia, and the severity of the clinical manifestations. The more serious the manifestations, the more aggressive the treatment. The goal of medical intervention is correction of the body water osmolality, with restoration of cell volume, by raising the ratio of sodium to water in the ECF. The increased ECF osmolality draws water from the cells, thereby decreasing cellular edema.

Restore Sodium Levels. Fluids are restricted to allow the sodium to regain balance. Intake of balanced diet is usually adequate therapy for mild hyponatremia, with sodium levels of 126 to 135 mEq/L. Fluids may be restricted to a range of 1000 to 1500 ml/day.

If the plasma sodium level declines below 125 mEq/L, sodium replacement is needed. For sodium levels of 125 mEq/L or less, intravenous (IV) therapy is the treatment of choice. Dietary supplementation may still be appropriate for a client who can ingest oral fluids or food. Foods high in sodium are listed in Box 14-1. For moderate hyponatremia, with sodium levels of 125 mEq/L, IV normal saline solution (0.9% NaCl) or lactated Ringer's solution may be ordered if the client is symptomatic. When the plasma sodium level is 115 mEq/L or less, a concentrated saline solution such as 3% NaCl may be indicated until the plasma sodium reaches 125 mEq/L. A diuretic such as furosemide is often given intravenously to prevent pulmonary fluid overload. Demeclocycline, an agent that antagonizes antidiuretic hormone (ADH), is the preferred agent for treatment of hyponatremia resulting from syndrome of inappropriate antidiuretic hormone (SIADH).

Rapid elevation of plasma sodium concentrations to more than 125 mEq/L increases intravascular fluid volume and may result in hypernatremia and CNS damage. Recommendations for IV replacement therapy include an infusion rate of 0.5 mEq/L/hr if the loss is chronic, not to exceed a total of 12 mEq of sodium in 48 hours, or of 1 mEq/L/hr if the loss is acute, not to exceed 25 mEq in 48 hours. To prevent fluid shifts and exacerbation of vasospasm in persons with subarachnoid hemorrhage, normal saline is usually the IV solution of choice.

■ Nursing Management of the Medical Client
Assessment

Take a complete history of risk factors and presenting manifestations. Collect complete and detailed information on the client's diet and medications, including over-the-counter and herbal medications. Older adults are especially susceptible to drug-drug interactions that may alter sodium balance. The client and family members should be asked about behavioral changes, headaches, increased weakness or sleepiness, dizziness, and palpitations.

Measure the client's body weight, because the stated weight may not be accurate. Compare the client's height and weight to the body mass index (BMI) chart. Measure the client's waist circumference and compare to recommendations of less than 35 inches for women and less than 40 inches for men. Assess intake and output, peripheral vein filling time, and vital signs every 4 to 8 hours. Also, monitor plasma sodium levels and estimate the plasma osmolality. It is important to remember that in hyponatremic conditions, such as hypervolemic hyponatremia, plasma sodium levels may appear to be normal to low.

Diagnosis, Outcomes, Interventions

Collaborative Problem: Risk for Hyponatremia. The collaborative problem of *Risk for Hyponatremia* can be used to label this client problem. State the problem as *Risk for Hyponatremia related to unreplaced loss or limited oral intake.* When actual hyponatremia is present, the collaborative problem is stated as *Hyponatremia related to* (e.g., *vomiting, diarrhea, gastric suctioning, burns, SIADH, surgery, or fluid overload*). The cause needs to be clear because it relates directly to the interventions.

Outcomes. The nurse will have a high index of suspicion for high-risk clients and will monitor clients who have had fluid losses or limited fluid intake for manifestations of hyponatremia. When assessment indicates an actual sodium deficit, restoration is the primary goal. An outcome may be as follows: The nurse will monitor laboratory sodium and chloride levels and will continue to monitor for clinical manifestations of hyponatremia.

Interventions

Reduce Sodium Loss in High-Risk Clients. If plasma sodium levels are greater than 125 mEq/L, encourage intake of 30 to 60 ml of clear liquids or more per hour as tolerated. If the client is on a low-sodium diet, do not be concerned about sodium restriction until the vomiting or diarrhea subsides and the client is taking whole foods.

BOX 14-1 *High-Sodium and Low-Sodium Foods*

High-Sodium Foods (approximately 250 mg/serving)

Breads
Cereals: most instant hot & cold cereals
Chips
Cheeses: all types
Meats: sausage, luncheon, frankfurters, bacon, ham
Convenience foods: pizza, pot pies, ravioli, soups (may have up to 5 times this amount)
Most fast food items have 1 to 5 times this amount

Low-Sodium Foods (<50 mg/serving)

Fruits: fresh, frozen, canned
Vegetables: fresh, frozen, canned
Low salt breads
Unsalted pastas
Oatmeal, cooked
Unsalted popcorn
Puffed rice
Shredded wheat
Fresh meat, chicken, fish (1 oz)

Data from Mahan, L.K., & Escott-Stump, S. (2000). *Krause's food, nutrition, and diet therapy* (10th ed.). Philadelphia: W.B. Saunders.

To prevent sodium loss, irrigate nasogastric tubes and wounds with isotonic saline and give only minimal ice chips, even if ordered, when a nasogastric tube is connected to suction. Never give more than three tap water enemas in succession without consulting the physician about converting the enema solution to normal saline. Treat nausea with prophylactic antiemetics. Consult the physician if (1) the sodium level is less than 125 mEq/L or sooner if the client is symptomatic or (2) the client is receiving nothing by mouth (NPO status) and has no intake of electrolytes or has an increased loss of electrolytes.

Restore Sodium Balance. Encourage the intake of a well-balanced diet. Give nutrient-dense supplements between meals. If the client is receiving nutrition only through tube feedings, it is sometimes necessary to add extra salt to the feeding to achieve the desired sodium level. If the hyponatremia is secondary to hypervolemia, consult with the physician and dietitian to coordinate therapeutic fluid restriction. Strict behavioral modification or psychiatric consultation may be necessary for a client who drinks water compulsively.

To decrease the thirst that accompanies fluid restriction, offer ice chips, cold fluids, and frequent oral care. Some clients feel less thirsty if they hold the fluids in their mouth first to fully moisten the oral mucous membranes before swallowing. Restricting fluids is contraindicated in persons with subarachnoid hemorrhage because it increases the risk of cerebral vasospasm and cell death.

When plasma sodium levels are 125 mEq/L or less and the client is symptomatic, notify the physician immediately. Administration of hypertonic IV saline (3% saline) is the most commonly prescribed therapy. *Caution:* Hypertonic saline must be given very slowly by IV piggyback infusion in a large vein to decrease the risk of hypernatremia, pulmonary overload, and phlebitis. If the client is confused or agitated, also initiate safety and seizure precautions.

Evaluation

Mild to moderate deficits are usually corrected in 8 to 24 hours. More severe deficits may take several days, especially in older adults. Evaluate the client's and family members' understanding of positive health behaviors that prevent further occurrences of sodium deficit.

■ Self-Care

Teach the client to consult the physician if vomiting or diarrhea persists for more than 48 hours, or sooner if extreme weakness, dizziness, palpitations, irregular pulse of new onset, cough or dyspnea, or CNS changes (such as headache, confusion, or seizures) develop. Anyone who has a chronic disease—such as renal, liver, or heart disease or diabetes mellitus—should consult a physician if any manifestations persist for more than 24 hours.

Teach clients to consult a physician before taking over-the-counter or herbal medications. Review the exercise precautions discussed in Chapter 13. Refer people with eating disorders to counseling and community support groups.

HYPERNATREMIA

Hypernatremia is defined as a plasma sodium level greater than 145 mEq/L. It occurs in about 1% of hospitalized clients and carries a high mortality rate, whether it has an acute or a chronic onset. Hypernatremia is usually associated with water loss or sodium gain. It can occur with increased, decreased, or normal total body sodium levels and decreased or increased TBW levels. The underlying cause of hypernatremia is a TBW deficit relative to the total body sodium content, which results in hyperosmolality.

Etiology and Risk Factors

Body fluid loss resulting in hypernatremia may be from renal or extrarenal causes, such as GI or skin problems. Hypernatremia can be classified as one of three types:

- Hypovolemic hypernatremia, in which TBW is greatly decreased relative to sodium (loss of hypotonic fluid)
- Euvolemic hypernatremia, in which TBW is decreased relative to the normal total body sodium
- Hypervolemic hypernatremia, in which TBW is increased but the sodium gain exceeds the water gain

Hypervolemic hypernatremia is the least common type of hypernatremia. Table 14-2 presents clinical conditions and disorders that may contribute to the development of hypernatremia. Older adults and debilitated people are at highest risk for development of hypernatremia. Major risk factors include inadequate water intake in conjunction with decreased thirst (hypodipsia), lack of access to drinkable water, physical or chemical restraint, mental confusion, and NPO status. Excessive water loss and insufficient fluid replacement associated with fever, vomiting, diarrhea, excess drainage, polyuria, tube feeding, or prolonged hyperventilation are also major risk factors.

Other factors that increase the risk for hypernatremia include increased sodium intake, such as with IV administration of hypertonic saline or hypertonic tube feedings. Retention of sodium occurs in heart, renal, or liver disease; Cushing's syndrome; hyperaldosteronism; corticosteroid therapy; and uncontrolled diabetes mellitus or diabetes insipidus. Uncontrolled diabetes mellitus results in polyuria, leading to dehydration and secondary hypernatremia. Hypernatremia from untreated diabetes insipidus tends to be mild. Although the ADH mechanism is altered, the thirst mechanism is intact and stimulates the client to drink water and fluids, which helps balance water losses and hypernatremia.

TABLE 14-2	*Clinical Conditions and Disorders That May Contribute to Hypernatremia*
Type of Hypernatremia	**Clinical Conditions and Disorders**
Hypovolemic hypernatremia	Renal losses, osmotic diuresis, diuretics, severe hyperglycemia Extrarenal losses: profuse diaphoresis, decreased thirst, diarrhea occurring with inadequate volume replacement or fluid replacement with hyperosmolar solutions, burns
Euvolemic hypernatremia	Excess fluid losses from the skin and lungs Hypodipsia in older adults and infants Diabetes insipidus
Hypervolemic hypernatremia	Administration of concentrated saline solutions; hypertonic feedings; excess mineralocorticoids Accidental or intentional salt ingestion; commercially prepared soups and canned vegetables

Pathophysiology

When sodium levels increase, water moves to maintain balance. However, the osmotic shift of water from the cells to the ECF in an attempt to dilute the hyperosmolar state only creates another problem: cellular dehydration. If the hypernatremia evolves slowly or is chronic, the brain develops its own osmotic particles, called *idiogenic osmoles,* to prevent fluid shifts into and out of the brain cells.

The heart is sensitive to the increasing sodium levels. Calcium must move through the calcium channels for cardiac muscle contraction to occur. However, in hypernatremia, sodium molecules compete with calcium in the slow calcium channels of the heart, resulting in decreased myocardial contractility. Myocardial depolarization, however, occurs more easily with the increased sodium levels.

Generally, the body responds to increased sodium levels by suppressing the effects of aldosterone and ADH. These two substances normally act to increase renal blood flow and cause excretion of sodium and water. In hypernatremia, the magnitude of the problem overwhelms the ability of these adaptive mechanisms to compensate.

Clinical Manifestations

In the early stages of hypernatremia, clinical manifestations are nonspecific because two thirds of body water is intracellular; primary water losses tend to cause only modest effects on circulating blood volume. Early manifestations include polyuria followed by oliguria, anorexia, nausea, vomiting, weakness, and restlessness. The anorexia, nausea, and vomiting are related to increased fluid retention in the gastric cells. Early neurologic manifestations of restlessness, agitation, irritability, and muscle weakness are related to the sensitivity of brain cells to fluid shifting.

The response of the kidneys varies with the type of hypernatremia. In a hypervolemic state, the kidneys excrete some of the excess water. In a hypovolemic state, oliguria is the method of renal compensation. As fluid levels decrease in the interstitial compartments, the skin becomes dry and flushed, the mucous membranes become dry and sticky, and tongue furrows develop. The person experiences increasing thirst and fever. Temperature elevation is from the decreasing amount of fluid available for dissipating heat.

Cardiovascular manifestations are related to the type of hypernatremia. In hypovolemic hypernatremia, orthostatic hypotension with compensatory tachycardia occurs. In hypervolemic hypernatremia, a hypertensive blood pressure, jugular venous distention, prolonged peripheral vein emptying, S_3 gallop, and generalized weight gain and edema are often present.

Dysrhythmia can result from the competition of sodium ions with calcium ions in the slow channels of the heart cells. Pulmonary manifestations, such as crackles, dyspnea, and pleural effusion, are also due to the increasing hydrostatic pressure seen in hypervolemic hypernatremia.

When sodium levels reach 155 mEq/L or more, cells (especially brain cells) shrink because of the increased ECF osmolality. More severe neurologic changes occur, manifested as confusion, seizures, or coma, in some cases with irreversible brain damage. Altered neuromuscular contractility and irritability lead to muscle twitching, tremor, hyperreflexia, and seizures. The development of rigid paralysis is a grave sign.

The diagnosis of hypernatremia is validated when plasma sodium levels are greater than 145 mEq/L and plasma osmolality is more than 295 mOsm/kg. Because chloride is the major ECF ion that balances sodium, it is common to find a plasma chloride level greater than 106 mEq/L. Unless the sodium elevation is an acute change, many clients are not symptomatic until plasma sodium reaches 155 mEq/L or more.

Outcome Management

Again, a thorough history and physical examination, including laboratory studies, are necessary for accurate diagnosis of hypernatremia. Awareness of demographic variables is essential for choosing the appropriate interventions for restoring sodium balance.

■ Medical Management

Medical management is determined by the type of hypernatremia. The goal of medical intervention is correction of the body water osmolality, with restoration of cell volume, by decreasing the ratio of sodium to water in the ECF.

For a client experiencing minor manifestations from hypovolemia or euvolemic hypernatremia, the focus is on correcting the underlying disorder and giving oral fluid replacement. However, clients with cardiovascular, pulmonary, or neurologic manifestations from severe hypernatremia usually require hospitalization and the more aggressive approach of IV hypotonic saline.

To decrease total body sodium and replace fluid loss, either a hypo-osmolar electrolyte solution (0.2% or 0.45% NaCl) or 5% dextrose in water (D_5W) is administered. These solutions do not cause a considerable dilution of body sodium; instead, the plasma sodium level gradually decreases as excess sodium is excreted. When administered continuously, D_5W is considered to be a hypo-osmolar solution because the dextrose is metabolized quickly and only water remains. If the plasma sodium level is lowered too rapidly, fluid shifts from the vascular fluid into the cerebral cells, causing cerebral edema. Slow administration of IV fluids with a goal of reducing plasma sodium levels, at a rate of not more than 2 mEq/L/hr for the first 48 hours, decreases this risk.

Hypernatremia caused by sodium excess may be treated with administration of D_5W and a diuretic, such as furosemide. When hypernatremia results from diabetes insipidus, desmopressin acetate, in the form of a nasal spray, is commonly ordered to slow the rate of diuresis.

Although dietary sodium restriction is useful in preventing hypernatremia in high-risk clients, it cannot bring a high sodium level down to normal. People with renal disease may need sodium intake restricted to 500 to 2000 mg/day (see Box 14-1). In hypervolemic hypernatremia, fluids must also be restricted. Clients with diabetes insipidus who are receiving antidiuretic medications must be taught to avoid excessive water intake. Drinking excess water defeats the purpose of the medication.

■ Nursing Management of the Medical Client

Assessment

Assess for the usual clinical manifestations, especially in head-injured and other high-risk clients. Obtain a thorough diet and medication history, including the use of corticosteroids and over-the-counter medications, such as cough medicine, herbals, food flavorings and spices (salt).

Depending on the client's condition, assess vital signs and peripheral vein filling time every 4 to 8 hours, measure intake and output every 8 hours, and monitor body weight daily. Use oral membrane and skin assessment tools to guide your interventions. Monitor for changes in plasma sodium and plasma osmolality (by estimated values). Report early signs of altered mental status, such as agitation, irritability, or confusion that may indicate progression of hypernatremia or hyponatremia. Monitor lung sounds every 2 to 4 hours, and notify the physician of increasing pulmonary overload.

Diagnosis, Outcomes, Interventions

Collaborative Problem: Hypernatremia. Use a collaborative problem, such as *Hypernatremia related to* (e.g., *decreased thirst, excessive administration of salt solutions,* or *impaired excretion of sodium and water*). The cause needs to be identified specifically, because it guides the choice of interventions.

Outcomes. The nurse will maintain a high index of suspicion for high-risk clients and will monitor plasma sodium and chloride levels and clinical manifestations of hypernatremia.

Interventions. Monitor the client for response to IV fluid replacement of hypo-osmolar electrolyte solutions, absence of clinical manifestations of hypernatremia, and return to normal sodium levels. Prevent osmotic diuresis from D_5W by maintaining the prescribed rate. Use IV pumps in high-risk clients. Initiate safety and seizure precautions if the client manifests weakness or cerebral changes.

Offer water and fluids hourly to clients with hypovolemic or euvolemic hypernatremia. Consult with the dietitian and the physician concerning the need for fluid and sodium restriction in those with hypervolemic hypernatremia. Teach the client and family members the food items that should be restricted as well as the rationale for these restrictions.

Give 1 ml of fluid per kilocalorie (kcal) of hypertonic feeding solution. Initiate new gastric feedings slowly. Increase the rate if the client tolerates the feeding, as evidenced by no diarrhea, with residuals less than half the amount of the feeding per hour, or up to 100 ml.

Consult the physician for manifestations that indicate worsening of the hypernatremia or fluid overload, such as increasing weight gain or pulmonary, cardiovascular, or neurologic manifestations.

Diagnosis: Impaired Oral Mucous Membrane. The problem statement *Impaired Oral Mucous Membrane related to lack of body water secondary to hypernatremia* can be used.

Outcomes. There are several options for outcome statements, depending upon the condition of the mouth initially. If the oral membranes are simply dry, but not open or cracked, an outcome of maintaining moist oral mucous membranes is appropriate. If the oral mucous membranes are cracked or open, the outcome should state that no further deterioration will occur and that the mouth will be moist. Additional nursing diagnoses for pain from oral ulcerations or inadequate nutrition related to mouth pain should be considered.

Interventions. Provide oral care every 2 hours with a nonalcoholic mouthwash. Avoid lemon-glycerin swabs because they dry the membranes and may cause pain. Dilute saline and nonalcoholic rinses have been found to be effective. Use a soft toothbrush to prevent injury to the mucosa. Moisten the client's lips every 1 to 2 hours. Offer cool, nonacidic fluids such as apple juice. Low-acid juices provide fluid while decreasing pain and irritation. Limited ice chips may also decrease the discomfort from dry mucous membranes.

Caregivers often feel uncomfortable about giving oral care, and often the client's mouth is simply rinsed or lightly "brushed" with foam toothbrushes. This "light touch" oral care is appropriate when clients are in pain from mouth ulcers. However, lack of thorough oral care also leads to mouth ulcers, dental decay, and malnutrition. Mucus can accumulate on the roof of the mouth and impair swallowing or even breathing. Assess the mouth before and after mouth care, and be aggressive in cleaning the mouth.

Evaluation

Even if the desired outcome of sodium maintenance has been met, continue to monitor clients at high risk. The key to evaluating health promotion strategies is evaluating not only whether the client and family members understand the health promotion activities but, more important, asking whether they have incorporated the necessary changes into their lifestyle. If change has not occurred, investigate the barriers and recommend alternatives or resources.

If the desired outcome of sodium restoration has been met or partially met, the manifestations of excess should be absent or at least lessened. Mild to moderate excesses are usually corrected in 8 to 24 hours. If the excesses are more severe or occur in very young or older clients, intervention must be more cautious, and 48 hours or more may be needed before positive outcomes are noticeable. Evaluate the client with altered oral mucous membranes every 8 to 12 hours. If improvement is not seen within a few hours, increase the frequency of oral care.

■ Self-Care

Teach clients the importance of taking hourly fluids—30 to 60 ml of clear liquids or more as tolerated—and avoiding excessive caffeinated beverages. Impress upon family members the importance of keeping fresh foods and a variety of fluids on hand, especially for the client who lives alone. Encourage the use of community resources, such as Meals on Wheels. Instruct the client on how to read food labels and to avoid foods with high "Na" (sodium) content and over-the-counter medications or herbals unless physician-approved. Fluid intake should reach 600 ml in 24 hours.

Teach the client to consult the physician if vomiting or diarrhea persists for more than 48 hours or sooner if extreme weakness, dizziness, palpitations, changes in mental state, new onset of cough, or increasing restlessness occurs. Persons with a concurrent chronic disease (such as diabetes mellitus or disease of the liver, heart, or kidneys) should consult a physician if any of these manifestations persist for longer than 24 hours. Explain the importance of reporting weight gains of more than 3 pounds in 1 week. Some clients are managed at home with IV fluids. Home health care nurses see their clients often (see the Bridge to Home Health Care feature on Managing Intravenous Therapy on the website).

■ POTASSIUM IMBALANCES
HYPOKALEMIA

Hypokalemia is defined as a plasma potassium level of less than 3.5 mEq/L. It is a common electrolyte disorder, especially in the older adult population.

Etiology and Risk Factors

The body does not conserve potassium; thus, potassium deficit commonly results from inadequate potassium intake. However, potassium is found in most foods and fluids. People at high risk for hypokalemia include those who are debilitated, confused, restrained, or lacking access to dietary sources for financial or other reasons, or who are malnourished, anorexic, or bulimic. Clients on potassium-restricted diets or some weight reduction diets, or those receiving potassium-free IV solutions compounded by lack of dietary potassium are also at risk.

Potassium levels can also decrease when the excretion or loss of potassium exceeds intake. People at high risk for loss include those with vomiting or diarrhea, nasogastric suctioning, intestinal fistulae, or ileostomy. Potassium is also lost with the osmotic diuresis that occurs with diabetic ketoacidosis. Often, hypokalemia develops in surgical clients as a result of the increased cortisol levels during the stress adaptation period and from the effects of general or spinal anesthesia. Some studies suggest that hypokalemia in alcoholic clients, as well as hypocalcemia, hypophosphatemia, and hypomagnesemia, is secondary to alcohol-induced nephrotoxicity. Alcohol abstinence often results in electrolyte levels returning to normal.

Medications that commonly cause hypokalemia include the potassium-wasting diuretics (thiazide, loop, and osmotic diuretics), cathartics, steroids, amino-glycosides, amphotericin B, digitalis preparations, beta-adrenergic drugs, cisplatin, and bicarbonate.

Several conditions cause redistribution of potassium. An increased level of sodium intake promotes potassium loss. Increased levels of insulin promote the movement of not only glucose but also potassium into the cell. In alkalosis, potassium exchanges with hydrogen across the cell wall, thus increasing the level of hydrogen but decreasing the level of potassium in the plasma. Clients who are in the healing phase after a severe tissue injury or burn also experience hypokalemia as a result of the shifting of potassium into the cell. An increase in catecholamines also promotes cellular uptake of potassium.

Other factors associated with an increased risk of hypokalemia include Cushing's syndrome, the diuretic phase of renal failure, hyperaldosteronism, liver disease, cancer, wounds, and Bartter's syndrome, a chronic electrolyte-wasting syndrome.

Pathophysiology

When plasma potassium levels decrease, a decrease in potassium gradient occurs between the ICF and the plasma. The decreased gradient causes the resting membrane potential to increase, thus increasing excitability. Therefore cell membranes are more responsive to stimuli. Almost all of the manifestations that occur with hypokalemia result from the changes in neuronal excitability and its consequent effect on muscle function.

Clinical Manifestations

 The clinical manifestations of hypokalemia include abnormal findings on the electrocardiogram (ECG) and GI, cardiac, renal, respiratory, and neurologic disturbances. Abnormalities may not be apparent with mild hypokalemia (3.3 to 3.4 mEq/L), especially if the decrease in the potassium concentration is gradual. Slowed smooth muscle contraction leads to early GI manifestations, which include anorexia, abdominal distention, and constipation. Slowed skeletal muscle contraction results in muscle weakness and leg cramps. Increased conduction of nerve impulses secondary to an increase in the transmembrane potential leads to the neurologic manifestations of fatigue, paresthesias, hyporeflexia, and irritability.

With severe hypokalemia, ECG changes may occur (see Figure 14-1). The depressed and prolonged ST segment, depressed and inverted T wave, and prominent U wave are due to the prolongation of myocardial repolarization. Dysrhythmias are common because of increased cellular excitability. Hypokalemia also leads to a decrease in myocardial contraction, which is manifested as hypotension and a slow, weakened pulse. Potassium levels of less than 2.5 mEq/L increase the risk for ventricular fibrillation and cardiac arrest. Pulmonary manifestations of shallow respirations, shortness of breath, and

apnea, culminating in respiratory arrest, are also from progressive deterioration of respiratory muscular contraction.

The progressive neurologic consequences of altered nerve conduction are manifested as dysphasia, confusion, depression, convulsions, areflexia, and coma. Extreme smooth muscle slowing leads to vomiting and an ileus as well as urinary retention. Skeletal muscle weakness may progress to paralysis. Hypokalemia also inhibits the ability of the kidney to concentrate urine, which leads to polyuria, nocturia, and a decreased plasma osmolality.

Although plasma potassium levels less than 3.5 mEq/L are diagnostic for hypokalemia, the ECG is the most reliable tool for identifying abnormalities in intracellular potassium level.

Outcome Management

A thorough history and physical examination with appropriate diagnostic studies are essential in accurate diagnosis and management of hypokalemia.

■ Medical Management

Medical management is focused on identifying and correcting the cause of the imbalance. The aggressiveness of the therapy is determined by the potassium level and the clinical manifestations. Extreme hypokalemia necessitates cardiac monitoring.

Restore Potassium Levels. Maintenance doses for clients not taking any source of potassium are 40 to 60 mEq/day in the IV solution. Larger amounts are needed with coexisting potassium losses.

For clients with minor potassium deficits or for those who have potassium-wasting conditions, administering foods high in potassium helps correct the deficit and offsets losses. The adult recommended allowance for potassium is 1875 to 5625 mg/day. Box 14-2 includes examples of foods that are high and low in potassium.

Mild to moderate hypokalemia is treated by correcting or controlling the cause of the loss or by supplementing potassium intake through the diet or with medication. Oral potassium replacement therapy is usually prescribed for mild hypokalemia (plasma potassium, 3.3 to 3.5 mEq/L) or for potassium-wasting conditions. Oral potassium (chloride or gluconate) is extremely irritating to the gastric mucosa and must be taken with a glass of water or juice or with meals.

Severe hypokalemia requires IV intervention. A client with a plasma potassium level between 3 and 3.4 mEq/L needs approximately 100 to 200 mEq of IV potassium for the potassium level to increase 1 mEq/L. If the plasma potassium level is less than 3 mEq/L, it takes approximately 200 to 400 mEq of IV potassium to increase the level 1 mEq/L. Potassium given intravenously *must always be diluted in IV fluids*. The usual concentration

---

BOX 14-2 *High-Potassium and Low-Potassium Foods*

High-Potassium Foods (approximately 7 mEq/serving)

Fish (not shellfish)

Whole grains, nuts

Vegetables: artichokes, broccoli, brussels sprouts, cabbage, carrots, celery, collards, cucumber, mushrooms, potatoes with skins, spinach, tomatoes

Fruits: apricots, banana, cantaloupe, guava, honeydew melon, nectarine, orange, prunes, strawberries, tangerines, watermelon

Beverages: brewed coffee, tomato juice, fruit juices

Low-Potassium Foods (approximately 3 mEq/serving)

Vegetables: corn, sweet potato, lima beans, french-fried potatoes

Fruit: apples, applesauce, apple juice, blueberries, cranberries

Beverages: instant coffee, cola, cranberry juice, ginger ale, noncarbonated drinks, root beer, lemon-lime soda

Data from Mahan, L.K., & Escott-Stump, S. (2000). *Krause's food, nutrition, and diet therapy* (10th ed.). Philadelphia: W.B. Saunders.

---

of IV potassium is 20 to 40 mEq/L. Potassium is *not* given intramuscularly and is *never* given as a bolus (IV push) injection. Giving potassium by IV push creates sudden, severe hyperkalemia, which may result in cardiac arrest.

For severe potassium deficits, 10 to 20 mEq of potassium can be given every hour if *diluted* in IV fluids; a cardiac monitor must be used to ensure safety. Use of saline as a diluent is recommended; avoid dextrose as a diluent, because it increases intracellular potassium shifting. Because potassium is irritating to the veins, concentrations greater than 20 to 40 mEq/L increase the risk of phlebitis, and large veins should be used for administration.

If hypokalemia is refractory to the usual treatments, assess for manifestations of hypomagnesemia. Many clients who are hypokalemic are also hypomagnesemic. Hypokalemia that does not respond to treatment is frequently associated with hypomagnesemia. Magnesium is necessary for the kidney to conserve potassium.

■ Nursing Management of the Medical Client
Assessment

Assessment focuses on identifying risk factors for hypokalemia through history-taking and a thorough physical examination. Obtain a history that focuses on dietary intake, conditions promoting potassium loss, and use of diuretics, cortisone, over-the-counter medications, and herbals. Review laboratory reports of potassium lev-

els. Report even borderline plasma potassium levels to the physician, especially in high-risk clients, particularly those about to undergo surgery. General anesthesia not only promotes potassium loss but, in combination with lower plasma potassium levels, synergistically increases the risk of cardiac dysrhythmia. Consult the physician about the need for potassium supplementation in anyone who has been on NPO status or who has an obvious cause of potassium loss or marked decrease in potassium intake.

Ongoing assessments of the client with hypokalemia include all the body systems, because the effect of low potassium is widespread. Assess cardiac function, including apical pulses, and renal function every hour in the client with severe hypokalemia, and progress to every 8 hours as the client's condition improves. Assess neuromuscular and bowel function every 4 to 8 hours. A urine output of 0.5 ml/kg/hr is necessary to prevent rebound hyperkalemia. Hypokalemia increases the risk of digitalis toxicity because low potassium levels increase the sensitivity of the myocardium to digitalis-induced dysrhythmia. If the client receives digitalis, monitor for nausea, anorexia, vomiting, diarrhea, headache, weakness, blurring or visual halos, or marked change in cardiac rate or rhythm. Nausea is the most common manifestation of digitalis toxicity in older adults.

If the apical pulse is irregular, assess for pulse deficits. Because this procedure is impractical for self-monitoring, at least ensure that the client or a family member is able to assess a radial pulse accurately for 1 minute and is aware of the need to notify the physician if the pulse is less than 60 beats/min.

Diagnosis, Outcomes, Interventions

Collaborative Problem: Hypokalemia. Use a collaborative problem format such as *Hypokalemia related to* (specific etiology). Causative factors often include vomiting, diarrhea, Cushing's disease, prolonged or intensive diuretic use, cortisone therapy, decreased intake, and NPO status.

Outcomes. The client's potassium level will be 3.5 to 5 mEq/L. Because the nurse cannot treat the problem independently, the outcome can also be written as follows: "The nurse will monitor potassium levels and report abnormal potassium levels or manifestations of potassium imbalance to the physician."

Interventions. Give oral or IV potassium as prescribed, ensuring that it is *diluted in IV fluids; it cannot be given as an IV push*. Always *agitate* IV bags before hanging them up to prevent giving a loading dose, which can cause cardiac arrest. Monitor IV sites hourly for phlebitis, infiltration, and rate of infusion. Change IV sites every 72 hours or sooner if the vein becomes tender to palpation. Tenderness indicates damage to the intima of the vein; this is an early sign of phlebitis.

Use the smallest IV catheter possible to allow maximum plasma flow around the site at which the potassium enters the vein. This promotes dilution of the potassium, thereby decreasing the risk of phlebitis. If an IV solution containing potassium infiltrates surrounding tissue, consult the physician for advice. Potassium infiltration can cause tissue sloughing. Give IV fluids with potassium chloride by a controlled infusion pump to ensure the correct flow rate.

Notify the physician if signs of hypokalemia persist or worsen, such as dysrhythmia of increasing severity, or if signs of overcorrection occur, such as manifestations of hyperkalemia. During the administration of IV potassium, consult the physician if the client's urine output is less than 0.5 ml/kg/hr for 2 consecutive hours, if the pulse deficit is greater than 20 beats/min, or if signs of impaired peripheral tissue perfusion are present. Anticipate the need for additional potassium with increased IV glucose, such as in total parenteral nutrition (TPN); increased insulin levels result in shifting of potassium into the cell.

Diagnosis: Risk for Injury. Because potassium is needed for normal nerve conduction and muscle function, low plasma potassium levels often lead to weakness and can lead to falls or seizures. The nursing diagnosis is stated as *Risk for Injury related to muscle weakness and hypotension or seizures secondary to hypokalemia.*

Outcomes. The client will be at reduced risk of injury, as evidenced by an absence of falls, near falls, bruises, contusions, and seizures.

Interventions. Employ safety and seizure precautions to reduce the risk of injury. Keep the bed in a low position with padded side rails up. Before the client walks, clear the path of obstacles and place nonslippery shoes and a gait belt on the client. Use restraints only after all other alternatives to prevent inadvertent harm to self or others have been tried. It is imperative that health care providers comply with the client's rights and follow the defined protocols for use of restraints. Side rails are considered restraints; thus, the rationale for use and reevaluation of need must follow your agency's policy and be thoroughly documented.

Diagnosis: Imbalanced Nutrition: Less than Body Requirements. If the main cause of the client's hypokalemia is inadequate consumption of foods rich in potassium, then use the nursing diagnosis *Imbalanced Nutrition: Less than Body Requirements related to insufficient intake of foods rich in potassium.* However, this diagnosis can be used *only* if the client can eat and drink.

Outcomes. The client will demonstrate improved nutrition, as evidenced by consumption of adequate amounts of food and fluid to maintain a normal potassium level.

Interventions. Instruct the client to choose and consume foods rich in potassium (see Box 14-2). Instruct the client to take potassium supplements with a glass or more of water or juice and food to decrease GI irritation.

Evaluation

If the desired outcome of potassium maintenance has been met, continue to monitor high-risk clients for evidence of deficit. Continue to reinforce strategies for prevention. If the outcome of potassium restoration has been met or partially met, the manifestations of deficit should be absent or at least lessened in severity. Mild to moderate deficits are usually corrected in 8 to 24 hours. Correction of more severe deficits may take several days, especially in the older adult. Continue to evaluate the client's and family members' understanding of positive health behaviors, and assess for barriers to achieving those behaviors.

■ Self-Care

Teaching is essential to the promotion and maintenance of potassium balance. Provide a copy of the list of food groups, and emphasize the importance of eating a well-balanced diet. Review alternative cooking methods, reinforcing that prolonged cooking of vegetables may result in potassium and vitamin wasting. Suggest steaming, microwaving, and, if possible, eating raw vegetables as methods to increase nutrient retention.

Teach the basic principles of sick care. These principles include ingestion of 30 to 60 ml hourly of fluids with electrolytes; for example, cola contains potassium and reduces nausea. Sick care also involves teaching clients when to consult a physician. People with chronic diseases, such as heart, liver, or kidney disease or diabetes mellitus, should consult a physician for any illness that interferes with food ingestion or causes loss of nutrients and persists for more than 24 hours. Anyone who becomes symptomatic—who develops weakness of sudden onset, irregular heartbeat, or change in mental status—should consult a physician.

Teach the importance of not taking over-the-counter medicine or herbals, especially laxatives, without physician approval. Encourage clients who are lactose-intolerant to avoid milk products or to take lactase. Reinforce the label instruction that potassium products should be taken with food to avoid GI irritation.

Encourage use of support services—first, the family or extended family and then the religious community as well as respite services, Meals on Wheels, food stamps, Alcoholics Anonymous, or other community services.

HYPERKALEMIA

Hyperkalemia is defined as an elevation of the potassium level greater than 5 mEq/L. Hyperkalemia is rare in clients with normal kidney function but affects more than half of people with acute and chronic renal failure.

Etiology and Risk Factors

The three major causes of hyperkalemia are as follows:

- Retention of potassium by the body because of decreased or inadequate urine output
- Excessive release of potassium from the cells during the first 24 to 72 hours after traumatic injury or burns, or from cell lysis or acidosis
- Excessive infusion of IV solutions that contain potassium or excessive oral intake, especially in a person who has renal disease

All three potential causes of hyperkalemia limit the ability of the kidneys to excrete the excess potassium. Because the kidneys are responsible for 80% to 90% of potassium excretion, the underlying cause of hyperkalemia is often related to decreased kidney function. People with as little as 5% glomerular function can maintain normal plasma potassium levels if urine output is at least 1 L/day. Shock compounds the problem because of a low volume of circulating vascular fluids and diminished kidney function. The GI tract and skin cannot excrete enough potassium to compensate for an acute state of hyperkalemia.

Most potassium is inside the cell. Therefore conditions that destroy cells release potassium into the circulation. People with fast-growing cancers, such as non-Hodgkin's lymphoma, acute leukemia, small cell carcinomas, and some metastatic cancers, are at risk for *tumor lysis syndrome* (TLS). TLS is the consequence of rapid destruction of tumor cells by chemotherapy or irradiation, which results in hyperkalemia, hyperphosphatemia, hypocalcemia, and hyperuricemia. Hyperkalemia can also result from burns, crush injuries, or severe infections involving extensive cell destruction. Potassium levels can also increase after the use of stored blood, and after open-heart surgery or other surgical procedures in which a perfusion pump is used.

Therapy with potassium-sparing diuretics or concurrent use of potassium supplements and angiotensin-converting enzyme (ACE) inhibitors may also cause hyperkalemia. Disorders that decrease or inhibit secretion of aldosterone, such as adrenal insufficiency, may also cause hyperkalemia. Acidosis also increases hyperkalemia owing to the compensatory shifting of potassium out of the cell in exchange for hydrogen; the exception is diabetic acidosis in which glucose-related osmotic diuresis promotes potassium wasting.

Pathophysiology

Hyperkalemia increases the excitation threshold of the cell membrane, causing the cell to become less excitable. As hyperkalemia becomes more severe, muscles become weak, flaccid, and paralyzed.

Clinical Manifestations

Acute hyperkalemia may cause manifestations when the plasma level is only moderately elevated, to 6 mEq/L. However, if the condition developed slowly, manifestations may not be present until the plasma level reaches 7 mEq/L. Clinical manifestations can involve many body systems, including GI, cardiac, renal, and neurologic systems. Mild to moderate hyperkalemia (a plasma level near 6 mEq/L) causes nerve and muscle irritability, resulting in paresthesia (numbness, tingling), tachycardia, and intestinal colic and diarrhea.

As the plasma potassium level approaches 7 mEq/L, sodium channels become progressively inactivated, which causes disturbances in nerve and muscle function. Impaired cardiac conduction and ventricular contraction, hypotension, cardiac arrest, convulsions, and severe neuromuscular weakness progressing to flaccid paralysis and respiratory muscle paralysis can develop. The acidosis that occurs with hyperkalemia has a synergistic effect on the progressive impairment of depolarization. The renal abnormalities oliguria and anuria are commonly precursors to hyperkalemia rather than consequences of the imbalance.

As noted previously, the key to the level of severity is the amount of time the body has had to adapt to the imbalance. Although a plasma potassium level greater than 5 mEq/L is diagnostic for hyperkalemia, the ECG is the most reliable tool for identifying an imbalance (see Figure 14-1). Blood studies may yield false-positive results when hemolysis of blood specimens has occurred, when tourniquets are applied too tightly, when multiple attempts are made to obtain a sample from the same site, or when excess force is used to transfer blood into tubes or to aspirate blood into a syringe. Under these conditions, the cell ruptures and releases potassium into the sample of blood.

Other useful laboratory studies include determination of blood urea nitrogen (BUN), plasma creatinine, and carbon dioxide levels. Elevated BUN and plasma creatinine levels, which reflect decreased renal function, are important predictors of hyperkalemia. If the total carbon dioxide levels in the venous blood are low, an arterial blood gas study should be done to rule out metabolic or respiratory acidosis as a possible cause of hyperkalemia.

Outcome Management
■ Medical Management

The goals of medical management are to correct the potassium level as quickly as possible to prevent life-threatening consequences. Although a thorough history and physical examination are desirable, if the client's state is critical, intervention may preempt a thorough assessment.

Restore Potassium Balance. If the plasma potassium level is less than 5.5 mEq/L, dietary restriction of potassium may be all that is needed (see Box 14-2).

If the level is higher or if the client is symptomatic, pharmacologic intervention is usually necessary. The onset of symptoms and the need for aggressive intervention are usually related to the suddenness of the development of hyperkalemia. Improving urine output by forcing fluids, giving IV saline, or giving potassium-wasting diuretics usually corrects mild hyperkalemia.

When hyperkalemia is severe, immediate action is needed to avoid lethal cardiac disturbances. Temporary corrective measures may include the following: infusion of IV calcium gluconate to decrease the antagonistic effect of the potassium excess on the myocardium; infusion of insulin and glucose or sodium bicarbonate to promote potassium uptake into the cells (useful in metabolic acidosis); and use of the beta-agonist albuterol (0.5 mg IV), which results in a decrease in plasma potassium level within 30 minutes, lasting for 6 hours. These are only temporary methods for decreasing plasma potassium; repeating these methods may not be effective.

As hyperkalemia persists or increases, a cation-exchange resin such as sodium polystyrene sulfonate may be given orally or rectally as a retention enema. When this medication is given, the potassium ion is exchanged for the sodium ion in the intestinal tract; the potassium ion is then excreted in the stool. To prevent the constipating effect of this drug, it is usually combined with sorbitol, and diarrhea often results. In marked renal failure, peritoneal dialysis or hemodialysis may be needed.

Prevention is central to the management of TLS. Adequate hydration is the key: 3000 ml of IV fluid is given 24 hours before therapy, during therapy, and for 48 hours after therapy. Diuretics (to decrease the risk of pulmonary overload) and a uric acid blocker (to increase the excretion of uric acid) are also given to prevent renal failure.

If hyperkalemia is secondary to respiratory acidosis, enhancing pulmonary function is the primary focus. If it is from metabolic acidosis, the immediate risks associated with the acidosis and hyperkalemia are addressed first, and then interventions are targeted at the system in which the acidosis originated.

■ Nursing Management of the Medical Client
Assessment

Assessment focuses on identifying risk factors for hyperkalemia through history-taking and a thorough physical examination. Review laboratory reports of potassium levels. Report even borderline plasma potassium levels

to the physician, especially in high-risk clients, such as those who have cancer or are undergoing chemotherapy.

Ongoing assessments include checking vital signs, bowel function, urine output, lung sounds (crackles), and peripheral edema every 4 to 8 hours. Monitor plasma levels of potassium and creatinine and BUN. In severe hyperkalemia, perform hourly checks of vital signs, including apical pulses. ECG changes should be monitored continuously. In the absence of ECG monitoring, apical pulses constitute the next most valuable indicator of abnormality in intracellular potassium concentration. Monitor urine output hourly if severe hyperkalemia or a history of renal insufficiency exists or if the urine output drops to less than 0.5 ml/kg/hr for 2 consecutive hours.

Monitor not only for a therapeutic response to treatment (improvement) but also for signs of overcorrection. Rapid correction places a client at risk for hypokalemia and metabolic alkalosis. In a client taking digitalis, the occurrence of hypokalemia is associated with a digitalis toxic response.

Diagnosis, Outcomes, Interventions

Collaborative Problem: Hyperkalemia. Use the following collaborative problem statement: *Hyperkalemia related* to (specify etiology). Consider the contribution of renal dysfunction, shock from traumatic injuries, or burns (tissue destruction).

Outcomes. Because nurses cannot treat the problem independently, the outcome can also specify the following; "The nurse will monitor potassium levels and report abnormal findings or manifestations of hyperkalemia to the physician."

Interventions. Administer fluids as ordered to promote renal excretion of potassium. Report manifestations indicating the development of hypokalemia and urine outputs of less than 0.5 ml/kg/hr for 2 consecutive hours, or less than 720 ml/day.

If the client is to receive a blood transfusion and is at risk for hyperkalemia, notify the blood bank so that "old" blood (more than 2 weeks old) is not supplied. Use a 19-gauge needle or 20-gauge catheter to deliver the packed cells, to prevent red blood cell (RBC) rupture with release of intracellular potassium. When obtaining blood specimens, use vacuum tubes when possible to avoid false-positive results on tests for hyperkalemia.

High potassium levels have the potential to induce life-threatening dysrhythmias. Treat them according to protocol, and report ECG changes that indicate worsening hyperkalemia or overcorrection resulting in hypokalemia. Set cardiac monitor alarms with narrow limits to ensure early detection of lethal dysrhythmias. *Remember, a machine cannot replace your bedside assessment.* Cardiopulmonary resuscitation may be required, but it is seldom successful in cases of severe hyperkalemia because the heart muscle cannot respond to medications or countershock. Consult the physician for any serious change, including progression of altered tissue perfusion, especially in the heart, lungs, brain, or kidneys.

Evaluation

Evaluate the client's responses to therapy every hour if severe hyperkalemia is present or every 8 hours if mild hyperkalemia exists. Hyperkalemia must be corrected quickly because of the risk of dysrhythmia.

■ Self-Care

Teaching still remains one of the primary interventions to promote and maintain normal potassium balance for those at high risk for hyperkalemia. Explain the significance of potassium restriction. Crucial elements of teaching include dietary potassium sources and the importance of reading labels, avoiding salt substitutes, which are usually made from a potassium salt, and avoiding over-the-counter medication not approved by a physician. Clients must also understand the importance of consulting a physician if renal function worsens or if an acute illness lasts more than 24 hours. Occasionally, a person with renal insufficiency is in a state of hypokalemia caused by an acute loss. Use a cardiac monitor to ensure safe administration of potassium to any client with renal insufficiency.

CALCIUM IMBALANCES
HYPOCALCEMIA

Hypocalcemia is defined as a plasma calcium level less than 4.5 mEq/L, or 9 mg/dl. Calcium levels are often reciprocal with phosphorus levels. Phosphate imbalances are discussed later in this chapter.

Low calcium levels are common in older adults because of inadequate intake. Hypocalcemia can also develop from an inadequate intake of vitamin D as a result of intentional changes in the diet or to diseases that impair absorption. Diets can be deficient in vitamin D in people with lactose intolerance, GI disease, liver disease, alcoholism, anorexia, and bulimia. Decreased intake for several days, such as with NPO status, or for longer periods, as in high-protein and other weight-reduction diets, has also been linked to hypocalcemia.

Parathyroid disease decreases plasma calcium levels. A deficiency of parathyroid hormone (PTH) results in a decrease in plasma calcium levels resulting from decreased bone resorption and GI absorption and increased urinary excretion of calcium. Unplanned removal of the parathyroid can occur when the thyroid is removed (Figure 14-2).

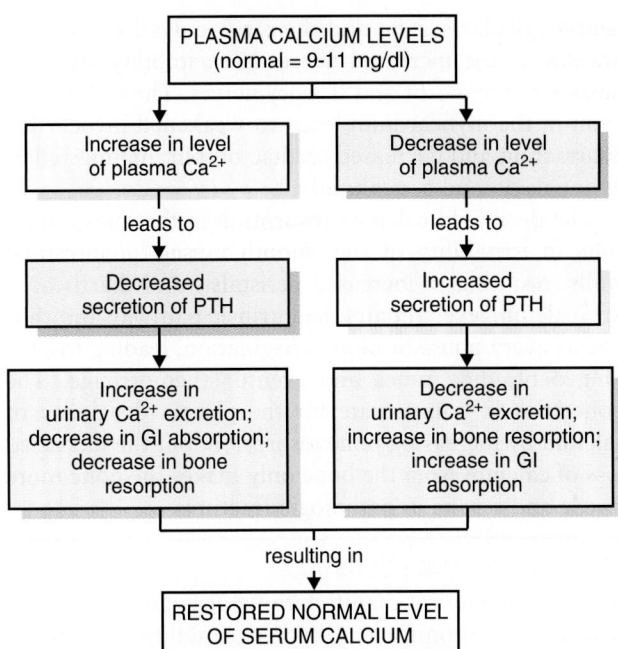

FIGURE 14-2 Parathyroid hormone (PTH) regulation of plasma calcium level. *GI*, Gastrointestinal.

Vitamin D must be activated by exposure to the sun; therefore hypocalcemia can develop in people who experience prolonged institutionalization. However, only a few minutes of sun exposure each week on the arms and face is enough to promote vitamin D synthesis.

Hypocalcemia can develop in persons with pancreatitis owing to a release of lipases into soft tissue spaces, with subsequent binding of free fatty acids to calcium. Open wounds are associated with increased loss of calcium. Excess sodium, as seen in Cushing's disease, promotes the excretion of calcium. Overcorrection of acidosis may also lead to hypocalcemia, because alkalosis causes decreased calcium ionization, leading to more calcium-protein binding. Clients receiving multiple transfusions of stored blood are at increased risk because of the binding of the preservative citrate with the calcium.

Several medications have been linked with hypocalcemia:

- Magnesium sulfate, colchicine, and neomycin inhibit PTH secretion.
- Aspirin, anticonvulsants, and estrogen alter vitamin D metabolism.
- Phosphate preparations impair reabsorption of calcium.
- Steroids increase calcium mobilization.
- Loop diuretics reduce calcium reabsorption.
- Antacids and laxatives decrease calcium absorption from the intestine.

Decreased calcium causes a partial depolarization of nerves and muscles because of a decrease in threshold potential. Therefore a smaller stimulus initiates the action potential. The manifestations expressed by the neuromuscular system and the cardiac dysrhythmias all are due to the increased neuronal excitability and irritability in the motor and sensory nerves. The lack of calcium in the myocardium leads to weakened myocardial contraction and decreased cardiac output, manifested as hypotension and a weak pulse.

The decreased calcium absorption in the intestine results in irritability of the smooth muscle in intestinal walls, resulting in increased peristalsis and diarrhea. A low calcium level impairs the intrinsic pathway and thus affects every phase of blood coagulation, leading to prolonged bleeding times and eventual hemorrhage. The bone tries to compensate for the plasma deficiency of calcium by increasing bone resorption, but the increased loss of calcium from the bone only makes the bone more brittle and results in pathologic fractures.

Clinical Manifestations

Most of the clinical manifestations of hypocalcemia are related to neuromuscular hyperexcitability. Numbness and tingling of the hands, toes, and lips; and emotional lability (e.g., irritability and anxiety) are manifestations of mild hypocalcemia. In the person with hypoparathyroidism, early signs of hypocalcemia resulting from overingestion of phosphate products or protein, or both, are cardiac palpitations and restlessness. Both phosphate and protein increase calcium binding. Findings in severe hypocalcemia are cardiac insufficiency, hypotension, dysrhythmias, a prolonged QT interval, Trousseau's and Chvostek's signs (Figure 14-3), and prolonged bleeding times; these abnormalities progress to seizures, laryngeal stridor, tetany, hemorrhage, cardiac collapse, and eventual death.

With prolonged hypocalcemia, cataracts may develop because of increased uptake of sodium and water by the lens. Trophic changes, such as dry, sparse hair and rough skin, may also be noted. Spontaneous fractures can occur when the bone is depleted of calcium.

A plasma calcium level less than 4.5 mEq/L, or 9 mg/dl, is considered diagnostic for hypocalcemia. This measurement and the clinical manifestations are the validating data used in most situations. Also, when clients have manifestations of hypocalcemia but have a normal plasma calcium, an ionized calcium level should be determined, because it is the only value that gives the true level of free (active, ionized) calcium. A level less than 1.18 mEq/L (<2.36 mg/dl) indicates hypocalcemia.

Also, abnormal plasma albumin and pH levels influence the interpretation of plasma calcium levels because of the effect on calcium binding. For example, when the albumin level is low, a falsely normal plasma calcium level can be present. Conversely, when plasma albumin is high, more calcium is bound, thus, the functional ionized calcium level is actually lower than the plasma level reveals. When albumin levels are abnormal, the total plasma calcium can be adjusted by adding or subtracting

Chvostek's sign   Trousseau's sign

FIGURE 14-3 Chvostek's and Trousseau's signs. A calcium deficit (hypocalcemia) or magnesium deficit (hypomagnesemia) increases the resting potential of nerves. This increase allows nerve stimulation and firing with less stimulus. Touching the facial nerve adjacent to the ear produces twitching of the client's upper lip (Chvostek's sign). The hand and fingers can also go into spasm (Trousseau's sign or carpal spasm). These spasms can occur spontaneously or when blood flow is decreased (e.g., during blood pressure cuff inflation).

0.8 mg/dl for every 1 g/dl decrease or increase, respectively, in plasma albumin. A basic pH causes an increase in calcium binding. The plasma level may appear normal, but the functional ionized calcium level is actually lower. The opposite is true with an acid pH. Therefore a plasma ionized calcium (iCa) assay should be done in clients who are critically ill, those with marginal calcium imbalances, or those with an abnormal albumin level or acid-base imbalance. A person with true hypocalcemia has an ionized calcium level less than 1.18 (normal equals 1.18 to 1.30 mEq/L).

Outcome Management

The goals of medical management are to determine and correct the cause of the hypocalcemia, restore calcium levels to normal values, and determine a method to reduce recurrence.

■ Medical Management

Restore Calcium Balance. Asymptomatic hypocalcemia is usually corrected with oral calcium gluconate, calcium lactate, or calcium chloride. For increased absorption, the calcium supplement should be given with a glass of milk with meals. The vitamin D in the milk promotes calcium absorption.

Chronic or mild hypocalcemia can be treated in part by having the client consume a diet high in calcium (Box 14-3). If hypocalcemia is secondary to parathyroid deficiency, the client must avoid high-phosphate foods, such

<table>
<tr><td>

BOX 14-3 *High-Calcium and Low-Calcium Foods*

High-Calcium Foods (>100 mg/serving)
Dairy Products: cheese, ice cream, milk, yogurt
Other: instant oatmeal, rhubarb, spinach, tofu

Low-Calcium Foods (<25 mg/serving)
Apples
Bananas
Chicken
Hamburger
Cooked oatmeal
Pasta
Vegetable juices

</td></tr>
</table>

Data from Mahan, L.K., & Escott-Stump, S. (2000). *Krause's food, nutrition, and diet therapy* (10th ed.). Philadelphia: W.B. Saunders.

as milk products and carbonated beverages, and excess protein. Protein binds with available calcium and only exacerbates the manifestations of hypocalcemia. Maintenance needs are met through calcium and vitamin D supplements.

Tetany from acute hypocalcemia needs *immediate* attention. IV calcium chloride or calcium gluconate must be given slowly to avoid hypotension and bradycardia and other dysrhythmias. Use D_5W solutions when dilution is necessary; avoid saline solutions, because they promote calcium loss. Calcium solutions can extravasate and lead to severe tissue damage. Infuse calcium slowly through a small IV needle in a large vein to quickly dilute the solution. If any blanching or pain is noted at the site of injection, stop *immediately.* Withdraw the remaining fluid from the needle and follow agency protocol for extravasation.

■ Nursing Management of the Medical Client

A thorough history of the client's current and chronic illnesses, diet intake, and medications, including over-the-counter medications and herbals, assists in identifying risks for calcium deficit and guides interventions for health promotion and maintenance. If digitalis and calcium are among the medications identified, assess for digitalis toxicity as well, because hypocalcemia increases the risk of this problem.

Check for Trousseau's and Chvostek's signs in high-risk clients (see Figure 14-3). *Trousseau's sign* is the occurrence of carpal spasm, or contraction of the fingers and hand, when a blood pressure cuff is kept inflated on the upper arm for 5 minutes at diastolic pressure. *Chvostek's sign* is occurrence of spasm of the muscles innervated by the facial nerve when the client's face is tapped lightly below the temple. Spasm of the face, lip, or nose is also evidence of tetany. In addition, assess for paresthesias (finger, toes, circumoral).

Assess the client's cardiac status by monitoring the ECG and vital signs, especially the apical heart rate and rhythm. Frequency of assessment varies from 1 to 4 hours, depending on the client's condition. Assess color, warmth, motion, and sensation (CWMS) and peripheral pulses to provide data for evaluation of the peripheral cardiac output.

Monitor also for bleeding in the gums and petechiae or ecchymosis in the skin. Assess for changes in the clarity of urine, because microscopic bleeding causes clear urine to become cloudy before frank bleeding is apparent. Also, note black or blood-streaked stool, which may signify occult GI bleeding. Be suspicious of an intracerebral hemorrhage when a client reports headaches of new onset. Monitor plasma calcium levels for improvement or worsening.

Monitor IV sites for infiltration or phlebitis when IV calcium is being infused. Calcium chloride is extremely irritating to the subcutaneous tissue. Notify the physician if the client's manifestations do not resolve or if signs of overcorrection (hypercalcemia) occur. When possible, use fresh blood for transfusions. Avoid giving calcium and bicarbonate in the same IV solution, because a precipitate will form. Use filters with TPN solutions.

To prevent pathologic fractures, use caution by obtaining adequate help to turn or move the client. Use gait belts and or extra personnel to walk or transfer the client to and from bed.

Instruct the client about foods that are rich in calcium, such as milk, cheese, yogurt, and green leafy vegetables. Encourage taking calcium supplements with meals and vitamin D milk for better absorption. *Exception:* For persons with hypocalcemia resulting from hypoparathyroidism, phosphorus intake should be decreased by *omitting* milk, milk products, and other high-phosphorus foods (e.g., carbonated beverages). Calcium and vitamin D supplements are prescribed for this population as well. Several types of vitamin D are available. Therefore clients with hypoparathyroidism must be advised not to take over-the-counter forms without first consulting with a physician to ensure that the right supplement is taken. These clients should also be advised to ingest protein only in amounts recommended by the American Dietetic Association (ADA). Increased intake of protein leads only to further binding of available calcium.

■ Self-Care

Reinforce intake of a well-balanced diet, avoiding high-protein diets or other nonprescribed weight-loss diets, and encourage weight-bearing exercises to prevent bone resorption. Consult the physician about the need for mineral and vitamin supplements for clients who consume less than half of their meals (e.g., the older adult population). Calcium carbonate is often recommended as an inexpensive supplement.

Older clients may have difficulty incorporating large amounts of food and fluids containing calcium into the diet. Part of the difficulty is in changing long-established eating habits. Many older adults drink very little milk because of habits formed in childhood. Suggest other forms of calcium that may be more appealing, such as yogurt, cheese, milkshakes made with ice milk, or green leafy vegetables.

HYPERCALCEMIA

Hypercalcemia is defined as a plasma level greater than 5.5 mEq/L, or 11 mg/dl. Hypercalcemia can occur in any age group. It is a common electrolyte disorder that can have serious physical complications.

Etiology and Risk Factors

The three most common causes of hypercalcemia are (1) metastatic malignancy, (2) hyperparathyroidism, and (3) thiazide diuretic therapy. The most common cancers that cause hypercalcemia are malignancies of the lung, breast, ovary, prostate, bladder, bone (multiple myeloma, leukemia), kidney, head and neck, and lymph tissues. Malignancy-induced hypercalcemia is the result of either bone destruction or an increased secretion of ectopic PTH.

Other causes of hypercalcemia include an excessive intake of calcium supplements with vitamin D or of calcium-containing antacids, prolonged immobilization, metabolic acidosis, and hypophosphatemia. Prolonged immobilization causes resorption of calcium from the bone. Recall that bone density is maintained by weight-bearing stress on bone. Metabolic acidosis promotes hypercalcemia by two mechanisms: decreased binding of calcium, which increases the plasma ionized calcium levels, and inhibition of calcium excretion from the kidney. Hypophosphatemia inhibits the ability of the kidney to excrete excess calcium.

Pathophysiology

Destruction of bone tissue results in an increased release of calcium into the vascular spaces. Excessive PTH production promotes calcium retention, which leads to hypophosphatemia. Hypophosphatemia compounds the problem by promoting more calcium retention.

When excess calcium is present, the cell membrane threshold potential becomes more positive, which results in membranes that are refractory to depolarization. This decreased cell membrane excitability requires a stronger stimulus for a response to occur. As a result, cardiac and smooth muscle activity is decreased. Excess calcium in the bloodstream also impairs renal function and precipitates as a salt, which often forms renal stones.

Clinical Manifestations

The clinical manifestations of hypercalcemia, which are generally nonspecific, are determined by the plasma calcium level. Mild hypercalcemia, with calcium levels at or slightly above 5.5 mEq/L, or 11 mg/dl, is usually asymptomatic. In mild cases, the plasma calcium level may increase momentarily when the client consumes calcium-containing antacids, or a large dose of an oral calcium supplement, and the kidneys are initially unable to eliminate the excess.

In moderate hypercalcemia, with calcium levels of 6.2 mEq/L, or 13 mg/dl, manifestations usually include anorexia, nausea, vomiting, polyuria, muscle weakness, fatigue, lethargy, dehydration, and constipation. Increased calcium stimulates the release of hydrochloric acid, gastrin, and pancreatic enzymes and slows bowel transit time, which leads to the anorexia, nausea, vomiting, abdominal distention, and constipation. The weakness, fatigue, depression, and difficulty concentrating are due to neurologic depression. Hypercalcemia also causes osmotic diuresis; the polyuria leads to dehydration and thirst and further exacerbates the constipation.

Calcium precipitates tend to form ureteral or kidney stones, which results in urinary blockage and severe colicky pain. Excess calcium also impairs glomerular blood flow, which can lead to renal failure. Bone pain is often associated with cancer of the bone and is due to the pressure on nerve endings from the tumor cells. Pathologic fractures are due to the decalcification of the bony matrix and can occur with cancer of the bone or with any condition that causes resorption of calcium. Calcium deposits can also occur on the skin.

Progressive neurologic depression from increasing hypercalcemia is manifested as extreme lethargy, a depressed sensorium, confusion, and eventually coma. Severe hypercalcemia may result in hypercalcemic crisis, which carries a 30% to 50% mortality rate. A hypercalcemic crisis occurs when calcium levels reach 7.1 mEq/L, or 15 mg/dl. The resultant increased conduction transmission, shortened repolarization (shortened QT interval, widened T wave), and severe cardiac depression can cause cardiac dysrhythmias, ECG changes, and cardiac arrest. Hypokalemia may occur as the body eliminates potassium rather than calcium.

Outcome Management
■ Medical Management

The goals of medical management are to determine and correct the cause of the hypercalcemia, restore calcium levels to normal values, and determine a method to reduce recurrence. Prevention and early detection of complications such as renal stones and fractures are also important. Benefits of treatment are evaluated against risk.

Restore Calcium Balance. Immediate correction of moderate and severe hypercalcemia is essential. IV normal saline, given rapidly with furosemide to prevent fluid overload, promotes urinary calcium excretion. Antitumor antibiotics that inhibit the action of PTH on osteoclasts in bone tissue, which reduces decalcification and the plasma calcium level, may be given.

Calcitonin decreases the plasma calcium level by inhibiting the effects of PTH on the osteoclasts and increasing urinary calcium excretion. Corticosteroid drugs decrease calcium levels by competing with vitamin D, resulting in decreased intestinal absorption of calcium, and by inhibiting prostaglandins, resulting in decreased bone resorption. IV phosphate decreases plasma calcium; however, it is used as a last resort because it may result in severe calcification of various tissues.

Thiazide diuretics should be changed to furosemide or to another diuretic that does not cause retention of calcium. If the cause of the hypercalcemia is excessive use of calcium or vitamin D supplements or calcium-containing antacids, these agents should be either avoided or used in a reduced dosage. If the client is not nauseated, encourage oral liquids. These actions are designed to lower the calcium level in 36 to 48 hours. Etidronate disodium reduces plasma calcium by inhibiting precursors to calcium mineralization and, secondarily, by reducing bone formation. The client needs to be hydrated with large volumes of normal saline before etidronate administration and must be given loop diuretics to enhance urine output and calcium excretion following drug administration.

Gallium nitrate has been effective in inhibiting bone resorption and in decreasing osteoclastic activity. The drug should be stopped if the urine output is less than 2 L/day or if the plasma creatinine level is greater than 2.5 mg/dl.

For client teaching, review high-calcium foods that should be restricted (see Box 14-3). Instruct the client that forcing fluids helps to lower plasma levels by flushing excess calcium through the kidney. If manifestations of renal calculi (stones) are present, teach that consumption of foods and fluids that increase urine acidity helps decrease stone formation. These include meat, eggs, whole grains, cranberry juice, and prune juice.

■ Nursing Management of the Medical Client

Because plasma calcium levels are not routinely assessed, it is essential that you identify high-risk clients. Screening assessment includes obtaining a thorough history, focusing on risk factors, medications (including over-the-counter calcium supplements or antacids), and diet history. Assess vital signs, apical pulses, and ECG every 1 to 8 hours, depending on the severity of the client's manifestations. Bowel sounds, renal function, and hydration status should be assessed every 8 hours. Also, recall that it is important to monitor for fluid volume depletion secondary to hypercalcemia.

Early treatment may prevent a hypercalcemic crisis. Unless fluids are contraindicated (as in clients with heart failure), increase fluid intake. If flank pain or renal colic is present, strain all urine to capture renal calculi for analysis. Report urine output of less than 0.5 ml/kg/hr for 2 consecutive hours. Report any manifestations that indicate worsening of the clinical status, such as an increase in severity of dysrhythmias, a decrease in sensorium, or manifestations of overcorrection (hypocalcemia).

Once the crisis is controlled, prevention of complications through teaching and safety interventions becomes the primary focus of health maintenance. Instruct the client to avoid calcium supplements. Sodium intake is increased, unless contraindicated, to promote calcium loss through the kidneys. Consumption of high-fiber foods and fluids should be increased to prevent constipation, and an acid-ash diet may be recommended to decrease the risk of stone formation. The client should also be taught to report clinical manifestations of renal calculi, such as flank pain, hematuria, or cardiac dysfunction (such as an irregular pulse or palpitations).

If the client has confusion, lethargy, or coma, institute safety precautions, including a low bed position. To prevent injury, turn and move the client with extreme caution and with adequate assistance. Gait belts, back braces, tripod canes, and walkers may be used to facilitate safer ambulation. Assist with resistive range of motion and weight-bearing activities to decrease calcium loss from the bone. Report clinical manifestations of fractures immediately, such as bone pain, deformity of limbs, or ecchymosis.

■ Surgical Management

Surgery may be used to remove an ectopic PTH-secreting tumor. Noninvasive or invasive lithotripsy or endoscopic removal of renal or ureteral calculi may be necessary.

▌ PHOSPHATE IMBALANCES
HYPOPHOSPHATEMIA

Hypophosphatemia is defined as plasma phosphorus levels less than 1.2 mEq/L. The overall major risk for hypophosphatemia is loss or long-term lack of intake, increased growth or tissue repair, and recovery from malnourished states. Failure to meet these increased needs results in a state of phosphorus depletion.

Phosphorus depletion can occur as a result of prolonged and excessive intake of antacids. Administration of high levels of glucose via tube feeding or IV line causes phosphorus to enter the cell for glucose phosphorylation. The increased sodium found in Cushing's syndrome, the increased calcium found in hyperparathyroidism, and the decreased arterial partial pressure of carbon dioxide ($PaCO_2$) in chronic respiratory alkalosis also cause phosphorus to move into the cell. Lead poisoning leads to a decreased availability of phosphate. Phosphate loss occurs in burns, and a mild renal loss occurs with metabolic alkalosis.

Pathophysiologic changes that occur with hypophosphatemia can affect every organ system because of the effect of hypophosphatemia on optimal adenosine triphosphate (ATP) and oxygen supply. Phosphate depletion impairs the conversion of glucose and many other intermediate substances to ATP. The ultimate result is a disruption in the sole mechanism responsible for regeneration of ATP.

The plasma level, whether normal or low, does not always reflect the total body phosphate content. Careful review of a client's history, laboratory data, medications, and clinical manifestations, with emphasis on nutritional health in people at high risk, increases the likelihood of identifying phosphate deficiencies. The primary manifestations of hypophosphatemia are decreased cardiac and respiratory function, muscle weakness, fatigue, brittle bones, bone pain, confusion, and seizures.

Mild hypophosphatemia can be treated with diet and dietary supplementation. Teach a well-balanced diet and help the client and family gain access to resources. Clients who have a serious phosphate imbalance are often deficient in many other nutrients. TPN is usually the intervention of choice until the plasma levels become stable.

HYPERPHOSPHATEMIA

Hyperphosphatemia, a plasma phosphate level greater than 3 mEq/L, is rare but serious. The most common causes are excessive intake of high-phosphate foods, excess vitamin D (especially with renal insufficiency), impaired colonic motility causing increased absorption, hypoparathyroidism, and Addison's disease. Clinical manifestations are related to the degree of hyperphosphatemia or to secondary hypocalcemia. Tachycardia, palpitations, and restlessness are among the earliest manifestations. Anorexia, nausea, vomiting, hyperreflexia, tetany, and more serious dysrhythmias may follow if the imbalance worsens.

In certain conditions, an increased intake or decreased excretion of phosphate or an increase in cell lysis results in high levels of phosphorus. In renal failure, the kidney is less able to excrete phosphate; the excess phosphate impairs calcium reabsorption. TLS results in a state of hyperphosphatemia from excess cell rupture. Women are at risk after menopause owing to a slight increase in phosphate secondary to a deficiency of estrogen. Exposure to lead increases the risk of phosphorus imbalances. Hyperphosphatemia leading to death has been associated with administration of phospho-soda enemas in the presence of altered renal or bowel function. Follow manufacturer recommendations when giving phospho-soda enemas.

In mild or asymptomatic hyperphosphatemia, treatment focuses on limiting high-phosphate foods, especially milk, ice cream, cheeses, large amounts of meat and fish, and carbonated beverages, or giving calcium or aluminum products that promote the binding and excretion of phosphate. Dialysis is the primary treatment for renal failure that is refractory to conservative approaches.

MAGNESIUM IMBALANCES
HYPOMAGNESEMIA

Hypomagnesemia is defined as a plasma magnesium level less than 1.5 mEq/L, or 1.8 mg/dl. Magnesium deficits are being identified more often as a result of increased knowledge about this ion. Twenty-two percent to 42% of clients with calcium, phosphate, sodium, and potassium imbalances have been found to have a coexisting magnesium imbalance. However, it is a rare imbalance in people who consume a well-balanced diet. As with other intracellular ions, plasma levels may be normal in the presence of intracellular depletion. Also, hypomagnesemia is often overlooked, because tests for plasma magnesium levels are not routinely ordered until a severe deficit has occurred. Plasma levels may be helpful in severe or acute changes, but a 24-hour urinalysis after an IV magnesium challenge, ion-selective imaging scan, or nuclear magnetic resonance imaging scan (to determine soft tissue levels) is more predictive of total body magnesium levels, but these studies are rarely done because they are expensive.

Hypomagnesemia is becoming recognized as a common cause of refractory (not responsive to treatment) hypokalemia and hypocalcemia. The hypomagnesemic state inhibits potassium reabsorption; the hypomagnesemia, therefore, needs to be corrected before potassium and calcium imbalances respond to treatment.

Magnesium deficits are often seen in critically ill and alcoholic clients. Alcoholism decreases intestinal absorption as a result of a decrease in enzymes that are normally produced by the liver. Alcoholism also promotes magnesium wasting as a result of nephrotoxicity and leads to malnutrition. Other causes of hypomagnesemia are severe or chronic malnutrition; malabsorption syndromes, such as Crohn's or celiac disease or pancreatitis; and GI losses from vomiting, GI suction, diarrhea, high-volume ileostomies, fistulae, laxative abuse, or radiation enteritis. Mechanisms for renal losses include the diuretic phase of acute renal failure and hyperphosphatemia. Prolonged IV or TPN therapy without magnesium replacement also increases the risk for hypomagnesemia. Excess calcium (as in hyperparathyroidism) and excess sodium (as in Cushing's syndrome or hyperaldosteronism) inhibit magnesium reabsorption. The hyperglycemia seen with diabetic acidosis causes osmotic diuresis and loss of magnesium. Alkalosis is also associated with hypomagnesemia.

Excessive amounts of phosphorus in the intestine (as from overuse of antacids) inhibit the uptake of magnesium from the intestinal villi. Some medications interfere with renal handling of magnesium as either a primary action or a side effect. These include diuretics (loop, osmotic, thiazide), antibiotics (such as aminoglycoside antibiotics), carbenicillin, amphotericin B, cisplatin, corticosteroids, and digitalis. Cocaine abuse has also been linked to hypomagnesemia.

The myocardial irritability that occurs with hypomagnesemia seems to be a result of changes in the resting membrane potential caused by alterations of both potassium and magnesium ions, which stimulates beta$_2$-adrenergic cells. It is often associated with digitalis use. Magnesium depletion and digitalis both promote potassium loss from myocardial cells. Digitalis uptake also seems to be increased in hypomagnesemia. GI changes from decreased contractility, such as anorexia, nausea, and abdominal distention, can occur. Psychological disorders, such as depression, psychosis, and confusion, may also develop.

Severe hypomagnesemia causes neuromuscular manifestations such as Chvostek's and Trousseau's signs, tetany, convulsions, and vasospasm leading to stroke. Cardiac abnormalities include premature ventricular contractions, atrial or ventricular fibrillation, and ECG changes (prolonged QT intervals, widened QRS complexes, and broadening of T waves). Other ECG changes are related to the concomitant low levels of potassium. Low magnesium levels have been linked with an increased incidence of ventricular dysrhythmias and decreased 1-year survival rates in clients with heart failure as well as with lethal dysrhythmias in clients who have had myocardial infarctions. Studies also suggest a link between estrogen therapy in postmenopausal women and increased coagulation risk; estrogen promotes tissue uptake of magnesium and hence hypomagnesemia.

Management

Treatment of hypomagnesemia includes oral magnesium replacement in the form of magnesium-containing antacids or parenteral magnesium sulfate. Increasing dietary intake of magnesium also helps ensure balance and stability.

IV magnesium reduces the tendency of the small airways to spasm and has been found useful in treating acute asthma that has been refractory to other therapy. The positive inotropic, negative chronotropic, and vasodilatory effects of magnesium have also been found to increase cardiac output and decrease oxygen consumption in people with shock and sepsis. Magnesium has also been successfully used as a mood stabilizer in clients with bipolar disease.

Nursing management includes monitoring vital signs every 4 to 8 hours and reviewing ECG readings hourly. Initiate safety and seizure precautions for clients who are extremely confused or at risk for seizures. Monitor plasma magnesium, potassium, and calcium levels. Also, many experts recommend assessing the client's deep tendon reflexes because normal reflexes suggest normal cellular magnesium levels.

Consult a physician about the need for magnesium maintenance or replacement if the client has severe malnutrition, is on NPO status for more than 3 days (especially in the presence of coexisting losses), or has manifestations of hypokalemia or hypocalcemia even after treatment. TPN may be necessary to correct coexistent nutrient imbalances, which is common. Maintaining glucose control in people with diabetes mellitus decreases the risk of magnesium loss from the glucose-related osmotic diuresis. Rapid infusion or undiluted magnesium sulfate can cause a hot or flushed feeling and phlebitis. Avoid giving magnesium in saline solutions.

Instructing clients and family members about foods rich in magnesium provides information that may be essential to prevent magnesium deficiency or to correct a mild deficit (Box 14-4). Caution clients about taking mineral supplements without the advice of a dietitian or pharmacist. The calcium-to-magnesium ratio should be maintained at 4:1; a higher ratio can lead to deposition of calcium in the soft tissues and vessels. Taking magnesium without potassium causes shifting of potassium into the cell. In the alcoholic client, magnesium should be given with thiamine to promote nerve regeneration.

HYPERMAGNESEMIA

Hypermagnesemia, a plasma magnesium level greater than 2.5 mEq/L, or 3 mg/dl, is a rare disorder. Hypermagnesemia may occur with renal insufficiency, excessive use of magnesium-containing antacids or laxatives, or administration of potassium-sparing diuretics. Many potassium-sparing diuretics conserve magnesium. Hypermagnesemia is also seen with severe dehydration from ketoacidosis, with decreased synthesis of aldosterone (such as in Addison's disease or after adrenalectomy), and with overuse of IV magnesium sulfate for controlling premature labor or pregnancy-induced hypertension.

Clinical manifestations are related to the blocked release of acetylcholine from the myoneural junction,

---

BOX 14-4	*High-Magnesium and Low-Magnesium Foods*

High-Magnesium Foods (>75 mg/serving)
Cashews
Chili
Halibut
Swiss chard
Tofu
Wheat germ

Low-Magnesium Foods (<25 mg/serving)
Chicken
Egg
Fruits
Green peas
Hamburger
White bread

Data from Mahan, L.K., & Escott-Stump, S. (2000). *Krause's food, nutrition, and diet therapy* (10th ed.). Philadelphia: W.B. Saunders.

which results in a decrease in muscle cell activity. With mild hypermagnesemia, peripheral vessels dilate, causing hypotension. ECG changes include prolonged PR and QT intervals. In extreme hypermagnesemia, profound sedative effects on the neuromuscular system lead to severe muscle weakness, lethargy, drowsiness, loss of deep tendon reflexes, respiratory paralysis, and loss of consciousness. Cardiac signs include delayed myocardial conduction manifested on the ECG as wide QRS complexes, elevated T wave, heart block, and premature ventricular contractions.

Management

Management of hypermagnesemia includes decreasing the use of magnesium sulfate. Saline infusions with a diuretic increases renal elimination of magnesium. However, a side effect of the treatment is a loss of calcium. Hypocalcemia may intensify the hypermagnesemia. IV calcium may be used to antagonize the effects of hypermagnesemia. Albuterol has also been used to reduce magnesium levels. The presence of severe respiratory distress requires ventilatory assistance. If renal failure is present, hemodialysis may be necessary.

Nursing management focuses assessment on vital signs, respiratory function, ECG recordings, urine output, and the level of sensorium; these should be checked every 1 to 4 hours, depending on the client's condition. Safety and seizure precautions should be initiated when confusion or seizure risk is present. Changes in deep tendon reflexes should be reported. Keep IV calcium salts in the code cart for emergency reversal of severe hypermagnesemia.

Teach clients to avoid constant use of laxatives and antacids containing magnesium, especially if urine output is decreased. Encourage eating foods that contain fiber and drinking adequate fluids to promote fecal elimination.

CONCLUSIONS

Electrolyte imbalances are found in all age groups in every type of health care setting. It is rare for a person to have only one electrolyte imbalance; more commonly, multiple electrolyte and fluid imbalances are present, especially in high-risk populations such as the very young, older adults, and people with chronic illnesses.

Nurses play an essential role in health promotion, health maintenance, and health restoration for clients at risk for or experiencing fluid and electrolyte imbalances.

Nursing management includes the following pivotal roles:
- *Teaching* clients and their families about positive health behaviors, about the importance of nutrient intake (even during nonacute illnesses), and about manifestations of fluid and electrolyte imbalance that necessitate physician consultation
- *Promoting* nutritional maintenance and replacement in clients who are at high risk for or who are experiencing fluid or electrolyte imbalance
- *Assisting* the physician in early detection of imbalances and of poor response to treatment or signs of overcorrection
- *Promoting* balanced nutrition in rehabilitation or extended care settings through family support, early physician referrals for supplements, dietary consultation, or management of imbalances

THINKING CRITICALLY *evolve*

1. An older, tube-fed resident from a nursing home is admitted with recent changes in level of consciousness. Her skin and mouth are very dry, and her urine is scant and dark yellow. Laboratory assessment reveals sodium, 150 mEq/dl; chloride, 106 mEq/dl; BUN, 52; and creatine, 1.2. Her family calls and wants to know "if she will make it." How would you respond?

Factors to Consider. What do these assessment findings suggest? What interventions would you expect to be prescribed? What precautions will be needed to prevent further fluid and electrolyte shifts?

2. A 45-year-old woman was admitted with a rapid heart rate. Her past medical history is negative for cardiac disease. One week ago, she started on a new weight loss program, which included furosemide. Could her heart rate be potentially lethal?

Factors to Consider. Why would a client take furosemide in a weight-loss program? What side effects may be occurring? What laboratory studies do you anticipate being ordered? Which electrolytes do you think will be abnormal?

Discussions for these questions can be found on the website and the CD-ROM.

BIBLIOGRAPHY
1. Bennett, J. (2000). Dehydration: Hazards and benefits. *Geriatric Nursing, 21*(2), 84-88.

1a. Cacchione, P.Z., et al. (2003). Clinical profile of acute confusion in the long-term care setting. *Clinical Nursing Research, 12*(2), 45-58.

2. Edwards, S. (2001). Regulation of water, sodium and potassium: Implications for practice. *Nursing Standard, 15*(22), 36-42.

 2a. Gennari, F.J. (2002). Disorders of potassium homeostasis. Hypokalemia and hyperkalemia. *Critical Care Clinics, 18*(2): 273-288.

3. Guyton, A., & Hall, J. (2001). *Textbook of medical physiology* (10th ed.). Philadelphia: W.B. Saunders.

4. Hamilton, S. (2001). Detecting dehydration malnutrition in the elderly. *Nursing, 31*(12), 56-57.

 4a. Hodgkinson, B. et al. (2003). Maintaining oral hydration in older adults: A systemic review. *International Journal of Nursing Practice, 9*(3), 519-528

5. Huether, S., & McCance, K. (2000). *Understanding pathophysiology* (2nd ed.). St. Louis: Mosby.

6. Iggulden, H. (1999). Dehydration and electrolyte disturbance. *Elderly Care, 11*(3), 17-23.

7. Innerarity, S. (2000). Hypomagnesemia in acute and chronic illness. *Critical Care Nursing Quarterly, 23*(2), 1-17.

8. Innis, J. (2002). Treating nephrogenic diabetes insipidus. *Dimensions of Critical Care Nursing, 21*(3), 98-99.

9. Kearney, K. (2000). Hyperkalemia. *American Journal of Nursing, 100*(1), 55-56.

10. McAulay, D. (2001). Dehydration in the terminally ill patient. *Nursing Standard, 16*(4),33-37.

11. Mentes, J. (2000). Hydration management protocol. *Journal of Gerontological Nursing, 26*(10), 6-15.

12. Mitchell, M. (2003). *Nutrition across the lifespan* (2nd ed.). Philadelphia: W.B. Saunders.

13. Mower-Wade, D., Bartley, M., & Chiari-Allwein, J. (2001). How to respond to shock. *Dimensions of Critical Care Nursing, 20*(2), 22-27.

14. Schmidt, T. (2000). Assessing a sodium and fluid imbalance. *Nursing, 30*(1), 18.

15. Schmidt, T. (2000). How to recognize hypokalemia. *Nursing, 30*(2), 22.

15a. Sheehy, C.M. et al. (199). Dehydration: Biological considerations, age-related changes, and risk factors in older adults. *Biological Research in Nursing, 1*(1), 30-37.

16. Smith, S., & Andrews, M. (2000). Artificial nutrition and hydration at the end of life. *Medsurg Nursing, 9*(5), 233-247.

16a. Uphold, C.R., & Graham, M.V. (2003). Clinical guidelines in family practice (4th ed.). Gainesville, Fla.: Barmarrae Books.

17. Zembrzuski, C. (2000). Nutrition and hydration. *Journal of Gerontological Nursing, 26*(12), 6-7.

Acid-Base Balance

Margie J. Hansen

evolve

Web Enhancements   http://evolve.elsevier.com/Black/medsurg/

Appendix A   **Appendix C**
Religious Beliefs and Practices Affecting Health Care   Laboratory Values of Clinical Importance in Medical-Surgical Nursing

Normal function of body cells depends on regulation of the hydrogen ion (H^+) concentration within very narrow limits. If H^+ levels exceed these normal limits, acid-base imbalances result and are recognized clinically as abnormalities of serum pH. Because acid-base imbalances may be caused by disorders of any body system, their incidence in clinical settings is quite high.[10] Along with other health care professionals, nurses are responsible for preventing, detecting, and intervening in acid-base imbalances.

REGULATION OF ACID-BASE BALANCE

The symbol *pH* refers to the negative logarithm of the H^+ concentration. It is used to express the acidity or alkalinity of a solution. A pH of 7.0 is *neutral*, having an equal number of acids and bases. An *acidic* solution has a pH less than 7.0, and an *alkaline* solution has a pH greater than 7.0. Because pH is a *negative* log (indicating a reciprocal relationship), a rise in pH reflects a drop in H^+. Conversely, a decline in pH indicates an increase in H^+.

Normal serum pH is 7.35 to 7.45. The function of cellular proteins is seriously impaired when pH falls to 7.2 or less or rises to 7.55 or higher. Rapid rates of change in pH are especially detrimental. Typically, a serum pH below 6.8 or above 7.8 is fatal.

Three physiologic systems act interdependently to maintain a normal serum pH:
- Chemical buffering of excess acid or base by buffer systems in the blood plasma and in cells
- Excretion of acid by the lungs
- Excretion of acid or regeneration of base by the kidneys

MODULATION OF SERUM pH BY BUFFER SYSTEMS

A buffer system consists of a weak acid (one that does not readily release H^+ into solution) and a salt of a base. For example, carbonic acid (H_2CO_3), a weak acid, and sodium bicarbonate ($NaHCO_3$), the salt of a base with which H^+ can combine, make up the clinically important bicarbonate buffer in the blood. The organic acids formed during cellular energy metabolism are strong acids; that is, they readily contribute free H^+ to body fluids, potentially producing large alterations in pH. The pH of buffered solutions tends to remain fairly stable despite the addition of strong acids or bases because buffer-system components combine with added acids or bases to convert them to weaker forms. Because only free H^+ contributes to pH, changes in pH are minimized. Examples of buffering reactions are presented next.

Strong acid buffered:

$$HCl + (H_2CO_3/NaHCO_3) \rightarrow H_2CO_3 + NaCl,$$
where HCl is hydrochloric acid and NaCl is sodium chloride.

Strong base buffered:

$$NaOH + (H_2CO_3/NaHCO_3) \rightarrow NaHCO_3 + H_2O,$$
where NaOH is sodium hydroxide.

Several buffer systems are present in the blood, both within red blood cells (RBCs) and in the plasma. The numerous negative charges on proteins permit the binding of large quantities of H^+ cations. Accordingly, proteins such as hemoglobin in RBCs and albumin in the plasma are quantitatively (judged according to amount) the most important blood buffers. Negatively charged ions, such as phosphate within body cells and carbonate within bones, are important intracellular buffers.

In clinical settings, however, the bicarbonate buffer is monitored because of its accessibility within the plasma as well as its physiologic importance as an *open* buffer system. In an open buffer system, the end products of acid-buffering reactions are continuously eliminated from the body by the lungs and kidneys, allowing these reactions to continue without being slowed by the accumulation of end products. When bases must be buffered, the carbon dioxide (CO_2) consumed by carbonic acid formation is readily replenished by normal metabolism. Furthermore, the dissociation constant (pKa) of this system is ideal for buffering fluids such as plasma, in which the addition of acids is more prevalent than the addition of bases. The *dissociation constant* (pKa) of a buffer is the pH at which half its components are in the acid form and half are in the base form. At normal serum pH, the bicarbonate buffer has about 90% of its components in base form.

Because all intracellular and extracellular buffer systems operate interdependently, the status of the bicarbonate buffer is representative of acid-base homeostasis within the body as a whole. Buffer systems act instantly to minimize the impact of adding strong acids or bases to body fluids; thus, these systems are the body's first line of defense against acid-base imbalance. Unlike the lungs and kidneys, however, buffers do not actually eliminate acid or base from the body.

REGULATION OF VOLATILE ACID BY THE LUNGS

Volatile acids are acids that can be converted to gases. During normal ventilation (breathing), the lungs exhale large quantities of "potential" acid in the form of CO_2 gas. CO_2 is continuously produced by body cells as an end product of complete oxidative metabolism of nutrients for energy. CO_2 diffuses from body cells into the blood, where it may combine with water to form H_2CO_3, which then dissociates, or separates, into its component ions: H^+ and HCO_3^- (bicarbonate). This *hydrolysis reaction,* which is reversible, is shown as follows:

$$H_2O + CO_2 \rightleftharpoons H_2CO_3 \rightleftharpoons HCO_3^- + H^+$$

It is apparent from this equation that CO_2 and H_2CO_3 are directly related. As serum CO_2 levels rise, H^+ production increases and pH falls, indicating increased acidity. Conversely, lower CO_2 levels are consistent with higher (more alkaline) pH values. The hydrolysis reaction further demonstrates that some of the CO_2 entering the blood forms the base HCO_3^-. Although some hydrolysis occurs in the plasma, most takes place in the cytoplasm of RBCs, where the enzyme carbonic anhydrase (CA) catalyzes the reaction at much more rapid rates than in the plasma. The presence of CA in other cells, notably the renal tubular cells, is also important to acid-base homeostasis (discussed later in this chapter).

Figure 15-1 demonstrates the hydrolysis reaction at the tissue level. Consistent with the *law of mass action,* the rate and direction of this reaction are determined by (1) the addition of substrate or (2) the removal of end product. In the tissues, the addition of CO_2 to the blood by metabolizing cells drives hydrolysis in the forward direction, forming H^+ and HCO_3^-, mostly in the RBCs. The H^+ formed by hydrolysis is buffered by hemoglobin, thereby minimizing changes in the pH of the RBC cytoplasm. The HCO_3^- formed in RBCs diffuses out into the plasma, while the chloride anion (Cl^-) moves in to maintain electroneutrality. This anion countertransport is known as the *chloride shift*. HCO_3^- formed in this way accounts for the major portion (80%) of CO_2 transported in the blood. Small amounts are transported while dissolved in plasma (8%) or are combined with he-

FIGURE 15-1 Tissue level hydrolysis. **A,** Carbon dioxide (CO_2) is formed during cellular energy metabolism. **B,** CO_2 diffuses into plasma, then into red blood cells. **C,** CO_2 enters hydrolysis catalyzed by carbonic anhydrase (CA), yielding hydrogen (H^+) and bicarbonate (HCO_3^-). **D,** HCO_3^- diffuses into plasma in exchange for Cl^- (chloride shift). **E,** H^+ is buffered by hemoglobin (Hb) and other intracellular buffers. *RBC,* Red blood cell; *ATP,* adenosine triphosphate.

moglobin (as carbaminohemoglobin) or other proteins (12%). The amount of carbonic acid in the blood at any time is negligible (0.0006%).

In the lungs, CO_2 diffuses along its concentration gradient from the plasma to the alveoli, from which it is exhaled. Removal of CO_2 drives the hydrolysis reaction in reverse, as shown in Figure 15-2. In a reversal of the chloride shift, HCO_3^- reenters the RBCs, and Cl^- exits. HCO_3^- combines with H^+, which has been released from its buffers, regenerating CO_2 and H_2O.

REGULATION OF FIXED ACIDS AND BICARBONATE BY THE KIDNEYS

Acids that cannot be converted to gases must be eliminated in the urine. These *fixed acids* include the following:

- Sulfuric, phosphoric, and other acids produced by protein metabolism
- Ketones produced by lipid metabolism and potentially accumulating with accelerated lipid metabolism, as in diabetic ketoacidosis
- Lactic acid produced by carbohydrate metabolism and potentially accumulating with increased metabolic rates and with accelerated anaerobic glycolysis, as in shock and hypoxemia
- Occasionally, ingested toxins, such as salicylate (aspirin), drugs, and methanol

The kidneys regulate serum pH by secreting H^+ into the urine and by regenerating HCO_3^- for reabsorption into the blood. At the glomerulus, HCO_3^- is filtered from the blood into the proximal convoluted tubule. Because HCO_3^- is a large, charged particle, it is poorly reabsorbed. Any HCO_3^- filtered in excess of H^+ is excreted in the urine. H^+ is actively secreted into the renal tubules, primarily by proximal tubular cells, but also in the distal tubule and collecting duct. This system operates only until tubular pH falls to about 4.5. At lower pH values, significant amounts of H^+ leak from the tubular lumen back into the blood. Secretion of large amounts of H^+ into the renal tubules would result in a rapid fall in tubular pH and would inhibit further H^+ secretion if not for the presence of *urinary buffer systems*. These systems permit the tubular fluid to accept large quantities of H^+ while limiting how much the urinary pH decreases.

Urinary Buffer Systems

The three principal buffer systems in renal tubules are the bicarbonate, ammonia, and phosphate (titratable acid) systems.

In the *bicarbonate buffer* (Figure 15-3), H^+ is secreted into the tubular lumen by tubular cells in countertransport with sodium (Na^+). The combination of H^+ with filtered bicarbonate regenerates CO_2 in a reversal of the hydrolysis reaction. This CO_2 is reabsorbed into tubular cells, where hydrolysis proceeds efficiently because of the presence of

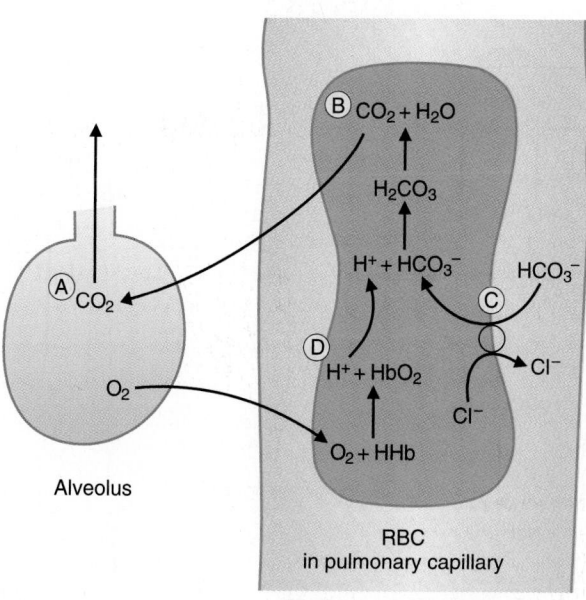

FIGURE 15-2 Reversal of hydrolysis in the lung. **A,** Carbon dioxide (CO_2) is exhaled, creating a gradient for diffusion of CO_2 from the blood to the alveolus. **B,** Removal of CO_2 drives reverse hydrolysis in the red blood cell (RBC). **C,** Bicarbonate (HCO_3^-) reenters the RBC in exchange for Cl^- (reverse chloride shift). **D,** Oxygen binding to hemoglobin (Hb) promotes H+ release (reverse Haldane effect). *HHb,* Combined hydrogen/hemoglobin.

FIGURE 15-3 Function of the urinary bicarbonate (HCO_3^-) buffer. **A,** Hydrogen (H^+) is actively secreted into the tubule in exchange for sodium (Na^+). **B,** HCO_3^- is filtered into the tubule at the glomerulus. **C,** H^+ and $H_2CO_3^-$ enter reverse hydrolysis, yielding water (H_2O) and carbon dioxide (CO_2). **D,** H_2O remains in the tubule as urine unless it is reabsorbed. **E,** CO_2 diffuses into tubular cells and enters hydrolysis, catalyzed by carbonic anhydrase (CA), yielding H^+ and HCO_3^-. **F,** HCO_3^- is reabsorbed, with Na^+, into the blood.

CA. The HCO_3^- formed is reabsorbed with sodium into the blood. Thus, for every molecule of H^+ secreted, a molecule of HCO_3^- is returned to the blood to restore components of the plasma bicarbonate buffer system.

The *ammonia buffer* depends on the generation of ammonia (NH_3) from amino acids, such as glutamine, in renal tubular cells (Figure 15-4). NH_3 diffuses into the tubular lumen, where it may combine with secreted H^+ to form ammonium (NH_{4+}), a large, charged particle that cannot be reabsorbed. H^+ in this form is thus trapped in the tubule. NH_{4+} is excreted in the urine in combination with Cl^- from NaCl. Na^+ is actively reabsorbed, along with tubular HCO_3^-.

The *phosphate buffer* operates similarly (Figure 15-5), resulting in the formation of weak acids that are excreted in the urine. Sodium and bicarbonate are reabsorbed.

Effects of Other Electrolytes

Although H^+ and HCO_3^- are critical determinants of acid-base balance, they are also electrolytes, subject to the *principle of electroneutrality*, which holds that total cations must equal total anions in any fluid compartment. Renal regulation of serum pH is greatly influenced by the concentrations of other electrolytes, particularly potassium (K^+), sodium (Na^+), calcium (Ca^{2+}), magnesium (Mg^{2+}), chloride (Cl^-), lactate$^-$, and protein (Pr^-).

When serum potassium is elevated (*hyperkalemia*), renal tubular cells secrete more K^+ but retain H^+ for electroneutrality. The opposite occurs in *hypokalemia*,

which promotes renal secretion of H^+. Similarly, H^+ imbalance influences both renal regulation and cellular shifts in potassium. In cases of serum H^+ excess, renal tubular cells secrete more H^+, but K^+ is retained, promoting hyperkalemia. At the tissue level, H^+ moves into cells to be buffered by intracellular proteins, and K^+ moves out into the blood to maintain electroneutrality. This shift does not represent true K^+ excess but does contribute to clinical manifestations of hyperkalemia, which include potentially lethal cardiac dysrhythmias. Treatment of the H^+ excess causes a shift in the opposite direction, promoting hypokalemia. In response to a deficit in serum H^+, renal cells retain H^+ and secrete more K^+, and cellular proteins release H^+ to the extracellular fluid while K^+ shifts intracellularly.

Na^+ and Cl^- are of particular importance in maintaining fluid balance, and the kidney is the principal site of their regulation. Active reabsorption of Na^+ from the renal tubules creates gradients that drive the secretion of H^+ and the reabsorption of anions such as Cl^- and HCO_3^-. The juxtaglomerular cells of the renal glomeruli sense a low extracellular volume, triggering the renin-angiotensin-aldosterone system. Release of the mineralocorticoid hormone aldosterone from the adrenal cortex stimulates renal reabsorption of Na^+ from the distal tubule and proximal collecting duct. Maintenance of electroneutrality requires concurrent increases in the secretion of H^+ and K^+ as well as reabsorption of HCO_3^-. The kidney's priority in such cases is to restore volume balance,

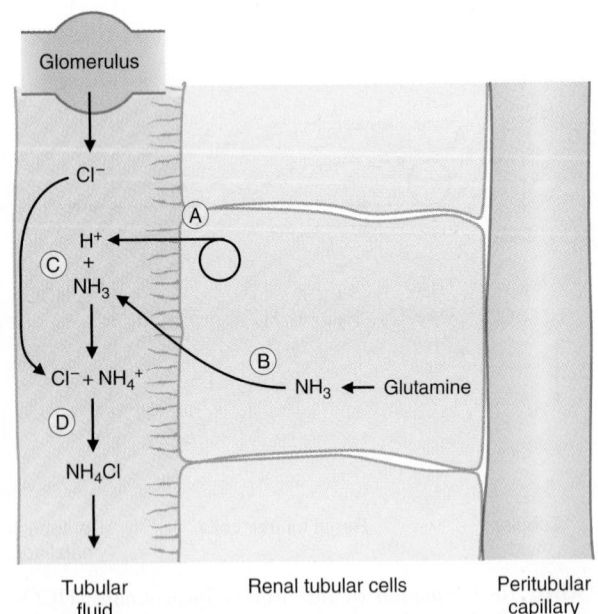

FIGURE 15-4 Function of the ammonia (NH_3) buffer. **A,** Hydrogen (H^+) is actively secreted into the tubular fluid. **B,** NH_3 is formed in the tubular cell and diffuses into the tubular lumen. **C,** Hydrogen (H^+) combines with NH_3 to form ammonium (NH_4^+), which cannot be reabsorbed. **D,** NH_4^+ combines with filtered chloride (Cl^-) for excretion in the urine. *NH₄Cl,* Ammonium chloride.

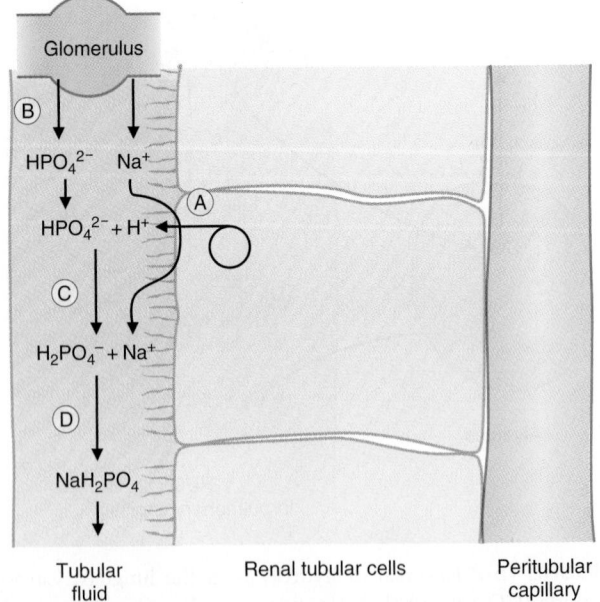

FIGURE 15-5 Function of the phosphate buffer. **A,** Hydrogen (H^+) is actively secreted into the tubule. **B,** HPO_4^{2-} (hydrogen phosphate) and Na^+ are filtered into the tubule at the glomerulus. **C,** H^+ and HPO_4^{2-} combine to form dihydrogen phosphate ($H_2PO_4^-$). **D,** $H_2PO_4^-$ combines with filtered Na^+ for excretion in the urine.

but this happens at the cost of worsening pH status. Clinical conditions that cause low serum Na⁺ *(hyponatremia)* almost invariably result in low Cl⁻ *(hypochloremia)*. In Cl⁻ deficit, the kidney reabsorbs more HCO_3^- to maintain electroneutrality. Conversely, in conditions in which excess HCO_3^- is lost in the urine, Cl⁻ is retained.

Although intracellular proteins are the most important buffers in whole-body acid-base homeostasis, serum proteins such as albumin are also significant. In H⁺ excess, for example, serum proteins bind circulating H⁺, displacing other cations, such as calcium. The level of free (ionized) Ca^{2+} thus rises, promoting clinical manifestations of hypercalcemia. In H⁺ deficit, a greater fraction of serum calcium is bound, decreasing levels of Ca^{2+}. Because H⁺ excess creates a need for more urinary buffers, including ammonia (which is derived from protein), increased buffering of acid promotes depletion of protein. Similarly, deficiency of serum albumin caused by renal disease or other disorders may promote H⁺ excess.

INTERACTION OF ACID-BASE REGULATORY SYSTEMS

Clinical evaluation of total acid-base homeostasis is aided by an understanding of the *Henderson-Hasselbalch equation*, which describes the relationships among pH, acid (H_2CO_3), and base (HCO_3^-):

$$pH = pKa + \log([HCO_3^-]/[H_2CO_3])$$

In this equation, pKa is a constant value (6.1). The base component is represented by serum HCO_3^- (normal value 24 mEq/L); because carbonic acid levels are negligible, the acid is represented by dissolved CO_2. Dissolved CO_2 is derived from the measurement of $PaCO_2$, the partial pressure of CO_2 in arterial blood (normal value 40 mm Hg, multiplied by a unit conversion factor of 0.03 to yield 1.2). When normal values are substituted, the equation becomes:

$$7.4 = 6.1 + \log \frac{24}{1.2}$$

This equation reveals that a ratio of 20 parts base to 1 part acid must be present to yield a normal pH. An increase in the numerator (base) promotes an increase in blood pH; a decrease in base lowers pH. An increase in the denominator (acid) lowers pH; a decrease in acid raises pH (Figure 15-6).

ACID-BASE COMPENSATION

When primary disease processes alter either the acid or the base component of the ratio, the lungs or the kidneys (whichever is unaffected by pathologic change) act to restore the 20:1 ratio and normalize pH. This process is known as *acid-base compensation*. When kidney disease impairs excretion of fixed acids, for example, the respiratory system can increase ventilation to "blow off" excess acid as CO_2. In respiratory failure, the kidneys can compensate for retention of acid (CO_2) by secreting H⁺ and regenerating HCO_3^-.

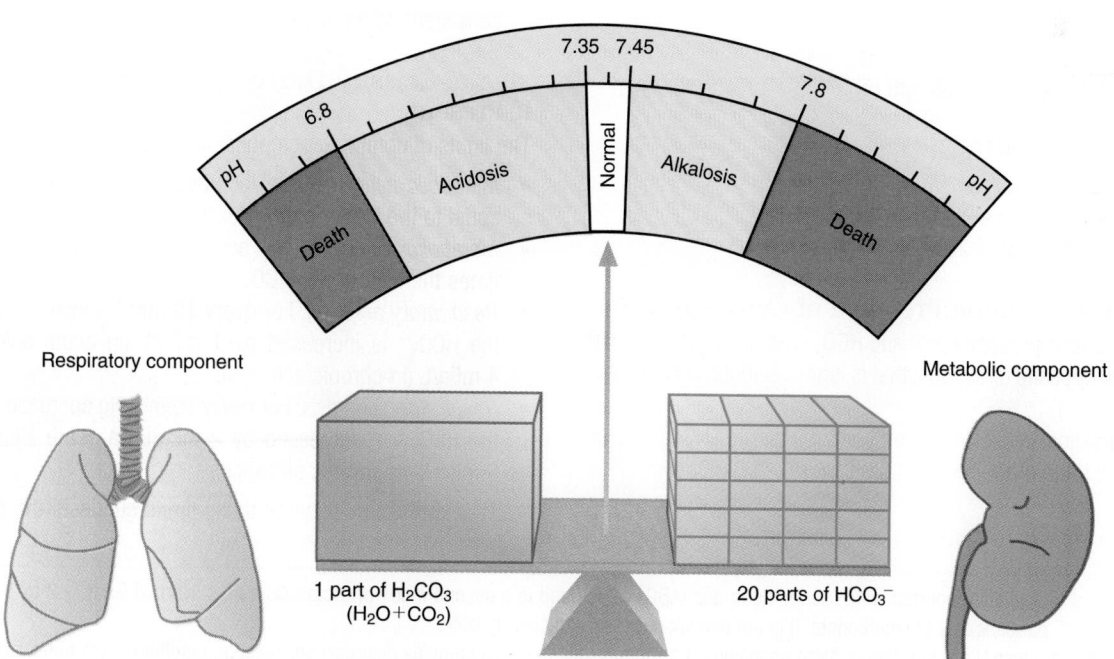

FIGURE 15-6 Regulation of acid-base balance. *H_2CO_3,* Carbonic acid; *H_2O,* water; *CO_2,* carbon dioxide; *HCO_3^-,* bicarbonate.

As stated, blood buffers act to modulate pH changes but do not eliminate acid or base from the body. The lungs or kidneys alter the actual amounts of acid and base, but regulation by these systems is not as fast. The lungs respond within minutes, but maximal compensation takes up to 24 hours. The kidneys may require up to 72 hours to achieve optimal compensation.

Except in mild, chronic respiratory alkalosis (see later discussion), compensation does not fully restore normal pH. Respiratory compensation is limited because reducing ventilation to compensate for a renal deficit of H^+ would eventually result in hypoxemia. Because hypoxemia is a respiratory stimulant, ventilation would again increase. Similarly, renal compensation for ventilatory disorders is potentially limited by many factors, including renal blood flow, tubular flow rates, and saturability of tubular transport processes.

ACID-BASE CORRECTION

Although compensatory responses for primary acid-base disorders may nearly restore the 20:1 ratio of base to acid, the actual amounts of acid and base remain abnormal. Thus, compensation must be differentiated from *correction*, in which the ratio is restored and the absolute quantities of dissolved CO_2 (as derived from $PaCO_2$) and HCO_3^- are returned to normal range. Correction occurs only with resolution of the underlying disorder.

ANALYSIS OF ARTERIAL BLOOD GASES

The status of acid-base homeostasis may be monitored clinically through the serial measurement of *arterial blood gases* (ABGs). Among the parameters reported are pH, $PaCO_2$, and HCO_3^-. As illustrated in Box 15-1, these values may be used to (1) determine the presence and type of acid-base imbalance and (2) evaluate the level of compensation.

DISORDERS OF ACID-BASE BALANCE

The four general classes of acid-base imbalance are (1) respiratory acidosis, (2) respiratory alkalosis, (3) metabolic acidosis, and (4) metabolic alkalosis.

BOX 15-1 *Analysis of Arterial Blood Gases*

Step 1: Classify the pH
Normal: 7.35-7.45
Acidemia: <7.35
Alkalemia: >7.45

Step 2: Assess $PaCO_2$
Normal: 35-45 mm Hg
Respiratory acidosis: >45 mm Hg
Respiratory alkalosis: <35 mm Hg

Step 3: Assess HCO_3^-*
Normal: 22-26 mEq/L
Metabolic acidosis: <22 mEq/L
Metabolic alkalosis: >26 mEq/L

Step 4: Determine Presence of Compensation
Compensation present: $PaCO_2$ and HCO_3^- are abnormal (or nearly so) in opposite directions; that is, one is acidotic and the other alkalotic.†
Compensation absent: One component ($PaCO_2$ or HCO_3^-) is abnormal, the other normal.

Step 5: Identify Primary Disorder, If Possible
If pH is clearly abnormal: The acid-base component most consistent with the pH disturbance is the primary disorder.
If pH is normal or near-normal: The more deviant component is probably primary.‡ Also, note whether pH is on acidotic or alkalotic side of 7.4. The more deviant component should be consistent with this pH.

Step 6: Classify Degree of Compensation, If Present
The limits of complete compensation are as follows:
• *Metabolic acidosis:* The decrease in $PaCO_2$ is approximately equal to the last two digits of the pH.
• *Metabolic alkalosis:* The $PaCO_2$ is approximately equal to 0.6 times the increase in HCO_3^-.
• *Respiratory acidosis:* For every 10 mm Hg increase in $PaCO_2$, the HCO_3^- is increased by 1 mEq/L (in acute acidosis) or 4 mEq/L (in chronic acidosis).
• *Respiratory alkalosis:* For every 10 mm Hg decrease in $PaCO_2$, the HCO_3^- is decreased by 2 mEq/L (in acute alkalosis) or 5 mEq/L (in chronic alkalosis).

"Compensation" beyond these limits suggests the presence of a complex disorder.

---

* Base excess (BE) is also reported with arterial blood gas (ABG) values and is a second index of metabolic status. Normal BE is −2 to +2. Because fluctuation in BE parallels that of bicarbonate, it is not usually necessary to classify both.
† It is possible, but less likely, that two or more opposing primary imbalances (i.e., a complex disorder) are present, resulting in the appearance of compensation. The detection of complex disorders is facilitated by the use of an acid-base map (see Figure 15-7) and by the use of the "formulas" described in Step 6, but a complex disorder cannot always be differentiated from compensation on the basis of laboratory values.
‡ It is unlikely that the more deviant component represents compensation, because except in rare cases the body does not overcompensate for imbalance. When pH approaches the normal range, compensatory mechanisms are no longer triggered.

These disorders are not clinical diagnoses or diseases in themselves; rather, they are clinical syndromes associated with a wide variety of diseases.

Acidosis refers to any pathologic process that causes a relative excess of acid (volatile or fixed) in the body. *Acidemia* is excess acid in the blood. The presence of acidemia does not necessarily confirm an underlying pathologic process; technically, it is merely a laboratory finding.

The same distinction may be made between the terms alkalosis and alkalemia. *Alkalosis* indicates a primary condition resulting in excess base in the body, and *alkalemia* refers more narrowly to elevation of serum pH. Care must be taken not to confuse these terms conceptually, and they must not be used interchangeably in clinical practice.

The incidence of acid-base imbalances in clinical settings is high. A study of 110 consecutive admissions to a general hospital revealed an overall incidence of acid-base imbalances of 56%. The most common disorder was respiratory alkalosis (26 cases), followed by respiratory acidosis (16), metabolic alkalosis (10), and metabolic acidosis (6). Eleven clients had more than one acid-base imbalance concurrently.[11]

RESPIRATORY ALKALOSIS

Respiratory alkalosis is a state of relative excess of base in body fluids resulting from increased respiratory elimination of CO_2. *Acute* respiratory alkalosis lasts for 24 hours or less; *chronic* respiratory alkalosis persists longer.

Etiology and Risk Factors

Respiratory alkalosis is caused by alveolar hyperventilation, in which excess CO_2 is eliminated. The most common cause of respiratory alkalosis is hypoxemia from such pulmonary disorders as pneumonia, pulmonary embolism, asthma, adult (acute) respiratory distress syndrome (ARDS), and pulmonary edema. Transient respiratory alkalosis may also occur secondary to acute anxiety or as a response to respiratory stimulant drugs such as epinephrine and salicylates. Neural disorders, such as stroke and intracranial lesions, may stimulate the central respiratory drive.

The most common causes of mild, chronic respiratory alkalosis are residence in high altitudes and pregnancy. Pulmonary fibrosis and other disorders that limit ventilatory volume result in an increased ventilatory rate, with a possible net excess of CO_2 elimination.

Pathophysiology

A low partial pressure of oxygen in arterial blood (PaO_2) is sensed by peripheral chemoreceptors in the carotid bodies and aortic arch. The rate at which these receptors fire then increases, stimulating the respiratory center in the medulla and increasing the rate and depth of ventilation. Peripheral chemoreceptors are also stimulated in states of low blood flow, such as shock.

Conditions that physically impede expansion of the lungs (such as pulmonary fibrosis) stimulate activation of the respiratory center via the Hering-Breuer, or stretch reflex. The J receptors, located in the alveolar-capillary membrane, are thought to stimulate increased ventilation in disorders such as ARDS, which causes thickening of this membrane.

The central chemoreceptors and respiratory center may be stimulated excessively by chemicals or toxins. In the case of salicylate overdose, it is interesting that adults usually exhibit respiratory alkalosis and that children more often have metabolic acidosis from the acid ingestion. The reason for this difference between children and adults is unknown. In severe alkalemia, changes in the ionization of structural and regulatory proteins result in widespread organ dysfunction. Cellular shifts and increased binding of Ca^{2+} to serum proteins induce electrolyte imbalance.

The buffering response in acute respiratory alkalosis results from (1) shifting of acid from intracellular fluid into the blood and (2) movement of HCO_3^- into cells in exchange for Cl^-. An adaptive increase in lactic acid production occurs secondary to stimulation of glycolysis. Renal compensation in chronic respiratory alkalosis involves decreased H^+ secretion as well as excretion of excess filtered HCO_3^-.

Clinical Manifestations

Manifestations of respiratory alkalosis in a client's ABG analysis include a high pH and a low $PaCO_2$. HCO_3^- levels fall with compensation in chronic respiratory alkalosis, and serum lactate dehydrogenase levels are often elevated. Compensated chronic respiratory alkalosis is the only acid-base imbalance in which serum pH may be returned to within normal limits despite persistence of the initiating cause. Hyperventilation, the underlying cause, is clinically apparent.

Central nervous system manifestations of altered blood flow and neurotransmission are usually predominant. They include paresthesias, lightheadedness, and confusion. Musculoskeletal and cardiac manifestations of hypokalemia and hypocalcemia (such as dysrhythmias and muscle weakness) may be present. Chest pain may occur secondarily to coronary artery spasm but is more often noncardiac in origin. Acute, but not chronic, respiratory alkalosis may cause gastrointestinal manifestations such as nausea, vomiting, and diarrhea due to sympathetic nervous system effects.

Outcome Management

Treatment of the Underlying Disorder

Treatment of mild, chronic respiratory alkalosis is usually not warranted because it produces little risk and few symptoms. Aggressive treatment of the underlying causes of hypoxemia is essential in cases of severe respiratory alkalosis. Electrolyte imbalances usually resolve with treatment of the underlying cause.

Respiratory Support

Oxygen therapy may be used to correct underlying hypoxemia. Rebreathing of CO_2 (as from breathing into a paper bag or other closed system) provides prompt but short-term relief in anxiety-related respiratory alkalosis.

RESPIRATORY ACIDOSIS

Respiratory acidosis is a state of relative excess of acid in body fluids resulting from retention or excessive production of CO_2. *Acute* respiratory acidosis develops and resolves within 3 days or less; *chronic* respiratory acidosis persists over a longer period.

Etiology and Risk Factors

Respiratory acidosis nearly always results from hypoventilation. Chronic respiratory acidosis is most commonly caused by chronic obstructive pulmonary disease (COPD). In end-stage COPD, pathologic changes lead to airway collapse, air trapping, and disturbance of ventilation-perfusion ($\dot{V}/\dot{Q}$) relationships. Acute respiratory acidosis also occurs when respiratory infection or concurrent cardiac disease increases the work of breathing. Hypoventilation with resulting respiratory acidosis is seen in diseases of the neuromuscular junction in which diaphragmatic movement is impaired (such as Guillain-Barré syndrome) and in depression of the medullary respiratory center by drugs or lesions of the central nervous system.

Respiratory acidosis may occur iatrogenically (as a result of treatment) from inadequate mechanical ventilation or from excessive oxygen administration to clients with chronic CO_2 retention (as in COPD). In the latter case, hypoventilation results from the following:

- Depression of the medullary respiratory center with removal of the hypoxemic stimulus
- Worsening of $\dot{V}/\dot{Q}$ relationships secondary to replacement of airway nitrogen (which helps keep airways open) with oxygen

Normally, the most important stimulus for ventilation is an increase in the acidity of cerebrospinal fluid (CSF) resulting from diffusion of CO_2 into the CSF from the blood; however, the higher level of HCO_3^- resulting from renal compensation for chronic respiratory acidosis minimizes the effect of increasing Pa_{CO_2} in these clients. Oxygen therapy may worsen $\dot{V}/\dot{Q}$ relationships because it displaces nitrogen, a much less soluble gas, in alveoli. As oxygen is absorbed, alveoli may collapse, contributing to hypoventilation.

The second, much less common cause of respiratory acidosis is excessive CO_2 production from hypermetabolism or from excessive metabolism of carbohydrate fuels for energy. Clinical use of enteral feedings or parenteral nutrition formulas that are disproportionately high in carbohydrate may contribute to elevated Pa_{CO_2} levels, particularly in clients who also have impaired ventilation.

Pathophysiology

CO_2 accumulates in the blood and diffuses readily into all body compartments. This *hypercapnia* drives the hydrolysis reaction forward, generating carbonic acid that dissociates into H^+ and HCO_3^-. Immediate buffering by nonbicarbonate buffers occurs. Renal compensation proceeds over 3 to 5 days, with greater secretion of H^+ and regeneration of bicarbonate. Renal ammonia production increases, enhancing the function of the ammonia urinary buffer but depleting protein stores. As serum HCO_3^- levels rise with compensation, Cl^- is excreted in greater amounts, potentially inducing hypochloremia in chronic respiratory acidosis. Renal retention of K^+ and cellular cation shifts may lead to hyperkalemia. Displacement of Ca^{2+} from albumin may result in hypercalcemia.

In acute respiratory acidosis, the rapid rise in Pa_{CO_2} results in hypoxemia in clients who are breathing room air because retained CO_2 displaces oxygen in alveoli. Hypoxemia poses a more serious threat to life than either acidemia or hypercapnia in severe acute respiratory acidosis. Acidemia alters the ionization of structural and regulatory proteins (enzymes, for example), resulting in widespread manifestations of organ dysfunction.

Clinical Manifestations

An arterial blood sample that has a low pH signifies that the client has acidemia, and a high Pa_{CO_2} signifies hypercapnia. The subject probably has hypoventilation, the usual underlying cause of respiratory acidosis; manifestations of hypoxemia may be present in severe cases. HCO_3^- levels are normal or, if renal compensation is occurring, elevated. Compensation is present to a greater extent in chronic respiratory acidosis than in acute respiratory acidosis.

Clinical manifestations of organ system dysfunction from acidemia include hypotension and cardiac dysrhythmias caused by decreased vascular tone, decreased myocardial contractility, and manifestations of electrolyte imbalance. Altered cerebral blood flow and depressed neurotransmission in acute respiratory acidosis may manifest as tremors, seizures, lethargy, stupor, and ultimately coma (hypercapnic encephalopathy). Because of compensation, clients with chronic hypercapnia have less dramatic manifestations and little alteration of cerebral blood flow.

Outcome Management

Treatment of the Underlying Disorder

Treatment of respiratory acidosis is focused primarily on resolving the underlying disorder. For example, you may give an antibiotic to treat pneumonia, an opioid antagonist to treat a drug overdose, or dialysis to clear toxins from the blood. Electrolyte imbalances usually resolve with such treatment; however, life-threatening hyperkalemia may require emergency treatment with dialysis or cation-exchange resins.

Respiratory Support

Mechanical ventilation and supplemental oxygen are often employed in conditions that cause respiratory acidosis. Currently, the trend is to use ventilation at lower tidal volumes than would be required to restore $PaCO_2$ completely to normal range. This *permissive hypercapnia* results in fewer airway injuries but comparable clinical outcomes; however, because the client's own ventilatory drive exceeds that provided by the ventilator, sedation is usually required. Oxygen therapy must be administered cautiously (at low flow rates or low percentages) to the client with chronic CO_2 retention to minimize the risk of worsening the client's respiratory status via nitrogen washout and blunting of the ventilatory drive.

Administration of Exogenous Alkali

If the subject has adequate renal function, administration of base (typically, sodium bicarbonate) to correct the pH partially is not warranted. Such treatment may actually worsen the client's condition because bicarbonate further raises CO_2 levels by driving reverse hydrolysis. An exception may be made if the client has severe bronchospasm because alkalinization may restore the responsiveness of the airways to beta-agonist drugs.[2]

METABOLIC ALKALOSIS

Metabolic alkalosis is a state of relative excess of base (or H^+ deficit) in body fluids resulting from a gain of bicarbonate or a loss of fixed acids.

Etiology and Risk Factors

Metabolic alkalosis develops through a two-phase mechanism. In the *generation phase,* the imbalance is first created by (1) loss of acid (as with HCl loss during vomiting) or gain of base (as with administration of $NaHCO_3$) or (2) loss of fluids containing more Cl^- than HCO_3^- (as with overuse of loop or thiazide diuretics). Metabolic alkalosis associated with fluid volume loss is referred to as *contraction alkalosis.* Another common type, *posthypercapnic metabolic alkalosis,* results from too-rapid correction of chronic respiratory acidosis, in which case a compensatory increase in HCO_3^- then persists as a primary disorder.

In the *maintenance phase,* alkalosis persists because renal excretion of HCO_3^-, which would otherwise correct the disorder, is impaired. This impairment may result from hypovolemia in contraction alkalosis or, much

less commonly, from aldosterone excess. In hypovolemia, greater Na^+ reabsorption by the distal tubule (stimulated by the renin-angiotensin-aldosterone system) increases both H^+ secretion and HCO_3^- regeneration. In primary aldosteronism (or with prolonged corticosteroid administration, in which aldosterone-like effects also arise), the hormone stimulates increased Na^+ reabsorption by the same distal tubular transport mechanism.

Metabolic alkalosis from fluid loss is referred to as *saline sensitive* because restoration of volume with fluid containing NaCl permits the kidneys to restore acid-base homeostasis. Alkalosis in cases of aldosterone excess is not correctable with administration of a saline solution and so is termed *saline resistant.*

Overcorrection of acidosis with $NaHCO_3$ may cause alkalosis, as can massive transfusion of whole blood. The citrate anticoagulant used for storing blood is metabolized to bicarbonate. Packed RBCs contain much less citrate; thus their use in multiple transfusion is preferred.

Loss of gastric fluid via nasogastric suction or vomiting further contributes to metabolic alkalosis because of loss of HCl. Additional HCl must be produced by gastric cells via the hydrolysis reaction. H^+ is secreted into the stomach with Cl^-; the HCO_3^- produced during the reaction is reabsorbed into the blood.

Pathophysiology

Respiratory compensation for metabolic alkalosis is limited by the hypoxemia that quickly develops with hypoventilation. Most buffering occurs in the extracellular fluid, where the buffers are much less effective for base loads than for acid loads. Severe alkalemia leads to widespread organ dysfunction because of altered ionization of body proteins as well as enhanced Ca^{2+} binding to serum proteins. Neurologic and cardiovascular systems are primarily affected. Hypokalemia, which occurs from cellular shifts and renal or intestinal losses, is more prominent in metabolic alkalosis than in respiratory alkalosis.

Clinical Manifestations

Metabolic alkalosis is manifested in ABG values by a high pH and a high HCO_3^-. $PaCO_2$ rises with compensation. Adaptive hypoventilation may be apparent and may induce some hypoxemia. Manifestations of volume deficit are often present in association with the underlying disorder. Hypokalemia and hypomagnesemia may manifest as cardiac dysrhythmias. Central nervous system manifestations include lethargy, confusion, and seizures.

Outcome Management

Treatment of the Underlying Disorder

Prompt treatment of the underlying disease process is the primary approach. Replacement of lost fluids and electrolytes (potassium and magnesium) and support of renal function (possibly with dialysis against a high-chloride, low-bicarbonate dialysate) are often the mainstays of therapy.

Administration of Acetazolamide

Acetazolamide (Diamox) is a diuretic that inhibits CA and promotes loss of bicarbonate in the urine. Losses of potassium and phosphate are also greater with the use of acetazolamide, however, and may lead to manifestations of electrolyte imbalance.

Administration of Exogenous Acid

In severe alkalemia, the intravenous administration of acid (HCl) or HCl precursors (ammonium chloride or arginine monohydrochloride) may be warranted to enhance physiologic compensation. Risks of acid infusion are substantial, however; they include local tissue injury (sclerosis of veins), hypervolemia, hyperosmolar imbalance (with HCl precursors), increased ammonia levels (with ammonium chloride), and hyperkalemia (with arginine monohydrochloride).

METABOLIC ACIDOSIS

Metabolic acidosis is a state of relative acid excess (or base deficit) in body fluids resulting from a gain of fixed acids or a loss of bicarbonate.

Etiology and Risk Factors

Metabolic acidosis may be caused by either of two mechanisms: accumulation of fixed acid or loss of base. These mechanisms often can be differentiated clinically by the presence or absence of a high *anion gap*. Normally, the anion gap is 10 ± 4 mEg/L.[12] It is calculated by subtracting the sum of the serum concentrations of the major anions, bicarbonate and chloride, from the serum concentration of sodium. The difference, or "gap," represents anions in the serum other than HCO_3^- and Cl^-, notably albumin, phosphate, sulfate, and organic anions such as ketones and lactate.

When acidosis results from addition of organic acid (as in lactic acidosis), bicarbonate is consumed in buffering but is not lost from the body. Unmeasured anions (primarily proteins) buffer most of the acid load, and the anion gap thus increases. Common causes of *high anion gap acidosis* include the following:

- Azotemic renal failure, in which acid end products of protein metabolism cannot be effectively excreted because of impaired glomerular filtration
- Diabetic ketoacidosis, in which ketoacids accumulate because of accelerated lipid metabolism in the absence of insulin
- Lactic acidosis, a consequence of an increase in anaerobic carbohydrate metabolism

- Ingestion of toxins with acid metabolites (less common)

Non–anion gap acidosis caused by loss of base is also called *hyperchloremic metabolic acidosis*. In this case, the kidneys retain chloride when excess bicarbonate is lost from the body, and the anion gap remains normal. Excess bicarbonate may be lost through either the kidneys or the intestinal tract. In renal tubular acidosis, the renal tubular cells cannot reabsorb bicarbonate, which therefore is lost in the urine. Intestinal secretions, high in bicarbonate, may be lost through enteric drainage tubes (such as an ileostomy tube) or diarrhea. Drugs that inhibit CA, such as acetazolamide, interfere with bicarbonate regeneration during urinary buffering. Critically ill clients who receive very aggressive fluid volume replacement with normal saline or other bicarbonate-free solution may develop a relative bicarbonate deficiency due to dilution of extracellular fluids. In non–anion gap acidosis caused by a gain of mineral acid (such as HCl), chloride is ingested with the acid, and bicarbonate is excreted proportionately.

Pathophysiology

Metabolic acidosis is accompanied by a compensatory increase in ventilation. Severe acidemia induces insulin resistance and depresses glycolytic enzymes, resulting in impairment of energy metabolism. The function of regulatory and structural proteins is impaired by altered ionization, leading to widespread organ dysfunction. Increased protein catabolism also occurs. Hyperkalemia occurs because K^+ shifts out of cells as excess H^+ enters. Insulin deficiency in diabetic ketoacidosis may worsen hyperkalemia because insulin normally promotes cellular uptake of K^+ along with glucose. Uptake of lactic acid by the liver is reduced, whereas hepatic lactate production is increased.

In metabolic acidosis caused by a gain of organic acids, buffering rapidly depletes bicarbonate stores. If renal function is not impaired, renal regeneration of HCO_3^- occurs with excretion of H^+; however, this response takes several days.

Clinical Manifestations

Metabolic acidosis is apparent in ABG values as a low pH and a low HCO_3^-. $PaCO_2$ drops as respiratory compensation occurs. Systemic manifestations of acidemia resulting from altered protein function and electrolyte imbalance are similar to those of respiratory acidosis except that compensatory hyperventilation is present.

Outcome Management

Treatment of the Underlying Disorder

Aggressive intervention aimed at resolving the underlying disorder is the primary form of treatment and usually involves restoration of normal tissue oxygenation and perfusion. Electrolyte imbalance is treated only if it is life threatening because it normally resolves with correction of the underlying disorder.

Respiratory Support

Assisted mechanical ventilation may be indicated for clients whose ability to hyperventilate in compensation is limited.

Administration of Exogenous Alkali

In metabolic acidosis associated with hyperkalemia or with toxin ingestion, administration of intravenous sodium bicarbonate or other alkalinizing substances may be warranted to minimize the detrimental effects of the acidosis until the underlying disorder is resolved or until physiologic compensation is effective. In the more common types, lactic acidosis and ketoacidosis, no evidence exists that alkali administration is beneficial; in fact, it may be detrimental. Fluid overload, hyperosmolar imbalance, and alkalosis attributable to excessive treatment are risks of this approach. As previously mentioned, administration of bicarbonate results in increased CO_2 levels, which may be detrimental in clients with respiratory disease or advanced cardiac failure. Alternative alkalinizing agents, such as tromethamine (Tham), produce less CO_2 but have not proved more effective than $NaHCO_3$ for the treatment of severe acidemia.

COMPLEX ACID-BASE DISORDERS

Mixed acid-base disorders, in which two primary acid-base imbalances coexist, are common. In cardiac arrest, for example, lactic acid quickly accumulates as a result of anaerobic metabolism; the carbonic acid level is elevated because of respiratory arrest. In COPD, underlying respiratory acidosis may be complicated by metabolic alkalosis secondary to diuretic or steroid therapy.

A *triple acid-base disorder* is present when metabolic acidosis and metabolic alkalosis coexist with either respiratory acidosis or respiratory alkalosis. (The two respiratory imbalances cannot coexist because they have opposite effects on ventilation.) As an example of a triple disorder, imbalances caused by ingestion of methanol (an exogenous toxin that produces metabolic acidosis), vomiting (which produces metabolic alkalosis), and respiratory arrest from aspiration (which produces respiratory acidosis) may occur simultaneously.

A complex acid-base disorder should be suspected when a client's $PaCO_2$ value and HCO_3^- level do not correlate with pH or when ABG evidence of compensation exceeds predicted levels (see Box 15-1). Use of an acid-base map may also facilitate detection (Figure 15-7). If the plotted ABG values converge at a point outside the usual range for a primary imbalance, a complex disorder is likely.

■ Nursing Management of the Medical Client Assessment

You must be alert for manifestations of acid-base imbalance in high-risk clients. These clients include those who:
- Have a known disease of the pulmonary, cardiovascular, or renal system
- Are in a hypermetabolic state, such as with fever, sepsis, or burns
- Are receiving total parenteral nutrition or enteral tube feedings high in carbohydrate
- Are receiving mechanical ventilation
- Have diabetes
- Are vomiting, have diarrhea, or have enteric drainage
- Are an older adult

Age-related decreases in respiratory and renal function may limit the client's ability to compensate for acid-base disturbances. The normal aging process results in decreased ventilatory capacity as well as loss of alveolar surface area for gas exchange; thus older adults are susceptible to respiratory acidosis from hypoventilation and to respiratory alkalosis from hypoxemia. Older adults commonly take multiple medications for hypertension or cardiovascular disease; these drugs may contribute to hypokalemia and metabolic alkalosis. Respiratory compensation in this condition is compromised because of the structural and functional changes mentioned.

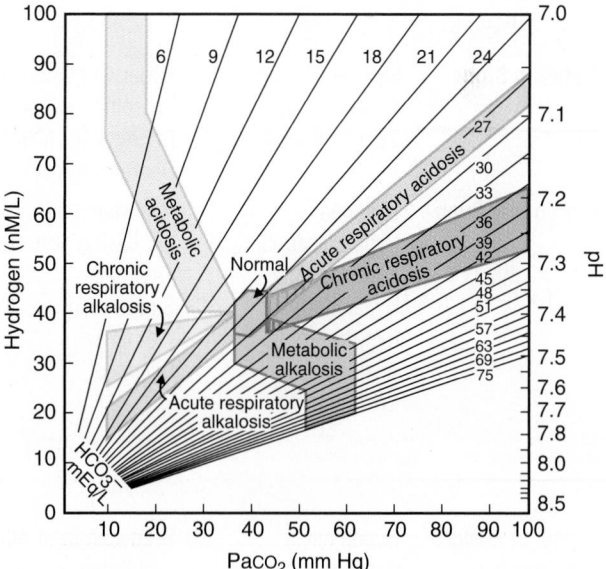

FIGURE 15-7 An acid-base map. To use the acid-base map, plot the pH on the vertical axis and the partial pressure of arterial carbon dioxide ($PaCO_2$) on the horizontal axis. Note the point at which the values intersect. If the result falls outside the normal area or the 95% confidence bands for the major primary disorders, the client probably has a complex acid-base imbalance; however, a point falling within one of the bands does not rule out a complex disorder. HCO_3^-, Bicarbonate.

Decreased cardiac output in the aging person diminishes renal perfusion and glomerular filtration. Aldosterone is less effective in older persons, as is ammonia buffering. These changes limit renal compensation for respiratory imbalances and may put an older client at higher risk for metabolic imbalance.

To assess for acid-base imbalances, document the findings of a comprehensive physical assessment of ventilatory status, cardiovascular function, and fluid-electrolyte balance, as described in the Critical Monitoring feature on Acid-Base Imbalances, below. Carefully analyze the trends you see. Consider laboratory values, including ABG, electrolyte, blood urea nitrogen, creatinine, and serum lactate dehydrogenase values.

Interpret Arterial Blood Gas Values. Knowledgeable interpretation of ABG values is critical for timely, appropriate intervention in acid-base disturbances. Often the nurse is the first to see a client's ABG results and becomes the communication link between respiratory therapists and physicians about potential changes in a client's status or treatment. In critical care units, many nurses are using bedside ABG analyzers to obtain these

results. Systems for continuous in vivo monitoring of blood gases have recently been developed. Although ABG interpretation is essential to diagnosis and treatment of acid-base imbalance, ABG findings are helpful only when they are considered as part of the total clinical picture.

Protect the Client. Preventing client injury during diagnostic procedures is one of your most important responsibilities. For example, perform Allen's test to ensure adequate circulation to the hand before a client receives a radial artery puncture for withdrawal of an arterial blood specimen. Perform this test as follows:
1. Have the client tightly close the intended test hand into a fist.
2. Apply pressure over the pulse points for both radial and ulnar arteries.
3. Ask the client to open the fist; the palm has a blanched look from a lack of blood.
4. Release pressure on the ulnar artery. If the artery has adequate circulation, the client's palm reddens within 10 or 15 seconds; it is safe to use the radial artery to obtain a blood specimen.

CRITICAL MONITORING
Acid-Base Imbalances

	Respiratory Acidosis	Metabolic Acidosis	Respiratory Alkalosis	Metabolic Alkalosis
Defining Signs	Hypoventilation Increasing $Paco_2$ Decreasing pH	Hyperventilation (Kussmaul's respirations, or air hunger) Decreasing HCO_3^- value Decreasing pH	Hyperventilation Decreasing $Paco_2$ Increasing pH	Increasing HCO_3^- value Increasing pH Hypoventilation
Commonly Seen	Dyspnea Hypercalcemia Hyperkalemia Hypochloremia Hypernatremia Anxiety Confusion	Hyperkalemia Increasing serum Cl^- and anion gap Stress response followed by lethargy Dyspnea	Confusion Hypocalcemia Hypokalemia Lightheadedness	Confusion Decreasing level of consciousness Hypocalcemia Hypochloremia Hypokalemia Hypomagnesemia Hypovolemia Numbness and tingling of limbs
Signs of Severe Imbalance	Hypotension Papilledema Seizures Dysrhythmias Muscle tremors Lethargy Coma Hypoxemia	Bradycardia or other dysrhythmia Decreased cardiac output Gastrointestinal distention Hypotension Nausea and vomiting	Dysrhythmias Numbness and tingling of limbs and around mouth Muscle weakness Chest pain Nausea, vomiting, diarrhea	Dysrhythmias Decreased cardiac output Hypotension Hypoxemia Muscle cramping or tetany Muscle tremors Seizures

Failure to assess collateral circulation may result in severe ischemic injury to the client's hand if the ulnar artery is compromised and the radial artery is injured by the puncture.

Critically ill clients commonly have femoral or radial arterial catheter systems from which blood specimens are drawn. Frequent sampling can result in significant blood loss if an open system is used. Nursing research has demonstrated that a minimal discard specimen of 2 ml is sufficient to clear the arterial line of heparinized solution before blood is aspirated for ABG testing.[13] Closed systems allow reinstillation of initially aspirated heparinized solution and blood. Nursing responsibilities for clients with arterial lines are discussed in Chapter 61.

You are responsible for minimizing errors in ABG analysis caused by faulty specimen collection and handling. Potential sampling errors, their consequences, and nursing implications are summarized in Table 15-1. Despite quality control procedures, erroneous blood gas data are sometimes reported. A sampling error or transcription error should be suspected when the reported values lack internal consistency or external congruity. *Internal consistency* means that the values make sense when considered as a whole. An alkalotic pH, for example, is inconsistent with excess $PaCO_2$ and deficient HCO_3^-. *External congruity* means that the ABG findings are consistent with other laboratory data and with clinical assessment findings. For example, a client with a pH of 7.10 should appear profoundly ill.

Diagnosis, Outcomes, Interventions

Nursing Diagnoses. Several nursing diagnoses may apply to the management of underlying causes and clinical manifestations of acid-base disturbances. For example, *Ineffective Breathing Pattern, Ineffective Tissue Perfusion,* or *Risk for Injury* may be appropriate. Acid-base imbalances are perhaps best conceptualized as collaborative problems, however, because the interventions of several health care professionals, including nurses, respiratory therapists, and physicians, are required for effective treatment.

Outcomes. When acid-base imbalances are approached as collaborative problems, the expected outcomes reflect timely resolution of underlying disorders and minimization of the detrimental effects of acidemia or alkalemia. Your role in promoting these outcomes includes implementing medical management and watching for clinical manifestations of the imbalances and the response to treatment.

Interventions. Corrective interventions address the underlying causes of acid-base imbalances and are the mainstay of treatment in such disorders. Compensatory imbalances are not treated but instead resolve spontaneously as the primary disorder is reversed. You should optimize the client's respiratory and renal function through positioning, pulmonary hygiene, and hydration.

TABLE 15-1   *Sources of Error in Sampling for Arterial Blood Gas Analysis*

Air bubbles in syringe	↑ PaO_2 ↓ $PaCO_2$ ↑ pH	Expel all air bubbles immediately. Do not agitate syringe. Do not use any sample that appears frothy.
Inadvertent venous sample or venous contamination of arterial sample	↓ PaO_2 ↑ $PaCO_2$ ↓ pH	Avoid use of femoral artery. Use short-beveled needle. Do not overshoot artery and then withdraw to "catch" it. Watch for autofilling of syringe with arterial puncture. Verify questionable results with new sample.
Anticoagulant effects Altered pH	↓ pH	Use lithium heparin, if possible. Use 1:1000 units/ml concentration. Use minimum 2-ml discard sample with arterial line aspiration.
Dilution of sample	↑ pH ↓ all other values	Use syringe with minimal dead space. Use dried heparin if available. Use at least 3-ml sample.
Effects of metabolism of white blood cells in sample	↓ PaO_2 ↑ $PaCO_2$ ↓ pH	Place sample in ice water immediately. Have sample analyzed within 20 min. Cool sample to 5° C if it cannot be analyzed quickly. Have sample analyzed immediately if client has leukocytosis.

Data from Malley, W.J. (1990). *Clinical blood gases: Application and noninvasive alternatives.* Philadelphia: W.B. Saunders; and Williams, A.J. (1998). ABC of oxygen: Assessing and interpreting arterial blood gases and acid-base balance. *British Medical Journal, 317*(7167), 1213-1216.
$PaCO_2$, Partial pressure of carbon dioxide in arterial blood; *PaO_2,* partial pressure of oxygen in arterial blood; ↑, increase in; ↓, decrease in.

Also, help clients cope with the anxiety that often accompanies—and may contribute to—acid-base imbalance. Collaborate in the administration of drug therapy, fluid and electrolyte replacement, oxygen therapy, and mechanical ventilation when indicated.

Provide Respiratory Support. Altered ventilation is a component of all significant acid-base imbalances, whether as a contributing cause or as a result of compensation. You can help to promote optimal ventilation through such measures as repositioning, airway management, hydration, and implementation of oxygen therapy and mechanical ventilation.

Administer Exogenous Acid or Alkali. In extreme circumstances that require intravenous administration of acid or base, you must be knowledgeable about the potential risks of this therapy, and you must carefully monitor administration rates and therapeutic response. For a detailed discussion of appropriate nursing interventions for specific disorders underlying acid-base imbalances, consult the appropriate chapters of this book.

Evaluation

Acid-base disorders can be acute and corrected quickly, with control of the underlying disorder, or they may be chronic and managed with compensation. Clients with chronic forms of acid-base imbalance must be assessed closely because they may decompensate quickly.

CONCLUSIONS

In collaboration with other health care professionals, you may reduce the client's risk for adverse outcomes resulting from acid-base imbalances. Because of the narrow homeostatic range of serum pH, the client at risk must be carefully monitored to detect imbalance as early as possible. Nursing interventions that promote optional respiratory and renal function are particularly important in prevention and treatment of acid-base imbalances.

THINKING CRITICALLY *evolve*

1. The client is a 65-year-old widow with a long history of type 2 diabetes mellitus. She was a heavy smoker for 40 years but has not smoked in the last 5 years. She is admitted to the general medical unit because of a 1-week history of profuse diarrhea, attributed to food poisoning. She appears to be in respiratory distress. Her admission ABG values are pH, 7.26; $PaCO_2$, 13 mm Hg; HCO_3^-, 5 mEq/L. What acid-base imbalance does she have? Should you encourage her to breathe more slowly? Other than ABGs, what laboratory values should you monitor closely in this case? Why?
Factors to Consider. What acids or bases are lost through diarrhea? Why might a respiratory change have developed if the client's primary problem is gastrointestinal (e.g., metabolic)?

2. A 19-year-old college student is brought to the emergency department at 4:30 AM by his friends. While studying for final examinations, he grew increasingly anxious during his "cram session," frequently voicing doubts about passing a particularly difficult course. His breathing became increasingly labored, and he seemed dazed and confused. He says his "face feels numb." His pulse is rapid (165 beats/min) and he is diaphoretic. He was seen with bleeding duodenal ulcers 2 years ago. ABG analysis of blood samples drawn in the emergency department reveals pH, 7.58; $PaCO_2$, 21 mm Hg; HCO_3^-, 20 mEq/L. What acid-base imbalance does the client have? What caused it? What bedside assessments should you perform and why? What interventions should you consider that might prevent future episodes?
Factors to Consider. Can rapid breathing alone alter the excretion of components needed for acid-base balance?

3. A 72-year-old retired college professor has a 55-pack-year history of cigarette smoking and advanced emphysema. He had an acute myocardial infarction 5 years ago, from which he recovered uneventfully. He sees his physician in the clinic, complaining of a "cold" that he "just cannot get rid of" and "soreness" in his chest. His blood pressure is 165/90 mm Hg, and he has inspiratory crackles in both lung bases. His ankles are edematous. ABG analysis of blood samples drawn during the visit revealed pH, 7.34; $PaCO_2$, 65 mm Hg; HCO_3^-, 34 mEq/L. What acid-base imbalance does he have? What is the probable cause? What additional information would be helpful in planning his care? What variables should you consider in determining priorities of care?
Factors to Consider. Consider that the client has developed heart failure. When the lungs fill with fluid, what happens to O_2/CO_2 exchange and, thereby, acid-base balance?

Discussions for these questions can be found on the website and the CD-ROM.

BIBLIOGRAPHY

1. Adrogue, H.E., & Adrogue, H.J. (2001). Acid-base physiology. *Respiratory Care, 46*(4), 328-341.
2. Epstein, S.K., & Singh, N. (2001). Respiratory acidosis. *Respiratory Care, 46*(4), 366-383.
3. Fall, P.J. (2000). A stepwise approach to acid-base disorders. *Postgraduate Medicine, 107*(3), 249-263.
4. Foster, G.T., Vaziri, N.D., & Sassoon, C.S.H. (2001). Respiratory alkalosis. *Respiratory Care, 46*(4), 384-391.
5. Hansen, M. (1998). *Pathophysiology: Foundations of disease and clinical intervention.* Philadelphia: W.B. Saunders.
6. Heitz, U.E., & Horne, M.M. (2001). *Pocket guide to fluid, electrolyte, and acid-base balance.* (4th Ed.). St. Louis: Mosby.
7. Horne, C., & Derrico, D. (1999). Mastering ABGs: The art of arterial blood gas measurement. *American Journal of Nursing, 99*(8), 26-33.
8. Khanna, A., & Kurtzman, N.A. (2001). Metabolic acidosis. *Respiratory Care, 46*(4), 354-365.
9. Kirksey, K.M., Holt-Ashley, M., & Goodroad, B.K. (2001). An easy method for interpreting the results of arterial blood gas analysis. *Critical Care Nurse, 21*(5), 49-54.
10. Kraut, J.A., & Madias, N.E. (2001). Approach to clients with acid-base disorders. *Respiratory Care, 46*(4), 392-403.
11. Palange, P., et al. (1990). Incidence of acid-base and electrolyte disturbances in a general hospital: A study of 110 consecutive admissions. *Recenti Progressi in Medicina (Roma), 81*(12), 788-791.
12. Swenson, E.R. (2001). Metabolic acidosis. *Respiratory Care, 46*(4), 342-353.
13. Wilkes, P. (1998). Hypoproteinemia, strong-ion difference, and acid-base status in critically ill patients. *Journal of Applied Physiology, 84*(5), 1740-1748.
14. Wong, F.W.H. (1999). A new approach to ABG interpretation. *American Journal of Nursing, 99*(8), 34-36.

Clients Having Surgery

Nancy J. Girard

Having surgery is a major event in any person's life. Clients faced with surgery want to know that someone is there with them and will look out for them during a time when they may have no control or self-protective abilities. The perioperative nurse is the member of the surgical team to whom clients are most likely to look for advocacy.

PERIOPERATIVE NURSING

The total surgical episode is called the *perioperative period*. This period in the health care continuum includes the time before surgery, or the *preoperative period;* the time spent during the actual surgical procedure, or *intraoperative period;* and the period after the surgery is completed, or *postoperative period*. In the broadest definition of perioperative nursing practice, care can range from home, through surgery and recovery, and back to home again. A *perioperative nurse* is a registered nurse who uses the nursing process to design, plan, and deliver care to meet the identified needs of a client whose protective reflexes or self-care abilities are potentially compromised because of the operative procedures to be performed. Surgery is performed in a multitude of settings, and the nurse's role as a surgical team member is partially defined by the practice setting. Thus perioperative nursing is client centered rather than task oriented. The perioperative nurse must possess and apply knowledge of anatomy, physiology, psychology, and sociocultural and spiritual beliefs and practices, in addition to knowledge of all aspects of the surgical procedure to be performed. The perioperative nurse must be a good communicator, delegator, and supervisor to ensure that the needs of the client are being met throughout the surgical experience.

BASIC CONCEPTS OF PERIOPERATIVE NURSING

Nursing care of the perioperative client takes place immediately before, during, and immediately after a surgical procedure. In each of these periods, specific assessments and interventions are performed by nurses acting both as independent clinicians and as members of the health care team. The goals of perioperative nursing practice are to assist clients and their significant others through the surgical episode, to help promote positive outcomes, and to help clients achieve their optimal level of function and wellness after surgery. The management of clients' needs, both unique and predictable, may be through direct or indirect interventions. These interventions are planned to assist the client in meeting the projected outcomes in an efficient and appropriate manner.

evolve *Be sure to check out the bonus material on the Evolve website and the CD-ROM, including free self-assessment exercises.*
http://evolve.elsevier.com/Black/medsurg/

Nursing Outcomes Classification (NOC)
for Nursing Diagnoses–Clients Having Surgery

Acute Pain
  Comfort Level
  Pain Control
  Pain: Disruptive Effects
  Pain Level
Anxiety
  Anxiety Control
  Coping
Deficient Knowledge
  Concentration
  Knowledge: Diet
  Knowledge: Disease Process
  Knowledge: Health Resources
  Knowledge: Illness Care
  Knowledge: Medication
  Knowledge: Prescribed Activity
  Knowledge: Treatment Procedure

  Knowledge: Treatment Regimen
  Information Processing
Disturbed Thought Processes
  Cognitive Ability
  Cognitive Orientation
  Concentration
  Decision Making
  Distorted Thought Control
  Identity
  Information Processing
  Neurologic Status: Consciousness
Hypothermia
  Thermoregulation
  Neurologic Status
  Vital Signs Status
Risk for Aspiration
  Cognitive Ability

  Endurance
  Immobility Consequences: Physiologic
  Infection Status
  Knowledge: Treatment (Procedures)
  Neurologic Status
  Respiratory Status: Gas Exchange
  Respiratory Status: Ventilation
  Risk Control
Risk for Injury
  Neurologic Status
  Risk Control
  Safety Behavior: Fall Prevention
  Safety Behavior: Home Physical Environment
  Safety Status: Physical Injury
  Symptom Control

Perioperative nursing care is implemented by registered nurses who strive to assist the client by functioning in various roles.

PREOPERATIVE PERIOD

Each client responds differently to surgery. Therefore for each client having surgery, a care plan based on the nursing process is developed. It is vital to identify potential risks and complications that may arise during the perioperative period. In addition, a care plan can also identify the need for supportive services at home or in the hospital after surgery.

Preoperative Assessment

Assessment is the first step in the nursing process and is designed to provide information that enables the nurse and the client to plan for optimal postoperative outcomes. Because of same-day admissions and limited time for interaction with the client, the perioperative nurse must be able to complete quickly and effectively a meaningful preoperative evaluation of the physical, mental, and emotional status. Preoperative assessment can take place in many different places, including the physician's office before admission to a health care facility, at home during the days before the operation and on admission, the night before surgery if the client is in the hospital, and on admission on the day of surgery. In the case of emergency surgery, time often does not permit complete preoperative assessment, care planning, and teaching. Nevertheless, preparation must be as thorough as possible.

Preoperative assessment includes the medical/health history, the psychosocial history, physical examination, cognitive assessment, and diagnostic testing. When surgery must be performed following a traumatic event (e.g., gunshot wound, stab wound, serious accident, or severe fall), a preoperative assessment must include details of the traumatic event described as precisely as possible. If the client was injured in a fall or a motor-vehicle accident, information about injury-related factors, such as the position in which the injury occurred or whether the accident caused the victim to lose consciousness, may help to assess surgical risk or identify underlying conditions related to the injurious event. Traumatically injured clients are usually admitted to the operating room from an emergency department. Emergency department staff will provide a detailed report with the transfer.

Medical/Health History

Obtaining a health history allows clients to explain their understanding of impending surgery and to establish rapport with the nurse conducting the interview. Reassurance by the nurse through this process may reduce anxiety in the client and family members or significant others. In most instances, the past medical history has been previously recorded and is found in the medical record. A complete medical history is critical, and the nurse reviews it to ensure that it is thorough, completing any missing pieces and validating information with the client. The purpose of reviewing the past medical history is to determine operative risk. The past medical history should include, but is not limited to, the following.

Previous Surgery and Experience with Anesthesia. Any untoward reactions to anesthesia (e.g., high fever, intraoperative death of family members, known malignant hy-

E B EVIDENCE-BASED PRACTICE IN ACTION

Latex Allergy in the Operating Room

Latex allergy is an abnormally high sensitivity to a protein in rubber, which causes a physical reaction. A latex allergy can be life-threatening. Anyone can develop a latex allergy, but people who undergo frequent surgeries are at higher risk because they are exposed to latex so often. The thin, highly stretchy rubber found in gloves, tubes, drains, and rubber bands are common sources of latex allergy. Thin latex gloves are often coated with cornstarch to make it easier to get the gloves on and off. When the gloves are removed, rubber particles that attach to the cornstarch may become airborne, causing an allergic reaction in those who have a latex sensitivity.

There are two types of allergic reactions to latex products. The first type is contact dermatitis, which is most commonly associated with chronic glove wear. Irritant dermatitis often appears as chapped hands, sometimes with cracking and scaling of the skin. Although this form of allergy is very irritating, it is not life-threatening. The second and more serious reaction is an immediate allergic reaction. As with other common forms of allergy, these reactions occur in people who have previously been exposed to latex and have become sensitized. Clients who are already allergic may develop respiratory manifestations when re-exposed to latex aerosols generated by powdered latex products. Anaphylaxis can develop.

Individuals who are allergic to latex products may experience allergic reactions resulting from cross-reactivity from a variety of fresh fruits, vegetables, and nuts, including avocado, banana, carrot, celery, chestnut, hazelnut, kiwi, melons, papaya, potato, and tomato.

Products containing latex are labeled. Latex exposure should be avoided whenever possible in those who show signs of latex allergy, because exposure is cumulative. Non-latex gloves are available, and powder-free surgical gloves are used to reduce airborne exposure. Admission questions are used to determine high-risk clients. Clients who are known to be allergic to latex are treated only with latex-free products.

Bibliography

1. American Academy of Dermatology. (1998). American Academy of Dermatology's Position paper on latex allergy. *Journal of American Academy of Dermatology, 39*(1), 98-106.
2. Elliott, B.A. (2002). Latex allergy: The perspective from the surgical suite. *Journal of Allergy and Clinical Immunology, 110*(2 Suppl.), S117-S120.
3. Hourihane, H., et. al. (2002). Impact of reported surgical procedures on the incidence and prevalence of latex allergy: A prospective study of 1263 children. *Journal of Pediatrics, 140*(4), 479-482.
4. Tesiorowski, C. (2003). Latex allergies in the healthcare worker. *Journal of Perianesthesia Nursing, 18*(1), 18-31.

---

perthermia, prolonged nausea and vomiting) by the client or anyone in the family must be reported to anesthesia personnel. These problems do not preclude surgery but often require a change in the type of anesthetics used.

Serious Illness or Trauma. This information should cover anything that might influence the surgery and recovery. An ABCDE mnemonic is often used to ascertain information:

- *A*—allergy to medications, chemicals, and other environmental products such as latex (see the Evidence-Based Practice in Action feature on Latex Allergy in the Operating Room, above). All allergies are reported to anesthesia and surgical personnel before the beginning of surgery. If allergies exist, an allergy band must be placed on the client's arm immediately. Latex-free medical supplies may be needed depending on the nature of the allergic response.

- *B*—bleeding tendencies or the use of medications that deter clotting, such as aspirin or products containing aspirin, heparin, or warfarin sodium. Herbal medications may also increase bleeding times or mask potential blood-related problems. See the Complementary and Alternative Therapy feature on Supplements That Should Not Be Taken During the Time of Surgery on p. 310).

- *C*—cortisone or steroid use.
- *D*—diabetes mellitus, a condition that not only requires strict control of blood glucose levels but is also known to delay wound healing.
- *E*—emboli; previous embolic events (such as lower leg blood clots) may recur because of prolonged immobility.

Clients whose immune system is suppressed are at a much higher risk for development of a postoperative infection and have a diminished capacity to fight that infection.

Alcohol, Recreational Drug, or Nicotine Use. The use of drugs signals a potential problem with the administration of anesthesia or analgesia and risk for withdrawal complications. Clients who use alcohol or drugs may experience withdrawal manifestations while the drugs are withdrawn during the postoperative course. In addition, clients addicted to alcohol often have malnutrition or unpredictable reactions to anesthetic agents. As little as two drinks per day can lead to withdrawal manifestations that may require dosage alterations in anesthesia and analgesia.

The abuse of tobacco or inhaled drugs reduces hemoglobin levels, making less oxygen available for tissue repair. Smokers may be more susceptible to thrombus (clot) formation because of the hypercoagulability secondary to nicotine use. Smokers are also much more likely to have damage to lung tissue. Clients are instructed to abstain from any nicotine product for at least 1 week before surgery. Nicotine is a potent vasoconstrictor, and the flow of blood to surgical sites is an important aspect of healing. The use of nicotine patches and nicotine gum is also inappropriate preoperatively because the body continues to receive nicotine.

Current Discomforts. Clients with pre-existing painful conditions may require alternate methods of pain reduction while they are receiving nothing by mouth (NPO). Clients who drink a considerable amount of caffeinated beverages such as coffee often develop headaches related to their NPO status, when their caffeine intake ceases abruptly. Without appropriate preoperative assessment, the headache may be misinterpreted as a surgical problem.

Chronic Illnesses. Arthritis of the neck or back is considered in positioning the client during surgery or in extending the neck during intubation.

Advanced Age. Older clients have specific perioperative needs that should be identified preoperatively and considered in developing and maintaining a plan of care.

Medication History. Many clients take prescription and over-the-counter (OTC) drugs that may increase operative risks (Table 16-1). Ask the client whether he or she is taking any medications and whether these have been brought to the hospital. Dosage and administration schedules for all medications should be noted on the chart.

Psychological History

Knowledge of cultural beliefs and practices is an important component of holistic nursing care. Some cultures practice traditional health care as well as alternative and complementary practices that may include use of candles, rituals, and herbs. Certain rituals are important to the client and should be respected by all members of the health care team. For example, in some cultures, the family makes decisions regarding health care as a unit. In other cultures, the oldest woman makes all medical decisions. The nurse must be accepting of each individual's beliefs and should play an active advocate role by supporting the client in any manner possible.

Ability to Tolerate Perioperative Stress

Physiologic stressors in the perioperative client include pain, tissue damage, blood loss, anesthesia, fever, and immobilization. The stressful stimuli imposed by surgery promote the physiologic stress response by combining both psychological factors (such as anxiety and fear of the unknown) and physiologic factors (including blood loss, anesthesia, pain, and immobility). The sympathetic nervous system is activated by any stressor. A person's age, physical condition, and duration of the stress determine the success of the stress response in maintaining homeostatic balance. The ability to tolerate the stress of surgery and anesthesia is decreased significantly in older and debilitated people. All body systems are affected by the stress response; therefore this assessment is crucial throughout the perioperative experience. The nurse must be able to assess stress and to plan and implement appropriate interventions to reduce or treat complications related to stress in an effective manner.

Lifestyle Habits

Sedentary lifestyles can complicate the surgical course because of poor muscle tone, limited cardiac and respiratory reserves, and decreased stress response. On the other hand, an overly active lifestyle may lead to postoperative compliance problems.

Social History

An important component of a social history on a preoperative client is the support system. Identification of client occupation and physical and mental requirements for job performance also provides important information that may prove useful for care planning.

Physical Examination

A physical examination is performed on all persons undergoing surgery to identify the present health status and to have baseline information for comparisons during and after surgery. These data are used to determine nursing diagnoses or to identify problems and to develop pertinent outcome goals. Perform a complete physical examination when possible. When perioperative time is brief, such as with same-day surgery admission or trauma cases, you may be required to complete the assessment in minutes. This assessment is of the utmost importance and must be accurate. Report any abnormal findings to the surgical team members immediately because such information might affect initiation of the surgery.

Review preoperative laboratory and diagnostic study results, and post them on the client's chart (Table 16-2). Missing laboratory data constitute a common problem in ambulatory surgery settings, especially if the client's tests were ordered days before the scheduled procedure or a preadmission clinic. Missing laboratory reports could lead to cancellation of the surgery.

First, examine the part of the body that will be operated on first. Next, complete a general systems assessment. Systems to be assessed include cardiovascular, pulmonary, renal, musculoskeletal, skin, and neurologic. Ask the client whether there are any particularly troublesome manifestations, and include this information in the written assessment for further investigation. Again,

TABLE 16-1	*Medications with Possible Effects on the Surgical Client*
Medication	**Possible Effects**
Antibiotics	
Gentamicin	Produces mild respiratory depression; may mask infection and affect metabolism of muscle relaxants
Penicillins	
Antidysrhythmic Agents	
Propranolol HCl	Affects tolerance of anesthesia; interacts with epinephrine used in local anesthesia
Quinidine gluconate	Depresses cardiac function
Procainamide HCl	Potentiates anesthetic agents that are neuromuscular blockers
Antihypertensive Agents	
Methyldopa	May alter response to muscle relaxants and narcotics
Captopril	May cause intraoperative or postoperative hypotensive crisis
Corticosteroids	
Dexamethasone	Delays wound healing
Hydrocortisone sodium	Masks infection
succinate	Increases risk of hemorrhage
Prednisone	Increases serum glucose
	Decreases stress response (steroid replacement needed during surgery)
Anticoagulants	
Heparin sodium	Increases risk of hemorrhage intraoperatively and postoperatively because of clotting abnormalities
Warfarin sodium	
Aspirin	
NSAIDs	
Glaucoma Medications	
Pilocarpine hydrochloride	May cause respiratory or cardiovascular collapse during surgery
Antidiabetic Agents	
Chlorpropamide,	Basil insulin needs remain when client receives nothing by mouth; glucose levels may fluctuate because of physiologic stress
glipizide, glyburide,	
insulin	Dosage alterations required; client may require injected insulin
Tricyclic Antidepressants	
Amitriptyline, amoxapine,	Lowers blood pressure, thus increasing risk of shock
doxepin	Potentiates the effects of narcotics and barbiturates
Thiazide Diuretics	
Hydrochlorothiazide,	Increases risk for dysrhythmias
Furosemide	Can deplete potassium and cause fluid and/or electrolyte imbalances
Beta-Adrenergic Blockers	
Atenolol, propranolol	Antidysrhythmics and antihypertensives, which can cause adverse effects when combined with anesthetic agents
Street Drugs	
Beer, whiskey, cocaine,	Alcohol and narcotic abuse increase tolerance to narcotics, requiring more anesthesia and analgesia, potential for delirium tremens during surgery or immediately postoperatively; may precipitate a medical crisis
heroin	

NSAIDs, Nonsteroidal anti-inflammatory drugs.

document all unusual findings, and communicate them to the surgical team.

The best way to organize a brief assessment in the immediate preoperative period is to develop a personal system for conducting the examination and use it consistently. Although each person will devise a particular method for gathering data, a head-to-toe examination is a common method (Box 16-1). Assess cognition throughout the examination by noting the client's demeanor and responses to directed questioning. For example, you can assess orientation to time, place, and person in "casual" conversation with the client during the

TABLE 16-2	*Common Preoperative Laboratory Tests*		
		Conditions Often Leading to Abnormal Findings	
Test	**Normal Range in Serum***	**Elevated in**	**Decreased in**
Potassium (K^+)	3.5-5.0 mEq/L or mmol/L	Renal failure Acidosis Traumatic crush injury Burns Massive hemolysis of test specimen Addison's disease	NPO status when K^+ not replaced through IV fluids Excessive use of non–K^+-sparing diuretics Vomiting Malnutrition Diarrhea Alkalosis Aldosteronism
Sodium (Na^+)	136-146 mEq/L or mmol/L	Dehydration Cardiac failure Renal failure Excessive infusion of fluids containing sodium Inadequate thirst Diabetic acidosis	GI fluid loss through NG tube drainage, vomiting, diarrhea Excessive use of laxatives or diuretics Excessive infusion of fluids without sodium SIADH
Chloride (Cl^-)	98-107 mEq/L or 98-107 mmol/L	Dehydration Excessive infusion of fluids containing $NaCl^-$ Mineralocorticoid deficiency Renal failure Respiratory alkalosis	Diabetic acidosis Excessive GI losses through NG drainage, vomiting, diarrhea Excessive use of diuretics
Calcium (Ca^{2+})	8.6-10 mEq/L or 2.15-2.5 mmol/L	Excessive intake of calcium Excessive intake of vitamin D Renal failure Hyperparathyroidism Bone cancer Immobility Steroid use Adrenal insufficiency	Lack of oral intake Lactose intolerance Inadequate intake of vitamin D End-stage renal disease Low serum protein Alkalosis Acute pancreatitis Damage to parathyroid glands
Glucose (fasting)	60-100 mg/dl or mmol/L	Diabetes mellitus Gluconeogenesis with stress response Steroid use Excessive administration of fluids containing glucose	Diabetes mellitus Excess insulin
Carbon dioxide	23-31 mEq/L or mmol/L†	Chronic obstructive lung disease Intestinal obstruction Vomiting or NG suction Metabolic alkalosis	Hyperventilation Diabetic ketoacidosis Diarrhea Lactic acidosis Renal failure Salicylate toxicity
Creatinine	0.6-1.2 mg/dl or 53-106 μmol/L‡	Acute or chronic renal failure End-stage renal disease Shock Rhabdomyolysis	Atrophy of muscle tissue Hyperthyroidism Muscular dystrophy Paralysis Lack of dietary protein

COPD, Chronic obstructive pulmonary disease; *GI,* gastrointestinal; *IV,* intravenous; *NaCl,* sodium chloride; *NG,* nasogastric; *NPO,* nothing by mouth; *SIADH,* syndrome of inappropriate antidiuretic hormone.

* Always refer to normal valves for the laboratory that processed the blood sample.
† Normal values vary slightly by age.
‡ Normal values vary slightly by age and gender.

TABLE 16-2	*Common Preoperative Laboratory Tests—cont'd*		
		Conditions Often Leading to Abnormal Findings	
Test	**Normal Range in Serum***	**Elevated in**	**Decreased in**
Blood urea nitrogen (BUN)	8-23 mg/dl or mmol/L†	Dehydration Renal failure Excessive dietary protein Liver failure	Overhydration Malnutrition
Albumin	3.5-5.0 g/dl	Acute burns Large open wounds Chronic liver disease Protein-calorie malnutrition Infection and fever	Dehydration
Prealbumin	18-40 mg/dl	Protein-calorie malnutrition	Dehydration
Hemoglobin	Females: 11.7-16 g/dl Males*: 13.1-17.2 g/dl	Dehydration Polycythemia Chronic pulmonary diseases Heart failure High altitude	Dehydration Polycythemia Chronic pulmonary diseases Heart failure
Hematocrit	35%-47%†	Dehydration Polycythemia Chronic pulmonary diseases Heart failure	Blood loss Anemia Renal failure with loss of erythropoietin
White blood cell count	4500-11,000 cells/μl	Acute infection Acute inflammation Stress Lymphoma Leukemia	Bone marrow dyscrasias Use of immunosuppressant medications Systemic lupus erythematosus
Differential count	Segmented neutrophils 50%-60%	Bacterial infection, especially streptococcal or staphylococcal Inflammation with tissue necrosis Malignancy of bone marrow, especially chronic myeloid leukemia	Depletion of available pool of neutrophils during severe infection Bone marrow damage
	Banded neutrophils 0%-3%	Overwhelming infection Early indicator of sepsis	
	Eosinophils 1%-4%	Allergy Inflammation of skin Parasitic infection	Bacterial infections
	Basophils 0.5%-1%	Healing phase of wounds Chronic inflammation	Acute infection Hyperthyroidism Stress
	Lymphocytes 20%-40%	Bacterial, viral, or other causes of infection Lymphocytic leukemia	Lymphatic drainage Advanced cancers Bone marrow disease Immune deficiency that decreases T-lymphocytes
	Monocytes 2%-6%	Infection (monocytes become macrophages) Granulomatous diseases Collagen disease	Bone marrow failure

Continued

TABLE 16-2	*Common Preoperative Laboratory Tests—cont'd*		
		Conditions Often Leading to Abnormal Findings	
Test	**Normal Range in Serum***	*Elevated in*	*Decreased in*
Prothrombin time (PT)	11-15 sec	Coagulation defect Liver disease Anticoagulant use (Coumadin)	Coagulation (clotting) disorder Extensive cancer
Partial thromboplastin time, activated (aPTT)	24-34 sec	Coagulation defect Liver disease Anticoagulant use (Heparin)	Coagulation (clotting) disorder Extensive cancer

COPD, Chronic obstructive pulmonary disease; *GI*, gastrointestinal; *IV*, intravenous; *NaCl*, sodium chloride; *NG*, nasogastric; *NPO*, nothing by mouth; *SIADH*, syndrome of inappropriate antidiuretic hormone.

* Always refer to normal valves for the laboratory that processed the blood sample.

† Normal values vary slightly by age.

‡ Normal values vary slightly by age and gender.

BOX 16-1	*Preoperative Head-to-Toe Assessment*

- Assess cognition throughout the examination by noting the client's demeanor and responses to directed questioning. For example, you can check the client's orientation to time, place, and person in the course of eliciting information during the physical assessment.
- Assess muscle strength and coordination, gait, and balance by watching the client walk and move while entering the preparation area. (This may not be possible with all clients.)
- Take a full set of vital sign measurements. Note the ease of respiration.
- Look at the client's eyes and nose, and assess the mobility of the neck.
- Listen to the heart and the lungs. Listen to the rate and rhythm of the heart. Note the character of the lung sounds, listening for any diminution of intensity or the absence of breath sounds. Shortness of breath on minor exertion should also be noted. Dyspnea, wheezing, clubbed fingers, chest pain, cyanosis, and coughing with expectoration of copious or purulent mucus should be reported to anesthesia personnel. Question the client carefully about smoking habits and recent illness with a cold or influenza. Obtain a history of respiratory allergies and infections.
- Assess range of motion of the shoulders and the strength of the arms and hand grip.
- Ask about the ability to urinate and whether the client has diabetes.
- Assess the ability to flex the spine (this is important if the client is scheduled to have spinal anesthesia).
- Examine the extremities for edema, coldness to the touch, and cyanosis.

- Assess the range of motion and strength of the legs and feet.
- Assess cognition preoperatively to determine whether any postoperative changes are the effects of surgery. This is particularly important in the older adult. The effects of the operation and of associated medications often cause temporary cognitive deficits that can be erroneously identified as a permanent condition by the health care team. Temporary deficits in memory and recall are normal and are seen in most clients, but these manifestations can persist in the older adult. Note equal movement of the face and shoulders on both sides of the body if a crude estimate of cranial nerve function is needed. Complete neurologic testing includes assessment of cranial nerve function, reflex response of the upper and lower extremities, and sensory reflexes, as well as cognitive assessment. This level of testing is performed before neurologic surgery.
- During the examination, observe the condition of the skin. Note and document lesions, pressure ulcers, necrotic tissue, skin turgor, erythema or other discoloration of the skin, and the presence of external devices. Record the approximate size, color, and location of any lesions for later comparison.
- Review the chart for results of laboratory and diagnostic tests. Commonly ordered for the client undergoing heart surgery include chest x-ray film, electrocardiogram, hemoglobin, hematocrit, serum electrolytes, and urinalysis.
- During the physical examination, pay attention to the client's verbal and nonverbal communication. Does the client complain of any pain unrelated to the impending surgical procedure?

physical assessment and, if possible, watch the client walk and move when he or she enters the preparation area. Include this information in the ambulatory status section of the examination.

Specific Body System Assessments

Cardiovascular Assessment. Pathologic cardiac conditions or events that increase operative risk include angina pectoris, the occurrence of a myocardial infarction within the last 6 months, uncontrolled hypertension, heart failure, and peripheral vascular disease. All cardiac conditions can lead to decreased tissue perfusion with impairment of surgical wound healing. In addition to the portion of the cardiovascular assessment completed as part of the head-to-toe assessment, note specific findings that warrant further work-up. Document shortness of breath on minor exertion, hypertension, heart murmurs or S_3 gallops, and chest pain. These manifestations may be present if the client is scheduled for heart or vascular surgery, but they may make the ability to tolerate anesthesia and blood loss questionable. Laboratory studies to measure the function of the cardiovascular system include an electrocardiogram (ECG), especially for clients over 40 years of age, and determinations of hemoglobin, hematocrit, and serum electrolytes.

Respiratory Assessment. Chronic lung conditions, such as emphysema, asthma, and bronchitis, increase operative risk because these disorders impair gas exchange in the alveoli, predisposing the client to postoperative pulmonary complications. Assessment of pulmonary conditions includes examining for the presence of shortness of breath, wheezing, clubbed fingers, chest pain, cyanosis, and coughing with expectoration of copious or purulent mucus. Question the client carefully about smoking habits. Obtain a complete history of respiratory allergies and infections. If a client demonstrates any respiratory distress at the time of the assessment, notify the surgeon before anesthesia is administered. Abnormal breath sounds may indicate the need for respiratory therapy both before and after surgery. Clients with severe respiratory disease are usually managed preoperatively with aerosol therapy, postural drainage, and antibiotics. Clients who smoke are strongly encouraged to stop smoking as early as possible before surgery. Nicotine patches are usually not an appropriate alternative because of vasoconstriction caused by the nicotine.

Laboratory studies performed before surgery to diagnose respiratory conditions include chest radiography and pulse oximetry. Chest radiography (or x-rays) detects abnormalities, if present, in the lungs, such as infections, collapsed alveoli or segments of the lung, tumors, fractures of the ribs, and size of the heart. The pulse oximeter is used to determine gross levels of tissue oxygenation. Explain the purpose of the oximeter to the client and why it is important to monitor oxygenation throughout the surgical experience. The definitive laboratory test for blood oxygenation is arterial blood gas (ABG) analysis. Although routine ABG analyses are not ordered preoperatively, a physician may order the test if the client has been determined to be at high risk for surgical complications. Additional pulmonary function tests may be ordered in specific situations (see Chapter 61).

Assess the presence of sleep apnea. If present, alert the surgery team and document it, including determination of whether the client uses an apnea assistance respiratory device at home and whether it will be continued postoperatively during hospitalization.

Musculoskeletal Assessment. A history of arthritis, fractures, contractures, joint injury, or musculoskeletal impairment is an important factor in surgical positioning and postoperative support. The physical examination should reveal any problems with joint mobility or deformities that may interfere with operative positioning as well as with the postoperative course. For example, if the preoperative assessment identifies arthritis of the neck and shoulder, the circulating nurse can incorporate this information into the care plan. Hyperextension of the arthritic neck during intubation for general anesthesia can cause postoperative pain and discomfort unrelated to the surgery. The musculoskeletal system can be assessed through passive and active range of motion and a history provided by the client, a family member, or the medical record. Documentation of impairment before the surgical procedure assists in the investigation of any impairment postoperatively.

Gastrointestinal Assessment. Gastrointestinal conditions associated with poor surgical outcomes include severe malnutrition and prolonged nausea and vomiting. The client's gastrointestinal system should be assessed if the planned operation is in the abdominal area or if the general physical examination reveals any abnormal data. Because opioid analgesics increase constipation, information about normal bowel patterns can help to ensure that postoperative expectations for return of function are appropriate. A client with a long history of constipation may have more difficulty postoperatively than that experienced by a client with regular bowel function.

Skin Integrity Assessment. Skin integrity must be assessed and documented preoperatively to establish a baseline for comparison postoperatively. The operative site must be clear of any rashes, blisters, or infectious processes. Document and report lesions, pressure ulcers, necrotic skin tissue, skin turgor, erythema or discoloration of the skin, and the presence of external devices. Note the size, color, and location of the skin impairment to determine whether the impaired skin remains stable or worsens during and after the surgical procedure.

Padding and positioning equipment should be used to maintain skin integrity and to prevent pressure ulcers. Any alterations in skin integrity that can occur intraoperatively and are not related to the actual surgical procedure are preventable by the nurse and other members of the surgical team with adequate padding and repositioning as needed during long procedures.

Tattoos and body piercings should also be noted. Incisions can be made through tattoos, but the design may be altered afterward. Piercings may need to be removed, based on the surgeon's preference.

Renal Assessment. Adequate renal function is necessary to eliminate protein wastes, to preserve fluid and electrolyte balance, and to remove anesthetic agents. Important renal and related disorders include advanced renal insufficiency, acute nephritis, and benign prostatic hypertrophy. If renal deficiency exists, the surgical team must be made aware of the problem. To assess renal status, ask about voiding patterns, such as frequency and dysuria. Also, if a urine sample is collected or an indwelling catheter is in place, note its appearance and document and report abnormal urine characteristics. Monitor fluid balance by recording intake and output throughout the surgical continuum.

The most common preoperative tests to assess renal function are determination of blood urea nitrogen (BUN) and serum creatinine and urinalysis. BUN and serum creatinine levels indicate the ability of the kidney to excrete urea and protein wastes. Elevated levels may reflect dehydration, impaired cardiac output, or renal failure. Elevated creatinine is associated with renal disease. Serious renal disease and urinary infections must be treated, if possible, before surgery. Urinalysis results may indicate urinary infection, diabetes, malnutrition, renal disease, or dehydration.

Liver Function Assessment. Liver disease such as cirrhosis increases a client's surgical risk because an impaired liver cannot detoxify medications and anesthetic agents. The client also may be unable to metabolize carbohydrates, fats, and amino acids. Liver disease may be manifested by decreased albumin levels, leading to decreased immunoglobulin and fibrinogen levels. Low albumin levels predispose the client to fluid shifts, surgical wound infection, and ineffective coagulation. Clients with a history of alcoholism or other substance abuse require a careful assessment of liver function before surgery. If evidence of risk factors for liver disease is uncovered during the immediate preoperative assessment, information must be shared immediately with other members of the surgical team. Because a client with liver disease is often malnourished and debilitated and may have clotting disorders, the surgeon generally orders a high-calorie diet or hyperalimentation during the preoperative and postoperative periods and corrects clotting abnormalities.

Cognitive and Neurologic Assessment. Serious neurologic conditions, such as uncontrolled epilepsy or severe Parkinson's disease, increase surgical risk. Important preoperative neurologic abnormalities include severe headache, frequent dizziness, light-headedness, ringing in the ears, unsteady gait, unequal pupils, and a history of seizures. Assessment of the client's orientation to time, place, and person can be accomplished by simple questioning. To determine baseline neurologic function, include testing of cranial nerves, reflex responses of the upper and lower extremities, sensory reflexes, and cerebral responses (see Chapter 69).

Assess cognition preoperatively to determine postoperative effects of surgery. This is particularly important in an older adult. The effects of the operation and of associated medications frequently lead to temporary cognitive deficiencies that can be erroneously identified as a permanent condition. Temporary deficits in memory and recall are considered normal and are seen in most clients, but the older adult can experience these manifestations for a longer time.

Endocrine Assessment. Diabetes mellitus is the most common pre-existing endocrine pathophysiologic disorder. In some ethnic groups, especially Hispanic populations, diabetes is rampant. Diabetes mellitus predisposes the affected client to poor wound healing and increased risk of surgical wound infection. Corresponding cardiovascular, peripheral vascular, neurologic, visual, and renal complications may be present as well. These factors can greatly increase the surgical risk for a client with diabetes. A client who has well-controlled diabetes (i.e., blood glucose levels are consistently monitored and kept within a normal range during the perioperative period) is less susceptible to infection. Chapter 47 describes the care of clients with diabetes mellitus.

Thyroid functioning may also need to be assessed preoperatively. Thyroid hormone replacement is usually continued throughout the perioperative period. Stopping thyroid medications may precipitate hypothyroidism, with manifestations of hypotension, bradycardia, and hypothermia. This event can be devastating if it occurs during surgery or immediately postoperatively.

Additional Assessments.
Other factors that may be considered during the planning of surgical intervention include (1) age, (2) nutrition, (3) fluid and electrolyte balance, (4) infection, and (5) hematologic conditions.

Age. Normal physiologic changes that occur with aging, along with the increased presence of disease, may adversely affect surgical outcomes. Chronic conditions commonly found in the older client that may increase surgical risk include malnutrition, anemia, dehydration, atherosclerosis, chronic obstructive pulmonary disease (COPD), diabetes mellitus, cerebrovascular changes, and peripheral vascular disease. Table 16-3 outlines major physiologic changes that occur in older adults and appropriate perioperative nursing interventions.

Pain. Pain is an important physiologic indicator that must be carefully monitored (see Chapter 22). During the preoperative nursing assessment, ask if the client is experiencing any pain (Box 16-2). If pain is present, obtain a full assessment of the pain. Determine whether the pain is chronic and unrelated to the pathologic condition necessitating surgery or whether it is acute and attributable to the need for the surgical procedure. Be aware that although most operations increase pain, older adults who have undergone joint replacement surgery often state that the postoperative pain is minor compared with the chronic pain of a disintegrating joint.

Nutritional Status. Nutritional status (positive nitrogen balance) is directly related to intraoperative success and postoperative recovery. The client who is well nourished preoperatively is better prepared to handle surgical stress and to return to optimal health after surgery. Improving nutrition is usually attended to in a clinic or physician's office weeks before surgery. However, if the operation is performed on an emergency basis or was not planned, nutritional status may be a risk factor through the perioperative period. In addition, some operations are completed to improve nutrition. For example, a client who is to undergo placement of a permanent feeding tube would be expected to have evidence of malnutrition. Likewise, one who is to have an intestinal bypass for obesity is also malnourished (in terms of excess intake).

Assessment of nutritional status preoperatively includes obtaining a diet history, observing the client's general appearance and laboratory diagnostic testing, and comparing current weight with ideal body weight. Laboratory tests that can assist in the assessment of nutritional status include determinations of serum albumin, prealbumin, hemoglobin and hematocrit, BUN, and creatinine clearance.

Protein-calorie malnutrition leads to delayed recovery, infection, and slow wound healing. Malnourished clients who have surgery may need aggressive nutrition after surgery to promote wound healing.

Obesity is also associated with poorer surgical outcomes. Adipose (fatty) tissue increases the technical difficulty of surgery. Fatty tissue is less vascular and more prone to postoperative infection, incisional hernias, and wound dehiscence or evisceration. The surgeon may use an alternative closure method for a client with excess adipose tissue at or around the incision.

Obese clients frequently suffer from hypertension, heart failure, and metabolic problems. They are more susceptible to postoperative pulmonary complications.

TABLE 16-3 Interventions for Physiologic Changes in Older Adults Undergoing Surgery

Physiologic Change	Nursing Interventions
Cardiovascular	
Decreased cardiac output	Know what anesthetic agents are being used.
Moderate increase in blood pressure	Monitor vital signs carefully.
Decreased peripheral circulation	Encourage early ambulation and leg exercises.
Dysrhythmias	Assess for hypotension or hypertension or hypothermia.
	Note changes in baseline ECG; note any changes.
Respiratory	
Decreased vital capacity	Assess for pulmonary aspiration.
Reduced oxygenation of blood	Monitor respirations carefully.
	Use vigorous pulmonary hygiene.
	Postoperatively, auscultate lung sounds.
	Monitor oxygen saturation using pulse oximeter.
Renal	
Decreased renal blood flow and glomerular filtration rate	Monitor urine output q 1-2 hr during immediate postoperative period.
Decreased ability to excrete waste products	Evaluate intake and output.
	Monitor fluid and electrolyte status.
Musculoskeletal	
Decrease in lean body mass	Assess level of mobility.
Increase in spinal compression	Position the client on operating table with padding to reduce trauma to bones and joints.
Increased incidence of osteoporosis and arthritis	Assist with early ambulation or exercises in accordance with client's ability.
	Provide adequate nutrition.
	Provide effective pain management.
Sensorimotor	
Decreased reaction time	Orient client to environment.
Decreased visual acuity	Plan individual teaching, allowing time to reinforce client learning.
Decreased auditory acuity	Maintain core body temperature.
Slowed thermoregulation	

BOX 16-2 *Preoperative Pain Assessment*

Many factors that are present before surgery can alter the experience of pain or the usual treatments of pain after surgery. These factors are commonly addressed in a preoperative assessment, with specific attention paid to the following aspects:

Chief Complaint. What is the planned surgical procedure? What are the circumstances under which the procedure is being performed? Is the procedure elective or emergent? Is the client currently in acute pain?

Past Medical History. What concurrent medical problems are present? Are there any known problems with coagulation that would prevent use of epidural analgesia? Are there congenital abnormalities? Are there concurrent neurologic diseases such as multiple sclerosis, muscular dystrophy, stroke, mental retardation or dementia, amyotropic lateral sclerosis, or peripheral neuropathy? Is there a history of prior trauma to the proposed surgical site? Is there a history of infection or respiratory difficulty?

Past Surgical History. Is there any history of surgery (e.g., spine surgery)?

Medications. What medications is the client currently taking? Is the client taking any anticoagulants that would alter choices for postoperative pain control? Is the client taking opiates on a chronic basis? Is the client taking any monoamine ox-

idase inhibitors (MAOIs)? Is the client using topical analgesic patches?

Allergies. Is the client allergic to any of the opiates, local anesthetics, nonsteroidal anti-inflammatory drugs, agonist-antagonists, corticosteroids, or any other medications commonly used to provide postoperative pain control?

Psychosocial History. Is there any history of drug or alcohol abuse or addiction?

Past Pain History. Does the client have chronic pain? How is the chronic pain currently being treated? What postoperative pain control methods were used successfully or unsuccessfully? Did the client develop side effects from the chosen method? Does the client have an implanted system for pain control?

Physical Examination. Are there physical or mental abnormalities that preclude the use of certain postoperative pain control techniques? Will the surgical procedure involve the insertion areas for regional or neuraxial analgesia techniques? Are there manifestations of infection at the site of proposed needle insertion?

Pain Assessment. If the client reports any pain, a pain assessment needs to be completed. This assessment may help in the evaluation of postoperative pain. Does the client understand how to rate pain numerically? If not, can the other tools for pain assessment be used effectively?

Modified from Veterans Health Administration. (2002). *Clinical practice guideline for the management of postoperative pain. Version 1.2.* Washington, DC: Department of Defense, Veterans Health Administration.

Obesity decreases the efficiency of coughing and deep breathing. The pressure of the abdominal contents on the diaphragm and lungs decreases expansion, which may lead to hypoventilation. An obese client is more prone to postoperative immobility, which increases the risk of venous stasis and deep vein thrombosis or pulmonary embolism. Immobility also increases the risk of pressure ulcers. Good preoperative teaching that describes turning, coughing, deep breathing, and moving after surgery is essential. Most complications related to obesity can be prevented, or the risk of their occurrence reduced, with appropriate interventions.

Fluid and Electrolyte Balance. Fluid volume deficits (dehydration/hypovolemia or fluid volume excess/hypervolemia) predispose a client to complications during and after surgery. Actual or potential fluid imbalance can be assessed by evaluation of skin turgor. A coated tongue can also be a manifestation of fluid volume deficit. A decrease in urine output or specific gravity is also diagnostic of decreased fluid volume. If dehydration is severe, irritability or confusion can be apparent. Dehydration results from limited fluid intake, prolonged vomiting, diarrhea, or bleeding. Fluids can be administered intravenously if dehydration is identified.

Electrolyte imbalances also increase operative risk. Preoperative laboratory results should be checked to determine whether serum sodium, potassium, calcium, and magnesium concentrations are within the normal range. In-depth assessment and management of fluid and electrolyte imbalances are discussed in Chapters 13 and 14, respectively.

Infection and Immunity. Any pre-existing infection can adversely affect surgical outcomes because bacteria may be released into the bloodstream during surgery. Their release may lead to infection elsewhere in the body. When the surgical site is near a lymph node or lymphatic vessel that is draining infectious material, the likelihood of surgical infection increases. During the preoperative assessment, documentation of any possible exposure to communicable diseases, the presence of skin lesions, or manifestations of an infection (such as coughing, sore throat, or elevated body temperature) is vital. An elevated white blood cell (WBC) count also suggests an infection and should be communicated immediately to the surgical team. Because infection greatly increases surgical risk, it may be necessary to reschedule elective surgery.

A low WBC count is also a danger sign and may indicate that the client is at risk for infection. A low WBC

TABLE 16-4	*Categories of Surgical Procedures*	
Category	**Purpose**	**Example**
Aesthetic	Improvement of physical features that are within the "normal" range	Breast augmentation
Constructive	Repair of a congenitally defective body part	Cleft palate and cleft lip repair
Curative	Removal or repair of damaged or diseased tissue or organs	Hysterectomy
Diagnostic	Discovery or confirmation of a diagnosis	Breast biopsy
Exploratory	Estimation of the extent of disease or confirmation of a diagnosis	Exploratory laparotomy
Emergent	Life-saving	Repair of traumatic punctured lung
Palliative	Relief of symptoms but without cure of underlying disease	Colostomy
Reconstructive	Partial or complete restoration of a body part	Total joint replacement
Urgent	Performed as soon as client is stable and infection is under control	Appendectomy

count may be a manifestation of immunosuppression. People with diabetes mellitus, those who are undergoing radiation therapy or chemotherapy, and those with chronic medical conditions are at high risk of immunosuppression. Steroid use also decreases the client's ability to fight infection; therefore the client taking steroids should be assessed and monitored for immunosuppression.

Hematologic Function. Clients with blood coagulation disorders are at risk for hemorrhage and hypovolemic shock during and after surgery. The following five factors should be assessed preoperatively to identify potential hematologic problems:

- A history of bleeding or a diagnosis of a pathologic condition such as hemophilia or sickle cell anemia
- Manifestations such as easy bruising, excessive bleeding following dental extractions and razor nicks, and severe nosebleeds
- Hepatic or renal disease
- Use of anticoagulants, aspirin, or other nonsteroidal anti-inflammatory drugs (NSAIDs)
- Abnormal bleeding time, prothrombin time, or platelet count

Remember that many clients take herbs, aspirin, and other OTC medications that may increase the risk of bleeding. The client may not consider nonprescription medications important and often may not include them in a medication history. Ask specific questions regarding all prescription and nonprescription medications. Specifically ask about the use of herbal preparations. Ginkgo biloba, garlic, ginger, and ginseng may prevent the formation of blood clots and may lead to excess blood loss in surgery. Two other popular herbs—St. John's wort, an antidepressant, and kava-kava, a relaxant—may prolong the sedative effect of anesthesia. Advise clients to stop taking herbal products at least 2 weeks before elective surgery. Ask how often the client takes the OTC medications and when the last dose of any of those drugs was taken.

For a variety of reasons, blood transfusions are used less frequently than in past years. Many clients fear the transmission of human immunodeficiency virus and hepatitis B. If possible, clients should be encouraged to donate their own blood for use during or after surgery (autologous transfusion). Blood substitutes or fluid volume expanders can also be used in some cases to replace lost blood until the body can produce new blood cells. Blood transfusions are discussed in Chapter 77.

Estimating Medical Risk for Surgery

Each surgeon determines the relative risk versus benefit from the operation for the specific client. In addition, the outcomes for many surgical procedures have been researched, and these figures can be presented to the client and family. The natural history of the condition requiring surgery (that is, the outcome if it goes untreated) is also presented. This information then can be considered by the client and his or her family members before consenting to surgery. The surgeon presents a frank but optimistic discussion of risks of the procedure. Well-intentioned friends and family may wish to shield the client from unpleasant facts. Although medical facts may be unpleasant, it is imperative that the client have full and complete information before consenting. Some clients (such as those with malnutrition or anemia) benefit from waiting for surgery.

The type of surgery to be performed also has some inherent risk. The types of operations by category are presented in Table 16-4.

Anesthesia and Anesthetic Risk

The anesthesia care provider visits the client before surgery to perform a complete respiratory, cardiovascular, and neurologic examination. The client's general surgical risk (i.e., his or her ability to withstand the surgery) is expressed according to the American Society of Anesthesia (ASA) grading system (Box 16-3). Generally, the topics discussed with the client during this examination include the type of anesthesia planned and the sensations the

---

BOX 16-3   *Classification of Physical Status*

ASA I
Healthy person with no systemic disease, undergoing elective surgery, and at no extremes of age.

ASA II
Client with one-system, well-controlled disease. Disease does not affect daily activities. Other clients classified in this level include those with mild obesity, alcoholism, and smoking.

ASA III
Client with multiple-system disease or well-controlled major system diseases. The disease status limits daily activities. However, there is no immediate danger or death due to any individual system disease.

ASA IV
Client with severe, incapacitating disease. Typically, the disease is poorly controlled, or end-stage disease is present. Danger of death related to organ failure is present.

ASA V
Client is very ill and in imminent danger of death. Operation is deemed to be a last resort attempt at preserving life. The client is not expected to live through the next 24 hours. In some cases, the client had been healthy up to a recent catastrophic event.

Data based on American Society of Anesthesiologists (ASA) classification.

---

client may experience when undergoing anesthesia. Fears about anesthesia are also addressed. The client's risk of side effects and complications is assessed at this time.

The pharmacologic preparation for anesthesia is based on many variables, including the client's age and physical and psychological condition, the type of surgery, and the type of anesthesia to be used. Preoperative and anesthetic medications are discussed later in the chapter.

Educational Assessment
The client's experience with previous surgery and level of anxiety should be noted. His or her education level, sensory impairments (e.g., loss of vision), expectations regarding the operation, and availability of support systems are used to guide plans for teaching. In general, clients who have undergone multiple operations need less educational preparation. However, do not assume that such clients need no reinforcement of preoperative and postoperative assessments and interventions.

The client undergoing elective surgery and planning to go home the same day requires some additional planning (see the Case Management feature on the Elective Surgery Client on the website).

Preoperative Nursing Diagnoses
Common psychosocial nursing diagnoses during the preoperative period include *deficit knowledge related to unfamiliar surgical experience, anxiety, and fear related to pain, death, disfigurement,* or *the unknown.* The outcomes for these problems must be achievable in a short preoperative time frame.

Immediate Preoperative Nursing Care

Physical Care
Preparation of the Skin. Explain shower and bathing protocols for the night before a planned surgical procedure. Usually the operative area is cleaned the night before surgery with soap and water or an antimicrobial solution to reduce the number of microbes on the skin. Allergies to chemicals (e.g., iodine) necessitate use of other cleansing agents. If the skin assessment has identified fragile and delicate skin in an older client, nursing care must involve a gentle method for cleansing skin and hair and for any necessary hair removal. Additional considerations may include the use of padding over pressure points and tape that will not irritate or rip the skin as well as lifting—rather than pulling or sliding—the client from bed to bed to prevent traumatizing the skin.

Preparation of the Gastrointestinal Tract. The gastrointestinal tract needs special preparation on the evening before surgery to (1) reduce the possibility of vomiting and aspiration, (2) to reduce the risk of possible bowel obstruction, (3) to allow visualization of the intestine during bowel surgery, and (4) to prevent contamination from fecal material in the intestinal tract during bowel or abdominal surgery. Preparation involves restricting food and fluid, administering enemas as needed, and inserting a gastric or intestinal tube when appropriate. Gastrointestinal tubes are usually inserted during surgery for drainage. This procedure is usually performed for clients undergoing major abdominal or intestinal tract surgery.

Traditionally, if a client undergoing surgery is to receive a general anesthetic, foods and fluids are restricted for 8 to 10 hours before the operation. This restriction significantly reduces the possibility of aspiration of gastric contents, which may lead to pneumonia. Because solid food must be withheld for 8 to 10 hours before surgery, clients who are to undergo anesthetic procedures must be instructed not to eat or drink anything after midnight. Therefore clients are assigned NPO status after midnight the night before surgery is scheduled. If a client scheduled for surgery has eaten or had something to drink after midnight, the surgery may be delayed or postponed. Preoperative care for hospitalized clients also includes the restriction of food and water if anesthesia is to be used. Research is bringing into question the need for prolonged periods of having the client NPO, but for the most part practice has not changed.

When a client is on NPO status, do the following:

- Explain the reason for the fluid and food restriction.
- Remove food and water from the bedside at midnight.
- Place "NPO" signs on the door and on the bed.
- Mark the care plan or Kardex with "NPO."
- Inform the diet and nutrition department about the client's NPO status.
- Inform other caretakers and family members that the client is NPO.

If the client has been instructed to take important medications orally, small sips of water are permitted. For example, a client with cardiovascular disease may need to take heart medications such as digoxin on the morning of surgery; however, the client may have been given preoperative instructions not to eat or drink anything. Make sure that the medication is taken with a sip of water and inform the client that this exception is permissible. Record this medication and the amount of fluid taken on the client's care record.

Enemas are not routinely ordered during the preoperative period except for surgical procedures that involve the gastrointestinal tract, perianal or perineal areas, and the pelvic cavity. The client may perform the enema at home, or the nurse may complete it at the hospital. Some clients may require further bowel cleansing on the morning of surgery. Clients who are to be admitted for same-day surgery are instructed before the surgical date about the need for enemas and whether they will be self-administered. If bowel cleansing is done by the client, ensure that directions are completely understood.

Nutritional Care

Nursing interventions for clients who are malnourished preoperatively include encouragement of high carbohydrate intake to increase energy, high protein intake to assist in wound healing, and supplementing the diet with vitamins to encourage healing. Vitamin C is beneficial in wound healing, whereas vitamin K will increase blood clotting times. Total parenteral nutrition can be used preoperatively to bolster the client's nutritional status.

Total parenteral nutrition solutions that contain lipids (fats) supply total nutritional replacement, including vitamin and mineral supplements. Tube feeding (enteral nutrition) can be administered through a tube placed in the stomach or small intestine. The tube is placed through the nose or directly into the stomach through a skin incision. Both enteral and parenteral feeding can improve a client's nutritional status, and either type of feeding can be continued postoperatively until satisfactory swallowing or gastrointestinal functioning returns (see Chapter 31).

Treatment of obesity before surgery calls for a reducing diet, mild exercise if possible, and assessing for and controlling conditions such as hypertension and diabetes mellitus. Obese clients are not placed on a weight-reduction diet after surgery while they are healing. Wound healing is delayed when protein intake is inadequate.

Preoperative Teaching

Preoperative teaching is important to ensure a positive surgical experience for the client. Numerous research studies support the value of preoperative instructions in reducing both the incidence of postoperative complications and the length of stay in the hospital. The client's learning needs, level of anxiety, and fears about surgery are assessed individually so that an individualized teaching plan can be formulated.

The timing of preoperative teaching is highly individualized. Ideally, there would be enough time for the client to be given instructions and time to answer questions. If teaching is done too far in advance, the client may forget important components of the education. On the other hand, a client who is taught immediately before surgery may be too anxious to comprehend what is being taught. In many cases, the client is admitted on the day of surgery. It is imperative that the client has received written or oral instructions before this time so that the nurse can simply reinforce these instructions and answer individual questions from the client and family members. Many ambulatory surgery or "same-day surgery" centers conduct telephone interviews before admission to educate and allow the client to ask questions.

Being aware of the effects of surgery on cognition, determine learning needs preoperatively and teach both the client and his or her family before surgery if at all possible. Only essential activities should be taught in the immediate preoperative period because of the client's total concentration on surviving the surgery. Assess the client's ability to see, hear, and understand verbal communication. Glasses and hearing aids can be worn until the actual surgical procedure to promote the client's learning necessary information and to reduce the client's apprehension and fear. As the client moves into surgery, these important items must be carefully stored or given to an accompanying adult. Add careful documentation of the location of items, such as hearing aids and glasses, to the client's record to ensure retrieval after surgery. If any items are lost, the institution will be responsible for replacing them.

The client should understand what the preoperative, intraoperative, and postoperative course entails. Consult with the physician before speaking to the client about specific or technical details so that you can clarify if needed. Explain all nursing care and any possible discomfort that may result as a consequence of nursing interventions. Tell the client what you will do to minimize any discomfort. If the client is scheduled to go to the surgical intensive care unit after the operation, ask what the client and family members already know or have heard about intensive care, taking time to address any misconceptions or incorrect information.

Preoperative Anxiety and Fear

All clients are anxious and fearful of surgery. The extent to which a client fears surgery depends on many factors, such as (1) how serious the operation is, (2) individual coping abilities, (3) cultural expectations, and (4) experiences with previous surgery. Well-meaning family members and friends often contribute to the fear level unintentionally. Fear of the unknown is one of the most prevalent causes of preoperative anxiety. During the preoperative phase, clients also fear postoperative pain, the discovery of cancer, the loss of an organ or limb, anesthesia, vulnerability while unconscious, the threat of loss of job or financial security, loss of social and familial roles, disruption of lifestyle, separation from significant others, and death.

Clients respond differently to fear. Some respond by becoming silent and withdrawn, childish, belligerent, evasive, tearful, or clinging. Most clients feel helpless to some extent when admitted to a health care facility. Although surgery may be commonplace for the health care professional, it is a frightening experience for clients and their families. Report extreme anxiety and fear to the anesthesia personnel so that a sedative can be administered. A surgical procedure can be canceled if fear is overwhelming.

Allow the client to take the lead in asking questions about surgery and the postoperative period. Provide only as much additional information as the client wants to know. Emphasize to the client that a nurse will be with him or her throughout the total surgical experience. In addition, stand close to the client when taking him or her into the operating room. If touch is culturally appropriate, it can be used to reassure the client.

If the surgical procedure to be performed has potential long-term effects, support groups may be contacted to offer support preoperatively. Cancer organizations, amputation support groups, and enterostomal therapist associations are examples of large national organizations that offer peer support for surgical and nonsurgical clients.

Components of Preoperative Teaching

Information provided to the client before surgery should be geared to individual needs. This information can be (1) sensory, (2) psychosocial, or (3) procedural.

Sensory information addresses the sights, sounds, and "feel" of the operating room. Instruct the client that the operating room and skin preparation fluids will be cold but that warm blankets are available. Many surgical suites are now incorporating music into their preoperative and intraoperative areas. Clients may be given headphones and can choose from a variety of music types to help them relax and to reduce external noxious sounds in the operating room environment. If the client wears a hearing aid and music is used, check with the anesthesia personnel to determine whether the hearing aid can remain in place during surgery.

Psychosocial information involves coping abilities and worries about family and similar concerns. Typical questions the client may have include the following: What if I die? Who is going to care for my children? What if I become an invalid? Who is going to earn enough money to care for my family? You can provide answers if this information is available or arrange for others, such as a social worker or a member of the clergy, to talk to the client.

Procedural information details activities during the preoperative period and postoperative care. It includes information that the client needs to know and wants to know about what is going to happen. For example, you can state, as appropriate, something like the following: "Your family can be in the presurgical area before you are taken into the operating room," or "There will always be a nurse with you during this time, and I will remain by your side throughout the entire operation." Provide explanations and printed information about the health care facility routines, visiting hours, mealtimes, the location of the chapel and waiting room, and so on. If you find that the client is unclear about what the operation entails, the physician must be notified (see later discussion). You can elaborate on or clarify information regarding surgery.

The client's role in postoperative care is taught before surgery. The nurse provides instructions on (1) deep breathing, (2) coughing, (3) turning, (4) ambulating, and (5) pain control, and the client's learning of some of these procedures is validated by return demonstration.

Deep-Breathing Exercises. To help prevent postoperative surgical complications, careful preoperative instructions and practice in deep breathing and coughing exercises should be completed and reinforced.

Breathing and coughing exercises help to expand collapsed alveoli in the lungs and to prevent postoperative pneumonia and atelectasis. It also promotes faster clearance of inhalation agents from the body. Demonstration of correct deep breathing can be done by inhaling slowly through the nose, distending the abdomen, and exhaling slowly through pursed lips. After demonstrating this method, ask the client to provide a return demonstration to ensure understanding (Figure 16-1). The client is instructed to use this breathing method as often as possi-

1. Have the client sit upright at the side of the bed or supported in bed in semi-Fowler's position.
2. Instruct the client to place his or her hands on the abdomen to feel whether the chest rises to indicate that the lungs are expanding.
3. Have the client inhale through the nose until the abdomen distends.
4. Instruct the client to exhale through pursed lips while contracting the abdominal muscles.
5. Have the client repeat this exercise every hour during the first postoperative day.

FIGURE 16-1 Deep (diaphragmatic) breathing after surgery.

ble, preferably 5 to 10 times every hour during the post-operative period of immobilization.

Coughing Exercises. Coughing removes retained secretions from the bronchi and larger airways. Coughing may be painful, and analgesia may be required.

For coughing exercise, the client may remain in a sitting or supine position. Teach the client how to splint the surgical incision, to minimize pressure, and to control pain during coughing. Splinting is accomplished by lacing the fingers and holding them tightly across the incision before coughing. A small pillow or folded towel held over the incision also facilitates splinting. For example, some institutions may provide a stuffed item such as a heart and teach the client to "hold the heart" when coughing. The client is instructed to take three deep breaths, exhaling through the mouth, before coughing from deep in the lungs. Encouragement to perform deep-breathing exercises before coughing is important because the deep breathing assists in stimulating the cough reflex and mobilizing retained secretions. Many clients simply clear their throats when coughing hurts. Encourage true coughing and use aggressive measures to control pain, reteaching the procedure as needed.

Low-tech breathing devices, such as incentive spirometers, are often used to promote expansion of the alveoli postoperatively by guiding the client to reach a predetermined level of lung inflation. Use of these aids promote alveolar inflation and strengthens respiratory muscles that were weakened during anesthesia administration. Clients should have the opportunity to practice the use of the breathing aids before surgery so that they can use

it appropriately after surgery. Most facilities teach clients to use them 5 or 10 times an hour after surgery. If the client has a television in the room, a good way to help the client remember to do breathing exercises is to tell them to do it every time a commercial comes on.

Turning Exercises. Preoperative clients also need to practice turning from side to side, using the bedside rails to assist movements. Turning helps to prevent venous stasis, thrombophlebitis, pressure ulcer formation, and respiratory complications. The client should be instructed to turn and reposition in bed every 1 to 2 hours during the postoperative period. Obese clients may require wider beds to facilitate movement.

Extremity Exercises. Postoperative extremity exercise helps to prevent circulatory problems, such as thrombophlebitis, by facilitating venous return to the heart. The client is taught to flex and extend each joint, particularly the hip, knee, and ankle joints, while lying supine; the lower back is kept flat as the leg is lowered and straightened. The feet can be moved in circular motions while the client is lying down or sitting. The client should be encouraged to practice these exercises before surgery to gain familiarity with the appropriate exercises to be used postoperatively.

Antiembolism stockings can be used on the lower extremities perioperatively and can be applied preoperatively or in the operating room. These stockings use a low-compression gradient to encourage venous blood flow. Sequential pressure stockings use compression that is applied sequentially up and down the lower extremities to massage the legs rhythmically for even more effective prevention of clot formation. Anticoagulation may also be prescribed.

Ambulation. Ambulation should be encouraged whenever appropriate because it helps to prevent many postoperative complications. Clients are taught an appropriate ambulation schedule preoperatively so that they have an idea of when they are allowed to get out of bed after surgery. Teaching of proper methods of arising from bed to prevent pain and to minimize orthostatic hypotension is important. With abdominal surgery, one way to minimize pain on movement is to have the client turn to the side before sitting up in bed. He or she can then push to a sitting position with his or her arm, which minimizes strain on the abdominal area. The client is instructed to sit up slowly and pause before attempting to stand. Teach the client to use the same splinting method for providing support to the incision that is used during coughing and deep-breathing exercises to decrease pain on arising and sitting.

Pain Control. Having uncontrolled pain postoperatively is a common concern among preoperative clients. It is important to reassure clients that their pain will and can be controlled after surgery. Undertreatment of postoperative pain is unacceptable (see Chapter 22). Fears of addiction are unfounded, and clients have suffered needlessly. Preoperatively, teach the client how to communicate their level of pain to the caregiver. For example, they can rate the intensity of a scale from 1 to 10, with 1 being no pain to 10 being the most severe possible. Explain the type of pain relief or reduction that will be used postoperatively. For example, some surgeons inject the surgical site with a long-acting local anesthetic before closing the wound so that the client will not feel any pain in the site until the medication wears off. The ambulatory surgery client probably will be home when the local anesthetic wears off. Because the stress of surgery or side effects of anesthesia can affect memory temporarily, give instructions about taking the postoperative pain medication before surgery to both the client and accompanying family members.

If the client is to be hospitalized after surgery, explain the type of pain medication used. During the immediate postoperative period, clients can receive medications orally, intravenously, intramuscularly, or epidurally. Clients on a demand schedule (intramuscular) ask for pain medications when they are beginning to feel uncomfortable. They frequently believe that they should be stoic, and they may hesitate to ask for relief. All clients need to be assured that they will not become addicted to pain medications in the short time for which the pain medication is required. In addition, anticipate pain when the client will be moving for the first time when he or she does breathing or ambulation exercises or when the analgesia has worn off. At such times, pain medication should be offered. If the client is to have a patient-controlled analgesia (PCA) pump after surgery, demonstrate how the machine operates, and emphasize that safety features will prevent overdosing and explaining Explain how they can administer their own pain medication as needed rather than wait for the nurse's assistance. Without preoperative teaching about these procedures, however, postoperatively the client will be groggy and sore and may not understand how to control pain.

Pain can also be controlled through continuous infusion of analgesic agents through an epidural or intravenous (IV) route. Explain the method of planned pain control and how adjustments can be made for comfort.

Equipment. Whenever possible, explain the equipment that will be used during the perioperative period. Depending on the type of surgery to be performed, various tubes, drains, and IV lines may be used. Discussion should focus on the purpose of specific pieces of equipment and how their use is related to the surgery.

Tubes. The most common type of tube used during the intraoperative period is an indwelling urinary catheter. Another commonly used tube is a nasogastric (NG) tube, which is used to decompress the stomach and upper bowel or to drain the stomach contents. These tubes are often inserted in the operating room.

Drains. Drains are inserted to promote evacuation of fluid from the dead space (tissue planes created during the operation) in the operative site. Many different types of drains are used. The Penrose drain works by wicking away fluid within the operative site, which then moves through the drain via gravity to an outside dressing or collection container. Drains are frequently attached to mild suction. Hemovac and Jackson-Pratt drains are commonly used low-suction devices.

Intravenous Infusion Devices. IV infusions are usually started before surgery. The purpose of the infusion is to administer medication, fluids, and nutrient solutions. The surgeon may request IV access for use in case of emergency even if the client is not expected to need IV medications.

Preoperative Teaching for Older Adults

Older clients usually desire the same basic operative information as that provided for younger clients. You must attend to this need in a sensitive and effective way. Preoperative teaching for older clients should include consideration of possible decreased sensory ability. Sit close to the client when teaching, speaking slowly and in a manner that results in a lower tone of voice. High-pitched sounds are frequently hard for older adults to discern. Because glare from lights may bother the older client's eyes, bright lights should be avoided while preparing the client preoperatively. Because the older client is more susceptible to hypothermia, blankets should be applied in the preoperative area if the client desires, and an appropriate method of warming in the operating room, where temperatures are usually cool, should be planned.

Informed Consent

Anyone undergoing any invasive procedure must give informed consent for that procedure to be performed. A *consent form* is the legal document that signifies that the client has been told about and understands all aspects of a specific invasive procedure. This document guards the client against unwanted invasive procedures. It also protects the health care facility and health care professionals when a client denies understanding the procedure that was, or is planned to be, performed. Once the operative permit—indicating the client's *informed consent*—is signed, it becomes a permanent part of the client's record. This document accompanies the record to the operating room (Figure 16-2).

Formal consent is necessary for each invasive procedure. The client or the client's legal surrogate must receive a full explanation of the operation before giving verbal and written consent. Pictures and diagrams may

619271 (CH Rev. 7-96)

I, _____ , hereby consent to the procedures outlined below, to be performed by

_____ , and his/her associates, assistants and appropriate hospital personnel.

The procedure proposed is _____

_____

_____

for diagnosis/treatment of _____ .

This procedure has been explained in terms understandable to me, which include the following:

1. The nature and extent of the procedure to be performed and risks involved, including those which, even though unlikely to occur, involve serious consequences.

2. Alternative procedures and methods of treatment.

3. The dangers and probable consequences of such alternatives (including no procedures or treatment).

4. The estimated period of hospitalization and/or incapacity and the estimated period of convalescence (assuming there are no complications).

5. The expected consequences of the procedure upon my future health.

6. I understand that there are other risks, such as the risks of infection and other serious complications, in the pre-operative and post-operative stages of my care, which can result in serious consequences such as loss of the use of parts of my body and life.

7. I have asked all of the questions which I thought were important in deciding whether or not to undergo treatment or diagnosis. Those questions have been answered to my satisfaction.

8. I understand that no assurance can be given that the procedure will be successful and no guarantee or warranty of success or cure has been given to me.

9. I have been advised that I may have anesthesia, which in rare instances has serious and even fatal complications.

10. I further authorize and request my physician and his/her associates, assistants and appropriate hospital personnel to perform such additional procedures which in their judgement are incidentally necessary or appropriate to carry out my diagnosis/treatment.

11. I have been afforded the opportunity to consult with other physicians to my complete satisfaction before signing this form and I understand that I have the right to refuse any medical and surgical procedures and treatment.

12. I authorize the hospital to dispose of or use for research any tissue or body parts which may be necessary to remove in a manner consistent with state and federal regulations for such disposal.

I certify that I have read and fully understand the above consent statement, that the explanations are understood by me, that all blanks or statements requiring insertion or completion were filled in prior to the time of my signature, that this consent was given freely, voluntarily and without reservation.

Patient's Signature:	Date:	Time:

In the event patient is a minor, unconscious or otherwise not competent to give consent: I, _____

the (relationship to patient) _____ , of _____ hereby give consent on his/her behalf.

Witness to Signature:	Date:	Time:

CONSENT FOR SURGERY OR DIAGNOSTIC/THERAPEUTIC PROCEDURES

FIGURE 16-2 Consent form for surgery or diagnostic/therapeutic procedures. (Courtesy of the Nebraska Medical Center, Omaha, NE.)

be necessary for a complete understanding of the surgical procedure. Moreover, the client or the surrogate must be told who will perform the surgery; anesthesia and anesthetic choices; the potential risks, complications, and risk of disfigurement or death; and whether organs or body parts may be removed. The client or the surrogate is also informed about alternative treatments. The surgeon must explain the procedure in terms and language the client or the surrogate can readily understand. You are responsible for ensuring that the client or the surrogate receives an honest, accurate, and fair statement of what to expect during and after surgery and that the client understands it before informed consent is given. If the client requires consent in a language other than that printed in the form and the person obtaining consent is not fluid in his or her language, an interpreter must be used. The presence of an interpreter during consent must be documented.

The procedure for obtaining an informed consent varies from state to state and according to the individual policy of each health care facility. Generally, the surgeon explains the surgical procedure, the possible risks and complications, and the alternatives. The nurse may obtain and witness the client's signature on the consent form and may help to reinforce what the client has been told by the surgeon. It is not appropriate for the nurse to explain the surgical procedure, risks, complications, and alternatives unless this is done for reinforcement or clarification. The consent must be signed before the client receives any medication that may alter consciousness.

Adults sign their own operative permit unless they are unconscious or mentally incompetent. In such cases a surrogate, such as a relative or a legal guardian, is responsible for consent. If the relative or the guardian is out of state, consent can be secured by telephone in the presence of one or two witnesses. If no relative or guardian can be found, one can be appointed by court order.

Children under legal age who are not emancipated minors must have consent from the child's parent or legal guardian. Emancipated minors are considered those who are under the legal age of emancipation but, because of marriage or other circumstances, are independent of the parents. If the child's parent or guardian cannot be present to sign the permit, consent can be obtained from an appropriate person by telephone, fax, or letter. When a minor child's relatives cannot be located, the state in which the surgery is to be performed provides written procedures that must be followed to obtain consent by court order.

Preparing the Client on the Day of Surgery

Many clients are admitted to the hospital or surgical center the morning of surgery. These clients can be admitted to the hospital after the procedure if their condition requires specialized observation or nursing care. For so-called ambulatory surgery or same-day surgery, clients arrive at the hospital or surgery suite the morning of surgery but go home the same day to the care of family members or significant others. The ambulatory surgery approach presents a dilemma in providing preoperative instruction to the client because time is limited during the admission period before the actual surgical event. Often the nurse will telephone the night before the procedure to remind the client of any preoperative instructions. Instructions about evening showers or baths, start-ing NPO status after midnight, wearing washable clothing that is easily removed and put back on, wearing flat shoes, not wearing pantyhose, and securing a ride home after the procedure should be reinforced. The nurse conducting the telephone educational session should convey a positive attitude about the planned surgical procedure and assist in allaying doubts or fears related to the surgery.

Preoperative Preparation Immediately Before Surgery

Final preoperative preparation begins 1 to 2 hours before surgery for clients in the hospital, having same-day admission, and on admission to have outpatient surgery. Ask the client if he or she has any unanswered questions or concerns. Make sure the client understands the operative procedure to be performed and continue to assess for manifestations of anxiety. Unexpected delays in performing the surgery should be communicated to the client and his or her family.

To prevent omissions in preoperative nursing interventions, most facilities supply nurses with a preoperative checklist. As each intervention on the list is completed, initial it on the form. An example of a preoperative checklist is provided in Box 16-4. Individual surgical centers may include various other actions on this form. You may need to give medications ordered preoperatively to the client before going to the operating room. You must know the approximate time the surgical procedure is scheduled and must begin the preoperative activities early enough to have them completed when the operating room is ready.

Preoperative Medications

Preoperative medications are given to allay anxiety, to decrease pharyngeal secretions, to reduce side effects of anesthetic agents, and to induce amnesia. Table 16-5 presents an overview of common preoperative medications. Specific drug choices are based on individual client variables, the goals of sedation, and the potential for undesirable side effects. Preoperative medications may be given in the preoperative holding area or on the nursing unit. Before administering preoperative medications, ensure that the operative permit is correctly signed because legal consent cannot be given by a medicated adult. Have the client void before medication is administered so that he or she will not need to get out of bed again. After administering preoperative medication, make sure the bed is in the lowest position and the side rails of the bed are raised to prevent inadvertent falls. Lower the window shades, and turn bright lights off to avoid glare. Instruct the client not to get up without assistance because the medications are likely to cause drowsiness or dizziness. Document all actions and reactions of the client during this time. Once the client is calm and drowsy, disruptions should take place

BOX 16-4 *Immediate Preoperative Activities*

Before the client enters the operating room, check to determine that:

- All known allergies are recorded and an allergy wristband is present if indicated.
- Vital signs are checked and recorded. Report marked differences from baseline to the surgeon or anesthesia personnel.
- The identification band is present and correct.
- The consent form is signed and the surgical procedure is listed correctly.
- Skin preparation is completed if ordered preoperatively.
- Any special orders, such as administering enemas or starting an intravenous line, are completed.
- The client has not eaten or had fluids by mouth for the last 8 hours.
- The client has just voided; measure and record the amount of urine (if indicated).
- Oral hygiene or other physical care is completed.

- The presence of dentures, bridgework, or other prostheses is noted, and the anesthesia personnel knows about it.
- Storage is arranged and documented for valuables according to health care facility policy, or valuables are given to family members.
- The client has removed jewelry. (Many facilities allow the client to keep the wedding band on as long as it is taped securely.) If jewelry is removed, it should be stored according to policy or given to the family. Assist with the removal of hairpins, wigs, and so on.
- The perioperative nurse is notified about the presence of a hearing aid. Leave it in place so that operating room personnel can communicate with the client.
- The client is wearing a hospital gown and protective cap. Elastic bandaging or antiembolic hose has been applied, if ordered.
- Make-up is removed so skin color can be observed.

TABLE 16-5 *Commonly Used Preoperative Medications*

Medication	Desired Effect	Undesired Effect(s)
Tranquilizers		
Diazepam (Valium)	Decreases anxiety	May cause dizziness, clumsiness, or confusion
Droperidol (Inapsine)	Decreases anxiety Produces an antiemetic effect	Anxiety/hypotension during and after surgery
Sedatives		
Midazolam HCl	Induces desired sleepiness Decreases anxiety	Hypotension, undesired respiratory depression
Promethazine HCl (Phenergan)	Same as for droperidol	Hypotension during and after surgery
Analgesics		
Morphine sulfate	Relieves pain Decreases anxiety Sedation	Respiratory depression Hypotension Circulatory depression Decreased gastric motility causing potential for vomiting
Fentanyl citrate (Sublimaze)	Is a short-acting analgesic for minor or outpatient surgery; adjunct to general anesthesia	Same as for morphine sulfate
Meperidine HCl (Demerol)	Same as for morphine sulfate	Same as for morphine sulfate
Anticholinergics		
Atropine sulfate	Controls secretions	Excessive dryness of mouth, tachycardia
Glycopyrrolate (Robinul)	Same as for atropine sulfate	Same as for atropine sulfate
Histamine H$_2$-Receptor Antagonists		
Cimetidine (Tagamet) (see Integrating Pharmacology feature on p. 748 for other H$_2$ antagonists)	Inhibits gastric acid production	Mild dizziness, diarrhea, somnolence, and rash
Antiemetics (Zofran)	Suppression of nausea	

only when necessary and then be brief. Observe the client for side effects (e.g., hypotension and respiratory distress).

Transporting the Client to Surgery

When surgical personnel call for the client, he or she is gently transferred to a stretcher. Adequate assistance for transfer must be obtained to reduce the possibility of injury to the client or staff. Appropriate covering is provided for the client, and side rails are raised. The medical record accompanies the client to the operating room. The trip to surgery should be as smooth as possible so that the sedated client does not experience nausea and dizziness.

Preparing the Client's Room for Postoperative Care

The client's room should be prepared so that the initial care on return from surgery can be orderly. Furniture should be arranged so that the stretcher can be brought easily to the bedside. The bed should be placed in high position and made with clean linen in an open position. Bed rails should be down on the receiving side, up on other side. An emesis basin should be located close to the bed. Blood pressure monitoring equipment, IV setup, suction, and oxygen should be nearby. All equipment should be tested to ensure that it is in working condition before the client returns.

Caring for Significant Others

A designated area is usually provided for family members to wait in during surgery. If family members plan to leave the facility during the procedure, ensure that there is a way to contact them and should supply them with the phone number of the nurses' station and client's room. Some institutions issue pagers to those waiting so that they can feel free to go to the cafeteria and yet remain in touch.

When discussing the surgical procedure with the client's significant others, be sure to provide answers congruent with the information that the surgeon already has provided, and remain cognizant of confidentiality issues. Family members should also be prepared for any equipment that may accompany the client postoperatively. A preoperative explanation will assist the family in understanding what equipment is attached to their loved one and why. Significant others need to be informed when surgery is completed or if any delays occur. The surgeon should speak with family members as soon as possible after completion of the procedure.

INTRAOPERATIVE PERIOD

Nursing care during the intraoperative phase focuses on the client's emotional well-being as well as on physical factors such as safety, positioning, maintaining asepsis, and controlling the surgical environment. The preoperative assessment assists the nurse in planning appropriate interventions for this phase of the surgical experience. The nurse remains the client's advocate during this period, anticipating and guarding against potential complications. Whereas the surgeon concentrates on performing the surgical procedure and the anesthesia provider concentrates on the client's breathing and on maintenance of the client's physiologic stability, the circulating nurse is responsible for all other activities that take place in the operating room.

Members of the Surgical Team

The surgical team is a group of highly trained and educated professionals who coordinate their efforts to ensure the welfare and safety of the client. Although the specifics of each type of surgical procedure may vary, certain key players must always be present, such as the surgeon, the anesthesiologist, the circulating nurse, and scrub personnel (Box 16-5).

The surgeon heads the surgical team and makes decisions about the surgical procedure. Depending on the surgical procedure to be performed, a second surgeon or a specially trained nurse may serve as an assistant. The anesthesiologist or nurse anesthetist alleviates pain and promotes relaxation with medications. The anesthesia provider maintains the airway, ensures adequate gas exchange, monitors circulation and respiration, estimates blood and fluid loss, infuses blood and fluids, administers medications to maintain hemodynamic stability, and alerts the surgeon immediately to any complications. The circulating nurse is a core member of the surgical team and maintains the coordination of all team members while always remaining the client's advocate. Scrub personnel organize the surgical equipment and hand the surgeon the appropriate instruments required for the operative procedure. Depending on the specific surgical procedure, the surgical team may include other members; for instance, a pathologist may be called in to examine specimens, an x-ray technician may be needed to perform various radiologic procedures, or a perfusionist may be required when cardiac bypass is necessary. The circulating nurse must control the traffic within the operating suite and know the designated responsibilities of each team member.

Anesthesia

Anesthesia is an artificially induced state of partial or total loss of sensation with or without loss of consciousness. Anesthetic agents can produce muscle relaxation, block transmission of pain nerve impulses, and suppress reflexes. It can also temporarily decrease memory retrieval and recall. The depth and effects of anesthesia are monitored by observing changes in respiration, oxygen saturation and end-tidal carbon dioxide (CO_2) levels, heart rate, urine output, and blood pressure.

BOX 16-5 *Roles of the Perioperative Nurse*

Perioperative nursing is performed preoperatively, intraoperatively, and postoperatively. Each of these periods is characterized by specific actions required by nurses, who participate both independently and as part of a health care team.

Many roles are available to the perioperative nurse. The ongoing shift from tertiary care practice to community-focused practice is continuing to create even more new roles. The role these nurses play in the perioperative environment depends on their academic preparation, extended specialty education, experience, career plan, and needs of the employer. The roles of the perioperative nurse include, but are not limited to, the following:

- Circulating nurse
- Scrub nurse
- Registered Nurse First Assistant (RNFA)
- Certified Registered Nurse Anesthetist (CRNA)
- Manager
- Educator
- Case Manager, and Clinical Nurse Specialist (CNS)

Circulating Nurse

The circulating role is a major one for perioperative nurses. A nurse functioning as a circulator should be a Registered Nurse (RN). He or she assesses the client preoperatively, planning for optimal care during the surgical intervention, coordinating all personnel within the operating room, delegating and monitoring unlicensed personnel, and monitoring responsible cost compliance associated with operating room procedures. The circulator does not wear sterile clothing and can go in and out of the operating room. In addition to caring directly for the client, the circulator has very defined activities during surgery. These include the following:

- Ensuring all equipment is working properly
- Guaranteeing sterility of instruments and supplies
- Assisting with positioning
- Performing surgical skin preparation
- Monitoring the room and team members for breaks in sterile technique
- Assisting anesthesia personnel with induction and physiologic monitoring
- Handling specimens
- Coordinating activities with other departments, such as radiology and pathology
- Documenting care provided
- Minimizing conversation and traffic within the operating room suite

Scrub Nurse

An RN or Surgical Technician (ST) can perform the role of scrub person. The duties include gathering all equipment for the procedure, preparing all supplies and instruments using sterile technique, maintaining sterility within the sterile field during surgery, handling instruments and supplies during surgery, and cleaning up after the case. During surgery, the scrub person maintains an accurate count of sponges, sharps, and instru-

ments on the sterile field and counts the same materials with the circulating nurse before and after the surgery.

Registered Nurse First Assistant

The RNFA role is relatively new. In 1980, the American College of Surgeons supported the use of qualified RNs as first assistants in place of second or assisting physicians during surgical procedures. The Association of Operating Room Nurses (AORN) published its official statement on the role of the RNFA in 1984. The RNFA is an experienced perioperative nurse who has had additional specialized education to perform this role. The RNFA works with the primary surgeon during the surgery. This is a role separate from that of the scrub person. Some of the activities of an RNFA include providing exposure of the surgical area, using instruments to hold and cut, retracting and handling tissue, providing hemostasis, and suturing. RNFAs must work with a surgeon and are not independent practitioners.

Certified Registered Nurse Anesthetist

The CRNA is a nurse who has a minimum of 2 years of additional education specializing in the administration of anesthetics. Entry into a CRNA program usually requires a Bachelor of Science degree in nursing or other appropriate field plus 1-2 years of acute or intensive care nursing experience. These nurses work under the direction of an anesthesiologist.

Manager

The manager of the operating room has extensive experience and has had additional education in management. It can be any RN, but hospitals today prefer candidates with a Bachelor of Science in Nursing (BSN). Many large hospitals now require a Master's (MSN) degree, with a major in acute care or management. This nurse has many names, depending on the institution, such as head nurse, clinical nursing director, operating room manager, and others.

Educator

The role of educator can be played by any RN, but usually nurses with a BSN or MSN who are experienced perioperative nurses are best qualified. They are responsible for staff continuing education, orientation of new staff, and working with staff to learn how to be preceptors to students. These nurses may also fulfill the role of circulator or Clinical Nurse Specialist outside their teaching responsibilities.

Case Manager

The perioperative case manager is also a new role for RNs. The role calls for extensive experience, an ability to communicate, and a knowledge of the total surgical episode from home before surgery to home care needs after surgery. These nurses may have different functions within their place of work depending on the need of the institution or employing agency. As with any role, the role of case manager should be investigated before nurses accept a position of employment.

Continued

BOX 16-5 *Roles of the Perioperative Nurse—cont'd*

Clinical Nurse Specialist
The Clinical Nurse Specialist is an Advanced Practice Nurse. These nurses must hold an MSN with a major reflecting their specialty. The major roles (depending on institutional needs) vary but incorporate direct client care; education of staff, clients, family members, people of other disciplines; consultation; and research. A perioperative or surgical Clinical Nurse Specialist may not always be in the operating room but may go on rounds with physicians; interact with clients in homes, clinics, or other sites; and monitor clients in hospital surgical units. These nurses have specialized skills in heart, transplantation, renal, and cancer fields.

Most clients are anxious about the anesthesia. Some are concerned about the adequacy of the pain-blocking effects, whereas others are concerned about being "put to sleep" with a drug. Some clients wonder whether they will talk during anesthesia or experience nausea and vomiting postoperatively. Nurses must respond to these concerns by providing reassurance about the capability of the anesthesia provider and about the availability of other drugs to reduce any unpleasant side effects of the anesthesia. The client needs frequent reminders to let the nurse or physician know immediately about any side effects experienced from the anesthesia, and the nurse must remain diligent in assessing for any possible complications. Bring any side effects noted to the immediate attention of the anesthesia provider.

The decision about the type of anesthesia to be used is made by the anesthesia provider in consultation with the surgeon and the client. The choice of anesthetic agent for a surgical procedure depends on many variables. The two major techniques in anesthesia are general and regional.

Agents for *general anesthesia* (general anesthetics) block pain stimulus at the cerebral cortex and induce depression of the central nervous system (CNS) that is reversed either by metabolic change and elimination from the body or by pharmacologic means. General anesthetic agents produce analgesia, amnesia, unconsciousness, and loss of reflexes and muscle tone. The neurologic, respiratory, and cardiovascular systems are affected by these agents. General anesthesia is best suited for surgery on the head, neck, upper torso, and back; for prolonged surgical procedures; or for use in clients who are unable to lie quietly for a long period. General anesthetic agents affect all tissues in the body to some degree.

In *regional anesthesia,* drugs are given to block the pain stimulus at its origin, along afferent neurons, or along the spinal cord. Unlike general anesthesia, regional anesthesia produces a loss of painful sensation in only one region of the body and does not result in unconsciousness. In addition to the regional anesthetic agent, the client also may receive sedative agents that produce drowsiness. The client can also receive epidural opioids, which have a systemic effect and produce some drowsiness.

General Anesthesia

Stages of General Anesthesia. General anesthesia has four stages (Table 16-6). Surgery is performed in stage III. These stages were identified many years ago when ether was the most common drug used for anesthesia. The effects of ether allowed these distinct stages to be easily differentiated. The stages were used to guide the surgeon in determining when surgery could begin. Ether, which is no longer used because of its unpleasant and explosive nature, has been replaced with greatly improved anesthetic agents that provide rapid induction of anesthesia. With the rapid action of these new drugs, the stages of anesthesia are not readily apparent; however, they still occur. Some signs may be noted if the anesthetic drug is given slowly as the nurse holds the hand of the client during induction. Mild tremors of the hand may be felt as the client moves through stages I and II to stage III.

Because the last sense to be depressed during induction is hearing, remember to maintain a quiet atmosphere during this time. The client can hear and may remember conversations on awakening. The nurse, always remaining the client's advocate, ensures that all conversation during induction and throughout the case is appropriate. Clients emerge into consciousness backward through all three stages of anesthesia after the anesthetic agents are discontinued. Therefore hearing is the first sense to return.

Administration of General Anesthesia. General anesthesia can be administered in a variety of ways. The most common method of administering anesthesia is to use a combination of agents based on the client's need with consideration of the type of surgery to be performed. This type of anesthesia is called *neuroleptic* or *balanced anesthesia.* Balanced anesthesia is typically achieved by using a combination of an inhalation agent, oxygen, an opioid, and a neuromuscular blocking agent. Inhalation and the IV route are the most common routes of administration. Table 16-7 describes the most commonly used general anesthetic agents and the implications for the delivery of nursing care associated with the use of each.

Neuromuscular Blocking Agents. Neuromuscular blocking agents are classified as *depolarizing* and *nondepolarizing.* These agents block the transmission of nerve

TABLE 16-6	*The Four Stages of Anesthesia*			
Stage	Start-Point	End-Point	Physical Reactions	Nursing Interventions
I: Onset	Anesthetic administration	Loss of consciousness	Client may be drowsy or dizzy; Possible auditory or visual hallucinations	Close operating room doors; keep room quiet; stand by to assist client
II: Excitement	Loss of consciousness	Loss of eyelid reflexes	Increase in autonomic activity; Irregular breathing; Client may struggle	Remain quietly at client's side; assist anesthetist, if needed
III: Surgical anesthesia	Loss of eyelid reflexes	Loss of most reflexes; Depression of vital functions	Client is unconscious; Muscles are relaxed; No blink or gag reflex	Begin preparation (if indicated) only when anesthetist indicates stage III has been reached and client is breathing well, with stable vital signs
IV: Danger (death)	Functions excessively depressed	Respiratory and circulatory failure	Client is not breathing; A heartbeat may or may not be present	If arrest occurs, respond immediately to assist in establishing airway; provide cardiac arrest tray, drugs, syringes, long needles; assist surgeon with closed or open cardiac massage

impulses to the muscle fibers. Neuromuscular blocking agents (Table 16-8) are administered via the IV route and are given mainly to facilitate intubation by easing laryngospasm and relaxing muscles for controlled ventilation. When general anesthetics are given with neuromuscular blocking agents, the latter can be given in smaller and thus safer doses. Common muscle relaxants are succinylcholine, tubocurarine, pancuronium, and vecuronium.

Types of General Anesthesia

Intravenous Anesthesia. When general anesthesia is administered intravenously, the client experiences an extremely rapid induction. Unconsciousness generally occurs about 30 seconds after the medication is administered. This process promotes a rapid transition from the conscious stage to the surgical anesthesia stage. It also prepares the client for a smooth transition to the surgical stage of anesthesia because the IV anesthetic can act as a calming agent. IV anesthesia is sufficiently potent to be used alone in such minor procedures as dental extractions and pelvic examinations. Examples of IV anesthetics are thiopental sodium and ketamine.

Inhalation Anesthesia. For inhalation anesthesia, a mixture of volatile liquids or gas and oxygen is used. These anesthetics are advantageous because of their ease of administration and elimination through the respiratory system. These are usually used to maintain the client in stage III anesthesia following induction. The mixture is given through a mask or through an endotracheal tube (Figure 16-3), which is inserted once the client is paralyzed and unconscious. Anesthesia intubation is often more dif-

ficult in an obese client because of the typically thickened neck and in the client with arthritis or a neck fracture.

When inhalation anesthetic agents are administered by mask, the gases generally flow into the mask via a finely calibrated vaporizer that is controlled by a machine. When an endotracheal tube is used to give the anesthetic, the gases flow directly into the client's tracheobronchial tree, resulting in a quick response. Many different liquids and gases are used in inhalation anesthesia. Two commonly used inhalation anesthetics are halothane and isoflurane. A commonly used gas anesthetic is nitrous oxide.

Regional Anesthesia

Regional anesthetics are useful in many clinical situations. Local anesthetic agents, which are used to obtain local anesthesia, can also be administered to function as a central, peripheral, IV, regional, retrobulbar, or transbronchial nerve block. (See Table 16-10 for a description of agents commonly used for local anesthesia.) These anesthetic agents block the conduction of impulses in the nerve fibers without depolarizing the cell membrane.

Epinephrine can be added to many of the local anesthetics in an effort to prolong the anesthetic effect. Epinephrine also causes local blood vessels to constrict, thus delaying absorption of the anesthetic agent. This factor also can reduce bleeding through vasoconstriction. Epinephrine should be used with caution in older adults who have cardiovascular or liver disease. Traditionally, epinephrine was not used in hand or foot surgery because of the small blood vessels in the area. Because the effect is vasoconstriction, use of epinephrine could com-

TABLE 16-7	*General Anesthetic Agents*		
Drug	**Action**	**Side Effects**	**Nursing Implications**
Inhalation Agents			
Nitrous oxide	Gas has very low anesthetic potency, so it must be used with other agents; highest analgesic effect of all agents; little or no effect on BP or P; no muscle relaxant properties	Minimal side effects; little or no hypotension or respiratory depression; low incidence of malignant hypothermia	Monitor vital signs, especially BP and P; monitor effects of CNS depressants for 24 hr after administration
Halothane (Fluothane)	Volatile liquid with high anesthetic potency, so it could be used alone; has weak analgesic effect; causes moderate decrease in BP and large decrease in respirations; only a mild muscle relaxant	Hypotension, depression of myocardium with decreased cardiac output, bradycardia, respiratory depression; sensitizes heart to catecholamines; malignant hyperthermia, hepatitis, postoperative mild nausea and vomiting, decreased urine output	Monitor all vital signs closely; monitor body temperature for signs of malignant hyperthermia; keep client warm during recovery, and watch for severe shivering; avoid use of catecholamines (epinephrine or norepinephrine); monitor liver function after surgery; monitor urine output closely
Enflurane (Ethrane)	Volatile liquid with fairly high anesthetic potential; has weak analgesic effect; causes moderate decrease in BP and large decrease in respirations; is a moderate muscle relaxant	Hypotension, respiratory depression; blocks labor; minimal sensitization of heart to catecholamines; seizures with high doses	Do not give to clients with history of seizures; monitor vital signs, especially BP, P, and respirations; not for use during labor
Isoflurane (Forane)	Volatile liquid with high anesthetic potential; has weak analgesic effect; causes moderate decrease in BP and large decrease in respirations; is a moderate muscle relaxant; produces profound vasodilation	Hypotension related to vasodilating effect; respiratory depression; suppresses uterine contractions	Does not sensitize heart to catecholamines, so it can be used with epinephrine and norepinephrine; monitor vital signs; avoid rapid position changes because it may lead to hypotension as a result of vasodilation
Intravenous Drugs			
Thiopental sodium (Pentothal)	Short-acting barbiturate that produces rapid unconsciousness; a weak analgesic and muscle relaxant	Respiratory depression with momentary apnea after injection, retrograde amnesia, myocardial depression, hypotension, headache, and shivering	Monitor for allergic reactions; monitor respiratory function closely, especially during induction; monitor vital signs; cannot be mixed with solutions containing atropine, tubocurarine, or succinylcholine; avoid extravasation
Fentanyl citrate–droperidol (Innovar)	A potent opioid (fentanyl) combined with a neuroleptic (droperidol); produces indifference to surroundings and insensitivity to pain; CNS depressant, which produces calming, analgesia, and reduced motor activity	Emergence delirium with hallucinations, hypotension, vasodilation, nausea and vomiting, laryngospasm, respiratory depression, shivering, and apnea	Use with caution in clients with head injuries, increased intracranial pressure, COPD, hepatic or renal dysfunction, or bradydysrhythmias, or in older clients; monitor vital signs; maintain patent airway; reduce narcotic doses to one fourth or one third for first 24 hr postoperatively; when Innovar is used for induction, fentanyl citrate (Sublimaze) alone is used for maintenance of anesthesia

BP, Blood pressure; *CNS,* central nervous system; *COPD,* chronic obstructive pulmonary disease; *CSF,* cerebrospinal fluid; *P,* pulse.

TABLE 16-7	*General Anesthetic Agents—cont'd*		
Drug	**Action**	**Side Effects**	**Nursing Implications**

Intravenous Drugs—cont'd

| Ketamine HCl (Ketalar) | Produces state of dissociative anesthesia; causes sedation, immobility, analgesia, amnesia, and unresponsivenss to pain; short-acting (no antagonist) | Delirium, hallucinations, disturbing dreams, tonic and clonic movements, respiratory depression, hypotension or hypertension, decreased or increased pulse, nystagmus, increased salivation, laryngospasms, and mild nausea and vomiting | Contraindicated in clients with history of stroke and severe hypertension; use with caution in clients with alcoholism or elevated CSF; maintain airway; do not give in same syringe as for barbiturates; minimize stimulation as client emerges from anesthesia; use diazepam if hallucinations occur or delusions are severe; excellent for anesthesia in young and older clients; pad side rails of gurney; place client in quiet dark area; do not stimulate client inadvertently; any sudden moves elicit hallucinations |

TABLE 16-8	*Neuromuscular Blocking Agents*		
Drug	**Action**	**Side Effects**	**Nursing Implications**
Pancuronium bromide (Pavulon)	Nondepolarizing agent; prevents acetylcholine from binding to receptors on muscle endplate, blocking depolarization	Tachycardia, hypertension, prolonged dose-related apnea, allergic reaction, and excessive sweating and salivation	Use carefully in older or debilitated clients or in clients with renal, hepatic, or pulmonary disease, myasthenia gravis, or thyroid disease; measure intake and output carefully; have resuscitation equipment available; do not mix in syringe or solution with barbiturates; neostigmine reverses effect
Vecuronium bromide (Norcuron)	Nondepolarizing agent; prevents acetylcholine from binding to receptors on muscle endplate, blocking depolarization	Transient tachycardia; prolonged dose-related apnea, redness, itching, and induration	Has no effect on cardiovascular system; use with caution in clients with hepatic disease, obesity, or neuromuscular disease; tolerated well in renal disease; reversed with anticholinesterase and neostigmine; have emergency resuscitation equipment available
Succinylcholine chloride (Anectine)	Nondepolarizing agent that prolongs depolarization of muscle endplate	Increased or decreased pulse rate and blood pressure, dysrhythmias, increased intraocular pressure, prolonged respiratory depression, malignant hyperthermia, postoperative muscle pain, excessive salivation, and hypersensitivity	Monitor vital signs; maintain patent airway; postoperative stiffness is normal; drug of choice for short procedures; keep emergency resuscitation equipment on hand; repeat infusions can prolong apnea; neostigmine reverses effect

promise tissue perfusion, leading to adverse outcomes such as poor circulatory response. Recently, however, the use of epinephrine in hand and foot surgery has been reevaluated.

Types of Regional Anesthesia. Regional anesthesia can be administered in a variety of different ways: spinal, epidural, caudal, topical, local infiltration, field block, peripheral nerve block, and IV regional block.

Spinal Anesthesia. Spinal anesthesia offers many advantages for clients undergoing surgical procedures involving the lower half of the body. It is often the anesthetic technique of choice for older adults because of its

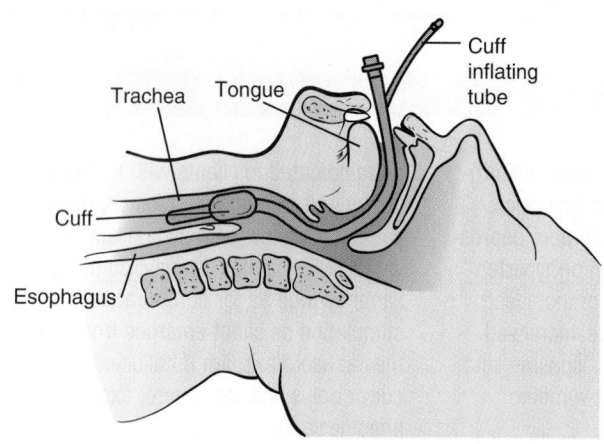

FIGURE 16-3 Correct placement of the endotracheal tube for anesthesia administration.

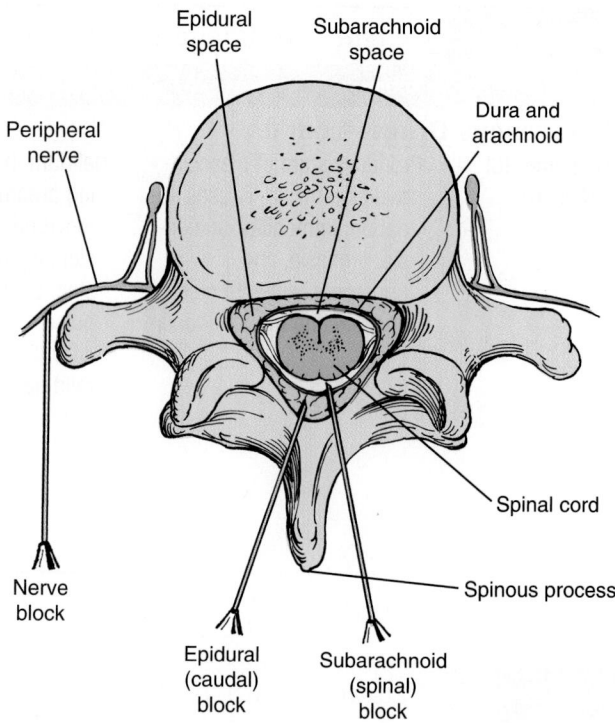

FIGURE 16-4 Cross-section of a lumbar vertebra showing injection sites for anesthesia.

overall advantages. Benefits of spinal anesthesia include its relative safety, excellent lower-body muscle relaxation, and absence of effect on consciousness; furthermore, its use does not require an empty stomach. Spinal anesthesia is achieved by injecting local anesthetics into the subarachnoid space (Figure 16-4). Autonomic nerve fibers are affected first and are also the last to recover. After blockade of the autonomic nervous system, spinal anesthesia blocks the following fibers in this order: (1) touch, (2) pain, (3) motor, (4) pressure, and (5) proprioceptive fibers. These fibers alert the brain of physical orientation. Recovery is in the reverse order.

Spinal anesthesia can be used for almost any type of major procedure performed below the level of the diaphragm, such as a hysterectomy or appendectomy. Figure 16-5 illustrates proper positioning for the injection of drugs for spinal anesthesia. Within minutes of administration the client experiences a loss of sensation and paralysis of the toes, feet, legs, and then abdomen. Most clients exhibit a slight hypotension initially as a result of the vasodilation that occurs with administration of the spinal anesthetic. The complications of spinal anesthesia are listed and described in Table 16-9, along with prevention and intervention suggestions for nurses. As with any anesthesia, the client who has undergone spinal anesthesia is at risk for neurologic, respiratory, or cardiovascular complications; however, the risk of spinal anesthesia in general is no higher than with general anesthesia.

Epidural Anesthesia. An epidural block is achieved by introduction of an anesthetic agent into the epidural space (see Figure 16-4). The epidural space is generally entered by a needle at a thoracic, lumbar, sacral, or caudal interspace. The needle is carefully positioned in the epidural space without penetrating the dura and without entering the subarachnoid space. When the needle is properly positioned, the cerebrospinal fluid cannot be

aspirated. An epidural block, like spinal anesthesia, produces a blockade of the autonomic nerves and hypotension can result. If the level of the block is too high and the respiratory muscles are affected, respiratory depression or paralysis may occur.

Caudal Anesthesia. Caudal anesthesia is produced by injection of the local anesthetic into the caudal or sacral canal. Caudal anesthesia is a variation of epidural anesthesia. This method is commonly used with obstetric clients.

Topical Anesthesia. Topical anesthetic agents may be applied directly on the area to be desensitized. The anesthetic may be a solution, an ointment, a gel, a cream, or a powder. This short-acting form of anesthesia can block peripheral nerve endings in the mucous membranes of the vagina, rectum, nasopharynx, and mouth. Topical anesthesia is used in minor procedures such as a rectal examination when painful hemorrhoids are present or before a bronchoscopic examination to desensitize the bronchi. Medications used for local and topical anesthesia are listed in Table 16-10.

One drug commonly used for topical anesthesia is a 4% to 10% solution of cocaine. This agent is for topical use only and is used primarily to anesthetize the eye and the mucous membranes of the nose, mouth, and urethra. Cocaine is highly toxic. If accidentally injected, it can cause severe excitement or seizures, followed by shock,

FIGURE 16-5 Proper positioning for spinal anesthesia administration flexes the client's torso to expand the space between the lumbar vertebrae.

TABLE 16-9	*Complications and Discomforts of Spinal Anesthesia*		
Complications and Discomforts	**Causes**	**Intervention**	**Prevention**
Hypotension	Paralysis of vasomotor nerves; usually occurs shortly after induction of anesthesia	Administer oxygen by inhalation Vasoactive drugs Trendelenburg's position if level of anesthesia is fixed, 10-20 min after induction	In clients not prone to heart failure, 500-800 ml of IV fluids, administered rapidly before block
Nausea and vomiting	Occurs mainly from abdominal surgery because of traction placed on various structures within abdomen or from hypotension	Ephedrine Antiemetics Oxygen Fluids	
Headache (can be extremely painful, may last a week)	Cerebrospinal fluid (which cushions the brain) is lost through dural hole; leakage of fluid with loss of cushioning effect increased by (1) use of a large spinal needle or (2) poor hydration	Apply tight abdominal binder Fluids Analgesics In severe cases, inject 10 ml of client's blood to plug hole (blood patch)	Use of very small spinal needle reduces incidence of spinal headache to 0.9% Administer IV and oral fluids before and after induction of spinal anesthesia Keep client flat and quiet 6-8 hr postoperatively
Respiratory paralysis	Occurs if drug reaches upper thoracic and cervical spinal levels in large amounts or in heavy concentrations	Artificial respiration	Avoid extreme Trendelenburg's position before level of spinal anesthesia set, i.e., 10-20 min after induction
Neurologic complications (e.g., paraplegia, severe muscle weakness in legs)	Paralysis postoperatively may be due to (1) unsterile needles, syringes, and anesthetic medications; (2) pre-existing diseases of CNS (e.g., multiple sclerosis and spinal cord tumors), which cause paralysis, rather than spinal anesthesia itself; (3) transient response to anesthetics; (4) position during surgery	Supportive care for transient forms related to medication Antibiotics and steroids for infectious causes Permanent paralysis will require rehabilitation	Strict sterile technique Heat-sterilized medications and instruments Careful preoperative neurologic examination to ascertain presence of neurologic disease

IV, Intravenous; *CNS,* central nervous system.

TABLE 16-10	*Local and Topical Anesthetic Agents*		
Drug	**Action**	**Side Effects**	**Nursing Implications**
Local Agents			
Bupivacaine HCl (Marcaine HCl)	Amide-type local anesthetic that blocks depolarization, preventing generation and conduction of nerve impulses; combined with epinephrine, it has prolonged action	Edema, anaphylaxis; rarely, anxiety, convulsions, respiratory arrest, cardiac arrest, blurred vision, and shivering	Contraindicated in children under 12 years of age, or for spinal or paracervical block or topical anesthesia; use with caution in older clients or in clients with hepatic disease or allergies; onset 4-15 min, duration 3-6 hr; keep resuscitative equipment available
Chloroprocaine HCl (Nesacaine)	Ester-type local anesthetic that blocks depolarization, preventing generation and condition of nerve impulses	Anaphylaxis, edema; rarely, anxiety, convulsions, respiratory arrest, cardiac arrest, blurred vision, and shivering	Contraindicated in clients with allergies to "caines," CNS disease; use cautiously in older adults; check solution for particles or discoloration; keep resuscitative equipment available; do not use solution with preservative for caudal or epidural blocks
Lidocaine HCl (Xylocaine)	Amide-type local anesthetic that blocks depolarization, preventing generation and conduction of nerve impulses; combined with epinephrine, it has prolonged action	Edema, anaphylaxis, dysrhythmias; rarely, anxiety, respiratory arrest, cardiac arrest, and tinnitus	Contraindicated in clients with hypersensitivity, severe hypertension, septicemia, spinal deformities, or neurologic disorders; use cautiously in older clients and those with heart block or general drug allergies or in severe shock; use solutions with epinephrine only in body areas with good blood supply; use preservative-free solution for spinal, epidural, and caudal blocks
Topical Agents			
Benzocaine (Americaine)	Blocks conduction of impulses at sensory nerve endings	Sensitization rash, possible tolerance	Contraindicated in clients with history of hypersensitivity to "caines"; discontinue if rash develops; avoid contact with eyes; avoid inhalation of spray; has short duration of action; do not use over infected area; if used rectally, clean area well first
Ethyl chloride spray	Produces local anesthesia by producing sensation of cold	Frostbite, tissue necrosis from prolonged use, muscle spasms, and increased pain	Do not apply over broken skin; protect adjacent skin; avoid contact with eyes; avoid inhalation; highly flammable, do not use near open flame; very short duration
Tetracaine HCl (Pontocaine HCl)	Blocks conduction of impulses at sensory nerve endings	Local sensitization and rash	Do not use in hypersensitive clients; clean rectal area well before applying; do not use if rash develops
Cocaine	Ester-type topical anesthetic that blocks uptake of norepinephrine by adrenergic neurons	CNS stimulation, euphoria, decreased fatigue, tachycardia, vasoconstriction, and hypertension	For topical use only; produces psychological dependence with prolonged or repeated use; schedule II narcotic; use cautiously in clients with history of severe hypertension or heart disease; combined with epinephrine, it can lead to cardiovascular toxicity; monitor vital signs closely

CNS, Central nervous system.

respiratory failure, and cardiac arrest. Emergency resuscitation equipment must be available when cocaine is used. Other agents commonly used for topical anesthesia include tetracaine, procaine, mepivacaine, bupivacaine, and lidocaine (Xylocaine). To avoid anaphylactic reactions from previous sensitization to anesthetic agents, check the client's drug allergies before applying any topical anesthetic agent.

Local Infiltration Anesthesia. Local infiltration anesthesia involves injection of an anesthetic agent such as lidocaine (Xylocaine) into the skin and subcutaneous tissue of the area to be anesthetized. Local anesthesia blocks only the peripheral nerves around the area of the incision. When local anesthetic is administered, the person injecting the drug must aspirate before injection to ensure that the needle is not in a blood vessel. If a local anesthetic agent is inadvertently injected into the bloodstream, it becomes systemic, and cardiovascular collapse or convulsions could result.

Field Block Anesthesia. The area proximal to a planned incision can be injected and infiltrated with local anesthetic agents to produce what is known as a *field block*. This block forms a barrier between the incision and the nervous system. This procedure differs from simple injection of local anesthesia, in which only the area of the incision is injected. A field block actually walls in the area around the incision and prevents transmission of sensory impulses to the brain from that area. The anesthesia provider must take precautions when performing a field block to avoid injection of the agent into a blood vessel.

Peripheral Nerve Block Anesthesia. A *nerve block* anesthetizes individual nerves or nerve plexuses rather than all the local nerves anesthetized by a field block. Nerve blocks can be obtained in a finger (digital nerve block), the entire upper arm (brachial plexus nerve block), or the chest or abdominal wall (intercostal nerve block). Nerves most commonly blocked are those within the brachial plexus and the intercostal, sciatic, and femoral nerves. Drugs commonly used as nerve block agents are lidocaine, bupivacaine, and mepivacaine. The anesthesia provider injects the anesthetic along the nerve rather than into the nerve in an effort to decrease the risk of nerve damage. Once the drug has been injected, it takes several minutes for onset of the anesthesia.

Nerve blocks, like local infiltration blocks, can produce severe systemic response if the drug is accidentally injected into a blood vessel. Because epinephrine causes vasoconstriction, particularly in the extremities, anesthetic procedures for surgery performed below the wrist or ankle typically use agents that do not contain epinephrine.

Intravenous Regional Extremity Block Anesthesia (Bier Block). Regional anesthesia of a limb can be achieved with an agent such as lidocaine when it is injected into a vein of the limb to be anesthetized. A pneumatic dual-cuff tourniquet applied to the anesthetized area prevents the lidocaine from circulating beyond the area undergoing the procedure. This type of anesthesia is used most commonly for procedures of the extremities that are of short duration. The tourniquet can be inflated only for 2-hour increments.

Monitored Anesthesia. Monitored anesthesia is used during an operation in which the surgeon infiltrates the surgical site with a local anesthetic and the anesthesia provider supplements the local anesthetic with IV drugs to provide sedation and systemic analgesia. The anesthesia care provider monitors the client's blood pressure, heart rate, and respiration while the local anesthesia and IV support are being provided. *Local standby* and *anesthesia standby* also refer to monitored anesthesia.

Other Methods of Regional Anesthesia and Analgesia

Acupuncture. Acupuncture is an ancient Chinese pain-killing technique that works by the insertion of long, thin needles into specific acupuncture points located on lines called *meridians* that connect anatomic sites on the body. Practitioners of acupuncture have named and numbered approximately 1000 acupuncture points, each about 0.25 cm in diameter. When performing major surgery, Chinese doctors use acupuncture as a form of anesthesia. Some advantages of acupuncture include (1) decreased anesthesia-related side effects during or after surgery, (2) less blood loss during surgery, and (3) reduced need for postoperative analgesia because acupuncture's pain-killing effects persist for several hours.

Several Western hypotheses have been postulated to explain why acupuncture works. One hypothesis is based on the outdated gate control theory of pain control and contends that the technique stimulates the larger sensory nerve fibers that carry non-pain impulses. Another theory suggests that acupuncture triggers the release of endorphins, endogenous polypeptides with analgesic properties. Some Western physicians remain skeptical about the technique's pain-killing capabilities.

Cryothermia. Cryothermia is the use of cold to induce anesthesia. Because a very low surface temperature reduces pain, the surgical site is treated with ice preoperatively. Although there are many acceptable alternatives to cryothermia, this technique can be used in extreme conditions that threaten life and when the client cannot tolerate conventional forms of anesthesia.

Intraoperative Nursing Care

Intraoperative nursing care is the second component of perioperative nursing. It is often called *operating room nurs-*

EB EVIDENCE-BASED PRACTICE IN ACTION

Avoiding Wrong Site Surgery

Surgeries on the wrong site or on the wrong client or performance of the wrong procedure on a client are completely preventable and should never happen. The error reporting database of the Joint Commission on Hospital Accreditation Organization (JCAHO) includes more than 150 such cases collected since 1996, of which 126 have root cause analysis information. Of the 126 cases, wrong site surgery is most common among orthopedic surgeries, second most common among urologic surgeries, and third most common among neurosurgical procedures. Fifty-eight percent of the cases occurred in either a hospital-based ambulatory surgery unit or a freestanding ambulatory setting, with 29% occurring in the inpatient operating room and 13% occurring in other inpatient sites such as the emergency department or intensive care unit. Seventy-six percent involved surgery on the wrong body part or site, 13% involved surgery on the wrong client, and 11% involved the wrong surgical procedure.

A number of factors contributed to the increased risk for wrong site, wrong person, or wrong procedure surgery, including emergency cases (19%); unusual physical characteristics, including morbid obesity or physical deformity (16%); unusual time pressures to start or complete the procedure (13%); unusual equipment or setup in the operating room (13%); the involvement of multiple surgeons in the case (13%); and the performance of multiple procedures during a single surgical visit (10%).[2]

The root causes identified by the hospitals usually involved more than one factor, but the majority involved a breakdown in communication between surgical team members and the client and family. Other contributing causes included policy issues such as not requiring the surgical site to be marked, not requiring verification in the operating room or a verification checklist, and incomplete client assessment, including an incomplete preoperative assessment. Staffing issues, distraction factors, avail-

ability of pertinent information in the operating room, and organizational cultural issues were also cited as contributing risk factors.[3]

The following activities are recommended:
- Ask the client to mark the surgical site with a permanent marker.[1]
- Ask the surgeon to sign the marked site and then actually operate through or next to the initials.
- Orally verify the surgery. Just before starting the operation in the operating room, each member of the surgical team should confirm the correct person, the correct surgical site, and the correct procedure.[4]
- Take a "time out" in the operating room. This gives the surgical team one last chance to double check among themselves about the impending procedure, to check charts, and to corroborate information with the client using active, not passive, communication techniques.[4]
- Create and use a verification checklist, including appropriate documents such as medical records, x-rays, and/or imaging studies in the operating room to verify the correct client, procedure, and site.

References
1. DiGiovanni, C.W., et al. (2003). Patient compliance in avoiding wrong-site surgery. *Journal of Bone and Joint Surgery, 85A*, 815-819.
2. Joint Commission on Accreditation of Healthcare Organizations. (2001). A follow-up review of wrong site surgery. *Sentinel Event Alert, (24)* at http://www.jcaho.org.
3. Saufl, N.M. (2002). Sentinel event: Wrong-site surgery. *Journal of Perianesthesia Nursing, 17*(6), 420-422.
4. Scheidt, R.C. (2002). Ensuring correct site surgery. *AORN Journal, 76*(15), 770-777.

ing. Intraoperative nurses see the client immediately before surgery, either in a holding area or in an admission unit. The intraoperative nurse completes an initial brief assessment. The care plans that were developed and planned preoperatively, along with the findings on the extensive admission examination, are used in this phase. Intraoperative nursing care plans incorporate safety, monitoring of the client, and control of operative resources along with considerations of the individual needs of each client.

Maintaining Safety and Preventing Injury

Safety is a major consideration in the perioperative nursing. Using data gathered from the preoperative assessment, the nurse implements care individually designed for each client. This care includes positioning, control-

ling equipment and supplies, maintaining surgical asepsis, monitoring the physiologic status, and monitoring for potential emergencies. It is imperative that the intended surgical site be marked and the site confirmed by the client (see the Evidence-Based Practice in Action feature on Avoiding Wrong Site Surgery, above).

Position the Client. Procedures vary among institutions, but after admission to the operating room, the client is identified and then moved to the operating room bed. At this time, the client is anesthetized and positioned, and the skin is prepared and any other procedures that must be completed before draping and creating the sterile field (such as catheterization or hair removal) are done. The perioperative nurse understands the various operative positions as well as the physiologic changes that occur when a

TABLE 16-11   *Guidelines for Positioning the Client During Surgery*

Nursing Action	Rationale
Explain to the client, in simple, understandable terms, why the positions and restraints are necessary.	Some clients feel that retraining straps are punitive. Some positions can be difficult or embarrassing.
Preserve the client's dignity and avoid undue exposure.	To promote a positive feeling that will encourage healing.
Place restraining straps 2 inches above the knees.	Most secure position on operating bed. Avoids pressure injury from strap on bony prominences.
Nerves, muscles, pressure points, and bony prominences are padded.	To prevent nerve and tissue damage; decrease pressure that will impair or slow circulation; prevent pressure sores during long surgical procedures.
Position the client to obtain or maintain adequate respiratory exchange and vascular circulation.	To ensure tissue perfusion, oxygenation, and minimize the pooling of blood. Slow blood flow predisposes to thrombus formation.
Avoid pressure on the chest and on body parts such as the female breast and male genitalia.	Prevent injury and minimize discomfort after surgery.
Do not allow the client's extremities to dangle over the sides of the table.	Hands or feet can be inadvertently compressed against the operating room bed by surgery team personnel as they lean over the client's body. Impairment of circulation or nerve and muscle damage may result.
When using an arm board, do not abduct the upper extremity more than 90 degrees.	Hyperextension can result in permanent nerve damage caused by stretching or crushing the brachial plexus between the first rib and scapula.
Avoid excessive strain on the client's muscles.	Postoperative strain and discomfort may result.
Be certain the client's ankles are not crossed when in the prone position.	Circulation may be occluded.
Always move both lower extremities at the same time when putting them up in stirrups and when lowering.	Hip joint could be dislocated or the muscles strained when extremities are positioned one at a time.
Monitor the total position throughout surgery.	Remember, the client may remain in one position for hours.

client is placed in a specific position. Table 16-11 reviews these positions and the changes that may occur. Essential factors to consider in positioning a client on the operating table are (1) the site of the operation, (2) the age and size of the client, (3) the type of anesthetic used, and (4) pain normally experienced by the client on movement, such as that from arthritis. The position must not hinder respiration or circulation, must not apply excessive pressure to skin surfaces, and must not limit surgical exposure. The following surgical positions are shown in Figure 16-6:

- *Dorsal recumbent (supine):* Commonly used for coronary artery bypass grafting, hernia repair, mastectomy, or bowel resection
- *Trendelenburg:* Permits displacement of the intestines into the upper abdomen and is often used during surgery of the lower abdomen or pelvis
- *Lithotomy:* Exposes the perineal and rectal areas and is ideal for vaginal repairs, dilation and curettage, and most types of rectal surgery
- *Prone:* Commonly used for cervical spine, posterior fossa craniotomy, back, rectal, and posterior leg surgery

- *Lateral:* Used for clients undergoing kidney, chest, or hip surgery

Many other positions can be used, depending on the type of surgery and the visualization of the site required by the surgeon. Laser techniques, endoscopy, or biopsy all may require different client positioning. Interventions may include gathering special supplies that can accommodate an obese client, arranging for an appropriate operating table to withstand excess weight, and providing extra padding to assist in skin integrity maintenance. Additional padding is applied to the operating table for the very thin client or the client with kyphosis.

Whatever the client's position on the operating table, general guidelines to promote safety are followed. Most clients feel stiff and sore after a long surgical procedure and may actually complain of the effects of positioning.

Provide Equipment Safety. Almost everything in the operating room can be a source of injury if careful control is not exercised. Every action is designed to prevent accidents. These procedures include counting surgical sup-

Dorsal recumbent/supine

Trendelenburg

Lithotomy

Prone

Lateral

FIGURE 16-6 Five surgical positions.

plies and equipment that could inadvertently be left inside the surgical incision, such as needles, sponges, and instruments. Counts are performed by two people, usually the circulating nurse and the scrub person, at three different times: (1) before the initial incision, (2) during the surgery, and (3) immediately before the incision is closed. A final correct count is announced to the surgeon and charted on the intraoperative chart.

Electrical safety is also controlled during surgery. All plugs and wires are inspected for correct attachment; all equipment is checked to ensure that it is in working order; and measures are taken to prevent electrical burns to the client. An *electrosurgical unit* (ESU) is used to sear the ends of capillaries and blood vessels to control bleeding during surgery. When unipolar cautery is used, place a grounding pad on a large body-surface area (thigh or back) to "ground" the client and to prevent sparking and burns. Grounding pads must be placed over intact skin, away from any bony prominences and not over scars or fragile tissue. Many ESUs have a safety feature that does not allow the unit to work if the grounding pad is placed inappropriately. Bipolar cautery does not require a grounding pad.

Maintain Surgical Asepsis. The perioperative nurse ensures the sterility of supplies and equipment. All members of the health care team use sterile technique to minimize postoperative infections. If a suspected or actual break in the sterile field occurs, the contaminated instruments and clothing are removed and replaced with new, sterile items. Members of the surgical team who are in the "sterile area" are those actively performing or assisting in the surgical procedure, including the surgeon and the assistants and scrub personnel. The circulating nurse is not sterile and monitors the sterile field to maintain the sterility of supplies and personnel. Surgical asepsis may be broken but must be rectified immediately. The nurse is the advocate of the client in maintaining a sterile surgical environment.

Assist with Wound Closure. After final counts are completed, the nurse anticipates the type of wound closure needed and obtains the supplies for the surgical team. The surgical wound may be closed with sutures, staples, or other materials or may be left open to heal by secondary intention. Common skin closures are illustrated in Figure 16-7. If a drain is needed, it is placed in a sep-

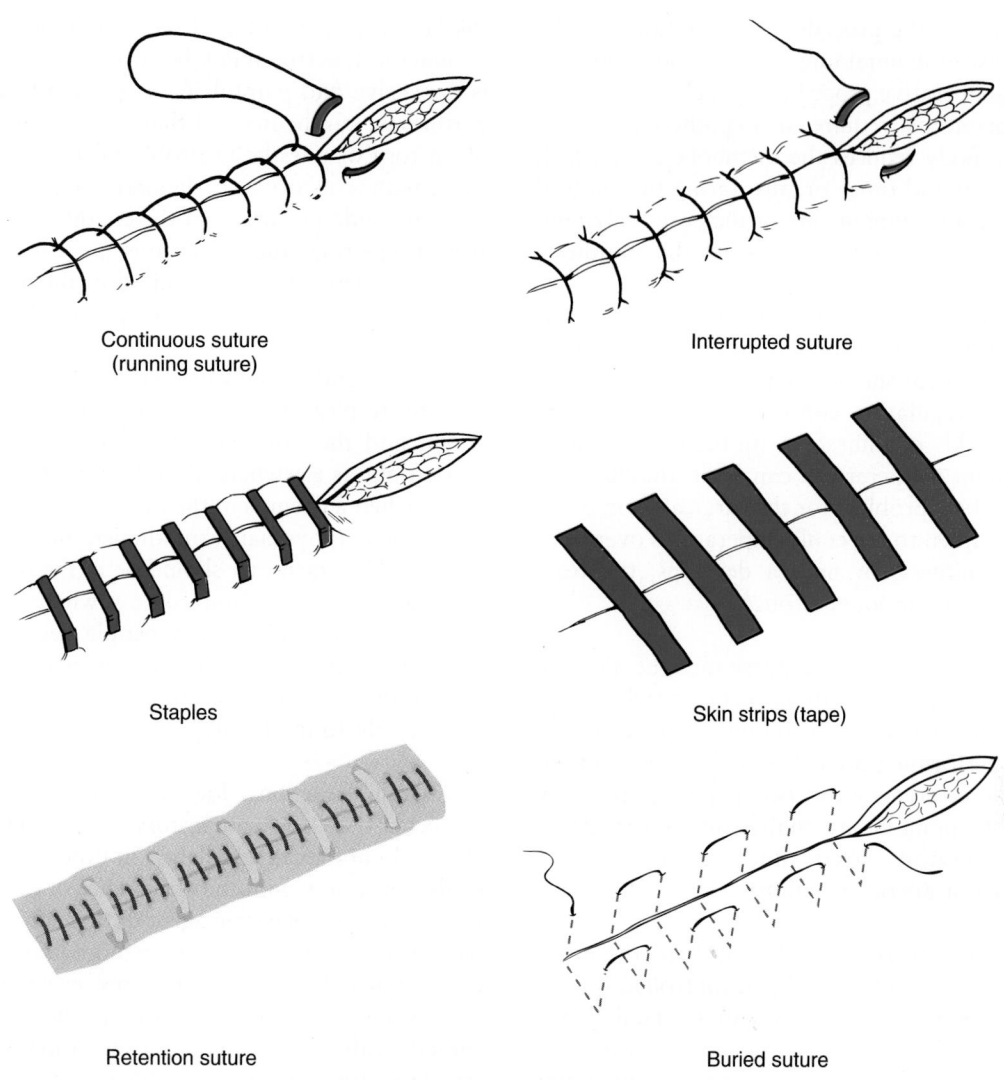

Continuous suture
(running suture)

Interrupted suture

Staples

Skin strips (tape)

Retention suture

Buried suture

FIGURE 16-7 Skin closures.

arate small incision parallel to the operative incisions to drain blood or serum from the operative site. The use of a surgical drain promotes wound healing and decreases the potential for infection. There are many types of surgical drains. The drain is chosen by surgeon preference and is based on the size of the wound and the type of drainage expected. Drains may be free draining, attached to a high-suction apparatus, or they may be self-contained with low suction. The intraoperative nurse and the postoperative nurse are responsible for assessing whether the drainage is flowing freely through the system. When the client is transferred out of the operative area, the responsible nurse continues to monitor the patency of the drain and the characteristics of the drainage.

Monitoring

Body Temperature. Hypothermia can occur easily in the operating room. The operating room temperature is maintained at a standard cool level of 60° to 75° F. Hu-

midity is regulated at 50% to 60%. Temperature control is set to allow optimal performance of the surgical team members, who must wear layers of clothing, and to inhibit bacterial growth. The client can become cold in the operating room if appropriate covering is not provided. Heat is lost from the skin and from the area open for surgery. When tissues that are not covered with skin are exposed to the air, heat loss is greater than normal. The client should be kept as warm as possible to minimize heat loss without causing vasodilatation, which may cause more bleeding. Most operating rooms have a cabinet that warms blankets, and unless the surgical procedure requires cooling, the nurse should offer the client a blanket immediately on transfer to the operating room bed. Some surgery centers allow the client to wear booties or socks during the operation to provide as much comfort as possible. The intraoperative nurse reports the lowest core body temperature to the postoperative nurse when transferring the client after surgery. Thermal blankets can also be used; these blow warm air over the client's body during the procedure. IV solutions can be warmed to assist in maintaining a warm body temperature during the operative procedure as well.

Certain operations require a hypothermic client. Cooling of the body reduces the metabolic rate, which protects the brain and other organs during the surgical procedures. Constant monitoring of the core body temperature is needed, and the nurse assists the anesthesia provider in this activity.

At other times a warm operating room is needed. A warm room is preferred for surgery for large body burns, for replantation, or for surgery in infants. Because of immature internal regulation controls, the infant's body temperature quickly equilibrates with the room temperature. Thus room temperatures can be in the 90s. Hyperthermia can be a problem for the surgical team member who has adapted to the cool temperatures over time. If weakness, faintness, or nausea develops, the team member must leave the room at once.

Emergencies. The perioperative nurse must be alert for potential emergencies. When these occur, knowledge, instant decision making, and critical thinking are essential, as is speed in performing needed skills. Although almost any imaginable emergency can occur during an operation, the most common are malignant hyperthermia, cardiac or respiratory arrest, uncontrollable hemorrhage, and drug or allergic reactions.

Malignant Hyperthermia. Malignant hyperthermia is a genetic disorder characterized by uncontrolled skeletal muscle contraction leading to potentially fatal hyperthermia. It occurs in predisposed clients when they receive a combination of succinylcholine and inhalation agents (especially halothane). Unless the triggering event is stopped and the body is cooled, death can result. This condition can occur within 30 minutes of anesthesia induction or several hours after surgery. The initial manifestation is increased end-tidal carbon dioxide, masseter (jaw) muscle rigidity, cardiac dysrhythmias, and a hypermetabolic state. The client's fever can rise to as high as 109° F (43° C).

Everyone in the operating room must know the protocol for treatment of malignant hyperthermia. Medications for the emergency treatment of malignant hyperthermia is on a cart that should be near or in the operating room suite. Nurses must know where the cart is and the procedure to follow if this event occurs. Dantrolene, a skeletal muscle relaxant, is used to decrease skeletal muscle rigidity. The nurse must know how to reconstitute this drug, supplied as a powder, and must be capable of assisting the surgeon or anesthesia personnel with its administration and with any other treatments needed to save the client's life.

There is a screening test for malignant hyperthermia. A muscle biopsy specimen must be taken from the vas-

tus lateralis or abdominal rectus muscle and sent to a malignant hyperthermia laboratory for testing. This test is expensive and painful. A diagnosis of malignant hyperthermia can be made if there is any personal or family history of anesthesia problems. High-risk clients or those with a history of malignant hyperthermia can successfully undergo surgery if the condition is known. The triggering drugs and conditions are carefully removed from the client care plan, and all members of the surgical team are made aware of the potential problem.

Cardiac and Respiratory Arrest. Although rare, cardiac or respiratory arrest can occur in the operating room, and the same emergency procedures should be carried out as elsewhere. A code blue status may not be called when a client is in the operating room because the key people (physician, anesthetist, nurse) are already present. The crash cart should be in the operating room suite, and everyone should know where it is kept. The nurse manager and any key people need to be notified immediately if cardiac or respiratory arrest occurs. In the case of death in the operating room, it is the surgeon's duty to talk to the family.

Allergic Reactions. Ideally, allergic reactions should not occur if an adequate history is taken; However, some clients do not recall an allergy; in other cases, the allergy is identified only with the occurrence of a second allergic reaction to the triggering agent during surgery. For example, latex allergies are becoming more frequent, and every client should be asked about latex sensitivity or allergy. Clients who are allergic to latex can successfully undergo surgery with latex-free equipment. In many surgery centers, latex-free carts are available for such situations.

Documenting Intraoperative Care

The intraoperative nurse documents every event and action in the operating room. Information concerning any drains, tubes, or other devices remaining in the client on completion of the surgical procedure, as well as the type of closure and dressing used, is given to the postoperative care nurse on transfer.

Moving and Transporting the Client

On completion of the operation, a member of the surgical team wipes off any excess blood, skin preparation, and debris from the client's skin and puts a clean gown and blanket on the client. There should always be enough personnel for moving or transferring a client postoperatively to prevent injuries. Avoid rapid movements when changing the client's position because this can predispose the development of hypotension. In particular, move the client gradually from whatever surgical position was used onto the transportation cart. During emergence (revival) from anesthesia, the client is prone to nausea, confusion, and hypotension. Care must be taken not to catch, kink, or dislodge IV or catheter tubing, drains or other equipment during the transfer. During transfer to the bed or stretcher, the client's modesty must be maintained. Avoid rough handling, which may damage fragile skin.

After being placed on the stretcher, the client is covered with warm blankets and secured with a safety belt. Make sure that the side rails of the stretcher are up to ensure the client's safety in case he or she becomes agitated during transport from the operating room. The anesthesia care provider, as well as another member of the operating room professional staff, and sometimes the surgeon or the assistant, should accompany the client to the postoperative care unit.

In some hospitals, certain clients are transferred directly from the operating room to the intensive care unit (ICU) for continued specialized care and constant nursing supervision. Possible candidates for immediate transfer to the ICU include the following:

- Clients at risk of severe complications who remain unstable for a long time after completion of the procedure and who will probably have a complicated postoperative course
- Clients who have undergone major surgery (e.g., resection of aortic aneurysm, open heart surgery, kidney transplantation)
- Clients who have suffered a cardiac or respiratory arrest during or immediately following surgery
- Clients who came to surgery from the ICU and will return there

Family members should always be notified of the client's status and where the client will go immediately after surgery. The surgeon usually discusses the surgical procedure, outcomes, and postoperative course with family members.

POSTOPERATIVE PERIOD

The postoperative period of surgery is the third and final stage of the perioperative period. Nursing care continues to be a critical element in returning the client to an optimal level of functioning. The postoperative period can be divided into three phases:

- The initial period of time for recovery from anesthesia, during which the client is monitored closely by post-anesthesia nurses
- The time from discharge from the post-anesthesia care unit (PACU) to the first day or so after surgery while the client is recovering from the effects of the surgery and is beginning to eat and ambulate
- The postoperative phase, the time of healing, which may last for weeks, months, or even years after surgery

There is certainly an overlap of these phases, but in the following discussion they are dealt with separately.

> **BOX 16-6** *Equipment Used in the Post-Anesthesia Care Unit (PACU)*
>
> The PACU nurse prepares and checks the function of the following equipment:
>
> - Sphygmomanometer or automatic blood pressure monitor
> - Pulse oximeter—a noninvasive device that measures oxygen saturation of arterial blood and the pulse rate; provides warning of hypoxemia
> - Stethoscope—to auscultate breath sounds and blood pressure
> - Cardiac monitor and electrodes
> - Intravenous equipment (e.g., insertion equipment, fluids, tubing, infusion pumps)
> - Suction equipment (e.g., catheters, sterile saline, sterile gloves)
> - Supplies to support respiration (e.g., artificial airways, oxygen, tongue depressors, oxygen tubing with masks and cannulas, intubation equipment, and anesthesia machine)
> - Medications (e.g., narcotics, narcotic antagonists, hypnotics, antihypertensives, neuromuscular blocking agents)
> - Emesis basin, mouth wipes, urinals, bedpans
> - Thermometers—oral, rectal, and tympanic membrane types
> - Warmed blankets or electric warming units to maintain body temperature
> - Emergency cart containing appropriate equipment and medications—drugs including cardiotonics, vasotonics, and respiratory agents; a tracheostomy tray; endotracheal tubes; a defibrillator; a cutdown tray; a ventilator; gastric suction equipment; and chest tube insertion equipment

---

Post-Anesthesia Care Unit Nursing

The goal of post-anesthesia nursing is to assist an uncomplicated return to safe physiologic function after an anesthetic procedure by providing safe, knowledgeable, individualized nursing care for clients and their family members in the immediate post-anesthesia phase. The immediate post-anesthesia period is a critical time for the client. Close and constant observation is essential. The client's vital physiologic functions must be supported until the effects of the anesthetic agents abate. Until then, the client is dependent and drowsy and may be unable to call for assistance. Equipment commonly used in PACU nursing care is listed in Box 16-6.

The client is received in the PACU on a bed or a stretcher, where he or she remains or is transferred to another bed or to a recovery chair. Proper positioning of a sedated, unconscious, or semiconscious client must ensure airway patency. For an unconscious adult client, extend the neck and thrust the jaw forward (Figure 16-8). The position may depend on the surgery performed. The preferred position is the lateral Sims position because side-lying allows the client's tongue to fall forward and mucus or vomitus to drain from the mouth. Regardless

FIGURE 16-8 So that the jaw can be moved forward after anesthesia, the operator's fingers are placed behind the angle of the jaw. As the jaw is moved, the tongue comes forward, opening the airway.

BOX 16-7 *Information Given to the Post-Anesthesia Care Unit Nurse by the Perioperative Team*

- Operative procedure performed
- Medical diagnosis, pertinent medical history, and daily medications
- Vital signs
- Blood loss, fluid replacements
- Urine output and presence of indwelling urinary catheters
- Anything eventful or complications during surgery
- Anesthetic agents, narcotics, neuromuscular blocking agents, or antibiotics
- Drains inserted and their locations and purpose
- Physician orders to be carried out immediately

of the position used, carefully monitor the client's respiratory status. Suction equipment must be ready to suction vomit or oral secretions.

After the client has been positioned safely and has been determined to be stable, the nurse receives a verbal, detailed report of events from members of the operating room team (Box 16-7). The PACU nurse reviews the client's record with the anesthesia provider present, noting specifically (1) the anesthesia record for IV medications and blood received during surgery; (2) any unanticipated complications; (3) significant preoperative findings; (4) presence of tubes, drains, and types of wound closure; and (5) the length of time the client was in surgery. Ideally, a preoperative nursing assessment and nursing history are available in the record for comparison with the postoperative assessment.

Immediate Assessments

After the transfer report from the operating room, the PACU nurse performs an assessment. The ABCs (airway, breathing, and circulation) are critical and must be assessed first. Included in the assessment are the following:

Airway: Patency; presence of tubes and respiratory assistance devices.

Breathing: Respiration rate and depth; presence of bilateral breath sounds, stridor, wheezes, hoarseness, or decreased breath sounds. Stay at the bedside until the client's gag reflex returns.

Circulation: Pulse, blood pressure, skin color, pulse oximeter, ECG tracing if attached, wound status and dressings (this may include checking underneath the client's body for oozing or frank bleeding). A slight increase in a client's heart rate after surgery, as the result of stress response, may be normal. A cardiac monitor is also recommended

for postoperative clients who have been under general anesthesia so that heart rhythm abnormalities can be diagnosed and treatment can be started immediately. Causes of postoperative cardiac dysrhythmias include hypovolemia, pain, electrolyte imbalances, hypoxemia, and acidosis. When dysrhythmias develop, the PACU nurse follows facility protocols if the disturbances are life threatening and monitors the client's blood pressure, oxygen saturation, and ventilation.

Other: Level of consciousness, muscle strength, ability to follow commands, IV infusions, dressings, drains, and special equipment, tubes, and drains that must be immediately attached to containers or suction, reddened or bruised areas on skin unrelated to surgery (inspect pressure points and tape and skin preparation sites; look for signs of cautery or thermal burns), temperature (assist the client to regain normal core body temperature or anticipate complications).

After receiving the admission report and reviewing the client's record, the PACU nurse documents all observations. Most PACUs use a flow-type method of charting, which includes a numerical rating scale measuring clients' respirations, level of consciousness, ability to move, body temperature or skin color, and blood pressure (Figure 16-9). As the client recovers from the anesthesia, the rating improves to a top score of 10.

Nursing Diagnoses

Nursing diagnoses most common during this period of care are *Risk for Injury, Hypothermia, Risk for Aspiration, Acute Pain,* and *Disturbed Thought Processes.* Most common potential complications are respiratory problems, hypovolemia or hypervolemia, hemorrhage, and cardiac problems.

Patient Identification (Stamp)

NAME

REG. NO.

LOCATION

DATE

NHS NEBRASKA HEALTH SYSTEM
CLARKSON HOSPITAL • UNIVERSITY HOSPITAL
A Partner with University of Nebraska Medical Center

NURSING NOTES:

Nurse Signatures	Nurse Initials

ALDRETE SCORE▲		Baseline		Post Recovery
	Time			
ACTIVITY				
Able to move four extremities voluntarily or on command. 2				
Able to move two extremities voluntarily or on command. 1				
Unable to move extremities voluntarily or on command. 0				
RESPIRATION				
Able to deep breathe and cough freely. 2				
Dyspnea or limited breathing. 1				
Apneic. 0				
CIRCULATION				
Baseline BP ...._____				
Systolic BP +/- 20% of preanesthetic level. 2				
Systolic BP +/- 20-49% of preanesthetic level. 1				
Systolic BP +/- 50% of preanesthetic level. 0				
CONSCIOUSNESS				
Fully awake. 2				
Arousable on calling. 1				
Unresponsive. 0				
OXYGENATION				
Able to maintain O2 saturation > 92% on room air. 2				
Needs O2 inhalation to maintain saturation > 90%. 1				
O2 saturation < 90% even with O2 supplement. 0				
	TOTAL			

▲Aldrete, J.A. & Kroulik, D.J., *Clinical Anesthesia*, Vol. 7, Feb. 1995
and *Anesthesia & Analgesia*, Vol. 49, No. 6, 1970

Potential alteration in fluid volume and/or urinary elimination
Expected outcome: Maintains fluid levels

INTAKE

				On	Off
IV	_____		Sequential Stockings		
Oral	_____		Support hose		
_____	_____		Ice		
TOTAL:	_____				

OUTPUT

Urine _____

Drain _____

_____

TOTAL: _____

☐ See extended Outpatient Flowsheet

IV DC'd at _____

CATHETER TIP INTACT? ☐ YES ☐ NO

Narcotic Waste____ mgs of _____ #1 _____ #2 _____

Potential for Knowledge Deficit: Expected Outcome: Patient or Significant Other will Verbalize Understanding of Instructions.

DISCHARGE CRITERIA   **N/A**

☐ RX GIVEN AND EXPLAINED.   ☐
☐ VITAL SIGNS STABLE_____   ☐
☐ NAUSEA, VOMITING, DIZZINESS MINIMAL   ☐
☐ POST ANESTHESIA RECOVERY SCORE 9-10   ☐
☐ SWALLOW, COUGH AND GAG REFLEX PRESENT   ☐
☐ ABSENCE OF RESPIRATORY DISTRESS   ☐
☐ DRESSING CHECKED c̄ MINIMAL DRAINAGE   ☐
☐ RESPONSIBLE ADULT PRESENT TO ESCORT HOME   ☐
☐ ALERT AND ORIENTED   ☐
☐ PAIN CONTROLLED   ☐

Time discharged _____ per _____

Accompanied by _____

NHS-914 (6/99)

Postoperative Phone Call:

Phone Number: _____ Date: _____ Time: _____

	Yes	No	☐ message left
Drsg dry/intact	☐	☐	Unsuccessful Attempts: _____
Nausea/Vomiting	☐	☐	Spoke With: _____
Pain	☐	☐	
Swelling	☐	☐	
Fever	☐	☐	
Voiding easily	☐	☐	☐ Unable to reach, chart
Surgeon/Anes. Contacted	☐	☐	returned to MR

_____
_____
_____
_____

Completed by _____ RN

OUTPATIENT PACU FLOWSHEET   PROCEDURES TAB

FIGURE 16-9 Post-Anesthesia Care Unit (PACU) documentation. (Courtesy of the Nebraska Medical Center, Omaha, NE.)

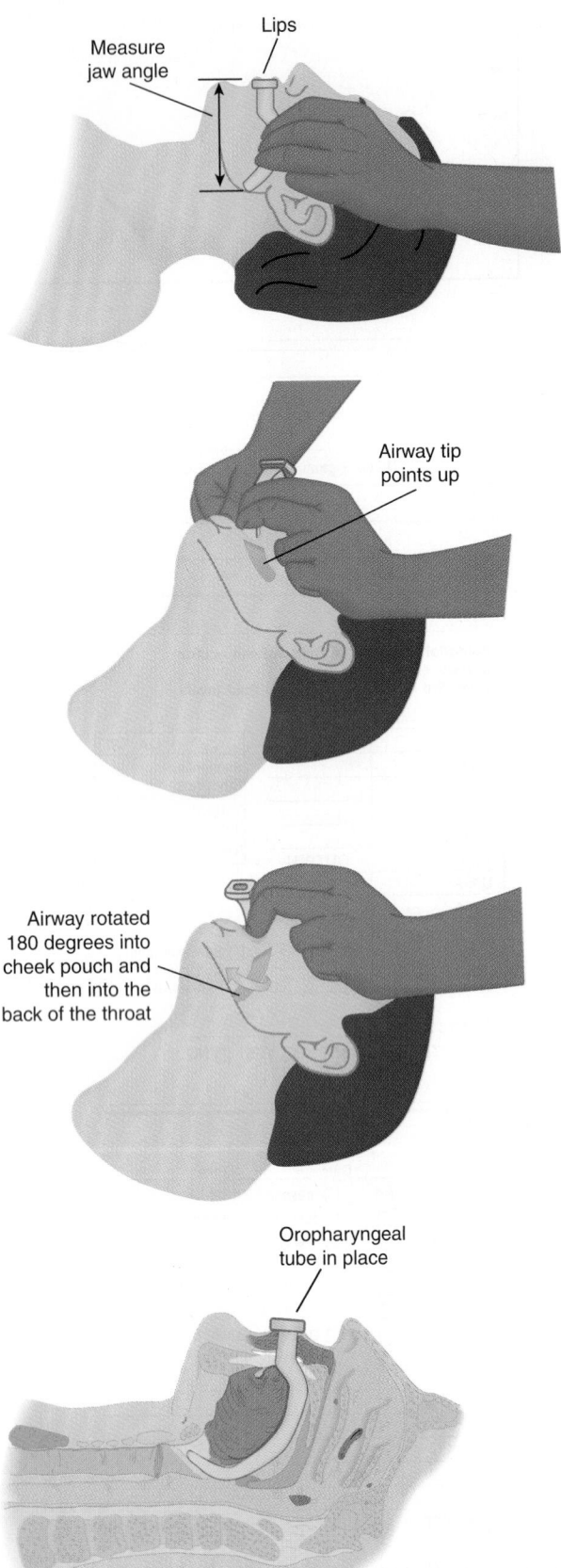

Measure jaw angle

Lips

Airway tip points up

Airway rotated 180 degrees into cheek pouch and then into the back of the throat

Oropharyngeal tube in place

FIGURE 16-10 Artificial airway. The flattened, hollow tube prevents the tongue from falling back and occluding the natural airway.

Nursing Care

Protect the Airway. One major complication that occurs in the PACU is airway obstruction or hypoventilation. The primary nursing intervention to protect the airway is to position the head of a minimally responsive client to the side with the chin extended forward to prevent respiratory obstruction. The client who is unable to clear mucus or vomitus from the throat requires suctioning immediately.

An oral or nasal airway may be in place to help maintain patency and control the tongue. The airway is a hollow rubber or plastic tube. It is inserted through the nose or mouth and passes over the base of the tongue to keep the tongue from falling back into the throat and obstructing the anatomic airway (Figure 16-10). Airways should not be taped in place. When clients awaken and the gag reflex returns, they may spit out the airway. The PACU nurse may also remove the airway for the responsive client who is unable to remove it unassisted. Left in place too long, it can irritate the tissue, stimulate vomiting, or cause laryngospasm.

When the client is extubated, observe for the development of crowing respirations. The client may be experiencing laryngospasm. If this problem develops, the client could progress to respiratory arrest. Immediately try to ventilate the client by using a face mask oxygen-delivery system, securing a tight fit over the mouth and nose. The use of positive pressure sometimes alleviates the laryngospasm. If the spasm does not abate, succinylcholine is given to paralyze the voluntary muscles temporarily, including the muscles that control respiration. Respiration must be supported by mechanical means (i.e., a ventilator) when muscle relaxants are used. Respiration in clients who have received muscle relaxants must be closely monitored for at least 1 hour after the relaxants appear to have worn off because of the possibility of paralysis recurrence. Some clients remain intubated and ventilated, such as those who have undergone open heart surgery. They require close monitoring and intermittent suctioning.

The nurse also consults with the surgeon and the anesthesia provider and administers prescribed medications as needed. Interventions may also include the continued administration of oxygen, positive-pressure airway support, and use of reversal medications. Reversal agents such as naloxone (Narcan) are administered to reverse the respiratory depression from anesthetic agents and opioids. Neostigmine with glycopyrrolate (Robinul) is given to reverse the effect of some neuromuscular blocking agents. Most clients receive oxygen. An oximeter will usually remain on the client to monitor tissue oxygenation. The flow rate of oxygen should be closely checked against physician orders. This may be administered by a respiratory therapist, but the nurse is responsible for assessment and monitoring of treatment. Oxygen levels will vary, depending on the method of delivery, such as nasal canula, simple face masks, or more controlled methods. Flow rates vary from 2 to 15 L/min with a positive pressure mask. Clients with COPD receive no more than 20%/2 L.

Maintain Normal Blood Pressure. Postoperative hypotension can have numerous causes, including inadequate ventilation, side effects of anesthetic agents or preoperative medications, rapid position change, pain, fluid or blood loss, and peripheral pooling of blood after regional anesthesia. A drop in blood pressure slightly below a client's preoperative baseline reading is common after surgery; however, a significant drop in blood pressure, accompanied by an increased heart rate, may indicate hemorrhage, circulatory failure, or fluid shifts. Do not diagnose impending hypovolemic shock on the basis of one low blood pressure reading. If you are concerned about a dropping blood pressure, measure pressure every 5 minutes for 15 minutes to determine the variability. Decreased blood pressure can also mean that the anesthesia is wearing off or that the client is experiencing severe pain.

In addition to hypotension, manifestations of shock include tachycardia; restlessness and apprehension; and cold, moist, pale, or cyanotic skin. When a client appears to be going into shock, the PACU nurse intervenes as follows: (1) administering oxygen or increasing its rate of delivery, (2) raising the client's legs above the level of the heart, (3) increasing the rate of IV fluids (unless contraindicated because of fluid excretion problems), (4) notifying the anesthesia provider and the surgeon, (5) providing medications as ordered, and (6) continuing to assess the client and response to interventions.

Hypertension may also develop. Older adults with a history of hypertension may exhibit hypertensive episodes after the stress of surgery. If the blood pressure rises above the baseline, the PACU nurse should consult with the anesthesia provider or the surgeon and administer antihypertensive medication as ordered.

Monitor for Return of Consciousness. The PACU nurse monitors the level of consciousness. Orientation to person is the first cognitive response to return after anesthesia. Level of orientation is assessed by noting whether the client responds to his or her name. Be certain that a client who normally wears hearing aids has them in place and turned on before any attempt is made to talk to the client. Orientation to place is also an important indication of postoperative return of cognitive function. Because of confusion from anesthesia and analgesia medications, the client is usually not oriented to time until after the nurse provides this information. Assessment of returning cognitive functioning includes the ability to remember facts after being told. Older adults and clients with liver or kidney impairment may take longer to regain orientation.

Postoperative delirium may occur with some procedures, such as open heart surgery; therefore do not assume that aberrations are due to age-related "senility." Rather, check the present cognitive status against that noted in the preoperative assessment to gain a truer picture of the client's level of consciousness and cognition.

Assess for Return of Sensation and Motion. In the PACU, the client is monitored carefully for return of sensation as the anesthetic agent wears off. Check return of motion to the extremities by asking clients to wiggle their toes; however, the ability to move the toes will be delayed if client had spinal anesthesia. In such cases, the toe movement signifies that the motor blockade is wearing off, but blockade of the autonomic nervous system may still be present. Clients who are still experiencing autonomic blockade are prone to hypotension despite the presence of ability to move their toes and extremities.

Assess for Normothermia. The client in the PACU is monitored for temperature and vital signs every 15 minutes until vital signs are stable or more often if they are unstable. The frequency of monitoring and length of time over which monitoring must be done are dictated by facility PACU policy. Clients are monitored until they are discharged from the PACU, usually at least 1 hour. Clients must have a minimum temperature greater than 96.8° F (36° C) before they are discharged from the PACU. The heat loss that occurs in the operating room can continue in the PACU if the client is not warmed sufficiently. Warming requires the maintenance of temperature without overwarming and causing excessive vasodilatation, which can cause fluid shifts and a decrease in blood pressure. The PACU nurse must also realize that malignant hyperthermia can also occur in the PACU and should repeatedly assess for manifestations of this condition.

Assess Perfusion. Assessment of skin color, warmth, and turgor provides evidence of tissue perfusion. Verify skin color in clients with dark or brown skin with another nurse to avoid making incorrect assumptions. Dusky, pale, cold, moist skin is an important assessment finding that may be a manifestation of shock. Because it is not possible to detect systemic conditions by skin color alone, assessment should include other pertinent data. For example, when impending shock is suspected, check the client's blood pressure, and inspect the lips and nails as well as the skin to detect pallor or cyanosis. Consider these findings in relation to oxygen saturation and hemoglobin before assuming a diagnosis of shock.

Assess the Surgical Site. The dressing over the surgical incision must be checked frequently. If it is soiled, note the color, type, and amount of drainage. Reinforce the dressing, but do not change it or open it without a physician's order. If seepage is noted, an outline of the fluid on the dressing is drawn and the date and time noted. If oozing continues, the estimation of the amount can be more easily determined by areas outside the previously marked borders. Sometimes bleeding is present but not visible on dressings. If bleeding is suspected, look for blood that may have leaked downward out of sight, under the operated extremity or under the back.

Promote Fluid and Electrolyte Balance. Assess intake and output hourly. Monitor all parenteral fluids to ensure that the proper amount and type of fluids are being infused. Intake can include solutions of IV fluids, medications, blood products, nutritional support, and colloid infusions. The amount of solution in the IV bottle should be checked on admission of the client to the PACU along with the rate of infusion. All types of delivery systems and lines must be considered: pumps, infusion machines, monitoring machines, IV lines, central venous lines, and arterial lines. Check the insertion sites for redness, soreness, and swelling because these may be indications of infiltration. Note medications that have been added to solutions, so that when the next dose is ready to be infused, a new bag of dilution fluid is present. This procedure ensures that there is no lapse in administration of ordered fluids or medications.

Changes in renal function and fluid and electrolyte balance may develop soon after surgery. The stress response to surgery stimulates the secretion of antidiuretic hormone and aldosterone, which cause fluid retention. Until the stress subsides, urine volume decreases regardless of fluid intake. Avoid fluid overload while maintaining the client's blood pressure, cardiac output, and urine output. If an indwelling bladder catheter is present, document the amount of output and compare it with the amount of intake via IV fluids.

Manage Drainage Systems. Drainage tubes, such as a T tube, gastric tube, urinary catheter, or wound drains must be constantly monitored. For example, urinary catheters and T tubes are unclamped and attached to gravity drainage systems. Gastric, chest, and intestinal tubes are attached to wall suction. Wound drainage systems are attached to self-contained suction devices. The PACU nurse must ensure that tubes are patent and draining freely. Check that there are no kinks in the tubes and that they are not occluded. Document the amount and characters of drainage on a regular schedule. Compare the type and amount of drainage with those expected for the surgical procedure.

Promote Comfort. Pain is an expected outcome postoperatively, and yet one of the most frequent postoperative problems is inadequate analgesic administration. You must carefully and regularly assess the client's level of pain. Pain may be caused by a factor unrelated to the surgical procedure, such as positioning that occurred during surgery. The discomfort of a full bladder can imitate abdominal pain even when appropriate doses of pain medication have been administered. The goal is to provide appropriate pain relief and/or reduction while not overmedicating. If there is any problem in making the postoperative client comfortable, call the anesthesia provider or surgeon to minimize the time the client is in pain.

Maintain Safety. Continue to be the client's advocate and to protect the client from injury that may be caused by equipment, medication, and postoperative risks. Side rails must remain in the up position to protect the client from falling out of the bed. Proper body alignment and frequent repositioning assist in maintaining circulation and relieving skin pressure. Postoperative equipment is checked to ensure that it is working properly before the client is received in the PACU. Place equipment in a safe location and electrical cords or lines out of the way so that they do not present a danger to the client or staff members.

Discharge

Common criteria for evaluating the client's readiness for discharge from the PACU are based on a general scoring system. The criteria that are scored include activity, respiration, circulation, consciousness, and skin color. A typical scoring system is shown in Box 16-8.

When the client is considered ready for discharge from the PACU, a report (via telephone or verbal) must be relayed to the receiving unit. The report must include the client's condition along with a summary of details of the operative procedure and events that may affect client care. Thorough documentation of the client's progress in the PACU is included in the client's permanent medical record and is an important source of information for use in providing appropriate care. If for some reason the client is to have an extended stay in the PACU, notify the family immediately, and explain the reasons for the prolonged stay.

BOX 16-8   *Criteria for Discharge from the Post-Anesthesia Care Unit (PACU)*

The vital signs must be stable or at near-preoperative levels. Each numbered entity is scored from 0 to 3. A score of 9 or 10 usually indicates that the client is ready for transfer out of the PACU.

1. There is only moderate or light drainage from any operative site.
2. All essential postoperative care has been completed.
3. Urine output is at least 0.5 ml/kg/hr for an adult.

"Same-day surgery" clients cannot be discharged until they are able to tolerate fluids by mouth, can ambulate with a steady gait and no orthostatic hypotension, and have voided. A responsible adult must accompany the client being discharged from the ambulatory care center. Taxicabs are not an appropriate means of transportation after a surgical procedure. Discharge instructions include written and oral information. It is best if this information is reviewed both preoperatively and postoperatively. The instructions usually include information about medications, how to care for the surgical wound, the amount and type of activity that is appropriate, when and how to seek help for any problems that may arise, and when and where follow-up appointments are scheduled. The client who has had a same-day procedure is telephoned by a RN the day after surgery to ensure that there are no complications or further questions.

Postoperative Nursing Care

After the client has been released from the PACU, the nursing assessments and interventions are similar to those performed in the PACU. The most common immediate postoperative complications are those related to spinal anesthesia and those affecting the respiratory, cardiovascular, and renal systems and fluid and electrolyte balance.

Establish Postoperative Goals

At this point, the postoperative care plan is expanded and revised. The plan should include an assessment of the client's needs and goals as well as nursing interventions. Nursing diagnoses are used to specify and define postoperative problems and to guide the plan of nursing care. Findings on the preoperative assessment constitute an important body of information at this time because the findings can be used as baseline values for comparison with those obtained in postoperative assessments. A general nursing care plan is prepared (see the Management and Delegation feature on Postoperative Care: Vital Signs on p. 306). Specific assessment and care measures are often based on the surgical procedure performed and the preoperative condition of the client.

Assess the Postoperative Client

Assess Respiratory Status. Assess for a patent airway. Observe the client and assess the breathing pattern at rest. Listen to sounds; breath respirations should be unlabored and quiet. As a result of the effects of general anesthetic agents and opioids, respiratory drive and depth may be reduced, leading to hypoxia. Clinical manifestations of hypoxia include confusion, restlessness, pale skin, pulse oximetry readings below 90%, and cool skin temperature. Although restlessness is an early man-

ifestation of hypoxia, there may be other causes such as pain. Cyanosis and finally respiratory arrest are very late manifestations of hypoxia.

Major complications following surgery are decreased lung expansion, atelectasis (collapse of alveolar sacs), or aspiration of retained secretions. Lung assessment should include auscultation in all lobes as well as assessment of rate and rhythm of respirations. Breathing assistance technology, such as incentive spirometry, that was demonstrated and practiced preoperatively should be used to increase lung expansion and keep alveoli open (Figure 16-11). A body temperature greater than 100° F (37.7 C) in the first 24 hours after surgery is frequently caused by atelectasis.

Assess Circulation. Assess vital signs, skin color, and temperature according to facility protocols. Vital signs are assessed frequently (e.g., every 30 minutes). Reassure the client that this pattern of assessment is a matter of routine and does not indicate anything is wrong. Because the client has been immobile during the operation and may have experienced pressure on body parts that diminished circulation, extremities must be evaluated for weakness, circulation, and numbness. Bony prominences should be assessed for deep tissue injuries, which look like bruises (see Chapter 51). Although all clients must be encouraged to get out of bed and walk as soon as possible after surgery to prevent the formation of thrombus

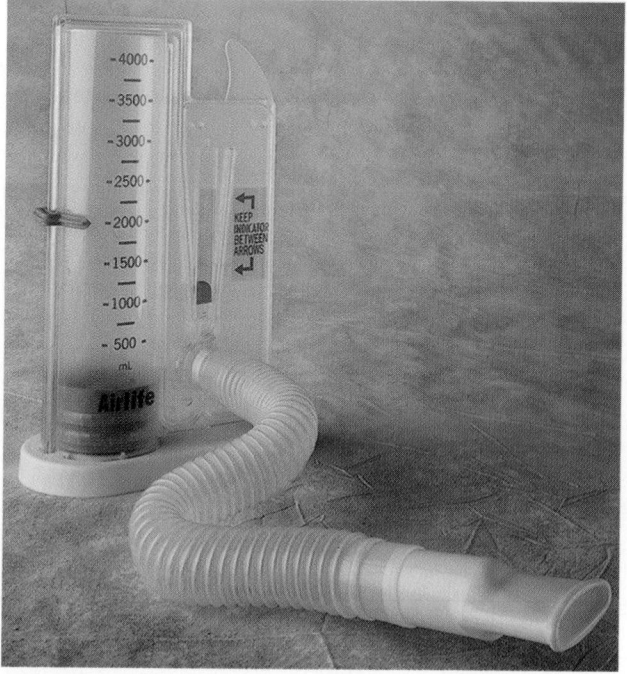

FIGURE 16-11 Use of an incentive deep-breathing exerciser promotes alveolar inflation, restores and maintains lung capacity, and strengthens the respiratory muscles. (Courtesy of Baxter Healthcare Corporation, Round Lake, IL.)

MANAGEMENT AND DELEGATION

Postoperative Care: Vital Signs

Delegation in consideration of measuring and recording vital signs and other client data is described in Chapter 4. The postoperative client requires special consideration with regard to delegation. Following your initial postoperative assessment you may determine that it is appropriate to delegate the measurement and recording of vital signs, urine output, drain or tube output, and the observation of surgical dressings to an unlicensed assistant.

In so doing, reassure the client that the frequency of observation and measurement by the unlicensed assistant is within normal parameters for their condition. Instruct your assistant as to the frequency with which the vital signs and observations are to occur. Review the vital sign measurements necessitating immediate notification to you. Reinforce the importance of timely measurement, recording and notification with your assistant.

Care of this client includes monitoring and observation of surgical dressings, drain tubes, and urine output. Instruct your assistant as to the location of any dressings and drains. Ensure the drains are appropriately secured and labeled and that the labels correlate with the output record or flow sheet before delegation of monitoring and recording drain output. Note the presence of any drainage on a new surgical dressing. Outlining the drainage with a waterproof marker at the time of your assessment establishes a baseline for comparison and progressive monitoring. The presence of drainage on a previously clean dressing is immediately reportable to you and bears further assessment and intervention. Ascertaining whether drainage may be expected is helpful information for you to have at the outset of the postoperative period.

Your knowledge of the type of surgical closure and the presence of a drain or packing below the dressing will allow you to anticipate whether drainage is expected. Your assessment should include a description of the quantity and quality of drain output or drainage on the surgical dressing. You may then delegate the continued observation of the drain or dressing to your assistant with explicit instructions that they alert you to any changes in the color, amount, or other characteristics of the drainage.

Urine output is closely monitored for 24 to 72 hours after surgery. The quantity and color of your client's urine are important indicators of their fluid and hydration status. In clients with normal renal function an average of 0.5 ml/kg/hr is desirable. Instruct the assistant as to the frequency with which urine is to be measured and recorded. Discuss your baseline assessment of urine color, quantity, and clarity. Instruct your non-catheterized

clients to collect their urine each time they void to allow measurement and observation. The assistant is to notify you of any changes from your baseline findings or a decrease in expected urine quantity.

Comfort and relief from pain are important considerations for your postoperative client. Your institution will have specific guidelines for the assessment and management of postsurgical pain. Unlicensed assistants may help in surveillance for adequacy of pain relief and/or reduction. Instruct your assistant to incorporate questions about pain at the time other vital signs are measured. They can then relay this information to you so that you can provide further assessment and intervene to ensure that the client is achieving adequate pain relief and/or reduction. Your assistant may also provide comfort measures for the client such as a back rub or turning and positioning to further promote pain relief and/or reduction.

Coughing, deep breathing, incisional splinting, and incentive spirometry are essential to minimize respiratory complications in the postoperative period. Following your respiratory assessment and initial client instruction in the proper use of the incentive spirometer with incisional splinting, your assistant may provide encouragement and reinforce proper use of the incentive spirometer with the client. Unlicensed assistants may not provide client teaching that remains your responsibility. Assistants may reinforce instruction and provide functional assistance to your client in this situation. Instruct your assistant to note the client's effort and frequency of spirometer use on the daily record or flow sheet. The client's responses to spirometer use (i.e., cough, sputum production, color, and consistency should be recorded). Variations from the client's baseline performance are immediately reportable to you. This includes a client's report or appearance of difficulty breathing, increased sputum production, discolored or bloody sputum, and inability to perform incentive spirometry as previously instructed or complaints of increased pain.

The unlicensed assistant is a vital extension of your eyes and ears in providing ongoing monitoring for the stable postoperative client. As a client's postoperative condition improves the frequency of observation may be reduced. In the event a postoperative client's condition deteriorates or becomes unstable, your delegation considerations change. You would assume responsibility to assess and monitor the client's condition personally, no longer delegating these tasks to your assistant. The frequency of your assessment and intervention increases and the role of the assistant becomes more supportive of your actions and less engaged in monitoring the client directly.

and devastating emboli, early ambulation is especially important after surgery of the abdominal area. The aorta and femoral arteries may have been manipulated during the procedure. In addition, the client may find that the dorsal recumbent position (as in a recliner chair) is most

comfortable because it reduces strain on the incision; however, this position slows venous return in the pelvis and can foster thrombus and pressure ulcer formation.

Thrombus can form in any blood vessel, and you should be especially alert to any complaints of extremity pain, unilateral edema, or warmth in the calf. If the thrombus dislodges and travels via the bloodstream, it can lodge anywhere in the body, producing emergency conditions that need to be treated immediately. It is obvious when a clot suddenly lodges in the lung, heart, or brain, but embolism in other body sites may be less apparent. Walking can nullify much of the threat of thrombus formation; however, most clients do not want to move after surgery. Leg exercises should have been taught preoperatively, and you should emphasize their importance in the prevention of thrombus formation to promote an optimal postsurgical outcome.

Assess Neurologic Status. Assess the client for level of consciousness, orientation, and lingering effects of anesthesia in the first 24 hours. In older adults, cognitive deficits may remain for days or even weeks after surgery. Compare present mental status with preoperative ability to define the client's neurologic status clearly. Medications are slower to clear through aging kidneys, and hypothermia and pain can also affect cognition. Clients need to know that impaired cognition is to be expected—especially older clients, in whom the fear of dementia may be marked. If they are not aware that the condition is temporary, clients may believe that during surgery they had a stroke from which they will never recover. This in turn can lead to depression with decreased coping ability. Nurses can facilitate recovery by promoting cognitive activity, repeating instructions often if needed, having patience with clients slow in recovery, and fostering hope. For every shift, changes that are noted need to be documented. If a decrease in cognition appears, notify the physician immediately. Most common is the slow, steady progress to preoperative status.

Obese clients also have a delayed return of consciousness after anesthetic procedures. Greater amounts of anesthetic agents are required for these clients. IV anesthetic agents are fat-soluble, and much of the drug dose is deposited from the blood into fatty tissue. In obesity, therefore excretion of these anesthetic agents is slower because of the increased amounts of drug retained.

Monitor the Wound. Assess the dressing and the amount and character of any drainage that is present. Be alert to the method of care that the surgeon prefers. Most surgeons prefer to do the first dressing change. Some surgeons leave the original surgical dressing intact for 24 to 48 hours. Others request that the dressing be changed as it becomes soiled. If the wound is closed and healing by first intention, dressings on the wound may be minimal, and the client may be allowed to shower after 24 hours. If the wound healing is to be by second or third intention, then it is left open to heal from the fascia to the skin, and special wound handling must occur. Measures can include wound packing, dressings, drains, ostomy bags, and so on, depending on wound size and location and drainage from the wound. Measure and record the amount of drainage every shift for comparison with earlier assessments to guide potential care plan changes (see Chapter 20).

Each client must have an individualized care plan to facilitate the most effective healing. Document the wound's appearance, drainage, and the client's reports of discomfort at least every shift. If you are in doubt about how to describe the wound, it is suggested that two nurses compare observations at each change of shift.

Although it is commonplace for nurses to look at wounds, the appearance of the surgical wound is frightening to many clients. It sometimes takes days before a client can even look at the wound. Assess the client's willingness to look at the wound. Do not force the client to look at the wound until he or she is ready. Look for subtle cues—for example, the client may continue to look away from the wound while dressings are being changed. Body image is altered in response to surgery, even surgery on internal organs. Body-image reintegration or restoration requires weeks or months to occur. Show acceptance of the client's appearance and assist the client in verbalizing feelings about the postoperative appearance and the reactions of others.

If wound infection develops, the clinical manifestations appear in the wound 3 to 4 days postoperatively. Clinical manifestations include redness beyond the incision line, edema that remains after the initial swelling, increasing pain, and increased drainage. Sometimes drainage becomes purulent or foul smelling. The client may also have fever, malaise, anorexia, and leukocytosis (increased WBC count with increased numbers of band WBCs). Notify the surgeon of any suspected wound infection. Wound cultures may be ordered to verify that organisms in the wound are sensitive to the antibiotics prescribed.

If collagen fibers are not mature enough to hold the incision closed without suture, the wound may open. An opening of a skin wound is called *dehiscence*. Wounds in which dehiscence has occurred are treated as open wounds—that is, they are kept clean, with application of packing or dressings and allowed to heal by secondary or tertiary intention (see Chapter 20).

If abdominal wounds become infected and the abdominal incision opens, the fascia or internal organs may be visible (Figure 16-12). This condition is called *evisceration* and constitutes an emergency. Return the client to bed. Do not attempt to replace the organs. Cover the wound with sterile dressings moistened with normal saline. Monitor the client's vital signs, keep the client as calm as possible, and notify the surgeon immediately for emergency surgery. In many clients, evisceration is preceded by a gush of serosanguineous drainage about 48 hours earlier. Notify the surgeon of this sudden increase in drainage, and plan to put an abdominal binder on the client's body for support.

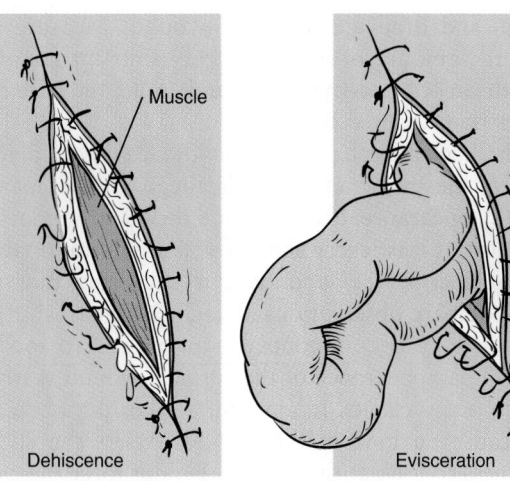

FIGURE 16-12 Clients with wound dehiscence and evisceration after surgery require immediate attention (see text).

Clients must learn to care for any dressing before discharge, so education must be a written intervention in the care plan on admission to the nursing unit. Training should proceed daily until the client or a family member feels comfortable with the wound-care skills necessary to promote healing.

Routine care of drains and dressings can be delegated to trained unlicensed assistive personnel (see the Management and Delegation feature on Postoperative Care: Dressings and Drains, below).

Monitor Intravenous Lines. All IV lines must be checked for patency, type of fluid to be infused, and rate. For any client with an IV infusion, intake and output monitoring must be completed. This is a nursing decision; although there may be a physician's routine order,

MANAGEMENT AND DELEGATION

Postoperative Care: Dressings and Drains

The assessment and care of postoperative wounds, including drain management and dressing changes, are your responsibility. The emptying, measurement, and recording of drainage from a postoperative wound may be delegated to unlicensed assistive personnel who have demonstrated competence in performing this task; the removal and application of some dressings may also be delegated to such personnel with special training and competence.

Before delegating the care of postoperative dressings and drains, consider the type of surgical procedure performed, the extent of the wound and dressing care requirements, and the nature of the drainage and type of drain present.

Drains

1. Initially, assess the quality, character, and volume of the drainage expressed via the drain. At this time, note the patency of the drain and any leakage of fluid at the drain insertion site.
2. Ensure that the drain is secured and labeled properly. Your documentation should reflect the appropriate labeling. For example, for a client having two abdominal drains (one a right upper quadrant drain and the second a midline drain) list these as such on the output record. The drains may be labeled by name or location at the time of placement by the physician.
3. Record the volume of drainage from each drain separately unless otherwise noted by the physician.
4. Perform the irrigation of any drain as ordered.
5. Specify the frequency with which the drain is to be emptied for the assistive personnel. A frequency of every 4 hours or once per shift may be delegated, whereas you may choose to perform more frequent measurement and recording of drainage as appropriate. For example, you might best perform hourly drain emptying with subsequent IV fluid replace-

ment of the volume measured, which requires an hourly adjustment in the IV infusion rate.
6. Perform the assessment for air leak at intervals throughout your shift. Chest tube drainage may be measured and recorded by assistive personnel.

Dressings

1. In many institutions, the physician changes the initial postoperative dressing.
2. Assistive personnel may perform subsequent dressing changes if the wound is closed and does not require special intervention. The physician orders the type and frequency of dressing changes.
3. Delegate the dressing change to assistive personnel after your assessment of the wound. It may also be appropriate to have the assistive personnel remove the dressing in preparation for your assessment and then reapply the dressing after you examine the wound. (*Note:* A registered nurse should assess any wound at least once per day, more frequently as guided by the type of wound and required intervention.)
4. Specify type of dressing (clean or sterile) for assistive personnel.

Describe findings immediately reportable to you for the assistive personnel, including changes in the color, character, and quantity of the drainage from a drain or around a drain site. Additionally, any sign of redness, swelling, tenderness, warmth, pain, bleeding, discharge, or separation of wound edges is reportable. The finding of new drainage or blood on a postoperative dressing is immediately reportable to you.

In summary, even though you have delegated the completion of these tasks, you remain responsible for assessment and evaluation of the client's postoperative wound and drains. Verify the competency of the assistive personnel in performing each of these tasks during orientation and annually thereafter.

none is required to monitor the client. If there have been no complications during surgery and the IV line is not needed for medication delivery, it is often capped with a "heparin lock," which allows infusions of IV medications without additional IV fluids. The heparin lock is usually maintained for potential emergency access until the client is considered stable. A heparin lock is usually more comfortable than an IV port attached to an infusion line. It also costs less and allows the client to move around and walk much more easily. Assess the insertion site for any signs of redness, swelling, or pain. If any problems are noted, the catheter may have to be removed from the vein; replacement may or may not be indicated. Application of mild heat to an insertion site that has been infiltrated with IV solution may help to decrease local pain.

Monitor Drainage Tubes. Assess drainage tubes (e.g., NG tubes) and checks the client's postoperative physician's instructions to determine whether to attach the tubes to suction or to use gravity drainage. Note the amount, color, and consistency of drainage and documents the findings. If the client has a low-suction NG tube, it must remain patent. Irrigate the tube with normal saline according to the surgeon's orders; some tubes cannot be irrigated because of the increased risk of injuring internal sutures. Make sure the tube is connected to suction if ordered.

If the tube has a dual lumen and if one side is for air, do not insert medication through the air vent. Medication can easily occlude this port. If the port gurgles, do not plug the port to quiet the system. By plugging up the air vent, the suction system becomes a closed system, thereby increasing the suction on the wall of the stomach, which can cause trauma and bleeding. NG tubes inserted for decompression and removal of intestinal secretions remain in place until peristalsis begins. The removal of an NG tube requires an order by the surgeon. Assess for bowel sounds, passage of flatus, and hunger as signs of peristalsis as long as the tube is in place. When peristalsis returns, the physician will probably order the NG tube to be clamped initially and then removed if the clamping was tolerated without nausea or vomiting.

Promote Comfort. All clients who have just had surgery will experience pain. Pain medication should be given when needed and before the pain becomes severe. When the "demand approach" (as-needed meds) is used for analgesia, it is crucial to medicate the client at the onset of the pain. When pain becomes too severe, more medication and a longer time are needed for the medication to take effect. Clients may return to the surgical unit with a PCA device for pain medication administration (Figure 16-13). Repeat instructions on how to use the device and assure the client that a "lock-out" function prevents inadvertent overdosing.

FIGURE 16-13 A patient-controlled anesthesia (PCA) device allows clients to control their own pain relief and/or reduction postoperatively. The printout allows the nurse to assess and record the amount of opioid analgesia. (Courtesy of Abbott Laboratories, Hospital Products Division, North Chicago, IL.)

Document the date and time of the medication, the amount given, and the route of administration. Also include a description of the pain the client is experiencing and the effectiveness of the pain medication in controlling it. Consider the time to onset of medication effect in determining when evaluation of pain control should be assessed. For example, reassess the client 30 minutes after oral pain medication is administered. Intravenous medications should control pain within 5 to 10 minutes. It is usually the nurse who determines whether the client is obtaining a sufficient dose of medication, whether pain is being controlled, or whether it is causing side effects such as nausea and vomiting. Communicating these details to the physician allows for a change to best suit the client's needs, leading to a positive outcome for pain relief and/or reduction. It is vital that pain be managed if the client is to comply with instructions for coughing, deep breathing, and ambulation. Chapter 22 addresses pain and pain management.

Reduce Nausea and Vomiting. Postoperative nausea and vomiting (PONV) do not occur frequently; however, the surgical experience for clients with PONV will remain uniquely unpleasant. Vomiting is a reflex, and the reflex is stimulated in many ways. Stimuli can arise from gastrointestinal tract distention on irritation, vagal stimulation, centers in the cerebrum, the chemoreceptor trigger zone (CTZ) located in the floor of the fourth ventricle in the brain, rotation or disequilibrium of the vestibular labyrinths of the ear, increased intracranial pressure, pain, or sensory perceptions (such as the sight of blood

TABLE 16-12	*Risk Factors for Postoperative Nausea and Vomiting*

Client Factors	Type of Surgery
Ambulation	Eye
Bowel obstruction/ileus	Intra-abdominal
Female gender	Intracranial
History of motion sickness	Laparoscopic
History of vomiting with	Middle ear
previous anesthetic	Testicular
procedure	**Medications**
Hypoglycemia	Anticholinesterases
Hypotension	Etomidate
Obesity	Isoflurane
Swallowed blood	Nitrous oxide?
Uncontrolled pain	Pentothal
Young age	Propofol
	Regional anesthetics above
	T5 spinal level

COMPLEMENTARY AND ALTERNATIVE THERAPY

Supplements That Should Not Be Taken During the Time of Surgery

A review of a variety of supplements has found that many of them may interact with anesthetics and/or may affect coagulation parameters. Some of the potential supplements include echinacea, ephedra, garlic, ginkgo, ginseng, kava, St. John's wort, and valerian. This list is expected to grow as more research is completed. Therefore, to be safe, clinicians should advise clients to eliminate all dietary supplements at least 2 to 3 weeks before any surgical procedure. When a client has recovered from surgery, an in-depth conversation with a health professional should be conducted to determine which supplements can be restarted.

Reference

Ang-Lee, M., Moss, J., & Yuan, C-S. (2001). Herbal medicines and perioperative care. *Journal of the American Medical Association, 286*, 208-216.

or an odor or a taste). Several medications stimulate the CTZ, including morphine, meperidine, cardiac glycosides, and amphetamines.

Risk factors are shown in Table 16-12. PONV can be prevented by reducing movement, controlling pain, and early intervention with antiemetics. Several categories of medications are used to control PONV and include (1) anticholinergics and histamine type 1 (H_1) receptor antagonists, which reduce excitability of the labyrinth receptors; (2) antidopaminergic drugs, which depress the CTZ; and (3) gastrointestinal antispasmodics, which promote forward peristaltic movement. PONV has also been controlled with acupuncture.

Discharge Instructions and Care

Regardless of the length of stay in the hospital or surgical center, when the client is ready to go home, ensure that the client and a family member as appropriate have the information and skills needed to continue a successful recovery. Teach skills over a period of days, with ample time for questions and "hands-on" practice. Give all information in writing to the client or family members. Most institutions provide a printed form filled out with specific postoperative information, such as instructions on medications and wound care, an appointment for a postoperative clinic visit, and names and telephone numbers in case there are further questions or an emergency arises. Drug prescriptions are also provided if medications are to be continued at home.

If the client has further health care needs after discharge, collaboration with other health care workers, such as those in social services, home nursing (see the Bridge to Home Health Care feature on Recovering from

Surgery on the website), or rehabilitation services is appropriate. Many resources are available in the community for clients, and most institutions have a list for the local area. Determine the resources available in your community for the clients, what each provides, and how they are contacted. A partial listing of the most common resources follows:

- Child Protection Services
- Emergency social services or hospital social services
- Emergency legal assistance
- Hospice
- Local chapters of organizations offering help (e.g., American Cancer Society, American Heart Association, American Diabetes Association)
- Local mastectomy, laryngectomy, or colostomy support groups
- Local senior citizens assistance program
- Medic Alert Foundation
- Local sexual assault center (by law, suspected sexual abuse of minors must be reported)
- Malignant Hyperthermia Hotline
- Substance abuse treatment programs or groups
- Visiting Nurse Association or home health care services

CONCLUSIONS

The nurse plays a critical role in the perioperative care of the client. Today surgery ranges from outpatient procedures to complex inpatient procedures. No matter what type of surgery is performed, however, the client needs expert nursing care. The quality of nursing care can determine whether the client has a successful perioperative experience.

THINKING CRITICALLY *evolve*

1. A young adult client in the emergency department has acute appendicitis. Surgery is scheduled in 30 minutes. What teaching should be completed before the client has the surgery? What interventions must be completed before the client is taken to the operating area? **Factors to Consider.** What important client teaching is completed before any surgery in which general anesthesia is used? Are possible complications discussed at the time? What measures usually appear on a preoperative checklist?

2. An older client has undergone major abdominal surgery under general anesthesia. At age 80 years, she is in relatively good health following a stroke about 8 years ago. Her only medication is a 325-mg aspirin tablet taken once a day. What complications are most likely in an 80-year-old client? How can these complications be prevented? How is pain tolerated by the older client? **Factors to Consider.** What complications are associated with general anesthesia? How do a thorough history and assessment help you in your plan to prevent complications after surgery? What age-related considerations must be made? Does the use of aspirin increase the risk of any complications?

Discussions for these questions can be found on the website and the CD-ROM.

BIBLIOGRAPHY

1. Anonymous. (2001). Clinical guideline for the prevention of unplanned perioperative hypothermia. *Journal of Perianesthesia Nursing, 16*(5), 305-314.
2. Association of Perioperative Nurses. (2003). *AORN standards, recommended practices, and guidelines.* (2002). Denver: Author.
3. Azhari, R. (1999). Advanced practice: perioperative clinical specialist/case manager opens doors to OR. *Nursing Spectrum (Greater Chicago/NE Illinois & NW Indiana Edition), 12*(3), 6.
4. Bailes, B.K. (2000). Perioperative care of the elderly surgical patient. *AORN Journal, 72*(2), 185-196.
5. Bailes, B.L. (2002). Clinical innovations: evidence-based practice guidelines—one way to enhance clinical practice. *AORN Journal, 75*(6), 1166-1167.
6. Balzer, M., et al. (2001). Assessment of the older female surgical patient. *Seminars in Perioperative Nursing, 10*(1), 38-42.
7. Barnes, S. (2001). Ambulatory surgery: preparing for surgery: providing the details. *Journal of Perianesthesia Nursing, 16*(1), 31-32.
8. Bergstrom, N. (2000). Review: specially designed products to prevent or heal pressure sores are more effective than standard mattresses . . . commentary on Cullum N, Deeks J, Sheldon TA et al. Beds, mattresses and cushions for pressure sore prevention and treatment. (*Cochrane Review,* latest version, 2000). Cochrane Library Oxford: Update Software. Evidence-Based Nursing.
9. Beyea, S.C. (2000). Clinical practice guidelines—an organizational effort . . . fifth of a series of articles. *AORN Journal, 71*(4), 852, 855-858.
10. Beyea, S.C. (2000). Research corner: why should perioperative RNs care about evidence-based practice? *AORN Journal, 72*(1), 109-111.
11. Bijur, P.E., et al. (2001). Reliability of the visual analog scale for measurement of acute pain. *Academic Emergency Medicine, 8*(12), 1153-1157.
12. Busen, N.H. (2001). Perioperative preparation of the adolescent surgical patient. *AORN Journal, 73*(2), 335, 337-338, 340-341.
13. Carpenito, L.J. (1999). *Nursing care plans and documentation: nursing diagnosis and collaborative problems* (3rd ed.). Philadelphia: J.B. Lippincott.
14. Collette, C.L. (2000). Clinical exemplar: understanding patients' needs is the foundation of perioperative nursing. *AORN Journal, 71*(3), 629-630.
15. Cu, A. ado Barrio, et al. (1999). The effect of a structured, individualized "nursing visit" on the anxiety of surgical patients: a randomized clinical study [in Spanish]. *Enfermeria Clinica, 9*(3), 98-104.
16. Davila, Y.R. (1999). Cultural considerations in perioperative nursing. *Seminars in Perioperative Nursing, 8*(3), 128-136.
17. Durel, Y.P., & Durel, J.B. (2000). A comprehensive review of thermoregulation and intraoperative hypothermia. *Current Reviews for Perianesthesia Nurses, 22*(5), 53-63.
18. Fortunato-Phillips, N. (2000). Malignant hyperthermia: update 2000. *Critical Care Nursing Clinics of North America, 12*(2), 199-210.
19. Harris, M.R. (2000). Searching for evidence in perioperative nursing. *Seminars in Perioperative Nursing, 9*(3), 105-114.
20. Girard, N. (2000). Care of the geriatric patient. In M.L. Phippen & M.P. Wells (Eds.), *Patient care during operative and invasive procedures* (pp. 675-695). Philadelphia: W.B. Saunders.
21. Haslego, S.S. (2002). Malignant hyperthermia: how to spot it early. *RN, 65*(7), 31-36.
22. Jones, D.A., et al. (1999). Nursing diagnoses and defining characteristics at 24 and 72 hours post-surgery with general anesthesia: preliminary results. In Rantz, M. (Ed.), *Classification of nursing diagnoses: proceedings of the thirteenth conference, North American Nursing Diagnosis Association. Celebrating the 25th anniversary of NANDA.* Glendale, Calif.: Cinahl Informational Systems.
23. Kee, C.C., and Miller, V. (1999). Perioperative care of the older adult with auditory and visual changes. *AORN Journal, 70*(6), 1011-1013, 1015-1016, 1018-1020.

24. Keller, C. (1999). The obese patient as surgical risk. *Seminars in Perioperative Nursing, 8*(3), 109-117.

25. Killen, A.R. (2002). Morality in perioperative nurses. *AORN Journal, 75*(3), 532-533, 537, 539-541.

26. Kleinbeck, S.V.M. (1999). Development of the perioperative nursing data set. *AORN Journal, 70*(1), 15-18, 21-23, 26-28.

27. Krouse, H.J., et al. (2001). Utility of video modeling as an adjunct to preoperative education. *Southern Online Journal of Nursing Research, 2*(8),14.

28. Larsen, P.D., & Martin, J.L.H. (1999). Elder care: polypharmacy and elderly patients. *AORN Journal, 69*(3), 619, 621-622, 625.

 29. Lee, S.D., et al. (2000). Clinical application of perioperative evidence-based practice. *Seminars in Perioperative Nursing, 9*(4), 188-192.

30. Leinonen, T., et al. (2001). The quality of perioperative care: development of a tool for the perceptions of patients. *Journal of Advanced Nursing, 35*(2), 294-306.

31. Martell, R. (1999). Too few nurses for post-op care of elderly patients. *Nursing Standard, 14*(10), 4.

32. Martin, J.H., & Haynes, L.C.H. (2000). Depression, delirium, and dementia in the elderly patient. *AORN Journal, 72*(2), 209-213, 216-221, 223.

33. McAuliffe, M.S., & Henry, B. (2000). Nurse anesthesia practice and research—a worldwide need. *CRNA—the Clinical Forum for Nurse Anesthetists, 11*(3), 89-98.

34. McCaffery, M. (2002). Controlling pain: teaching your patient to use a pain rating scale. *Nursing, 32*(8), 17.

35. Miller, J., & Ingram, L. (2000). Perioperative nursing and animal-assisted therapy. *AORN Journal 72*(3), 477-479, 481-483.

36. Mitchell, M. (2000). Nursing intervention for pre-operative anxiety. *Nursing Standard, 14*(37), 40-43.

37. Morrison, J.D. (2000). Evolution of the perioperative clinical nurse specialist role. *AORN Journal, 72*(2), 227-232.

38. Murphy, J.M. (1999). Preoperative considerations with herbal medicines. *AORN Journal, 69*(1), 173, 175, 177-178.

 39. Newman, B., & Lim, F.P. (2001). An evidence based approach to a perennial problem: pressure ulcers. *Contemporary Nurse, 10*(1/2), 102-109.

40. Nicoll, L.H., & Beyea, S.C. (2000). Working with staff around evidence-based practice: the next generation of research utilization. *Seminars in Perioperative Nursing, 9*(3), 133-142.

 41. Paavilainen, E., et al. (2001). Family involvement in perioperative nursing of adult patients undergoing emergency surgery. *Journal of Clinical Nursing, 10*(2), 230-237.

42. Polomano, R.C., et al. (2001). Evidence for opioid variability, part 1: a biological perspective. *Seminars in Perioperative Nursing, 10*(1), 3-16.

43. Power, H. (2000). Patients who saw an information video 1 week before colonoscopy had reduced anxiety and better knowledge immediately before the procedure . . . commentary on Luck A, Pearson S, Maddern G et al. (1999). Effects of video information on precolonoscopy anxiety and knowledge: a randomised trial. *Lancet, 11*(354), 2032-2035. *Evidence-Based Nursing 3*(3), 79.

44. Ramsbottom, L. (2001). But the patient has MRSA!! A simple infection control model for the operating suite, based on transmission. *AORN Journal, 14*(1), 28-31.

45. Renaud, K.L. (2002). Cardiovascular surgery patients' respiratory responses to morphine before extubation. *Pain Management Nursing, 3*(2), 53-60.

46. Rosenberg, H. (2001). Malignant hyperthermia in the ambulatory setting. *Seminars in Anesthesia, 20*(4), 270-274.

47. Schouchoff, B. (2002). Pressure ulcer development in the operating room. *Critical Care Nursing Quarterly, 25*(1), 76-82.

48. Schroeter, K. (1999). Ethical perception and resulting action in perioperative nurses. *AORN Journal, 69*(5), 991-995, 997-1002.

49. Schroeter, K. (2002). Ethics in perioperative practice—patient advocacy . . . second in a nine-part series. *AORN Journal, 75*(5), 941-944, 947-949.

50. Schroeter, K. (2002). Ethics in perioperative practice—principles and applications . . . first in a nine-part series. *AORN Journal, 75*(4), 818, 820-824.

 51. Schultz, A., et al. (1999). Etiology and incidence of pressure ulcers in surgical patients. *AORN Journal, 70*(3), 434, 437-440, 443-444.

52. Seifert, P.C. (2002). Ethics in perioperative practice—commitment to the patient . . . fourth in a nine-part series. *AORN Journal, 76*(1), 153-154, 156-160.

53. Spath, P. (2000). Guest column: find out what's causing unplanned admissions: research shows the reasons why. *Hospital Case Management, 8*(8), 117-118, 127-128.

 54. Steelman, V.M. (1999). Prion diseases—an evidence-based protocol for infection control. *AORN Journal, 69*(5), 945-947, 949-951, 953-954.

55. Watson, K., & Rinomhota, S. (2002). Preoperative fasting: we need a new consensus. *Nursing Times, 98*(15), 36-37.

56. Wertheim, W.A. (2000). Perioperative risk: review of two guidelines for assessing older adults. *Geriatrics, 55*(7), 61-66, 109.

Physiologic Foundations of Medical-Surgical Nursing

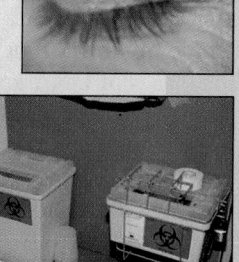

Anatomy and Physiology Review

Physiologic Genomics
Robert G. Carroll

Physiologic genomics is a field of research that links gene expression to biological function. This field studies topics such as cell replication, development, metabolic function, tissue and organ function, and whole organism function. The previous unit introduced the basics of DNA and cellular replication. This unit examines these processes in which appropriate control allows growth and repair, but disordered control is the basis for cancer. Importantly, manipulation of the human genome could allow correction of diseases at the genetic level and will likely emerge as an important therapeutic adjunct to improve the care of clients.

GENES

In humans, DNA consists of 23 pairs of chromosomes. Each chromosome contains many genes, with humans having an estimated 30,000. Only about 2% of the DNA is transcribed into the blueprint for protein synthesis, or messenger RNA (mRNA). The segment of mRNA that codes for the protein is called an *exon*. Most mRNAs are composed of many exons that are interrupted by non-coding sequences termed *introns*. The introns are then spliced out and only the exons are used for translation into proteins. About 98% of the DNA is not transcribed, and the function of these regions is not yet fully established.

CONTROL OF GENE TRANSCRIPTION

Although each cell (except reproductive cells) contains the same genome, cells appear and function differently from one another. The selective expression of only part of the genome in each cell accounts for these differences. In humans, gene transcription is complex and is controlled by a variety of factors, including cell type, chemical composition of the extracellular environment, and signals from other cells. Hormones are an example of a signaling molecule from another cell that alters the transcription of the genome in the target cell.

The genetic code for the synthesis of all proteins made by humans is contained in each cell's DNA. However, each cell expresses only a fraction of these genes.

Regulatory proteins interact with specific DNA sequences called *response elements* to alter gene expression and to determine which genes are transcribed. These regulatory proteins are called *transcription factors*, which can increase or decrease the transcription of specific genes.

DIFFERENTIATION

Stem cells are undifferentiated cells, such as those of a fertilized ovum. Under specific conditions, stem cells will differentiate into specific types of tissue. Consequently, stem cells are valuable potential building blocks for tissue repair and regeneration. During fetal development, most cells of the body undergo terminal differentiation, and cannot return to the stem cell status. Certain stem cell populations persist through fetal development and possibly into adulthood.

One characteristic of differentiated cells is that they show selective gene expression. This accounts for why a liver hepatocyte and a cardiac myocyte have such different appearance and function. Despite these differences, both the hepatocyte and the myocyte still possess the same genes.

Cancerous cells show partial loss of differentiation (dedifferentiation) and can synthesize proteins not normally produced by that tissue. For example, 2.8% of clients with oat cell carcinoma of the lung have manifestations of adrenocorticotropic hormone (ACTH) excess. In this type of cancer, the gene encoding ACTH production is inappropriately transcribed and is not subject to the normal ACTH negative feedback regulation.

FUNCTION

Ongoing DNA transcription is responsive to both endocrine signals and a changing environment. Steroid-based hormones bind to perinuclear receptors and act primarily by altering transcription. Peptide hormones generally bind to cell membrane receptors, but also exert genomic effects. Separate from this, the extracellular environment and basement membrane help regulate DNA transcription.

DNA SEQUENCING: THE HUMAN GENOME PROJECT

In June 2000, researchers announced the completion of a working draft of the human genome. This information provides a starting point for study of mutations that can cause disease. In the future, knowledge of an individual's genetic makeup may help identify individuals at risk for certain diseases as well as those individuals susceptible to drug side effects.

ABNORMAL GROWTH

Normally, cell growth and replication is regulated by a series of "checkpoint" genes. Mutations in checkpoint genes can lead to unrestricted growth, or cancer. A gene in which this type of mutation causes unrestricted growth is termed a *proto-oncogene*. If changes in expression of this gene result in cancer, the gene is then called an *oncogene*. In general, cancers are an imbalance between normal growth repression and stimulation. At the genetic level, this is caused by underexpression of genes that inhibit growth (the tumor suppressor genes) or overexpression of genes that enhance growth, or some combination of the two. Most cancers require both a genetic susceptibility and an environmental trigger to occur.

Cancer is abnormal replication of cells, in which the normal controls over cell cycling and programmed cell death have been disrupted. One characteristic of cancerous cells is an alteration in the cell membrane and the ability to adhere to both other cells and the extracellular glycoprotein matrix. Consequently, cancerous cells are more susceptible to break free from their original location and spread through the lymphatics and circulatory system to other parts of the body (metastasize).

BIBLIOGRAPHY

1. Berne, R., et al. (2004). *Physiology* (5th ed.). St. Louis: Mosby.
2. Kierszenbaum, A.L. (2002). *Histology and cell biology: An introduction to pathology.* St. Louis: Mosby.
3. Guyton, A., & Hall, J. (2001). *Textbook of medical physiology* (10th ed.). Philadelphia: W. B. Saunders.
4. Silverthorn, D. (2001). *Human physiology* (2nd ed). Saddle River, NJ: Prentice Hall.
5. Starr, C.& Taggart, R. (2004). *Biology: The unity and diversity of life* (10th ed.). Stamford, CT: Thompson Brooks/Cole Australia.

Chapter 17

Perspectives in Genetics

Mira Lessick
Lindsay Ann Middelton

---

evolve

Web Enhancements

http://evolve.elsevier.com/Black/medsurg/

Appendix A
Religious Beliefs and Practices Affecting Health Care

There is a substantial body of knowledge about genetics in nursing literature written by nurse researchers, clinicians, policy makers, and national nursing organizations. Nurses are among the few professions contributing knowledge about how clients and families are using genetic technology to improve health and quality of life.

THE GENETICS REVOLUTION AND NURSING

Revolutionary discoveries in molecular genetics that have occurred through the Human Genome Project (HGP) during the past decade are greatly influencing health care and the practice of nursing. These discoveries are bringing forth new ways of thinking about the concepts of health and disease and new approaches to the assessment, diagnosis, treatment, management, and prevention of illness. Nurses in all specialty practice areas and health care settings must become genetically literate if they are to effectively incorporate this burgeoning knowledge into client care. Not only will advances in genetics significantly impact nursing practice, but widespread integration of genetics into nursing education and research will be expected as well.

The HGP began in 1990 as an international effort to **EB** analyze the structure of human DNA and determine the location of all human genes on chromosomes. In April 2003, scientists announced completion of the sequencing of the human genome, which includes approximately 3 **EB** billion base pairs (DNA building blocks) that make up the estimated 30,000 to 35,000 genes of the human genome. The products of the HGP will benefit medicine and health care by increasing knowledge about human growth and development and understanding of the role of genes in both health and disease.

Areas of clinical practice affected by the genetics revolution include the potential application of pharmacogenomics to predict individual responsiveness to drugs, prenatal diagnosis, carrier screening for select genetic disorders, diagnostic genetic testing for adult-onset disorders, presymptomatic genetic testing, and predisposition testing for complex trait disorders. In addition, gene therapy holds promise for the future treatment of many conditions, including inherited and noninherited disorders. These advancements in genetic knowledge and technology also carry significant ethical, legal, and social implications that affect all levels of practice.

BASIC CONCEPTS OF GENES, CHROMOSOMES, AND DNA

Genes are the basic units of heredity; they comprise the blueprint that directs the development and structure of the human body. Genes also direct the many thousands of chemical processes required for cellular metabolism.

---

evolve Be sure to check out the bonus material on the Evolve website and the CD-ROM, including free self-assessment exercises.
http://evolve.elsevier.com/Black/medsurg/

Within the nucleus of every cell, it is estimated that there are between 30,000 and 35,000 genes in a person's genome, packaged on microscopic rod-like structures called *chromosomes* (Figure 17-1). Humans share 99.9% of their DNA sequence in common, and the 0.1% difference accounts for the vast variability and diversity of mankind. Each chromosome is a tightly coiled DNA (deoxyribonucleic acid) helix containing hundreds to thousands of genes. Genes can be thought of as functional segments along the helix, interspersed with noncoding DNA, much like "beads on a string." (See Box 17-1 for a glossary of genetic terms.)

Humans have 23 pairs of chromosomes. At the time of fertilization, one of each pair is inherited from the mother's ovum and the other one of the pair is inherited from the father's sperm. As demonstrated in Figure 17-2, chromosomes are arranged in a karyotype and designated by number according to their size and shape. Chromosome pairs 1 to 22 are called *autosomes,* which are present in both males and females, and the 23rd pair consists of the sex chromosomes. Females have two X chromosomes and males have an X and a Y chromosome.

Human chromosomes consist of a short and long arm separated by an area of constriction known as the *centromere*. The short arm of the chromosome is referred to as the p-arm and the long arm of the chromosome is referred to as the q-arm. For example, the designation 8q

refers to the long arm of the eighth chromosome. Chromosomes are stained to reveal alternating light and dark horizontal bands. Because the banding patterns are unique to each chromosome, the bands assist in the identification of individual chromosomes and serve as geographical landmarks for localization of genetic markers and genes. In the cytogenetics laboratory, the chromosomes are stained and analyzed for number, structure, and missing (deleted) or additional (duplicated) genetic material. By convention, the chromosomes are arranged in descending order of size, and oriented such that the short arm is on top and the long arm is on the bottom.

Just as there are maternal and paternal copies of each chromosome, there are also maternal and paternal copies of each gene. The sequence, or *spelling*, of the maternal and paternal gene pair may be identical (homozygous) or different (heterozygous). For example, an individual with blood type AB inherited the type A allele (gene copy) from one parent and the type B allele from the other parent, and thus is considered to be heterozygous for the gene pair.

DNA is made up of two long, twisted strands (see Figure 17-1), and each strand is composed of smaller chemical units called *nucleotides*. Each nucleotide, in turn, is made up of three components: a sugar, a phosphate, and a nitrogenous base. The sugar and phosphate molecules bond tightly into two strands, providing the structural backbone of DNA. The third component of the nucleotide is one of four nitrogenous bases: A (adenine), T (thymine), G (guanine), and C (cytosine). The two DNA strands line up next to each other like two sides of a zipper with the bases acting like interlocking teeth. The two sides of the zipper fit together in only one-way: A always pairs with T and G always pairs with C. The partnership of two nucleotides is referred to as a *base pair,* and the only shape that accommodates the exact matching of bases is the DNA helix. DNA must undergo replication, transcription, and translation before a functional protein is produced. Before cell division, a new DNA strand must be synthesized. To do this, the two strands separate and unwind, with each strand becoming a template for a new strand.

DNA is formed and replicated in the cell nucleus, whereas protein assembly takes place in the cytoplasm of the cell. The transportation of the genetic code from the nucleus to the cytoplasm, and the interpretation of the code involves two basic processes: transcription followed by translation. Ribonucleic acid (RNA) is the nucleic acid involved in these two processes. Although similar in structure to DNA, RNA differs in that it is comprised of only one strand, and the nitrogenous base thymine (T) is replaced by uracil (U). Transcription is the process by which RNA is synthesized from the DNA template. Genes are comprised of both coding (exons) and noncoding (introns) regions. Transcription is the process whereby the noncoding regions (introns) that are

FIGURE 17-1 From cell nucleus to DNA base pairs. (From Lea, D. [2000]. A clinician's primer in human genetics: What nurses need to know. *Nursing Clinics of North America, 35*[3], 583-614.)

BOX 17-1   *Glossary of Genetic Terms*

allele An alternate form of a gene or DNA segment. Of a gene pair, one allele is inherited from the father and the other allele from the mother. Sometimes the maternal and paternal alleles are identical (homozygous); other times they are different forms of the same gene (heterozygous).

aneuploidy An abnormal number of chromosomes in a cell; a number other than 46 chromosomes in somatic (body) cells or other than 23 chromosomes in germ cells (eggs and sperm).

autosome A single chromosome from any of 1 to 22 pairs of the chromosomes not involved in sex determination (XX or XY). A disease caused by mutation in an autosomal gene or gene pair shows *autosomal* inheritance.

chromosome Structures found in the nucleus of the cell that contain the genes. Chromosomes occur in pairs, and a normal human cell contains 46 chromosomes, 22 pairs of autosomes, and 2 sex chromosomes.

consultand The person referred for genetic counseling.

DNA sequencing Determining the exact order of the base pairs in a segment of DNA.

dominant A genetic trait expressed when a person has a gene mutation on one of a pair of chromosomes and the wild-type form of the gene on the other chromosome. A person who has a dominant gene usually expresses the trait.

familial Any trait that is more common in relatives of an affected individual than in the general population, whether the cause is genetic or environmental, or both.

first-degree relatives Parents, siblings, children.

gene A functional unit of inheritance consisting of DNA.

gene mapping Assignment of genes to specific sites on specific chromosomes.

genetic condition Variations, disorders, birth defects, or diseases that are caused or influenced by genes that may or may not be transmitted from parent to offspring.

genetic counseling A communication process that deals with the human problems associated with the occurrence, or risk of occurrence, of a genetic condition in a family. Genetic professionals help the individual or family to (1) comprehend the medical facts, (2) appreciate the way heredity contributes to the condition and appreciate the risk of recurrence in specified family members, (3) understand the alternatives for dealing with the risk of recurrence, (4) choose the course of action that is appropriate for them, and (5) make the best possible adjustment to the condition.

genetics The study of inherited variation.

genome The totality of the DNA of an organism.

genomics Translation of the sequence of the human genome into health benefits. Molecular analysis of the functioning organisms in health and disease.

heterozygote A person who has different alleles at a given location on a specific chromosome.

homozygote A person in whom the two alleles at a given location on a chromosome are the same.

Human Genome Project An international research project to map each human gene and to completely sequence human DNA.

multifactorial Describes traits or diseases that are due to the interaction of multiple genes and environmental factors.

mutation Any change in DNA that alters a gene, which can produce deformity or disease, or have a neutral or beneficial effect. Mutations occur spontaneously during cell division or may be caused by environmental influences, such as radiation or chemicals.

nucleotide One of the building blocks of DNA and RNA. A nucleotide consists of a nitrogenous base (one of four chemicals: adenine, guanine, cytosine, thymine) as well as one molecule of sugar and one molecule of phosphoric acid.

pedigree Also referred to as a *family tree;* a pictorial family history diagram that traces genetic characteristics and health conditions in a family.

predisposition Having increased susceptibility to a health condition (e.g., cancer) as determined by genetic analysis.

proband The affected family member through whom the family is ascertained.

recessive A genetic trait that is expressed only when a person has two copies of a mutant autosomal gene or a single copy of a mutant X-linked gene in the absence of another X chromosome.

second-degree relatives Grandparents, aunts, and uncles.

syndrome A characteristic pattern of anomalies, presumed to be causally related.

transcription The process by which complementary mRNA is synthesized from a DNA template.

translation The synthesis of amino acids, which then become proteins, from the mRNA template.

translocation Transfer of all or part of a chromosome to another chromosome.

wild-type The common allele of the gene; considered to be the "normal" allele.

X-linked Genes located on the X chromosome. One altered gene on an X chromosome in a male can produce disease, such as hemophilia.

An extensive glossary of genetic terms has been developed by the National Human Genome Research Institute and is available at the website http://www.genome.gov/glossary.cfm.

interspersed throughout most genes are spliced out (or removed). This process results in an mRNA (messenger RNA) transcript that is then able to move across the nuclear membrane into the cytoplasm. It is within the cellular cytoplasm that a protein is manufactured based on the sequence of mRNA.

Genes direct the production of all the body's proteins. Twenty essential amino acids assemble together in an infinite number of ways to create the larger, more complex proteins. Three nucleotides comprise a triplet, called a *codon,* for example, CCG. Each codon specifies the production of one amino acid. Proteins (polypeptides) are

FIGURE 17-2 Normal male chromosome karyotype. (Courtesy of the Clinical Cytogenetics Section, Laboratory of Pathology, National Cancer Institute, National Institutes of Health, Bethesda, MD.)

then formed, comprised of many amino acids. The four letters of this genetic code (A, T, G, and C) are used to write an infinite combination of instructions for the many thousands of proteins.

Translation is the process whereby the codon sequence of the RNA transcript is converted into a sequence of amino acids. This is accomplished by a cytoplasmic particle called the *ribosome,* which reads the code and assembles the prescribed amino acids, thereby constructing a complete polypeptide. Thus the production of complex proteins is directed, or coded, by a gene. Gene function and expression are influenced by regulatory genes located either in close vicinity to the gene or at some distant location. Examples of regulatory elements are promoters, which enhance gene expression, and repressors, which downregulate or slow gene expression.

Genes do not act alone; rather they are influenced by the genetic background of an individual and by the external or internal environment. A person's genetic constitution, or genome, is referred to as the *genotype.* How these genes express themselves as in height, hair color, body chemistry, and so on, is referred to as the *phenotype.* With this background to the structure and function of normal genes, it is possible to consider molecular pathology and how these errors relate to human disease.

In general, genes are generally stable and are passed from one generation to the next without change or alteration. However, genes occasionally change, referred to as *mutation.* Between the structural genes are long segments of noncoding DNA, the function of which is not completely understood. Within this DNA are mutations or variations in nucleotide sequence, which have no apparent impact on the structure and function of human bodies. These normal variations are relatively fre-

quent in the population and are referred to as *polymorphisms.*

Mutations can occur in the germ line (sperm and egg) cells or may occur in the somatic (body) cells after fertilization. It has been determined that 2% of the DNA is comprised of sequences that code for specific proteins, so that a change or alteration in the remaining 98% of noncoding regions often may not be detected. However, if a mutation occurs within the coding sequence of a structural gene, the final gene product, a protein, may not be formed correctly. The protein may not be produced at all, or the quantity and quality and the function may be significantly altered.

PRIMARY CATEGORIES OF GENETIC CONDITIONS

The three primary categories of genetic conditions are chromosomal, single gene (mendelian), and multifactorial (complex trait). Disorders categorized as chromosome abnormalities involve an entire chromosome or a significant portion of a chromosome, which is comprised of many genes. Conditions that are categorized as "single gene" are caused by a mutation or alteration in a single gene. This category is also referred to as mendelian, named after the Austrian monk and founding father of modern genetics, Gregor Mendel. Finally, conditions categorized as multifactorial are due to the inheritance of one or more mutant genes interacting with the environment, other genes, or other factors to produce the trait or disease.

Chromosomal Disorders

The field of cytogenetics pertains to the study of chromosomes, how they are transmitted from parents to offspring, and the mechanisms by which aberrations occur. The two main classes of chromosome anomalies are abnormal chromosome number (aneuploidy) and structural rearrangements. The usual process by which an individual possesses an abnormal chromosome number in every cell (aneuploidy) is typically due to an error occurring during meiosis. Meiotic cell division is the process by which the sperm and egg receive one half of the genetic material, or 23 chromosomes. At conception, the sperm and egg fuse to produce a fertilized egg with the restored number of 46 chromosomes.

Aneuploidy results from errors in meiotic cell division, creating a sperm or egg with too many or too few chromosomes. This abnormal chromosome number is passed on to the child at conception. One of the most common chromosome disorders in live-born infants is Down syndrome (or trisomy 21). Most individuals with Down syndrome have three copies of chromosome 21. This syndrome is characterized by typical physical features, mild to severe mental retardation, and an increased risk for other health problems including congenital heart disease and thyroid dysfunction.

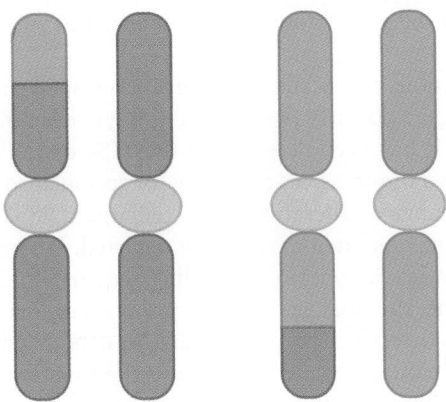

FIGURE 17-3 Reciprocal translocation.

The risk of having a child with chromosomal aneuploidy increases with maternal age. Women older than 35 years of age are offered prenatal diagnosis by amniocentesis or chorionic villus sampling to detect changes in chromosome number. For couples who have a child with a chromosomal aneuploidy, the chance of having another child with an abnormal number of chromosomes is slightly higher (0.5% to 1%) than would be expected based on the mother's age.

The second category of chromosomal errors is the structural rearrangement of one or more chromosomes. Several types of structural abnormalities are observed, but the most common abnormality involves the breaking and rearrangement of two or more chromosomes. In these situations, usually two chromosomes break somewhere along their length and the free chromosome pieces exchange places. This is referred to as a *reciprocal translocation* (Figure 17-3). If the chromosomal break occurs in a section of the DNA that does not contain a structural gene and there is no gain or loss of chromosomal material (balanced translocation), there most likely will be no impact on the health of the individual. However, when carriers of balanced translocations conceive, the embryo may receive an unbalanced amount of chromosomal material, resulting in an increased risk of miscarriage or a child with physical or mental abnormalities.

Single Gene Disorders and Patterns of Inheritance

Conditions that are categorized as "single gene" are conditions caused by a mutation or alteration in a single gene, transmitting in a mendelian pattern of inheritance. More than 8500 conditions are caused by a single gene that does not function at all or does not function as well as it should. Typically, single gene disorders are rare, occurring in 1 in 5000 to 100,000 live births. There are three primary single gene or mendelian inheritance patterns: autosomal recessive, autosomal dominant, and X-linked recessive. The term *autosomal* refers to conditions

that are caused by mutated or altered genes on one of the chromosome pairs 1 to 22 (autosomes). Genetic conditions that follow an X-linked recessive pattern of inheritance are caused by gene alterations located on the X chromosome.

Autosomal Recessive Inheritance

Cystic fibrosis (CF) is an example of a common autosomal recessive genetic disorder in the Caucasian population. The lungs and pancreas are the primary organs affected in CF. Chronic pulmonary infection resulting from thickened secretions leads to obstructive lung disease. Thick secretions in the pancreatic ducts prevent enzymes from reaching the gastrointestinal tract, thereby interrupting proper digestion.

CF is caused by the inheritance of two copies of an altered or nonfunctioning CF gene. Parents of children with cystic fibrosis are heterozygous carriers for the CF gene, meaning they have one copy of the gene mutation and one copy of the wild-type (normal) gene. Carriers of the altered gene are usually asymptomatic, with no increased risk for other health problems. With each pregnancy, however, carriers may either transmit the mutated CF gene or transmit the wild-type gene.

Each child of heterozygous parents who are carriers of an autosomal recessive condition, such as CF, have a 25% chance of inheriting two copies of the mutated gene and therefore being affected, a 50% chance of being a carrier and unaffected, and a 25% chance of neither having the disorder nor being a carrier. These risks are independent of the gender of the child; that is, males and females can be equally affected by autosomal recessive conditions. Figure 17-4 demonstrates a pedigree that is characteristic of an autosomal recessive condition in which a horizontal pattern of inheritance involving affected siblings is observed. (Refer to Figure 17-9 for a key to common pedigree symbols.)

When considering whether an individual is affected with an autosomal recessive condition, it is often helpful to know the ethnic background of the individual's parental ancestors. The carrier frequency of a few childhood-onset recessive disorders is known for particular ethnic groups. For example, approximately 7% of individuals of Ashkenazi Jewish ancestry are carriers of Tay-Sachs disease; 5% to 7% of African Americans are carriers of sickle cell disease; and 1 in 25 Caucasians of Northern European ancestry are carriers of CF. The carrier frequency of these and other conditions provides the basis for offering carrier screening of adults in their childbearing years.

It is also helpful to know whether the parents are biologically related (consanguineous). In general, parents who are biologically related have a higher chance of carrying a copy of the same recessive gene than two unrelated individuals. For example, first cousins have a 1 in

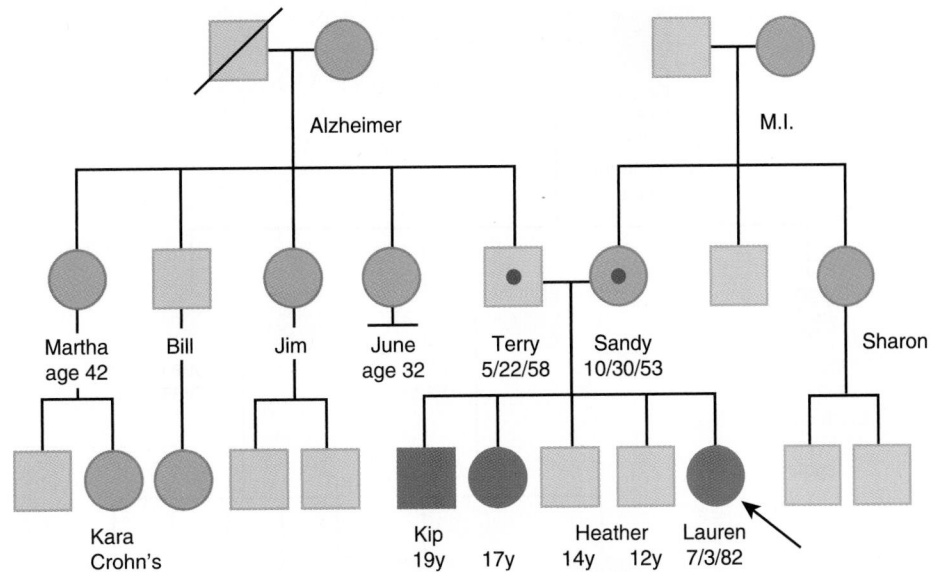

FIGURE 17-4 Autosomal recessive pedigree.

8 chance of carrying the same mutated gene and therefore have an increased risk for having a child with an autosomal recessive condition. A couple need not be related nor of a certain ethnic background to have a child affected with an autosomal recessive condition.

Autosomal Dominant Inheritance

In contrast to autosomal recessive inheritance, an individual with an autosomal dominant condition needs only to have one mutated gene to be affected. The one mutated gene of the pair dominates the other parental allele. As shown in Figure 17-5, each child of an individual who has an autosomal dominant condition has a 50% chance of inheriting the gene mutation and being affected and a 50% chance of inheriting the wild-type gene and being unaffected. Similar to autosomal recessive inheritance, gender has no bearing on whether an offspring is affected by an autosomal dominant condition; that is, males and females are equally affected.

Variable expressivity and incomplete penetrance are features observed frequently in autosomal dominant conditions. An altered or mutated gene may not always be expressed (incomplete penetrance) or, if expressed, may vary widely in different individuals (variable expressivity). An example of the application of these concepts is depicted in the pedigree of a family with neurofibromatosis (NF) (Figure 17-6). NF is an autosomal dominant disorder characterized by cutaneous and internal neurofibromas, café-au-lait spots (light brown, flat skin lesions), Lisch nodules (benign, small tumors of the iris), an increased risk of malignancy, and other less common manifestations. From analysis of this pedigree, it can be postulated that Mary must carry the NF gene, because both her father and son are affected. However,

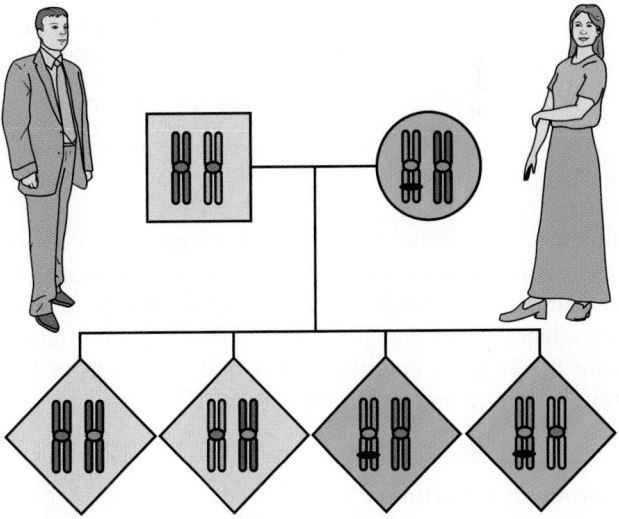

FIGURE 17-5 Autosomal dominant mating outcomes. The four possible combinations of parental chromosomes in a mating between a mother with a dominant genetic condition (highlighted symbol) and a father who has two functional copies of the dominant gene. The genetic mutation is noted by a horizontal black symbol on the affected chromosome. Gender of the offspring is not specified because either gender can be affected. (Courtesy of Betty Wolf.)

she does not demonstrate clinical features of the disorder. Therefore neurofibromatosis is considered to be nonpenetrant in Mary.

This family also demonstrates the phenomenon of variability of expression. The clinically affected members of this family all have NF, but their clinical features vary both in their severity and organs of involvement. Mary's father, Chuck, has multiple café-au-lait spots, multiple disfiguring cutaneous neurofibromas, and had ab-

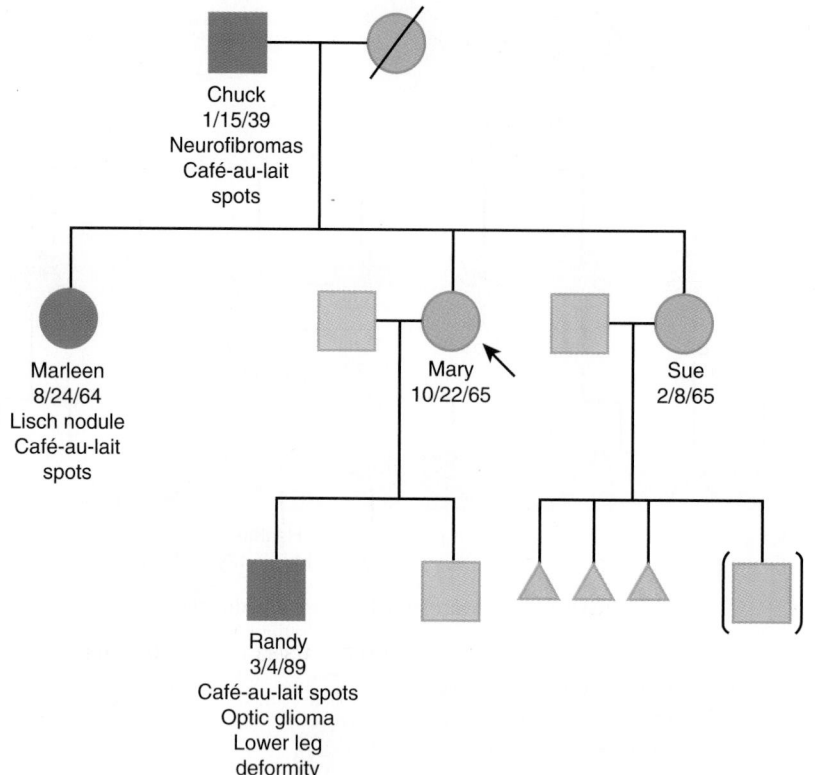

FIGURE 17-6 Neurofibromatosis pedigree. (Refer to Figure 17-9 for key to symbols.)

dominal surgery due to invasion of a large neurofibroma within the peritoneal cavity. Mary's sister, Marlene, has 15 café-au-lait spots and one Lisch nodule. Randy, Mary's son, has clinical manifestations consisting of multiple café-au-lait spots, an optic glioma, and a lower leg deformity (a less common manifestation of NF).

X-Linked Inheritance

In some cases, the gender of an individual does have relevance as to whether an individual will be affected with a particular genetic condition. For example, Duchenne muscular dystrophy (DMD) is an X-linked recessive condition with onset in early childhood and is characterized by progressive muscular weakness until death, typically in their teens. DMD preferentially affects males, because it is caused by an alteration of a gene carried on the X chromosome.

Whereas males and females have two copies of autosomes (chromosomes 1 to 22), they differ in their sex chromosomes. Females have two X chromosomes, whereas males have one X chromosome and one Y chromosome. Thus males have only one copy of each of the genes carried on the X chromosome, whereas females have two copies. A deleterious mutation in a recessive gene on the X chromosome is always expressed in males because they do not have a functional copy of the gene on a second X chromosome. An alteration in a gene on

one of the two X chromosomes in a female generally produces no manifestations, because the wild-type gene on the second X chromosome produces sufficient protein product to prevent clinical disease.

The mother of a boy affected with an X-linked recessive condition may be a carrier of the condition or the son may be affected as a result of a new mutation that occurred during the periconceptual period. A male child inherits his X chromosome only from his mother and his Y chromosome only from his father. With each pregnancy, women who are carriers of a deleterious mutation on one of their two X chromosomes face the following possible mating outcomes: each son of a woman who is a carrier of an X-linked condition has a 50% chance of inheriting the X chromosome with the gene mutation and being affected, and a 50% chance of inheriting the X chromosome with the wild-type (functional) gene and thus being free of the disease. Each daughter of a carrier female has a 50% chance of inheriting the X chromosome with the gene mutation and being an unaffected carrier, and a 50% chance of inheriting the X chromosome with the wild-type gene and being neither a carrier nor affected or at risk for having an affected son. Figure 17-7 demonstrates a pedigree that is characteristic of an X-linked recessive condition.

Because a man passes his X chromosome to his daughters, all daughters of a man affected with an X-linked genetic condition are carriers of the condition, but

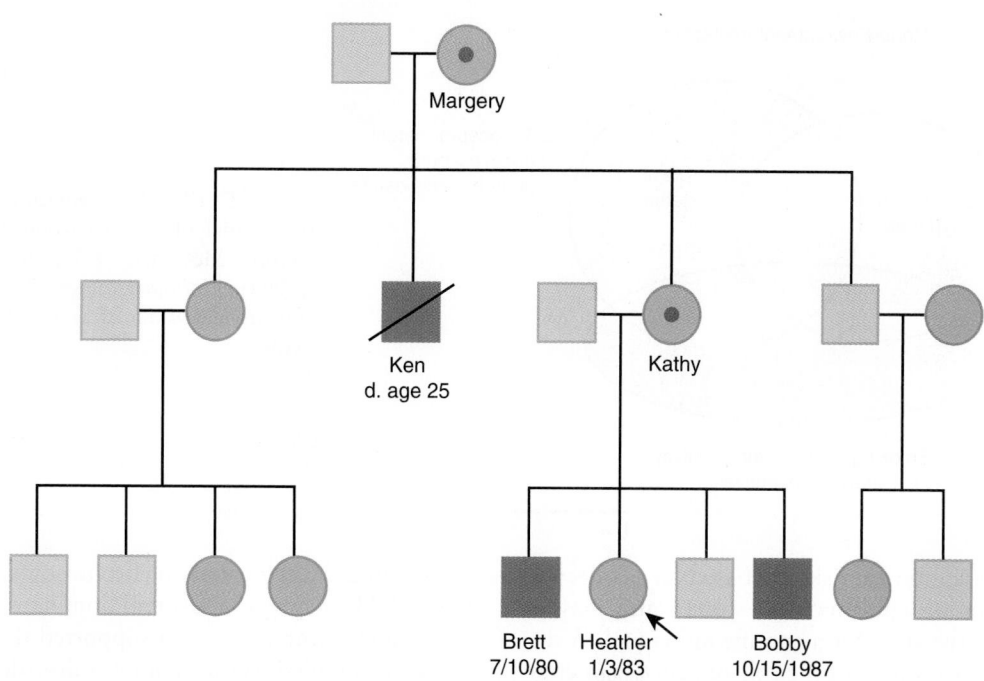

FIGURE 17-7 X-linked recessive pedigree. (Refer to Figure 17-9 for key to symbols.)

generally are unaffected. Sons who receive their father's Y chromosome are neither carriers of nor are they affected by the condition. An affected father can never pass an X-linked recessive condition to his sons.

Multifactorial (Complex Trait) Inheritance

The third category of genetic conditions is one in which disorders are attributed to an interaction between one or more genes (polygenic) or between one or more genes and environmental influences. Genes do not function in isolation, but rather in concert with other genes, and they are influenced by the surrounding environment. Most human traits, including disease, are determined by the interaction of many genes and environmental influences rather than the function of a single gene. When environmental factors and gene-gene interactions are known to influence the expression of a genetic trait or disease, the term *multifactorial* or *complex inheritance* is used.

Complex inheritance is believed to be the basis for most, if not all common diseases such as diabetes, essential hypertension, multiple sclerosis, coronary artery disease, and cancer, as well as some of the common isolated birth defects of childhood including cleft lip and cleft palate, congenital heart disease, and neural tube defects. These conditions occasionally occur in more than one member of an extended pedigree, but they do not follow clear mendelian inheritance patterns.

Every individual has genes that predispose or increase susceptibility to particular traits or disease. The presence of a predisposing gene alone may not result in the trait or disease, but confers susceptibility to that particular characteristic. The likelihood of developing a disease or having a trait increases when a person who possesses a predisposing gene also carries other genes that influence the function of that gene or provides added predisposition to that particular trait or disease. This risk is further amplified when specific environmental influences are present.

An example of the interplay between genes and environment is presented in Figure 17-8, which illustrates the multiple factors involved in coronary artery disease. An individual who carries the polygenic (multiple genes) traits of hypertension, obesity, or elevated cholesterol/ triglyceride as individual conditions may not be destined to develop coronary artery disease. However, if that person possesses a major gene mutation for defective cholesterol metabolism and leads an unhealthy lifestyle, the risk of coronary artery disease is substantially increased because of this combination of factors. Alternatively, if an individual carries a major predisposing gene to coronary artery disease but is lean, normotensive, and a nonsmoker, the predisposing genetic mutation in cholesterol metabolism may not impact the health of that individual. An understanding of the genetic and environmental contributions to the pathophysiology of a particular disease may lead to more effective prevention, earlier detection, and targeted treatment modalities of these diseases.

Risks to other family members often can be provided with confidence in single gene inheritance; however, it is more difficult to assess the risk in multifactorial conditions. Empiric risks are generally provided for conditions that are derived from complex inheritance

Gene-Environment Interaction

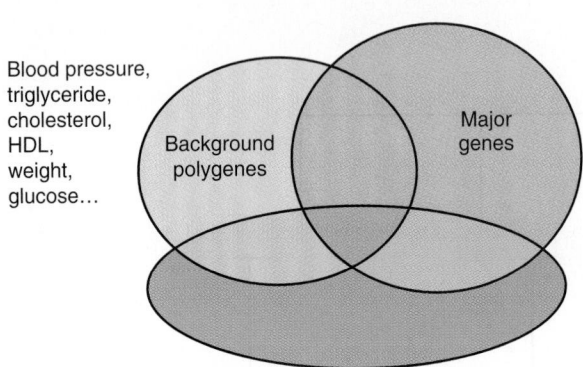

Blood pressure, triglyceride, cholesterol, HDL, weight, glucose...

LDL receptor defect, defective Apo B, type III hyperlipidemia, diabetes...

Smoking, stress, diet, inactivity, oral contraceptives...

FIGURE 17-8 Gene-environment schematic for model of gene-environment interactions. (From McCance, K.L., & Huether, S.E. [1994]. *Pathophysiology: The biologic basis for disease in adults and children.* St. Louis: Mosby.)

(multifactorial). Empirical risks are based on a collection of large population epidemiologic studies and may or may not reflect the risks for a specific individual. A discussion of three examples of the role of genetics in common diseases follows.

Alzheimer's Disease

Alzheimer's disease (AD) is a chronic neurodegenerative disorder characterized by adult-onset, slowly progressive dementia involving personality changes, memory loss, deterioration of cognitive functions with neuronal cell loss, deposition of amyloid neuritic plaques, and intraneuronal neurofibrillary tangles in the cerebral cortex. AD is the most common cause of dementia in late life; it is most commonly inherited in a multifactorial manner. The disorder can be categorized as either familial or sporadic. *Familial* AD accounts for about 25% of all cases of AD and is associated with a positive family history (multiple affected family members) and early- or late-onset disease. The *sporadic* form of AD accounts for the majority (approximately 75%) of all cases of AD, and is usually associated with a negative family history and onset of disease at any time in adulthood. Sporadic AD is considered a multifactorial condition and is thought to result from a combination of aging, genetic predisposition, and exposure to environmental agents (e.g., head trauma, viruses, toxins).

Much progress has been made during the past decade in determining the role of genetics in AD. The strongest evidence for a genetic contribution to AD is found in early-onset familial AD. This category comprises less than 5% of all cases of AD and refers to families in which multiple cases of AD occur with age of onset usually in the 40s or 50s (mean age of onset before age 65 years). Three gene mutations have been identified as a cause of early-onset familial AD, including the amyloid precursor protein (APP) gene located on chromosome 21, presenilin-1 (PS1) located on chromosome 14, and

presenilin-2 (PS2) located on chromosome 1. Early-onset familial AD displays autosomal dominant transmission.

Genetic research has also supported the concept that late-onset familial AD is a complex disorder that may involve multiple susceptibility genes. The diagnosis of this type of AD is typically made in families with multiple affected AD members, most of whom have onset of dementia after the age of 60 or 65 years. There is a well-documented association of late-onset familial AD with the e4 allele of Apolipoprotein E (APOE) located on chromosome 19. The e4 allele, by unknown mechanisms, appears to shift the age of onset curve toward an earlier age. It has been estimated that the e4 allele of APOE is a susceptibility gene for as much as one half of cases of AD in the general population.

Diabetes Mellitus

Progress is being made in understanding the molecular and genetic basis of diabetes mellitus. Diabetes has two major clinical subtypes: type 1, or insulin-dependent diabetes mellitus (IDDM), and type 2, or non–insulin-dependent diabetes mellitus (NIDDM). Both types of diabetes mellitus demonstrate multifactorial inheritance in that both genetic and environmental factors are necessary for expression.

Type 1 diabetes mellitus tends to run in families: the risk to siblings of an affected individual with type 1 diabetes mellitus or to the offspring of a diabetic father is more than 10 times the population risk. In addition, twin studies show a concordance rate of 30% to 50% in monozygotic (identical) twins with lower rates in dizygotic (fraternal) twins. Two chromosomal locations have a well-established association with type 1 diabetes mellitus. These are the HLA region, which is the major histocompatibility complex in humans located on chromosome 6, and the insulin gene located on chromosome 11. The HLA system is estimated to contribute about 40% of the familial clustering of type 1 diabetes mellitus, and inherited genetic variations in the insulin gene region contribute about 10% of the familial clustering.

Type 2 diabetes mellitus accounts for most cases (over 90%) of diabetes. Two major risk factors for this condition are positive family history and obesity; the latter increases insulin resistance, which is a feature of type 2 diabetes mellitus. In contrast to type 1 diabetes mellitus, there is no HLA association and monozygotic twin concordance rates are substantially higher (often exceeding 90%) than in type 1 diabetes mellitus. A subset of type 2 diabetes mellitus, called maturity onset diabetes of the young (MODY) can be inherited as an autosomal dominant trait. MODY accounts for approximately 2% to 5% of clients with type 2 diabetes mellitus and typically occurs before age 25 years. Studies have shown that about one half of cases of MODY are due to mutations in the glucokinase gene located on chromosome 7.

Cancer

Cancer is a common disease that occurs as a sporadic event in most cases. All cancer can be thought of as a genetic disease, because most cancers result from an accumulation of random mutations that occur over time in somatic (body) cells. In sporadic cancers, the cancer typically develops in a single cell. The cell progresses from a normal to a malignant cell through a series or sequence of mutations. Each of these mutations promotes uncontrolled cellular growth, which is the hallmark of cancer development.

Occasionally pedigrees demonstrate the presence of one or more cancers in a family, suggesting familial tendency. Familial cancer clustering can occur as a result of multiple genetic effects, shared environmental factors, culturally transmitted risk factors (e.g., ethnicity, diet), or coincidence. However, in 5% to 10% of cases, the cancer may occur as a result of inheriting, from a parent, a major gene predisposing to cancer. Inheriting a major cancer-causing gene generally does not confer a 100% risk that cancer will develop, but it may confer a significant risk that at some point in a person's lifetime, a particular cancer may develop. Having this information allows for implementation of a rigorous surveillance program that will identify cancer early, which may decrease morbidity and mortality.

Nurses should become familiar with the several clinical hallmarks associated with an inherited susceptibility to cancer as listed in Box 17-2. For example, inherited cancers often occur at a younger age than sporadic cancers, and they are often bilateral in paired organs (e.g., breasts, kidneys) and multifocal (multiple sites within a single organ). In addition, relatives in multiple generations are generally affected, revealing an autosomal dominant pattern of transmission. The nurse should look for the presence of these "red flags" to identify and

---

BOX 17-2   *Clinical "Red Flags" Suggestive of Inherited Susceptibility to Cancer*

- Early age of onset (<50 years)
- Bilateral cancer in paired organs
- Multifocality, the presence of multiple distinct tumors in one organ
- Evidence of autosomal dominant inheritance
- Cancer in two or more first- or second-degree relatives
- Multiple primary cancers in one individual
- Constellation of cancers in a client or family recognized as part of an identified cancer genetic syndrome

---

BOX 17-3   *Statement on the Scope and Standards of Genetics Clinical Nursing Practice*

The International Society of Nurses in Genetics, Inc., (ISONG) is responsible for defining and establishing the scope of professional nursing practice in genetics and identifying the characteristics of this unique specialty area. These characteristics pertain to standards of clinical care and standards of professional performance.

Genetic conditions are defined as variations, disorders, birth defects, or diseases that are caused or influenced by genes; these conditions may or may not be transmitted from parent to offspring.

Genetic nursing focuses on providing nursing care to clients who have, or are at risk for, known genetic conditions.

The scope of genetic nursing practice has two levels: basic and advanced. These levels of practice are distinguished by educational preparation, professional experience, practice focus, specific roles and functions, and credential status.

---

refer clients and their families to a cancer genetic clinic for evaluation, diagnosis, and counseling.

NURSING ROLE IN CLINICAL GENETIC CARE

The role of the nurse in providing genetic health care varies and is dependent upon several factors, including the client's health concerns, the client's needs, and the nurse's education, expertise, role and job description. In all roles, nurses practice within an ethical framework providing care that supports truth-telling, disclosure, privacy, nondiscrimination, and confidentiality. The nurse provides care that preserves and protects client autonomy, dignity, and rights (Box 17-3).

The nurse is often the first health professional to assess the client's medical history. Obtaining a personal and family health history is an essential component to a nursing health assessment, and a thorough family history is often the first clue that a familial disorder is present or may identify health problems to which the client may be multifactorially predisposed. Nurses should be able to provide a basic assessment of the client and family, construct a pedigree, identify potential genetic concerns, and provide basic genetic education. The nurse should also assess psychosocial aspects, including coping and adaptation styles, the client's support system, and the client's health beliefs and practices.

When the reproductive, family, or health histories in individuals suggest indications for referral to genetic professionals, the nurse makes appropriate referrals. The nurse ensures client comprehension of the health care plan, supports client autonomous decision-making, and provides emotional support for the client and family. Nurses practicing at the advanced practice level in genetic health care are involved in a variety of responsibilities. Advanced Practice Nurses in Genetics perform physical examinations and provide genetic counseling, including pedigree interpretation, risk assessment, and communication of genetic test results. Some nurses provide case management, refer clients to appropriate health care providers or community resources, collaborate with other health professionals, or manage home care and therapy. Advanced Practice Nurses in Genetics administer state genetic screening programs, conduct genetic research, and serve as integral staff members in genetic testing laboratories (Box 17-4).

GENETIC DISEASE AND FAMILY ASSESSMENT

An expanded three-generation family medical history, in a pedigree format, is an invaluable tool for health care providers concerned not only about the identification of health risks for individual clients, but also about the health status of the entire family. The pedigree is a pictorial description of the family structure and provides the family medical history in such a manner that can be quickly accessed by all health care providers throughout the care of a client and his or her family. In addition to identifying familial health concerns, the process of pedigree development provides an opportunity to build or enhance rapport with clients. By carefully listening to a client's response to questions about the medical history of family members, a nurse can assess the social relationship between family members and the client's health practices.

An expanded family history usually consists of health information about the client, his or her children, the client's siblings, parents, aunts, uncles, and grandparents. Documented information should include diagnosis, age at diagnosis, and age at death, if applicable. As shown in Figure 17-9, circles in the diagram represent females, squares represent males, and diamonds represent

BOX 17-4 *Advanced Practice Nurse in Genetics (APNG) and Genetics Clinical Nurse (GCN) Credentials*

The ISONG-awarded APNG and GCN credentials demonstrate evidence of competence and clinical expertise based on the Scope and Standards of Genetics Clinical Nursing Practice. It provides recognition to professional colleagues of the nurse's ability to provide genetic health care. It provides the nurse with a sense of pride in accomplishment of advanced practice knowledge and skills in genetic health care or generalist practice knowledge and skills that every qualified nurse can attain.

The APNG and GCN credentials are awarded upon successful completion of a professional portfolio that is scientifically evaluated using carefully designed rating scales based on criteria defined in the ISONG Scope & Standards of Genetics Clinical Nursing Practice.

Requirements include the following:
- Clinical Practice experience in a genetic health setting
- Education
  APNG requires a Master's in Nursing or equivalent; GCN requires a Baccalaureate in Nursing or equivalent.
- Basic, advanced, or continuing education in genetics
- Teaching of clients, families, communities, health professionals, and the public

individuals for which the gender is unknown. An arrow identifies the client who is commonly referred to as the *consultand*. An arrow may also designate the proband, the affected family member through whom the family is ascertained. Information, such as name, date of birth, medical history, and other medical problems about the various family members are noted below each symbol. A diagonal line through a symbol signifies that the represented person is deceased. A single horizontal line between two symbols represents a mating relationship. A vertical line attached to the mating line at the top and the horizontal sibship line at the bottom represents the line of descent. Symbols attached to the sibship line with an individual vertical line represent the offspring of the couple. A shaded or solid symbol represents an affected individual. In order to condense a pedigree, nonbiologically related individuals are often not displayed. For a more comprehensive discussion of pedigree development, refer to Bennett, et al. (1995). There are several purposes for constructing a pedigree that go beyond determining health risks. The construction of a pedigree assists with determining the following:
- Statistical probability of developing a disease
- Degree of familial relationship or percentage of shared DNA
- Pattern of transmission of diseases in the family

- Likelihood of a hereditary versus nonhereditary component of disease causation
- Increased risk of disease for different family members

GENETIC TESTING

Rapid advances in genetic science and technology have dramatically increased the number of available genetic tests. In every health care setting, nurses encounter genetic issues among their clients and are increasingly called upon to understand and effectively respond to concerns surrounding genetic testing for families. Accordingly, nurses have a responsibility to become knowledgeable about the basics of genetic testing and the accompanying ethical and psychosocial implications.

Genetic testing refers to the analysis of a person's DNA, chromosomes, proteins, and/or certain metabolites obtained from a sample of blood or other body tissue in order to detect changes that indicate the presence or absence of a genetic condition or a predisposition to develop one. Genetic tests are performed to (1) confirm or rule out a present condition, (2) determine whether an individual is a carrier of a genetic condition, (3) detect fetal abnormalities, and (4) predict diseases in asymptomatic individuals through presymptomatic or predisposition testing.

Screening for Carriers of Genetic Disease

The main purpose of carrier screening is the identification of individuals who are themselves healthy but carry a disease-causing gene and thus are at risk for transmitting a particular genetic condition to future offspring. Carrier screening is generally performed for autosomal recessive and X-linked recessive conditions. Examples of disorders in which carrier testing is available are Tay-Sachs disease, sickle cell disease, CF, thalassemia, and fragile X syndrome. Carrier testing is voluntary and focuses on individuals with a positive family history of a disorder and those who identify themselves as being members of a particular high-risk ethnic group (e.g., Tay-Sachs disease in the Ashkenazi Jewish population and sickle cell disease in the African-American population). Knowing one's carrier status may provide (1) relief from fear of the unknown and (2) information that could be useful in making life and family planning decisions.

Presymptomatic and Predisposition Testing

Both presymptomatic and predisposition (or susceptibility) tests are forms of predictive testing. In presymptomatic testing, individuals known to be at high risk for a genetic disorder because of family history can be tested to determine whether they have inherited a disease-causing genetic mutation before they develop clinical manifestations of the disorder. A classic example of presymptomatic testing is detection of the gene for Huntington's disease (HD), a progressive adult-onset neurologic disorder. Because the HD

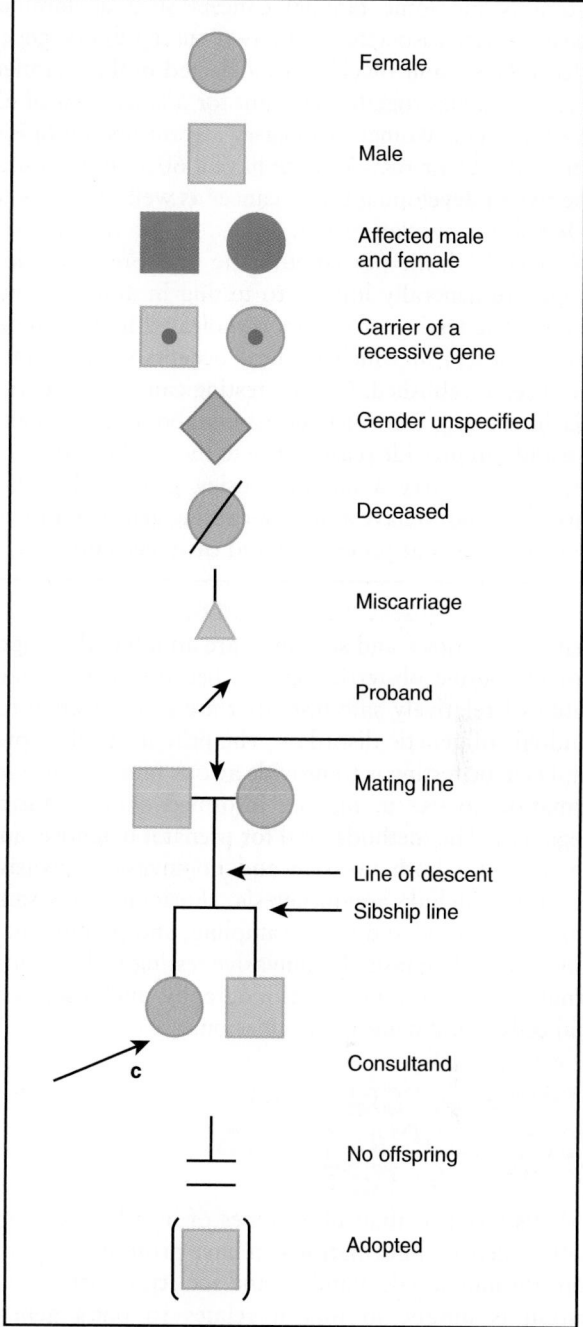

FIGURE 17-9 Commonly used pedigree symbols.

gene shows complete penetrance, a person who tests positive for the mutation has essentially a 100% chance of developing the disorder at some age.

Recent discoveries are also making it possible to test for the presence of a genetic component that contributes to the predisposition of many common diseases such as diabetes, heart disease, and cancer. Predisposition (or susceptibility) testing is used to identify a genetic mutation that makes a person more likely, but not definitely certain, to develop a disorder. For example, gene mutations for some familial cancers such as familial breast cancer, associated with two susceptibility genes called BRCA1 and BRCA2, are detected in this manner. These two genes together account for 5% to 10% of all breast cancers. Women who carry a germ line mutation in the BRCA1 or BRCA2 gene have a 60% to 90% lifetime risk of developing breast cancer as well as a 20% to 60% risk for ovarian cancer.

Currently, both presymptomatic and predisposition testing are generally limited to testing in adults. However, genetic testing of minors is indicated in certain genetic disorders in which medical benefits to the minor have been established. Genetic testing can assist individuals in making informed decisions about their health care and can provide reassurance to those who learn that they do not carry a disease-causing gene. Individuals who are found to have a disease-causing gene can pursue strategies aimed at prevention and early detection.

Prenatal Diagnosis and Screening

Prenatal diagnosis and screening are an integral component of routine obstetric practice because of the availability of relatively safe tests that are cost effective for hundreds of genetic disorders. The primary goal of prenatal genetic testing is to provide at-risk families with information to use in making informed choices during pregnancy. The methods used for prenatal diagnosis and screening are both invasive and noninvasive. Invasive techniques include amniocentesis, chorionic villus sampling, fetal blood and tissue sampling, and preimplantation genetic diagnosis. Noninvasive testing includes maternal serum screening, ultrasonography, and analysis of fetal cells in the maternal circulation.

ETHICAL, LEGAL, AND PSYCHOSOCIAL ISSUES IN GENETIC TESTING

Perhaps more so than other types of health care information, genetic information can have profound implications for individuals, families, and society. Genetic information is unique in that it relates to one's genetic identity, provides highly personal data about an individual, predicts one's future health risks, and is relevant to other family members. Issues that challenge nurses in the context of genetics and genetic testing include privacy and confidentiality, informed consent, stigmatization, potential for discrimination, and disruption of family and social relationships.

Nurses have a critical role in assuring privacy and confidentiality of genetic information obtained from such sources as family history assessments, genetic tests, and other interventions. The inadvertent loss of privacy and confidentiality with regard to genetic information can result in potential harm to clients. For example, disclosure of genetic test information to third parties, such

as insurance companies or employers, may result in higher insurance rates, cancellation or denial of insurance policies, or loss of job opportunities. Because of the potential for misuse of information, it is imperative that genetic testing centers have policies and procedures in place that protect the rights of privacy and confidentiality for clients. Clients need to know that test results will not be shared with anyone other than the person being tested, unless the person gives explicit consent to disclose such information. Both federal and state legislation aimed at providing protections against discrimination has been, and continues to be, developed.

The process of informed consent (Box 17-5) is a critical component of pretest counseling, and nurses are expected to actively participate in this process. The decision to undergo a genetic test should be an autonomous decision, made on the basis of the client's consideration of the physical, psychological, or social risks and benefits, and the person's values and beliefs. Individuals should be aware that they have a right to accept or decline testing. Nursing actions in the informed consent process may include ensuring that written consent is obtained before testing, serving as a client advocate, assisting in providing education about testing, and ensuring that the client's autonomy is protected in making testing decisions.

The possibility of stigmatization is another ethical issue associated with genetic testing. Impairment of one's self-esteem is a potential harm that may occur with testing. Little is known about the effects of genetic informa-

---

BOX 17-5 *Components of Informed Consent for Genetic Testing*

- Purpose of the test
- What can be learned from both a positive and negative test, including information on health risks associated with test results
- Possibility that test results will be ambiguous or noninformative
- Options for risk assessment without genetic testing
- Risk of transmitting a mutation to offspring
- Options for medical follow-up based on test results
- Technical accuracy of the test
- Risks of psychological distress, family disruption, and genetic discrimination following disclosure of test results
- Discussion of rules of disclosure of test results to others (family members, third parties)
- Confidentiality standards
- Risks that nonrelatedness may be discovered and policy for disclosure
- Fees associated with the genetic test as well as preventive procedures

tion upon one's view of oneself and the emotional burden of knowing about one's own genetic makeup.

Genetic testing also carries the risk of producing psychological harm. Individuals with positive genetic test results may experience a wide range of emotions, including anger, anxiety, depression, or psychological distress. In addition, the finding among family members that one is a carrier of a genetic condition and others are not can alter their relationships with each other. Family members may also have guilt feelings regardless of their genetic status. Guilt feelings for transmitting a disorder such as HD may be experienced by individuals who carry the HD gene mutation. On the other hand, individuals who have not inherited a disease-causing genetic mutation may experience feelings of survivor guilt.

Families may also develop patterns for managing disease risk in mutation carriers. An example is the pressuring of a female relative found to have a BRCA1 mutation to undergo prophylactic mastectomy. Another potential consequence of genetic testing is the discovery of misidentified paternity. This occurs when test results of both parents are inconsistent with paternity. Discussion about this possibility is an important component of the informed consent process.

FUTURE DIRECTIONS

The Genomic Era

The Genomic era continues to unfold upon completion of a comprehensive sequence of the human genome. The future holds many exciting challenges for scientists in order to translate genome-based knowledge into health benefits. Although the genome is characterized chemically, its function is not well understood. The next phase of genomics is to catalogue and comprehend the functional elements, such as the protein-coding sequences, and to understand how genes interrelate to one another through pathways. Moreover, the genome holds much variation, and how these variations impact health and illness is yet to be understood. With enhanced knowledge of genes and their pathways, development of genome-based approaches to prediction of disease susceptibility and drug response, early detection of illness, and development of powerful new therapeutic approaches to disease is envisioned.

Gene Therapy

Because of the influx of information from molecular genetic technology and the HGP, both the scientific and public communities anticipate that gene therapy will revolutionize disease treatment modalities. At the onset of the new millennium, approximately 500 clinical gene therapy trials have been conducted with approximately 3000 enrolled clients. Ninety percent of the studies relate to human immunodeficiency virus or cancer and the remainder involve rare recessive disorders. To date, only a small handful of clients have benefited from gene therapy.

Many questions need to be answered before gene therapy becomes a viable option in the treatment of disease. Will gene transfer result in adequate protein production at the correct sites? Will the transferred gene relate to or have an association with its regulatory genes or will random insertion of a transferred gene upset or negatively impact the activities of other proteins? Many scientific obstacles need to be overcome before gene therapy becomes a practical modality for treatment of disease.

Pharmacogenomics

Perhaps the most immediate and significant impact of the molecular knowledge gained in the recent past is in the field of pharmacogenomics. It has long been recognized that drugs that are safe in one individual may cause harm in another. Pharmacogenomics is the concept of individualized and rational drug selection based on the genotype of a particular client that will optimize safety and increase drug effectiveness. The science is based on genotype variations (polymorphisms) that influence an individual's response to a drug. The outcome will be customized drug therapy, that is, prescribing the right drug at the correct dose for the individual client.

A small number of metabolic pathways degrade the vast majority of drugs by means of enzymes in the liver and small intestine, and it is the family of P450 enzymes that may be responsible for degradation of a significant number of drugs. The functional differences between variants of these enzymes may, in large part, be due to genetic polymorphisms inherited as genetic traits. The allelic differences may abolish, alter, or enhance drug metabolism.

One P450 enzyme, CYP2D6 is essential in the metabolism of antidepressants and neuroleptics. The CYP2D6 genotype may be predictive as to expected side effects. Individuals who lack functional CYP2D6 genes may not be able to clear drugs well and may demonstrate adverse effects resulting from increased drug plasma levels.

Another example is CYP2C9, a member of the P450 family whose genotype may be considered for optimal warfarin therapy. The clearance of warfarin in individuals who inherit two copies of the CYP2C9 allele has been shown to be reduced by 90% compared to individuals who have the wild-type allele. The differences in these two genotypes may have significant implications in the dose and schedule of warfarin treatment.

Nurses are likely to have a significant role in the application of pharmacogenomics in client care. Nurses may need to explain to clients why certain medications are being prescribed to some but not to others with the same disease. In addition, nurses will need to educate clients about the potential benefits and limitations of genotyping and implications for therapy.

CONCLUSIONS

It is essential that nurses have a basic understanding of molecular genetics and principles of human genetics in order to function effectively in the modern health care arena. This knowledge is relevant in assisting nurses to understand the mechanisms and treatment of disease, assess genetic risk for disease, provide a scientific foundation for nursing care, and promote, retain, and restore health and wellness among clients and families.

THINKING CRITICALLY *evolve*

1. *Cancer Genetic Clinical Situation:* A 46-year-old woman is informed that she carries a mutation in the dominant familial adenomatous polyposis (FAP) gene that is responsible for her colon cancer. Her physicians ordered the gene test without pretest genetic counseling. Individuals who inherit the FAP gene mutation are predisposed to development of many hundreds of colon polyps with almost 100% risk of cancer. Onset of polyps may occur in adolescence. She inquires about genetic testing of her 17-year-old son and 10-year-old daughter.
Factors to Consider. Is genetic testing of the children appropriate? Who should make the decision to be tested? What is the nurse's role in this situation? Identify several psychosocial issues the family and adolescent might consider before deciding to have children tested. What options are available relative to the parents' concern?

2. *Huntington's Disease Clinical Situation:* A 33-year-old woman inquires about the possibility of genetic testing for Huntington's disease (HD). Her father is in advanced stages of HD, and the genetic mutation is known. HD is a chronic, progressive, neurodegenerative disease of the central nervous system with onset typically between 30 and 50 years of age. Both the client and her fiancé believe knowledge of her genotype would be helpful in their family planning.
Factors to Consider. What are some of the personal issues that may be considered by the client? What are potential ramifications to the couple's future relationship? What are the concerns if the client and her fiancé think differently about genetic testing? Is there external family pressure for the client to be tested? What is the implication to their potential offspring?

3. *Diabetes Mellitus Clinical Situation:* The client is a 24-year-old woman who has a 12-year history of type 1 diabetes mellitus. She has had a difficult time in managing her diabetes and has been hospitalized several times over the years for diabetic ketoacidosis. It has not been easy to maintain ideal blood glucose levels, and her insulin requirement has gradually changed. She did not adhere to dietary restrictions during her adolescent years. Having been recently married, she and her husband are thinking about starting a family.
Factors to Consider. What are the risks of having a child with diabetes? Is genetic testing available? What concerns during pregnancy should be considered for this client?

Discussions for these questions can be found on the website and the CD-ROM.

BIBLIOGRAPHY

1. Bennett, R.L., et al. (1995). Recommendations for standardized human pedigree nomenclature. *American Journal of Human Genetics, 56*, 745-752.
2. Campion, D., et al. (1999). Early-onset autosomal dominant Alzheimer disease: Prevalence, genetic heterogeneity, and mutation spectrum. *American Journal of Human Genetics, 65*, 664-670.
3. Collins, F.S., et al. (2003). A vision for the future of genomics research: A blueprint for the genomic era. *Nature, 422*(6934), 835-847.
4. Cruts, M., et al. (1998). Estimation of the genetic contribution of presenilin-1 and -2 mutations in a population-based study of presenile Alzheimer's disease. *Human Molecular Genetics, 7*, 43-51.
5. Cummings, J.L., et al. (1998). Alzheimer's disease: Etiologies, pathophysiology, cognitive reserve and treatment opportunities. *Neurology, 51*(suppl.), 2-17.
6. Cuthbert, A.L. (2002). Disease genes: Flattery and deception. *Trends in Pharmacologic Sciences, 23*, 504-509.
7. Editorial. (1999). Gene therapy for rare disorders. *Nature Genetics, 22*(4), 313-314.
8. Emilien, G., et al. (2000). Impact of genomics on drug discovery and clinical medicine. *Quarterly Journal of Medicine, 93*, 391-423.
9. Farlow, M.R. (1997). Alzheimer's disease: Clinical implications of the apolipoprotein E genotype. *Neurology, 48*(suppl. 6), S30-S34.
10. Fearon, E., & Vogelstein, B. (1990). A genetic model for colorectal tumorigenesis. *Cell, 61*, 759-767.
11. Gelehrter, T.D., Collins, F.S., & Ginsburg, D. (1998). *Principles of medical genetics* (2nd ed.). Baltimore: Williams & Wilkins.
12. Geller, G., et al. (1997). Genetic testing for susceptibility to adult-onset cancer: The process and content of informed consent. *Journal of the American Medical Association, 277*, 1467-1474.
13. Guttmacher, A.E., & Collins, F.S. (2002). Genomic medicine: A primer. *New England Journal of Medicine, 347*, 1512-1520.

14. Human Genome Program, U.S. Department of Energy. (2001). Genetics and its impact on society: A 2001 primer. Available: http://www.ornl.gov/hgmis/publicat/primer

 15. International Society of Nurses in Genetics. (1998). *Statement on the scope and standards of genetics clinical nursing practice.* Washington, DC: American Nurses Association.

16. International Human Genome Sequencing Consortium. (2001). Initial sequencing and analysis of the human genome. *Nature, 409,* 860-921.

17. Jones, K.L. (1997). *Recognizable patterns of human malformation* (5th ed.). Philadelphia: W. B. Saunders.

18. Jorde, L.B., et al. (1999). *Medical genetics* (2nd ed.). St. Louis: Mosby.

19. Lashley, F.R. (1998). *Clinical genetics in nursing practice* (2nd ed.). New York: Springer.

20. Lea, D.H. (2000). A clinician's primer in human genetics: What nurses need to know. *Nursing Clinics of North America, 35*(3), 583-614.

21. Lea, D.H., Jenkins, J.J., & Francomano, C.A. (1998). *Genetics in clinical practice: New directions for nursing and health care.* Sudbury, MA: Jones & Bartlett.

22. Lessick, M., et al. (2001). Advances in genetic testing for cancer risk. *MEDSURG Nursing, 10*(3), 123-127.

23. McKusick, V.A. (1998). *Mendelian inheritance in man: A catalog of human genes and genetic disorders* (12th ed.). Baltimore: The Johns Hopkins University Press.

24. Meyer, M.R., et al. (1998). ApoE genotype predicts when—not whether—one is predisposed to develop Alzheimer disease. *Nature Genetics, 19,* 321-322.

25. Middelton, L., & Lessick, M. (2003). Inherited urologic malignant disorders: Nursing implications. *Urologic Nursing, 23*(1), 15-30.

26. Middelton, L.A., & Peters, K.F. (2001). Genes and inheritance. *Cancer Nursing, 24*(5), 357-370.

27. Middelton, L.A., et al. (2001). The role of the nurse in cancer genetics. *Cancer Nursing, 24*(5), 357-369.

28. Nussbaum, R.L., McInnes, R.R., & Willard, H.F. (2001). *Thompson & Thompson genetics in medicine* (6th ed.). Philadelphia: W. B. Saunders.

29. Phillips, K.A., et al. (2001). Potential role of pharmacogenomics in reducing adverse drug reactions: A systematic review. *Journal of the American Medical Association, 286,* 2270-2279.

30. Rushnak, J.M., et al. (2001). Pharmacogenomics: A clinician's primer on emerging technologies for improved patient care. *Mayo Clinical Proceedings, 76,* 299-309.

31. Scanlon, C., & Fibison, W. (1995). *Managing genetic information: Implications for nursing practice.* Washington, DC: American Nurses Association.

32. Steele, C.D. (2000). The genetics of Alzheimer's disease. *Nursing Clinics of North America, 35*(3), 687-694.

33. Sundberg, M.I., Oscarson, M., McLellan, R.A. (1999). Polymorphic human cytochrome P450 enzymes: An opportunity for individualized drug treatment. *Trends in Pharmaceutical Science, 20,* 342-349.

34. Tinkle, M.B., & Cheek, D.J. (2002). Human genomics: Challenges and opportunities. *Journal of Obstetric, Gynecologic, and Neonatal Nursing, 31,* 178-187.

35. Venter, J.C., et al. (2001). The sequence of the human genome. *Science, 291,* 1304-1351.

36. Williams, J., & Lessick, M. (2001). Historical evolution of nursing in genetics. *MEDSURG Nursing, 10*(6), 301-307.

Perspectives in Oncology

Patricia Meier

Web Enhancements

http://evolve.elsevier.com/Black/medsurg/

Figures

Age-Adjusted Cancer Death Rates, Males by Site, United States, 1930-1999

Age-Adjusted Cancer Death Rates, Females by Site, United States, 1930-1999

Tables

Estimated New Cancer Cases and Deaths by Sex, United States, 2003

Appendix A

Religious Beliefs and Practices Affecting Health Care

The face of health care, including scientific knowledge and care delivery systems, is ever changing. Likewise, the experience of cancer is changing for our clients and families. Today a person confronted with a new diagnosis often knows someone who has survived cancer; yet cancer remains a frightening unknown for many. Some clients, especially older ones, still associate the word with death. Cancer nursing requires a clinical knowledge of the disease and its treatment as well as the skills to care for and support clients and their families. The pathophysiology and scientific advances discussed in this chapter provide a foundation for promoting positive outcomes for clients with cancer, discussed in the next chapter.

Approximately 1.3 million new cancers are diagnosed in the United States each year. Survival rates and quality of life for people living with the disease have improved. Yet each year about 556,000 Americans die of cancer. Cancer remains the second leading cause of death in the United States.[2,16]

The National Cancer Institute (NCI) estimates that 8.9 million Americans alive today have a history of cancer. This number includes disease-free survivors who are considered "cured," persons living with cancer as a chronic disease, and those currently receiving treatment. Sixty-two percent of clients with cancer diagnosed this year are expected to be alive 5 years after the diagnosis.

This statistic is based on clients diagnosed and treated 5 years ago. It does not take into account an estimation of survival resulting from evolving detection methods and newer treatment modalities.[2]

TERMINOLOGY

The terms *cancer, neoplasm, malignant neoplasm,* and *tumor* are often used interchangeably by both professionals and the lay public. Strictly speaking, these words are not interchangeable. Although generally used as a synonym for cancer, the word *tumor* simply refers to a lump, mass, or swelling. That swelling can be a neoplastic mass, or it may be only an accumulation of fluid.

The word *neoplasm* (derived from the Greek *neos,* "new," and *plasis,* "molding") is defined as an abnormal mass of tissue that serves no useful purpose and may harm the host organism. A neoplasm can be either *benign* or *malignant.* A benign neoplasm is *usually* a harmless growth that does not spread or invade other tissues. A benign tumor does occupy space. Consequently, if it is located near a vital tube or organ, it can be fatal, as with a benign brain tumor. A malignant neoplasm is a harmful mass, capable of invasion of other tissues and *metastasis* ("spread") to distant organs.

The term *cancer* is used to refer to malignant neoplasms. Cancer is a disease of the cell in which the normal mechanisms of the control of growth and prolifera-

---

Be sure to check out the bonus material on the Evolve website and the CD-ROM, including free self-assessment exercises.

http://evolve.elsevier.com/Black/medsurg/

tion have been altered. It is invasive, spreading directly to surrounding tissue as well as to new sites in the body.

The term *oncology* refers to the medical specialty that deals with the diagnosis, treatment, and study of cancer. An *oncologist* is a physician who specializes in cancer therapy. There are surgical, radiation, and medical oncologists. A *medical oncologist* is a physician with expertise in treating cancer with chemotherapy or biotherapy and in handling general medical problems related to the disease or side effects of cancer treatment. Table 18-1 lists other important terms.

EPIDEMIOLOGY

Epidemiology is the study of the distribution and determinants of diseases and health problems in specified populations. The goal of epidemiologic study is the prevention or control of the health problem. One who uses an epidemiologic approach to cancer evaluates patterns of the disease, identifies possible causes, and infers relationships between patterns of disease and determining factors. Although the causes of many cancers remain unknown, epidemiologic studies have helped to identify factors that underlie theories of causation. Nurses can use their knowledge of the factors associated with cancer causation in promoting positive outcomes for their clients through nursing assessment and interventions.

The NCI established the Surveillance, Epidemiology, and End Results (SEER) program in 1973 as a way to report population-based data in site-specific incidences of cancer, mortality, and survival rates (See SEER WebLink). This report is based on a sample of 14% of the U.S. population from 11 registries. Currently these include six metropolitan areas (Atlanta, Detroit, San Francisco/Oakland, Seattle/Puget Sound, Los Angeles, and San Jose-Monterey). It also contains data from five states (Connecticut, Hawaii, Iowa, New Mexico, and Utah) and the Commonwealth of Puerto Rico. With the 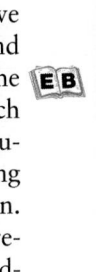 addition of supplemental and expansion registries such as the Alaska Native Tumor Registry, 26% of the population are included in SEER data. The SEER reporting areas reasonably represent the subsets of the population. Data are gathered from hospital medical records. Therefore, the accuracy of the data recorded in clients' med-

TABLE 18-1	*Cancer Terminology*
Terms	**Definitions**
Adenocarcinoma	Cancer that arises from glandular tissues. Examples include cancers of the breast, lung, thyroid, colon, and pancreas.
Anaplastic	Tumor cells that are completely undifferentiated and bear no resemblance to cells of tissues of their origin.
Aneuploid	Tumor cells that do not have the normal 46 chromosomes in a human cell. Aneuploid tumors often have a worse prognosis.
Antigens	Substances that cause activation of the immune system.
Carcinoma	A form of cancer that is composed of epithelial cells; develops in tissues covering or lining the organs of the body, such as the skin, uterus, or breast.
Carcinoma in situ	The earliest stage of cancer in which the tumor is still confined to the local area, before it has grown to a significant size or has spread.
Cytokine	A substance secreted by immune system cells, usually to send messages to other immune cells.
Differentiation	The process of maturation of a cell line of cancer cells. When they are fully differentiated or well differentiated, they more closely resemble the normal cells in the tissue of origin.
Dysplasia	An alteration in the size, shape, and organization of differentiated cells. Cells lose their regularity and show variability in size and shape, usually in response to an irritant. Cells may revert to normal when the irritant is removed but may transform to a neoplasia.
Hyperplasia	An increase in the number of normal cells in a normal arrangement in a tissue or organ; usually leads to an increase in the size of the part and an increase in functional activity.
Metaplasia	The replacement of one type of fully differentiated cell by another fully differentiated cell that is not normal for that part of the body.
Oncogenes	Specific segments of cellular deoxyribonucleic acid (DNA) that, when inappropriately activated, contribute to the transformation of normal cells into malignant cells.
Sarcoma	A cancer of supporting or connective tissue such as cartilage, bone, muscle, or fat.
Tumor markers	Chemicals in the blood that are produced by certain cancers.

ical records by physicians, nurses, and others can affect the accuracy of the SEER data. This ongoing project provides a great deal of information about cancer incidence, prevalence, and mortality for different geographic areas and ethnic groups.[25]

Incidence and Prevalence

The *incidence* rate for cancer reflects the number of new cases occurring in a specified population during a year, expressed as the number of cancers per 100,000 people. For the year 2003, about 1,334,100 new diagnoses of cancer were expected (see the table on the website for estimated new cancer cases and deaths).[2] The incidence gives perspective on the current magnitude of the problem and provides a source for establishing future priorities in cancer control programs. The *prevalence* of cancer is the total number of people alive today whose cancer has been diagnosed in the current year (incidence) and those whose cancer has been diagnosed previously. The 8.4 million Americans living with a history of cancer (prevalence) include the 1,334,100 people whose cancer has been diagnosed in the current year (incidence).

The reported incidence of cancer appears to have increased since 1900 for several reasons. First, diagnostic methods have become more precise. Utilization of diagnostic tests, such as mammograms for breast cancer and the prostate-specific antigen (PSA) blood test for prostate cancer has led to earlier detection than previously.

Second, data collection and analysis of cancer statistics have become more sophisticated over the years. Therefore, reported rates of incidence and mortality that are due to cancer are more accurate. Both can result in an increase in the *reported* incidence of cancer but not a true increased incidence of cancer.

Third, Americans are living longer than even a few decades ago. Most cancers take many years to develop. More people are now living long enough for cancer to develop. Therefore the apparent rise in cancer rates can be somewhat misleading. These factors simply reflect more precise diagnostic and statistical methods combined with the trend toward a longer life span rather than a true increase in the rates of cancer. Many lifestyle behaviors associated with cancer causation, however, such as smoking, alcohol intake, and multiple sex partners, are risk factors linked to true changes in cancer rates.

Mortality

The mortality rate is the number of deaths caused by cancer that occur in the specified population in a given year, expressed as the number of deaths that are due to cancer per 100,000 persons. Figures from the American Cancer Society (ACS) show changes in the mortality rates for lung cancer for both males and females (see the figures illustrating death rates by site in males and in fe-

males on the website).[2] A decline in lung cancer deaths for males is a reflection of the decline in smoking by American men. Meanwhile, in the words of a long-running tobacco company advertisement, women have "come a long way baby"—all the way to increased incidence of and mortality from lung cancer. In 1987, for the first time, more women died of lung cancer than of breast cancer.[8] An increasing incidence of lung cancer in women reached a plateau of 52.4 per 100,000 in 1997 and 1998.[27] After several decades of increasing female mortality from lung cancer, mortality rates have leveled off among whites, but not among African-American women. The prevalence of smoking by women has declined, although more recently and more gradually than in men. Fortunately, since 1997 tobacco use by youth has again begun to decline after increasing considerably during the early 1990s.[2]

Trends

Incidence rates in males stabilized between 1995 and 1999, whereas incidence rates in females have increased 0.3% per year between 1987 and 1999.[2,16] Mortality rates for all cancers, excluding lung cancers, have been declining since the 1950s. Mortality rates for all cancers, including lung cancers, have been declining since 1991. Mortality rates from cancer declined 1.5% per year in males and 0.6% per year in females from 1992 to 1999. Factors that may explain this decline include the decrease in tobacco use, better cancer research and treatment, and earlier cancer detection and prevention. Lung cancer incidence in men, who began quitting smoking earlier than women, is declining significantly from 102.1 per 100,000 in 1984 to 81.1 in 1999.[2,27] Cancer is not just being treated earlier. Through cancer screening, for example, precancerous colon polyps can be removed before they become cancerous.

Although overall cancer rates inched down, declines were not seen in all areas. The incidence of deadly melanoma from chronic exposure to ultraviolet radiation is actually rising about 3% per year. Incidence rates for non-Hodgkin's lymphoma have increased nearly two-fold since the early 1970s. Although 5% to 35% of cancers are associated with diet and physical activity, di- etary patterns likely did not have an impact on the decline in overall cancer incidence.[2,6] Obesity in Americans is actually increasing. Also, cancer rates did not improve for some minority populations. Overall the incidence and mortality of cancer remain higher for African Americans than for any other racial or ethnic group. The good news for African-American men is that mortality has declined more in this group between 1992 and 1999 than in any other group.[2,16] Figure 18-1 reflects the rates of cancer incidence and mortality by race or ethnicity.[2]

Thirty percent of all cancers are associated with smoking. Lifestyle choices are responsible for most ex-

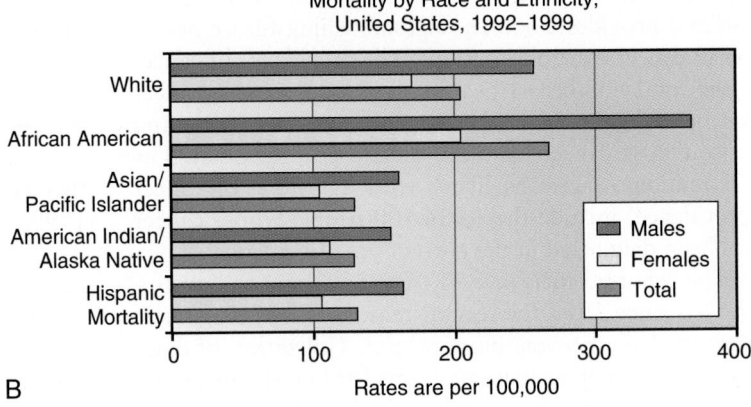

FIGURE 18-1 **A,** Average annual incidence and death rates for selected cancer types, by race and ethnicity, United States, 1992-1999. **B,** Mortality by race and ethnicity, United States, 1992-1999. Rates are per 100,000 and are age-adjusted to the 2000 U.S. standard population. (Data from American Cancer Society. [2003]. *CA: A Cancer Journal for Clinicians, p. 22.* Atlanta.)

posure to environmental carcinogens. The considerable increase in tobacco use by teenagers during the early 1990s has fortunately begun to decline since 1997.[2] Recent gains are fragile. Lifestyle choices resulting in severe sunburn from ultraviolet radiation, especially in children, are associated with a greatly increased risk of melanoma in later life. Another concern related to melanoma is the use of tanning beds. Long-term exposure to ultraviolet radiation is associated with basal cell and squamous cell skin cancers.[36] Prevention, early detection, and treatment of cancer remain significant health care concerns.

PATHOPHYSIOLOGY

Knowledge about the pathophysiology of cancer will help you better understand the significance of clinical observations and plan interventions, including client teaching, for outcomes management. A common misconception is that cancer is *one* disease. Cancer is many diseases.

Cancers comprise all diseases of cells that are altered or transformed in some way but are able to multiply, grow, and spread. Cancer development begins at the molecular level and may begin with mutations or damage of one or more genomes. Cancerous cells differ from normal cells in appearance, growth, and function. The change from normal to neoplastic cells is a process, not a single event or a single alteration in

cells. The development of a cancer is a series of events that generally occur over many years. Clinical manifestations are only the final stages in the natural history of a cancer.

Carcinogens

Carcinogens (factors associated with cancer causation) may be (1) radiation, (2) chemicals, (3) viruses, or (4) other physical agents (Table 18-2).[37] In addition, hormones play a significant role in the development of many cancers.[13]

Radiation

More than 80% of exposure to radiation is from natural sources,[32,36] including ionizing radiation from cosmic rays and radioactive minerals, such as radon gas, radium, and uranium. Sunlight and tanning beds are two sources of ultraviolet radiation, a complete carcinogens.

About 15% of radiation exposure comes from diagnostic or therapeutic procedures, including radiographs, radiation therapy, and radioisotopes used in diagnostic imaging. Individual doses vary widely with the numbers and types of procedures done.[36] The levels of radiation emitted by equipment for a given procedure have been falling significantly since the 1980s. Physicians commonly avoid ordering unnecessary procedures for clients. The amount of risk of a second malignancy

TABLE 18-2	*Known or Suspected Chemical Carcinogens in Humans**		
Target Organ	**Agent**	**Industry**	**Tumor Type**
Lung	Tobacco smoke, arsenic, asbestos, crystalline silica, benzo[*a*]pyrene, beryllium, bis(chloromethyl)ether, 1,3-butadiene, chromium VI compounds, coal tar and pitch, nickel compounds, soots, mustard gas	Aluminum production, coal gasification, coke production, hematite mining, painters	Squamous, large cell, and small cell cancer and adenocarcinoma
Pleura	Asbestos, erionite	—	Mesothelioma
Oral cavity	Tobacco smoke, alcoholic beverages, nickel compounds	Boot and shoe production, furniture manufacturing, isopropyl alcohol production	Squamous cell cancer
Esophagus	Tobacco smoke, alcoholic beverages	—	Squamous cell cancer
Gastric	Smoked, salted, and pickled foods	Rubber industry	Adenocarcinoma
Colon	Heterocyclic amines, asbestos	Pattern makers	Adenocarcinoma
Liver	Aflatoxin, vinyl chloride, tobacco smoke, alcoholic beverages, thorium dioxide	—	Hepatocellular carcinoma, hemangiosarcoma
Kidney	Tobacco smoke, phenacetin	—	Renal cell cancer
Bladder	Tobacco smoke, 4-aminobiphenyl, benzidine, 2-naphthylamine, phenacitin	Magenta manufacturing, auramine manufacturing,	Transitional cell cancer
Prostate	Cadmium	—	Adenocarcinoma
Skin	Arsenic, benzo[*a*]pyrene, coal tar and pitch, mineral oils, soots, cyclosporine A, PUVA	Coal gasification, coke production	Squamous cell cancer, basal cell cancer
Bone marrow	Benzene, tobacco smoke, ethylene oxide, antineoplastic agents, cyclosporine A	Rubber workers	Leukemia, lymphoma

 From Yuspa, S.H., & Shields, P.G. (2001). Etiology of cancer: Chemical factors. In V. T. DeVita, S. Hellman, & S. A. Rosenberg (Eds.), *Cancer: Principles and practices of oncology* (6th ed., p. 186). Philadelphia: Lippincott Williams & Wilkins.

*These carcinogen designations are determined by regulatory or review agencies based on public health needs. They do not imply proof of carcinogenicity in individuals. This table is not all-inclusive. For additional information, see agency documents and publications.

 caused by radiation therapy is still open to debate. At most, about 5% of all secondary cancers are clearly linked to radiation therapy for a previous cancer.[36]

Chemicals

Tobacco, a chemical carcinogen, remains the most important known cause of cancer in the United States, accounting for almost 30% of cancer deaths. It has been linked not only with lung cancer but also with oropharyngeal, bladder, pancreatic, cervical, and kidney cancers. Cole and Ralu state that **"smoking causes more cancer in the USA than do all other known causes combined."**[6] Because there is a clear linear relationship between the amount and number of years of smoking and cancer risk, a nurse can often find in a physician's history the number of pack-years a client has smoked. (A *pack-year* refers to the number of packs of cigarettes smoked per day times the number of years the client has smoked. It provides a measure of the client's cigarette abuse.)

Smokeless tobacco (chewing tobacco, snuff) is linked to oral cancers. Cancer risks associated with smokeless tobacco products may be decreasing because the suspected carcinogens, naturally occurring tobacco-specific nitrosamines, have been removed.[6]

In addition to lifestyle exposure to the chemicals in tobacco products, people can be exposed to chemicals in the workplace. Occupational exposure causes 2% to 8% of all human cancers. The risk estimates are much higher among the subpopulation of persons actually exposed to carcinogens in the workplace. These occupationally occurring cancers are, for the most part, preventable.[29] Health care workers wear radiation badges to ensure that they do not receive unsafe levels of exposure. Most chemotherapeutic agents bind directly to genetic material or affect cellular protein synthesis.[7,26,33] Before safe handling practices were instituted by the Occupational Safety and Health Administration (OSHA), the urine of pharmacists and nurses mixing or administering chemotherapy agents was found to show mutagenic changes from cumulative exposure. Today pharmacists mix chemotherapeutic agents under laminar flow hoods. The hood draws away air that contains aerosolized drug and prevents the pharmacist from breathing in the chemicals. Oncology nurses must wear gowns and gloves to administer chemotherapy and use special procedures to clean up any spills to prevent absorbing the chemicals through the skin or mucous membranes. Whereas personal protective equipment (PPE) is being used by pharmacy staff, there is limited use of PPE by nurses administering chemotherapy.[26,33] This is a potential health concern for nurses.

Viruses

Some viruses are strongly associated with cancer. Over the past century, one microbe after another was identified to have a possible causal relationship with cancer in humans but was later disproved. Only nine biologic agents are known to be associated with cancer causation. Of these, the hepatitis B and C viruses, the human papilloma viruses (HPV), and *Helicobacter pylori* are considered public health problems in the United States.[6] In the 1970s and early 1980s, many lay persons thought cancer was contagious and therefore often shunned those with cancer. Occasionally, yet today, a client or family member expresses this fear. Even when there is a viral link, the cancer is not contagious. Rather, a virus at some point infected the cell, causing genetic damage to the cell's deoxyribonucleic acid (DNA), thus leading to the development of cancer.

Age, Gender, Genetics, Ethnicity

Host characteristics that influence cancer susceptibility include age, gender, genetic predisposition, and ethnicity or race. Age is a factor because the person has had more years of potential exposure to carcinogens. Females have a generally lower risk of cancer incidence. Hormonal status is associated with an increased risk of neoplasia in tissues that are responsive to hormones, including breast, endometrium, prostate, ovary, thyroid, bone, and testes. In addition to biologic or genetic differences, cultural and socioeconomic factors may put an ethnic or racial group at increased or decreased risk of a specific cancer.[21]

For persons who do not smoke, dietary patterns and physical activities become the most important cancer risk factors that they can modify. The ACS estimates that one third of cancer deaths in the United States are related to diet and physical activity.[2] Research into the relationship of diet and cancer is ongoing.[32] Changes in the 2001 ACS guidelines to decrease cancer risk include an emphasis on physical activity and weight control as well as an addition of a physical activity recommendation for youth.[2] A balanced, healthy diet that includes a high proportion of plant foods (fruits, vegetables, grains, and beans), limited intake of high-fat foods, a balance of caloric intake and physical activity, and limited consumption of alcoholic beverages can reduce cancer risks and maintaining a healthy weight throughout life.[2,23]

Carcinogenesis: Transformation of Normal Cells into Cancer Cells

The process through which normal cells are transformed into malignant or cancer cells is called *carcinogenesis*. Figure 18-2 depicts the multistage model of carcinogenesis and stages of cancer using the TNM (tumor, node, metastases) system.[29,37] Four broadly identified stages of the process of carcinogenesis are as follows:

1. *Initiation* occurs when a carcinogen damages DNA. Carcinogens cause changes in the structure and function of the cell at the genetic or molecular level. This damage may be reversible or may lead to genetic mutations if not repaired; however, the mutations may not lead immediately to cancer.
2. *Promotion* occurs with additional assaults to the cells, resulting in further genetic damage.
3. At some point, these genetic events result in a *malignant conversion*.
4. With *progression*, the cells are increasingly malignant in appearance and behavior and develop into an invasive cancer with metastases to distant body parts.

Clinicians are already using their broad understanding of this process of transformation from normal cells to malignancy. Through health-promotion programs, the outcome goal of smoking cessation classes is to decrease lung cancer through prevention. Regular Papanicolaou (Pap) smears are a means of health maintenance through early detection of cervical dysplasia, a precancerous lesion. Likewise, precancerous colon polyps can be removed by colonoscopy before they progress to malignancy. Monitoring moles for early changes can allow a potentially lethal melanoma to be removed while it is still a localized, surgically curable disease.

Increased knowledge of the underlying biology of the process of carcinogenesis is coming quickly. In the 1980s, the identification of oncogenes led to the recognition that cancer is largely a genetic disease. Research shifted from carcinogenesis and mutagens to oncogenes and tumor suppressor genes. In less than a decade, researchers have clarified critically important mechanisms that control cell growth and division, regulate embryologic development, and cause disease.[32] With this knowledge, scientists are developing better treatments. Powerful new chemotherapy drugs and new ways of delivering these drugs are becoming available. *Biotherapy* is now recognized as a fourth treatment modality in addition to surgery, radiation therapy, and chemotherapy. Biotherapy is moving from research to standard treatment.[3,24]

The process of carcinogenesis transforms normal cells into cancer cells. The Unit 4 Anatomy and Physiology

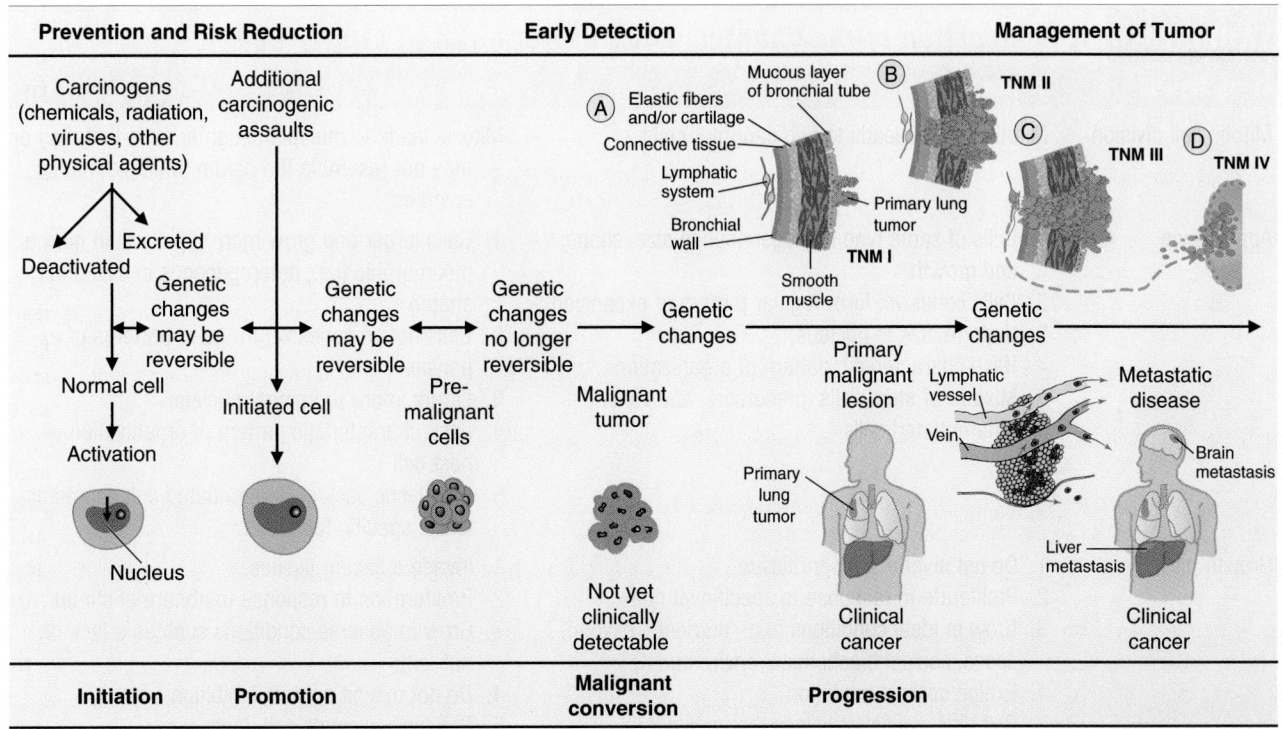

Prevention and Risk Reduction   **Early Detection**   **Management of Tumor**

FIGURE 18-2 Multistage model of carcinogenesis. The stages of cancer in the progression stage follow the T (tumor), N (node), and metastasis (M) system. **A,** Primary malignant lesion illustrates where the cancer is confined to lung tissue or the mucosa of the bronchial tube (TNM I). **B,** The cancer extends into bronchial muscle, serosa, and connective tissue (TNM II). **C,** The cancer penetrates the bronchial tube and tissue and adheres to or invades adjacent organs; or the lymphatic nodes are positive for cancer. **D,** Cancer metastasizes to distant organs such as the brain from the original lung tumor.

Review explores the characteristics of normal cells. They differ from cancer cells in many key ways (Table 18-3). Specific concepts that help us to understand changes that occur in the neoplastic transformation of cells are (1) the cell cycle, (2) altered differentiation, (3) altered growth characteristics, and (4) metastasis.

The Cell Cycle

The concept of the cell cycle has increased researchers' understanding of how both normal and neoplastic cells replicate (Figure 18-3). The cell's replication cycle is divided into the following intervals, or steps, with the letter G standing for "gap"—the interval separating cell division, or *mitosis (M)* and *synthesis (S)*.

In the normal mature organ, cell cycling is carefully controlled so that the organ maintains its function. Cells that die are replaced, but no extra cells are produced. Researchers are investigating the mechanisms of this control, which are not fully understood.

G_0 Phase. This phase is the interval in which the cell is at rest from cell division until a trigger in the immediate environment signals the beginning of the G_1 phase. Some cells do not replicate, or they replicate so infrequently that they are said to always be in a G_0 or resting state.

G_1 Phase. This phase is the interval in which ribonucleic acid (RNA) and protein are synthesized. The period the cell is in G_1 varies, depending on the type of cell and the proliferation activity of the tissue. With high activity, the G_1 interval is short. The interval lengthens when activity is low. There is a point in the G_1 phase known as the *restriction point,* after which the cell is committed to progressing into the S phase. One to 3 hours after passing the restriction point, cells initiate DNA synthesis. The acquisition of the ability to begin DNA synthesis marks the termination of the G_1 phase.

S Phase. Synthesis of both DNA and proteins of new chromosomes occurs during the S phase. The interval is probably 6 to 8 hours, although it varies in certain cell populations and under different conditions. Cell proliferation can be measured in the laboratory by flow cytometry. In reading a pathology report, you may find a reference to the percentage of cells in S phase. Only a small percentage of cells should be synthesizing DNA. An increase in S-phase fraction is a negative predictor of long-term survival.[4]

TABLE 18-3	*A Comparison of the Characteristics of Normal and Cancer Cells*	
Characteristic	**Normal Cells**	**Cancer Cells**
Mitotic cell division	Mitotic division leads to two daughter cells	Mitosis leads to multiple daughter cells that may or may not resemble the parent. Multiple mitotic spindles
Appearance	1. Cells of same type homogeneous in size, shape, and growth 2. Cells cohesive, form regular pattern of expansion 3. Uniform size to nucleus 4. Have characteristic pattern of organization 5. Mixture of stem cells (precursors) and well-differentiated cells	1. Cells larger and grow more rapidly than normal; pleomorphic (i.e., heterogeneous in size and shape) 2. Cells not as cohesive; irregular patterns of expansion 3. Larger, more prominent nucleus 4. Lack characteristic pattern of organization of host cell 5. Anaplastic, lack of differentiated cell characteristics, specific functions
Growth pattern	1. Do not invade adjacent tissue 2. Proliferate in response to specific stimuli 3. Grow in ideal conditions (e.g., nutrients, oxygen, space, correct biochemical environment) 4. Exhibit contact inhibition 5. Cell birth equals or is less than cell death 6. Stable cell membrane 7. Constant or predictable growth rate 8. Cannot grow outside specific environment (e.g., breast cells grow only in breast)	1. Invade adjacent tissues 2. Proliferation in response to abnormal stimuli 3. Grow in adverse conditions such as a lack of nutrients 4. Do not exhibit contact inhibition 5. Cell birth exceeds cell death 6. Loss of cell control a result of cell membrane changes 7. Growth rate erratic 8. Able to break off cells that migrate through bloodstream or lymphatics or seed to distant sites and grow in other sites
Function	1. Have specific, designated purpose 2. Contribute to the overall well-being of the host 3. Function in specific, predetermined manners (e.g., cells in the thyroid secrete thyroid hormone)	1. Serve no useful purpose 2. Do not contribute to the well-being of the host; parasitic, actually feed off host without contributing anything 3. If cells function at all, they do not function normally, or they may actually cause damage (e.g., lung cancer cells secrete ACTH and cause excessive stimulation of adrenal cortex)
Other	1. Develop specific antigens, characteristic of the particular cell formed 2. Chromosomes remain constant throughout cell division 3. Complex metabolic and enzyme pattern 4. Cannot invade, erode, or spread 5. Cannot grow in presence of necrosis or inflammation	1. Develop antigens completely different from a normal cell 2. Chromosomal aberrations occur as cell matures 3. Have more primitive and simplified metabolic and enzyme pattern 4. Invade, erode, and spread 5. Grow in presence of necrosis and inflammatory cells such as lymphocytes and macrophages 6. Exhibit periods of latency that vary from tumor to tumor 7. Have own blood supply and supporting stroma

ACTH, Adrenocorticotropic hormone.

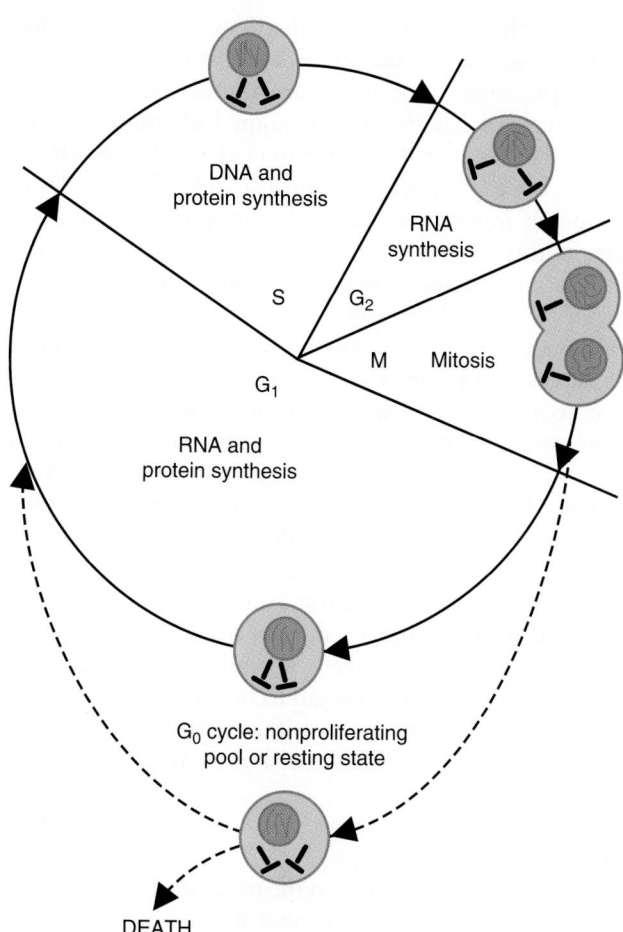

FIGURE 18-3 The cell cycle. Periods of DNA synthesis (S) and mitosis (M) are divided by gaps (G) in which the cell is in a resting state (G$_0$), producing substances in preparation for DNA synthesis (G$_1$), or producing proteins and some RNA in preparation for mitosis (G$_2$).

G$_2$ Phase. Biochemical processes, including the synthesis of some RNA, occur in preparation for mitosis. Little is known about this phase, which lasts only a few hours.

M Phase. Actual division of the cell *(mitosis)* occurs during this phase, producing two daughter cells. The M phase usually ranges from less than an hour to a few hours.

Altered Cell Differentiation

Cells that were genetically identical in the embryo eventually assume varying structures and functions. One muscle cell looks like all the other muscle cells but not like a kidney or liver cell. In normal growth, cells become more specialized or committed to a particular cell line as they mature. This process of development is called *differentiation*. Most cells contain the entire genome. The growth and function of a particular cell line result from the expression of certain genes and the

suppression of others. Transformation of a normal cell to a cancer cell can occur at any point in the process of differentiation. Changes in the appearance of the cell, the presence of tumor-specific antigens that are suppressed on the normal cell, and the loss of normal function can result from altered differentiation.

Appearance. An obvious difference from normal cells is in the appearance of cancer cells. Normal cells have well-organized cellular components. Cancer cells have variable sizes and shapes. Nuclei may be disproportionately large, or there may be multiple nuclei. A variety of abnormal mitotic features may be present. There may be an abnormal number of chromosomes *(aneuploidy)* or an abnormal arrangement of chromosomes.[29] The detection of aneuploidy in a pathology report is an unfavorable prognostic factor.

A pathology report generally describes the grade of the cancer cells. When the cells are well differentiated, or low grade, they are more mature in appearance and more like the normal cells from which they have arisen than poorly differentiated cancer cells. Anaplastic (undifferentiated) cells appear so disorganized under the microscope that they have no resemblance to the tissue of origin. Poorly differentiated and anaplastic cancers tend to be more aggressive—an unfavorable prognostic factor. During the natural history of many malignant neoplasms, as the cancer cells grow and divide, they often lose more and more of their mature characteristics. As a result, a malignant neoplasm can be heterogeneous with more than one variation of the malignant cell line. This heterogeneity is caused by random mutations during tumor progression.[34]

At times, a neoplasm initially responds to therapy. You may read in a radiology report that the tumor has shrunk back, with a partial remission (PR) or a complete remission (CR) of all radiologic evidence of the neoplasm; then the neoplasm may come back and grow aggressively. A likely explanation is that the treatment successfully eliminated one variant of the cancer cells, causing those cells to die and the overall size of the tumor to shrink. Then other variants of the cancer cells, which were resistant to the treatment, grew and multiplied, so that the tumor increased in size.

Biochemical studies may reflect differences resulting from altered cell metabolism. The cell's surface membrane is the interface between the cell and extracellular components. Cell membrane changes may result in the production of enzymes that aid in cancer spread. A loss of glycoproteins results in a loss of cell-to-cell adhesion. Loss of antigens that identify the cell as "self" or production of tumor-specific antigens can alter the immune system's ability to mount a response.[29]

Tumor cell membranes have a greater fluidity than normal cell membranes do. This may be due to changes in the lipid composition of the membrane of tumor cells. Scientists are trying to take advantage of this difference.

Some chemotherapy drugs are now being delivered in *liposomes* (spheres with an outer lipid layer and internal core of drug). The tumor cells take in more of the liposomal drug than is taken in by the normal cells. The result is a better treatment effect with fewer harmful effects on the normal cells.

Tumor-Specific Antigens. Cell surfaces express antigens. Some tumors express more of an antigen than is expressed by normal cells. These tumor-specific antigens can be used as a diagnostic tool in the detection of cancer or in monitoring the effectiveness of cancer treatment. One example is the PSA test. Normally, a man's blood level of PSA is low (i.e., 0 to 2 ng/ml). In the presence of prostate cancer, this antigen can be elevated. The PSA blood test is now being used as one early detection tool, along with the digital rectal examination, to detect prostate cancer in men who are still asymptomatic.[2] During treatment, a decline in the PSA level is an indicator of the effectiveness of the treatment. During follow-up after treatment ends, a rise in the PSA level can be an early indicator that the cancer has recurred.

Function. Unlike normal cells, cancer cells typically serve no useful purpose. The result of neoplastic growth is an abnormal tissue mass that does not contribute in any way to the well-being of the host. The mass occupies space and draws nutrition and sustenance from the host. If the cancer cells function at all, they often do not function normally and may even act in a way that causes damage to the host. For example, a functional tumor of the thyroid gland produces excess amounts of thyroid hormone, leading to a hypermetabolic state.

Altered Growth Characteristics

Another obvious difference from normal cells is the uncontrolled growth of cancer cells. Because of changes in their cell surfaces, neoplastic cells differ from normal cells in growth patterns and mobility. Cancer cells lose the contact inhibition of normal cells, can establish metastasis, avoid normal regulation by hormones, and avoid being recognized by the immune system as altered.

Contact Inhibition and Doubling Time. When normal cells are cultured in the laboratory, they exhibit a behavior known as *contact inhibition*. This means the cells continue to divide until they cover the bottom of the Petri dish and stop dividing when they touch the edges of the dish. Cancer cells continue to divide, piling up on the other cells. In human tissues, the growth of normal cells is carefully regulated. Cells divide to produce new cells only when needed to replace cells that have died. Cancer cells do not stop dividing and multiplying. A common misconception is that neoplastic cells replicate faster than the normal cells from which they arise. They do not necessarily go through the cell cycle at a faster

rate than the normal cells of the tissue from which they have arisen. Rather, the abnormality is that they do not stop replicating. Cancer cells are almost continuously in the process of cell division, spending little time in the G_0 phase. This appears to be due to (1) lack of responses to signals to stop replicating, and (2) lack of responses to cell death *(apoptosis)* signals.[18] (Apoptosis is discussed later in this chapter.)

This continuous growth results in a phenomenon referred to as *doubling time*. The doubling time of a human malignant tumor can vary from weeks to months. As depicted in Figure 18-4, it may take 10 years for a tumor to reach 1 cm in size. In only another year, that same tumor may grow to 8 cm. The smallest clinically detectable mass weighs about 1 g, or 1 cm³ in size. A *tumor burden* (amount) of 1 kg, which requires only about 10 more doublings, is potentially lethal.[29]

Clients sometimes ask whether exposing the tumor to air during surgery can cause it to grow more rapidly. More likely, if the surgeon did not see evidence of tumor in other areas, it had already spread, but the size of the tumor mass was still too small to be seen or felt. Then in a few more doubling times, without effective treatment, it became evident and proceeded to enlarge.

Metastasis

Normal cells are adherent to the other normal cells from which they have arisen. Normal breast tissue cells, for example, are never found anywhere in the body except in the breast. Malignant or cancer cells are less adherent and more mobile than normal cells. They have the ability to spread from the original site of the tumor to distant organs. This phenomenon is called *metastasis* (from the Greek *meta,* beyond, and *stasis,* standing).

The capacity of a neoplastic tumor to metastasize to other sites is a major characteristic of malignancy—and the most frequent reason why cancer treatment fails. It is the characteristic that distinguishes malignant from benign growths. Neoplastic cells must progress through a sequence of complex stages to overcome multiple barri-

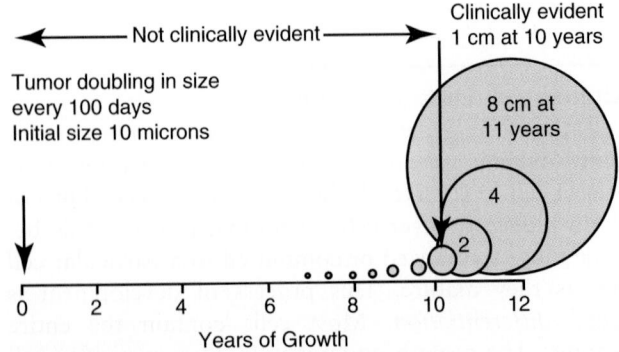

FIGURE 18-4 Depiction of tumor growth showing doubling time related to tumor size.

ers and successfully spread to other sites. Failure to complete any stage in the metastatic cascade disrupts formation of metastases.[34]

No single gene product is solely responsible for the highly complex processes in the metastatic cascade. Progressive alterations in cellular oncogenes and inactivation of tumor suppressor genes result in uncontrolled growth and development of metastatic potential. For the purposes of this discussion, the metastatic cascade is divided into three stages (see Figure 18-2).

Stage 1. The progressive alteration of malignant cells with additional genetic changes results in a heterogeneous population of malignant cells with varying degrees of metastatic potential. Increasing tumor size, leading to tissue pressure and mechanical expansion, may cause neoplastic invasion; however, the size of the primary tumor is not the sole predictor of metastasis. Tumors with identical size and histologic cell type can vary markedly in metastatic spread. As the malignant tumor grows, the cells at the center become hypoxic, and it begins to seek its own blood supply. Neoplastic cells from the primary tumor invade surrounding tissue and penetrate blood or lymph vessels. Vascularization *(angiogenesis)* of the tumor dramatically increases its metastatic potential.[29,34]

Loss of tumor cell cohesiveness with increasing motility is an important factor in the metastatic cascade. These cells can detach from the primary tumor and create defects in the basement membranes with resulting stromal invasion and spread into the circulation. Tumors, even when very small, shed cells. As many as 10^7 to 10^9 cells per day may be found circulating in the bloodstream of clients with cancer.[29,34] Although surgery, for example, can cure most early breast cancers, some eventually recur because of these shed cells. Adjuvant chemotherapy or hormonal therapy, given when no visible tumor remains, may therefore be considered for clients with early-stage breast cancer to decrease the risk of recurrence. Yet fewer than 1% of circulating cancer cells successfully metastasize.[34] In the future, new scientific knowledge may allow oncologists to identify the clients with early-stage breast cancer who would benefit from adjuvant chemotherapy. This would allow most women for whom surgery alone was curative to avoid the adverse effects of chemotherapy.

Benign neoplasms and cancer in situ do not cause destruction of the host stroma (the supporting tissues of an organ). With progression to invasive disease, the neoplasm penetrates the epithelial basement membrane and invades the interstitial stroma at multiple stages in the metastatic cascade.[4] A client's pathology report often indicates whether there was invasion of the neoplasm into surrounding tissue or into lymphatic, perineural, or vascular tissues. Such invasion may be an indication of occult (as yet undetected) metastatic disease.

Cancer cells that successfully metastasize represent a subpopulation of the primary tumor's cells. Not all cells in the primary mass share the unique genetic and biologic properties necessary for metastasis.[29]

Stage 2. Cancer cells migrate via the lymph or blood circulation or by direct extension. The lymphatic system provides the most common pathway for the initial spread of malignant cancer cells. There may be spread to the lymph nodes draining the region of the primary tumor site. Lymph node involvement is seen in about 50% of all fatal cancers. The blood vessels (both veins and arteries) carry cancer cells from the primary tumor to the capillary beds of the lungs, liver, and bones. Metastatic spread to distant organs and tissues is almost always the result of cells moving through the bloodstream.

Direct extension of tumors to adjacent tissues also occurs. For example, a breast cancer may spread directly to the chest wall. In body cavities, cells may spread by gravity, resulting in new growths on other serosal surfaces. Cells shed by cancers of the ovary are often found to have fallen onto and "seeded" the entire peritoneal cavity with metastatic sites of the tumor.

To complete this stage in the metastatic cascade, tumor cells must survive a variety of hemodynamic and immunologic challenges.

Stage 3. Cancer cells are established at the secondary site. This may result from entrapment due to the size of the tumor clump, adherence to cells at the new site through specific interactions, or by binding to exposed basement membrane. Continued growth and proliferation at the metastatic site are also dependent on the development of its own blood supply *(angiogenesis)* and ability to evade eradication by immune responses. Cells from the metastatic site may then go on to disseminate to form additional metastatic lesions.[34]

Researchers have observed that certain tumor cells have, for unknown reasons, an affinity for certain sites. Although the exact mechanism of metastasis is unclear, the metastatic sites of many cancers are fairly predictable. The predilection of certain malignant neoplasms for particular sites may be due to the ability of the tumor to live within only certain tissues or to some other unknown factor. The most common site of metastasis is lymphatic tissues; the next most common sites are the liver, lungs, bones, and brain.[29]

Angiogenesis. The metastatic cascade begins and ends with *angiogenesis.* A tumor cannot grow more than 0.5 mm without a blood supply to transport nutrients to the tumor. Very tiny tumors can receive oxygen and nutrients by diffusion. Proliferation beyond 0.5 mm requires a vasculature blood supply. Angiogenesis is the ability of cancer cells to secrete substances that stimulate blood vessel growth.[6,11] The angiogenic process involves a series of sequential steps that result in a shift in the balance between stimulators and inhibitors of angiogenesis. When the ratio of proangiogenic molecules exceeds the antiangiogenic molecules new blood vessels are formed. Scientists are studying various anti-angiogenesis strategies.[29,34] Cutting off development of new blood supplies could halt the growth of a tumor. The destruction of a single tumor capillary may be able to kill many cancer cells that rely on that vessel for nutrition. Benign tumors are sparsely vascularized and grow slowly, whereas malignant tumors are highly vascular and grow rapidly. If angiogenesis is inhibited, cancer progression may be halted or slowed by preventing metastasis. Several types of anti-angiogenic agents are currently under investigation.[11,29,34]

The growth of metastatic tumors puts severe stress on the affected person, both physiologically and psychologically. As the *tumor burden* (the amount of tumor in the body) increases, fewer metabolic resources are available for normal cells. As mentioned earlier, when the total burden of tumor in the body approaches 1 kg, the sheer burden of the tumor is potentially lethal.

When a client's cancer metastasizes to other sites, clients and family members may erroneously believe that the client has multiple cancers; it is one cancer spread to other organs. For example, cells that have spread to the bone from a breast cancer are breast cancer cells, not malignant variants of bone tissue cells; however, a client may have two different cancers at one time. In the process of making a new diagnosis of colon cancer, for example, a clinician may also discover a previously undetected prostate cancer.

Knowing the natural history and the most likely pattern of spread can be very helpful to the clinician. If the cancer is likely to spread to the liver, bone, or brain, the clinician will want to rule out evidence of such spread in making treatment decisions and in monitoring for recurrence following treatment.

Inability of the Immune System to Recognize Cancer Cells

Role in Preventing Carcinogenesis

The immune system usually defends against bacterial or viral invaders and plays a key role in controlling the growth of cancer cells. There are two critical components of the immune response: (1) the ability to recognize a pathogen as foreign and (2) the ability to mount a response to eliminate the pathogen.[3,4] This section addresses the role of the immune system in preventing carcinogenesis. The Unit 17 Anatomy and Physiology Review discusses the immune system.

Cancer cells arise continually as a result of somatic (nonreproductive cell) mutations. The immune system—specifically the T-cell lymphocytes, macrophages, and antigens—recognizes these cells as non-self and destroys them. Immune surveillance theory, as yet unproved, proposes that immune responses, particularly cell-mediated responses, provide a defense against cancer cells by recognizing the antigens on the surface of some neoplastic

cells as foreign. These cells are killed by cytotoxic T cells that have receptors for specific tumor antigens and by interferon-activated natural killer (NK) lymphocytes and macrophages.[3]

Macrophages, the important first line of defense, phagocytize the pathogen and present it as antigen to T and B lymphocytes. T-cell recognition of antigen stimulates proliferation of T and B cells, with B-cell production of antibodies against the pathogen and T-cell secretion of cytokines. Cytokines, hormone-like peptides or glycopeptides, regulate activation of the immune system against cancer cells. Cytokines both enhance and suppress complex immune interactions.

Antigens on cancer cells can take various forms, resulting in T-cell recognition of the cells as abnormal. The cancer cells may express antigens that are not present on normal cells. Cancer cells may have antigens that are "unmasked" and thus visible to the immune system. These same antigens when present on normal cells are masked and thus are not recognized by the immune system. Cancer cells may also express antigens that are only present during oncofetal or embryonic development of normal cells. Cytotoxic T cells that have receptors for specific tumor antigens and interferon-activated NK lymphocytes and macrophages can then destroy these cancer cells.

Failure of Immune Defenses

Unfortunately, the immune defenses are not always effective. The immune system may be unable to recognize cancer cells as foreign or to mount an immune response for several reasons.

An immature, old, or weak immune system may contribute to this. People who are malnourished or chronically ill may also be immunocompromised. The tumor burden (number of cancer cells) may be too small to stimulate an immune response. Alternatively, the tumor burden may be so great as to overwhelm the immune system.

Some cancer cells escape detection because they resemble normal cells. Other cancer cells produce substances that shield them from recognition. Cancer cells may also escape detection by becoming coated with fibrin. Tumor invasion of the bone marrow can result in decreased production of lymphocytes needed to destroy the tumor mass.

The incidence of malignancy increases with the use of immunosuppressive drugs after organ transplantation to counteract rejection. Chemotherapeutics or radiation used to treat cancer can also induce suppression of the immune response.[3,29]

Apoptosis

With the development of molecular biology in the 1980s, scientists began to understand another important step in the process of carcinogenesis: the failure of cells to die.[1,10,14,20,28] In normal physiology, a damaged cell sacrifices itself for the greater good. There are two pathways to cell death:

1. *Necrosis* is cell death resulting from injury. The dead cells swell, lyse, and release their cellular contents into the intercellular spaces, causing the inflammatory response.

2. In *apoptosis* (from the Greek word for "falling off"), cellular "suicide" results in cells rapidly shrinking with loss of their intercellular contents.[29] They are quickly phagocytized and digested by macrophages and other cells in the vicinity. Inflammation is not triggered. Figure 18-5 depicts this programmed cell suicide. The morphologic changes of apoptosis can be completed in less than an hour.[10,14]

Most, if not all, cells manufacture a set of proteins that serve as weapons of self-destruction. As long as a cell is useful to the body, it restrains its death machinery. If the cell becomes infected or malignant or otherwise threatens the health of the organism, however, the lethal proteins are unleashed.[10]

Increasingly, scientists view cancer as both a disease of excessive cell growth and a lack of normal cell death. In the process of carcinogenesis, cells accumulate enough damage to genes that control cell growth and survival that the mutation seems irreparable. The affected cell usually kills itself rather than risk becoming deranged and potentially dangerous. If the cell does not die, it or its daughter cells may live long enough to accumulate mutations that make it possible to divide uncontrollably and to metastasize to distant sites.

When a death signal, such as tumor necrosis factor (TNF), is initiated, a survival signal is also initiated. The balance between cell survival and cell death signals de-

termines cell fate.[20] Apoptosis may not be induced in response to a cancer cell because there has also been damage to a tumor suppressor gene. In many cancers, genetic damage apparently fails to induce apoptosis because there has been damage to the gene that codes for the p53 protein. The p53 protein is a suppressor gene that can prompt activation of cell suicide. It is estimated that as many as half of solid cancers, including lung, colon, and breast cancers, have damage to the p53 protein.[10]

Still other apoptotic triggers can lead to programmed death of cancerous cells. Normal cells also tend to self-destruct when deprived of their usual growth factors or contact with other like cells. This is probably a built-in defense mechanism against metastasis. Part of the reason some cancers are resistant to the effects of radiation therapy or chemotherapy may be due to the lack of cell death through apoptosis even after cancer treatment. Researchers are investigating genetic therapies that might overcome this resistance to apoptosis.

GENETICS AND CANCER

Medical genetics has rapidly evolved into a full-fledged scientific field, and oncology is at the forefront in utilizing these scientific strides. The Human Genome Project, a federally funded, multibillion-dollar international initiative, was begun in 1990, with the goal of locating, mapping, and sequencing the genes of a human's genetic composition. Scientists have completed a draft mapping the estimated 30,000 to 40,000 genes on the human chromosome. Over the coming decade, work will continue to apply this knowledge toward identifying genes associated with disease and developing modalities to prevent or treat disease.[4,17,23] A powerful new technology combining biology with computers is emerging. This

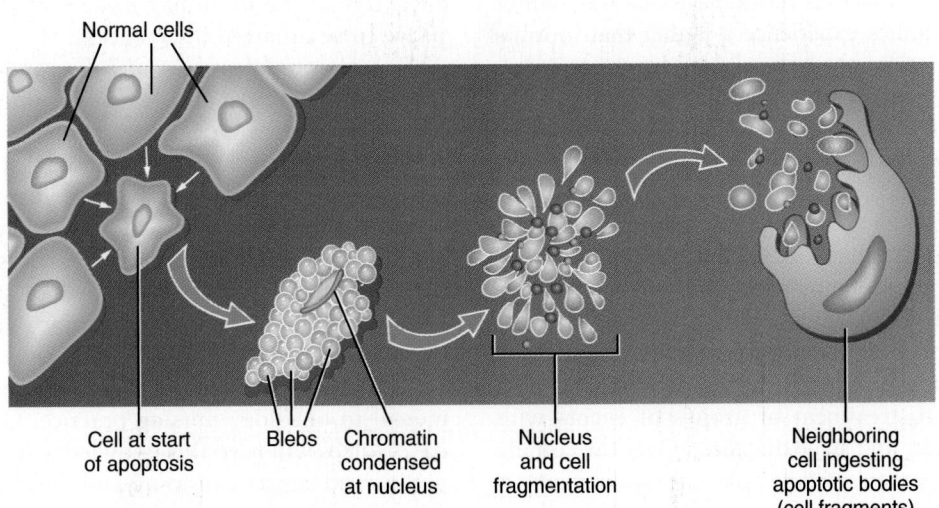

FIGURE 18-5 Programmed cell death resulting from apoptosis. With apoptosis (cell suicide), the cell shrinks and pulls away from surrounding cells. Blebs appear on the surface of the cell. Chromatin condenses on the edge of the nucleus. The nucleus and then the cell itself break up. Cell fragments are ingested by other cells. (From Duke, R.C., Ojcius, D.M., & Young, J.D. [1996]. Cell suicide in health and disease, *Scientific American, 275*[6], 81.)

gene chip analysis technology will make possible the screening of vast numbers of genes. The potential payoff is great.[19]

Cancer is a genetic disease. Clinically, cancer comprises 100 or more diseases. On the molecular level, cancer may result from different combinations of a few similar gene mutations.[22] Two neoplasms that are morphologically indistinguishable can have different gene profiles. In clinical practice, two women can have breast cancers with the same histology, grade, and stage and receive the same therapy and yet have different outcomes. With gene profiling comes the ability to recognize areas of genetic abnormalities on the chromosome. Different combinations of genetic mutations and environmental influences can cause a normal cell to become malignant. This can result in two seemingly identical cancers responding very differently to therapy. On the other hand, an area of genetic mutation, such as damage to the *p53* suppressor gene, can be seen in the profiles of clinically very different cancers.[15] Another person whose genetic profile carries this same abnormality may develop cancer or may never develop cancer but might pass the abnormality on to offspring. The reader is referred to Chapter 17 for a more complete discussion of the biology of genetics.

Up to 30% of rare childhood cancers result from genetic predisposition. In adults, about 34% of cancers have a *familial* basis; only 5% to 10% of adult cancers are *hereditary*. Hereditary cancers result from a single inherited gene disorder. Patterns of occurrence are clearly predictable. These cancers usually occur at an early age, in unusual sites, and in paired organs (both breasts, for example). There also may be multiple primary (versus metastatic) sites. Hereditary cancers include some breast, colorectal, melanoma, ovarian, and renal cell cancers as well as retinoblastoma and Wilms' tumor.[3] Some families experience a higher than normal rate of cancer that cannot be explained by environmental exposure or general risk. Inherited susceptibility to cancer may not be rare at all. The cancers may be all of one type or of two or more types. There is no predictable pattern of inheritance because the cancers are probably not linked to a single gene disorder. Cancers that may have a potential familial link include breast, ovarian, colorectal, prostate, melanoma, uterine, leukemia, sarcomas, and primary brain tumors.

At present oncologists select treatments and give clients a statistical prognosis based on research data about response to treatment of groups of clients with similar type, grade, and stage of cancer. Over the coming decade, medical genetics will be able to provide scientists new tools to answer more specifically questions about cancer causation and response to treatment.[19,30] As we come to understand how treatments work at the genetic level, oncologists will be able to customize a treatment plan to the specific areas of genetic damage resulting in

a client's cancer. New biologic agents being developed have an additive effect when combined with chemotherapy and radiation therapy.[15]

Genetic discoveries are expected to have a profound impact on nursing practice in several areas and no doubt will change the traditional perspective on screening, identifying, preventing, and treating cancer.[5] Most nurses are already performing some genetics-related activities. Do you know the genetic basis for the recommendation to use sunscreens? Has a client ever expressed concern about their familial experience of cancer? Has a client ever asked you about a vaccine for melanoma or pancreatic cancer? As clients become more aware that genetics has a role in cancer causation, nurses will need to be able to provide client teaching or referrals to professionals who can address these concerns.[17] Precise identification of cancer-causing genetic abnormalities will significantly improve the accuracy of cancer prediction and thus the capacity to target preventive interventions to at-risk populations.[30] As a result, the perspective of nursing will shift from symptomatic clients with cancer to counseling asymptomatic clients. CA125, a tumor marker that has already been identified, is useful in monitoring the response of ovarian cancer to therapy; however, it has not been sufficiently sensitive for detecting early stage disease. Higher levels of a new biomarker, osteopontin, may prove to be valuable in early detection tool for ovarian cancer. Likewise, molecular profiling of prostate cancer has led to the identification of new biomarkers that may have value in analysis of prostate biopsy specimens.[31] Counseling and support are vital for any client considering genetic testing. Genetic testing may reveal cancer risks for which the efficacy of measures to reduce risk is unknown. A prophylactic mastectomy to prevent breast cancer for a woman with a *BRCA* gene mutation may in light of future knowledge prove to be a flawed intervention.

Issues of confidentiality and discrimination, as well as the dilemma of predicting as yet incurable illnesses, may have an enormous negative effect on the client's and family's quality of life and psychological state. Learning one's genetic test results may cause distress, sadness, depression, anxiety, or anger and may affect one's relationship with other family members. Clients considering genetic testing need to be informed of state and federal laws protecting them from insurance and job discrimination and the limitations of these laws.[12,13]

Knowledge of genetics is rapidly becoming fundamental to oncology nursing practice. Genetics is oncology. Nurses will need this knowledge to help their clients understand cancer causation and their customized treatments, to recognize risk factors, and to promote effective prevention/early detection strategies. The diffusion of our evolving science of cancer genetics will be dependent on health professionals, including nurses, applying that knowledge in our clinical practices.[5] For more information on genetics, refer to Chapter 17 and the genetic boxes throughout the textbook.

CLASSIFICATION OF NEOPLASMS

Benign Versus Malignant

As stated, neoplastic tumors can be either benign or malignant. The word *benign* comes from the Latin *benignus*, meaning "kind." A benign tumor expands in size as it grows, but it does not infiltrate or metastasize. Because it occupies space, it may be fatal if it is located near a vital tube or organ. As a rule, though, the person with a benign neoplasm has a good prognosis because the tumor can be readily excised. Malignant neoplasms, on the other hand, represent a serious threat to the life and well-being of the host. Table 18-4 compares the characteristics of benign and malignant neoplasms.

TABLE 18-4	*Comparison of the Characteristics of Benign and Malignant Neoplasms*	
Characteristic	**Benign Neoplasm**	**Malignant Neoplasm**
Speed of growth	Grows slowly Usually continues to grow throughout life unless surgically removed May have periods of remission	Usually grows rapidly Tends to grow relentlessly throughout life Rarely, neoplasm may regress spontaneously
Mode of growth	Grows by enlarging and expanding Always remains localized; never infiltrates surrounding tissues	Grows by infiltrating surrounding tissues May remain localized (in situ), but usually infiltrates other tissues
Capsule	Almost always contained within a fibrous capsule Capsule does not prevent expansion of neoplasm but does prevent growth by infiltration Capsule advantageous because encapsulated tumor can be removed surgically	Never contained within a capsule Absence of capsule allows neoplastic cells to invade surrounding tissues Surgical removal of tumor difficult
Cell characteristics	Usually well differentiated Mitotic figures absent or scanty Mature cells Anaplastic cells absent Cells function poorly in comparison with normal cells from which they arise If neoplasm arises in glandular tissue, cells may secrete hormones	Usually poorly differentiated Large numbers of normal and abnormal mitotic figures present Cells tend to be anaplastic (i.e., young, embryonic type) Cells too abnormal to perform any physiologic functions Occasionally a malignant tumor arising in glandular tissue secretes hormones
Recurrence	Recurrence extremely unusual when surgically removed	Recurrence common following surgery because tumor cells spread into surrounding tissues
Metastasis	Metastases never occur	Metastases very common
Effect of neoplasm	Not harmful to host unless located in area where it compresses tissues or obstructs vital organs Does not produce cachexia (weight loss, debilitation, anemia, weakness, wasting)	Always harmful to host Causes death unless removed surgically or destroyed by radiation or chemotherapy Causes disfigurement, disrupted organ function, nutritional imbalances May result in ulcerations, sepsis, perforations, hemorrhage, tissue slough Almost always produces cachexia, which leaves person prone to pneumonia, anemia, and other conditions
Prognosis	Very good Tumor generally removed surgically	Depends on cell type and speed of diagnosis Poor prognosis if cells are poorly differentiated and evidence of metastatic spread exists Good prognosis indicated if cells still resemble normal cells and there is no evidence of metastasis

Tissue of Origin

Besides being classified as benign or malignant, neoplasms are also classified according to the tissue from which they arise. Almost all names for neoplasms end in the suffix *-oma*, meaning "tumor" (Table 18-5). This suffix is usually attached to a term for the parent tissue of the neoplasm. Thus, adenoma comes from the Greek *aden-*, or gland, plus-*oma*. When more than one parent tissue enters into the formation of a neoplasm, the names of the tumors are even more descriptive. For example, an adenomyoma is a benign neoplasm that contains both glandular and muscle (Greek genitive *myos*) cells.

Because epithelial tissues vary greatly, benign tumors of epithelial origin are classified according to either their *microscopic* appearance (e.g., adenoma) or their *macroscopic* appearance (e.g., polyp, from the Greek *polys* for "many" plus *pous* for "foot").

TABLE 18-5 *Classification of Neoplasms by Tissue of Origin*

Tissue of Origin	Benign	Malignant
Connective tissue		Sarcoma
Embryonic fibrous tissue	Myxoma	Myxosarcoma
Fibrous tissue	Fibroma	Fibrosarcoma
Adipose tissue	Lipoma	Liposarcoma
Cartilage	Chondroma	Chondrosarcoma
Bone	Osteoma	Osteogenic sarcoma
Epithelium		Carcinoma
Skin and mucous membrane	Papilloma	Squamous cell carcinoma
Glands		Basal cell carcinoma
		Transitional cell carcinoma
	Adenoma	Adenocarcinoma
	Cystadenoma	Cystadenocarcinoma
Pigmented cells (melanocytes)	Nevus	Malignant melanoma
Endothelium		Endothelioma
Blood vessels	Hemangioma	Hemangioendothelioma
		Hemangiosarcoma
		Kaposi's sarcoma
Lymph vessels	Lymphangioma	Lymphangiosarcoma
		Lymphangioendothelioma
Bone marrow		Multiple myeloma
		Ewing's sarcoma
		Leukemia
Lymphoid tissue		Malignant lymphoma
		Lymphosarcoma
		Reticulum cell sarcoma
Muscle tissue		
Smooth muscle	Leiomyoma	Leiomyosarcoma
Striated muscle	Rhabdomyoma	Rhabdomyosarcoma
Nerve tissue		
Nerve fibers and sheaths	Neuroma	Neurogenic sarcoma
	Neurinoma	
	Neurilemoma	
	Neurofibroma	Neurofibrosarcoma
Ganglion cells	Ganglioneuroma	Neuroblastoma
Glial cells	Glioma	Glioblastoma
Meninges	Meningioma	Malignant meningioma
Gonads	Dermoid cyst	Embryonal carcinoma
		Embryonal sarcoma
		Teratocarcinoma

The following are three of the most common benign neoplasms:

1. *Fibromas:* Fibromas may grow anywhere in the body, but they frequently make their home in the uterus. Fibromas are generally small but occasionally grow to great size. These encapsulated, relatively harmless neoplasms cause no manifestations unless, because of their location, they press on a bone or nerve. Fibromas are easily removed surgically.

2. *Lipomas:* Lipoma, a common benign neoplasm, arises in adipose tissue. Lipomas rarely cause manifestations, but they are poorly encapsulated and may exert pressure on surrounding tissues as they expand.

3. *Leiomyomas:* The leiomyoma, a benign neoplasm of smooth muscle origin, is the most common benign tumor in women. Leiomyomas may develop anywhere in the body, but most often they grow in the uterus. Rarely (~1% cases), these neoplasms become malignant.

Malignant neoplasms are also categorized by tissue origin. A malignant neoplasm that arises from epithelial tissue is called a *carcinoma;* a malignant neoplasm that arises from mesenchymal origins (i.e., blood vessels, lymphatic tissue, nerve tissue) is called a *sarcoma* (from Greek *sarx,* or flesh).

The following are three representative examples of malignant neoplasms or cancers:

1. *Carcinoma in situ:* This is a neoplasm of epithelial tissue that remains confined to the site of origin. In situ carcinoma can occur in the cervix, and it may occur in squamous epithelium in other parts of the body. This form of cancer is, by definition, localized and thus can be removed surgically; however, in situ carcinoma can become invasive, eroding into surrounding tissues.

2. *Malignant fibrosarcomas:* These tumors are similar to benign fibromas. Fibrosarcomas tend to grow in the same sites and may originate as benign fibromas, later becoming malignant. These bulky, well-differentiated tumor masses are usually responsive to surgery. Fortunately, they rarely metastasize.

3. *Bronchogenic carcinomas:* These tumors account for 90% of all cases of lung cancer. Bronchogenic carcinomas usually develop in the lower trachea and lower bronchi. Surgical excision of the tumor is the intervention of choice; however, this type of cancer readily gives rise to metastasis; if this occurs, surgery is contraindicated.

CONCLUSIONS

Effective nursing care and client teaching to achieve outcome goals require that you understand the pathophysiology of the cancer. You should know the natural history of the disease, such as the normal course of disease progression, likely sites of metastasis, potential for effective treatment, and side effects and complications of both the disease and the treatments. With a basic understanding of cancer, you can build on that knowledge base by listening to the client's history, reviewing the information provided in the medical record, and consulting with colleagues, including nursing peers, nursing leaders, physicians, and oncology nurses, both locally and nationally.

BIBLIOGRAPHY

1. Ameisen, J.C. (1996). The origin of programmed cell death. *Science, 272,* 1278-1279.

2. American Cancer Society. (2003). *Cancer facts and figures—2003.* Atlanta: Author.

3. Appel, C. (2001). Biotherapy. In S. Otto (Ed.), *Oncology nursing* (4th ed., pp. 684-730). St. Louis: Mosby.

4. Appel, C. (2001). Genetics. In S. Otto (Ed.), *Oncology nursing* (4th ed., pp. 21-40). St. Louis: Mosby.

5. Calzone, K.A., & Tranin, A.S. (2003). The scope of cancer genetics nursing practice. In A.M. Tranin and J. Jenkins (Eds.), *Genetics in oncology practice: Cancer risk assessment* (pp. 13-22). Pittsburgh: Oncology Nursing Society.

6. Cole, P., & Ralu, B. (2001). Analytic epidemiology: Cancer causes. In V.T. DeVita, S. Hellman, & S.A. Rosenberg (Eds.), *Cancer: principles and practices of oncology* (6th ed., pp. 241-252). Philadelphia: Lippincott, Williams & Wilkins.

7. Connor, T.H., et al. (1999). Surface contamination with antineoplastics in six cancer treatment centers in Canada and the United States, *ASHP, 56,* 1427-1432.

8. Crane-Okada, R. (2001). Breast cancer. In S. Otto (Ed.), *Oncology nursing* (4th ed., pp. 113-167). St. Louis: Mosby.

9. DeVita, V.T., Hellman, S., & Rosenberg, S.A. (Eds.). (2001). *Cancer: principles and practices of oncology* (6th ed.). Philadelphia: Lippincott, Williams & Wilkins.

10. Duke, R.C., Ojcius, D.M., & Young, J.D. (1996). Cell suicide in health and disease. *Scientific American, 275*(6), 80-87.

11. Fidler, I.J., Kerbel, R.S., & Ellis, L.M. (2001). Biology of cancer: Angiogensis. In V.T. DeVita, S. Hellman, & S.A. Rosenberg (Eds.), *Cancer: principles and practices of oncology* (6th ed., pp. 137-147). Philadelphia: Lippincott, Williams & Wilkins.

12. Greco, K. (2003). How to provide genetic counseling and education. In A.M. Tranin & J. Jenkins (Eds.), *Genetics in oncology practice: cancer risk assessment* (pp. 189-224). Pittsburgh: Oncology Nursing Society.

13. Groopman, J. (1998, February 9). Decoding destiny, *The New Yorker,* pp.42-47.

evolve *Did you remember to check out the bonus material on the Evolve website and the CD-ROM, including free self-assessment exercises?*
http://evolve.elsevier.com/Black/medsurg/

14. Hetts, S.W. (1998). To die or not to die. *Journal of the American Medical Association, 279*(4), 300-307.

15. Ishii, H., et al. (2001). Potential cancer therapy with the fragile histidine triad gene. *Journal of the American Medical Association, 286*(19), 2441-2449.

16. Jemal, A., et al. (2003). Cancer statistics, 2003, *CA: A Cancer Journal for Clinicians, 53*(1), 5-26.

17. Jenkins, J., & Masny, A. (2003). Why should oncology nurses be interested in genetics? In A.M. Tranin & J. Jenkins (Eds.), *Genetics in oncology practice: Cancer risk assessment* (pp. 1-12). Pittsburgh: Oncology Nursing Society.

18. Kastan, M.B., & Skapek, S.X. (2001). Molecular biology of cancer: The cell cycle. In V.T. DeVita, S. Hellman, & S.A. Rosenberg (Eds.), *Cancer: principles and practices of oncology* (6th ed., pp. 122-134). Philadelphia: Lippincott, Williams & Wilkins.

19. King, H.C., & Sinha, A.A. (2001). Gene expression profile analysis by DNA microarrays: Promise and pitfalls, *Journal of the American Medical Association. 286*(18) 2280-2288.

20. Korsmeyer, S.J., & Zinkel, S.S. (2001). Molecular biology of cancer: Apoptosis. In V.T. DeVita, S. Hellman, & S.A. Rosenberg (Eds.), *Cancer: principles and practices of oncology* (6th ed., pp. 111-121). Philadelphia: Lippincott, Williams & Wilkins.

21. Liotta, L., & Liu, E. (2001). Essentials of molecular biology: Basic principles. In V.T. DeVita, S. Hellman, & S.A. Rosenberg (Eds.), *Cancer: principles and practices of oncology* (6th ed., pp. 3-15). Philadelphia: Lippincott, Williams & Wilkins.

22. Loescher, L.J., & Whitesell, L. (2003). The biology of cancer. In A. M. Tranin and J. Jenkins (Eds.), *Genetics in oncology practice: cancer risk assessment* (pp. 23-56). Pittsburgh: Oncology Nursing Society.

23. McKusick, V.A. (2001). The anatomy of the human genome: A neo-vesalian basis for medicine in the 21st century, *Journal of the American Medical Association, 28*(18), 2289-2295.

24. Miaskowski, C. (1999). *Oncology nursing: an essential guide for patient care.* Philadelphia: Saunders.

25. National Cancer Institute Surveillance, Epidemiology and End Results. (2003). About SEER. Retrieved August 12, 2003, from http://seer.cancer.gov/about.

26. Occupational Safety and Health Administration (OSHA). (1995). Controlling occupational exposure to hazardous drugs. *ASHP, 53,* 1669-1685.

27. Otto, S. (2001). Lung cancers. In S. Otto (Ed.), *Oncology nursing* (4th ed., pp. 380-415). St. Louis: Mosby.

28. Otto, S. (Ed.). (2001). *Oncology nursing* (4th ed.). St. Louis: Mosby.

29. Pfeifer, K. (2001). Pathophysiology. In S. Otto (Ed.), *Oncology nursing* (4th ed., pp. 3-20). St. Louis: Mosby.

30. Rieger, P.T. (2003). The impact of genetic information in the management of cancer. In A. M. Tranin, & J. Jenkins (Eds.), *Genetics in oncology practice: Cancer risk assessment* (pp. 139-188). Pittsburgh: Oncology Nursing Society.

31. Rubin, M.A., et al. (2002). Methylacyl coenzyme A racemase as a tissue biomarker for prostate cancer. *Journal of the American Medical Association, 287*(13), 1662-1670.

32. Schulmeister, L. (2001). Epidemiology. In S. Otto (Ed.), *Oncology nursing* (4th ed., pp. 42-52). St. Louis: Mosby.

33. Sessink, P.J., & Bos, R.P. (1999). Drugs hazardous to healthcare workers. *Drug Safety, 20*(4), 347-357.

34. Stetler-Stevenson, W.G., & Kleiner, D.E. (2001). Molecular biology of cancer: invasion and metastasis. In V.T. DeVita, S. Hellman, & S.A. Rosenberg (Eds.), *Cancer: Principles and practices of oncology* (6th ed., pp. 123-136). Philadelphia: Lippincott, Williams & Wilkins.

35. Tranin, A.M., Masny, A., & Jenkins, J. (Eds.) (2003). *Genetics in oncology practice: cancer risk assessment.* Pittsburgh: Oncology Nursing Society.

36. Ullrich, R.L. (2001). Etiology of cancer: Physical factors. In V. T. DeVita, S. Hellman, & S. A. Rosenberg (Eds.), *Cancer: Principles and practices of oncology* (6th ed., pp. 195-206). Philadelphia: Lippincott, Williams & Wilkins.

37. Yuspa, S.H., & Shields, P.G. (2001). Etiology of cancer: Chemical factors. In V.T. DeVita, S. Hellman, & S.A. Rosenberg (Eds.), *Cancer: principles and practices of oncology* (6th ed., pp. 179-193). Philadelphia: Lippincott, Williams & Wilkins.

Clients with Cancer

Patricia Meier

Web Enhancements

http://evolve.elsevier.com/Black/medsurg/

The continuum of disease progression begins with the precancerous and cellular level changes discussed in the previous chapter on the pathophysiology of malignant neoplasms. The goal of health promotion is to prevent cancer or to detect it early, in its most treatable stage. After a new diagnosis of cancer, the client may experience remission, stable disease, recurrence, progressive disease, end-stage or terminal disease, or long-term survivorship. Treatment modalities depend on the type and extent of the cancer but often include some combination of surgery, radiation therapy (RT), chemotherapy, and biotherapy. Bone marrow transplantation (BMT) may be part of the treatment plan. Clinical trials offer the hope of new treatments for clients.

Complementary approaches are being used in combination with other cancer treatments. The disease process and the effects of treatment on normal tissue present common complications or oncologic emergencies that require effective nursing management to achieve desired outcomes. Cancer care is not just about the disease and treatment; it comes in the midst of people's lives. Therefore an important role of the nurse in managing outcomes is to recognize, intervene, and provide support for the human responses to living with cancer.

HEALTH PROMOTION AND MAINTENANCE

Cancer Prevention and Control

The downward trend in the rates of cancer deaths in the United States is due in part to the prevention and detection of early stage cancers. Between 1973 and 1997 cancer deaths from prostate and lung cancer declined for men. Deaths of women from breast and colorectal cancer have increased. Recognizing the role of health professionals in motivating clients to alter lifestyle behaviors, the National Cancer Institute (NCI) set an objective to have at least 75% of primary care providers routinely

Nursing Outcomes Classification (NOC)
for Nursing Diagnoses—Clients with Cancer

Fatigue
  Activity Tolerance
  Endurance
**Imbalanced Nutrition: Less Than Body
Requirements**
  Nutritional Status: Food and Fluid
    Intake
Ineffective Coping (Individual)
  Coping

Decision Making
Role Performance
Social Support
Risk for Infection
  Immune Status
  Risk Control
  Risk Detection
  Tissue Integrity: Skin and Mucous
    Membranes

Risk for Injury
  Knowledge: Personal Safety
  Neurologic Status
  Risk Control
  Risk Detection
  Symptom Control

---

counsel clients about cessation of tobacco use, modifications of diet and exercise, and guidelines for screening.[35,82] These goals have been difficult to achieve from the outset, given that (1) 20% to 30% of Americans smoke; (2) 90% eat too few fruits, vegetables, and grains while consuming too much fat; and (3) more than half have sedentary lifestyles.

Prevention, Screening, and Early Detection

The three interrelated activities involved in cancer prevention and control are prevention, screening, and early detection. Primary prevention involves measures to avoid or reduce exposure to carcinogens. Screening programs help to identify high-risk populations and individuals. Early detection involves finding a precancerous lesion or a cancer at its earliest, most treatable stage.

Primary prevention activities are aimed at intervention before pathologic change has begun.[35,82] They can help to reduce cancer risk through alteration of lifestyle behaviors to eliminate or reduce exposure to carcinogens. Many cancers are associated with smoking, dietary habits, and alcohol consumption.[35,76,82] All the cancers caused by combined tobacco and alcohol consumption could be avoided. Adapting a more healthful diet and physically active lifestyle, limiting exposure to sun and other sources of ultraviolet radiation, modifying sexual practices, and decreasing exposure to environmental and occupational carcinogens would lead to further reduction in cancer incidence. (See the Complementary and Alternative Therapy feature on Physical Activity and Cancer Prevention and on Obesity and Mortality from Cancer on the website. Also see the Complementary and Alternative Therapy feature on Mediterranean Diets and Death from Cancer at right.) Exposure to carcinogens can vary widely among population segments. In lower socioeconomic, medically underserved, and nonwhite segments of the population, the incidence of cancer is increased, and cancer is usually diagnosed at more advanced stages (see the table on Cancer Problems by Ethnic Groups on the website).[79]

Secondary prevention,[35,82] also referred to as *early detection,* provides the opportunity to detect precancerous lesions or early stage cancers before manifestations become readily apparent to the client and to treat them promptly. Screening efforts facilitate early detection. Methods of early detection are (1) inspection, (2) palpation, and (3) the use of tests or procedures. Inspection is useful in identifying lesions of the skin, lip, mouth, larynx, external genitalia, and cervix. Lumps or nodules in the breast, mouth, salivary glands, thyroid, subcutaneous tissue, anus, rectum, prostate, testes, ovaries, and

COMPLEMENTARY AND ALTERNATIVE THERAPY

Mediterranean Diets and Death from Cancer

A traditional Mediterranean diet may reduce the risk of dying from cardiovascular disease and cancer. Researchers evaluated more than 22,000 apparently healthy individuals 22 to 86 years of age in Greece. Participants were rated on how closely they followed a Mediterranean diet. This type of diet is traditionally high in fruits and vegetables, legumes, nuts, cereal grains, and olive oil (monounsaturated fat) and contains moderate amounts of fish, dairy (mostly cheese and yogurt), alcohol, and low in saturated fat. Adherence to the diet was measured on a scale of 0 (did not follow the diet closely) to 9 (strictly followed the diet). After about 4 years of follow-up, the researchers found that the more closely individuals adhered to the diet, the lower their risk of death, including death from cardiovascular disease and cancer (about a 25% decrease for every 2-point increase on the scale). Thus a greater adherence to the traditional Mediterranean diet was associated with a significant reduction in total mortality.

Reference

Trichopoulou, A., et al. (2003). Adherence to a Mediterranean diet and survival in a Greek population. *New England Journal of Medicine, 348,* 2599-2608.

uterus as well as enlarged lymph nodes can be detected through palpation. Mammograms, Papanicolaou (Pap) smear, occult blood testing of feces, endoscopy, and radiologic imaging studies are some of the tests or procedures that can be used. As a result of early detection, (1) premalignant lesions may be arrested, removed, or reversed; or (2) cancer treatment can be started earlier, often while the cancer is in a stage more amenable to treatment.

Screening identifies high-risk groups of people more likely to have cancer or precancerous lesions. (For current American Cancer Society (ACS)[2,82] recommendations for screening, see the ACS WebLink on the website.) It is estimated that 75% of all cancers in the United States could be cured if all available screening tests and self-examination methods were practiced routinely.[35] Criteria for screening are as follows[35,82]:

- The population to be screened has a high incidence of the disease.
- The disease is detectable in its presymptomatic stage.
- Prognosis is poor if diagnosis is delayed until manifestations appear.
- An effective treatment is available for disease that is diagnosed early.
- There is an effective test for screening.
- The potential benefits of screening outweigh its potential risks and costs.

Approaches to Cancer Prevention

Three main approaches to cancer prevention are (1) education, (2) regulation, and (3) host modification.[35,82] A client's health beliefs can be vital determinants of learning readiness when information is made available.

The beliefs that influence the effectiveness of *education* consist of the client's perception of susceptibility to developing cancer, beliefs about the harmful or beneficial consequences of lifestyle behaviors, and perceptions about the benefits of prevention and early detection.

Methods of *regulation* used in the United States include prohibiting the sale of tobacco and alcohol to minors, limiting smoking in public places, imposing excise taxes, regulating the use of manufactured carcinogens such as asbestos, and prohibiting carcinogens in foods.

Host modification aims to alter the body's internal environment to decrease the risk of cancer or to reverse a carcinogenic process. Clinical trials of possible vaccines to immunize against some cancers, including melanoma, kidney cancer, colon cancer, and pancreatic cancer, have begun. Yet another avenue for host modification being studied in clinical trials is *chemoprevention*. This process involves the use of noncytotoxic (non–cell-destroying) nutrients, pharmacologic agents, or both to prevent or reverse carcinogenesis. Individuals who use chemopreventive agents or who participate in studies of potential

chemopreventive agents must be willing to accept the side effects and adverse risks of the agents.[25]

Prevention and Early Detection of Common Cancers

Breast Cancer

Breast cancer is the most commonly diagnosed cancer in American women, second only to lung cancer for cancer mortality. Risk factors (early menarche, late menopause, or being either nulliparous or older than 30 years at the birth of a first child) relate to their effect on circulating hormones. Incidence increases with age; more than 77% of women diagnosed with breast cancer are older than 50 years of age at diagnosis. Having first-degree relatives with or a previous personal history of breast cancer also are indicators of higher risk. Many women diagnosed with breast cancer have no known risk factors.

Breast cancer mortality could be reduced by 30% through early detection using routine screening mammography alone or together with an annual clinical breast examination by a primary health care provider beginning between 40 and 50 years of age. The ACS also recommends that women perform monthly breast self-examination (BSE) beginning at 20 years of age. The data are insufficient to determine the role of BSE in decreasing mortality; however, clients who perform BSE generally present with smaller tumors.[2,35,82] Previous studies have shown tamoxifen to be an effective chemopreventive for breast cancer. STAR (Study of Tamoxifen and Raloxifene), a national study conducted by the National Surgical Adjuvant Breast and Bowel Project (NSABP) and supported by the NCI, is currently being conducted for postmenopausal women at high risk for breast cancer. The study is comparing the effectiveness of the osteoporosis drug, raloxifene, with tamoxifen as a chemopreventive.

Lung Cancer

One in two Americans who continue to smoke will ultimately die as a result of their cigarette addiction.[2] Lung cancer is the leading cause of cancer deaths among Americans. More than 80% of lung cancers result from tobacco abuse. Other risk factors are tuberculosis (scar tumor), asbestos, exposure to radiation, and air pollution. To prevent lung cancer, clients should be counseled not to smoke. A healthy diet with at least five servings of fruits and vegetables is an added preventive step. Previous clinical trials have not found chemopreventives effective in preventing lung cancer. Spiral computed tomography (CT) scanning is being investigated for use in mass screening for lung cancer in high-risk groups. The National Lung Screening Trial, initiated in 2002, will enroll 50,000 current or former smokers.[28,82]

Colorectal Cancer

Colorectal cancer has the third highest incidence of all cancers in both men and women; the incidence is greater in men. Risk factors include familial polyposis, familial nonpolyposis syndromes, cancer family syndrome, hereditary site-specific colon cancer, and ulcerative colitis. The incidence of colorectal cancer increases with age after 50 years. Alcohol consumption, smoking, and a sedentary lifestyle are also contributing risk factors. A weaker risk factor associated with colorectal cancer may be a high-fat, low-fiber diet. There is no known prevention, although a healthy diet (high fiber, low fat, vitamins C and E, calcium, and folic acid) and a physically active lifestyle may be of benefit. Research suggests that some pharmaceutical agents such as cyclooygenase-2 (COX-2) inhibitors and aspirin may provide some protection.[2,50,80] Emerging technologies such as CT "virtual colonoscopes" and immunochemical fecal occult blood testing are being investigated. To date evidence is insufficient to recommend such technologies for routine screening.

Early detection through routine screening is the key to decreasing mortality. The ACS recommends that people with an average risk for colon cancer be screened annually with digital rectal examinations and fecal occult blood tests begin at 40 years of age, with sigmoidoscopy every 3 to 5 years beginning at 50 years of age. For people with a high risk for colon cancer, the ACS recommends discussing the frequency of monitoring with their physician.[2,35,51]

Prostate Cancer

Age is the greatest risk factor for prostate cancer; 70 years is the median age at diagnosis. The incidence increases with each decade of life beginning at age 50. African-American men have the highest incidence of prostate cancer in the world. Another risk factor is family history; almost 25% of men with prostate cancer have two first-degree relatives with the disease. An occupationally related risk factor is exposure to cadmium. Prevention strategies include limiting exposure of workers handling cadmium batteries and keeping the intake of dietary fat low.

The ACS recommends that men at age 50 years and high-risk clients at age 40 years begin receiving a digital rectal examination as part of their annual physical examination in addition to a prostate-specific antigen (PSA) blood test. The role of PSA findings in early detection is still unsettled. Early stage prostate cancer is more amenable to treatment; however, the controversy centers on whether the PSA leads to the diagnosis and treatment of prostate cancers that would never progress if not detected.[2,90] The ACS has updated their guidelines on prostate screening to recommend men be informed of the benefits and limitations of screening.[2,68] A clinical trial sponsored by the NCI is currently investigating the benefits of selenium or vitamin E supplements as chemoprotection for prostate cancer.[57]

Cervical Cancer

Risk factors for cervical cancer are closely linked to sexual behavior and sexually transmitted infections. First intercourse at an early age, multiple sexual partners, or a sexual partner who has had multiple sexual partners put a woman at increased risk. The human papillomavirus and the acquired immunodeficiency syndrome (AIDS) are also risk factors, as are low socioeconomic status and cigarette smoking. Other than changing sexual behavior and avoiding tobacco use, there are no known preventive actions the client can take to avoid cervical cancer.

The Pap smear detects cancer in a premalignant stage, which is very amenable to treatment. With adequate screening, cervical cancer should not exist; however, cultural and social barriers to prevention and early detection of this disease persist.[2,35] The ACS has updated their guidelines for the early detection of cervical cancer. They now recommend that cervical cancer screening begin 3 years after the onset of vaginal intercourse but no later than age 21. The evidence now shows there is little risk of missing a cervical cancer until 3 to 5 years after exposure to the human papilloma virus (HPV). The harm in beginning screening earlier is from inappropriate interventions because of overdiagnosis of cervical lesions that would have regressed spontaneously. After the age of 30, women who have had two normal tests can be screened every 2 to 3 years.[2,75]

Head and Neck Cancer

Men are at greater risk of head and neck cancer than are women. A synergistic effect of alcohol and tobacco use increases the risk for cancer of the head and neck. Poor oral hygiene, long-term sun exposure, and occupational exposures (asbestos, tar, nickel, textile, wood or leather work, and machine tool operation) are additional risk factors. Southern Chinese clients are also at greater risk. All clients who smoke or combine smoking with drinking alcohol should be counseled to stop these behaviors. Retinoids have been used as a chemopreventive. The evidence does not support the value of routine screening programs, although early detection by dentists and dental hygienists can identify precancerous lesions.[2]

Skin Cancer

About one million new diagnoses of basal cell and squamous cell skin cancers are made each year. These highly curable cancers are not included in overall cancer statistics. The incidence of the most serious form of skin cancer, melanoma, has been increasing by about 4% each year since 1973. Individuals with a fair complexion; a family history; multiple or atypical nevi (moles); and occupational exposure to coal tar, pitch, creosote, arsenic, or radium are at greater risk. Prevention involves avoiding ultraviolet radiation as well as limiting midday sun exposure, wearing a hat or clothing to protect the skin, using sunscreen with a sun protective factor (SPF) of 15 or higher, and avoiding severe sunburns, especially in childhood.

Early detection, especially for melanomas, is critical. Annually 37,700 melanomas are detected at a curable in situ stage. Screening programs should include teaching clients how to inspect their own skin. Moles can be mapped as a baseline for future inspections. Basal and squamous cell skin cancer frequently appears as a pale, wax-like, pearly nodule or a red, scaly patch. Note should be made of any changes, such as new moles or a sore that repeatedly scabs over but fails to heal. Moles that are asymmetrical, that have irregular borders or uneven variations in color, or that change in diameter or height should be checked by a physician. A change in the color, surface appearance, or sensation of a mole should also be reported. Clients should be taught the importance of regular self-inspection and of seeking medical attention.[2]

HEALTH RESTORATION

Maintaining Wellness During Treatment

For clients with cancer, tertiary prevention[35] consists of limitation of disability and rehabilitation. For any client who must undergo cancer treatment, maintaining optimum wellness is important to both treatment outcome and quality of life in the midst of cancer. The nurse's role in caring for clients undergoing cancer treatment to maintain optimum wellness is addressed in the later discussion of outcome management during cancer treatments.

Rehabilitation

In addition to disease treatment, rehabilitation therapy is often important to the client's quality of life. Rehabilitation may consist of reconstructive surgery after breast cancer or surgery to reverse a temporary colostomy after colon cancer treatment. An important opportunity for rehabilitation may be an exercise program to help a client counteract chemotherapy-related fatigue.

A client whose treatment has resulted in lymphedema is most grateful for the improved quality of life after a rehabilitation referral for lymphedema management. Clinicians often think of lymphedema management as benefiting only clients with breast cancer; however, professionals may overlook the possible secondary effect of lower-extremity lymphedema after treatment for prostate cancer or after treatment for other cancers that affects the lymph nodes, such as surgery for melanoma

or metastatic colon cancer. Additional rehabilitation strategies, such as speech therapy and prosthetic devices, are described in various chapters of this book in the discussions of specific disorders.

OUTCOME MANAGEMENT

Diagnosis of Cancer

Accurate diagnosis is paramount to effective cancer treatment. The vital first step in the diagnostic process is obtaining a complete history and physical examination. The history and physical assessment, together with diagnostic tests, can be highly predictive of a cancer diagnosis. Further, your careful attention to a client's history and physical status will result in accurate nursing diagnoses and interventions.

Obtain History

Because some cancers are known to be linked with certain genetic and environmental factors, you will be concerned with cancer histories of blood relatives, the client's work history, and the environmental factors that may be associated with cancer causation. (See Chapter 4 for a discussion of health history and physical assessment. Genetic history taking is discussed in Chapter 17.) You should also listen for the client's previous life experiences with cancer—whether it was of a blood relative, the client's own history, or a friend's experience. This information will be useful in assessing both the client's previous knowledge and his or her perceptions about cancer and the client's readiness for teaching.

Assess Clinical Manifestations

When cancer is in its early stages, manifestations are few. Clinical manifestations usually appear once the cancer has grown sufficiently large to cause one or more of the following problems:

- Pressure on surrounding organs or nerves
- Distortion of surrounding tissue
- Obstruction of the lumen of vessels, intestines, ureters, and so on
- Interference with the blood supply of surrounding tissues
- Interference with organ function
- Disturbance of body metabolism
- Parasitic use of the body's nutritional supplies
- Mobilization of the body's defensive response

A localized tumor usually produces manifestations related to increased pressure or obstruction in a single region. Metastatic disease and extensive tumors of major organs may display a variety of local and systemic manifestations.

Common clinical manifestations that may arise secondary to cancer include weight loss, weakness or fatigue, central nervous system (CNS) alterations, pain, and hematologic and metabolic alterations. Close assessment of such manifestations may reveal that these manifestations are directly or indirectly related to cancer.

Anorexia, weight loss, weakness, and fatigue are related to the body's inability to consume and use nutrients appropriately. Mechanical interference by tumors, malabsorption, paraneoplastic endocrine secretions (such as excessive secretion of thyroid hormones), and a tumor's use of nutrients may all contribute to a process that must be interrupted to avoid general physical debility.

The client who has difficulty with vision, speech, coordination, or memory may be experiencing primary or metastatic CNS disease. Increased intracranial pressure caused by tumor growth may cause headache, lethargy, nausea, and vomiting.

Although pain is not a common manifestation of early stage cancer, it may occur as a result of obstruction or destruction of a vital organ, pressure on sensitive tissues or bone, or involvement of nerves. Pain that is not adequately treated may become constant and progressively severe. Bone cancer is particularly painful because the rigidity of bone allows little or no expansion as the tumor cells proliferate.[52] The pain worsens when pathologic fractures produce instability and muscle spasms. Even though pain is usually a late manifestation in cancer, it may be the manifestation that brings the client to a health care provider.

Complete Diagnostic Evaluation

In addition to the history and physical assessment, laboratory and imaging studies may provide further data to support a cancer diagnosis. Many of the diagnostic laboratory and imaging studies utilized to detect other diseases are used to detect cancer. (See Chapter 4 for a discussion of diagnostic assessment.)

A variety of blood tests can be performed to help diagnose cancer (Table 19-1). Some of the more routine tests, such as the complete blood count (CBC) and differential count, do not test for specific types of cancer but indicate the presence of nonspecific problems. These tests are also vital to monitoring the side effects of treatment. Other blood tests, such as tumor marker measurements and biochemical tests, identify the extent of a particular type of cancer. Tumor markers such as PSA can be indicators of cancer; tumor markers are often even more useful as "barometers" demonstrating the effectiveness of treatment.

Unexplained anemia often indicates a malignancy. Hematologic changes include leukopenia, leukocytosis, and bleeding disorders, which in some cancers may occur before local manifestations. Metabolic manifestations, such as Cushing's syndrome, hypercalcemia, syndrome of inappropriate antidiuretic hormone (SIADH)

secretion, and carcinoid syndrome, also signify the possibility of cancer.

Basic x-rays, CT, magnetic resonance imaging (MRI), ultrasound, and other imaging studies are used in the diagnosis of cancer (see Chapter 4). When measurable amounts of tumor remain after surgery, imaging studies such as CT scans are repeated at regular intervals to evaluate the effectiveness of chemotherapy or radiation therapy.

Grading and Staging of Cancer

Microscopic evidence of malignant cells from the tumor tissue is the *only* definitive evidence of cancer. When a neoplastic growth is definitely diagnosed, it must be further defined in terms of its degree of malignancy *(grade)* and extent *(stage)*. After tissue has been obtained through a *biopsy* or the surgical removal of tumor, it is sent to the pathologist for microscopic examination. The pathologist prepares a section of the tissue to examine the specimen. The tumor *grade* is an evaluation of the extent to which tumor cells differ from their normal precursors. In low numerical grades, grades 1 and 2, the cells are well differentiated and deviate minimally from normal cells. High grades, grades 3 and 4, refer to cells that are poorly differentiated and the most aberrant compared with normal cells. Tumor grading involves a histologic and anatomic description of the cancer. The pathologist also evaluates the biopsy specimen for other characteristics that help identify the cell type of the malignancy or provide important indicators of prognosis.

Once the diagnosis has been made and the microscopic cell type and grade of the tumor have been determined, the extent of spread *(staging)* of the tumor also needs to be identified. Cancer staging is the process of determining the extent of disease as the basis for treatment decisions. *Staging* involves a systematic search for the characteristics of the primary tumor (T), involvement of lymph nodes (N), and evidence of metastasis (M), on the basis of knowledge of the natural history of the disease. The TNM system is the primary accepted system for cancer staging today (Table 19-2).

Clinical staging is based on evidence acquired before treatment and is obtained from physical examination, imaging, endoscopy, biopsy, laboratory tests, surgical exploration, and other diagnostic tests. It is based on all the information that is gathered. *Pathologic staging* is based on the microscopic evidence acquired before treatment, which is supplemented or modified by information obtained at surgery and from the pathologic examination of resected specimens, including the primary tumor, regional lymph nodes, and metastatic nodules. For example, the true stage of colon cancer is usually determined after surgery, when the regional lymph nodes are examined for the presence of tumor cells. Staging of ovarian cancer is based on the extent and location of disease found by the surgeon.

TABLE 19-1	*Laboratory Blood Tests for Cancer*	
Test	**Reference Values**	**Conditions in Which Levels May Be Altered**
Hematologic (CBC)		
Hemoglobin	M: 14-18 g/dl F: 12-16 g/dl	↓ Anemia; nonspecific; may indicate malignancy
Hematocrit	M: 40-54 ml/dl F: 37-47 ml/dl	↓ Anemia; nonspecific; may indicate malignancy
Leukocytes (WBC count)	4500-11,000/mm³	↑ Leukemia, lymphomas ↓ Leukemia, metastatic disease to bone marrow
Platelets	150,000-300,000/mm³	↑ Myeloproliferative disorders, CML, Hodgkin's disease ↓ ALL, AML, multiple myeloma, bone marrow suppression
Blood or Serum		
Acid phosphatase	0.11-0.60 mU/ml	↑ Metastatic prostate cancer
ACTH	10-80 pg/ml (in AM)	↑ Lung cancer
Alkaline phosphatase	20-90 mU/ml	↑ Cancer of bone or bone metastasis, liver cancer, lymphoma, leukemia
Calcitonin	Undetectable	↑ Medullary thyroid cancer if >100 pg/ml
Calcium	9.0-11.0 mg/dl	↑ Bone metastasis, breast cancer, leukemia, lymphoma, multiple myeloma, and lung, kidney, bladder, liver, and parathyroid cancers
Gastrin	<200 pg/ml	↑ Gastric and pancreatic cancers
LDH	100-190 mU/dl	↑ Liver cancer, liver metastasis, lymphoma, acute leukemia
Parathyroid hormone	430-1860 ng/L	↑ Squamous cell lung, kidney, pancreatic, and ovarian cancers
Serotonin	50-200 ng/ml	↑ Carcinoid syndrome
SGPT (AST)	5-35 mU/ml	↑ Metastatic cancer to the liver
SGOT (ALT)	740 mU/ml	↑ Metastatic cancer to the liver
Testosterone	M: 275-875 ng/dl F: 23-75 ng/dl	↑ Adrenal and ovarian cancers
Uric acid	M: 2.5-8.0 mg/dl F: 1.4-7.0 mg/dl	↑ Leukemia, multiple myeloma ↓ Hodgkin's disease, multiple myeloma, lung cancer
Tumor Markers		
AFP	<10 ng/ml	↑ Lung, nonseminomatous testicular, pancreatic, colon, and gastric cancers, choriocarcinoma
CA-125	<35 units	↑ Ovarian and pancreatic cancers
Calcitonin	<100 pg/ml	↑ Medullary thyroid, small cell lung, and breast cancers, carcinoid
CEA	0-2.5 ng/ml nonsmokers <3.0 ng/ml smokers	↑ Colorectal, breast, lung, stomach, pancreatic, and prostate cancers
Estrogen receptors	Positive >10 fmoles/mg	↑ ER + breast cancer
HCG	0-5 international units/L	↑ Choriocarcinoma, germ cell testicular cancer; ectopic production in lung, liver, gastric, pancreatic, and colon cancers
Progesterone receptor assay	Positive >10 fmoles/mg	↑ PR + breast cancer
Prostatic acid phosphatase	0.26-0.83 units/L	↑ Metastatic prostate cancer
PSA	0-4 ng/ml	↑ Prostate cancer
CA-19–9		↑ Pancreatic, colon, and gastric cancers
CA-15–3		↑ Breast cancer

ACTH, Adrenocorticotropic hormone; *AFP,* alpha-fetoprotein; *ALL,* acute lymphocytic leukemia; *ALT,* alanine transferase; *AML,* acute myelogenous leukemia; *AST,* aspartate transaminase; *CBC,* complete blood count; *CEA,* carcinoembryonic antigen; *CML,* chronic myelogenous leukemia; *ER,* estrogen receptors; *F,* female; *f,* femto-; *HCG,* human chorionic gonadotropin; *LDH,* lactic acid dehydrogenase; *M,* male; *mU,* milliunits; *PSA,* prostate-specific antigen; *SGOT,* serum glutamic-oxalo-acetic transaminase; *SGPT,* serum glutamate pyruvate transaminase; *U,* units; *WBC,* white blood cell; ↑, increase; ↓, decrease.

TABLE 19-2	*TNM Staging System*
Stage	**Characteristics**

Primary Tumor (T)

TX	No primary tumor can be assessed
T0	No evidence of primary tumor
TIS	Carcinoma in situ
T1, T2, T3, T4	Increasing size and extent of the primary tumor

Regional Lymph Nodes (N)

NX	Cannot be assessed
N0	No regional lymph node involvement
N1, N2, N3	Increasing involvement of regional lymph nodes

Distant Metastasis (M)

MX	Presence of metastasis cannot be assessed
M0	No distant metastasis
M1	Distant metastasis

From Miaskowski, C., & Buchsel, P. (1999). *Oncology nursing assessment and clinical care.* St. Louis: Mosby.

According to the TNM classification, cancers can be grouped into one of four stages (I to IV) or indicated as stage 0 for carcinoma in situ (without spread). Higher stages signify more extensive disease, with stage IV consistently representing distant metastasis and the worst prognosis. Grading and staging information guides the physician in choosing the intervention and estimating the client's prognosis.

Instead of the TNM classification system, other established classifications may be used for particular malignancies, such as Clark's classification for malignant melanomas and Dukes' classification for colorectal cancer. *Clark's classification* considers the level of invasion of melanomas, and *Dukes' system* refers to the depth of invasion of colorectal cancer.

Identifying Treatment Goals

The major objective of cancer therapy is to treat the client effectively with appropriate therapy for a sufficient duration so that a cure (or control) of the cancer results with minimal functional and structural impairment. *Cure* is a controversial word because of the chronic nature of most cancers; for this reason, many health care providers prefer the term *control*. If a cure is not possible, the following are important alternative goals:

- *Control* of the cancer by slowing disease progression
- *Palliation,* or alleviation of manifestations
- *Rehabilitation* to maintain a high quality of life for as long as possible or even when cure results

Decisions made at the time of first diagnosis are crucial because early aggressive intervention usually offers the best hope of cure. Even when cure is not possible, many clients with cancer have benefited from an extended life span and an improved quality of life as a result of cancer treatment.

Determining Treatment Modalities

Methods of treating clients with cancer are surgery, RT, chemotherapy, biotherapy, and bone marrow transplantation (BMT). The choice of method depends on the type of tumor, the extent of disease, and the client's comorbid conditions (such as cardiac disease), performance status, and wishes.

Performance status is a way of evaluating a client's overall health status and ability to tolerate treatment. See the table on the website for a description of two common performance status scales. In most cases, a client is treated with a combination of methods rather than a single therapy. This approach is called *combined modality* or *multimodal* therapy. Combined modality therapy is used in most cancer treatment regimens because it is more effective in destroying cancerous cells. For example, first surgically debulking (removing as much tumor as possible) an ovarian cancer increases the potential for the chemotherapy to be effective on the remaining tumor volume.

TREATMENT MODALITIES

Surgery

Surgery plays a major role in the diagnosis, staging, and treatment of cancer. It is also an integral part of the rehabilitation and palliation for clients with cancer. Surgery is used less frequently as a method of cancer prevention.

Although many aspects of surgical care of the client with cancer are similar to those for all clients undergoing surgery for any reason (see Chapter 16), some differences do exist. Several disorders chapters address surgery of a specific part of the body affected by cancer. In addition to providing expert physical care, it is important that, preoperatively, you evaluate the client's understanding of the proposed procedure and the changes it involves. The emotional impact of the diagnosis may affect the client's expectations, coping, and ability to learn. Preoperatively, clients with cancer may be nutritionally compromised and may require nutritional therapy before surgery. Those who have undergone adjuvant (treatment after removal of all detected cancer) or palliative (comfort care) chemotherapy or RT may have side effects of a low red blood cell (RBC) or white blood cell (WBC) count, which would need correction before surgery.

Diagnostic Surgery

As mentioned, the diagnosis of cancer is established by microscopic identification of malignant cells from tumor tissue. A variety of methods, most involving a surgical procedure, are used to obtain tissue for diagnostic purposes. The biology of the tumor, its size and location, and the proposed method of treatment determine which biopsy method should be used.

Cytologic specimen collection and needle biopsy are relatively simple procedures. A negative biopsy result does not prove the absence of cancer but rather might indicate inadequate or misplaced tissue sampling. Negative needle biopsy results generally must be followed by additional specimen collections to obtain an accurate diagnosis.

Cytologic Specimens. Cytologic specimens can be obtained from tumors that tend to shed cells from their surface. Tumor cells can often be obtained from cytologic examination of fluids aspirated from effusions or ascitic fluid. The physician may obtain cytologic brushings or tissue biopsy specimens while using an endoscope to examine a questionable area. An endoscopy involves direct visualization of the gastrointestinal (GI) tract, bronchoscopy of the lungs, laryngoscopy of the larynx, colposcopy of the cervix and vagina, cystoscopy of the bladder, or laparoscopy of the pelvic or abdominal cavity. During these tests, questionable areas can be examined, tissue samples and aspirates taken for biopsy, the extent of the disease staged, and pathologic processes excised.

Needle Biopsy. Needle biopsy is a simple method of obtaining tissue samples. In a *fine-needle aspiration,* tumor cells are withdrawn from the tumor with a needle and syringe. A *core-needle biopsy* is essentially the same procedure; however, the needle is larger, and a core or barrel of tissue is obtained. Core-needle biopsy allows the pathologist to examine the cells with their spatial relationships intact, whereas fine-needle aspiration provides individual cells or clumps of cells for review.

Excisional Biopsy and Incisional Biopsy. The size of the tumor and the purpose of the biopsy are determinants of whether an excisional or incisional biopsy is performed. If the suspected tumor is small, the entire tumor is excised for examination; this is called a *total* or *excisional* type of biopsy. It is used for small tumors (2 to 3 cm) for which the biopsy also may serve as the treatment if the tissue margins contain no tumor cells. If tumor cells remain, a wider excision is required.

If the tumor is large, only a part of the neoplasm is excised. This procedure is termed a *subtotal* or *incisional* type of biopsy. Stereotactic breast biopsy is a radiography-guided method for localizing and sampling small, nonpalpable breast lesions that are discovered on mammography and that suggest malignancy.

Surgery as Treatment

Surgery is performed in 55% of clients with cancer.[68] Of the clients who undergo cancer surgery, 40% are treated with surgery alone. Cancers that are localized to the or-

gan of origin and the regional lymph nodes are potentially curable by surgery, although multimodal treatment is more likely to be used to control any submicroscopic spread.

Historically, the generally accepted concept of tumor growth was an orderly sequence of growth from the organ of origin to adjacent tissue, regional lymph nodes, and eventually distant sites in a systematic fashion. The logical surgical approach to this type of growth was the widest excision possible of the tumor, surrounding tissue, and regional lymph nodes. Thus radical surgery became the standard for cancer treatment. Analysis of treatment results, however, demonstrated that, despite radical excisions, tumors recurred. Current concepts of tumor biology hold that tumors probably shed cells into the systemic circulation throughout their growth and that therefore local therapies (surgery and radiation) generally must be combined with systemic therapies (biotherapy and chemotherapy) to improve client survival.

When surgery is performed with curative intent, the type of tumor determines the extent of the excision. For slow-growing tumors, such as squamous cell carcinoma and adenocarcinoma of the skin, a wide local excision may be sufficient. Tumors of the colon and breast that spread to the regional lymph nodes are removed with an en bloc excision of the tumor and regional lymph nodes. Sentinel node mapping for breast cancer is discussed in Chapter 42 (the procedure is also used for melanoma). Large tumors, such as sarcomas, which tend to spread locally without metastasis, are removed with radical excisions, such as amputations. In all surgical procedures, various operative techniques, such as glove changing, instrument cleaning, and wound irrigation with cytotoxic agents, are used to prevent dissemination of tumor cells into and beyond the operative field.

Surgery for Recurrence and Metastasis

Cancer that recurs locally can be resected, resulting in occasional cure, remission, or both. Local recurrences of sarcomas as well as colon, breast, and skin cancers have been successfully excised. Solitary metastatic lesions that appear in the lungs, liver, or brain can sometimes be removed to effect a surgical cure. Excision of metastatic lesions is considered if (1) no other evidence of disease exists and (2) the metastatic lesion has appeared after a relatively long disease-free interval. The metastatic lesion must exhibit some stability and must be refractory (unresponsive) to chemotherapy and RT. Metastatic renal cell carcinomas, sarcomas, melanomas, and colon carcinomas have been removed in selected clients, resulting in cures or prolonged survival times.

Palliative Surgery

Because surgical procedures carry an inherent potential for morbidity, the use of surgery in palliative care is carefully considered and is used only if the risk-benefit ratio is favorable. Examples of palliative surgery that can benefit the client with cancer and improve quality of life include procedures that (1) reduce pain by such means as interrupting nerve pathways or implanting pain-control pumps, (2) relieve airway obstructions, (3) relieve obstructions in the GI and urinary tracts, (4) relieve pressure on the brain or spinal cord, (5) prevent hemorrhage, (6) remove infected and ulcerating tumors, and (7) drain abscesses.

Reconstructive Surgery

Advances in reconstructive surgery offer a different perspective on rehabilitation to the client who has experienced curative surgery. Restoration of form and function is possible to varying degrees, depending on the site and extent of surgery. Reconstructive surgery may be performed concurrently with the radical procedure, or it may be delayed. The major goal of reconstructive surgery is to improve the client's quality of life by restoring maximal function and appearance.

Preventive Surgery

The client at unusually high risk for cancer may elect to undergo a preventive *(prophylactic)* surgical intervention. Certain conditions or diseases increase the risk of cancer occurrence so significantly that removal of the target organ is justified to prevent cancer development. Clients with familial polyposis, for example, have a 50% risk of having colon cancer by age 40 years. By the time they are 70 years old, all clients with this inherited trait have colon cancer. Clients with ulcerative colitis also have a greater risk for colon cancer. Prophylactic subtotal colectomies may be indicated for this group.

Clients with multiple high-risk factors may consider preventive surgery. Prophylactic *mastectomy* (breast removal) or *oophorectomy* (ovary removal) are controversial preventative therapies. The advent of genetic testing has added further complexity to the controversy. The decision to have genetic testing can have far-reaching psychological implications for the client and other family members. Women with *BRCA1* and *BRCA2* mutations need to be counseled on the strengths and limitations of risk assessment in predicting their own likelihood of developing breast cancer.[22,33]

■ Nursing Management of the Surgical Client

Cancer operations tend to be more complex than similar procedures for benign conditions. This tendency can lead to the potential for more complications. For the most part, the postoperative care (such as wound care and prevention of infection) of the client with cancer is similar to that of any client having the same surgical procedure for a non-cancer diagnosis. The difference lies in what follows. With a benign condition, although there is certainly a period of healing and perhaps rehabilitation, the surgery usually concludes the active treatment.

With cancer surgery, however, the client often has begun only one phase of multimodal treatment. Surgery is not always the first phase of treatment because many treatment protocols begin with chemotherapy or RT to shrink the tumor mass and decrease the likelihood of micrometastasis. In the midst of the emotional impact of the diagnosis, the client and family are confronted with an often overwhelming amount of information about the diagnosis, necessary tests, treatment alternatives, and decisions to be made. The client will probably be seen or treated in multiple health care settings by many different health professionals. To help the client manage outcomes effectively, the medical-surgical nurse must not only provide excellent care during the hospitalization but also proactively assist the client with continuing care. The value of home nursing care for cancer clients is well documented. Hughes et al. found that home care nurses use a variety of interventions, especially teaching, to respond to complex problems for older postsurgical cancer clients.[38]

Assess Discharge Needs. Questions you can ask as a guide to discharge planning are as follows:

- What does the client need to know, and what does the client need to be able to do?
- Does the client know how to get to the medical oncologist's office or the clinic?
- Will the client need assistance with transportation, such as an ACS "Road to Recovery" volunteer driver?
- Would the client benefit from initial information about chemotherapy or from talking with someone who has "been there"?
- Would the client benefit from a referral for home health nursing?
- If the client or family members have questions you cannot answer, is there a social worker, oncology nursing colleague, or chaplain who can provide assistance?

See the Case Management feature on The Client with Cancer on the website.

No one person or profession can meet all the needs of the client with cancer and his or her family. To manage outcomes effectively requires teamwork involving the client, the family, the nurse, and other health professionals.

Radiation Therapy

More than 60% of all clients with cancer receive RT at some point during the course of their disease. RT may be used as a primary, an adjuvant, or a palliative treatment. When RT is used as a *primary* modality, it is the only treatment used and aims to achieve local cure of the cancer (e.g., early-stage Hodgkin's disease, skin cancer, prostate cancer, carcinoma of the cervix). For clients with laryngeal cancer, the potential for cure with RT is equal to the cure rate with surgery—but without the client's loss of the voice box.

As an *adjuvant* treatment, RT can be used either pre-operatively or postoperatively to aid in the destruction of cancer cells (e.g., colorectal cancer, early breast cancer). In addition, it can be used in conjunction with chemotherapy to treat disease in sites not readily accessible to systemic chemotherapy, such as the brain. In some situations, chemotherapy is used as a radiosensitizer. It is combined with RT and is administered before the RT dose in an attempt to enhance the effects of RT. For example, a client with rectal cancer may receive the drug 5-fluorouracil (5-FU) by continuous infusion via an ambulatory pump while receiving RT to kill residual cancer cells left behind after the surgery. Cells in the S-phase, which are relatively radioresistant, can be killed by the 5-FU.[23,40]

As a *palliative* treatment modality, RT can be used to reduce pain caused by obstruction, pathologic fractures, spinal cord compression, and metastasis. When the cancer is widespread, RT cannot be used to treat all areas of cancer spread because too much normal tissue would be harmed. RT may be used to destroy tumor in a localized area to relieve a distressing manifestation. A few radiation treatments can be quite effective in relieving pain from a metastatic bone lesion.

How Radiation Therapy Works

Radiosensitivity, the relative susceptibility of tissues to radiation, depends on the individual cells and the characteristics of the tissue itself. A highly radiosensitive tumor is greatly affected by radiation because it divides rapidly, is well vascularized, and has high oxygen content.

Radiation therapy is the use of high-energy ionizing radiation to treat a variety of cancers. Ionizing radiation destroys a cell's ability to reproduce by damaging its DNA, delaying mitosis to repair DNA or inducing apoptosis. Rapidly dividing cells are more vulnerable to radiation than more slowly dividing cells. Normal cells have a greater ability than cancer cells to repair sublethal DNA damage from radiation. Therefore the radiation oncologist may deliver a sufficient dose of radiation to kill the cancer cells while sparing normal cells from excessive cell death.

In addition to the DNA effects, a complex chain of chemical reactions occurs in the extracellular fluid, resulting in the formation of free radicals. Well-oxygenated tumors show a much greater response to radiation than poorly oxygenated tumors. Oxygen free radicals formed during ionization interact readily with nearby molecules, causing cellular damage. A well-

vascularized tumor may therefore be more responsive to RT than the same type of tumor if it is larger and, as a result, more poorly vascularized.

Types of Radiation Therapy

Radiation therapy can be administered by a variety of methods. The RT may be delivered as external-beam therapy or via a radiation source placed close to the surface of the body or inside the body. Advances in radiation therapy include (1) increased knowledge of radiation physics, (2) the use of computers making three-dimensional treatment planning possible, (3) enhancements of treatment machines to allow more precise conformal therapy of the tumor with less effect on adjacent normal tissue, and (4) stereotactic radioneurosurgery.[40]

External-Beam Radiation Therapy. External beam RT, or *teletherapy,* is the delivery of radiation from a source placed at some distance from the target site. It is administered in the RT department by high-energy x-ray or gamma-ray machines (e.g., linear accelerator, cobalt, betatron, or a machine containing a radioisotope). The major advantage of high-energy radiation is its skin-sparing effect; that is, the maximum effect of radiation occurs at tumor depth in the body and not on the skin surface. Neutron-beam therapy delivered from a cyclotron particle accelerator is currently used to treat many types of cancers, including salivary gland tumors, sarcomas, and tumors of the prostate and lung. Therapists do not remain in the room with the client during the treatment; rather, they monitor the client via closed-circuit television and remain in voice contact via an intercom.

Advances in radiation therapy include (1) increased knowledge of radiation physics, (2) the use of computers for three-dimensional treatment planning, (3) enhancements of treatment machines that allow for precise conformal therapy of the tumor with minimal effect on adjacent normal tissue, and (4) stereotactic radioneurosurgery.[40]

Internal Radiation Therapy. Internal RT involves placement of specially prepared radioisotopes (radioactive isotopes) directly into or near the tumor itself *(brachytherapy)* or into the systemic circulation. The two major types of internal RT are (1) sealed-source RT, in which the radioactive material is enclosed in a sealed container; and (2) unsealed-source RT, in which the radioactive material is administered systemically, such as by injection or orally.

Sealed-Source Radiation Therapy. Sealed-source RT is used for both intracavity and interstitial therapy. In *intracavity* therapy, the radioisotope, usually cesium 137 or radium 226, is put in an applicator, which is then placed in the body cavity for a carefully calculated time, generally 24 to 72 hours. Intracavity RT is used to treat cancers of the uterus and cervix.

In *interstitial* therapy, the radioisotope of choice (e.g., iridium 192, iodine 125, cesium 137, gold 198, or radon 222) is placed in needles, beads, seeds, ribbons, or catheters, which are then implanted directly into the tumor. For example, clients with prostate cancer may receive implanted seeds as therapy. Implants may be left in the tumor either temporarily (when ribbons, needles, or catheters are used) or permanently (when prostatic seeds are used), depending on the half-life of the isotope.

With sealed sources of internal radiation, the radioisotope is completely enclosed by nonradioactive material. Thus the radioisotope cannot circulate through the client's body, nor can it contaminate the client's urine, sweat, blood, or vomitus. Consequently, the client's excretions are not radioactive. Radiation exposure can result from direct contact with the sealed radioisotope, however, such as touching the container with bare hands or from lengthy exposure to the sealed radioisotope.

Afterloading devices have been developed in which an empty applicator (the product that holds the radiation source) is placed during an operative procedure, and the radioactive source is not loaded until the client returns to the hospital room or the radiation treatment department. The technique of remote afterloading may be used to deliver frequent, short-term, high doses of radiation directly to a selected tumor. Generally, hollow applicators are surgically placed. The radioactive source is inserted into the applicator and left in place for a specific time afterward. After a treatment, the radioactive source is removed, but the applicator is left in place if more than one treatment is planned. The client is returned to the hospital room until the next treatment. When brachytherapy is used in the hospital room, the radioactive source can be returned to the brachytherapy device while you are in the client's room providing care. Thus the use of afterloading devices has helped to decrease radiation exposure for staff but lengthens the total time needed to deliver the dose for the client.

Unsealed-Source Radiation Therapy. Unsealed sources of internal radiation are used in systemic therapy. Unsealed sources used for internal RT are colloid suspensions that come into direct contact with body tissues. The radioisotopes can be administered intravenously, orally, or by instillation directly into a body cavity. For example, iodine 131 is given orally in very low doses to treat Graves' disease (see Chapter 45) or in high doses to treat thyroid cancer. Strontium chloride 89 (Metastron) is administered intravenously for relief of painful bony metastases.

With unsealed sources of internal radiation, the radioisotope circulates through the client's body. Therefore the client's urine, sweat, blood, and vomitus contain the radioactive isotope.

Radiation Safety Standards

Three key principles you should follow to protect yourself and others from excessive radiation exposure are (1) distance, (2) time, and (3) shielding.[23]

The greater the *distance* from the radiation source, the less the exposure dose of ionizing rays. Distance and radiation exposure are inversely related. Thus the intensity of radiation decreases inversely with the square of the distance from the source. For example, if you stand 4 feet from a source of radiation, you are exposed to about one fourth the amount of radiation you would receive at 2 feet (Figure 19-1). When providing care to a client with a uterine implant, you will receive less radiation exposure if you stand at the head of the client's bed rather than directly beside the client.

You should aim to minimize the amount of *time* you are exposed to the radiation source, although you must still meet the client's care needs. Your exposure time should generally be limited to 30 minutes of direct care per 8-hour shift.[23,40] You need to plan your time in the client's room so you can spend it efficiently while providing care to the client. Time required to organize supplies should be spent outside the room. Care for the client should be rotated among available nursing staff to limit exposure for each employee. Pregnant nurses should not be assigned to care for clients receiving RT.

The use of *shielding* devices whenever possible reduces radiation exposure. The dose of x-rays and gamma rays is reduced as the thickness of the lead shield is increased. In practice, nurses have found that working with lead shielding can be cumbersome. When shielding is not feasible, you should maintain maximum distance from the radioactive source and limit the duration of exposure.

1 meter
2 meters (1/4 of exposure)
3 meters (1/9 of exposure)
4 meters (1/16 of exposure)

FIGURE 19-1 Inverse relationship of distance and radiation exposure.

With sealed-source internal radioactive implants, clients require a private room and bath because of the risk of implant dislodgment and consequent exposure of other people to the radiation. Rooms at the ends of halls or stairwells may be designated for use by such clients because their location lessens the chance that others will be exposed to the radiation. Institutions with a high volume of radiation implants may have specially designed rooms with lead-shielded walls. Shields, a lead container called a *pig*, and a pair of long-handled forceps should always be present in the client's room. If the radiation source becomes dislodged, forceps are used to pick it up and place it immediately in the pig. Generally, the radiation therapist and the radiation safety officer are notified *immediately* of the situation.[40] They retrieve and secure the radiation source.

The staff members caring for clients with radioactive implants are rotated to limit the amount of exposure of each employee. Pregnant staff should be assigned to other clients. Staff members must wear their own film badges or dosimeters while in the client's room. Because the visiting policy is restricted, the client may experience feelings of isolation.[23,40] To maintain contact while keeping distance from radiation exposure, talk with the client from the doorway of the room. Encourage family and friends to telephone. Prepare the client ahead of time for limited employee contact. Before the radiation source is inserted, the client should be provided with ways to pass the time, such as reading and handwork. Such clients usually feel well but are isolated and confined to their beds as a safety measure to prevent the appliance from being dislodged when the client is to have radioactive implants inserted in the abdominal cavity. The client has a Foley (indwelling) urinary catheter and should be eating a low-fiber diet after evacuation of the colon before insertion of the radioactive implant. The client should not have a bowel movement before the device is removed in 2 to 3 days.

The client receiving internal RT with an unsealed source also needs to have a private room and bath. Further precautions must be taken because all body secretions are radioactive. All surfaces, including the floor area the client will be walking on, are covered with Chux, paper, or other protective covering. Foods are served on disposable plates with disposable utensils. Trash and linens are kept in the client's room and are not removed until after the client is discharged. To decrease further the risk of radiation exposure of caregivers, bed linens are generally not changed unless they are grossly soiled. Instruct the client to flush the toilet several times after each use.

Visitor and staff contact is limited, as already described for sealed-source RT. Anyone entering the room wears a new pair of booties each time to avoid tracking the radioactive isotope out into the hallway. You must wear gloves to avoid exposure if you are handling body fluids. Any emesis (vomiting), especially that occurring shortly after the client has ingested an oral isotope, should be covered with absorbent pads, and the radiation safety officer should be called immediately. Additional precautions may be necessary, depending on the radioisotope used and the policies and procedures of the individual practice setting.

Before the client is discharged, instruct him or her about any precautions that should be continued at home. The radiation safety officer will scan the client to ensure that the radiation has decreased to a safe level. All precautions for the room should be continued even after the client has been discharged, until the radiation safety officer has lifted restrictions.

The U.S. Nuclear Regulatory Commission requires that radiation exposure of people be kept as low as reasonably achievable. All institutions using radioactive materials must have written policies concerning radiation protection. In addition, a radiation safety officer licensed by the U.S. Atomic Energy Commission to work with radioactive material must be available at all institutions that use radioactive materials.[23,40]

The law also requires monitoring devices, such as film badges, for health care workers exposed to radiation and the keeping of a record of each worker's exposure. Do not share your film badge with anyone. The film badge provides a measure of whole-body exposure. The general precautions—distance, time, and shielding—apply for all forms of external and internal RT. Sealed and unsealed sources of internal RT require additional precautionary measures for their safe use.

Treatment Considerations for Radiation Therapy

The goal of RT is to destroy the cancer while keeping dosages within the normal tissue tolerance to avoid harming surrounding normal tissues. Several factors determine the treatment effects and side effects of RT:

1. Tumor location in relation to surrounding normal tissue affects both treatment effects and side effects. Certain normal tissues are more sensitive to radiation and may incur permanent damage as a result of radiation. The spinal cord and the GI, integumentary, and myeloproliferative systems are at greatest risk for damage. If the spinal cord lies in the treatment field, the maximum safe dose of RT is lower than if the RT can be delivered from directions (ports) that avoid the spinal cord. Additionally, customized shielding "blocks" may be created to protect normal tissues from ionizing rays. Multileaf collimators and computer-controlled treatment machines allow precisely conforming the treatment field to the shape of the tumor and delivering the treatment dose through multiple ports.[23,40]

2. The size of the treatment field affects the dose of RT. If a small area is treated, the client can tolerate a higher dose of radiation than if a larger area is treated. RT is a regional treatment. Widespread or metastatic disease likely extends beyond the treatment field; in such situations, RT would not be an effective curative treatment modality.

3. The client's overall health or performance status affects the ability to tolerate RT. For example, a client who already has severe chronic obstructive pulmonary disease is less able to tolerate RT to the lung.

4. The therapeutic ratio of the treatment effects on the tumor to the side effects on normal tissue is an important cost-benefit determinant in decision-making about RT.

5. The side effects a client may experience are related to the total dose of radiation. Radiation dose is prescribed in units called *grays* (Gy). This term has replaced the unit of dose known as the *rad* (radiation absorbed dose): 1 Gy equals 100 rad; 1 cGy (centigray) equals 1 rad. The RT dose is higher when the goal is curative eradication of the cancer than when the goal is pain control or palliation. A client receiving 5000 cGy for cure experiences more side effects than a client receiving 2000 cGy to the same body area for palliation.

6. In general, only the area in the treatment field is affected by the radiation. For example, hair loss occurs only in the area being treated with radiation. Therefore a client receiving RT to the chest experiences hair loss on the chest but usually not on the scalp.

7. Administering the radiation in divided (fractionated) rather than single doses minimizes the side effects by allowing the normal cells time to recover. *Fractionation* refers to dividing the total radiation dose into small, frequent doses. A common dosage schedule for external RT is 150 to 200 cGy, 5 days per week, for a total of 4 to 5 weeks. Fractionation also increases the probability that tumor cells will be in a vulnerable phase of the cell cycle when treated; cells are more sensitive to RT during the late G_2 and early M phases. Fractionation allows normal cells time to repair themselves. At times, an RT dose is *hyperfractionated* (divided into smaller doses given two or three times daily rather than once a day).

Some complementary therapies are also used during RT (see the Complementary and Alternative Therapy feature on Oral Glutamine Supplements versus Placebo for the Prevention of Acute Diarrhea in Clients Receiving Pelvic Radiation Therapy at right. Also see the Complementary and Alternative Therapy feature on Low-Residue Diet for Reducing the Complications of Pelvic Radiotherapy for Cancer on the website.

■ **Nursing Management of the Client Receiving Radiation Therapy**

The staff of most RT departments includes a nurse to meet the learning and manifestation management needs of the client. Yet nurses in the chemotherapy clinic, inpatient unit, or home care setting may be faced with concerns of or questions from clients and family members about the side effects of RT.

Provide Education. In addition to the emotional impact of the cancer diagnosis, RT can be a source of fear and misunderstanding. Clients may experience fears of being burned or becoming radioactive. Because RT cannot be seen or felt during treatment, the client may also fear that the treatment is not effective. Education can dispel such common fears and misconceptions.

Comparing RT with the effects of the sun can be helpful. One generally does not notice the full effect of the sun immediately after coming indoors; so many manifestations of RT do not develop until about 10 to 14 days of treatment, and some do not subside until several weeks after treatment. If the cancer was not causing physical manifestations, the client may not have evi-

COMPLEMENTARY AND ALTERNATIVE THERAPY

Oral Glutamine Supplements versus Placebo for the Prevention of Acute Diarrhea in Clients Receiving Pelvic Radiation Therapy

A total of 129 clients were enrolled from 14 institutions for this study. Clients received 4 g of glutamine or placebo, twice a day, beginning with the first or second day of radiation treatment and continuing for 2 weeks after radiation treatment. The median age of the clients was 69 years (range, 34 to 86 years). Quality of life scores and the average number of problems reported on the bowel function questionnaire were similar for both treatment groups. The incidence of grade 3 or higher diarrhea was 20% for the glutamine group and 19% for the placebo arm. The maximum number of stools per day was 5.1 for the glutamine group and 5.2 for the placebo group. Thus no evidence of any beneficial effect of glutamine at 8 g/day was found compared with placebo during pelvic radiation therapy for cancer. Clients in this study had to be at least 18 years of age or older and have histologically confirmed adenocarcinoma or squamous cell carcinoma. Other trials are needed that use higher doses of glutamine.

Reference

Kozelsky, T., et al. (2003). Phase III double-blind study of glutamine versus placebo for the prevention of acute diarrhea in patients receiving pelvic radiation therapy. *Journal of Clinical Oncology, 21,* 1669-1674.

dence (like seeing a suntan) of the treatment's effect. If, however, the tumor was obstructing air flow, the client may realize a few weeks into the RT that breathing is easier or coughing is diminished—even before imaging studies are performed to verify tumor shrinkage. Likewise, if RT is being delivered for painful bone metastases, the client will probably note a decrease in pain or diminished need for pain medications 1 to 2 weeks into the RT.

Minimize Side Effects. In general, skin reactions and fatigue may occur with RT to any site, whereas other side effects occur only when specific areas are involved in the treatment field. The response of normal skin to RT varies from mild erythema to moist desquamation similar in appearance to a second-degree burn.[23,40] The term *burn* should not be used to describe these skin reactions, however, because doing so may frighten the client unnecessarily. Because megavoltage and cobalt deliver the maximum dose beneath the skin, skin reactions have become less significant than in years past. See the Client Education Guide feature on Skin Care Within the Treatment Field, below.

Site-specific manifestations of RT include mucositis, *xerostomia* (dry mouth), radiation caries, esophagitis, *dysphagia* (difficulty swallowing), nausea and vomiting, diarrhea, *tenesmus* (straining at stool or in urination), cystitis, urethritis, *alopecia* (hair loss), and bone marrow suppression. These may be the result of acute changes associated with inflammation or chronic changes associ-

ated with fibrosis. During RT, a CBC is usually performed weekly. The degree of myelosuppression varies with the amount of bone marrow within the treatment field. Areas at greatest risk are the pelvic region, sacrum, skull, lumbar and thoracic spine, ribs, shoulder region, and sternum.

In women of childbearing age, RT may cause prolonged or permanent infertility. In prostate brachytherapy, when radioactive seeds have been permanently implanted, there is a low, weakly penetrating radiation exposure for others. Therefore the client should use a condom for sexual intercourse in the first weeks after the procedure. Also, the client should avoid close (<6 feet) contact with pregnant women and young children (younger than 3 years) for more than 5 minutes a day during the first 2 months after implantation.[23,30]

Many of the manifestation management strategies for side effects of RT are similar to those for the side effects of chemotherapy, described later in this chapter. Information on nursing management of the general side effects of RT is included in the Oncology Nursing Society's *Manual for Radiation Oncology Nursing Practice*.[15] The NCI offers a free client education booklet, *Radiation Therapy and You: A Guide to Self-Help*.[56] A nurse or therapist in the RT department is a readily accessible source of information. Furthermore, you can alert the RT staff about the client's concern and thus help the client manage outcomes of the RT side effects.

Chemotherapy

As with surgery and RT, the goals of chemotherapy can be cure, control, or palliation of manifestations. Chemotherapy is a systemic intervention and is appropriate when the following occur:

- Disease is widespread
- The risk of undetectable disease is high
- The tumor cannot be resected and is resistant to RT

The client who is at high risk for recurrence but shows no evidence of current disease may be a candidate for *adjuvant chemotherapy;* in this type of therapy, after initial treatment with either surgery or RT, chemotherapeutic drugs are used to eliminate any remaining submicroscopic cancer cells that are suspected to be still present. Adjuvant therapy is now well established in the treatment of breast cancer.

Neoadjuvant chemotherapy refers to the preoperative use of chemotherapy to reduce the bulk and lower the stage of a tumor, making it amenable to surgery or possibly even cure with subsequent local therapy.

The objective of chemotherapy is to destroy malignant tumor cells without excessive destruction of normal cells. Several types of cancer are now considered curable with chemotherapy, even in advanced stages. Unfortunately, these tumors account for only about 10% of all cancers.

CLIENT EDUCATION GUIDE
Skin Care Within the Treatment Field

- Keep your skin dry.
- Do not wash the treatment area until you are instructed to do so. When permitted, wash the treated skin gently with mild soap, rinse well, and pat dry. Use warm or cool water, *not* hot water.
- Do not remove the lines or ink marks placed on your skin.
- Avoid using powders, lotions, creams, alcohol, and deodorants on the treated skin.
- Wear loose-fitting clothing to avoid friction over the treatment field.
- Do not apply tape to the treatment site if dressings are applied.
- Shave with an electric razor. Do not use pre-shave or after-shave lotions.
- Protect your skin from exposure to direct sunlight, chlorinated swimming pools, and temperature extremes (e.g., hot water bottles, heating pads, ice packs).
- Consult your radiation therapist or nurse about specific measures for individual skin reactions.

How Chemotherapy Works

The phases of the cell cycle are common to all cells (see Chapter 18). Normally, cells respond to the body's need for growth, repair, or regeneration in an orderly manner and cease production by entering a resting phase or slowing growth when the need is met. At any given time, normal cells are found in all phases of growth. Cancer cells reproduce in the same manner as normal cells; however, growth occurs in an uncontrollable manner and may not enter the resting phase. In general, cells that are actively dividing are the most sensitive to chemotherapy.

Chemotherapy directly or indirectly disrupts reproduction of cells by altering essential biochemical processes. The desired outcome is control or eradication of all malignant cells. Experiments and clinical experience suggest that most types of chemotherapy do not kill all cancer cells during one exposure. According to the cell kill hypothesis, only a percentage of cancer cells are killed with each course of chemotherapy. Repeated doses—or cycles—of chemotherapy must therefore be used.

The use of drugs in combination, known as *combination chemotherapy,* has consistently been far superior to single-agent therapy. Drugs selected to be used in combination must each be effective against the type of cancer being treated. When combined, chemotherapeutic agents destroy more malignant cells and produce fewer side effects because each drug strikes the cancer cells at a different point in the cell cycle. Combination chemotherapy is now the standard in most situations. The regimens are complex, cyclic, and individualized for the client and the type of cancer.

Classification of Chemotherapeutic Agents

Chemotherapeutic agents generally are classified according to their pharmacologic actions and effects on the cell generation cycle; however, the method by which cancer cells are inhibited or destroyed is not always known. A classification of common chemotherapeutic agents is shown in Box 19-1.

■ Nursing Management of the Client Receiving Chemotherapy

Only adequately prepared registered professional nurses who are skilled in the administration of chemotherapeutic agents should assume responsibility for performing it.[65] At a minimum, the nurse should have completed chemotherapy administration classes. Ideally, nurses providing oncology care are also oncology certified nurses (OCNs), who have the specialized knowledge and skills to manage potential outcomes of cancer and its treatment. It is vitally important that the bedside nurse be aware of the oncology issues of the agent being administered. Nurses who have not received education in chemotherapy administration may incorrectly believe that one will need only a

chemotherapy-trained nurse to come to the bedside long enough to hang the chemotherapeutic agent; however, careful monitoring for potential adverse reactions and side effects is required during and even after completion of the infusion. When the bedside nurse does not have the requisite knowledge, the institutional policies can ensure that a nurse with expertise in cancer care is responsible for supervising care and guiding the bedside nurse in the assessment and administration issues to give safe, effective care to the individual client. It is vitally important that the bedside nurse be aware of the oncology issues of the agent being administered. Careful monitoring for potential adverse effects during or following infusion of a chemotherapeutic agent is essential. Recommendations for course content, clinical practicum, and nursing practice can be found in the Oncology Nursing Society's *Cancer Chemotherapy Guidelines.*[14]

Assessment

A thorough client evaluation is necessary before cytotoxic drugs can be administered. Review the client's medical history to identify potential risk factors for chemotherapy toxicity, such as a history of impaired cardiac, pulmonary, or renal function. Carefully assess the severity and duration of side effects experienced since the previous course of therapy. Abnormal laboratory values may indicate organ-specific toxicities of chemotherapeutic agents. Before a subsequent course of chemotherapy, a CBC with differential count is vital in ensuring adequate bone marrow recovery since the last chemotherapy treatment. The differential count is used to calculate the absolute neutrophil count (ANC) (see later discussion), a means of determining the percentage of mature white cells. Drug doses may have to be modified or delayed on the basis of these results.

The client's chart should contain either a copy of the formal drug protocol or a written summary of the planned chemotherapy regimen. Chemotherapy doses are usually based on body surface area in square meters (m^2), which is determined by the client's height and weight. Clear and complete chemotherapy prescriptions consist of (1) the name of the drug, (2) dose/m^2 and total dose, (3) route of administration, (4) administration rate for intravenous (IV) infusions, and (5) frequency of administration. Plans for antiemetic therapy, hydration, diuresis, and electrolyte supplementation are frequently included as well. It is vital that clients know what side effects to watch for and what to do when side effects arise. See the Care Plan feature on Side Effect Management for the Client Receiving Chemotherapy on pp. 368 to 371.

Most serious side effects of the treatment do not occur in the chemotherapy clinic but develop after the client has returned home. Knowing about the expected side effects of cancer treatment and appropriate interventions increases your ability to give prompt, effective

Text continued on p. 372

BOX 19-1   *Classification of Chemotherapeutic Agents*

Cell-Cycle Specific Groups	Cell-Cycle Nonspecific Groups
Antimetabolites cytosine arabinoside or cytarabine (Ara-C, Cytosar) 5-fluorouracil (5-FU) floxuridine (FUDR) 6-mercaptopurine (6-MP, Purinethol) methotrexate (MTX) 6-thioguanine (6-TG) capecitabine (Xeloda) pentostatin (Nipent) gemcitabine (Gemzar) **Vinca Alkaloids** vinorelbine (Navelbine) vincristine (Oncovin) vinblastine (Velban) **Epipodophyllotoxins** etoposide (VP-16, VePesid) teniposide (VM-26, Vumon) **Taxanes** paclitaxel (Taxol) docetaxel (Taxotere) **Camptothecins** topotecan (Hycamtin) irinotecan (Camptosar) **Miscellaneous** L-Asparginase (Elspar) hydroxyurea (Hydrea) pegaspargase (Oncaspar) procarbazine (Matulane) imatinib mesylate (Gleevec)	**Alkylating Agents** busulfan (Myleran) melphalan (Alkeran) carboplatin (Paraplatin) cisplatin (CDDP, Platinol) cyclophosphamide (Cytoxan) dacarbazine (DTIC) ifosfamide (Ifex) mechlorethamine hydrochloride (nitrogen mustard, Mustargen) thiopeta (Thioplex) chlorambucil (Leukeran) **Antitumor Antibiotics** bleomycin (Blenoxane) dactinomycin (actinomycin D, Cosmegen) daunorubicin (Cerubidine) doxorubicin (Adriamycin) idarubicin (Idamycin) mitomycin-C (Mitomycin) mitoxantrone (Novantrone) plicamycin (Mithracin) **Hormonal Therapy** **Glucocorticoids** prednisone, hydrocortisone, methylprednisolone (Solu-Medrol) dexamethasone (Decadron) **Estrogens** chlorotrianisene (TACE), diethylstilbestrol (DES), esterified estrogen (Estratab), estradiol (Estrace) **Aromatase Inhibitor** anastrozole (Arimidex) **Anti-Estrogens** tamoxifen (Nolvadex) **Progestins** medroxy progesterone (Depo-Provera) megestrol acetate (Megace) **LHRH Analogs** leuprolide (Lupron) goserelin acetate (Zoladex) **Nitrosureas** carmustine (BCNU) lomustine (CCNU) streptozocin (Zanosar)

Data from Brown, K.A., et al. (2001). *Chemotherapy and biotherapy: Guidelines and recommendations for practice.* Pittsburgh, PA: ONS Publishing Division.

CARE PLAN

Side Effect Management for the Client Receiving Chemotherapy

Nursing Diagnosis. Risk for Injury related to side effects secondary to chemotherapy.

Outcomes. Client will experience minimal side effects of chemotherapy, will demonstrate knowledge of rationale for chemotherapy and treatment plan, and will demonstrate knowledge about potential side effects of drugs and related self-management strategies.

Interventions	Rationales
1. Monitor client during clinic or home visits or when taking phone calls for potential side effects of the drugs—while reinforcing client education of manifestations to report.	1. Some side effects, such as drug extravasation and nausea and vomiting, may occur immediately; others are more likely to occur between treatment cycles.
2. Identify and monitor for known side effects of the drugs used in the treatment regimen, including leukopenia, nausea and vomiting, diarrhea or constipation, stomatitis, hair loss, and drug-specific side effects.	2. Early detection and intervention can minimize the morbidity of adverse side effects.
3. Perform more in-depth assessment and additional nursing interventions as indicated for the symptoms identified.	3. See No. 2.

Client Education	Rationales
1. Assess client's learning readiness, including previous life experience related to cancer and expectations related to chemotherapy.	1. A family member's or friend's cancer experience—whether it has any bearing on the client's cancer experience or not—can have a major effect on the client's expectations, anxiety, and even willingness to proceed with treatment.
2. Identify family members and other support persons whom client wished to be included in education; document this information for taking phone calls from support persons.	2. Protects client confidentiality while involving client's support persons.
3. Develop a teaching plan appropriate to the client's individual needs and the specific chemotherapy regimen.	3. Each client's experience will depend on the cancer, the treatment regimen utilized, co-morbid conditions, and ability to cope.
4. Verify client's understanding of the cancer diagnosis, treatment regimen, and informed consent.	4. The information is often overwhelming to hear, and the terminology and content are often unfamiliar.

5. Provide client and family caregivers with oral and written information regarding:
  a. Chemotherapy
  b. Each drug used in the treatment regimen.
  c. Anticipated schedule of administration.
  d. Rationale for follow-up procedures, including laboratory tests, office visits, and imaging studies.
  e. Potential side effects—when they may occur, self-care management, and manifestations to report to the physician or nurse.
	5. Written information that reinforces teaching is vital. Recall alone is not likely to be efficient. Because most care is provided in outpatient settings, health professionals generally are not present when potentially life-threatening side effects appear.

Evaluation. Client will rebound quickly from side effects of chemotherapy and return to pre-chemotherapy activities.

Nursing Diagnosis. Risk for Infection related to leukopenia secondary to chemotherapy.

Outcomes. Client will remain free of infection, as evidenced by temperature remaining within normal limits. Client demonstrates knowledge related to prevention of infection.

Interventions	Rationales
1. Practice good hand-washing, especially between caring for clients.	1. These interventions will decrease the risk of exposure to a nosocomial infection. Good hand-washing is the most important means of preventing the spread of a nosocomial infection.

Data from McNally, J.C., et al. (Eds.). (1991). *Guidelines for oncology nursing practice.* Philadelphia: W.B. Saunders; and from Otto, S. (2001). *Oncology nursing* (4th ed.). St. Louis: Mosby.

CARE PLAN

Interventions	Rationales
2. Keep neutropenic clients separate from others exposed to infections.	2. When neutropenic, a client is at greater risk for infection.
3. Care for neutropenic clients before caring for other clients.	3. This helps prevent nosocomial spread of an infection to client.
4. Use aseptic technique in client care and treatments.	4. See No. 2.
5. Check baseline vital signs.	5. Baseline vital signs provide a basis for early detection of manifestations of infection.
6. Monitor hematologic laboratory results, especially complete blood count, white blood cell count, differential, and absolute neutrophils count.	6. See No. 5.
7. Monitor for signs of infection, including respiratory, urinary, oral mucosal, and skin.	7. See No. 5.
8. Administer Neupogen as ordered.	8. Neupogen decreases infection and increases WBCs in clients receiving chemotherapy who develop neutropenia.

Client Education	Rationales
1. Explain purpose of chemotherapy, how it works, and reason for potential side effects.	1. Because the client is generally home when adverse side effects arise, it is vital that the client be an involved member of the health care team.
2. Explain relationship between effects of treatment on white blood cell (granulocyte) count and potential for infection.	2. See No. 1.
3. Teach measures for preventing infections, including meticulous hand-washing and good oral hygiene.	3. Infection in the neutropenic client is potentially life-threatening.
4. Discuss necessity of avoiding crowds and people who have infection or have recently been vaccinated.	4. See No. 3.
5. If applicable to client, note the need to avoid cleaning cat litter boxes, fish tanks, and canine or human excreta.	5. These are high-risk potential sources of infection.
6. Teach the manifestations that must be reported immediately (e.g., fever, chills, sore throat, burning or pressure with voiding, purulent drainage).	6. When the client is neutropenic, an infection can become rapidly life-threatening.
7. Verify that client has, and is able to read, a thermometer.	7. See No. 6.
8. Verify that client knows how to reach the health professionals after hours.	8. The consequences of not knowing how to reach professionals in an emergency can be both serious and frightening.

Evaluation. Client will remain free of infection or seek treatment promptly if manifestations of infection appear.

Nursing Diagnosis. Imbalanced Nutrition: Less Than Body Requirements related to disease process and treatment.

Outcomes. Client will identify measures to prevent nutritional deficits and will maintain adequate nutritional status, as evidenced by body weight within preset parameters.

Interventions	Rationales
1. Evaluate nutritional status: a. Measure height and weight. b. Compare with prediagnosis weight. c. Assess laboratory values (e.g., serum albumin, complete blood count). d. Obtain anthropometric measurements when indicated.	1. Weight loss over time is an indicator of malnutrition. With significant decrease in weight, chemotherapy dosages must be decreased.
2. Monitor oral cavity for stomatitis, infection, and pain.	2. Client may avoid nutritional intake if it is painful to eat.
3. Arrange for assistance in obtaining and preparing food, if needed.	3. Adequate hydration and a high-protein, high-calorie diet that includes foods high in electrolytes (e.g., Gatorade, fruit juices, salty broths, soups, milk, green leafy vegetables) are vital to recovery of normal cells from the adverse effects of chemotherapy.
4. Refer client to the dietitian if indicators of malnutrition are present.	4. See No. 3.

Continued

CARE PLAN

Side Effect Management for the Client Receiving Chemotherapy—cont'd

Client Education	Rationales
1. Discuss relationship of adequate nutrition to disease process and treatment.	1. The client who understands the vital role nutrition plays in the treatment is more likely to make an effort to ensure an adequate intake in spite of the loss of appetite and alterations in the sense of taste.
2. Discuss the elements of a nutritional diet.	2. See No. 1.
3. Help client identify foods that are tolerated and those that cause discomfort or have become distasteful.	3. See No. 1.
4. Discuss strategies for counteracting the loss of appetite or alterations in taste and for ensuring adequate nutritional intake.	4. Suggestions specific to the client's experience (e.g., extra sweetener if foods taste bitter, popsicles for fluid intake) can be very helpful.
5. Emphasize good oral hygiene.	5. Pain and alteration of taste can impair nutritional intake.

Evaluation. Client will maintain ideal body weight and will consume adequate nutrients.

Nursing Diagnosis. Fatigue related to cancer treatment.

Outcomes. Client will demonstrate knowledge about methods that may prevent transient states of tiredness from progressing to the more intransigent states of acute or chronic fatigue and will be able to engage in a certain percentage of desired activities.

Interventions	Rationales
1. Include evaluation of fatigue in nursing assessment. Obtain data on physical performance status, response to treatments over time, and impact on activities of daily living.	1. The first step in treatment is recognition of the problem. Unfortunately, cancer treatment—related fatigue is often not recognized, and its effect not appreciated, by health professionals.
2. Review laboratory and other clinical data (e.g., oxygen saturation levels) for physiologic manifestations.	2. Fatigue is multidimensional and comprises neuromuscular, attentional, and perceptual factors.
3. Assist client in identifying aggravating and alleviating factors.	3. See No. 2.
4. Administer erythropoietin or blood transfusions as ordered.	4. Anemia is a common cause of fatigue in clients receiving myelosuppressive therapy. Erythropoietin stimulates RBC synthesis to prevent or treat anemia.
5. Carry out treatments for dehydration or electrolyte imbalance.	5. Dehydration and electrolyte imbalance can contribute to fatigue and weakness.
6. Promote sleep and rest.	6. Clients with cancer report that sleep and rest are helpful but not completely effective in addressing cancer-related fatigue.
7. Assist referrals to community resources that will reduce fatigue (e.g., physical therapy, home health services, transportation services).	7. This step allows the client to conserve energy for activities that maintain quality of life.

Client Education	Rationales
1. Inform client of the relationship of the therapy with fatigue.	1. Understanding that the fatigue can result from the therapy rather than solely from the disease can alleviate undue anxiety.
2. Prepare client to anticipate periods during chemotherapy treatments when acute fatigue is more likely to be experienced.	2. Client can plan activities related to anticipated energy levels.
3. Encourage the client to report fatigue and its effect on activities of daily living.	3. Professionals may be able to offer additional interventions.

Data from McNally, J.C., et al. (Eds.). (1991). *Guidelines for oncology nursing practice.* Philadelphia: W.B. Saunders; and from Otto, S. (2001). *Oncology nursing* (4th ed.). St. Louis: Mosby.

CARE PLAN

Client Education	Rationales
4. Help client identify strategies that may prevent transient tiredness from progressing to more intransigent fatigue: a. Vary activities. b. Use distraction techniques. c. Use relaxation techniques to dissipate the negative effects of stressors. d. Maintain good nutritional and fluid intake. e. Schedule activities to balance rest and activity in order to conserve energy.	4. An intervention before fatigue becomes intransigent is more effective. a. A variety of activities prevents boredom. b. Use of distraction helps the client focus on something besides fatigue. c. Relaxation techniques relieve fatigue by reducing effects of stressors. d. Nutrition provides a source of energy, and hydration promotes excretion of cell destruction end products/toxins. e. Results of studies of exercise programs are quite promising, whatever the exercise (bicycle ergometry, walking, or personal).

Evaluation. Client will alternate rest and activity to minimize fatigue or will not experience fatigue if erythropoietin administration prevents anemia from developing.

Nursing Diagnosis. Ineffective Coping related to cancer diagnosis.

Outcomes. Client begins process of adapting to psychoemotional stressors. Client demonstrates functional adaptive behaviors and problem-solving capacity.

Interventions	Rationales
1. Develop rapport; use active listening skills. 2. Assess coping by directly asking the client how he or she is coping with the cancer and the treatment. 3. Provide consistent, empathetic, and positive regard. 4. Support client's expression of feelings. 5. Guide the client to community resources such as support groups. 6. Refer client to appropriate and qualified professional for further intervention as indicated.	1. Client will know that you are concerned about his or her well-being as a person. Listening often is the best source of data on the depth of the impact of the cancer experience. 2. When asked, the client may share fears or concerns. The professional can offer support and suggest related interventions. 3. See No. 1. 4. See No. 1. 5. Provides client opportunity to share feelings with and to learn from others who experience cancer. 6. For some clients, the emotional impact of the cancer experience—often combined with other life issues—can be overwhelming.

Client Education	Rationales
1. Explain relationship between coping and the perception of stressors. 2. Help client identify problems, factors over which one has control, and coping methods that have worked for the client during previous life experiences. 3. Teach problem-solving as needed. 4. Teach client about keeping a journal for identification of events, feelings, and strategies used for particular problems. 5. Emphasize the importance of social network and community resources for dealing with concerns.	1. The first step in the problem-solving process is to under stand the problem. 2. Many clients experience a sense of loss of control and feelings of helplessness when confronted with a cancer diagnosis. 3. The client may not recognize that coping strategies from other life experiences can be used in coping with a cancer experience. 4. Keeping a journal can help the client identify specific concerns; possible solutions can then be identified. 5. A social network of support counteracts feelings of isolation.

Evaluation. Client will cope with cancer diagnosis by maintaining interpersonal relationships and activities.

care. In a medical-surgical or home care setting, you should be able to recognize variations from normal, perform a complete assessment of the client's status, and then report that information in a timely manner to the client's oncology caregivers. You can therefore communicate pertinent data to the oncology professional as a basis for a medical or nursing diagnosis. Nurses in all practice settings must work together, sharing information and knowledge, to ensure continuity of care for the client who is undergoing chemotherapy for cancer.

Administration of Chemotherapy

Before administering antineoplastic agents, consult with the pharmacist and review chemotherapy drug handbooks and investigational drug protocols for detailed information regarding drug actions, dosages, administration guidelines, and potential side effects. A critical step in the administration of chemotherapeutics is verification of the drug, dose, and schedule.[14,17] Chemotherapy calculations and drugs should be checked by two nurses against the written orders. Errors in chemotherapy orders may result from such factors as the misplacement of a decimal point or the dispensing of the wrong drug. An overdose of an antineoplastic agent could result in profound toxicity and death.

Educating the client and his or her family about chemotherapy and the identification, prevention, and management of side effects are primarily nursing functions. As mentioned, the Care Plan in this chapter offers an example of a plan for managing side effects of chemotherapy. The NCI provides an excellent booklet, *Chemotherapy and You*, free of charge for client teaching.[54] Hypersensitivity reaction and extravasation, discussed later in this chapter, can occur during the administration of chemotherapy. Other side effects are most likely to occur after the client is discharged from the outpatient clinic or inpatient unit. Potentially life-threatening side effects, such as infection during neutropenia (see later discussion), are more likely to occur while the client is at home, when no health professionals are available.

Routes of Administration

Two routes are discussed: IV and regional. Other routes of administration of chemotherapeutic agents include oral, subcutaneous, and intramuscular. As new chemotherapeutic agents become available in oral form, increasing numbers of clients are self-administering these drugs at home. An in-depth discussion of safe administration of oral chemotherapeutics can be found elsewhere.[11]

Intravenous Chemotherapy. Most chemotherapeutic agents are administered intravenously. *Extravasation* (escape from the vein) of some chemotherapeutic agents can cause significant harm to the surrounding tissue. Therefore you must always know before administering a drug whether it is a *vesicant* (an agent capable of causing tissue damage).

Great care should be taken in vein selection and in venipuncture technique. Large veins in the fleshy part of the forearm are the preferred peripheral access sites. Avoid areas of impaired lymphatic drainage, phlebitis, invading neoplasm, hematoma, inflammation, sclerosis, impaired venous circulation, the lower extremities, and sites distal to a recent venipuncture site. Also avoid veins that are on the dorsal aspect of the hand or over an area of flexion, such as the wrist or elbow. When administering a vesicant drug, you must be prepared ahead of time to deal with a potential extravasation to limit tissue damage. Preparation includes having immediate availability of an antidote, if there is one.[14]

In the past, vascular access devices (VADs) were placed as a last resort in clients with poor venous access. Today, because chemotherapy regimens are complex and supportive care is extensive, VADs are being used during the initial treatment of clients requiring continuous chemotherapy, multiple access, parenteral fluids, antibiotics, and frequent blood testing. Chemotherapy clients are generally satisfied with their VADs and find that they improve the quality of their lives.[22]

Implanted and external vascular access catheters are usually inserted into one of the major veins of the upper chest. Centrally implanted VADs are placed by a surgeon, generally during a brief outpatient procedure. The brachial or cephalic vein in the forearm is used for peripherally inserted central catheters (PICCs), which are often placed by specially trained nurses. The distal catheter tip is advanced to the level of the superior vena cava at or above the junction of the right atrium. Proper catheter tip placement of both central and peripheral VADs is confirmed by fluoroscopy or radiography. Various types of VADs are depicted in Figure 19-2.

In addition to VADs, arterial, peritoneal, and intraventricular access devices permit regional delivery of chemotherapy to the liver or peritoneal cavity or into the cerebrospinal fluid of the brain.[67,68] Each type of device has advantages and disadvantages, including factors such as maintenance requirements, ease of use, cost, ease of insertion, longevity, and effect on body image.

The most commonly reported complications are infection and catheter occlusion.[89] The prevention of VAD infections centers on catheter care, daily assessment for manifestations of infection, and client education. Intraluminal occlusion may occur secondary to a blood clot or precipitate. Prevention strategies include proper flushing, vigilance for drug incompatibilities, and adherence to proper drug dilutions. Other complications can also occur with VADs.[89] Nurses need to be aware that the potential for extravasation is not eliminated by using a VAD rather than a peripheral IV site. When administering a vesicant agent, diligent observation is still required to ensure early intervention if an extravasation occurs. Procedures for the care and maintenance of VADs vary

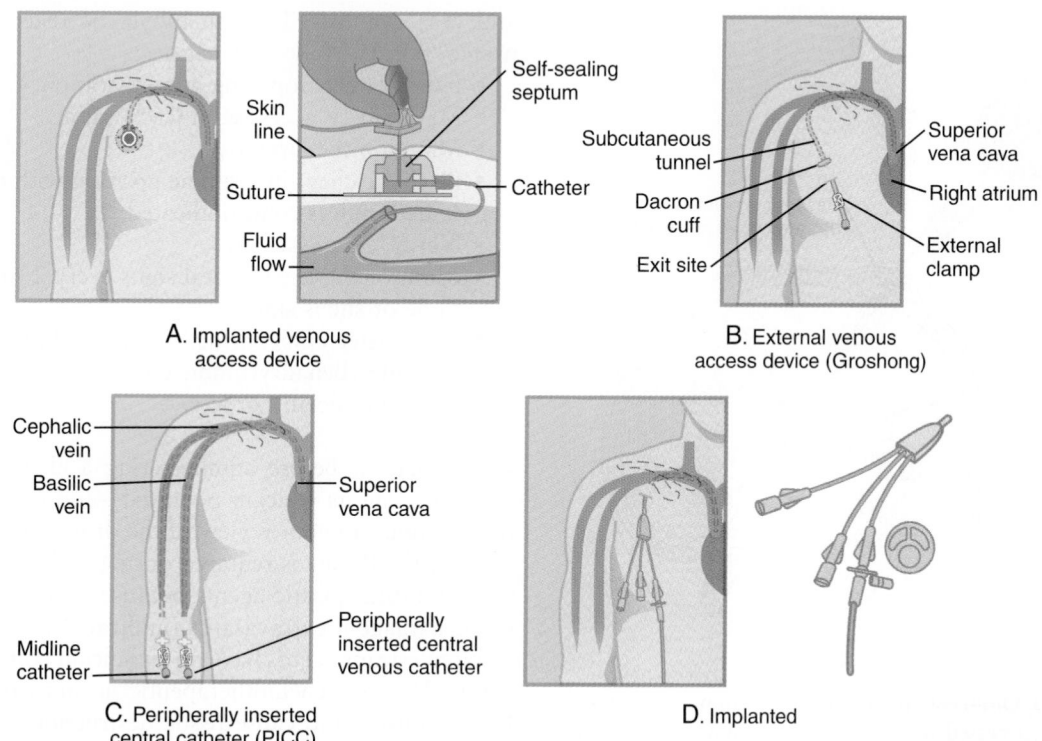

FIGURE 19-2 Catheters for administration of antineoplastic medications. **A,** Implanted venous access device or port. **B,** Tunneled external venous access device (Groshong). These can be single-, double-, or triple-lumen catheters. **C,** Peripherally inserted central catheter (PICC). **D,** Subclavian catheter. These can be single-, double-, or triple-lumen catheters.

with each clinical setting and type of device. Nursing management strategies for VADs are extensively described elsewhere.[18,47,89]

When the procedure for accessing a VAD is performed according to institutional policy and goes as expected, use of a VAD is relatively easy. Major, even life-threatening, problems can arise, however, if the VAD is not accessed correctly or the nurse does not know how to recognize a problem and the corrective action to take. Nurses who access VADs infrequently should review their institution's procedure before doing so.[89] If the procedure in any way varies from the expected, obtain the advice of a nurse who is more experienced in VADs before proceeding.

Regional Chemotherapy. Regional chemotherapy via alternative routes allows high concentrations of drugs to be directed to localized tumors. Methods are (1) topical, (2) intra-arterial, (3) intracavitary, (4) intraperitoneal, and (5) intrathecal.

Topical. Fluorouracil cream can be applied to the skin to treat actinic keratoses (sun keratoses). Squamous cell carcinoma can arise from these precancerous lesions if they are left untreated.

Intra-Arterial. *Intra-arterial* infusions involve some risk but enable major organs or tumor sites to receive maximal exposure with limited serum levels of medications. As a result, systemic side effects are lessened.

Intracavitary. *Intracavitary* therapy instills the medication directly into an area such as the abdomen, bladder, or pleural space.

Intraperitoneal. *Intraperitoneal* chemotherapy is an option for cancer involving the intra-abdominal area, such as ovarian cancer. With this method, a high concentration of a chemotherapeutic agent is delivered to the actual tumor site with minimal exposure of healthy tissues, thereby decreasing toxic side effects.

Intrathecal. Most medications given systemically are not effective against CNS tumors because they cannot cross the blood-brain barrier. The physician may instill chemotherapeutic agents into the CNS through an implanted reservoir placed in the ventricle (Ommaya reservoir—see Figure 19-3) or via a lumbar puncture. Kosier and Minkler[44] and Otto[65] provide an excellent review of the nursing management of clients with an implanted Ommaya reservoir.

Adverse Reactions

Two potentially serious adverse reactions, the seriousness of which depends on the chemotherapeutic agents,

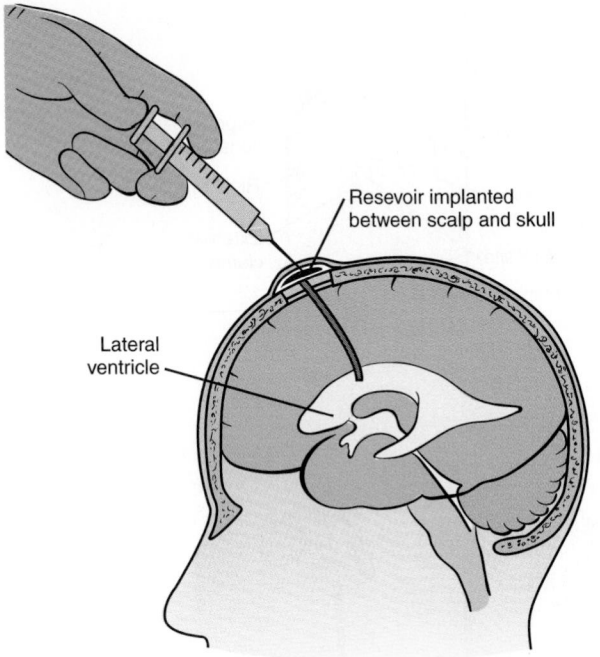

FIGURE 19-3 Ommaya reservoir. An Ommaya reservoir should only be accessed with a small-gauge non-coring or butterfly needle.

may occur during administration: hypersensitivity reactions and extravasation.

Hypersensitivity Reaction. Hypersensitivity reaction (an exaggerated immune response to a foreign substance) to chemotherapy, although uncommon, can be serious and life-threatening.[1] The antineoplastic agents most commonly implicated in the development of hypersensitivity reactions are L-asparaginase (Elspar), carboplatin (Paraplatin), cisplatin (Platinol-AQ), paclitaxel (Taxol), bleomycin (Blenoxane), rituximab (Rituxan), and teniposide (Vumon).[14] When administering a drug with anaphylactic potential (i.e., the potential to cause a possibly fatal hypersensitivity reaction), take the following precautions to ensure client safety:

- Obtain an allergy history from the client.
- Administer a test dose if ordered by the physician.
- Stay with the client the entire time the drug is being administered.
- Have emergency equipment and drugs readily available.
- Obtain baseline vital signs.
- Establish a free-flowing IV line for the administration of fluids and emergency drugs in case they are needed.

The manifestations of an immediate hypersensitivity reaction are (1) dyspnea, (2) chest tightness or pain, (3) pruritus (itching), (4) urticaria (wheals), (5) tachycardia, (6) dizziness, (7) anxiety, (8) agitation, (9) inability to speak, (10) abdominal pain, (11) nausea, (12) hypotension, (13) cloudy mental status, (14) flushed appearance,

and (15) cyanosis. If an anaphylactic reaction is suspected, take the following actions:

- Immediately stop drug administration.
- Maintain IV access with 0.9% saline.
- Maintain the airway.
- Place the client in a supine position with the feet elevated, unless contraindicated.
- Notify the physician.
- Monitor the client's vital signs every 2 minutes until he or she is stable.
- Administer epinephrine, aminophylline, diphenhydramine (Benadryl), and corticosteroids according to the physician's orders.

Extravasation. Before administering a chemotherapeutic drug, note its vesicant potential—and its antidote, if there is one—in your review of the drug. Careful assessment of the IV site is required during and after the infusion of antineoplastic agents because some agents cause tissue damage if extravasated (infiltrated).

Nonvesicant agents have no significant soft tissue toxicities. Vesicant chemotherapeutic agents can cause or form a blister and cause tissue destruction. Commonly used vesicant drugs are doxorubicin (Adriamycin) and vincristine (Oncovin). Cisplatin (Platinol-AQ) and paclitaxel (Taxol) are also vesicant drugs. Because they are commonly mixed in large volumes of fluid, the extravasation can be detected more easily before serious tissue damage occurs. Irritant drugs can produce venous pain at the site and along the vein, with or without an inflammatory reaction. Pain, erythema, swelling, and lack of a blood return indicate an extravasation.[1]

Procedures for management of extravasation are controversial and unique to each clinical setting. Institutionally approved guidelines for the management of extravasation should be readily available. Guidelines for the management of extravasation are included in the Oncology Nursing Society's *Cancer Chemotherapy Guidelines*.[14] The following are general recommendations:

- Stop drug administration.
- Leave the needle in place, and attempt to aspirate any residual drug from the tubing, needle, and site.
- Administer an antidote, if appropriate, then remove the needle.
- Do not apply direct manual pressure to the site.
- Apply warm (for vinca alkaloid) or cold compresses as indicated.
- Observe the site regularly for pain, erythema, swelling, induration, and necrosis.
- Document the appearance of the site before and after chemotherapy.

Safe Preparation, Handling, and Disposal

The safe administration and disposal of chemotherapeutic agents decreases the risk of undue exposure for the health care provider. Most chemotherapeutic agents bind directly to genetic material in the cell nucleus or affect cellular protein synthesis. The toxic potential of significantly high workplace exposure to these agents varies and is difficult to assess. The potential risks include genotoxicity, carcinogenicity, teratogenicity, and serious organ damage. Undue exposure to antineoplastic drugs can occur from three major routes:

- Inhalation of aerosols
- Absorption through the skin
- Ingestion of contaminated materials

Several organizations, including the U.S. Occupational Safety and Health Administration (OSHA), the National Study Commission on Cytotoxic Exposure, and the Oncology Nursing Society, have prepared guidelines for the safe preparation, handling, and disposal of antineoplastics.[14,23,62,63,77] These guidelines call for (1) the wearing of gloves and gowns during preparation and administration and (2) the use of a biologic safety or laminar-flow cabinet for preparation. Antineoplastic agents and their metabolites are found in the excreta and body fluids of clients undergoing chemotherapy. For this reason, you should wear gloves and disposable gowns when handling body secretions, such as blood, vomitus, or excreta, of clients who have received chemotherapy within the previous 48 hours.

Biotherapy

Biotherapy is the use of agents to affect a biologic response. The effort to understand and manipulate the human immune system has engaged scientists for decades. The observation of interactions between the immune system and malignant cells, such as spontaneous tumor remissions, continues to fuel the quest to isolate and identify effective biologic agents. Immune response remains at the core of biotherapy. Biotherapy now also includes agents that affect biologic responses in other ways (Box 19-2). In the last decade, four major technological advances have assisted scientists in their search[4,35,72]:

- A greater understanding of the complex cellular nature of the immune system

---

BOX 19-2   *Classification of Biologic Agents*

Adoptive Immunotherapy
lymphokine-activated killer (LAK) cells
tumor-infiltrating lymphocytes (TILs)

Hematopoietic Growth Factors: Erythropoietin
epoetin alfa (Epogen, Procrit)

Hematopoietic Growth Factors: Granulocyte-Colony Stimulating Factor (G-CSF)
filgrastim (Neupogen)
pegfilgrastim (Neulasta)

Hematopoietic Growth Factors: Granulocyte Macrophage-Colony Stimulating Factor (GM-CSF)
sargramostim

Hematopoietic Growth Factors: Macrophage-Colony Stimulating Factor (M-CSF)
Under investigation

Hematopoietic Growth Factors: Interleukin 11 (IL 11)
oprelvekin (Neumega)

Interferons: Interferon Alfa (IFN-α)
interferon alfa (Roferon-A)
interferon alfa-2b (Intron-A)
pegylated interferon (Pegasys)
interferon alfa-n3 (Alferon N)
charferon alfacon-1 (Infergen)

Interferons: Interferon Beta (IFN-β)
interferon beta-1a (Avonex)
interferon beta-1b (Betaseron)

Interferons: Interferon Gamma (IFN-γ)
interferon gamma-1b (Actimmune)

Interleukins: Interleukin-2 (IL-1)
interleukin 1-alpha
interleukin 1-beta

Interleukins: Interleukin-2 (IL-2)
aldesleukin (Proleukin)

Interleukins: Interleukin-3 (IL-3), Interleukin-4 (IL-4), Interleukin-6 (IL-6), Interleukin-12 (IL-12)
Under investigation

Levamisole
levamisole (Ergamisol)

Monoclonal Antibodies
satumomab pendetide (OncoScint)
capromab pendetide (Prosta-Scint)
trastuzumab (Herceptin)
rituximab (Rituxan)
gemtuzumab ozogamicin (Mylotarg)

Gene Therapy
Under investigation

Data from Brown, K.A., et al. (2001). *Chemotherapy and biotherapy: Guidelines and recommendations for practice.* Pittsburgh, PA: ONS Publishing Division.

- Progress in genetic engineering, enabling the development of recombinant biologic agents
- Advances in molecular biology
- Refined and improved laboratory equipment and computer systems

Hematopoietic Growth Factors

Hematopoietic growth factors are a family of glycosylated proteins that mediate *hematopoiesis* (the formation and development of blood cells). They are used to stimulate bone marrow recovery after courses of chemotherapy. Generally, they are named for the major cell lineage they mediate: Granulocyte and macrophage colony-stimulating factor (GM-CSF) affects both the granulocyte and macrophage lineage; granulocyte colony-stimulating factor (G-CSF) (filgrastim, Neupogen) affects only granulocytes. GM-CSF is approved for myeloid (bone marrow) reconstitution after autologous BMT and for use in clients experiencing BMT failure or engraftment delay. G-CSF and GM-CSF are approved for the treatment of chemotherapy-associated neutropenia. GM-CSF is generally well tolerated. Filgrastim is now available in a pegylated form, pegfilgrastim (Neulasta), which can be administered once per chemotherapy cycle rather than as a daily subcutaneous injection.[8] GM-CSF is currently approved by the U.S. Food and Drug Administration (FDA) for use for bone marrow recovery in BMT. It is being investigated for additional potential therapeutic benefits including anti-tumor activity, wound healing, and treatment of mucositis.[16]

Side effects of these growth factors are (1) mild to moderate flu-like manifestations, such as fever, myalgia (muscular pain), bone pain, fatigue, and headache; (2) rash, (3) a transient increase in liver enzymes, and (4) *thrombocytopenia* (reduced platelets). The most commonly reported side effect of G-CSF is bone pain. Clients report pain in bone areas that have large marrow reserves, such as the pelvis, sternum, and long bones. This pain may be the result of the marrow expansion that occurs from the rapid increase in the neutrophil pool that G-CSF causes.

Erythropoietin, another hematopoietic growth factor, is approved by the FDA for use in treating anemia secondary to end-stage renal failure and in treating anemia associated with cancer chemotherapy (epoetin alfa [Procrit, Epogen]). Clients with serum erythropoietin levels greater than 200 mU/ml are unlikely to show a response to therapy. It is important to maintain adequate levels of iron, folic acid, and vitamin B_{12} because these components are essential for the development of RBCs. The most commonly reported side effect is transient flu-like manifestations, such as *arthralgias* (joint pain) and myalgias.

Oprelvekin (Neumega) is a hematopoietic growth factor for chemotherapy-induced thrombocytopenia. Its most common side effects are edema, dyspnea, tachycardia, and conjunctival redness. More experience with the use of this treatment is needed before broad generalizations can be made about its usefulness. Oprelvekin reduces the need for platelet transfusions and allows clients to receive the desired doses of chemotherapy as scheduled.[74]

Biologic Response Modifiers

Biologic response modifiers (BRMs), which either are derived from biologic sources or affect biologic responses, are another form of biotherapy. BRMs change the relationship between the tumor and the host by altering the host's biologic response to the tumor. Many of these naturally occurring substances are hormone-like proteins or *glycoproteins* (proteins with a sugar attached). BRMs have multiple biologic actions, including production of immunologic or other biologic effects. They may augment, modulate, or restore the immune response; they may have direct cytotoxic effects; or they may produce other biologic effects, such as maturation of cells and interference with a tumor's ability to metastasize. In addition to hematopoietic growth factors, BRM agents include interferons, interleukins, monoclonal antibodies, immunomodulators, and tumor necrosis factor.[71]

Some biologic agents have already received FDA approval and are being used as part of standard therapy. Many others are being investigated in clinical trials. Rituximab (Rituxan) has been approved since 2001 for treatment of non-Hodgkin's lymphoma. Ongoing studies will help to determine whether combining rituximab with chemotherapy or interferon will lead to a significantly longer time before disease progression than with using rituximab as single-agent therapy. Trastuzumab (Herceptin) is being used in combination with paclitaxel (Taxol) for treatment of *Her*-2-positive breast cancer. Trastuzumab is being investigated as a treatment option in other solid tumors (ovarian, pancreatic, prostate) that overexpress the Her-2 protein. Tositumomab (Bexxar) and ibritumomb (IDEC-Y2B8), two agents currently being investigated, combine a radioisotope with a monoclonal antibody (MoAb).[45,83]

Interferons

Interferons (IFNs) are small proteins that have cellular activity in three areas: antiviral, immunomodulatory, and antiproliferative. Interferon-alpha received FDA approval for use in hairy cell leukemia in 1986. The drug's clinical indications have been broadened to include AIDS-associated Kaposi's sarcoma. Clinical trials are being conducted to investigate its use in other hematologic malignancies, including chronic leukemias, multiple myeloma, cutaneous T-cell lymphoma, and low-grade non-Hodgkin's lymphoma.

Toxicities appear to be dose related, with lower doses of IFN associated with few side effects and high doses having side effects that may require therapy to be interrupted or stopped. A flu-like syndrome, a common side effect of IFN therapy, may consist of fever, chills, tachycardia, muscle aches, malaise, fatigue, and headaches. Continued use of IFN produces a tachyphylactic response (rapidly decreasing response after administration of a few doses) such that these manifestations decrease in intensity over time. Premedication with acetaminophen (Tylenol) and diphenhydramine (Benadryl) is helpful in reducing the client's discomfort.

Interleukins

Most *interleukins* (proteins that serve as regulators of the immune system) are capable of inducing multiple biologic activities. A number of interleukins have been identified. Thus far, only interleukin-2 (IL-2) has received FDA approval. It is derived from T cells, augments various T-cell activities, and enhances the function of natural killer cells. Success has been seen in renal cell carcinoma and melanoma. Other areas of interest for its use are hematologic malignancies and BMT.

Major toxic responses with IL-2 therapy are due to increased capillary permeability, which may produce hypotension, ascites, pulmonary edema, fatigue, and generalized weight gain. Additionally, integumentary changes occur and may include generalized redness, rash, pruritus, and occasionally skin desquamation. Toxicity resulting from IL-2 varies greatly with the dose of drug administered. Higher doses produce greater toxicity, necessitating astute clinical management.

Monoclonal Antibodies

Monoclonal antibodies are specific antibodies directed against single antigenic determinants on the cell surface.[4] MoAbs provide high specificity lacking in other types of treatment modalities. They can be used either diagnostically or therapeutically. Diagnostic uses of these agents include the early detection of cancer by identification of surface markers on tumor cells and as a delivery agent of radioisotopes to the tumor site to aid in tumor visualization. Therapeutically, MoAbs may be used to deliver immunotoxins, such as ricin, chemotherapeutic agents, and radioisotopes, directly to the tumor site. To date, MoAbs have demonstrated limited success as a therapeutic option, and clinical trials continue for a variety of cancers.

Vaccines

The use of vaccines to treat cancer was first proposed more than 100 years ago. With a better understanding of the mechanisms of the immune response, new vaccine approaches are being investigated that are targeted toward specific antigens. Whereas the aim of vaccines for other diseases is to prevent contracting the disease, the goal of cancer vaccines is also to bolster the body's immune system to destroy cancer cells. Through clinical trials, vaccines are being investigated for several cancers, including B-cell lymphomas, multiple myeloma, melanoma, renal, breast, colon, ovarian, prostate, and head and neck cancers.[83]

Anti-Angiogenesis Agents

As discussed in Chapter 18, tumors are dependent on the angiogenesis development of blood vessels for continued growth and metastasis. Thalidomide (Thalomid) is already being used to treat relapsed and refractory multiple myeloma. Thalidomide was first marketed in the 1960s in Canada and Europe as a sedative. It was pulled off the market because of phocomelia birth defects (absence of limbs) of children born to women who had used the drug. The anti-angiogenesis effect of the drug, which limited the normal growth of limbs in the neonate, is now being exploited to limit tumor growth and metastasis. Clinical trials using thalidomide in the treatment of other solid tumors are likely to yield other therapeutic applications of this agent. Many other anti-angiogenesis agents are also being investigated.[83,85]

Emerging Targeted Therapies

New approaches in cancer therapies are based on the recognition of the abnormality in the malignant cell and developing a treatment that targets the agent. Imatinib mesylate (Gleevec) is an orally administered gene directed therapy already approved by the FDA for the treatment of chronic myelogenous leukemia (CML). It selectively blocks the abnormal *BCR-ABL* fusion gene (Philadelphia chromosome) that is vital to the survival and proliferation of CNL cells.[72]

Bone Marrow Transplantation

Bone marrow transplantation is discussed in Chapter 81. Although it is used as a primary treatment modality in leukemia, BMT may be used to counter the toxic effects of chemotherapy or RT in the treatment of breast cancer, lymphoma, and other cancers. BMT allows the client to receive lethal and potentially more effective doses of chemotherapy and RT without regard to hematopoietic toxicity. With BMT the damaged bone marrow is replaced by healthy marrow.

The client's own marrow can be harvested before treatment (*autologous* BMT). An *allogeneic* BMT involves the use of marrow from a matching donor. If the client's own marrow was harvested, the marrow may or may not have been chemically treated to destroy any cancer cells. It is then stored (frozen) to be reinfused after the chemotherapy or RT to "rescue" the bone marrow from the lethal effects of the treatment.

Clinical Trials

A *clinical trial* is a study conducted to evaluate a new treatment. The process of clinical trials provides for translation of the scientific discoveries of the past decades into safe, effective new therapies.[58] New drugs or treatment modalities are first evaluated through basic research studies in the laboratory and with animals. The most promising of these treatment approaches are then further assessed in clinical trials with human subjects. There are four phases of clinical trials[58]:

- *Phase 1:* Only a small number of clients are used as subjects in phase 1 clinical trials. The purpose of the study is to determine the maximum tolerated dose of a drug or treatment. The researchers are also watching carefully for harmful side effects. Although the treatment has been tested in the laboratory and in animals, it is not yet known how humans will respond. No direct benefit in terms of disease remission can be guaranteed. Because phase 1 studies involve significant risk without any promise of benefit, participation is offered only to people with advanced disease and for whom there are no other known treatment options. Safety, comfort, and ethical considerations are primary nursing concerns during this phase of clinical drug trials.

- *Phase 2:* Phase 2 studies are developed from the information gained from the phase 1 studies. The treatment now is offered to people with types of cancer that responded to the treatment in the phase 1 studies. The purpose of a phase 2 study is to determine the effectiveness of the treatment against those cancers while continuing to learn more about the harmful effects of the treatment. As with phase 1 studies, participation in phase 2 studies is offered only to people for whom there are no known treatment alternatives.

- *Phase 3:* In a phase 3 study, a promising new treatment is compared with a standard treatment. On the basis of scientific evidence, the researchers believe that the new treatment is likely to be as good as or better than the current standard treatment. Clients who participate in clinical trials are the first people to benefit from new, more effective treatment modalities.

- *Phase 4:* In phase 4 post-marketing surveillance studies, newly introduced drugs are monitored for adverse effects. Such studies may also compare two standard treatments. For example, surgery and RT may be compared to determine whether the survival rate following RT is similar to that after surgical treatment. Clinical trials are carried out on a nationwide basis, and the pooled results of these investigations are used to determine and validate the effectiveness of treatment regimens.

Nurses have a major role to play in these research trials. The following are nursing responsibilities associated with caring for a client who is participating in a clinical trial:

- Client education
- Documentation of treatment benefits and side effects
- Anticipation of adverse reactions and early recognition of toxicity
- Management of side effects

Research nurses have even greater responsibilities for monitoring of clients, recruitment of participants, and dissemination of data.

Once the physician or a clinical trials nurse has identified a candidate to participate in a study, the candidate can be invited to participate. A process to ensure informed consent could include a letter of invitation, informed consent education, and follow-up contact for additional questions.[58] Written informed consents for participation in a clinical trial are often lengthy and can be overwhelming. In most settings, nurses are responsible for reviewing the written consent and the physician's verbal teaching with the client. You can often help by highlighting key information in the consent form, such as the purpose of the study, the treatments being compared, and whom to contact for more information. An NCI pamphlet[101] describes important questions a client should ask when considering participation in a clinical trial.

■ Self-Care

Complementary and Alternative Approaches

Use by the public of complementary and alternative medicine (CAM) therapies is growing.[36] Estimates suggest that up to 82% of clients have used CAM therapies sometime in their lives.[84] Complementary approaches often combine one or more elements, such as (1) spiritual, psychological, nutritional, physical, pharmacologic, herbal, electromagnetic, or psychic approaches; (2) traditional medicines; (3) unconventional uses of conventional therapies; (4) unconventional instruments; and (5) humane approaches. (See the Complementary and Alternative Therapy feature on Antioxidant Vitamins to Reduce Cancer on the website and the Complementary and Alternative Therapy features on Green Tea Supplements and Cancer and on Vitamin E Supplements and Cisplatin Chemotherapy for Cancer on p. 379.

In research, prayer has been found to be a coping mechanism that correlates with perceptions of well-being.[79] Spirituality was a primary coping strategy for many persons. (See the Evidence-Based Practice in Action feature on Cancer Coping Strategies on p. 380.) Al-

COMPLEMENTARY AND ALTERNATIVE THERAPY

Green Tea Supplements and Cancer

A small study of 49 clients with a variety of cancers (mostly non–small-cell lung cancer), were given a large dose of green tea supplements (1 g/m²) for a median of 2 months. The green tea supplements were equivalent to taking 21 to 24 cups of green tea a day. No major responses occurred in any of the clients over a 6-month study period.

Reference

Pisters, K., et al. (2001). Phase 1 trial of oral green tea extract in adult patients with solid tumors. *Journal of Clinical Oncology, 19*(6), 1830-1838.

COMPLEMENTARY AND ALTERNATIVE THERAPY

Vitamin E Supplements and Cisplatin Chemotherapy for Cancer

A small study may have provided some insight into the possible benefits of certain supplements to reduce the risk of side effects from some chemotherapeutic drugs. Researchers recruited 47 clients who were randomly allocated to receive 300 mg/day of vitamin E supplements during cisplatin chemotherapy for cancer or clients received cisplatin chemotherapy alone. Most of these clients were being treated for lung cancer, but some clients were being treated for ovarian, rhinopharynx, urethral, gastric, testicular, esophageal, ethmoidal, or tongue cancer. A total of 27 clients completed the cisplatin therapy (13 clients in the vitamin E group and 14 clients in the non–vitamin E group). The incidence of neurotoxicity (a side effect of cisplatin) was significantly reduced in the vitamin E group (30.7%) compared with the non–vitamin E group (85.7%, $p < 0.01$). The severity of neurotoxicity was also significantly reduced in the vitamin E group versus non–vitamin E group. Animal studies using a human tumor cell line also suggested that this combination does not inhibit treatment with cisplatin, but more clinical studies are needed. In addition, a placebo in combination with cisplatin would have been a better study. Regardless, it could be that vitamin E supplements reduce the risk of peripheral neurotoxicity associated with cisplatin chemotherapy for prostate cancer.

Reference

Pace, A., et al. (2003). Neuroprotective effect of vitamin E supplementation in patients treated with cisplatin chemotherapy. *Journal of Clinical Oncology, 21,* 927-931.

though Sparber et al.[84] had not anticipated the high degree of importance of spirituality for clients, they concluded that there is a growing demand for integration of spirituality into health care. They also found that the use of CAM therapies increased clients' sense of control and well-being.[84]

Psychological approaches that are widely recognized yet underutilized include support groups, psychotherapy, imagery, biofeedback, and hypnosis. When used with antiemetic drugs, music can be an effective diversional therapy to decrease the frequency of nausea and vomiting.[23] Guided imagery also can help control nausea and vomiting, create a relaxation response, and control pain.[65] Art therapy can be used to help an adult with cancer gain insight into his or her situation.[79] See Chapter 5 for an overview of other complementary therapies and the NIH classifications.

Home Management of Side Effects

Aggressive, complex, and sophisticated cancer therapies are now being delivered in the ambulatory, office, and home care settings. This shift in care settings presents additional challenges for clients, family members, and health care providers. A high level of commitment is required from the client and family caregivers for the successful management of care in the outpatient setting. Clients and family members require education regarding complex treatment regimens. They must know how to recognize manifestations of side effects or adverse events, how to prevent side effects, and what they can do to treat the manifestations. Most important, they must know when to report manifestations and how to reach the physician—especially after office hours. When chemotherapy is administered in the home setting, provisions must be made for the safe handling and disposal of cytotoxic drugs to minimize client, family, and nurse exposure.[14]

Financial Concerns

Cancer care can place a financial burden on the client and family. First are the direct costs of deductibles and coinsurance. Unless the client has a prescription card, some medications, such as the serotonin (5-HT₃ [5-hydroxytryptamine]) antagonist antiemetics or oral chemotherapeutics, can be more costly than the client can afford.

In addition, cancer and its treatment often involve many hidden costs. Examples are transportation and meals for travel to clinic appointments, new clothing to accommodate weight loss or gain, medical supplies, special foods or nutritional supplements, long-distance telephone calls, and loss of income for the client or family caregiver. Ten percent, or $104 billion, of the $1 trillion spent on health care annually is used for cancer care; of this amount, $35 billion is used for direct medical care, $12 billion for lost productivity, and $57 billion for mortality costs.[46]

📖 EB EVIDENCE-BASED PRACTICE IN ACTION

Cancer Coping Strategies

Spirituality, hope, positive attitude, and support are factors reported in research studies to affect a person's ability to cope with cancer.[1-7] A research review determined that spiritual coping strategies and relationships with others and an ultimate other/God or nature were found to help individuals cope with ailments.[1] Following a review of nursing research from 1987-1999, Holt concluded the factors supporting hope for clients and families were social and professional support, cognitive strategies, spiritual or religious activities, relying on inner resources, and setting goals.[5] Ferrell determined spirituality as the main coping mechanism of women survivors of ovarian cancer.[3] The major coping strategies for young adults with cancer were social support, belief in recovery, and getting back to normal life as soon as possible.[6] The family was the most important source of emotional support.[6] Gaining knowledge about cancer and its treatment was a also good coping strategy.[6] Moreover, a positive life attitude, belief in one's own resources, belief in God, earlier life experiences, and a willingness to fight against the disease were resources for coping with cancer.[6] Variables of self-esteem, social support, and helpfulness of religious beliefs were significant in determining levels of hope in women during breast cancer treatment.[2] A positive attitude was defined as optimism for the day and getting through everyday events by taking control rather than focusing on the future. Factors that affected clients' positive attitude were their relationships with their specialists, people around them being positive and supportive, and having a pleasant environment at home and at the treatment center.[7]

Specific nursing interventions improved clients' perceptions of hope.[4,5] Nurses used interventions to support clients and families, assist with goal setting and distraction, affirm client worth, and provide symptom relief.[5] A quasi-experimental study sought to determine whether a specific nursing intervention program designed to enhance hope would positively influence levels of hope and quality of life in a convenience sample of 115 people with a first recurrence of cancer. The treatment group differed significantly (positively) from the control group with regard to level of hope and quality of life (QOL) immediately after intervention and across time.[4]

Implications

The onset of illness may render the individual being a believer or nonbeliever to realize the lack of control over his or her life. The use of spiritual coping strategies may enhance self-empowerment, leading to finding meaning and purpose in illness.[1-3] Clients with cancer must be positive for the present rather than the future. Nurses need to inspire and support client's positivity and hope while undergoing treatment for cancer.[7] Nurses should continue current practices to nurture hope in their clients. In addition, nurses need to provide spiritual care as an intervention that supports hope. Further research on nursing interventions is needed to stimulate hope as is research to understand the differences and relationships among hope, hopelessness, coping, courage, well-being, and spirituality across cultures.[5] Knowledge about the effectiveness of specific interventions designed to enhance hope is vital if nurses are to influence significantly hope in those in their care.[4]

References

1. Baldacchino, D., & Draper, P. (2001). Spiritual coping strategies: A review of the nursing research literature. *Journal of Advanced Nursing, 34*(6), 833-841.
2. Ebright, P., & Lyon, B. (2002). Understanding hope and factors that enhance hope in women with breast cancer. *Oncology Nursing Forum, 29*(3), 561-568.
3. Ferrell, B., et al. (2003). Meaning of illness and spirituality in ovarian cancer survivors. *Oncology Nursing Forum, 30*(2), 249-257.
4. Herth, K. (2000). Enhancing hope in people with a first recurrence of cancer. *Journal of Advanced Nursing, 32*(6), 1431-1441.
5. Holt, J. (2001). A systematic review of the congruence between people's needs and nurses' interventions for supporting hope. *Online Journal of Knowledge Synthesis Nursing, 8*(1), 10-20.
6. Kyngs, H., et al. (2001). Coping with the onset of cancer: Coping strategies and resources of young people with cancer. *European Journal of Cancer Care, 10*(1), 6-11.
7. Wilkes, L., et al. (2003). Positive attitude in cancer: Patient's perspectives. *Oncology Nursing Forum, 30*(3), 412-416.

EVALUATION OF TREATMENT RESPONSE

During and after treatment, the client is monitored for tumor response. Just as with diagnosis, listening carefully to the client's history and the physical examination are fundamental sources of data. If the client's cancer was symptomatic, the client may be able to predict that the treatment is working because the pain has lessened, breathing requires less effort, or other manifestations are subsiding.

When known disease remained after surgical intervention or diagnostic studies, repeating the imaging studies that were performed at the time of the diagnosis can be used to determine treatment effectiveness. Imaging studies are generally repeated after every two to three cycles of chemotherapy. If the tumor was associated with an elevated tumor marker at the time of diagnosis, testing for the marker again can be both a guide to the effectiveness of the chemotherapy and, later, a means of early detection of recurrence of the cancer. With ovarian cancer, a "second-look" surgical procedure may be performed after completion of the chemotherapy to verify that no detectable disease remains.

After treatment is completed, the client continues to be monitored for manifestations of disease recurrence and for delayed or long-term aftereffects of the treatment. Depending on the type of cancer, follow-up appointments may initially be at 3-month intervals, eventually extending to 6-month and then 1-year intervals.

■ Nursing Management of Oncologic Treatment and Emergencies

Comprehensively and successfully managing cancer-related manifestations—whether they are from the cancer itself or are side effects of treatment—is essential for achieving high-quality outcomes in cancer care. For some clinical manifestations, urgent intervention is required to prevent undue morbidity or even mortality. For example, infection, a potentially life-threatening complication in the client with neutropenia, is an oncologic emergency. When a person has few white cells, infection can progress quickly to septicemia and death unless aggressive intervention is instituted immediately. Failure to recognize, diagnose, and intervene for new-onset back pain can result in paralysis if the pain is secondary to spinal cord compression. Uncontrolled pain, discussed in Chapter 22, is often considered an oncologic emergency for the client with cancer because it so greatly interferes with the client's relationships and activities of daily living.

Both antineoplastic medications and RT can damage and destroy not only cancer cells but also certain normal cells. See the website for a box that summarizes the side effects of antineoplastic drugs. Side effects on normal cells are evaluated or graded according to the degree of severity. Mild to moderate side effects generally do not warrant discontinuation of treatment or a decrease of the dose. More severe or unexpected toxicities require careful evaluation and dose reduction.

The onset of the side effects of chemotherapy may be acute or delayed. *Acute* toxicities (1) tend to occur in tissues composed of rapidly dividing cells (bone marrow, hair, mucosa), (2) are frequently intermittent, and (3) generally resolve with complete recovery. In contrast, *delayed* or *late* effects can produce lifelong problems. Such effects include organ-specific treatment toxicities resulting in cardiac, renal, pulmonary, hepatic, reproductive, and neurologic dysfunction.

Because many of these problems appear after the client has returned home rather than in the clinical setting, the client as well as the health care providers must be aware of, monitor for, and report side effects. When taking a telephone call from a client, you must be prepared to anticipate the potential complications related to the concern that led to the call. Telephone triage is a particularly challenging aspect of ambulatory care because you must depend almost entirely on a verbal report to formulate an accurate picture of the client's situation and its urgency.

Myelosuppression

Neutropenia. Infection and bleeding, often resulting from diminished production of WBCs and platelets (thrombocytopenia) secondary to treatment, are two common causes of death in clients with cancer. The time after chemotherapy administration when the WBC or platelet count is at the lowest point is referred to as the *nadir*. For most chemotherapeutic agents, the nadir occurs within 7 to 14 days after drug administration. Knowledge of the blood count nadirs helps the health professional predict when the client is at greatest risk for infection and bleeding. Monitoring the CBC and differential count can identify when the nadir occurs and whether the client has adequate numbers of blood cells; it can also demonstrate evidence of impending bone marrow recovery.

The etiology of infections associated with cancer is multifactorial. Some cancers cause specific defects in the immune response. Side effects of treatment can result in myelosuppression (decreased RBCs, WBCs, and platelets). An impaired integumentary system can increase vulnerability to infection. Corticosteroids, which are used in many treatment protocols, suppress immune functions. Neutropenia predisposes the client to infection, especially infection by *opportunistic endogenous* (normally resident in the client's body or surroundings) organisms. More than half of the infections in clients with neutropenia are associated with organisms from the local environment. Major sources are food (raw fruits and vegetables), water, inhaled organisms, and organisms passed through direct contact. The client with neutropenia can quickly become septic; the mortality rate with septicemia can range from 30% to 80%.[66] For this reason, a CBC with differential count must be performed before administration of myelosuppressive (most chemotherapeutic) drugs and repeated periodically between treatments.

The two major types of WBCs are granulocytes (which include neutrophils) and agranulocytes. *Neutrophils* are the first and most numerous type of cell to arrive at any area of disease or tissue injury. When the number of neutrophils is substantially reduced, one of the body's prime defenses against infection is impaired. Therefore it is important to know what proportion of WBCs are neutrophils. The ANC is calculated by multiplying the WBC by the percentage of segmented and banded neutrophils in the CBC differential count:

$$ANC = WBC \times Neutrophils\ (\%)$$

On a CBC laboratory report, the neutrophils are often listed as *segs* (for segmented neutrophils) and as *bands* (banded neutrophils); the percentages of these two cells are added together to obtain the total percentage of neutrophils. For example, if the WBC count is 1200/mm³ and the percentage of neutrophils (sum of the percentages of segmented and banded neutrophils) is 34%, the ANC is 408 (1200 × .34 = 408).

Neutropenia is commonly defined as an ANC of less than 1000/mm³. The frequency of infection increases (1) as the ANC decreases below 500/mm³; and (2) with duration of the neutropenia. In the client with neutropenia, the usual manifestations of infection can be absent because of the lack of neutrophils to produce an adequate inflammatory response to the infection. Therefore fever is the cardinal, and often the only, manifestation of infection. Three oral temperature readings exceeding 38° C (100° F) in 24 hours or one temperature reading exceeding 38.5° C (101.3° F) is considered diagnostic of a fever.

Because infections are associated with greater morbidity and mortality, the development of fever in a client with neutropenia should be treated as an oncologic emergency that mandates prompt assessment, diagnosis, and intervention. Prompt initiation of antibiotic therapy for a client with neutropenic fever will increase the likelihood of a positive outcome.[66] Measures to be taken generally consist of (1) cultures, chest x-ray, and physical evaluation to attempt to identify the source; (2) broad-spectrum antibiotic therapy; and (3) monitoring of vital signs. G-CSF or GM-CSF (see earlier discussion) may be prescribed to reduce the duration and severity of neutropenia. Nursing management of outcomes begins with teaching clients the measures to protect against infection and reinforcement of such teachings as WBC counts reach their nadir. These measures are as follows[61]:

- Practice good personal hygiene, especially handwashing.
- Perform oral care daily and frequently rinse the mouth with an alcohol-free mouthwash, such as water or saline four to six times per day. Saline and baking soda (1 tsp baking soda to 1 L of normal saline) may also be used.
- Maintain adequate nutrition and fluid intake.
- Do not share eating utensils with anyone.
- Avoid raw or uncooked foods during nadir period. (There are few published studies on dietary restrictions to prevent infections.[81])
- Avoid crowds, people with infections, and children who have been recently vaccinated with live or attenuated vaccines.
- Avoid contact with animal excrement (e.g., bird, cat, or dog feces).
- Either avoid having cut flowers in the home, or change the water of fresh flowers daily, adding 1 tsp of chlorine bleach to the new water.
- Get adequate rest and exercise.
- Avoid indiscriminate use of antipyretics (e.g., acetaminophen, aspirin) because they can mask fever.

Clients should also be taught that, even with the best precautions, infections cannot always be prevented. The importance of immediately reporting any manifestations of infection must be stressed; these manifestations include the following: (1) temperature reading greater than 38° C (100.4° F), (2) cough, (3) sore throat, (4) chills or sweating, and (5) frequent or painful urination. Prompt initiation of antibiotic therapy will increase the likelihood of a positive outcome.[5]

Thrombocytopenia. Thrombocytopenia resulting from chemotherapy can cause subtle to life-threatening bleeding. A high risk of hemorrhage exists when the platelet count is less than 20,000/mm³. In the client with a solid (versus a hematologic) tumor, a platelet count greater than 10,000/mm³ puts the incidence of bleeding at less than 12%; however, fatal CNS hemorrhage or massive GI hemorrhage can occur.[33] The platelet count usually recovers within 2 to 6 weeks after the recovery of the WBC count following chemotherapy. Chemotherapy is usually withheld until the platelet count rises to 100,000/mm.[26,52]

Nursing measures to manage outcomes are used to prevent bleeding or detect early clinical manifestations of bleeding. Instruct the client to do the following:

- Avoid injury by being cautious with sharp objects and using an electric razor rather than a blade razor.
- Use lotions to prevent dryness and cracking of the skin.
- Use lubrication (women) during sexual intercourse (if sexual activity is advisable during treatment).
- Maintain good oral hygiene, and use either a soft toothbrush or, if the platelet count is very low, sponge oral swabs, and report excessive bleeding of gums.
- Avoid constipation; use stool softeners if needed.
- Avoid enemas or rectal suppositories, and report any rectal bleeding.
- Refrain from taking aspirin or nonsteroidal anti-inflammatory drugs (NSAIDs) without the doctor's permission.
- If nosebleeds or other external bleeding occurs, put pressure on the source of bleeding for 10 to 15 minutes.
- Avoid taking temperatures rectally at all times and orally if there is oral soreness or bleeding; take tympanic temperatures.
- Avoid intramuscular or subcutaneous injections; central lines can be used for parenteral medications.
- Notify the nurse or physician of manifestations of bleeding: petechiae (small red spots) or increased bruising, tarry stools, hypermenorrhea (heavy uterine bleeding), blood in urine or vomit, visual changes, and changes in level of consciousness (an early indication of intracranial hemorrhage).

Most oncologists use transfusions to keep a client's platelet count above 20,000/mm³ unless the client is known to have a platelet antibody. As previously mentioned, the thrombopoietic growth factor oprelvekin (Neumega) is now available to prevent severe thrombocytopenia following myelosuppressive chemotherapy in clients with nonmyeloid malignancies.[74]

Anemia. Anemia experienced by half of all clients with cancer can have multiple causes. There may be blood loss secondary to the disease. Abnormal destruction of RBCs is commonly a secondary disorder, arising from such causes as liver or spleen disease, BMT, nephrotoxic therapies or myelosuppressive effects of chemotherapy and RT.[29] The most common cause of anemia in the client with cancer is inadequate production of RBCs, which can result from infiltration of the bone marrow by tumor or suppression of bone marrow production of RBCs by cancer therapy.[52] Anemia leads to an impairment of oxygen delivery that is a common and predictable sequela of many cancer therapies.[52] It can cause fatigue, headache, dizziness, fainting, pallor, dyspnea, palpitations, and tachycardia.

Anemia is an important component of cancer-related fatigue, which is one of the most common and distressing manifestations experienced by the oncology client. Fatigue is poorly understood; no one definition describes all experiences. Research on cancer-related fatigue is still in its infancy. It is difficult to predict with certainty which interventions will have therapeutic benefit for which clients.[6] In addition to fatigue, anemic clients often experience decreased motivation, depression, and fatigue that interferes with normal activities. More clients identify fatigue as having more of a negative impact on their lives than cancer-related pain.[29] As advances are made in the scientific understanding of cancer-related fatigue, recommendations for interventions will very likely be altered.

Careful evaluation of exacerbating and relieving factors, the effect of fatigue on daily life, and personal and cultural influences as well as review of laboratory data add depth to the assessment of a client's fatigue and help to guide interventions.[6] Transfusions of packed RBCs can be used to relieve anemia that is producing manifestations. Erythropoietin may be prescribed to elevate or maintain the erythrocyte level and decrease the need for transfusions (see earlier discussion). Adequate levels of vitamin B₁₂, folic acid, and iron are also essential for erythropoiesis.[29] Other interventions can be grouped into three categories: (1) education, (2) exercise, and (3) attention-restoring activities. Clients who are taught that fatigue is expected report less fatigue than those who are not. Clients who balance exercise (such as walking) with rest report less fatigue. Engaging in activities that are interesting to the client may restore attention and the ability to think clearly.[6]

Gastrointestinal Effects

Nausea and Vomiting. Gastrointestinal effects of chemotherapy include nausea and vomiting, anorexia, alteration in taste, weight loss, oral mucositis, diarrhea, and constipation. The vomiting center in the medulla can be stimulated by any of five different afferent pathways or by arousal of the chemotherapy trigger zone located in the fourth ventricle of the brain. The emetic potential of a particular chemotherapeutic regimen depends on the drugs given, the dose and route of administration, and the client's susceptibility to emesis. RT to the chest, abdomen, or back can stimulate afferent pathways. Radiation-related emesis is related to the area and size of the treatment field and the dose delivered.

Adequate control of nausea and vomiting is an essential factor in a client's compliance with treatment. Uncontrolled nausea and vomiting, among the most feared treatment-related side effects, are experienced by as many as 60% of people receiving chemotherapy and can result in anorexia, malnutrition, dehydration, metabolic imbalances, psychological depression, and decreased immunity.

Three types of nausea and vomiting have been described. After the client has experienced nausea and vomiting, *anticipatory* nausea and vomiting may occur before the administration of further therapy. *Acute posttherapy* nausea and vomiting occur within minutes of the first 24 hours following therapy. *Delayed* nausea and vomiting consist of manifestations that persist or develop 24 hours after chemotherapy.[52]

Management of nausea and vomiting has greatly improved because of heightened interest and research. The addition of serotonin receptor antagonists (5-HT₃) (e.g., ondansetron [Zofran], granisetron [Kytril], dolasetron [Anzemet]) to the drug armamentarium has greatly improved the control of acute nausea caused by moderately to highly *emetogenic* (causing nausea and vomiting) chemotherapeutic agents. (See the Evidence-Based Practice in Action feature on Oral Complications of Cancer Treatment on pp. 384 and 385.) These 5-HT₃ antagonists are particularly useful for acute nausea and vomiting in the first 24 hours. They control afferent pathway stimulation from the effects of the chemotherapy on the GI tract. Ongoing evaluation is essential to find the most effective dose, schedule, and combination of these drugs.[3]

Nonpharmacologic interventions for nausea and vomiting related to chemotherapy include adjustment of oral and fluid intake, relaxation, exercise, hypnosis, biofeedback, guided imagery, and systemic desensitization. The client and caregivers should avoid offensive odors, such as those from flowers or foods. Food servings should be kept small and offered four to six times per day.

Anorexia. Anorexia and weight loss occur as a result of the disease process as well as the treatment. The client

EB EVIDENCE-BASED PRACTICE IN ACTION

Oral Complications of Cancer Treatment

In the past, nausea and vomiting and neutropenia were the most common dose-limiting toxicities of cancer therapy. The advent of serotonin receptor antagonists (ondansetron [Zofran], granisetron [Kytril], dolasetron [Anzemet]), and the hematopoietic growth factors (G-CSF [Neupogen] and erythropoietin [Procrit]) have allowed for improved control of these treatment-related side effects. Mucositis is now the principal dose-limiting toxicity of cancer treatments.[5,8]

Mucositis is inflammation with erythema or ulceration of the mucous membrane resulting from cancer therapy. It often involves not only the oral cavity but also the mucous membrane of the entire GI tract. Pain and infection often accompany mucosal injury. The prevalence of mucositis varies widely with the multiple treatment protocols that use different chemotherapeutic agents or ionizing radiation utilized. Of clients receiving chemotherapy, 30% to 40% experience oral complications. Up to 75% of clients receiving the agent 5-FU and 80% of clients undergoing hematopoietic stem cell transplant experience mucositis. Oral complications of head and neck radiation are often more severe than the complications of chemotherapy and can lead to permanent tissue changes.[2,3,5,7,8,12]

Oral complications can greatly affect morbidity and mortality and increase health care costs. Oral complications often necessitate dose reductions or treatment delays, which affects treatment outcomes, and prognosis. Along with the impact on the client's overall health and quality of life, this is a strong impetus for aggressive efforts to prevent or treat oral complications.[1,5,8,9,11] Because of pain and difficulty swallowing, nutritional intake can be impaired, resulting in dehydration and weight loss or cachexia. Mucositis may be further complicated by infection or bleeding. Mucosal atrophy of salivary glands secondary to radiation therapy can cause xerostomia. Oral pain, which can be severe, interferes with one's ability to talk, smile, or kiss a loved one.[2,5,8]

Recommendations gleaned from the current literature addresses the importance of an oral care standard. Systematic oral care is more important than any specific agent. This begins with identifying clients at risk and doing regular oral assessments.[5,6,8,11,13] Ideally involvement of a dentist beginning before treatment may reduce the risks of oral complications.[12] The importance of hand-washing before beginning oral assessment or care is understood. Use of a tool such as the "Oral Assessment Guide" by Eilers and colleagues is helpful in ensuring a comprehensive oral assessment.[4,11] A soft toothbrush has been found to be better than foam brushes and preferred by clients. A foam brush soaked in chlorhexidine can effectively remove plaque.[11] Electric toothbrushes may result in improved mouth care but may harm tender gums and cause bleeding.[10,12] Clients should also avoid whitening toothpastes.[5] Research dating back to the 1960s showed lemon-glycerin swabs do more harm than good because they decalcify the teeth, make the pH of the mouth more acidic, and dry mucous membranes. Yet it has taken decades to eliminate this nursing practice gradually.[3,5,10,11]

Dilute hydrogen peroxide was once routinely used as an oral rinse; however, studies have shown that it can harm new tissue and interfere with healing and promote fungal overgrowth. It should be used only for short periods as a cleansing agent.[11,12] Sodium bicarbonate or saline is often recommended as a mouthwash agent. Saline aids in the formation of granulation tissue. Sodium bicarbonate, however, creates an alkaline environment that can allow bacteria to multiply.[3,10,11] Chlorhexidine mouthwashes have the best antibacterial, antifungal effect, but it has an unpleasant taste and causes burning and stinging.[10,11] Fluoride rinses may be particularly beneficial for head and neck RT clients by preventing dental caries.[8] Clients should avoid most commercial mouthwashes because they contain 6% to 27% alcohol, which can dry the mucous membranes.[5,10,12] Frequent rinsing, however, is more important than the agent used. If clients do not like the taste of these agents, rinsing with plain water would be better than infrequent rinsing.[5] Recommendations for frequency of rinsing the mouth range from every 2 to 6 hours. Benefits of rinsing are diminished if the intervals are longer than 6 hours.[11-13]

Studies have shown conflicting findings on flossing. Flossing aids in the control of dental plaque; however, some cancer centers recommend not brushing or flossing if the platelet count falls below 30,000.[12] Artificial salivas, often prescribed for clients with xerostomia, have short-lived action. Based on clinical experience, some clinicians recommend sugar-free gum, ice lollies, or sipping on water.[11] Pain associated with oral complications often is mild to moderate, but can be severe. It is most often described as tender, sore, burning, dull, aching, or irritating. Systemic analgesics may be necessary when topical agents such as viscous lidocaine are not sufficient for pain reduction. Clients may not experience oral pain until the mucositis or stomatitis is quite severe.[6,7,12] Teaching the client to do his or her own oral assessments and the importance of regular mouth care are important because most cancer treatment is provided in the outpatient setting.[1,11]

Implications

Effective oral care must be a priority component of nursing care of the client receiving cancer treatment. Goals of oral care include cleanliness, comfort, and prevention of infection. Most research to date has focused on specific agents such as saline or other mouthwashes. Results have generally shown little difference and conflicting findings. Research and the experience of oncology professionals lends credibility to their recommendations.[9-11]

With our improved understanding of the biology of tissue injury, the potential for research is at a pivotal point. In addition to traditional agents, researchers are now looking at the potential for growth factors to reduce incidence of mucositis. Outcomes

E B EVIDENCE-BASED PRACTICE IN ACTION

Oral Complications of Cancer Treatment—cont'd

that could be studied include the extent or severity of tissue injury, pain, infection, impairment of nutritional status, impact on health care costs or hospital length of stays, and quality of life. As new research is reported, nurses who want to provide great care must update their knowledge and adapt their caregiving to incorporate the latest scientific knowledge.[1,2,8]

References

1. Coleman, E.A., et al. (2002). Symptom management and successful outpatient transplantation for patients with multiple myeloma. *Cancer Nursing, 25*(6), 452-460.

2. Dodd, M.J., et al. (2000). Factors influencing oral mucositis in patients receiving chemotherapy. *Cancer Practice, 8*(6), 291-297.

3. Dose, A.M. (1995). The symptom experience of mucositis, stomatitis and xerostomia. *Seminars in Oncology Nursing, 11*(4), 248-255.

4. Eilers, J., Berger, A., & Peterson, M. (1998). Development, testing, and application of the oral assessment guide. *Oncology Nursing Forum, 15,* 325-330.

5. Eilers, J. (2003). When the mouth tells us more than it says—The impact of mucositis on quality of life. *Oncology Supportive Care, 1*(4), 31-43.

6. Ganley, B.J. (1996). Mouth care for the patient undergoing head and neck radiation therapy: A survey of radiation oncology nurses. *Oncology Nursing Forum, 23*(10) 1619-1623.

7. McGuire, D.B., et al. (1998). Acute oral pain and mucositis in bone marrow transplant and leukemia patients: Data from a pilot study. *Cancer Nursing, 21*(16) 385-393.

8. McGuire, D.B. (2002). Mucosal tissue injury in cancer therapy. More than mucositis and mouthwash. *Cancer Practice, 10*(4), 179-191.

9. Madeya, M.L. (1996). Oral complications from cancer therapy: Part 1 - Pathophysiology and secondary complications. *Oncology Nursing Forum, 23*(5), 801-807.

10. Madeya, M.L. (1996). Oral complications from cancer therapy: Part 2—Nursing implications for assessment and treatment. *Oncology Nursing Forum, 23*(5), 808-819.

11. Miller, M., & Kearney, N. (2001). Oral care for patients with cancer: A review of the literature. *Cancer Nursing, 24*(4), 241-254.

12. National Cancer Institute (2003). Oral complications of chemotherapy and head/neck radiation. Retrieved August, 2003 from http://www.cancerinfo/pdg/supportivecare/oralcomplications/professionals

13. Yeager, K.A., et al. (2000). Implementation of an oral care standard for leukemia and transplantation patients. *Cancer Nursing, 23*(1), 40-48.

with cancer is at risk for protein-calorie malnutrition, which can lead to potentially severe consequences, including (1) diminished activity tolerance, (2) lowered survival rates, and (3) diminished quality of life.[92] Many variables, in addition to the effects of chemotherapy, can alter the client's ability to ingest food via the oral route. Common problems that may interfere with oral intake are anorexia, nausea and vomiting, early satiety, alterations in taste, dry mouth, stomatitis, esophagitis, viscous saliva, lactose intolerance, pain, diarrhea, and constipation.

Nursing management to prevent a compromised nutritional state is based on assessment. Weight loss of 5% or more of body weight in a 1-month period is considered significant. In assessing the client, you can begin by identifying potential interventions appropriate to the client's situation. If indicated, a referral can be made to a dietitian for a more comprehensive assessment. When medically appropriate, oral nutrition can be enhanced by relaxing dietary restrictions and emphasizing the need for a high-protein, high-calorie diet with fortification from natural food sources or commercial supplements. An excellent source of helpful tips and recipes for nutritious foods can be found in the booklet *Eating Hints,* which can be obtained free of charge from the NCI.[55]

Enteral and parenteral feedings for the client with protein-calorie malnutrition are discussed in Chapter 31.

Stomatitis. *Stomatitis,* or *oral mucositis,* is the term used to describe inflammation and ulceration of the mucosal lining of the mouth. The inflammation seen in the mouth is also present throughout the GI tract of a client with cancer or receiving cancer treatment. The severity of the stomatitis can affect the client's quality of life. Consequences of stomatitis include pain, decreased nutritional and fluid intake, infections, malabsorption, diarrhea, and delay of chemotherapy and RT treatments. Candida or other fungal infections that ordinarily live in the GI tract and environment are generally harmless to individuals with healthy immune systems, but can become pathogenic to immunocompromised clients. Candida species are associated with mortality as well as significant morbidity and debility.

Nursing assessment and interventions are discussed in Chapter 32. An oral hygiene program should start before therapy and should continue throughout treatment. Such a program consists of the following:

- A dental examination and treatment before therapy begins

- Thorough and gentle cleaning to avoid further trauma
- Moisturization if saliva is scanty or absent
- Avoidance of alcohol and smoking
- Culture analysis and antimicrobial therapy for infections
- Topical anesthetics and analgesics for pain or discomfort

Dietary modifications include (1) avoiding extremely hot or cold foods, spices, and citrus fruits and juices; (2) eating soft foods; and (3) taking nutritional supplements.

Diarrhea and Constipation. Most clinicians define *diarrhea* as an increase in stool liquid or frequency. It can result from GI mucosal damage secondary to RT or chemotherapy. A low-residue or liquid diet is usually advised. Electrolytes and intake and output should be carefully monitored. Scrupulous perineal hygiene is encouraged, especially in the client with neutropenia. Antidiarrheal agents may be prescribed.

Constipation is frequently described as hard, dry stool with straining; a decrease in the number of defecations; or both. Causes include (1) a decrease in either fluid and fiber intake or mobility of clients; (2) changes in usual bowel routines; (3) mechanical changes, such as tumor pressure on the bowel; and (4) metabolic changes, such as hypokalemia or hypercalcemia. The vinca alkaloid chemotherapeutic agents (vinblastine, vincristine) can slow bowel peristalsis. Other causes of constipation are opioid use, tumor invasion of the GI tract, and depression. Preventive measures may be taken for constipation, such as increasing fluid and bulk intake, using stool softeners prophylactically, increasing physical activity, and using laxatives when necessary.

Integumentary Effects

Alopecia. Alopecia is a common side effect of many antineoplastic agents. The extent of hair loss depends on the specific drug, dosage, and method of administration. Alopecia tends to begin 2 to 3 weeks after the first treatment; it is temporary. New hair growth tends to begin 4 to 6 weeks after the completion of chemotherapy and 8 to 9 weeks after RT. Hair color and texture may change, but the hair usually returns to its former condition within a year.[88] There can also be loss of body hair, including eyelashes, eyebrows, and pubic hair.

To help the client manage this side effect, which can be a traumatic change in body image and a constant reminder of the cancer, prepare the client for its occurrence. Begin by first allowing the client to grieve for the hair loss. Having information available about where to obtain attractive wigs or turbans is helpful. Many ACS units offer a program called "Look Good, Feel Better," which involves the assistance of a volunteer beautician.

Remember, hair loss bothers many men more than they acknowledge. Wigs are available for both men and women. Alternatively, many men choose to wear baseball caps to conceal the hair loss and for warmth. Hearing the experience of others with hair loss can often be helpful to both men and women.

Skin Reactions. The type of skin reactions that may occur in the client receiving chemotherapy depends on the drug administered. Red patches (*erythema*) or hives (*urticaria*) may appear at the drug injection site or on other body parts. (The extravasation of vesicant drugs was discussed earlier in this chapter.) These reactions generally disappear within several hours.

Darkening of the skin (*hyperpigmentation*) in the nail beds and mouth, on gums or teeth, and along the veins used for IV chemotherapy usually occurs within 2 to 3 weeks after administration of chemotherapy and continues for 10 to 12 weeks after the end of therapy. Sensitivity to sunlight (*photosensitivity*) may result in an acute sunburn after just a short exposure to the sun. The sensitivity disappears once treatment stops. Teach the client to use sunscreen or protective clothing before sun exposure.

A skin reaction called *radiation recall* may occur in clients who received RT before the administration of chemotherapy. When chemotherapy is given several weeks or months later, a recall reaction occurs in the previously irradiated skin area. RT skin effects range from redness, shedding, or peeling to blisters and oozing. After the skin heals, it is permanently darkened. It is important to maintain meticulous hygiene to avoid a superimposed infection in the area of radiation recall. Antibiotic therapy should be initiated at the first manifestation of infection.

Effects on the Reproductive System

Surgery, RT, and chemotherapy each can have effects on sexual health and sexual self-image. Up to 25% of women undergoing modified radical mastectomy for breast cancer report problems with sexual functioning. Surgery can affect sexual functioning through impairment of the vascular supply, removal of organs, or reduction of circulating hormone levels. Of women treated with RT for cervical cancer, 55% to 78% report sexual impairments. Body image, sexual functioning, and fertility can be affected by chemotherapy.[78] Not all clients experience these effects to the same degree, however. Preliminary studies suggest that the effects of chemotherapy on gonadal function vary with respect to the client's age at the time of therapy, the drugs administered, and the total drug dosage.[78]

Administration of antineoplastic agents during the first trimester of pregnancy increases the risk of spontaneous abortion and fetal malformations. Second- and third-trimester chemotherapy exposures may result in low birth weight or prematurity.[78] A pregnancy begun after cytotoxic chemotherapy has about the same chance of a successful outcome as a normal pregnancy.[78] The genetic effects of chemotherapy may not be evident for several generations of offspring, however. Therefore you should discuss the unpredictability of occurrence, degree, and duration of genetic damage with the client and his or her spouse or significant other.

Although initially you may not be comfortable with sexuality issues, you can still be an important source of support by giving the client permission to express concerns about this aspect of cancer therapy. Begin simply by asking open-ended questions about how the cancer experience has changed the client's relationships. Beyond providing information yourself, offer to seek further information or to consult with a colleague who may have additional information or suggestions to alleviate or at least ease the concern.

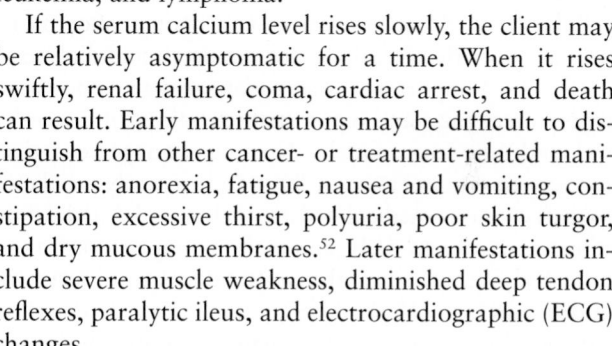 The PLISSIT (*p*ermission, *l*imited *i*nformation, *s*pecific *s*uggestions, *i*ntensive *t*herapy) model for evaluation of sexual function can be used for assessment purposes.[78] Pretreatment sperm banking offers the possibility of retaining reproductive capacity for some clients. Use of vaginal lubricants, methods of dilating the vagina after RT for cervical cancer (see Chapter 41), and penile prostheses (see Chapter 40) are topics you can discuss with the client. Counseling with a sexual therapist may be indicated.

Oncologic Emergencies

Infection, pain, spinal cord compression, hypercalcemia, SIADH, cardiac tamponade, superior vena cava syndrome, tumor lysis syndrome, and disseminated intravascular coagulation (DIC) are oncologic emergencies. If not identified early and treated, oncologic emergencies can result in severe morbidity and death. Each oncologic emergency is discussed only briefly here. The focus is on your role in appreciating and urgently reporting sometimes subtle manifestations to ensure the best possible outcome for the client. Consult other cancer nursing texts for further information on oncologic emergencies. Oncologic emergencies can be grouped as follows:

- Metabolic (infection and pain, hypercalcemia, tumor lysis syndrome, SIADH, DIC)
- Structural (spinal cord compression, superior vena cava syndrome, cardiac tamponade)

Infection and Pain. Infection, which can quickly progress as a life-threatening emergency in the client with neutropenia, was discussed in an earlier section. Although pain does not usually arise suddenly or unexpectedly, it is often regarded as an oncologic emergency because it is such a pervasive problem. As many as a third of clients in active treatment and 60% to 90% of people with advanced cancer have pain.[46] Pain can interfere with a per-

son's ability to enjoy activities and relationships that are meaningful. When pain is uncontrolled, the goal of enabling the client to live fully cannot be met. For nursing management of pain, see Chapter 22.

Hypercalcemia. After infection, hypercalcemia is the most commonly occurring oncologic emergency, and it can be a potentially fatal condition. Hypercalcemia is due to bone resorption (*demineralization*) and is defined as a serum calcium level greater than 11 mg/dl. If the client also has decreased serum albumin, a common finding with cancer, a corrected serum calcium value should be used. Of cases of cancer-related hypercalcemia, 80% occur with solid tumors, including breast, lung, head, neck, and renal cancers. The remaining 20% of cases occur in hematologic cancers, such as multiple myeloma, leukemia, and lymphoma.

If the serum calcium level rises slowly, the client may be relatively asymptomatic for a time. When it rises swiftly, renal failure, coma, cardiac arrest, and death can result. Early manifestations may be difficult to distinguish from other cancer- or treatment-related manifestations: anorexia, fatigue, nausea and vomiting, constipation, excessive thirst, polyuria, poor skin turgor, and dry mucous membranes.[52] Later manifestations include severe muscle weakness, diminished deep tendon reflexes, paralytic ileus, and electrocardiographic (ECG) changes.

Nursing management begins with the recognition of clients at risk for hypercalcemia, including people with (1) cancer of the breast, lung, head, neck, or kidney; (2) multiple myeloma; (3) leukemia; (4) lymphoma; and (5) potential or actual bone metastases. Maintaining adequate hydration and mobility is an important preventive measure in the at-risk client. Limiting dietary intake of calcium has little or no effect. Clients and family caregivers should be instructed on manifestations to report.

Medical management of hypercalcemia is aimed at controlling the growth of the tumor causing the hypercalcemia and, possibly, administration of drugs to lower serum calcium levels, such as calcitonin (Miacalcin) and oral glucocorticoids. For the client with advanced disease, for whom other interventions are no longer effective, treatment is aimed at comfort care.

Tumor Lysis Syndrome. Tumor lysis syndrome is a potentially fatal metabolic emergency that can develop as a tumor responds to treatment. When a large, bulky tumor is responsive to treatment, especially chemotherapy, the destruction of a large number of malignant cells may rapidly release intracellular potassium, phosphorus, and nucleic acid into the circulation. Electrolyte imbalances and acute renal failure usually begin 1 to 2 days after treatment starts and end within a week following the completion of therapy. Clients with malignancies that are very responsive to treatment are at highest risk, especially if they have a large tumor burden. Such malignancies include aggressive lymphomas, acute leukemias, or other bulky chemosensitive solid tumors such as small cell carcinoma of the lung. Clients with pre-existing renal compromise are also at greater risk.[13,52]

Medical management focuses on prevention in high-risk clients. Aggressive IV hydration is started before treatment begins and is continued until after treatment ends. Allopurinol (Zyloprim) is administered to decrease uric acid concentration. Sodium bicarbonate may be given in conjunction with the IV hydration to promote fecal excretion of excess phosphate.

Despite preventive measures, tumor lysis syndrome may occur. If so the goal is to remove potassium from the extracellular fluid with medications, retention enemas, or IV 50% dextrose, which acts to increase plasma insulin and thereby forces potassium back into the intracellular fluid. When preventive and maintenance measures are not effective, the client requires renal dialysis.[52]

The most important nursing management responsibility is to recognize and report manifestations of tumor lysis syndrome immediately. Nursing management then focuses on maintenance of fluid and electrolyte balance by carrying out medical orders, including IV hydration, monitoring weight daily, and maintaining a record of intake and output. Clinical manifestations to observe for and report are (1) weakness, (2) nausea, (3) diarrhea, (4) flaccid paralysis, (5) ECG changes, (6) muscle cramps or twitching, (7) oliguria (diminished urine output), (8) hypotension, (9) edema, and (10) altered mental status. Especially when treatment is provided in the outpatient ambulatory setting, the client and family must be taught about which manifestations to report immediately.[52]

Syndrome of Inappropriate Antidiuretic Hormone. The syndrome of inappropriate antidiuretic hormone results from the abnormal production of antidiuretic hormone (ADH). The incidence of SIADH is relatively low, occurring in only about 1% to 2% of clients with cancer. Of clients with cancer-related SIADH, 80% have an underlying diagnosis of small-cell lung cancer. Other causes of SIADH are infection, pulmonary disorders, emotional stress, CNS disorders, and some drugs, including such antineoplastic agents as cyclophosphamide (Cytoxan), vincristine (Oncovin), vinblastine (Velban), and cisplatin (Platinol-AQ). Manifestations, which are related to the rates of onset of the decrease in sodium and the increase in water retention, include (1) confusion, (2) irritability, (3) headache, (4) muscle weakness, (5) lethargy, (6) decreased urine output, (7) edema, (8) nausea and vomiting, and (9) anorexia.[52]

Syndrome of inappropriate antidiuretic hormone is not a preventable complication. It is a medical emergency only when the hyponatremia is severe (<120 mEq/L) and the client experiences manifestations. Mild SIADH is treated conservatively with fluid restriction

(<500 to 1000 ml/day). In about 7 to 10 days the body should be able to normalize the serum sodium concentration and osmolality. An IV infusion of hypertonic saline (3% to 5%) is given in severe cases to prevent pulmonary edema. Monitor intake and output. Pharmacologic agents given for SIADH include demeclocycline (Declomycin), lithium (Lithane), and urea. Beyond symptomatic treatment, the goal of medical management is to treat the underlying disease causing the SIADH.[52]

Disseminated Intravascular Coagulation. Disseminate intravascular coagulation involves the development of extensive, abnormal clots throughout small blood vessels. The widespread clotting consumes all circulating clotting factors and platelets, leading to excessive bleeding from several sites. The bleeding can be minimal or life-threatening. Also, clots that are blocking blood vessels decrease blood flow to major organs, which can cause pain, stroke-like manifestations, dyspnea, tachycardia, oliguria, and bowel necrosis. The mortality rate is near 70% despite appropriate treatment.

In clients with cancer, DIC is often caused by gram-negative infection or sepsis, release of thrombin or thromboplastin (clotting factors) from cancer cells, or blood transfusions. DIC is most commonly associated with leukemia and adenocarcinomas of the lung, pancreas, stomach, and prostate. Management involves treating the cancer and other measures as discussed in Chapter 77.

Spinal Cord Compression. Even for the terminally ill client in a hospice setting, early detection of and intervention for spinal cord compression are vital. Failure to intervene in this emergency can leave the client with permanent neurologic disabilities. Spinal cord compression is caused by direct pressure on or compromise of the vascular supply to the spinal cord. Back pain is often the only early presenting clinical manifestation, occurring in 95% of clients. Other early manifestations are motor weakness and decreased sensation. Depending on the rate of tumor growth, it may take only hours or days for the spinal cord compression to progress to irreversible neurologic damage with paralysis and loss of bowel and bladder control. Late manifestations are motor loss, additional sensory loss, constipation, and urinary hesitancy.[27,52]

In a client with known cancer, new-onset back pain should be a "red flag" signaling immediate evaluation. Pain localized over the involved area of the spine or radicular (belt-like) pain is present in more than 90% of clients with spinal cord compression. Carefully assess new-onset back pain; have the client point to the location of the pain and show you the areas of spread. Also carefully assess for any other clinical manifestations of neurologic deficit, such as numbness, tingling, constipation, and voiding hesitancy.

Data from the medical record can be helpful in determining whether the client has known bone metastasis. Give the physician a complete assessment of the pain, with a description of the location and characteristics. These data will provide the physician with the information needed to consider spinal cord compression in the differential diagnosis.

Treatment is usually with RT unless the tumor is resistant to RT or the client has already received the maximum RT dose in the involved area. A laminectomy for spinal cord decompression is an alternative. For the client in a hospice setting whose life expectancy is limited to days or weeks, administration of steroids to lessen the inflammation and swelling around the spinal cord can be a less aggressive but effective short-term alternative.

Superior Vena Cava Syndrome. Distressing but rarely life-threatening, superior vena cava (SVC) syndrome is a disorder that results from internal or external obstruction of the SVC. The obstruction reduces venous blood return to the heart and compromises cardiac output. SVC syndrome should be evaluated as an emergency because of concern for respiratory compromise. The onset of manifestations is usually gradual; however, if SVC syndrome was the presenting manifestation of cancer, time should be taken to diagnose accurately the underlying disease before treatment is initiated.

Typically, SVC syndrome is secondary to lung cancer, usually small-cell carcinoma (65%) or lymphoma (8%). The classical presenting manifestations are dyspnea (63%) and facial swelling (50%) with jugular vein distention. The client is often sitting up and leaning forward to breathe. Other manifestations are swelling of the arms, pain in the chest, and dysphagia.

The goals of medical management are to provide rapid palliation of the distressing manifestations and to treat the underlying cancer. External-beam RT continues to be the standard of care for palliation; however, clients with small-cell carcinoma of the lung or lymphoma may be palliated with the appropriate curative chemotherapy regimen with or without the addition of RT.[40]

Cardiac Tamponade. With cardiac tamponade (acute compression of the heart), early detection and proper management are critical to preventing cardiovascular collapse and death. When fluid collects in the pericardial sac (pericardial effusion), it affects the heart's ability to function properly and leads to cardiac tamponade. Normally the pericardium contains 15 to 50 ml of fluid; the pericardial sac may contain as much as 200 to 1800 ml of fluid before the heart begins to decompensate. The fluid prevents the heart from filling and contracting normally. The onset may be insidious.

The most common manifestations are tachycardia, severe dyspnea, cough, chest pain, edema, and hypoten-

sion. You may notice a narrowing of the pulse pressure (the difference between systolic and diastolic readings) or pulsus paradoxus (decreased or absent amplitude of the pulse with inspiration). Heart sounds may be muffled by the fluid. Jugular venous distention may be prominent. A chest x-ray is a cost-effective screening tool, although it cannot always visualize cardiac tamponade. An ECG shows a number of changes that could indicate tamponade.

Medical management of cardiac tamponade is individualized for the client. A *pericardiocentesis* (insertion of an 18-gauge needle into the chest to draw off the fluid) may be performed. Because the fluid can accumulate again, a pericardiotomy may be performed; this surgical procedure creates a window or opening in the pericardial sac for subsequent drainage of fluid. Even then, the pericardial fluid can accumulate again. Nursing management consists of carefully assessing clinical manifestations and teaching the client and family caregiver to watch for manifestations that may herald impending cardiac tamponade.[52]

PSYCHOSOCIAL ASPECTS OF CANCER CARE

When cancer becomes a part of life's journey, it is hard work. (See the Bridge to Home Health Care feature on Dealing with Grief Related to a New Cancer Diagnosis on the website.) The diagnosis of cancer affects not only the individual client but also the client's family. Because cancer is not just a physical disease, it compels the clients—and health care professionals—to face the meaning of their lives and their relationships. Just as life experiences affect the perceptions a client brings to the cancer experience, so do your life experiences affect the perceptions you bring to the client's care. It is therefore valuable for you to reflect on your beliefs and values about life and death and their meaning.

Providing Support for Clients

The most valuable intervention you can offer a client with cancer is your presence as a caring person. The dimensions of your presence consist of verbal expressions of empathy, positive regard, and availability of practical support.[79] Fellow clients can have a significant impact on clients with cancer. One practical source of support is taking this into consideration when making inpatient room assignments.[79]

Hearing the stories of colleagues, clients, their families, and survivors can be a vehicle for a novice nurse to learn the art of cancer nursing. Storytelling is becoming recognized for its value.[21,34,48,49] A story can be a means of providing comfort by offering social comparisons (helping clients know how others have fared and felt in a similar situation) or lessons from others' experiences.

There is great variability in the distress, changes, and other effects of cancer in the lives of clients and their families. Responses to cancer depend on the following:
- The disease and the disabilities and disfigurements it may cause
- Pre-existing medical conditions that may limit treatment options
- The client's psychological make-up and spiritual well-being
- The client's family and social community
- Availability of medical and financial resources

Providing Support for the Family

The diagnosis of cancer has an effect on the client's entire family. The daily life of the family is changed. Other family members may need to assume the role or responsibilities of the client or to serve as the family caregiver. Nursing often views the family as the context of caring for the client with cancer; the family needs to be the unit of care. A family's resources, perceptions of the cancer, functioning patterns, coping strategies, and stressors are factors affecting their ability to respond to the crisis of cancer.[20,46,79] Much of the distress for the client and the family can be lessened with minimal assistance from the health care team. Without these services, even highly functioning families struggle.

Promoting Positive Self-Concept

Cancer affects all levels of functioning. Physical and psychological distress, medication, or the disease itself can cloud the client's intellectual function. The client's self-concept is affected by physical changes as well as changes in role or function. A breadwinner in the family may become dependent on others and become a consumer of family savings and resources. The young adult, striving for independence, may need to revert to an earlier level of dependency.

Body image also changes for most clients. Weight loss, hair loss, and skin changes can result from treatment. Radical surgical procedures can make devastating and permanent changes in appearance and function. Procedures such as laryngectomy, glossectomy, mastectomy, and prostatectomy may result in physical changes that humiliate and overwhelm the client.

Promoting Coping Throughout the Cancer Continuum

Although each cancer experience is unique, people with cancer have some common problems. Strategies for outcome management to help clients cope with the disease and its treatment are addressed for each phase of the *cancer continuum:* diagnosis and treatment, survivorship, recurrent disease and progression, and terminal illness.

Diagnosis and Treatment

Clients reach the point of cancer diagnosis in many ways. A client may have had vague manifestations, such as weight loss and fatigue, that may have been ignored or a cause of some anxiety for weeks or months. Another client may have manifestations, such as pain or abdominal bloating, that evaded diagnosis. Many times, cancer is found incidentally during a routine examination. Often the client suspects cancer, but many people are shocked when the diagnosis is made. The diagnostic period may be long and extremely stressful. This period is filled with anxiety about each test result, especially when staging procedures are performed. More than 70% of clients consider the time of diagnosis and treatment as the most stressful in the cancer experience.[91]

Most clients fear death during the first few months of the cancer experience. Weisman[91] called this stage "the existential plight." Whether clients can express their fears or not, it is an underlying cause of distress. During diagnosis the magnitude of the client's problems becomes apparent. The client wonders: Is my disease curable? Will my disabilities be temporary or permanent? What types of physical impairment will occur? What will be the side effects of treatment? Will my manifestations be relieved? Will I be able to return to work? What adjustments have to be made in family life or work? Will finances be adequate? What plans need to be abandoned? Which changes in lifestyle will be temporary and which permanent?

Clients must deal not only with specific problems but also with the emotional distress they experience throughout this time. They may feel angry and frustrated because their lives have been changed; they may feel isolated or may worry about being abandoned by family and friends. They may be shocked and unbelieving that they are the ones with cancer. They may also feel guilty if they believe they have contributed to their disease through behavior, such as by smoking, drinking, or putting themselves at risk for sexually transmitted diseases.

Clients' reactions vary greatly. The initial response to the diagnosis of cancer may be profoundly influenced by previous life experiences with the disease. When the disease is advanced at the time of diagnosis, the client and family are likely to experience more psychological distress because they are confronted with the dual stressors of a cancer diagnosis and a terminal illness.[79] Some have minimal distress, whereas others may be overwhelmed and devastated. You may sometimes feel, on the basis of your own personality and experience, that a client is responding inappropriately (i.e., too little or too much) to a cancer diagnosis. It is crucial, however, to acknowledge every client's response as acceptable and unique for that client.

Weisman[91] identified coping styles used by many clients with cancer (Box 19-3). *Denial,* which is a part of coping, allows a client to "repudiate what cannot be avoided, by substituting a more favorable or agreeable idea."[53] Denial can be useful as a healthy coping mechanism in the diagnostic phase, when the number of problems may be overwhelming. Denial is harmful when it prevents the client from seeking appropriate treatment. Awareness and denial can exist at the same time.

Clients who are good problem-solvers or who cope effectively tend to confront reality, avoid excessive denial, remain flexible, accept support, and remain hopeful and optimistic. Clients who cope poorly use avoidance and excessive denial; they are pessimistic and feel hopeless.[53] Every client uses a variety of strategies to cope with cancer.

Families also should be assessed for their coping abilities. Use of a specific family assessment tool may not be possible, but often you will be readily able to identify "high-risk" families from your interactions with them. Unresolved past problems may affect a family's ability to cope with cancer in the present. Families who use excessive denial, exhibit strong anger and guilt, or are unreasonably demanding may be at increased risk for dysfunction. When the client is the pivotal person in the family or when the family has had a previous experience of cancer with a negative outcome, their need for ongoing psychosocial support systems may be increased.

Actively listen for remarks that describe the meaning and effect of cancer as experienced by the client. Often time limitations do not permit you to provide support separate from physical caregiving. Consequently, while giving care, take the opportunity to initiate social interactions, such as chatting about family, sharing stories, or greeting visitors. Consider these actions a professional intervention. What did you learn about the client's perceptions of cancer? What coping mechanisms did the client or significant others use with past lifestyle changes? How will the client's and the family's life be affected? What needs for teaching or community resources did you note? Would referrals to other members of the health care team, such as the chaplain and social worker, be helpful?

Providing social support and improving the client's sense of control help to reduce anxiety. Stress reduction or relaxation techniques can be taught. Speaking with cancer survivors encourages many clients. Support groups and one-to-one visitation programs such as Reach to Recovery or CanSurmount (ACS) provide this opportunity. Internet support groups offer the same opportunity for clients who are uncomfortable with the face-to-face interactions of a traditional support group.

Informational needs of the client and family are great during the diagnostic and treatment periods. Tests, procedures, and treatments, which are often technical and complicated, must be explained. Present consistent, accurate information in as much detail as the client wants. Be sure that all health care providers are telling the client the same thing. When clients from a cancer clinic were surveyed, information and support from family, friends, and caregivers were identified as a high-priority needs (Box 19-4).[46]

Address specific problems by (1) helping the client identify them, (2) providing information when necessary, and (3) referring the client to appropriate resources. Both the NCI and the ACS provide useful written

---

BOX 19-3   *General Coping Strategies*

- Seek more information (rational inquiry).
- Share concern and talk with others (mutuality).
- Laugh it off; make light of the situation (affect reversal).
- Try to forget; put it out of your mind (suppression).
- Do other things for distraction (displacement, redirection).
- Take firm action on the basis of present understanding (confrontation).
- Accept but find something favorable (redefinition, revision).
- Submit to the inevitable (fatalism, passive acceptance).
- Do something—anything—however reckless or impractical (impulsivity).
- Consider or negotiate a feasible alternative (if *x*, then *y*).
- Reduce tension with excessive drink, drugs, danger (life threats).
- Withdraw into isolation; get away (disengagement).
- Blame someone or something (externalization, projection).
- Seek direction; do what you are told (cooperative compliance).
- Blame yourself; sacrifice or atone (moral masochism).

Modified from Weisman, A. (1979). *Coping with cancer* (p. 23). New York: McGraw-Hill.

BOX 19-4   *Needs of Clinic Patients with Cancer*

The following needs were identified and rank-ordered by a sample of clinic patients. The last three items were ranked of equal importance.

- Information about operating special equipment
- Information about radiation
- Information provided in a way that is understandable
- Ways to be active in decision making
- Adequate preparation before discharge from hospital
- Support from family
- Support from friends
- Information about chemotherapy
- Time off from work to recuperate
- Information about what to expect in the future
- A patient caregiver
- Time off work for treatment

Modified from Gates, M.F., Lackey, N.R., & White, M.R. (1995). Needs of hospice and clinic patients with cancer. *Cancer Practice, 3*(4), 226-232.

materials to reinforce teaching. Site-specific information can be obtained from the NCI via the Internet (http://www.nci.nih.gov or http://www.cancer.gov), fax (301-402-5874), or telephone (1-800-4-CANCER). Other key Internet websites may be bookmarked on a computer in the clinical area or in a patient library.

Survivorship

Clients who have completed successful treatment enter an indeterminate period of long-term survivorship. Survivorship has been divided into a time of acute survival followed by a period of extended survival. Transition between these periods is not precise but evolves as time passes and the cancer does not recur.

Depending on the extent of treatment, the period of extended survival may still be one of physical fatigue and limitation. Physical rehabilitation to improve functioning may dominate the client's energy in this early period. Efforts focus on restoring the client's previous level of functioning.

The long-term physical effects of cancer treatment are now becoming apparent as data accumulate, especially from clients with pediatric cancer. The physical effects may range from minimal restriction to life-threatening complications. The effects can be organ-specific, such as cardiomyopathy or pulmonary fibrosis, or general, such as fatigue.

The potential for development of a second malignancy as a result of primary treatment is always a possibility. Although this possibility is usually rare, some studies have reported up to a 20% occurrence of another cancer after treatment of Hodgkin's disease and other cancers with alkylating agents.

Psychologically, the period of extended survival is one in which clients must take up previous roles or adjust and reorganize their lives. The possibility of recurrence may dominate their lives. Plans may be suspended. Decisions about changing jobs, buying a house, starting a family, or beginning retirement may be difficult in the face of the uncertainty of recurrence or concerns about insurance coverage.

Making sure the client carries through with routine follow-up and long-term health care with attention to prevention and early detection (health promotion) is vital to early detection of recurrent cancer and second primary sites as well as early intervention for late effects of treatment. Follow-up appointments and events such as National Cancer Survivors Day celebrations (which are held in many communities each June) are opportunities for obtaining emotional support, alleviating fears of recurrence, and enabling clients to know that they are not alone in their feelings and concerns.

Employment discrimination has been a problem for cancer survivors. Clients with a cancer history have proved themselves to be dependable and productive. Yet studies show that as many as 84% of blue-collar work-

ers and 38% of white-collar workers with cancer experience some type of discrimination in employment.[79] Over the years, these issues have been partially rectified by state laws protecting the rights of the disabled.

Obtaining insurance coverage for a client with a history of cancer has also been difficult, ruinously expensive, and sometimes impossible. Legislative efforts have corrected some of these problems. Insurance discrimination can be legally appealed. Federal programs such as COBRA (Consolidated Omnibus Budget Reconciliation Act) protect the insurance coverage of an employee for 18 months after termination of employment but at an increased monthly premium. A client, spouse, or parent may be trapped in an unrewarding job to maintain the employer-funded group insurance. Direct clients who have difficulty with insurance coverage to contact the National Coalition for Cancer Survivorship (see the website for a box on Cancer-Related Resources), the ACS, their state department of human rights, or their state insurance department. The NCI booklet *Facing Forward* provides detailed information about resources.[87]

With time, these problems usually recede and clients move into a period of extended survival. The experience of cancer is nonetheless indelibly imprinted on their lives. Amazingly, most clients cope well and face the difficulties in their lives with courage. For many clients the experience brings about a reappraisal of goals and values, making life richer and more meaningful.

Recurrent Disease and Progression

Most clients with cancer live with the threat or reality of recurrent disease. Weisman[91] describes the effect that this phase has on the client as "the hope for a cure" becoming the "struggle for existence." With recurrent cancer, therapy may once again be used to eradicate or stabilize the disease process.

Although subsequent recurrent disease may occur, it is usually the first recurrence that causes surprise, shock, and disbelief in the client. Physical impairment may be greater, and quality of life may be limited because of disease or treatment. The client who previously projected an optimistic outlook may now express a more guarded attitude. Maintain open communication and be sensitive to the informational and support needs of the client and family.

Clients at this stage in the cancer continuum are usually not in imminent danger of dying. They are generally aware of the likely eventuality of death. Often they still want to continue treatment. Surgery, RT, or chemotherapy may still be of value for palliation of manifestations regardless of whether the treatment extends life. Surgery, RT, or chemotherapy may be used to palliate complications caused by persistent tumor growth. For example, surgery may be used to manage a malignant obstruction, or RT may be used to prevent paralysis from spinal cord compression. Palliative treatment is not curative but rather is aimed at improving the quality of the remainder of the client's life, however long or short.

Although clients at this stage may not qualify for traditional hospice care, they could benefit from the supportive services and management of manifestations offered by hospice programs. Increasingly hospitals are developing supportive care programs or palliative care teams to meet these needs. *Palliative care* is the provision of management of manifestations and psychosocial support, best offered by a multidisciplinary health care team. Palliative care can be added gradually as the cancer and its manifestations progress. Clients can participate in evaluating when the side effects of treatment modalities such as chemotherapy outweigh the benefits of palliating cancer manifestations. Increasingly today, professionals are recognizing the value of incorporating quality-of-life outcomes for clients throughout the course of their illness. Palliative care programs combine the medical model's goal to prolong life with hospice goals to relieve manifestations and improve the quality of clients remaining time.[19,24,46] See Chapter 23 for further discussion of palliative care.

Terminal Illness

About 50% of clients with cancer eventually die of their disease. The time from diagnosis to death ranges from weeks to years. Not all clients with cancer become terminally ill. Some clients die during the initial treatment; others die of complications of treatment. Many, however, reach an end-point at which their cancer no longer responds to treatment and progression of the disease cannot be controlled. Then the goal of treatment is directed toward providing supportive care and minimizing distress until death occurs. See Chapter 23 for an overview of hospice and palliative care.

CONCLUSIONS

Cancer therapy has progressed rapidly in the last half of the 20th century. Many cancers once considered incurable are now controlled with a variety of combination therapies. Even when cancer is not cured, length of life may be extended. The quality of the extended length of life has also greatly improved. Professionals have greater knowledge of and skills in controlling pain and managing nausea and vomiting resulting from chemotherapy, and more options are available for helping clients cope with hair loss.

The hospice movement has demonstrated that there is still much that can be done for a client with cancer, even when cure is no longer possible. The survivorship movement has made visible the hopeful side of cancer as well as being a resource to clients in dealing with insurance, workplace, and other issues.

New treatment modalities are showing promise in clinical trials, with some already becoming standard care. The nurse in the 21st century needs to stay abreast of new developments in this rapidly expanding field.

THINKING CRITICALLY *evolve*

1. You are a nurse working in a health clinic that focuses on prevention of disease. This month, the featured goal is cancer prevention. How will you assess each client for cancer risk factors?
Factors to Consider. How would you develop an assessment tool for the clinic nurses to use? How would you adapt teaching strategies to the cultural group being served? What teaching can help clients to avoid factors that increase their risk of cancer?

2. The client is a 22-year-old man who comes to the neighborhood health clinic with concern that his companion, who has pain and a lump in the right testicle, may have testicular cancer. The companion is at home. What teaching should be completed during this visit? What psychosocial concerns would the client and the companion have?
Factors to Consider. What diagnostic studies should you anticipate? What care should be given to the client awaiting diagnosis after cancer testing?

3. C.H. is a 54-year-old engineer responsible for grading, paving, and asphalting of county road surfaces. He is admitted for evaluation of chest pain and increasing shortness of breath. Because of a history of quadruple bypass surgery when he was 44, he assumes that he has additional coronary artery blockage. He has continued to smoke despite his cardiac history. Several members of his mother's family and his father died of cancer. He has lung cancer that has metastasized to the brain. He will be treated with chemotherapy and radiation therapy. What risk factors does C.H. have for lung cancer? What teaching should the nurse plan for him? What long-term plans should the nurse consider for him?
Factors to Consider. How will this client's cardiac history affect his chemotherapy regimen? What oncologic emergencies does C.H. face? Why is he not a surgical candidate?

Discussions for these questions can be found on the website and the CD-ROM.

BIBLIOGRAPHY

1. Albanell, J., & Baselga, J. (2000). Systemic therapy emergencies. *Seminars in Oncology, 27*(3), 347-361.

2. American Cancer Society. (2003). *Cancer facts and figures—2003.* Atlanta: Author.

 3. Anastasia, P.J. (2000). Effectiveness of oral 5-HT3 receptor antagonists for emetogenic chemotherapy. *Oncology Nursing Forum, 27*(3), 483-493.

4. Appel, C. (2001). Biotherapy. In S. Otto (Ed.), *Oncology nursing* (4th ed., pp. 684-730). St. Louis: Mosby.

5. Baltic, T., Schlosser, E., & Bedell, M. (2002). Neutropenic fever: One institution's quality improvement project to decrease time from patient arrival to initiation of antibiotic therapy. *Clinical Journal of Oncology Nursing, 6*(6), 337-346.

6. Barnett, M. (2001). Fatigue. In S. Otto (Ed.), *Oncology nursing* (4th ed., pp. 787-801). St. Louis: Mosby.

7. Barrett, R. (2002). A nurse's primer on recruiting participants for clinical trials. *Oncology Nursing Forum, 29*(7), 1091-1098.

8. Bendell, C. (2003) Pegfilgrastim for chemotherapy-induced neutropenia. *Clinical Journal of Oncology Nursing, 7*(1), 55-56, 63-64.

9. Berger, A., Portenoy, R.K., & Weissman, D.E. (2002). *Principles and practice of supportive oncology* (2nd ed.). Philadelphia: Lippincott Williams & Wilkins.

10. Berlin, J. (2002). Targeting vascular endothelial growth factor in colorectal cancer. *Oncology, 16*(8, suppl. 7), 13-15.

11. Birner, A. (2003) Safe administration of oral chemotherapy. *Clinical Journal of Oncology Nursing, 7*(2), 158-162, 170-172.

12. Blash, J.L. (2002). Systemic candida infections in patients with leukemia: An overview of drug therapy. *Clinical Journal of Oncology Nursing, 6*(6), 323-331.

13. Brant, J.M. (2002). Rasburicase: An innovative new treatment for hyperuricemia associated with tumor lysis syndrome. *Clinical Journal of Oncology Nursing, 6*(1), 12.

14. Brown, K.A., et al. (2001). *Chemotherapy and biotherapy: Guidelines and recommendations for practice.* Pittsburgh, PA: ONS Publishing Division.

15. Bruner, D.W. (2001). *Outcomes in radiation therapy: Multidisciplinary management.* Sudbury, MA: Jones & Bartlett.

16. Buchsel, P., et al. (2002). Granulocyte macrophage colony-stimulating factor: Current practice and novel approaches. *Clinical Journal of Oncology Nursing, 6*(4), 198-204.

17. Burke, M.B., et al. (Eds.). (2001). *Cancer chemotherapy: A nursing process approach* (3rd ed). Sudbury, MA: Jones & Bartlett.

18. Camp-Sorrell, D. (2004). *Access device guidelines: Recommendations for nursing practice and education* (2nd ed.). Pittsburgh, PA: Oncology Nursing Press.

19. Carson, M.G. (2000). Measuring patient outcomes in palliative care: A reliability and validity study of the support team assessment schedule. *Palliative Medicine, 14,* 25-36.

20. Carter, P., & Chang, B. L. (2000) Sleep and depression in cancer care givers. *Cancer Nursing, 23*(6), 410-415.

21. Chelf, J., et al. (2000). Storytelling: A strategy for living and coping with cancer. *Cancer Nursing, 23*(1), 1-6.

22. Chernecky, C. (2001). Satisfaction vs. dissatisfaction with venous access devices in outpatient oncology: A pilot study. *Oncology Nursing Forum, 28*(10), 1613-1616.

23. Dunne-Daly, C. (1999). Principles of radiotherapy and radiobiology. *Seminars in Oncology Nursing, 15*(4), 250-259.

24. Esper, P., et al. (1999). A new concept in cancer care: The supportive care program. *American Journal of Hospice & Palliative Care, 16*(6), 713-722.

25. Foltz, A.T., & Mahon, S.M. (2000). Application of carcinogenesis theory to primary prevention. *Oncology Nursing Forum, 27*(9), 5-11.

26. Fukuyama, S.N., & Itano, J. (1999). Thrombocytopenia secondary to myelosuppression. *American Journal of Nursing,* April supplement, 5-12.

27. Garner, C.M. (1999). Cancer-related spinal cord compression. *American Journal of Nursing, 99*(7), 34.

28. Giarell, D. (2002). To screen or not to screen: Using spiral computerized tomography in the early detection of lung cancer. *Clinical Journal of Oncology Nursing, 6*(4), 223-227.

29. Gillespie, T.W. (2002). Effects of cancer-related anemia on clinical and quality-of-life outcomes. *Clinical Journal of Oncology Nursing, 6*(4), 206-211.

30. Gray, M. (2002). A prostate cancer primer. *Urologic Nursing, 22*(3), 151-169.

31. Greco, F.A. (Ed.). (1996). *Handbook of commonly used chemotherapy regimens.* Chicago: Precept Press.

32. Greene, F. (Ed.). (2002). *AJCC cancer staging manual.* (6th ed.). New York: Springer-Verlag.

33. Groopman, J. (1998). Annals of medicine: Decoding destiny—what it is like to know your genes contain a deadly mutation. *The New Yorker,* February 9, 42-45.

34. Groopman, J. (1997). *The measure of our days: New beginnings at life's end.* New York: Viking.

35. Gullatte, M. (2001). Prevention, screening, and detection. In S. Otto (Ed.), *Oncology nursing* (4th ed., pp. 53-81). St. Louis: Mosby.

36. Hawks, J., & Moyad, M. (2003). CAM: Definition and classification overview. *Urologic Nursing, 23*(3), 221-223.

37. Houshamand, S., et al. (2000). Prophylactic mastectomy and genetic testing: An update. *Oncology Nursing Forum, 27*(10), 1537-1547.

38. Hughes, L.C., et al. (2002) Describing an episode of home nursing care for elderly post-surgical cancer patients. *Nursing Research 51*(2), 110-118.

39. Isaksen, A.S., & Gjengedal, E. (2000). The significance of fellow patients for the patient with cancer. *Cancer Nursing, 23*(5), 382-391.

40. Iwamotto, R. (2001). Radiation therapy. In S. Otto (Ed.), *Oncology nursing* (4th ed., pp. 606-637). St. Louis: Mosby.

41. Jennings-Dozier, K., & Mahon, S.M. (2000). Cancer prevention and early detection—From thought to revolution. *Oncology Nursing Forum, 27*(9), 3-4.

42. Klemm, P., & Nolan, M.T. (1998). Internet cancer support groups: Legal and ethical issues for nurse researchers. *Oncology Nursing Forum, 25*(4), 673-676.

43. Kolcaba, K., & Fox, C. (1999). The effects of guided imagery on comfort of women with early stage breast cancer undergoing radiation therapy. *Oncology Nursing Forum, 26*(1), 67-72.

44. Kosier, M.B., & Minkler, P. (1999). Nursing management of patients with an implanted Ommaya reservoir. *Clinical Journal of Oncology Nursing, 3*(2), 63-67.

45. Kosits, C., & Callaghan, M. (2000). Rituximab: A new monoclonal antibody therapy for non-Hodgkin's lymphoma. *Oncology Nursing Forum, 27*(1), 51-59.

46. Kuebler, K., Berry, P., & Heidrich, D. (2002). *End-of-life care: Clinical practice guidelines.* Philadelphia: W.B. Saunders.

47. Larouere, E. (1999). The art of accessing an implanted port. *Nursing, 29*(5), 56-58.

48. Lehna, C. (1999). Storytelling in practice: Part one—mothers' stories. *Journal of Hospice and Palliative Nursing, 1*(1), 21-25.

49. Lehna, C. (1999). Storytelling in practice: Part two—professional storytelling. *Journal of Hospice and Palliative Nursing,* 1(1), 27-30.

50. Levin, B., et al. (2003). Emerging technologies in screening for colorectal cancer: CT colonography, immunochemical fecal occult blood tests, and stool screening. *Cancer Nursing,* 23(2), 117-121.

51. Mahon, S.M. (2002). Cancer prevention and early detection. *Clinical Journal of Oncology Nursing,* 5(3) 105-107.

52. Meyers, J. (2001). Oncologic complications. In S. Otto (Ed.), *Oncology nursing* (4th ed., pp. 498-581). St. Louis: Mosby.

53. Mullan, F. (1985). Seasons of survival: Reflections of a physician with cancer. *New England Journal of Medicine,* 313, 270-273.

54. National Cancer Institute. (1999, reprinted 2002). *Chemotherapy and you: A guide to self help during cancer treatment.* (NIH Pub. No. 99-1136). Washington, D.C.: U.S. Government Printing Office.

55. National Cancer Institute. (Revised 1998, Reprinted 2002). *Eating hints for cancer patients.* (NIH Pub. No. 98-2079). Washington, D.C.: U.S. Government Printing Office.

56. National Cancer Institute. (Revised 1999, Reprinted 2002). *Radiation therapy and you: A guide to self-help during cancer treatment.* (NIH Pub. No. 99-2227). Washington, D.C.: U.S. Government Printing Office.

57. National Cancer Institute (2001). SELECT: Selenium and vitamin E cancer prevention trial. NIH Publication No. D1-4978.

58. National Cancer Institute. (1998). *Taking part in clinical trials: What cancer patients need to know.* (NIH Pub. No. 97-4250). Washington, D.C.: U.S. Government Printing Office.

59. National Cancer Institute. (1997). *Taking time: Support for people with cancer and the people who care about them.* (NIH Pub. No. 97-2059). Washington, D.C.: U.S. Government Printing Office.

60. Nelson, N.J. (1997). Studies show prophylactic surgeries seem to reduce cancer risk. *Journal of the National Cancer Institute,* 89(11), 762-763.

61. Nunez, A.M., & Liebman, M.C. (1999). Febrile neutropenia. *American Journal of Nursing,* April Supplement, 9-12.

62. Occupational Safety and Health Administration (OSHA). (1995). Controlling occupational exposure to hazardous drugs. *American Journal of Health-System Pharmacology,* 52(6), 1669-1683.

63. Occupational Safety and Health Administration (OSHA). (1995). *Work-place guidelines for personnel dealing with cytotoxic (antineoplastic) drugs.* (OSHA Instruction CPL 2-2.20B CH-4, 21-1-21-34). Washington, D.C.: U.S. Government Printing Office.

64. Oncology Nursing Society. (1992). *Cancer chemotherapy guidelines: Recommendations for the management of vesicant extravasation, hypersensitivity and anaphylaxis.* Pittsburgh, PA: Author.

65. Otto, S. (2001). Chemotherapy. In S. Otto (Ed.), *Oncology nursing* (4th ed., pp. 638-683). St. Louis: Mosby.

66. Otto, S. (2001). Protective mechanisms. In S. Otto (Ed.), *Oncology nursing* (4th ed., pp. 917-947). St. Louis: Mosby.

67. Otto, S., & Johnston, L. (2001). Home care, alternative care settings, and cancer resources. In S. Otto (Ed.), *Oncology nursing* (4th ed., pp. 802-842). St. Louis: Mosby.

68. Pfeifer, K. (2001). Surgery. In S. Otto (Ed.), *Oncology nursing* (4th ed., pp. 585-605). St. Louis: Mosby.

69. Pickett, M., et al. (2000). Prostate cancer elder alert: Living with treatment choices and outcomes. *Journal of Gerontological Nursing,* 26(2), 22-34.

70. Potter, K.L., & Schafer, S.L. (1999). Nausea and vomiting: One of the most distressing chemotherapy-related symptoms. *American Journal of Nursing,* April Supplement, 2-4.

71. Rieger, P. (2001). Biotherapy: The fourth modality. In M.B. Burke, et al. (Eds.), *Cancer chemotherapy: A nursing process approach* (3rd ed., pp. 43-73). Sudbury, MA: Jones & Bartlett.

72. Rieger, P. (2003). The impact of genetic information in the management of cancer. In A. Tranin, A. Masny, & J. Jenkins (Eds.), *Genetics in oncology practice: Cancer risk assessment* (pp. 139-187). Pittsburgh, PA: Oncology Nursing Society.

73. Rumsey, K.A., & Richardson, D.K. (1995). Management of infection and occlusion associated with vascular access devices. *Seminars in Oncology Nursing,* 11(3), 174-183.

74. Rust, D.M., Wood, L.S., & Battiato, L.A. (1999). Oprelvekin: An alternative treatment for thrombocytopenia. *Clinical Journal of Oncology Nursing,* 3(2), 57-62.

75. Saslow, D. et al. (2002). American Cancer Society guidelines for the early detection of cervical neoplasia and cancer. *CA: A Cancer Journal for Clinicians,* 52(6), 342-362.

76. Schulmeister, L. (2001). Epidemiology. In S. Otto (Ed.), *Oncology nursing* (4th ed., pp. 42-52). St. Louis: Mosby.

77. Sessink, P., & Bos, R.P. (1999). Drugs hazardous to healthcare workers: Evaluation of methods for monitoring occupational exposure to cytostatic drugs. *Drug Safety,* 20(4), 347-359.

78. Shell, J. (2001). Impact of cancer on sexuality. In S. Otto (Ed.), *Oncology nursing* (4th ed., pp. 973-999). St. Louis: Mosby.

79. Shell, J., & Kirsch, S. (2001). Psychosocial issues, outcomes, and quality of life. In S. Otto (Ed.), *Oncology nursing* (4th ed., pp. 948-972). St. Louis: Mosby.

80. Shelton, B.K. (2002). Introduction to colorectal cancer. *Seminars in Oncology Nursing,* 18(2), Supplement 2, 2-12.

81. Smith, L.H., & Besser, S.G. (2000). Dietary restrictions for patients with neutropenia: A survey of institutional practices. *Oncology Nursing Forum,* 27(3), 515-531.

82. Smith, R., Cokkiniles, V., & Eyre, H.J. (2003). American Cancer Society guidelines for the early detection of cancer, 2003. *CA: A Cancer Journal for Clinicians,* 53(1), 27-43.

83. Sorokin, P. (2002). New agents and future directions in biotherapy. *Clinical Journal of Oncology Nursing,* 6(1), 19-24.

84. Sparber, A., et al. (2000). Using complementary medicine by adult patients participating in cancer clinical trials. *Oncology Nursing Forum,* 27(4), 623-630.

85. Tariman, J. (2003). Thalidomide: Current therapeutic uses and management of its toxicities. *Clinical Journal of Oncology Nursing,* 7(2), 143-147.

86. Tranin, A., Masny, A., & Jenkins, J. (2003). *Genetics in oncology practice.* Pittsburgh, PA: Oncology Nursing Society.

87. U.S. Department of Health and Human Services. (1996). *Facing forward: A guide for cancer survivors.* (NIH Pub. No. 96-2424). Washington, D.C.: National Cancer Institute.

88. Vanderhoof, D.D., & Brant, J.M. (1999). Alopecia: The forgotten side effect? *American Journal of Nursing,* April Supplement, 17-19.

89. Viale, P. (2003). Complications associated with implantable vascular access devices in the patient with cancer, *Journal of Infusion Nursing,* 26(2), 97-103.

90. Weinrich, S.P., et al (2000). Barriers to prostate cancer screening. *Cancer Nursing,* 23(2), 117-121.

91. Weisman, A. (1979). *Coping with cancer.* New York: McGraw-Hill.

92. Wilkes, G. (2000). Nutrition: The forgotten ingredient in cancer care. *American Journal of Nursing,* 100(4), 46-51.

93. Yamamoto, D.S., & Viale, P.H. (2003). Cyclooxygenase-2: From arthritis treatment to new indications for the prevention and treatment of cancer. *Clinical Journal of Oncology Nursing,* 7(1), 21-29.

Clients with Wounds

Joyce M. Black

evolve

Web Enhancements

http://evolve.elsevier.com/Black/medsurg/

Concept Map
Understanding Inflammation and Its Treatment
Appendix A
Religious Beliefs and Practices Affecting Health Care

Appendix C
Laboratory Values of Clinical Importance in Medical-Surgical Nursing

Healing is a fundamental property of living tissue. If healing did not occur, all species would eventually become extinct. Unfortunately, many health care practices seem to lack respect for this critical attribute of healing and accept the process as passive, inevitable, and unimprovable. Popular literature assumes that if people survive, they heal, and if people are healthy, they heal.

Healing activities have always formed the basis of nursing practice. Florence Nightingale defined the nursing role as preparing the client for the most favorable conditions for healing. Nurses today still serve as a crucial link in the process of wound healing. They educate clients about disease management and wound care and support them through the physical and psychological processes of healing.

Wound healing is most apparent on the skin but occurs in all areas of the body. Bones, tendons, organs, and tissues all heal by regenerating cells to restore function. The most favorable outcome of healing is the complete return to normal structure and function. Such an outcome is possible if tissue damage is minor, no complications occur, and the destroyed tissues can regenerate. Body tissues have varying capabilities for regeneration. For example, mucous membrane is completely regenerated. Deep skin injury regenerates with a scar, which restores only a barrier. It has been thought that the central nervous system (CNS) cannot regenerate its damaged cells. Although new information is challenging that belief, today the knowledge does not exist to promote CNS tissue regeneration.

This chapter focuses on tissue injury and repair. Tissue injury is common and is seen in clients who sustain trauma as well as in those who have undergone surgery. Because tissue injury is common, the body is well equipped with mechanisms of defense and healing.

NORMAL WOUND HEALING

Wound healing has been defined as "a complex and dynamic process that results in the restoration of anatomic continuity and function."[11] Wound healing has been seen as analogous to building a house. Adequate supplies must be available to build a house, which is analogous to adequate nutrition, blood flow, and oxygen for wound healing. Cells come together, like the electrician, plumber and painter to do a specific task. Building the house requires a blueprint; in the body the communication must go on chemically. The work of the cells is organized and coordinated by growth factors, or cytokines, which communicate to provide an orderly sequence to the work.

Healed wounds constitute a spectrum of repair. An *ideally healed* wound is one that has returned to normal anatomic structure, function, and appearance. In humans, this degree of healing can occur only in epidermal tissue, mucous membrane, and bone. Once there is injury through the dermis, normal appearance cannot

evolve *Be sure to check out the bonus material on the Evolve website and the CD-ROM, including free self-assessment exercises.*
http://evolve.elsevier.com/Black/medsurg/

Nursing Outcomes Classification (NOC)
for Nursing Diagnoses—Clients with Wounds

Impaired Skin Integrity Tissue Integrity: Skin and Mucous Membranes	**Wound Healing: Primary Intention** **Wound Healing: Secondary Intention**	**Ineffective Tissue Pefusion** Peripheral Perfusions

return because scar tissue replaces missing dermis and epidermis. On the other end of the spectrum, a *minimally healed* wound has anatomic continuity (the wound has closed), but it does not have sustained functional result. Hence the wound can recur. Between these two extremes of healing, an *acceptably healed* wound is characterized by restoration of sustained function and anatomic continuity.

The type of injury has considerable influence on the form of repair. Clean, approximated incisions heal with minimal synthesis of new tissue and barely test a client's resources. In sharp contrast, major burn wounds require complete regeneration of tissue and stimulate massive responses from all body systems to sustain life. The location of the wound also influences healing. Perineal wounds are likely to become infected, wounds over joints are subject to motion and therefore increased scarring, and wounds in peripheral areas or those that do not receive adequate blood supply heal slowly, if at all.

Phases of Wound Healing

Regardless of the cause of the wound, healing follows a predictable course, and many actions occur simultaneously. Events can be described in four phases (Figure 20-1):

- Vascular response
- Inflammation
- Proliferation or resolution
- Maturation, or reconstruction

Vascular Response Phase

Within seconds after an injury, regardless of the type, blood vessels constrict to stop bleeding and reduce exposure to bacteria. The clotting process begins. Platelets form a clot and stop bleeding. At the same time, the plasma protein system begins to form a fibrous meshwork. When the platelets come in contact with the fibrin meshwork across the open vessel wall, they become sticky and adhere (aggregate) to the fibers, forming a plug. This meshwork of clotted blood and serum covers the wound while it heals and prevents further loss of blood and plasma. Platelets also release various proteins and growth factors to stimulate healing (see later discussion).

Capillaries dilate 10 to 30 minutes after injury and remain dilated for some time because of serotonin released by the platelets. Plasma is able to flow into the wounded

area to dilute toxins secreted by the organisms, bring oxygen and nutrients necessary for tissue repair, and carry phagocytes into the area. The wounded area becomes warm and red; these changes are considered classic manifestations of inflammation, and the wound begins the inflammatory phase of healing.

Inflammation Phase

Inflammation, the second phase of wound healing, is essential for wound healing. Inflammation occurs whenever the cells have been injured. Cellular injury can occur from trauma, oxygen or nutrient deprivation, chemical agents, microorganism invasion, temperature extremes, or ionizing radiation. Inflammation also occurs when dead cells are present. Inflammation begins at the moment of injury and may extend for 4 to 6 days, depending on the extent of the injury. The mustering of the inflammatory response is so necessary to healing that

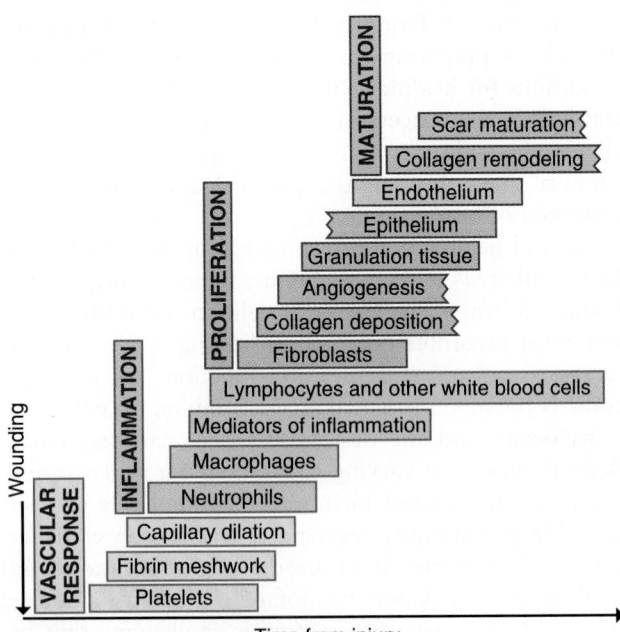

FIGURE 20-1 Normal wound healing. The wound-healing proceeds through four phases: (1) the vascular response, (2) inflammation, (3) proliferation of cells to heal the wound, and (4) maturation of the wound. Each step has many components. The jagged edge depicts an ongoing process. (Modified from Cohen, I., et al. [Eds.]. [1992]. *Wound healing.* Philadelphia: W.B. Saunders.)

it is commonly said, "no inflammation, no healing."

The purpose of inflammation is to limit the effects of harmful bacteria or injury by destroying or neutralizing the organism and by limiting its spread throughout the body. The inflammatory response thereby sets up proper conditions to promote tissue repair (see the Concept Map on Understanding Inflammation and Its Treatment, below). Unlike the *immune response*, which uses specific antibodies for a slow and deliberate response, the effects of inflammation are immediate. Unfortunately, health care terminology uses the word *inflamed* to describe a wound that is not healing normally. Do not be confused between the normal process of inflammation and the term *inflamed*, which means exaggerated inflammation and possible infection.

"Walling-Off" Effect. A walling-off effect occurs in the damaged area to prevent the spread of injurious agents to other body tissues. Fibrinogen clots block the lymphatic channels and spaces in the tissues so that fluid barely flows through the area. The process of walling off the area depends partly on the invading agent. For example, staphylococci invade and destroy nearby tissues quickly, and therefore the process of walling off also develops quickly to control the spread. In contrast, streptococci can digest the walls, which allows the

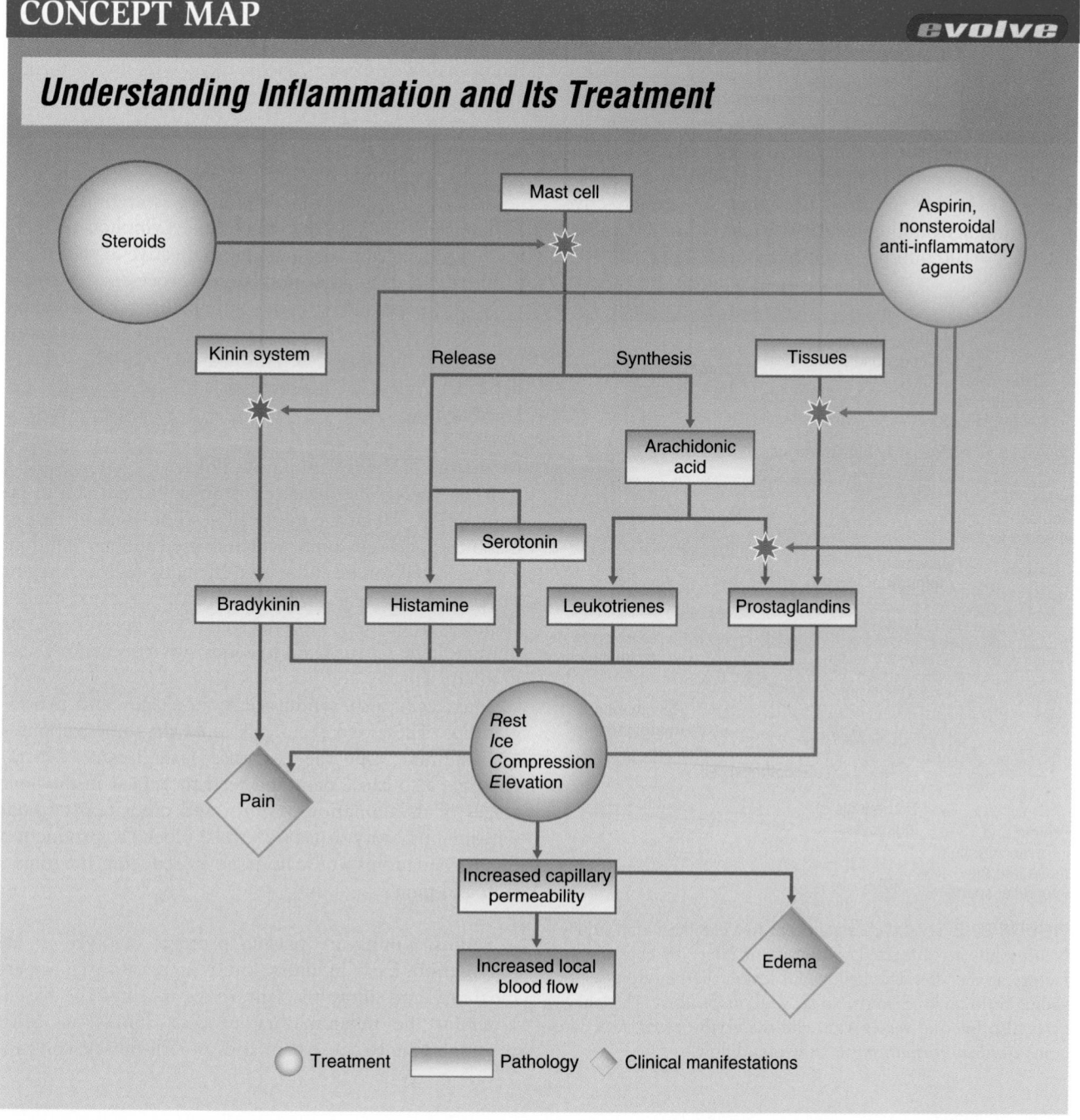

CONCEPT MAP   *evolve*

Understanding Inflammation and Its Treatment

streptococci to multiply and spread. As a result, streptococcal infections have a much greater tendency to invade other organs (e.g., heart valves) and are associated with a higher mortality rate.

White Blood Cell Activity. During the inflammation phase, the white blood cells (WBCs) become active to clean up the wound and initiate further healing processes.

Neutrophils. Neutrophils are vital defense mechanisms because they are both the first and the most numerous cell types to arrive at any area of disease or injury. The slowed flow of blood allows the neutrophil to leave the center of the bloodstream and line the walls of the capillaries, a process called *pavementing,* or *marginating,* because the cells line up like bricks on a sidewalk. Histamine stimulates the cells that line the capillary to constrict, creating spaces in the wall. Neutrophils, which are normally too large to squeeze through the lining, can pass through the capillary wall and enter the site of tissue injury to begin phagocytosis, through a process called *diapedesis* (Figure 20-2). Neutrophils phagocytose bacteria, dead cells, and cellular debris. These cells are short lived, but they are effective in clearing a wound of debris if bacteria are not excessive (i.e., >100,000 per gram of tissue).

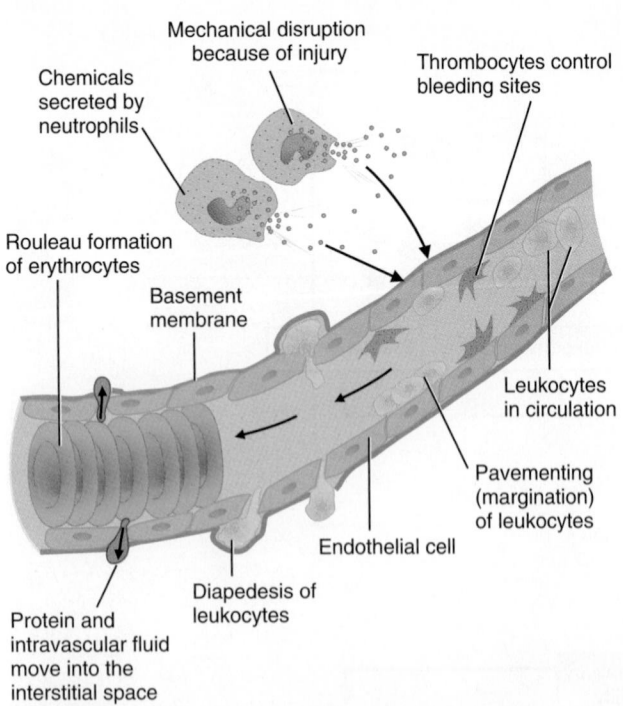

Mechanical disruption because of injury

Chemicals secreted by neutrophils

Thrombocytes control bleeding sites

Rouleau formation of erythrocytes

Basement membrane

Leukocytes in circulation

Pavementing (margination) of leukocytes

Endothelial cell

Diapedesis of leukocytes

Protein and intravascular fluid move into the interstitial space

FIGURE 20-2 Several changes occur in a capillary after injury. Neutrophils are attracted to the site of injury by chemotactic factors at the site. The neutrophil leaves the blood vessel by sliding through holes in the vessel wall *(diapedesis).* The leukocytes also line the vessel wall, and the erythrocytes stack like coins *(rouleau formation)* to slow blood flow.

Neutrophils are sometimes called *polymorphonuclear neutrophils* (PMNs), or polys, because of their irregularly shaped nuclei. Neutrophils compose about 60% of the circulating WBCs. Mature neutrophils appear segmented and are called *segs*. Immature cells are "banded" and called *bands*. Bands are not effective in phagocytosis. The presence of an increase in segmented WBCs indicates a bacterial invasion. The presence of increased band neutrophils indicates more severe infection because the bone marrow has released immature cells. Leukocytes are also the major producers of interferon.

The amount of oxygen in the wound influences the effectiveness of phagocytic cells. Both macrophages and neutrophils can function in an anaerobic environment, but their ability to digest bacteria effectively is slowed. Macrophages are inactivated when tissue levels of oxygen are below 30 mm Hg. (Normal tissue oxygen levels are not the same as levels of oxygen bound to hemoglobin or dissolved oxygen. Tissue oxygen levels are normal at or above 30 mm Hg.)

Other White Blood Cells. Eosinophils and basophils may also migrate to the injured area. Eosinophils help to control the inflammatory response by secreting antihistamine. Basophils secrete histamine. Lymphocytes help the macrophages to become more effective at the site of local injury through a number of processes. Lymphocytes are controlled by the adrenocortical hormones. Therefore clients receiving steroid therapy have reduced numbers of lymphocytes. This change places the steroid-dependent client at increased risk for infection and delayed healing.

Mediators of the Inflammation Phase

Mast Cells. The mast cell is an important cell in inflammation. When the mast cell is stimulated, it releases histamine and serotonin, which cause capillary dilation. The mast cell can be stimulated by many factors, such as physical injury (e.g., wounds, burns, x-ray exposure), chemical injury (e.g., toxins, snake and bee venom), or immunologic means (e.g., hypersensitivity reactions seen in allergies).

Mast cells also synthesize leukotrienes and prostaglandins. These two chemicals cause the same responses as histamine, but the response lasts longer. Prostaglandins also cause pain and tend to appear in the later stages of inflammation. Aspirin and other nonsteroidal anti-inflammatory drugs (NSAIDs) block the production of prostaglandins and can assist in reducing inflammation and pain.

Kinins. Kinins are plasma proteins involved in inflammation. Early in injury, kinins increase vascular permeability and allow the leukocytes to enter the tissue. Later in the inflammatory process, kinins act with prostaglandin to cause pain and smooth-muscle contraction and to increase leukocyte chemotaxis. Kinins increase vascular permeability, fluid in the wound, and the number of leukocytes available to assist with phagocytosis. The primary kinin is bradykinin.

Cytokines. Cytokines regulate the mobility, differentiation, and growth of leukocytes. Among the best understood cytokines are interleukins and interferon. *Interleukins* promote the growth and function of several cells. Interleukin can account for many of the clinical manifestations of both acute and chronic inflammation, such as fever, anorexia, cachexia, and movement of PMNs to the site of injury. Interferons augment immunity through several processes, especially the promotion of B-cell maturation and moderating of suppressor T-cell function.

The Complement System. The complement system is composed of a group of plasma proteins that normally lie dormant in the blood, interstitial fluid, and mucosal surfaces. Microorganisms (or antigen-antibody complexes) activate the complement system. Complement activation promotes inflammation and induces movement of leukocytes into the area of injury. The final aspect of complement activation is the coating of microbes to make them vulnerable to phagocytosis. Many bacteria have an outer capsule that resists phagocytosis. (Complement is fully discussed in the Unit 17 Anatomy and Physiology Review.)

Proliferative Phase

The third phase of wound healing, the proliferative or resolution phase, contains overlapping processes of collagen deposition, angiogenesis (formation of new blood vessels), granulation tissue development, and wound contraction. This phase ends about 2 weeks after injury, but the processes of healing are not complete and continue for 1 to 2 years.

The fibroblast is the most important cell in this phase. Fibroblasts synthesize collagen and granulation tissue. Tissue macrophages continue to patrol the wounded tissue for foreign material. The macrophage also secretes *angiogenesis factor* (AGF), which stimulates the formation of new blood vessels at the end of injured vessels. The macrophage also secretes other cytokines such as platelet-derived growth factor (PDGF), transforming growth factor (TGF), interleukin-1 (IL-1), and basic fibroblast growth factor (bFGF). This cell has a major role in wound healing. Wounds can heal without leukocytes, but wound healing is significantly impaired without macrophages.

Myofibroblasts in the wound cause the wound to contract. Wound contraction is crucial for survival. If a wound from an acute injury did not contract, infections would be lethal complications in all acute injuries. Contraction is undesirable in some wounds because of the

cosmetic deformities that result. Contracture of the scar can produce profound deformities; contracture of the scar at the neck can pull the chin onto the chest. Wounds over joints can also contract severely. Contracture also occurs in internal organs, such as the intestine, breast, and liver.

Epithelialization. *Epithelialization* is the migration of epithelial cells from the edges of the wound of hair follicles within the wound. When epithelium covers a wound, the wound is considered to be closed, or healed. Large wounds or full-thickness wounds may require skin grafting because epidermal migration is normally limited to about 3 cm. Epithelialization can be hastened if a wound is kept moist.

Mediators of the Proliferative Phase

Growth Factors. Growth factors communicate between cells in the wound bed. Dozens of growth factors and cytokines govern wound healing. They can prime other cells to enter a growth phase, or they can move a cell from a growth phase to a DNA production phase. Wounds that fail to heal may be lacking growth factors, and clinical research is ongoing to determine which factors could be topically applied to stimulate wound healing.

Matrix Metalloproteases. Matrix metalloproteases (MMPs) are a group of enzymes that degrade the wound bed. Normally, a balance of wound repair and wound destruction goes on as a wound heals. Chronic wounds that are not healing have a greater amount of MMPs than wounds that are healing in a timely manner.

Maturation Phase

The final phase of wound healing (maturation or reconstruction) is marked by remodeling of the scar. This phase occurs for a year or longer after the wound is closed. During the maturation phase, the scar is remodeled, capillaries disappear, and the scar tissue regains about two thirds of its original strength. The remodeling is the process of collagen synthesis and lysis. Remodeling provides tensile strength to the wound.

Scar tissue is never as strong or as durable as normal tissue. Tensile strength never reaches more than 80% in scar tissue. Over the 12 months after injury, the scar becomes mature and appears thin and white instead of the red, raised appearance seen with granulation tissue. Scarring is a normal part of wound healing. Some scars are barely visible, whereas others remain quite visible throughout the client's lifetime.

Wound Healing Intention

Wound healing intention refers to the probable process of healing for any wound. Wounds can heal by (1)

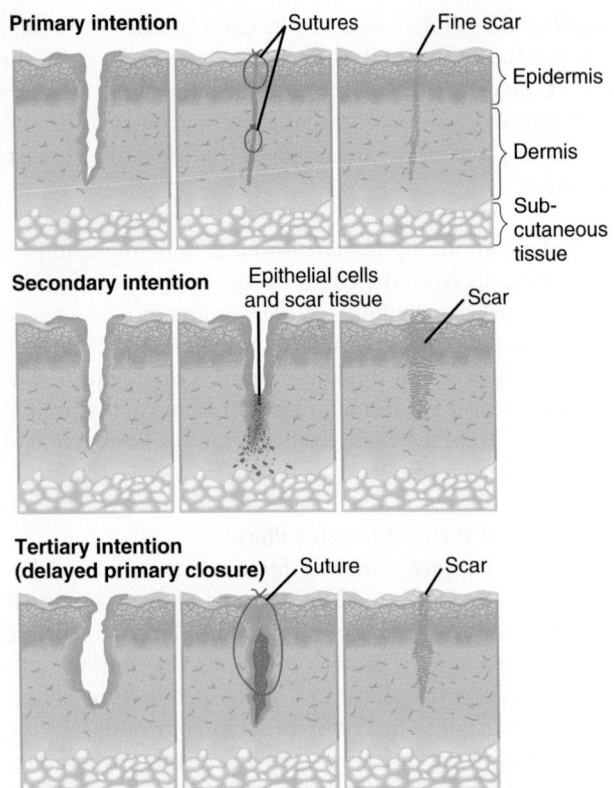

FIGURE 20-3 Wound healing by primary, secondary, and tertiary intention (delayed primary closure).

primary, (2) secondary, or (3) tertiary (delayed primary) intention (Figure 20-3).

Primary Intention

Primary intention is the use of suture (stitches) or other wound closures to *approximate* (place close together) the edges of an incision or clean laceration. Healing is primarily through collagen synthesis, and little scarring or contraction is needed. The risk of infection and tissue defects is minimal. The eventual scar is usually thin and flat.

Secondary Intention

Wounds healing by secondary intention are left open rather than closed with sutures and heal by the generation of tissue. Consider open wounds to be like pressure ulcers or abrasions. Open wounds require the regeneration of much more tissue than does the wound healing by primary intention, and the risk of infection also increases. Wounds healing by secondary intention have a prolonged phase of inflammation because more time is required for phagocytosis of necrotic tissue. The ability of epithelial cells to migrate is limited, and epithelialization may not heal the wound. Therefore the wound is

characterized by longer phases of proliferation and maturation, leading to healing by contraction and the formation of scar tissue. Sometimes healing of is hastened by the application of skin grafts or musculocutaneous (myocutaneous) flaps (see Chapter 51).

Tertiary Intention

Certain wounds may be contaminated, and although they can be closed by primary intention, they are not. Because of the increased risk of infection, these wounds are closed later, when they are free of debris. This type of wound closure is called *healing by tertiary intention*, or *delayed primary closure*.

Intrinsic and Extrinsic Factors in Wound Healing

Factors in the wound itself *(intrinsic)* and within the client *(extrinsic)* can have a profound effect on how quickly a wound heals. These factors are described in Table 20-1.

CLIENTS WITH ACUTE INFLAMMATION

Inflammation occurs in all clients who have sustained any form of tissue trauma. Because the response to inflammation is the same regardless of the cause, the manifestations of inflammation are relatively consistent.

Fever, leukocytosis (an increase in the number of WBCs), increased plasma proteins (e.g., fibrinogen, C-reactive protein), and malaise are the systemic reactions to inflammation: Fever is caused by a *pyrogen* (a fever-causing chemical) released from leukocytes, macrophages, and tumor necrosis factor (TNF). Prostaglandins also act on the hypothalamus to reset the internal thermostat. Fever is usually adaptive because bacterial reproduction is sensitive to even slight increases in temperature. WBC and plasma protein levels increase as the body responds to the invasion. Plasma proteins are collectively called *acute phase reactants*. They provide components of coagulation, transportation, and complement production. The *erythrocyte sedimentation rate* (ESR, or "sed rate"), the rate at which cells settle to the bottom of a glass test tube, also rises with inflammation. Increased levels of fibrinogen cause the red blood cells to stack (like coins) and therefore settle more quickly.

Outcome Management
■ Medical Management

Goals of medical management of a client with acute inflammation include (1) minimizing complications of the edema accompanying inflammation, (2) reducing the inflammatory response, and (3) monitoring systemic responses. Because the inflammatory response is a desired

TABLE 20-1	*Intrinsic and Extrinsic Factors in Wound Healing*	
Factors	**Effect on Wound Healing**	**Treatment**

Intrinsic Factors: Local Factors in the Wound Itself That Can Alter Healing

Infection	Prolongs the inflammatory response Wounds will not heal until infection is controlled	Diagnosed with wound cultures; wounds considered infected when more that 100,000 bacteria are present in 1 g of tissue Systemic or topical antibiotics, debridement
Foreign bodies	Increases the risk of wound infection	Removal of foreign body if infected
Inadequate blood supply	Reduced fibroblast function, increased risk of infection Wounds cannot heal without adequate arterial flow	Restore blood flow with surgery or improve blood flow with medications Protect ischemic skin from injury
Smoking	Reduces arterial flow because nicotine is a vasoconstrictor Carbon monoxide in cigarette smoke reduces tissue oxygen	Abstinence from tobacco Use of smoking cessation programs, but not nicotine patches to control urge to smoke
Neuropathy	Unintentional injury of wounded or previously healed wounds Unregulated blood flow to injured tissues	Protection from injury Daily inspection to detect wounds in early stages

Extrinsic Factors: Characteristics of the Client That Have an Effect on Wound Healing

Protein malnutrition	Reduces collagen deposition and WBC function	Supplements to the diet Tube feeding or hyperalimentation if acceptable to the client/family
Carbohydrate malnutrition	All wound healing phases slowed, protein is used for energy	Same as above
Lack of vitamin C intake	Impaired collagen synthesis	Vitamin C supplementation
Diabetes	Increased risk of infection when blood glucose not controlled Accelerated atherosclerosis, which impairs blood supply	Monitor and regulate blood glucose to less than 200 mg/dl Monitor for methicillin resistant *Staphylococcus aureus* (MRSA) infections
Glucocorticoid steroids	Impair all aspects of wound healing, especially the inflammatory phase. Also impair contraction and epithelialization	Protect paper thin skin from injury Limit use of topical steroids on incisions Vitamin A can reverse some of the effects

WBCs, White blood cells.

response to promote wound healing, the client with inflammation often requires only supportive care.

Control the Effects of Edema. *R*est, *I*ce, *C*ompression, and *E*levation (RICE) is a mnemonic that can be used to guide care to reduce the effect of edema. If an extremity is inflamed, it is elevated and wrapped to reduce edema. Ice is used to control the inflammatory response in the extremities, especially when edema and pain are present. Some physicians order ice for 24 to 72 hours to control inflammation and then apply heat to remove the accumulated waste products. When ice is

ordered, be certain that the cold reaches the wound and that it is not rendered ineffective by bulky dressings. To prevent tissue injury, do not apply ice directly to unprotected skin.

If edema is causing a detrimental alteration of tissue perfusion, anti-inflammatory agents may be required. In certain areas of the body, such as the brain and extremities, the edema that accompanies inflammation can be detrimental to tissue perfusion. These clients may require surgery to release pressure in the area or restore blood flow. Fasciotomy and burr holes are examples of these operations (see Chapters 29 and 75, respectively).

The degree of inflammation is monitored to determine whether it is leading to healing. Analgesics may be required for pain control.

Reduce Inflammation. Anti-inflammatory agents may be prescribed to stabilize the mast cell and reduce edema in the area. Medications in this category range from NSAIDs to corticosteroids. Foreign bodies may be removed to reduce the cause of the inflammation.

Monitor Systemic Responses. Temperature is monitored, and fever is treated with antipyretics (e.g., acetaminophen) when it reaches detrimental levels (i.e., >38.3° C or 101° F. Low-grade fever should not be treated with antipyretics because the high temperature retards bacterial growth; however, fever can be detrimental if it is extreme or prolonged. Therefore the client's temperature is monitored closely to prevent harm. The client with a fever may also experience malaise, nausea, anorexia, weight loss, tachypnea, and tachycardia. The diet of the client with inflammation should be high in vitamin C, protein, calories, and fluids. Vitamin C supports WBC function, production of collagen, and angiogenesis. Protein aids in the formation of blood cells and tissue. Carbohydrates supply needed energy for fuel for healing. Additional fluids are needed to remove metabolic waste and rehydrate the client, especially if the client has been febrile. If the inflammation is

in response to a probable invasion by organisms, antibiotics may be prescribed.

Leukocytosis is due to the increase in the number of leukocytes in circulation to combat infection. Sometimes, in an effort to combat infection, the bone marrow releases immature leukocytes (banded neutrophils or bands). When the number of immature neutrophils is high, the client is said to have a "left shift." At times, the release of immature cells means that the body is having difficulty combating the infection with mature cells. Interpretation of the WBC differential is shown in Table 20-2.

■ Nursing Assessment of the Medical Client
Assessment

The clinical manifestations of inflammation in acute wounds include redness, swelling, heat, pain, and loss of function. Tissues are red, warm, painful, and swollen and have limited mobility. In addition, an inflammatory exudate is formed. The exudate dilutes the toxins released by bacteria, brings certain nutrients to the wound, and carries phagocytes for defense. Various types of exudate are present, depending on the stage of inflammation and its cause.

Serous exudate is seen in early inflammation and is composed of water with a small amount of colloids, ions, and phagocytic cells. A *blister* is a common exam-

---

TABLE 20-2	*Interpretation of Differential Counts Within a Complete Blood Count*		
Cell Type	**Function**	**Normal Value**	**Significance of Change**
Segmented neutrophils (segs)*	Mature neutrophils act as phagocytes	50%-60%	Elevated with infection; a "left shift" means that many band (immature) cells are present as the body fights infection; "right shift" is the presence of more mature cells, as seen with liver disease and pernicious anemia
Band neutrophils	Immature neutrophils	3%-8%	Elevated in acute stages of infection
Lymphocytes	Produced by lymphoid tissue, participate in humoral response	25%-40%	Elevated in infectious mononucleosis, cytomegalovirus infection, and infectious hepatitis; decreased in acquired immunodeficiency syndrome (AIDS), Cushing's syndrome, chronic uremia, and following trauma (e.g., burn injury)
Monocytes	A second line of defense, increasing in chronic infections	2%-8%	Elevated in chronic bacterial infection, viral disease, Hodgkin's disease, multiple myeloma, and some forms of leukemia
Eosinophils	Phagocytic, destroy antigen-antibody complexes before they can harm the body	1%-4%	Elevated in allergic disorders and parasitic infections; decreased in infectious mononucleosis, congestive heart failure, pernicious anemia, and during the use of steroids, epinephrine, and thyroxine

*To calculate the absolute neutrophils count (also called an absolute granulocyte count):

$$\text{Absolute neutrophil count} = \frac{\text{Total \% of neutrophils (segs + bands)} \times \text{WBC count (cells/mm}^3)}{100}$$

When the absolute neutrophil count falls below 1000/mm^3, the client is said to be "neutropenic," and precautions must be taken to prevent infection.

ple of serous exudate. Hemorrhagic or sanguineous exudate is composed of blood. Drainage is bright red or dark red. Serosanguineous exudate is drainage composed of both serous fluid and blood. It is pink and usually fairly thin. Purulent exudate is filled with more leukocytes *(pus)* and is common in chronic inflammation from walled-off lesions.

The type of drainage present in the wound is indicative of the phase of healing. For example, a surgical wound initially presents with sanguineous drainage. As hemostasis progresses, the drainage becomes serosanguineous and finally advances to serous drainage (Table 20-3).

Monitor the level of WBCs, differential counts, and fever as indicators of infection. Expect the WBC level to rise in clients with known infections and after acute injury, such as a surgical incision. Monitor also older clients, who often have infection but not necessarily elevated WBC counts.

Diagnosis, Outcomes, Interventions

Diagnosis: Ineffective Tissue Perfusion.
Edema from the inflammatory response may restrict blood vessels and entrap nerves in the traumatized area. The nursing diagnosis *Ineffective Peripheral Tissue Perfusion related to edema* is an appropriate diagnosis.

Outcomes.
The client will have adequate tissue perfusion as evidenced by the usual skin color, the presence of pulses in areas distal to the edema, skin warmth, lack of paresthesias, and lack of escalating pain.

Interventions.
Assess clients with visible injury causing inflammation for resolution of bleeding in the area, adequate blood flow, and nerve conduction distal to the affected site. Frequent assessments (every 2 hours) of the edematous area are needed. Measurement of the circumference of the area also enables the examiner to determine whether the area is becoming markedly edematous. To measure the same site, mark the area on the client with a pen to ensure appropriate location of serial measurements.

In addition to assessing the circumference, assess pulses, skin temperature, capillary refill, sensation, and movement in areas distal to the inflammation. Compare the involved side to the other side, using the client's uninvolved side as a baseline. Dressings or casts over the affected area can also form a constriction. This response can be called *compartment syndrome.* Clients who have been injured or had orthopedic surgery are at highest risk for compartment syndrome (see also Chapter 29).

Objects that may become entrapped in edematous tissues, such as rings, should be removed because they can cause serious damage. The inflamed area should be elevated. Application of cold compresses causes vasoconstriction and decreases the amount of edema. Prolonged use of cold compresses can lead to rebound vasodilation and increase the risk of tissue injury. Vasoconstriction can also decrease the inflow of new blood and thereby slow the removal of toxins and waste from the site of injury.

If the extremity is edematous, it should be elevated. Distal circulation and sensation should be assessed often for the first 48 hours after injury or surgery. Edematous skin is more likely to break down. Keep the skin lubricated and protected from injury. Factors that impede venous flow should be controlled. For example, rolled stockings that constrict venous return should not be worn. Compression bandages may be used to reduce edema by promoting lymphatic and venous drainage. Explain the appropriate way to apply these bandages (from distal to proximal) and when to rewrap them to maintain compression.

Evaluation

The outcome of the inflammatory response is usually time dependent. Most edema subsides over 72 hours

TABLE 20-3	*Inflammatory Exudates*	
Type	**Appearance**	**Significance**
Hemorrhagic, sanguineous	Bright red or bloody	Small amounts expected after surgery or trauma; large amounts may indicate hemorrhage; sudden large amounts of dark-red blood may indicate a draining hematoma
Serosanguineous	Blood-tinged yellow or pink	Expected for 48-72 hr after injury or trauma; a sudden increase may precede wound dehiscence
Serous	Thin, clear, yellow	Expected for up to 1 week after trauma or surgery; a sudden increase may indicate a draining seroma
Purulent	Thin, cloudy, foul-smelling; may be thick if filled with dead cells	Usually indicates infection; may drain suddenly from an abscess (boil)
Catarrhal	Thin, clear mucus	Seen with upper respiratory infection

with appropriate RICE measures. If the edema has not subsided in that time frame, consider another cause of the edematous process, such as infection.

■ Self-Care

Clients who are capable of caring for a wound or area that is likely to become inflamed need instructions on how to elevate the extremity, how to use heat or ice, how to follow the medication regimen, and how to change dressings. Clinical manifestations of edema and infection must be reported, such as changes in color, pulse, and pain. For clients going home, creative problem solving is needed to find a mechanism to elevate arms or legs while sleeping or sitting in a chair. The edematous extremity must remain higher than the heart to reduce edema, and this degree of elevation is hard to achieve at home and even more so while asleep.

CLIENTS WITH CHRONIC INFLAMMATION

Chronic inflammation is differentiated from acute inflammation by its duration and the cells that mediate the response. If the invading organisms were not controlled or eliminated during the acute stage of inflammation, the body attempts to protect surrounding tissues from further invasion by building a wall around the infected site called a *granuloma*. Some forms of infection, such as fungi, parasites, and perhaps antibody-antigen reactions (autoimmune disease), result in granuloma formation. Tuberculosis is a good example. When tuberculosis develops, a thick wall forms around the mycobacteria. The bacteria continue to live in the walled-off area, and it is soon filled with dead tissue. As the tissue dies, the cellular enzymes are released and the fluid leaves the granuloma. The empty sac remains.

Unlike an acutely inflamed wound, the appearance of a chronically inflamed wound often does not appear red, warm, and tender. The tissue often appears pale and **EB** odorous if infected and fails to heal.[5]

Outcome Management

The chronically inflamed wound has purulent drainage *(suppuration)* and does not heal completely. A common example of chronic inflammation is seen when foreign objects are not removed from tissues (e.g., splinter, glass, dirt). Chronic inflammation can also occur when certain forms of bacteria cannot be killed by phagocytes. For example, the organisms that cause tuberculosis, syphilis, and leprosy have cell walls with a very high lipid and wax content, which makes them impermeable to the phagocyte.

Care of the client with chronic infection is focused on determining the source of the problem. Wounds may be *debrided* (cleaned and freed of dead tissue), and the client may be given antibiotics or anti-inflammatory agents.

CLIENTS WITH INCISIONS

Outcome Management

Wounds made intentionally with a scalpel and closed with sutures, staples, or strips of tape are called *incisions*. Incisions are the most common example of wounds healing by primary intention. An incision should be assessed every 8 hours. If the incision is not visible, check the dressings for drainage and odor. The incision normally appears somewhat pink and swollen; small areas of induration around the suture marks are common. Erythema should not extend beyond a half-inch from the incision. If the wound was closed primarily, you should be able to palpate the presence of newly synthesized collagen just under an intact suture line. This internal scar is known as a *healing ridge*. When this ridge is not present 5 to 7 days after suturing, suspect slowed collagen synthesis. The client may need additional protection of the nonhealing area to prevent infection.

A wound that is healing by primary intention should be protected from further trauma, including external pressure. Keep the wound free of pulling forces that stretch the sutured skin. Keep the wound clean, but do not wash the suture line because water carries microorganisms into the wound along the sutures. Protect it from the external environment and drainage with dressings.

Apply dressings using an aseptic or sterile technique. Sterile gloves are usually not required. Hold the side of the dressing that will not touch the client's incision by the clean or gloved hands, and tape it in place. The type of dressing used changes as the wound responds to treatment. Use dressings that best suit the wound. Gauze dressings are used most often on a wound that is healing by primary intention. Dressings for open wounds are discussed in the following section.

Wound drainage tubes can be placed in the dead space created during exposure of the operative area. Drainage of a wound is indicated when actual or potential fluid accumulation threatens the healing process. The drain facilitates removal of blood from the wound. Assess the volume and type of fluid hourly immediately after surgery. If a reservoir is attached to the drain, measure the volume of drainage by markings on the reservoir. If the drainage is emptied from the reservoir, follow standard precautions for its disposal. In addition, if the drainage is caustic (e.g., bile), the skin around the site must be protected with skin barriers.

Teach the client how to care for the incision, the clinical manifestations of wound infection, how to care for and empty the drain reservoir, and when to return for suture removal. Sutures in areas where scarring must be controlled (e.g., on the face) are usually removed in 4 to 7 days; in other areas, sutures are usually removed in 7 to 10 days. Sutures in the hand and foot are removed in 1 to 2 weeks or longer.

CLIENTS WITH OPEN WOUNDS

Outcome Management
■ Medical Management

The goal of medical management of an open wound is to prepare the client and the wound for the quickest and most durable form of healing. The treatment of a wound includes the removal of its cause, the correction of underlying problems that are delaying healing, and the initiation of topical (or systemic) treatments to facilitate healing.

Control the Cause of the Wound. Open wounds are common in clients with diseases that impair blood flow to the legs (arteriosclerosis, venous insufficiency, diabetes) or that reduce sensation (paralysis, diabetes). If wound healing is delayed because of lack of venous return, the extremity requires compression and elevation. If the cause of the wound is lack of arterial flow, the extremity should be positioned flat. If pressure is a causative or contributing factor, repositioning and proper support surfaces must be considered.

Protein-calorie malnutrition may be present, which delays healing of all wounds because the protein needed to manufacture new cells is not available. The client's diet should be high in carbohydrates, protein, iron, and vitamins. In addition, the client may remain at risk of further skin breakdown, such as pressure ulcers.

Remove Devitalized Tissue from the Wound: Debridement. Wound healing is optimized and the risk of infection is reduced when all necrotic (dead) tissue, exudate, and metabolic wastes are removed from the wound. Moist, devitalized tissue supports bacterial growth. Various forms of debridement are used to remove these tissues (see later discussion). Systemic and topical antibiotics alone seldom stop infection because they cannot penetrate the avascular tissues.

Before a wound can heal, necrotic tissues must be removed. Debridement can be accomplished by means of a variety of techniques: (1) surgical or sharp, (2) mechanical, (3) enzymatic, and (4) autolytic (these last three are described later). Timely debridement is necessary to remove the devitalized tissue and reduce the risk of infection and the physical obstacles dead tissue places on the process of granulation. In addition, the true size and stage of the wound cannot be known until the necrotic tissue is removed.

Surgical or Sharp Debridement. Wounds covered with dead tissue, called *eschar* or *slough,* need to be cleaned to promote healing and reduce infection (Figure 20-4, *A*). *Sharp debridement* is performed by the physician or trained nurses and is the quickest method. This procedure is used for large wounds, a wound that involves a thick eschar that would not be permeated by

any topical agent, and a wound that is acutely infected. The eschar or slough is removed to the level of bleeding tissues. The wound size, depth of the wound, contamination, and the client's status influence whether the client is in satisfactory condition to tolerate sharp debridement, which may call for general anesthesia or sedation. Pain medications should be used for clients undergoing sharp debridement.

Sharp debridement is carried out under sterile conditions, usually in an operating room, a treatment room, or an outpatient surgical setting. Risks associated with general anesthesia, blood loss, and infections are a major concern. After sharp debridement, the client is

FIGURE 20-4 A, A wound on the sacrum with eschar that needs debridement. **B,** Diabetic foot ulcers are an example of a wound with yellow, soft slough that needs cleaning. **C,** Healing venous stasis ulcers have a clean wound filled with granulation tissue that needs protection.

monitored for manifestations of bleeding and bacteremia (sepsis). Sepsis is suspected if unexplained fever, tachycardia, hypotension, or deterioration in mental status develops. The physician should be notified of these changes. Sepsis can be fatal if it is not recognized early and treated aggressively (see septic shock in Chapter 83). Once the wound is clean, surgery may be used to speed healing and to reduce the risk of infection and contracture. Skin grafts are commonly used to replace the epidermis. The partial-thickness burn wound is the best example of a wound that could heal by secondary intention but is often grafted to speed healing and reduce infection and scarring. Cutaneous or musculocutaneous flaps can also be used to close a large wound (see Chapter 51).

■ Nursing Management of the Medical Client

Assessment

The client's history must be taken, including a history of the wound itself. The wound history includes causative intrinsic and extrinsic factors, duration of the wound, and current and previous methods of treatment and their corresponding success. Sometimes wound treatments are used that actually impair healing, such as hydrogen peroxide or Dakin's solution. This information is important when one is obtaining a complete wound history. Assessments should be thorough and should focus on the whole client, not just the wound.

Psychosocial assessment should include the client's age, occupation, living situation, financial status, health care benefits, roles and responsibilities, cultural and spiritual beliefs, body image and self-esteem, and ability to learn self-care and comply with the treatment plan. Also note compliance with treatment of underlying disorders, such as diabetes and collagen diseases.

A complete physical assessment should be performed. Focus the data collection on height and weight; degree of range of motion; muscle wasting and level of activity; circulation, such as peripheral pulses, color, edema, and the temperature of extremities; lung sounds; and level of pain. A complete wound assessment is needed (Box 20-1). Clearly document wound assessments to allow for an objective evaluation at a later date. Describe the actual size of the ulcer by measuring its length, width, and depth. If the wound is a pressure ulcer, use the staging system to further describe it (see Chapter 51). Describe the color, type of drainage, presence of undermining, and condition of periwound skin in the assessment data for later comparison. A photograph is an excellent means of documentation and determination of the progress in healing. Obtain consent before photographs are taken. Photographs should be taken with a consistent method that includes reproducible distance, color, and grid film or a ruler in the photo so that size can be determined.

Examine laboratory values for hemoglobin, hematocrit, albumin, prealbumin, and WBCs, specifically lym-

---

| BOX 20-1 | *Wound Assessment* |

When assessing an open wound, obtain the following information:
1. Is the wound painful?
2. What is the size of the wound? Use objective measures to indicate the length and width (such as centimeters or millimeters). Avoid terms such as "the size of a grape." Use a sterile gloved finger or cotton swab to measure depth. Consider using photographs to provide a baseline and serial evaluations.
3. Where is the wound located anatomically?
4. What is the color of the wound? Estimate the percentage of each color when more than one color is noted.
5. Is there granulation tissue or epithelial tissue? Granulation tissue is red, shiny, and bumpy; epithelial tissue looks like pale skin.
6. Are there sinus tracts, or are the edges undermined? Use a gloved hand or swab to measure the extent. Indicate the location and direction of tunneling.
7. Are there signs of infection in the wound? Look for erythema extending beyond the edges of the wound as well as warmth, edema, odor, and purulent exudate. (Also consider systemic signs.)
8. Is there any drainage? Note the color, odor, consistency, and approximate amount by the number of dressings saturated.
9. What is the condition of the surrounding skin? Is it intact, red, indurated, or macerated?

---

phocytes. These values indicate the degree of nutritional impairment that might contribute to the wound's lack of healing. Generally, the risk of delayed healing correlates with low serum albumin levels; however, albumin levels are a slow-to-change indicator of nutritional state. A pre-albumin level is more indicative of current nutritional status.

Diagnosis, Planning, Interventions

Diagnosis: Impaired Skin Integrity. The nursing diagnosis should be used to indicate an actual loss of skin. The actual statement might be phrased *Impaired Skin Integrity related to delayed wound healing secondary to impaired circulation, to infection, or to malnutrition.*

Outcomes. The client will experience improved skin integrity, as evidenced by a cleaner wound within 1 week, less drainage from the wound, no odor from the wound and no manifestations of infection in the wound. A long-term goal might be a smaller wound in 3 weeks.

Interventions. Many agencies have wound care nurses who should be contacted for up-to-date information and

TABLE 20-4	*Topical Agents Used in Treatment of Open Wounds*	
Agent	**Indications**	**Impact on Wound Healing**
Antiseptic Solutions		
Normal saline	Used to moisten dry eschar; keep a clean wound healing by secondary intention	Speeds healing because solution is iso-osmolar, and it keeps the wound bed moist
Hydrogen peroxide	Used to dissolve clotted blood in a wound	Retards healing; do not use as a dressing on an open wound
Providone-iodine (Betadine)	Used for preparation of intact skin; may be used to clean very contaminated wounds	Retards healing; does not penetrate eschar
Dakin's solution	Used $\frac{1}{2}$ to $\frac{1}{4}$ strength to clean contaminated wounds	Retards wound healing
Acetic acid	Used to treat wounds contaminated with *Pseudomonas*	Retards wound healing slightly
Antibiotic Solutions and Ointments		
Neomycin-bacitracin-polymyxin B (Neosporin)	Used to clean wounds contaminated with gram-negative and gram-positive bacteria	Increases epidermal healing but may sensitize tissues; high incidence of allergy
Polymyxin B-bacitracin (Polysporin)	Treatment of gram-negative organisms	None known
Silver sulfadiazine	Used in wounds with eschar (e.g., burns); effective against gram-negative and gram-positive organisms	Enhances epidermal healing; penetrates eschar
Gentamicin	Most effective against gram-negative organisms, but its use may promote resistance in hospital flora	None known
Bacitracin	Effective against gram-positive and gram-negative organisms	May enhance epidermal healing

for assistance with complex wounds. Every nurse, however, must properly identify basic concepts of wound assessment and treatment.

Keep the Wound Moist. Wound healing is optimized when the wound is kept moist. A moist environment promotes collagen synthesis, granulation tissue formation, and epithelial cell migration. This moist environment, however, can create a medium conducive to infection, and a clean technique must be used for wound care. Heat lamps or treatments that dry the wound must be avoided.

Wet-to-moist or continuously moist dressings are used in clean and granulating wounds. Insert dressings into the wound or place them on all surfaces of the wound while they are moist, making certain to protect normal intact skin. Remove the dressings while they are still moist to avoid disrupting the granular bed. Bleeding should not occur when the dressing is removed. If the dressing is too dry to pull off, moisten it with sterile normal saline before attempting to remove it. Foam and hydrocolloid dressings can also be used to keep a clean wound moist. The wound bed should be gently cleansed

with normal saline to remove debris before replacing the dressings.

Prevent Injury to Healing Tissues. Normal saline is the only solution for wound care recommended by the Agency for Health Care Policy and Research (AHCPR). Normal saline is physiologic, does not harm tissues, and adequately cleans most wounds. Avoid applying solutions on and in the clean wound that may impair healing. For example, full-strength iodine, hydrogen peroxide, and Dakin's solution were once commonly used for wound care; however, these solutions damage the wound. (Table 20-4). If they are used for infected wounds, it is important to limit their use to the shortest time possible.

Protect the Periwound Skin. Moisture on normal, intact skin makes the skin more prone to breakdown. The cardinal rule is to keep the wound bed moist and surrounding skin dry.

Select Dressings. Dressings can protect a healing wound; absorb exudate, or debride a necrotic wound.

Dressings are chosen based on the appearance of the wound bed (see Figure 20-4). Gauze still remains the most commonly used dressing. Gauze is used as a dry cover for surgical wounds or for wounds that heal by primary intention (Table 20-5). Only mesh gauze should be used in a wound because cotton dressings are likely to leave fibers behind. Use cotton-filled gauze as an outer dressing. If the wound edges are friable or if the wound will be injured when the dressing is removed, a nonadherent dressing can be used to avoid injury to the wound or periwound skin. If gauze is used to pack the wound, hydrocolloid dressings can be placed like a window frame around the wound. The tape can be applied to the window rather than the skin.

Clean, granulating wounds do not require daily dressing changes (Figure 20-4, C). Granulating wounds should be dressed with occlusive, moisture-retaining dressings, such as foam, moist gauze, hydrocolloid or hydrogel. If the wound is shallow, a thin layer of antibi-

otic ointment and nonadhering dressing (or synthetic dressing) may be used to cover it. If the wound is deep, saline-moistened gauze can be used to pack the wound, but the dressing should not be allowed to dry out before it is changed. When a dressing adheres to a wound bed, granulation tissue and new epithelium are also removed when the dressing is changed. Continue to observe for infection. If purulent drainage develops, do not apply occlusive dressings. Allow the wound to drain by using gauze or alginates. Debriding dressings, like wet to dry dressings, should not be used on granulating wounds. Debridement removes new tissues, leads to bleeding and slows healing.

Excessive exudate can delay healing. If the wound produces exudate, several absorptive dressings can be used. Absorptive dressings, calcium alginates, and hypertonic saline dressings are appropriate choices for moderate or highly exudative wounds. Foams can also be used for absorption and autolytic debridement. Table

TABLE 20-5	Wound Dressings		
Type	Product	Indications for Use	Nursing Implications
Nonadhering, nonimpregnated	Telfa	Shallow, open wounds	Second dressing or tape needed; it is nonadhesive; can lead to maceration
Impregnated	Adaptic gauze, Vaseline gauze, Xeroform	Moist wounds	Nonabsorbent, occlusive, not traumatic to remove
Gauze	Adaptic gauze, Kling gauze, NuGauze, Primapore	Wet-to-dry debridement, wound packing	Moderately absorbent; can be used as wound packing for shallow wounds; use long strips of gauze to pack deep wounds; gauze does not provide a bacterial barrier; if allowed to dry on a wound, it may remove viable tissue when removed
Transparent films	Bio-occlusive, OpSite, Tegaderm	Coverage of shallow wounds, intravenous sites, blisters, abrasions	Adhesive; therefore no secondary dressing is needed; retain moisture, semipermeable, water-resistant; facilitate autolytic debridement
Hydrocolloids	Comfeel, Duoderm, Intrasite, Restore, Tegasorb, Intact	Shallow ulcers, donor sites, second-degree (partial-thickness) burns; do not use on infected wounds	Retain moisture, occlusive or semipermeable, water-resistant, adhesive; require replacement because the dressing melts; reduce pain
Hydrogels	Elastogel, wound gel, Spenco, Vigilon	Pressure ulcers, dermal ulcers, partial-thickness burns, abrasions, blisters	Have a cooling effect; maintain moist environment, relieve pain, permit autolytic debridement; easily removed unless they dry out
Exudate absorbers	Bard absorption dressing, Envisan	Deep wounds with eschar	Retain moisture, absorbent, promote autolytic debridement
Calcium alginates	Sorbsan, Kaltostat, Algiderm	Clean wounds with profuse drainage	Retain moisture, absorbent, left intact for several days
Foams	Reston, Flexan, Lyofoam, Polymen, Tielle	Full-thickness wounds with moderate to heavy drainage, skin tears	Moisture, absorbent, nonadherent, left intact for several days

20-5 describes the actions, indications, and nursing implications for various categories of wound dressings.

Necrotic wounds cannot be covered with occlusive dressings. Microorganisms cannot drain from the wound bed and become invasive, quickly leading to sepsis.

The selection of dressing type changes as the wound responds to treatment. Careful assessment and reassessment will indicate progress, or lack of progress, in wound healing. As the wound changes, variations in the dressing materials are made so that healing is maximized. No single dressing provides the optimal atmosphere required during all healing stages of the wound.

Fill Dead Space. *Dead space* is empty space within a wound. In an ulcer, it is the space between the base of the ulcer and the underside of the dressing around its perimeter. If this space is closed, empty pockets may develop anaerobic infection. Long-acting normal saline gel and alginate wound packing are good media to fill a clean wound and the pockets of empty space before a topical dressing is applied.

Deep wounds with tunnels or undermining are at high risk of infection. These wounds can also heal with "false floors," which trap bacteria and lead to further infection. It is important that an open wound heal from the inside out. Deep wounds are often packed with gauze strips soaked in saline or an antibiotic solution to debride the wound or prevent abnormal healing. Strips of gauze must be used to avoid having soiled single dressings lost in the wound. The gauze is packed into the wound with enough force to hold the edges of the wound open, but not so much force that the wound is under tension. Wounds packed too tightly compromise blood flow and delay healing. The outer edge of the dressing is covered with dry dressings. Packing is usually changed every 4 to 6 hours. Some gel packing strips are changed less often. Skin surrounding the wound should be assessed for breakdown from frequent tape removal, and dressings should be secured with other methods if needed (e.g., Montgomery straps).

Remove Necrotic Tissue. Debridement is needed to remove nonviable tissue in the wound. Ulcers cannot heal with necrotic tissue present. Necrotic tissue becomes a breeding ground for microorganisms and increases the risk of septicemia, osteomyelitis, limb amputation, and death. Yellow or tan adherent material in the wound base is called *slough* (see Figure 20-4, *B*). Black, leathery material in the wound base is called *eschar*. This necrotic tissue must be removed for the wound to heal. (The only exception is dry eschar on the heel, which should not be routinely removed.) The risk of infection rises in proportion to the amount of necrotic tissue present.

Several techniques can be used to debride necrotic tissue; sharp debridement (discussed earlier), mechanical debridement with irrigation and dressings, enzymatic debridement, and autolytic debridement.

Irrigation. Irrigation between 4 and 15 pounds per square inch (psi) removes debris, bacteria, and necrotic tissue without damaging tissues; 8 psi is the most pressure that should be used on a wound. High-pressure devices, such as a WaterPik, create excessive force and trauma and may cause bacteria to be driven into the wound. Wound irrigation is safe and effective with a 35-ml syringe and a 19F angiocatheter, small syringes of saline, or outer plastic tubing from an intravenous (IV) needle. Hydrotherapy by use of a whirlpool is also an option for wound cleaning.

When irrigating around a wound, use barrier precautions with masks or goggles, gowns, and gloves because you may be sprayed by contaminated solutions. The client may also need protection with a pad or container to collect the contaminated irrigation solution.

Wet-to-Dry Dressings. An all-gauze dressing is moistened with the prescribed solution and wrung out until the dressing is just moist. The moist dressing should be gently packed into all crevices in the wound and left long enough to begin to dry (4 to 6 hours) (Figure 20-5). As the dressing dries, debris, necrotic tissue, exudate, and drainage adhere to it. The wound is debrided as the dressing is gently removed. The dressings are not remoistened to make removal easier because this practice defeats the purpose of the dressing, which is to debride the wound. The process is often painful, and clients should have adequate analgesia before the dressing is changed. Topical skin protectant can be used to protect surrounding intact skin from exposure to moisture. Wet-to-dry dressings are a nonselective form of debridement and can inadvertently remove new granulation tissues as well as necrotic tissue, creating an environment that retards healing. Therefore they are used only until the wound is clean and granulating.

Enzymatic Debridement. Proteolytic enzymes can be applied to necrotic tissue to digest them. Enzymatic

FIGURE 20-5 Wet-to-dry dressings are placed into a wound with the use of strip gauze.

debridement should be considered when the client cannot tolerate surgical excision; has soft, stringy slough; or is at home or in long-term care. Enzymatic debridement is relatively slow and should not be used on wounds that appear infected. Medicate clients before the use of enzymatic agents, which cause burning. Apply the enzymatic ointment to only about 2 to 4 square inches of necrotic tissue at one time. Enzymes work best in a moist environment; use moist gauze and cover the wound with dry gauze. Enzymatic agents should not be placed on viable tissue because they cause tissue necrosis. They also cannot be used on wounds communicating with major body cavities, wounds with exposed nerves, or neoplastic ulcers. They must be used with caution around the eyes.

Dry eschar is best removed with a scalpel. If this is not an option, dry eschar should be *scored* (should have small cuts made into it) before the enzymatic ointment is applied to enhance penetration.

Autolytic Debridement. Autolytic debridement is the use of the body's own digestive enzymes to break down necrotic tissue. With this method, an occlusive dressing is placed over the ulcer and the eschar or devitalized tissue is allowed to self-digest. This is a slow process; however, autolytic debridement may be appropriate for clients who cannot tolerate other methods and are not susceptible to infection. Autolytic debridement is contraindicated for infected wounds.

 Provide Nutritional Support. In addition to local wound care, the client must be provided with a diet that is high in protein, fat, carbohydrates, vitamins, and minerals to facilitate healing. Regardless of the client's actual body weight (e.g., obesity), healing a wound is not the time to begin a weight-loss diet. The wound must be healed first. Review the nutritionist's recommendations for caloric, protein, and fluid intake. Determine whether the client is receiving the needed nutrients. If the client can eat, offer supplements or adjust the diet so that the meal is more palatable. If the client cannot or will not eat, the use of tube feeding or hyperalimentation should be considered. Many clients report that they do not have an appetite and therefore do not feel like eating. Clients and family should be encouraged to eat anyway; an appetite is not needed to consume food.

Reduce Interface Pressure. If the client has pressure ulcers, pressure reduction is key to management and prevention. Turning and repositioning constitute the oldest form of reducing pressure on body surfaces. Clients should be turned and repositioned every 2 hours if they do not move spontaneously. If the client cannot be moved or refuses to turn, consider changing the surface of the bed to one that creates less interface pressure. Chair cushions must also be used to reduce pressure on the ischia when sitting. Four inches of foam is adequate for most clients. Over time, however, foam develops a "memory," which reduces its effectiveness. If an imprint of the client's buttocks remains in the foam after rising from the chair, the foam needs to be replaced. Other seat cushions are also available. All clients who sit in chairs need to be repositioned hourly regardless of the surface on which they sit.

Evaluation

In hospital settings, wounds should be assessed with each dressing change. Wounds at risk of infection should be assessed every 24 hours. Clean, granulating wounds can be evaluated every 3 to 5 days, provided the dressings remain intact and clean. If the dressings appear stained or surrounding skin is red, swollen, or painful, the dressings should be removed and the wound closely assessed for infection. If the wound shows no signs of healing after 2 weeks, a 2-week trial of topical antibiotics is recommended, including quantitative bacterial cultures and a bone scan to assess for osteomyelitis.

■ Self-Care

The client with open wounds often requires long-term care or community resources for safe self-care. Planning for discharge should begin several days before the client is released so that the home situation can be appraised and the necessary support, supplies, and equipment obtained. Appropriate referral to the home health agency or wound healing clinic should be made before discharge. Social services, home health care, or a discharge planner should be involved in the plan of care. The client's financial status, home environment, and support systems must be evaluated. Third-party reimbursement may cover supplies, equipment, and nursing care.

Several areas of client education are needed. The client or family should demonstrate dressing removal, wound cleaning, and dressing application before discharge. Detailed written instructions on wound care should be provided to the client, family, and home health care nurse. Videotaping the dressing change may be helpful once the client is home. Explain what changes should be expected and what changes should be reported to the health care provider. Fever, a change in drainage, or the development of an odorous drainage should be instructed as being a reportable change.

The average cost of skilled nursing services for treating wounds in the home is $1600 per healed wound. Some cost-cutting measures for saline and gloves have been designed, and it is now possible to make normal saline for home use on wounds. Use to 1 gallon of distilled water or 1 gallon of tap water boiled for 5 minutes; do not use well water or sea water. Add 8 teaspoons of table salt. Mix the solution well and cool to room temperature before use. This solution can be stored for up to 1 week.

In the home, rather than purchasing gloves for dressing changes, soiled dressings can be removed using a plastic sandwich bag (Figure 20-6). The inside of the bag

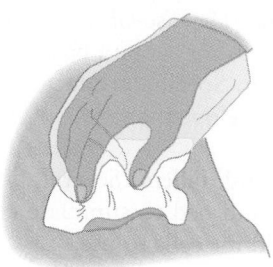

Place a small, clean bag over your hand like a mitten.
Carefully lift the dressing off the sore.

Turn the bag inside out to enclose the dressing.
Seal the bag before throwing it away.

FIGURE 20-6 Plastic bags used as gloves to remove a dressing in the home. (Modified from Agency for Health Care Policy and Research. [1994]. *Treating pressure sores.* Bethesda, MD, U.S. Department of Health and Human Services, AHCPR Pub. No. 95-B0654.)

is used as a glove to remove the dressing, and the dressing is disposed of in the same bag. Methods of obtaining needed wound care supplies should also be discussed with the client and his or her family.

A balanced diet with frequent high-protein snacks should continue until the wound and contributing factors have been resolved. A vitamin and mineral supplement should be taken as directed. The client is often required to incorporate lifestyle changes into activities of daily living (ADL) in an effort to promote healing.

DISORDERS OF WOUND HEALING

DELAYED WOUND HEALING

Not all wounds heal in a timely manner or stay healed. Both intrinsic and extrinsic factors delay wound healing. When assessing wounds and clients with wounds, be aware of the factors that can delay healing. Some factors are controllable and some are not. The factors mentioned here are just a few of the conditions that can impede wound healing. Recent research indicates that wounds that do not heal have high levels of protein-degrading enzymes in the wound bed and low levels of growth factors.

WOUND INFECTION

Wound infection is a serious consequence and a common cause of delayed wound healing. Infection is often due to

lack of blood supply, lack of oxygen, autocontamination, or exposure to environmental pathogens. Clinical manifestations of wound infection include increased drainage, purulent drainage, odor from the wound or drainage, erythema around the entire wound (not just the edges), increasing pain, fever, leukocytosis, and general malaise. The infected wound is slow to heal and may open (see later discussion on evisceration and dehiscence).

Cultures can be used in the diagnosis of wound infection. A swab culture of wound drainage can be obtained. When obtaining a swab culture, remove the excess visible drainage first, and then swab the wound bed. A quantitative culture (an actual sample of tissue) is usually needed to study open wounds. All open wounds are colonized, and using a swab culture does not reveal the true offending organisms within the wound; rather, it reveals only organisms growing on the wound's surface. Methicillin-resistant *Staphylococcus aureus* (MRSA) has become a common organism infecting wounds in high-risk persons, such as those with several chronic illnesses, those in institutions for prolonged periods, and those with diabetes. A precise technique of wound care is needed to reduce the risk of cross-contamination.

Chronically infected wounds have friable granulation tissue and a foul odor and fail to heal; in addition, the client has increasing pain. The surface of the wound is colonized with bacteria. Therefore a qualitative tissue culture should be used—not swab cultures of the surface.

Outcome Management

Topical antimicrobial agents can be used as the primary treatment. The ideal antimicrobial is a broad-spectrum agent and preserves regenerating tissues. All antimicrobials compromise wound healing to some degree by having low efficacy against a particular organism or by interfering with healing. A variety of topical agents can be used either to clean or disinfect the wound (see Table 20-4).

Hydrogen peroxide breaks down into water and oxygen. When hydrogen peroxide is used in a wound, H_2O_2 must be rinsed off the wound bed with normal saline to remove any trapped oxygen before the tissues can absorb it. Povidone-iodine, acetic acid, and sodium hypochlorite are used only in debris-contaminated, infected, and malodorous wounds. These agents are cytotoxic and inhibit granular tissue growth and damage endothelial cells and fibroblasts. Therefore their use is usually short term only.

■ Medical Management

The goal of medical management of clients with wound infection is to eradicate the infection. The extrinsic and intrinsic factors that lead to nonhealing are examined. Not all of these factors can be eliminated, however. Clients cannot be made younger, and some clients refuse to stop smoking, even though their nonhealing is due to inadequate circulation. At times, bypass surgery may be required to restore adequate blood flow. Cultured epithelial grafts, wound fillers, and hyperbaric oxygen are relatively new treatments in the care of nonhealing wounds. Most chronic nonhealing wounds are managed by a team of health care providers that may include a wound care physician, vascular or orthopedic surgeons, a wound-care nurse, a nutritionist, a physical therapist, hyperbaric medicine specialists, and social workers and psychologists. Even for these teams, chronic nonhealing wounds are a challenge.

Adjunctive Wound Healing Treatments

Electric Stimulation. Pulsed galvanic stimulation (Diapulse) is a form of electricity applied to the skin's surface. The electric currents stimulate DNA synthesis, increase blood flow, enhance fibroblast proliferation, and promote cell migration across the wound. This modality appears to be effective in promoting healing in wounds that have been refractory to other forms of treatment. Clients who are considering the use of electrotherapy should seek centers that have proper equipment and trained personnel.

Hyperbaric Oxygen Therapy. Hyperbaric oxygen (HBO) is the administration of oxygen at greater than atmospheric pressure. When oxygen is inhaled under pressure, the level of tissue oxygen is greatly increased. The high levels of oxygen promote the action of phagocytes and promote healing of the wound by increasing the action of fibroblasts. HBO is effective in clients with complex wounds, especially clients with osteomyelitis and other types of infection. HBO is becoming more available in the United States. As with electric stimulation, a properly trained staff is critical. Clients who have inner ear problems and claustrophobia require pretreatment care.

Growth Factors. The same growth factors that are found in the wound bed naturally can be grown in a laboratory and applied to the wound bed. Research is ongoing to determine the biologic activity and the potential benefits of topical application of these growth factors. Determining the timing and proper combinations of the growth factors is a subject of research. Becaplermin (Regranex), a platelet-derived growth factor, for use in diabetic foot ulcers, has gained approval by the Food and Drug Administration.

Negative-Pressure Wound Therapy. The application of controlled negative pressure in a clean wound bed can assist and accelerate wound healing. A sterile, reticulated foam sponge is placed in the wound bed. A connecting evacuation tube is attached to external suction and removes excess fluid in the wound and peripheral edema. The foam and tube are secured with transparent adhesive dressing. A small electrical unit controls pressure, and drainage is collected in a canister attached to the unit and to the sponge. Negative pressure wound therapy increases healing rates by up to 40%.

Normothermia. The use of warming devices to improve blood flow to the wound has also been shown to aid wound healing. Specific products and programs are currently being developed.

Dynamic Wound Fillers. Several fillers can be inserted into a wound bed to stimulate cell growth or to provide a scaffold for cells to use.

■ Nursing Management of the Medical Client

The nurse's role in the care of the client with a nonhealing wound is to provide ample information for self-care, including how to change dressings, the disease process underlying the wound, and how to return to work or activities without increasing the risk of nonhealing. For example, a woman with venous stasis ulcers may need to return to work but can do so safely only when the ulcer is healed. She also needs to know how to apply bandages, how long to elevate her legs while at work, and how to move her legs while working (e.g., walking rather than standing). Nurses serve a vital role in determining whether these requirements are feasible for the client and employer.

PALLIATIVE CARE OF FRAIL CLIENTS WITH NONHEALING WOUNDS

For frail clients with little hope of recovery, wounds may never heal. Defining care for these clients is the subject of intense debate, including a change in approaches to the wound that support the client's and family's goals and promote comfort rather than aggressively promote wound healing. Palliative care that addresses pain control, odor management, drainage control, and quality of life should be the main concerns. The wound should be protected to prevent deterioration and infection. The client's health should also be maintained so that the risk of infection or spread of infection or sepsis is minimized.

WOUND DISRUPTION

Dehiscence is the interruption of a previously intact suture line (see Chapter 16). A sharp pain in the suture line or a cough and increased serosanguineous drainage from the wound frequently will precede dehiscence. *Evisceration* is the opening of a wound with exposure of internal organs. It is obviously more serious than dehiscence. If a client experiences evisceration, cover the exposed organs with sterile wet dressings, notify the physician, and prepare the client for surgery. Also notify the physician about dehiscence, although it is not an emergency.

ALTERED COLLAGEN SYNTHESIS

Hypertrophic scars are scars that are raised above the suture line. They may be painful and itch. In general, hypertrophic scars tend to regress over time. *Keloids* are scars that extend well beyond the suture line (Figure 20-7). These scars tend to occur in African Americans

FIGURE 20-7 Keloid formation. Keloids are overgrowths of scar tissue above and beyond the normal boundaries of the scar. They are fairly resistant to treatment.

and clients of Mediterranean descent. The scars can be excised from a wound but unfortunately tend to recur. Newer treatments include the use of topical forms of heat.

CONCLUSIONS

Wound healing is a complex process but often goes on with little effort on the part of the client. Only when the wound does not heal or pressure ulcers develop are the many steps in wound healing evident. Wound care follows some basic principles: debride the wound of nonviable tissues, keep the wound bed moist, protect the surrounding skin, apply the proper dressings, use safe topical agents, and fill dead space.

THINKING CRITICALLY *evolve*

1. You are caring for a man with large venous stasis ulcers on his lower legs. When he was admitted, the ulcers were covered with soft, yellow, devitalized tissue. He has been treated with wet-to-dry dressings for the past 7 days. Today you notice that the ulcers are red and wet with a lumpy appearance. What should be done?

Factors to Consider. Is the appearance of red and lumpy tissue in a wound good or bad? What might be happening? What type of dressing is best used on this red and lumpy tissue?

2. You are caring for an older homeless man after he has undergone emergency abdominal surgery. He has had a nasogastric tube in place for 3 days for ileus and is receiving 1 L of IV fluids of 5% dextrose with 0.45 normal saline with 20 mEq of potassium every 8 hours. Before surgery, his serum albumin was 3.2 g/dl, hemoglobin was 9.6 g/dl, and WBC was 17,000/mm^3. His weight was 104 pounds and height 5 feet 5 inches. What are this client's chances of recovery? What interventions should be considered?

Factors to Consider. Does this client have evidence of malnutrition? If so, what effect does malnutrition have on wound healing? What short-term and long-term interventions may need to be initiated? Does this client have a risk of fluid or electrolyte imbalance? If so, which ones, and what can be done (or is being done) to reduce the risk?

Discussions for these questions can be found on the website and the CD-ROM.

BIBLIOGRAPHY

1. Alvarez, O., et al. (2002). Chronic wounds: Palliative management for the frail population. *Wounds: A Compendium of Clinical Research and Practice, 14*(8 Suppl), 5s-27s.
2. Childress, B.B., & Stechmiller, J. (2002). Role of nitric oxide in wound healing. *Biological Nursing Research, 4*(1), 5-15.
3. Collins, N. (2003). Obesity and wound healing. *Advances in Skin and Wound Care, 16*(1), 45-47.
4. Cuzzell, J. (2002). Wound healing: translating theory into clinical practice. *Dermatology Nursing, 14* (4), 257-261.
5. Gardner, S. et al. (2001). The validity of clinical signs and symptoms used to identify localized chronic wound infection. *Wound Repair and Regeneration, 9*(3), 178-186.
6. Greenhalgh, D.G. (2003). Wound healing and diabetes mellitus. *Clinics in Plastic Surgery, 30* (1), 37-45.
7. Hart, J. (2002). Inflammation: Its role in the healing of acute wounds. *Journal of Wound Care, 11*(6), 205-209.
8. Hunt, T.K., Hopf, H., & Hussain, Z. (2000). Physiology of wound healing. *Advances in Skin and Wound Care, 13* (2 Suppl), 6-11.
9. Kloth, L.C. (2002). How to use electrical stimulation for wound healing. *Nursing, 32* (12), 17.
10. Monaco, J., & Lawrence, W. (2003). Acute wound healing: an overview. *Clinics in Plastic Surgery, 30* (1), 1-12.
11. Lazarus, G., et al. (1994). Definitions and guidelines for assessment of wounds and evaluating healing. *Archives of Dermatology, 130*, 489-493.
12. Wood, Z. (2002). Hyperbaric oxygen in the management of chronic wounds. *British Journal of Nursing, 11* (16 Suppl) S16, 18-19, 22-24.

 evolve **Did you remember to check out the bonus material on the Evolve website and the CD-ROM, including free self-assessment exercises?**

http://evolve.elsevier.com/Black/medsurg/

Perspectives on Infectious Disorders

Carol Weber

For one brief moment in human history (circa 1950 to 1980), management of infectious disease did not dominate health care practice. By the close of that era, sickness and death caused by infectious diseases had plummeted as a result of multifaceted social, public health, and medical control efforts. Environmental sanitation had curbed such killers as yellow fever, cholera, typhus, malaria, typhoid fever, and plague.

International vaccination programs had eradicated smallpox. Organized efforts to vaccinate all children lowered the occurrence of vaccine-preventable diseases, particularly measles, mumps, rubella, diphtheria, tetanus, and poliomyelitis. Improved living conditions and personal hygiene had diminished parasitic diseases and gastrointestinal (GI) infections. The widespread availability of antibiotics quelled the fear of deadly tuberculosis, syphilis, gonorrhea, bacterial meningitis, scarlet fever, and rheumatic fever. Nosocomial (hospital-acquired) infections, which had already responded to medical asepsis, responded further to antibiotics, and medical technology continued to produce anti-infective agents to match the newly developing antibiotic-resistant organisms. As a result, health professionals could focus on the prevention and management of chronic disease.

This brief moment in history did not last. The 1980s and 1990s brought new infectious agents, such as *Legionella*, the human immunodeficiency virus (HIV), and the Ebola virus (which actually first appeared in 1976), all reminders of human vulnerability to infectious disease. In the spring of 2003, a previously unknown organism—a coronavirus—caused a worldwide outbreak of severe acute respiratory syndrome (SARS). (See Chapter 64 for a further discussion of SARS.) Hepatitis, tuberculosis, sexually transmitted diseases, and many vaccine-preventable diseases persist, spread, and continue to kill. Nonpathogenic organisms continue to create devastating disease in immunocompromised people and in those with chronic diseases or malnutrition. Antibiotic-resistant organisms have developed with chronic misuse and improper prescription of antibiotics. In addition, many of the major killers of the past, such as cholera and yellow fever, continue to cause death and destruction in parts of the world where poor sanitation, poor hygiene, and poverty are endemic. Use of biologic agents such as anthrax are potential bioterrorism threats (see the Terrorism Alert feature on Preparing for Bioterrorism on p. 418).

All people, particularly health care professionals, must maintain vigilance to infectious diseases—to prevention rather than simply treatment. Prevention requires an understanding of the infectious process and the control measures needed. This chapter describes the process of infection and selected aspects of prevention and control. Other chapters explain the nursing care of clients with specific infectious diseases.

THE PROCESS OF INFECTION

Infection is a process by which an organism establishes a parasitic relationship with its host. The process begins with transmission of an infectious organism. Infection may end in infectious disease, a condition that depends on the response of the host to the invader. The entire

TERRORISM ALERT
Preparing for Bioterrorism

The recent terrorist events in the United States and the intentional spread of anthrax in the mail in the fall of 2001 have heightened our awareness about the need to prepare for acts of bioterrorism. Many biologic agents can cause illness in humans, but not all are capable of large-scale impact. The U.S. Department of Defense has identified those bacteria, viruses, and toxins that are good candidates for use as effective biologic weapons.[37] Anthrax is the leading candidate on the list because it can exist as a spore and remain viable under a variety of environmental conditions. An aerosol release of *Bacillus anthracis* can be widely dispersed and remain suspended in the air for extended distances. Once inhaled, the resultant pneumonia can be highly fatal, especially with delayed treatment; and early diagnosis is difficult because few physicians have experience with anthrax. A vaccine for anthrax exists, but it requires six doses over a 2-year period, and supplies of the vaccine are limited.

The lead agency for overall public health planning for response to acts of biological terrorism is the CDC. The CDC has identified the biologic warfare agents most likely to be involved in a terrorist attack and has grouped them into three categories.[43] Category A agents have the greatest potential for mass casualties and require broad-based public health preparedness efforts. These agents are easily disseminated and include anthrax, botulism, plague, smallpox, tularemia, and viral hemorrhagic fevers. Category A agents are being given the highest priority for preparedness, including improved surveillance and

laboratory diagnosis, and stockpiling of specific medications. Category B agents have some potential for large-scale dissemination but generally cause less illness and death. These agents would require fewer special public health preparedness efforts than those in Category A. Examples include Q fever, brucellosis, glanders, ricin toxin, epsilon toxin, and *Staphylococcus* enterotoxin B. Several biological agents of concern for food and water safety are also included in this category. Category C agents do not currently present a high bioterrorism risk to public health but could emerge as future threats.

The CDC has established a bioterrorism program to upgrade national public health capabilities to detect and communicate different health threats, including not only bioterrorism but also chemical attacks (see Chapter 84 for further discussion of chemical warfare). The program coordinates state and major local public health departments in efforts to improve preparedness and response capabilities. Many legal and administrative strategies are being developed to maximize coordination of available resources in the community.[31] The American Nurses Association is working closely with the U.S. Department of Health and Human Services to establish teams of nurses, National Nurse Response Teams, who would be trained in disaster response and be ready to deploy in the event that administration of vaccines or prophylactic antibiotics is required.[26] As the single largest health care professional group, nurses will be an important link in a fully developed bioterrorism response system.

process and its outcome hinge on a complex interaction of (1) the *infectious agent,* (2) an *environment* conducive to transmission of the organism, and (3) a susceptible *host.* The agent, the host, and their environmental interactions are prerequisites to infectious disease.

Agent

Humans coexist with many microorganisms in complex, mutually beneficial relationships. Many organisms establish residence on or in the host and usually cause no harm. Other organisms are parasitic, maintaining themselves at the expense of their host. Some parasites arouse a pathologic response in the host and are called *pathogens* or *pathogenic agents.* In one sense, pathogens are ineffective parasites because they stimulate an inflammatory response, leading to a disease that may harm the host and eventually kill the pathogen.

All microorganisms can be distinguished by certain intrinsic properties. These properties provide the basis for identifying and classifying bacteria, viruses, fungi, and helminths. An organism's properties include its shape, size, structure, chemical composition, antigenic

make-up, growth requirements, viability under adverse environmental conditions, and ability to produce toxins. Viability is a particularly important property to health care professionals because it determines the pathogen's ability to survive outside its host. Organisms that can survive drying, sunlight, heat, or other adverse environmental conditions require more aggressive tactics to prevent transmission.

Environment

Transmission of an infectious agent from a source to a susceptible host occurs within an environment. Organisms live and multiply in a *reservoir,* which can be a person, animal, plant, soil, food, or other organic substance or combination of substances. The reservoir provides what the organism needs for survival at specific stages in its life cycle. Infected persons are the reservoirs for most bacteria and viruses that affect humans.

Both human and animal reservoirs may be infected and, therefore, may also be hosts. An infected host may be asymptomatic—a *carrier* of the pathogen. A carrier maintains an environment that promotes growth, multiplication, and shedding of the parasite without exhibiting manifestations of disease.

Organisms can have one or more than one *route of transmission* from the reservoir to a new host. In fact, transmission can occur through five mechanisms:

1. *Contact transmission:* Through *direct* transmission, an organism moves from an infected person (or *carrier*) to an uninfected person via direct contact between their body surfaces. Through *indirect* transmission, an uninfected person picks up an infectious organism from an intermediate object, such as contaminated gloves, a used needle, or a dirty dressing.

2. *Droplet transmission:* An uninfected person picks up an infectious organism when an infected person coughs, sneezes, or talks. These activities propel droplets a short distance through the air, and they may land on an uninfected person's conjunctivae, nasal mucosa, or oral mucosa. Certain procedures, such as suctioning and bronchoscopy, can generate droplets as well.

3. *Airborne transmission:* Droplets can evaporate into airborne nuclei, or microbes can become attached to floating dust particles. Unlike droplets, dry nuclei and dust particles can float a long way in the air. Relatively few organisms remain viable as airborne nuclei, but those that do can be transmitted in the air and breathed into the lungs.

4. *Common vehicle transmission:* Many uninfected persons can pick up an infectious organism from the same contaminated source, such as food, water, a medication, or a device.

5. *Vector transmission:* An infected creature, such as a mosquito, fly, rat, or flea, transmits an infectious organism by biting an uninfected host (Box 21-1).

The *portal of exit* is the place whence the parasite escapes the reservoir. Generally, this site corresponds to the *portal of entry* into the next host. For example, the portal of exit for GI parasites is generally the feces and the portal of entry into a new host is the mouth. As is the case with other links in the transmission chain, variability exists. Hookworm eggs, for example, are shed in the feces, but hookworm larvae enter through the skin of a person walking barefoot in soil containing hatched eggs. Common portals of exit include secretions and fluids (respiratory and vaginal secretions, blood, tears, semen, breast milk), excretions (urine and feces), open lesions, and exudates. Some organisms, such as HIV, have more than one portal of exit. Knowledge of the portal of exit is essential for preventing transmission of a pathogen.

A pathogen may enter a new host by ingestion, inhalation, contact with mucous membranes, percutaneously, or transplacentally. Infectious diseases vary as to the number of organisms and the duration of the exposure required to start the infectious process in a new host.

BOX 21-1   *West Nile Virus*

West Nile virus has been commonly found in humans and birds and other vertebrates in Africa, Eastern Europe, West Asia, and the Middle East, but it was not documented in the United States until 1999. The virus can infect humans, birds, mosquitoes, horses, and some other animals.

The principal route of human infection with West Nile virus is through the bite of an infected mosquito. Mosquitoes become infected when they feed on infected birds. When the virus is injected into humans by a mosquito, it can multiply and possibly cause illness. Most people who become infected with the virus will not have any type of illness. Those who develop West Nile fever will have flu-like manifestations, lasting only a few days and without any long-term health effects. It is estimated that 1 in 150 persons infected with West Nile virus will develop encephalitis or meningitis, a more severe form of the disease. Even in areas where the virus is circulating, however, very few mosquitoes are infected with the virus. The chances of becoming severely ill from any one mosquito bite are extremely small.

One cannot get West Nile Virus from casual contact such as touching or kissing a person who has the disease. However, in a small number of cases, the virus has been transmitted through blood transfusion, organ transplantation, breastfeeding, and pregnancy (from mother to fetus).

You can reduce your risk of becoming infected with West Nile virus by applying insect repellent to exposed skin. Choose an insect repellant that contains diethyltoluamide (DEET) and one that provides protection for the amount of time you will be outdoors. Also spray your clothing because mosquitoes can bite through thin clothing. Wearing long-sleeved shirts, long pants, and socks while outdoors can also reduce your risk. Take special precautions from April to October, the months when mosquitoes are most active.

Data from Centers for Disease Control Division of Vector-Borne Infectious Diseases (2003). West Nile Virus. Retrieved August 6, 2003, from http://www.cdc.gov/ncidod/dvbid/westnile/index.htm.

Host

Some humans are more susceptible to infectious disease than others. A susceptible host has characteristics and behaviors that increase the probability of infectious disease. Factors such as age, gender, ethnicity, heredity, altitude, and temperature influence the likelihood of infection. For example, the ethnic custom of eating raw fish may increase the risk of exposure to pathogens. General health and nutritional status, hormonal balance, and the presence of concurrent disease also play a role. Living conditions and personal behaviors—such as drug use, diet, hygiene, and sexual practices—also influence the risk of exposure to pathogens and resistance once exposure has occurred. Susceptibility is also influenced by

TABLE 21-1 *Agents and Sites of Selected Infectious Diseases*

Disease	Infectious Agent	Site of Infection	Reservoir	Mode of Transmission
Bacteria				
Cholera	*Vibrio cholerae*	Gastrointestinal tract	Humans	Ingestion of water contaminated with feces
Diarrhea	*Escherichia coli*	Gastrointestinal tract	Humans	Ingestion of contaminated food or water
Giardiasis	*Giardia lamblia*	Gastrointestinal tract	Water, humans, wild animals	Ingestion of cysts in fecally contaminated water and food
Gonorrhea	*Neisseria gonorrhoeae*	Genitourinary tract	Humans	Sexual contact
Lyme disease	*Borrelia burgdorferi*	Skin, joints, systemic	Wild rodents and deer	Tick bite
Malaria	*Plasmodium* spp.	Red blood cells, liver	Mosquito	Bite from infected mosquito
Meningitis	*Neisseria meningitidis*	Meninges	Humans	Direct contact with droplets from respiratory passages
Pneumonia	*Streptococcus pyogenes*	Lung	Humans	Inhalation; aspiration of gastric contents
Rocky Mountain spotted fever	*Rickettsia rickettsii*	Vascular endothelium	Ticks	Tick bite
Toxoplasmosis	*Toxoplasma gondii*	Eye, lung, brain	Cats	Ingestion of cysts on fecally contaminated fingers or in food; transplacental
Tuberculosis	*Mycobacterium tuberculosis*	Lung	Humans	Inhalation of droplet nuclei
Wound infection	*Staphylococcus aureus*	Connective tissue	Humans	Contaminated hands, surgical instruments
Fungi				
Candidiasis	*Candida albicans*	Skin, mucous membranes, genital tract	Humans	Overgrowth associated with damaged skin or mucosal or use of antibiotics
Histoplasmosis	*Histoplasma capsulatum*	Lung	Bat or bird feces	Inhalation of spores
Helminths				
Trichinosis	*Trichinella spiralis*	Gastrointestinal tract, muscle	Animals	Ingestion of raw or undercooked meat
Viruses				
Acquired immunodeficiency syndrome (AIDS)	Human immunodeficiency virus	Helper T lymphocyte	Humans	Contaminated needles, blood transfusions, sexual contact, transplacental
Hepatitis B	Hepatitis B virus	Liver	Humans	Contaminated needles, blood transfusions, sexual contact, perinatal
Influenza A	Influenza A virus	Respiratory tract	Humans	Direct contact by aerosol droplets; airborne spread
Measles (rubeola)	Paramyxoviridae	Skin, respiratory tract, systemic	Humans	Direct contact with nasal or throat secretions; airborne spread
Rabies	*Lyssavirus*	Systemic	Dogs, wild animals	Animal bite

anatomic and physiologic defenses, sometimes called *lines of defense.* Even though an infectious disease is said to be caused by an etiologic (causal) agent, infection results from interactions among a variety of factors related to agent, host, and environment (Table 21-1).

The host's first-line defenses are external and act to bar invasion by pathogens. These defenses are nonspecific in that they act against any invading pathogen. First-line defenses include (1) *physical* and *chemical barriers* and (2) the body's own natural flora.

Physical barriers include intact skin and mucous membranes; oil and perspiration on skin; cilia in respiratory passages; gag and cough reflexes; and peristalsis in the GI tract; and the flushing action of tears, saliva, and mucus. All act to remove organisms before they have an opportunity to infect. The chemical composition of body secretions such as tears and sweat, together with the pH of saliva, vaginal secretions, urine, and digestive juices, further prevents or inhibits the growth of organisms. Compromise of any of these natural defenses increases host susceptibility to pathogen invasion.

Another important first-line defense is the *normal flora* of microorganisms that inhabit the skin and mucous membranes of the oral cavity, GI tract, and vagina. These microorganisms are indigenous to (occur naturally in) specific tissue. They typically coexist with their host in a mutually beneficial relationship as long as they do not migrate from the specific site. Through a mechanism called *microbial antagonism,* they control the replication of potential pathogens. The importance of this mechanism is evident when the mechanism is disturbed. An example of disturbance is the overgrowth of *Candida albicans* (thrush) that results from extensive antibiotic therapy that destroys normal flora in the GI tract or vagina.

Some normal flora can become pathogenic under specific conditions, such as immunosuppression or displacement of the pathogen to another area of the body. The opportunistic infections experienced by clients with symptomatic HIV infection are an example of immunosuppression. Displacement is seen when *Escherichia coli,* normally found in the GI tract, invades the urogenital tract and becomes pathogenic. Displacement of normal flora is a common cause of nosocomial infections. Invasive procedures increase the risk of displacing these organisms. For this reason, it is essential to maintain meticulous hand-washing and asepsis.

The *second line of defense* (the inflammatory process) and the *third line* (the immune response) share several physiologic components. These include the lymphatic system, leukocytes, and a multitude of proteins and enzymes.

Even after successful transmission of a pathogen, there may be more than one possible outcome. The pathogen may merely contaminate the body surface. The process ends there if the host's first-line defenses, such as

intact skin or mucous membranes, block the pathogen from further invasion. Successful invasion with replication of a pathogen that does not lead to clinical manifestations or a detectable immune response is referred to as *colonization.*

When microorganisms in or on the host cause an immune response, an infection is said to be present. The period during which the pathogen is replicating but before it is shed from the host is called the *latent period.* During latency, host inflammatory and immune responses may ward off the organism or its by-products, thus preventing tissue damage, or the pathogen or its products may begin to destroy undefended or poorly defended tissue, producing infectious disease. Disease manifestations herald the end of the *incubation period,* which is defined as the time from invasion of the disease to the appearance of manifestations. By definition, *infectious disease* is the pathophysiologic response of a host to the destructive action of the pathogen, to its toxic products, or to the host immune responses to fight the pathogen. This pathophysiologic response is generally symptomatic. An asymptomatic pathologic response is called a *subclinical infection.*

An important point is that an asymptomatic host can still transmit a pathogen. The host may harbor the pathogen in sufficient quantities to shed it at any time after latency and toward the end of the incubation period. The time during which an organism can be shed is called the *period of communicability.* It usually precedes manifestations and coincides with part or all of the clinical disease, sometimes extending to convalescence. The communicable period, like the incubation period, varies with the pathogen and the disease.

RISKS OF HOSPITALIZATION

Nosocomial infections (those that arise in a hospital or other health care facility) are a leading cause of death in the United States and are associated with significant morbidity. The rate of hospital-acquired infections has increased by 36% in the last 20 years, and 25% of the clients who develop a nosocomial infection receive care in intensive care units (ICUs).[47] Infections present or incubating at the time of admission to the hospital are referred to as *community acquired.* Occupationally acquired infections among the staff of a hospital are also considered nosocomial.

The source of nosocomial pathogens in health care facilities varies, but both health care workers and clients are reservoirs in most instances. For example, *Staphylococcus aureus* is often carried on the skin and in the nasopharynx. Respiratory secretions, feces, urine, and blood are reservoirs for some nosocomial organisms. Liquids and inanimate objects in the hospital environment may also serve as sources of nosocomial infections. The most important means of transmission is via the hands of health care workers. Hand-washing, combined with principles of asepsis and proper use of gloves, is the best method of preventing nosocomial infections.

The most common sites of nosocomial infections in clients are the urinary tract, lower respiratory tract, surgical wounds, and the bloodstream.[37] Various pathogens can cause nosocomial infections in multiple sites. For example, *Pseudomonas aeruginosa* is the organism that causes most cases of nosocomial pneumonia, but it also causes urinary tract and surgical site infections. *S. aureus* is a common cause of surgical site infection, pneumonia, and bloodstream infection. Table 21-2 lists common nosocomial pathogens.

Urinary Tract Infections

 Urinary tract infections (UTIs) are the most common nosocomial infections in both acute and long-term health care facilities, and more than 80% stem from urethral catheterization.[37] Major risk factors for catheter-related UTIs include female gender, increased duration of catheterization, and breaks in the closed catheter system.[1,35]

In most catheter-related infections in women, bacteria enter the bladder by the periurethral route.[35] Organisms originating primarily from the fecal flora and found at the meatal and perineal areas may be introduced into the bladder during insertion of the catheter, or they may migrate along the external surface of the catheter into the bladder. In men, catheter-related infections usually result from *cross-infection* (transmission between clients), with bacteria introduced into the collection system at the junction of the catheter and drainage tube or at the outflow spigot; they then migrate to the bladder in 24 to 48 hours. Most nosocomial UTIs are easily managed but can lead to bacteremia and death.[1,48]

Pneumonia

Pneumonia is the second most common nosocomial infection and is associated with more deaths than any other nosocomial infection.[1,37] Nosocomial pneumonia is defined as pneumonia that occurs 48 hours or longer after admission to the hospital. Most nosocomial pneumonias are caused by gram-negative bacteria. Aspiration of oropharyngeal or stomach organisms is the predominant mechanism by which nosocomial pneumonia develops. Airborne transmission is usually not the cause.

Stasis (lack of movement) of respiratory secretions caused by immobility and a decreased cough also contributes to nosocomial pneumonia. Postoperative clients, particularly those who have had thoracic and upper abdominal surgery, and clients who require ventilatory support are at high risk of aspiration. Clients with diminished consciousness, impaired gag reflex, intubation, or tracheostomy are also at increased risk for aspiration of oral secretions. Other risk factors include old age, decreased mobility, and severe disease, such as chronic lung disease, cardiovascular disease, renal insufficiency, and malignancies.

Nosocomial pneumonia is difficult to prevent because in most cases the microorganisms are derived from the client's own flora. Soon after hospitalization, the oropharynx of many clients becomes colonized with gram-negative bacteria that may be aspirated into the lungs. The use of histamine (H_2) blockers, antimicrobial therapy, and enteral nutritional therapy have been found to promote colonization of the oropharynx with gram- negative bacteria.[48] Contaminated respiratory therapy equipment can serve as a source of pathogens as well.

Surgical Site Infections

Surgical site infections are a major source of hospital morbidity and account for nearly 55% of extra hospital days.[37] These infections usually result from *endogenous* (inside the host) or *exogenous* (outside the host) microorganisms that enter the site at the time of an operation. The most common source of infecting bacteria is the client's own flora. Although the physical environment of the operating room is an uncommon source of infection, operating room personnel may shed bacteria-laden skin particles that travel through the air to the open wound.

TABLE 21-2	The Most Common Causes of Nosocomial Infection*
Site of Infection	**Pathogen**
Bloodstream	Coagulase-negative staphylococci
	Enterococcus spp.
	Staphylococcus aureus
	Candida albicans
	Enterobacter spp.
Lung	*Staphylococcus aureus*
	Pseudomonas aeruginosa
	Enterobacter spp.
	Klebsiella pneumoniae
	Haemophilus influenzae
Surgical site	*Staphylococcus aureus*
	Coagulase-negative staphylococci
	Enterococcus spp.
	Escherichia coli
	Pseudomonas aeruginosa
Urinary tract	*Escherichia coli*
	Candida albicans
	Enterococcus spp.
	Pseudomonas aeruginosa
	Klebsiella pneumoniae

Data from Centers for Disease Control and Prevention. (1999). Guideline for prevention of surgical site infection—1999. *Am J Infect Control, 27,* 97-134; and Centers for Disease Control and Prevention. (1999). National Nosocomial Infections Surveillance (NNIS) System report; data summary from January 1990-May 1999, issued June 1999. *Am J Infect Control, 27,* 520-532.

*Organisms are listed by major site and order of importance.

Factors that influence the development of surgical site infections include (1) the number and types of organisms present in the wound, (2) the type of operation, (3) the surgeon's technique, and (4) the duration of the operation.[15] Old age, diabetes mellitus, obesity, malnutrition, and underlying immunocompromise are client-related factors that increase the risk of surgical site infection.

The risk of surgical site infection also increases with the length of the client's preoperative hospital stay.[15] Shortening the preoperative stay tends to reduce the risk of infection by decreasing the opportunity for colonization with nosocomial bacteria.[48] Proper preparation of the surgical site is also important. Shaving the operative site—once a common practice—is now known to damage the epithelium, impair the skin's defense mechanism, and raise the risk of infection.

Device-Related Infections and Bacteremias

Rates of nosocomial infection of the bloodstream are increasing, particularly in ICUs, where there is a concentrated population of seriously ill clients.[49] The increase is due partly to the increased use of intravascular devices in these settings. Intravascular devices may include intravenous lines; intra-arterial infusion lines; and devices used for diagnostic, therapeutic, and hemodynamic monitoring. Catheter-related bloodstream infections are associated with increased morbidity, mortality rates of 10% to 20%, prolonged hospitalization, and increased medical costs.[7] The risk of infection is influenced by factors related to the device itself, the site of insertion, the technique used to place the device, and the duration of catheterization. Short peripheral catheters inserted into the veins of the hand or forearm have rarely been associated with bloodstream infections. Central venous catheters account for up to 90% of all catheter-related bloodstream infections. Multilumen catheters are associated with a higher risk of infection than single-lumen catheters. Partially implantable catheters and totally implanted injection ports are associated with lower infection rates.[7]

Device-related infections and bacteremias are usually caused by microorganisms found on the client's skin or on the hands of health care workers. These microorganisms invade disrupted tissue and migrate around the site of insertion and along the device into the intravascular space. The use of semipermeable membrane dressings over the insertion site facilitates the growth of skin flora. Dressing changes following institution-specific protocols must be done at regularly scheduled intervals under aseptic conditions. Colonization of skin flora can also occur around the hub of the device, the tubing-device junction, or other connectors attached to the system. Although liquids given through the device may become contaminated, infusion-related infection is relatively uncommon.

Client factors that contribute to the risk of device-related infections include age, nutritional status, type and severity of underlying illness, skin condition, and immunosuppressive therapy. Bacteremia is especially common in clients with chronic diseases, malnutrition, and cancer.[28,50]

Other Nosocomial Infections

Effective screening and processing of donated blood and blood products have greatly reduced the risk of HIV transmission to clients in health care settings. The risk of provider-to-client transmission of HIV is remote, although the matter has created much public anxiety. The risk of occupational exposure to HIV in the health care setting has been associated primarily with parenteral exposures to blood from clients infected with HIV.[12] Infection after exposure of mucous membranes to infected blood is much less common.

Nosocomial infection with *hepatitis B virus* (HBV) is another concern in hospitals because the source of a typical nosocomial HBV infection is never identified. Provider-to-client transmission of HBV does not occur with routine client contact. Client-to-provider transmission is a much larger problem and is why health care workers must be vaccinated against HBV.

The resurgence of *tuberculosis* is another major concern in health care facilities. Two factors responsible for this resurgence are (1) poor compliance with therapeutic drug regimens and (2) the emergence of drug-resistant strains of *Mycobacterium tuberculosis*. When clients infected with susceptible strains of the pathogen receive appropriate therapy, sputum smears begin to clear by the third week of treatment. Clients with resistant strains, however, continue to cough up large numbers of viable organisms, exposing many health care workers. Respiratory isolation must be closely followed with high-risk clients until adequate treatment has been given.

Acute GI infections can be caused by a variety of agents, including bacteria, viruses, and protozoa, but nosocomial transmission of agents such as *Clostridium difficile* is on the rise.[12] See Chapter 35 for further discussion of this problem.

Nosocomial infections tend to occur more frequently and with more severity in ill, debilitated, malnourished, immunocompromised, and older clients (Box 21-2). Susceptibility to infection increases when invasive procedures and indwelling devices are used. With the expanding use of invasive devices, more exposure to antimicrobial therapy, and more severely ill hospitalized clients, the risk of nosocomial infections will probably increase. Furthermore, the emergence of resistant organisms is likely to continue, resulting in infections that are more difficult to treat. Although resistance to infection is enhanced by vaccines and immune globulin, manipulation of the physical environment must be used as a supplementary measure to reduce the risk. This means that nurses must be ever more vigilant in administering care and in supervising those providing care.

Antibiotic-Resistant Microorganisms

Among researchers and health care professionals, concern is increasing over the frequent, widespread use of antimicrobial drugs in hospitals and long-term care facilities (LTCFs). Studies in hospitals have demonstrated that 23% to 37.8% of clients receive antibiotics, of which half are used inappropriately.[37] For example, antimicrobial drugs are used routinely as prophylaxis for invasive and even noninvasive surgical procedures. Although prophylaxis may be helpful when applied wisely, many drugs are used inappropriately. In the ICU, 80% of clients receive antimicrobials.[30]

In LTCFs, antimicrobials are among the most frequently prescribed medications. Studies have shown that antibiotics account for nearly 40% of all systemic drugs used in LTCFs.[50] Nursing home studies have revealed frequent orders for antibiotics, often without adequate evidence of underlying infection. Worse, many of these drugs were prescribed for infections not responsive to antibiotic therapy, such as viral respiratory tract infections.

The most important factor in the development of antimicrobial resistance is antimicrobial use.[28,44] Areas within the hospital that have the highest rates of antimicrobial resistance also have the highest rates of antimicrobial use. In ICUs, where clients are usually undergoing intensive antibiotic therapy, the rates of antimicrobial resistance are significantly higher than in other areas of the hospital,[28] and the transfer of infected or colonized clients from hospital to LTCF is believed to be the primary way resistant bacteria have been introduced into LTCFs.[50] Once endemic to a hospital or LTCF, the antibiotic resistance genes can be transferred from one client to another and from one bacterial species to another.

Resistance to an antibiotic by a pathogen develops by spontaneous genetic mutation or genetic transfer of plasmids or chromosomal DNA. This genetic information allows bacteria to develop resistance by producing an enzyme that will inactivate or destroy the antibiotic by altering the antibiotic target site to evade action of the antibiotic or by preventing antibiotic access to the target site.[44] Some resistance can be acquired by a single genetic change; others require a series of changes.[44] Unfortunately, resistance tends to occur to multiple antibiotics.

BOX 21-2   *Infectious Disease in Older Adults*

More than any other population, older clients are at risk for infection. Infection often leads to hospitalization for nursing home residents, and it is one of the top 10 causes of death in older adults. Many common infectious diseases, such as pneumonia, urinary tract infection (UTI), sepsis, skin and soft tissue infection, tuberculosis, and herpes zoster, become more common with advancing age.

Older adults have an increased risk of infection, partly as a normal consequence of growing older. With aging, mechanical barriers—such as skin and mucosal—undergo structural and functional decline. The physiologic reserve capacity of organ systems dwindles, and the immune system falters. When these defense mechanisms are compromised, infection can progress locally and even spread systemically.

Many older adults have chronic diseases that further jeopardize their host defenses. Conditions associated with aging, such as diabetes mellitus and malnutrition, probably exert more influence on immunity than age itself.

Not only do older people contract more infections, they also tend to experience more complications of those infections. For example, an older client with pneumonia or a UTI is more likely to develop bacteremia than a younger client with the same infection.

To make matters worse, infection can be more difficult to detect and diagnose in the older client. Older people often do not manifest typical signs and symptoms of infectious diseases. Instead, they may have worsening cognition, an abnormal mental status, lethargy, agitation, loss of appetite, incontinence, or an increased tendency to fall.

Fever—the cardinal sign of infection—may be absent in infected older clients, even those who have bacteremia or pneumonia. Many older people have a low baseline temperature. Suspect infection in any older client with an oral temperature of 99° F or higher or an increase in baseline temperature of 2° F or more. Coexisting diseases may mask the signs of infection even further.

Even drugs used to treat infections are less successful when given to older clients. The drugs produce a slower or delayed response in the older person's body while producing even more adverse reactions. Age-related changes in gastrointestinal, cardiac, and renal function alter the way in which antimicrobial agents are absorbed, distributed, and excreted.

Researchers are looking for better ways to detect and better drugs to treat infections in older adults. While these agents are being investigated in the older population, you can help already infected clients by encouraging individualized dosage regimens and monitoring these clients carefully.

Data from Yoshikawa, T. T., & Norman, D. C. (Eds.). (2001). *Infectious disease in the aging: A clinical handbook.* Totowa, NJ: Humana Press.

In other words, once an organism is resistant to one antibiotic in a class, it usually is resistant to all antibiotics in that class.

S. aureus, one of the pathogens most frequently reported to cause nosocomial infections, has a remarkable ability to develop resistance to antibiotics. Before the advent of penicillin in the early 1940s, the fatality rate for bacteremia caused by *S. aureus* was about 90%.[36] The use of penicillin dramatically reduced that rate, but within a few years resistant strains of *S. aureus* evolved that produced a penicillin inactivator. New antibiotics, such as methicillin, were effective in the 1960s, but they provided only a temporary solution to the problem. In the 1980s epidemics of infections with methicillin-resistant *S. aureus* (commonly called MRSA) forced operating rooms and ICUs to close. In recent years, MRSA has accounted for approximately 80% of all *S. aureus* isolates reported to the National Nosocomial Infections Surveillance System.[12] MRSA is the etiologic agent in many cases of conjunctivitis, skin and soft-tissue infections, pneumonia, infected pressure ulcers, and catheter-associated urinary tract infections. Once introduced into a hospital or LTCF, MRSA is difficult to eliminate because it acquires resistance to multiple antimicrobial agents.[36] The most important reservoirs of MRSA are infected or colonized clients, and the main mode of transmission of MRSA is via the hands of health care workers.[14]

With the emergence of MRSA, vancomycin became the only drug available to treat MRSA infections; however, widespread use of vancomycin has now contributed to the emergence of vancomycin-resistant organisms, including vancomycin-intermediate-sensitive *S. aureus* (VISA) and vancomycin-resistant enterococci (VRE). The first case of VISA occurred in 1997,[14] indicating the development of a strain of *S. aureus* with reduced susceptibility to vancomycin. In June 2002, the first case of an infection with vancomycin-resistant *S. aureus* (VRSA) was reported after VRSA was isolated from a swab obtained from a client's catheter exit site.[22] When MRSA began showing resistance to vancomycin, two new agents became available to treat MRSA: the combination of quinupristin and dalfopristin (Synercid) in 1999 and linezolid (Zyvox) in 2000.[30] It will only be a matter of time before resistant strains of pathogens emerge for these new drugs.

Enterococci are now the second most common pathogen in nosocomial infections.[50] Their emergence in the past two decades can be attributable to their resistance to many commonly used antimicrobial agents (aminoglycosides, aztreonam, cephalosporins, clindamycin, ampicillin, nafcillin, oxacillin, and trimethoprim-sulfamethoxazole). Strains of VRE began appearing in 1986, most likely as the result of the use of orally administered vancomycin for treating antibiotic-associated diarrhea in hospitals.[42] Enterococci are normal inhabitants of the GI tract and cause nosocomial urinary tract, bloodstream, wound,

and intraabdominal infections.[37] Treatment of VRE infections poses a major challenge because these organisms are resistant to a wide variety of antimicrobials. Synercid and Zyvox are the only drugs currently available for treatment of VRE, and for some strains there are no longer any effective antimicrobial agents.[30] Environmental cultures in hospital rooms have identified VRE-contaminated client gowns, bed rails, floors, door handles, blood pressure cuffs, stethoscopes, glucose meters, and telephones. It appears that VRE is transmitted directly by client-to-client contact and indirectly by the hands of health care workers, contaminated environmental surfaces, and client care equipment. Residents in LTCFs are a major reservoir for VRE, which can be transmitted to other residents, and when these clients are admitted to a hospital, to other clients.[27]

Streptococcus pneumoniae is a gram-positive bacterium that colonizes the nasopharynx and oropharynx and causes respiratory infections, otitis media, sinusitis, bloodstream infections, and meningitis.[37] Pneumonia caused by *S. pneumoniae* is one of the most frequent causes of lower respiratory tract infections. Penicillin has been the drug of choice for treating infections with *S. pneumoniae,* but penicillin-resistant pneumococci (PRP) have now emerged.[50] What is worrisome is that PRP are also resistant to erythromycin, tetracycline, and other antibiotics.

Widespread use of trimethoprim/sulfamethoxazole for UTIs, upper respiratory infections, and GI infections has resulted in the emergence of resistance. Major organisms resistant to this combination of antibiotics include *S. pneumoniae, H. influenzae,* and many enteric gram-negative bacilli (*Escherichia coli, Klebsiella* spp.).[50]

Other strains of bacteria have developed resistance to third-generation cephalosporins, fluoroquinolones, and imipenem. Although 90% of nosocomial infections are caused by bacteria, *Candida albicans* is the seventh most common pathogen associated with nosocomial infection in ICU clients.[37] Recent data suggest that *C. albicans* is developing resistance to some of the few antifungal agents available for treatment.[28]

Tuberculosis is an example of a resistance problem that has spread globally. Resistant *Mycobacterium* has been identified in 35 countries and regions.[2] Some *M. tuberculosis* strains are resistant to one drug, but other strains have become multidrug resistant. For tuberculosis, as well as many other infections, multi-drug resistance can result in treatment failure and death.

These are just a few of the increasing problems associated with antibiotic resistance. In fact, nearly all organisms have acquired resistance to some therapeutic agents.[2]

Misuse of antimicrobial drugs can alter a client's normal flora and encourage resistance of pathogenic organisms. To help avoid growing resistance to antimicrobial drugs, obtain appropriate specimens for culture before starting antibiotic therapy. In addition, check sensitivity reports to ensure that the client receives an appropriate antibiotic.

Controlling the spread of antimicrobial resistance is difficult and requires appropriate selection and administration of antimicrobials, use of antibiotic combinations, and strict asepsis and infection control efforts. Finally, although infection control practices, such as handwashing, aseptic techniques, and barrier precautions, do not directly limit the emergence of resistant strains, they do prevent transmission of resistant organisms from one client to another.

PREVENTING AND CONTROLLING INFECTION

To be effective, strategies to prevent and control infection must be based on knowledge of agent-host-environment interactions. The goal in developing and implementing interventions is to prevent the spread of an infectious agent from its reservoir or source to susceptible hosts.

Methods for controlling the transmission of infectious disease vary with the characteristics of the organism, its reservoirs, the type of pathologic response it produces, and technology available for control. In general, the aim is to intervene at the point where the greatest number of people can be protected and using the least amount of resources.

The simplest and most effective way to prevent transmission is meticulous *hand-washing and the use of alcohol-based hand rubs.*[21] The hygienic hand rub is a technique that involves rubbing a fast-acting antiseptic preparation onto the hands until they are dry. Hand hygiene is an absolute necessity, even when gloves are worn. Wash your hands with soap and water or use an alcohol-based hand rub before donning gloves and after removing them, and before and after each client contact. Teach this procedure to all personnel and continually monitor for compliance. These simple, inexpensive techniques, used appropriately, are potent weapons against the spread of infection.

Another method to prevent and control infectious disease involves environmental measures. Some pathogens, such as *S. aureus,* can be controlled by disinfection, sterilization, or anti-infective drugs. Other pathogens can be controlled best by eradicating their non-human reservoirs via environmental sanitation measures, such as water treatment; food safety programs; and control of animals, vectors, sewage, and solid wastes.

Transmission from the portal of exit can often be prevented by detecting and treating clients who are shedding pathogens, such as gonococci. Antimicrobials are among the drugs most frequently prescribed in the United States to treat infections, although the use of antibiotics is not without problems. Another example of prevention is the use of prophylactic antitubercular medications for clients who are exposed to tuberculosis and whose skin test result is positive.

Immunization Programs

Several infectious diseases have been dramatically reduced by maximizing host defenses through active and passive vaccinations that stimulate the immune system to counteract the infectious agent:

Active vaccination refers to the deliberate administration of a modified infecting agent, called a *vaccine,* or a modified toxin, called a *toxoid,* to stimulate an immune response. Protection is not immediate: some time is needed to achieve protective antibody levels; however, induced active immunity usually results in long-lived protection against disease.

Passive vaccination refers to the administration of antibodies to a nonimmune person to provide temporary protection against a pathogenic agent or toxin. Passive immunity provides immediate but short-lived protection that lasts a few weeks.

Vaccination programs in the United States have resulted in a significant reduction in childhood infectious diseases. A major resurgence of measles occurred from 1989 to 1991, however, signaling a major problem with childhood vaccination programs.[25] Baseline data from 1989 indicated that the immunization level of preschool children was approximately 70% to 80%, with some segments of the population having levels below 50%.[46] Urban minority populations, particularly African-American and Hispanic-American children, had much lower immunization levels than those in the general population.[25] The goal of the Department of Health and Human Services is to vaccinate at least 90% of all children in the United States by age 2 years.[46,47] Entry requirements for school and day care has been one of the most effective interventions in increasing vaccination rates.[47]

An entire population does not have to be immune for prevention of a disease epidemic. When a large proportion of individual members of a community becomes immune to a disease, the chance of contact between susceptible persons and infected persons decreases. This type of immunity is called *herd immunity.* For example, epidemics of measles are less likely to occur when herd immunity increases and the number of susceptible persons in the community decreases.

Vaccination schedules and recommendations are established by the Advisory Committee on Immunization Practices (ACIP) of the Centers for Disease Control and Prevention (CDC). ACIP recommends that all children be vaccinated against measles, mumps, rubella, diphtheria, pertussis, tetanus, poliomyelitis, *Haemophilus influenzae* type b, HBV, pneumococcal, and varicella virus.[23] Hepatitis A (HAV) vaccines are recommended for high-risk children.

Vaccinations are as important for adolescents and adults as they are for children (Table 21-3). Infections seen primarily in children are now occurring in adolescents and adults who never developed active immunity. Adolescents and adults who escaped natural infection or who were not adequately immunized as children are at risk for childhood diseases and their complications. In 1996 the ACIP recommended establishing a routine vac- cination visit to a health care provider for adolescents 11 to 12 years old to review their vaccination status and to administer needed vaccines for measles, mumps, rubella, HAV and HBV infections, tetanus, diphtheria, and vari- cella.[8]

Adolescents older than 12 years and adults through age 64 should complete a primary series of diphtheria and tetanus toxoids, plus measles-mumps-rubella vac- cines if they did not receive them as children.[4] Adults 65 years and older should complete a primary series of diphtheria and tetanus toxoids but are generally consid- ered immune to measles, mumps, and rubella. Most peo- ple born before 1957 are likely to have been infected naturally with these diseases. Persons who have a reli- able history of varicella are considered immune; those

who do not can be tested to determine their immune sta- tus or can be vaccinated without testing.[18] Vaccination for other diseases, such as influenza, pneumococcal pneumonia, HAV, and HBV, is recommended for persons in certain age, occupational, environmental, and lifestyle groups and for those with special health problems.

The older adult population and persons with chronic diseases are at particular risk for infectious diseases be- cause of a decline in their immune system. More than 90% of all deaths from influenza A and B viruses occur in people 65 years and older.[20] The most effective way to reduce the impact of influenza is to vaccinate people at high risk each year before the influenza season. The ACIP recommends that influenza vaccine be adminis- tered annually to adolescents and adults at high risk and to all people age 65 and older. For persons living in nurs- ing homes and other chronic care facilities, annual vac- cination can reduce the risk of influenza outbreaks by in-

TABLE 21-3	*CDC Recommendations for Vaccination of Older Adolescents and Adults in the United States*
Disease	**Recommendation**
Polio	Primary series of oral poliovirus vaccine in childhood is sufficient. If no childhood series, vaccine need not be given except to persons at risk because of health care occupation or foreign travel.
Tetanus, diphtheria	Booster dose of tetanus and diphtheria toxoids (Td) every 10 years after primary series of Td; tetanus toxoid may be repeated in 5 years if a dirty wound is sustained. If no childhood series, initiate series of three doses within 1 year.
Pertussis	Primary series of pertussis vaccine is given in childhood only.
Measles	Documented immunity or two doses of MMR* vaccine at least 1 month apart. People who have received only one dose of vaccine since their first birthday should receive a second dose, particularly on enrolling in college, traveling to a foreign country, or entering a health care field.
Mumps	Documented immunity or two doses of MMR vaccine at least 1 month apart.
Rubella	Documented immunity or two doses of MMR vaccine at least 1 month apart. Vaccine particularly recom- mended for previously unimmunized women of childbearing age and susceptible health care providers.
Hepatitis A	Two doses of vaccine at least 6 months apart for persons who reside in a community that has a high rate of hepatitis A virus infection, who are at risk because of foreign travel, or who have chronic liver disease.
Hepatitis B	Complete series of three doses within 6 months for high-risk individuals, including health care providers, susceptible dialysis clients, people with hemophilia, intravenous drug abusers, and sexual and household contacts of hepatitis B virus carriers.
Varicella	Documented immunity or two doses of vaccine separated by 4 to 8 weeks. Recommended for health care providers, teachers of young children, day care employees, and others at high risk for exposure and for transmitting disease.
Influenza	Annually for people older than 65; residents of nursing homes and other chronic care facilities; people with chronic cardiac or pulmonary disease, diabetes or other metabolic disorders, renal disease, severe ane- mia, or immunosuppression; health care providers and others in close contact with people in high-risk groups.
Pneumococcal	Single dose of vaccine for people older than 65; those with chronic cardiac or pulmonary disease, cirrhosis, alcoholism, diabetes, Hodgkin's disease, nephrosis, renal failure, cerebrovascular fluid leaks, immunosup- pression, sickle cell anemia, and asplenism. Revaccination should be considered after 5 years for people at highest risk.

Data from Centers for Disease Control and Prevention, Atlanta.[4,8,9,11,13,17-20]
*MMR, Measles-mumps-rubella vaccine.

ducing herd immunity. Annual vaccination with the current vaccine is necessary because new variants of influenza continue to occur; vaccination against one strain may not confer immunity to another.

Pneumococcal pneumonia, caused by *Streptococcus pneumoniae,* is an important cause of morbidity and mortality in the very young, in older adults, and in others with certain high-risk or chronic conditions. The ACIP recommends that these persons receive a single dose of pneumococcal polysaccharide vaccine.[11]

Nurses can be instrumental in ensuring that all children, adolescents, and adults are properly immunized. Every visit to a health care provider should be an opportunity to obtain a history of vaccination status and to provide vaccinations as needed. In addition, you and other health care providers should be concerned about improving your own resistance to infectious diseases. One important approach is to maintain your immunization status by being vaccinated against HBV infection, measles, mumps, rubella, polio, tetanus, diphtheria, varicella, and influenza.

For all health care providers, HBV infection is a major occupational hazard because of the likelihood of contact with blood and blood-contaminated body fluids from infected clients. The Occupational Safety and Health Administration (OSHA) has developed regulations that require employers to offer at-risk employees the HBV vaccine at the employers' expense. Influenza vaccination is recommended yearly for health care providers in hospital, chronic care, and outpatient settings to reduce the risk of illness and to reduce the possibility of transmitting the virus to clients. The vaccinations you receive protect not only you but also your clients.

Infection Control in Hospitals

Many nosocomial infections can be prevented if health care personnel adhere to infection control practices. The CDC and the Joint Commission on Accreditation of Healthcare Organizations (JCAHO) issue guidelines and establish standards for control of hospital infection. The CDC develops and updates guidelines related to the control and prevention of nosocomial infections, and JCAHO requires hospitals to establish infection control programs that meet accreditation standards. The JCAHO standards require hospital infection control committees to establish surveillance programs, implement infection control policies and procedures, and conduct continuing education for all hospital employees regarding infection control.[34] Most hospitals employ an infection control nurse or infection control practitioner who is responsible for the coordination of a hospital-wide infection control program.

Infection control programs in hospitals address two major areas related to nosocomial infection: (1) surveillance and reporting and (2) control and prevention. The purpose of surveillance is to establish and maintain a database to track the rates of nosocomial infections. Surveillance activities include early detection of infections in clients and personnel and reporting of relevant data to designated persons for appropriate action. Surveillance systems to detect both organisms and diseases are necessary components of prevention and control strategies. National data on nosocomial infections are obtained from selected hospitals in the United States by the CDC and are used to estimate rates and trends.[16]

The focus of infection control strategies is on barrier precautions to reduce infection risk for all clients and personnel and on occupational health practices to protect health care staff from infection.

Barrier Precautions

Barriers are intended to prevent the transfer of an infective organism to a susceptible host. By placing a clean layer of plastic or fabric between a susceptible site and a potential source of pathogenic organisms, the likelihood of transmitting an infection can be reduced. The prevented transmission can be from client to caregiver or caregiver to client. The risk for a client increases when caregivers have contact with the client's mucous membranes and nonintact skin. The risk for caregivers increases whenever they are in contact with a client's moist body substances. Protective barriers include gloves, gowns, masks, and protective eyewear.

None of the protective barriers is intended to replace hand-washing. *The most important means of preventing the spread of microorganisms is hand-washing.* Hands become soiled during client care, particularly after contact with moist body sites and substances. Soiled hands have played a major role in transferring organisms to new client hosts. Unfortunately, gloves provide a false sense of security because hands can become contaminated even when gloves are used. The use of gloves is not a substitute for hand-washing.

In the past, most barrier precautions were instituted after a client's infection was diagnosed. When an infection was suspected or recognized, a system of barrier precautions, referred to as *isolation procedures,* was instituted to prevent transmission of pathogens among hospitalized clients, health care personnel, and visitors. Depending on the diagnosis, one of several isolation strategies was used. Precautions varied, depending on the methods needed to interrupt transmission of the infection. For the isolation strategy to be effective, the diagnosis of infection had to be made or suspected early; however, most infections are communicable for some period when manifestations are absent and the infection is undetected.

In the early 1980s, unrecognized cases of HBV and HIV infection were identified as important sources of disease. Health care workers could potentially become infected through needle-sticks and body fluids contaminated with clients' blood. In response to this problem, the CDC recommended "universal precautions" as a means of preventing transmission of HIV, HBV, and other blood-borne pathogens.[3] Universal precautions focused on preventing transmission of blood-borne pathogens from infected or potentially infected clients to susceptible caregivers. Universal precautions required the use of protective barriers with all clients regardless of their presumed infection status. These precautions emphasized (1) the use of gloves and gowns to reduce contamination of skin and clothing; (2) the use of masks and goggles to reduce contamination of the mucous membranes of the mouth, nose, and eyes; and (3) prevention of needle-stick injuries. Used needles were not to be recapped by hand, and puncture-resistant containers were to be used for disposal of sharps.

In 1987 the practice of *body substance isolation* (BSI) was proposed as a system to isolate all moist and potentially infectious body substances from all clients, regardless of their presumed infection status.[32] Personnel used clean gloves during contact with nonintact skin and mucous membranes and when anticipating contact with blood, feces, urine, sputum, saliva, wound drainage, and other body fluids. BSI was based on the assumption that the blood and body substances of all clients might contain potentially infectious, transmissible organisms.

In 1996 the Hospital Infection Control Practices Advisory Committee (HICPAC) of the CDC synthesized the various isolation systems into one new set of guidelines.[29] The new guidelines recommend two tiers of isolation strategies: (1) standard precautions and (2) transmission-based precautions.

Standard precautions are the more important tier and are designed for the care of all clients in hospitals regardless of their diagnosis or presumed infection status. These precautions synthesize the major components of universal precautions and BSI. Standard precautions apply to nonintact skin, mucous membranes, blood, and all body fluids, secretions, and excretions except sweat.

Transmission-based precautions form the second tier and are designed only for the care of clients who have known or suspected infections or have been colonized with transmissible pathogens. These are *additional* precautions needed to interrupt transmission of a nosocomial infection and are used with standard precautions. The three types of transmission-based precautions can be combined for infections that have more than one route of transmission:

1. *Contact precautions* are designed to reduce direct and indirect contact transmission of microorganisms.
2. *Droplet precautions* are for infections transmitted by large-particle droplets such as those generated during coughing, sneezing, speaking, or suctioning.
3. *Airborne precautions* are designed to reduce the transmission of pathogens on airborne droplet nuclei.

In many cases, the risk of transmitting a nosocomial infection is highest before a diagnosis can be made. Certain clinical syndromes and conditions warrant the addition of transmission-based precautions while the definitive diagnosis is anticipated. For example, contact precautions should be implemented for incontinent or diapered clients who have acute diarrhea with a likely infectious cause such as HAV infection. Clients with infected draining skin lesions or wounds that cannot be covered warrant contact precautions because the wound may be infected with *S. aureus*. Droplet precautions should be implemented for clients with meningitis until infection with *Neisseria meningitidis* is ruled out.

Other examples include clients admitted with rashes or respiratory infections with possible etiologic agents that require additional precautions beyond standard precautions. Additional precautions should also be taken with clients who have a history of infection or colonization with multi-drug–resistant organisms or who had a recent hospital or nursing home stay in a facility where multi-drug–resistant organisms were prevalent.

Control of the spread of nosocomial infections depends on meticulous attention to infection control practices. The CDC has provided excellent institutional infection control guidelines that can be tailored to meet the needs of specific situations or environments. In addition to standard and transmission-based precautions, the CDC has issued special guidelines for preventing nosocomial transmission of tuberculosis,[5] VRSA,[10] and VRE[6] in health care facilities. See the Management and Delegation feature on Infection Control on p. 430.

Occupational Health Practices

The second major component of an infection prevention and control program is to protect health care workers from infection. Occupational health practices include evaluating personnel for existing infections, administering vaccinations, keeping records, managing exposures, educating employees, and developing and enforcing infection control procedures.

When it was recognized that health care workers who had contact with clients' blood were at increased risk for infection by blood-borne pathogens, infection control efforts focused on preventing employee exposure to blood. By 1989 most hospitals had implemented the universal precautions guidelines to protect employees at risk of transmission of HIV and HBV. In addition, efforts focused on HBV vaccination of employees at risk for blood exposure. New employees are screened for susceptibility to tuberculosis, HBV, measles, mumps, rubella, and chickenpox. Annual influenza vaccinations are strongly encouraged, and periodic tuberculin skin testing is recommended for employees at risk for exposure to tuberculosis.

In 1991 OSHA published guidelines—the *blood-borne pathogens standard*—to protect employees exposed to blood and other potentially infectious materials.[38] One of the most important components of the

MANAGEMENT AND DELEGATION
Infection Control

Regulatory agencies have developed specific and complete guidelines for infection control to protect clients and staff from the transmission of infectious diseases. All health care providers must receive training and education on their role in maintaining infection control practices, including standard precautions. Your role in providing and delegating care of clients on isolation for known or suspected organisms includes assessment of clients and their environment. Note the level of precaution required according to your institution's system. Ensure that strict attention to isolation techniques is maintained by all who interact with the client. For the newly isolated client, you are responsible for client and family assessment and education regarding infection control measures. Unlicensed assistive personnel may then reinforce your teachings.

Some components of infection control practice may be delegated to unlicensed assistive personnel, such as room setup and maintenance of supplies and equipment. Consider delegating the following tasks:

- Stocking of gloves, gowns, and masks
- Stocking of client-specific equipment, such as thermometers, stethoscopes, and sphygmomanometers
- Cleaning of equipment after use, such as oxygen saturation machines and wheelchairs
- Removal of linen and unused equipment from the client's room

Delegation of direct care provision for clients in isolation to unlicensed assistive personnel should include reinforcement of the outlined precautions. *Note:* Care of a client in isolation does not change the practice parameters for what unlicensed assistive personnel may provide to the client or what you can delegate. Emphasize the ways in which the isolation status might affect delivery of care. For example, a client isolated because of methicillin-resistant *Staphylococcus aureus* (MRSA) is routinely cared for with gown, gloves, and mask. If that client is actively incontinent, you may need to give unlicensed assistive personnel additional instruction to change gloves between tasks.

Describe findings that are immediately reportable to you for the unlicensed assistive personnel. Such findings may include a disruption of isolation technique or any difficulty the unlicensed assistive personnel experience while providing care.

---

guidelines is the requirement that all health care employees at risk for exposure to blood and body fluids be offered an HBV vaccination free of charge. In addition, OSHA requires all care providers to wear protective attire when they are likely to have contact with blood and other moist body substances that may contain pathogens. Because a third of occupational exposures to HIV result from recapping needles after use, OSHA standards urged the use of needle-less or recessed needle systems. Injuries from contaminated needles and other sharps are also associated with hepatitis B and hepatitis C viruses.[40] The OSHA blood-borne pathogens standard incorporates most elements of universal precautions plus barrier precautions and sharps disposal systems that must be available at the point of use. Since publication of the standard, a wide variety of medical devices have been developed to reduce the risk of needle-sticks and other sharps injuries. In response to growing concern about employee protection, Congress passed the Needlestick Safety and Prevention Act in 2000 requiring OSHA to revise the standards to mandate the use of new safer medical devices.

Another major area of concern has been the role and selection of respiratory protection equipment to prevent transmission of tuberculosis in hospitals. OSHA has proposed standards for respiratory protection programs to protect hospital personnel from pathogens spread by the airborne route. In particular, surgical masks have not been effective in preventing inhalation of droplet nuclei, and the use of disposable particulate respirators has been recommended instead. Regulations and recommendations are continually being updated by OSHA as health care methods and techniques evolve.[39]

Infection Control in Long-Term Care Facilities

Nosocomial infections are common among residents of LTCFs and are a major source of morbidity and mortality. UTIs, respiratory infections (influenza, pneumonia), infected pressure ulcers, gastroenteritis, and conjunctivitis are the most common infections found in long-term care facilities.[45] Many LTCFs are becoming reservoirs for antimicrobial-resistant organisms, including MRSA and VRE.[50]

Many hospital-oriented infection control guidelines are relevant to LTCFs, but they must be adapted, depending on the acuity of residents, facility size, resources, and other factors. The LTCF is a home to residents, one in which they usually reside for months or years. Strict barrier approaches used in hospitals can have a negative effect on the residents and the facility's social and rehabilitative goals. Infection control programs must be designed to balance the medical and social needs of long-term care residents. The Association for Practitioners in Infection Control (APIC) has addressed this problem in its guidelines for infection control programs in long-term care facilities.[45]

Infection Control in Community-Based Settings

Today health care is provided to clients in their homes, in physicians' offices, in ambulatory care centers, and in outpatient specialty clinics. Intravenous infusions, hemodialysis, and mechanical ventilation are provided in the home, and nearly half of all surgical procedures are performed in outpatient settings.[48] Venipuncture, wound care, suturing, skin biopsy, bone marrow aspiration and biopsy, plastic and reconstructive surgery, and other minor surgical procedures are commonly performed in physicians' offices. Same-day surgery centers accommodate both minor and major ambulatory surgeries and procedures. Outpatient specialty clinics are available to provide hemodialysis and peritoneal dialysis.

Infections arise during the provision of care in home and outpatient settings, but identifying a break in infection control practices can be difficult. Infection control surveillance programs in community-based settings have been limited, and specific data about infections occurring in homes and outpatient settings are not readily available.[33] Infection control guidelines from the usual resources, such as the CDC, have been written primarily for hospitals. Until setting-specific guidelines are published, commonsense adaptations of hospital infection control practices are recommended.[41,48] As the shift to managed care continues, it can be expected that infection surveillance and control issues will become more important as a basis for measuring the quality of care and as a requirement for agency certification.

Home care has grown to encompass services provided by family members, partners, and friends as well as health care professionals. Lay caregivers must be given simple guidelines for infection control in the home. Hand-washing, use of gloves, and appropriate methods for disposal of contaminated sharps and other waste are examples of infection control practices that must be taught by the home care provider. Clients and their caregivers should be taught about safe food handling, health concerns about pets, and sanitation issues. See the Bridge to Home Health Care feature on Infection Control on the website.

Protecting the health care worker is a critical component of infection control in any health care setting, and the employee health plan should be similar to that used in hospitals. You should not assume that health care workers who work in outpatient settings are at lower risk for infectious diseases than those employed by hospitals. Policies should be developed that meet the requirements of OSHA and other regulating agencies and that acknowledge the unique requirements of the health care setting.

CONCLUSIONS

Infectious diseases have been killers of humans throughout recorded history. For most of this time, conquering infection has been the focus of health care. The nurse's role in preventing, detecting, and treating infectious disease is a vital one. You must be aware of agent-host-environment interactions and take appropriate steps to prevent accidental transmission in all health care settings.

BIBLIOGRAPHY

1. Baddour, L.M., & Gorbach, S.L. (2003). *Therapy of infectious diseases*. Philadelphia: Saunders.
2. Benin, A.L., & Dowell, S.F. (2001). Antibiotic resistance and implications for the appropriate use of antimicrobial agents. In A.G. Mainous III & C. Pomeroy (Eds.), *Management of antimicrobials in infectious diseases: Impact of antibiotic resistance*. Totowa, NJ: Humana.
3. Centers for Disease Control. (1988). Update: Universal precautions for prevention of transmission of human immunodeficiency virus, hepatitis B virus, and other bloodborne pathogens in health-care settings. *Morbidity and Mortality Weekly Report, 37*(24), 377-387.
4. Centers for Disease Control. (1991). Update on adult immunization: Recommendations of the Immunization Practices Advisory Committee (ACIP). *Morbidity and Mortality Weekly Report, 40*(RR-12), 1-94.
5. Centers for Disease Control and Prevention. (1994). Guidelines for preventing the transmission of *Mycobacterium tuberculosis* in health-care facilities. *Morbidity and Mortality Weekly Report, 43*(RR-13), 1-132.
6. Centers for Disease Control and Prevention. (1995). Recommendations for preventing the spread of vancomycin resistance: Recommendations of the Hospital Infection Control Practices Advisory Committee (HICPAC). *Morbidity and Mortality Weekly Report, 44*(RR-12), 1-13.
7. Centers for Disease Control and Prevention. (1996). Guideline for prevention of intravascular device-related infections. *American Journal of Infection Control, 24*, 262-293.
8. Centers for Disease Control and Prevention. (1996). Immunization of adolescents: Recommendations of the Advisory Committee on Immunization Practices, the American Academy of Pediatrics, the American Academy of Family Physicians, and the American Medical Association. *Morbidity and Mortality Weekly Report, 45*(RR-13), 1-13.
9. Centers for Disease Control and Prevention. (1997). Immunization of health-care workers: Recommendations of the Advisory Committee on Immunization Practices (ACIP) and the Hospital Infection Control Practices Advisory Committee (HICPAC). *Morbidity and Mortality Weekly Report, 46*(RR-18), 1-42.
10. Centers for Disease Control and Prevention. (1997). Interim guidelines for prevention and control of staphylococcal infection associated with reduced susceptibility to vancomycin. *Morbidity and Mortality Weekly Report, 46*(27), 626-628, 635.
11. Centers for Disease Control and Prevention. (1997). Prevention of pneumococcal disease: recommendations of the Advisory Committee on Immunization Practices (ACIP). *Morbidity and Mortality Weekly Report, 46*(RR-8), 1-24.
12. Centers for Disease Control and Prevention. (1998). Guideline for infection control in health care personnel, 1998. *American Journal of Infection Control, 26*, 289-354.

13. Centers for Disease Control and Prevention. (1998). Measles, mumps, and rubella—vaccine use and strategies for elimination of measles, rubella, and congenital rubella syndrome and control of mumps: Recommendations of the Advisory Committee on Immunization Practices (ACIP). *Morbidity and Mortality Weekly Report, 47*(RR-8), 1-57.

14. Centers for Disease Control and Prevention. (1999). Antimicrobial resistance: MRSA-methicillin resistant *Staphylococcus aureus. Issues in Healthcare Settings,* CDC online: http://www.cdc.gov/ncidod/hip/Aresist/mrsahcw.htm.

15. Centers for Disease Control and Prevention. (1999). Guideline for prevention of surgical site infection, 1999. *American Journal of Infection Control, 27,* 97-134.

16. Centers for Disease Control and Prevention. (1999). National Nosocomial Infections Surveillance (NNIS) System report, data summary from January 1990-May 1999, issued June 1999. *American Journal of Infection Control, 27,* 520-532.

17. Centers for Disease Control and Prevention. (1999). Prevention of hepatitis A through active or passive immunization: Recommendations of the Advisory Committee on Immunization Practices (ACIP). *Morbidity and Mortality Weekly Report, 48*(RR-12), 1-37.

18. Centers for Disease Control and Prevention. (1999). Prevention of varicella. Update recommendations of the Advisory Committee on Immunization Practices (ACIP). *Morbidity and Mortality Weekly Report, 48*(RR-6), 1-5.

19. Centers for Disease Control and Prevention. (2000). Poliomyelitis prevention in the United States: Updated recommendations of the Advisory Committee on Immunization Practices (ACIP). *Morbidity and Mortality Weekly Report, 49*(RR-5), 1-22.

20. Centers for Disease Control and Prevention. (2001). Prevention and control of influenza: Recommendations of the Advisory Committee on Immunization Practices (ACIP). *Morbidity and Mortality Weekly Report, 50*(RR-4), 1-44.

21. Centers for Disease Control and Prevention. (2002). Guideline for hand hygiene in healthcare settings: Recommendations of the Healthcare Infection Control Practices Advisory Committee and the HICPAC/ SHEA/APIC/IDSA Hand Hygiene Task Force. *Morbidity and Mortality Weekly Report, 51*(RR 16), 1-44.

22. Centers for Disease Control and Prevention. (2002). *Staphylococcus aureus* resistant to vancomycin—United States, 2002. *Morbidity and Mortality Weekly Report, 51,* 565-567.

23. Centers for Disease Control and Prevention. (2003). Recommended childhood and adolescent immunization schedule—United States, 2003. *Morbidity and Mortality Weekly Report, 52*(4), Q1-Q4.

24. Centers for Disease Control Division of Vector-Borne Infectious Diseases. (2003). West Nile virus. Retrieved August 6, 2003, from http://www.cdc.gov/ncidod/dvbid/westnile/index.htm.

25. Cochi, S.L., et al. (1994). Meeting the challenges of vaccine-preventable diseases in child day care. *Pediatrics, 94*(6, Part 2), 1021-1023.

26. Couig, M.P. (2002). Remarks by Rear Admiral Mary Pat Couig, MPH, RN, FAAN, Chief Nurse Officer, U.S. Public Health Service, ANA Convention Opening Session, June 30, 2002. Retrieved January 23, 2003, from the World Wide Web: http://nursingworld.org/conventn/2002/news/couig.htm.

27. Elizaga, M.L., Weinstein, R.A., & Hayden, M.K. (2002). Patients in long-term care facilities: A reservoir for vancomycin-resistant enterococci. *Clinical Infectious Diseases, 34,* 441-446.

28. Fridkin, S.C., & Gaynes, R.P. (1999). Antimicrobial resistance in intensive care units. *Clinics in Chest Medicine, 20,* 303-316.

29. Garner, J.S., & Hospital Infection Control Practices Advisory Committee. (1996). Guideline for isolation precautions in hospitals. *Infection Control and Hospital Epidemiology, 17,* 54-80.

30. Hamilton, D.C., & Ludlam, H. (2001). New anti-Gram-positive agents. *Current Opinion in Critical Care, 7,* 232-237.

31. Hoffman, R.E. (2003). Preparing for a bioterrorist attack: Legal and administrative strategies. Emerging Infectious Diseases [serial online] 2003 Feb [cited 2003 Feb 14]; 8. Available: http://www.cdc.gov/ncidod/EID/vol9no2/01-0538.htm.

32. Jackson, M.M., & Lynch, P. (1991). An attempt to make an issue less murky: A comparison of four systems for infection precautions. *Infection Control and Hospital Epidemiology, 12,* 448-450.

33. Jarvis, W.R. (2001). Infection control and changing health-care delivery systems. *Emerging Infectious Diseases, 7,* 170-173.

34. Joint Commission on Accreditation of Healthcare Organizations. (2002). *2002 Hospital Accreditation Standards (HAS).* Chicago: Author.

35. Maki, D.G., & Tambyah, P.A. (2001). Engineering out the risk of infection with urinary catheters. *Emerging Infectious Diseases, 7,* 342-347.

36. Maranan, M.C., et al. (1997). Antimicrobial resistance in staphylococci: Epidemiology, molecular mechanisms, and clinical relevance. *Infectious Disease Clinics of North America, 11*(4), 813-849.

37. Nelson, K.E., Williams, C.M., & Graham, N.M.H. (2001). *Infectious disease epidemiology: Theory and practice.* Gaithersburg, MD: Aspen.

38. Occupational Safety and Health Administration. (1991). Occupational exposure to bloodborne pathogens: Final rule. *Federal Register, 56,* 64003-64182.

39. Occupational Safety and Health Administration. (1997). Occupational exposure to tuberculosis: Proposed rule. *Federal Register, 62*(201), 54159-54209.

40. Occupational Safety and Health Administration. (2001). Occupational exposure to bloodborne pathogens: Needlestick and other sharps injuries; Final rule (2001, January 18). *Federal Register 66,* 5317-5325.

41. Rhinehart, R. (2001). Infection control in home care. *Emerging Infectious Diseases, 7, 208-211.*

42. Rice, L.B. (2001). Emergence of vancomycin-resistant enterococci. *Emerging Infectious Diseases, 7, 183-187.*

43. Rotz, L.D., et al. (2002). Public health assessment of potential biological terrorism agents. *Emerging Infectious Diseases, 8* (2).

44. Shlaes, D.M., et al. (1997). Society for Healthcare Epidemiology of America and Infectious Diseases Society of America Joint Committee on the Prevention of Antimicrobial Resistance: Guidelines for the prevention of antimicrobial resistance in hospitals. *Infection Control and Hospital Epidemiology, 18,* 275-291.

45. Smith, P.W., & Rusnak, P.G. (1997). SHEA/APIC position paper: Infection prevention and control in the long-term-care facility. *Infect Control and Hospital Epidemiology, 18* (12), 831-849.

46. U.S. Department of Health and Human Services. (1990). *Healthy people 2000.* Washington, DC: U.S. Government Printing Office.

47. U.S. Department of Health and Human Services. (2000). *Healthy People 2010: Understanding and Improving Health.* (2nd ed.) Washington, DC: U.S. Government Printing Office.

48. Wenzel, R.P. (Ed.). (1997). *Prevention and control of nosocomial infections* (3rd ed.). Baltimore: Williams & Wilkins.

49. Wenzel, R.P., & Edmond, M.B. (2001). The impact of hospital-acquired bloodstream infections. *Emerging Infectious Diseases, 7,* 174-177.

50. Yoshikawa, T.T., & Norman, D.C. (Eds.). (2001). *Infectious disease in the aging: A clinical handbook.* Totowa, NJ: Humana Press.

Unit 5

Psychosocial Foundations
of Medical-Surgical Nursing

Anatomy and Physiology Review

Arousal, Pain, and Conscious Awareness

Robert G. Carroll

Awareness and response to dangerous settings are key to the survival of an organism. Humans have a variety of distance senses (smell, sight, hearing) that can be used to identify potentially dangerous situations and allow an individual to avoid them. If avoidance fails and damage occurs, pain results.

Pain is a conscious perception that results from environmental stress. *Nociceptors*, often called *pain receptors*, are free nerve endings activated by stimuli that can cause (or already have caused) tissue damage. Neuronal transmission of nociceptors is redundant and is subject to only minor filtering before reaching the somatosensory cortex.

The reticular activating system (RAS) controls the degree of filtering of afferent sensory inputs (including pain) and therefore helps determine conscious perception. The activity of the cortex is superimposed on a normal sleep-wake cycle and can interact with this cycle.

This section uses the perception of pain to introduce the concepts of neuronal transmission, the processing of information, arousal, and conscious awareness. Unit 16 provides additional details about neuron action potential, synaptic transmission, and other somatosensory modalities.

To understand the mechanisms by which one can facilitate pain reduction, one must understand the neurologic contributions to pain perception. Pain is a perceptual interpretation of nerve activity that reaches consciousness. It depends on activation of neurons that transmit the noxious information to the central nervous system. Pain perception is initiated by activation of neurons along a pathway, which eventually terminates in a sensory cortex in the brain. The pathway involves both peripheral and central nervous system components and can be activated at any point along its trajectory.

NEURONAL COMMUNICATION

At the single neuron level, action potentials generally arrive at the dendrites or cell body and initiate an action potential at the beginning of the axon; then an action potential travels along the axon to the next synapse in the sequence. Neurons in sensory pathways rarely make a 1:1 synaptic connection. The diversity of synaptic connections allows sensory information to be coded and processed before arriving at the cerebral cortex. Neuronal interconnections generally fall into a diverging or a converging pattern.

Divergence occurs when an action potential from one axon activates synapses with multiple other neurons. This arrangement allows a single stimulus to have multiple effects. One advantage of this arrangement is that the information becomes redundant, meaning that one synaptic failure will not result in loss of the message.

Convergence occurs when one neuron receives afferent connections from multiple other axons. This is important because activity at a synapse from one neuron is not sufficient to generate an action potential in the post-synaptic neuron. The generation of an action potential in the post-synaptic neuron requires simultaneous activity at a number of synapses *(spatial summation)* or repetitive activation of a single synapse *(temporal summation)*.

The flexibility of neuronal interconnections is enhanced by having some neurons exciting the post-synaptic neuron and other neurons inhibiting the post-synaptic neuron. Excitation or inhibition is determined by the type of neurotransmitter released from the pre-synaptic neuron, and the receptor specificity of the post-synaptic neuron.

THE PHYSIOLOGY OF PAIN
PAIN AS AN INTEGRATIVE EXPERIENCE

Nociceptor Activation

Nociceptors are free nerve endings that are widely distributed throughout the body. Nociceptors can be found in the periphery in skin, fascia, bone periosteum, skeletal muscle, ligaments, and mucous membranes. In the viscera, nociceptors are found in the capsules of most organs. Chemically mediated activation of nociceptors can be initiated by (1) cell wall destruction as a result of events such as tissue injury, ulceration, tumor invasion, and cell necrosis; (2) inflammation; (3) infection; (4) nerve injury; and (5) extravasation of plasma from the circulatory system associated with edema, ischemia, or occlusion of vasculature. Mechanically mediated activation of nociceptors is accomplished by noxious stretch or pressure due to (1) distention of viscera, fascia or periosteum; (2) occlusion of gastrointestinal or genitourinary structures; or (3) obstruction of ducts/viscus. These receptors are activated by a variety of mechanical, thermal, and chemical stimuli.

Chemicals that mediate nociception in the periphery include bradykinin, prostaglandins, substance P, histamine, serotonin, leukotrienes, and nerve growth factor. Bradykinin is the most potent pain-producing chemical. It is released into tissues when cell walls are destroyed and when plasma leaks from the vasculature. Bradykinin initiates a pain-producing signal by increasing the ability of Na^+ to flow across the membrane.

Prostaglandins result from cell wall destruction. They most likely contribute to the pain experience by sensitizing receptors, making them more responsive to other chemical, thermal, and mechanical stimuli. They are also potent vasodilators, resulting in an increase of bradykinin release into the tissues. The resulting edema may also contribute by stimulating pressure receptors. Pressure from edema is not typically painful because the pressure is usually not strong enough to stimulate nociceptors. Prostaglandins depolarize these receptors, making them responsive to the relatively weak stimulus provided by the swelling of edema.

Substance P is released into peripheral tissues when nociceptive neurons are activated. This chemical facilitates the release of plasma by increasing vascular permeability, resulting in bradykinin availability. Substance P further enhances pain responses by contributing to prostaglandin release.

Histamine is released from mast cells when inflammation is a component of the pain-producing event. In the periphery, histamine increases vascular permeability contributing to bradykinin activity and edema. Substance P facilitates the release of histamine from mast cells.

Serotonin is released in the periphery by platelets and mast cells. Therefore any event that influences the presence of blood products in tissues or inflammation contributes to serotonin release. Serotonin causes pain directly by altering Na^+ flow in the receptive neuron membrane causing the neuron to fire. Receptors are indirectly facilitated by serotonin as the chemical also sensitizes receptors to the effect of bradykinin.

Leukotrienes are produced by cell-wall destruction during the same process that produces prostaglandins. They contribute to pain perception by attracting neutrophils to an area of injury. Cell-wall destruction is a component of neutrophil activity to combat infection re-

sulting in bradykinin release. Thermal and mechanical receptors have also been shown to be sensitized by leukotrienes.

Hydrogen ions are released as a result of ischemia and hypoxia. They cause Na^+ channels to open resulting in activation of neurons in the pain pathway. Hydrogen ions also facilitate Ca^{2+} channel opening enhancing neurotransmitter release.

Nerve growth factor (NGF) is released when neurons are injured. It is similar to bradykinin in activating nociceptive neurons. It causes injured nerves to sprout new axons and dendrites in greater numbers than existed before the injury. As a result, the area responsive to nociceptive activation is increased in the periphery. Substance P production is also increased by NGF increasing the nociceptive effect the neurotransmitter. In addition, the number of Na^+ and K^+ channels are increased, making it easier to generate an ion flow which will cause the neuron to "fire."

Pain may follow direct activation of free nerve endings, or they may become sensitized, rendering them more susceptible to nociceptive activation. Sensitizing chemicals are released into tissues as a result of cell-wall destruction and the release of plasma from the circulatory system as seen with edema, inflammation, ischemia, and infection. Cells may be damaged by trauma and by the events that accompany inflammation and infection, including mast-cell destruction during the release of histamine in inflammation and the effect of neutrophil activity in the presence of infection. Chemicals that sensitize receptors and nerve fiber membranes render events that do not typically produce pain sensations now capable of initiating pain-producing signals. Sunburned areas produce a burning sensation when one showers with water that normally produces a pleasant warm sensation. Areas of injury are painful in response to touch and mild pressure that would not normally be painful. Normal peristalsis of the gut, which is typically undetectable, produces painful abdominal cramping in the presence of inflammation within the abdominal cavity.

The complexity of pain perception is illustrated by examination of the response to touching a hot stove with your hand. The extreme heat activates the nociceptors and generates action potentials in two different types of neurons, resulting in the perception of fast pain and slow pain.

Fast pain is carried by small myelinated nerves (A-delta fibers). These neurons make multiple synaptic connections in the spinal cord. One connection activates the motor neurons that initiate a withdrawal reflex. This spinal reflex serves to remove the hand from the damaging environment, even before there is any cortical awareness of the injury. Other synaptic connections activate neuron sequences passing through the thalamus and terminating in the sensory cortex, the limbic system, and the hypothalamus. Fast pain is generally described as sharp and well localized and is generally associated with damage to the skin and muscles. A-delta fiber activity typically results in activation of the sympathetic nervous system to prepare the individual to engage in "fight or flight" behaviors that will allow him or her to react to the pain-producing event. As a result, heart rate, respiratory rate and blood pressure may be increased. These sympathetic reactions may or may not be observed in people with pain because these reactions are relatively rapidly adapting, often short-lived responses.

In contrast, *slow pain* is carried by small, unmyelinated nerves (C fibers). These neurons make multiple connections in the spinal cord, and ascending information goes to the midbrain and the reticular formation and contribute to the emotional, cognitive, and situational components of pain. Slow pain is characteristic of damage to the skin, muscles, and internal organs and is characterized by dull, burning, suffering sensations. The poorly localized aspect of slow pain leads to the observation that pain originating in internal organs is perceived in areas with related dermatomes; that is, slow pain associated with myocardial ischemia is often perceived as being in the left arm.

Spinal Cord

The dorsal horn of the spinal cord is the first synaptic relay of the nociceptor-pain pathway. Afferent sensory neurons enter the spinal cord and make multiple synapses in the dorsal horn. This is the first point of divergence of the nociceptor sensory information. Here the nociceptive signal is transferred to the next neuron in the pain pathway and transmitted to the thalamus and brain stem structures by means of spinal tracts. The thalamic signal is involved in the ability to determine the location and intensity of the pain-producing event. The signal is transmitted from the thalamus to the sensory cortex, where the pain is perceived as a sensation. Interneurons that synapse in the spinal cord use substance P and glutamate as neurotransmitters.

Electrical activity resulting in pain perception can be modified at the synapse by manipulating the release of neurotransmitters. An event that inhibits neurotransmitter release decreases the potential for transmission of the nociceptive signal. The inhibition may occur to an extent that extinguishes the pain-producing signal, resulting in total pain reduction. Conversely any event that facilitates release of the neurotransmitter will enhance the transmission of the signal. For example, an event that prohibits the opening of the Ca^{2+} channels inhibits the pain response.

Secondary responses to the signal are initiated throughout the brain, including the limbic system, where the emotional response to pain is generated. Signals transmitted to brain stem structures contribute to the response the individual has to the pain experience and to endogenous (naturally occurring) pain modulation systems. (Figure U5-1)

Brain

Nociceptive sensory information is transmitted to the brain by multiple ascending pathways. Sensory information is carried through the spinothalamic tract and the spinoreticular tract to the thalamus and the RAS, system, respectively. Neurons from the thalamus project to the cerebral cortex (for the conscious perception of pain) and also the limbic system (controlling the emotional response to pain). The amygdala receives nociceptive stimulation via the spinomesencephalic tract. Finally pain elicits an autonomic response, directly via the spinohypothalamic tract, and also indirectly through activity of the thalamus and cerebral cortex.

Conscious Perception of Pain

The diversity of target sites for ascending nociceptive tracts indicates the complexity of the pain perception. Fast pain is a somatosensory sensation, with the origin of the involved nociceptors being precisely localization on the somatic map of the body. In contrast, localization of slow pain is much less precise and may actually be referred from C fibers of the same dermatome (as when myocardial ischemia is "sensed" as pain radiating down the left arm). Nociceptive afferents also synapse in the RAS, where they can regulate conscious awareness and attention. Pain elicits a sympathetic autonomic nervous system response (the "flight-or-fight response"), including an increase in pulse and respiratory rate. Finally

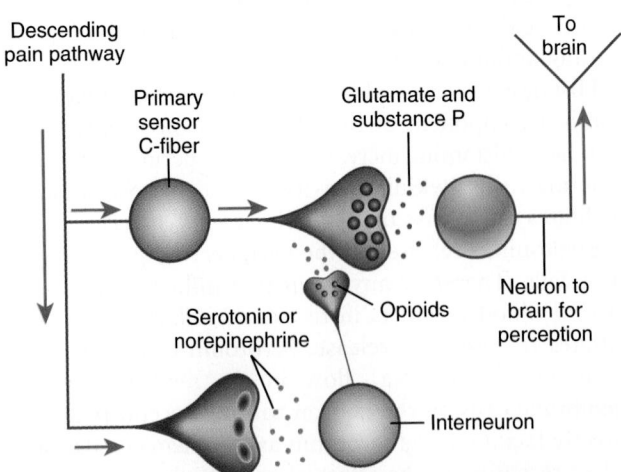

FIGURE U5-1 Endogenous inhibition in a synapse in the spinal cord. As the pain impulse enters the dorsal horn, it has the potential of being modified by interneurons in the synapse containing endogenous opioids.

there is a significant emotional aspect of pain, mediated through the limbic system and insular cortex.

Hyperalgesia

Hyperalgesia is an enhancement of the perception of pain. This event can be mediated both at the tissue level and at the spinal cord. Stimuli that do not originally activate nociceptors may do so after repeated application of noxious stimuli, a process called *sensitization*. Substances released from damaged cells act to decrease the threshold for nociceptors. At the spinal cord level, repetitive afferent input from C fibers cause the dorsal horn cells to become more easily excitable, a process thought to underlie the phenomenon of "phantom limb pain."

PAIN SUPPRESSION APPROACHES

Pain is the conscious interpretation of stimuli associated with nociceptor activity. Pain management remains one of the most significant challenges in nursing. A variety of approaches are currently used to diminish the suffering from pain.

Nociceptor

Diminished stimulation of the free nerve endings will reduce the perception of pain. One approach is to use ice to cool the injured area, which diminishes the activity of the nociceptors. A second approach uses a local anesthetic (Novocain, Xylocaine) injected at the site of injury or along the nerve pathway to completely but reversibly block action potential transmission. This eliminates both sensory and motor neuron activity. In extreme cases the sensory nerves can be severed to block permanently nociceptor action potential transmission.

Synaptic Interruption

The dorsal horn cell in the spinal cord is the first of the multiple synapses involved in nociceptive transmission. Glutamate, acting on AMPA-type glutamate receptors, is the major neurotransmitter. The response of the postsynaptic cell, however, is enhanced by substance P and a variety of neuropeptides released from the nociceptor axons. Blocking the NMDA receptor diminishes both nociceptor afferent transmission and also prevents the hypersensitivity caused by repetitive activity of nociceptors.

Gate Theory of Pain

Nociceptor transmission can be regulated by neurons not directly involved in the afferent pain transmission pathways (Figure U5-2). Non-nociceptive afferents diminish the sensitivity of dorsal horn neurons involved in nociception. The non-nociceptive afferents include sensory neurons that encode vibration. This mechanism is used to explain the effectiveness of transcutaneous electrical nerve stimulation (TENS) in modulating the sensation of pain. In addition to inhibition from sensory af-

FIGURE U5-2 The gate-control theory: Mark II. The new model includes excitatory *(white circle)* and inhibitory *(black circle)* links from the substantia gelatinosa (SG) to the transmission (T) cells as well as descending inhibitory control from brain stem systems. The round knob at the end of inhibitory link implies that its action may be presynaptic, postsynaptic, or both. All connections are excitatory, except the inhibitory link from SG to T cell. *L*, Large-diameter fibers; *S*, small-diameter fibers. (From Melzack, R., & Wall, P.D. [2001]. *The challenge of pain.* London: Penguin Books.)

ferents, descending inhibitory pathways can diminish the effectiveness of the pain transmission pathways at the spinal cord and thalamic levels.

Brain Chemicals and Analgesics

The importance of pain reduction led to early identification of morphine (opium) and codeine as significant analgesics. Injection of morphine into the brain inhibits the activity of the spinal cord dorsal horn cells, indicating that morphine activates descending inhibitory pathways. The localization of opiate receptors in the brain and spinal cord led to the identification of endogenous compounds that bind those receptors. Three major classes of peptides—enkephalins, endorphins, and dynorphins—are produced by the body and activate the opiate receptors and consequently have significant analgesic actions.

The three groups of non-opioid analgesics are salicylates, acetaminophen, and nonsteroidal anti-inflammatory drugs (NSAIDs). These drugs generally have both local and central analgesic effects that are tied to the inhibition of prostaglandin synthesis.

FACTORS AFFECTING PAIN

The perception of pain is shaped by emotional state and past experiences. A variety of factors can cause pain perception to be a subjective experience. The person-to-person variability in the perception of pain contributes to the clinical difficulty in clinical management of pain.

THE PHYSIOLOGY OF SLEEP AND AROUSAL

Humans structure activities around a daily (circadian) rhythm. The timing of the sleep-wake cycle and other circadian rhythms such as body temperature is controlled in part by the suprachiasmatic nucleus in the anterior hypothalamus. Located above the optic chiasm, this area receives input from the retina, which provides information about darkness and light. The suprachiasmatic nucleus controls the production of the hormone melatonin, which is believed to be a potent sleep inducer.

The RAS controls arousal from sleep, wakefulness, and the ability to respond to stimuli. The RAS is located in the brain stem and contains projections to the thalamus and cerebral cortex. The diffuse network of neurons in the RAS is in a strategic position to monitor ascending sensory inputs and descending stimuli. The neurotransmitters of the RAS serve as chemical messengers regulating the sleep-wake cycle and the stages of sleep. The onset of sleep and of each subsequent sleep stage is an active process involving delicate shifts in the balance of several of these neurotransmitters.

The transition from the awake state to a non-rapid eye movement (NREM) sleep is marked by decreases in the concentrations of serotonin, norepinephrine, and acetylcholine. The later transition to rapid eye movement (REM) sleep is marked by a dramatic increase in acetylcholine and further decreases in serotonin and norepinephrine. As REM sleep continues, the concentrations of serotonin and norepinephrine increase eventually stopping REM sleep. The release of acetylcholine seems to reestablish REM sleep. The continuous interaction of these two systems produces the normal alterations between NREM and REM sleep. Other neurotransmitters such as gamma aminobutyric acid (GABA) and dopamine contribute to the reciprocal processes involved in shift in sleep state.

All of these neurotransmitters are also actively involved in the waking process. For example, neurons that produce serotonin and norepinephrine play a role in the modulation of sensory input, mood, energy, and information processing, including attention, learning, and memory. Imbalances in these neurotransmitters induce sleep pattern disturbances. Medications or diseases may reciprocally affect not only sleep but also aspects of sensory processing, mood, and cognition.

THE NEED FOR SLEEP

The structure of the sleep cycle is well studied and offers clues about the need for sleep. Sleep is believed to have a restorative and protective function. During sleep sympathetic activity decreases while parasympathetic activity may increase. Hormonal shifts facilitate anabolic processes. Selective deprivation of "slow-wave" sleep is associated with vague physical complaints.

Rapid eye movement sleep may be especially important for maintaining mental activities, such as learning, reasoning, and emotional adjustment. Sleep also appears to serve as an energy-conserving measure for most of the body except for the brain.

SLEEP STAGES

Sleep can be defined behaviorally, functionally, and electrophysiologically. Electrophysiological monitoring of sleep is called *polysomnography* and includes at least three parameters: (1) brain-wave activity, (2) eye movements, and (3) muscle tone. Polysomnography shows that sleep can be divided into REM and NREM. NREM sleep can further be divided into stages 1 through 4. The stages vary in depth but are characterized by slow, rolling eye movements, low-level and fragmented cognitive activity, maintenance of moderate muscle tone, and slower but generally rhythmic respiration and pulse rates. As a person progresses from stage 1 to stage 4 sleep, the wave forms recorded by electroencephalography (EEG) become more synchronized, slower, and higher in amplitude. See Figure 24-1.

The stages of sleep are characterized as follows:
- *Stage 1* is very light. Respirations begin to slow, and muscles relax. At sleep onset, some erratic breathing may occur as well as sudden myoclonic jerks (sleep starts) as the body shifts from an awake to a sleep state. Stage 1 is such a light stage sleep that persons awakened from it often claim that they were not asleep at all.
- *Stage 2* is still light sleep. The brain waves are frequently mixed and low voltage in pattern, with bursts of activity called *sleep spindles* and large-amplitude waves called *K complexes*. More than 50% of sleep occurs as stages 1 and 2.
- *Stages 3 and 4* are slow-wave sleep, named for the characteristic high-voltage, low-frequency delta waves. Respirations become slow and even. The pulse and blood pressure fall. Oxygen consumption by muscle tissues and urine formation decreases. Dreams that occurred during the NREM stage of sleep are generally thought-like ruminations about recent events and current concerns with little story line.

As in stage 1, REM sleep is characterized by low-voltage, random fast waves, as in stage 1 NREM. People in REM sleep have characteristic rapid eye movements, erratic respirations, changes in heart rate, and very low muscle tone. During REM sleep, ventilation depends primarily on the movements of the diaphragm because intracostal and accessory muscle tone is markedly diminished and all postural and nonrespiratory muscles are essentially paralyzed. The ventilatory response to hypoxia and hypercapnia is decreased, and thermoregulation is significantly reduced. Dreams in REM sleep are vivid, story like, emotional, and bizarre.

Most people move through an orderly progression of NREM sleep from stages 1 to 4 and back through stages 3 to 2 before initiating a period of REM sleep. Although this is the typical progression, it is not essential or always seen. Atypical progressions are characteristic of some sleep disorders, such as narcolepsy, in which REM sleep is entered almost immediately after sleep onset.

In adults each sleep cycle through the stages lasts about 90 minutes. During the first few cycles, more time is spent in slow-wave sleep. The percentage of REM sleep increases later in the sleep period.

Wide variations in sleep patterns exist among individuals. By explaining the range of these variations, the nurse can help clients seek a pattern that leaves them feeling reasonably refreshed and alert. Eight hours of undisturbed sleep at night with no daytime naps has become the assumed ideal pattern in North American society. Some adults, however, do well with 6 hours or less, and other normal adults require 10 hours or more of nighttime sleep. Even young adults often awaken once or twice at night, and with aging such awakenings are more frequent. Humans may be physiologically inclined to have a long and short sleep period every 24-hour day, such as is common in warmer climates, where the siesta is a normal part of the day's schedule.

CHANGES IN SLEEP PATTERNS IN OLDER ADULTS

Older people take longer to fall asleep, have increased nocturnal wakefulness, and experience more sleepiness during the day than do younger adults. With aging the percentage of stage 4 decreases considerably and REM sleep decreases somewhat, with more time spent in stage 1. REM sleep is more evenly distributed through the night. *Sleep latency,* the time it takes to get to sleep, increases, as does the average time it takes to get back to sleep after arousal. Age-related respiratory dysfunction may be responsible for sleep fragmentation. Other problems, such as pain, the need to void, and nocturnal dyspnea, can also decrease effective sleep.

Hospitalization affects the quality of nocturnal and other sleep time, especially for older adults. The hospital environment often lacks light and dark cues. Confinement curtails activity or exercise that normally causes fatigue. In addition, unfamiliar sights and sounds and frequent awakenings for the assessment of vital signs and other interventions can disturb sleep. Institutionalization in a long-term care facility may perpetuate the environmental impact of noise, caregiver interruptions, inactivity, and lack of day-night cues.

CONCLUSIONS

Awareness is a neural construct based on activity of the cerebral cortex. Afferent sensory information provides a framework for constructing this awareness. The perception of pain is an example of the complexity of neuronal transmission and modulation that is applied to sensory information as it travels toward the cerebral cortex. Sleep is another example of the range of awareness experienced during the course of the day.

BIBLIOGRAPHY

1. Berne, R., et al. (2004). *Physiology* (5th ed.). St. Louis: Mosby.
2. Guyton, A.C., & Hall, J.E. (2001). *Textbook of medical physiology* (10th ed.). Philadelphia: W.B. Saunders.
3. Hanson, M. (1998). *Pathophysiology.* Philadelphia: W.B. Saunders.
4. Kandel, E.R., Schwartz, J.H., & Jessel, T.M. (2000). *Principles of neural science* (4th ed.). New York, McGraw-Hill.
5. Thibodeau, G., & Patton, K. (1999). *Anatomy and physiology* (4th ed.). St. Louis: Mosby.

Chapter 22
Clients with Pain

Karen A. Sikorski
Donna M. Barker

Pain is a complex, multifaceted phenomenon. It is an individual, unique experience that may be difficult for clients to describe or explain and is often difficult for others to recognize, understand, and assess. Unrelieved acute pain leads to debilitation, diminished quality of life, and depression. Unrelieved acute postoperative pain leads to development of chronic pain syndromes and increased complications. In fact, unrelieved pain can kill.[28a] Pain management challenges every health care team member, because there is no single, universal treatment.

Nurses are probably the most important component of the team, because they are the client's primary advocate for pain reduction and/or relief. Listening to concerns, assessing pain intensity and distress levels, planning for care, educating the client about pain, promoting use of nonpharmacologic pain techniques, and evaluating the process for promoting positive outcomes are nursing responsibilities. An attentive nurse can identify discomfort in clients often without verbal confirmation from the client (Figure 22-1). Nurses can relieve pain merely by acknowledging the discomfort and confirming that measures will be taken to reduce and/or relieve the pain. This commitment and statement of caring establish trust and rapport with the client.

This chapter summarizes what is currently known about the physiology of pain, how to assess and diagnose aspects of pain, how to implement a variety of both pharmacologic and nonpharmacologic techniques to manage the discomfort, and how to evaluate outcomes appropriately.

THE PROBLEM OF PAIN

In the natural environment, pain serves as a mechanism to warn us about the potential for physical harm. Thus pain is the body's protective mechanism to prevent further tissue damage by providing the impetus to withdraw from the pain-producing situation. The discomfort and distress associated with pain often last far beyond the tissue-damaging experience. Pain is the primary reason people seek health care and is associated with increased length of hospital stay, longer recovery time, and poorer client outcomes.[1,21] Pain is typically undertreated.[7] In the early 1970s, researchers reported that pain was seriously undertreated after surgery.[31] Thirty years later, this situation has changed little, even though there have been immense advances in knowledge of the causes of pain and the mechanisms that contribute to pain reduction and/or relief. New medications and the

Nursing Outcomes Classification (NOC)
for Nursing Diagnoses—Clients with Pain

Activity Intolerance
  Endurance
  Energy Conservation
  Self-Care; Activities of Daily Living
Acute Pain and Chronic Pain
  Comfort Level
  Pain Control
  Pain: Disruptive Effects
  Pain Level
  Symptom Control
  Symptom Severity
  Well-Being

Anxiety
  Anxiety Control
  Coping
  Symptom Control Behavior
Deficient Knowledge
  Knowledge: Health Behaviors
  Knowledge: Treatment Regimen
Disturbed Sleep Pattern
  Comfort Level
  Pain Level
  Rest

  Sleep
  Well-Being
Fear
  Fear Control
  Comfort Level
Ineffective Coping
  Coping
  Decision-Making
  Quality of Life
Powerlessness
  Health Beliefs: Perceived Control

FIGURE 22-1 The nurse asks the client about pain. The client is the expert regarding her pain.

recognition of complementary pain management strategies have contributed to the improved ability to manage pain and to provide satisfactory pain reduction and/or relief. If the existing knowledge and resources were used to manage pain, 90% of people with pain would receive satisfactory reduction and/or relief.[33] Barriers to adequate pain management may involve health care professionals, including nurses; clients, physicians, and the health care system.[12,33] These barriers are presented in Box 22-1.

Physicians tend to underprescribe, recommending over longer periods of time doses lower than those considered therapeutic. Typically, medications are prescribed with a range of allowable doses and time periods. For example, acetaminophen with codeine may be prescribed as one or two tablets taken every 3 to 4

BOX 22-1 *Barriers to Pain Management*

Problems Related to Health Care Professionals
Inadequate knowledge of pain management
Poor assessment of pain
Concern about regulation of controlled substances
Fear of pain
Fear of client addiction
Concern about side effects of analgesics
Concern about clients becoming tolerant to analgesics
Continuing myths regarding pain

Problems Related to Clients
Reluctance to report pain
Concern about distracting physicians from treatment of underlying disease
Fear that pain means disease is worse
Concern about not being a "good" client
Reluctance to take pain medications
Fear of addiction or of being thought of as an addict
Worries about unmanageable side effects
Concern about becoming tolerant to pain medications

Problems Related to the Health Care System
Low priority given to cancer pain treatment
Inadequate reimbursement (the most appropriate treatment may not be reimbursed or may be too costly for clients and families)
Restrictive regulation of controlled substances
Problems of availability of treatment or access to it

Modified from Jacox, A., et al. (1994). *Management of cancer pain. Clinical practice guidelines No. 9.* AHCPR Pub. No. 94-1592. Rockville, MD: Agency for Health Care Policy and Research, U.S. Department of Health and Human Services, Public Health Service.

The authors would like to thank Juanita Fogel Keck and Susan Baker for their contribution to this chapter in the sixth edition of *Medical-Surgical Nursing*.

hours. Many nurses tend to routinely administer the smallest prescribed dose of medication over the widest time frame (e.g., one tablet every 4 hours). Health care providers need to learn more about the mechanisms and treatment of pain. A nurse's inaccurate beliefs, values, attitudes, or expectations lead to misunderstandings about the client's pain experience. Often a client's statement of pain is ignored or not believed if that client's experience does not match the nurse's expectation.

Clients contribute to the problem of inadequate pain management. They may be reluctant to take pain medications due to fear of addiction, fear of being labeled a "drug user," or fear of taking strong medications that will render them unable to be adequately medicated in the future if their pain becomes worse. They may believe that some degree of pain is normal and cannot be relieved. Health care providers and people in pain may believe that some degree of pain is expected and is not treatable, especially after surgery and in the presence of cancer. Pain can be relieved, or nearly so, with appropriate strategies.

Nurses and clients do not know enough about combination medications for pain reduction and/or relief. These situations generated by nurses can lead to frustrated, angry, uncooperative clients as a result of unrelieved pain. Education of client and health care providers is a primary action to begin to remedy this problem.

DEFINITION OF PAIN

How is *pain* defined? Does the definition include feelings of agony, distress, or suffering? Is pain defined in a structural, physiologic manner only? Does the definition include individual perception of the painful stimulus? Do cultural and ethnic backgrounds, gender, or age affect pain perception?

Pain is a multidimensional phenomenon and is thus difficult to define. It is a personal and subjective experience, and no two people experience pain in exactly the same manner. You may find pain control a difficult task when caring for individual clients, but it is one of the most important areas of care because people cannot function adequately when they are in pain. Pain is best viewed as a personal experience, not merely as a manifestation of a medical condition.

Health care practitioners have defined pain in many ways. It is generally related to some type of tissue damage, which serves as a warning signal, but it is much more. The International Association for the Study of Pain (IASP) offers the accepted medical definition of pain as "an unpleasant sensory and emotional experience associated with actual or potential tissue damage, or described in terms of such damage."[20]

Margo McCaffery, one of nursing's pain pioneers, defined pain as "whatever the experiencing person says it is and existing whenever the person says it does."[33] This definition makes each person the expert about his or her own pain. Because clinical pain is subjective, the only people who can accurately define their own pain are those who are experiencing that pain. Despite its subjective nature, the nurse is charged with accurately assessing and helping to reduce and/or relieve pain and McCaffery's definition helps nurses achieve this goal. All pain is real even if the cause cannot be ascertained. The nurse is not to presume to judge the presence of pain.

PERCEPTION OF PAIN

Pain *perception,* or *interpretation,* is an important component of the pain experience. Because we perceive and interpret pain based on our own individual experience, pain is different for each person. Pain perception does not depend solely on the degree of physical damage. Both physical stimuli and psychosocial factors can influence our experience of pain. Although few agree about the specific effects of these factors, *anxiety, experience, attention, expectation,* and the *meaning of the situation* in which injury occurs affect pain perception. Cognitive functions, such as distraction, may also affect the severity and quality of the pain experience.

In the past, pain was viewed primarily as a sensation, with motivational and cognitive processes believed to influence only the reaction to pain. However, it has become apparent that mechanisms within the pain pathway can modify pain-related neural impulses before they are transmitted to the brain. Thus pain perception is likely to be determined by a relative balance between sensory peripheral input and mechanisms of central control in the brain.

Pain perception is influenced by one's tolerance for pain. To understand tolerance, one must differentiate between *pain threshold* and *pain tolerance*. The pain threshold is defined as the lowest intensity of a painful stimulus that is perceived by a person as pain. The pain threshold may vary according to physiologic factors (such as inflammation or injury near pain receptors), but essentially it is similar for all people if the central nervous system (CNS) and peripheral nervous systems are intact.

Tolerance is defined as the amount of pain a person is willing to endure. It is different for each person who experiences pain, based on subjective factors such as the meaning of the pain and the setting. Some people have a high tolerance; that is, they can tolerate a lot of pain without distress, whereas others have a very low tolerance. Tolerance also varies for a given person, depending on a variety of factors associated with each specific pain incidence, such as nausea, fatigue, meaning of the pain, coping ability, sensory input, and genetic makeup. Only the person, not the health care team, can determine the person's tolerance level.

Another aspect that can alter one's perception of pain is past experience with pain. Expectations regarding the new pain experience may be based on previous pain episodes. For example, when a person has had a bad experience with pain, the anticipation that future pain may be as bad can make subsequent pain episodes worse. If the person has had a good experience with pain management, future pain episodes may be more positively experienced. Therefore it is important for nurses to facilitate adequate pain reduction and/or relief that will result in positive client outcomes.

MISCONCEPTIONS AND MYTHS

Many misunderstandings exist about pain (Table 22-1). If nurses continue to believe these myths, adequate pain assessment and relief are hampered. For example, many health care providers believe that it is possible to predict the amount of pain people should have, based on their medical condition. However, the diagnosis or type of surgery is *not* an effective fundamental basis for deter-

mining the amount of pain the person should be experiencing or the analgesic required to relieve that pain.

Both children and older adults experience unrelieved pain because health professionals incorrectly assume that age predicts pain.[55] The fact that clients do not visibly exhibit physiologic or behavioral signs of pain often leads to the belief by the health care provider that they do not have pain. A more likely explanation is that the client has adapted to the pain. The adaptive psychological responses include the following:

- A shifting away from the pain or guarding of the painful area
- Reporting pain only if asked directly
- Exhibiting sleepiness (which may also be due to insomnia secondary to the pain or may be used as a coping mechanism)

TABLE 22-1	*Common Misconceptions About Pain*
Myth or Misconception	**Fact**
Addiction occurs with prolonged use of morphine or morphine derivatives.	The incidence of addiction is less than 0.1%.
The nurse or physician is the best judge of a client's pain.	Only the client can judge the level and distress of the pain; pain management should be a team approach that includes the client.
Pain is a result, not a cause.	Unrelieved pain can create other problems such as anger, anxiety, immobility, respiratory problems, and delay in healing.
It is better to wait until a client has pain before giving medication.	Playing "catch-up" is not an effective way to manage pain; it is better to routinely administer analgesia, thus maintaining a low pain level.
Real pain has an identifiable cause.	There is always a cause of pain, but it may be very obscure and must be assessed carefully. Pain of a psychological origin is just as real as pain of physiologic origin.
The same physical stimulus produces the same pain intensity, duration, and distress in different people.	Intensity, duration, and distress vary with each individual.
Some clients lie about the existence or severity of their pain.	Very few people lie about pain.
Very young or very old people do not have as much pain.	All clients with an intact neurologic system experience pain; age is not a determinant of pain, but it may influence expression of pain.
Pain is a part of aging.	Pain does not accompany aging unless a disease process or ailment is present.
If a person is asleep, they are not in pain.	People in pain become exhausted and may truly be asleep or merely trying to sleep. Some people sleep as an escape mechanism.
If the pain is relieved by nonpharmaceutical pain relief techniques, the pain was not real anyway.	Nonpharmaceutical pain relief methods can be effective. A client's method of relief should be acknowledged as long as it does not harm.
Nurses should rely on their own definitions of pain and cultural beliefs about pain.	It is a mistake to impose one's own definitions, cultural beliefs, and values to another person's pain. Let the client tell you what the pain means.

- Exhibiting decreased physical activity
- Showing a blank facial expression

These manifestations do not mean that the person is not experiencing pain but that the person is exhibiting adaptive responses to pain that continues to be present.

A major barrier to adequate pain management is concern about addiction to pain medications, particularly to opioids, which results in undermedication for clients.[55] *Addiction* is a behavioral pattern of drug use characterized by (1) overwhelming involvement with the use of a drug (compulsive use) and securing a supply of it and (2) a tendency to relapse after withdrawal from the drug (to begin taking it again whether or not pain is present). This behavior is sometimes described as the "four Cs": *c*ompulsive, *c*raving for the drug, seeking and using the drug despite the *c*onsequences, and loss of *c*ontrol. Most people who take opioid analgesic medication for pain do not become addicted; in actuality, psychological addiction rarely occurs. (The incidence of addiction is less than 0.1%.[26]) Never use the term *addict* unless a medical diagnosis has been established, because many individuals exhibiting "drug-seeking behavior" are simply seeking better pain reduction and/or relief, not the medication itself (see Chapter 24).

Pseudoaddiction is a term that has been used to describe client behaviors that may occur when pain is undertreated.[6] Clients begin to exhibit behaviors that are similar to behaviors commonly seen in persons with addiction (i.e., seeking medications), calling for prescriptions earlier, and using prescriptions from multiple sources. These behaviors are eliminated when the pain is relieved.

Education is the primary means of removing the effect of these myths on pain management. By knowing the facts about pain, pain assessment, pharmacology, and pain treatment, the nurse can provide more complete care (Box 22-2).

Misinformation About Pain

One of the major blocks to accurate assessment of a person's pain is the person. If the health care team members still believe myths and have misconceptions about pain, it is likely that the client has also been misinformed about pain and pain control. People sense the expectations of the health care team about their own pain. They have learned that they are expected to tolerate certain levels of pain and not to complain excessively. People have also learned to be afraid of pain medications, especially opioids. A major nursing responsibility, therefore, is to educate clients about pain and pain control. The nurse needs to help people understand that they, not the health care team, are the true experts about their pain. The nurse is also responsible for helping clients provide an accurate pain history and assessment data.

When documenting pain, avoid saying that the client "complains" of pain. This term tends to invalidate or minimize the client's experience, as if the client is fussing

---

BOX 22-2 *Dependence, Addiction, and Tolerance*

Dependence

Psychological dependence, also known as addiction, is a pattern of continual craving for opioid drugs when not experiencing pain. The pattern of drug seeking is compulsive and without control. There is continued use despite physical, social, or financial harm. The client also seeks the drug without concern for the consequences of continued use.

Physical dependence is seen when a client is abruptly taken off of opioids. The client has anxiety, chills alternating with hot flashes, irritability, vomiting, abdominal cramps, and insomnia. These same manifestations are seen when the client is given opioid antagonists.

Tolerance

Tolerance to opioids develops when the liver becomes efficient at metabolizing the medications and higher doses are required to achieve the same level of pain control or comfort. The development of tolerance for opioids in clients who have received these medications for weeks does not mean that the client is addicted or psychologically dependent upon them.

---

unnecessarily. It is more accurate and helpful simply to use the word "states" or "reports." When discussing pain (e.g., with clients) or when documenting pain, avoid using the phrase "pain attack." Feeling that one is "under attack" may increase the feeling of powerlessness, creating the perception that the client is a victim. Use the term "episode" or "pain flare" to promote self-control and a sense that the client can do something to manage the episode.

Negative Effects of Pain

A barrier to adequate pain management has been the belief that pain, while uncomfortable, has few negative physiologic effects. Unrelieved pain can affect the major organ systems—pulmonary, cardiovascular, gastrointestinal, endocrine, and immune. Unrelieved pain has resulted in untoward effects that have resulted in increased costs that affect all of society. Costs are increased because of longer hospital stays, the need to treat the negative effects of pain, and the client's loss of productivity. Pain prevents coughing, deep breathing, and sighing, leading to pulmonary complications with significant associated morbidity and mortality. Pain may also prevent ambulation, contributing to the development of deep vein thrombosis and potential life-threatening pulmonary emboli. Pain of any type induces release of catecholamines and stress hormones. Cardiovascular complications (tachycardia, hypertension) and decreased immune activity may result.

Reflex muscle contraction may be enhanced, resulting in increased muscle tension and spasm. Abdominal wall muscle tension and spasm reduce the ability of the chest wall to expand. As a result, clients take short, shallow, frequent breaths. Oxygen and carbon dioxide exchange is less effective with this breathing pattern. Vital capacity has been reported to decrease to 40% of presurgery capacity when pain was not relieved and to only 70% of presurgery values when pain was totally relieved. Although respiratory depression in response to opioids is rare, hypoventilation resulting from untreated pain is not.

Intestinal and bladder smooth muscle tone is affected such that peristalsis and bladder motility are decreased. Bowel and bladder distention may result. The decreased motility of the bowel contributes to constipation. If distention is severe enough, the abdominal contents may interfere with the ability of the diaphragm to expand. It appears as though constipation may be a complication of either opioid administration or unrelieved pain. Given the negative effects of pain, it is better to give the opioid and treat the constipation.

Catecholamine secretion in response to pain leads to increased myocardial oxygen demand and consumption. Clients with atherosclerosis may be impaired to the point of myocardial ischemia, dysrhythmias, infarction, cardiac failure, and death. Older adults—at greatest risk for atherosclerotic vascular changes—are at greatest risk for receiving inadequate pain reduction and/or relief. On the basis of the negative effects of pain, relieving pain is a priority.

STANDARDS AND GUIDELINES FOR PAIN MANAGEMENT

Agency for Health Care Policy and Research
In 1992, the Agency for Health Care Policy and Research (AHCPR)[1] released its first set of Clinical Practice Guidelines for acute pain resulting from surgery or trauma. The guidelines were intended to serve as a resource to help health care providers and clients facilitate positive pain management outcomes. The following are the four major pain management goals:

- Reduce the incidence and severity of acute postoperative or post-traumatic pain
- Encourage clients to communicate unrelieved pain so that they can receive prompt evaluation and effective treatment
- Enhance comfort and satisfaction
- Contribute to fewer postoperative complications and shorter hospital stays after surgical procedures

These guidelines were designed to help the individual, family, and health care professionals work *together* to promote better reduction and/or relief of acute pain. These guidelines can be used to guide pain assessment and management to improve control of acute pain for all clients. Complete guidelines are available from the Agency for Health Care Research and Quality (AHRQ). The guidelines emphasize the following[1]:

- A collaborative, interdisciplinary approach to pain control, including all members of the health care team and input from the client and client's family, when appropriate
- An individualized proactive pain control plan developed preoperatively by clients and practitioners (pain is easier to prevent than to bring under control, once it has begun)
- Assessment and frequent reassessment of the client's pain
- Use of both drug and non-drug therapies to control or prevent pain
- A formal, institutional approach to management of acute pain, with clear lines of responsibility

American Pain Society
The American Pain Society, in its *Principles of Analgesic Use in the Treatment of Acute Pain and Cancer Pain*, have set the standard for pain management[5]:

- Individualize the route, dosage, and schedule
- Administer analgesics on a regular schedule
- Know the dose and time course of several opioid analgesic preparations
- Give infants and children adequate doses of opioids
- Follow up clients closely
- Use care when changing to a new opioid or route
- Recognize and treat side effects
- Do not use meperidine and be aware of potential hazards of mixed agonist-antagonists
- Do not use placebos
- Monitor for development of tolerance and treat appropriately
- Expect physical dependence and prevent withdrawal
- Do not diagnose an opioid addiction based only on the presence of opioid dependence
- Be alert to the psychological state of the client

Joint Commission on Accreditation of Healthcare Organizations
The Joint Commission on Accreditation of Healthcare Organizations (JCAHO) expanded its scope of pain management standards in 2000. The new standards include the following key elements[23]:

- Recognize and treat pain promptly
- Make information about analgesics readily available to clinicians
- Promise attentive analgesic care
- Define explicit policies
- Examine processes and outcomes with goal of continuous improvement

Overall, the standards require organizations to do the following[23]:

- Recognize the individual's right to appropriate pain assessment and management
- Identify persons with pain in initial assessments and ongoing (as needed) reassessments
- Educate clients, residents, laypersons, and their families about pain management as appropriate

American Geriatrics Society

Many specialty health professional organizations have position statements and guidelines for pain management in their respective specialties. The American Geriatrics Society developed guidelines for the Management of Persistent Pain in Older Adults offering recommendations and guidelines for the management of pain in older clients including assessment, pharmacologic and non-pharmacologic management, and management of pain in older adults with cognitive impairment.[4]

TYPES OF PAIN

Acute Pain

Acute pain is usually of short duration (less than 6 months) and has an identifiable, immediate onset, such as incisional pain after surgery. It is also regarded as having a limited and often predictable duration, such as postoperative pain, which usually disappears as the wound heals. Acute pain is often described in sensory terms, such as "sharp," "stabbing," and "shooting." It is considered a useful and limiting pain, in that it indicates injury and motivates the person to obtain relief by treatment of the cause. Acute pain is usually reversible or controllable with adequate treatment. People suffering from acute pain often come to terms with it because of the meaning or the limited nature of the pain, as in the pain of childbirth. When the pain is relieved, the person returns to the pre-pain state.

Acute pain may be accompanied by observable physical responses, including (1) increased or decreased blood pressure, (2) tachycardia, (3) diaphoresis, (4) tachypnea, (5) focusing on the pain, and (6) guarding the painful part. The cardiovascular and respiratory responses are due to stimulation of the sympathetic nervous system as part of the *fight or flight response*. These responses are often interpreted as positive evidence of a person's pain. Such interpretation is not reliable, however, because these sympathetic responses are temporary and may not be present in clients with continuing acute pain. Unrelieved acute pain leads to chronic pain states.

Chronic Pain

Chronic pain is a major health concern. The pain may have originally been acute in nature or may have been so obscure that the person does not know when it first developed. Chronic pain syndromes are often defined in vague terms, and many of their causes remain unknown.[56] Therefore a diversity of treatment modalities has been used to treat the manifestations.

Chronic pain may be divided into three types:
1. Chronic nonmalignant pain, such as from low back pain or rheumatoid arthritis
2. Chronic intermittent pain, such as from migraine headache
3. Chronic malignant pain, such as from cancer

Chronic pain lasts for long periods of time and is not readily treatable.[34] A person's response to pain depends on its duration and, possibly, its intensity. Pain that is constant, continuous, and moderate is often described as far more difficult to bear than pain that is intense but relatively short in duration. The course of chronic pain includes months and years of pain, not minutes or hours.

Chronic pain is associated with withdrawal and despair. Anxiety may give way to depression. Some clients learn to adapt and cope with the pain, adjusting their lives. However, absence of the expected expression of severe pain does not mean that the pain is gone; therefore the client's description of pain, not the manifestations one expects to see, is very important. Intractable, prolonged, and intense pain is difficult to endure. Most people undergo major affective and behavioral changes when experiencing pain for prolonged periods. Such changes may be compounded, and chronic pain syndrome can develop. Characteristics of clients experiencing chronic pain syndrome include the following:

- Depression
- Increased or decreased appetite and weight
- Drastically restricted activity level, leading to reduced work capacity, poor physical tone, and increased depression
- Social withdrawal and life role changes
- Preoccupation with physical manifestations
- Poor sleep and chronic fatigue, which may result from inactivity, analgesics, and depression as well as from pain
- Decreased concentration

Once these changes take place, the pain may become more complicated to treat than the pain's original physical source.

Chronic Nonmalignant Pain

Chronic pain is usually considered to be pain that lasts more than 6 months (or 1 month beyond the normal end of the condition causing the pain) and has no foreseeable end unless it is associated with very slow healing, as with burns. It is continuous or persistent and recurrent. There is some disagreement whether acute recurrent pain (as in migraine and sickle cell crisis) should be classified as chronic pain with acute flares, but such pain is usually referred to as chronic.

Chronic pain may or may not have an identifiable cause, or the cause may be difficult to determine. However, chronic pain is like any other chronic illness with periods of exacerbations and remissions. Chronic pain is frequently associated with concomitant disability as a result of the pain experience. For example, a client immobilized by the pain of severe rheumatoid arthritis may be further compromised by the effects of the immobility.

Chronic pain is a frustrating condition, making it difficult for the person to live a normal life. Clients experiencing continuous or continually recurring chronic pain tend to become increasingly engrossed in their illness. They may seem fearful, tense, fatigued, and tend to become withdrawn and isolated. Their pain is exhausting both physically and emotionally for themselves and their families. Health care providers may also feel frustrated and incompetent when their attempts to relieve chronic pain are ineffective. However, if nurses understand the anatomy, physiology, and psychosocial aspects of chronic pain, they can be very helpful to the client and family. Professionals may be able to intervene before extreme suffering occurs.

Chronic Intermittent Pain

Chronic intermittent pain refers to exacerbation or recurrence of the chronic condition. The pain occurs only at specific periods; at other times, the client is free from pain. Typical conditions include migraine and cluster headache, sickle cell crisis, and the intermittent abdominal pain associated with chronic gastrointestinal disorders, such as irritable bowel syndrome and Crohn's disease. Pain management is directed toward reduction and/or relief of pain in much the same manner as that for individual acute pain episodes. However, chronic recurrences render the condition more difficult to control. The client anticipates continual exacerbation of the situation and is intensely influenced by psychosocial factors that are difficult to manage.

Chronic Malignant (Cancer-Related) Pain

Malignant pain is considered to have qualities of both acute and chronic pain. The category encompasses neuropathic, deep visceral, and bone pain, among others (Table 22-2). Each type of pain is best managed by strategies specific to it. Therefore the nurse needs to carefully assess each type of pain and treat it appropriately. A diagnosis of cancer adds an additional psychological component associated with potential physical deformity and the potential for impending death, preceded by agonizing suffering. The mental anguish may intensify the perception of pain.

SOURCES OF PAIN

Classification

The human body is typically classified by systems. Systems involved in pain production include the following:
- *Superficial cutaneous* regions encompassing skin and subcutaneous tissues
- *Somatic* tissues of the body wall, including muscle, bone, periosteum, cartilage, tendons, deep fascia, ligaments, joints, blood vessels, and nerves
- *Visceral* structures, including organs and their capsules

The characteristics of a person's pain experience depend, in part, on the source of the noxious stimulation.

TABLE 22-2 Sources of Noxious Stimuli for Clients with Cancer

Source of Stimuli	Cause
Cell destruction	Chemotherapy Cell necrosis Ulceration Tumor invasion Tissue injury
Inflammation	Products of cell destruction
Infection	Bacterial invasion
Nerve injury	Direct injury through incising nerve structures Tumor invasion of peripheral nerves, plexes, spinal cord, brain Chemotherapy/radiation injury
Ischemia/hypoxia	Edema Hematoma Occlusion of vessels by tumor
Noxious stretch or pressure	Distention of thoracic and abdominal viscera, fascia, periosteum Occlusion of gastrointestinal and genitourinary structures Obstruction of ducts and viscus

Therefore it is helpful to understand the typical characteristics of each pain type.

Cutaneous (Superficial) Pain

Cutaneous pain may be characterized by an abrupt onset and a sharp or stinging quality or by a slower onset and a burning quality, depending upon the type of nerve fiber involved. Cutaneous pain tends to be easily localized. The skin surface is readily divided into areas called *dermatomes*. Each dermatome is served by one spinal nerve and dorsal root. When the skin is stimulated by a noxious stimulus, the nerve serving that dermatome is activated. The signal is transmitted to the one specific area of the sensory cortex serving the dermatome. As a result, the stimulus is perceived to occur within that dermatome. The boundaries of dermatomes may appear to be distinct in anatomic drawings, but nerve distribution actually overlaps. Excitation of one nerve may produce pain that is perceived to originate from adjacent dermatomes.

Deep Somatic Pain

Somatic structures are those of the body wall, such as muscles and bone. Table 22-3 displays a comparison of deep somatic pain with cutaneous pain. Deep somatic pain is poorly localized, may produce nausea, and may be associated with sweating and blood pressure changes. Deep somatic pain is generally diffuse and less

TABLE 22-3 Cutaneous and Deep Pain

Characteristic	Cutaneous Pain	Deep Pain
Quality	Sharp, bright sensation or burning; felt superficially	Primarily dull and aching; may be described as boring, crushing, throbbing, or cramping; if less intense, described as soreness
Duration	Typically short	Often fairly long
Localization	Tends to be precise Pain is often experienced as a point, surface, or line	Often diffuse and inaccurate; seems to originate in a fairly broad area Pain frequently felt as if it were three-dimensional and occupying space
Hyperalgesia (excessive sensibility to pain)	May occur as a primary problem	May exist as secondary problem; occurring at a distance from the original noxious stimulus In referred pain, a superficial hyperalgesia may be associated with deep pain
Nausea	Rarely occurs	Sickening pain found only when deep structures are involved, as in renal and intestinal colic, gallstones, and angina
Associated symptoms	May be hyperalgesia, paresthesia, tickling, burning, or itching Also associated with brisk movements, a quick pulse, and a sense of invigoration	Resulting from autonomic responses, including pallor, sweating, nausea, vomiting, bradycardia (at times), lowering of blood pressure, syncope, faintness, and perhaps even death in shock Muscle contraction and tenderness often present Segmental spread of pain often noted; pain may not remain confined to original spinal segment but may spread into one or more adjacent segments

localizable than cutaneous pain. Pain from deep structures frequently radiates from the primary site (e.g., pain from a lumbar disk is felt along the sciatic nerve).

Somatic structures vary in their sensitivity to pain. Highly sensitive structures include tendons, deep fascia, ligaments, joints, bone periosteum, blood vessels, and nerves. Skeletal muscle is sensitive only to stretching and ischemia. Bone and cartilage respond to extreme pressure and chemical stimulation (e.g., rheumatoid arthritis, osteomyelitis).

Visceral Pain

Visceral pain refers to pain coming from body organs. It tends to be a diffuse, poorly localized, vague, dull pain. Nerve fibers innervating body organs follow the sympathetic nerves to the spinal cord. This may be the reason why autonomic manifestations (e.g., diarrhea, cramps, sweating, hypertension) frequently accompany visceral pain. Visceral pain typically includes acute appendicitis, cholecystitis, and inflammation of the biliary and pancreatic tracts, gastroduodenal disease, cardiovascular disease, pleurisy, and renal and ureteral colic. Often visceral pain is manifested as sweating, restlessness, nausea, emesis, pallor, and agitation.

Most viscera are not sensitive to stimuli that cause pain in somatic structures (e.g., cutting, burning, or pressure). This is understandable, because viscera are not normally exposed to such traumas, and the body thus does not "need" a response system. Although these types of stimuli do not produce pain in most viscera, other stimuli may cause severe pain, for example, violent or abnormal contractions of hollow viscera, such as the ureters and alimentary tract.

In the chest, the parietal pleura is richly supplied with pain endings through the intercostal nerves and through the phrenic nerve, on the surface of the diaphragm. The visceral pleurae in the chest, however, are insensitive to pain. The bronchi, on the other hand, are sensitive to pain. Elsewhere and throughout its serous surfaces, the visceral pericardium is insensitive to pain, except for the lower portion of the fibrous pericardium, which appears to have pain fibers from the phrenic nerve.

Pain in the gastrointestinal tract is common. It appears to arise mainly from the tract's muscular and serous lining. Gastrointestinal pain seems to occur when intestinal mucosa is inflamed, ulcerated, or otherwise abnormal or when the visceral muscles contract strongly or develop spasm. Even though the wall of the intestine is not sensitive to cutting, burning, or crushing, it does produce pain under other conditions, such as widespread ischemia and distention. Abdominal pain may also occur when body organs are perforated and their contents drain into the peritoneal cavity.

Visceral pain differs from cutaneous pain, in that highly localized damage to the viscera rarely causes severe pain but such damage to the body surface would cause pain. For example, a surgical cut in the gut does not cause pain but a cut in the skin would cause severe pain. If the stimulus to the viscera causes diffuse stimulation of nerve endings, the resulting pain is severe, as in ischemia (lack of oxygen) of the gut. Visceral pain is known to produce referred pain.

Referred Pain

Referred pain is felt in an area distant from the site of the stimulus. It occurs when nerve fibers serving an area of the body distant from the site of the stimulus pass in close proximity to the stimulus. The referred pain sensation may be intense, and there may be little or no pain at the point of noxious stimuli. For example, myocardial ischemia typically is not felt as pain in the heart but most often as left arm, shoulder, or jaw pain. The fibers innervating these areas are close to those innervating the myocardium, resulting in the referred pain.

Identification of the segment of the spinal cord that is involved in transmitting referred pain is helpful diagnostically. Pain arising from a deep structure, whether a viscus or a deep somatic structure, has a referred segmental distribution, or a pattern of pain, determined according to the spinal cord segment supplying the structure. Referred pain is often baffling, warranting careful assessment. Examples of common patterns include pleural pain from the diaphragm referred to the shoulder and the pain of cholecystitis referred to the back and in the angle of the scapula. Figure 22-2 illustrates common sites of referred pain.

Inflammation

Inflammation is one of the most common pathologic conditions influencing pain sensitivity. Numerous harmful substances, such as bacterial and chemical agents, can cause inflammation. Inflammatory responses may result from stressors, such as heat, cold, or trauma. Gross assessment findings associated with the inflammatory process are redness, swelling, heat, and pain. Inflammatory pain is secondary to the distention of stretch-sensitive tissue (periosteum, pleura) and the direct effect of released neuroregulators on afferent nerve endings. Principal chemical mediators of the inflammatory response are histamine, substance P, bradykinin, prostaglandins, and leukokinins.

Neuropathic Pain

Neuropathic pain is caused by damage or injury to nerve fibers in the periphery or by damage to the CNS. Nox-

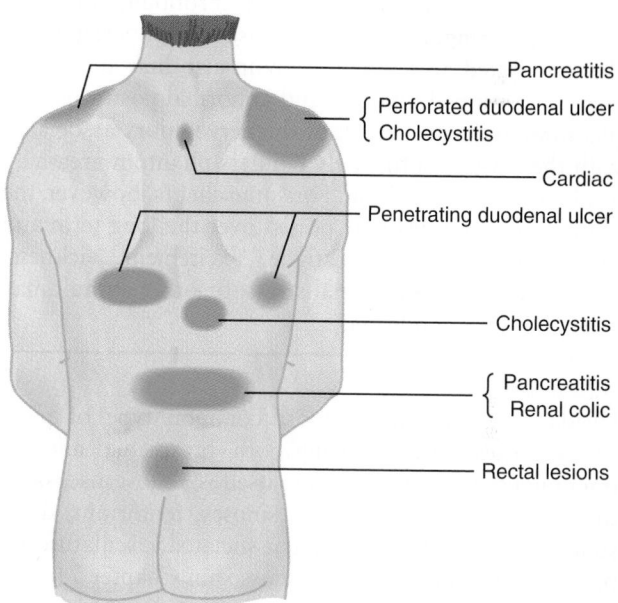

FIGURE 22-2 Areas of referred pain.

ious electrical impulses are generated at the site of the injury. Therefore the pain is felt as numbness, burning, stabbing, "needles," and electric shock. Clients may experience allodynia, "pain due to a stimulus that does not normally provoke pain."[7] The pain is perceived to occur in the area served by the nerve. For example, an injury to a nerve that serves the hand would be perceived as pain in the hand even though the injury may be at the spinal cord level. Such pain is particularly problematic for the individual, because there is no obvious pathologic process corresponding to the pain sensation (e.g., the hand). Therefore the person may not be believed. Neuropathic pain is difficult to manage because it responds poorly to typical pain medications, particularly to nonsteroidal anti-inflammatory drugs (NSAIDs)[61] and opioids.[45,61]

Phantom Limb Sensation

Following amputation of a body part (e.g., limb, breast), a person may continue to experience sensations in the part amputated as if that part were still present or attached. The nerve fibers that served the part continue to extend to the periphery, ending at the incision site. The nerves have been injured by the surgery. As the cut nerve endings attempt to regenerate, they may form small neuromas at the incision cite. When nerve fibers are stimulated as a result of injury or neuroma, they continue to mediate the sensations associated with their original location. As a result, neuropathic sensations may be generated. These abnormal sensations may be perceived as presence of the limb, paresthesia, or pain.

Sensations associated with paresthesia may consist of itching, pressure, tingling, numbness, or "pins and needles." Painful sensations include throbbing, burning, stabbing, boring, and vise-like sensations experienced in the amputated area. Phantom pain also may be experienced as cramped, twisted, and abnormal posturing of a phantom limb. As a result of the nerve injury associated with the surgery, a formerly painless phantom area may gradually become painful. For some clients, however, the abnormal sensations may persist over the long term and may never go away. Fatigue, excitement, sickness, weather changes, emotional stress, or other stimuli may exacerbate the condition.

Headache

Headache results in the most common type of pain. Many causes exist, involving both intracranial and extracranial structures. The brain itself is almost insensitive to pain, although the venous sinuses, tentorium, dura, some of the cranial nerves, and associated vasculature are pain-sensitive. Headache is discussed in Chapter 71.

Malignancy

Pain occurs in 40% to 70% of people with solid tumors.[14] The Oncology Nursing Society issued a three-part position paper on cancer pain addressing the scope of nursing practice regarding cancer pain, ethical issues, practice issues, education of staff and clients, research recommendations, and sections on nursing administration, social policy, and pediatric cancer pain.[52] The paper also lists cancer and pain management resources and is an excellent reference for the nurse caring for clients with cancer.

Treatment of cancer pain is difficult because of its many causes. Bone pain usually responds to a combination of radiation therapy and NSAIDs, whereas other pain may require opioid analgesics, such as morphine. The client and the nurse must believe that cancer pain is controlled if the correct medications and modalities are used in adequate amounts and in adequate combinations. In fact, 90% of cancer pain can be controlled with oral medications. In 1994, the AHCPR developed clinical practice guidelines with 10 goals for the management of cancer pain (Box 22-3).[21]

Human Immunodeficiency Virus Infection

Pain is common in clients with active human immunodeficiency virus (HIV) infection. Reports on the prevalence of pain in this population range from 25% to 40% in early and ambulatory stages to 60% to almost 100% in end-stage disease.[28,53] The sources of pain in this population include (1) gastrointestinal or abdominal pain from colitis, esophagitis, gastritis, herpes, and cytomegalovirus (CMV); (2) peripheral neuropathy; (3) headache; (4) pleuritic pain from pneumonia; (5) oropharyngeal pain from

---

BOX 22-3   *Clinical Practice Guidelines for the Management of Cancer Pain*

1. Inform clinicians and clients and their families that most cancer pain can be relieved by available methods.
2. Dispel unfounded fears that addiction results from the appropriate use of medications to control cancer pain.
3. Inform clinicians that cancer pain: (a) accompanies both disease and treatment, (b) changes over time, (c) may have multiple simultaneous causes, (d) if unrelieved, can affect the physical, psychological, social, and spiritual well-being of the client.
4. Promote prompt and effective assessment, diagnosis, and treatment of pain in clients with cancer.
5. Strengthen the ability of clients with cancer and their families to communicate new or unrelieved pain in order to secure prompt evaluation and effective treatment.
6. Provide clinicians with a synthesis of the literature and expert opinion for application to the management of cancer pain.
7. Familiarize clients and their families with options available for pain relief, and promote their active participation in selecting among these.
8. Provide a model for cancer pain management to guide therapy in selected painful, life-threatening conditions such as AIDS.
9. Provide information and guidelines on the use of controlled substances for the treatment of cancer pain that distinguishes the use of these drugs for legitimate medical purposes from their abuse as illegitimate drugs.
10. Identify health policy and research issues that affect cancer pain management.

Modified from Jacox, A., et al. (1994). *Management of cancer pain. Clinical practice guidelines No. 9.* AHCPR Pub. No. 94-1592. Rockville, MD: Agency for Health Care Policy and Research, U.S. Department of Health and Human Services, Public Health Service.
AIDS, Acquired immunodeficiency syndrome.

oral candidiasis or herpes; and (6) pain from Kaposi's sarcoma lesions, which causes lymphatic obstruction. Approximately 40% of clients with HIV experience neuropathic pain, which is particularly difficult to manage pharmacologically.

Pain management is made more difficult in this population by the psychosocial correlation of the pain experience. Clients often lack the social support and resources of persons with chronic, malignant pain in other populations.[53] The multidimensional character of the pain in HIV infection and the client's personal situation requires a multidisciplinary team that can establish an open, trusting relationship in order to provide the best pain reduction and/or relief.[28]

Pain associated with HIV infection is usually under-treated, even in late stages.[1,28,53] A health care provider's opinion about the client with HIV and acquired immunodeficiency syndrome (AIDS) may be negative, resulting in lack of desire to help manage pain. The health care professional may believe that pain is an appropriate punishment for the behavior that led the person to contract HIV. Clients may be reluctant to report pain, fearing that increasing pain indicates a worsening of disease. Pain management may be complicated by a previous history of drug abuse or addiction. Prior addiction should not alter the way in which pain is treated. Clients may require higher doses of analgesics because they may have a high tolerance to opioids. Third-party payers present an additional barrier because they have considered pain management a low priority.[28]

Pain management for clients with HIV infection or AIDS is often difficult. It has been recommended that pharmacologic treatment be accomplished using cancer pain as a model incorporating the World Health Organization (WHO) cancer management "ladder."[21,28] The ladder, depicted as a pyramid, shows that most pain can be controlled with noninjected forms of medications (see Figure 22-10). However, caution must be taken with the use of NSAIDs because of reports of cross-reaction between acetaminophen and drugs used to treat HIV infection. In addition, clients with cancer are at risk for gastrointestinal and renal diseases, which contraindicate the use of NSAIDs.[28] Recommended oral analgesics for mild to moderate pain in AIDS include aspirin and ibuprofen, choline magnesium trisalicylate (Trilisate), and weaker opioids (codeine, oxycodone, propoxyphene [Darvon]).[28] Adjuvant medications are also suggested for this population at any step in the WHO ladder.[28] It is imperative that pain of HIV infection and AIDS be treated vigorously, using the model of cancer pain treatment as the foundation and giving attention to the unique aspects of pain associated with this disease.

FACTORS AFFECTING PAIN

A client's reaction to pain is intensely personal and accounts for the great variability in pain experiences from person to person. Numerous factors contribute to this variability (Figure 22-3). Some of these are discussed as examples to indicate the means by which one person's pain experience can be expected to differ from that of another person's.

Situational Factors

The situation associated with the pain influences the person's response to it. A response to pain experienced in a formal or crowded situation may differ greatly from the response of a client who is alone or in a hospital. A woman who has had a hysterectomy for cancer may perceive her pain as more severe than that of a woman who has undergone removal of a benign cyst even though the surgical trauma is similar. Pain perception is influenced by the diagnosis in addition to the tissue trauma. A client

PHYSIOLOGIC FACTORS

Organic origin
Integrity of nervous system,
  including endogenous opioids
Concomitant physical influences
  (stress, fatigue)
Age
Type of pain
Location
Intensity
Duration
Frequency
Quality
Threshold
Tolerance
Genetics

AFFECTIVE FACTORS

Distress of pain
Depression
Mood
Anxiety, fear, worry

PSYCHOSOCIAL INFLUENCES

Family and occupational roles
Personal beliefs
Spiritual belief system
Cultural/societal influences
Sexual identity and
  stereotypes
Demographic factors

COGNITIVE

Past experience
Meaning of pain
  experience
Attention paid to
  sensation/distraction
Expectations
Coping mechanisms
Knowledge
Values/attitudes
Communication skills

FIGURE 22-3 Considerations of the pain experience.

with a cancer diagnosis may require more aggressive pain management and additional emotional support than a client with a noncancer diagnosis.

Sociocultural Factors

Race, culture, and ethnicity are critical factors in one's response to pain.[11] These factors influence all sensory responses, including responses to pain. We learn how to respond to pain and other experiences from our family and ethnic group. Pain responses tend to reflect the mores of our culture. Within this framework, we learn what is appropriate and acceptable for our peer group. For example, verbally voicing pain may be considered appropriate within the Italian community and unacceptable within the German community, which values stoicism. In the Mexican culture, moaning or crying is used to help alleviate the pain rather than communicating a need for intervention.[24] Cultural mores of some Hispanic groups view health as the absence of illness. If a person is not convinced that the pain is related to an illness, he or she might refuse treatment for it. See the Diversity in Health Care feature on Cultural Perspectives on Pain on the website.

Problems may also arise because of a person's view of health care team members. Members of various cultural groups may have difficulty communicating feelings to physicians and nurses who are from different backgrounds or ethnic groups.[11] Health care providers may have difficulty appreciating the pain experiences of clients from unfamiliar cultural groups, because they tend to adopt white, middle-class cultural mores surrounding pain expectations and avenues for treatment.

People from different cultures may handle pain in various ways. A problem arises when the nurse does not recognize the person's way of dealing with pain or when the nurse does not accept it. Researchers found that nurses' judgments about the pain their clients experienced were affected by the nurses' own beliefs and those of their culture.[11] Nurses may also misinterpret expressions of pain from clients who do not speak English as a first language.[29] Health care providers must be sensitive to the contribution of cultural factors and language barriers in order to facilitate adequate pain management.

Age

Age may play a significant role in perception and expression of pain. There are some variations in pain threshold associated with chronologic age, but no clear trends have been established.[15] Adults may not report pain for fear that it indicates a poor diagnosis. Pain may also mean weakness, failure, or loss of control for the adult.

There is controversy regarding pain perception in the older adults. There is no reason to assume that pain perception is altered in older adults unless some damage has occurred in the CNS. The transmission and perception may be slowed with aging, but intensity of the pain is

not diminished. Health care providers may underestimate the pain of older people as a result of impaired ability to express pain. Physical factors, such as paralysis and aphasia, may interfere with the ability to communicate.[54] Confused older adults may be unable to articulate their pain experience. Altered expression does not mean absence of pain.

Age is considered an important factor in dosing of medications. Metabolic changes in older adults affect their response to opioid analgesics. Drugs are metabolized and excreted more slowly in older people. In addition, older adults frequently take combinations of medications for a variety of ailments, making them more susceptible to drug interactions.

Older people may assign different meanings to their pain. Pain may be considered a natural manifestation of aging. This may be interpreted in two ways. First, older people may think pain is simply something to be endured as a normal part of the aging process. Second, it may be seen as a sign of aging and, therefore, something to be denied because it means they are getting old. Many older people are hesitant to express pain for fear of being labeled as "complaining." These misconceptions serve to cause these people to experience pain unnecessarily. Careful assessment of the older person's pain is essential to prevent unnecessary suffering.

Few assessment instruments have been tested in the geriatric population, and visual, auditory, and motor impairments, common among older adults, make typical assessment tools difficult to use.[1] The FACES Pain Rating Scale, which is commonly used in children, has been shown to be accurate in older adults, even those with mild dementia.[30a] Therefore pay particular attention to verbal and nonverbal clues of pain in this population. Pain may be indicated by lack of appetite, sleeping disorders, tearing of the eyes, moaning, or splinting of a body part. Pain in older adults may result in increased falls and social isolation.

Gender

Gender is an important factor in response to pain.[9] In one study, gender was a significant factor in the pain response, with men reporting less pain than women regardless of ethnicity. In some cultures in the United States, boys and men are expected to express pain less than women do. This does not mean that men feel pain less, only that they are assumed to show it less. Yet health care providers who value bearing pain without complaint may view women as "complainers" and may ignore or devalue their pain expressions. Both men and women may experience pain unnecessarily if the nurse is not aware of gender biases in pain expression.

Meaning of Pain

The meaning of a person's pain influences his or her response to the pain.[29,59] Pain caused by childbirth may be responded to differently than pain caused by surgery. If the cause of pain is known, the person may be better able to interpret meaning and to deal with the experience. If the cause is unknown, more negative psychological factors (e.g., fear, and anxiety) may be evoked, intensifying the degree of pain perceived. If the meaning of the experience is negative, then the pain may be perceived more intensely than pain perceived in situations with positive outcomes. For example, pain that is associated with a threat to body image may be much worse than pain that is not associated in this way. If the meaning of pain is not considered, you may make inappropriate assessments of the client's pain experience, resulting in inadequate pain control.

Anxiety

The degree of anxiety experienced by the client may also influence the response to pain. Anxiety intensifies pain perception.[22] Anxiety is often related to the meaning of the pain. If the cause is unknown, anxiety is likely to be higher and the pain worse.

Past Experience with Pain

Past experience with pain affects the way current pain is perceived. People who have had negative experiences with pain as children have reported greater difficulties with managing pain.[47] The impact of past experiences, however, is not predictable. The person with a miserable experience in the past may perceive the next episode more intensely even though the medical conditions may be similar. Conversely, a person may view the next experience more positively because it is not as bad as the previous one. However, it is *not* true that the more pain we experience, the more accustomed we become to it. One might expect that the more pain we have experienced, the less anxious and more tolerant we may be. In actuality, we may be more anxious and desire rapid pain relief to avert a familiar and unpleasant painful experience.

Earlier pain experience allows one to adopt coping mechanisms that may or may not be used with subsequent episodes with pain. Discuss the client's past experiences with pain, including how the client managed the pain. In addition to methods that provided pain reduction and/or relief in the past, assess which measures did not have a positive outcome. Allow the client to use familiar positive intervention when possible.

Expectation and the Placebo Effect

Client expectations play a major role in a person's pain experience, including perception of pain and the effectiveness of interventions for pain reduction and/or relief.[2,58] The severity of pain experienced, in addition to the emotional and cognitive overtones generated by the experience, is influenced by the client's expectations. Positive expectations engender positive outcomes; negative expectations lead to negative outcomes. Similarly,

one's belief in the ability of an intervention to be effective affects the degree of pain reduction and/or relief attained. For example, it is not uncommon for a client to proclaim that the pain reliever Motrin is effective while Advil is not, even though the two medications are pharmaceutically identical.

The messages you deliver regarding pain and pain management strategies can affect the client's expectations. The confidence that you display regarding potential effectiveness of intervention strategies will have a significant effect on the client's ability to obtain positive pain reduction and/or relief outcomes. Clients must be assured that pain can be effectively treated.

Placebos have been administered when health care providers doubted that clients were truly in pain. Placebos are pills that look like medications but that have no medicinal properties. Historically, they have been made of sugars and inert materials. When clients are given placebos, they are told that the pills contain pain medication. It was not uncommon for these clients to obtain pain reduction and/or relief. It has been reported that 30% to 70% of people receiving placebos report short-lived pain reduction and/or relief, which in some research studies has been reversed by naloxone (Narcan).[2,58] The most likely explanation for the effect of placebos is the initiation of the body's endogenous opiate systems activated by the expectation of relief.[2] The response tends to be temporary, because the endogenous response is brief. A placebo response does not indicate absence of real pain; it indicates a person's ability to produce a positive outcome of pain reduction and/or relief internally via a real physiologic mechanism.

Health care providers have incorrectly concluded that positive responses to placebos indicate that clients did not have real pain. However, a placebo response indicates that the client believes that the pill will "work" and has responded to the positive attitude portrayed by the nurse administering the pill. *Placebos should not be given.*[8] The client's response to placebos provides no data about the nature or severity of pain. *Placebo use is deceitful and unethical. It compromises the nurse-client relationship and the confidence the client has in the nurse's ability and desire to help with pain reduction and/or relief.* Use of placebos is costly because the client is charged for an ineffective medication, which often needs to be followed with a true pain reduction and/or relief preparation. Clients receiving placebos may be reluctant to report continued pain or to ask for additional pain medication, leaving them at risk for the negative physical effects of unrelieved pain.

■ Nursing Management of the Client in Pain Assessment

The primary goals of pain assessment are to identify the cause of the pain, to understand the client's perception of the pain, and to measure the characteristics of the pain to implement pain management techniques. To assess a client's pain, obtain a pain history, a daily account of the current pain history, which includes pain aggravating and alleviating factors, and a collection of subjective and objective data through use of measurement tools. Perform the assessment in an unbiased, caring manner. Assessment is a constant and ongoing task, which may occur every 15 minutes for the acute, postoperative client to every 4 hours for the acute, stable client with adequate pain relief. The AHCPR Clinical Guidelines for acute pain management recommend that pain be assessed every 2 hours for the first 48 hours after surgery or trauma and every 4 hours thereafter as a standard routine and more often if indicated. In addition, reassessment should occur within 20 to 30 minutes after administration of any medication given for pain reduction and/or relief and 5 to 15 minutes after intravenous (IV) medication administration at the time of the drug's peak effect.[1] All clients should be screened for pain, and if pain is present, a comprehensive pain assessment should be completed.

History and Physical Examination. A complete medical history and physical examination (H&P) focuses on basic questions about physical, behavioral, and psychological factors (Box 22-4). This H&P helps the nurse to understand the unique pain experience of the client and to formulate a plan to resolve the pain. The H&P also provides baseline data to allow assessment of the client's progression through a pain experience.

Data Collection. Data collection by use of well-tested measurement tools is essential in assessing pain for appropriate management interventions.[50] Multidimensional assessment tools (e.g., McGill-Melzack Pain Questionnaire, Initial Pain Assessment Tool by McCaffery and Pasero[1]) are useful to obtain the initial H&P data and to provide information regarding the multifaceted nature of the pain experience (Figures 22-4 and 22-5).

Single-item assessment tools include the Visual Analog Scale (VAS), numerical scales (0-10), and visual descriptor scales. These scales can be used to measure both physical pain intensity and psychological distress (Figures 22-6 and 22-7). The tools are easy to use and provide the client and nurse with a simple means to quantify pain. They are also cost-effective when used in clinical settings because they are easily copied and can be reproduced cheaply. They do require a relatively high level of cognitive ability.

Pictorial scales measure pain in small children, such as the widely used Faces Pain Rating Scale developed by Wong and Baker[60] (Figure 22-8). Clients with impaired

---

BOX 22-4 *Subjective and Objective Assessment Data*

History
Age
State of consciousness
Medications currently taken/medication for allergies
Physical state (fatigue, debility, lack of sleep, and prolonged suffering reduce a client's ability to tolerate pain)
Emotional state (worry, fear, and anxiety reduce a person's ability to tolerate pain)
Pain expectancy (the anticipation of pain)
Pain acceptance (willingness to experience pain)
Pain apprehension (generalized desire to avoid pain)
Pain anxiety (the anxiety pain provokes because of its associated mystery, loneliness, helplessness, threat)
Effects on activities and quality of life
Methods of pain relief
    What do you do to relieve the pain?
    What has *not* worked to relieve your pain?

Physical Examination
Sympathetic Responses
Pallor
Increased blood pressure
Increased pulse
Increased respiration

Skeletal muscle tension
Dilated pupils
Diaphoresis

Parasympathetic Responses
Decreased blood pressure
Decreased pulse
Nausea, vomiting
Weakness
Pallor
Loss of consciousness

Behavioral Characteristics
Assumes a posture that minimizes pain (lying rigidly, guarding, drawing up the legs, or assuming the fetal position)
Moans, sighs, grimaces, clenches the jaws or fist, becomes quiet, or withdraws from others
Blinks rapidly
Crying, appears frightened, exhibits restlessness
Has a drawn facial expression
Has twitching muscles
Withdraws when touched
Holds or protects affected area or remains motionless

McGill - Melzack Pain Questionnaire

Person's Name_____ Date_____ Time_____ am/pm

Analgesic(s)_____ Dosage_____ Time Given_____ am/pm

_____ Dosage_____ Time Given_____ am/pm

Analgesic Time Difference (hours):   +4   +1   +2   +3

PRI: S_____   A_____   E_____   M(S)_____   M(AE)_____   M(T)_____   PRI(T)_____
   (1-10)   (11-15)   (16)   (17-19)   (20)   (17-20)   (1-20)

1 FLICKERING QUIVERING PULSING THROBBING BEATING POUNDING	11 TIRING EXHAUSTING	PPI_____
	12 SICKENING SUFFOCATING	COMMENTS:
2 JUMPING FLASHING SHOOTING	13 FEARFUL FRIGHTFUL TERRIFYING	
3 PRICKING BORING DRILLING STABBING LANCINATING	14 PUNISHING GRUELLING CRUEL VICIOUS KILLING	
	15 WRETCHED BLINDING	
4 SHARP CUTTING LACERATING	16 ANNOYING TROUBLESOME MISERABLE INTENSE UNBEARABLE	
5 PINCHING PRESSING GNAWING CRAMPING CRUSHING	17 SPREADING RADIATING PENETRATING PIERCING	
6 TUGGING PULLING WRENCHING	18 TIGHT NUMB DRAWING SQUEEZING TEARING	CONSTANT PERIODIC BRIEF
7 HOT BURNING SCALDING SEARING	19 COOL COLD FREEZING	
8 TINGLING ITCHY SMARTING STINGING	20 NAGGING NAUSEATING AGONIZING DREADFUL TORTURING	
9 DULL SORE HURTING ACHING HEAVY	PPI 0 NO PAIN 1 MILD	ACCOMPANYING SYMPTOMS: NAUSEA HEADACHE DIZZINESS DROWSINESS CONSTIPATION DIARRHEA COMMENTS:
10 TENDER TAUT RASPING SPLITTING	2 DISCOMFORTING 3 DISTRESSING 4 HORRIBLE 5 EXCRUCIATING	

SLEEP: GOOD FITFUL CAN'T SLEEP   COMMENTS:

FOOD INTAKE: GOOD SOME LITTLE NONE   COMMENTS:

ACTIVITY: GOOD SOME LITTLE NONE   COMMENTS:

FIGURE 22-4 The McGill-Melzack Pain Questionnaire, adapted for the study of opioid drugs. The descriptors listed at left comprise four groups: 1 to 10, sensory; 11 to 15, affective; 16, evaluative; 17 to 20, miscellaneous. The rank value for each descriptor is based on its position in the words set. Total rank values comprise the pain-rating index (PRI). The present pain intensity (PPI) is based on a scale from 0 to 5. The drawings are used to designate the site of pain (From Bonica, J.J. [1980]. *Pain* [p.145]. New York: Raven Press.)

Initial Pain Assessment Tool

Date _____

Patient's Name _____ Age _____ Room _____

Diagnosis _____ Physician _____

Nurse _____

I. Location: Patient or nurse mark drawing.

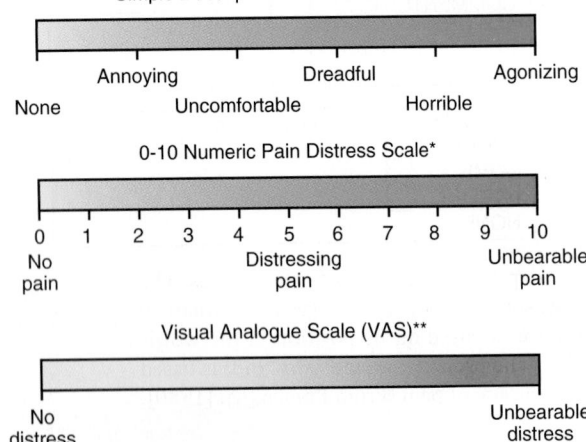

II. Intensity: Patient rates the pain. Scale used _____
    Present: _____
    Worst pain gets: _____
    Best pain gets: _____
    Acceptable level of pain: _____

III. Quality: (Use patient's own words, e.g., prick, ache, burn, throb, pull, sharp) _____
_____

IV. Onset, duration variations, rhythms: _____
_____

V. Manner of expressing pain: _____
_____

VI. What relieves the pain? _____
_____

VII. What causes or increases the pain? _____
_____

VIII. Effects of pain: (Note decreased function, decreased quality of life.) _____
    Accompanying symptoms (e.g., nausea) _____
    Sleep _____
    Appetite _____
    Physical activity _____
    Relationship with others (e.g., irritability) _____
    Emotions (e.g., anger, suicidal, crying) _____
    Concentration _____
    Other _____

IX. Other comments: _____
_____

X. Plan: _____
_____

FIGURE 22-5 Initial pain assessment tool. (From McCaffery M., & Pasero, C. [1999]. *Pain: Clinical manual* [2nd ed.]. St. Louis: Mosby.)

Simple Descriptive Pain Distress Scale*

None   Annoying   Uncomfortable   Dreadful   Horrible   Agonizing

0-10 Numeric Pain Distress Scale*

0   1   2   3   4   5   6   7   8   9   10
No pain   Distressing pain   Unbearable pain

Visual Analogue Scale (VAS)**

No distress   Unbearable distress

   * If used as a graphic rating scale, a 10-cm baseline is recommended.
  ** A 10-cm baseline is recommended for VAS scales.

FIGURE 22-6 Pain distress scales.

cognitive ability may be better able to report their pain with the use of pictorial scales.[30a]

Clients may experience several types of pain during one medical episode. After surgery, one may experience pain due to poor body position, incisional pain, and deep visceral pain. The client may also have a condition that produces chronic pain such as arthritis, that continues to be painful, or a secondary complication may be developing, such as pain due to myocardial infarction or pulmonary emboli. When planning interventions, learn to distinguish among the causes of pain. Each assessment for acute pain includes location, intensity, quality, and duration to aid in making intervention decisions. In addition, assessment for chronic pain includes sleep, appetite, function, concentration, and relationships.

Intensity. The single most important indicator of pain intensity is the client's self-report of the pain. Many health care facilities have incorporated *pain rating scales* for use with standard practice. These scales are used to assess current levels of pain but can be used to determine the amount of pain the client finds acceptable. This information is essential for both the client and nurse in planning and evaluating pain interventions. The AHCPR recommends the Brief Pain Inventory (Short Form) (Fig-

ure 22-9) as a means of conducting ongoing assessments of pain intensity.[21]

You can obtain the client's self-report of pain intensity by asking clients to rate pain on a scale that they must mentally visualize or by showing the scale to the client. People in pain may have trouble concentrating on mental tasks and may find it particularly difficult to respond to a scale they must visualize. In some hospitals, it has been beneficial to provide a copy of the intensity scale in plain view of each client, typically taped to the bedside wall.

Location. Location of pain may be ascertained by verbal description or by marking the location on a drawing of the body. Use of body drawings provides an opportunity for the client to report multiple sites of pain using a self-report document that can be included in the medical record. The document is then available for use by any member of the health care team caring for that client.

Quality. Quality of the pain is typically indicated by descriptive adjectives such as "stabbing like a knife" or "throbbing" (Box 22-5). Some clients may have difficulty describing the quality of painful sensations, or they may have problems using the term "pain" to indicate their discomfort. Showing clients a list of words to describe pain may facilitate their ability to report pain quality.

Duration. Duration refers to the time of onset, duration, and intervals of the pain. Terms used to classify the

FIGURE 22-7 Pain intensity scales.

PAIN INTENSITY MEASURES

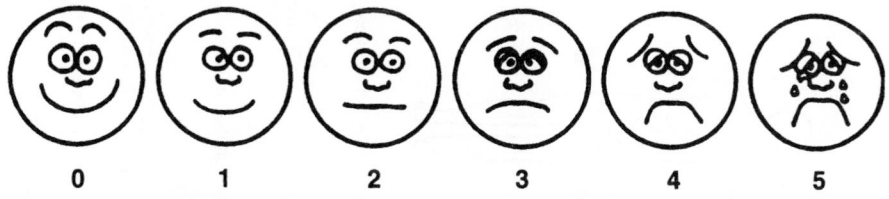

When using the Faces, explain to the person that each face is for a person who feels happy because he has no pain (hurt for young children) or sad because he has some or a lot of pain. Face 0 is very happy because he doesn't hurt at all. Face 1 hurts just a little bit. Face 2 hurts a little more. Face 3 hurts even more. Face 4 hurts a whole lot. Face 5 hurts as much as you can imagine, although you don't have to be crying to feel this bad.

Word:

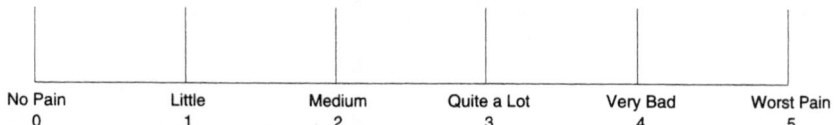

FIGURE 22-8 Faces Pain Rating Scale. Explain to the person that each face is for a person who feels happy because he or she has no pain (hurt) or sad because he or she has some or a lot of pain. Face 0 is very happy because he or she doesn't hurt at all. Face 1 hurts just a little bit. Face 2 hurts a little more. Face 3 hurts even more. Face 4 hurts a whole lot. Face 5 hurts as much as you can imagine, although you don't have to be crying to feel this bad. Ask the person to choose the face that best describes how he or she is feeling. This rating scale is recommended for persons age 3 years and older. (From Wong, D.L., et al. [2001]. *Wong's essentials of pediatric nursing* [6th ed.]. St. Louis: Mosby. Copyrighted by Mosby.)

Pain Inventory

Date: _____ / _____ / _____   Time: _____

Name: _____
        Last   First   Middle Initial

1) Throughout our lives, most of us have had pain from time to time (such as minor headaches, sprains, and toothaches). Have you had pain other than these everyday kinds of pain today?   1. Yes   2. No

2) On the diagram, shade in the areas where you feel pain. Put an X on the area that hurts the most.

3) Please rate your pain by circling the one number that best describes your pain at its **worst** in the past 24 hours.

0   1   2   3   4   5   6   7   8   9   10
No   Pain as bad as
pain   you can imagine

4) Please rate your pain by circling the one number that best describes your pain at its **least** in the past 24 hours.

0   1   2   3   4   5   6   7   8   9   10
No   Pain as bad as
pain   you can imagine

5) Please rate your pain by circling the one number that best describes your pain on the **average.**

0   1   2   3   4   5   6   7   8   9   10
No   Pain as bad as
pain   you can imagine

6) Please rate your pain by circling the one number that tells how much pain you have **right now.**

0   1   2   3   4   5   6   7   8   9   10
No   Pain as bad as
pain   you can imagine

7) What treatments or medications are you receiving for your pain?

8) In the past 24 hours, how much **relief** have pain treatments or medications provided? Please circle the one percentage that most shows how much relief you have received.

0%   10%   20%   30%   40%   50%   60%   70%   80%   90%   100%
No   Complete
relief   relief

9) Circle the one number that describes how, during the past 24 hours, pain has **interfered** with your:

A.   General activity

0   1   2   3   4   5   6   7   8   9   10
Does not   Completely
interfere   interferes

B.   Mood

0   1   2   3   4   5   6   7   8   9   10
Does not   Completely
interfere   interferes

C.   Walking ability

0   1   2   3   4   5   6   7   8   9   10
Does not   Completely
interfere   interferes

D.   Normal work (includes both work outside the home and housework)

0   1   2   3   4   5   6   7   8   9   10
Does not   Completely
interfere   interferes

E.   Relations with other people

0   1   2   3   4   5   6   7   8   9   10
Does not   Completely
interfere   interferes

F.   Sleep

0   1   2   3   4   5   6   7   8   9   10
Does not   Completely
interfere   interferes

G.   Enjoyment of life

0   1   2   3   4   5   6   7   8   9   10
Does not   Completely
interfere   interferes

UC950340GEN NP-2395EN

FIGURE 22-9 Pain Inventory, Short Form. (From Pain Research Group, Department of Neurology, University of Wisconsin—Madison. Used with permission.)

<table>
<tr><td colspan="2">BOX 22-5 Descriptive Terms for Pain</td></tr>
<tr><td>Descriptive Word</td><td>How Pain Makes Person Feel</td></tr>
<tr><td>Sharp</td><td>Horrible</td></tr>
<tr><td>Piercing</td><td>Annoyed</td></tr>
<tr><td>Shooting</td><td>Miserable</td></tr>
<tr><td>Crushing</td><td>Frightened</td></tr>
<tr><td>Tender</td><td>Suffocated</td></tr>
<tr><td>Hurting</td><td>Tortured</td></tr>
<tr><td>Aching</td><td>Overwhelmed</td></tr>
<tr><td>Dull</td><td>Depressed</td></tr>
<tr><td>Sore</td><td>Defeated</td></tr>
<tr><td>Cramping</td><td>Anxious</td></tr>
<tr><td>Prickly</td><td>Victimized</td></tr>
</table>

TABLE 22-4 *Pain-Related Nursing Diagnoses*

Diagnosis	Etiology
Activity Intolerance	Related to unrelieved pain
Ineffective Coping	Related in lack of knowledge of possible methods of coping
Powerlessness	Related to lack of participation in decision-making process
Anxiety	Related to past experiences of poor pain control
Disturbed Sleep Pattern	Related to unrelieved pain at night
Deficient Knowledge	Related to lack of exposure to informational resources
Fear	Related to anticipation of a pain experience

pattern include "constant, steady, intermittent, periodic, brief, or momentary."

Distress. The psychological reactions to pain contribute to the overall pain experience. The emotional component may serve to intensify or diminish pain perception. Pain management strategies may need to be directed toward modifying the distress aspect of a pain episode.

Diagnosis, Outcomes, Interventions

Diagnosis: Acute Pain. The primary nursing diagnosis is *Acute Pain related to tissue injury from an incision, ischemia, or tumor encroachment in organs or bone.* Nurses have an impact on pain, discomfort, or suffering, no matter what the cause. In some situations, the client may be experiencing unrelieved pain. Unrelieved pain may be related to the following:

- Underadministration of ordered medication doses
- Administering medications in inappropriate time frames
- Not providing stronger medications when indicated
- Not providing combinations of medications when indicated
- Inadequate use of nonpharmaceutical management strategies

Pain may contribute to additional diagnoses as clients respond to the pain episode. Examples of such nursing diagnoses are presented in Table 22-4.

Outcomes and Goals. Outcomes and goals should be determined as a team consisting of the client, physicians, nurses, and often the extended family. A realistic outcome should be established to control or maintain the client at desired levels of pain and functioning. Desirable outcomes are that the client will (1) report freedom from pain, (2) request analgesia, and (3) perform daily activities without limitation related to pain.

A widely used method of providing effective care is through use of clinical care plans or clinical pathways. Care plans and pathways provide nurses with aids to diagnose the problem, plan for expected outcomes, implement interventions, state the rationale for the interventions, and evaluate the outcome. Many health care facilities provide standard care plans or clinical pathways that are part of the department protocol. Standard plans provide the beginning basis for client care. They are then modified as indicated based on the needs of each client.

Interventions. Effective pain reduction and/or relief is best achieved through the combination of both pharmaceutical and nonpharmaceutical therapies. Historically, pharmaceutical management has been the primary means of providing relief from pain, particularly acute pain. Although medications continue to serve as a major component of pain management, nonpharmaceutical techniques are being increasingly used to provide pain reduction and/or relief. Nonpharmacologic interventions are particularly useful (1) as adjuncts to pain reduction and/or relief, (2) while the client is waiting for medications to take effect, or (3) when side effects or client concerns make use of medications problematic.

Administration of Pain-Relieving Medication. Numerous medications are used for pain reduction and/or relief. They are administered in a variety of ways: by mouth, rectally, topically, sublingually, by inhalation, or by injection, which is the least effective and most painful route and should be avoided. Medications may be injected by subcutaneous, intramuscular, or IV routes. Some medications may be injected spinally or paravertebrally or into selected nerves to produce nerve blocks. Physicians perform the latter types of injections, with nurses assisting with the procedures and providing aftercare. Too often nurses view the administration of pain-relieving medications as all they need to do for pain management. However, medication may be more effective when combined with other pain reduction and/or relief techniques such as music, massage, and biofeedback. When administering medication and repositioning the client, give a back rub or simply interact with a client; the effectiveness of the drug may be increased. Simply providing an intervention or a pill does not replace thoughtful, comprehensive pain management.

Therapeutic interaction with someone experiencing pain may include the following:

- Facilitating the client's expression of feelings, which imparts a sense of being cared for
- Providing support, reassurance, and understanding, which allows the client to develop confidence in the nurse
- Teaching the client self-management strategies to reduce and/or relieve pain

Pain management strategies, including medications, are more effective when clients believe they are in control of the situation. A nurse who actively involves the client in the planning, intervention, and assessment of pain management strategies provides the client with enhanced potential to obtain satisfactory pain reduction and/or relief.

Managing Chronic Intractable Pain. Chronic intractable pain (pain that cannot be satisfactorily relieved by typical pharmaceutical means) causes additional difficulties for those experiencing it. Clients may require a combination of nursing interventions (cognitive, behavioral, physical, pharmaceutical). Nursing and medical therapeutic regimens must be coordinated and consistent to ensure a unified approach. Use of balanced or preemptive analgesia is necessary.[42] Complete pain relief may be unrealistic, however, and should not be promised.

Managing Progressive Pain. People with progressive pain, such as that seen in malignancies, may require pain-relieving medications routinely as a preventive measure, in the same way that vasodilators are regularly taken by people with ischemic heart disease. As the disease progresses, clients may require increasingly stronger drug doses. Some people hesitate to take pain-relieving medications routinely for fear of addiction. They may believe that they must avoid increasing dosages because they are afraid that they will "use up" the medication's pain relief potential and will not be able to obtain adequate medication in the future. Education of the unlimited ceiling dosage of morphine is necessary. Clients may also be concerned that they will be labeled as "drug users" if they take opioids over the long term.

In reality, people experiencing pain due to widespread cancer require routine pain-relieving medications in order to function. Help is needed for clients and their significant others to understand the need for regular, often strong medications. Clients should be reassured that adequate pain reduction and/or relief will be possible in the future and that routine use of the medications means only that the condition warrants it, much like the routine use of medication for hypertension.

Many conditions associated with pain are managed at home. The treatment of acute postoperative, chronic, and malignant pain is often performed by clients and family members. See the Bridge to Home Health Care on Controlling Pain on the website.

MEDICATIONS TO CONTROL PAIN

Anesthetic Agents

An *anesthetic* is a pharmacologic substance that, in addition to abolishing pain, generally causes loss of feeling and sensation. Many *analgesics* (pharmacologic substances that diminish or eliminate pain without producing unconsciousness), depending on their mode of action and route of administration, act as anesthetics when given in larger doses. There are many different types of anesthesia. *General anesthesia* is usually accompanied by loss of consciousness and reflexes along with amnesia regarding the experience. *Local anesthetics* produce anesthesia in a restricted area of the body without loss of consciousness.

A technique frequently used in minor surgery and other procedures is infiltration of a local anesthetic into the skin and subcutaneous tissue to produce loss of sensation, or local anesthesia. The same agent injected near a sensory nerve causes anesthesia in the distribution of the nerve *(regional anesthesia)*. Nerves are often mixed in function; that is, they carry both sensory and motor fibers. Hence, a *nerve block* may cause motor weakness or temporary paralysis, in addition to loss of sensation, in the innervated area. A nerve block is the application of a pharmacologic substance that inhibits nerve conduction (e.g., numbing the mouth for dental procedures).

Local anesthetic agents may be applied topically (on the skin or mucous membranes), infiltrated locally, used for specific nerve blocks (e.g., spinal anesthetic for surgery), or administered intravenously, depending on the reason for their use. Local anesthetic agents act by temporarily blocking nerve impulses between the peripheral structures and higher centers. Such blocks are reversible because the nerves regain their function over a period of minutes to hours.

Neurolytic agents (e.g., phenol, alcohol) produce prolonged nerve blocks, which destroy the nerves. Neurolytic blocks may not be truly permanent because nerve fibers regrow after several months. However, the growth is often disorganized. Hence, the sensation from these nerve fibers is often abnormal or painful. Consequently, neurolytic blocks are generally used only in terminally ill persons with a short life expectancy, such as those with cancer-related pain.

Local Anesthesia

Chemically, local anesthetics are divided into two classes:

1. The *esters* (e.g., procaine [Novocain]) are metabolized in the plasma, are less heat-stable than the amides, and account for most of the rarely occurring allergic reactions to local anesthetics.
2. The *amides* (e.g., lidocaine [Xylocaine] and bupivacaine [Marcaine, Sensorcaine]) are metabolized in the liver.

Lidocaine is one of the most commonly used local anesthetics. It acts within 5 to 10 minutes and lasts about 2 hours. It has a wide range of applications, including topical and intravascular block. Allergy to lidocaine is rare.

Bupivacaine is long-acting (4 to 8 hours) but has a slow onset. It is four times more potent than lidocaine and four to six times more toxic. Therefore a lower concentration is used. Bupivacaine appears to block sensory nerves in preference to motor nerves when used in low concentration. Thus effective analgesia may result without accompanying motor weakness.

Local anesthetics are usually vasodilators, increasing blood flow into the area in which they are injected. Thus they shorten the duration of their own action by enhancing their own vascular absorption. Adding epinephrine, a vasoconstrictor, to local anesthetic solutions prolongs the anesthetic effect by decreasing the vascular uptake of the anesthetic, allowing it to stay in contact with the nerve tissue for a longer period. The recipient may sense an increased heart rate from the epinephrine.

NOTE: Epinephrine-containing solutions are *not* typically used for nerve blocks of the penis, fingers, or toes, where vasoconstriction could cause inadequate blood flow and necrosis of the distal extremity.

In addition to prolonging anesthesia, epinephrine-containing local anesthetic solutions offer other advantages. The supplementary use of a vasoconstrictor reduces the possibility of the anesthetic reaching a toxic blood level. The toxicity of local analgesic medication depends on its concentration in the blood. This, in turn, depends on the speed of absorption. Vasoconstricting medications delay absorption of a local analgesic solution and thus prevent a suddenly high blood concentration, which gives the body more time to metabolize and detoxify them. Vasoconstrictors also inhibit bleeding in the area of the injection. Larger doses of epinephrine containing local anesthetic should be used cautiously in people with coronary artery disease. Care of clients given anesthesia is discussed in Chapter 15.

Topical Local Anesthesia

Dilute solutions of local anesthetics may be applied topically in the form of pastes, sprays, or other preparations. They may reduce the severe pain of burns, abrasions, and necrosis of the mucous membranes and skin. Remember, once an area is anesthetized, it does not transmit painful sensation and the area is thus at greater risk for injury. If topical anesthetic agents are applied to burned or abraded skin or mucous membranes, absorption of the medication is almost as rapid as that following IV administration.

A relatively new agent, EMLA cream, is a mixture of lidocaine and prilocaine. It is useful in preventing pain from venipuncture, injections, heel sticks, and minor plastic surgery. It must be applied in advance to the area (45 minutes to 1 hour) and covered with an occlusive dressing. EMLA cream is an excellent strategy for eliminating the pain associated with penetration of the skin and should be encouraged.

Analgesics

Various factors are considered in selecting the most effective analgesic for a specific client. These factors include the cause, quality, intensity, duration, and distribution of the pain. The World Health Organization (WHO)[62] has suggested that decisions regarding pain medications may be aided by use of a "pain ladder" (Figure 22-10). The ladder was originally designed to guide the care of persons with cancer pain, but its use has been extended to apply to acute pain. Non-opioids, such as acetaminophen and NSAIDs, are suggested by the first ladder step. If the pain persists or increases, step 2 suggests mild opioids (such as codeine) plus non-opioid analgesics. If the pain continues to persist or increases, step 3 suggests strong opioids (such as morphine) with or without non-opioids. Adjuvant medications may be added at any step in the ladder.

Systemic analgesic medications are the most frequently used means of pain control. Analgesics are the most commonly prescribed, and thus widely used, medications. They are also purchased extensively over the counter. This is not unexpected, because pain is usually the first manifestation of injury, and most diseases begin with or include pain at some time during their course.

Pharmaceutical Considerations

Some analgesics have a *ceiling effect*, which occurs when medications have a maximum effective dose; increasing the dose cannot increase pain relief but may increase side effects. Medications with a ceiling effect may be combined with other analgesics when additional pain relief is needed. Pure opiates have no ceiling dosage.

Tolerance. Tolerance, a physiologic phenomenon, occurs when larger doses of medications are needed to

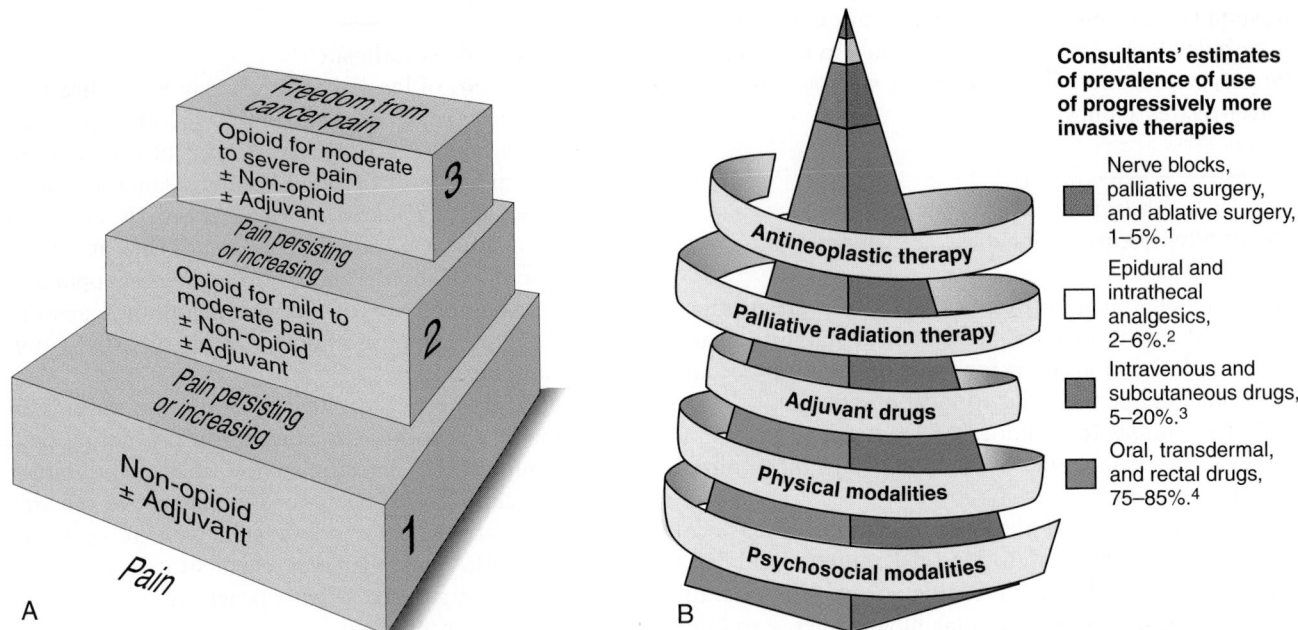

FIGURE 22-10 **A,** World Health Organization (WHO) analgesic ladder describes the steps in treating cancer pain. **B,** Pain management strategies: A hierarchy. NOTE: The pyramid depicts a hierarchy of pain management strategies from least invasive (at the base) to most invasive (at the apex). Therapies depicted on the ribbon may benefit many patients who are receiving concurrent treatments at any level of invasiveness. Estimates presented in the sidebar are based on published data and consultants' estimates for various clinical populations in industrialized nations but may not reflect all settings and do not necessarily reflect what is optimal. ([1]Hiraga, Mizuguchi, and Takeda, 1991; Portenoy, 1993; Ventafridda, Caraceni, and Gamba, 1990. [2]Hiraga, Mizuguchi, and Takeda, 1991; Ventafridda, Caraceni, and Gamba, 1990. [3]Keller, 1984; Paice, 1993; Portenoy, 1993. [4]Goisis, Gorini, Ratta, et al, 1989; Hiraga, Mizuguchi, and Takeda, 1991; Scug, Zech, and Dorr, 1990; Takeda, 1986; Ventafridda, Caraceni, and Gamba, 1990; Walker, Hoskin, Hanks, et al., 1988.) (**A** from World Health Organization. [1996]. *Cancer pain relief* [2nd ed.]. Geneva: Author; **B** from Jacox, A., et al. [1994]. *Management of cancer pain. Clinical practice guidelines No. 9.* AHCPR Publication No. 94-1592. Rockville, MD: Agency for Health Care Policy and Research, U.S. Department of Health and Human Services, Public Health Service.)

provide the same amount of pain relief as the previous smaller dose. It may occur in people who require long-term pain management with opioids. The person becomes tolerant to these medications because the opiate receptors become less sensitive to them. Tolerance may be managed by continuing the dose of the opioid and adding a non-opioid analgesic or adjuvant medication or by switching to an alternate drug.

Tolerance should not be confused with *addiction*, which is rare. Concern about addiction in cases of tolerance has led health care providers to modify opioid prescriptions by ordering smaller doses over longer periods of time. Client response to the modification may lead one to conclude that addiction was the underlying problem, because these people may be forced to display behaviors often associated with psychological addiction.[5] This is called *pseudoaddiction*. The client no longer receives adequate pain relief and may attempt to manipu-

late the provider into providing adequate medication. Such behavior is understandable but is often viewed as "medication-seeking," a classic definition of one psychologically addicted. Clients may "act out" their pain in the belief that if they look as if they have severe pain, their need for medication will be recognized by the health care provider. The client does not receive adequate pain relief in response to these behaviors and rationalizes that health care providers are no longer dependable. The health care provider concludes that the client's behavior is inappropriate and no longer values or believes the client. This atmosphere of mistrust creates a situation in which adequate pain relief for the client becomes increasingly unlikely. Addiction is discussed in Chapter 24.

Dependence. Physical dependence commonly occurs when medications are taken over a long term. Physical manifestations associated with sudden termination of the medication include anxiety, irritability, chills alternating with hot flashes, salivation, lacrimation, rhinorrhea, diaphoresis, piloerection, nausea and vomiting, abdominal cramps, and insomnia.[5]

Physical dependence is not a problem unless opioids are to be discontinued. The effects of withdrawal can be avoided by weaning the client from the medication slowly. It is essential that health care providers, clients, and their significant others realize that physical dependence is not synonymous with psychological addiction. Client and family education regarding this matter is an expected nursing function.

Types of Analgesics

Analgesics are medications developed to provide pain relief. The discussion is organized according to the WHO analgesic ladder, which is based on the notion that pain medication decisions are based in part on the intensity and controllability of the pain.[62] The three steps reflect mild, moderate, and severe degrees of pain intensity.

Non-Opioid Analgesics. Non-opioid analgesics fall into four primary categories[5]:
- Aspirin
- Salicylate salts
- Acetaminophen
- NSAIDs

As a group, these drugs have a ceiling effect but do not cause physical dependence or tolerance. Their site of action is primarily in the periphery at the receptor site, where they serve an anti-inflammatory function and prevent the production of prostaglandins. They may have a central role in pain relief, in that prostaglandins inhibit the production or the release of serotonin, removing the pain reduction and/or relief effect of the neurotransmitter. Preventing prostaglandin production would maintain the inhibitory effect of serotonin in the dorsal horn. An exception is acetaminophen, which produces pain reduction and/or relief but is not an anti-inflammatory agent and does not appear to affect prostaglandins. The physical means by which acetaminophen produces pain relief is not known.[5]

The American Pain Society recommends that a non-opioid medication be included with any analgesic regimen, even when opioids are prescribed.[5] Opioids act centrally, within the brain and spinal cord. Non-opioids add peripherally mediated pain reduction and/or relief to the central effects of opioids when they are given in combination. Parenteral and rectal forms of non-opioids have been developed for individuals who cannot take oral medications. Refer to Table 22-5 for dosing information for non-opioid medications.

Aspirin. Historically, aspirin (acetylsalicylic acid, ASA) has been the primary non-opioid medication for pain. It is one of the most effective non-opioid medications available. Aspirin is available in many forms, including tablets (plain, chewable, enteric coated, sustained-release), capsules, rectal suppositories, and topical creams. As with most nonsteroidal analgesics, aspirin has an antiplatelet effect and is a gastric irritant. Side effects include bleeding associated with prolonged clotting time and gastric disturbances. Enteric-coated tablets reduce the gastric reactions because the coating remains intact until the product reaches the small intestine, where the tablet dissolves and is absorbed. Because of the association of aspirin with Reye's syndrome, a potentially fatal condition seen primarily in young children, it is not used in children younger than age 12 years with viral illnesses. Recent cases of adults with Reye's syndrome–like manifestations and negative outcomes suggest that aspirin may pose a risk for people of any age when administered to those with viral infections.

Salicylate Salts. These salts are similar to aspirin but produce fewer gastric side effects. Choline magnesium trisalicylate (Trilisate) and diflunisal (Dolobid) are typical examples. Platelet aggregation remains functional when salicylate salts are used in people with normal clotting abilities.

Acetaminophen. Acetaminophen is similar to aspirin in its ability to provide pain reduction and/or relief, but it does not affect the gastric mucosa. It has no effect on platelet aggregation and does not affect bleeding time. Its anti-inflammatory effect is much less than that of other non-opioids. It is tolerated well by most people of any age, and it is the drug of choice when given for pain to people with viral infections.

NSAIDs. NSAIDs are nonsteroidal anti-inflammatory agents other than aspirin and acetaminophen. NSAIDs are present in numerous preparations, providing alternative medication choices. If one form is ineffective, another can be tried. NSAIDs were originally developed to treat arthritis, but they are also effective for mild to moderate pain of nonarthritic origin. NSAIDs act to decrease inflammation, but it is their ability to block prostaglandin synthesis that is credited for most of their pain-relieving properties.[10,43] NSAIDs are particularly helpful for clients with cancer or postoperative pain, because a major contributing factor to pain in these clients is cell destruction.

NSAIDs potentiate the effects of opiates and are often given in combination preparations that incorporate codeine or codeine derivatives. Tylenol with codeine is used widely for moderate pain. NSAIDs are particularly effective for pain resulting from bone insult, including

TABLE 22-5 Dosing Information for Acetaminophen and Nonsteroidal Anti-Inflammatory Drugs (NSAIDs) *

Chemical Class	Generic Name	Half-Life (hr)	Dosing Schedule	Recommended Oral Starting Dose (mg)	Maximum Oral Dose Recommended (mg/day)	Comments
P-Aminophenol derivatives	Acetaminophen	2	q 4-6 hr	650	6000	Overdosage produces hepatic toxicity. No GI or platelet toxicity. Available as liquid and for rectal administration.
Salicylates	Aspirin	3-12	q 4-6 hr	650	4000	Standard for comparison. May not be as well tolerated as some of the newer NSAIDs. Available for rectal administration.
	Diflunisal	8-12	q 12 hr	500	1500	Less GI toxicity than aspirin.
	Choline magnesium trisalicylate	9-17	q 12 hr	500-1000	4000	Minimal GI toxicity. No effect on platelet aggregation. Available as liquid.
	Choline salicylate	2-3	q 3-6 hr	870	5352	Liquid. Minimal effect on platelet function.
	Magnesium salicylate		q 4-6 hr	1000	4000	
	Salsalate	16	q 12 hr	500-1000	4000	
Proprionic acids	Ibuprofen	2	q 6 hr	400	3200	Available as a suspension.
	Naproxen	13	q 12 hr	250	1025-1375	
	Fenoprofen	2-3	q 6-8 hr	200	3200	
	Ketoprofen	2-3	q 6-8 hr	25	300	Available for rectal administration and as a topical gel.
	Flurbiprofen	5-6	q 12 hr	100	300	
	Oxaprozin	400	q 24 hr	600	1800	
Acetic acids	Indomethacin	4-5	q 8 hr	25	150	Higher incidence of GI and CNS side effects than proprionic acids. Available in slow-release preparations and for rectal administration.
	Tolmetin	2-5	q 8 hr	200	2000	
	Sulindac	14	q 12 hr	150	400	Not recommended for prolonged use because of increased risk for GI toxicity.
	Diclofenac	2	q 8 hr	25	150	
	Ketorolac	4-7	q 6 hr	10	40	Use limited to 5 days. Recommended parenteral dose ≤30 mg; total daily dose ≤120 mg.
Oxicams	Piroxicam	50	q 24 hr	20	40	
Fenamates	Mefenamic acid	2	q 6 hr	250	1000	Use limited to 7 days.
	Meclofenamate	2	—	—	400	Not recommended for analgesia.
Pyranocarboxylic acids	Etodolac	7	q 8 hr	200	1200	
Other	Nabumetone	24	q 24 hr	1000	2000	Minimal effect on platelet aggregation.

From McCaffery, M., & Pasero, C. (1999). *Pain: Clinical manual* (pp. 139-140). St. Louis: Mosby.
GI, Gastrointestinal; *CNS*, central nervous system.
*May be duplicated for use in clinical practice.

bone metastases of malignancy and fractures. Degradation of bone tissue in these conditions produces prostaglandins. The ability of NSAIDs to prevent prostaglandin production significantly decreases pain produced by these lesions.[44] Ketoprofen and ketorolac (Toradol) also block production of leukotrienes.[43]

The most common side effects associated with NSAIDs are gastrointestinal upset and bleeding. These agents also inhibit platelet aggregation, increasing the risk of hemorrhage. Clients taking NSAIDs must be monitored closely for the development of peptic ulcers. In clients who are taking high doses for long periods of time (as for arthritis) a histamine H_2-receptor antagonist such as ranitidine (Zantac) or misoprostol (Cytotec) may be used.

NSAIDs may also have negative effects on the renal system, particularly in clients with heart failure, chronic renal disease, lupus, blood volume depletion, diuretic use, atherosclerosis, and multiple myeloma.[5] Clients may experience sudden decreased urine output associated with water and sodium retention.

New forms of NSAIDs appear to prevent the negative side effects and to broaden the routes available for administration. For example, ketorolac was developed to provide an injectable form. The recently available cyclooxygenase (COX-2) inhibitors were developed in response to the negative gastrointestinal side effects of aspirin and NSAIDs.[19] Celecoxib (Celebrex) and rofecoxib (Vioxx) disrupt the synthesis of prostaglandins by interfering with the cyclooxygenase portion of the arachidonic acid cascade. Two types of cyclooxygenase predominate. COX-1 is found primarily in the stomach and has a protective function. COX-2 is usually assumed to be associated with pain initiated by inflammation. It was therefore assumed that development of an NSAID that spares the gastric protection function of COX-1 but disrupts COX-2 activity would provide pain reduction and/or relief while preventing the negative gastric consequences associated with existing NSAIDs.[19] Although this concept is not totally supportable, COX-2 inhibitors have provided pain relief and/or reduction with little gastric consequence.[16,19] Nurses need to continuously upgrade their knowledge regarding these medications. NOTE: Clients allergic to sulfa should not take celecoxib. NSAIDs should be administered on a scheduled basis.

Opioid Analgesics. Opioid analgesics are derived from natural opium alkaloids and their synthetic derivatives. They tend to be grouped as opioids because their effects resemble those of opium. Opioids are typically categorized from weak to strong to aid health care providers in selecting the correct medication (Table 22-6). Opioids are added to the medication regimen when pain is moderate to severe and non-opioids are insufficient to manage pain effectively. Tolerance and physical dependence seen in long-term administration are not associated with short-term opioid treatment.

Opioids bind with receptors that can be engaged by endogenous opioids, including mu (μ), kappa (κ), and delta (δ) receptor types.[45] Binding with receptors in the spinal cord renders the presynaptic membrane of nociceptor fibers incapable of opening Ca^{2+} channels, inhibiting nociceptive neurotransmitter release. Opiate binding with the postsynaptic membrane hyperpolarizes the membrane by altering the ability of K^+ ions to flow across the membrane. Opiate receptors are found in the

TABLE 22-6 *Analgesic Step Pain Ladder*

Step One		Step Two	Step Three
NSAIDs and Others		**Opioid-Agonist Drug**	**Agonist Drugs**
Acetaminophen	Carbamazepine	Codeine	Morphine sulfate
Acetylsalicylic acid	Celecoxib	Oxycodone (with aspirin and with	Methodone
(aspirin)	Meloxicam	acetaminophen)	Hydromorphone
Ibuprofen	Phenytoin	Hydrocodone	Oxymorphone
Choline	Amitriptyline	Meperidine	Levorphanol
magnesium	Doxepin	Propoxyphene HCl	Fentanyl
trisalicylate	Imipramine	Propoxyphene napsylate (with aspirin and	
Diflunisal	Trazodone	with acetaminophen)	**Agonist-Antagonist Drugs**
Ketoprofen	Hydroxyzine		Butorphanol
Naproxen	Lidocaine	**Agonist-Antagonist Drugs**	Nalbuphine
Ketorolac	Mexiletine	Pentazocine HCl	Dezocine
tromethamine	Tocainide		
Piroxicam	Dexamethasone		**Partial Agonist Drugs**
Sulindac	Dextroamphetamine		Buprenorphine
Indomethacin	Methylphenidate		

From the World Health Organization (1996). *Cancer pain relief* (2nd ed.). Geneva: Author.

periaqueductal gray (PAG) matter and the periventricular gray (PVG) matter in the midbrain. Activation of these receptors by opioids initiates the descending effect of serotonin and norepinephrine.[63]

All opioids produce side effects to some degree. The side effects are determined, in part, by the receptor type engaged by the medication and by the location of the receptor. The three receptor types have very different distributions and locations with the CNS. Side effects may be managed by discontinuing one form of opiate medication with untoward side effects and replacing it with another that binds to a different receptor type.

Opioid Agonists. Opioid agonists are opiate derivatives that bring about pain relief by producing the maximum degree of receptor binding. Agonists bind fully to their corresponding receptor type and do not affect the ability of other opioid preparations to engage their specific receptor. They are typically associated with mu receptors and have no ceiling effect.

Examples of opioid agonists are displayed in Table 22-7. They include morphine-like medications, which differ from morphine in rate of onset, duration of action, route of administration, adverse side effects, and chemical configuration. The mechanisms by which they produce pain reduction and/or relief are similar. (See Chapter 23 for further discussion on analgesic and rescue dosing.)

Opioid Antagonists. These agents reverse the side effects and analgesia of opioids. They have no agonist effects and thus produce no analgesia. They are used to counteract a negative effect of an opioid, typically respiratory depression. Naloxone is the most common example (Box 22-6).

Opioid Agonist-Antagonists. These medications engage one receptor type while inhibiting receptor binding of another. When they are given following use of the opioid they inhibit, they precipitously reverse the medication's effects and can precipitate acute withdrawal. When the combination agents are given alone, they produce analgesia and the positive effects of opioids with fewer side effects. Respiratory depression is a less likely effect, although psychomimetic effects are more probable. Examples are listed in Table 22-7.

Methadone. A potent, long-acting opioid analgesic, methadone gained popularity in the management of cancer pain before the development of the long-acting forms of morphine. Unlike most morphine preparations, methadone has a long plasma half-life. This long plasma half-life, when repeated doses are given, may account for methadone's longer duration of analgesic action, but it also poses certain problems. This medication is not recommended for older people and people with compro-

mised hepatic and renal function. The long plasma half-life necessitates close monitoring of any client receiving repeated doses because cumulative effects develop over 1 to 2 weeks. If the client becomes oversedated, the dosage should be reduced or the intervals between administration lengthened.

Meperidine. Meperidine (Demerol) is a popular analgesic medication but has many limitations. It should not be used on a prolonged basis, no longer than 48 hours or more than 600 mg in 24 hours, because of the potentially toxic metabolite by-product normeperidine, which is produced during its biotransformation. Meperidine does not provide effective pain reduction and/or relief with repeated doses and causes untenable CNS side effects. The metabolic by-product is toxic to the CNS and can lead to anxiety, tremors, myoclonus, and seizure activity. Nerve injury from diffusion of medication can also occur. Meperidine should not be used in clients with altered renal function or in older adults.

Propoxyphene. Propoxyphene (Darvon) also has a toxic metabolite, norpropoxyphene, which accumulates and causes confusion, depression, and cardiac dysrhythmias.

Adverse Effects of Opioid Analgesics. Some side effects of opioid analgesics—constipation in particular—last as long as the medication is administered. Others, such as nausea and vomiting and drowsiness, decrease as the administration is continued. Other side effects (e.g., respiratory depression) are rare, and the incidence decreases precipitously with longer administration.

Constipation. Constipation is the most common side effect seen with opioid use[58,63] and results from increased smooth muscle tone and decreased motility of the gastrointestinal tract. Opioids diminish the propul- sive peristaltic contractions in the small and large intestine and delay the passage of gastric contents through the duodenum. Tolerance does not develop to constipation as it does to the other side effects of opioids. Clients taking opioid analgesics need to follow a bowel regimen to prevent constipation. A diet high in fiber with plenty of fluids and stool-softening medications, such as docusate sodium (Colace) or docusate sodium casanthranol (Peri-Colace), is a common prophylactic treatment. A senna-based bulk laxative, such as Senokot-S, is also often needed.[33,58] Constipation is treatable and is not a side effect mandating that opioid medications be discontinued. A bowel program should be instituted with both a stool softening agent and a peristaltic (motility) agent. Reports have indicated that some clients may indeed discontinue opiates because of constipation.

TABLE 22-7	*Equianalgesic Dose Chart for Selected Opioid Drugs*

A Guide to Using Equianalgesic Dose Charts
- Equianalgesic means approximately the same pain relief.
- The equianalgesic chart is a guideline. Doses and intervals between doses are titrated according to individual's response.
- The equianalgesic chart is helpful when switching from one drug to another or switching from one route of administration to another.
- Dosages in this equianalgesic chart are not necessarily starting doses. They suggest a ratio for comparing the analgesia of one drug to another.
- The longer the client has been receiving opioids, the more conservative the starting doses of a new opioid.

Opioid	Parenteral (SC/IV) (Over ~ 4 hr)	Oral (PO) (Over ~ 4 hr)	Onset (min)	Peak (min)	Duration[1] (hr)	Half-life (hr)
Mu Agonists						
Morphine	10 mg	30 mg	30-60 (PO)	60-90 (PO)	3-6 (PO)	2-4
			30-60 (CR)[b]	90-180 (CR)[b]	8-12 (CR)[a,c]	
			30-60 (R)	60-90 (R)	4-5 (R)	
			5-10 (IV)	15-30 (IV)	3-4 (IV)	
			10-20 (SC)	30-60 (SC)	3-4 (SC)	
			10-20 (IM)	30-60 (IM)	3-4 (IM)	
Codeine	130 mg	200 mg NR	30-60 (PO)	60-90 (PO)	3-4 (PO)	2-4
			10-20 (SC)	UK (SC)	3-4 (SC)	
			10-20 (IM)	30-60 (IM)	3-4 (IM)	
Fentanyl	100 µg/hr parenterally and transdermally ≅ 4 mg/hr morphine parenterally; 1 µg/hr transdermally ≅ morphine 2 mg/24 hr PD	—	5 (OT)	15 (OT)	2-5 (OT)	3-4
			1-5 (IV)	3-5 (IV)	0.5-4 (IV)	
			7-15 (IM)	10-20 (IM)	0.5-4 (IM)	
			12-16 h (TD)	24 hr (TD)	48-72 (TD)	13-24 (TD)
Hydrocodone (as in Vicodin, Lortab)	—	30 mg[e] NR	30-60 (PO)	60-90 (PO)	4-6 (PO)	4
Hydromorphone (Dilaudid)	1.5 mg[f]	7.5 mg	15-30 (PO)	30-90 (PO)	3-4 (PO)	2-3
			15-30 (R)	30-90 (R)	3-4 (R)	
			5 (IV)	10-20 (IV)	3-4 (IV)[a,c]	
			10-20 (SC)	30-90 (SC)	3-4 (SC)	
			10-20 (IM)	30-90 (IM)	3-4 (IM)	
Levorphanol (Levo-Dromoran)	2 mg	4 mg	30-60 (PO)	60-90 (PO)	4-6 (PO)	12-15
			10 (IV)	15-30 (IV)	4-6 (IV)[a,c]	
			10-20 (SC)	60-90 (SC)	4-6 (SC)	
			10-20 (IM)	60-90 (IM)	4-6 (IM)	

Modified from McCaffery M., Pasero C. (1999). *Pain: Clinical manual* (pp. 241-243). St. Louis: Mosby.

ATC, Around-the-clock; *CR*, oral controlled-release; *hr*, hour; *IM*, intramuscular; *IV*, intravenous; *µg*, microgram; *mg*, milligram; *min*, minute; *NR*, not recommended; *NS*, nasal spray; *OT*, oral transmucosal; *PO*, oral; *R*, rectal; *SC*, subcutaneous; *SL*, sublingual; *TD*, transdermal; *UK*, unknown.

[a]Duration of analgesia is dose-dependent; the higher the dose, usually the longer the duration.

[b]As in MS Contin, for example.

[c]IV boluses may be used to produce analgesia that lasts approximately as long as IM or SC doses. However, of all routes of administration, IV produces the highest peak concentration of the drug, and the peak concentration is associated with the highest level of toxicity (e.g., sedation). To decrease the peak effect and lower the level of toxicity, IV boluses may be administered more slowly (e.g., 10 mg of morphine over a 15-minute period) or smaller doses may be administered more often (e.g., 5 mg of morphine every 1-1.5 hr).

[d]At steady state, slow release of fentanyl from storage in tissues can result in a prolonged half-life of up to 12 hr.

[e]Equianalgesic data not available.

[f]The recommendation that 1.5 mg of parenteral hydromorphone is approximately equal to 10 mg of parenteral morphine is based on single-dose studies. With repeated dosing of hydromorphone (e.g., PCA), it is more likely that 2 to 3 mg of parenteral hydromorphone is equal to 10 mg of parenteral morphine.

Continued

TABLE 22-7	Equianalgesic Dose Chart for Selected Opioid Drugs—cont'd					
Opioid	**Parenteral (SC/IV) (Over ~ 4 hr)**	**Oral (PO) (Over ~ 4 hr)**	**Onset (min)**	**Peak (min)**	**Duration[1] (hr)**	**Half-life (hr)**
Mu Agonists—cont'd						
Meperidine (Demerol)	75 mg	300 mg NR	30-60 (PO) 5-10 (IV) 10-20 (SC) 10-20 (IM)	60-90 (PO) 10-15 (IV) 15-30 (SC) 15-30 (IM)	2-4 (PO) 2-4 (IV)[a,c] 2-4 (SC) 2-4 (IM)	2-3
Methadone (Dolophine)	10 mg[g]	20 mg[h]	30-60 (PO) UK (SL) 10 (IV) 10-20 (SC) 10-20 (IM)	60-120 (PO) 10 (SL) UK (IV) 60-120 (SC) 60-120 (IM)	4-8 (PO) UK (SL) 4-8 (IV)[a,c] 4-8 (SC) 4-8 (IM)	12-190
Oxycodone (as in Percocet, Tylox)	—	20 mg	30-60 (PO) 30-60 (CR)[i] 30-60 (R)	60-90 (PO) 90-180 (CR)[i] 30-60 (R)	3-4 (PO) 8-12 (CR)[i] 3-6 (R)	2-3 4.5 (CR)
Oxymorphone (Numorphan)	1 mg	(10 mg R)	15-30 (R) 5-10 (IV) 10-20 (SC) 10-20 (IM)	120 (R) 15-30 (IV) UK (SC) 30-90 (IM)	3-6 (R) 3-4 (IV)[a,c] 3-6 (SC) 3-6 (IM)	2-3
Propoxyphene[j] (Darvon)	—	—	30-60 (PO)	60-90 (PO)	4-6 (PO)	6-12
Agonist-Antagonists						
Buprenorphine[k] (Buprenex)	0.4 mg	—	5 (SL) 5 (IV) 10-20 (IM)	30-60 (SL) 10-20 (IV) 30-60 (IM)	UK (SL) 3-4 (IV)[a,c] 3-6 (IM)	2-3
Butorphanol[k] (Stadol)	2 mg	—	5-15 (NS)[l] 5 (IV) 10-20 (IM)	60-90 (NS) 10-20 (IV) 30-60 (IM)	3-4 (NS) 3-4 (IV)[a,c] 3-4 (IM)	3-4
Dezocine (Dalgan)	10 mg	—	5 (IV) 10-20 (IM)	UK (IV) 30-60 (IM)	3-4 (IV)[a,c] 3-4 (IM)	2-3
Nalbuphine[k] (Nubain)	10 mg	—	5 (IV) <15 (SC) <15 (IM)	10-20 (IV) UK (SC) 30-60 (IM)	3-4 (IV)[a,c] 3-4 (SC) 3-4 (IM)	5
Pentazocine[k] (Talwin)	60 mg	180 mg	15-30 (PO) 5 (IV) 15-20 (SC) 15-20 (IM)	60-180 (PO) 15 (IV) 60 (SC) 60 (IM)	3-4 (PO) 3-4 (IV)[a,c] 3-4 (SC) 3-4 (IM)	2-3

Modified from McCaffery M., Pasero C. (1999). *Pain: Clinical manual* (pp. 241-243). St. Louis: Mosby.
ATC, Around-the-clock; *CR,* oral controlled-release; *hr,* hour; *IM,* intramuscular; *IV,* intravenous; μg, microgram; *mg,* milligram; *min,* minute; *NR,* not recommended; *NS,* nasal spray; *OT,* oral transmucosal; *PO,* oral; *R,* rectal; *SC,* subcutaneous; *SL,* sublingual; *TD,* transdermal; *UK,* unknown.
[g]In opioid-tolerant clients converted from continuous IV hydromorphone to continuous IV methadone, start with 10% to 25% of the equianalgesic dose.
[h]In opioid-tolerant clients converted to methadone, start PO dosing PRN with 10% to 25% of the equianalgesic dose.
[i]As in OxyContin (oxycodone), for example.
[j]65-130 mg = approximately one-sixth of all doses listed in this chart.
[k]Used in combination with mu agonists, may reverse analgesia and precipitate withdrawal in opioid-dependent clients.
[l]In opioid-naïve clients who are taking occasional mu agonists, such as codeine or oxycodone, the addition of butorphanol nasal spray may provide additive analgesia. However, in opioid-tolerant clients, such as those receiving ATC morphine, the addition of butorphanol nasal spray should be avoided because it may reverse analgesia and precipitate withdrawal.

BOX 22-6 *Naloxone Administration*[a,b]

1. Patients who require naloxone (Narcan) usually meet all of the following criteria:
   - Unresponsive to physical stimulation
   - Shallow respirations or respiratory rate <8 breaths/min
   - Pinpoint pupils
2. Stop the administration of the opioid and any other sedative drugs. If given IV, maintain IV access.
3. Summon help. Ask a co-worker to prepare naloxone (see No. 4) and bring it to you. Remain with the patient and continue to attempt to arouse him or her.
4. Mix 0.4 mg (1 ampule) of naloxone and 10 ml of normal saline in a syringe for IV administration.[c]
5. Administer the dilute naloxone solution IV[d] very slowly (0.5 ml over 2 min)[e] while you observe the patient's response (titrate to effect).
6. The patient should open his or her eyes and talk to you within 1 to 2 minutes. If not, continue IV naloxone at the same rate up to a total of 0.8 mg or 20 ml of dilute nalox-

one. If no response, begin looking for other causes of sedation and respiratory depression.

7. Discontinue the naloxone administration as soon as the patient is responsive to physical stimulation and able to take deep breaths when told to do so. Keep the syringe nearby. Another dose of naloxone may be needed as early as 30 minutes after the first dose because the duration of naloxone is shorter than the duration of most opioids.
8. Assign a staff member to monitor sedation and respiratory status and to remind the patient to deep breathe every 1 to 2 minutes until the patient becomes more alert.
9. Notify the primary physician and pain service. Document your actions.
10. Provide a nonopioid for pain relief.
11. Resume opioid administration at one-half the original dose when the patient is easily aroused and respiratory rate is >9 breaths/min.

May be duplicated for use in clinical practice. From McCaffery M, Pasero C: *Pain: Clinical manual,* p. 270. Copyright © 1999, Mosby.
Data from American Pain Society. (1992). *Principles of analgesic use in the treatment of acute and cancer pain* (3rd ed.). Glenview, IL: Author, Brimacombe, J., et al. (1991). Two cases of naloxone-induced pulmonary oedema: The possible use of phentolamine in management. *Anesthesia and Intensive Care, 19*(4), 578-580; Deglin, J.H., & Vallerand, A.H. (1995). *Davis' drug guide.* Philadelphia: F.A. Davis; Passero, C., & McCaffery, M. (1994). Preventing and managing opioid induced respiratory depression. *American Journal of Nursing, 94*(4), 25-31; Reisine, T., & Pasternak, G. (1996). Opioid analgesics and antagonists. In J.G. Hardman & L.E. Limbird (Eds.). *Goodman & Gilman's the pharmacological basis of therapeutics* (9th ed.). New York: McGraw-Hill.

Box 22-6 provides the recommended titrate-to-effect procedure for administering naloxone (Narcan) to reverse clinically significant respiratory depression. Giving too much naloxone or giving it too fast can precipitate severe pain, which is extremely difficult to control, and increase sympathetic activity leading to hypertension, tachycardia, ventricular dysrhythmias, pulmonary edema, and cardiac arrest. In physically dependent patients withdrawal syndrome can be precipitated; patients who have been receiving opioids for more than 1 week may be exquisitely sensitive to antagonists.

[a]For infants and children, follow the same procedure outlined in Box 22-6, with the following exceptions: (1) Respiratory rate that requires naloxone will vary according to infant's/child's usual rate; (2) Naloxone dose for children weighing >40 kg, follow dosing recommendations in Box 22-6, for children weighing <40 kg, dilute 0.1 mg naloxone in 10 ml of saline to make a 10 μg/ml solution. Administer IV at 0.5 μg/kg every 2 minutes until desired effect is achieved.

[b]Physicians' orders for opioids should include an order for naloxone administration according to APS recommendations, or a protocol incorporating the APS recommendations can be adopted for use by any nurse who suspects a patient is experiencing clinically significant opioid-induced respiratory depression.

[c]If naloxone is available only in a prefilled syringe, 10 ml of saline can be drawn into a 12 ml syringe, leaving enough room to accept the transfer of naloxone from the prefilled syringe. This procedure would ensure correct dilution.

[d]If IV route is inaccessible, administer undiluted naloxone, 0.4 mg, subcutaneously or intramuscularly. The patient should respond within 5 minutes. If not, repeat dose up to a total of 2 mg.

[e]This is the recommended amount and rate for administering naloxone to reverse opioid-induced respiratory depression. Administering a larger amount in a shorter period of time than this risks reversing more than opioid-induced respiratory depression (e.g., analgesia).

Nausea and Vomiting. Opioids may precipitate nausea and vomiting because of their action on the brain stem centers. Morphine-like medications also affect the vestibular system, which can produce these manifestations. Changing the type of opioid used may eliminate the side effect. Antiemetic agents may also be administered. This side effect decreases with analgesic use. Clients should not be denied pain relief because of this effect. Instead, they should receive treatment for the nausea and vomiting until it subsides.

Respiratory Depression. Respiratory depression is caused by diminished sensitivity of the respiratory center

to carbon dioxide. All opioids have the potential to produce respiratory depression, which can be rapidly reversed with an opioid antagonist, typically naloxone. The reaction is relatively rare, occurring primarily following the initial doses of opioid among those who never received the medication or whose last dose was a long time ago. It rarely occurs in awake individuals.[5]

This potential for respiratory depression should not discourage the proper use of opioids to reduce and/or relieve pain in people of all ages. The development of respiratory depression is not necessarily dose-related. Most clients do not respond with depressed respiratory rates regardless of dose. Another person may react with decreased respiration to relatively small doses. Rather than limit the use of opioid analgesics, carefully assess and reassess each client after giving the medication for the occurrence of respiratory depression. Because sedation precedes respiratory depression, sedation scales should be used to assess and reassess clients.

Deaths that occur secondary to opioid overdose are usually due to respiratory depression and usually occur in people who have not received opioids in the past. With morphine, maximal respiratory depression usually occurs within 15 minutes of IV administration, within 30 minutes of intramuscular (IM) administration, within 90 minutes of subcutaneous (SC) administration, and within 4 to 12 hours of epidural administration. Remember these time ranges when assessing the respiratory status following administration of opioids. For an overdose to occur, however, doses well above the therapeutic level would have to be given. Accumulated doses, especially in clients with liver or renal failure and in older clients, can cause an overdose.

It is also important to clearly diagnose respiratory depression. The presence of pain may result in increased respiratory rates among clients taking frequent, shallow breaths. Providing an opioid may relieve the pain, allowing one's respiratory pattern to return to a more normal breathing pattern. A respiratory rate of 30 breaths/min may be reduced to 15. Such a decrease has been interpreted as medication-caused respiratory depression, and the pain reduction and/or relief achieved has been reversed by naloxone administration. Assess respiratory depression in conjunction with normal functioning rather than the decrease in breaths per minute. Is the resulting respiratory rate life-threatening?

Treatment of respiratory depression includes arousing the client, establishing a patent airway, administering an opioid antagonist such as naloxone, and providing artificial ventilation as necessary.

Circulatory Depression. In some clients, circulatory depression may produce hypotension.[30] In a supine client, therapeutic dosages of morphine or synthetic opioids have little effect on blood pressure and cardiac rate or rhythm. However, some people experience orthostatic hypotension when moving from a supine position to a head-up or standing position. This hypotension is secondary to a direct dilating action on the peripheral blood vessels, caused by the opioids, which reduces the capacity of the cardiovascular system to respond to gravitational shifts. Advise the client to avoid abrupt body position changes. For this reason, opioids are used cautiously in people with reduced blood volume, because the effect is more pronounced. Increasing fluid volume decreases the orthostatic changes.

Cutaneous Effects. Opioid medications may facilitate histamine release resulting in pruritus, flushing, and sweating. The client becomes tolerant to this effect with repeated administration of the opioid.[40] In the meantime, the clinical manifestations may be alleviated by ingestion of antihistamines.

Urinary Retention. Urinary retention may occur as the result of the increase in smooth muscle tone of the detrusor muscle of the bladder and the bladder sphincter.[33] The hypertoned muscle fibers resist opening and prevent adequate bladder emptying. Urinary retention and urgency may result, necessitating catheterization.

Adjuvant Medications. Adjuvants are medications developed for other conditions but they also have pain-reducing properties. Adjuvant medications may be used in combination with analgesics or may be used alone. A wide variety of medications can be classified as adjuvant analgesics.[5] Tricyclic antidepressants (TCAs), such as amitriptyline (Elavil), are effective for neuropathic pain. They can be given daily at bedtime so that the drowsiness associated with them promotes sleep. Other effective medications for neuropathic pain are phenytoin (Dilantin), carbamazepine (Tegretol), and gabapentin (Neurontin). Nerve compression and bone pain may respond to dexamethasone (Decadron). Muscle relaxants, such as baclofen (Lioresal) and diazepam (Valium), are used to treat muscle spasm associated with pain.

TCAs are used with opiates and anticonvulsants for the treatment of neuropathic pain. Phenothiazines are not appropriate for pain relief. They are good antiemetics, but, when given for pain, phenothiazines simply increase sedation, hypotension, and respiratory depression. A phenothiazine such as promethazine (Phenergan) should never be used for pain relief. Promethazine actually *increases* the perception of pain.[59]

Antidepressants. TCAs contribute to pain relief via the descending pain inhibitory system by blocking cellular reuptake of serotonin and epinephrine. They may also potentiate the effect of opiates at synapses and increase their plasma bioavailability. The analgesic effect occurs with doses lower than needed to produce an antidepressant effect. TCAs are used to enhance pain reduction and/or relief regardless of a depression diagnosis. However, relief of depression in clinically depressed clients with pain is a positive outcome. TCAs can be given as a single daily dose at bedtime or in divided doses. Analgesic effects usually begin within a week of initiation of the TCA.

Anti-Anxiety Agents. Drugs such as diazepam and chlordiazepoxide (Librium) are believed to mediate pain by contributing to Cl^- channel opening. Movement of Cl^- ions hyperpolarizes the postsynaptic membrane, making it less receptive to incoming nociceptive stimuli. Diazepam is particularly effective for relief of painful muscle spasm.

Anticonvulsants. Anticonvulsant agents are used in situations associated with nerve injury. Nerve fibers may generate electrical activity at the site of injury causing the nerve membrane to fire with a pain-producing signal. Agents such as phenytoin (Dilantin), gabapentin (Neurontin), topiramate (Topamax), tiagabine (Gabitril), and zonisamide (Zonegran), which stabilize the membrane, help prevent the ectopic generation of pain-producing activity, resulting in lancinating, shooting, shock-like pain.

Corticosteroids. These drugs are used to facilitate relief for various types of pain. In the periphery, they reduce edema and inflammation, reducing the compression caused by swelling and the availability of chemical mediators of nociception. They may also inhibit the production of prostaglandins and leukotrienes. In the CNS, they function similarly to anti-anxiety agents by modifying the flow of Cl^- ions. Corticosteroids provide pain reduction and/or relief from bony metastasis of cancer.

Local Anesthetic Agents. Local anesthetics, when administered orally, are membrane stabilizers that produce analgesia by suppressing aberrant electrical activity in central neurons or peripheral axons. Membrane-stabilizing agents include mexiletine (Mexitil), lidocaine, bupivacaine, and tocainide (Tonocard). These agents appear to be effective against lancinating and continuous neuropathic pain. They operate to inactivate Na^+ or K^+ channels, preventing generation of the electrical pain-producing signal. Membrane-stabilizing agents are used primarily for their antidysrhythmic effect, and clients with heart disease must be carefully assessed before these medications are started.

Miscellaneous Agents. *Baclofen,* a gamma-aminobutyric acid (GABA) antagonist, is used as an analgesic for lancinating or paroxysmal neuropathic pain. *Capsaicin* is a topical medication that depletes peptides (such as substance P) in small primary afferent neurons that mediate nociceptive transmission. It appears useful for postherpetic neuralgia and for postmastectomy pain in some clients.

Factors Influencing the Effectiveness of Analgesics

Relative Analgesic Potency. Relative analgesic potency refers to the ratio of the doses of two analgesics required to produce the same effect. Analgesics are compared with therapeutic doses of morphine. Estimates of relative analgesic potency provide a basis for prescribing the dose when the client is being switched from one analgesic to another or from one route of administration to another. The route used to provide pain reduction and/or relief affects the potency of the medication.

The availability of the analgesic is determined in part by the events encountered before the drug enters the circulatory system. Orally administered medications must be dissolved in stomach contents and absorbed by the gut before the agent can contribute to pain reduction and/or relief. Using the IM or SC routes necessitates that the medication be absorbed from muscle or subcutaneous tissues before it becomes available. IV medications enter the circulatory system directly. Oral and SC doses must be higher than IV doses. Doses are equally effective when equianalgesic dosing is used.

Duration of Action. The duration of action of an analgesic agent is the result of factors such as pain intensity, dose size, and the client's ability to absorb, biotransform, and eliminate the medication. The duration of action for the analgesics (see Table 22-7) is based on a dose that produces a peak effect equivalent to that of morphine. The time of peak effect and the duration of action of a particular opioid vary with the route of administration. For instance, the peak analgesic effect of IV morphine occurs between 15 minutes and 40 minutes after administration. The peak analgesic effect of orally administered morphine occurs from 2 to 12 hours after administration. The duration of action of orally administered opioids is usually somewhat longer than that of IM analgesics. *Duration* of analgesia may not be the same as the *effect* of analgesia. Learn about peak and duration of analgesic effect so that activities that might produce pain can be planned to coincide with peak periods of action. For example, if a client is scheduled for physical therapy at 10:00 AM, give pain medication that will reach its peak effect around 10:00 AM.

Several new forms of morphine have been developed. An oral liquid can be given for more rapid but short-acting effects. A controlled-release form is also available. With long-acting morphine, the onset is somewhat slower but the duration ranges from 8 to 12 hours. Fentanyl, which is available as a patch for transdermal delivery of medication, is effective for 48 to 72 hours. Fentanyl is also available for transmucosal delivery. Oral transmucosal fentanyl citrate is available in "lollipop" form. The medication is delivered systemically directly through the transmucosal route and partially by the amount of the medication that is swallowed.

Oral Potency. As opioids are absorbed from the intestine and pass through the liver and into the systemic circulation, they differ in the degree to which they are active. This difference in absorption accounts, in part, for the oral doses listed in Table 22-7 for various forms of oral morphine. Preparations with lower bioavailability require higher doses per pill. More recently developed forms of morphine have greater bioavailability, and therefore the dosages of these are lower than those of the older oral form. Opioids are available in various forms, with varying onset, peak effect, duration, and half-lives; become aware of these variations. The different equianalgesic doses are based on a single dose of IV morphine (see Table 22-7). An equianalgesic dose is expected to provide the same degree of pain reduction and/or relief as the single IV morphine dose. Dose requirements may decrease after the client has received a loading dose. Failure of health care providers to recognize differences in the oral and intramuscular potencies of opioids and the concept of equianalgesic doses can lead to undertreatment of a person's pain.

Administration of Analgesics

Principles of administration of analgesics are listed in Box 22-7. The goal of analgesic administration is to provide pain reduction and/or relief while maintaining the ability of the client to be in control of the environment, participate in care, and reduce side effects. Assessment of the client before and after analgesic administration is necessary to ensure safe and adequate pain reduction and/or relief. Assess the following factors before analgesic administration:

- Medication allergies or sensitivities
- Previous response to analgesics
- Other medications being taken
- Body weight
- Individual pain experience
- Age, general state of health, mental status
- Cardiac, respiratory, renal, hepatic, and CNS status

Allergies or Sensitivities to Medications. Before administering an analgesic such as morphine, ensure that the client does not have a history of untoward reactions to the medication. When possible, ask the client or significant others, and review the chart or other documentation for such information. Allergies to opioids are rare and clients often consider side effects to be allergies.

Concomitant Medications. Clients taking monoamine oxidase (MAO) inhibitor antidepressants should not receive meperidine. Medications that cause sedation, constipation, or orthostatic hypotension must also be considered when the client is receiving opioids.

Body Weight. The standard morphine dose is 10 mg parenterally. This dose produces satisfactory analgesia in approximately 70% of people with moderate to severe postoperative pain. The analgesic effect is dose-related. Analgesics tend to be prescribed according to a standard protocol applied to all clients with similar disease, however, rather than being based on physical characteristics, including body weight. Therefore the standard dose may be too high for small adults and too low for obese adults. One cannot assume that the standard dose will produce adequate pain relief in all adults. Routinely assess degree of pain relief to ensure that adequate doses are being delivered.

BOX 22-7	*Principles of Pharmaceutical Pain Management*

- Provide medications in adequate doses.
- Utilize a preventive approach to pain relief. Predictable and chronic pain is managed more effectively if the client maintains a therapeutic blood level of analgesics. Use around-the-clock dosing with rescue medication available.
- Closely assess clients with particular diligence with first doses or when the medication dose or the type is changed.
- Medication doses are specific as to type and route. For example, the dose for an oral preparation is higher than that for an intravenous dose of the same medication.
- Combinations of analgesics may be more effective than those given singularly.
- Additions of adjuvant medications enhance pain relief produced by analgesics and are not intended to replace analgesics.
- Understand and be prepared to treat side effects of medications.
- Do not consider avoidance of non–life-threatening side effects (such as constipation, nausea, pruritus) more important than providing pain relief. These concomitant conditions are easily treated.
- Recognize that respiratory depression is a rare occurrence, occurring most commonly among clients who are sedated.

Respiratory depression rarely occurs after the first few doses of an opioid.
- Asking for pain medication reflects the need for pain relief in 99.9% of people with pain and does not reflect an addictive personality.
- Do not use placebos for pain. The placebo response usually indicates that the responder has an effective endogenous opiate system and had obtained opiate-mediated pain relief.
- Believe the client's report of pain.
- Maintain a therapeutic relationship that facilitates mutual trust. Your attitudes and beliefs do affect the client's ability to respond to pain management strategies.
- Incorporate the goal of total pain relief into the pain management regimen for most clients.
- Operate as a team to provide the most effective pain relief outcomes. Include the client and significant others in pain interventions, allowing the client to maintain an adequate degree of personal control in the experience.
- *Only the client, and no one else, can determine the amount of pain experienced. There is no objective indicator of pain that can be observed by another.*

Individual Differences. Given the multitude of factors that contribute to any one person's pain experience, the characteristics of one client's pain may differ from those of another client. It is not possible to design a pain management regimen that will be equally effective for all people with similar pathologic processes. For example, a person's age determines, to some extent, the length of time during which an analgesic will be effective. Age may influence the amount of relief obtained from medications. While there is most likely little difference in the ability of the CNS of an older adult to respond to stimuli, decreases in muscle mass, increases in gastric pathology, and changes in circulatory characteristics may result in a decreased ability to absorb and utilize analgesics. An older person tends to receive pain reduction and/or relief from an opioid for a longer time compared with a younger person. This difference in duration of action may relate to the speed with which an opioid is cleared from the body. Opioid clearance is faster in younger people than in older people.

People with debilitating diseases, regardless of age, also have a heightened sensitivity to the effects of opioids. Because of individual differences in responses to pain medications, you must become diligent in assessing the client's responses to the medications.

Body System Assessment. Because all analgesics have the potential to produce mild to severe side effects, it is important to assess a client's cardiac, respiratory, renal, and CNS status before administering analgesics. Hepatic function is also assessed because of the important role of the liver in detoxifying analgesics. The presence of increased intracranial pressure is cause for concern. The physician typically conducts a body system assessment before ordering a specific medication regimen. You must report changes in physical status that may place the client at risk if given the analgesic. The physician may then determine that an alternative regimen is needed.

Methods of Administration

Nurse-Administered (Demand) Analgesia. The traditional method of treating pain is by nurse-administered pain medication on a schedule, or on a *prn* (as needed) basis. This system does the following:

- Allows you to assess the pain and evaluate effectiveness of the medication
- Facilitates your ability to detect or avoid untoward reactions or side effects
- Permits dose adjustment

However, pain is often significantly undertreated with the prn system. Undertreatment may occur because (1) nurses assume authority for pain management, including determination of the amount of pain experienced by the client, and (2) the nurse, client, or significant others are overconcerned about possible opioid side effects and

fear inducing opioid addiction. The concern about negative effects of pain results in medications ordered in inadequate doses in overly long intervals. When given a range of doses over a range of times, nurses tend to give the smallest dose over the longest time.

The primary inhibitory factor is couched in the belief by the nurse that he or she is in the best position to determine pain medication needs. However, studies have shown that nurses routinely underestimate the amount of pain being experienced. Because there is no objective indicator of pain, the only one who can determine pain medication needs is the client. Nurses who have been taught to treat medication-seeking behavior as a sign of addiction may be uncomfortable with this situation. The problem is particularly severe when medications are ordered on a prn basis. We have typically interpreted the order as "when the client asks for medication." When the client does ask, our fears about addictive personalities surface and the client is seen as medication-seeking and may be labeled as a potential addict. The situation is especially severe when the client is young or belongs to a social or ethnic group devalued by the nurse.

Asking for nonscheduled medications is often the only means provided to clients to obtain pain medications. In most cases, the request is based on need for pain relief and nothing else. Clients must be valued and believed in order to receive adequate pain relief. The prn system also deprives the client of the ability to control the situation. Lack of control over pain experiences increases the pain endured during the episode. The pain may be worsened by anxiety about whether the next dose will be given in time to prevent the return of severe pain.

Intermittent dosing, such as occurs with prn medication orders, causes wide swings in the client's blood levels of the analgesic, which may result in sedation following one dose and unacceptable pain levels preceding the next dose. The prn dosing leads to a "hill and valley" pattern of pain relief. Clients receive a dose of medication sufficient to produce adequate pain relief. They are then expected to wait until the pain is again intense before asking for the subsequent dose.

We have been encouraged by values germane to our work environment to encourage clients to hold out as long as they can so as not to risk addition and undesirable side effects. The hill and valley approach requires that each succeeding dose be maximum strength to bring the client's blood level back to a therapeutic level. Pain relief is more efficiently and effectively achieved if the valleys are avoided. If the prn schedule is to be maintained, clients need to be encouraged to request pain medication when their pain begins to return. This problem is lessened if prn medications are offered on a regular, scheduled basis for clients with acute pain. If the medication is administered regularly, by the clock, pain relief is enhanced.

Patient-Controlled Analgesia. Patient-controlled analgesia (PCA) entails use of an IV or SC infusion pump that contains the analgesic and that is controlled by the client. A bolus dose may be given at the onset of PCA use to provide immediate pain relief. The client can then self-administer subsequent doses by pressing a button that releases a preset dose delivered intravenously. The pumps are programmed to deliver preset demand doses of analgesic until a maximum dose is reached. Then there is a minimal interval during which no further analgesic can be administered (i.e., a lock-out period). With this system, clients control the administration of their own pain medication within the limits prescribed by the physician.

There are many advantages to PCA:

1. The client usually reports good pain control.
2. PCA helps to relieve the client's anxiety about waiting for the nurse to administer the medication, thereby lowering the dose needed to reduce and/or relieve pain.
3. PCA promotes the client's independence and control over the situation.
4. Clients administer lower doses of opioids compared with traditional prn formats.
5. Clients can adjust their analgesic doses to a near-constant blood concentration.
6. Clients report superior analgesia with a lower incidence of side effects compared with the traditional nurse-administered method.
7. As the pain lessens, clients adjust to lower doses and eventually stop taking the analgesic.

Some problems are associated with PCA. Some clients complain of inadequate analgesia at night, requiring frequent wakening to redose themselves. At some institutions, a basal rate is added at night by continuous delivery at a low but constant dose through the PCA pump to avoid this situation. Frequent assessment by the nurse is necessary for the success of PCA. The success of this method depends on one's understanding of the system and on how well the client is taught to use it. Failure can often be traced to a poor understanding on the part of the client, the nurse, or both.

Oral Route. Oral (PO) dosing is usually preferred. It is noninvasive, convenient, and cost-effective and allows for the greatest flexibility in medication choices. Oral preparations may be in tablet, capsule, liquid, or sublingual forms. Some tablet preparations can be crushed and added to suspensions (e.g., to applesauce) that are more easily swallowed. Oral opioids are available in immediate and sustained-release forms. Sustained-release medications are designed to be metabolized slowly in the gastrointestinal system and must not be crushed or modified. The entire dose is released at one time if the integrity of the tablet is compromised. The peak effect of oral medications is 1½ to 2 hours for immediate-release

preparations. Availability of the medication is delayed until the tablet is degraded and the medication is absorbed, passed through the liver, and made available to the circulatory system.

Intramuscular Route. *IM dosing is common but is the least desirable route and should be avoided.* IM injections are painful, and some people find the injections so objectionable that they are reluctant to seek relief for their pain if the medications are to be administered this way. Additional disadvantages include wide variability and unreliable absorption from muscle and subcutaneous tissues. Peak effects occur within 30 to 60 minutes and are accompanied by a rapid "fall-off" of medication effectiveness. Additional side effects of IM injections include *trauma-induced fibrosis of muscle and soft tissues, nerve damage from chemical injury, and development of sterile abscesses.*[3]

Intravenous Route. IV dosing provides the most rapid pain reduction and/or relief. Medications may be provided in bolus doses or by continuous infusions. Bolus doses are given in one administration and provide the most rapid onset of pain reduction and/or relief. Bolus hydromorphone reaches peak effect in 5 to 15 minutes, morphine in 15 to 20 minutes.[3] Continuous infusion provides a steady delivery of IV pain medication. It is usually preferred because plasma levels of the medication are maintained and the occurrence of side effects is lessened. Bolus doses may be needed if pain relief falls below acceptable levels with continuous infusion. The infusion dose may then need to be increased to maintain adequate relief.

Rectal Route. Rectal suppositories provide an alternative route to parenteral administration for people unable to take oral medications. They are provided in doses similar to those of oral preparations. Medications appropriate for the rectal route include morphine, hydromorphone (Dilaudid), oxycodone, and methadone.

Transdermal Route. Transdermal analgesia is provided by means of a skin patch. The most common opioid administered transdermally is fentanyl, which is potent. It is available in a variable-dosing transdermal application system that the client or family member can apply independently. The patch delivers specified amounts of medication over 48 to 72 hours. This system provides an easy means of maintaining independence and avoids the inconveniences of frequent dosing.

Analgesia from the first application may take up to 24 hours to reach an adequate blood level. During this period, supplemental analgesia is maintained. The patch is typically applied to clean, dry skin on the chest or upper back. These areas are less vulnerable than other areas to dislodgment of the patch. The patch may be applied to any convenient location with intact skin as long as the client can protect it. Excessive hair should be carefully clipped, not shaved, before application. The patch should not be applied over irritated or broken skin. The patch is left in place for up to 72 hours, and then is removed. A new patch is applied at a different site to prevent skin irritation.

Transmucosal Analgesia. Transmucosal analgesia is achieved either sublingually (methadone and buprenorphine [Buprenex]) or by means of a lozenge (Oralet) or a lollipop (Actiq). The transmucosal route is particularly effective for breakthrough pain in clients with scheduled opioid medications around the clock. Up to two thirds of clients with chronic or malignant pain who are treated around the clock with opioids have episodes of breakthrough pain.[46]

Continuous Subcutaneous Analgesia. Pain reduction and/or relief is achieved through an infusion setup using a pump device. A 25- or 27-gauge needle is used, or a special SC needle device can be implanted subcutaneously. The client wears a medication reservoir that can be refilled. The needle site is rotated every 3 to 7 days according to the type and volume of medication administered. The volume delivered ranges from 2 to 4 ml/hr.

Observe the site for redness, excessive swelling, leakage of fluid around the infusion site, or edema. If an extremity is used, carefully assess it for the presence of edema, which interferes with absorption of the medication. Closely monitor the client for adequacy of analgesic effect. If the medication is ineffective and sufficient medication is available in the reservoir, a higher concentration may be required.

Intraspinal and Epidural Analgesia. Opioids are injected intrathecally or epidurally. The epidural space is outside the dura mater of the spinal cord and brain; the intrathecal (spinal) space is inside the dura mater and contains the spinal fluid. The dorsal horns of the spinal cord contain receptors for endogenous opioid substances. By means of the intraspinal analgesia route, medication is delivered directly into the areas with the intended receptor sites. These receptors bind opioids and provide excellent pain reduction and/or relief of long duration (8 to 24 hours) without causing sympathetic and motor nerve blockade. Relatively small doses provide high opioid concentrations in the spinal fluid that bathes the dorsal columns. These concentrations are far higher than those in the spinal fluid after similar doses given by standard parenteral routes. Local anesthetics can be combined with opioids, thus using multiple pain pathways.

Repeated bolus doses, PCA, or a constant infusion via an implanted refillable infusion pump of the opioid may be given through a small catheter placed in the epidural or intrathecal space. Catheters have been left in place for days to months without adverse effects.

Possible side effects include pruritus, urinary retention, and delayed respiratory depression occurring 6 to 12 hours after a dose. Low doses of naloxone may reverse these side effects without reducing analgesia.

Nerve Blocks. Neuroblockade is achieved through injection of various substances (e.g., local anesthetics) close to the nerves, thereby blocking their conductivity. Blockade may be used to produce a complete, reversible interruption of nerve pathways for the following purposes:

- To eliminate a local focus of pain-producing stimulation or nervous irritation
- To interrupt the perception of pain, either at the source of the pain or anywhere along the peripheral afferent neurons
- To interrupt reflex mechanisms that are maintaining abnormal activity in blood vessels, glands, or skeletal or smooth muscle
- To eliminate reflex responses to pain (e.g., tachycardia, hypertension) by directly infiltrating skeletal muscle and other involved structures

Irreversible nerve-blocking procedures, which permanently block the pain pathway, are often used in managing pain associated with cancer. The effect of the block may be short-lived, however. The nerves may regenerate to some extent, with an associated return of sensory and motor functions.

Nerve blocks given for pain relief are called *analgesic blocks*. The analgesia is generally produced by injection of a local anesthetic agent. The anesthetic agent relieves pain and thus allows treatment that might otherwise be extremely uncomfortable, such as manipulation of a painful joint or wound debridement. Sometimes, by interrupting reflexes that are causing sustained pain, analgesic blocks can produce a beneficial effect that is prolonged beyond the effective duration of the agent injected.

Analgesic blocks are useful in various acute and chronic disorders. They often reduce the amounts of analgesic medication that might otherwise be needed. Injecting local anesthetics into tender points of muscle or skin *(trigger point injection)* causes a type of analgesic block that may modify pain and break the pain cycle, allowing manipulation and stretching of a joint. However, the pain may not be permanently eliminated unless the primary afferent impulses are either chemically or surgically terminated or until the underlying pathologic condition causing the pain is corrected.

Clients with Addictive Disease

Clients with addictive disease or who are in recovery often receive less than optimal pain relief due in part to the value judgments by health professionals. These persons may be involved in more acute pain episodes due to

---

BOX 22-8 *Recommendations for All Patients with Addictive Disease*

- Identify and use resources available to assist with the diagnosis and treatment of both addiction and pain.
- Encourage the patient to use support systems (e.g., family, significant others, or rehabilitation sponsor); offer additional resources (e.g., addictions counselor).
- Involve the patient in pain management planning and, with the patient's consent, include family and significant others.
- Provide the patient with verbal and written information about the pain management plan, including what the patient can expect from caregivers and what the patient's responsibilities are.
- Ensure consistency in the implementation of the pain management plan.
- Educate the patient, family, and significant others about the differences between addiction, physical dependence, and tolerance.
- Help the patient make informed choices about medications by educating the patient, family, and significant others about medication options.
- Select and titrate analgesics based on pain assessment, side effects, and function, as well as sleep and mood.

- Be prepared to titrate opioid analgesics and benzodiazepines to doses higher than usual. The patient may have developed tolerance to some medications, or drug use may have caused increased sensitivity to pain.
- Benzodiazepines, phenothiazines, or other sedating medications that do not relieve pain should not be used as substitutes for analgesics.
- If pain is present most of the time, provide analgesics around-the-clock (ATC).
- Use the oral route and long acting analgesics when possible.
- Consider the use of IV or epidural patient-controlled analgesia (PCA) for acute pain management.
- Record and discuss with the patient any behavior suggestive of inappropriate medication use, especially of controlled substances.
- When opioids, benzodiazepines, or other medications with a potential for physical dependence are no longer needed, taper them very slowly to minimize the emergence of withdrawal symptoms.
- Consider nonpharmacological methods of treatment for pain but do not use them in place of appropriate pharmacological approaches.

Reprinted with permission of the American Society of Pain Management Nurses, 7794 Grow Drive, Pensacola, FL 32514. Copyright 2002. American Society of Pain Management Nurses.

---

increased traumatic events, such as injuries. Persons with addictive disease are often challenging to staff who are struggling to advocate for pain relief. However, clients with addictive disease have the right to be treated with respect and to receive the same quality of pain management as all other clients. Nurses are in an ideal position to advocate and intervene for these clients across all treatment settings."[6] Box 22-8 lists recommendations for all clients with addictive disease and recommendations for clients in recovery.

NONPHARMACEUTICAL INTERVENTIONS

Activities such as cutaneous stimulation, acupuncture, acupressure, massage, listening to music, progressive relaxation, guided imagery, rhythmic breathing, meditation, hypnosis, humor, biofeedback, Therapeutic Touch, distraction, and magnets have been used clinically with positive results. The therapies are thought to cause physiologic changes. For example, peripheral blood vessels may be dilated, muscle tension is decreased, the immune system is strengthened, and brain chemicals are activated or modified. Techniques such as these can be used to manage pain and to promote healthy living. It may be possible to teach clients a combination of these techniques to maximize their opportunities for self-control

over manifestations of pain. Figure 22-11 presents modalities for pain reduction and/or relief.

Cutaneous Stimulation
Cutaneous stimulation activates the large-diameter (A-beta) fibers, which stimulate inhibitory neurons in the spinal cord and engage the descending analgesic system. Pain reduction and/or relief is achieved by endogenous opiate activity.

Cutaneous stimulation can decrease the intensity of pain the client perceives and, in some instances, may eliminate it.[37] It also can help in changing the sensation in a painful or noxious area to a more pleasant sensation, such as warmth. This process may also be seen as a form of distraction because the client may focus on the sensation being created rather than the pain. Cutaneous stimulation can be applied to the unaffected side and still elicit positive benefits because the stimulated fibers cross within the spinal cord. This method is particularly useful when an area is too painful to be directly stimulated, as with burns.

Transcutaneous Electrical Nerve Stimulation
Transcutaneous electrical nerve stimulation (TENS) delivers electrical bursts through the skin to superficial and deep nerves. TENS is used most often for clients with chronic pain, such as muscle pain from arthritis.

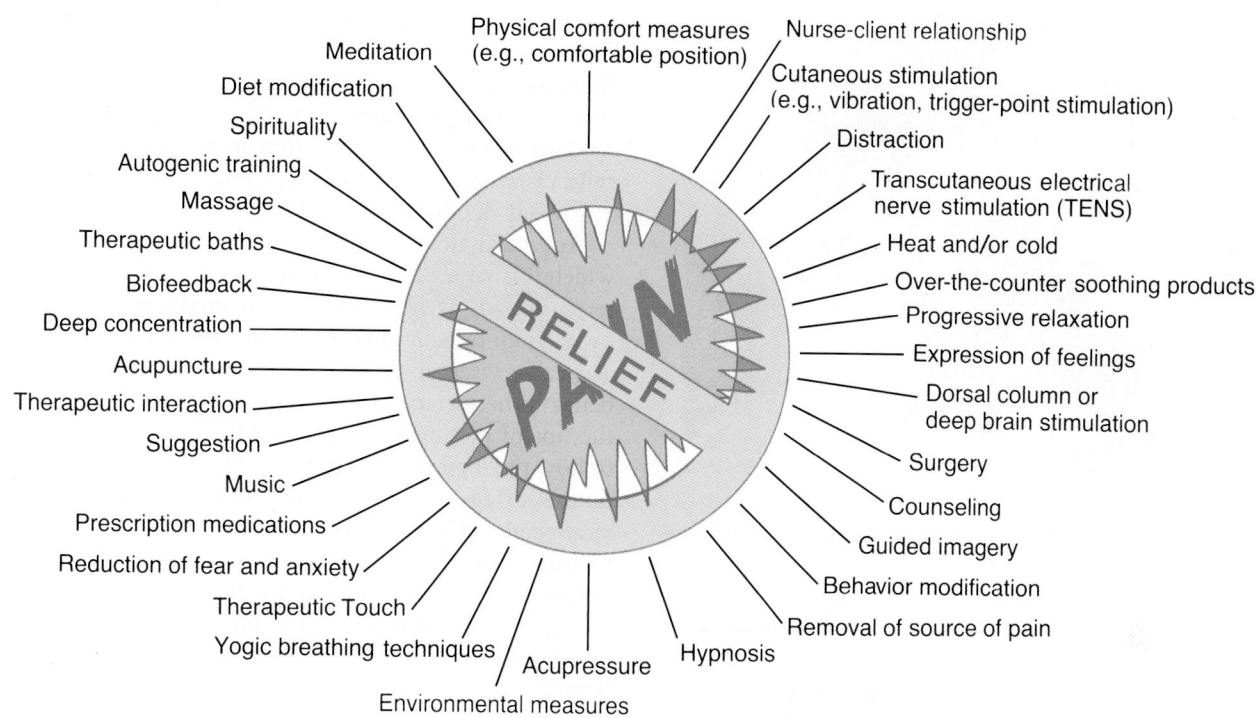

FIGURE 22-11 Measures of pain relief and/or reduction.

TENS has been shown to reduce and/or relieve pain effectively in many people.[61] Success with TENS depends on the client's understanding of, interest in, and motivation to use the apparatus as well as the clinician's skillfulness in applying the device. The client needs to learn to adjust placement of the surface electrodes and the intensity and timing of the stimuli to maximize pain reduction and/or relief (Figure 22-12). Involve significant others as appropriate in learning and teaching sessions. The client may need their help in applying the electrodes to areas that are difficult to reach. Electrode placement depends on the site of the pain. Positive and negative poles are usually placed within several inches of each other. Voltage and pulsation are controlled by the person wearing the device. Battery packs make the device portable.

Massage

Massage may be effective when applied to various sites. A back rub is a good method of providing cutaneous stimulation (Figure 22-13). It is particularly relaxing at bedtime and may block pain so as to promote more comfortable sleep. However, you should be knowledgeable in massage techniques so as not to increase discomfort; for example, too deep or rough massaging may actually increase a client's pain. A nurse administers a massage by stimulating the client's skin by lightly kneading, pulling, or pressing with fingers, palms or knuckles.

Foot massage is particularly helpful and cost-effective. The feet are easily accessible, and the intervention can be applied to people in any body position.

FIGURE 22-12 Surface patches are used for transcutaneous electrical nerve stimulation (TENS) treatment.

FIGURE 22-13 Back rub provides cutaneous sensation to reduce pain.

Heat and Cold Applications

Cold and *warmth receptors* that activate A-beta fibers respond to changes in skin temperature. Temperature changes adequate to provide pain reduction and/or relief are within 4 to 5 degrees of body temperature. Stimuli that feel cool or warm are sufficient to engage A-beta fibers. The receptors are rapidly adapting, requiring that the temperature be readjusted at frequent intervals ranging from 5 to 15 minutes.

Heat is an excellent means of pain reduction and/or relief that is amenable to nursing autonomy. Warm applications may be achieved by warming devices (e.g., heating pads, warming towels). In the clinical setting, warm applications may be achieved by warming damp disposable bed pads in the microwave. Incontinence pads can be cut to desired sizes, are inexpensive, and are disposable. Take care to avoid heat temperatures that will burn. Remember, painful areas may be hypersensitive to skin stimuli. Heat temperatures that are typically perceived as nonpainful may become painful when applied to the sensitive area.

Cold application also brings pain reduction and/or relief, and nurses can consider this treatment.[36] *Ice* may also be used to provide pain reduction and/or relief and to prevent or reduce edema and inflammation. The effectiveness of ice applications does not depend on A-beta fiber stimulation; however, ice decreases the conduction velocity of nociceptive nerve fibers, rendering the fiber incapable of transmitting the pain signal to the spinal cord. The client perceives the application area as numb.

Thermal stimuli are most effective when applied directly to the painful area. When direct application is not possible, relief may be achieved by applying the intervention to a point proximal or distal to the painful area. A cold compress wrapped around the wrist may alleviate pain in the hand.

Acupuncture

Acupuncture has been practiced in Asian cultures for centuries and produces pain reduction and/or relief in modern health care.[13] Very thin metal needles are skillfully inserted into the body at designated locations and at various depths and angles.

Approximately 1000 known acupuncture points are widely distributed over the surface of the body in patterns known as *meridians*. Each meridian contains its own group of acupuncture points and is associated with a specific visceral organ. Meridians run bilaterally just beneath the surface of the skin and begin or terminate at the tips of the fingers or toes. "Vital energy" is believed to flow through these meridians. The acupuncture points on the surface of the body provide external access to this vital energy. Through needle insertion at specific points, various physiologic processes can be influenced or controlled and are determined by the specific pathologic condition and the desired physiologic effect.

Acupressure

Acupressure is a noninvasive method of pain reduction and/or relief based on the principles of acupuncture.[25] Pressure, massage, or other cutaneous stimulation, such as heat or cold, is applied over acupuncture points.

Music

Music has been used to reduce or relieve pain in a number of settings.[17,27] The exact physiologic mechanisms have not been determined; however, several possible theories include distraction, release of endogenous opioids, or disassociation. All three mechanisms are probably involved. Music clearly provides distraction and disassociation by focusing on the characteristics of the musical selection. The auditory pathway interacts with endogenous opiate systems at several foci within the brain, including the hypothalamus and the limbic system. These areas are known to project to PAG/PVG, providing a mechanism to contribute to pain reduction and/or relief through both cerebral activity and spinal cord responses mediated by descending fibers from nucleus raphe and locus ceruleus. **EB**

People in pain may find music to be relaxing. Pain reduction and/or relief may also be achieved through physiologic responses to relaxation. The relaxation response is mediated through the hypothalamus.

When using music for pain reduction and/or relief, allow clients to choose the type of music most suited to them. Some people find the use of a radio, cassette, or compact disc players with headphones a quiet way to listen to music without bothering others. This allows the client to increase the music volume or to play it softly. Encourage the family members to bring in the client's favorite selections. This also gives the family a sense of doing something to help.

Progressive Relaxation Training

Progressive relaxation training is used to treat various physical and psychosocial problems, including pain. The client is taught to gradually tighten, then deeply relax, various muscle groups, proceeding systematically from one area of the body to the next. The deep relaxation produced by this method can decrease anxiety and excessive muscle contraction and promote the onset of sleep. Audiotape cassettes are available.

Deep Breathing for Relaxation

Deep breathing for relaxation is easy to learn and contributes to pain relief and/or reduction by reducing muscle tension and anxiety.[33] First, the client clenches the fists while taking a deep breath. The client then holds his or her breath for a moment, and exhales while letting oneself "go limp." The cycle is followed by a slow, deep breath mimicking a yawn.

Guided Imagery

Guided imagery helps a client visualize a pleasant experience. The client is coached to visualize a scene (e.g., relaxing on a beach). The coach instructs the client to imagine the sensory aspects of the scene: the sounds, sights, and emotions expressed. The more vivid the image, the more effective the intervention. Visualization may be combined with soft, lyrical, relaxing music. Audiotapes for guided imagery are available.

Imagery relieves pain through several mechanisms.[57] It is a way to help people distract themselves from their pain, which may increase their pain tolerance. Imagery may also produce a relaxation response, thus relieving pain. Last, the image can be a healing one, designed not only to relieve the pain but possibly to diminish the source of the pain[55] (e.g., a tension headache may be alleviated).

Imagery is often combined with relaxation and biofeedback to produce a multifocal technique for pain reduction and/or relief. The image used in this technique can be a complex scene that requires the person to think of each detail. This image would increase distraction. The image might be a relaxing scene, such as a beach or meadow, which would help with the relaxation response, or the image might consist of visualizing the pain being worn away until it is so small that it can be "blown away." When introducing an image setting, ask the client what setting is relaxing for him or her. Avoid using an image that may provoke anxiety, such as using a beach for someone who is afraid of water or a meadow for someone with severe allergies to pollen.

Rhythmic Breathing

Rhythmic breathing is typically considered a method of both relaxation and distraction. It may also provide effective pain reduction and/or relief by stimulating baroreceptors in the atria and carotid sinuses. Stimula-

tion of these receptors initiates activity in a neuropathway that sends projections to the periaqueductal and periventricular gray matter, resulting in opioid-mediated pain inhibition. This method can be combined with rhythms such as music, a ticking clock, or a metronome. Little concentration is necessary because once the individual begins the process, it takes on an automatic quality. This method focuses attention away from the pain and on the breathing and the rhythm. The Lamaze method of childbirth is a good example of a pain control method that incorporates this technique.

Meditation

Meditation focuses one's attention away from pain. It also provides energy and peace to the person who is meditating. The client simply sits comfortably and quietly with focused attention. The focus may vary. Examples include flow of the breath, a mantra, and a picture or mental image of a great spiritual being or peaceful place. Sometimes the person who is meditating communicates with a spiritual being. There are many meditation techniques, some with a spiritual base, such as Siddha meditation. Meditation is easily practiced anywhere, and no special equipment is required. The positive experiences available through meditation are available to anyone, including people in pain.

Hypnosis

A person's reaction to pain can be significantly altered by hypnosis. Hypnosis is based on suggestion, dissociation, and the process of focusing attention.[48]

Various procedures may be used to reduce pain following induction of a hypnotic state, including the following:

- Suggestion to alter the character of the pain or one's attitude toward it
- Body disorientation and dissociation
- Anesthesia and analgesia for superficial and deep sensation

In situations of chronic pain, a posthypnotic suggestion may be used in combination with *autohypnosis* (self-hypnosis) to provide prolonged relief. Many hypnotic subjects successfully learn to use deliberate spontaneous trance induction or autohypnosis.

Although hypnosis cannot change organic lesions that are producing pain, it can often reduce discomfort.[48] The procedure itself is fairly simple and innocuous compared with the administration of many anesthetic and analgesic medications; however, take care not to probe any fears or unpleasant memories. A hypnotherapist must be skilled and informed and the client carefully selected to avoid negative effects. Increasingly nurses are being certified to provide clinical hypnotic therapies in the United States.

Hypnosis may be used as an adjunct to other pain-relieving therapies. Alteration of pain by hypnosis should be performed by those who are aware of the possible diagnostic implications of pain in the medical management of disease.

Humor

Research in the use of humor in the clinical setting has revealed that the intervention actually increases the number of NK (natural killer) cells of the immune system.[32] This is particularly important for implementation in clients with cancer. It has been postulated that humor elevates endogenous opioids or endorphins. Regardless of the physiologic advantages, use of humor simply makes people feel better, more relaxed, and in less pain. Clients may find some degree of pain reduction and/or relief by watching comedic videotapes, listening to audiotapes and compact discs they find funny, or reading humorous books. The nurse might suggest that hospitalized clients bring humorous materials with them to use during their inpatient experience.

Biofeedback

Biofeedback refers to a wide variety of techniques that provide a client with information about changes in bodily functions of which the client is usually unaware, such as blood pressure. Biofeedback equipment provides immediate, continuous information. Some people learn to use this information to control previously involuntary functions. The purpose of biofeedback in pain management is to teach self-control over physiologic variables that relate to the pain, such as muscle contraction and blood flow.

Information used to reduce muscle contraction is obtained by an electromyogram (EMG) recorded from body surface electrodes. (Needle EMG electrodes are not used.) Changes in blood flow are produced by monitoring skin temperature, which increases with increased blood flow. Depending on the equipment used, clients can self-monitor their changes through *auditory displays* (decreases in muscle contractions are heard as decreases in the pitch of a tone) or *visual displays* (increases in skin temperature are seen as increases on a dial). The client tries to change the display of information in the desired direction, such as to reduce muscle contraction (relax muscle tension) and reduce blood flow. The continuous, precise information received shows the effectiveness of the effort and often helps the client learn physiologic control of these functions.[51]

Biofeedback can be performed at home with purchased or rented equipment under the guidance of a suitably prepared health care worker. Alternatively, it may be performed in an office or clinic setting with a biofeedback therapist or other specialist, such as a nurse trained in biofeedback. The equipment is expensive.

Therapeutic Touch

Therapeutic Touch is a type of pain management that has been used for disorders such as tension headaches.[49]

It is a derivative of the "laying on" of hands. The human body is believed to have energy fields that express aberrant patterns when body systems are insulted. Therapeutic Touch is thought to realign aberrant fields. Education and practice are required on the part of the nurse.

Therapeutic Touch involves three steps:

1. Becoming centered or focused in a meditative state. This helps you become aware of the vibrations in the surrounding energy fields.
2. Assessing the client's energy field. Pass your hands over the client's body at a distance of 2 to 6 inches to sense changes in the field.
3. During the treatment step, using your hands to re-arrange the client's energy field and return it to normal.

Distraction

Cognitive strategies to modify pain perception have been effective in numerous research studies. The most effective cognitive strategy involves distraction. Attention is directed away from the painful sensation or the negative emotional arousal associated with the pain episode. The primary theoretical explanation is that a person is able to focus attention on a limited number of foci. Actively focusing attention on a cognitive task is thought to limit one's ability to attend to the noxious sensation.

To be effective, the distraction task requires considerable cognitive effort. Distraction exercises that are too easy rapidly become automatic or engage monotonous repetitive responses and are likely to be ineffective.

Interventions may be administered by a multitude of modalities that require the client to engage in highly focused interesting mental exercises. Typical techniques used in hospital settings include videotapes of favorite movies, audiotapes of favorite music, craft activities, and interacting with others. The distraction technique may be more effective if it involves action on the client's part. For example, listening to music and tapping one's fingers to the rhythm may be more effective than passive listening alone. Cognitive strategies need to be tailored to the client's personal preferences. Techniques used should be self-selected. People may want to bring their own tapes, videos, books, or craft items. If the items are supplied by an agency, a library of materials is needed to allow clients to select what is pleasing to them.

Magnets

Magnets have been used to relieve a variety of painful disorders.[41] It is speculated that the pull of the magnet increases blood flow to the region, opening the Na^+ and Cl^- channels in the cells. Magnet therapy has been a mainstay in pain management in Eastern Asian countries and is gaining popularity in Western medicine. (See the Complementary and Alternative Therapy feature on Magnet Therapy for Plantar Heel Pain on p. 651.)

EVALUATION AND DOCUMENTATION

Evaluation

Evaluation is most effective when a formal evaluation protocol is used throughout a health care agency "across all stages of the disease and across all practice settings."[21] A formalized process within the institution provides a unified methodology that can be learned and used by every member of the health care team. According to the Clinical Practice Guidelines,[21] key items to consider include the following:

- Client satisfaction with pain management and its impact on the client's quality of life
- Satisfaction with pain management and its impact on the client's quality of life (particularly in chronic illness or when clients require home health care)
- The designation of who is responsible for pain management
- The systematic assessment of pain in all settings where people receive care
- The accuracy of diagnostic approaches for common pain syndromes

- The range and appropriateness of pain management options available within a particular practice setting
- The effectiveness of pain management options used to prevent and treat pain
- The prevalence and severity of side effects and complications associated with pain management
- The quality of pain management across points of transition in the provision of services

The effectiveness of pain management protocols needs to be evaluated frequently and throughout the course of treatment. Figure 22-14 illustrates a sample plan used to determine pain management needs for clients having surgery.[1] The example includes the three phases of a surgical experience (preoperative, intraoperative, and postoperative).

During an evaluation, both the process used to manage pain and the outcomes achieved are assessed. Assessment and evaluation are ongoing components of the plan. There are no objective indicators of a person's pain. The only means to determine pain intensity and associated emotional discomfort accurately is to ask the person. Sometimes direct measurement of a client's

A   B

FIGURE 22-14 Pain treatment flow chart.

MM#17986

3/97

Clarian Health
Methodist·IU·Riley

F = Faces
W = Word
I = Infant Assessment Tool
A = Adult & Child Assessment Tool

PAIN MANAGEMENT FLOW SHEET

Initials	Name & Title	Initials	Name & Title

☐ In-Patient   ☐ Out-Patient

Date Time	Scale Rating	Resp. LOS	Location/Type	Drug Administered Dosage/Route	Other Interventions	Comments/Response	Initials

LEVEL OF SEDATION	DEGREE OF SOMNOLENCE (Patient Awakens/Responds to:)	INTERVENTIONS		COMMENTS EXAMPLES
0	Caregiver entering room	R = repositioning	M = massage	diarrhea
1	Soft verbal stimulation	F = feeding	CS = cutaneous stimulation	constipation
2	Loud Verbal Stimulation	VS = verbal support	GI = guided imagery	depressed
3	Mild Physical Contact	HR = holding/rocking	MT = music therapy	crying
4	Vigorous Physical Contact	T = toileting/diapering	HA = hot application	vomiting
		D = distraction	CA = cold application	nausea
		A = adjust environment	SO = significant other present	anxious
		E = emotional support	=	agitated
		P = play	=	itching
		S = sucking/pacifier	=	

Adapted from: Gwirtz, K.H. (1992). Single dose intrathecal opioids in the management of acute postoperative pain. In Sinatra, R., Hord, A., Ginsberg, R., & Preble, L. (Eds.). Acute Pain: Mechanisms and Management (pp.253-268). St. Louis: Mosby.

19058

MEDICAL RECORDS COPY	PAIN MANAGEMENT FLOWSHEET							W-37
B-CLIN. NOTES	E-LAB	G-X-RAY	K-DIAGNOSTIC	M-SURGERY	Q-THERAPY	T-ORDERS	W-NURSING	Y-MISC.

FIGURE 22-15 Pain management flow sheet. (Courtesy of Clarian Health Partners, Indianapolis, IN.)

report of pain is not possible, and someone else must estimate pain by observation. These assessments may or may not be accurate. Ongoing evaluation of the effectiveness of pain management interventions is essential when the client is not verbal. The pain management strategy employed for the client is based on an interpretation of need. These clients cannot provide data regarding effectiveness of the strategy. The health care provider must ascertain whether the pain was indeed relieved by the intervention they selected.

Evaluation requires the identification of a standard against which practice process and outcomes can be compared.[21] For example, the health care provider consults with the client to determine the degree of pain reduction and/or relief desired by the client. An evaluation criterion must consider whether the desired outcome has been achieved. If the criterion is not met, the evaluation helps determine the reason. Modifications in the pain management program may be needed to achieve the desired outcome. These modifications should be documented to allow for evaluation of outcomes achieved by the new interventions. Some institutions have used a standard for all clients based on the knowledge that unrelieved pain has negative physical effects. For example, a standard may mandate that medication for pain be administered if a client reports a pain intensity of 3 or greater on an 11-point numerical scale.

Although the primary focus of evaluation is directed toward effectiveness of management strategies for clients, it is also necessary to periodically evaluate the treatment protocols incorporated into hospital procedure manuals and pain management standards accepted by the clinicians. As the knowledge base underlying practice interventions increases, the standard procedures for pain management may also need to change. Conducting periodic evaluation of practice, based on research, enhances the potential for providing the best care possible. A few questions to consider are as follows:

- Is the client still in pain? If so, is progress being made to minimize or relieve the pain?
- Are the client's beliefs and values being considered?
- Are the client and family active participants in pain management planning?
- Have pain management nonpharmaceutical interventions been given ample time to be effective? Can the client try the strategy one more time?
- Are a variety of pain measures being used?
- Do new data indicate a new diagnosis or complication?

Documentation

Data gathered through evaluation must be documented. Documentation data are to be recorded in a manner that makes the information available to all members of the health care team. This may be best done by means of a pain document record or flow sheet (Figure 22-15) that allows visualization of the client's pain experience throughout a hospitalization experience and that can follow the client from one health care setting to another. The flow sheet should be entered into the client's permanent hospital record.

CONCLUSIONS

The most effective pain management program may depend on use of a combination of medications and nonpharmaceutical interventions. Clients may benefit from the incorporation of several nonpharmaceutical interventions used simultaneously. Research has supported the efficacy of numerous nonpharmaceutical techniques. These findings plus the wide variability in the strength and types of medications make it possible (1) to design a pain program that can be individualized and (2) to modify a pain management protocol if a component of the program is ineffective. One ineffective strategy can be replaced by another strategy until a successful combination of treatments is determined.

The variety of potential treatments also benefits clients for whom progression of the pain experience is a component. The protocol can be modified to meet changing needs when the pain increases or abates. Box 22-3 summarizes possible interventions posited by the Clinical Practice Guidelines for Management of Cancer Pain and Pain due to Trauma, Surgery, and Painful Procedures.[21]

THINKING CRITICALLY *evolve*

1. An 80-year-old client, Mrs. Parker, is terminally ill with cancer. An opiate analgesic has been prescribed for her pain. She is being cared for at home by family members who are concerned about pain control for their loved one. What should the client and family be taught about complications associated with use of opiate analgesia? Who would be the ideal person to assess and coordinate the client's response to dosing of a particular opiate or combination of opiate and non-opiate medications?

Factors to Consider. What complications are associated with the use of opiate analgesia? What factors contribute to the dosing schedule of a client with cancer-related pain? How much control over analgesia is given to the client? How should the caregiver and family monitor the response of the individual to the prescribed medication regimen?

A discussion for this question can be found on the website and the CD-ROM.

BIBLIOGRAPHY

1. Acute Pain Management Guideline Panel. (1992). *Acute pain management in adults: Operative procedures. Quick reference guide for clinicians.* AHCPR Publication. No. 92-0019. Rockville, MD: Agency for Health Care Policy and Research, Public Health Service, U.S. Department of Health and Human Services.

2. Ader, R.W. (1997). The role of conditioning in pharmacotherapies: The placebo effect? *Proceedings of the American Pain Society,* 16th Annual Scientific Meeting, New Orleans, p. 53.

3. Albers, R.W., & Siegal, G.J. (1999). Membrane transport. In G.J. Siegal, et al. (Eds.), *Basic neurochemistry: Molecular, cellular, and medical aspects* (6th ed., pp. 95-118). Philadelphia: Lippincott Williams & Wilkins.

4. American Geriatrics Society. (2002). The management of persistent pain in older persons. *Journal of the American Geriatrics Society,* 50(6), S205-S224.

5. American Pain Society. (2003). *Principles of analgesic use in the treatment of acute pain and cancer pain* (5th ed.). Glenview, IL: Author.

6. American Society of Pain Management Nurses. (2002). *ASPMN Position statement: Pain management in patients with addictive disease.* Pensacola, FL: Author.

7. American Society of Pain Management Nurses. (2002). In B. St. Marie (Ed.), *Core curriculum for pain management nursing.* Philadelphia: W.B. Saunders.

8. American Society of Pain Management Nurses. (1996). ASPMN Position statement: Use of placebos for pain management. Pensacola, FL: Author.

9. Berkley, K.J., & Holdcroft, A. (1999). Sex and gender differences in pain. In P.D. Wall & R. Melzack (Eds.), *Textbook of pain* (4th ed., pp. 951-965). Edinburgh: Churchill Livingstone.

10. Brune, K., & Zeilhoffer, H.U. (1999). Antipyretic (non-narcotic) analgesics. In P.D. Wall & R. Melzack (Eds.), *Textbook of pain* (4th ed., pp. 1139-1153). Edinburgh: Churchill Livingstone.

11. Cleeland, C.S., et al. (1997). Pain and treatment of pain in minority patients with cancer: The Eastern Cooperative Oncology Group minority outpatient pain study. *Annals of Internal Medicine,* 127, 813-816.

12. Edwards, M. (1998, March/April). Barriers to effective pain/symptom control. *American Journal of Hospice and Palliative Care,* 15(2), 107-111.

13. Filshie, J., et al. (1996). Acupuncture for the relief of cancer-related breathlessness. *Palliative Medicine,* 10(2), 145-150.

14. Foley, K.M. (1995). Pain relief into practice: Rhetoric without reform. *Journal of Clinical Oncology,* 13, 2149-2151.

15. Gagliese, L., Katz, J., & Melzack, R. (1999). Pain in the elderly. In P.D. Wall & R. Melzack (Eds.), *Textbook of pain* (4th ed., pp. 991-1006). Edinburgh: Churchill Livingstone.

16. Geis, G.S. (1999). Update on clinical developments with celecoxib, a new specific COX-2 inhibitor: What can we expect? *Journal of Rheumatology,* 26(Suppl. 56), 31-36.

17. Gerdner, L.A., & Buckwalter, K.C. (1999). Music therapy. In G.M. Bulecheck & J.C. McCloskey (Eds.), *Nursing interventions: Effective nursing treatments* (3rd ed., pp. 451-468). Philadelphia: W. B. Saunders.

18. Gordon, D. (1998). Assessment and management of pain. In Maher, A.B., Salmond, S.W., & Pellino, T.A. (Eds.), *Orthopaedic nursing.* Philadelphia: W.B. Saunders.

19. Hawkey, C.J. (1999). COX-2 inhibitors. *The Lancet,* 353, 307-314.

20. International Association for the Study of Pain. (1986). Pain terms: A current list with definitions and notes on usage. *Pain, 3,* S216-S221.

21. Jacox, A., et al. (1994). *Management of cancer pain. Clinical practice guidelines No. 9.* AHCPR Publication No. 94-1592. Rockville, MD: Agency for Health Care Policy and Research, U.S. Department of Health and Human Services, Public Health Service.

22. Janssen, S.A., & Arntz, A. (1996). Anxiety and pain: Attentional and endorphinergic influences. *Pain, 66,* 145-150.

23. Joint Commission on Accreditation of Healthcare Organizations. (2000). Pain Assessment and management: An organizational approach. Oakbrook Terrace, IL: Joint Commission on Accreditation of Healthcare Organizations.

24. Juarez, G., Ferrell, B., & Borneman, T. (1998). Influence of culture on cancer pain management in Hispanic patients. *Cancer Practice,* 6(5), 262-269.

25. Kovacs, F.M., et al. (1997). Local and remote sustained trigger point therapy for exacerbations of chronic low back pain: A randomized, double-blind, controlled, multicenter trial. *Spine, 22*(7), 786-797.

26. Lander, J. (1990). Fallacies and phobias about addiction and pain. *British Journal of Addiction,* 85, 803-809.

27. Laurion, S. & Fetzer, S.J. (2003). The effect of two nursing interventions on the postoperative outcomes of gynecologic laparoscopic patients. *Journal of PeriAnesthesia Nursing,* 18(4), 254-261.

28. Lefkowitz, M. (1998). Pain management in the HIV-positive patient. In M.A. Ashburn and L.J. Rice (Eds.), *The management of pain,* New York: Churchill Livingstone.

28a. Liebskind, J.C. (1996). Editorial. *Pain,* 44(1), 3-4.

29. Linton, S.J. (1999). Psychological factors. In I.K. Crombie, et al. (Eds.), *The epidemiology of pain.* Seattle: IASP Press (pp. 25-42).

30. Lundeberg, T. (1995). Pain physiology and principles of therapy. *Scandinavian Journal of Rehabilitation Medicine Supplement, 32,* 13-42.

30a. Manz, B., et al. (2000). Pain assessment in the cognitively impaired and unimpaired elderly. *Pain Management Nursing,* 1(4), 106-115.

31. Marks, R.M., & Sacher, E.J. (1973). Undertreatment of medical inpatients with narcotic analgesics. *Annals of Internal Medicine,* 78, 173-181.

32. Matz, A., & Brown, S.T. (1998). Humor and pain management. *Journal of Holistic Nursing,* 16(1), 68-75.

33. McCaffery, M., & Pasero, C. (1999). *Pain: Clinical manual* (2nd ed.). St. Louis: Mosby.

34. Merskey, H., & Bogduk, N. (1994). *Classification of chronic pain: Descriptions of chronic pain syndromes and definitions of pain terms.* Seattle: IASP Press.

35. Michlovitz, S. (1996). The use of heat and cold in the management of rheumatic diseases. In S.L. Michlovitz (Ed.), *Thermal agents in rehabilitation* (2nd ed., pp. 258-274). Philadelphia: F. A. Davis.

36. Michlovitz, S. (1996). Cryotherapy: The use of cold as a therapeutic agent. In S.L. Michlovitz (Ed.), *Thermal agents in rehabilitation* (2nd ed., pp. 88-108). Philadelphia. F. A. Davis.

 37. Mobily, P.R., Herr, K.A., & Nicholson, A.C. (1994). Validation of cutaneous stimulation interventions for pain management. *International Journal of Nursing Studies, 31*, 533-544.

38. Moore, R., & Brodsgaard, I. (1999). Cross-cultural investigations of pain. In I.K. Crombie, et al. (Eds.), *Epidemiology of pain* (pp. 53-80). Seattle: IASP Press.

39. *NIH [National Institutes of Health] Technological Assessment Statement* (1995, October 16-18). Integration of behavioral and relaxation approaches into the treatment of chronic pain and insomnia. (pp. 1-34.)

40. Paice, J.A. (1999). Pain. In C.H. Yarbo, et al. (Eds.), *Cancer symptom management* (2nd ed., pp. 118-144). Boston: Jones & Bartlett.

41. Papi, F., et al. (1995). Exposure to oscillating magnetic field influences sensitivity to electrical stimuli: II. Experiments on humans. *Bioelectromagnets, 16*, 295-300.

42. Pasero, C. (2003). Multimodal balanced analgesia in the PACU. *Journal of PeriAnesthesia Nursing, 18*(4), 265-268.

43. Payne R. (1998). Nonopioid analgesics for cancer pain: Update on clinical pharmacology. In R. Payne, et al. (Eds.), *Assessment and treatment of cancer pain: Progress in pain research and management* (Vol. 12, pp. 289-307). Seattle: IASP Press.

44. Payne, R., & Janjan, N. (1998). Management of metastatic bone pain. In R. Payne, et al. (Eds.), *Assessment and treatment of cancer pain: Progress in pain research and management* (Vol. 12, pp. 269-273). Seattle: IASP Press.

45. Portenoy, R.K. (1996). Opioid therapy for chronic nonmalignant pain: A review of the critical issues. *Journal of Pain and Symptom Management, 11*, 203-217.

46. Portenoy, R.K., & Lesage, P. (1999). Management of cancer pain. *The Lancet, 353*, 1695-1700.

47. Porter F.L., Grunau R.E., & Anand K.J. (1999). Long-term effects of pain in infants. *Journal of Developmental and Behavioral Pediatrics, 20*(4):253-261.

48. Price, D.D. (1999). Mechanisms of hypnotic analgesia. In *Psychological mechanisms of pain: Progress in pain research and management* (Vol. 15, pp. 183-204). Seattle: IASP Press.

49. Ramnarine-Singh, S. (1999). The surgical significance of therapeutic touch. *AORN Journal, 69*(2), 358, 360-365, 367-369.

50. Sloan, P.A., et al. (1996). Cancer pain assessment and management by housestaff. *Pain, 67*, 475-481.

51. Spence, S.H., et al. (1995). Effects of EMG biofeedback compared to applied relaxation training with chronic, upper extremity cumulative trauma disorders. *Pain, 63*(2), 199-206.

52. Spross, J.A., McGuire, D.B., & Schmitt, R.M. (1990). Oncology Nursing Society position paper on pain. Pittsburgh: Oncology Nursing Society.

53. Stephenson, J. (1996). Experts say AIDS pain "dramatically undertreated." *Journal of the American Medical Association, 276*, 1369-1370.

54. Sternbach, R. (1968). *Pain: A psychophysiological analysis.* New York: Academic Press.

55. Stimmel, B. (1997). *Pain and its relief without addiction: Clinical issues in the use of opioids and other analgesics.* New York, Haworth Medical Press.

56. Turk, D.C., & Okifuji, A. (1998). Directions in prescriptive chronic pain management based on diagnostic characteristics of the client. In P.J. Vincent (Ed)., *American Pain Society Bulletin, 8*(5), 5-11.

57. Tusek, D., Church, J.M., & Fazio, V.W. (1997). Guided imagery as a coping strategy for perioperative clients. *AORN Journal, 66*(4), 644-649.

58. Wall, P. (1999). Placebos. In P.D. Wall & R. Melzack (Eds.), *Textbook of pain* (4th ed., pp. 1419-1430). Edinburgh: Churchill Livingstone.

59. Weisenberg, M. (1999). Cognitive aspects of pain. In P.D. Wall & R. Melzack (Eds.), *Textbook of pain* (4th ed., pp. 345-358). Edinburgh: Churchill Livingstone.

60. Wong, D., & Baker, C. (1988). Pain in children: Comparison of assessment scales. *Pediatric Nursing, 14*(1), 9-17.

61. Woolf, C.J., & Mannion, R.J. (1999). Neuropathic pain: Aetiology, symptoms, mechanisms, and management. *The Lancet, 353*, 1959-1964.

62. World Health Organization (WHO). (1990). Cancer pain relief and palliative care. *Report of a WHO expert committee. Technical report series 804.* Geneva: Author.

63. Yaksh, T.L. (1999). Central pharmacology of nociception. In P.D. Wall & R. Melzack (Eds.), *Textbook of pain* (4th ed., pp. 253-308). Edinburgh: Churchill Livingstone.

FURTHER REFERENCES

American Academy of Pain Medicine and American Pain Society. (1997). *The use of opioids for the treatment of chronic pain.* Glenview, IL: Author.

American Society of PeriAnesthesia Nurses. (2003). ASPAN Pain and comfort clinical guideline. *Journal of PeriAnesthesia Nursing, 18*(4), 232-236.

Defining key terms in pain management. (2002). Stamford, CT: Purdue Pharma, L.P.

Perspectives in Palliative Care

Kim K. Kuebler
Debra E. Heidrich

evolve

Web Enhancements

http://evolve.elsevier.com/Black/medsurg/

Bridge to Home Health Care
  Providing Hospice Care
Diversity in Health Care
  Cultural Aspects of Death and Dying

Appendix A
  Religious Beliefs and Practices Affecting Health Care

Nurses caring for clients with advanced diseases will ultimately witness the final stage of life—dying. The dying process is often accompanied by a myriad of psychological, spiritual, and physical needs, and nurses are in the ideal position to identify and address them. Nurses must be knowledgeable about the normal dying process, the control of pain and other symptoms, and the role of the interdisciplinary team to provide optimal support and symptom management for dying clients and their families. "Nurses spend more time with patients and their families than do any other health professionals and are in the most immediate position to provide care, comfort, and counsel at the end-of-life, when critical decisions must be reached and compassionate and highly specialized care provided."[42]

Note: In this chapter, *symptom* is used instead of *clinical manifestations*, the term used elsewhere in the text. Common symptoms associated with dying differ from clinical manifestations that accompany specific medical problems. *Symptom management* is the preferred term often used in the care of clients with advanced illness and is the primary focus within the specialty of palliative care.

EVOLUTION OF HOSPICE AND PALLIATIVE CARE

The terms *hospice care*, *palliative care*, and *end-of-life care* sometimes are used interchangeably and at other times are used to differentiate various models of care; however, palliative care should be considered early in the course of advanced illness rather than restricted to the end of life.[22,67] The following discussion briefly identifies the evolution of the hospice movement, the development of palliative care, and the current unmet needs of end-of-life care in the United States.

The hospice movement began in the late 1960s in the United Kingdom when Dame Cicely Saunders identified that the complex needs of dying clients were not being addressed within the traditional health care system. Her vision and understanding of the unmet needs of the dying prompted the development of the first hospice, St. Christopher's Hospice in London, England.[17] Saunders believed that the dying required the multiple skills of an interdisciplinary team to provide "patient-centered care." The precepts of the hospice movement in the United States are a direct result of the work at St. Christopher's Hospice.[5,20]

Another pioneer whose work greatly influenced the hospice movement is Elizabeth Kübler-Ross. Her theoretical framework for the death and dying process brought forth recognition of the psychological and existential needs of the dying.[33] Her life work was to help clients and society to view terminal illness not as a destructive, negative force but as one of the "windstorms" in life that can enhance inner growth.[33,34] Kübler-Ross is most noted for identifying and defining the phases of the normal death and dying experience: (1) denial, (2) anger,

evolve Be sure to check out the bonus material on the Evolve website and the CD-ROM, including free self-assessment exercises.

http://evolve.elsevier.com/Black/medsurg/

(3) bargaining, (4) depression, and (5) acceptance (Table 23-1).[33,34] After spending many years at the bedside of the dying, Kübler-Ross recognized the importance of the interdisciplinary team in providing support to the client and family as they experience the various phases of the dying process.[33,34]

While Kübler-Ross was advocating for the dying and St. Christopher's Hospice was successfully caring for terminally ill clients, Florence Wald, then the dean of graduate nursing studies at Yale University, expressed interest in bringing the hospice movement to the United States. Wald recognized the tremendous need in America to improve the care of the dying and helped to integrate the British hospice movement into the first home care hospice in New Haven, Connecticut, in 1974.[5,17]

During this same period, Canadians also recognized a need to address better care at the end of life. Balfour Mount defined *palliative care* and opened the first hospital-based palliative care service at the Royal Victoria Hospital of McGill University in Montreal in 1975.[17] The McGill model used the interdisciplinary team approach of client- and family-centered care and yet differed as the first program to include research and education in the area of pain and symptom management.[5,20]

All these pioneers advocated for improved care for the terminally ill and their families. They believed that professionals trained to provide physical comfort through pain and symptom management as well as psychosocial and spiritual support could promote a healthy,

TABLE 23-1	*Kübler-Ross's Stages of Dying*
Stage	**Clinical Manifestations**
Denial	"This can't be true." "I'll be just fine after surgery (or radiation or chemotherapy)." Client and family may search for health care providers who will give more favorable opinion or may seek alternative therapies.
Anger	"Why me?" Client and family have feelings of resentment, envy, or anger directed at client, family, health care providers, God, and others.
Bargaining	"I just want to see my daughter's graduation, then I'll be ready . . ." Client (or family) asks for more time to reach an important life event and may make promises to God.
Depression	"I just don't know how my wife will get along after I'm gone." Family and client may grieve and mourn for impending losses.
Acceptance	"I have no regrets—I've done everything I've wanted to in my life and am proud of what I've accomplished. Client and family are neither angry nor depressed.

From Kübler-Ross, E. (1969). *On death and dying.* New York: Macmillan.

normal dying experience and include supportive bereavement services.

During the 1970s, the hospice concept of care continued to grow as a grassroots movement throughout the United States. Citing the cost-effectiveness of and client and family satisfaction with this level of care, Congress approved a Medicare Hospice Benefit in 1982.[44,48] With a solid source of reimbursement available, the number of hospice programs grew markedly over the next several years.[5,32,44]

Dying in America

Hospice care has steadily expanded since its inception. In 1985 about 160,000 clients were served. In 1999 about 700,000 received hospice care. Yet, despite this increase, only 29% of all clients who died in the United States in 1999 were enrolled in a Medicare hospice program.[56] Problems in the care of the dying and their families in the United States have been extensively documented and widely publicized.[32,67] Hospice care was initiated on the basis of a quality-oriented alternative to the traditional biomedical model of health care with the intent to ensure that clients and their families could have appropriate care at the end of life.[28] The genesis for Hospice initially was in protest against the aggressive use of science to battle disease and choose instead the "quality-of-life alternative" offered by hospice.[28] Hospice care was enacted in part to a change in climate that rejected aggressive biotechnical interventions and allowed clients to die at home with the support of a skilled interdisciplinary team.[22,26,28]

For two decades the Medicare Hospice Benefit has provided full coverage for terminally ill older Americans; however, fewer than one third of dying clients use these services.[23] Most Americans still die in hospital or nursing home beds rather than in their own homes.[23,39] The limited use of hospice care in the United States is multifactorial and includes the following:

- Western society is a "death-denying" culture in which many clients and health care professionals desire life-prolonging care.
- Clients and families often lack knowledge regarding the availability of hospice services.
- Physicians have difficulty in determining prognoses in terms of 6 months or less.

Some leaders in the field believe that the underutilization of hospice care continues to be a public health issue in the United States.[56] (See the Bridge to Home Health Care feature on Providing Hospice Care on the website.)

The SUPPORT Study

A significant study that has since spurred national interests in end-of-life issues is a result of the findings from SUPPORT (Study to Understand Prognoses and Preferences for Outcomes and Risks of Treatments),[72] which revealed that Americans were often dying in moderate to severe pain and without regard to their advance directives. This 28-million-dollar study, funded by the Robert Wood Johnson Foundation and conducted at five medical centers nationwide over 10 years, found that 80% of Americans die in institutional settings, often with unmanaged pain, in isolation, connected to mechanical ventilators, and in intensive care units. The utilization of living wills, health care proxies, and communication efforts between clients and their physicians often proved futile.[43,52,72]

The results of the SUPPORT study, the Institute of Medicine's influential report, and numerous studies have identified that end-of-life care in the United States suffers from serious deficiencies.[12] These studies indicate that good end-of-life care is not the standard and that there is a great need for improvement in many areas of health care delivery.[8,12]

A more recent study that examined palliative practices across the country rated all states on eight criteria as a means for assessing the state of end-of-life care in the United States.[6] Despite all that we learned from the SUPPORT Study, this new report found that Americans can currently expect at best a fair chance of finding good care for their loved ones or themselves when diagnosed with advanced illness.[39]

Palliative Care

Palliative care is an emerging and well-defined specialty that combines an interdisciplinary approach to promote competent and compassionate care.[50] Palliative care does not emphasize cure but rather provides relief of suffering by managing symptoms and maximizing quality of life.[53] Palliative care provides a longitudinal continuum of care and is not offered in only the last 6 months of life as reflected in the Medicare Hospice Benefit.[53] Palliative care should be available and integrated into the beginning of the disease process until death.[53,67]

The World Health Organization (WHO) recently expanded the definition of palliative care to include earlier integration of its precepts into the course of illness and provided the following definition[81]:

> Palliative care is an approach that improves the quality of life of patients and their families facing the problems associated with life-threatening illness, through the prevention and relief of suffering by means of early identification and impeccable assessment and treatment of pain and other problems, physical, psychosocial and spiritual.

Like hospice care, palliative care recognizes that dying is a normal process that should be neither hastened nor postponed. The provision of symptom management that includes emotional and spiritual support for clients and their families is considered when developing the plan of care to promote an optimal dying experience followed by family bereavement.[7,17,43,50,52]

Palliative philosophy identified from the Last Acts Palliative Care Task Force and the National Hospice and Palliative Care Organization includes the following:

- Palliative care provides support and care for persons facing life-limited illness across all care settings.
- Palliative care identifies death as normal and natural.
- The dying process is profoundly individualized and occurs within the dynamics of family.
- Palliative care enhances the quality of life and integrates the physical, psychological, social, and spiritual aspects of care.
- The interdisciplinary team addresses the multidimensional needs of the dying clients and his or her family.
- Palliative interventions affirm life and neither hasten nor postpone death.
- Appropriate palliative care and a supportive environment promote quality of life and health closure for the client and family.[4]

Disease Trajectory

The leading causes of death in the United States include heart disease, cancer, stroke, chronic obstructive pulmonary disease, and dementia.[75] All these diseases have a relatively predictable course. The disease trajectory is identified from the onset of a life-limited diagnosis until death. Some terminal diagnoses have a long disease trajectory with a gradual decline in functional status over time; others have a very short trajectory with a sharp decline; still others have variable trajectories with periods of remission and exacerbation.[45,47] The vast majority of Americans, however, who die each year are older adults with a median age of 77 years, and they typically suffer from a slow, progressive chronic disease.[10] Women will average about 3 years at the end of life with progressively debilitating illness, whereas men will often have 2 years with a serious progressive disability, all of whom could benefit from palliative care.[30]

Determining specific interventions to improve each client's quality of life is determined largely by his or her position on the disease trajectory. A comprehensive assessment is essential when determining the client's disease trajectory to guide identification of appropriate palliative interventions. This assessment comprises the following actions:

1. Defining the nature of the clinical finding and symptoms.
2. Performing a thorough history and physical examination, reviewing current and tried medications, and evaluating a minimal set of diagnostic procedures to differentiate underlying pathophysiologic disorders from a reversible symptom.
3. Evaluating the problem within the context of the client's situation and allowing for prioritization.

For example, the priority assigned a urinary tract infection (UTI) in a cognitively impaired, dehydrated, and bedridden client will be different from that given to a UTI in a cognitively intact client with good symptom control.

4. Defining the "cost" of diagnostic and therapeutic interventions and the varying differences between clients—for example, what may be considered appropriate therapy for one client may be inappropriate for another—when evaluating the risk versus benefit of treatment and the financial burden of unnecessary interventions.

5. Discussing the various care options with the client and the family and encouraging informed decision making.[43]

Quality of Life

Palliative care is offered when a progressive illness is symptomatic and interferes with the quality of life. Many variables go into defining quality of life, including (1) socioeconomic status, (2) physical health, (3) relationships with friends and family, and (4) satisfaction with self.[31,63] Quality of life is defined as "a personal statement of the positivity or negativity of attributes that characterize life."[31]

A person's quality of life is often linked to the experience of symptom distress and the meanings that the person assigns to these physical sensations.[31,63] Nurses caring for clients who are experiencing distressing symptoms, such as pain, fatigue, constipation, and nausea, should understand that each client responds differently. The effect of a symptom on life routines varies from client to client, depending on overall functional status, coping abilities, and social supports. A palliative plan of care must be based not only on symptom management but also on the effect of the symptom and the burden of the intervention on the client's overall quality of living.

SYMPTOMS AT THE END OF LIFE

Scientific palliative care is assessment driven and evidence based to promote the integration of rational decision making and treatment in the management of common symptoms.[19] Dr. MacDonald, a palliative care leader, recognized that inadequate symptom control throughout the trajectory of illness not only produces suffering but also has a negative effect on the course of illness.[47] Clients with advanced diseases experience multiple symptoms, some of which are more severe than others.[47,72] It is important to assess and diagnose the cause of each symptom and base the appropriate interventions on the underlying cause.[47] In one study, pain was found to be the most prevalent symptom among clients with advanced cancer (89% of respondents). In 87% of clients with pain, the severity of the pain was

rated as moderate to severe. In addition to pain, the symptoms of weakness, anorexia, dyspnea, constipation, early satiety, fatigue, and dry mouth were experienced by more than 40% of clients.[47,72]

Symptoms vary not only in frequency and intensity but also in the distress experienced by clients. Although pain may be prevalent, it is not always identified as the most distressing symptom. Some studies have found that dyspnea, asthenia (lethargy, generalized weakness, and fatigue), dry mouth, anorexia, depression, and insomnia may actually be more distressing than pain for clients with terminal illnesses.[19,47,72] The management of symptoms includes nonpharmacologic and pharmacologic interventions. When using medications, care should always be given to titration of the dose to effect. Oftentimes, complex palliative care clients encounter polypharmacy with the idea of "one symptom, one drug," whereas the ideal is to use one medication that palliates multiple symptoms.[19,47] See the Case Study feature on Cancer of the Prostate at the End of Life in Chapter 40 for application of many concepts that follow.

Pain

Pain is a multidimensional phenomenon. Not only is a person's pain experience a physical response to an underlying disorder or disease state, but various emotional, intellectual, behavioral, sensory, and cultural dimensions also influence the pain experience.[21,62] When a client is nonresponsive and unable to report pain, the nurse should observe for the behavioral indicators of pain (Table 23-2). Communication within the entire health care team is essential for optimal pain management. Chapter 22 describes types of pain, subjective and objective assessment of pain, and pain management strategies.

Opioid Analgesics

Opioids are the mainstay of treatment for moderate to severe pain.[1,21,81,82] These medications bind with opiate receptors in the central nervous system (CNS) and block the transmission of pain impulses to the higher brain centers. Most opioid medications bind to the mu receptor and are called *mu agonists*. Morphine (MS Contin), hydromorphone (Dilaudid), fentanyl (Duragesic), and oxycodone (Oxycontin) are examples of mu-agonist opioids frequently used in the treatment of pain.[1,21,61] There is no ceiling to the analgesic effect of mu-agonist opioids.[13,77] See Chapter 22 for further discussion of opioid therapy.

In addition to modulating the transmission and perception of the pain impulse, opioids may bind with receptors in other tissues, leading to the potential for side effects. For example, opioid receptors are present in the gastrointestinal tract. When opioids bind with these receptors, intestinal motility is decreased and gastric emp-

TABLE 23-2	*Behavioral Indicators of Pain in the Nonresponsive Client*
Restlessness	Agitation, frequent moving, an inability to get comfortable, fidgety, picking at things
Vocalizations	Moaning, groaning, crying out
Muscle tension	Tense muscles, not relaxed, clenched teeth, tightened fists, guarded movements
Facial expression	Frowning, grimacing, distressed
Physiologic indicators	Fast heart rate, frequent and labored breathing, sweating

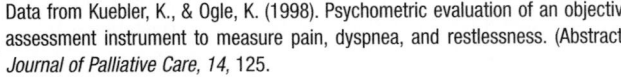 Data from Kuebler, K., & Ogle, K. (1998). Psychometric evaluation of an objective assessment instrument to measure pain, dyspnea, and restlessness. (Abstract). *Journal of Palliative Care, 14*, 125.

tying is delayed, leading to constipation. Prophylactic treatment of constipation with both a stool softener and a stimulant is essential and should be initiated along with the first opioid dose. The clinician should not wait for the client to complain of constipation before beginning treatment. Constipation is the only side effect of opioids to which a person does not develop tolerance. A bowel protocol must be continued for the duration of treatment with opioids.

Other potential side effects of opioids are respiratory depression, nausea and vomiting, and sedation. Clinically significant respiratory depression is rare during treatment of pain if the opioid dose is increased slowly and decreased if sedation is noted. In addition, some persons develop tolerance to the respiratory-depressive side effects of opioids after the first several days of treatment. The client who has taken the same dose of an opioid for several weeks is not at risk for a clinically significant opioid-induced respiratory depression.[21,62,74]

Although nausea and vomiting may not be problems for all clients, many clients do experience these problems as a side effect of opioids. Nausea and vomiting occur when the chemoreceptor trigger zone of the brain is stimulated by these medications. A client is less likely to experience nausea when opioids are administered orally than when they are administered parenterally. As with respiratory depression, tolerance to this side effect of opioids develops over time. Clients who experience nausea and vomiting should be treated with antiemetics for the first 2 to 3 days after the opioid is initiated until tolerance develops. A small number of clients experience persistent nausea from the opioids. These clients may benefit from either changing to a different opioid or continuing to use antiemetics.[13]

A client who has been in pain and receives an initial dose of an opioid may experience some degree of sedation, in part as a result of the direct effect of opioids on the brain. In addition to the sedative side effect of the opioid, however, the client is probably exhausted from not sleeping well while in pain. Teach the client that some sleepiness is expected and that it is probably not due entirely to the new medication. As with the other side effects of opioids, tolerance to the sedation develops after the first 2 to 3 days. If, however, the client is difficult to arouse or the sedation lasts more than 2 to 3 days, the opioid dose may be too high for the intensity of the pain.

Clients who are sedated by an opioid and still are experiencing pain probably have pain syndromes that are not completely responsive to opioids. These clients require the addition of adjuvant medications to achieve comfort. Recognize that *there is no ceiling to the amount of opioid analgesic* required for each client to achieve a satisfactory level of analgesia. Hence, clients may require very high doses of opioids to achieve pain reduction.

Adjuvant Analgesics

Adjuvant medications have a primary action other than pain reduction but also can serve as analgesics for some painful conditions.[13] They are often used in combination with other analgesic medications. At each step of the WHO analgesic ladder (see Chapter 22), adjuvant medications may be added, depending on the type of pain experienced. Several classes of medications are essential to optimal management of pain (Table 23-3).

Nonsteroidal anti-inflammatory drugs (NSAIDs) can be helpful when the inflammatory process is involved and is initiating the pain impulse, such as in bone or soft-tissue damage. Clients with metastatic bone disease often require the combination of an opioid and an NSAID for comfort.

Tricyclic antidepressants (TCAs) and anticonvulsants can be effective analgesics in the management of pain syndromes that have a neurologic component.[13,58,61] TCAs appear to be most helpful for pain described as burning or aching; anticonvulsants are useful in the treatment of shooting and shock-like neurologic pains. The effective analgesic dose of a TCA is much lower than the dose required for an antidepressant effect.[1,13,58,61] Some clients are aware that these medications are used to treat depression and may be suspicious that the clinician "thinks the pain is in my head." Explain to clients that these medications are used to manage pain at low doses. Because it takes 5 to 7 days for TCAs to reach the desired plasma level, inform the client that it may take several days for this new medication to be effective.

Clients who report "colicky" pain may be experiencing the discomfort of smooth-muscle spasm. This type of pain is best treated with an anticholinergic medication.

Anxiety is a complex symptom that is caused by physical, emotional, and spiritual concerns. Clients who are

TABLE 23-3	*Adjuvant Analgesics*		
Pain Source	**Pain Character**	**Medication Class**	**Examples**
Bone or soft tissue	Tenderness over bone or joint Pain on movement	Nonsteroidal anti-inflammatory drugs	Ibuprofen Naproxen Indomethacin
Nerve damage/neuropathic	Burning, shooting, shock-like, or aching pain	Tricyclic antidepressants	Amitriptyline Doxepin
		Anticonvulsants	Carbamazepine Phenytoin Valproic acid Gabapentin
Smooth muscle spasms	Cramping or grabbing pains (intermittent)	Anticholinergics	Scopolamine Hyoscyamine Oxybutynin Dicyclomine
Anxiety	Generalized restlessness and discomfort	Benzodiazepines	Lorazepam Diazepam
		Butyrophenones	Haloperidol

in pain often experience some anxiety, and it may be helpful to treat the anxiety to achieve comfort.[57,58,60,61] Benzodiazepine medications are frequently used for anxiety in the palliative care setting. Haloperidol, a butyrophenone, may also be used. Management of anxiety is covered in Chapter 25.

Analgesic Dosing

The initial analgesic dose is determined based on the type and intensity of pain as well as response to current analgesics. Medication doses are titrated up or down to achieve effectiveness, both at the beginning of therapy and during the course of treatment. For example, a client receiving morphine for bone pain may find that a lower dose of morphine is possible when a NSAID is added to the regimen. Gradual escalation of the dose is required if pain reduction is inadequate. For unrelieved opioid-responsive pain problems, the opioid dose can be safely increased by 25% for mild pain (rating of 1 to 3 on a 0 to 10 scale); by 50% for moderate pain (rating of 4 to 7 on a 0 to 10 scale); and by up to 100% for severe pain (rating of 8 to 10 on a 0 to 10 scale).[49] The goal is to use the smallest dose that reduces the pain so that it causes the fewest side effects.

Therapeutic levels of analgesics must be maintained at all times for clients with persistent or chronic pain to manage the pain. Therefore, an around-the-clock (ATC) schedule (see next section) is most appropriate.[1,58,61] The frequency of doses to maintain therapeutic levels is determined by the route of administration and the duration of action of the medication. *Immediate-release* (short-acting) oral morphine requires dosing every 4 hours; oral hydromorphone (Dilaudid) may need to be given every 3 hours. *Controlled-release* medications offer the benefit of more convenient dosing schedules (every 8, 12, or 24 hours).

Rescue Dosing

The goal of ATC dosing is to keep the level of the analgesic in a range high enough to manage the pain but below the point at which a client experiences avoidable or unmanageable side effects. Unfortunately, pain does not stay at the same intensity 24 hours a day. Many clients experience pain above the normal baseline pain; this pain is often labeled *breakthrough pain*. The pain may spike above (break through) the therapeutic blood level of analgesia, and additional medications are required to manage such episodes. A short-acting (or immediate-release) dose of an opioid should be administered to "cover" the spike in the client's pain.[1,58,61]

For clients taking oral opioids, the recommended rescue dose is in the range of 5% to 15% of the total daily ATC dose of opioid.[1,20] The rescue dose should be made available every 1 to 2 hours because most immediate-release opioids reach peak effectiveness in 60 to 90 minutes. After that point, the level of the opioid in the system begins to decrease. A client experiencing pain 2 hours after a rescue dose should not be made to wait for additional medication because the level of analgesia will continue to decrease and the client will become increasingly uncomfortable. As a rule, a client who requires more than four rescue doses during a 24-hour period or is awakened from sleep experiencing pain should have the pain experience reevaluated.[14] An increase in the

ATC dose is often appropriate under these circumstances.

Dyspnea

Dyspnea is a subjective experience described as difficult breathing or an "uncomfortable awareness" of breathing that accounts for a high proportion of the client's inability to carry out activities of daily living (ADL) and gravely affects the perceived quality of life.[11,18,40,79,80] Dyspnea occurs in as many as 50% to 70% of persons at the end of their life.[79,80] Clients also mention labored breathing, shortness of breath, and feelings of suffocation.[36] The continuous exhaustion that accompanies breathlessness can be one of the most devastating symptoms for both the client and the observing family members.[36,79,80]

Etiology

Dyspnea generally results from a greater awareness of normal breathing, an increased workload of breathing, or abnormalities in the ventilatory system.[11,79,80] In a 1999 consensus statement, the American Thoracic Society[3] emphasized that many factors can contribute to the symptom of breathlessness, including pathophysiologic changes as well as clients' emotional and spiritual evaluation of the changes in their functional status and quality of living.

Disease processes commonly associated with dyspnea include (1) acute and chronic pulmonary disorders, (2) heart failure, and (3) neuromuscular disorders. In the terminally ill population, anemia and generalized weakness also can contribute to dyspnea. In addition, emotions play a major role. The fear associated with the inability to "catch one's breath" can lead to panic and worsen the sensation of dyspnea.[3,11,18,19,36,79,80]

Assessment

Assessment of clients with dyspnea includes subjective and observational data. Clients should be asked to rate dyspnea on a scale. The scale must make sense to the client, and all persons caring for that client must use the same scale. A visual analog scale with "not at all breathless" at the low end of the scale and "severely breathless" at the high end may be helpful for quantifying this symptom.[35] This information can help determine the severity of the symptom and provides a baseline to evaluate the effectiveness of interventions.[68] Clients' evaluations of their own functional status and the effect of dyspnea on ADL provide helpful information about both the physical and emotional responses to dyspnea.[3,79,80]

An objective assessment of the client provides additional information about dyspnea.[35] Observe for an increased respiratory rate, use of accessory muscles, gasping or labored breathing, restlessness, and diaphoresis.

Management

The underlying cause of dyspnea should be treated as appropriate for the client's position in the disease trajectory. For example, pneumonia in a client who is alert and oriented and has a good quality of life (as determined by the client) should be treated. It may be appropriate, however, *not* to treat pneumonia in a client who is clearly near the end of the disease trajectory if treatment of the pneumonia will not improve the quality of life. All treatment options should be reviewed with the client and family, including the option of *no* treatment.[11,35,79,80]

Although it may not be possible to treat the underlying cause of dyspnea at the end of life, many effective interventions can be used to manage the distress and uncomfortable sensations associated with dyspnea.[11,35,79,80] Interdisciplinary team support is essential in the management of dyspnea. The psychosocial and existential issues that contribute to the symptom of dyspnea require the support of professionals trained in these areas.

Opioids. Morphine is widely used for the relief of dyspnea.[11,34,76,77] Data from several clinical studies reveal that 80% to 95% of clients with terminal cancer find significant relief from the use of morphine. Exactly why opioids alleviate dyspnea is not known, but they are believed to blunt the perceptual response to dyspnea or to reduce the respiratory drive.[3,11,18,40] There is no standard optimal dose of morphine for the treatment of dyspnea, but the following recommendations are based on clinical experience:

- For the client who is already taking morphine for pain and who is dyspneic, the morphine dose should be increased by 50%.
- The dyspneic client who has not been receiving morphine should be started on 5 to 6 mg of morphine every 4 hours as needed.[40]

It may be appropriate to consider ATC dosing of morphine if the client is requiring frequent "as needed" doses. Sustained-release preparations may be more convenient and effective in this situation.[18,40]

Anti-Anxiety Agents. Both benzodiazepines and phenothiazines have been effective in the management of dyspnea. Each class of drugs has the potential to depress hypoxic or ventilator responses and to alter the emotional responses to dyspnea.[18,63] Both classes of medications have the potential for side effects, but given the prevalence of anxiety associated with the experience of breathlessness, it is considered good palliative care to try anxiolytic therapy on an individual basis.[18,63]

Bronchodilators. Bronchodilators help to decrease the effort of breathing, and several studies cite their effects on breathlessness. The significant decrease in dyspnea after theophylline use is believed to result from an improvement in the length-tension relationship in the diaphragm.[18,79,80]

Corticosteroids. Corticosteroids are commonly used in the palliative care setting to treat dyspnea. These medications are believed to influence the symptom of dyspnea by decreasing inflammation in the pulmonary tissue and increasing bronchodilation.[11,18,79,80] Corticosteroid therapy is indicated when bronchodilators have been ineffective. A trial of corticosteroids is justified in almost all clients with problematic chronic airway disease, pointing out that the dose of steroid should be high enough to work efficiently but low enough not to cause potential gastric irritation or fluid retention.[18]

Oxygen Therapy. Palliative care literature does not support the use of oxygen therapy for the relief of dyspnea. Oxygen (O_2) therapy should be used only for clients who are hypoxic or who tend to have pulmonary hypertension. If O_2 saturation is less than 90% with room air, the clinician may want to (1) consider O_2 by nasal cannula at 1 to 3 L per minute, (2) recheck the client's O_2 saturation in 20 to 30 minutes, and (3) titrate the O_2 therapy up to 6 L per minute by nasal cannula if necessary.[11,18,36,79]

Nonpharmacologic Interventions. Nurses are frequently the care providers who introduce nonpharmacologic interventions to clients and families and ensure, through education and support, that the interventions are being used to maximal effectiveness. Some interventions that nurses can initiate that will contribute to the comfort of clients experiencing dyspnea are (1) pursed-lip breathing, (2) breathing exercises, (3) positioning, (4) having a fan blowing in the room, (5) coping techniques, (6) a calming presence, (7) relaxation therapy, (8) massage, (9) acupuncture, (10) hypnosis, and (11) visualization.[11,18,36,79]

Delirium

Incidence

Delirium has been found in up to 77% to 85% of terminally ill clients with cancer and in 57% of terminally ill clients with acquired immunodeficiency syndrome (AIDS).[9] Some clinicians consider delirium the "hallmark" of dying. Studies have indicated, however, that 25% to 35% of episodes of delirium are reversible.[9,19] As many as 80% of clients with advanced cancer develop delirium during the last week of life, with many of these clients experiencing several prior episodes of delirium that resolved.[19] In the palliative care setting, early detection and assessment are likely to improve outcomes.[15]

Various terms have been used to describe delirium, such as acute brain failure, acute confusional state, acute

secondary psychosis, exogenous psychosis, sundown syndrome, and organic brain syndrome.[9,15] According to the criteria of the American Psychiatric Association's *Diagnostic and Statistical Manual of Mental Disorders (DSM-IV-TR)*,[2] *delirium* is defined as "an etiologically non-specific, global, cerebral dysfunction characterized by concurrent disturbances of level of consciousness, attention, thinking, perception, memory, psychomotor behavior, emotion, and the sleep-wake cycle." It is often identified as a sudden and significant decline in a previous level of functioning and is conceptualized as a reversible process. Delirium can also affect sleep, psychomotor activity, and emotions.[15,29,37,73]

DSM-IV-TR criteria for delirium are as follows[2]:
1. Disturbance of consciousness with reduced ability to focus, sustain, or shift attention
2. A change in cognition (such as memory deficit, disorientation, language disturbance) or the development of a perceptual disturbance that is not better accounted for by pre-existing, established, or evolving dementia
3. Development of the disturbance over a short time (usually hours to days) and a tendency to fluctuate over the course of the day

Assessment

The diagnosis of delirium is based on careful observation and awareness of its key features. Because the clinical manifestations are nonspecific, the clinician must (1) look for manifestations of a disturbance in consciousness and a change in cognition, (2) identify the rapidity of onset, and (3) assess for associated medical and environmental risks that lead to a definitive diagnosis. Delirium is commonly unrecognized by clinicians and hence is misdiagnosed.[15,29]

The most commonly used assessment instrument for identifying cognitive changes is the Mini-Mental State Examination (MMSE), a systematically scored method of evaluating cognitive function. The examination can indicate early changes in cognition as it relates to the cortical function of the brain.[15,29] The MMSE evaluates orientation, attention, recall, and language. Scores below 24, of a maximum of 30, are indicative of cognitive changes.[15,29] The MMSE relies heavily on client cooperation, however, and does not account for the abrupt changes that often occur in a client's cognitive status.[15,29]

Management

The prognosis for the client experiencing delirium is often poor. Delirium shortens the survival of cancer clients, makes the assessment of pain and symptoms difficult, and is a main cause of distress among clients, family, and health care providers.[19] This fact, however, should not deter the clinician from looking for the underlying cause because a significant number of cases are reversible. Frequently cited reversible causes of delirium are (1) medications (e.g., opioids, sedatives, anticholinergics, and steroids), (2) hypoxia, (3) dehydration (see the Evidence-Based Practice in Action feature on Dehydration, below), (4) metabolic causes (e.g., hypercalcemia, hyponatremia), (5) sepsis, (6) polypharmacy, and (7) intercranial pressure from metastatic disease.[15,29,73] Potentially helpful interventions for these reversible causes are listed in Table 23-4.

First-line pharmacologic treatment of delirium usually involves the butyrophenone class of neuroleptics when the client is agitated; however, they are *not* recommended in delirium associated with alcohol or benzodiazepine withdrawal. Haloperidol (Haldol) is the drug of choice for hallucinations and agitation in the medically ill. In addition to relieving psychotic symptoms, haloperidol is useful as an antiemetic agent. A benzodiazepine can be added to the regimen if haloperidol alone is not effective. Caution should be considered when us-

ing benzodiazepines that have a long half-life, such as diazepam (Valium), because the active metabolites can accumulate in the dehydrated and dying client and create agitation. Lorazepam (Ativan) may be considered to reduce episodes of severe distress and anxiety. Transdermal clonidine (Catapres), an alpha-adrenergic agonist, may be useful for clients suffering from autonomic symptoms such as anxiety and tachycardia. If the agitation does not respond to these pharmacologic agents, sedation may be achieved with chlorpromazine (Thorazine) or midazolam (Versed).[15,29,57]

Depression

The prevalence of depression in clients with cancer ranges anywhere from 10% to 25%; the prevalence appears to increase in the presence of functional losses, advancing illness, and unmanaged symptoms.[57] It is believed that many cases of depression in the terminally ill go unrecognized by clinicians because many of the clinical manifestations of depression (e.g., fatigue, anorexia

EVIDENCE-BASED PRACTICE IN ACTION

Dehydration

Historically the standard care in the management of dehydration is replacing fluids or hydrating the client. Traditional hospice models, however, have promoted the lack of parenteral hydration. Evidence can be found to support both approaches.[1-4] Near the end of life, it is important for the nurse to recognize that dehydration may actually exacerbate symptoms and create suffering. Symptoms such as confusion, delirium, and renal failure can create the accumulation of active drug metabolites. An example of drug accumulation from opioid therapies can create nausea, confusion, restlessness, delirium, and myoclonus and possibly lead to hyperalgesia. There is a fine line between hydration and dehydration in the terminally ill client, and the emphasis should be placed on comfort measures and the reduction of symptoms.[1]

Terminally ill clients require less fluid than the gravely ill client, and yet the nurse should not confuse edema and thirst as indicators of dehydration. Edema can be the result of underlying pathophysiology, for example, advanced cancer. Edema in this client is more likely a result of tumor blockage accompanied by impaired venous or lymphatic drainage. Thirst or dry mouth may also be the result of specific medications frequently used in palliative care (e.g., anticholinergic medications, opioids, tricyclic antidepressants).

Implications

When making the decision to hydrate the client, the health care provider considers the various options that are available based on the client's setting. Clients able to take fluids by mouth should be encouraged to do so because oral consumption is considered the preferred route. Clients who are unable to maintain adequate

fluid intake by mouth should be considered for parenteral fluid replacement. Clients in the acute care setting usually have intravenous (IV) lines inserted, which allow for replacement of fluids. Several studies have demonstrated that if the client cannot tolerate an IV or resides in the home care setting, the preferred route for hydration is a subcutaneous route also known as *hypodermoclysis* or *clysis*.[1-4]

Hypodermoclysis is easily accomplished by inserting a 25-gauge butterfly subcutaneously; the site can be used for up to 7 days.[2-4] Rehydration is accomplished with the infusion of normal saline at 70 to 100 ml/hr via continuous infusion. Hypodermoclysis is also used when providing fluid maintenance or augmentation with infusions of $\frac{2}{3}$ dextrose and $\frac{1}{3}$ normal saline via a continuous infusion of 40 to 80 ml/hr. Other rates can include 1000 ml by gravity overnight or 500 ml bolus bid infused over 1 hour.

References
1. Bruera, E., & Sweeny, B. (2001). Hydrate or dehydrate. *Supportive Care Cancer, 9*(3), 177-186.
2. Cerchietti, L., et al. (2000). Hypodermoclysis for control of dehydration in terminal stage cancer. *International Journal of Palliative Nursing, 6*(8), 370-374.
3. Frisoli, J., et al. (2000). Subcutaneous hydration by hypodermoclysis. A practical and low cost treatment for elderly patients. *Drugs and Aging, 16*(4), 313-319.
4. Moriarty, D., & Hudson, E. (2001). Hypodermoclysis for rehydration in the community. *British Journal of Community Nursing, 6*(9), 437-443.

TABLE 23-4	Reversible Causes of Delirium	
Cause	**Intervention**	
1. Medications		
a. Opioid metabolites may accumulate, especially in the presence of renal insufficiency.	a. Consider switching to an equianalgesic dose of a different opioid.	
b. Benzodiazepine metabolites may accumulate in the presence of hepatic disease.	b. Hydration may be helpful to assist in eliminating these metabolites. If antianxiety medications are needed, consider switching the client to a butyrophenone.	
2. Hypoxia	2. Intervene to improve oxygenation with bronchodilators, mucolytics, and breathing techniques. Consider oxygen therapy if O_2 saturation is <90%.	
3. Dehydration	3. Consider oral or parenteral hydration.	
4. Metabolic		
a. Hypercalcemia	a. Evaluate the benefits of hydration and use of bisphosphonates.	
b. Hyponatremia	b. Encourage moderate alcohol intake before meals and encourage sodium intake.	
5. Sepsis	5. Consider anti-infective therapy.	
6. Polypharmacy	6. Use medications that have more than one action to treat symptoms (e.g., Haldol to decrease delirium and nausea).	
7. Increased intercranial pressure from metastatic disease	7. Use corticosteroids to decrease cerebral edema.	

or weight loss, insomnia) can be attributed to the disease process itself. Key indicators of clinical depression in the terminally ill are (1) alterations in mood; (2) feelings of hopelessness, worthlessness, or excessive guilt; and (3) recurrent death wishes, including thoughts of suicide.[57] The *DSM-IV-TR* defines a major depressive syndrome when five of the following symptoms have been present for 2 weeks or longer: depressed mood, anhedonia, weight loss or gain, insomnia or hypersomnia, agitation

or motor retardation, fatigue or loss of energy, depreciation or guilt feelings, concentration difficulties, or thoughts of death or suicide.[2,4,46]

Etiology

A terminal diagnosis potentiates both anxiety and depression. A client with a family or personal history of previous depressive episodes is at even higher risk for depression than the general population. Interestingly, some cancer diagnoses, such as pancreatic cancer, have been associated more strongly with depression. It is not clear whether psychological or physiologic factors are involved in this higher risk.[2,9,46]

Depression is thought to be a direct result of abnormal serotonin (5-hydroxytryptamine [5-HT]) neurotransmission in the CNS. This abnormal secretion may be genetic, or it may be induced by some unknown mechanism. Other neurotransmitters, such as gamma-aminobutyric acid (GABA) and norepinephrine, have also been closely linked in anxiety and may be associated with depression.[57]

Assessment

Nurses play a pivotal role in identifying clients with depression. An important question you can ask is, "Are you depressed?" or "How has your mood been lately?" Although feeling sad and anxious at times is a normal response to a terminal diagnosis, do not ignore these symptoms. Persons with clinical depression should be referred to skilled health care professionals for evaluation and treatment.

Management

Optimal therapy is achieved with the combination of supportive psychotherapy, cognitive-behavioral techniques, and pharmaceutical management. This approach requires coordination of the interdisciplinary team. Antidepressant medications can be effective in treating depression. There are several classes of antidepressants. The newer selective serotonin re-uptake inhibitors (SSRIs) cause fewer side effects and are at least as effective as the TCAs.[57] A trial of antidepressant therapy is warranted in the terminally ill client because it may greatly enhance the quality of life. See Chapter 25 for further discussion of anxiety, depression, medications, and treatments.

Fatigue and Weakness

Fatigue is among the most prevalent symptoms of persons with advanced illnesses and is universally associated with advanced malignancy. It is a distressing, subjective experience that impedes functioning and impairs quality of life. Clients describe fatigue as tiredness, exhaustion, generalized weakness, diminished energy, increased need to rest or sleep, diminished motivation, diminished capacity to pay attention, or a disturbed mood.[16,54,59,71]

Etiology

Although the etiology of fatigue is not clearly understood, many physiologic, psychoemotional, and spiritual factors are recognized as contributing factors to the phenomenon of fatigue.[16,54,59,71] Fatigue may result from any one or combination of the following problems:

- *Disease/treatment-related:* Disease process, disease treatments (surgery, radiation therapy, chemotherapy, biologic therapy), infection, anemia, malnutrition or cachexia, chronic hypoxia, metabolic or electrolyte disorders, endocrine disorders, neuromuscular disorders, medication side effects (e.g., excessive sedation from opioids).
- *Physiologic:* Overexertion, immobility or lack of exercise, poor sleep, pain, or other discomfort.
- *Psychoemotional:* Stress, anxiety, grief, depression.
- *Spiritual:* Fear, distress.

Assessment

Because of the multidimensional nature of fatigue and the potential for several contributing factors to be present at any one time, a comprehensive assessment is required. It is important to identify and treat reversible causes of fatigue. All medications should be reviewed and any unnecessary centrally acting drugs eliminated. If the clinician suspects that opioids are contributing to fatigue, reduction of the opioid dose by 25% should be considered, followed by evaluation of the client's cognition if pain is still controlled and fatigue is lessened.[54] If pain returns with the reduction in dose, the opioid dose should be returned to the previous level.

NOTE: For the client who is still in pain and is sedated from opioids has an opioid-resistant pain syndrome, an adjuvant medication will be required (see Adjuvant Analgesics earlier in this chapter). Stress, fear, and spiritual distress are best addressed through counseling.

Management

If anemia is contributing to fatigue, transfusion with packed red blood cells may be appropriate. It appears there is no threshold hemoglobin level below which persons universally experience fatigue.[54] Because so many factors contribute to fatigue, persons with low hemoglobin levels who receive transfusions may still feel fatigued. In end-of-life care, a transfusion is not appropriate if the client's quality of life does not improve. Some persons with advanced diseases may have significant anemia but have few clinical manifestations.[24,50] These

persons also would not receive a transfusion. Erythropoietin is helpful in treating the fatigue associated with chemotherapy-induced anemia,[55] but there is little research to show its effectiveness in persons with advanced diseases.

Nurses can initiate many interventions to help clients cope with fatigue. Strategies to manage stress include counseling, education, relaxation, and massage. Instituting a regular exercise program can be effective in lessening fatigue in clients undergoing chemotherapy. Although no studies on the effect of an exercise program on fatigue in the palliative care setting have been published, this strategy should be considered for clients who are able to participate in some form of exercise. In addition, for clients who can eat and take in fluids, you can encourage adequate nutrition and hydration.[24,54,71]

Although no studies have been reported on the effects of energy-conservation techniques for persons with fatigue,[55] modifications of activity and rest patterns are often included as intervention strategies. The nurse encourages clients to (1) incorporate rest times into their daily schedules, (2) plan their most strenuous activities for the time of day when energy levels are highest, and (3) capitalize on saving energy by accepting the assistance of others, delegating tasks, and using equipment such as a bedside commode or a portable telephone.

Medications may be helpful in treating fatigue in some clients. Corticosteroids are sometimes used to treat fatigue in persons with advanced cancer. The exact mechanism of action is not clear, but some researchers believe that corticosteroids may lessen fatigue by inhibiting tumor and tumor-induced substances that contribute to the symptom. Others suggest that fatigue is relieved by the central euphoric effect of these medications. If anorexia or cachexia is a contributing factor in fatigue, the appetite-stimulating effect of corticosteroids may be helpful.

Psychostimulants have also been used to treat people with fatigue (see Chapter 24). Pilot studies using these medications are promising.[27] The largest experience in people with cancer has been with methylphenidate (Ritalin). Dextroamphetamine (Dexedrine) and pemoline (Cylert) have also been used.[51,54,71]

Sleep Disturbances

Etiology

Impaired sleep is a common, and often overlooked, problem in clients with advanced illnesses. Insomnia occurs in up to 59% of persons with advanced cancer. Many times a disturbance in sleep is accepted as "part of being sick"; however, it is important to recognize the importance of sleep. Sleep is associated with tissue restoration; sleep deprivation alters immune function. Although people with a terminal illness are not going to "recuperate" from their underlying disease, they can benefit from the healing and protective functions of sleep when dealing with tissue injury and infection. Excessive sleepiness is also emotionally disabling, resulting in an inability to participate in treatment, comprehend information, and share in social interactions. Furthermore, impairment of sleep may lead to depression, irritability, and withdrawal.[41,65]

Assessment

Evaluation of the amount and quality of sleep is an important component of the overall assessment of a client in the palliative care setting.[41,65] This evaluation covers the following:

- Usual bedtime
- How long it takes to fall asleep
- Any wakefulness during the night
- Usual waking time
- Subjective feeling of being "refreshed" in the morning
- Frequency and length of daytime naps
- Use of sleep medications
- The cause of any sleep problems as identified by the client

There are many potential causes of sleep disturbances. Physiologic factors contributing to impaired sleep include pain, nausea and vomiting, itching, respiratory problems, medications (e.g., corticosteroids, bronchodilators, antihypertensives), metabolic disturbances, and delirium. Sometimes medication dosing schedules interrupt sleep. Controlled-release medications provide the advantage of not needing to be awakened during the night for dose administration.

Psychoemotional factors, such as depression and anxiety, also interfere with sleep. The client's environment definitely influences the amount and quality of sleep; unfamiliar surroundings, frequent interruptions, noise, bright lighting, and unpleasant odors can all lead to a disturbance in sleep. In addition, lack of exercise, inactivity, and boredom may lead to excessive napping during the day, resulting in poor sleep at night.

Management

Treatable causes of sleep disturbance must be addressed with appropriate interventions and discontinuation of medications that interfere with sleep when possible. General sleep hygiene strategies include the following[41,65]:

- Establishing a regular sleep schedule
- Staying out of bed during the day
- Napping only when necessary
- Keeping active (mentally or physically) during the day
- Minimizing nighttime disruptions
- Avoiding stimulants at night (caffeine, nicotine)

Persons who have difficulty falling asleep may benefit from establishing a relaxing bedtime routine. Depending on individual preferences, this relaxation routine may consist of massage, progressive muscle relaxation, imagery, music, and warm milk or herbal tea.

When other interventions are not effective in promoting or maintaining sleep, medications may be appropriate. Benzodiazepines are the main group of medications used to promote sleep. Some controversy remains about the long-term effectiveness of the benzodiazepines, and most are recommended for short-term use. Thus, the need for sleep medications must be reevaluated on a regular basis. In general, benzodiazepines are used intermittently, at the lowest effective dose, and are never discontinued abruptly.[77] Benzodiazepines used for sleep disturbances include the following:

- *Short half-life (2 to 4 hours):* Triazolam (Halcion), zolpidem (Ambien). Because of their quick onset of action, these medications are helpful for clients who have difficulty falling asleep. They do not, however, benefit clients with sleep maintenance problems. Rebound insomnia is common if the medication is abruptly stopped. Triazolam, which is associated with adverse drug reactions, has been removed from the market in some countries.
- *Intermediate half-life (6 to 15 hours):* Lorazepam (Ativan), oxazepam (Serax), temazepam (Restoril). These medications are helpful for promoting sleep onset and maintenance.
- *Long half-life (29 to 100 hours):* Flurazepam (Dalmane), quazepam (Doral). Although these agents help to promote sleep onset and maintenance, daytime sedation is common because of their long half-lives. Also, drug accumulation may occur in older adults. (See Chapter 24 on sleep management.)

Cachexia-Anorexia Syndrome

Incidence

Cachexia is derived from the Greek words *kakos and hexis,* meaning "poor condition." The term *cachexia-anorexia syndrome* is often used loosely to define weight loss, wasting, or loss of appetite.[25] Cachexia-anorexia syndrome is, however, one of the most common problems afflicting clients with advanced cancer and AIDS. Its associated symptoms of debility, chronic nausea, and constipation represent the most common constellation.[25]

The incidence in clients with cancer varies with the type of primary tumor. The client who has adenocarcinoma of the breast is less likely to exhibit cachexia-anorexia syndrome than the client who has adenocarcinoma of the lung or pancreas. Wasting is not commonly observed in clients with a hematologic malignancy, and yet it is prevalent in clients with myelodysplastic syndromes.[47]

Etiology

Several studies have identified chemical factors (due to tumor burden) that contribute to cachexia-anorexia syndrome. Numerous cytokines have been identified to produce this syndrome, including tumor necrosis factor, interleukin-1 and interleukin-6, and interferon. Other causes are metabolic abnormalities, a decrease in nutritional intake, and eventual loss of appetite.[19] Correctable causes are found in clients who have obstruction of the upper or lower bowel as a result of tumor invasion. A simple diagnostic indicator suggests a 5-pound weight loss in the previous 2 months or an estimated daily caloric intake of fewer than 70 calories per kilogram of body weight.[19,25]

Other contributing factors in cachexia-anorexia syndrome are presented in Table 23-5. Clinical manifestations commonly observed in this syndrome are (1) muscle loss, (2) impaired immunity, (3) loss of body fat, (4) glucose intolerance, (5) fluid retention, (6) vitamin deficiencies, and (7) fatigue and weakness (asthenia).[19,25]

Management

Interventions are as varied as the contributing factors. Some clients may not respond favorably to the replacement of dietary supplements and require more aggressive intervention, such as a progestational (hormonal) agent. Progestational agents can improve the client's appetite in up to 80% and often induce weight gain.[19]

 These are the only agents that have demonstrated the ability to induce weight gain after several weeks of treatment at maximal doses (e.g., megestrol acetate (Megace) 160 mg three times daily).[19,25]

TABLE 23-5	*Factors Contributing to Cachexia-Anorexia Syndrome*

- Tumor involvement of gastrointestinal tract
- Antitumor therapy
- Infections
- Taste change
- Medications
- Food aversions
- Pain
- Psychological factors
- Changes in metabolism
- Hormonal changes
- Fatigue, weakness
- Increased metabolic rate; altered fat, protein, or carbohydrate metabolism; fluid-electrolyte abnormalities; hormonal changes
- Malabsorption
- Tumor metabolism

The following pharmacologic strategies are suggested for the client with cachexia-anorexia syndrome:

1. Progestational agents
2. Corticosteroids
3. Dietary interventions involving omega-3 fatty acids and branched-chain amino acids
4. Combination approaches:
   a. Cannabinoids
   b. Dietary supplements
   c. Prokinetic agents
   d. CNS stimulants (methylphenidate)

Remember, the loss of appetite often assessed in the dying client is a normal process that should not be confused with cachexia-anorexia syndrome.

INDICATORS OF IMMINENT DEATH

Certain physical, cognitive, and behavioral changes occur as a person enters the active dying process. Family members must be informed about the changes to expect so that they feel as prepared as possible and can recognize when death is approaching.[77] The following are common nursing diagnosis of imminent death:

- Impaired urinary elimination due to renal failure or decreased perfusion of the kidneys.
- Total urinary incontinence caused by changes in perception or lack of muscular control.
- Urinary retention due to medications or sensory changes causing inability to relax urinary sphincter.
- Ineffective tissue perfusion: peripheral resulting from shunting of circulation to vital organ systems, leading to tachycardia, mottling, and peripheral cyanosis.
- Impaired gas exchange and ineffective breathing pattern due to pulmonary compromise or compensation for metabolic alterations, leading to tachypnea, dyspnea, apnea, or Cheyne-Stokes respirations.
- Ineffective airway clearance resulting from weakness, leading to congested breathing (sometimes referred to a "death rattle").
- Impaired physical mobility due to generalized weakness.
- Impaired swallowing resulting from weakness and loss of gag reflex.
- Disturbed sensory perception due to altered perfusion to sensory organs and to brain itself and metabolic alterations; may progress to coma. Hearing is believed to remain intact throughout the dying process.
- Acute confusion from delirium or decreased circulation to the brain.
- Disturbed thought processes resulting from biochemical alterations.
- Anxiety, death anxiety, or fear due to physical discomfort (e.g., pain, dyspnea), unfinished business, or spiritual concerns.

TABLE 23-6	*Common Objective Body System Indicators of Imminent Death*
Cognition/orientation	Not always nonresponsive, may be agitated or restless, cannot subjectively respond to verbal stimuli
Cardiovascular	Tachycardia, irregular heart rate, lowered blood pressure or significant widening between systolic and diastolic pressures, dehydration
Pulmonary	Tachypnea, dyspnea, use of accessory muscles, acetone breath, Cheyne-Stokes breathing, pooling of secretions or noisy respirations
Gastrointestinal	Diminished appetite, smaller amounts of feces (despite not eating), incontinence
Renal	Diminished urine output, incontinence, concentrated urine
Mobility	Limited mobility, bedbound, and requires frequent position changes

Table 23-6 highlights the indicators of impending death.

COMMUNICATION ISSUES

The dying process can be a time of emotional crisis for many clients and their families. The nurse can help lead clients and families down a less threatening path to what is often termed "the unknown." To do so, however, it is important to develop a level of comfort when communicating with dying clients and their families. Self-examination and articulation of personal feelings about death and dying are essential to providing emotional support and guidance to the dying. Uncomfortable emotions expressed by a nurse can impede the ability of clients and families to finish important issues and accomplish healthy closure.

Clients and families facing the last days of life should be given the opportunity to express any or all concerns about issues that matter the most to them. The nurse can serve as a listener, a friend, and an advocate for the client. Being available in a nonjudgmental and nonthreatening manner allows the client and family to trust the nurse. Once trust is established and the client believes that the nurse will effectively manage his or her symptoms, the client may begin to open up emotionally and discuss many concerns about the illness and death.[66] Each client is unique, and so are the conversations that occur between nurse, client, and family. The nurse can provide the therapeutic use of self through the following interventions[69,70]:

- Provide listening skills that encourage the client or family to tell their "story."
- Encourage a mutual participatory relationship that is not dominated by controlling conversations.
- Use less directive skills such as silence, paraphrases, reflections, and sincerity.
- Offer structure to the conversation and yet empower the client or family to express his or her needs.
- Promote opportunities for discussion and demonstrates a willingness to listen to difficult and painful concerns.

Communicating with dying clients and their families takes into account the multidimensional nature of people. See the Diversity in Health Care feature on Cultural Aspects of Death and Dying on the website. Sensitivity and knowledge surrounding culture, spirituality, lifestyle, and emotional connections are essential when supporting clients and their families at the end of life.

One of the most important tasks of the bedside nurse is to empower clients and families to participate in the final act of living. Through ongoing assessment, communication, and skilled physical care, you can communicate reassurance, confidence, and support for the vulnerable client and family. The seasoned hand of a skilled professional supporting and guiding the client can change the journey through dying and death from a frightening process to one of peace and comfort.

CARE FOR CAREGIVERS

The families of terminally ill clients commonly serve as primary caregivers in the home care environment and are often highly involved in providing care in other palliative care settings (e.g., extended care facility, acute care setting). This "intensive caring" is physically and emotionally exhausting. To provide and maintain this level of care, these caregivers need education and support from all members of the interdisciplinary health care team. Coping tasks for families caring for a loved one who is dying and suggested interventions are described in Table 23-7.

Even though this intensive caring is difficult, most family caregivers are able to provide appropriate levels of care for their loved ones. Nurses play a pivotal role in assessing their educational and support needs, providing information and support, and referring caregivers to other team members and community agencies to address their needs.

SUPPORT OF THE GRIEVING FAMILY

Bereavement care is an important component of any palliative care program.[64,78] Providing bereavement care requires an understanding of the normal grieving process and the tasks of grief work. Grief is a normal and expected reaction to a loss. Family members will grieve the loss of their loved ones. One role of the health care team is to reinforce the understanding that grieving is healthy, a necessary process that the family must go through to be able to move on in their lives. Nurses need to validate

TABLE 23-7 *Family Coping Tasks in Terminal Illness*	
Coping Task	**Support or Interventions**
1. Promote acceptance versus denial	1. Provide realistic information about the illness and treatment options. Encourage open and honest communication among family members.
2. Establish a relationship with the health care team	2. Explain the roles of all interdisciplinary team members. Establish trust and maintain open lines of communication.
3. Meet the needs of the dying person a. Physical needs	a. Provide information about pain and symptom management, use of equipment, skin care/position, rest and nutrition, infection control, and safety. Reassure caregivers that they are doing a good job. Assess the need for assistance, such as home health aide. Assess the need for transfer to a different care setting.
b. Emotional needs	b. Encourage caregivers to take time to sit and listen to their loved one and to share each other's feelings and concerns. Assess the need for additional support/counseling from the interdisciplinary team.
4. Maintain functional equilibrium (i.e., the family must maintain some sense of normalcy to continue to function as a family unit)	4. Assist family to identify and prioritize activities that must be continued (e.g., going to work or school, doing laundry, buying groceries). Assist family to identify support persons to help with these tasks. Encourage caregivers to use respite care services to care for themselves and to attend family events outside of direct caregiving.
5. Regulate family affect	5. Allow caregivers the opportunity to express their feelings. Give them permission to have whatever feelings they have (i.e., "feelings just are—there's no right or wrong"). Acknowledge that normally joyful times, such as holidays, may not feel as joyful. Encourage formal counseling, if needed. Encourage caregivers to address their own needs and to care for themselves, too.
6. Negotiate relationships outside the family	6. Give permission to take time to maintain friendships. Discuss options for maintaining jobs while caring for a dying loved one.
7. Cope with the post-death phase (healthy grieving)	7. Support family while they accept the finality of their loss. Discuss the functioning of the family unit without the loved one. Encourage using available bereavement supports/counseling.

as normal the manifestations that the bereaved may be experiencing (Table 23-8).

In addition to knowing the normal responses to grief, it is helpful for those working with the bereaved to understand the tasks of the grieving process. Four tasks of mourning that must be accomplished for the bereavement to reach a satisfactory conclusion include the following:

- Accepting the reality of the loss
- Experiencing the pain of the loss
- Adjusting to the environment in which the deceased is missing

• Finding a way to remember the deceased while moving forward with life[78]

Most people adjust to bereavement adequately, but for some bereavement can be complicated. It is important for health care providers to identify people with abnormal or complicated grieving and refer them for skilled counseling and support. The following are examples of complicated grieving[64,78]:

• *Chronic grief*: prolonged grieving; the sense that person is "stuck" in the grieving process

• *Delayed grief*: a previously insufficiently mourned loss that becomes evident later
• *Exaggerated grief*: intensification of the normal grief response to the point of dysfunction
• *Masked grief*: grief hidden at the time of loss; and manifests itself later as a physical or psychiatric problem

Health care providers play a pivotal role in assisting families throughout the grieving process. Table 23-9 identifies strategies helpful to persons experiencing grief.

TABLE 23-8   *Manifestations of Normal Grief*

Behaviors	Cognitions	Feelings	Physical Sensations
1. Sleep disturbances 2. Appetite disturbances 3. Absent-minded behavior 4. Social withdrawal 5. Dreams of the deceased 6. Avoiding reminders of the deceased 7. Searching and calling out 8. Restless overactivity 9. Sighing 10. Crying 11. Carrying objects as reminders 12. Visiting places as reminders	1. Disbelief 2. Confusion 3. Preoccupation/Obsessiveness 4. Visual and auditory hallucinations 5. Sense that loved one is nearby	1. Sadness 2. Anger 3. Guilt 4. Anxiety 5. Loneliness 6. Fatigue 7. Helplessness 8. Yearning 9. Emancipation 10. Relief 11. Numbness	1. Hollowness in the stomach 2. Chest and throat tightness 3. Over-sensitivity to noise 4. Sense of unreality 5. Feeling shortness of breath 6. Muscle weakness 7. Lack of energy 8. Dry mouth

Data from Roberts, K.F., & Berry, P.H. (2002). Grief and bereavement. In K.K. Kuebler, P.H. Berry, & D.E. Heidrich (Eds.). *End-of-life care: Clinical practice guidelines* (pp. 53-63). Philadelphia: W.B. Saunders.

TABLE 23-9   *Interventions for Grieving Persons*

Task	Interventions
Accept the reality of the loss	Listen actively. Encourage gentle exploration of what the future may look like without person who has died. Assess and encourage the development of a support system. Encourage time with the body of the deceased at the time of death. Offer opportunities to repeat the story of the death. Normalize feelings through personal contacts and written materials about grief and loss. Avoid the use of platitudes. Attend the funeral or visitation if possible; send a personal card to the family. Respect survivors' feelings without judgment.
Experience the pain of the loss	Assist in identifying feelings or behaviors and normalize them. Assist the survivor in placing meaning on the death.
Adjust to the environment in which the deceased is missing	Assist the survivor in further identifying the meaning of loss in practical terms (e.g., role changes). Provide practical assistance with developing needed skills. Advise the survivors to minimize change and to grieve where things are familiar; discourage moving or any similar large life change.
Remember the deceased with moving forward with life	Listen actively without judgment. Validate and normalize feeling. Encourage attendance at grief and loss support or educational groups.

Data from Roberts, K.F., & Berry, P.H. (2002). Grief and bereavement. In K.K. Kuebler, P.H. Berry, & D.E. Heidrich (Eds.). *End-of-life care: Clinical practice guidelines* (pp. 53-63). Philadelphia: W. B. Saunders.

CONCLUSIONS

The nurse who is able to offer compassion, assess the multitude of symptoms, and participate in their management from an interdisciplinary team is a vital link for the client and family experiencing the final phase of life. The skilled and knowledgeable nurse is the bearer of light along the path of the unknown as the client and family attempt to make sense of life's greatest mystery: death. The nurse can promote a healthy and positive dying experience for all involved.

THINKING CRITICALLY *evolve*

1. T.S., a 57-year-old man, has stage IV squamous cell carcinoma of the right lung with metastatic bony involvement. You find that he is in excruciating pain and is so sedated that he is unable to rate his pain subjectively. He is nauseated, has not had a bowel movement in 6 days, and is anorexic and dehydrated. His current medications include sustained-release morphine 60 mg every 6 hours, a transdermal opioid of 75 μg, and immediate-release morphine 20 mg every 2 hours, which have not provided relief. What can you do to make this client more comfortable?

Factors to Consider. Besides poor pain control, what other problems need attention? Consider the addition of an adjuvant analgesic, the dosing of the opioids, and the client's hydration status.

2. F.T., a 43-year-old man, entered the emergency department with complaints of severe dyspnea. The chest x-ray revealed pleural effusion of the right lung. The results of the thoracentesis, which drained 1500 ml of fluid, were positive for adenocarcinoma. After several diagnostic studies were performed, no primary site for the tumor was identified. He was referred to an oncologist for palliative chemotherapy. You are asked to make a home visit to change the dressing on his chest tube. Your first assessment reveals a very cachectic, dehydrated, constipated, dyspneic client whose pain is well managed. The chest tube drainage totals 450 ml daily. The client and his wife are questioning the relevance of the chemotherapy, given the poor prognosis as well as his continued weight loss, loss of appetite, and weakness. He informs you that he does not want to be hospitalized and would like to remain at home and comfortable. After learning about this client's status and wishes, what actions should you take?

Factors to Consider. What actions should be taken to facilitate the client's request? Is 24-hour care needed now or in the future? What additional needs might the client or his wife have?

3. J.K. is a 38-year-old, unmarried teacher who has diabetes mellitus and polycystic kidney disease (PKD). Her most recent kidney-pancreas transplant has been rejected, and she is undergoing hemodialysis again. She has not been compliant with her diet and fluid restrictions, and multiple dialysis access sites have become infected. She states that she does not want to continue dialysis. What should you do next? Should her parents be told of her request?

Factors to Consider. How can you be certain that the client understands the ramifications of ending the hemodialysis? What can you do to keep her comfortable once dialysis is discontinued?

Discussions for these questions can be found on the website and the CD-ROM.

BIBLIOGRAPHY

1. Agency for Health Care Policy and Research. (1994). *Managing cancer pain*. Washington, DC: Department of Health and Human Services. Authors.

2. American Psychiatric Association. (2000). *Diagnostic and statistical manual of mental disorders (DSM-IV-TR)* (4th ed., text revision). Washington, DC: Author.

3. American Thoracic Society Standards. (1999). The diagnosis and care of patients with chronic obstructive pulmonary disease. *American Journal of Respiratory Critical Care Medicine, 159*, 321-340.

4. Bednash, G., & Ferrell, B. (2002). Nursing care at the end-of-life. *ANCC/AACN Continuing Education for Nurses*. Washington, DC: ANCC.

5. Bennahum, D. (2003). The historical development of hospice and palliative care. In D. Sheehan & W. Forman (Eds.), *Hospice and palliative care: Concepts and Practices* (2nd ed., pp. 3-13). Sudbury, MA: Jones & Bartlett.

6. Billings, A., Gardner, M., & Putnam, A. (2002). A one-day, hospital-wide survey of dying inpatients. *Journal of Palliative Medicine, 5*(3), 363-374.

7. Blacksher, E., & Christopher, M. (2002). On the road to reform: Advocacy and activism in end-of-life care. *Journal of Palliative Medicine 5*(1), 13-22.

8. Block, S. (2002). Medical education in end-of-life care: The status of reform. *Journal of Palliative Medicine, 5* (2), 243-248.

9. Brietbart, W., Chochinov, H., & Passik, S. (2003). Psychiatric symptoms in palliative care. In D. Doyle, G. Hanks, N. Cherny, & K. Calman (Eds.), *Oxford textbook of palliative medicine* (3rd ed., pp, 746-774). Oxford: Oxford University Press.

10. Brumley, R. (2002). Future of end-of-life care" the managed care organization perspective. *The Journal of Palliative Medicine 5*(2), 263-270.

11. Carrieri-Kohlman, V., & Stalbarg, M. (2003). Dyspnea. In V. Carrieri-Kohlman, A. Lindsay, & C. West (Eds.). *Pathophysiological phenomena in nursing* (3rd ed., pp. 177-207). Philadelphia: W. B. Saunders.

evolve Did you remember to check out the bonus material on the Evolve website and the CD-ROM, including free self-assessment exercises?

http://evolve.elsevier.com/Black/medsurg/

12. Casarett, D., et al. (2002). Does a palliative care clinic have a role in improving end-of-life care? Results of a pilot program. *Journal of Palliative Medicine, 5*(3), 387-396.

13. Cherny, N., & Portenoy, R.K. (1999). Practical issues in the management of cancer pain. In P.D. Wall & P. Melzack (Eds.). *Textbook of pain* (4th ed., pp. 1479-1522). New York: Churchill Livingstone.

14. Coyle, N., & Layman-Goldstein, M. (2001). Pain assessment and management in palliative care. In M. Matzo & D. Sherman (Eds.). *Palliative care nursing: quality care to the end of life* (pp. 362-486). New York: Springer Publishing Company.

15. Culp, K. (2003). Acute confusion. In V. Carrieri-Kohlman, A. Lindsay, & C. West (Eds.), *Pathophysiological phenomena in nursing* (3rd ed., pp. 155-171). Philadelphia: W. B. Saunders.

16. Dean, G., & Anderson, P. (2001). Fatigue. In B.R. Ferrell & N. Coyle (Eds.). *Textbook of palliative nursing* (pp. 91-100). New York: Oxford University Press.

17. Doyle, D., et al. (2003). Introduction. In D. Doyle, G. Hanks, N. Cherny, & K. Calman (Eds.), *Oxford textbook of palliative medicine* (3rd ed., pp. 1-12). Oxford: Oxford University Press.

18. Dudgeon, D. (2002). Managing dyspnea and cough. *Hematology Oncology Clinics of North America, 16*(3), 557-577.

19. Driver, L., & Bruera, E. (2002). *The M.D. Anderson palliative care handbook.* Houston: Department of Symptom Control and Palliative Care, The University of Texas M.D. Anderson Cancer Center.

20. Finn-Paradis, L. (1985). *The development of hospice in America: The hospice handbook.* Rockville, MD: Aspen.

21. Fink, R., & Gates, R. (2001). Pain assessment. In B.R. Ferrell & N. Coyle (Eds.). *Textbook of palliative nursing* (pp. 53-75). New York: Oxford University Press.

22. Ferrell, B., & Coyle, N. (2002). An overview of palliative nursing care. *American Journal of Nursing, 102*(5), 26-33.

23. Friedman, B., Harwood, K., & Shields, M. (2002). Barriers and enablers to hospice referrals: An expert overview. *Journal of Palliative Medicine 5*(1), 73-81.

 24. Given, B., et al. (2002). Pain and fatigue management: Results of a nursing randomized clinical trial, *Oncology Nursing Forum, 29*(6), 949-956.

25. Grant, M., & Dean, G. (2003). Anorexia. In V. Carrieri-Kohlman, A. Lindsay, & C. West (Eds.). *Pathophysiological phenomena in nursing* (3rd ed., pp. 35-47). Philadelphia: W. B. Saunders.

26. Homant, S. (2002). Hospice care. In K. Kuebler, & P. Esper (Eds.), *Palliative practices from A-Z for the bedside clinician* (pp. 147-150). Pittsburgh, PA: Oncology Nursing Press.

27. Homsi, J., Walsh, D., & Nelson, K.A. (2000). Psychostimulants in supportive care. *Supportive Care in Cancer, 8,* 385-397.

28. Hoyer, T. (2002). Hospice and future of end-of-life care: Approaches and funding ideas. *Journal of Palliative Medicine, 5*(2), 259-270.

29. Ingham, J., & Caraceni, A. (2002). Delirium. In A. Berger, R. Portenoy, & D. Weissman (Eds.), *Principles and practice of supportive oncology* (2nd ed., pp. 555-576). Philadelphia: Lippincott, Williams & Wilkins.

30. Introcaso, D., & Lynn, J. (2002). Systems of care: Future reform. *Journal of Palliative Medicine 5*(2), 255-262.

31. Kassa, S., & Loge, J. (2003). Quality of life in palliative medicine. In D. Doyle, G. Hanks, N. Cherny, & K. Calman (Eds.), *Oxford textbook of palliative medicine* (3rd ed., pp. 195-206). Oxford: Oxford University Press.

32. Kinzbrunner, B. (1998). Hospice: 15 years and beyond in the care of the dying. *Journal of Palliative Medicine, 1,* 127-137.

33. Kübler-Ross, E. (1969). *On death and dying.* New York: Macmillan.

34. Kübler-Ross, E. (1995). *Death is of vital importance: On life, death and life after death.* New York: Station Press.

35. Kuebler, K. (1996). *Hospice and palliative care practice protocol: Dyspnea.* Pittsburgh, PA: Hospice Nurses Association.

36. Kuebler, K. (2002). Dyspnea. In K. Kuebler, P. Berry, & D. Heidrich (Eds.). *End of life care: clinical practice guidelines* (pp. 301-315). Philadelphia: W. B. Saunders.

37. Kuebler, K., English N., & Heidrich, D. (2001). Delirium, confusion, agitation and restlessness. In B. Ferrell & N. Coyle (Eds.). *Textbook of palliative nursing* (pp. 290-308). New York: Oxford University Press.

38. Kuebler, K., & Ogle, K. (1998). Psychometric evaluation of an objective assessment instrument to measure pain, dyspnea and restlessness (Abstract). *Journal of Palliative Care, 14,* 125.

39. Last Acts (2002). *Means to a better end: A report on dying in America today.* Washington DC: Authors.

40. LeGrand, S., et al. (2003). Opioids, respiratory function, and dyspnea. *American Journal of Hospice and Palliative Care, 20*(1), 57-61.

41. Lee, K. (2003). Impaired sleep. In V. Carrieri-Kohlman, A. Lindsay, & C. West (Eds.). *Pathophysiological phenomena in nursing* (3rd ed., pp. 363-385). Philadelphia: W. B. Saunders.

42. Lindell, A. (2000). Personal quote. *Journal of the American Medical Association 284*(19), 2442.

43. Lo, B. (1995). End-of-life care after termination of SUPPORT. *Hastings Center Report Special Supplement, 25,* S6-S8.

44. Lynn, J. (1998). Complaints about hospice: Growing up or going wrong? *ABCD Exchange, 1,* 2-7.

45. Lynn, J. (2000). Learning to care for people with chronic illness facing the end of life. *The Journal of the American Medical Association 284*(9), 2508-2511.

46. Lucas, B. (1999). Coping with psychiatric emergencies in the office: Patient care for the nurse practitioner. *Clinician Reviews, 2,* 31-42.

47. MacDonald, N. (2002). Redefining symptom management. *Journal of Palliative Medicine, 5*(2), 301-304.

48. Mahoney, J. (1998). The Medicare hospice benefit—15 years of success. *Journal of Palliative Medicine, 1,* 139-146.

49. McCaffery, M., & Pasero, C. (1999). *Pain: clinical manual (2nd Ed.).* St. Louis: Mosby.

50. McHale, H. (2002). Palliative care. In K. Kuebler & P. Esper (Eds.). *Palliative practices from A-Z for the bedside clinician.* Pittsburgh, PA: Oncology Nursing Press 193-195.

51. McKinnon, S. (2002). Fatigue. In K. Kuebler, P. Berry, & D. Heidrich (Eds.). *End of life care: clinical practice guidelines* (pp. 317-326). Philadelphia: W. B. Saunders.

52. Marshall, P. (1995). The SUPPORT Study: Who's talking? *Hastings Center Report Special Supplement 25,* S9-S11.

53. Melvin, T. (2001). The primary care physician and palliative care. *Primary Care 28*(2), 239-248.

54. Miaskowski, C., & Portenoy, R. (2002). Assessment and management of cancer-related fatigue. In A. Berger, R. Portenoy, & D. Weissman (Eds.), *Principles and practice of supportive oncology* (2nd ed., pp. 141-153). Philadelphia: Lippincott, Williams & Wilkins.

55. Nail, L. (2002). Fatigue in patients with cancer. *Oncology Nursing Forum, 29,* 537-544.

56. Ogle, K., Mavis, B., & Wyatt, G. (2002). Physicians and hospice care: Attitudes, knowledge and referrals. *Journal of Palliative Medicine, 5(1),* 85-92.

57. Paice, J. (2002). Managing psychological conditions in palliative care. *American Journal of Nursing, 102*(11), 36-43.

58. Panke, J. (2002). Difficulties in managing pain at the end of life. *American Journal of Nursing, 102*(7), 26-34.

59. Piper, B. (2003). Fatigue. In V. Carrieri-Kohlman, A. Lindsay, & C. West (Eds.). *Pathophysiological phenomena in nursing* (3rd ed., pp. 209-234). Philadelphia: W. B. Saunders.

60. Pollack, M. (1999). New treatments for panic disorders, psychiatric illness in primary care. *Clinician Reviews, 9*(3), 4-9.

61. Portenoy, R. (2001). *Contemporary diagnosis and management of pain in oncologic and AIDS patient* (3rd ed.). Newton, PA: Handbooks in Health Care Company.

62. Puntillo, K., Miaskowski, C., & Summer, G. (2003). In V. Carrieri-Kohlman, A. Lindsay, & C. West (Eds.). *Pathophysiological phenomena in nursing* (3rd ed., pp. 235-254). Philadelphia: W. B. Saunders.

63. Rhodes, V., & McDaniel, R. (1998). The symptom experience and its impact on quality of life. In C. Yarbo, M. Frogge, & M. Goodman (Eds.), *Cancer symptom management* (2nd ed., pp. 3-8). Sudbury, MA: Jones & Bartlett.

64. Roberts, K., & Berry, P. (2002). Grief and bereavement. In K. Kuebler, P. Berry, & D. Heidrich (Eds.). *End of life care: Clinical practice guidelines* (pp. 53-63). Philadelphia: W. B. Saunders.

65. Sateia, M., & Santulli, R. (2003). Sleep. In D. Doyle, G. Hanks, N. Cherny, & K. Calman (Eds.), *Oxford textbook of palliative medicine* (3rd ed., pp. 731-745). Oxford: Oxford University Press.

66. Scanlon, C. (2003). Ethical concerns in end-of-life care. *American Journal of Nursing, 103*(1), 48-56.

 67. Sepulveda, C., et al. (2002) Palliative care: The World Health Organization's global perspective. *Journal of Pain and Symptom Management 24*(2), 91-96.

68. Shepherd, S., & Geraci, S. (1999). The differential diagnosis of dyspnea: A pathophysiological approach. *Clinician Reviews, 9*(3), 52-71.

69. Stanley, K. (2000). Silence is not golden: Conversations with the dying. *Clinical Journal of Oncology Nursing 4*, 34-40.

70. Stanley, K. (2002). Communication. In K. Kuebler & P. Esper (Eds.). *Palliative practices from A-Z for the bedside clinician* (pp. 47-50). Pittsburgh, PA: Oncology Nursing Press.

71. Sweeney, C., Neuenschwander, H., & Bruera, E. (2003). Fatigue and asthenia. In D. Doyle, G. Hanks, N. Cherny, & C. Calman MacDonald (Eds.), *Oxford textbook of palliative medicine* (3rd ed., pp. 560-567). Oxford: Oxford University Press.

72. The SUPPORT Principal Investigators. (1995). A controlled trial to improve care for seriously ill hospitalized patients: The Study to Understand Prognoses and Preferences for Outcomes and Risks of Treatments (SUPPORT). *Journal of the American Medical Association, 274*, 1591-1598.

73. Trzepacz, P., et al. (1999). American Psychiatric Association Guidelines: Practice guidelines for the treatment of patients with delirium. *American Journal of Psychiatry, 156*, S1-S20.

74. Twycross, R.G. (1999). Opioids. In P. D. Wall & P. Melzack (Eds.). *Textbook of pain* (4th ed.) (pp. 1187-1214). New York: Churchill Livingstone.

75. von Gunten, C., et al. (2002). Recommendations to improve end-of-life care through regulatory change in U.S. health care financing. *Journal of Palliative Medicine, 5*(1), 35-41.

76. Walsh, D. (1998). The Medicare hospice benefit: A critique from palliative medicine. *Journal of Palliative Medicine, 1*, 147-149.

77. Waller, A., & Caroline, N. (2000). *Handbook of palliative care in cancer* (2nd ed.). Boston: Butterworth Heinemann.

78. Weaver, S., & Eutsey, D. (Eds.). (1998). *Palliative care: Patient and family counseling manual.* Gaithersburg, MD: Aspen.

79. Wickam, R. (2002). Dyspnea: Recognizing and managing an invisible problem. *Oncology Nursing Forum, 29*(6), 925-933.

80. Wood, L., & Harwood, K. (1999). Dyspnea. In C. Yarbro, M. Frogge, & M. Goodman (Eds.), *Cancer symptom management* (3rd ed., pp. 29-46). Sudbury, MA: Jones & Bartlett.

81. World Health Organization (WHO). (2002). *National cancer control programmes: policies and managerial guidelines* (2nd ed.). Geneva: Authors.

82. World Health Organization (WHO) (1986, 1990, 1996). *Cancer pain relief and palliative care.* Report of a WHO Expert Committed (WHO Technical Support Series, No. 804). Geneva: Authors.

Clients with Sleep and Rest Disorders and Fatigue

Marlene Reimer

Most of us experience occasional problems of disturbed sleep, unwanted drowsiness, and fatigue. As a nurse, you will frequently be involved with clients in whom these disturbances interfere with health, healing, and daily activities. Contributing factors may include personal lifestyle habits, environmental features, internal rhythms, and changes associated with episodic or chronic illness.

SLEEP AND SLEEP PATTERN DISTURBANCES

Sleep can be defined as a normal state of altered consciousness during which the body rests; it is characterized by decreased responsiveness to the environment, but a person can be aroused from sleep by external stimuli. Almost a third of the general population has some problems with sleep during any given year.

These disturbances may be secondary to situational, environmental, or developmental stressors, or they may be associated with illness or with pre-existing disorders. The relationship is often reciprocal in that the disorder decreases sleep and the decreased sleep affects the disorder. Sleep pattern disturbance also contributes to sensory disorders, such as intensive care unit psychosis.

Sleep pattern disturbance is a nursing diagnosis that is defined as a disruption of sleep time that causes discomfort or interferes with a desired lifestyle.[20,34] A sleep pattern disturbance may be related to one of more than 80 sleep disorders identified in the International Classification of Sleep Disorders.[12] Intermittent sleep-related problems are also of concern for nursing diagnosis and intervention.

Chronobiology

Chronobiology refers to the study of biologic changes as they occur in relation to time. Knowledge of chronobiology as it relates to sleep is important to nurses in planning client care and teaching.

Circadian rhythms follow an approximate 24-hour cycle through a complex process linked to light and dark. The *sleep-wake cycle* is one of the circadian rhythms of the body. The effects of illness and hospitalization may disrupt these rhythms, particularly in older persons, who are especially vulnerable to such changes. Nurses can minimize this effect by encouraging a regular schedule with appropriate environmental cues.

Ultradian cycles are circadian rhythms of less than 24 hours. The recurrent pattern of sleep stages, repeating approximately every 90 minutes in adults, is an example. Recognizing this cycle, nurses can arrange care to avoid waking clients more often than absolutely necessary.

Chronopharmacology refers to the study of how biorhythms affect the absorption, metabolism, and excretion of drugs. As an example, the blood level achieved by a continuous infusion of heparin varies throughout the

---

Nursing Outcomes Classification (NOC)
for Nursing Diagnoses—Clients with Sleep and Rest Disorders and Fatigue

Disturbed Sleep Pattern	Well-Being	Energy Conservation
Anxiety Control	**Fatigue**	Nutritional Status: Energy
Rest	Activity Tolerance	Psychomotor Energy
Sleep	Endurance	

day. The risk of clotting is greater in the morning, and the risk of bleeding is greater in the evening. Effectiveness of anticancer drugs varies according to the time of administration. Further, steroid medications should be administered in the morning to approximate most closely the natural elevation in cortisol levels.

Physiology of Sleep and Arousal

The timing of the sleep-wake cycle and other circadian rhythms, such as body temperature, is controlled, at least in part, by the suprachiasmatic nucleus in the anterior hypothalamus. Located above the optic chiasm, this area receives input from the retina, which provides information about darkness and light. The suprachiasmatic nucleus controls the production of melatonin, which is believed to be a potent sleep inducer.[28]

Arousal from sleep, wakefulness, and the ability to respond to stimuli rely on an intact *reticular activating system* (RAS).[29] The RAS is located in the brain stem and contains projections to the thalamus and cortex. The diffuse network of neurons in the RAS is in a strategic position to monitor ascending and descending stimuli through feedback loops.

Although the RAS provides the anatomic framework for arousal, it is the neurotransmitters that serve as the chemical messengers. The onset of sleep and of each subsequent sleep stage is an active process involving delicate shifts in the balance of several of these neurotransmitters.

The transition from the awake state to *non–rapid eye movement* (NREM) sleep occurs through increased concentrations of serotonin (5-hydroxytryptamine [5-HT]) and gamma-aminobutyric acid (GABA). The later transition to *rapid eye movement* (REM) sleep is marked by a dramatic increase in acetylcholine and decreases in serotonin and norepinephrine. As REM sleep continues, the concentrations of serotonin and norepinephrine increase, eventually stopping REM sleep. Cholinergic activation with the release of acetylcholine seems to reestablish REM sleep. The continuous interaction of these two systems is thought to produce the normal alterations between NREM and REM sleep. Cytokines are also intimately linked to sleep-wake cycles.[13,48]

All these neurotransmitters are actively involved in waking processes as well. For example, neurons that produce serotonin and norepinephrine play a role in the modulation of sensory input, mood, energy, and information processing, including attention, learning, and

memory. Thus imbalances in these neurotransmitters induced through sleep pattern disturbances, medications, or diseases may reciprocally affect not only sleep but also aspects of sensory processing, mood, and cognition. Travel across time zones can alter the usual sleep structure by changing light cues and eating times associated with sleep. (See the Complementary and Alternative Therapy feature on Oral Melatonin Supplements for Jet Lag on p. 520.)

The Need for Sleep

Much is known about the architecture of the sleep cycle, but much less is known about the need for sleep.[33] It is commonly held that sleep has a restorative and protective function. In sleep, sympathetic activity decreases, whereas parasympathetic activity may increase. Hormonal shifts facilitate anabolic processes. Selective deprivation of slow-wave sleep is associated with vague physical complaints. REM sleep may be especially important for maintaining mental activities, such as learning, reasoning, and emotional adjustment (see the Complementary and Alternative Therapy feature on Lack of Sleep and Health Problems on p. 520). Sleep is also believed to serve as an energy-conserving measure for most of the body except the brain.[23,24]

Sleep Stages

Sleep can be defined behaviorally, functionally, and electrophysiologically. Electrophysiologic monitoring of sleep, called *polysomnography,* includes at least three parameters: (1) brain-wave activity, (2) eye movements, and (3) muscle tone. Polysomnography shows that sleep can be divided into REM and NREM, and NREM sleep can be further divided into stages 1 through 4. The stages vary in depth but are characterized by slow rolling eye movements, low-level and fragmented cognitive activity, maintenance of moderate muscle tone, and slower but generally rhythmic respirations and pulse rate. As a person progresses from stage 1 to stage 4 sleep, the waveforms recorded by electroencephalography (EEG) become more synchronized, slower, and of higher amplitude (Figure 24-1).

The following are characteristics of NREM sleep:

- *Stage 1* is very light. Respirations begin to slow, and muscles relax. At sleep onset, some erratic breath-

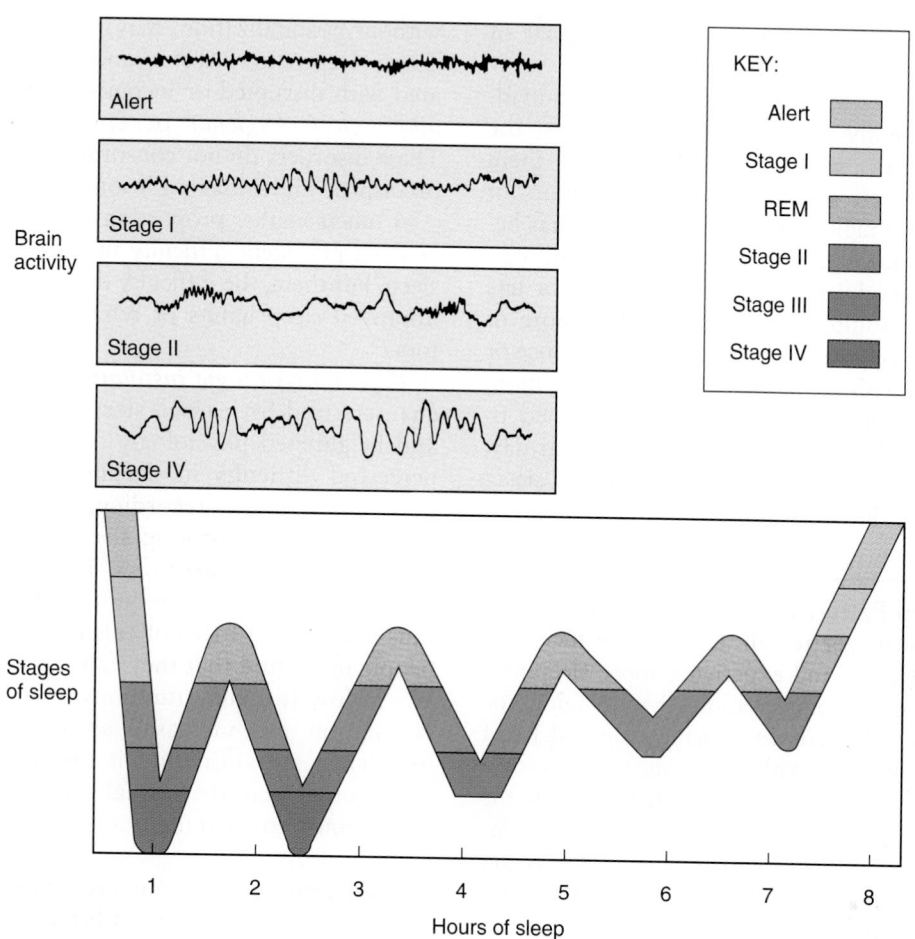

FIGURE 24-1 The electrical activity of the brain during various stages of sleep can be shown on electroencephalograms. During the night, people go through three to five 90-minute sleep cycles. Each cycle includes a sequence of sleep stages. REM, rapid eye movement. (From Solomon, E.P., Schmidt, R.R., & Adranga, P.J. [1990]. *Human anatomy and physiology* [2nd ed.]. Philadelphia: Saunders College.)

ing may occur as well as sudden myoclonic jerks (sleep starts) as the body shifts from an awake to a sleep state. Stage 1 is such a light stage of sleep that persons wakened from it often claim that they were not asleep at all.

- *Stage 2* is still light sleep. The brain waves are frequently mixed and low voltage in pattern, with bursts of activity called *sleep spindles* and large-amplitude waves called *K complexes*. More than 50% of sleep occurs as stages 1 and 2.
- *Stages 3 and 4* are known as *slow-wave sleep,* named for the characteristic high-voltage, low-frequency delta waves. Respirations become slow and even. The pulse and blood pressure fall. Oxygen consumption by muscle tissues and urine formation decreases. Dreams that occur during the NREM stages of sleep are generally thought-like ruminations about recent events and current concerns with little story line.[29]

Rapid eye movement sleep is characterized by low-voltage, random fast waves, as in stage 1 NREM. Peo-

ple in REM sleep have characteristic rapid eye movements, erratic respirations, changes in heart rate, and very low muscle tone (see Figure 24-1). During REM sleep, ventilation depends primarily on the movement of the diaphragm because intercostal and accessory muscle tone is markedly diminished and all postural and nonrespiratory muscles are essentially paralyzed.[29] The ventilatory response to hypoxia and hypercapnia is decreased, and thermoregulation is significantly reduced. Dreams in REM sleep are vivid, story-like, emotional, and bizarre.

Most people move through an orderly progression of NREM sleep from stages 1 to 4 and back through stages 3 to 2 before initiating a period of REM sleep (see Figure 24-1). Although this is the typical progression, it is not essential or always seen. Atypical progressions are characteristic of some sleep disorders, such as narcolepsy, in which REM sleep is entered almost immediately after sleep onset.

In adults, each sleep cycle through the various stages lasts about 90 minutes. During the first few cycles, more time is spent in slow-wave sleep, and the percentage of REM sleep increases later in the sleep period.

Wide variations in sleep patterns exist among individuals. By explaining the range of these variations, the nurse can help clients seek a pattern that leaves them feeling reasonably refreshed and alert. Eight hours of undisturbed sleep at night with no daytime naps has become the assumed ideal pattern in North American society, although some adults do well with 6 hours or less and other healthy adults require 10 hours or more of nighttime sleep. Even young adults often awaken once or twice a night, and with aging such awakenings are more frequent. Humans may be physiologically inclined to have a long and a short sleep period each 24-hour day, such as is common in warmer climates, where the siesta is a normal part of the day's schedule.

Changes in Sleep Patterns of Older Adults

Older adults take longer to fall asleep, have increased nocturnal wakefulness, and experience more sleepiness during the day than do younger adults.[18] With aging, the percentage of stage 4 decreases considerably and REM sleep decreases somewhat, with more time spent in stage 1. REM sleep is more evenly distributed through the night. *Sleep latency,* the time it takes to get to sleep, increases, as does the average length of time it takes to get back to sleep after arousal. Age-related respiratory dysfunction may be responsible for sleep fragmentation. Other problems, such as pain, the need to void, and nocturnal dyspnea, may also decrease effective sleep.

Hospitalization affects the quality of nocturnal and other sleep time, especially for older adults. The hospital environment often lacks light and dark cues. Confinement curtails activity and exercise. In addition, there are unfamiliar sights and sounds and frequent awakenings for assessment of vital signs and other interventions that disturb sleep. Institutionalization in a long-term care facility may perpetuate the environmental impact of noise, caregiver interruptions, inactivity, and lack of day-night cues.[3,36,42]

SLEEP DISORDERS

Dyssomnias

The dyssomnias include sleep disorders characterized by difficulty initiating or maintaining sleep *(insomnia)* or by excessive sleepiness. These disorders may arise predominantly from within the body *(intrinsic)*, from external sources *(extrinsic)*, or from disruptions of circadian rhythm.[2,12]

Intrinsic Sleep Disorders

Insomnia. Many people experience transitory periods during which they have difficulty initiating or maintaining sleep. The onset or exacerbation of illness, with or without hospitalization, may precipitate such difficulty. These sleep pattern disturbances are most often associated with disrupted or inconsistent sleep habits *(inadequate sleep hygiene)* or environmental disruptions. These disorders do not constitute insomnia, but they do predispose individuals to insomnia.

A much smaller proportion of the population has developed persistent difficulty in initiating or maintaining sleep. For them, the difficulty does not respond readily to improved sleep habits or removal of precipitating factors.[12]

Psychophysiologic insomnia is a primary insomnia characterized by learned sleep-preventing associations and heightened physiologic responses to stress.[12] The perceived difficulty in sleeping can be confirmed by polysomnographic recording, which usually shows the same pattern of long sleep latency or fragmentation that the client describes. The total sleep time is often within normal range but is considered inadequate, thus becoming a focus of concern for the client. These people often find that they can fall asleep unintentionally in low-stimulus situations, such as watching television, but feel increased arousal when they go to bed. They may also find it easier to get to sleep in places other than their usual bedroom, having become conditioned to their bedroom as a place of sleepless nights.

Management of insomnia is complex, but there is increasing evidence to support behavioral and pharmacological interventions (see the Evidence-Based Practice in Action feature on Insomnia p. 511). Clients often feel that they have already tried the usual interventions to promote sleep. Sleep habits can become increasingly erratic if the client tries to sleep during the day to compensate for sleeplessness at night. Sleep should be consolidated or restricted by curtailing time in bed to the minimum believed necessary, and rising time should be consistent.[32] Relaxation exercises can be helpful, but initially they should be practiced at times other than bedtime; in this way, by the time these exercises are introduced at bedtime, they are effective. Referral to a sleep specialist or mental health professional who can work with the client over a period of time should be considered.

Narcolepsy. Narcolepsy is one of the disorders characterized by excessive daytime sleepiness.[41,45,47] The client also experiences disturbed nocturnal sleep and repeated episodes of almost irresistible daytime drowsiness followed by brief periods of sleep, especially when engaged in monotonous activities. Many narcoleptic clients also experience *cataplexy,* a sudden loss of muscle tone at times of unexpected emotion (e.g., fright). On initial wakening, they may experience *sleep paralysis* for one to several minutes, during which time they cannot move. This condition, like the other manifestations of narcolepsy, is thought to be linked to malfunc-

E B EVIDENCE-BASED PRACTICE IN ACTION

Insomnia

The evidence to support different interventions and combinations of interventions for insomnia is providing increasing direction for nursing practice. Furthermore, the interventions shown to be effective for the management of insomnia can also be applied in helping clients with less severe sleep disturbances.

Intervention research for insomnia has focused on three types of nonpharmacologic interventions:

- *Sleep hygiene* (an educational intervention in which clients are taught about normal sleep, effects of caffeine, stress, exercise, sleeping environment, etc., on sleep)
- *Stimulus control* (a more intensive educational and behavioral intervention in which clients are also encouraged to establish a regular sleep-wake schedule and learn to associate their bedroom with sleep rather than arousal)
- *Sleep restriction* (a behavioral intervention in which time in bed is restricted to actual sleep time to improve *sleep efficiency,* that is, the percentage of time in bed when a client is actually sleeping)

Early studies usually focused on one intervention, with or without a control group. For example, in 1987, Spielman and others demonstrated that teaching people to restrict the time they spent in bed but not sleeping improved their sleep quantity and quality up to 3 years later.[4] Relaxation training has been a popular intervention for some time. In a 1992 study involving 53 adults between 47 and 76 years of age, sleep hygiene instructions and support, essentially an educational intervention, was compared with progressive relaxation training and stimulus control. All three groups showed improvement in sleep quality over a control group with no intervention; but 2 years later, it was the stimulus control group who had sustained the most improvement in their sleep quality.[1] Relaxation training continues to be used as an adjunct to improving sleep and rest but is no longer recommended as a sole intervention for insomnia.

Many more studies have been done now that essentially replicated the results of the earlier ones and extended the research to testing combination therapies. Cognitive behavioral therapy (CBT) has become an established approach for treating people with psychophysiological insomnia. By combining sleep hygiene education, stimulus control, sleep restriction, and cognitive restructuring of beliefs about sleep over a 6- to 8-week series of individual or group sessions, Morin and others have

shown that 70% to 80% of participants will take less time to fall asleep and will have fewer awakenings than nonparticipants.[3] They then went on to compare CBT, drug therapy, and combined CBT and drug therapy with a no treatment control group. As in earlier studies, all groups except the no treatment group showed initial improvement, but the group with the most sustained improvement 2 years later comprised those who were treated with CBT only (Morin). McLeod and Reimer demonstrated that nurses and other workers could implement basic CBT for community living seniors in a non-medical environment.[2]

Implications

Given the strength of this research evidence for the value of CBT and its components in helping people with insomnia get better sleep, nurses can use these interventions to help people with more transitory sleep disturbances as well. Teaching clients about reducing their caffeine intake, getting daily exercise, and maintaining a regular sleep-wake schedule can be done in hospital or community environments. The nurse can also help people examine their beliefs about sleep. Even young adults often wake up once or twice a night, and yet some people hold the belief that if they wake up at all during the night they have not had a "good sleep." Likewise, the nurse can help even hospitalized clients be cued that it is time to go to sleep (i.e., stimulus control) by doing things like assisting them to brush their teeth if that is a typical before-bed activity, turning down the lights, and removing unnecessary equipment at the bedside.

References

1. Engle-Friedman, M., et al. (1992). An evaluation of behavioral treatments for insomnia in the older adult. *Journal of Clinical Psychology, 48*(1), 77-90.
2. MacLeod, M.A., et al. (2002). Results from a community-based sleep program for seniors in Calgary, Alberta. *Sleep,* 25, A397-398.
3. Morin, C.M., et al. (1999). Behavioral and pharmacological therapies for late-life insomnia: A randomized controlled trial. *Journal of the American Medical Association, 281*(11), 991-999.
4. Spielman, A.J., Saskin, P., & Thorpy, M. (1987). Treatment of chronic insomnia by restriction of time in bed. *Sleep, 10*(1), 45-56.

tioning of the mechanism controlling REM sleep. The REM sleep that is experienced is normal, but it occurs at different times.

Another REM-like manifestation is *hypnagogic hallucinations,* which occur at sleep onset or awakening.[41] Some people experience sleep paralysis or one of the other associated manifestations without narcolepsy. When these manifestations are seen together with excessive sleepiness,

however, they constitute the classic auxiliary manifestations of narcolepsy. Automatic behaviors during which there is a lapse of awareness are also frequent.

On polysomnography, the most characteristic finding is sleep-onset REM periods. A multiple sleep latency test, to measure how long it takes to fall asleep during normal waking hours, shows a sleep latency of less than 5 minutes over four or five testing periods. Occurrence of REM periods at sleep onset at least twice during the test periods is another criterion for the diagnosis.[12] Narcolepsy is a genetically related condition with autosomal dominance in some cases. The prevalence is about 1 in 1000 people in the United States.[41] Genetic transmission of narcolepsy may be multifactorial and may involve a human leukocyte antigen (HLA) and another gene that is not HLA-related. Environmental factors may also have a role.

The effects of the disease on lifestyle are significant, with 60% to 80% of clients reporting episodes of having fallen asleep at work, while driving, or both. The associated disruption of social and occupational roles and self-esteem may be a major factor contributing to depression and decreased quality of life frequently seen in clients who have narcolepsy.

Impaired release of neurotransmitters such as dopamine may also be a factor in both the narcolepsy and the associated depression. Medical management of narcolepsy usually consists of low doses of stimulants such as modafinil (Provigil) or methylphenidate (Ritalin) to improve alertness and tricyclic antidepressants to control cataplexy.[41]

Emphasize good sleep hygiene in counseling clients who experience narcolepsy. It is important that they maintain a regular schedule with adequate nocturnal sleep. Recommend regular naps at times when clients are prone to increased sleepiness. Safety is a major issue for these clients. Assistance may be needed in coping with the disruptive effects of narcolepsy on family, work, and social roles.

Sleep-Disordered Breathing. Sleep apnea is characterized by cessation of breathing for 10 seconds or longer occurring at least five times per hour.[12] Sleep apnea can be classified as obstructive or central apnea or mixed. More recently other syndromes of upper airway resistance (UARS) and obesity hypoventilation syndrome have been added to the cluster of conditions known as sleep disordered breathing.[7] Sleep disordered breathing with associated recurrent nocturnal hypoxia can contribute to memory and cognitive deficits, depression, erectile dysfunction, and decreased quality of life.

Obstructive Sleep Apnea Syndrome (OSAS). In OSAS, respiratory efforts of the diaphragm and intercostal muscles are apparent but ineffective against a collapsed or obstructed upper airway. Snoring indicates partial obstruction. Escalating snoring followed by a silent pause that ends with a gasp or snort probably indicates complete airway obstruction. As hypoxia ensues, the person eventually awakens to breathe. The frequent awakenings impair the normal sleep cycle. With sleep, the muscles of the upper airway relax and may occlude an airway that is already narrowed by enlarged soft tissue structures, jaw structure, or obesity. Partial obstruction may result in UARS with or without snoring.

Repeated microarousals lead to excessive daytime sleepiness in most clients. A few, particularly older people, may present with insomnia.

Obstructive sleep apnea syndrome affects 2% to 4% of the adult population.[7] Prevalence is much higher among obese adults and people over 65 years of age. Women are less likely than men to develop OSAS, particularly before menopause.[12] A much smaller percentage progress to the classic pickwickian syndrome, characterized by obesity, severe sleep apnea, daytime hypercapnia, and cor pulmonale. It is now recognized that prevalence rates of OSAS in children may be 1% or higher, contributing to poor school performance and hyperactivity. Among children the most common predisposing factors are obesity, large adenoids, and tonsils.

Consider referral to a sleep disorders center for clients observed to have repeated periods of apnea (one a minute or more than 15 to 20 periods an hour) lasting longer than 10 seconds, whether or not these periods are associated with snoring. Because OSAS is particularly common among men who are obese with short, thick necks and who are heavy snorers, these clients should be observed during sleep for apneic periods. During assessment, question clients regarding the degree of daytime sleepiness and sudden nighttime awakening, with particular concern about safety in relation to driving and occupational activities.

Milder cases of OSAS, in which excessive daytime sleepiness is not yet a concern, may respond to weight reduction, measures to promote sleeping in positions other than supine, and avoidance of alcohol. Research has shown, however, that more definitive treatment should be considered even in mild OSAS.[40]

The application of continuous positive airway pressure (CPAP) by means of a face mask covering the nose is the treatment of choice. The CPAP device provides room air under increased pressure, essentially providing a pressure splint to keep the upper airway open. Bilevel positive airway pressure (BiPAP) operates by the same principle but uses lower pressure during expiration.

The CPAP mask should be applied securely over the nose and held in place by the head gear. It should be turned on whenever the client is ready to go to sleep and should be maintained throughout the sleep period. Additional humidification may be necessary, especially in dry climates. Clients may experience nasal congestion, air leaks, pressure marks on the face, or pressure intolerance. Such problems are not uncommon and may lead to discontinuation of the therapy if they are not effectively managed. It is therefore important that nurses have a working knowledge of the therapy, the importance of regularity in its use, and sources available for technical assistance (e.g., sleep disorders center, respiratory equipment supplier). CPAP units are portable and have features such as battery operation and voltage conversion to accommodate travel requirements.

People who regularly use CPAP should bring their units to the hospital with them. These clients need to be closely monitored when recovering from anesthesia and when receiving opioids because they are at risk for ineffective breathing patterns.[21]

A note should be made on the health record at the time of admission that the client has OSAS. If the client is scheduled for surgery, the anesthetist and recovery room staff must be alerted. The CPAP unit may be requested to accompany the client to the recovery room.

Question orders for benzodiazepines or other hypnotic drugs for clients with OSAS, chronic obstructive pulmonary disease (COPD), or loud snoring because of possible respiratory depression. Teach clients with such conditions that alcohol may also worsen their manifestations because of its selective effect in relaxing the muscles of the upper airway and depression of arousal (see the Client Education Guide on Living with Obstructive Sleep Apnea Syndrome on the website).

Uvulopalatopharyngoplasty (UPPP) is a common surgical procedure for reducing snoring. Resecting the uvula, the posterior portion of the soft palate, tonsils, and any excessive pharyngeal tissue can reduce the propensity to obstruction in some clients.[15] Concern has arisen, however, that reducing or eliminating snoring may place clients at unknown risk for OSAS. Therefore preoperative assessment, including respiratory pattern during sleep, is recommended before UPPP or the a laser-assisted UPPP procedure, which is done in stages in a physician's office.[46] Somnoplasty is another surgical procedure for removal of excessive tissue through the use of high radiofrequencies that spare the mucosa. Tracheostomy may be required in severe OSAS.

Oral or dental appliances are being used increasingly as another treatment for sleep apnea.[16] Essentially, they act by keeping the jaw forward and the upper airway open.

Central Sleep Apnea Syndrome. Central sleep apnea is characterized by apneic periods during which no apparent respiratory effort occurs.[7,12] It may be seen with central nervous system (CNS) lesions, such as in stroke or brain stem involvement, but it is most commonly mixed with obstructive sleep apnea. Cheyne-Stokes respirations are common with this syndrome, and CPAP is the usual treatment. As with obstructive sleep apnea, sedative-hypnotic drugs should be avoided. In severe cases with CNS involvement, the use of diaphragmatic pacemakers or mechanical ventilation may be required.

Periodic Limb Movement Disorder. Periodic limb movement disorder may also contribute to daytime sleepiness and frequent nocturnal awakenings. Originally described as nocturnal myoclonus, it is characterized by periodic episodes of repetitive, stereotypic leg (or arm) movements that occur during sleep, causing partial arousals.[12,49] The

diagnosis can be confirmed during polysomnography with surface electromyography (EMG) of the anterior tibial muscles.

Periodic limb movement disorder is common in the older population.[22] Clonazepam, a benzodiazepine, or baclofen, a skeletal muscle relaxant, may be ordered to diminish the magnitude of the movement and the frequency of arousals. The anti-parkinsonian drug carbidopa-levodopa (Sinemet) and the tricyclic antidepressant imipramine seem to act more directly and almost eliminate the movements. Most of the other tricyclic antidepressants aggravate the condition. Iron and magnesium supplements may be beneficial if deficiencies are suspected.[49] Anticonvulsant medications such as carbamazepine and valproic acid have brought relief for some clients.

Restless Legs Syndrome. Restless legs syndrome involves annoying "crawling," itching, or tingling sensations of the legs while at rest and causes an almost irresistible urge to move.[12] The syndrome is often most severe before sleep onset. Clients almost always have periodic limb movements during sleep. Treatment is similar to that for periodic limb movements.

Extrinsic Sleep Disorders

The extrinsic sleep disorders encompass a range of factors, from environmentally to chemically induced. Some environmental factors that are present temporarily during hospitalization are discussed under Hospital-Acquired Sleep Disturbances later in this chapter.

Circadian Rhythm Sleep Disorders

In the general population, the circadian rhythm sleep disorders, such as *time-zone-change syndrome* and *shift-work sleep disorder,* are not uncommon.[2] In taking a nursing history, be alert to a history of long-time shift work because these people may have developed altered sleep schedules.

Older and chronically ill clients who live alone may be vulnerable to *irregular sleep-wake patterns*. In this disorder, prolonged ignoring or absence of external cues to time, such as regular mealtimes, work periods, and daylight, leads to erratic periods of sleeping and wakefulness. Internal circadian cues may also be damped as a result of aging or diffuse brain disease.[12,28,29]

Management strategies for circadian rhythm disorders include maintenance of a regular schedule (e.g., people who regularly work the night shift are encouraged to maintain the same sleep schedule on nights off) and exposure to natural sunlight. Light therapy is being used to facilitate adjustments in circadian rhythms as well as in the treatment of *seasonal affective disorder* (SAD). SAD refers to the onset of a major depressive episode corresponding to a particular period of the year, usually late fall and early winter. Some seasonal variation in mood, activity level, and appetite is common in latitudes where climate and length of daylight change markedly.

Administration of bright light in the early morning is most effective in treating SAD or resetting habitual wakening to an earlier hour. Exposure to bright sunlight at those times can also be effective, but conventional indoor lighting is inadequate. Dosage of light is measured in units of illuminance (lux). The usual dosage is about 5000 lux-hours, which may be taken as 2500 lux for 2 hours, 5000 lux for 1 hour, or 10,000 lux for 30 minutes. This level of illumination requires special light boxes, a variety of which are now available.

Help clients to realize that light therapy should begin only under the guidance of a clinician experienced in its use. Teaching should include appropriate positioning of the head in relation to the light source. The most common side effects are eyestrain and headache. Too much light may contribute to irritability and insomnia. The long-term risk of exposure of the eyes to bright light therapy is under investigation. Until more is known, the presence of retinopathy, glaucoma, or cataract is generally considered a contraindication.

Parasomnias

The parasomnias are disorders that occur during sleep but usually do not produce insomnia or excessive sleepiness.[12] The underlying pathologic mechanism may involve partial arousal or abnormalities in sleep-wake transition.

Arousal Disorders

Partial arousals typically occur during slow-wave sleep.[15] *Sleepwalking*, also known as *somnambulism*, may include semi-purposeful behavior, such as dressing. The behavior may be lacking in coordination and appropriateness, however, such as voiding in the closet. The occurrence of sleepwalking in adults is often associated with anxiety. *Sleep terrors* are sudden arousals from slow-wave sleep accompanied by screaming, tachycardia, tachypnea, diaphoresis, and other manifestations of intense fear.[12] If awakened, the person is often disoriented and has little recall of the nature of the dream image. Sleep terrors typically occur in young children but may develop in adults.

Sleep-Wake Transition Disorders

Sleep-wake transition disorders are common in the general population, rarely causing enough disruption to be legitimately called disorders. As mentioned earlier, *sleep starts* refer to the sudden jerking movement of the legs

that often occurs just as a person is falling asleep. Nocturnal leg cramps are also common. The frequency and intensity may be greater with high caffeine intake, stress, or intense physical activity before going to bed. *Sleeptalking* may also occur more frequently during times of stress.

Parasomnias Associated with Rapid Eye Movement Sleep

Like the other parasomnias, those associated with REM sleep may be distressing but are seldom serious. *Nightmares* are frightening dreams that arise in REM sleep and are often vividly recalled on awakening. In contrast, night terrors occur in slow-wave sleep, and there is little recall. *Sleep paralysis* is one of the classic manifestations of narcolepsy but can occur in isolation. At sleep onset or on awakening, people experience episodes of one to several minutes during which they are unable to move.[15] This effect may be an extension of the normal state of low muscle tone during REM sleep.

Other Parasomnias

Other parasomnias are not specifically associated with a particular sleep stage. *Sleep bruxism* refers to grinding of the teeth during sleep and may lead to dental damage. *Sleep enuresis*, or bed-wetting, may occur in adults in association with other disorders, such as OSAS.[12] *Primary snoring* is distinguished from OSAS by its rhythmic nature without episodes of apnea or hypoventilation.

Sleep Disorders Associated with Medical and Psychological Disorders

Secondary sleep disorders are of particular relevance in considering problems common to medical-surgical clients. Whereas some clients have a pre-existing sleep disorder of the dyssomnia or parasomnia type, others develop a sleep disorder secondary to disease or its manifestations. By remaining aware of the physiology of normal sleep, you can anticipate the risk of sleep pattern disturbances in medical-surgical clients.

Neurotransmitter Imbalances

Neurotransmitter imbalances predispose to sleep pattern disturbances. These imbalances may be disease related or drug induced.

More than 70% of people being treated for Parkinson's disease, which results from a deficiency of the neurotransmitter dopamine, report sleep pattern disturbances.[12,30] Insomnia is the most frequent initial concern, followed by sleep fragmentation, disturbances in the sleep-wake schedule, and visual hallucinations.

Depression is accompanied by sleep disturbance in at least 90% of people who suffer from it.[12] Milder forms of depression and those that occur in young people are often associated with sleep-onset insomnia; more severe depressions are characterized by broken sleep and early morning wakening. Some relationship appears to exist between the pathogenesis of depression and REM sleep mechanisms in that depressed people who are deprived of REM sleep often show improved mood. The action of tricyclic antidepressants in suppressing REM sleep has been proposed as the primary mechanism underlying their effectiveness in treating depression.[5,37]

Neurotransmitter imbalances may also contribute to the sleep disturbances frequently seen with Alzheimer's disease and other dementias. The most typical pattern with dementias is frequent awakenings, with agitation progressing to loss of sleep-wake consolidation. Assessing sleep patterns, minimizing caregiver-initiated awakenings (e.g., for toileting), and ensuring a regular bedtime may help to reduce nocturnal and daytime agitation.[36] The sleep-wake cycle may be reversed in a client with Alzheimer's disease. The client may nap during the day and be awake at night, restless, agitated, and wandering. The incidence of sleep apnea is higher in people with Alzheimer's disease, possibly as a result of associated neuronal degeneration in the brain stem. Therefore the nocturnal respiratory patterns of these clients should be carefully assessed, with referral to a sleep disorders center if apnea is suspected.

Brain Injury

Brain injury of all degrees of severity affects sleep patterns. The appearance of differentiated sleep stages on EEG in comatose clients with severe brain injuries is a favorable prognostic indicator.[31] Sleep stages indicate that connections between the brain stem, diencephalon, and telencephalon are intact and allow shifts to occur between NREM and REM sleep. Even after mild brain injury, however, some degree of sleep disturbance may persist for several months.[11] Teaching clients and their families that this unsettled sleep is a typical part of *postconcussion syndrome* can allay anxiety and hasten functional recovery.

For clients in the confused, agitated stage of recovery that results from more severe brain injury, use of environmental cues (e.g., light and darkness), regularity of daily schedule, and appropriate daytime exercise and activity can help to restore the sleep-wake cycle.

Hormonal Imbalances

Hormonal imbalances also contribute to sleep pattern disturbance. Clients with *hyperthyroidism* tend to have fragmented, short sleep periods with an excess of slow-wave sleep. *Hypothyroidism* is characterized by excessive sleepiness, and polysomnographic recordings show a reduction in the proportion of slow-wave sleep.

Clients with *diabetes mellitus*, particularly type 1, may experience hypoglycemic attacks during the night. Besides the usual clinical manifestations of sweating, palpitations, hunger, and anxiety, which the client may recognize as a hypoglycemic reaction, you should be alert to complaints of nightmares and early morning headaches. If these manifestations are present, check blood glucose levels at regular intervals during the night. Insulin dosage or timing may need to be changed. Diabetic clients who have autonomic neuropathy have a higher prevalence of breathing abnormalities during sleep because of the associated dysfunction of autonomic respiratory control; thus their nocturnal breathing patterns should be assessed.

Sleep patterns normally vary across the menstrual cycle in response to estrogen and progesterone levels.[14,43] During the latter part of the cycle, when progesterone levels are higher, the first REM sleep period occurs earlier, and some studies have shown sleep disturbances to be more frequent. Women with *premenstrual syndrome* tend to have less slow-wave sleep throughout the menstrual cycle than their asymptomatic peers. With *menopause*, many women experience poorer sleep quality that may result in mood changes.[6] Estrogen replacement therapy may help to reduce these manifestations. *Postmenopausal* women are also at higher risk for experiencing snoring and obstructive sleep apnea.[27,43]

Respiratory Disorders

Nocturnal asthma attacks contribute to frequent awakenings in up to 70% of people with asthma.[12] Bronchial resistance increases during the early morning hours, even in healthy people, as does sensitivity to histamine.

Chronic airway limitations, such as asthma and emphysema, contribute to difficulty initiating sleep, frequent arousals with shortness of breath or cough, and chronic fatigue. Oxygen saturation may fall, particularly during REM sleep, when ventilation depends on the diaphragm, which is often flattened and inefficient in clients with advanced chronic airflow limitation. In addition, ventilation and perfusion are altered. Dysrhythmias are common during sleep in clients with advanced respiratory disease, especially when oxygen saturation falls below 60%.[12] Pulmonary artery pressure increases as a result of the pulmonary vascular constriction induced by the low oxygen desaturation and the destructive processes of the underlying disease.

Ventilatory responses to hypoxia and hypercapnia are decreased during sleep, even in people with normal respiratory functioning. Clients with advanced respiratory disease are even more vulnerable; therefore hypnotics and other CNS depressants that damp arousal should be given with greater caution.

Some of the medications used in the treatment of chronic airway limitations, such as theophylline preparations, can contribute to insomnia. Anxiety and depression associated with effects of the disease may exacerbate the tendency toward fragmented sleep. Try to provide a calm, secure, and relaxed environment for clients. Stimulants such as caffeine may need to be avoided.

The recumbent posture for sleeping is problematic for many people with respiratory disorders. Encourage clients to use several pillows or to have the head of the bed elevated; during acute episodes, they may find it more comfortable to sleep in a reclining chair.

Cardiovascular Disorders

Up to 25% of people with hypertension have been found to have OSAS.[44] An association between snoring and hypertension has also been documented. Thus it is important that you assess clients who have hypertension or who snore while having repeated apneic periods during sleep.

In clients with severe heart failure, periodic breathing of the Cheyne-Stokes type occurs. This pattern may result in significant hypoxemia, frequent arousals, increased stage 1 sleep, and reduced total sleep time.

The variability of heart and respiratory rates during REM sleep may be a factor in nocturnal angina.[44] Clients recovering from myocardial infarction are often deprived of sleep during their stay in a critical care unit and may experience REM rebound on transfer to a stepdown or standard unit. The greater cardiac demands during REM sleep may put some additional strain on the recovering heart, which makes continued nursing surveillance during this period particularly important.

Gastrointestinal Disorders

Gastric acid secretion normally decreases during sleep, but people with duodenal ulcers have higher than average levels of secretion.[44] Recurrent awakenings with epigastric pain are common, especially in the first 4 hours after sleep onset,[12] and antacids or histamine antagonists may need to be administered.

Gastroesophageal reflux (heartburn) can be more serious when it occurs during sleep because the longer exposure of the esophagus to gastric acid can lead to esophagitis. Hypnotics should be used cautiously with such clients because the suppression of arousal makes them more vulnerable to esophagitis and pulmonary aspiration. You may suggest that these clients avoid eating within 3 hours of bedtime, consider use of antacids or histamine antagonists, and raise the head of the bed on blocks (reverse Trendelenburg position) to decrease the likelihood of reflux and subsequent aspiration.

Other Disorders

Numerous other disorders seem to have an effect on or an association with sleep. Any condition that results in pain, discomfort, or impaired mobility has the potential to disrupt sleep.[35] Various skin conditions, such as atopic eczema, are associated with decreased REM sleep. Unrefreshing sleep, chronic fatigue, and diffuse musculoskeletal pain are among the diagnostic criteria for fibromyalgia. The EEG tracing of clients with this condition often shows a unique pattern of intrusion of alpha waves into slow-wave sleep, producing *alpha-delta activity*.[12] The clinical manifestations tend to be vague, and clients are often discouraged about the inability of health care professionals to diagnose and treat this condition. The nurse may be in a position to encourage referral to a sleep disorders center.

The effect of sleep or sleep deprivation on some disorders can be useful for diagnostic purposes. For example, the typical occurrence of erections in healthy men during REM sleep is used as a diagnostic measure in differentiating sources of impotence.[50] REM-associated erections are also the reason the nurse must be careful when securing an indwelling urinary catheter in a male client and allow a sufficient amount of slack in the tubing to accommodate an erection.

Sleep deprivation and erratic sleep patterns reduce the seizure threshold, which you should consider in assessment and teaching of clients with seizure disorders. Seizure activity may also be a cause of sleep disturbance. Partial and focal seizures can arise in all phases of sleep, including REM; generalized tonic-clonic seizures are more likely to occur during slow-wave sleep than during REM. The tendency of sleep deprivation to trigger seizure activity is used diagnostically in that clients may be required to stay awake all night before they undergo sleep-deprivation EEG. Some treatment regimens for clients susceptible to nocturnal seizures involve selective medication-induced suppression of sleep stages in which the client's seizures most frequently occur.

HOSPITAL-ACQUIRED SLEEP DISTURBANCES

Clients in the hospital may report difficulty getting to sleep, awakening frequently with difficulty getting back to sleep, or early morning awakening. The etiologic mechanism and interventions range with the type of difficulty.

Sleep Onset Difficulty

Sleep onset difficulty is a common problem in hospitals because of the strange environment and the anxieties associated with illness and hospitalization. A sleep latency time of 20 to 30 minutes is within normal range for most adults. Environmental controls, such as reduction of noise and interruptions, and conservative relaxation measures, such as a back rub, should be tried before resorting to a hypnotic agent. The rapid-acting hypnotics, such as zolpidem (Ambien), are most effective with this type of insomnia.

If a hypnotic is given, monitor the client's safety in getting up at night. Most hypnotics cause some degree of antegrade amnesia, meaning that otherwise cognitively intact clients may become disoriented and forget where they are. The longer-acting hypnotics also result in some "hangover" effect. An increased risk of hip fractures from falls has been documented in people who are taking long-acting benzodiazepines.[39]

Sleep Maintenance Disturbance

Sleep maintenance disturbance may be associated with sustained use of or withdrawal from a variety of medications and related substances. Alcohol hastens sleep onset but leads to awakening later in the night. In acute intoxication, REM sleep is suppressed. Abrupt withdrawal, as occurs with hospitalization, may trigger massive REM rebound. In chronic alcoholics, sleep architecture remains disturbed even several years after abstinence. Sustained use of or withdrawal from antidepressants, monoamine oxidase inhibitors, propranolol, and phenytoin can also contribute to insomnia.

Other factors that contribute to sleep fragmentation include stimuli that tend to awaken people in the middle of the night. Internal stimuli, such as pain, discomfort, and the urge to void, are frequent disturbers of sleep. Sleep disorders, such as sleep apnea and periodic limb movement, are more frequently associated with excessive somnolence, but they do trigger awakenings, after which some people have difficulty getting back to sleep. Hospitalization provides an opportunity for nursing surveillance, which may be instrumental in detecting these disorders as distinct from disturbances triggered by natural or transitory stimuli.

External stimuli include environmental factors, such as light, noise, and temperature, as well as disruptions by other people. You can reduce nocturnal stimuli by darkening the client's room; turning lights off, except for a small night light for safety purposes; and closing curtains. To reduce nocturnal stimuli, reduce as much noise as possible by avoiding unnecessary conversation, minimizing equipment noise, and closing the client's door, if possible. You can adjust the temperature by providing bed coverings according to the client's preference and by modifying room temperature (directly by adjusting the thermostat or air conditioner or indirectly, by closing curtains and adjusting ventilation). Remove disturbing objects, such as equipment associated with painful procedures, to create a pleasant, tidy environment.

You can also reduce nocturnal stimuli by spacing necessary caregiving activities (e.g., turning, taking vital signs) to allow periods of 90 minutes or more of undisturbed sleep and, when possible, synchronizing these activities with periods during which the client is already awake. Finally, coordinate the nature and timing of interruptions by other caregivers (e.g., for laboratory testing or chest physiotherapy) to preserve periods of undisturbed sleep.

Early Morning Awakening

Early morning awakening occurs frequently among older clients. Sensitivity to environmental disturbances increases toward morning in people of all ages but even more so in older adults. Clients who are disturbed by early morning awakening should be screened for indications of depression.

Sleeplessness and agitation may be associated with an acute confusional state (i.e., delirium). Especially among older people, this transient cognitive disorder may be associated with acute illness and admission to the hospital. Unlike that of dementia, onset is rapid and is associated with a fluctuating level of consciousness. Thinking is disorganized and fragmented, memory is impaired, and delusions and hallucinations are common. Sleep is grossly disturbed with frightening dreams, disorientation, and restlessness. Delirium is usually precipitated by a treatable systemic illness such as dehydration, infection, drug toxicity, or renal failure. It is important that you identify delirium and pursue treatment possibilities. When the cause is removed, recovery is rapid.

Sleep Deprivation

Sleep deprivation is of particular concern for clients in critical care units. The noise level, 24-hour lighting, and frequency of caregiver interruptions create sensory overload and sleep deprivation, which is thought to be a major factor contributing to postoperative psychosis.[4]

Clients who have had surgery are also at risk for sleep pattern disturbance because of disruptions in circadian rhythms. The cause is unclear, but the disruptions may be related to the length and type of anesthesia, postoperative analgesia, or mechanisms associated with the procedure itself. REM sleep and slow-wave sleep are suppressed. It may take 4 to 6 weeks for the client's sleep patterns to return to normal after open heart surgery with cardiopulmonary bypass. Specific assessment of sleep quality and quantity should be incorporated into the care of all surgical clients.

DIAGNOSTIC ASSESSMENT

The primary diagnostic test for sleep disorders is polysomnography. Clients may be referred to a sleep disorders center for overnight EEG, electro-oculography (EOG), and submental EMG with surface electrodes.

Clients may also have continuous recording of arterial oxygen saturation by ear or finger oximeter, air flow as detected by monitoring expired carbon dioxide, respiratory movements by means of transducers placed around the chest and abdomen, and an electrocardiogram (ECG) and heart rate determination with standard limb leads. Ambulatory monitoring systems are also available to facilitate studies in the natural home environment.

A multiple sleep latency test (MSLT) may also be performed to assess impairment of daytime alertness. The MSLT is performed the day after a standard overnight polysomnogram. The time required for clients to fall asleep when in a relaxed state is evaluated at 2-hour intervals, with each nap limited to 20 minutes. The type of sleep is also assessed, making the test particularly useful in diagnosing narcolepsy, a condition in which clients typically have sleep-onset REM periods.

■ Nursing Management of Disturbed Sleep Pattern
Assessment

Include a brief assessment of the client's usual sleep habits and recent sleep quality as part of the initial nursing history. On the care plan, note the usual bedtime and rising times as well as any preferences or rituals that may enhance sleep quality. For example, clients with ineffective breathing patterns associated with conditions such as COPD and hiatal hernia may be accustomed to sleeping with several pillows or with the head of the bed elevated.

If sleep quality is reported to be poor, explore the nature of the disturbance by noting the following:

- Usual activities in the hour before retiring
- Sleep latency
- Number and perceived cause of awakenings
- Regularity of sleep pattern (e.g., shift work)
- Consistency of rising time
- Frequency and duration of naps
- Events associated with initial onset of sleep disturbance
- Ease of falling asleep in places other than the usual bedroom
- Situations in which client fights sleepiness
- Daily caffeine intake
- Use of alcohol, sleeping pills, and other medications
- Incidence of morning headache
- Frequency of snoring, apparent pauses in breathing (apneas), and kicking movements; this last information is best obtained from the sleeping partner or from your observation while the client is in the hospital

Objective data may include visible signs of fatigue and lack of sleep, such as circles under the eyes, lack of coordination, drowsiness, and irritability.

Diagnosis, Outcomes, Interventions

Diagnosis: Disturbed Sleep Pattern. Disturbed sleep pattern is a common nursing diagnosis (e.g., *Disturbed Sleep Pattern related to changes in routine secondary to hospitalization and pain*). It may be related to change in sleeping environment, shift work schedule, recurrent pain, or many other possibilities. Other nursing diagnoses may also be applicable (e.g., *Risk for Injury related to excessive daytime sleepiness*).

Outcomes. The client will have improved sleep patterns within 3 nights as evidenced by sleeping for 6 to 8 hours at one time, stated feeling of lessened fatigue, and decreased irritability.

Interventions. The client's usual bedtime routine should be followed as closely as possible. For example, if the client usually watches television before sleeping, attempt to make this possible. Schedule nursing assessments and interventions in blocks of time to allow 90 to 120 minutes of uninterrupted sleep. The environment should mimic nighttime, with lights dimmed and quiet maintained. Offer extra blankets for external warmth. Provide a light complex carbohydrate snack, such as whole wheat crackers, if the client's condition allows.

Other techniques used to promote sleep include back massage, relaxing music, and progressive relaxation techniques. Medications to promote sleep should be used judiciously because they can alter the architecture of sleep, often reducing the REM sleep and eventually leading to REM rebound. If the client is in pain, analgesics rather than sleeping medications should be given. Clients in pain do not sleep restfully.

Sleep medications may be useful during short periods of sleep disturbance (e.g., hospitalization, bereavement, relocation). These medications are usually given at bedtime, and administration may be repeated once if they are not effective. Consider the drug's half-life and the time of night before repeating administration. To avoid prolonged drowsiness, do not repeat sleeping medications after 3:00 AM. Try other measures to promote sleep, such as offering milk, analgesia, music, or back massage.

The client should be awakened with the least obtrusive stimulus possible, such as a soft touch or a soft voice. Startling the client may make it difficult for the client to go back to sleep. Many assessments and interventions can be performed without the client's being completely awake.

Evaluation

Some sleep disturbances are temporary and related to the stress of hospitalization. Clients with sleep disturbances may need follow-up care with repeated assessments to determine whether the problem was corrected. Clients with long-term sleep disorders may need ongoing support to maintain the effectiveness of treatment.

CHRONIC FATIGUE

Fatigue is a manifestation commonly associated with most acute and chronic illnesses but also experienced with normal, healthy functioning and everyday life.[1,38] Fatigue can be defined as a subjective state in which a client experiences a sustained sense of exhaustion and diminished capacity for physical and mental work that is not relieved by rest.[10] It is often the first indication of an abnormal process[9,17] and may become a chronic and debilitating condition. Fatigue differs from tiredness or sleepiness in that sleepiness is a temporary state that results from lack of sleep, sleep disorders, improper nutrition, sedentary lifestyle, or a temporary increase in work or social responsibilities.[8]

Chronic fatigue has no recognized function and often has no apparent relation to activity or exertion.[1] The affected person perceives it as being abnormal, unusual, or excessive. It typically has an insidious onset, persists over time, and is not generally relieved by usual restorative techniques. Chronic fatigue has a major effect on one's activities of daily living and quality of life.

Nurses have an important role in helping fatigued clients manage and cope effectively, whether they are in the hospital or in their own home. Understanding the debilitating effects of fatigue on individuals is an important component of effective nursing care.[9]

■ Nursing Management of Chronic Fatigue
Assessment

The major defining characteristics of chronic fatigue syndrome are as follows[10]:
- Verbalization of an unremitting and overwhelming lack of energy
- Inability to maintain usual routines
- Perceived need for additional energy to accomplish routine tasks
- Increase in physical complaints
- Emotional lability or irritability
- Impaired ability to concentrate and decreased performance
- Lethargy or listlessness
- Disinterest in surroundings
- Decreased libido
- Accident proneness

Fatigue, like pain, must be understood as multidimensional aspects that include physiologic, psychological, social, and spiritual components.[15] Physiologic fatigue has been associated with sleep disturbances, infection, fever, pregnancy, anemia,[1] acquired immunodeficiency syndrome (AIDS), hyperthyroidism or hypothy-

roidism, menopause,[10] stroke,[25] multiple sclerosis,[19] cancer and its treatments, and hepatitis.[38]

Psychological fatigue has been described as a state of weariness related to diminished motivation and can be associated with stress, depression, and anxiety.[1,10]

Chronic fatigue syndrome (CFS) refers to a medical diagnosis of profound fatigue lasting at least 6 months and causing a 50% or greater reduction in physical activities not explainable by other causes.[26] Impaired concentration and generalized aching are commonly associated. It is closely related to fibromyalgia, with about 75% of people with CFS exhibiting the same characteristic tender points. They, too, frequently report sleep disturbances. As with any clients reporting manifestations of chronic fatigue, take a detailed sleep history. Coexistence of treatable sleep disorders is not uncommon, and improved sleep hygiene may reduce the overwhelming sense of fatigue.

Diagnosis, Outcomes, Interventions

Diagnosis: Fatigue. The nursing diagnosis may be written as *Fatigue related to altered body chemistry secondary to chemotherapy.* Because of the complexity of chronic fatigue, a clear etiology may not be evident; in those cases, an etiology of unknown cause is used.

Outcomes. The goals of management are to improve the quality of sleep, reduce pain, and help the client regain control of his or her life.[26] This diagnosis will require long-term goals, such as the client reporting a moderate reduction in fatigue within 3 weeks.

Interventions. Much of the management of fatigue is based on relief of manifestations, with an emphasis on the whole person, mind, and body.[26] An excellent approach to understanding the fatigue is to have the client keep a diary of his or her fatigue. If a pattern is evident, plans can be made to perform routine activities when energy levels are high or to "save" or "bank" energy to use for more complex activities.

A prudent, well-balanced diet is the foundation of good health. Some people with CFS report varying degrees of intolerance to refined sugar, caffeine, alcohol, and tobacco, all of which should be minimized to promote optimum health.

The manifestations of CFS tend to worsen with physical or mental activity, and a prolonged relapse can be triggered by overexertion. Clients are best advised to balance gentle activity with frequent rest periods. Discourage excess rest and social withdrawal. Recommended activities include stretching, light calisthenics, light weights (1 to 2 pounds), walking, bicycling, or swimming. Most clients will need to start with 2 or 3 minute periods of exercise with frequent rest periods. The exercise should not make the individual tired. Careful planning of duration

COMPLEMENTARY AND ALTERNATIVE THERAPY

Oral Melatonin Supplements for Jet Lag

An analysis of past studues of melatonin for jet lag was conducted, and in this analysis a total of 10 trials met the inclusion criteria. All trials compared the use of oral melatonin versus a placebo. Participants took the melatonin either at the same time after arrival at the destination or close to bedtime at the destination. All trials evaluated treatment for more than 2 days.

A meta-analysis demonstrated a reduction in jet lag with oral melatonin. Daily doses between 0.5 and 5 mg/day were similar in effectiveness, but participants who took the higher doses fell asleep more quickly. Doses greater than 5 mg were not more effective than doses of 5 mg or less. Slow-release melatonin was less effective than fast-release pills. Adverse effects were minimal but were not generally or adequately measured. Clients with epilepsy, clients taking oral anticoagulants, or clients who develop a rash are not good candidates for melatonin. Whether melatonin was better or worse than prescription agents for sleep was not tested.

References

Herxheimer, A., & Petrie, K. (2001). Melatonin for preventing and treating jet lag. *Cochrane Database System Retrieved (1):CD001520.*

COMPLEMENTARY AND ALTERNATIVE THERAPY

Lack of Sleep and Health Problems

A small study may have provided some insight into the unhealthy behavior of getting too little sleep. A total of 11 healthy young men (ages 18 to 27 years) were allowed to sleep only 4 hours a night for 6 nights. They then were allowed to sleep up to 12 hr/day for another 6 nights. When the men were deprived of sleep, they experienced major imbalances in carbohydrate metabolism and hormone levels. These changes were similar to those observed in older men. These negative changes were reversed when the participants were allowed to sleep more. The researchers concluded that a lack of sleep has an effect similar to an accelerated aging process.

References

Leproult, R., Spiegel, K., & Van Cauter, E. (1999). Impact on sleep debt on metabolic and endocrine function. *Lancet, 354,* 1435-1439.

---

and distance allows the client to stop the activity before becoming tired. The exercise duration is then increased slowly over time but might have to be reduced or withheld temporarily during periods of relapse.

A supportive counselor can help clients cope with the prospects of long-term illness as well as family issues, anxiety, depression, grief, anger, and guilt, which frequently accompany any chronic illness. Cognitive behavioral therapists are specifically trained to provide both the guidance and the support that is helpful in CFS and other chronic illnesses, focusing on realistic goals, symptom management, and strengthening coping mechanisms.

The pain of CFS may be in muscles (sometimes described as "deep pain") or joints (arthralgias). Clients may also complain of headaches (typically pressure-like) and allodynia, which is generalized hyperalgesia or soreness of the skin to touch. Although it is advisable to avoid opioids whenever possible, therapy should begin with simple analgesics like acetaminophen, aspirin, or NSAIDs. Low doses of tricyclic antidepressants can also be helpful in tempering muscle pain. Clients with severe chronic pain should be advised to seek counseling about adjunctive pain management techniques, such as meditation, deep breathing, biofeedback, gentle massage, physical therapy, and others.

As a result of the loss of functional abilities and changes in brain chemistry, depression is a common symptom in clients with CFS and should be treated when present. You can support clients in understanding the causes of their fatigue and offer support in identifying energy patterns and the need for scheduling activities.[8] An understanding of the effects of conflict and stress on energy levels can help the client learn new fatigue coping skills. Allowing the expression of feelings regarding the effects of fatigue on one's life is important. Monitor for factors contributing to fatigue on a daily basis, and intervene in a timely manner. Intervention may include carefully planning activities of daily living and daily exercise schedules with appropriate rest periods. Assistance with self-care activities should be offered when needed, and attempts should be made to minimize sensory overload or sensory deprivation.

Evaluation

Fatigue may not resolve completely, depending on underlying factors. Thus evaluation of outcomes and revisions to interventions should be based on mutual planning with the client and family to reduce manifestations and to improve management and quality of life. Balance is needed so that strategies to reduce fatigue, such as avoidance of stress, do not preclude activities that are important to the client.

CONCLUSIONS

The adequacy of sleep and rest is important to consider in caring for clients with acute or chronic illness. Disorders of sleep and fatigue have been discussed with consideration of the reciprocity among these processes, illness, and hospitalization. The nurse can play a pivotal role in environmental modification and client teaching to minimize the impact of sleep, fatigue, and sensory disturbances.

THINKING CRITICALLY *evolve*

1. The client has just been given a prescription for zolpidem (Ambien) to treat insomnia. She confides to you that she has been using a product from a health food store, recommended by a friend. Now she asks you whether it is safe to continue taking the herbal remedy as well as her new prescription.

Factors to Consider. What is zolpidem? Can it interact with other medications? How could you find more information about the herbal medication the client is taking?

2. A late-middle-aged client who has had a stroke and is unable to move or speak is placed in a room at the end of the hall, away from the nurses' station. This client was assigned a window bed. He has few visitors. His roommate is a young man recovering from a mild head injury. The roommate has many visitors and uses the radio and television loudly and frequently. Which client is more likely to develop sensory deprivation? Sensory overload? What nursing assessments and interventions would help prevent sensory disturbances?

Factors to Consider. What factors (age, environmental, physical, psychological) affect sensory functioning? How do clients receive and interpret incoming stimuli? Does the room assignment contribute to the development of sensory disturbance in either client?

3. A young adult comes to the neighborhood health clinic. She is unkempt, has circles under her eyes, and yawns frequently. She gives a history of being unable to sleep for any length of time since she gave birth recently to twin sons. She took a variety of prescription "sleeping pills" before she became pregnant and wants a new prescription to help her sleep. What might be causing her sleeplessness? What sleep assessments should be completed? What impact might lack of sleep have?

Factors to Consider. What measures might help this young mother sleep naturally? How would her lack of sleep affect the health of her children? How normal is it for a young adult to experience difficulty with sleep and to take medications to assist with sleep?

Discussions for these questions can be found on the website and the CD-ROM.

BIBLIOGRAPHY

1. Aaronson, L.S., et al. (1999). Defining and measuring fatigue. *Image: Journal of Nursing Scholarship, 31*(1), 45-50.
2. Akerstedt, T. (1998). Shift work and disturbed sleep/wakefulness. *Sleep Medicine Reviews, 2*(2), 117-128.
3. Alessi, C.A., & Schnelle, J.F. (2000). Approach to sleep disorders in the nursing home setting. *Sleep Medicine Reviews, 4*(1),45-56.
4. Ancoli-Israel, S. (1997). Sleep problems in older adults: Putting myths to bed. *Geriatrics, 52*(1), 20-30.
5. Armitage, R. (2000). The effects of antidepressants on sleep in patients with depression. *Can J Psychiatry, 45*,803-809.
6. Baker, A., Simpson, S., & Dawson, D. (1997). Sleep disruption and mood changes associated with menopause. *Journal of Psychosomatic Research, 43*(4), 359-369.
7. Baldwin, C.M., & Quan, S.F. (2002). Sleep disordered breathing. *Nursing Clinics of North America, 37*, 633-654.
8. Carpenito, L.J. (1999). *Handbook of nursing diagnosis* (8th ed.). Philadelphia: J.B. Lippincott.
9. Cook, N.F., & Boore, J.R.P. (1997). Managing patients suffering from acute and chronic fatigue. *British Journal of Nursing, 6*(14), 811-815.
10. Cox, H.C., et al. (1997). *Clinical applications of nursing diagnosis* (3rd ed.). Philadelphia: F. A. Davis.
11. Deb, S., Lyons, I., & Koutzoukis, C. (1998). Neuropsychiatric sequelae one year after a minor head injury. *Journal of Neurology, Neurosurgery and Psychiatry, 65*(6), 889-902.
12. Diagnostic Classification Steering Committee. (1997). *International classification of sleep disorders: Diagnostic and coding manual* (Rev. ed.). Rochester, MN: American Sleep Disorders Association.
13. Dickstein, J.B., & Moldofsky, H. (1999). Sleep, cytokines and immune function. *Sleep Medicine Reviews, 3*(3), 219-228.
14. Driver, H.S., & Baker, F.C. (1998). Menstrual factors in sleep. *Sleep Medicine Reviews, 2*(4), 213-229.
15. El-Ad, B., & Korczyn, A.D. (1998). Disorders of excessive daytime sleepiness: An update. *Journal of Neurological Sciences, 153*(2), 192-202.
16. Ferguson, K.A. et al. (1997). A short term controlled trial of an adjustable oral appliance for the treatment of mild to moderate obstructive sleep apnea. *Thorax, 52*, 362-368.
17. Ferrell, B.R., et al. (1996). "Bone tired": The experience of fatigue and its impact on quality of life. *Oncology Nursing Forum, 23*(10) 1539-1547.
18. Floyd, J. (2002). Sleep and aging. *Nursing Clinics of North America, 37*, 719-731.
19. Ford, H., Trigwell, P., & Johnson, M. (1998). The nature of fatigue in multiple sclerosis. *Journal of Psychosomatic Research, 45*(1), 33-38.
20. Gordon, M. (2002). Manual of nursing diagnoses (10th ed.). St. Louis: Mosby.
21. Gupta, R.M., et al. (2001). Postoperative complications in patients with obstructive sleep apnea syndrome undergoing hip or knee replacement: A case control study. *Mayo Clinic Proceedings, 76*, 897-905.
22. Hening, W., et al. (1999). The treatment of restless legs syndrome and periodic limb movement disorder. *Sleep, 22*(7),970-999.

evolve **Did you remember to check out the bonus material on the Evolve website and the CD-ROM, including free self-assessment exercises?**

http://evolve.elsevier.com/Black/medsurg/

23. Hodgson, L.A. (1991). Why do we need sleep? Relating theory to nursing practice. *Journal of Advances in Nursing, 16,* 1503-1510.

24. Horne, J.A. (1988). *Why we sleep.* New York: Oxford University Press.

25. Ingles, J.L., Eskes, G.A., & Phillips, S.J. (1999). Fatigue after stroke. *Archives of Physical Medicine and Rehabilitation, 80,* 173-178.

26. Kenner, C. (1998). Fibromyalgia and chronic fatigue: The holistic perspective. *Holistic Nursing Practice, 12*(3), 55-63.

27. Krystal, A.D., et al. (1998). Sleep in peri-menopausal and post-menopausal women. *Sleep Medicine Reviews, 2*(4), 243-253.

28. Labyak, S. (2002). Sleep and circadian schedule disorders. *Nursing Clinics of North America 37,* 599-610.

29. Lee, K. (2003). Impaired sleep. In V. Carrieri-Kohlman, A.M. Lindsey, & C.M. West (Eds.), *Pathophysiological phenomena in nursing* (3rd ed., pp. 363-385). St. Louis: W.B. Saunders.

30. Lowe, A.D. (1998). Sleep in Parkinson's disease. *Journal of Psychosomatic Research, 44*(6), 613-617.

31. Mahowald, M.W. (2000). Sleep in traumatic brain injury and other acquired CNS conditions. In A. Culebras (Ed.), *Sleep disorders and neurological disorders* (pp. 365-385). New York: Marcel Dekker.

32. Mion, L.C. (1992). Environmental structuring. In G.M. Bulechek & J.C. McCloskey (Eds.), *Nursing interventions* (2nd ed., pp. 254-264). Philadelphia: W.B. Saunders.

33. Morin, C. et al. Nonpharmacologic treatment of chronic insomnia. *Sleep, 22*(8), 1134-1156.

34. North American Nursing Diagnosis Association (NANDA). (2001). *Nursing diagnoses: Definitions and classification 2000-2001.* Philadelphia: Author.

35. Ohayon, M.M., et al. (1997). How sleep and mental disorders are related to complaints of daytime sleepiness. *Archives of Internal Medicine, 157*(22), 2645-2652.

36. O'Rourke, D.J., Klaasen, K.S., & Sloan, J.A. (2001). Redesigning nighttime for personal care residents care. *Journal of Gerontological Nursing 27*(7), 30-37.

37. Partonen, T. (1998). A developmental approach to severe depression. *Medical Hypotheses, 51*(2), 165-166.

38. Piper, B.F. (2003). Fatigue. In V. Carrieri-Kohlman, A.M. Lindsey, & C.M. West (Eds.), *Pathophysiological phenomena in nursing* (3rd ed., pp.209-234). St. Louis: W.B. Saunders.

39. Ray, W., Griffen, M., & Downey, W. (1989). Benzodiazepines of long and short elimination half-life and the risk of hip fracture. *Journal of the American Medical Association, 262*(23), 3303-3307.

40. Redline, S., et al. (1998). Improvement of mild sleep disordered breathing with CPAP compared with conservative therapy. *American Journal of Respiratory Critical Care Medicine 157,* 858-865.

41. Rogers, A.E., & Dreher, H.M. (2002). Narcolepsy. *Neurology Clinics of North America, 37*(4), 675-692.

42. Schnelle, J.F., et al. (1998). Sleep hygiene in physically dependent nursing home residents: Behavioral and environmental intervention implications. *Sleep, 21*(5), 515-523.

43. Shaver, J. (2002). Women and sleep. *Nursing Clinics of North America 37,* 707-718.

44. Smith, R.P., et al. (1998). Obstructive sleep apnea and the autonomic nervous system. *Sleep Medicine Reviews, 2*(2), 69-92.

45. Standards of Practice Committee of the American Academy of Sleep Medicine. (2001). Practice parameters for the treatment of narcolepsy: An update for 2000. *Sleep, 24*(4), 451-461.

46. Standards of Practice Committee of the American Sleep Disorders Association. (1994). Practice parameters for the use of laser-assisted uvulopalatoplasty. *Sleep, 17*(8), 744-748.

47. Stansbury, T.T. (2001). Narcolepsy: Unveiling a mystery. *American Journal of Nursing, 101*(8), 50-53.

48. Steriade, M. (1994). Brain electrical activity and sensory processing during waking and sleeping states. In M.H. Kryger, T. Roth, & W.C. Dement (Eds.), *Principles and practice of sleep medicine* (3rd ed., pp. 105-124). Philadelphia: W.B. Saunders.

49. Sleasny, K., et. al. (2002). Clinical symptomatology and treatment of restless legs syndrome and periodic limb movement disorder. *Sleep Medical Review, 6*(4), 253-265.

50. Ware, J.C., & Hirshkowitz, M. (1994). Monitoring penile erections during sleep. In M.H. Kryger, T. Roth, & W.C. Dement (Eds.), *Principles and practice of sleep medicine* (3rd ed., pp. 967-977). Philadelphia: W.B. Saunders.

Clients with Psychosocial and Mental Health Concerns

Nancy Shoemaker

---

evolve

Web Enhancements

http://evolve.elsevier.com/Black/medsurg/

Care Plan
The Client with Degenerative Joint Disease and Concurrent Panic Disorder: Mrs. James
The Client with Hiatal Hernia and Concurrent Schizophrenia: Mr. Barnes
The Client with Diabetic Ketoacidosis and Concurrent Depression: Mrs. Conners

Diversity in Health Care
The Significance of Cultural Assessment

Boxes
NANDA International 2003-2004 Nursing Diagnoses Related to Adult Psychosocial Concerns
Psychosocial Dimension: Spirituality and Mental Illness

Psychosocial Dimension: Culture and Mental Illness
Psychosocial Dimension: Sexuality and Mental Illness
Emotional, Physical, and Spiritual Manifestations of Anxiety
Medications for Anxiety Disorders
Selected Standardized Tools for Assessment of Psychiatric Disorders
Medications for Schizophrenia
Medications for Mood Disorders

Tables
Characteristics of People with High and Low Self-Esteem
Levels of Psychiatric Treatment Services

Appendix A
Religious Beliefs and Practices Affecting Health Care

A sound knowledge base for responding to psychosocial and mental health concerns of clients and their families is vital in all settings where medical-surgical nursing is practiced. Psychosocial components are defined as the psychological and social aspects of the client's health status. Psychological factors include thinking, feelings, motivation, and personal strengths and weaknesses. Social issues are related to patterns of interaction with others (see Chapter 4). For all clients seeking health care for a physical problem, there is a potential for alteration in their mental or emotional status because of the stress of illness and navigating the health care system. The North American Nursing Diagnosis Association (NANDA) currently lists 156 approved nursing diagnoses; approximately 41% are related to psychosocial functioning (see the box on NANDA International 2003-2004 Nursing Diagnoses Related to Adult Psy-

chosocial Concerns on the website). To promote successful health outcomes, the nurse must address the psychosocial and mental health concerns of each client.

Some clients have a pre-existing mental disorder that may complicate or adversely affect the outcome of their medical treatment. Within a 12-month period, 23 million people suffer from anxiety disorders, 11 million more are affected by major depression, and more than 3 million are afflicted with schizophrenia.[3,5,6,8,23] For these clients, nursing attention to psychosocial needs makes the difference between compliance with treatment and noncompliance with resulting complications.

This chapter focuses on the psychosocial concerns of clients and families who require nursing care across various treatment settings. Basic principles regarding communication are outlined, and nursing interventions to reduce anxiety are presented. Concepts of anxiety,

---

evolve Be sure to check out the bonus material on the Evolve website and the CD-ROM, including free self-assessment exercises.

http://evolve.elsevier.com/Black/medsurg/

Nursing Outcomes Classification
for Nursing Diagnoses-Clients with Psychosocial and Mental Health Concerns

Anxiety
   Acceptance: Health Status
   Aggression Control
   Anxiety Control
   Coping
   Impulse Control
   Psychosocial Adjustment: Life Change
   Self-Mutilation Restraint
   Social Interaction Skills
   Symptom Control
Chronic Low Self-Esteem
Deficient Knowledge
   Cognitive Ability
   Communication Reception: Receptive
      Ability
   Concentration
   Information Processing
   Knowledge: Disease Process
   Knowledge: Health Resources
   Knowledge: Medication
   Knowledge: Treatment Regimen
   Memory
Disturbed Body Image
   Acceptance: Health Status
   Distorted Thought Control
   Self-Esteem
   Self-Mutilation Restraint
   Social Involvement
Disturbed Thought Processes
   Cognitive Ability
   Cognitive Orientation
   Communication Ability
   Concentration
   Decision Making
   Distorted Thought Control
   Identity
   Information Processing
   Memory

   Risk Control: Alcohol
   Risk Control: Drug Use
   Safety Behavior: Personal
Hopelessness
   Comfort Level
   Coping
   Decision Making
   Depression Control
   Depression Level
   Hope
   Mood Equilibrium
   Quality of Life
   Sleep
   Spiritual Well-Being
Ineffective Coping
   Aggression Control
   Caregiver Emotional Health
   Caregiver-Patient Relationship
   Caregiver Well-Being
   Depression Control
   Depression Level
   Family Coping
   Family Environment: Internal
   Family Normalization
   Family Health Status
Risk for Other-Directed Violence
   Abuse Protection
   Abusive Behavior Self-Control
   Aggression Control
   Cognitive Ability
   Depression Control
   Distorted Thought Control
   Impulse Control
   Quality of Life
   Risk Control
   Risk Control: Alcohol Use
   Risk Control: Drug Use
   Risk Detection

Risk for Self-Directed Violence
   Cognitive Ability
   Depression Control
   Depression Level
   Distorted Thought Control
   Impulse Control
   Loneliness
   Mood Equilibrium
   Quality of Life
   Risk Control
   Risk Control: Alcohol Use
   Risk Control: Drug Use
   Risk Detection
   Self-Mutilation Restraint
   Suicide Self-Restraint
   Will to Live
**Self-Care Deficit (Feeding,
   Bathing/Hygiene, Toileting)**
   Self-Care: Activities of Daily Living
      (ADL)
   Self Direction of Care
Situational Low Self-Esteem
   Body Image
   Hope
   Mood Equilibrium
   Role Performance
   Self-Esteem
   Social Interaction Skills
Spiritual Distress
   Anxiety Control
   Hope
   Quality of Life
   Spiritual Well-Being
   Suicide Self-Restraint
   Well-Being
   Will to Live

stress, coping mechanisms, and self-esteem are reviewed. Three clients with concurrent medical disorders and serious mental illness are discussed to illustrate the challenge that these individuals present for holistic nursing care. In each case, the role of the medical-surgical nurse is presented along with a suggested nursing care plan. Finally, the dimensions of culture and spirituality are addressed (see the boxes on Psychosocial Dimensions: Spirituality and Mental Illness, Culture and Mental Illness, and Sexuality and Mental Illness on the website). Chapter 4 describes how to obtain a psychosocial history as part of the comprehensive nursing assessment.

CLIENT SCENARIOS

Picture yourself as the nurse responsible for the clients in the following scenarios. The following scenarios help illustrate the later discussion of psychosocial and mental health issues and their application in nursing care across a variety of clinical settings:

1. You work the 3 to 11 PM shift in the emergency department (ED). You are assigned to Mrs. Barbara James, a 51-year-old black woman admitted several hours ago with acute chest pain and respiratory distress. Although diagnostic tests rule out myocardial infarction, she is crying and afraid to go home.

TABLE 25-1	Manifestations of Four Levels of Anxiety		
Anxiety Level	Physical Manifestations	Emotional Manifestations	Cognitive Manifestations
Mild	Increased pulse and blood pressure	Positive affect	Alert, can solve a problem, prepared to learn new information
Moderate	Elevated vital signs, tense muscles, diaphoresis	Tense, fearful	Attention focused on one concern, may be able to concentrate with direction
Severe	Fight-or-flight response, dry mouth, numb extremities	Distressed	Decreased sensory perception, can focus only on details, unable to learn new information
Panic	Continued as in severe level	Totally overwhelmed	Ignores external cues, focused only on internal stimuli, unable to learn

2. While on duty in a busy university medical clinic, you see a client with a recently diagnosed hiatal hernia. Gregory Barnes is a 32-year-old, slightly obese black man who smiles pleasantly as you introduce yourself and shakes your hand. He tells you that he has a problem with the elves who live in his basement and who take all his food.

3. You are a staff nurse on a medical acute care unit and are assigned to Mrs. Mary Conners, a 59-year-old West Indian woman admitted the previous day with diabetic ketoacidosis. Entering her room, you notice that the lights are off, and she does not look up when she responds to your greeting.

UNIVERSAL ISSUES

Universal psychosocial concepts include anxiety, stress, coping mechanisms, and self-esteem. Additional factors that influence reactions to stress are cultural and family background, exposure to similar stressors, and repeated exposure to stressors.

Anxiety

Before addressing the psychosocial concerns of clients with concurrent mental disorders, the nurse must first develop skills to manage the anxiety that is common to all clients. *Anxiety* is a universal human phenomenon, defined as a strong feeling of fear or dread with an unknown cause. All clients (and their loved ones) are vulnerable to feeling anxiety as they seek care for medical problems. Everyone may feel anxiety at times, especially when facing an unknown situation (changing schools, starting a new job). Under normal conditions, this discomfort is short-lived and may be helpful for problem solving (see the box on Emotional, Physical, and Spiritual Manifestations of Anxiety on the website).

Stress

Anxiety is part of the human reaction to stress. *Stress* is defined as "a particular relationship between the person and the environment that is appraised by the person as taxing and/or exceeding his or her resources and endangering his or her well-being."[19] Resources can include one's coping skills. In the case of potential physical danger, one is mobilized for self-protection with the fight-or-flight response. Most people would experience strong reactions in the face of crisis situations such as an imminent car accident or a tornado. In addition to external stressful events, people may define stress in different ways because it is the perception of the event, not the event itself, that stimulates the response. For example, one student may feel extreme stage fright when giving a speech, whereas another may feel only mild tension. Table 25-1 describes the levels of anxiety with implications for client teaching.

Coping Mechanisms

Most people respond to anxiety by using *coping skills* that are learned external behaviors or internal thought processes consciously used to decrease discomfort. Coping behavior can be classified as follows[9]:

- *Emotion-focused* behaviors to alter one's response to the stressor, such as thinking, saying, or doing something to make oneself feel better (crying, sharing feelings with someone)
- *Problem-focused* behaviors to directly alter the stressor, such as seeking facts about a problem or making a plan to overcome the obstacle (family member asking multiple questions over and over)

Chapter 1 discusses these behaviors in more detail.

Another common response to anxiety is the use of *ego defense mechanisms,* originally defined by Freud.[10] These thought processes are not deliberate or voluntary, like coping mechanisms. Instead, they exist at an unconscious level to disguise the real threat, protecting the person from feeling anxious about the real issue. One defense mechanism frequently seen in clients with serious illness is *denial.* See Box 25-1 for definitions and examples of selected defense mechanisms.

Assess the level of anxiety in all clients, and intervene as early as possible to reduce the anxiety to a manageable level. To achieve compliance with treatment, the client or family must be calm enough to understand the

BOX 25-1	*Selected Defense Mechanisms: Definitions and Examples*
Definition	**Example**
Denial—avoiding a problem by ignoring it or refusing to recognize it	A client with a cardiac condition tells his family that he has a "little problem" after the physician explains his diagnosis of heart attack.
Displacement—transferring feelings for a threatening topic or person to another more neutral topic or person	After a client is told that he cannot be discharged today as planned, he spends the whole shift complaining that his breakfast was cold.
Intellectualization—showing excessive thinking and logic to avoid uncomfortable feelings	After a leg amputation, a client shows great interest in the details of the surgery and even requests a textbook to identify the muscles and bones, but he does not watch while the nurse changes the dressing.
Projection—assigning one's own uncomfortable feelings or motivation to another person	A client tells the nurse, "Please explain about the operation again to my wife; she is so afraid that I won't wake up."
Rationalization—giving an apparently logical and acceptable explanation to cover up a feeling or motive that may not be socially acceptable	The nurse finds a client eating breakfast when he is on NPO status (nothing by mouth) for a diagnostic test. The nurse specifically told him about the procedure yesterday. When asked what happened, the client states, "Well, the aide brought me this tray so I thought it was okay."
Regression—demonstrating behavior characteristics of an earlier stage of development	An adult client insists on keeping multiple stuffed animals on her bed and bursts into tears when the nurse moves one to check her arm for IV access.

BOX 25-2	*Nursing Interventions to Decrease Client Anxiety*
Nonverbal Interventions	**Verbal Interventions**
Listen with full attention, looking at the client with unbroken eye contact. Maintain a calm, unhurried approach. Speak slowly in a clear, firm voice (not loud). Offer or use touch (e.g., hold a hand or give a back rub). If possible, decrease the noise and bright light.	Answer questions honestly. Explain all procedures in simple terms. Give reassurance based on the data. Give information about tests, medicines, and treatments as requested. Explain the reasons for limitations on activity or other restrictions. Acknowledge the client's anxiety, and encourage him or her to explore the reasons. Include family members in discussions unless the client requests otherwise. If necessary, repeat directions patiently.

Self-Esteem

Another universal concern that affects the client's reaction to the stress of illness is self-esteem. *Self-esteem* is defined as "the individual's personal judgment of his or her own worth."[14] The client's pre-existing level of self-esteem influences the adjustment to illness. A person with high self-esteem has positive expectations even in stressful situations. In contrast, a person with low self-esteem consistently demonstrates pessimism (see the table on Characteristics of People with High and Low Self-Esteem on the website for characteristics of self-esteem with implications for nursing care).

ADDITIONAL NEEDS OF CLIENTS WITH CONCURRENT MENTAL ILLNESS

After recognizing the psychosocial concerns of clients in general, you should become aware of additional needs for successful care of clients with concurrent mental illness. These needs consist of (1) comprehensive nursing assessment, (2) your self-awareness regarding communication, (3) basic mental health teaching for the client and family, and (4) referral for specialized services.

Comprehensive Nursing Assessment

As soon as you realize that the client is presenting with an altered mood or thought process, review the nursing database to ensure that it is complete. In many admis-

teaching. You can use several simple communication techniques to decrease anxiety in clients; see Box 25-2 for nursing interventions.

You must also be able to recognize positive coping efforts by clients and their families. As noted previously, these behaviors may be emotion focused or problem focused, but they function to decrease anxiety. Failure to understand these behaviors may lead to nontherapeutic staff reactions that impede recovery.

TABLE 25-2	*Commonly Used Terms to Describe Abnormal Mental Status Findings*
Term	**Mental Status Findings**

Mood

Depressed	Feeling sad, decreased energy and interest in usual activities
Elated	Feeling euphoric, overly optimistic, and energetic
Labile	Rapidly changing from one state to another (e.g., happy to sad or irritable)

Affect

Blunted	Overall decrease in emotional tone compared with a normal reaction to a situation
Flat	No expression of feelings, regardless of variation in topics
Inappropriate	Nonverbal signs of feelings do not match the verbal report of the person (e.g., person smiles when reporting a sad event)

Motor Activity

Agitation	Physically restless, unable to sit still
Psychomotor retardation	Physically slowed down, including all movements and speech

Perception

Hallucination	Sensory perception originating from within the brain but attributed to external sources (e.g., hearing voices)
Illusion	Incorrect interpretation of external sensory input (e.g., seeing a shadow in the closet and thinking it is a person)

Speech

Loose association	Speech pattern in which the listener cannot follow the connections between the speaker's ideas, seems illogical to listener
Pressured speech	Rapid flow of speech with intense undercurrent of feeling, may refuse to be interrupted

Thought Process

Delusion	A fixed, false belief that is strongly defended by the individual (e.g., may be paranoid [suspicious] or grandiose [unrealistically wonderful])
Psychosis	Severe impairment in reality testing, with distortion in perception and analysis of external and internal stimuli

sion situations, limited data are obtained before treatment is initiated. Make sure that you gather a complete psychosocial history (see Chapter 4). Table 25-2 lists definitions of commonly used terms to describe abnormal findings.

Psychosocial risk factors, such as a history of self-destructive, aggressive, or socially inappropriate behavior, must also be identified. Secondary sources, such as family and medical records, are often helpful. A complete medication history also provides data about concurrent mental illness if the client names psychotropic medications.

Awareness of Communication

The second requirement in caring for psychiatric clients is to pay extra attention to all communication with them. Under ordinary circumstances, communication with clients seems fairly routine and predictable: the nurse provides necessary physical care and teaching, which the client accepts or rejects.

Human communication is complex and built upon many assumptions and unspoken rules inherent in a given culture. Communication between two participants involves all of the verbal and nonverbal behavior that they perceive in each other.[25] In addition to using selected words, we send involuntary nonverbal signals. Nonverbal communication includes tone and volume of voice, eye contact, facial expression, body posture, and other body language. We expect to find congruence between the words and nonverbal cues; the words match the feeling and tone of the body (see the Diversity in Health Care feature on The Significance of Cultural Assessment on the website).

When the words and the nonverbal signs from a sender do not match, the receiving person must pause to analyze the situation. Psychiatric clients consistently have difficulty with communicating their needs. It is generally agreed that when the verbal and the nonverbal communication are incongruent, the nonverbal communication reflects the person's true feelings.

When communicating with clients who have concurrent psychiatric problems, pay attention to the communication process. Collect thorough data to determine the nursing diagnoses and to communicate with the treatment team. Monitor your own nonverbal behavior to prevent sending negative nonverbal messages to the client. Mental illness in our society still carries a considerable stigma: clients and their families feel ashamed because of an emotional problem; staff may have biases based on personal experience.[21]

Client and Family Teaching

The third important requirement for all clients with concurrent psychiatric disorders is basic client and family teaching. Basic teaching for all clients includes a definition of the illness, medications and treatment options, and relapse prevention.[7,12] This information is readily available in written teaching materials, which can be kept on file along with medical-surgical teaching guides. Whenever possible, include a family member in the instruction because he or she has a significant role in caring for the client (see the WebLinks on the website for resources to educate and support clients and their families).

Specialized Referrals

The fourth important requirement to consider when caring for clients with concurrent mental disorders is the need for specialized referrals. If manifestations are severe or risk factors are significant, additional evaluation is necessary and you are in a key position to advocate for appropriate services. In the hospital or institutional environment, consulting psychiatric staff can be called for an in-depth assessment and disposition. Likewise, in the community setting, referrals can be made to specialized outpatient services.

Summary

The medical-surgical nurse has a clear role to play with clients who have concurrent psychiatric disorders. The four steps just outlined do not require training beyond that of a generalist. They do require a professional commitment to provide holistic care to all clients and to fully use the multidisciplinary team available in the health care setting. In the sections that follow, the three psychiatric clients introduced in this section are revisited in more detail. An overview of their psychiatric disorders is presented along with specific nursing care plans for management in the medical-surgical setting.

ETIOLOGY OF MENTAL DISORDERS

The causes of psychiatric disorders are not yet fully understood. Ongoing brain research has identified biologic alterations and psychological theories have been used as a framework for treatment.

Biologic

Biologic evidence shows a genetic influence for the mental disorders: first-degree relatives have an increased risk for the same manifestations. Studies with medications and diagnostic imaging techniques have shown abnormalities in brain structures and neurotransmitters. For example, the ventricles are enlarged and brain volume is decreased in frontal and temporal lobes in schizophrenia. With mood disorders, the limbic system is altered. For anxiety disorders, frontal and temporal lobes and the brain stem are affected. Dysregulation in the following neurotransmitter systems is the target of the psychotropic medications: dopamine, serotonin, norepinephrine, gamma-aminobutyric acid (GABA), and glutamate.[18]

Psychological

Psychological approaches relate mental disorders to faulty defenses, or thinking and learning processes.[10] Psychoanalytic theory proposes that anxiety results from inability to control painful impulses, thoughts, or memories. Cognitive theory suggests that a person consistently distorts reality to see the world in a negative way. Behavioral theory explains abnormal behavior as a learned response to specific reinforcement in the environment.

ANXIETY

Mrs. James presents with a classic case of panic attack. The acute manifestations can create severe physical distress: palpitations, chest pain, elevated vital signs, dizziness, nausea, and distinct fear that one is dying. The cardiac work-up does not reveal abnormal cardiac enzymes or electrocardiogram (ECG), and the manifestations subside spontaneously. After additional diagnostic testing to rule out other medical disorders, panic disorder can be identified.

Panic disorder is one of the eight subtypes of anxiety disorders identified by the *Diagnostic and Statistical* *Manual of Mental Disorders*, fourth edition, text revision (*DSM-IV-TR*).[1] Anxiety disorders as a group are the most common psychiatric disorders in the United States and affect one of four people in a given year.[3,24] Box 25-3 describes each diagnosis.

Manifestations may range from mild to severe. Many of these clients never request treatment because of their feelings of shame. However, clients with panic disorder, post-traumatic stress disorder, or acute stress disorder may seek emergency care.[17]

Outcome Management

All of the anxiety disorders can be effectively treated through a combination of medication and psychotherapy. Several different classes of drugs that alter levels of neurotransmitters can be helpful (see the box on Med-

BOX 25-3	*Key Features of the Anxiety Disorders*

Panic Disorder—recurrent panic attacks followed by a change in behavior to try and avoid another attack persisting over more than 1 month

Generalized Anxiety Disorder (GAD)—excessive anxiety for 6 or more months that is uncontrollable, often focused on health or money concern

Phobia—severe, persistent fear of an object or situation that the person recognizes as irrational but cannot overcome

Obsessive-Compulsive Disorder (OCD)—preoccupation with disturbing thoughts (obsessions) or repetitive actions (compulsions) that interferes with normal activities of daily living

Post-Traumatic Stress Disorder (PTSD)—reexperiencing a real, horrifying event in nightmares or flashbacks, with a duration of manifestations more than 1 month; may be an immediate or a delayed reaction

Acute Stress Disorder—similar to PTSD except that manifestations occur within 1 month of the event and last only for approximately 1 month

Anxiety Disorder due to General Medical Condition—severe anxiety in the presence of clear physical findings of a somatic disorder (e.g., hypoglycemia)

Anxiety Disorder Not Otherwise Specified—showing some anxiety or phobic manifestations, but not severe enough to warrant a specific diagnosis

---

ications for Anxiety Disorders on the website for a list of commonly prescribed anti-anxiety medications).[2] These medicines may be prescribed for short-term or long-term use but usually are not needed permanently. Medication may offer some immediate benefit to reduce the discomfort of anxiety, but some form of psychotherapy (individual, group, or family) is necessary to achieve lasting positive outcomes. Clients have often adopted negative patterns of thinking or avoidance behaviors that are not easily given up.

Intervention

Returning to Mrs. James, the ED nurse needs to quickly devise a care plan with a discharge plan (see the Care Plan feature on The Client with Degenerative Joint Disease and Concurrent Panic Disorder on the website).[16]

Comprehensive Assessment

As the nurse explores the client's current psychological and social functioning, Mrs. James reports that she has had four episodes of respiratory distress in the past 6 months. She cannot relate the attack to any particular stressor but has started to avoid all places where she feels anxious. She also describes difficulty sleeping, increased appetite, crying spells, and decreased sexual interest.

When asked about her past level of functioning, Mrs. James states that, until 1 year ago, she was working as a nurse's aide and was independent. She drove, helped to care for her mother, and enjoyed going out with friends to church and social events. After a fall resulting in a knee injury, she never recovered full ambulation and recently applied for disability. In relation to her family history for emotional problems, Mrs. James explains that her mother is alcoholic and her daughter takes antidepressants, but she has always been "too strong for that kind of problem."

Communication Awareness

Throughout the interview, the nurse provides a private, supportive atmosphere. Initially, the nurse closes the curtain and moves the chair so that there is continuous eye contact. It is explained that they may have only 15 minutes before an interruption, but the nurse wants to learn as much as possible about Mrs. James. As the client talks, the nurse encourages her with nonverbal cues such as nodding her head. When the client becomes tearful at times, the nurse calmly pauses and offers her a tissue. The nurse shows no surprise or disapproval when Mrs. James mentions mental illness in her family. At the end of the assessment, the nurse explains that the discharge plan must be developed with the physician and she advises Mrs. James to call a family member to pick her up.

Client and Family Teaching

The nurse reports the findings on Mrs. James' anxiety and mood to the attending physician and recommends that the psychiatric consultant for the ED be called. The physician agrees, noting that all laboratory findings are normal. The probable diagnosis is panic disorder. As the physician goes to speak with the client, the nurse obtains material on panic attack and coping skills for families. The nurse gives these pamphlets to Mrs. James and her daughter, telling them that anxiety is a common, treatable problem. The nurse also explains the role of the psychiatric consultant and asks them to wait to talk with her. The client is uncertain, but the daughter encourages her to agree.

Specialized Referrals

In choosing the appropriate referral for discharge planning for Mrs. James, the nurse is aware that the medical center offers several levels of psychiatric care (see the table on the Levels of Psychiatric Treatment Services on the website). Because the client is not at immediate risk to harm herself or others, referral to the inpatient unit is not indicated. If an appointment is given to the outpatient clinic for next week, she may not follow up. Thus the nurse selects the resource person who can make an immediate, specialized assessment and disposition, namely, the ED consultant.

The psychiatric consultant (social worker, advanced practice nurse, or psychologist) performs a full, diagnostic interview, including appropriate standardized tests for anxiety and depression (see the box on Selected Standardized Tools for Assessment of Psychiatric Disorders on the website for a list of commonly used rating scales for mental health assessment). The ED nurse shares the nursing database with the consultant.

After meeting with the client and her daughter, the psychiatric consultant recommends referral to the Partial Hospital Program on the following day because of the severity of manifestations. The nurse communicates this recommendation to the physician and strongly supports this treatment in the discharge instructions to Mrs. James and her daughter.

SCHIZOPHRENIA

Mr. Barnes demonstrates clear manifestations of *schizophrenia* with fixed delusions and hallucinations. He represents a generation of young, chronically mentally ill people who have been cared for primarily in the community instead of being institutionalized. Schizophrenia is an incurable, severe mental illness that usually strikes between the ages of 17 and 25.[22] *DSM-IV-TR* lists five subtypes (Box 25-4).

BOX 25-4	*Types of Schizophrenia and Manifestations*
Type	**Manifestations**
Paranoid	Presence of hallucinations and delusional thinking; fairly organized in speech and behavior; may show some range in affect
Disorganized	Dominant manifestations of disorganized speech and behavior, with flat or inappropriate affect; may also have hallucinations and delusions
Catatonic	Presence of bizarre motor activity, either excessive and purposeless or immobilized as if in a stupor; may be mute or show incoherent speech
Undifferentiated	Presence of two or more of the following manifestations, but without a dominant feature as in the above three types: hallucinations, delusions, disorganized speech or behavior, and flat affect
Residual	Behavior does not show obvious hallucinations, delusions, or disorganization, but alterations persist in range of affect and thinking patterns

In all cases, a person's thinking and communication skills are profoundly affected. Manifestations are generally classified as positive or negative.[22] *Positive* manifestations include the most obvious signs of psychosis (auditory or visual hallucinations, delusions, disorganized thinking and speech). *Negative* manifestations refer to the lack of usual emotional or social responses (blunted affect, avoidance of social contact, lack of attention to hygiene).

Outcome Management

The positive manifestations of schizophrenia can be controlled by antipsychotic medication, but the negative manifestations and severe social impairment require supportive psychotherapy. Antipsychotic medicines have been used since the 1950s, and several classes of drugs have evolved over time in an effort to reduce unpleasant side effects (see the box on Medications for Schizophrenia on the website).[11] These medications usually must be taken for a lifetime to control the manifestations. With medication, some clients report a total absence of hallucinations but for others, internal voices become a permanent experience.

A major concern for most clients is the presence of side effects related to sedation and abnormal movements.[2] Because typical antipsychotics affect all dopamine receptors, including those for movement, muscle side effects known as *extrapyramidal symptoms* (EPS) are extremely common. Manifestations of EPS may include stiffness or tremor in arms and legs, extreme restlessness with subjective discomfort, drooling, and acute muscle spasms of the tongue, neck, or face.[2] These side effects are usually short-term and treatable with an anticholinergic agent such as benztropine or trihexyphenidyl. However, a long-term side effect of typical antipsychotics, called *tardive dyskinesia* (TD), occurs in approximately one third of clients and is usually irreversible.[2] Common manifestations of TD are obvious, involuntary movements of the tongue, face, hands, or legs. The main benefit of the newer, atypical antipsychotics is the lower incidence of EPS and TD because the drugs are more selective in affecting neurotransmitters.[2]

One final side effect of antipsychotics should be noted. *Neuroleptic malignant syndrome* is a rare but serious condition that may appear suddenly with extreme muscle rigidity, high fever, sweating, and fluctuations in consciousness. The client requires emergency hospitalization with supportive treatment to prevent seizures, coma, or even death.

Treatment of impaired social functioning involves long-term supportive therapy and psychosocial rehabilitation. Social withdrawal and lack of interest in school or work often signal the onset of the illness and may persist throughout treatment. To develop and maintain maximal level of functioning, schizophrenic clients need individual counseling and support, psychoeducation, organized rehabilitation services, and family psychoeducation.[13]

As with any chronic illness, the client experiences episodes of remission and exacerbation. Medication noncompliance, denial of illness, and stressful events may lead to multiple, short-term hospitalizations over a lifetime. With the consistent support of family and community resources, however, many clients can progress toward higher levels of independence.

Intervention

Returning to the case of Mr. Barnes, the nurse immediately recognizes that the client has abnormal thinking (see the Care Plan feature on The Client with Hiatal Hernia and Concurrent Schizophrenia on the website). The nurse notes that he is well groomed and shows appropriate social skills for the clinic environment. Uncertain about his reliability as a historian, the nurse asks Mr. Barnes to include his mother in the interview.

Comprehensive Assessment

While completing the nursing assessment, the nurse evaluates the client's knowledge of his medical illness, his psychosocial functioning, and his current level of compliance with psychiatric care. Despite his bizarre speech, Mr. Barnes offers accurate dates and descriptions of his medical manifestations. He firmly repeats his belief in the elves in the basement that talk to him at night and cause him to feel hungry all the time.

His mother adds that Mr. Barnes' mental illness was first diagnosed in his last year of high school. Before that, she had not noticed any problems. He has been hospitalized 10 times for severe paranoia and hostile threats toward his family. The most recent stay was 6 months ago and he is more compliant with his medication since his doctor switched to a long-acting intramuscular form.

Exploration of daily activities reveals that Mr. Barnes is constantly supervised by his mother. He stays at home watching television, reading, and doing chores. He has no contact with peers and never worked. He states, "My brother and his friends don't like me anymore. My schizophrenia makes me stupid."

Communication Awareness

Throughout the interview, the nurse takes care to include Mr. Barnes in the conversation, even though his mother tends to dominate. The nurse maintains a calm facial expression when the client discusses his delusions and respectfully records his answers. No attempt is made to challenge the reality of his remarks, but the nurse does not agree with his distortions. The nurse is also careful not to invade the client's personal space without asking for permission.

Client and Family Teaching

Although the client and his mother seem to be familiar with the term *schizophrenia,* it is not clear how much teaching they have received. Before giving them material about hiatal hernia, the nurse asks whether they would like to learn more about schizophrenia. They both are interested. The nurse explains that schizophrenia is a chronic illness that can be controlled and praises the client for his knowledge of his medication and medical care.

Specialized Referrals

Before setting up the next clinic appointment, the nurse considers whether any other mental health resource is indicated. Mr. Barnes' condition is stable at this time, with monthly psychiatrist appointments; however, he feels stigmatized and he is totally dependent on his mother. To promote the best overall health outcomes for Mr. Barnes, the nurse must consider *tertiary prevention* with regard to his mental illness. (See Chapter 1 for a review of primary, secondary, and tertiary prevention.) The nurse believes that additional professional support could improve his level of community functioning.

The nurse recommends a referral to the psychiatric clinical specialist in the outpatient clinic at the medical center to explore community resources. The nurse offers to introduce them to the psychiatric nurse at their next clinic visit. The nurse calls the clinical specialist, who explains several referrals could be made for Mr. Barnes: to a young adult supportive therapy group, a psychosocial rehabilitation program, or a mental health support group for clients and families. The clinical specialist will also call the attending psychiatrist to coordinate the treatment plan.

MOOD DISORDERS

Mrs. Conners shows the most common manifestations of a serious mood disorder. Mood disorders are classified into three major categories: (1) depressive disorders, (2) bipolar disorder (formerly called manic-depressive illness), and (3) mood disorder due to general medical condition or substance use.[1] Manifestations of all depressions include a sad mood, which may be accompanied by crying spells; persistent negative thinking with hopelessness; possible suicidal thinking; decreased energy and motivation; and changes in sleep, appetite, and sexual interest.

In clients with bipolar disorder, mood can fluctuate from depression to the other extreme, mania. *Manic manifestations* include excessive cheerfulness or irritability; an unrealistic, optimistic attitude toward one's accomplishments; overabundance of energy; and decreased sleep with increased physical appetite. Box 25-5 describes mood states.

BOX 25-5	*Manifestations of Mood Disorders*

Depression (Major or Bipolar)

Sad mood, but may be irritable
Crying spells
Negative thinking, continuously pessimistic
Feelings of guilt and hopelessness
Preoccupation with usually minor somatic complaints
Loss of pleasure in usual activities and decreased socialization
Decreased ability to concentrate and remember current events
Decreased energy level
Change in sleep, increased or decreased
Change in appetite, increased or decreased
Decreased libido and sexual activity
May feel suicidal
May develop psychosis with delusions about a negative future (e.g., fatal illness)

Mania

Elated mood, not attributable to a reality event
Denial of having an emotional problem
Impulsive acts that may be dangerous or socially inappropriate (e.g., promiscuity)
Increased energy level
Increased socialization to the point of becoming intrusive
Excessive, rapid speech
Change in appetite, increased or decreased
Decreased need for sleep
Increased libido

BOX 25-6	*Risk Factors for Suicide*

- Depressed mood
- Psychosis
- Hopelessness
- Serious medical disorder
- Substance abuse
- Male gender
- Caucasian race
- Family history of substance abuse
- Living alone
- Previous attempted suicide

COMPLEMENTARY AND ALTERNATIVE THERAPY

St. John's Wort for Major Depression

Previous randomized studies have found that St. John's wort may reduce the manifestations of mild to moderate depression. However, its effect on major depression had not been tested until recently. A randomized, blinded, and placebo-controlled trial was conducted at 11 academic centers in the United States. A total of 200 physically healthy outpatients 18 years of age or older with major depression and without psychotic features were recruited (mean age 42.4 years, 64% women). Clients received either St. John's wort (one 300-mg tablet 3 times daily, $n = 98$) or placebo ($n = 102$) for 8 weeks. The dose was increased to 4 tablets (1200 mg) daily for individuals who did not sufficiently improve by week 4 of the study. Interestingly, both groups significantly improved over time ($p < 0.001$), but the groups did not differ significantly from each other. More clients responded to St. John's wort, but the difference was not statistically different from the placebo. This study would have been better if a standard treatment arm had been included. Regardless, this initial study demonstrated minimal to no benefit of this herb over the placebo for the reduction of major depression.

Reference

Shelton, R., et al. (2001). Effectiveness of St. John's wort in major depression: A randomized controlled trial. *Journal of the American Medical Association, 285*, 1978-1986.

The key element in mood disorders is that the person cannot control the severity of the feeling. There may or may not be a clear precipitant for the reaction. Unlike a healthy person with transient mood changes, a depressed person cannot "just get over it" and the client with mania does not wish to give up the euphoria that characterizes this mood.

Major depressive disorders usually start between the ages of 20 and 50 years, and up to 75% of clients suffer a recurrence within 5 years.[8,23] Adolescent and adult women are two times more likely to have depression than their male counterparts. Mood disorders frequently co-occur with other psychiatric or medical illnesses. Clients may show depression with substance abuse, an anxiety disorder, or an eating disorder. Medical problems often associated with depression include cardiovascular, endocrine, neurologic, and autoimmune disorders, as well as certain cancers. Whenever depressive manifestations are mixed with physical complaints, close collaboration between a psychiatrist and primary care provider is necessary for appropriate treatment.

The most serious adverse outcome for mood disorders is suicide.[4] Take all verbal expressions of suicide intent or threat seriously and act accordingly (see later in this chapter). Up to 15% of clients who are hospitalized for major depression eventually commit suicide. The period of greatest risk is during psychiatric hospitalization or just after release.[4] There are known risk factors associated with suicide in the United States (Box 25-6).[15] Older adults and adolescents are at special risk. Chapter 3 discusses depression in older adults.

COMPLEMENTARY AND ALTERNATIVE THERAPY

St. John's Wort and Drug Metabolism

St. John's wort is one of the most popular antidepressant supplements sold around the world. However, this supplement has a profound effect on inducing the activity of cytochrome P450 3A4 in the liver. This observation suggests that long-term administration of this supplement could result in a decreased effectiveness or an increased dosage requirement for all drugs affected by this pathway. The biggest concern about this supplement is that at least 50% of all marketed medications are affected by this liver pathway. Therefore the ability of this supplement to affect numerous medications should be a major concern to health professionals.

Reference

Markowitz, J., et al. (2003). Effect of St. John's wort on drug metabolism by induction of cytochrome P450 3A4 enzyme. *Journal of the American Medical Association, 290*, 1500-1504.

COMPLEMENTARY AND ALTERNATIVE THERAPY

Exercise versus a Prescription Medication for Major Depressive Disorder

A study from Duke University used 156 adult volunteers with major depressive disorder (MDD). Interesting results were found 6 months after completion of the study, in which volunteers were randomly assigned either a 4-month course of aerobic exercise (30 minutes 3 times per week), sertraline therapy, or a combination of both. All groups exibited significant improvement during the initial study, but at the 6-month follow-up period the exercise group had significantly lower relapse rates than the medication group. In fact, exercising on one's own during 6 months after the actual intervention was associated with a 51% lower risk of depression diagnosis.

Reference

Babyak, M., et al. (2000). Exercise treatment for major depression: Maintenance of therapeutic benefit at 10 months. *Psychosomatic Medicine, 62*, 633-638.

Outcome Management

Mood disorders can almost always be managed effectively through a combination of medication and psychotherapy. In some cases, electroconvulsive therapy (ECT) is indicated. Antidepressant medication is used for up to 1 year or for a lifetime, depending on the client's potential for relapse. Particularly for bipolar disorder, mood stabilizers may be needed for long-term treatment. Several classes of antidepressant drugs affect neurotransmitters in different ways (see the box on Medications for Mood Disorders on the website and see the Complementary and Alternative Therapy features on St. John's Wort for Major Depression, on St. John's Wort and Drug Metabolism, and on Exercise versus a Prescription Medication for Major Depressive Disorder on p. 532 and above).[11] If a client does not respond to one medication after a fair trial, the physician may switch to another class or try a combination. Antidepressants and mood stabilizers do not produce effects immediately as the antianxiety drugs do. Thus the depressed client often suffers for 3 to 6 more weeks after starting treatment. Hopelessness about treatment, especially if the first medication is ineffective, compounds the risk for suicide.

Several types of psychotherapy may be helpful for mood disorders. In all cases, client education is important to explain the course of the illness and the benefits of treatment, despite the delay in improvement. Often, short-term therapy is beneficial with a focus on learning to manage current stressors and relationships. Marital therapy may be indicated because a mood disorder frequently causes marital discord, and conflict with loved ones often precipitates a depressive episode.

ECT is a viable treatment alternative for some clients with depression and may be provided in an inpatient or outpatient setting. An electrical shock is administered to a specific region of the brain to induce a seizure. General anesthesia is required, and the client does not remember the experience. The mechanism of action is not entirely understood but its effect on the neurotransmitter receptors may be similar to that of the tricyclic antidepressants. The client experiences short-term memory loss, but improvement is faster than with medication treatment.[23]

Intervention

After meeting Mrs. Conners (in diabetic ketoacidosis), the nurse is concerned about two major problems. First, the client's mental status appears altered and she is in distress. Second, the average length of stay for this medical diagnosis is only 1 more day, and much teaching must be done before discharge. Returning to the nursing database, the nurse notes that the psychosocial section is incomplete. It is documented that the client is a native West Indian, lives with her daughter, and has a history of depression. She has been hospitalized three times in the past year, twice on the psychiatric unit and once for ketoacidosis (see the Care Plan feature on The Client with Diabetic Ketoacidosis and Concurrent Depression on the website).

Comprehensive Assessment

The nurse decides to complete the psychosocial history, even though Mrs. Conners may not seem cooperative. Mrs. Conners speaks in a soft voice, with just a few words at a time. The client says that she has had diabetes for 2 years and depression for 35 years. She has been going to the same psychiatrist for 20 years and asks the nurse to notify him. When asked about her medication, Mrs. Conners knows the name and dosage of her antidepressant and admits that she occasionally misses a dose. The nurse specifically asks about suicidal thoughts. See Box 25-7 for assessment questions.

The client describes her mood as sad and becomes tearful. She denies current suicidal ideation but admits to one overdose in the past. She expresses guilt about the overdose because of her religion. Then she says that she is too tired to talk. The nurse returns at lunch time and finds Mrs. Conners dressed in a long gown and wearing a colorful turban wrapped around her hair. Her daughter is coaxing her to eat some homemade soup. The daughter states that her mother has a pattern of medication noncompliance followed by diet noncompliance, which results in rehospitalization.

Communication Awareness

During the interview, the nurse is careful to respect Mrs. Conners' low energy level. The nurse uses questions that require only short answers and speaks clearly and softly.

When the client talks about feeling sad, the nurse does not try to cheer her up but reminds her that her depression has been successfully treated in the past.

After the input from the daughter, the nurse realizes how important the client's cultural background is for the care plan. In the West Indian culture, an older person may be uncomfortable around authority figures and strangers. Respect and good manners are important; people expect to be greeted with "Good morning" or "Good afternoon" and are always addressed by the last name. Personal issues are discussed only with family members who comprise the main support system. Religious beliefs are important and folk foods are considered medicinal.[20]

Client and Family Teaching

Although the client and her daughter openly discuss the diagnosis of depression, the nurse emphasizes that this is a medical illness that can be treated just like the diabetes. Reassurance may be needed about a possible change in medication or dosage. The nurse collects information on depression, the medications, and community support groups. This information is given to the client and her daughter to review and determine whether they have any questions.

BOX 25-7 Screening Assessment of Suicidal Risk

Interview Questions
1. Have you been thinking about death or hurting yourself?
2. If yes, do you have a plan?
3. Have you ever tried to hurt yourself before?
4. If yes, what did you do?
5. What would stop you from hurting yourself now?
6. Can you sign a written contract with me that you will not harm yourself for the next _____ (time period until next evaluation)?

Additional Indications of Higher Risk for Suicide
1. Has a specific plan that is available and dangerous (e.g., hanging, shooting, or jumping from a high location)
2. History of previous attempts
3. Cannot identify person or religious belief that would prevent action
4. Refusal to sign a safety contract
5. Living alone or estranged from loved ones
6. Use of alcohol or drugs
7. Presence of psychosis with command hallucinations to harm self (cannot safely contract)

Results of Screening
1. If the client shows no positive risk factors, no action is necessary except continued monitoring of behavior.

2. If the client shows positive risk factors but agrees to a written contract not to harm self, the nurse:
   a. Co-signs the contract, defining the time period from now until the next visit
   b. Notifies the attending physician (e.g., by telephone) in front of the client to report the assessment and to request a psychiatric nurse evaluation; if the physician orders other actions, these are shared with the client
   c. Strongly seeks the client's permission to share the contract with a family member, if available
   d. Contacts the psychiatric nurse to give a report and schedule a visit for the following day

3. If the client shows positive risk factors but refuses to sign a "no harm contract," the nurse must take emergency action. The nurse:
   a. Instructs the client, and family if available, that this condition is a mental health emergency and requires immediate evaluation by a physician in an emergency department
   b. Calls 911 for assistance, explaining that there is a psychiatric emergency
   c. Provides brief information to the police and emergency medical team upon arrival, with a follow-up telephone report to the appropriate emergency department
   d. Notifies the attending physician of the emergency actions

Specialized Referrals

As soon as the nurse observes that the mood disorder is complicating the client's medical condition, the discharge planner is contacted along with the attending physician. Discharge planning for Mrs. Conners requires a coordinated effort between medical and psychiatric clinicians. The attending physician asks the discharge planner to arrange for a consultation with the treating psychiatrist.

When the discharge planner calls the psychiatrist, he states that he can visit the client later that day. He adds that he may need to transfer her to the psychiatric unit because of her suicidal history. The nurse introduces the discharge planner to the client and her daughter and tells them to expect the psychiatrist that evening.

CONCLUSIONS

The medical-surgical nurse has a vital role in caring for the psychosocial needs of all clients. Sensitivity to client and family anxiety improves the nurse's communication skills and increases the probability that clients will achieve the desired outcomes. For clients who have concurrent mental illness, the nurse must consider several additional needs in order to provide comprehensive nursing care:

- Increased attention to completing the comprehensive nursing assessment
- Heightened awareness of verbal and nonverbal communication
- Basic teaching about illness and treatment options
- Referral to appropriate specialized resources available in the health care system

To provide holistic care to clients with concurrent mental illness does not require specialized training beyond the generalist level. But nurses must learn about the range of multidisciplinary services available at their health care facility in a particular community. The nurse is in a prime position in the health care team to advocate for appropriate mental health services for clients. Recognition of mental health needs supports the accomplishment of general health outcomes while reducing the pain and suffering of preventable adverse events.

BIBLIOGRAPHY

1. American Psychiatric Association. (2000). *Diagnostic and statistical manual of mental disorders (DMS-IV-TR)* (4th ed., text revision). Washington, DC: Author.
2. Antai-Otong, D. (2003). Adverse drug reactions associated with antipsychotics, antidepressants, and mood stabilizers. *Nursing Clinics of North America, 38*(1), 161-176.
3. Antai-Otong, D. (2003). Anxiety disorders: Treatment considerations. *Nursing Clinics of North America, 38*(1), 35-44.
4. Antai-Otong, D. (2003). Suicide: Lifespan considerations. *Nursing Clinics of North America, 38*(1), 137-150.
5. Antai-Otong, D. (2003). Treatment considerations for patients with borderline personality disorders. *Nursing Clinics of North America, 38*(1), 101-110.
6. Bailey, K.P., Sauer, C.D., Herrell, C. (2002). Mood disorders. In M.A. Boyd (Ed.), *Psychiatric nursing contemporary practice* (2nd ed., pp. 410-451). Philadelphia: Lippincott Williams & Wilkins.
7. Bostrom, A.C., Boyd, M.A. (2002). Schizophrenia. In M.A. Boyd (Ed.), *Psychiatric nursing contemporary practice* (2nd ed., pp. 332-383). Philadelphia: Lippincott Williams & Wilkins.
8. Costell, S. (2003). Mood disorders. *Nursing Clinics of North America, 38*(1), 21-34.
9. Boyd, M.A. (2002). Stress management and crisis intervention. In M.A. Boyd (Ed.), *Psychiatric nursing contemporary practice* (2nd ed., pp. 920-948). Philadelphia: Lippincott Williams & Wilkins.
10. Boyd, M.A. (2002). Theoretic basis of psychiatric nursing. In M.A. Boyd (Ed.), *Psychiatric nursing contemporary practice* (2nd ed., pp. 64-92). Philadelphia: Lippincott Williams & Wilkins.
11. Brown, A. (2002). New psychiatric medications in development in 2002. *NARSAD Research Newsletter, 14*(2), 27-32.
12. Carson, V.B. (2000). Basic interventions. In V.B. Carson (Ed.), *Mental health nursing the nurse-patient journey* (2nd ed., pp. 286-335). Philadelphia: W.B. Saunders.
13. Fordyce, E., & Taylor, D. (2000). Thought disorders. In V.B. Carson (Ed.), *Mental health nursing the nurse-patient journey* (2nd ed., pp. 635-678). Philadelphia: W.B. Saunders.
14. Fuhrmann, J.S. (2000). Shared attributes of every traveler. In V.B. Carson (Ed.), *Mental health nursing the nurse-patient journey* (2nd ed., pp. 163-186). Philadelphia: W.B. Saunders.
15. Hauenstein, E.J. (2002). Case finding and care in suicide: Children, adolescents and adults. In M.A. Boyd (Ed.), *Psychiatric nursing contemporary practice* (2nd ed., pp. 1006-1030). Philadelphia: Lippincott Williams & Wilkins.
16. Jensen, L. (2003). Managing acute psychotic disorders in an ED. *Nursing Clinics of North America, 38*(1), 45-54.
17. Katerndahl, D.A. (2002). Factors influencing care seeking for a self-defined worst panic attack. *Psychiatric Services, 53*(4), 464-470. **EB**
18. Laraia, M.T. (2001). Biological context of psychiatric nursing care. In G.W. Stuart, & M.T. Laraia (Eds.), *Principles and practice of psychiatric nursing* (7th ed., pp. 88-119). St. Louis: Mosby.
19. Lazarus, R., & Folkman, S. (1984). *Stress, appraisal and coping.* New York: Springer.
20. Leininger, M.M. (2001). *Culture care diversity and universality a theory of nursing.* Boston: Jones and Bartlett Publishers.
21. Link, B., et al. (2001). The consequences of stigma for the self-esteem of people with mental illnesses. *Psychiatric Services, 52*(12), 1621-1626. **EB**

22. Moller, M.D., & Murphy, M.F. (2001). Neurobiological responses and psychotic disorders. In G. Stuart, & M.T. Laraia (Eds.), *Principles and practice of psychiatric nursing* (7th ed., pp. 402-437). St. Louis: Mosby.

23. Scott, C.M. (2000). Mood disorders. In V.B. Carson (Ed.), *Mental health nursing the nurse-patient journey* (2nd ed., pp. 679-720). Philadelphia: W.B. Saunders.

24. Stuart, G. (2001). Anxiety responses and anxiety disorders. In G. Stuart, & M.T. Laraia (Eds.), *Principles and practice of psychiatric nursing* (7th ed., pp. 274-298). St. Louis: Mosby.

25. Watzlawick, P., Beavin, J.H., & Jackson, D.D. (1967). *Pragmatics of human communication*. New York: W.W. Norton.

Clients with Substance Abuse Disorders

Linda Carman Copel

evolve

Web Enhancements

http://evolve.elsevier.com/Black/medsurg/

Bridge to Home Health Care
Addressing Substance Abuse
Ethical Issues in Nursing
What Considerations Should Be Made for Substance Abusers
Who Are Being Treated for Other Medical Problems?

What Ethical Issues Surround Your Relationship to an Impaired Nurse?
Appendix A
Religious Beliefs and Practices Affecting Health Care

As the client passed through the hospital door, it was the beginning—the first step of many on the journey back from the world of drugs and alcohol. No longer did this person need to be entangled in the cycle of pain, ineffective coping with addictive substances, more pain, and more drugs. The client, struggling to think clearly, had the following thoughts: "I must be dying. My body hurts. Where am I? What is going on here? How did this happen? I can't stand it. What are they doing to me? They can't help me. I can't help me. No one can help me. My life has always been a mess. There is nothing I can do."

Clients with psychoactive substance abuse disorders struggle with an inability to solve problems. They are unable to use adaptive behaviors to handle life stresses, traumas, and demands. *Ineffective Coping, Defensive Coping, Ineffective Denial, Imbalanced Nutrition: Less than Body Requirements, Risk for Injury,* and *Risk for Infection* are a few of the nursing diagnoses specific to the assessment data obtained from these clients. Nurses are challenged by the myriad of physical and emotional health problems faced by clients with addiction. Their health histories and at-risk behaviors culminate in problems ranging from liver and cardiovascular disease to depression and human immunodeficiency virus (HIV) infection. The client's physical condition is further compromised by nutritional deficits and fluid and electrolyte imbalances. In addition, many clients suffer from injuries, either self-inflicted trauma or violence at the hands of others. Often, multiple injuries in various stages of healing are evident upon examination.

Underlying the physical problems are the emotional wounds from both past and present life situations. Without effective coping skills, clients tend to continuously repeat their self-destructive pattern of behavior. The inability to perceive reality accurately and to develop and maintain supportive relationships hinders successful lifestyle changes. Accelerating bouts of depression and feelings of powerlessness continue, perpetuating a sense of incompetence. A pervasive sense of failure may be overwhelming.

Studies consistently show that substance-abusing clients need both medical and psychiatric nursing care to achieve their highest level of functioning and to maintain sobriety. Nurses have the challenge of dealing not only with the addicted client's many physiologic problems but also with the effects and withdrawal symptoms of the drugs involved. Even as you seek to assess and diagnose the physiologic effects of abused substances, clients typically offer defensiveness and may remain in denial. These clients' lack responsibility for their personal behavior. Constant blaming and manipulation of others is typical behavior that requires your attention and intervention along with the physiologic issues. As much as

evolve *Be sure to check out the bonus material on the Evolve website and the CD-ROM, including free self-assessment exercises.*
http://evolve.elsevier.com/Black/medsurg/

Nursing Outcomes Classification
for Nursing Diagnoses—Clients with Substance Abuse Disorders

Acute Confusion
Cognitive ability
Disturbed Thought Processes
Information Processing
Impaired Memory
Neurologic Status: Consciousness
Acute Pain
Comfort
Anxiety
Aggression Control
Anxiety Control
Coping
Impulse Control
Self-Mutilation Restraint
Chronic Low Self-Esteem
Self-Esteem
Body Image
Deficient Knowledge (specify)
Knowledge: Substance Abuse Control
Disturbed Personal Identity
Identity
Self-Mutilation Restraint
Disturbed Sensory Perception (spec-ify: visual, auditory, kinesthetic, gus-tatory, tactile, olfactory)
Anxiety Control
Body Image
Rational Thought Process
Sleep
Disturbed Thought Processes
Cognitive Orientation
Concentration
Decision Making
Identity
Information Processing
Memory
Dysfunctional Grieving
Concentration
Coping
Family Coping

Grief Resolution
Psychosocial Adjustment: Life Change
Fatigue
Activity Tolerance
Endurance
Fear
Fear Control
Hopelessness
Decision Making
Hope
Mood Equilibrium
Quality of Life
Imbalanced Nutrition: Less Than Body Requirements
Nutritional Status: Nutrient Intake
Impaired Social Interaction
Role Performance
Social Interaction Skills
Social Involvement
Impaired Verbal Communication
Communication Ability
Communication: Expressive Ability
Communication: Receptive Ability
Ineffective Coping
Aggression Control
Depression Control
Depression Level
Ineffective Denial
Fear Control
Health Beliefs: Perceived Threat
Coping
Ineffective Role Performance
Abuse Protection
Ineffective Sexuality Patterns
Abuse Recovery: Sexual
Body Image
Self-Esteem
Sexual Identity: Acceptance
Interrupted Family Processes
Family Coping
Family Environment: Internal

Family Functioning
Family Normalization
Noncompliance (specify)
Adherence Behavior
Compliance Behavior
Treatment Behavior: Illness or Injury
Powerlessness
Depression Control
Depression Level
Family Participation in Professional Care
Risk for Impaired Skin Integrity
Self-Mutilation Restraint
Risk for Injury
Risk Control
Safety Behavior: Personal
Safety Status: Physical Injury
Risk for Other-Directed Violence
Abuse Protection
Abusive Behavior Self-Control
Aggression Control
Distorted Thought Control
Impulse Control
Risk Control: Alcohol Use
Risk Control: Drug Use
Risk Detection
Risk for Poisoning
Risk Control: Drug Use
Risk for Trauma
Risk Control
Safety Status: Physical Injury
Social Isolation
Mood Equilibrium
Social Interaction Skills
Social Involvement
Social Support
Spiritual Distress
Hope

any client population, this one challenges the entire health care team to provide holistic treatment for physical, emotional, and spiritual needs.

FRAMEWORKS FOR EXPLAINING ADDICTIVE BEHAVIORS

Over the past 100 years, clinicians and researchers have attempted to develop and refine the knowledge base on substance-abusing people. Early studies of alcoholism noted generational patterns of alcoholism in families.

On the basis of this observation, it was suggested that alcoholism might have a genetic component. However, there is no evidence to support this supposition with other commonly abused drugs.[10,18,22,31]

Various explanations of the causes of substance abuse have focused on three conceptual frameworks:

- Biologic
- Psychological
- Sociocultural

However, there is no one identifiable cause of substance use. Rather, a combination of factors typically coalesces to produce drug use patterns. A person may be at risk for substance abuse because of a complex combination of biologic, psychological, and sociocultural variables. All aspects of the client's background must be considered when treatment is initiated. In addition to what the client brings to the treatment setting, the theoretical approach used by the team to view the underlying dynamics of substance abuse influences the process of recovery.

Biologic Framework

The biologic theory, or disease concept, of substance abuse views addiction as a physiologic condition that can be identified and treated. The emphasis is on a physiologic cause, such as genetic predisposition, defects in metabolism, neurobiologic abnormalities, and abnormal levels of chemicals in the body.[38] Historically, studies attempting to link genetic transmission of alcoholism have been unable to identify a target gene.

Present research focuses on examining the inherited biochemical abnormalities that may predispose an individual to alcoholism.[5] It is believed that alcohol dependence is a combination of interwoven social and psychological variables in people who are physiologically vulnerable.[30] For example, people of East Asian ancestry tend to experience a physical reaction to alcohol characterized by tachycardia, a sensation of warmth and flushing, and generalized discomfort. The response is believed to be related to the lack of activation of the enzyme aldehyde dehydrogenase, resulting in the accumulation of acetaldehyde, a toxic product of alcohol metabolism.[25,37] This physiologic process may be the reason that Asian Americans tend to have the lowest rate of alcohol consumption and associated substance use problems compared with other racial groups.[30] Hence, an examination of biologic differences associated with the use of alcohol warrants continued investigation.

Psychological Framework

Psychological theories attempt to explain the variables that may predispose someone to substance use. According to the psychoanalytic model, the person is viewed as being fixated at the oral stage of development, seeking gratification of needs through behaviors such as drinking. With the psychodynamic approach, a person experiences both interpersonal and intrapersonal difficulties that provide the foundation for the addiction.

Behavioral theories regard addiction as a learned behavior that can be unlearned in a manner similar to that of changing negative habits or dysfunctional behaviors. A *family systems approach* emphasizes that relationships, roles, and unhealthy communication patterns among family members contribute to addictive behaviors; this dysfunctional lifestyle is transmitted to future generations.[13,21]

For years, researchers and clinicians have sought, without success, to discover an addictive personality

type. Some common characteristics noted in clients who abuse substances are low self-esteem, low frustration tolerance, inability to cope with physical and emotional pain, depression, lack of healthy relationships, and involvement in high-risk behaviors. Proponents of the psychological theories believe that people engage in substance use in an attempt to feel better about themselves and to meet their emotional needs. Thus, the use of a psychoactive substance becomes reinforced and eventually evolves into an addiction.

Sociocultural Framework

With the sociocultural theories, substance use is viewed from the perspective of cultural and social norms within various groups in society. The issues of whether to use drugs, what type of drugs to use, and how and when to use them are determined by factors in a person's background. Such factors may include values, belief systems, spiritual orientation, ethnicity, gender, family standards, or the contemporary social environment. The relationships between these variables can contribute to a person's susceptibility to drug use and potential for addiction treatment and ongoing recovery.

DEFINITIONS AND TERMINOLOGY

According to the *Diagnostic and Statistical Manual of Mental Disorders,* fourth edition, text revision *(DSM-IV-TR),*[2] the substance-related disorders comprise the range of substance use from taking a drug of abuse, to the adverse effects of any medication, to exposure to toxic substances. *DSM-IV-TR* lists 11 types of substances commonly abused: alcohol, amphetamines, caffeine, cannabis, cocaine, hallucinogens, inhalants, nicotine, opioids, phencyclidine (PCP), and the group "sedatives, hypnotics, or anxiolytics."[2] Polysubstance dependence and other substance-related disorders, particularly toxins or prescribed and over-the-counter medications, are also included.[2]

To understand and assess substance abuse, you must learn the associated terminology (Table 26-1). In working with clients who are actively using substances, you must also know the types of drugs commonly used, the major routes of administration, and side effects (Table 26-2). The order and severity of manifestations are influenced by the size of the dose and the length of time the drug has been used.

GENERAL ASSESSMENT

The purposes of a drug and alcohol assessment are to do the following:

- Determine whether substance abuse exists
- Evaluate the relationship between substance abuse and other health care problems
- Implement effective health promotion and health restoration interventions

All clients must be assessed for the use and misuse of chemical substances. Clients who struggle with addiction

TABLE 26-1	*Substance Abuse Terms and Definitions*
Term	**Definition**
Psychoactive substance	A substance that affects a person's mood or behavior
Substance abuse	Continued use of a psychoactive substance despite the occurrence of physical, psychological, social, or occupational problems
Substance dependence	A range of physiologic, behavioral, and cognitive symptoms indicating that a person persists in using the substance, ignoring serious substance-related problems
Physiologic dependence	The body's physical adaptation to a drug, whereby withdrawal symptoms occur if the drug is not used
Psychological dependence	The emotional need or craving for a drug either for its effect or to prevent the occurrence of withdrawal symptoms
Addiction	A compulsion, loss of control, and progressive pattern of drug use; characterized by behavioral changes, impaired thinking, unkept promises to stop usage, obsession with the drug, neglect of personal needs, decreased tolerance, and physiologic deterioration
Polysubstance abuse	Concurrent use of multiple drugs
Intoxication	An altered physiologic state resulting from the use of a psychoactive drug
Overdose	Accidental or deliberate consumption of a drug in a dose larger than is ordinarily used, resulting in a serious toxic reaction or death
Tolerance	A state resulting from metabolic changes in cell functions, whereby the tissue reaction to a drug declines and the person needs to take increasing amounts to achieve the same effect
Cross-tolerance	A state whereby the effect of a drug is decreased and greater amounts are required to achieve the desired effect because the person has become tolerant to a similar drug
Predisposition	Any factor that increases the likelihood of an event occurring
Potentiation	The ability of one drug to increase the activity of another drug when taken at the same time
Drug misuse	Any use of a drug that deviates from medical or socially acceptable use
Dual diagnosis	The coexistence of a major psychiatric illness and a psychoactive substance abuse disorder
Blackout	An acute situation in which a person experiences a period of memory loss for actions as a direct result of using drugs or alcohol
Withdrawal	Discontinuation of a substance by a person who is dependent on it
Detoxification	The process of withdrawing a person from an addictive substance in a safe manner
Toxic dose	The amount of a drug that produces a poisonous effect
Recidivism	The tendency to relapse into a former pattern of substance use and associated behaviors
Recovery	The return to a normal state of health, whereby the person does not engage in problematic behavior and continues to meet life's challenges and personal goals
Sobriety	Complete abstinence from drugs while developing a satisfactory lifestyle
Abstinence	Voluntarily refraining from activities or the use of substances that cause problems in the physiologic, psychological, social, intellectual, and spiritual arenas of a person's life

are found at all stages of life and therefore in all clinical specialties. It is common for a client who abuses drugs to be hospitalized for an injury, illness, or surgical procedure. The nurse-generalist must identify clients with actual or potential substance problems and institute a collaborative team approach to provide health care (see Bridge to Home Health Care on Addressing Substance Abuse on the web *evolve* site).

The ability of nurses to provide care is influenced by the personal thoughts and feelings about substance abuse and the people who become addicts. Self-awareness about substance use and abuse is essential if the nurse is to establish a therapeutic relationship and provide treatment. The Seaman-Mannello Scale, a Likert-type scale that assesses nurses' attitudes toward al-

cohol and alcoholism, and the National Council on Alcoholism and Drug Dependence Scale can provide insight about personal values and beliefs regarding substance use.[29] Nurses can also examine their attitudes and their own use of drugs and alcohol by considering the questions of how, when, where, and under what conditions they use them.

Individual beliefs about drug and alcohol use come from the nurse's family background and previous knowledge about and experience with addicted people. This information allows nurses to anticipate their response patterns toward this group of clients. If nurses know their feelings and beliefs, they can recognize a judgmental attitude, rejecting behaviors, or enabling behaviors. This knowledge can prevent the nurse from being drawn into

TABLE 26-2 | *Characteristic Effects of Abuse of Major Substances*

Drug Classification and Street Names (Route of Administration)	Effects*	Drug Classification and Street Names (Route of Administration)	Effects*
Alcohol (Oral) "Booze" "Brew"	Relaxation and sedation Decreased inhibition Lack of coordination Unsteady gait Slurred speech Nausea and vomiting Transient visual, tactile, or auditory hallucinations Anxiety Psychomotor agitation High risk of permanent liver or brain damage	**Cocaine—cont'd**	Muscle twitching Respiratory depression Hallucinations, paranoid delusions, or paranoia Formication (sensation of insects crawling on the skin) Personality changes Antisocial behavior Euphoria followed by depression and feeling let down
Amphetamines (Oral, injected, smoked) Dexedrine Methamphetamine "Ice" "Uppers" "Crank" "Speed"	Grandiosity Hypervigilance Hypertension or hypotension Tachycardia or bradycardia Mydriasis (dilated pupils) Euphoria Appetite suppression Personality changes Antisocial behavior Psychosis similar to paranoid schizophrenia	**Hallucinogens** (Oral, inhaled) Lysergic acid diethylamide (LSD) "Acid" Peyote Psilocybin Mescaline	Intensified perceptions and feelings Synesthesia (seeing sounds or hearing colors) Visual, auditory, or tactile hallucinations Fear of losing one's mind Mydriasis Tachycardia Palpitations Blurred vision Dizziness, weakness, and tremors Altered perceptions (flashbacks) Impaired judgment and bizarre behavior Mood swings and psychosis-like symptoms
Caffeine (Oral)	Stimulation of senses Alertness and enhanced performance Anxiety and restlessness Flushed face Talkativeness Tremors or muscle twitching Tachycardia or cardiac dysrhythmias Insomnia Irritation of the stomach		
Cannabis (Smoked, oral) Marijuana "Grass" "Pot" "Hash" "Weed"	Mild intoxication Increased appetite Dry mouth Lack of coordination Impaired judgment and memory Sexual arousal Tachycardia Visual hallucinations	**Inhalants** (Inhaled) Spray can propellants Paint Paint thinner Glue Gasoline Cleaning fluid	Euphoria and giddiness Headache Dizziness, fatigue, or drowsiness Nystagmus (involuntary rapid eye movements) Unsteady gait or tremors Slurred speech Blurred vision or diplopia (double vision) Damage to major organs: lungs, liver, and kidneys Cardiac arrest
Cocaine (Oral, injected, inhaled) "Coke" "Crack" "Snow" "Blow" "Lady" "Powder"	Talkativeness Grandiosity Hypervigilance Anxiety Impaired judgment Tachycardia or bradycardia Hypertension or hypotension Mydriasis	**Nicotine** (Inhaled, oral)	Tachycardia Vasoconstriction Irritation of oral mucosa Persistent cough Damaged alveoli and bronchioli Emphysema High risk of oral, laryngeal, or lung cancer

From Copel, L.C. (2000). *Nurses' clinical guide to psychiatric and mental health care.* (2nd ed). Springhouse, PA: Springhouse.

*Drug effects are arranged in order of severity of effect, with prolonged use or a high dose of the drug associated with appearance of the later effects.

Continued

TABLE 26-2   *Characteristic Effects of Abuse of Major Substances—cont'd*

Drug Classification and Street Names (Route of Administration)	Effects*	Drug Classification and Street Names (Route of Administration)	Effects*
Opioids (Oral, injected, inhaled) Morphine Codeine Methadone Hydromorphone (Dilaudid) Heroin "Smack" "Horse" "Fine China"	Immediate euphoria followed by dysphoria Psychomotor retardation or agitation Slurred speech Impaired judgment and memory Sedation and respiratory depression Constricted pupils Decreased sexual and aggressive drives	**Phencyclidine—cont'd**	Decreased sensory awareness Hypertension and tachycardia Unsteady gait and lack of coordination Nystagmus Mood swings and paranoia
Phencyclidine (PCP) (Oral, injected, inhaled) "Angel dust" "Hog"	Grandiosity and illusions of strength Impulsiveness Psychomotor agitation Assaultive behavior	**Sedatives, Hypnotics, and Anxiolytics** (Oral, injected) Benzodiazepine (e.g., diazepam [Valium], alprazolam [Xanax], chlordiazepoxide [Librium]) Secobarbital (Seconal) Pentobarbital (Nembutal) Methaqualone (Quaalude)	Incoordination and unsteady gait Slurred speech Nystagmus Sedation Inappropriate sexual behavior and aggressive drives Impaired judgment Mood swings

From Copel, L.C. (2000). *Nurses' clinical guide to psychiatric and mental health care.* (2nd ed). Springhouse, PA: Springhouse.
*Drug effects are arranged in order of severity of effect, with prolonged use or a high dose of the drug associated with appearance of the later effects.

BOX 26-1   *Examples of Substance Use Screening Tools*

For Use with Adults
- Michigan Alcoholism Screening Test (MAST)[33]
- Short Michigan Alcoholism Screening Test (SMAST)[34]
- Addiction Severity Index[23]
- CAGE Questions[11]
- T-ACE (a modified version of the CAGE used with pregnant women)[36]
- Alcohol Use Disorders Identification Test (AUDIT)[28]
- Alcohol Dependence Scale[35]
- Self-Administered Alcoholism Screening Test (SAAST)[39]
- Alcohol Use Inventory[17]

For Use with Adolescents
- Guide's Rational Adolescent Substance Abuse Profile (GRASP)[1]
- Problem Severity Scales for Assessment of Alcohol and Drug Abuse[16]

power struggles regarding the client's manipulative behavior.

In addition to self-assessment measures for nurses, some instruments allow the nurse to gain information about the client's drug and alcohol use (Box 26-1). To use a tool as part of the assessment process, the nurse must know how to score the instrument and how to correctly interpret the findings.

Interviewing the substance abuse client presents a challenge because of the client's tendency to deny or minimize the problem. A comprehensive assessment includes the client's history and physical examination. The previously mentioned screening tools can be helpful. Laboratory studies address cardiac, liver, kidney, and respiratory functioning as well as urine toxicology. A thorough mental status assessment is a requisite part of the examination. The major components of this assessment are listed in Table 26-3.

Attention is paid to the psychosocial evaluation, especially the components that address difficulties in family, occupational, social, or leisure functioning. Some clinicians recommend that after the history and physical examination are completed, the health care provider should take a specific drug and alcohol history that asks about drug usage for the 11 major psychoactive substances in addition to other prescription and over-the-counter substances.[8] Components of a drug and alcohol history are listed in Box 26-2.

Although all clients need to be assessed for substance abuse, of special concern are those who by virtue of lifestyle or social conditions may be at increased risk. Adolescents, women (particularly pregnant women), racial and ethnic minorities, homosexual women and men, clients with HIV infection or acquired immunodeficiency syndrome (AIDS), homeless people, older adults, and health care professionals are identified as populations requiring special prevention, treatment, and education about substance abuse.[4,6] Extra attention

TABLE 26-3	*Components of the Mental Status Assessment*
General appearance	Appearance versus stated age
	Grooming and hygiene
	Posture, gait, and station
	Interaction during the interview
	Facial expressions
	Orientation or level of consciousness
Motor behavior	Restlessness
	Agitation
	Lethargy
	Tremors
Speech	Clarity and coherence of speech
	Rate of speech
	Volume and intonation
	Barriers to communication, such as confusion or delusions
	Vocabulary appropriate to socioeconomic background
Affect	Flat or labile
Mood	Euphoric, anxious, fearful
Thought processes	Thoughts presented as normal, concrete, scattered, or illogical
	Delusions—a false belief that is firmly maintained despite evidence to the contrary
Perception	Awareness of self and environment
	Illusions—misinterpretation of external stimuli
	Hallucinations—sensory experiences with no external stimuli present
Memory	Memory for remote, recent, and immediate past
	General knowledge level
	Ability to calculate
	Ability to think abstractly
	Insight
	Judgment or problem-solving ability

BOX 26-2   *Components of a Drug and Alcohol History*

- How often the drug was used (past and recent use)
- Age at first use
- Duration of use
- Age at last use
- Method of use
- Quantity used
- Initial and current reactions to the drug
- How the drug was obtained or how use of the drug was supported
- What has been done to reduce drug use
- Client's perception of use of the drug as a problem
- Use of drug related to any health problems

ASSESSMENT AND MANAGEMENT OF SUBSTANCE-ABUSING CLIENTS

The immediate result of overconsumption of any psychoactive substance is acute intoxication. Nurses in an emergency department or a medical-surgical setting may care for clients suffering from trauma as a direct result of acute intoxication. In addition to treating the client's injuries, the nursing care of intoxication consists of monitoring vital signs, especially respiratory status, because respiratory depression or arrest can occur. Be vigilant for manifestations of shock, cardiac dysrhythmias, electrolyte imbalances, or subdural hematomas. Typically, intravenous (IV) fluids are given to prevent dehydration. Some people become intoxicated but do not seek medical intervention because no injuries or emergencies bring them to health care facilities.

When a person sharply reduces or stops use of a psychoactive substance, the process of *withdrawal* occurs. Depending on the drug, withdrawal may begin within 8 to 12 hours or be delayed for 1 to 3 days. Prompt recognition of withdrawal symptoms can promote client safety and prevent complications. Factors that influence the withdrawal process include (1) the specific drug used, (2) the dose taken, (3) the method of intake, (4) the time of last use, and (5) the length of time during which the drug has been used. You must also consider the client's overall health, particularly the functioning of the kidneys, lungs, and liver—the principal organs that metabolize and excrete drugs. Table 26-4 lists an overview of common withdrawal symptoms for alcohol and other substances.

Alcohol

Ethyl alcohol (ethanol), a central nervous system (CNS) depressant, is found in alcoholic beverages. The ingested alcohol is absorbed directly into the bloodstream from the stomach and proximal part of the small intestine. Because alcohol is water-soluble, it circulates easily throughout the

must be given to clients with chronic physical or mental illnesses.

Self-medication can occur in vulnerable populations as a coping strategy to relieve physical and emotional pain associated with a chronic illness. After obtaining a comprehensive assessment, you may discover that a client struggles with polysubstance abuse. Examples of polysubstance abuse can include cocaine with alcohol, alcohol and sedatives, hypnotics, and anxiolytics, and nicotine and alcohol. Such clients require specialized care during the withdrawal process according to the combination of drugs used.

TABLE 26-4   *Common Withdrawal Symptoms Associated with Psychoactive Drugs*

Drug Classification	Major Withdrawal Symptoms	Drug Classification	Major Withdrawal Symptoms
Alcohol	Nausea and vomiting Tremors and weakness Sweating Tachycardia Hypertension Delusions Agitated behavior Hallucinations and nocturnal illusions	Inhalants	Symptoms appear over varying time periods following withdrawal Central nervous system damage (cerebral atrophy or peripheral neuropathies) Acute or chronic renal failure Bone marrow depression Cardiac dysrhythmias Respiratory damage (lung or sinus damage, pneumonitis, emphysema, respiratory depression) Liver disease (hepatitis, cirrhosis)
Amphetamines	Dysphoria Disorientation Fatigue and depression with suicidal potential Disturbed sleep and unpleasant dreams Hallucinations or delusions	Nicotine	Irritability and nervousness Headache Inability to concentrate Craving for cigarettes Fatigue and dizziness Tremors and palpitations
Caffeine	Irritability and nervousness Inability to concentrate Headache Tremors Lethargy	Opioids	Dysphoria Anxiety Insomnia Increased respirations and yawning Sweating Lacrimation and rhinorrhea (nasal discharge) Tremors and muscle twitching Mydriasis (dilated pupils) Piloerection (erection of the hair) Nausea, abdominal cramps, and vomiting
Cannabis	No acute withdrawal symptoms; other symptoms appear over varying time periods following withdrawal Amotivational syndrome (inability to concentrate or complete tasks) Chronic respiratory problems Memory and learning difficulty Suppressed prolactin and testosterone levels		
Cocaine	Severe craving for drug Severe depression ("postcoke blues") Fatigue Psychomotor agitation or retardation Anxiety Insomnia or hypersomnia Increased appetite	Phencyclidine (PCP)	Symptoms may appear over varying time periods following withdrawal Anxiety Withdrawn, catatonic state Hypertension Seizures Bizarre behavior and speech associated with temporary psychosis
Hallucinogens	Symptoms appear over varying time periods following withdrawal Apprehension, fear, or panic Hyperactivity Sweating Tachycardia Altered perceptions (flashbacks) Perceptual distortions, especially hallucinations	Sedatives, hypnotics, and anxiolytics	Anxiety Sweating Tachycardia Tremors Nausea and vomiting Insomnia and disturbing dreams Transient visual, auditory, or tactile hallucinations Seizures

From Copel, L.C. (2000). *Nurses' clinical guide to psychiatric and mental health care.* (2nd ed.). Springhouse, PA: Springhouse.
See WebLinks for links to resources.

body and readily passes through the blood-brain barrier. Approximately 95% of alcohol is metabolized in the liver, with the remaining 5% being excreted through the lungs, kidneys, and skin.[25] The body's mechanism for oxidizing alcohol is accomplished through the liver enzyme alcohol dehydrogenase. This process breaks down the alcohol to acetaldehyde, which is further broken down to acetic acid. Acetic acid then goes through the citric acid cycle to become carbon dioxide and water. From this chemical process, it is evident that alcohol can affect every aspect of the body. A growing number of young people may be using alcohol to enhance a drug's effect.

A blood alcohol level (BAL) test is used to measure the concentration of alcohol in the blood. The purpose of the test is to detect and estimate the level of alcohol in the brain. The legal intoxication level in most states is 100 mg/dl (0.10%); in a few states, it is 0.08%.

Although some studies suggest that small amounts of alcohol can be harmless or even healthful, large amounts produce a predictable series of deleterious effects. After drinking one or two alcoholic beverages, a person experiences a depression of the inhibitory regions of the brain that manage judgment, self-control, speech, and motor coordination. Alcohol is classified as a CNS depressant that affects all levels of the brain, starting with the reticular activating system and the cerebral cortex. Alcohol suppresses the inhibitory neurotransmitter gamma-aminobutyric acid (GABA). When the release of GABA is decreased, the initial results are an excitement or euphoric response.

With acute alcohol intoxication, alcohol continues to accumulate in the brain, resulting in depression of the cerebral cortex, cerebellum, and midbrain. In severe brain depression, disruption of the spinal reflexes, respiratory system, cardiac functioning, or temperature regulation occurs. At this point, the intoxicated person may become unconscious, and, without treatment, death may occur.

Early clinical manifestations of alcohol withdrawal (e.g., tremors, anorexia, anxiety, restlessness, insomnia) tend to occur within 6 to 8 hours after the last drink is ingested. During the next 2 to 3 days, the client may further experience disorientation, nightmares, abdominal pain, nausea, diaphoresis, and elevations in temperature, pulse, and blood pressure along with visual and auditory hallucinations. *Delirium tremens* (DTs) is a manifestation of severe alcohol withdrawal or its life-threatening complications. The client with DTs is at risk for cardiac dysrhythmias, hypertension, increased respirations, profuse sweating, delusions, and hallucinations.

Many clients are given medications to decrease the incidence of withdrawal manifestations and to prevent DTs. The benzodiazepines are commonly used because they cause less respiratory depression and hypertension compared with other drugs. Typically, the physician or-

ders either a long-acting benzodiazepine (diazepam [Valium] or chlordiazepoxide [Librium]) or a short-acting benzodiazepine (lorazepam [Ativan] or oxazepam [Serax]). The long-acting benzodiazepines are often used to facilitate the withdrawal process; the short-acting benzodiazepines are used for clients with severe liver dysfunction or a high degree of cognitive impairment.

Since 1995, the drug naltrexone hydrochloride (ReVia) has been approved for the treatment of alcoholism. It has been successful in decreasing the craving for alcohol and, together with the client's participation in a recovery program, facilitates client compliance with treatment. The drug was originally intended to treat clients undergoing opioid detoxification. According to the manufacturer, the mechanisms of action for naltrexone in alcoholism are not completely known. However, because the drug is an opioid receptor antagonist, it blocks the effects of opioid drugs by its competitive site binding. The relatively few side effects of the drug are nausea, fatigue, dizziness, headache, anxiety, and insomnia. Contraindications include hepatitis, liver disease, and liver failure.[12,13]

Treatment with naltrexone is controversial because taking the drug conflicts with the Alcoholics Anonymous (AA) model of total abstinence from alcohol and being "drug-free." The use of any drug is seen as a "crutch" or a substitution for the alcohol. For philosophical and political reasons, some clients taking naltrexone are excluded from receiving support and the other benefits of participating in AA.

There are also nonpharmacologic approaches to treating withdrawal. The *social model*, or the nonmedicinal treatment model, incorporates the use of an extensive physical examination, followed by close medical supervision during therapy. Several studies have shown that approximately 75% of the clients enrolled in these programs improve.[14,26,27]

The major nursing interventions for a client experiencing withdrawal focus on the continuous monitoring of manifestations and promoting a safe, calm, and comfortable environment. During the withdrawal period, clients need reassurance and support because they may feel that they will not survive the ordeal of detoxification. In the immediate period after the withdrawal syndrome has ceased, you can refer the client for further assessment and treatment of addiction or its complications. At this time, especially after what the client has been through, address with the client the relationship between drug use and the concomitant acute or chronic physical health problems. Common medical consequences of alcohol abuse are identified in Table 26-5.

Amphetamines

Amphetamines have been used to treat *narcolepsy* (sudden sleep) and *attention deficit hyperactivity disorder* (ADHD). People often use amphetamines illegally to

TABLE 26-5	*Medical Consequences of Alcohol Abuse*
Body System	**Consequences**
Cardiac	Dysrhythmias Hypertension Cardiomyopathy Heart failure Beriberi heart disease
Gastrointestinal	Gastritis Gastric or duodenal ulcers Perforated gastrointestinal ulcers Esophageal varices Pancreatitis Interference with absorption of vitamin B_{12}, thiamine, and folic acid Malabsorption syndrome Alteration in nutrition, with potential for malnutrition Wernicke-Korsakoff syndrome Enlarged or fatty liver Liver enzyme changes Cirrhosis Alcoholic hepatitis Portal hypertension Ascites Hepatic encephalopathy
Hematopoietic	Anemia Thrombocytopenia Leukopenia Capillary fragility Spider nevi Palmar erythema
Neurologic	Peripheral neuropathy Brain atrophy
Musculoskeletal	Myopathy Decreased bone density with risk of fracture Fractured bones related to trauma
Immune	Depressed immune system Increased susceptibility to infections
Respiratory	Altered respirations Chronic obstructive pulmonary disease Pneumonia Tuberculosis
Endocrine	Testicular atrophy Gynecomastia Irregular menses Decreased libido Hypoglycemia Alcoholic ketoacidosis

remain awake and alert, to increase their ability to perform physical tasks, or to produce a state of euphoria (a "high"). The abuse of amphetamines, according to the National Institute on Drug Abuse, is most common in the 18- to 34-year-old age group.[18] The pattern of abuse tends to be one of daily chronic use or periodic binges that end with the user being overwhelmed by exhaustion ("crashing").

Amphetamines stimulate the CNS and accelerate heart and brain activity. Amphetamines block the reuptake of dopamine and norepinephrine by interfering with the transport protein, ultimately causing accumulation of dopamine and norepinephrine at the synapses.[20] Amphetamines are metabolized by the liver enzymes and excreted in the urine. In some cases, after continual drug use, half of the drug may be excreted from the body unchanged.[6]

With amphetamine intoxication, the clinical findings may include cardiac dysrhythmias, hypertension, fever, labile emotions, paranoia, delusions, panic reactions, and psychosis. For client management, perform frequent assessment of vital signs and basic body functioning and provide safe, supportive care. Closely monitor the client for changes in cardiac or neurologic status, because myocardial infarction and cerebral hemorrhage have occurred after amphetamine use. Antipsychotic agents may be used to decrease CNS stimulation, or sedatives may be given. IV amino acids may be given to speed up the detoxification process of stimulant drugs.[3]

Amphetamines commonly cause psychological dependence, often with craving behavior. Abrupt cessation of the drug can precipitate anxiety, agitation, severe depression, hyperphagia, and hypersomnolence. An amphetamine psychosis may occur after continuous high doses. Nursing care focuses on (1) providing rest, (2) orienting the client as necessary, (3) monitoring for both physical and emotional changes, and (4) intervening to prevent complications of adverse effects or withdrawal symptoms.

Caffeine

In the United States, caffeine—a CNS stimulant—is the most commonly used psychoactive substance. Products containing caffeine include coffee, tea, chocolate, cola beverages, and prescription and nonprescription medications. People rely on caffeine to promote wakefulness, elevate their sense of well-being, decrease fatigue, and facilitate motor activity.

The mode of action within the body is stimulation of the CNS, thereby exciting the respiratory system and increasing body metabolism.[5] Caffeine is absorbed from the gastrointestinal tract, broken down in the liver, and excreted in the urine. The intake of a large quantity of caffeine can cause intoxication, manifested by cardiac dysrhythmias, sleep disturbances, mood changes, increased production of urine, gastrointestinal discomfort, and anxiety, especially panic attacks. Caffeinism and caffeine withdrawal syndrome are seen only with long-term use of caffeine, usually a documented intake of more than 500 mg/day.[18] Lack of caffeine can lead to severe headache. This problem can be seen in clients placed on NPO (nothing by mouth) status (e.g., before surgery).

Nursing care begins with recognition of the clinical manifestations of excessive caffeine use and withdrawal. Monitoring the manifestations and observing for additional problems (such as whether the caffeine is exacerbating known health problems) are appropriate.

Cannabis

Marijuana, a cannabis derivative, is the most widely used illegal drug in the United States, with more than 55% of young adults reporting personal use.[18] The mode of action of marijuana is not clearly understood, and researchers continue to try to identify the mechanism that accounts for its effects on the CNS and cardiovascular system.[6]

Tetrahydrocannabinol (THC) is the active ingredient in marijuana and the agent responsible for the psychological effects. The amount of marijuana that crosses the blood-brain barrier depends on the method of intake used. THC is absorbed in fatty tissues, primarily the brain and testes, and is slowly released back into the bloodstream, where it is eventually excreted in urine and feces.[18]

Clients who use marijuana experience manifestations of intoxication, such as euphoria, mood changes, memory impairment, tremors, decreased body temperature, dry mouth, lack of coordination, elevated blood pressure and heart rate, and injected conjunctivae (bloodshot eyes). The CNS and cardiac, immune, and reproductive systems are affected. Long-term use also influences respiratory functioning. Marijuana residues in the lungs are considered more carcinogenic than tobacco residues.

Withdrawal from marijuana is typically an uncomfortable but not a life-threatening process. Nursing care includes monitoring the client's physical and emotional responses to the drug. It is often helpful for a nurse, family member, or friend to stay with the client, provide reassurance, and talk the client through the anxiety. Usually the client is not hospitalized unless pre-existing medical conditions or the coexistence of another psychoactive substance complicates the withdrawal process. For most clients, the initial effects of the drug dissipate within 4 to 6 hours; however, the effects of drug intoxication may last as long as 5 days.[30]

Cocaine

Cocaine is an opioid obtained from the leaves of the coca plant; it was originally used by the Indians of the Andes to alleviate feelings of hunger and fatigue and to promote endurance. Today cocaine is readily available on the illicit market in the form of cocaine hydrochloride, which is soluble in water and used intravenously, inhaled (snorted), or smoked as "crack," a form of concentrated (freebase) cocaine.

Cocaine stimulates the CNS and blocks the conduction of peripheral nerve impulses. Continued use of cocaine increases the amount of dopamine in the synapses of nerve cells by preventing dopamine reuptake. Cocaine also decreases the breakdown of dopamine and other catecholamines, thereby increasing the level of catecholamine activity at the nerve cell synapses. Cocaine is metabolized in the liver and excreted in the urine. Evidence of cocaine use can be extracted from a urine sample for up to 72 hours after use.

In assessing for the effects of cocaine, remember that cocaine stimulates the CNS and the cardiovascular system. Cocaine abuse has led to myocardial infarctions in young, presumably healthy individuals. An overdose causes tremors, seizures, and delirium. Death can also result from cardiac or respiratory failure. Intervention is based on treating these identified problems and acting to prevent cardiac and respiratory complications. Cocaine intoxication may not be common in medical-surgical settings, because the half-life of cocaine is approximately 60 minutes.[3] Nursing management of a cocaine overdose focuses on preventing or handling cardiovascular collapse, respiratory distress, delirium, and hyperthermia.

Withdrawal from chronic use of cocaine ("binging") results in an exhausted state known as crashing. Clients experience a profound sense of depression, have memories of the cocaine-induced feelings of euphoria, and have cravings for the drug. Often, clients are hospitalized if there is severe depression with suicidal risk, if coexisting medical problems necessitate intense monitoring or treatment, or if there are medical problems directly related to complications of IV use. Besides providing the physical care required for the cocaine-dependent client, the nurse helps the client become aware of the need to develop effective coping skills.

Hallucinogens

Hallucinogens, also known as *psychedelic drugs,* are both natural and synthetic substances that produce illusions, delusions, hallucinations, and alterations in thoughts, perceptions, and feelings. The effects of hallucinogens differ among individuals and are therefore unpredictable. An individual's personality may influence the reaction that occurs after hallucinogen use. Characteristic of lysergic acid diethylamide (also called LSD) and other psychedelic drugs are a subjective sensation of heightened awareness, an ability to look inward, and a feeling of oneness with the universe.

The mechanism of action is unknown. Hallucinogens are usually ingested and then absorbed from the gastrointestinal tract, metabolized in the liver, and excreted in the bile and feces.[6] The length of action is usually between 6 and 12 hours.[9]

The effects of hallucinogens are similar to those of other stimulants. The user experiences euphoria, dilated pupils, anxiety, and increased respirations, blood pressure, and heart rate. Panic attacks occur while the user is in a state of intoxication, accompanied by feelings of paranoia, confusion, hallucinations, possible dissociation, and loss of contact with reality. The resulting inability to perceive the environment accurately, impaired judgment, and feeling of having special powers make the person susceptible to dangerous activities. Suicide, homicide, and other acts of violence have been reported in people under the influence of hallucinogenic drugs. Some users also experience flashbacks. During a period of intoxication, or because of a flashback experience or the reliving of a "bad trip," a person may be brought to a health care setting.

Carefully assess the client for both physiologic and psychological problems. Nursing care focuses on attending to the panic that the client is experiencing as well as providing for client safety and creating a nonstimulating environment. Someone should stay with the client until the side effects have worn off. In the case of a severe overdose, be prepared to intervene for possible seizures, extremely high temperatures, and cardiac distress.[35] Because withdrawal symptoms may occur over a period of time, be vigilant for possible neurologic abnormalities and psychiatric manifestations.

Inhalants

Inhalants are chemicals that give off fumes or vapors that readily pass through the blood-brain barrier to produce an alteration in consciousness. Commonly used inhalants are (1) solvents (glue, gasoline, nail polish remover, lighter fluid, paint thinner), (2) aerosols (hair spray, insecticides), and (3) anesthetic agents used for recreational purposes (nitrous oxide, chloroform, ether).

The probable mechanism of action is that these volatile substances alter the biologic membranes of the cells of the CNS and affect the metabolism of neurotransmitters in the brain.[18] Inhalants are metabolized in the liver and kidneys. Low doses of inhalants cause initial CNS excitement within minutes of use. Immediately after inhaling a volatile substance through the nose or mouth ("huffing"), the user experiences a "high," accompanied by feelings of giddiness and euphoria. There is a decrease in inhibitions and a slowing of the heart rate, respiratory rate, and overall mental activity. With inhalant intoxication, physical manifestations include delirium, cardiac dysrhythmias, irritation of the mucous membranes of the nose and mouth, cough, and depression of brain waves. Depending on the substance inhaled, the effects may last from a few minutes to several hours.[20]

Continuous use of volatile substances results in brain, lung, liver, kidney, and bone marrow damage. Withdrawal symptoms associated with inhalants vary with the specific substance used. Sudden death related to the use of inhalants can occur from life-threatening dysrhythmias and hypoxia.

Nursing care concentrates on prompt intervention in emergency situations (seizures, loss of consciousness, respiratory arrest). Effective management of the client's acute and chronic physiologic problems remains your primary goal.

Nicotine

Nicotine is an alkaloid substance present in tobacco leaves. Using nicotine in the form of cigarettes, cigars, or chewing or pipe tobacco is an addictive habit practiced throughout the world. It is the leading cause of preventable death in the United States. Nicotine is absorbed through the lungs and within seconds crosses the blood-brain barrier and acts to stimulate the CNS. It is metabolized in the liver and excreted in the urine. Nicotine adversely affects the cardiovascular, respiratory, and gastrointestinal systems.

An overdose of nicotine is not a common occurrence. If intoxication develops, administration of oxygen and the treatment of symptoms are the nurse's priorities. Nicotine withdrawal occurs within 24 hours of smoking cessation. The withdrawal symptoms are uncomfortable, and the nurse can support the client through this process and assist with developing effective strategies for dealing with the manifestations.

Opioids

Opioids comprise drugs produced from opium along with manufactured or semisynthetic narcotics. The human body also produces natural opiates, which facilitate feelings of well-being. Chemicals known as *endorphins* are neurotransmitters that connect with opiate receptors in the brain. When a person uses opiates or other narcotics, an interference is created in the natural opioid system and the functions of the neurotransmitters in the brain are disrupted.[15] Opioids are metabolized in the liver and excreted in the bile and urine.

An opioid overdose constitutes a life-threatening situation as a result of seizures, shock, respiratory depression, or cardiac dysrhythmias. The client is usually in an unconscious or lethargic state and may die without appropriate medical treatment. The nurse assesses and intervenes with the health care team to provide the required emergency care. Establishing an airway, monitoring cardiac functioning and treating dysrhythmias, maintaining hydration, and administering an opioid antagonist such as naloxone (Narcan) are the nursing care priorities. The client should be hospitalized, with close monitoring of all body systems, for at least 24 hours.

For the client experiencing opioid withdrawal, focus on assessing and intervening for a variety of physiologic, psychological, and behavioral symptoms; these tend to occur within 72 hours of last drug use. Nursing care consists of constantly monitoring withdrawal symptoms along with providing rest, nutrition, and a comfortable environment. The initiation of a methadone program as a useful approach for treating opioid addiction is now recommended by the National Institutes of Health. Methadone therapy is useful for both detoxification and maintenance therapy. Clients often are referred to residential treatment programs to learn how to develop new, drug-free lifestyles.

Phencyclidine

PCP is a synthetic drug with stimulant, depressant, and hallucinogenic properties.[6,9] PCP not only increases the production of dopamine but also blocks its reuptake, thus causing increased blood pressure, heartbeat, and respiratory rates. PCP also increases acetylcholine in the CNS, thereby generating cholinergic effects manifested as diaphoresis, drooling, and pupillary constriction. Serotonin is also believed to be altered by the presence of PCP, resulting in a lack of coordination, slurred speech, and nystagmus.[19] PCP is metabolized in the liver and excreted in the urine.

Intoxication from PCP lasts up to 6 hours, and the effects of the drug are unpredictable. A person may experience euphoria, disorientation, or the racing or slowing of thoughts. In emergency departments, the client may be confused, hostile, violent, paranoid, or panicked. Nursing assessment of PCP intoxication often reveals severe cardiac or respiratory distress, which can lead to cardiac arrest. Clients under the influence of PCP can be in a psychosis-like state and can have nystagmus, abnormal muscle movements, and severe hypertension.

Nursing care concentrates on the assessment of subtle changes in vital signs and level of consciousness, gastric lavage if PCP has been ingested, and acidification of the urine.[18] In PCP withdrawal, you may see variable presentations of manifestations, particularly abnormal muscle movements. Carefully monitor the client's physical and mental condition to minimize health problems.

Sedatives, Hypnotics, and Anxiolytics

Sedative, hypnotic, and anxiolytic agents are considered to be CNS depressants. These medications are directly absorbed from the gastrointestinal tract into the bloodstream, where they enter the brain, are metabolized in the liver, and are eliminated via the kidneys. In cases of overdose, clients experience decreased CNS

functioning along with the slowing of the cardiac and respiratory systems. Monitor vital signs and initiate emergency procedures based on the clinical manifestations presented. An overdose of any of these depressant drugs constitutes a medical emergency, with some clients requiring hospitalization in an intensive care unit (ICU).

Nursing care focuses on maintenance of adequate respiratory and cardiovascular status, hydration, and possible gastric lavage if the drugs were taken within the previous 4 to 6 hours.[33] For clients undergoing withdrawal, promote safety and rest while treating both physical and emotional manifestations. Nursing care priorities are awareness of the possibility of delirium, seizures, fever, and changes in cardiac and respiratory status as well as the interaction between adverse effects of the drug and pre-existing medical problems. Table 26-6 summarizes common health problems observed in clients who abuse drugs other than alcohol.

■ Nursing Management of Substance-Abusing Clients

The nurse plays a vital role in the care of clients experiencing intoxication and withdrawal. Nurses also meet basic needs, develop a therapeutic relationship, and teach both the client and family about addiction and its effect on the entire family. Nursing strategies for meeting actual or potential health problems are implemented for nursing diagnoses generated from assessment data. Nursing diagnoses commonly applied to the substance abuse population are listed in Box 26-3.

Education is an essential component of care to help the client understand the need for lifestyle changes. The main components of a drug education plan for clients and families are outlined in Box 26-4. Sometimes clients who abuse alcohol are referred for various treatment options and given disulfiram (Antabuse) to deter drinking. Clients receiving disulfiram must be carefully instructed about the drug. Information to include in a teaching plan is provided in Box 26-5.

Substance abuse has a major impact on family members. The family often tries to deal with a substance-abusing member by altering his or her behavior and compensating for the addict's unfilled responsibilities. Often the family inadvertently isolates itself from others as it focuses most of its energy on the addict. Personal needs of the caregiver, other adults, and children go unmet. Family members are strongly affected by the addiction and must be involved in the recovery process. A caring, supportive, and educative response from the nurse conveys that the family's concerns are understood and will be included in the treatment program. A major role of the nurse is education of client and family. The educative responsive is detailed in Box 26-4.

TABLE 26-6 *Health Consequences of Commonly Abused Drugs*

	Amphetamines	Caffeine	Cannabis	Cocaine	Hallucinogens	Inhalants	Nicotine	Opioids	Phencyclidine (PCP)	Sedatives, hypnotics, and anxiolytics
Abrupt withdrawal symptoms (similar to alcohol withdrawal)										X
Agitation										
Angina		X					X			
Acquired immunodeficiency syndrome (AIDS)				X				X		
Anemia								X		
Atelectasis								X		
Arthritis								X		
Aspiration				X						
Bone marrow depression						X				
Brain damage						X				
Bronchitis				X			X			
Cancer (laryngeal)							X			
Cancer (lung)							X			
Cancer (oral cavity)							X			
Cerebrovascular accident (stroke)				X			X			
Confusion									X	
Dysrhythmias	X	X			X	X		X		
Emphysema							X			
Endocarditis (bacterial)				X				X		
Excoriations (from scratching nonexistent bugs)	X									
Flashbacks					X					
Gastrointestinal distress/ulcers						X	X			
Hallucinations									X	
Hepatitis (bacterial, viral)				X		X		X		
Hypergammaglobulinemia								X		
Hypertension	X	X		X	X				X	
Immune dysfunctions								X		
Insomnia		X								
Judgment, impaired									X	
Lung abscess								X		
Lung irritation			X			X				
Lymphadenopathy								X		
Mental slowness										X
Motor function, impaired										X
Muscle weakness						X				
Myocardial infarction				X			X			
Myositis ossificans (drug user's elbow)								X		
Nasal septal damage				X						

TABLE 26-6   Health Consequences of Commonly Abused Drugs—cont'd

	Amphetamines	Caffeine	Cannabis	Cocaine	Hallucinogens	Inhalants	Nicotine	Opioids	Phencyclidine (PCP)	Sedatives, hypnotics, and anxiolytics
Nephritis								X		
Neuropathy (peripheral)						X				
Osteomyelitis								X		
Paranoid psychosis	X									
Peptic ulcers		X								
Pharyngitis (chronic)			X							
Phlebitis								X		
Pneumonia								X		
Pulmonary emboli				X						
Pulmonary fibrosis								X		
Renal failure				X		X		X		
Respiratory arrest/failure						X				
Seizures	X			X					X	X
Skin ulcers or abscesses				X						
Sinusitis (chronic)			X							
Splenomegaly								X		
Testosterone (lowered levels)			X							
Tremors		X								
Tuberculosis								X		
Visual loss (from adulterants in street drugs)								X		

BOX 26-3   Common Nursing Diagnoses for Clients Who Abuse Substances

- Acute Confusion
- Anxiety
- Impaired Verbal Communication
- Ineffective Denial
- Dysfunctional Family Processes
- Fatigue
- Fear
- Dysfunctional Grieving
- Hopelessness
- Ineffective Coping
- Risk for Infection
- Risk for Injury
- Deficient Knowledge (specify)
- Noncompliance (specify)
- Imbalanced Nutrition: Less than Body Requirements
- Pain
- Impaired Parenting

- Disturbed Personal Identity
- Risk for Poisoning
- Powerlessness
- Ineffective Role Performance
- Chronic Low Self-Esteem
- Disturbed Sensory Perception (Specify: visual, auditory kinesthetic, gustatory, tactile, olfactory)
- Ineffective Sexuality Patterns
- Risk for Impaired Skin Integrity
- Disturbed Sleep Pattern
- Impaired Social Interaction
- Social Isolation
- Spiritual Distress
- Disturbed Thought Processes
- Risk for Trauma
- Risk for Self-Directed Violence, Risk for Other-Directed Violence

BOX 26-4	*Components of a Client and Family Education Plan*

- Concept of addiction
- Physical health problems associated with addiction
- Nutritional status
- Feelings and behaviors of all family members associated with addiction
- Areas of life affected by substance use: family, social, spiritual, sexual, occupational, financial, legal, and leisure
- Roles family members play in addiction
- Treatment options and treatment process
- Aftercare and self-help support groups or 12-Step programs
- Community resources
- Skill building in the areas of communication, expression of feelings, socialization, and coping strategies
- Impact of both addiction and the recovery process on the roles and responsibilities of all family members
- Client confidentiality and right to privacy protected under the 1975 Federal Drug and Alcohol Abuse Act and the Health Insurance Portability and Privacy Act (HIPPA)

DRUG AND ALCOHOL INTERVENTION

Confrontation About Drug Abuse

In medical-surgical settings, nurses and other members of the health care team may receive a request for assistance from family members who believe that the client needs to obtain drug and alcohol treatment. To confront the client about drug abuse, a carefully orchestrated format (a *therapeutic intervention*) can be implemented to force the client to participate in treatment.[8] The intervention must be planned in advance and executed under the guidance of a health care provider with a drug and alcohol counseling background. To prepare for the intervention, all participants compose a list of situations in which they have personal knowledge about the client's drug and alcohol behaviors.

During the therapeutic intervention, a group of family and friends gather together and bring the client face to face with the addiction problem. In an objective and nonjudgmental manner, the group states its concerns about the client, its observations about the client's substance abuse behavior, and its overall caring about the client's well-being. A plan for obtaining help from these significant people is presented to the client. This plan includes treatment recommendations and may contain a reservation for a particular treatment facility. It is believed that this loving and open confrontation can break through the abuser's denial and defensiveness. The client's family and friends must also state the consequences that will immediately ensue if help is refused.

BOX 26-5	*Information to Include in a Teaching Plan About Disulfiram (Antabuse)*

- Inform the client that disulfiram is not a cure for alcoholism; it only discourages drinking.
- Before initiating disulfiram therapy, ask whether the client has had any allergic reactions to substances such as sulfites, preservatives, or dyes.
- Ask whether the client has a history of seizures; severe mental illness, particularly psychosis; serious cardiac disease; kidney disease; diabetes mellitus; hypothyroidism; or skin allergies.
- Ask whether the client is taking anticoagulants (↑ effects), isoniazid (INH) (↑ CNS effects), metronidazole (Flagyl) (↑ toxicity), or phenytoin (Dilantin) (↑ toxicity).
- Instruct the client not to ingest any alcohol or use any products containing alcohol within 12 hours before taking disulfiram, while taking disulfiram, and for at least 14 days after discontinuing disulfiram.
- Explain to the client that it is necessary to read the labels on all products because alcohol is found in many foods, medicines, and personal hygiene products (e.g., sauces, vinegars, cough syrups, tonics, elixirs, mouthwash, colognes, after-shave lotions).
- Tell the client not to inhale chemicals that may contain alcohol (e.g., paints, varnish, shellac).
- Encourage the client not to use alcohol-containing products that are applied topically. Alcohol absorbed through the skin can cause redness, itching, headache, and nausea.
- Identify common side effects (e.g., headache, fatigue, a metallic or garlic-like aftertaste, skin rash) that may be experienced during the first 2 weeks of taking disulfiram. Inform the client that these manifestations resolve as the body adjusts to the medication.
- If the client ingests alcohol while taking disulfiram, blurred vision, chest pain, confusion, dizziness or fainting, palpitations, flushing, diaphoresis, nauseas, vomiting, headache, and dyspnea may occur. These symptoms last as long as alcohol is in the body. If the client drinks a large amount of alcohol, seizures, myocardial infarction, unconsciousness, or death may result.
- Instruct the client to carry a card that specifies that he or she is taking disulfiram, lists the side effects of alcohol use and states whom to contact in an emergency.

Treatment Options

After completing a comprehensive health history and providing care for the client, you are in an optimal position to recommend a treatment modality that corresponds to the needs of the client and family members. Activities that you are involved in range from primary prevention (education), to secondary prevention (outpatient services), to tertiary prevention (inpatient or outpa-

TABLE 26-7	*Levels of Treatment Strategies*	
Level of Prevention	**Activities**	**Resources**
Primary prevention	Education to prevent substance abuse Risk factor identification Lifestyle guidance	School programs Community programs Health promotion activities
Secondary prevention (outpatient)	Assessment and intervention of early physical and emotional issues and problems Educational interventions Pharmacologic interventions Self-management strategies Support and self-help groups Psychotherapy	Medical facilities as appropriate Individual, family, or group therapy Psychoeducational groups Self-help groups (e.g., AA, NA, CA, Al-Anon, Ala-teen, Naranon, ACOA)*
Tertiary prevention (inpatient or outpatient)	Interventions to monitor withdrawal and prevent or treat complications Focusing on relapse prevention Determining plan for aftercare and methods of obtaining support Individual, family, or group therapy	Medical services, such as detoxification Aftercare, such as partial programs, supervised living, or halfway house Individual, family, or group therapy Psychoeducational groups Self-help groups (e.g., AA, NA, CA, Al-Anon, Ala-teen, Naranon, ACOA)*

AA, Alcoholics Anonymous; *ACOA*, Adult Children of Alcoholics; *CA*, Cocaine Anonymous; *NA*, Narcotics Anonymous.
*See WebLinks for links to resources.

tient detoxification and rehabilitation). The common interventions for all three levels of care are listed in Table 26-7. A list of community resources that can provide education and support to substance-abusing clients and their families appears on the website.

Prevention of Relapse

Clients in the recovery process may be at risk for relapse or a return to substance abuse. Anticipate the possibility of *relapse* (slipping back into substance use after a period of abstinence) and prepare clients with strategies to prevent it. This regression can occur any time and may be defined as one-time use, brief intermittent use, or daily long-term use. Relapse should be viewed as a potential part of the illness process, much like the potential course of any other chronic illness. Seeing relapse as client failure sets the client up for defeat instead of recovery.

Physiologic, emotional, and social variables all contribute to relapse. Clients must be taught ways to assess their strengths and to identify situations that can distract them from their recovery. Peer pressure, stress, and negative feelings may trigger a relapse. Some relapse prevention strategies to include in educational programs are listed in Box 26-6.

Surgery and Substance Abuse

Clients who abuse substances often experience accidents, injuries, or illnesses that require surgical intervention. In fact, many injuries seen by nurses in emer-

---

BOX 26-6   *Strategies to Prevent Relapse*

- Assess and build on the client's coping skills.
- Take opportunities, such as role-playing, that help the client practice coping methods.
- Assist the client in identifying personal risks of relapse.
- Identify people, places, and things that can interfere with maintaining sobriety, and encourage the client to minimize contact with these obstacles and develop ways to handle them.
- Change environmental variables when possible.
- Discuss the concept of craving, how to identify it, what may trigger it, and how to handle it.
- Focus on the client's physiologic feelings and sensations, and develop methods to handle them.
- Teach strategies that promote a healthy lifestyle, such as exercise, nutrition, stress management, and relaxation techniques.
- Encourage participation in support groups or self-help groups.
- Recommend group or individual therapy if the client has problems with the family of origin, struggles with daily functioning, or mental illness.

---

gency departments are directly related to drug and alcohol use. Become skillful in observing for subtle changes, and perform frequent assessments to intervene immediately and prevent the escalation of manifestations. Traumatized clients usually require immediate surgery; hence, a thorough drug and alcohol assessment may not be done. It is a challenge for the nurse to distinguish medical problems, psychiatric disorders, and substance abuse disorders in a timely manner.

Alcoholic clients who are admitted for a surgical procedure require special attention. They are told not to drink for several days before surgery, but in reality they may have been drinking up to the night before. Postoperatively, the client begins to develop withdrawal and must be actively restrained. The challenges facing the nursing staff caring for a postoperative client with DTs are great. Client safety is a serious matter, as are wound healing and adequate nutrition. The client may be treated to reduce symptoms. In other cases, the client may be simply left to detoxify "cold turkey," a method that stops the substance abruptly. Your role as a client advocate is imperative for these clients.

If a client is addicted to CNS depressant drugs, a larger amount of an anesthetic may be needed to produce the desired effects. This situation occurs because the client has a higher tolerance to the anesthetic drug. For clients with liver impairment and overall poor health, anesthetics cannot be properly metabolized and the effect of sedation is prolonged. While undergoing surgery, the addicted client is at risk for cardiac dysrhythmias, respiratory depression, hemorrhage, and depletion of catecholamines.

In the postoperative period, these clients are susceptible to cardiac, respiratory, urinary, hemorrhagic, and wound complications. The experience of pain may be intensified because the clients often have tolerance to the pain medication. Carefully assess whether the client requires increased doses of medication for pain reduction and needs to be slowly weaned from the medication during recovery. Some addicted clients may experience drug withdrawal postoperatively because withdrawal has been delayed by the use of anesthetics.

THE IMPAIRED HEALTH CARE PROFESSIONAL

Just like other people, health care professionals can become addicted to drugs and alcohol. Research on the prevalence of substance abuse among nurses has revealed no difference between nurses and other health professionals. Furthermore, the prevalence of substance abuse among health professionals overall does not differ from that in the general population.[40] Many addicted health care professionals first start using drugs and alcohol in response to physical illness and pain, emotional difficulties, or work pressures.

The requirements of the professional nurse's role make nursing a stressful occupation. On a daily basis, the nurse is responsible for coordinating and directly providing care for clients who are in pain and crisis. The pressure of handling resources, making decisions, interfacing with med-

---

BOX 26-7 *Signs of a Chemically Impaired Colleague*

- Alcohol on breath
- Mood changes or confusion
- Difficulty making judgments and impaired memory
- Red eyes with flushed face
- Unsteady gait
- Tremors or impaired eye-hand coordination
- Irritability or hyperactivity
- Lethargy or dozing on breaks
- Disheveled appearance
- Wearing long sleeves or a sweater constantly, even in hot weather
- Incorrect drug counts
- Accidents, spillages, or drugs frequently being wasted
- Frequently found in the bathroom, nurses' lounge, or off the unit
- Recurrent unfinished assignments or client care mistakes

---

ical and other personnel, working long hours, often with inadequate staff, and being responsible for the daily operation of the medical-surgical unit can be overwhelming. In addition, nurses have access to opioids and operate on the premise that medications are a useful vehicle for relieving or reducing pain and altering states of feelings. Specialized knowledge about drugs and experience with administering them and watching their efficacy may lead health care providers to view drugs as a "pharmacologic coping method."[7,24] It is a method that can ultimately backfire.

The signs of a chemically impaired colleague are subtle and easily overlooked by peers and supervisors. Even other health care professionals may deny and avoid the problem rather than confront the person suspected of being chemically dependent. It is essential that nurses be aware of the manifestations of chemical dependence in peers (Box 26-7). Document questionable or problematic incidents, and be willing to participate in an intervention if deemed appropriate. Remember, a peer who suffers from addiction cannot meet the requirements of your state nurse practice act. Some states have a law that mandates reporting of an impaired colleague.

As with clients, steps must be taken to assist an impaired nurse to obtain treatment. The use of an employee assistance program (EAP) and peer support or assistance groups from the state nurses' association can facilitate referrals to treatment and can assist with recovery. Although peer assistance programs vary from state to state, most programs offer support, referral services, monitoring during recovery, and educational programs targeted to the health care professional.

CONCLUSIONS

Substance abuse remains a major health issue, affecting clients, families, and communities. Even so, many clients with substance abuse disorders are not identified and, therefore, do not obtain treatment. A lack of knowledge about addiction can perpetuate stigmatization of the client. Your challenge is to become informed about both the effects of drugs and appropriate strategies for treatment. Keen assessment skills, decision-making skills, and compassion are the prerequisites for comprehensive nursing care of the myriad physiologic and psychological needs presented by these clients.

Nurses play a vital role in developing and implementing drug and alcohol prevention strategies. Teaching how to use effective coping strategies, how to handle crises, and how to develop support systems are the primary steps that must be incorporated into the care. For you, as a nurse, it is important to spend time cultivating relationships and to allow yourself to engage in leisure activities that decrease feelings of frustration, hopelessness, and burnout.

THINKING CRITICALLY *evolve*

1. A group of young college students celebrated the end of the semester with a week-long party. Alcoholic beverages were plentiful; food was not a priority. A young couple brought their friend to the emergency department. They report their suspicions that she might have a drinking problem (e.g., erratic behavior, presence of alcoholic beverages in the dormitory room, smell of alcohol on her breath). They were unable to awaken her for any length of time and are worried that she drank too much. She has not had a drink for about 6 hours. What assessment is required? What nursing actions are appropriate?

Factors to Consider. How likely is it for the client to experience DTs? How will the client be treated?

2. You are a registered nurse in the local "Driving Under the Influence of Alcohol" teaching program. Your topic is "Alcohol and the Human Body." The audience is made up of clients mandated by the court to attend. After the presentation, which focuses on the complications associated with long-term drinking, the clients ask, "If alcoholism is a disease, why are we treated as criminals?" "I didn't drink so much, why did they pull me over?" What might these questions indicate?

Factors to Consider. Is alcoholism a disease of addiction? What psychological factor is evident in such questions?

Discussions for these questions can be found on the website and the CD-ROM.

BIBLIOGRAPHY

1. Addiction Research Corporation. (1986). *GRASP: Guide's rational adolescent substance abuse profile.* Piscataway, NJ: Rutgers University Center of Alcohol Studies.
2. American Psychiatric Association. (2000). *Diagnostic and statistical manual of mental disorders* (4th ed., text revision). Washington, DC: Author.
3. American Psychiatric Association. (1995). Practice guidelines for the treatment of patients with substance use disorders: Alcohol, cocaine, opioids. *American Journal of Psychiatry, 152*(11), Supplement 4-19.
4. Bellenir, K. (Ed). (1996). *Substance abuse sourcebook.* Detroit, MI: Omnigraphics.
5. Blum, K., et al. (1990). Allelic association of human dopamine D2 [EB] receptor gene in alcoholism. *Journal of the American Medical Association, 15*(263), 2055-2060.
6. Burns, E.M., Thompson, A., & Ciccone, J.K. (1993). *An addictions curriculum for nurses and other helping professionals* (Vol. 2). New York: Springer-Verlag.
7. Coombs, R.H. (1997). *Drug impaired professionals.* Cambridge, MA: Harvard University Press.
8. Copel, L.C. (2000). *Nurses' clinical guide to psychiatric and mental health nursing* (2nd ed.). Springhouse, PA: Springhouse.
9. Dodgen, C.E., & Shea, W.M. (2000). *Substance use disorders.* San Diego, CA: Academic Press.
10. Doweiko, H. (2002). *Concepts of chemical dependency.* Pacific Grove, CA: Brooks/Cole Publishing.
11. Ewing, J.A. (1984). CAGE. *Journal of the American Medical Association 252*(14):1906.
12. Freed, P.E., & York, L.N. (1997). Naltrexone: A controversial therapy for alcohol dependence. *Journal of Psychosocial Nursing and Mental Health Services, 35*(7), 24-28.
13. Freeman, E.M. (Ed.). (1993). *Substance abuse treatment: A family systems perspective.* Newbury, CA: Sage.
14. Galanter, M., & Kleber, H.D. (1999). *Textbook of substance abuse treatment* (2nd ed.). Washington, DC: American Psychiatric Press.
15. Goldstein, A. (2001). *Addiction: From biology to drug policy* (2nd ed.). New York: W. H. Freeman.
16. Henly, G.A., & Winters, K.C. (1988). Development of problem severity scales for the assessment of adolescent alcohol and drug abuse. *International Journal of the Addictions, 23*, 65-85.
17. Horn, J.L., et al. (1984). *Alcohol use questionnaire (AUQ).* [EB] Toronto, Canada: Addiction Research Foundation.
18. Jaffe, J. (Ed.). (1995). *Encyclopedia of drugs and alcohol.* New York, Macmillan.
19. Jefferson, L.V. (2001). Chemically mediated responses and substance-related disorders. In G.W. Stuart & M. Laraia (Eds.), *Principles and practices of psychiatric nursing* (pp. 485-625). St. Louis: Mosby.
20. Karch, S.B. (2002). *Karch's pathology of drug abuse.* Boca Raton, FL: CRC Press.
21. Lewis, J.A., Dana, R.Q., & Blevins, G.A. (2002). *Substance abuse counseling* (3rd ed.). Pacific Grove, CA: Brooks/Cole Publishing.

22. Lowinson, J., et al. (Eds.). (1997). *Substance abuse: A comprehensive textbook* (3rd ed.). Baltimore, MD: Williams & Wilkins.

23. McLellan, A.T., et al. (1992). The fifth edition of the addiction severity index. *Journal of Substance Abuse Treatment, 9*(3), 199-213.

 24. Mynatt, S. (1996). A model of contributing risk factors to chemical dependency in nurses. *Journal of Psychosocial Nursing and Mental Health Services, 34*(7), 13-22.

25. Nace, E.P., & Isbell, P.I. (1991). Alcohol. In R.J. Frances & S.I. Miller (Eds.), *Clinical textbook of addictive disorders* (pp. 43-68). New York: Guilford Press.

26. Naegle, M.A., & D'Avanzo, C.E. (2000). *Addictions and substance abuse: Strategies for advanced practice nursing*. Upper Saddle River, NJ: Prentice Hall.

27. Naranjo, C.A., Sellers, E.M., & Chater, M. (1983). Nonpharmacologic intervention in acute alcohol withdrawal. *Clinical Pharmacology and Therapeutics 34*, 814-819.

28. National Institute on Alcohol Abuse and Alcoholism. (1984). *Alcohol abuse curriculum guide for nurse practitioner faculty* (DHHS Pub. No. ADM 84-1313, Vol. 3). Rockville, MD: Health Professions Education Curriculum Resources Series.

29. National Institute on Alcohol Abuse and Alcoholism. (1990). *Seventh special report to the U.S. Congress on alcohol and health: From the secretary of health and human services* (DHHS Pub. No. ADM 90-1656). Rockville, MD: Author.

30. Ott, P.J., Tarter, R.E., & Ammerman, R.T. (1999). *Sourcebook on substance abuse: Etiology, epidemiology, assessment, and treatment*. Boston, MA: Allyn & Bacon.

31. Peele, S. (1986). The implications and limitations of genetic models of alcoholism and other addictions. *Journal of Studies on Alcohol, 47*, 63-73.

32. Pokorney, A.D., Miller, B.A., & Kaplan, H.B. (1992). The brief MAST: A shortened version of the Michigan Alcoholism Screening Test. *American Journal of Psychiatry, 129*, 342-348.

33. Selzer, M.L. (1971). The Michigan Alcoholism Screening test: The quest for a new diagnostic instrument. *American Journal of Psychiatry, 127*, 1653-1658.

34. Selzer, M., Vinokur, A., & van Roojan, L. (1975). A self-administered short alcohol screening test (SMAST). *Journal of Studies on Alcoholism, 36*(1), 86.

35. Skinner, H.A., & Horn, J.L. (1984). *Alcohol Dependence Scale (ADS): User's guide.* Toronto, Canada: Addiction Research Foundation.

36. Sokol, R.J., Martier, S.S., & Ager, J.W. (1989). The T-ACE questions: Practical prenatal detection of risk-drinking. *American Journal of Obstetrics and Gynecology, 160*, 863-870.

37. Sue, D. (1987). Use and abuse of alcohol by Asian Americans. *Journal of Psychoactive Drugs, 19*, 57.

38. Sullivan, E. (1995). Nursing care of clients with substance abuse. St. Louis: Mosby.

39. Swenson, W., & Morse, R. (1973). The use of self-administered alcoholism screening test (SAAST) in a medical center. *Mayo Clinic Proceedings, 50*, 204-208.

40. Trinkoff, A.M., Eaton, W.W., & Anthony, J.C. (1991). The prevalence of substance abuse among registered nurses. *Nursing Research, 40*(3), 172-175.

Mobility Disorders

Anatomy and Physiology Review

The Musculoskeletal System

Robert G. Carroll

The musculoskeletal system consists of the bony skeleton and three types of muscles: (1) skeletal, (2) cardiac, and (3) smooth. The muscle types are distinguished based on the presence of striations, the source of innervation, and the mechanism of contraction.

Physiologically, the musculoskeletal system enables changes in movement and position. The bony skeleton provides support, protection, and a movable frame. Skeletal-muscle contraction generates movement of this frame. The skeleton provides a storage pool for calcium and other ions. Skeletal muscle, which accounts for 40% to 50% of body weight, plays a major role in metabolism and temperature regulation.

STRUCTURE OF THE MUSCULOSKELETAL SYSTEM
MUSCLE

Skeletal Muscle

Skeletal muscle attaches to bones of the skeleton. Skeletal muscles are named according to the following properties: (1) action (e.g., flexor, extensor), (2) shape (e.g., quadrilateral, pennate), (3) origin (i.e., stationary attachment of muscle to skeleton), (4) insertion (i.e., movable attachment of the muscle), (5) number of divisions, (6) location, or (7) direction of fibers (i.e., transverse). The principal muscle groups are shown in Figure U6-1.

The contraction of skeletal muscle exerts force on bones or skin and moves them (Figure U6-2). Most skeletal muscles are under voluntary control of the nervous system, but some are controlled by the somatic division of the peripheral nervous system, such as those used to maintain balance.

Skeletal muscle is composed of many individual muscle cells called *muscle fibers*. These fibers are held together by thin sheets of fibrous connective tissue *(fascia)*. Fascia also penetrates the muscle, separating it into bundles *(fasciculi)*. Skeletal muscle is attached to the bones of the skeleton by very thin extensions of fascia or by tendons. *Tendons* (fibrous cords) make strong connections to bone.

Under microscopic examination, many nuclei of muscle cells are visible and are grouped into thread-like *myofibrils*. A close look at the myofibrils reveals alternating bands of light and dark *(striations)*. Muscle cells can be further divided into smaller segments called *sarcomeres,* delineated by Z bands. The sarcomere is the structure in the muscle where the actual contraction occurs. Two primary myofilaments are present in the sarcomere: thick myosin filaments and thin actin filaments. The *filaments* are proteins that briefly attach and ratchet or slide across one another to cause the muscle to contract.

Cardiac Muscle

Cardiac muscle *(myocardium)* is involuntary and exists only in the heart. It is composed of branched, striated muscle cells connected by gap junctions. Cardiac muscle is controlled by intrinsic factors (e.g., the amount of venous return to the right atrium), hormones, and signals from the autonomic nervous system. Cardiac muscle is discussed in the Unit 13 Anatomy and Physiology Review.

Smooth Muscle

"Smooth" muscle has no visible striations. It is involuntary and is present in the walls of hollow organs (e.g., digestive tract, blood vessels, urinary bladder) and in other areas (e.g., the eye). It is controlled by the autonomic nervous system, hormones, and intrinsic factors in the organ (e.g., stretch caused by food in the intestine). The electrical connections between smooth-muscle cells (gap junctions) allow the smooth muscle cells to function in a coordinated manner.

SKELETAL SYSTEM

Humans have an *endoskeleton* (i.e., it lies *within* the soft tissues of the body). It is composed of living tissue that is capable of growth, adaptation, and repair. The adult body contains 206 bones, which are divided into two major categories by position: axial and appendicular. The *axial skeleton* (80 bones) consists of the skull, vertebral column, and thorax. The *appendicular skeleton* (126 bones) includes the bones of the extremities, shoulders, and pelvis (Figure U6-3). Bones can also be classified by their shape:

1. *Long bones* are all longer than they are wide and are found in the upper and lower extremities. The hum-

ANTERIOR

Temporalis

Orbicularis oculi

Masseter

Sternocleidomastoid

Orbicularis oris

Pectoralis major

Pectoralis minor

Serratus anterior

Intercostals

Biceps brachii

Rectus abdominis

External oblique

Transversus abdominis

Brachioradialis

Internal oblique

Flexors of wrist and digits

Sartorius

Rectus femoris

Adductor muscles

Vastus intermedius

Patella

Vastus lateralis

Vastus medialis

Tibialis anterior

Fibularis longus

POSTERIOR

Splenius

Levator scapuli

Trapezius

Rhomboideus

Deltoid

Infraspinatus

Serratus posterior

Triceps brachii

Intercostals

Latissimus dorsi

Olecranon process

Lumbodorsal fascia

Extensors of wrist and digits

Gluteus maximus

Adductor muscles

Biceps femoris

Iliotibial band

Semitendinosus

Semimembranosus

Soleus

Gastrocnemius

Achilles tendon

FIGURE U6-1 Principal muscles.

erus, radius, ulna, femur, tibia, fibula, metatarsals, metacarpals, and phalanges are the long bones.

2. *Short bones* (e.g., carpals, tarsals) do not have a long axis; they are cubical.

3. *Flat bones* (e.g., ribs, cranium, scapula, and portions of the pelvic girdle) protect soft body parts and provide large surfaces for muscle attachments.

4. *Irregular bones* have various shapes, such as vertebrae, ear ossicles, facial bones, and pelvis. Irregular bones are similar to other bones in structure and composition.

Gross Anatomy of Bone

A typical long bone (Figure U6-4) has a shaft *(diaphysis)* and two ends *(proximal* and *distal epiphyses)*. The diaphysis is a hollow cylinder of compact bone that surrounds a medullary cavity *(marrow)*. It is lined with a thin connective tissue layer called *endosteum*. In children and young adults, the epiphyses are separated from the diaphysis by *epiphyseal cartilage* or plates, where bone grows longer. When bone growth is complete, the epi-

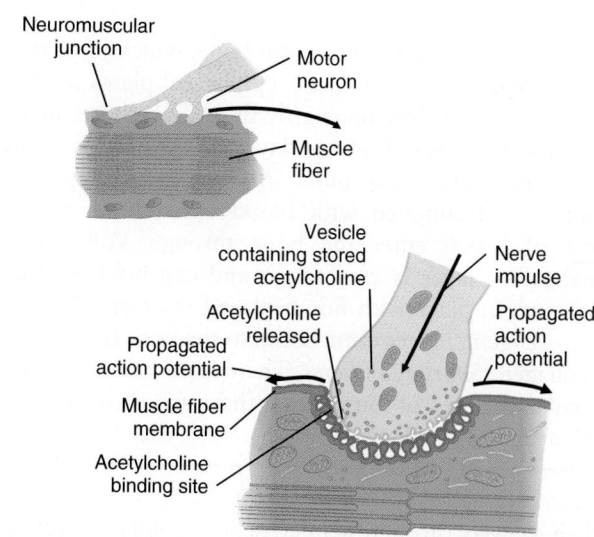

Neuromuscular junction

Motor neuron

Muscle fiber

Vesicle containing stored acetylcholine

Nerve impulse

Acetylcholine released

Propagated action potential

Propagated action potential

Muscle fiber membrane

Acetylcholine binding site

FIGURE U6-2 The neuromuscular junction. When a stimulus, such as a nerve impulse, travels to the neuromuscular junction, acetylcholine is released from storage in vesicles. The acetylcholine diffuses across the cleft and stimulates the muscle to contract.

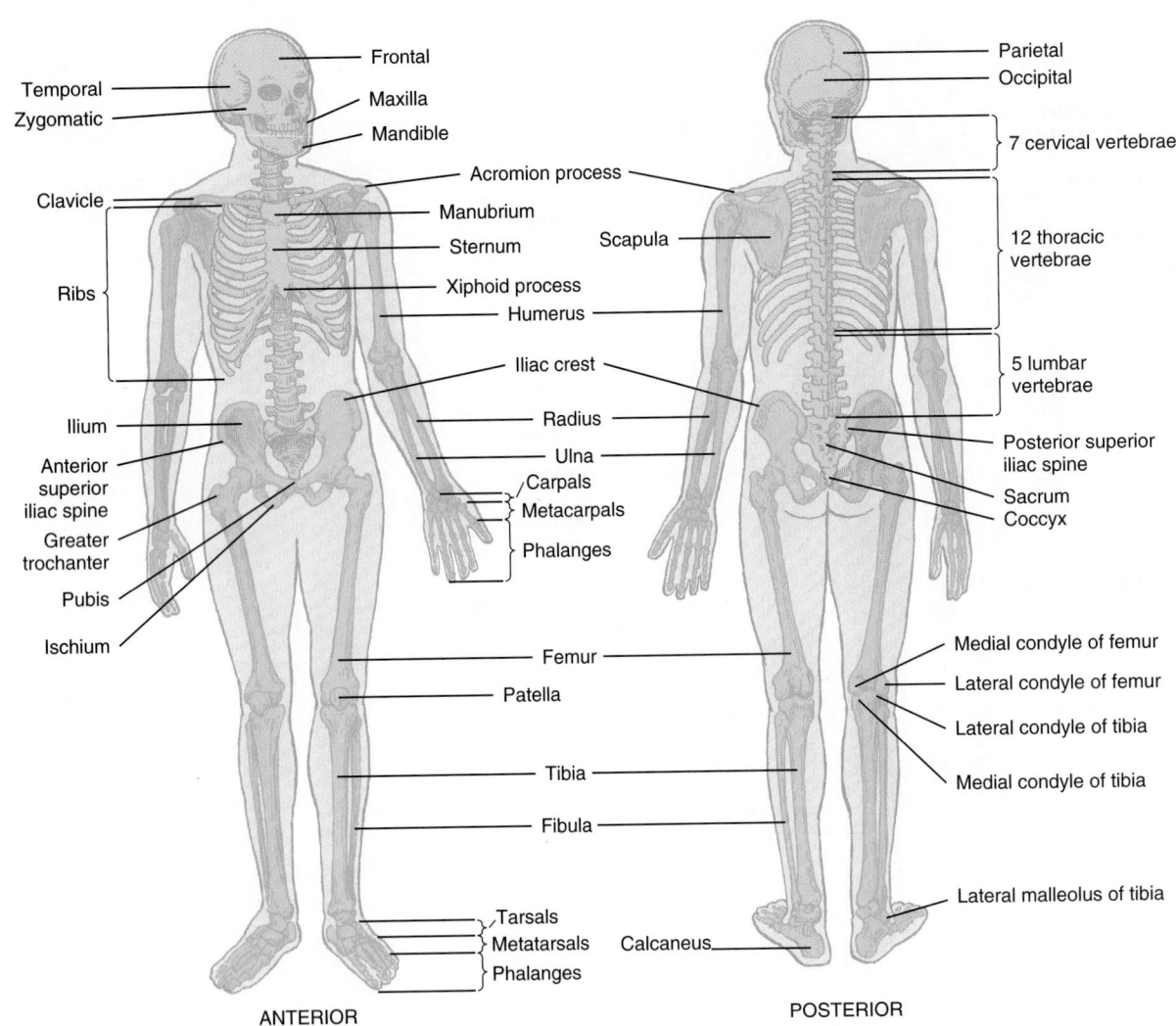

FIGURE U6-3 The adult human skeleton is composed of 206 bones. The axial skeleton is shown in blue, and the appendicular skeleton is shown in beige.

physeal cartilage is replaced with bone, which joins it to the diaphysis. Fractures of the epiphyseal plates in children can lead to slow bone growth or limb shortening.

Bones are covered with a layer of connective tissue called *periosteum*. The outer *(fibrous)* layer of periosteum is well supplied with blood vessels and nerves, some of which enter the bone through Volkmann's canals. This layer is very tough and can hold fracture fragments in place with nondisplaced fractures. The inner *(osteogenic)* layer is anchored to the bone by bundles of collagen *(Sharpey's fibers)*. There is no periosteum on articular surfaces of long bones; these areas are covered with articular cartilage.

Microscopic Anatomy of Bone

When viewed through a microscope, *compact bone* is highly organized and solid. It is organized into structural units called *osteons* or *haversian systems*. An osteon is essentially a cylinder of bone. Each osteon contains (1) vessels in a central canal *(haversian canal)*; (2) concentric layers of bone matrix *(lamellae)*; (3) tiny spaces between

the lamellae *(lacunae)*, which contain osteocytes; and (4) small channels *(canaliculi)*. The blood vessels transport nutrients to the bone and carry wastes away from the bone.

Spongy bone does not have such an organized structure. The lamellae are not arranged in concentric circles but rather in directions that correspond to the lines of maximum pressure or tension placed on the bone. Spongy bone has osteocytes embedded in lacunae, and lacunae intercommunicate via canaliculi. Blood reaches the osteocytes by passing through spaces in the bone marrow.

Composition of Bone

Bone's organic framework is formed from protein complexes and fibers, especially collagen (similar to the collagen found in other connective tissues). *Collagen* provides bone with great tensile strength so that it can withstand stretching and twisting. The inorganic salts (calcium and phosphate in crystalline form, termed *hydroxyapatite*) allow bone to withstand compression. The

FIGURE U6-4 Longitudinal section of a long bone. **A,** Magnified view of compact bone. **B,** Section of an osteon (haversian canal).

combination of collagen and salt makes bone exceptionally strong without being brittle. The composition of bone is analogous to that of reinforced concrete, in which steel rods (the collagen) provide tensile strength, and cement, sand, and gravel (the salts) provide compression strength.

Bone contains three types of cells. *Osteoblasts* are bone-forming cells; they lay down new bone by catalyzing reactions that take calcium and phosphate from the blood and form it into bone matrix in a collagen meshwork. *Osteocytes* are osteoblasts that are found in the bone matrix. *Osteoclasts* are cells that resorb (remove) damaged or old bone cells during periods of growth or repair. They are also critical in returning inorganic salts from bone to the bloodstream. These bone cells allow bone to grow, repair itself, and change shape. Even mature bone constantly changes, with new cells being formed and old cells being destroyed.

ARTICULATIONS

Articulations (joints) are places of union between two or more bones. Not all joints permit movement. Joints may be synovial, fibrous, or cartilaginous.

Synovial Joints

Most of the joints in the body are synovial. They are freely movable, permitting position and motion changes. Synovial joints are capable of various movements, de-

pending on the type of joint. Synovial joints have four characteristics:

1. Each joint is enclosed by an articular *capsule*, resulting in a joint cavity (Figure U6-5).
2. Synovial membrane produces *synovial fluid*, which fills the cavity for lubrication and cartilage nourishment.
3. Bone surfaces in the joint are covered by *hyaline cartilage* (articular cartilage).
4. Synovial joints have additional *support* features. *Ligaments* and *tendons* reinforce the capsule and help to limit motion. *Articular disks* are located between the bones in some synovial joints to buffer forceful impact.

Fibrous Joints

Fibrous joints are articulations in which bones are held together by fibrous connective tissue. Very little material separates the ends of the bone, and minimal movement is possible.

Suture Joints

Suture joints include the bones of the skull and sometimes the sutures between the ilium, ischium, and pubic bones. At birth the bones of the skull are separated to facilitate birth. The bones usually fuse by the time a child is 2 years of age. The edges of these bones have grooves *(interdigitations)* that fit firmly together and look somewhat like a suture.

Syndesmosis Joints

Syndesmosis (ligamentous) joints are held together by ligaments (bands of fibrous tissue) or membranes. Syndesmosis joints allow some "give." The joints at the distal end of the tibia and fibula are examples of syndesmosis joints.

Cartilaginous Joints

Bones are held together by cartilage (dense connective tissue; see Cartilage later in this chapter). Slight movement is possible in these joints. They are of two types: synchondrosis and symphysis.

Synchondroses

Synchondroses are held together by hyaline cartilage. Joints between the epiphyses and diaphyses of long bones are replaced by bone *(ossification)* at maturity. In the ribs, this form of cartilage also is temporary and eventually is replaced by bone. In the costal cartilages, synchondroses between ribs and sternum are not usually replaced by bone.

Symphyses

Symphyses are articular surfaces that have a fibrocartilaginous pad or disk connecting the articulating bones. Slight movement is allowed. Within the joint, the surfaces act as shock absorbers. The vertebrae are separated by symphyses.

CUSHIONING AND SUPPORTIVE STRUCTURES

Bursae and Tendon Sheaths

Bursae are small sacs lined with synovial membrane and filled with synovial fluid (Figure U6-5). They act as cushions between structures. The body has hundreds of bursae. Some are subcutaneous, lying between bone and skin (e.g., the bursa between the olecranon process of the elbow and the skin).

Tendon sheaths are cylindrical synovial structures similar to bursae. They are found where tendons cross joints and may be subject to constant friction. The sheath wraps around the tendon, forming a fluid-filled cushion through which the tendon can slide.

Ligaments

Ligaments are bands of fibrous tissue that connect bones at joints and provide stability during movement. Some commonly injured ligaments are the coracohumeral and the glenohumeral ligaments, which maintain shoulder stability; and the medial, collateral, patellar, and anterior and posterior cruciate ligaments, which support the knee (Figure U6-6).

Cartilage

Cartilage is a type of dense connective tissue that is prevalent throughout the musculoskeletal system. It can resist forces of tension and compression with consider-

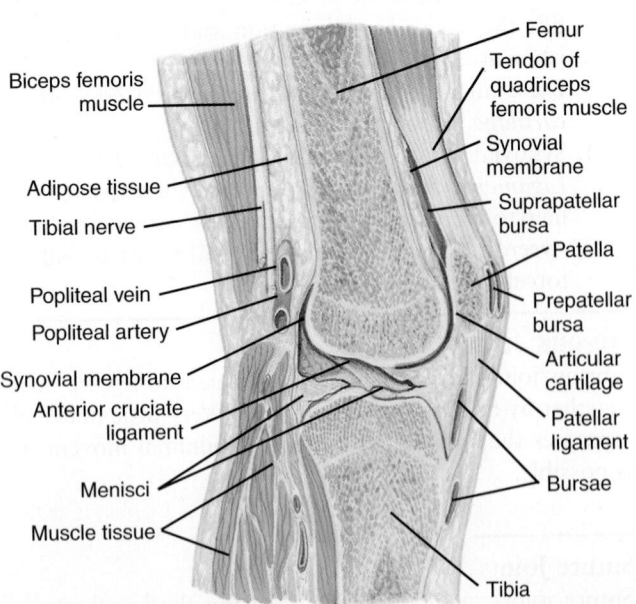

FIGURE U6-5 Anatomy of a synovial joint (knee). (From Thibodeau, G., & Patton, K. [2003]. *Anatomy and physiology* [5th ed.]. St. Louis: Mosby.)

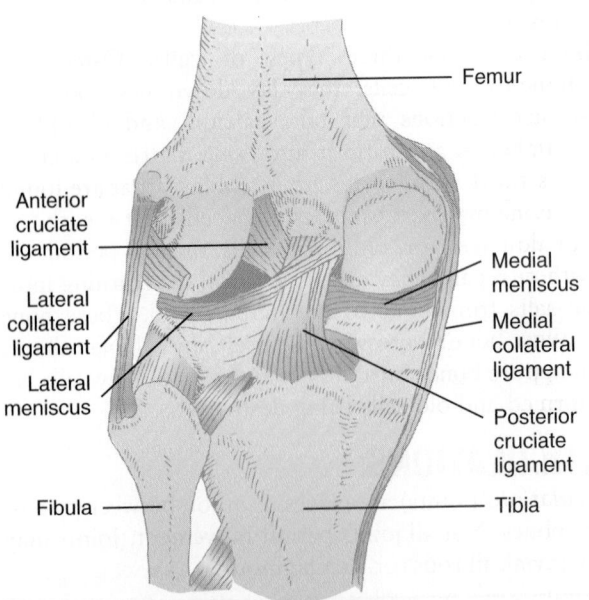

FIGURE U6-6 Posterior view of the knee. When the knee is extended, the taut anterior cruciate ligament prevents overextension. When the knee is flexed, the posterior cruciate ligament prevents the tibia from slipping posteriorly.

able resilience. It is semi-opaque (bluish white or gray) and has limited nerve and blood supply. Most of the skeleton of an embryo is cartilage that gradually changes into bone *(ossification)*.

Three types of cartilage are found in the body:

- *Hyaline cartilage,* found in respiratory tract, developing bones, and ends of articulating bones
- *Fibrocartilage,* found in ligaments and intervertebral disks
- *Elastin cartilage,* found in the external ear

FUNCTION OF THE MUSCULOSKELETAL SYSTEM
MUSCLE

Movement

Skeletal muscle contraction occurs when a stimulus excites an individual muscle fiber (see Figure U6-2). The stimulus, a nerve impulse, releases stored acetylcholine (ACh) from the end of the motor neuron. ACh crosses the neuromuscular junction and elicits an action potential by binding to a receptor on the muscle cell membrane (e.g., stimulatory electrical impulse). The action potential triggers contraction of the sarcomeres by releasing calcium inside the cell. Nerve fibers can supply more than 100 individual skeletal muscle cells. A continuous flow of stimuli maintains muscle tone (i.e., keeps muscles partially contracted, in a state of readiness for movement).

Calcium binding exposes the active sites on the actin protein. This actin binds to myosin, and the myosin filament heads pivot using previously hydrolyzed adenosine triphosphate (ATP) as an energy source. The movement releases adenosine 5'-diphosphate (ADP) and allows new ATP to bind to the myosin, detaching the myosin from the actin. Muscle fibers relax between contractions because calcium ions that are released during the action potential are free for only a short time. Calcium quickly returns to storage in the sarcoplasmic reticulum in the muscle. If nerve impulses arrive in rapid succession so that calcium remains free, the muscle will continue to contract (called *spasm* or *tetany*).

To generate power, muscle cells require large amounts of oxygen and glucose. Muscles thus have a rich vascular supply. An oxygen debt develops during exercise if oxygen cannot be delivered to muscles in concentrations great enough to meet the immediate metabolic needs of the cell. After exercise increased oxygen consumption is necessary to relieve oxygen debt.

Skeletal muscle exhibits a length-tension relationship. Before a contraction, stretching the muscle can alter the alignment of the actin and myosin proteins *(preload)*. The maximum tension generated by the contracting muscle comes when the greatest overlap between the actin and myosin proteins occurs, and this is close to the normal resting length of the skeletal muscle.

It is possible to stimulate a muscle but to exert a force so that the muscle does not shorten. This is called *isometric* ("same length") contraction. In contrast, during weight lifting, the muscle generates tension until the tension is sufficient to move the weight, allowing an *isotonic* ("same tension") contraction.

Motor Units and Summation

The *motor unit* is defined as the motor neuron and all skeletal muscle fibers it supplies. The number of muscle fibers involved in each motor unit reflects the degree of control. Small motor units allow fine control, such as in the muscles of the fingers. Large motor units coordinate the response of large muscles, such as those of the trunk.

Strength of contraction is increased by temporal or spatial summation. Temporal summation increases the rate of individual motor unit activity. Spatial summation increases the number of motor units activated. Both spatial and temporal summations result in *tetany,* a sustained contraction of skeletal muscle.

Propulsion

Smooth muscle is found in the walls of hollow conduits in the body, and its contraction applies pressure that may mix, break up, or move substances forward. For example, smooth muscle of the gastrointestinal (GI) tract propels food through the tract during digestion. Smooth muscle in arterioles regulates arterial blood flow by causing vasodilation and vasoconstriction. Smooth muscle in the uterus contracts during labor, and smooth muscle in the airways can constrict *(bronchospasm)* or dilate to promote air movement.

Heat Production

The activity of skeletal muscle produces heat, some of which can be used to maintain body temperature. During exercise, excess heat is released through sweating and vasodilation. When the body is cold, heat is generated by shivering.

SKELETAL SYSTEM

Bones give form to the body: they support various tissues and organs and permit movement by providing attachments for tendons and ligaments. The skeleton is also protective. The skull and rib cage, for example, protect the brain and special senses and the lungs, respectively.

Hematopoietic Function

Bone houses the hematopoietic tissues, which manufacture blood cells. In adults, blood cells form in marrow cavities in the skull, vertebrae, ribs, sternum, shoulder, and pelvis. The two types of bone marrow are *yellow* and *red*. Some investigators have noted a third type of bone marrow: brown. *Brown* marrow is generally found in older adults; it is similar to yellow marrow in that it is inactive but lacks adipose tissue. *Yellow* marrow (connective tissue composed of fat cells) is found in the shafts of long bones and extends into the haversian systems. Yellow marrow does not produce blood cells except during times of increased blood cell need. *Red marrow* has a hematopoietic function; it manufactures red and white blood cells. It is located in the cancellous bone spaces, found in flat bones (see the Unit 17 Anatomy and Physiology Review).

Role of Bone in Homeostasis

Bones also provide a crucial portion of mineral balance; they store calcium, phosphorus, sodium, potassium, and other minerals and release them for cellular metabolism and use by other body systems. When blood levels of calcium fall, the parathyroid gland senses the decrease and releases *parathyroid hormone* (PTH). PTH increases the movement of calcium from bone into the extracellular fluids by stimulating the osteoclasts to break down bone and free calcium. PTH also decreases renal excretion of calcium, increases the excretion of phosphate, and increases the metabolic transformation of vitamin D_3 to its active form to increase calcium absorption from the intestine.

Bone Remodeling

Throughout life, the bone mass continuously undergoes well-regulated processes of bone formation and bone resorption. The process of bone turnover is called *remodeling*, and it is one of the major mechanisms for maintaining calcium balance in the body. As much as 15% of the total bone mass normally turns over each year in a *three-phase process:*

- *Phase 1.* The cycle begins when a stimulus (such as a hormone, drug, or stressor) activates the bone cell precursors to become osteoclasts.
- *Phase 2.* Osteoclasts gradually resorb the bone. They leave behind an elongated cavity *(resorption cavity)*, which matches the general structure of the haversian system or trabeculae.
- *Phase 3.* New bone is laid down by the osteoblasts. The osteoblasts follow the path of the osteoclasts to create new haversian systems and trabeculae.

The entire process takes about 4 months. Rebuilding of bone requires normal plasma concentrations of calcium and phosphate and is dependent on vitamin D.

Bone Repair

The remodeling process enables repair of small bony injuries, but breaks *(fractures)* and other wounds of bone heal in a different manner. Initially, the bone heals by forming a hematoma. The fibrin of the hematoma provides a meshwork, which is the initial framework for healing. Granulation tissue *(pro-callus)* is produced, and a fibrocartilaginous callus develops before bony *(osseous)* depositions develop. Osteoblasts deposit disorganized clumps of bone matrix *(callus)*. The trabeculae and haversian systems follow. Finally, the bony edges are remodeled to the size and shape of the bone before injury.

EFFECTS OF AGING

Aging affects bone, muscle, and tendons. Bone tissue is lost because the rate of loss exceeds the rate of growth. The haversian systems in compact bone erode. The lacunae enlarge, and cortical bone becomes thin and porous. *Osteoporosis,* a condition of decreased calcium in bone, leads to weak, brittle bones and an increased risk of fracture.

Eventually cartilage becomes more rigid and fragile and muscle bulk decreases. As muscle mass decreases, so does maximal strength, which can decline by 50% between the ages of 20 and 50 years. Several theories have been offered to explain these changes, including changes in activity, reduced circulation, cardiovascular disorders, and nutritional problems.

CONCLUSIONS

The muscles of the body provide movement, propel substances, and produce heat. The three types of muscle—skeletal, cardiac, and smooth—perform distinct functions. Bone provides a framework and a protective structure for the body. The haversian system is the structural unit of bone. The major minerals in bone are calcium and phosphate, which are regulated by parathyroid hormone. Bone is constantly remodeled, and every 4 months it is completely replaced. Joints (articulations) provide connections between bones and allow movement involving more than one bone. Joints may be synovial, fibrous, or cartilaginous.

Musculoskeletal disorders are common. Fractures can occur at any age because of forces applied to the bone that exceed its tensile or compressive strength. Disorders seen in the articular surfaces (e.g., rheumatoid arthritis, osteoarthritis) develop when the articular cartilage degenerates, leading to pain and decreased movement. Muscle disorders include such conditions as muscular dystrophy (progressive muscle degeneration) and myasthenia gravis (loss of receptors on the muscle for ACh, leading to profound muscle weakness).

BIBLIOGRAPHY

1. Berne, R., et al. (2004). *Physiology* (5th ed.). St. Louis: Mosby.
2. Kierszenbaum, A.L. (2002). *Histology and cell biology: An introduction to pathology.* St. Louis, Mosby.
3. Guyton, A., and Hall, J. (2001). *Textbook of medical physiology* (10th ed.). Philadelphia: W.B. Saunders.
4. Silverthorn, D. (2001). *Human physiology* (2nd ed.). Upper Saddle River, NJ: Prentice Hall.

Assessment of the Musculoskeletal System

Peggy Doheny
Carol A. Sedlak

Assessment of the musculoskeletal system begins with a health history and provides direction for further assessment. The musculoskeletal physical examination can be either general (as in a screening examination) or local (for a specific problem or injury). Similarly, diagnostic tests can be either general or specific. The resulting data provide information to make judgments about the client's musculoskeletal status. Musculoskeletal assessment can also include the client's functional status and ability to perform activities of daily living (ADL) and to meet self-care needs. This aspect of the assessment involves evaluation of the client's exercise habits and leisure activities that promote health.

HISTORY

The musculoskeletal history consists of the following:
- Biographical and demographic data
- Chief complaint (including symptom analysis)
- Past health history
- Family health history
- Psychosocial history
- Lifestyle data
- Review of systems

Collect information to help determine the nature and extent of the client's current disorder. If the chief complaint is related to trauma, keep the history interview brief and focus on the cause of injury. If the injury is extensive, the interview may need to be delayed. Once the client's condition is stable, a more complete history can be obtained.

Biographical and Demographic Data

Personal information enables individualized care planning. For example, knowing where the client lives and the kind of transportation used helps to understand the energy required for the client to keep an appointment. Knowing the client's significant others is essential in planning care as well.

The client's age and gender may suggest possible causes of musculoskeletal problems. For example, 85% of people older than 70 years have some osteoarthritis. Osteoporosis (porous bone) occurs most often in postmenopausal women. Reiter's syndrome is most common in men between 20 and 40 years of age. Osteogenic sarcoma is rare after age 40 years. Carpal tunnel syndrome occurs more often in women than in men.

Current Health

Chief Complaint

Ask the client to describe the reason for seeking health care. Common musculoskeletal clinical manifestations are pain, tenderness, muscle tightness or weakness, joint stiffness, cramps, muscle spasms, swelling, redness, deformity, reduced movement or joint range of motion (ROM), sensory changes, and other abnormal sensations. ADL may be affected. Ask the client and significant others to recount their perceptions of the problem and its cause. Their answers often provide not only information about areas for further assessment but also clues about personal fears and concerns.

Symptom Analysis

Conduct a symptom analysis for each manifestation the client reports (see Chapter 4). Common musculoskeletal manifestations are pain, joint stiffness, swelling, deformity and immobility, and sensory changes.

Pain. Ask the client to point to the exact location of the pain. Poorly localized pain usually stems from problems in blood vessels, joints, fascia, or periosteum.

Ask the client to describe the pain: Is it an ache, a sharp pain, a throbbing? Aches are commonly muscular, sharp pain may be caused by a fracture or bone infection, and throbbing pain is usually bone-related. Ask the client to rate the pain on a scale of 0 to 10, on which 0 is no pain and 10 is the worst pain possible.

What makes the pain worse: Temperature changes? Movement? Lifting or carrying something heavy? Pain from osteoarthritis is worse in cold, damp weather. Pain that occurs with movement is typical of joint problems. Degenerative hip conditions produce pain during weight-bearing and during and after walking. Degenerative knee problems produce pain during and after walking. Vertebral disk herniation produces pain on bending or lifting and may radiate down one leg.

Is the pain worse at a particular time of day? Does it wake the client or prevent sleep and rest? Inflammation of bursae or tendons is worse at night. Degenerative joint pain is often worse at the end of a day.

Does rest reduce the pain? Most musculoskeletal pain is helped by rest.

Which medications help to reduce the pain? Pain from inflammation is usually helped by aspirin or non-steroidal anti-inflammatory drugs (NSAIDs). Opioid analgesics are usually required for traumatic injury.

Have there been any recent injuries? Sometimes a client does not associate a fall or other injury with current pain manifestations.

Is the pain associated with chills, fever, rash, or a sore throat? Joint pain occurring 10 to 14 days after a sore throat may be from rheumatic fever.

Joint Stiffness. Ask the client to point to joints that are stiff. Are they always stiff? How long does the stiffness last? Some conditions, such as ankylosing spondylitis, have remissions and exacerbations.

At what time of day is the stiffness worst? With degenerative joint disease, stiffness is often most severe in the morning after a night in bed.

What relieves the stiffness? Temperature changes? Exercise? Coldness and lack of use typically increase joint stiffness. Heat may reduce muscle spasm. Heat applied to a recently injured joint may worsen stiffness by increasing bleeding into and swelling of the joint.

Does the joint lock so it cannot move? Does the client hear or feel bones rubbing together? Bone malalignment within a joint causes locking. *Crepitus* (the sound of bone ends rubbing together) indicates fractures or joint destruction.

Does the client have pain or weakness in muscles with certain movements? Weakness in muscles may result from various neuromuscular disorders. If weakness is present, does it interfere with the client's usual activities?

Swelling. Ask how long the client has had swelling. Is there pain? Swelling and pain commonly accompany bone and muscle injury. With degenerative joint disease, swelling may not develop for some time, maybe weeks, after pain is present—or it may not develop at all.

Does swelling limit the client's movement? Limited movement may stem from soft tissue damage and swelling in a joint.

Does rest or elevating the part give relief? Elevation reduces swelling in acute injuries.

Ask whether the body part was casted recently. Removing a cast can result in temporary swelling. A casted limb also may have muscle atrophy.

Has the area been hot or red? Redness and heat indicate inflammation, infection, or recent injury and are not usually present with degenerative conditions.

Deformity and Immobility. Has the deformity developed suddenly or gradually? A gradually developing mass may be a tumor.

Is movement limited? Is this limitation always present? Is it worse after activity? Does any body position make it worse or better? Immobility from degenerative joint disease varies with the severity of the condition.

Ask how the deformity affects the client's daily activities. Does the client use any supportive equipment, such as crutches, a walker, or bandages? Use of such aids offers clues to the severity of the disability.

Sensory Changes. Does the client have a history of back pain or injury? If so, where is the pain located? Does the pain travel, for example, down the back of the leg? Does the client have trouble walking? Is there a loss of feeling anywhere? If so, is the loss of feeling associated with any pain? Does the client have any tingling or burning sensation? Pressure on nerves or blood vessels can occur from swelling, tumors, or fractures, causing loss of sensation. Sensory changes may be associated with pain in an arm or hand.

Past Health History

Carefully assess previous trauma, accidents, or surgery involving bones or joints. The client may have sustained fractures, dislocations, strains, or sprains. Previous accidents resulting in fractures may predispose to degenerative changes.

Question the client about a range of past health problems because many diseases can affect the musculoskeletal system. Explore both childhood and adult-onset disorders because of their possible long-term effects.

Childhood and Infectious Diseases

Health conditions may affect the musculoskeletal system directly or indirectly. For example, diabetes mellitus may predispose a client to degenerative joint disease. Blood dyscrasias, such as hemophilia, may cause bleeding in joints that produces pain, swelling, tenderness, and deformity. Psoriasis may precede psoriatic arthritis. Cartilage damage from trauma may precipitate degenerative changes in a relatively young person. Ask about a history of tuberculosis, sickle cell disease, poliomyelitis, inflammatory or degenerative arthritis, scurvy, rickets, osteomyelitis, soft tissue infection, fungus infection of bones or joints, and streptococcal and neuromuscular disorders.

Major Illnesses and Hospitalizations

Besides inquiring about diseases, such as diabetes mellitus, tuberculosis, poliomyelitis, and arthritis, ask about hospitalizations related to musculoskeletal disorders or trauma. If the client or significant others cannot remember details, ask for permission to obtain the medical records. Ask about past or present minor and major injuries, including (1) circumstances of the injury, (2) diagnosis of the injury, (3) treatment received, (4) duration of treatment, and (5) current problems resulting from the injury.

Musculoskeletal injury involves fractures, sprains, strains, and joint dislocations. Minor injuries may be treated on an ambulatory basis, whereas major injuries may require prolonged hospitalization, surgery, or rest and immobilization. Ask whether the client has residual impairment from the injury, such as a need to use an assistive device (cane, crutches, or walker). Ask whether the client has had to change or adjust ADL because of lingering limitations.

Medications

Question the client about past and present prescription and over-the-counter medications as well as herbal remedies. For each medication, find out (1) the reason for taking it, (2) the dose and frequency, (3) how long the client has taken it, and (4) any observed side effects. Ask about specific medications used for musculoskeletal problems, such as muscle relaxants, salicylates, NSAIDs, and steroids. Some medications may affect the musculoskeletal system adversely.

For example, corticosteroid therapy can lead to necrosis of the femur head, septic arthritis, and muscle weakness. High doses of anticoagulants can produce hemarthrosis (blood in joints). Anticonvulsants may cause osteomalacia. Phenothiazines may produce gait disturbances. Potassium-depleting diuretics may produce cramps and muscle weakness. Amphetamines and caffeine cause a generalized increase in motor activity. Hormone replacement therapy with estrogen has been shown to modify the effects of osteoporosis in postmenopausal women.

Use of NSAIDs for more than 4 weeks can lead to bleeding problems—especially in the gastrointestinal (GI) tract—because of decreased platelet aggregation. Renal and hepatic changes can also develop. Long-term use of NSAIDs requires follow-up laboratory assessments to monitor for side effects. Complete blood count and serum assays of liver enzymes, potassium, and creatinine, and urinalysis are usually assessed.

Herbal preparations may cause unwanted effects. For example, the use of glucosamine and chondroitin have gained popularity as a remedy for arthritis pain; however, glucosamine can increase insulin resistance and chondroitin may enhance the effects of anticoagulants. The herb cayenne *(capsicum)* or capsaicin applied topically reduces the ache and pain of arthritis. If taken internally, however, capsaicin can cause GI distress and, at high doses, may damage unmyelinated and small-diameter myelinated nerve fibers. White willow *(Salix alba)* has analgesic properties and contains salicin, which may have adverse effects similar to those of salicylate.

Family Health History

Some musculoskeletal problems with a familial predisposition are arthritis, osteoporosis, ankylosing spondylitis, gout, Heberden's nodes in osteoarthritis, muscular dystrophy, and scoliosis. Thirty percent of people with psoriatic arthritis have a family history of psoriasis.

Psychosocial History

The integrity of the musculoskeletal system enables a person to function effortlessly. However, many problems can disrupt that integrity, thus disrupting the coping ability of both the client and significant others. Ask about daily activities and habits. When assessing a client with a chronic illness or degenerative process, ask whether the disorder has affected the client's interactions with others or view of self and others. Crippling illnesses often curtail social activity and result in lower self-esteem.

Occupation

Ask whether heavy lifting or strenuous activity is common in the client's life. Such activity can cause muscle strain, degenerative vertebral disk problems, and other trauma. Low back pain can arise from jobs involving extensive driving. Habitually carrying heavy objects, such as a mailbag, shoulder bag, attaché case, or other equipment, can place uneven pressure on the spinal column. Prolonged use of computers and keyboards can cause orthopedic injuries from repetitive strain (see Chapter 29).

Activities of Daily Living

Are there everyday activities that are difficult or impossible, such as (1) opening containers, pouring liquids, and cutting up food, (2) dressing, using zippers, and fastening or unfastening buttons, snaps, or hooks, (3) grooming, combing hair, and applying makeup, (4) running a bath and testing water temperature, washing hair, and shaving, (5) writing, and (6) getting out of the house, climbing stairs, or getting in and out of chairs or cars?

Ask whether physical limitations prevent performance of daily activities. Assess the client's attention to safety and ask about safety practices used at work and at home. Does the client use recommended equipment, such as safety shoes or safety guards on power tools? There is a high incidence of accidental injury among people who pay little attention to safety practices.

Exercise

Document the details of the client's typical recreational activities and exercise pattern. Lack of exercise produces poor muscle tone, which leads to muscle strain. Sporadic exercise of poorly toned muscles is more likely to cause muscle injury and spasm. Lack of warm-up exercises increases the likelihood of injury as well.

Fractures and other trauma can arise from contact sports. Achilles tendon damage can occur from improperly landing on heels while jogging. Pain in arm joints can be caused by racket sports, such as tennis and squash, which require a strong grasp, wrist extension, and forearm rotation.

Ask about typical footwear. High-heeled shoes can shorten the Achilles tendon and pitch the center of gravity forward, leading to lordosis.

Nutrition

A well-balanced diet helps maintain the structure of the bones and muscles and a dietary history can provide clues to musculoskeletal problems (see Chapter 30). For example, obesity stresses weight-bearing joints and predisposes to ligament instability, particularly of the lower back. Poor calcium intake can lead to bone decalcification and fractures. Ask about foods eaten on a typical day. Assess for use of nutritional supplements. Adequate dietary intake of vitamins A and D, calcium, and protein are important for musculoskeletal health.

Inquire about recent weight changes. Excessive weight gain can place stress on the musculoskeletal system.

Habits and Safety

Health promotion habits and a positive lifestyle can reduce the risk for development of musculoskeletal disorders. Increasing dietary calcium and weight-bearing activities, such as walking, can help prevent osteoporosis and improve strength and flexibility. Maintaining musculoskeletal health enhances a person's ability to perform ADL. Moreover, early detection of conditions such as scoliosis through screening programs can help with early intervention.

Review of Systems

Ask about musculoskeletal problems such as (1) muscle pain, spasm, or tenderness; (2) joint pain, stiffness, other discomfort, swelling, or redness; (3) weakness; (4) limited movement; (5) clumsiness; (6) crepitus; (7) backache; and (8) changes in joints or bones. Investigate each reported problem. Inquire about the effect of the problem on the client's ability to perform ADL.

Assessment findings from other body systems may indicate musculoskeletal problems. The following are examples:

- Pain or burning when urinating, which is associated with Reiter's syndrome
- Tachycardia and hypertension, which may accompany gout
- Chronic diarrhea, which may occur when arthritis is associated with colitis or other GI problems
- Conjunctivitis, which may indicate Reiter's syndrome, and nongranulomatous uveitis, which may occur with ankylosing spondylitis
- Skin changes, which may indicate musculoskeletal problems (dry skin over the thumb and the first two

fingers suggests carpal tunnel syndrome, for example)

- Cramping leg pain with activity, which may signal intermittent claudication
- Generalized muscle cramping, which may result from electrolyte imbalances
- Joint pain with recent chills, fever, or sore throat, which may result from rheumatic fever

Detailed questions for the review of systems are found on the website for this book.

PHYSICAL EXAMINATION

Assessment of the musculoskeletal system should proceed systematically to avoid missing hidden problems. Use an examining room big enough for the client to move around. Natural lighting is best for assessing skin color changes and swelling. Artificial light distorts some assessment findings. During the examination, have the client sit, stand, and walk unless a position is contraindicated by the client's condition.

Musculoskeletal assessment consists of inspecting and palpating (1) muscle masses for symmetry, involuntary movements, tenderness, tone, and strength, (2) joints for symmetry, crepitus, tenderness or pain, and ROM, and (3) bones for deformity and limb length discrepancy. Assessment of muscle-stretch and deep tendon reflexes is discussed in Chapter 69.

General Musculoskeletal Examination

Use inspection and palpation to examine each body part. First, examine the body at rest, then assess ROM and muscle strength. Look for normal findings such as those outlined in Physical Assessment Findings in the

Healthy Adult feature on The Musculoskeletal System, below.

When the client enters the examination room, assess the gait, body mobility, posture, general joint motion, and balance. While observing movement and gait, watch for (1) gait patterns associated with specific disorders (see Chapter 69), (2) objective evidence of discomfort, and (3) indications of joint stiffness or muscle weakness, lack of coordination, and deformities. Then have the client sit on the edge of the examination table. Observe general appearance and body build. Examine the head, neck, shoulders, and upper extremities.

Have the client stand, and examine the chest, back, and ilium. Observe posture, body build, body contours, body alignment, and the cervical, thoracic, and lumbar spine. Observe the relationships of various body parts to one another, such as the relationship of feet to legs, legs to hips, and hips to pelvis (Figure 27-1).

Observe the client's stance and note spinal deformities or other abnormalities (Figure 27-2), such as the following:

- *Kyphosis,* an abnormally increased roundness of the thoracic curve or hump-back
- *Scoliosis,* a lateral deformity of the spine
- *Lordosis,* an abnormal increase in the lumbar curve, or swayback
- *Genu varum,* or bowleg
- *Genu valgum,* or knock-knee

FIGURE 27-1 When performing a musculoskeletal assessment, have the client stand and walk if possible. Observe the client's stance, joint mobility, and posture. If you were to assess this man only while he was reclining, you might not notice his posture, the curvature of his spine, and his limited range of motion.

PHYSICAL ASSESSMENT FINDINGS IN THE HEALTHY ADULT

The Musculoskeletal System

Inspection

Joints in alignment; posture straight; gait smooth.
Extremities symmetrical and of equal length.
Muscle groups symmetrical, without atrophy or fasciculations.
Joints without erythema, swelling, or deformities.
Full range of motion (active and passive) in all major joints.

Palpation

Muscle groups firm, symmetrical, nontender; without masses or spasms.
Joints stable and nontender, without heat, crepitus (palpable or audible), bogginess, or nodules.
Muscle strength in all major muscle groups rated 5/5.

FIGURE 27-2 Musculoskeletal deformities observable during assessment. **A,** Kyphosis. **B,** Scoliosis. **C,** Lordosis. **D,** Genu varum. **E,** Genu valgum.

The terms *varus (varum)* and *valgus (valgum)* refer to the direction in which the deformity lies in relationship to the midline where the distal aspect of the joint is angled toward the midline of the body. With a varus deformity, the deformity points toward the midline. With a valgus deformity (knock-knee), the deformity is bent or twisted away from the midline.

Last, with the client supine, examine the hips, knees, ankles, and feet for alignment, symmetry, and deformities. Determine any discrepancy between leg lengths by measuring from the anterior iliac spine to the medial malleolus. Measurements should be within 1 cm of each other. If a discrepancy is noted, determine whether it exists above or below the knee.

Muscles

Compare each muscle group with its contralateral side. Muscles should be free of *fasciculations* (fine muscle twitches) and smooth, without bulges or lumps. Palpate muscle groups gently, from proximal to distal, feeling the *muscle tone* (the state of tension in a muscle at rest, which is felt as firmness). Muscles should feel firm and smooth and should be bilaterally equal in size and nontender. A slight increase in mass, or *hypertrophy*, on the dominant side is normal, whereas *atrophy*, or decrease in muscle mass, on either side is abnormal. If muscle groups are noticeably unequal in size, use a tape measure to assess limb circumferences. Differences of 1 cm or less between the two sides are considered within normal variation.

Assess *muscle strength* while putting joints through active ROM. If a detailed assessment is necessary, each major muscle group can be assessed separately (Table 27-1). The sternocleidomastoid and trapezius muscles

TABLE 27-1	*Assessing Muscle Strength*
Muscle Group	**Technique**
Deltoid	Push down client's arm while it is held up and client resists.
Biceps	Hold client's arm in extension while it is fully extended and client flexes arm.
Triceps	Keep client's arm in flexion while it is flexed and client extends arm.
Wrist and finger muscles	Push client's fingers together while client spreads them and resists.
Grip strength	Pull your own crossed index and middle fingers from the client's grasp.
Hip muscles	Hold down client's leg while it is fully extended and while client lifts it off the table (client is supine).
Hip muscles (abduction)	Prevent client from spreading legs apart against resistance applied to the lateral surfaces of the knees (client is supine with legs extended).
Hip muscles (adduction)	Prevent client from bringing legs together against resistance applied to the medial surfaces of the knees (client is supine with legs extended).
Hamstrings	Straighten client's knees while client is supine with knees flexed and resists.
Quadriceps	Flex client's knee while client is supine with knee partially in extension and resists.
Ankle and foot muscles	Dorsiflex client's foot while client resists. Plantiflex client's foot while client resists.

are tested as part of the head and neck (cranial nerve) examination (see Chapter 69). Test muscle strength by asking the client to repeat ROM while applying resistance. Note the strength exerted against the resistance. If a weakness is detected, decrease the resistance. Because the dominant arm is usually stronger, ask whether the client is right-handed or left-handed. Rate muscle strength numerically as follows:

0 = Muscle is paralyzed with no visible or palpable contraction (zero)

1 = Contraction is palpable but muscle does not move (trace)

2 = Full ROM is present with the joint supported to eliminate gravity (poor)

3 = Full ROM is present with gravity as the only resistance (fair)

4 = Full ROM is present against moderate resistance (good)

5 = Full ROM is present against normal resistance and gravity (normal)

Include the muscle strength rating scale as part of the client's record to ensure understanding and consistency with other health care providers.

Joints and Bones

Inspect the client's joints and bones, and compare findings bilaterally. Symmetry should be found without redness, swelling, enlargement, or deformity. Palpate each joint and bone for edema and tenderness, which should be absent. Palpate joints during movement for crepitus, which is abnormal. Joints should feel smooth as they move, and nodules should be absent.

ROM is the maximum range of movement attainable by a healthy joint. ROM is measured with a goniometer,

FIGURE 27-3 Use of a goniometer to measure joint range of motion. This knee is flexed at 60 degrees.

a flexible protractor-type instrument placed on a joint to measure the angles created by joint movement (Figure 27-3). As needed, assess ROM in all joints (Figure 27-4).

Special Tests of Joint Function

Advanced practitioners may use special assessments to determine whether an injury has occurred in a joint. Some common tests are listed in Table 27-2. Two tests are shown in Figure 27-5.

Neurovascular Assessment

A neurovascular assessment is essential for clients with a past musculoskeletal injury because of the high risk of ischemia, deformity, or loss of function in the affected limb.

Components of Neurovascular Assessment

A neurovascular assessment involves checking for (1) pain, (2) pallor, (3) temperature, (4) pulses, (5) capillary refill, (6) paresthesia, and (7) mobility of affected joints.

If the client has pain, using an intensity rating scale of 0 to 10, as previously described, can help determine whether the pain is getting worse—a possible result of edema and nerve compression.

Pallor, coolness, or cyanosis can indicate circulatory compromise in the limb. Check pulses and capillary refill bilaterally to determine the adequacy of blood supply to small peripheral vessels. Capillaries should refill within 2 or 3 seconds.

Loss of sensation and motor function in a limb can signal nerve injury.

Peripheral Nerve Assessment

Test sensation and motor function in major peripheral nerves (Figure 27-6). Check sensation with the client's eyes closed. Light touch should be perceptible if sensation is normal. If a "pins and needles" sensation is reported, assess further (see Chapter 69). The client should be able to demonstrate active motion of a specific joint upon request. Inability to move a joint and the presence of pain with passive ROM may indicate compartment syndrome.

Perform further assessments, such as capillary refill, pulses, color, and warmth (see Chapter 29). When casts prevent full neurovascular assessment, observe for edema, capillary refill, and joint movement.

DIAGNOSTIC TESTS

Diagnostic tests of musculoskeletal structures are grouped by whether they are invasive or noninvasive. See Chapter 4 for a more detailed discussion of many of these tests and the necessary client preparation.

FIGURE 27-4 Joint range of motion (ROM). All joints are at 0 degrees when in anatomic position. ROM begins at 0 degrees, as shown by the *solid lines*. Attainment of average normal ROM is shown by *dotted lines* and the number of degrees in the angle formed by the two lines.

TABLE 27-2   *Assessing Joint Function*

Test or Sign	Purpose	Technique	Findings	Comments
Shoulder				
Adson's maneuver	Evaluates blood flow in subclavian artery; tests for thoracic outlet syndrome	Palpate radial artery while abducting, extending, and externally rotating the arm; have client take a deep breath and turn head toward arm being tested	*Negative:* Pulse remains strong *Positive:* Marked decrease or loss of radial pulse during the test	Blood flow can be compromised by cervical rib, tumor, hematoma, or infection that has tightened neck muscles
Apley's scratch test	Evaluates shoulder ROM	Have the client reach behind the head and touch the top of the opposite scapula Then have the client reach behind the back and touch the bottom of the opposite scapula	Inability to perform as instructed indicates less than normal ROM for shoulder	Limited ROM decreases functional ability for activities such as combing hair, pulling up a zipper, and placing something in a back pocket
Drop arm test	Evaluates for rotator cuff tear	Abduct client's shoulder to 90 degrees, and instruct client to slowly lower the arm to the side	*Negative:* Able to comply with instructions *Positive:* Arm drops suddenly or severe pain is felt in the shoulder as arm is lowered	Positive finding indicates tear in rotator cuff
Elbow				
Tennis elbow test	Evaluates for lateral epicondylitis	Hold the client's elbow (thumb on lateral epicondyle), pronate the client's forearm, flex the wrist fully, and extend the elbow	*Negative:* No pain *Positive:* Pain over lateral epicondyle of the humerus	Lateral epicondylitis is commonly seen in people who work at computers (word processing, data entry)
Wrist and Hand				
Finkelstein's test	Test for de Quervain's disease (tenosynovitis of the thumb)	Have the client make a fist with the thumb inside the fingers, then hold the client's forearm steady and deviate the wrist toward the ulnar side	*Negative:* No pain with maneuver *Positive:* Client feels pain over abductor pollicis longus and extensor pollicis longus tendons	Test may cause some discomfort in normal persons; therefore compare pain caused on the "affected" side with that on the normal side
Phalen's test	Evaluates for pressure on median nerve (carpal tunnel syndrome)	Have the client hold the backs of hands together with wrists flexed 90 degrees; position is held for 60 seconds	*Negative:* No symptoms *Positive:* Tingling or burning in area of hand innervated by median nerve	
Lumbar Spine				
Straight leg raising (Lasègue's sign)	Evaluates for presence of HNP	*Involved leg:* With client supine, passively raise the client's leg with the knee extended until pain is felt, then extend the leg slowly until there is no pain or tightness; dorsiflex the client's foot *Uninvolved leg:* With client supine, raise the leg as described for the involved leg	*Negative:* No pain *Positive:* Pain with dorsiflexion of the foot *Positive:* Pain in opposite leg (not test leg) strongly suggests HNP	Pain in posterior thigh indicates hamstring tightness Pain down entire leg indicates sciatic nerve involvement

Modified from Maher, A.B., Salmond, S.W., & Pellino, T.A. (2002). *Orthopaedic nursing* (3rd ed.). Philadelphia: W.B. Saunders.
ACL, Anterior cruciate ligament; *HNP,* herniated nucleus pulposus; *PCL,* posterior cruciate ligament; *ROM,* range of motion.

Continued

TABLE 27-2	*Assessing Joint Function—cont'd*			
Test or Sign	**Purpose**	**Technique**	**Findings**	**Comments**
Knee				
Drawer test (anterior)	Evaluates stability of ACL	Have client lie on back with knee flexed to 90 degrees and hip to 45 degrees; hold the foot of the test leg in place, and then draw the tibia forward on the femur (Place your hands around the tibia with the thumbs on the medial and lateral joint lines of the knee, as shown in Figure 27-5)	*Negative:* Movement 6 mm or less *Positive:* Movement more than 6 mm indicates tear in ACL	If PCL is injured, result may be false-positive If PCL injury is suspected, check for posterior "sag" sign (gravity and drawer test)
Drawer test (posterior)	Evaluates stability of PCL	Position client as described for anterior test and push tibia back on femur	*Negative:* Tibia does not move back *Positive:* Backward movement of tibia (felt or observed) indicates injury to PCL	
Gravity test (posterior sag sign)	Evaluates integrity of PCL	Have client lie supine with hips flexed to 45 degrees and knees to 90 degrees	*Positive:* Tibia "sagging" back on the femur indicates that PCL is torn	With minimal swelling, sag is very evident, as is obvious concavity distal to the patella
Lachman's test	Evaluates injury to the ACL	Have client lie supine with the knees between full extension and 30 degrees; then use one hand to stabilize the femur and the other hand to move the tibia forward (see Figure 27-5)	*Positive:* When tibia moves forward, the infrapatellar tendon slope disappears	This test is the best indicator of ACL injury
McMurray's test	Evaluates for medial and lateral meniscus injury	Have client lie supine with the injured leg fully flexed; then cup the heel with one hand and place your other hand on the knee (fingers on the medial joint line, thumb on the lateral joint line); first rotate the tibia medially, changing degrees of flexion; then rotate the tibia laterally, repeatedly changing degrees of flexion	*Positive:* If a snap or click is heard, there is probably a meniscal tear	Evaluation of meniscal injuries is difficult and requires considerable experience; because menisci have no blood or nerve supply, there may be no pain or swelling with injury

Modified from Maher, A.B., Salmond, S.W., & Pellino, T.A. (2002). *Orthopaedic nursing* (3rd ed.). Philadelphia: W.B. Saunders.
ACL, Anterior cruciate ligament; *HNP,* herniated nucleus pulposus; *PCL,* posterior cruciate ligament; *ROM,* range of motion.

FIGURE 27-5 Special advanced tests of joint function. **A,** The drawer test for instability of the knee ligaments. **B,** Lachman's test for anterior cruciate instability.

NONINVASIVE TESTS OF STRUCTURE

Radiography

Radiography (x-ray study) is the most widely used non-invasive musculoskeletal diagnostic procedure. X-ray examinations are used to do the following:

- Establish the presence of a musculoskeletal problem
- Follow its progress
- Evaluate the effectiveness of treatment

A plain film is obtained, usually an anteroposterior (AP) or lateral view, possibly both. Other common views include a notch (posterior or less commonly anterior) view of the knee in flexion, an oblique (45-degree angle) view, and a sunrise or patella view of the underside of the patella.

Tomography

Tomograms (body-section radiographs) show tissue at various planes through the body as though slices had been made. Tomography can be used to locate bone destruction, small cavities, foreign bodies, and lesions overshadowed by other structures and to evaluate whether a bone graft has united.

Assessment Technique

Nerve	Sensation	Motion

Radial	Prick web space between the thumb and index finger	Client hyperextends thumb then wrist and hyperextends the four fingers at the MCP joints
Ulnar	Prick distal fat pad of the small finger	Client abducts all fingers
Median	Prick distal surface of the index finger	Client opposes thumb and small finger; note whether client can flex wrist
Peroneal	Prick web space between the great toe and second toe	Client dorsiflexes ankle and extends toes at the metatarsal phalangeal joints
Tibial	Prick medial and lateral surfaces of the sole of the foot	Client plantar flexes ankle and toes

FIGURE 27-6 Assessment of peripheral nerves: radial, ulnar, median, peroneal, and tibial nerves. *MCP,* Metacarpophalangeal. (Modified from Stearns, G.M., & Brunner, N.A. [1987]. *Operative care* [Vol. 1, p. 89]. Rutherford, NJ: Howmedica.)

Fluoroscopy

Fluoroscopy may be used in conjunction with myelography to verify the location of the lumbar puncture. Fluoroscopy can be used to monitor the progress of contrast dye injected into the subarachnoid space during myelography. See Chapter 69.

Dual-Energy X-Ray Absorptiometry

Methods to measure bone density are performed to diagnose osteoporosis because the condition is not evident in x-ray studies until 30% to 50% of bone mass is lost. One method of measuring bone mass is with dual-energy x-ray absorptiometry (commonly called a DEXA scan). An x-ray tube is used to generate dual-energy photons. DEXA causes less radiation than an x-ray exposure and takes about 10 minutes. It can detect osteoporosis in sites such as the wrist, spine, and hips. No preparation is required, although the client may require teaching about osteoporosis once the findings are known.

Computed Tomography

Computed tomography is useful for assessing some bone and soft tissue tumors and spinal fractures.

Magnetic Resonance Imaging

Magnetic resonance imaging, or MRI, facilitates the early diagnosis of many conditions that affect tendons, ligaments, cartilage, and bone marrow (Figure 27-7).

INVASIVE TESTS OF STRUCTURE

Specialized radiographic procedures that are invasive and allow more precise visualization include arthrograms, sinography, and myelography. Other invasive tests of structure are radionuclide scanning, arthrocentesis, arthroscopy, electromyography, and biopsy. All are discussed here.

Radiography

Arthrography

Arthrography is a radiographic examination of soft tissue joint structures. It is used to diagnose trauma to joint capsules or supporting ligaments, especially those of the shoulder, wrist, hip, ankle, and knee. After local anesthesia has been achieved, a contrast agent or air is injected into the joint cavity with the use of aseptic precautions. A series of x-ray films is obtained as the joint is moved through ROM.

Before arthrography, explain the procedure, answer any questions, and obtain the client's informed consent to the procedure. Explain that the procedure may take up to an hour (follow-up x-ray studies are sometimes ob-

FIGURE 27-7 Magnetic resonance image of the right knee. *F,* Femoral condyle; *M,* meniscus; *P,* patella; *PT,* patellar tendon; *QT,* quadriceps tendon; *S,* synovial capsule; *T,* tibial plateau.

tained 30 minutes after the injection) and that the client must remain as still as possible except when asked to reposition. Ask whether the client has any allergies, especially to local anesthetics, iodine, or contrast dyes. Suggest that the client void before the procedure. Advise the client that the joint may be uncomfortable for 1 to 2 days afterward and the client should thus avoid strenuous exercise for that time.

Sinography and Myelography

Sinography and myelography are similar to arthrography in that both modalities involve injection of contrast agents and the taking of x-ray films. Sinography is used to examine sinus tracts (deep draining wounds). Myelography is discussed in Chapter 69.

Radionuclide Imaging

Bone Scans

In bone scanning, images of the skeleton are obtained after a radioisotope, usually technetium 99m (^{99m}Tc), is injected intravenously and allowed to migrate to bone. The whole body is usually scanned, although just a limb may be scanned (pinhole scan) if a stress fracture is suspected. Bone scanning is used to detect malignancies, osteomyelitis, osteoporosis, and some fractures, especially pathologic ones. The radioisotope concentrates in these areas, indicating abnormal bone metabolism. The radioisotope does not accumulate in poorly perfused bone.

Explain the procedure to the client and family, answer their questions, and obtain consent. The procedure takes about an hour, during which time the client lies supine. Reassure the client that the procedure is not painful and that there are no harmful effects from the isotopes. Suggest that the client void before the procedure.

After the scan, no special precautions are required except that the client should drink large amounts of water for 24 to 48 hours to help eliminate the radioisotope. Because the radioisotope carries minimal radioactivity, there is no hazard to others.

Gallium Scans

Gallium scans are similar to bone scans but are more specific to bone disorders. Gallium also migrates to brain, liver, and breast tissue. Because it is taken up by bone more slowly than ^{99m}Tc, gallium is given to the client by a nuclear medicine technician 2 to 3 hours before the scan. The scan takes 30 to 60 minutes to complete. Mild sedation may be needed for clients who are in pain, are restless, or are older. No special follow-up care is required.

Indium Imaging

Indium imaging is the use of indium 111, tagged to (connected to) leukocytes to detect bone infection. The client's leukocytes are separated from a sample of blood and labeled (tagged) with indium. Then the tagged cells are reinjected. Because leukocytes naturally accumulate in areas of bone infection, the tagged leukocytes can be detected by imaging. No special preparation or follow-up care is necessary.

Other Tests

Arthrocentesis

Joint aspiration, or *arthrocentesis,* is a method of aspirating synovial fluid, blood, or pus via a needle inserted into the joint cavity. It is used to diagnose rheumatoid arthritis and other inflammatory conditions or to remove fluid to reduce pain. Normal synovial fluid is clear to straw-colored and is present in minute amounts. Inflamed joints produce increased amounts. In normal joints, synovial fluid is usually thick and has a string-like appearance when expressed from a syringe.

Arthrocentesis is performed with the use of aseptic precautions after local anesthesia has been achieved and with or without fluoroscopy. Medication may be instilled into the joint, if necessary, to alleviate inflammation in septic arthritis. Apply a compression bandage after arthrocentesis, and advise the client to rest the joint for 8 to 24 hours.

Arthroscopy. A fiberoptic arthroscope allows endoscopic examination of various joints (hip, knee, shoulder, elbow, wrist) without making a large incision. Arthroscopy can be used for (1) obtaining a biopsy specimen, (2) assessing articular cartilage, (3) removing loose bodies, and (4) trimming cartilage. It usually is an outpatient procedure performed with the use of local anes-

thesia. The client recovers more quickly than after an *arthrotomy* (opening of the joint).

Arthroscopy is contraindicated in the client whose joint flexion is less than 50% or in whom a skin or wound infection is present at the site. Complications are rare but include infection, hemarthrosis (blood in the joint), swelling, synovial rupture, joint injury, and thrombophlebitis.

Instruct the client to fast from midnight the night before the test. Make sure that consent forms are signed. If local anesthesia is to be used, tell the client that there may be mild discomfort as it is administered and when the endoscope is inserted.

Teach the client to watch for signs of postprocedure infection, such as temperature elevation and local inflammation at the incision site, and to report them promptly. Ensure necessary postprocedure pain reduction. A normal diet may be resumed as soon as desired. Tell the client that unless a surgical incision is made and the surgeon gives specific instructions to the contrary, walking is usually permitted once sensation has returned. The client should avoid strenuous exercise for a few days.

Electromyography

Electromyography is used to assess such problems as muscle weakness, altered gait, and lower motor neuron lesions. Chapter 69 discusses this test in more detail because it is used for clients with neurologic disorders.

Biopsy

Biopsy (removal and examination of a sample of tissue) is used to detect disorders such as infection, cancer of the bone, and atrophy or inflammation of the muscle. Bone or muscle biopsy specimens may be collected either during surgery or through a needle or bore not requiring a surgical incision (aspiration, punch, or needle biopsy). Aspiration biopsy sampling may be performed under radiographic control, such as for sampling of the spine. Bone biopsy specimens are collected with the use of local anesthesia and aseptic technique in either the radiology department or the operating room to prevent osteomyelitis. Bone or muscle biopsy sampling takes about 30 minutes.

After the procedure, monitor the site for bleeding, swelling, and hematoma development. Because dressings usually cover the biopsy site, analyze the client's pain level to monitor for complications. Mild to moderate discomfort is expected; more severe levels of pain may signal complications. Elevate the biopsy site for 24 hours to reduce edema. Monitor the client's vital signs every 4 hours for 24 hours. Mild analgesia is often required. Instruct the client to assess the site on a regular basis (at least daily) after discharge for signs of infection.

TABLE 27-3   *Common Laboratory Studies Used in the Diagnosis of Musculoskeletal Conditions*

Test	Normal Value	Significance of Results
Antinuclear antibody (ANA)	Negative or at a titer ≤1:32	Positive results are associated with systemic lupus erythematosus, rheumatoid arthritis, rheumatic fever, and Raynaud's disease
C-reactive protein (CRP)	Trace amounts	Positive in acute inflammation, such as rheumatoid arthritis
Erythrocyte sedimentation rate (ESR)	*Westergren method:* Males: 0-15 mm/hr Females: 0-20 mm/hr *Wintrobe method:* Males: 0-9 mm/hr Females: 0-15 mm/hr	Elevations common in arthritic conditions, infection, inflammation, cancer, and cell or tissue destruction

Mineral Metabolism

Calcium	8.0-10.5 mg/dl or 4.5-5.5 mEq/L	Decreased levels found in osteomalacia, osteoporosis. Increased levels found in bone tumors, Paget's disease, and healing fractures
Alkaline phosphatase	30-90 units/L	Elevations found in bone cancer, osteoporosis, osteomalacia, and Paget's disease
Phosphorus	2.5-4.0 mg/dl	Increased levels found in healing fractures and osteolytic metastatic tumor diseases

Muscle Enzymes

Aldolase A	1.3-8.2 units/dl	Elevations in muscular dystrophy and dermatomyositis
Aspartate aminotransferase	10-50 units/L	Found in skeletal muscle but primarily in heart and renal cells
Creatine kinase	15-150 units/L	Increased levels found in traumatic injuries, progressive muscular dystrophy, and polymyositis
Lactate dehydrogenase (LDH$_4$, LDH$_5$)	60-150 units/L	Elevations in skeletal muscle necrosis, extensive cancer, and progressive muscular dystrophy

LABORATORY STUDIES

Table 27-3 lists the most common laboratory tests for clients with musculoskeletal disorders. Chapter 79 describes laboratory tests specific for rheumatic problems.

CONCLUSIONS

Assessment of the musculoskeletal system consists of a complete history, including symptom analysis and physical examination. Diagnostic studies commonly include x-rays and, in recent years, arthroscopy has evolved to allow the diagnosis and treatment of joint disorders during one procedure.

BIBLIOGRAPHY

1. Altizer, L. (2002). Neurovascular assessment. *Orthopaedic Nursing, 20*(4), 48-50.
2. Bascom, A. (2002). *Incorporating herbal medicine into clinical practice.* Philadelphia: F. A. Davis.
3. Jarvis, C. (2000). *Physical examination and health assessment* (3rd ed.). Philadelphia: W. B. Saunders.
4. Maher, A.B., Salmond, S.W., & Pellino, T.A. (2002). *Orthopaedic nursing* (3rd ed.). Philadelphia: W. B. Saunders.
5. O'Hanlon-Nichols, T. (1998). Basic assessment series: A review of the adult musculoskeletal system. *American Journal of Nursing, 98*(6), 48-52.
6. O'Malley, P., Trimble, N., Browning, M. (2002). Herbal therapies update: Implications for the clinical nurse specialist, *Clinical Nurse Specialist, 16*(4), 173-177.

evolve Did you remember to check out the bonus material on the Evolve website and the CD-ROM, including free self-assessment exercises?
http://evolve.elsevier.com/Black/medsurg/

Management of Clients with Musculoskeletal Disorders

Dottie Roberts
Joan M. Lappe

The musculoskeletal system allows the human body to maintain its upright posture, to move freely, and to function independently. Bone is a vital, dynamic connective tissue that serves three major functions: (1) it provides a framework for movement and protection of internal organs, (2) it performs a major role in metabolism and mineral homeostasis, and (3) it serves as the primary site of hematopoiesis. Disorders of the musculoskeletal system cause considerable morbidity, lead to decreased quality of life, and often result in reduced life expectancy.

DEGENERATIVE BONE DISORDERS
OSTEOARTHRITIS

Osteoarthritis (OA), or degenerative joint disease, is one of the oldest and most common types of arthritis. With research continuing on all arthritic disorders, OA is no longer believed to be a wear-and-tear disease that is a normal consequence of aging. Although aging does lead to decreasing quality and quantity of the proteoglycans in articular cartilage, the changes seen in the cartilage of asymptomatic adults are quite different from those found in people with OA. OA is now recognized as a chronic, progressive process in which new tissue is produced in response to joint insults and cartilage deterioration. Systemic involvement and inflammation are not typical of OA, although changes in the joint space may cause a localized inflammatory response that leads to transient joint effusion.

Etiology and Risk Factors

Osteoarthritis has been classified as either *idiopathic* (formerly primary) or *secondary*. *Idiopathic* OA affects people with no history of joint injury, joint disease, or systemic illness that might be associated with the development of arthritis. The most prevalent articular disease in adults 65 years of age and older, idiopathic OA occurs more commonly in women than in men. It accounts for substantial disability in the lower extremities as a result of its effects on the large weight-bearing joints.

Although OA has not historically been considered a genetic disease, a strong familial disposition exists for the development of idiopathic disease. Evidence now suggests the existence of an autosomal-recessive trait

---

Nursing Outcomes Classification (NOC)
for Nursing Diagnoses—Clients with Musculoskeletal Disorders

Acute Pain and Chronic Pain
Comfort Level
Pain Control
Pain: Disruptive Effects
Pain Level

Deficient Knowledge
Knowledge: Treatment Procedures

Impaired Physical Mobility
Ambulation: Walking
Joint Movement: Active
Mobility Level
Transfer Performance

Risk for Impaired Skin Integrity
Immobility Consequences: Physiologic
Peripheral Tissue Perfusion

Risk for Ineffective Tissue Perfusion
Tissue Perfusion: Peripheral

Risk for Infection
Immobility Consequences: Physiologic
Knowledge: Infection Control
Tissue Integrity: Skin and Mucous
  Membranes
Wound Healing: Primary Intention

Risk for Injury
Risk Control
Risk Detection

**Risk for Peripheral Neurovascular
Dysfunction**
Circulation Status
Joint Movement: Active
Mobility Level
Muscle Function
Neurologic Status
Peripheral Tissue Perfusion

with gene defects that contribute to early cartilage destruction. A genetic link has also been found in the occurrence of Heberden's nodes associated with OA of the distal interphalangeal (DIP) joints of the hands. In addition, sex hormones and other hormonal factors are believed to play an active part in the development and progression of OA.

Secondary OA occurs more frequently in men than in women. It results from trauma, other inflammatory joint disease, avascular necrosis, or neuropathic disorders such as Legg-Calvé-Perthes disease. Traumatic arthritis can develop after fracture or open joint injury. It can also stem from repetitive injury related to the person's occupation or sport (e.g., wrist arthritis in a keyboard operator, shoulder manifestations in a baseball pitcher).

Because OA is a chronic, incurable disorder, health care providers have focused instead on identifying modifiable risk factors that can decrease the impact of the disease. For example, studies have consistently shown that overweight people have higher rates of OA of the knee than peers of normal weight. Although overweight people also appear to be at higher risk for OA of the hip, the association is not as strong or as consistent as for OA of the knee. This risk variation is due to the different amount of force exerted across these joints when a person stands or walks. Up to six times the body's weight is exerted across the knee, whereas only three times the body's weight is exerted at the hip. Weight loss or maintenance is important to minimize the effects of OA.

Clients with OA are also encouraged to follow a regular exercise regimen, which offers benefits in several ways:

- Weight-bearing exercise leads to increased joint mobility and strengthens the joint's supporting muscles, tendons, and ligaments.
- Exercise stimulates cartilage growth by driving synovial fluid through the cartilage matrix. Because articular cartilage lacks blood vessels, the mechanical

process of joint movement is essential to cartilage regeneration and continued joint mobility.
- Exercise protects joints indirectly by aiding in weight control, in addition to other benefits.

Pathophysiology

Healthy articular cartilage appears smooth, glistening, and white. It possesses unique viscoelastic and compressive properties that contribute to its shock-absorbing characteristics. *Chondrocytes,* the cellular components of cartilage, constantly remodel and maintain the integrity of articular cartilage that protects the bone ends in a joint. Chondrocytes actually create the cartilage matrix by producing type 2 collagen and proteoglycans. The hydrophilic (water-attracting) properties of the proteoglycans in particular add to the ability of cartilage to resist wear with heavy joint use.

In simplest terms OA can be described as a process of cartilage matrix degradation accompanied by the body's ineffectual attempts at repair. Early pathologic changes include a decrease in proteoglycan content in the matrix, which leads to a softening and loss of elasticity by the cartilage. As the body attempts to compensate, chondrocytes initially proliferate and increase their synthesis of proteoglycans and collagen. Progressive destruction by lysosomal enzymes eventually outweighs production, however, and the cartilage becomes increasingly susceptible to joint friction. Changes in collagen synthesis also occur, minimizing the compressibility of the cartilage. Factors that cause these changes are not clearly understood, but the effect on cartilage is the loss of its ability to resist wear with heavy use.

Fibrillation, erosion, and cracking appear in the superficial layer of cartilage as collagen fibers rupture. Cartilage becomes yellowed and worn over articular surfaces, and bone growth increases at the joint margins and bony outgrowths (osteophytes) develop (Figure 28-1). Central loss of cartilage, accompanied by buildup of cartilage and bone peripherally, produces inequality in the joint surfaces. The normal distribution of joint stress is changed, resulting in pain and restricted motion. The synovium may also respond with excessive secretion of synovial fluid, creating an inflamed distended joint capsule.

Clinical Manifestations

The diagnosis of OA may be confirmed by radiographic changes that include the presence of osteophytes and of a narrowed joint space caused by erosion of articular cartilage. Because the severity of manifestations does not always correlate with joint changes, however, the American College of Rheumatology (ACR) has established classification criteria for OA that do not rely solely on radiographic findings.

A   Normal   B   Degenerated

FIGURE 28-1 Pathologic changes seen with osteoarthritis. **A,** Normal cartilage-covered bony surfaces for articulation. **B,** Articular cartilage and bony surfaces are altered with loss of joint space and osteophyte formation.

Typical clinical manifestations that help in the diagnosis of OA include worsening pain and stiffness that increase with activity and relieved by rest. Affected joints may exhibit crepitus, mild tenderness in the area of joint wear, deficits in range of motion (ROM), and possibly some joint enlargement. One or more joints may be affected, but joint discomfort is not usually symmetrical. The client may describe weight-bearing joints that "lock" or "give way" as a result of advancing disease. New bone growth in the hands may be evident in the appearance of Heberden's nodes (DIP joints) or Bouchard's nodes (proximal interphalangeal [PIP joints]) (Figure 28-2).

Although no laboratory test has the capacity to confirm the presence of OA, specific tests may be performed to rule out other conditions such as rheumatoid arthritis (RA), infection, gout, and tendinitis or bursitis. Differentiation between OA and RA is especially important (Table 28-1). Orders may include a test for rheumatoid factor or a serum uric acid determination. Aspiration and analysis of synovial fluid allow the practitioner to rule out infection or crystal deposition. An erythrocyte sedimentation rate (ESR) is useful only if systemic manifestations are present. Depending on the client's clinical presentation, magnetic resonance imaging (MRI) may be ordered to rule out meniscal injury. In practice, the possible diagnoses are usually narrowed greatly after completion of the history and examination.

Outcome Management
■ Medical Management

Goals for medical management of OA include (1) pain management with improvement or maintenance of mobility, (2) functional independence, and (3) maintenance of quality of life. Most people with early OA can be suc-

FIGURE 28-2 Osteoarthritis of the distal and proximal interphalangeal joints. (From Moskowitz, R.W., & Bluestone, R. [2001]. General aspects of differential diagnosis. In R.W. Moskowitz et al. [Eds.], *Osteoarthritis: Diagnosis and medical/surgical treatment* [3rd ed.]. Philadelphia: W.B. Saunders.)

TABLE 28-1	Differentiation of Osteoarthritis and Rheumatoid Arthritis	
	Osteoarthritis	**Rheumatoid Arthritis**
Pathology	Progressive process of central cartilage (spurs) destruction Peripheral bone growth in joint	Progressive process marked by exacerbations and remissions Inflammation of synovial membrane with cartilage damage and bone destruction Ligament, tendon, and joint capsule damage
Affected joints	Weight-bearing joints (hips, knees, ankles), spine, DIP and PIP joints Asymmetric	Small joints (PIP, MCP), wrists, knees Symmetric
Joint effusions	Mild swelling possible from localized inflammatory response	Common
Clinical manifestations	Localized pain and stiffness, mild swelling possible Pain with activity, improves with rest Heberden's and Bouchard's nodules	Pain, swelling, tenderness, redness, and warmth Nodules over extensor surfaces Anemia, fatigue, and muscle aches Pain at rest, especially at night Elevated ESR, often positive rheumatoid factor
Other affected systems	None	Lung, heart, skin
Body size	Possibly overweight	Usually average to below average weight for size
Age at onset	Fourth to fifth decade of life	Young to middle age
Gender	2:1 female-to-male ratio	3:1 female-to-male ratio
Heredity	Genetic factors contribute	Familial tendency
Diagnostic tests	X-rays	Rheumatoid factor (80% positive); x-rays; joint fluid analysis; negative Lyme disease titer
X-ray evidence	Osteophytes, subchondral cysts	Erosions, osteoporosis
Treatment	Exercise and weight control, maintenance of activity level with joint protection Heat or cold applications Relaxation strategies Medication and/or surgery	Inflammation reduction Balanced diet and exercise program with joint protection Relaxation strategies; heat or cold applications Medication and/or surgery

Modified from Roberts, D. (2002). Degenerative disorders. In A. B. Maher, S. W. Salmond, & T. A. Pellino (Eds.), *Orthopaedic nursing* (3rd ed.). Philadelphia: W. B. Saunders.
DIP, Distal interphalangeal; *ESR,* erythrocyte sedimentation rate; *PIP,* proximal interphalangeal; *MCP,* metacarpophalangeal.

cessfully treated with a conservative approach that involves the simultaneous use of several modalities.

All clients benefit from a careful balance between rest and exercise. A sedentary lifestyle can lead to weight gain, which exacerbates arthritic manifestations. Low-impact aerobic exercise, such as brisk walking, does not cause further harm to damaged joints. In fact, walking can relieve pain and improve joint mobility. It also increases muscle tone and enhances joint stability. Exercise can help with weight loss, which should be encouraged in the obese client because obese people face more rapid destruction of joints in the lower extremities.

When even a short exercise session leaves the OA client with sore joints, movement therapies such as tai chi may be suggested as a low-impact alternative to increase fitness and flexibility within the client's own limits. Instead of pushing the joints to the point of overexertion, the client learns to consider the internal effects of

balance and stress reduction to be more important than the physical exercise. Because it gradually increases joint flexibility and muscle strength without loading joints, doctors now recommend tai chi for people with varied musculoskeletal conditions.

The client with OA needs to understand the importance of rest if an affected joint becomes painful. The client's use of a cane in the contralateral hand can decrease joint stress during episodes of severe hip or knee pain. A neoprene or elastic brace may also reduce pain and help to stabilize the joint in a functional position. A collar, sling, or corset may be useful for manifestations in the neck, shoulder, or back; however, immobilization should be limited to 1 week to avoid increased joint stiffness.

Some clients also obtain relief by applying heat to affected joints or by alternating applications of heat and cold (contrast baths). Heat applications help with stiffness by increasing collagen elasticity and flexibility. Cold applications are used less frequently than heat but may be beneficial during episodes of acute inflammation, immediately after exercise, or for relief of muscle spasms.

Many people with OA report good results from topical application of capsaicin cream to affected joints several times a day. The cream is available over-the-counter or can be prescribed in greater concentrations. It can be used alone or as an adjunct to oral medications. Capsaicin is especially effective for OA of the knees and hands. About 50% of capsaicin users describe a cutaneous burning, but this reaction usually declines with continued use.

Until recently nonsteroidal anti-inflammatory drugs (NSAIDs) were the mainstay of pharmacologic management of OA. Because OA has only a minor inflammatory component, NSAIDs may not be the best first-line choice. Furthermore, research suggests that NSAIDs actually disrupt articular cartilage metabolism. Many deaths among older adults are also attributed to NSAID use each year, usually because of gastrointestinal bleeding. Acetaminophen is the drug of first choice for those with hip or knee OA because of its effectiveness, safety, and low cost. It is less likely than NSAIDs to cause gastrointestinal, hepatic, or renal damage. The recommended maximum dose of acetaminophen is 1 g every 6 hours, not to exceed 4 g in a 24-hour period.

According to ACR guidelines,[2] a person with OA should be switched to an NSAID when severe pain persists despite the maximum acetaminophen dose. Acetaminophen use often continues on an as-needed (PRN) basis as an adjunct to the NSAID, which should be started in an over-the-counter (OTC) strength. Progression to prescriptive strengths only occurs when clinical manifestations worsen. To minimize gastrointestinal effects, the NSAID can be prescribed with a synthetic prostaglandin such as misoprostol (Cytotec). The client with a history of gastroesophageal reflux disease (GERD) or peptic ulcer disease may benefit from the use of cyclooxygenase-2 (COX-2) selective anti-inflammatory drugs. Results of the Celecoxib Long-Term Arthritis Safety Study (CLASS), however, prompted the U.S. Food and Drug Administration (FDA) to approve labeling changes for celecoxib (Celebrex) that should include new information about the risk of serious gastrointestinal and renal effects in older adults.[25] See the Integrating Pharmacology feature on Medications for Osteoarthritis at right.

Viscosupplementation is a unique treatment option for knee OA. Hyaluronan, a polysaccharide that is a major component of synovial fluid, can be administered by intraarticular injection into the knee. After injection the joint can produce normal hyaluronan and synovial fluid independently for several months. As it helps to restore the elastoviscosity of the synovial fluid, hyaluronan also provides some relief of arthritic pain. The FDA currently approves Hyalgan and Synvisc as medical devices rather than as drugs.

INTEGRATING PHARMACOLOGY
Medications for Osteoarthritis

Conservative management of osteoarthritis typically focuses on relieving pain and any accompanying inflammation. In early disease in particular, adequate pain management allows the client to continue usual activities.

Unlike aspirin, acetaminophen does not relieve the redness, stiffness, or swelling caused by inflammatory conditions such as rheumatoid arthritis. As a simple analgesic, however, it is now recommended as a first-line treatment for mild osteoarthritis pain. It causes analgesia by inhibiting prostaglandin synthesis by the CNS. Because of the minimal effects on peripheral prostaglandin synthesis, however, it has no anti-inflammatory effects. Acetaminophen is contraindicated for clients with hepatic disease, and it can cause hepatic toxicity in excess doses in clients without previous liver disorders. Because of the hepatic effects of acetaminophen, clients who will be using it regularly for arthritis pain management should be encouraged to avoid alcoholic beverages. The combined effects of acetaminophen and alcohol may be especially damaging to the liver. The client should also be instructed to check the labels of the other over-the-counter medications commonly taken; if acetaminophen is an ingredient in a cold preparation, for example, the client should clarify with a health care provider the amount of additional acetaminophen that may be taken for arthritis pain.

The other major class of medications used for management of arthritis pain is the nonsteroidal anti-inflammatory drugs (NSAIDs). NSAIDs work by interfering with the cyclooxygenase (COX) pathway, ultimately inhibiting prostaglandin synthesis. Prostaglandin causes vasodilation, which allows more blood flow to an affected area and results in the heat and redness of inflammation. Prostaglandin also prolongs pain. By inhibiting prostaglandin synthesis, NSAIDs can decrease inflammation and pain associated with arthritis. The COX-1 enzyme in the stomach wall continuously produces prostaglandins that stimulate mucous formation and protect the stomach lining. Traditional NSAIDs such as ibuprofen and naproxen interfere with the COX-1 enzyme pathway, leading to increased risk of gastrointestinal side effects for clients taking these drugs. In contrast, production of the COX-2 enzyme is induced by macrophages as part of the inflammatory process. Newer NSAIDs are selective for the COX-2 enzyme pathway, decreasing inflammation while potentially having fewer gastrointestinal effects. COX-2 inhibitors include rofecoxib (Vioxx), celecoxib (Celebrex), meloxicam (Mobic), and valdecoxib (Bextra.)

Numerous dietary supplements offer popular alternative therapies for the treatment of OA. Glucosamine provides the building blocks for the body to make and repair cartilage, and chondroitin is believed to contribute to cartilage elasticity. The client who wishes to take glucosamine and chondroitin must have a realistic approach because results may be weeks in coming. The supplements do not work for everyone, and the client who has taken them consistently for 2 to 3 months without results may in fact receive no benefit from continued therapy. (See the Complementary and Alternative Therapy feature on Arthritis and Glucosamine Supplements, below.)

SAM-e (s-adenosylmethionine) is a popular European supplement that reached U.S. markets in 1999. SAM-e, which occurs naturally in all living cells, contributes to the production of proteoglycans for cartilage repair. The human body usually makes all the SAM-e it needs, but levels decrease with aging, depression, or deficiencies of B vitamins or methionine. Early research in the United States has shown positive effects on arthritis pain for people with early OA only. More research is needed to determine long-term effects of the supplement. (See the Complementary and Alternative Therapy feature on SAM-e Supplements and Osteoarthritis on the website.)

Herbal products are commonly taken by clients with arthritis either to treat their disease or to assist with memory and energy. Many of the most popular herbal products affect platelet aggregation and can prolong bleeding time. They may also interact with various prescribed medications. Assessment of the client's use of herbal products is important, particularly if surgery is anticipated. Clients should be cautioned to stop taking herbal products before surgery because of the risk of changes in heart rate, blood pressure, or hemostasis.[4]

■ Nursing Management of the Medical Client

The goal of nursing management is promotion of a healthy, positive adaptation in the client with OA. Education is the key to successful treatment of the disease, and the nurse plays a major role as a client educator. Clients and their families need accurate information about the disease and about steps to take to minimize its impact. Effective education can alter behavior, empowering clients to make a positive change in their health status. Important areas in client education include (1) pain management, (2) rest-activity balance, (3) nutrition and weight loss, and (4) self-care strategies.

Teaching clients about their medications is an important part of your role in successful long-term pain management. For example, a client who is taking an NSAID must be informed of the manifestations of gastrointestinal bleeding, such as abdominal pain, tarry stools, and hematemesis. Reinforce the client's need to notify the physician immediately if these manifestations occur. Also encourage the client to keep a pain journal to help focus on manifestations and identify cues that signal the need for rest or activity. Suggest nonpharmacologic pain management strategies (e.g., relaxation techniques, guided imagery) to decrease the feelings of anxiety or powerlessness that accompany disease progression. Other modalities, such as transcutaneous electrical nerve stimulation (TENS), can also be considered to reduce pain.

The client who chooses to use dietary supplements also needs information about known risks and benefits as well as any interactions with established therapies. Although supplements may have a place in arthritis management, the client must understand the implications of delaying medical care or choosing unproven remedies in place of proven treatments.

To assist with self-care deficiencies related to OA, collaborate with an occupational therapist in providing assistive devices to maintain independence with dressing and hygiene. Self-fastening tape (Velcro) closures, zipper pulls, or elastic shoelaces can make dressing easier. Long-handled combs or thick-barreled toothbrushes can also help clients with basic self-care tasks. The client with OA can learn to maintain affected joints in a neutral position at rest to avoid flexion contractures that will affect functional ability.

Also recognize the possible influence of OA on the client's sexual role functioning. Pain and stiffness, along with limited ROM, can create problems with sexual expression. Joint deformities can also negatively affect self-image, leading to reduced libido and depression. Inform the client about alternative sexual positions (e.g., side-by-side) that promote comfort during intercourse, and encourage the client to use analgesics or to take warm baths to alleviate pain and stiffness before sexual activity.

COMPLEMENTARY AND ALTERNATIVE THERAPY

Arthritis and Glucosamine Supplements

The largest randomized trial of glucosamine supplements for osteoarthritis of the knee included 212 clients. This study involved clients taking glucosamine sulfate (not chondroitin, another popular form) 1500 mg/day for 3 years versus placebo. Clients (average age, 65 years) taking glucosamine experienced a significant reduction in pain and a significant improvement in function versus placebo. In addition, objective measures of improvement were also found to be significantly higher in the glucosamine group. None of the clients in this trial were obese (body mass index [BMI] ≥30); so the potential for this supplement to improve osteoarthritis in heavier clients (a group that commonly experiences this condition) is unknown. In addition, the potential side effects of glucosamine are unknown at this time. It is important to note that glucosamine sulfate was the only form of glucosamine tested in this large trial.

Reference
Reginster, J.Y., et al. (2001). Long-term effects of glucosamine sulfate on osteoarthritis progression. *Lancet, 357,* 251-256.

■ Surgical Management of Hip Osteoarthritis

Osteotomy. Osteotomy is a surgical fracture, a cut across a bone with resection of a bone fragment either to correct a valgus (knock-kneed) or varus (bow-legged) deformity or to alter stresses on a joint. In early hip OA, when joint congruency still exists and motion is relatively normal, proximal femoral osteotomy may be performed. A wedge of bone is removed from the region of the lesser trochanter to realign the angle of the femoral neck and shaft. Partial weight-bearing is required for at least 3 months after surgery to allow healing of the osteotomy site. Because manifestations of OA generally progress despite this procedure, a large number of clients will require additional surgery. Osteotomy is more frequently performed on clients in their 40s, with the full expectation that total joint replacement will be needed in the future.

Arthrodesis. In an arthrodesis (joint fusion) procedure, the articular joint surfaces, which hold the bone ends together, are removed so that the bone edges unite like a fracture. Initial fixation may be provided with pins, braces, or casts. Arthrodesis is indicated for irreparable joint damage or instability. The procedure produces a sound, painless limb, but the resulting loss of movement may be a serious disadvantage in large joints such as the hip or knee.

Hip arthrodesis remains the operation of choice for the active client less than 55 years of age with advanced unilateral OA, severe post-traumatic arthritis, or septic arthritis. Hip arthroplasty would require lifestyle alterations, whereas arthrodesis allows a more normal lifestyle. Hip fusion can result in shortening of the affected extremity by 1 to 1.5 inches, and the client commonly needs a shoe lift postoperatively to help maintain a normal gait. Knee arthrodesis is often seen as a salvage procedure in response to conditions such as infection, malignant or aggressive tumors, painful Charcot or neuropathic arthropathy, or severe ligamentous instability. Knee fusion results in shortening of the affected leg by about 0.5 inch, which usually does not create significant postoperative dysfunction.

Total Hip Arthroplasty (Replacement). Total hip arthroplasty (THA) or replacement (THR) is performed to restore joint motion by replacing arthritic bone with metal components. (See Chapter 79 for a discussion of shoulder, elbow, and hand arthroplasty.)

Indications. Indications for THA include (1) failure of conservative treatments, (2) severe compromise of the client's functional ability, and (3) significant pain. The client's subjective complaints frequently have a greater impact on the decision for surgery than do radiologic changes of the joint. THA may also be performed for complications of femoral neck fractures, congenital disease or deformity, and failure of previous fixations or arthroplasties.

Both *cemented* and *noncemented* hip arthroplasties can be performed. Use of polymethyl-methacrylate (PMMA) bone cement allows immediate intraoperative fixation of femoral and acetabular components. Cemented prostheses are used for older clients or for those with compromised bone strength resulting from conditions such as osteoporosis. In younger, active, or heavier clients, loosening of the component at the bone-cement interface may become a problem. For these clients, use of prostheses with porous surfaces allows fixation without cement. Instead, bone grows into the porous surface as the client remains on limited weight-bearing status for a number of weeks after surgery. Although short-term outcomes of the two procedures are equivalent, long-term results must be determined to justify the cost of noncemented surgical technology. Many hospitals and orthopedic surgeons currently use a "demand matching" system to choose appropriately between cemented or noncemented components based on client needs.

Contraindications. Contraindications to THA include (1) recent or active joint sepsis (except in joint revision due to infection), (2) neutrotrophic joints, or (3) an inability to cooperate with immediate postoperative requirements or long-term joint rehabilitation. In addition, the client's general health must allow tolerance of anesthesia, blood loss, and surgical stress. Heart, lung, liver, and metabolic disorders should be stable before surgery.

Surgical Techniques. A common prosthesis currently in use is a three-component set: (1) the femoral neck and stem, (2) a slide-on femoral head, and (3) a metal acetabulum with or without fixation screw holes. Hip prostheses may be made of several different metal alloys that contribute to the relative lightness and durability of the components (Figure 28-3).

Depending on physician preference and on the type of exposure needed for the procedure, the surgical approach may be (1) anterolateral, (2) direct lateral, (3) transtrochanteric, or (4) posterolateral. The nurse must know the surgical approach to understand the leg position used to dislocate the operative hip. If that position is replicated after surgery, the client's risk for dislocating the hip prosthesis increases.

With an *anterolateral* position, the client lies supine on the table. The operative hip is externally rotated and extended, and the knee is flexed. With the *posterolateral* position, the client lies on his or her side with the operative hip internally rotated, flexed, and adducted. Many orthopedic surgeons use the posterolateral position for the anterior and posterior approaches.

Once the hip has been exposed, the surgeon performs an osteotomy of the femoral neck to expose the

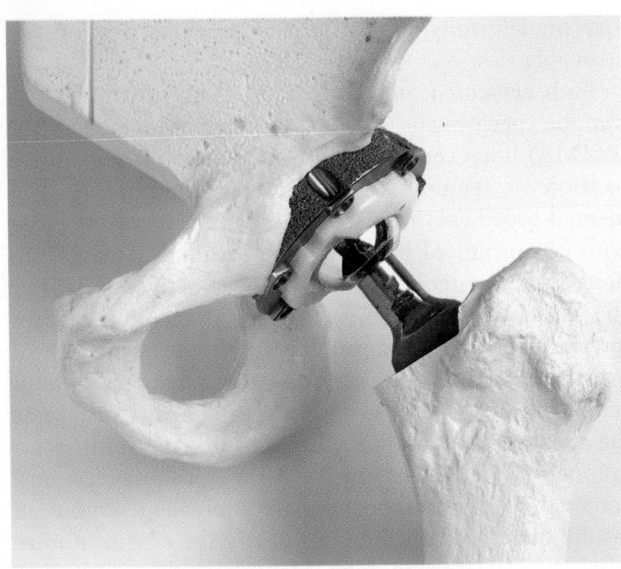

FIGURE 28-3 Hip prostheses. (Courtesy of Biomet Orthopedics, Inc., Warsaw, IN.)

acetabulum. Osteophytes and cysts are removed from the acetabulum to prepare it for reaming and for the prosthesis. Trial prostheses are placed, and their fit is evaluated before the final choice of appropriately sized components. If the prosthesis is to be *press-fit (noncemented)*, the bone is prepared for pegs or spikes. The surgeon presses the cup firmly into place and evaluates its apposition to the bone. If a *cemented* prosthesis is used, anchor holes are drilled into the iliac subchondral bone. After cleaning the bone thoroughly with pressure-pulsed lavage, the surgeon cements the cup into position.

To prepare the femur, the surgeon forms a tunnel by reaming the bone's intramedullary canal. After placement of a trial prosthesis, the hip is reduced to assess for motion, stability, and length. If the results are acceptable, the surgeon removes the trial components. For a press-fit prosthesis, the femoral stem is pressed into the reamed intramedullary canal. For a cemented prosthesis, the femur is cleaned and the canal is plugged to prevent the cement from traveling too far distally. The surgeon fills the canal with cement, inserting the femoral stem and then placing the femoral head. After the hip is reduced, the surgeon evaluates the extremity for motion, stability, and length.

Before closing the incision (~10 inches long), the surgeon may place a closed wound drainage system, such as a Hemovac, to help prevent hematoma, which can increase the risk of infection. The use of wound drainage systems has decreased in recent years, however, because they have been found to be ineffective in preventing hematomas while possibly increasing the risk of blood loss and contamination of the surgical wound. Instead, wound drainage may be collected for a limited time through a cell-saving device such as an OrthoPAT or a suctioned autotransfusion device such as the Autovac.

The collected blood is returned to the client as a postoperative transfusion, and then the device is discontinued.

A recent trend in THA is to perform the surgery through much smaller incisions. This procedure allows the client to ambulate more quickly with less pain.

Complications. The in-hospital mortality rate after THA is very low. Many other postoperative complications are short-lived and reversible, but some of them can have a great impact on the client's physical and psychological recovery from surgery. The most common and most serious complication is venous thromboembolism, which can occur in as many as 57% of clients if anticoagulant therapy is not administered.[33] Prevention **EB** of deep vein thrombosis (DVT) or pulmonary embolism (PE) requires early mobilization, often with a combination of pharmacologic and nonpharmacologic methods (see also Chapter 53).

Infection following a THA is a serious concern because of the possible development of osteomyelitis. Prophylactic antibiotics are considered essential, and careful wound assessment must begin immediately after surgery. Bladder or urinary tract infection is also possible because of urinary stasis or the presence of an indwelling urinary catheter. Because any localized infection can also spread to the wound, prompt recognition and treatment of clinical manifestations are imperative.

Postoperative joint instability increases the risk for dislocation or subluxation. The risk is even greater after revision arthroplasty because of the extended surgical exposure and soft tissue deficiencies. All clients require monitoring and education about the positions that should be avoided while soft tissues heal around the new joint. Positioning precautions are continued for about 6 weeks, until the surgical incision has healed and the client's periarticular muscle tone has improved.

After surgery with the commonly used posterolateral approach, the client must avoid positions of extreme hip flexion (>90 degrees), adduction, or internal rotation. Appropriate postoperative positioning requires an extended hip that is maintained in external rotation and abduction, often by using a foam wedge. An anterolateral approach is used less often. The client must maintain the hip in hyperflexion, adduction, and internal rotation. After this surgical approach, the client can sit up at 90 degrees of hip flexion without increasing the risk of dislocation.

Outcomes. A THA commonly results in immediate reduction of the client's pain. Surgical or incisional pain is often described as substantially less than the "bone-on-bone" pain of OA, and it is frequently more manageable with postoperative analgesia. The client's functional status improves over the course of rehabilitation and usually reaches its optimal level by 1 year after surgery. With the current emphasis on wellness, an increased number of clients now desire to resume sports activities after hip surgery. High activity levels are associated with decreased longevity for replacement components; however, low-impact activities, such as walking or hiking, swimming, bicycling, intermediate snow skiing, doubles tennis, golf, and bowling, are considered fairly safe for client participation and contribute greatly to improved quality of life after surgery.

Revision surgery may be a future consideration because of prosthetic loosening or other complications such as fracture of the femoral shaft, repeated dislocation, osteolysis, or heterotrophic bone formation. Because of improved techniques for cement insertion and the increased use of press-fit prostheses, loosening now occurs less commonly following THA.

■ Nursing Management of the Surgical Client: Total Hip Arthroplasty

In the current managed care environment, clients who have undergone THA typically do not remain in the acute care hospital setting for more than 4 or 5 days after a THA. They may be discharged to a rehabilitation unit, extended care facility, or even home. Although there is no universally accepted rehabilitation program after THA, coordination of care in the perioperative period speeds the client's recovery and return to independent living.

Preoperative Care
Assessment

Because most clients are admitted to the hospital on the day of surgery, the preadmission assessment of their physical and psychological readiness is currently accomplished in a variety of ways. Telephone interviews may be used, but many hospitals invite clients into a preoperative clinic for nursing assessment and for laboratory tests or x-rays. Some programs also arrange home visits to allow a physical therapist or nurse to assess the client's ambulation and the safety of the home. Discharge needs can often be identified based on the home environment and the extent of support available to the client.

Diagnosis, Outcomes, Interventions

Diagnosis: Deficient Knowledge. The client's previous inexperience with hospitalization and surgery in general, or with THA and its postoperative restrictions, may be described with the nursing diagnosis of Deficient Knowledge. The diagnosis can be written *Deficient Knowledge related to prior inexperience with surgery (total hip replacement).*

Outcomes. The client will demonstrate understanding of the proposed surgery, postoperative restrictions, and rehabilitation as evidenced by statements and adherence to the postoperative regimen.

Interventions. A common strategy for providing information about the details of hospitalization for THA is the use of a group class or "total joint camp." Clients receive information about various topics, from preoperative strengthening exercises and nothing-by-mouth (NPO) requirements to postoperative pain management and dietary advances. Topics include autologous blood donation and other transfusion options. Clients also often have the opportunity to use a walker or crutches for the first time as they are coached by a nurse or physical therapist. Instructors emphasize appropriate positioning precautions to prevent postoperative hip dislocation. Because poor dentition is also a potential infection source, the client should be encouraged preoperatively to achieve and maintain good oral hygiene.

Evaluation

Clients will provide a simple explanation of the surgery and verbalize their role in recovery. Mild anxiety may heighten the client's receptiveness to information, but severe anxiety can be a powerful barrier to learning. Provide frequent reinforcement of teaching, and encourage the client to ask questions about unclear information.

Postoperative Care

General care of clients after THA does not differ greatly from the usual care provided for any postoperative client. (For a review of general postoperative care, see Chapter 16.) After a THA, however, the client cannot assist with turning and repositioning. Prop up the client with pillows to maintain a side-lying position, and then return the client to a supine position on a 2-hour schedule. Do not turn the client to the operative side unless ordered by the physician. Because of the client's impaired mobility, pay careful attention to maintenance of skin integrity. A pressure-reduction mattress overlay may be indicated, especially if the client is frail or malnourished. Heels should be floated off the bed to reduce pressure ulcers.

Indwelling urinary catheters are not routinely used because of the risk of infection, but women are still likely to have a catheter because of the difficulty of positioning on a bedpan or transferring to a bedside commode in the immediate postoperative period. Perform perineal and catheter care carefully, recognizing the client's surgical pain and positioning precautions. Men will need assistance to sit or stand at the bedside to void.

Assessment

Frequent assessment of neurovascular status is imperative after a THA. Assess both legs for color, warmth, capillary refill, pedal pulses, movement, and sensation. Compare the surgical leg with the unaffected lower extremity. Report any deficits promptly to the surgeon.

Ensure that the client's postoperative position is maintained in accordance with specified hip precautions.

The surgical dressing applied at the end of the procedure, used to create pressure and promote hemostasis, is often bulky. It is left in place until removed by the surgeon or with a surgeon's specific order, usually 1 to 3 days after surgery. It should be regularly assessed for excessive drainage, however, and may be reinforced according to the surgeon's preference. After removal of the original dressing, the wound is covered with a light dressing or left open to air as ordered by the surgeon. Incisions left open to air do need to be covered for showering; use a transparent occlusive dressing. Afterward, carefully examine the wound to be certain that no water has seeped through the dressing because excessive wetness can interfere with wound healing.

In addition, a closed wound drainage system, such as a Hemovac, may be in place. Drainage is usually less than 200 ml/8 hr (or 600 ml/24 hr), but this amount can be increased if the client has been heavily hydrated. Measure drain output, and promptly report excessive drainage to the surgeon. If a cell-saver or autotransfusion device has been used, postoperative transfusion will be accomplished in accordance with hospital and surgeon protocols.

Diagnosis, Outcomes, Interventions

Diagnosis: Acute Pain and Chronic Pain.

Acute pain is expected after any surgery, including THA. The diagnosis can be written as *Acute Pain and Chronic Pain related to local tissue trauma from surgical incision.*

Outcomes. The client will demonstrate comfort as evidenced by reporting a tolerable level of pain, using decreasing amounts of analgesia, being able to move without grimacing, and stating that the pain is not interfering with rest or physical therapy.

Interventions. In the immediate postoperative period, the client may experience intense pain and may require injected opioid analgesics to attain acceptable control. Common interventions include patient-controlled analgesia (PCA) or epidural analgesia. Within 24 to 48 hours, the client should be tolerating fluids and able to take oral analgesics. Because pain is intensified with movement, the client may attempt to limit activity because of the expected increase in discomfort. Medicate the client before physical therapy or activities such as showering, and reinforce the importance of ambulation in decreasing risk for postoperative complications. Although THA can reduce pain in the operative joint, the client with arthritis in other joints continues to experience chronic pain. Once postoperative hemostasis has been achieved, the client's usual NSAID may be ordered to address chronic pain in nonsurgical joints.

Regularly assess for side effects of opioid analgesics. Respiratory depression is more likely with PCA or epidural analgesia than with oral opioids. Use pulse oximetry and regular assessment of vital signs to assess the client's respiratory status. Constipation, a common problem after THA, is related to the client's impaired mobility, opioid use, and slow progression to a regular diet. Encourage the client's intake of fluids and dietary fiber. In addition, stool softeners or laxatives may be indicated. If the client regularly uses a bulk-forming laxative or other strategy to maintain bowel regularity at home, assist the client in continuing that program in the hospital. Regular assessment and implementation of a proactive bowel program are important to minimize client concerns about bowel elimination. Interventions should ensure that the client has had a bowel movement before discharge from the acute hospital setting.

Diagnosis: Impaired Physical Mobility.

The client's degree of immobility after a THA will be affected by pain and fear of movement as well as by arthritic limitations in other joints. The diagnosis can be written as *Impaired Physical Mobility related to pain or fear of movement.*

Outcomes. The client will demonstrate improved physical mobility as evidenced by the need for less assistance in transfers (bed to chair, bed to standing), by safe use of a walker or crutches, and by the ability to ambulate a functional distance (150 feet).

Interventions. Moving the client after a THA can create much anxiety for both the client and the nursing staff. First, be aware of any weight-bearing limitations ordered for the client before transfer. Following a THA with a cemented prosthesis, the client is often allowed to put as much weight as desired on the operative extremity. This order is written as WBAT (weight-bearing as tolerated) or FWB (full weight-bearing). Although incisional pain may keep the client from putting full body weight on the operative extremity, he or she can safely put weight through the leg without harming the prosthesis. If the surgery was accomplished with a noncemented prosthesis, the physician may order NWB (non–weight-bearing), TTWB (toe-touch weight-bearing), or PWB (partial weight-bearing with a percentage specified, e.g., 25%). If the client is not allowed to bear full weight, pay careful attention to the operative extremity during transfers to ensure that the client avoids placing any weight on the leg.

In addition to postoperative limitations, the client may suffer from arthritis in other joints that increases pain and affects the ability to transfer from the bed to the chair. While in-bed exercises may begin the day of surgery, the client is not usually ready to attempt transfer to a bedside chair until the morning after surgery. When the client stands and transfers for the first time, the assistance of at least two staff members will be required. Use of appropriate technique will ensure a safe transfer for the client and will minimize the risk of injury to the staff member's lower back.

Transfer the Client. All intravenous (IV) lines, urinary catheters, wound drains, and oxygen tubing should be freed for ready movement. Although typically you will determine the side of the bed for transfer, the client usually moves away from the operative side. If the bedside chair has brakes, they should be locked before client transfer is made. The client should also be wearing shoes or slippers with non-skid soles. Staff should assist the client to the edge of the bed, maintaining the operative leg position in accordance with appropriate hip precautions. Encourage the client to push off the bed with his or her arms to reach a sitting position; however, because of weakness in the hip abductors and upper arms, the client may need help to pivot in bed and to sit up.

Once the client is seated at the edge of the bed, apply a gait belt to the client's waist to help with transfer. Use of the gait belt allows you to help with standing and transfer without risking injury to yourself. If the client becomes dizzy or starts to fall, the gait belt also helps you to control the client's movement to the floor or back onto the bed. Place the walker directly in front of the client, ready for use once he or she is standing; however, do not use it to help the client to a standing position because it is not stable.

To help the client to stand, first position your foot in front of the client's foot to keep it from slipping on the floor. Standing close to the client, grasp the gait belt and encourage the client to push off the bed with his or her hands. Once the client is standing, he or she can grasp the walker and pause for a moment to take slow, deep breaths as needed.

Remain aware of the risk for falling, and ask the client about dizziness—a manifestation of orthostatic hypotension—before attempting the final transfer to the chair. To help increase awareness of surroundings, encourage the client to stand erect when using the walker rather than stooping over and looking at the floor. With coaching about weight-bearing status, the client should need no more than a few pivoting movements with the walker to reach the chair. Remind the client not to attempt to sit until he or she can feel the chair seat against the back of his or her legs. Then the client should reach back to grasp the arms of the chair and lower himself or herself slowly to a sitting position. You can assist the client by grasping the gait belt and guiding descent into the chair. Pay close attention to maintaining flexion restrictions. For example, keeping the client's operative leg in a relaxed position, with the knee slightly lower than the hip, allows maintenance of precautions regarding hip flexion related to a posterolateral surgical approach. The

gait belt can be loosened after the client is safely settled in the chair.

When the client is ready to return to the bed, coach him or her to slide forward to the edge of the chair, and tighten the gait belt around the client's waist. Again, remind the client to keep the knee slightly lower than the hip as a positioning precaution. With the walker in position in front of the chair, the client uses the arms of the chair to push to a standing position before grasping the walker. Using the same ambulation process, return the client to bed and help him or her to a supine position. Maintain leg position according to individual hip precautions.

Introduce Additional Client Exercises. If the client is alert postoperatively, in-bed exercises are often begun the afternoon of surgery. Coach the client in the use of ankle pumps and quadriceps and gluteal isometrics ("quad sets" or "glute sets"). Transfers and ambulation with a physical therapist generally begin the morning after surgery. In addition, the therapist may perform gentle active and assisted ROM exercises. The client will continue exercises that improve ROM and strengthen hip muscles, occasionally receiving physical therapy at home or on an outpatient basis after discharge from the acute hospital setting.

Because of its stability, a walker is often used by older clients to assist with ambulation. If the client has arthritis in the shoulders or hands, a special walker with arm platforms may be indicated. Walkers also necessitate less energy expenditure for the client who has respiratory disease. Crutches may be used if the client has no balance problems.

Diagnosis: Risk for Peripheral Neurovascular Dysfunction. Surgery on any joint carries a risk for neurologic or vascular impairment. Be aware of the potential for compartment syndrome and nerve injury related to edema or extremity positioning that places pressure on the peroneal nerve. The diagnosis can be written as *Risk for Peripheral Neurovascular Dysfunction related to lower extremity edema or positioning.*

Outcomes. The client will demonstrate normal neurovascular status as evidenced by adequate peripheral pulses with capillary refill time of 3 seconds or less and by the absence of sensory impairments and motor weakness in the operative extremity.

Interventions. Assess the neurovascular status of the operative extremity at least every 4 hours or as directed by the surgeon. More frequent monitoring may be indicated by the client's condition. Assess the presence and quality of bilateral pedal pulses, skin color and temperature of the extremities, capillary refill in the toes, sensation and movement of the toes, and the client's ability to perform dorsiplantar flexion of the feet. As part of your assessment of motor function, flex and extend the client's toes yourself. If the client feels more pain from passive stretch than active motion, you should be suspicious of compartment syndrome. Compare current assessments to baseline data. Report any new pallor or coolness, numbness or tingling, or inability to move the extremity promptly to the surgeon.

Diagnosis: Risk for Injury.
Because the hip is unstable as the surgical incision heals, the risk for dislocation of the prosthesis is a significant concern after a THA. Client education and attention to hip positioning precautions are essential. The diagnosis can be written as *Risk for Injury related to prosthesis dislocation.*

Outcomes.
The client will have reduced risk of injury (hip dislocation) as evidenced by demonstrating understanding of the risk for hip dislocation, verbalizing and following positioning precautions while at bed rest, and during ambulation or transfers.

Interventions.
After a THA, assess the client's position frequently to ensure that precautions related to the specific surgical approach are maintained. Remind the client of appropriate precautions through the use of instructional handouts or fliers that can be posted at the head of the bed. Performance of prescribed exercises, such as gluteal isometrics, also strengthens muscles surrounding the joint capsule and decreases the risk for dislocation.

If the surgeon has used a posterolateral approach, the client should not flex the hip beyond a 90-degree angle, should not bend over to tie or slip on shoes, and should not reach for sheets that are fan-folded at the bottom of the bed. Special attention should be given to precautions when the client is getting in and out of bed or a chair. To avoid extremes of flexion, the client will need an elevated toilet seat (at least 21 inches high). The client should not cross his or her legs and should not inwardly rotate the operative leg.

To help maintain precautions after the posterolateral approach, the client may use a triangular foam abduction pillow placed between the legs and secured with straps (Figure 28-4). Use of the pillow prevents adduction and flexion of the operative hip; however, you must carefully position the straps to avoid placing pressure on the client's peroneal nerve. Instead of an abduction pillow, some surgeons order a knee immobilizer to be worn on the surgical leg. It serves primarily as a reminder to the client of mobility restrictions for that extremity. When using a walker, the client should be coached to point toes outward slightly. This position avoids internal rotation, particularly when the client is turning toward the operative side. Hip precautions must also be followed when the client is turned from back to side. The abductor pillow is left in place, and the client's side-lying position is maintained through the use of pillows at his or her back. Special precautions are needed to prevent the heel from developing a pressure ulcer. Be certain that the heels are free from pressure when the abductor pillow is attached to the legs.

If the surgeon has used an anterolateral approach, precautions are almost the opposite of those for the posterolateral approach. Because the client should avoid active abduction, the legs should be maintained side by side without a pillow or wedge between them. When the client walks, he or she should avoid turning the toes and knee outward. The operative leg should not be extended backward. To help maintain anterolateral precautions, place the tray table and phone on the client's operative side.

To help the client maintain appropriate hip precautions, an occupational therapist may suggest several assistive devices. Long-handled shoe horns, sock donners, and reachers help the client avoid extreme hip flexion and provide more independence in dressing. The therapist or case manager can also assist the client in acquiring bathroom equipment, such as an elevated toilet seat and shower chair, for use after discharge. Reinforce the importance of using these devices to decrease the risk of hip dislocation.

Diagnosis: Risk for Infection.
After a THA, the client is at increased risk for joint infection that may lead to the development of osteomyelitis. Although the inci-

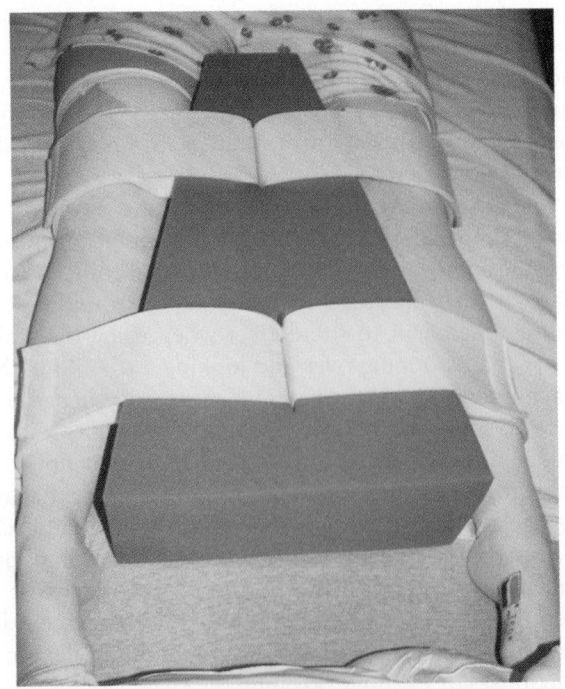

FIGURE 28-4 Abduction wedge is used to prevent hip adduction and flexion after a total hip arthroplasty using a posterior surgical approach.

dence of infection is low, it is a great concern as a factor in possible surgical failure, leading to removal of the prosthetic components. Joint replacements that are close to the skin surface or that have limited soft tissue coverage, as in a thin client, are at increased risk for infection. *Revision* THR carries an increased infection rate compared with *primary* THR because of the longer operative time and the larger surgical exposure. The diagnosis can be written as *Risk for Infection related to surgical procedure (total hip replacement)*.

Outcomes. The client will have reduced risk of wound infection as evidenced by normal temperature and white blood cell (WBC) count, the absence of purulent drainage from the wound, and the absence of redness or inflammation at the surgical site.

Interventions. Prophylactic IV antibiotics are routinely ordered immediately before surgery because of the risk of infection following a THA. The first dose is typically given before the surgical incision is made, and antibiotics are continued for 2 to 3 days postoperatively. If surgical drains are used to remove wound exudate, they should be emptied at least once each shift using aseptic technique. Because the drainage can harbor pathogens, note its color and odor and promptly report any abnormalities to the surgeon. Also routinely assess the surgical site for redness or purulent drainage. Use of staples is associated with a lower infection rate, but delays in wound healing can suggest superficial infection. Perform dressing changes using strict aseptic technique. Take the client's temperature at regular intervals, and perform careful assessments to determine the cause of any fever.

Increasing joint pain after superficial wound healing is also a possible manifestation of delayed deep infection. Instruct the client to report this manifestation promptly to the physician and to inform other health care providers of the surgery.

Diagnosis: Risk for Impaired Skin Integrity.
After a THA, the client is at high risk for pressure ulcers as a result of decreased physical mobility. Clients are often unable to change positions in bed without a great deal of assistance. Clients are also at risk for tape injury with dressing changes. This risk is due to (1) skin changes that occur in older adults, (2) intraoperative positioning and joint manipulation that lead to soft tissue edema, (3) the type of tape used to secure postoperative dressings, and (4) the method and direction of tape application. The diagnosis can be written as *Risk for Impaired Skin Integrity related to decreased physical mobility or to the application of tape with dressing changes*.

Outcomes. The client will demonstrate intact skin as evidenced by an absence of ulcers over bony prominences

and an absence of epidermal stripping beneath the tape used to secure postoperative dressings.

Interventions. To decrease the risk of pressure ulcer development, assist the THA client with position changes on a regular schedule in the immediate postoperative period. As the client regains mobility, he or she will also regain independence in position changes. Carefully assess the skin over bony prominences such as the sacrum and coccyx, scapulae, elbows, and heels. In addition to using a regular turning schedule, assess the need for a pressure-reducing mattress on the client's bed. Pressure on heels can be relieved, depending on surgeon preference, by using a towel roll for brief periods under the Achilles tendon or elevating the calf on a thin pillow.

Avoid epidermal stripping by placing postoperative dressings over a skin sealant that is applied wherever the tape touches the skin. Elastic tape should be placed vertically (superior to inferior) without tension to allow for stretching related to postoperative edema. Evaluate any redness, blistering, or epidermal stripping, and consult an enterostomal nurse specialist about the client's care as appropriate.

Collaborative Problem: Risk for Deep Vein Thrombosis.
Venous thromboembolism, the most common complication after a THA, can be manifested as DVT. Risk factors include a surgical procedure longer than 30 minutes, advanced client age, previous history of thromboembolism, venous stasis, cardiac conditions such as heart failure or dysrhythmias, lower extremity trauma, obesity, use of oral contraceptives, sepsis, malignancy, long-term immobilization, stroke, and pregnancy. Clots may form in the calf and travel to the popliteal fossa or the thigh. This collaborative problem can be written as *Risk for Deep Vein Thrombosis related to surgical procedure and immobility* (or other identified risk factors).

Outcomes. The nurse will monitor for the early manifestations of DVT: unilateral calf or thigh pain, redness, or edema.

Interventions. Routinely assess the client for evidence of thrombophlebitis: excessive pain, unilateral edema, or a red vein track. Homans' sign is a more nonspecific indicator. The client may have thrombophlebitis but have a negative Homans' sign. Conversely, a positive Homans' sign can result from other conditions, such as shin splints. Many clients have asymptomatic blood clots.

To decrease the risk of DVT, various pharmacologic and nonpharmacologic interventions are used. Early mobilization is a key factor in decreasing DVT risk. Encourage the client to perform ankle pumps regularly because they contract the calf muscles, simulating the movements of ambulation and encouraging venous blood return to the heart. Physical agents such as pneumatic compression devices and elastic compression stockings are commonly used; these modalities may be used individually or together, and they should be applied **EB** to both legs to promote adequate venous return (see Chapter 55). Compression devices or stockings should be worn until the client is fully ambulatory and should be removed only for brief periods for bathing and skin assessment. The pneumatic devices should be applied even when the client is sitting in a chair at the bedside because the dependent position of the lower extremities can contribute to increased venous stasis.

Pharmacologic agents used to decrease the risk of DVT include aspirin, low-dose heparin, low-molecular-**EB** weight heparin (LMWH), and warfarin sodium. A new synthetic anticoagulant, fondaparinux (Arixtra), was approved in early 2002 for reducing the risk of blood clots following THA, TKA, and hip fracture. LMWH, which does not require laboratory monitoring, works quickly to bring about anticoagulation. Warfarin is slower to reach therapeutic blood levels but is less expensive and easier for the client to take after discharge. A prothrombin time, with results reported as an International Normalized Ratio (INR) is ordered to monitor the effects of warfarin. Promptly report laboratory results to the surgeon to allow timely ordering of the current day's dose.

Extensive education about anticoagulants is essential to maximize their effectiveness and to minimize the likelihood of complications. Inform the client of manifestations of internal bleeding, such as tarry stools, rust-colored or tea-colored urine, hematemesis, and abdominal or flank pain. Explain that even a minor cut will bleed for a longer time. Instruct the client to apply direct pressure, for example, following a shaving cut or a cut with a kitchen knife. Urge clients to seek immediate evaluation for any head injury because significant intracranial bleeding can occur in response to even minor trauma if an anticoagulant is being taken. If the client is to take warfarin, reinforce the importance of consistent intake of foods that contain vitamin K (e.g., green leafy vegetables). Many of these foods are nutritionally important and should not be totally avoided, particularly by clients with a history of heart disease who follow a low-fat diet. If the client will be discharged with a prescription for LMWH, start instruction on injection technique early enough in the hospital to allow ample time for practice and reinforcement.

If you suspect a blood clot, notify the surgeon immediately. Venography or Doppler ultrasound of the leg is commonly used in the diagnosis of DVT. If the test reveals the presence of a clot, the client will be placed on bed rest with the leg elevated to promote venous return. A continuous heparin infusion and warfarin are often initiated at the same time, with the infusion continuing until shortly before discharge, and a warfarin prescription is written for home use. The surgeon may order calf measurements to aid in the detection of increased swelling related to DVT.

Because of the risk of pulmonary embolism, you must frequently assess the client's respiratory status. A clot in the leg can dislodge and move to the lung, typically causing dyspnea, anxiety, and a pleuritic chest pain. Because pulmonary embolism is often fatal, address suspicious manifestations immediately.

Evaluation

Goals should be mutually established by the client and an interdisciplinary care team that includes a surgeon, a nurse, physical and occupational therapists, and case manager. A list of goals can be posted in the client's hospital room as a reminder of the focus for each postoperative day. Clinical pathways are commonly used to map the care of clients after a THA because of the consistent postoperative needs of this population. Pathways help providers limit the number of tasks, such as laboratory orders, that may be forgotten or overlooked. Outcomes are often also indicated on the clinical pathway to track client progress consistently. Pathways often extend from admission through acute care to client rehabilitation in another setting. They also allow for later review of discrepancies or "outliers," that is, those clients whose experiences do not conform to the usual postoperative course. See the Clinical Pathway feature on Total Hip Replacement on the website.

evolv

■ Self-Care

The typical acute hospital stay after THA is 4 to 5 days. Because many clients require additional rehabilitation, they are sent from the hospital to rehabilitation centers or extended care facilities until they regain functional independence. Clients can be discharged home if they can transfer independently to and from the bed, walk alone a functional distance of 150 feet on a flat surface, and safely negotiate stairs.

Provide discharge instructions to the client and any family members or friends who will serve as support persons during the recovery period. The client must understand the hip precautions indicated by the surgical approach (anterolateral or posterolateral) to avoid dislocation. Precautions may continue for 6 months to a year after surgery, depending on the surgeon's assessment of soft tissue healing around the joint capsule.

Assistive devices, such as a walker or crutches and bathroom equipment, should be available for immediate use at home. The client will progress from walker to crutches or cane as muscle strength increases, perhaps within 4 to 6 weeks after surgery if a cemented prosthesis was used. Clients with a noncemented prosthesis may have limited weight-bearing (e.g., TTWB) for 6 weeks, followed by WBAT with the use of a crutch for another 6 weeks.

Clients frequently have questions about driving or returning to work. Clients with sedentary occupations may be cleared by the surgeon to drive and to return to work within 6 to 8 weeks. They may be counseled, however, to take regular breaks to avoid extended periods of sitting. It may be 3 months before a client can return to an occupation that requires lifting and bending, and activity will remain limited even after going back to work. Low-level physical activity, such as walking or swimming, is usually approved by the surgeon.

Depending on surgeon preference, the client may be allowed to shower after discharge. Safety measures, such as a nonslip mat and handrails in the shower area, are important. The client should not soak in a tub because water can enter the incision, increasing the risk of infection. Getting in or out of a tub may also violate hip precautions. The client can consume a regular diet but should also continue to be aware of any bowel elimination needs. Sexual activity typically can be resumed without discomfort as long as the client observes hip precautions.

The client should understand any medications, such as anticoagulants, that will be taken after discharge and should note follow-up laboratory and surgeon appointments. If the surgeon has ordered home care services or outpatient therapy, provide agency telephone numbers or locations for appointments. After a THA, prophylactic antibiotics are recommended whenever a transient bacteremia is expected, such as with dental work or a minor surgical procedure. The health care provider prescribes oral antibiotic coverage before the procedure.

In addition to bathroom safety features, the client may need other home modifications to aid independent recovery. Ramps, for example, may allow easier access to entrances. If the client lives in a multilevel home, encourage him or her to remain on a ground level until recovery is complete.

■ Surgical Management of Knee Osteoarthritis

After the hip and the spine, the knee is the third most common site of arthritic involvement. The knee, an extremely complex joint, actually demonstrates movement in three separate planes (Figure 28-5). Biomechanical stress during normal walking allows three times a person's body weight to be transmitted through the knee. Going up and down stairs increases the force to four or five times the body weight. The force is unevenly distributed, with the medial side of the knee often receiving the larger amount of stress. OA of the knee is better tolerated than OA of the hip, however, because the knee is not usually painful at rest.

Conservative treatment of OA of the knee is similar to that for the hip. Weight loss, activity modification, use of assistive devices, and use of analgesics or anti-inflammatory medications all help to decrease disease manifestations. Physical modalities such as idea of heat may also offer some pain reduction. Alternative therapies are also similar.

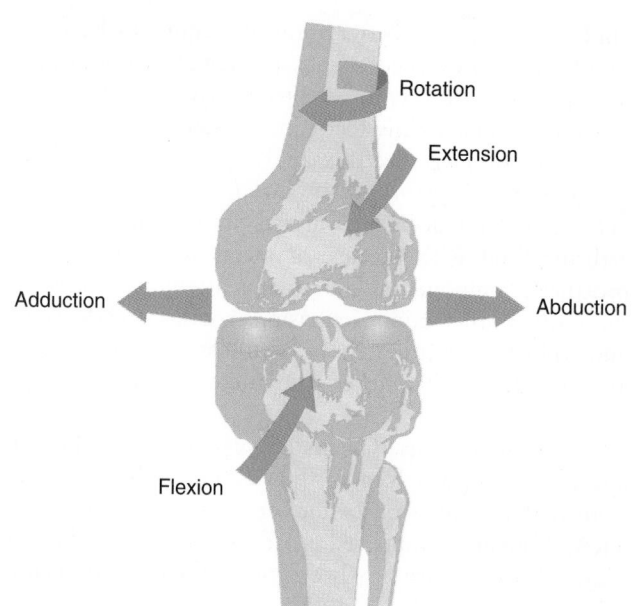

FIGURE 28-5 The knee is not just a simple hinge joint. Movement of the knee occurs in three separate planes. During normal gait, the knee moves through 70 degrees of flexion and extension, 10 degrees of abduction and adduction, and 10 to 15 degrees of internal and external rotation. (From Canale, S.L., & Canale, S.T. [2003]. *Campbell's operative orthopaedics.* [10th ed.] St. Louis: Mosby.)

Indications. If conservative interventions no longer control the client's manifestations, surgery may be appropriate. Options for OA management include (1) osteotomy, (2) arthrodesis, (3) unicompartmental knee arthroplasty (UKA), and (4) total knee arthroplasty (TKA). A tibial *osteotomy* may relieve the pain of knee OA by correcting the varus deformity (bow-leg) that follows wear of the medial compartment. Knee *arthrodesis* or fusion is indicated for young, active clients who are poor candidates for joint replacement surgery; fusion results in an immobile joint fixed in extension.

A recently introduced alternative to tibial osteotomy for the client with medial compartment osteoarthritis of the knee is the UniSpacer. For the client who has intact posterior and anterior cruciate ligaments and meets other clinical criteria, the UniSpacer can be inserted arthroscopically to restore normal knee alignment. An overnight hospital stay may be indicated, but recovery of motion is much quicker than with other invasive procedures.

Unicompartmental knee arthroplasty (UKA) is another alternative to osteotomy for clients who are 60 years of age or older, not obese, and relatively sedentary. Candidates for UKA must have an intact anterior cruciate ligament, no significant inflammation, and unicompartmental OA with no disease in other compartments of the knee. UKA was actually introduced more than 30 years ago and until recently has been a controversial surgical alternative. More precise client selection, improved implant design, and better surgical techniques have led to a higher initial success rate and fewer complications for UKA compared with osteotomy. The surgery generates less blood loss, and recovery is faster compared with osteotomy or TKA. See Box 28-1.

Total Knee Arthroplasty. Total knee arthroplasty (TKA), or replacement, allows resurfacing of the arthritic joint with the use of metal and polyethylene prosthetic components. The surgeon attempts to recreate the motions of flexion, extension, rotation, abduction, and adduction that may have been lost with progressive arthritis. TKA also relieves pain and corrects deformity.

Contraindications. Clients 65 years of age and older and those who weigh more than 200 pounds or are extremely active may be better served by alternatives to TKA, if possible. Improved prostheses and surgical techniques, however, are slowly extending the indications for

this procedure with younger clients. Conditions such as diabetes mellitus and peripheral vascular disease increase the client's risk for infection and delayed wound healing. Other contraindications are similar to those for prospective THA candidates.

Surgical Technique. Knee prostheses most commonly include three components: the femoral component, the tibial plate, and the patellar button (Figure 28-6). These tricompartmental prostheses vary in size to ensure the most accurate fit for each client. Some parts may also be specific for the right or left knee. A unicompartmental prosthesis, which is rarely used, replaces the femoral and tibial surfaces on only one side of the knee.

The surgical incision for TKA extends from 4 or 5 inches above the patella to 2 or 3 inches below it. The approach is either medial parapatellar or lateral parapatellar. Soft tissue is balanced across the joint, and the proximal tibia and distal femur are trimmed to fit the chosen prosthesis. Any flexion contractures or deformities (varus or valgus) may also be corrected. After os-

---

BOX 28-1	*Arthroscopic Surgery versus Placebo for Osteoarthritis of the Knee*

A recent randomized, blinded, placebo-controlled trial with a 2-year follow-up was conducted. The setting of the study was a Veterans Affairs medical center in Houston, Texas. A total of 180 clients who were less than or equal to 75 years of age (mean age 52 years, 93% men) had osteoarthritis of the knee as defined by the American College of Rheumatology, reported at least moderate knee pain despite maximal medical treatment for 6 or more months, and had not received arthroscopy in the previous 2 years were included in this unique study. Clients were allocated to 1 of 3 groups: lavage (n = 61), debridement (n = 59), or placebo (n = 60). The placebo group received three 1-cm skin incisions after first taking a short-acting tranquilizer and an opioid and while spontaneously breathing oxygen-enriched air.

Interestingly, lavage and debridement did not differ from placebo for pain in the study knee at 1 or 2 years or for any secondary outcome measure. Thus in clients with osteoarthritis of the knee, arthroscopic surgery did not relieve pain or improve function more than a placebo procedure. It should be noted that 44% of the eligible participants declined to participate, which raises the possibility of selection bias. The authors noted that, compared with those who declined, participants were younger, more likely to be Caucasian, and had more severe arthritis. It would have been valuable to observe follow-up data on those who declined to be randomized but who subsequently had either debridement or lavage. Regardless, this investigation does question the value of arthroscopic lavage and debridement in active men younger than 65 years of age with osteoarthritis of the knee.

Data from Moseley, J., et al. (2002). A controlled trial of arthroscopic surgery of the knee. *New England Journal of Medicine, 347,* 81-88.

FIGURE 28-6 Total knee prostheses. (Courtesy of Biomet Orthopedics, Inc., Warsaw, IN.)

teotomy the surgeon prepares the bone surfaces to accept the prosthesis based on the use of cemented or press-fit (noncemented) components. The patella is resurfaced with a polyethylene button after the surgeon ensures that the patellar prosthesis will track normally during flexion and extension of the knee.

Wound drains may be placed before closure of the incision, and a bulky pressure dressing applied. If the client is to start *continuous passive motion* (CPM) immediately, a lighter dressing is used. See the Evidence-Based Practice in Action feature on the Use of CPM After Total Knee Arthroplasty, below.

Complications. Infection, a potentially severe complication, occurs in 1% to 3% of TKA clients.[42] If it oc-
curs, venous thromboembolism can cause significant morbidity or death. Other complications may include patellar subluxation or dislocation, impaired wound healing, knee stiffness (inability to regain ROM), and loosening of the prosthesis.

■ Nursing Management of the Surgical Client: Total Knee Arthroplasty

Preoperative assessment and care are the same as for the client undergoing THA. Postoperative care concerns are also similar, but emphasis on knee exercise is greater because dislocation is not a significant risk. The goal of knee rehabilitation—to obtain maximal ROM with good muscle control—can be accomplished with consistent physical therapy or use of a CPM machine (Figure

---

EB EVIDENCE-BASED PRACTICE IN ACTION

Use of CPM After Total Knee Arthroplasty

One of the concerns following total knee arthroplasty (TKA) has been achieving optimal range of motion (ROM) for the client. Continuous passive motion (CPM) machines have been a popular intervention since their development. In recent years, however, research has examined the benefits of CPM versus rehabilitation through physical therapy.

In a study that compared three treatment modalities, the researchers wanted to determine which method of mobilization achieved the maximum ROM in the first 6 months following TKA.[1] Three treatment groups ($n = 40$/group) were established: standardized exercise and CPM, standardized exercise and slider board therapy, or standardized exercise alone. The three groups were similar with respect to age, gender, and diagnosis at the start of the study. Subjects were examined preoperatively, at the time of hospital discharge, and at 3 and 6 months after surgery. No differences were noted among the groups in knee ROM or in the WOMAC Osteoarthritis Index or the SF-36 scores. Researchers concluded that it is difficult to justify the use of adjunct ROM therapy such as the CPM or sliding board in addition to exercise sessions. As hospital stays continue to decrease for clients who have undergone TKA, their rehabilitation should emphasize active knee movement rather than passive therapy to promote functional independence.

Other researchers examined the effectiveness of CPM in improving postoperative function and ROM after TKA.[2] A group of clients was divided among three postoperative treatment regimens: no CPM ($n = 19$), CPM at 0 to 40 degrees ($n = 18$), and CPM at 0 to 70 degrees ($n = 20$). Those clients in the CPM groups used the machines for 48 hours; all clients had identical physical therapy treatment. Clients were assessed preoperatively, at 1 week, and at 1 year postoperatively. Although clients with CPM at 0 to 70 degrees did experience a significant increase in flexion and ROM at 1 week, no significant differences among the groups were noted at 1 year. In addition, researchers noted that those clients who had CPM had a significant increase
in analgesic requirement and in mean postoperative blood drainage. They concluded that CPM had no significant advantage in terms of improving knee function or ROM.

A third group of researchers had similar findings regarding the effects of CPM for clients transferred to a rehabilitation setting following TKA.[3] Knee ROM was measured on admission, on the third and seventh days of hospitalization and on discharge. One group of clients received CPM for 5 consecutive hours a day plus physical therapy; the other group received only physical therapy. The researchers found neither statistical nor clinical difference between the two groups. They concluded that the use of CPM in a rehabilitation setting has no benefit to clients admitted after a single TKA.

Implications

With decreased lengths of acute hospital stay for clients following TKA, the nurse must be prepared to assist them to regain functional independence by using strategies that promote knee ROM. The nurse can supplement physical therapy interventions by encouraging early and frequent ambulation to maximize ROM.

References

1. Beaupre, L.A., et al. (2001). Exercise combined with continuous passive motion or slider board therapy compared with exercise only: A randomized controlled trial of patients following total knee arthroplasty. *Physical Therapy, 81* (4), 1029-1037.

2. Pope, R.O., et al. (1997). Continuous passive motion after primary total knee arthroplasty. Does it offer any benefits? *Journal of Bone and Joint Surgery. British volume, 79* (6), 914-917.

3. Chen, B., et al. (2000). Continuous passive motion after total knee arthroplasty: A prospective study. *American Journal of Physical Medicine & Rehabilitation, 79* (5), 421-426.

28-7). This apparatus moves the knee slowly through its arc of motion, with settings determined by physician order. The machine, which is placed in a slightly abducted position on the bed, is frequently initiated at 0 degrees of extension and 10 to 40 degrees of flexion. Settings should be gradually and regularly increased, with the client and nurse working collaboratively to achieve the goal of 90 degrees of flexion.

According to surgeon preference, the client may be placed in the machine immediately after surgery. Some physicians delay initiation of CPM until the evening of surgery or the morning after surgery. The CPM machine should be used a minimum of 6 to 8 hours a day. The client must be supine during use of the CPM machine, with the head of the bed elevated no more than 15 degrees, and should thus be removed from the machine for meals. The client may also find it uncomfortable to use the CPM machine during sleep; this concern should be discussed with the surgeon.

When the client is out of the CPM, a knee immobilizer may be ordered to promote knee extension. Make sure that the immobilizer is of the correct length for the client and that it does not rub on the heel or groin. No pillows should be placed under the client's knee while in bed because this promotes flexion contracture.

Both ROM and strengthening exercises are an important part of functional recovery after TKA. Ankle pumps decrease the risk for blood clots in the lower extremities. The physical therapist may lead the client in active ROM exercises or may perform gentle passive ROM and stretching to increase knee flexion or extension. Isometric exercises to strengthen the quadriceps, hamstrings, and gluteal muscles are an important part of the regimen. Straight-leg raises also help with muscle strengthening. A home exercise program after hospital discharge includes ROM exercises and isometrics, with weekly increases in resistance as tolerated without producing joint irritation. To obtain optimal knee function, the client should continue exercises for at least 6 weeks after surgery.

FIGURE 28-7 A continuous passive motion exerciser allows the client to achieve early ROM. (Courtesy of the Chattanooga Group, Inc., Hixson, TN.)

The client is usually allowed to transfer from bed to chair within 24 hours after TKA. Carefully supporting the operative extremity, help the client move to a sitting position on the side of the bed. Coach the client to push off from the bed to stand in front of the walker before gripping it. Weight-bearing status is determined by surgeon order based on the use of cemented or noncemented components. The client with a cemented prosthesis is often allowed to bear weight as tolerated; NWB or TTWB is ordered for the client with a noncemented prosthesis. Once the client is in the chair, the operative leg can be elevated slightly for comfort or gently flexed to the floor. When the client has regained enough muscle strength to move the operative leg without assistance, crutch-walking can begin if desired. Use of the assistive device continues until the client has sufficient quadriceps function to ambulate independently.

METABOLIC BONE DISORDERS

Inappropriate functioning of the metabolic processes results in disorders manifested by changes in both physical and chemical structure of the bone. Disorders that alter bony equilibrium and affect bone turnover can be due to estrogen deficiency, parathyroid gland abnormalities, vitamin deficiency, malabsorption, or physical inactivity.

OSTEOPOROSIS

Osteoporosis is defined as a systemic skeletal disorder characterized by compromised bone strength predisposing to an increased risk of fracture. A fracture results when the osteoporotic bone encounters a force greater than it can withstand (e.g., trauma from a fall). The two components of bone strength include bone density and bone quality.

The term *osteopenia* refers to a low *bone mineral density* (BMD) compared with that expected for the person's gender and age. Persons with osteopenia have a greater risk for osteoporotic fracture than persons with normal or above-average density. Osteopenia is a risk factor for fracture just as hypertension is a risk factor for stroke.

In an attempt to assess the risk of osteoporotic fracture, the World Health Organization (WHO) has developed several general categories to clarify the definition of osteoporosis. The categories include the following:

1. *Normal*—a value for BMD or *bone mineral content* (BMC) that is not more than 1 standard deviation (SD) below the young adult mean value (Figure 28-8, *A*)
2. *Low bone mass (osteopenia)*—a value for BMD or BMC that lies between 1.0 and 2.5 SD below the young adult mean value
3. *Osteoporosis*—a value for BMD or BMC that is more than 2.5 SD below the young adult mean value (Figure 28-8, *B*)

4. *Severe (established) osteoporosis*—a value for BMD or BMC more than 2.5 SD below the young adult mean value *and* the presence of one or more fragility fractures

Osteoporosis is a major public health problem in many parts of the world, and its scope will increase as the population ages. It affects about 20% of postmenopausal white women in the United States. An additional 52% have osteopenia at the hip. One of every two women will experience a fracture at some point during her life. Nonwhite women and men are also at risk for osteoporotic fractures, although their risk is lower than that for white women.

Osteoporotic fractures also create a heavy economic burden. The annual cost to the health care system associated with osteoporotic fractures has been estimated at $17 billion (2001 dollars). A single hip fracture is estimated to cost $40,000. The number of hip fractures may increase three-fold by the year 2040. Thus any reduction in hip fractures would have a large impact on health care expenditures. (See the Complementary and Alternative Therapy feature on Vitamin A and an Increased Risk of Osteoporosis at right.)

Etiology and Risk Factors

Many factors, both genetic and environmental, are involved in the development of osteoporosis. Bone mass, which is measured by bone densitometry and reported as BMC or BMD, is an important risk factor in osteoporosis. To understand the relationship of bone density and risk of fracture, it is helpful to review some facts about bone mass.

Peak bone mass is the highest bone mass attained. Although longitudinal growth usually is complete by about age 20 years, consolidation of bone continues so that peak bone mass is not attained until about age 30 years

in both men and women. This is noteworthy because it indicates that interventions to increase peak mass can be effective up until about age 30.

What happens to bone mass in women between age 30 and menopause is uncertain. Most likely, bone mass plateaus until menopause or decreases slightly during

COMPLEMENTARY AND ALTERNATIVE THERAPY

Vitamin A and an Increased Risk of Osteoporosis

Several laboratory and epidemiologic studies have suggested an increased risk of fractures in people with a high vitamin A intake. Therefore a recent study enrolled 2322 men, 49 to 51 years of age, in a population-based cohort study. Fractures were found in 266 men during 30 years of follow-up. The risk of fracture was highest among men with the highest serum vitamin A (retinol) levels. Men with the highest levels of retinol had an overall risk of fracture that was greater than in men with the lowest levels of retinol by a factor of seven ($p < 0.001$). The level of serum beta-carotene was not associated with the risk of fracture. These initial data in men and previous data in women suggest that megadoses of vitamin A may be associated with a substantially higher risk of fracture. The results of this study and others should encourage immediate normal intakes of vitamin A, especially from supplements, until more clinical studies are completed. In laboratory studies vitamin A in large doses has been associated with the inhibition of bone-forming cells.

Reference
Michaelsson, K., et al. (2003). Serum retinol levels and the risk of fracture. *New England Journal of Medicine, 348,* 287-294.

A   B

FIGURE 28-8 Electron micrographs of normal (**A**) and osteoporotic (**B**) bone. (From Dempster, D.W., et al. [1986]. A simple method for correlative light and scanning electron microscopy of human iliac crest bone biopsies: Qualitative observations in normal and osteoporotic subjects. *Journal of Bone and Mineral Research, 1,* 15-21.)

this period. Bone loss in the hip probably starts as early as age 20 years. Although it is debated as to when bone loss naturally begins, during perimenopause women experience a marked acceleration in bone loss because of the loss of natural estrogen. Women start to lose bone about 1.5 to 2 years before their last menstrual period and continue rapid loss until about 1.5 years after their last menses. They may lose as much as 15% of their total mass during the perimenopausal period, after which the rate of bone loss slows to a rate of about 1% per year. Rapid bone loss also occurs in women whose ovaries have stopped functioning, such as women being treated for the prevention and treatment of ovarian and breast cancer.

Although men have larger and stronger skeletons than women, they can experience a marked loss of bone as they age, possibly resulting in fragility fractures. Bone loss in men starts later in life and progresses more slowly. Men do not experience the rapid bone loss associated with the perimenopausal decline in estrogen production seen in women. There are several reasons for loss of bone in men, including declining testosterone levels. In addition, estrogen may play a crucial role in men's bone health and changes in estrogen levels with age may be as important, if not more so, as changes in testosterone levels.

Those who have not gained their maximum peak bone mass have less bone "in the bank" to draw upon once the inevitable bone loss begins. Thus peak bone mass as well as later bone loss is a major determinant of osteoporotic fracture. For this reason, osteoporosis has been described as a pediatric disorder. Strong adult skeletons are built during childhood.

From 60% to 80% of the risk for this disorder is inherited. A history of fracture in a first-degree relative is a risk for fragility fracture. Factors other than heredity known to influence development of osteoporosis are listed in Box 28-2.

Osteoporosis can also result from underlying medical conditions, such as thyrotoxicosis, hyperparathyroidism, anorexia nervosa, and Cushing's syndrome, and from long-term use of medications such as thyroid hormone, anticonvulsants, furosemide, and corticosteroids. A person who has had one osteoporotic fracture is five times more likely to suffer another fracture than a person without a fracture. Thus history of a low-trauma fracture is an important risk factor.

Pathophysiology

Bone is a dynamic tissue that undergoes continuous *remodeling*, the process by which old bone is replaced by new (Figure 28-9). Bone remodeling serves two principal functions:

1. It replaces old bone with new so that the biomechanical properties of the skeleton are not compromised by continuous use.
2. It plays a role in mineral homeostasis by transferring calcium and other ions into and out of the skeletal reservoir.

The remodeling sequence starts with activation of *osteoclasts*, which resorb a small portion of bone over a relatively short period (as short as 7 to 10 days). Bone formation then takes place as *osteoblasts* form an organic matrix that is subsequently mineralized.

Peak bone mass and the subsequent rate and duration of bone loss are important determinants of whether skeletal integrity will be compromised to the degree that a fragility fracture will result. In addition, as bone tissue is lost, other alterations in the skeleton (e.g., changes in architecture, aging of the bone tissue, accumulation of microdamage) contribute to fracture risk. The supporting structures become so weak that even minimal stress can cause fractures. Spinal fractures occurring with osteoporosis are usually compression fractures that occur when one or more vertebrae collapse from carrying the weight of the upright body.

Clinical Manifestations

In many people, the diagnosis of osteoporosis is made after a fracture, often a vertebral compression fracture. Clinical manifestations of vertebral compression fracture include sudden onset of severe back pain that worsens on movement and is relieved by rest. This acute pain usually subsides within 2 to 6 weeks. Most compression fractures, however, are discovered accidentally on routine x-ray. Progressive vertebral deformities lead to shortened stature and progressive dorsal kyphosis (Figure 28-10). The lower ribs eventually rest on the iliac crests, and downward pressure on viscera causes ab-

---

BOX 28-2   *Risk Factors for Osteoporosis*

Major Risk Factors

Personal history of fracture as an adult
History of fragility (low trauma) fracture in a first-degree relative
Low body weight (less than about 128 pounds)
Current cigarette smoking
Use of oral corticosteroid therapy for more than 3 months

Additional Risk Factors

Impaired vision
Estrogen deficiency at any age
Dementia
Poor health/frailty
Recent falls
Inadequate physical activity
Low intake of dietary calcium (lifelong)
Suboptimal levels of serum vitamin D
Alcohol in amounts of more than two drinks per day

dominal distention and bloating. Respiration may also be impaired by restricted lung expansion.

Bone loss can also occur in the mandible, which may lead to loss of teeth or poorly fitting dentures as well as changes in the appearance of the face. Unfortunately, fractures of the wrist in postmenopausal women are often not recognized as osteoporotic fractures. (See the Complementary and Alternative Therapy feature on Cal-

cium Supplements to Prevent Postmenopausal Osteoporotic Fractures on p. 600.)

The many changes in appearance and the difficulty in finding clothing that fits can have a profound negative effect on self-esteem. Quality of life may be affected by chronic pain and functional disability. Fear of subsequent fracture may cause people to reduce their activity.

FIGURE 28-9 Bone remodeling is a process of bone resorption and bone formation. These two processes are controlled by systemic factors (the need for calcium) and local cytokines, some of which are found in the bone matrix. Cytokines are of key importance in communication between the osteoblasts and the osteoclasts. (Modified from Cotran, R.S., Kumar, V., & Robbins, S.L. [1999]. *Robbins pathologic basis of disease* [6th ed.]. Philadelphia: W.B. Saunders.)

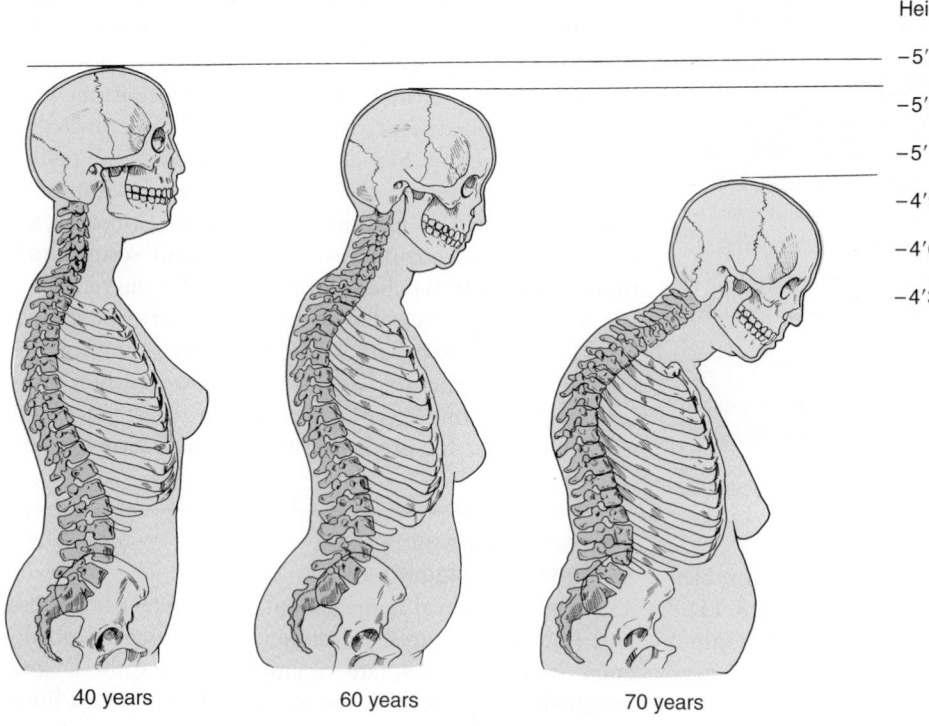

FIGURE 28-10 Osteoporotic changes: A normal spine at 40 years of age and osteoporotic changes at ages 60 and 70 years. These changes can cause a loss of height and may result in dorsal kyphosis.

Collimated x-ray detector

X-ray source

Dual-energy
x-ray beam

FIGURE 28-11 Dual-photon absorptiometry. (Modified from an original illustration in *Clinical Symposia*, illustrated by Frank Netter, M.D., copyright by Ciba-Geigy Corporation.)

COMPLEMENTARY AND ALTERNATIVE THERAPY

Calcium Supplements to Prevent Postmenopausal Osteoporotic Fractures

A recent analysis of the past clinical trials on calcium supplements for women found that they were effective. In other words, calcium supplementation (1000 to 1200 mg/day of elemental calcium) reduced menopause-related bone loss and reduced the rate of vertebral and non-vertebral fractures. Calcium was more effective when vitamin D was also taken at a dosage of 700 to 800 international units daily, especially in older clients, who have a high rate of vitamin D deficiency. Health professionals need to remember that some clients get a large portion of calcium through diet, and this should be determined first. Both calcium citrate and calcium phosphate are absorbed well, even in older adults, if taken with food. Also, keep in mind that calcium or vitamin D supplements or both have been a part of almost every drug clinical trial. Thus calcium and vitamin D supplements can be taken alone or in conjunction with drug therapy when approved by a doctor. Supplements of calcium and vitamin D enhance the effect of drug therapy for osteoporosis. Finally, if men qualify, they may be candidates for calcium and vitamin D because evidence supports the use of these supplements in men at high-risk for fractures.

Reference
Campbell, B. (2003). Do calcium supplements prevent postmenopausal osteoporotic fractures? *Journal of Family Practice, 52,* 234-237.

The "gold standard" for measuring BMD is full-table dual-energy x-ray absorptiometry (DXA) (Figure 28-11). This technique carries low risk and takes only a few minutes. The most commonly measured sites with DXA are the spine and the hip. BMD is commonly reported as a "T-score," which is the difference between the client's BMD and the BMD of "young normal adults" of the same gender. The difference between the client's score and the young adult norm is expressed as standard deviation (SD) below or above the average. Thus a person with a T-score of –2.0 would have a BMD that is 2 SD below the average for a young adult of the same gender. Under the WHO criteria, this person would be considered *osteopenic*. Guidelines for BMD testing are shown in Box 28-3.

In recent years, the number of peripheral densitometers has increased dramatically. These devices measure BMD at peripheral sites such as the heel or finger. They include *quantitative ultrasound* (QUS) devices and peripheral DXA. These devices are smaller and less expensive than full-table DXA, and the QUS devices involve no radiation exposure. Criteria for interpreting results with peripheral devices are not well developed, however.

Laboratory tests may be performed to rule out secondary osteoporosis or other metabolic bone diseases. These tests include blood count, urine calcium, multichannel screen, serum alkaline phosphatase, serum 25-hydroxyvitamin D, parathyroid hormone, ionized calcium, protein electrophoresis in urine and serum, and thyroid function. Biochemical markers of bone remodeling, such as urinary collagen cross-links, are sometimes used in conjunction with DXA or QUS to monitor the effectiveness of therapy. At this time, however, biochemical markers alone are not appropriate for diagnosis of osteoporosis or for predicting the risk of fracture in the future.

Outcome Management
■ Medical Management
The goal of medical management is to prevent bone loss and fragility fractures. Lifestyle changes focused on dietary intake of adequate calcium and vitamin D and weight-bearing exercise are prescribed to prevent bone

BOX 28-3	*Bone Mineral Density (BMD) Testing Guidelines*

BMD testing is recommended for the following:

- All postmenopausal women under age 65 years who have one or more additional risk factors for osteoporosis (besides menopause)
- All women age 65 years and older regardless of risk factors
- Younger postmenopausal women with one or more risk factors (other than being white, postmenopausal, and female)
- Postmenopausal women who present with fractures (to confirm diagnosis and determine disease severity)
- Estrogen deficient women at clinical risk for osteoporosis*
- Individuals with vertebral abnormalities*
- Individuals receiving, or planning to receive, long-term glucocorticoid (steroid) therapy*
- Individuals with primary hyperthyroidism*
- Individuals being monitored to assess the response or efficacy of an approved osteoporosis drug therapy.*

From the National Osteoporosis Foundation. (1999). *Physician's guide to prevention and treatment of osteoporosis.* Hillsborough, NJ: Excerpta Medica.

* Medicare covers BMD testing for the following individuals age 65 and older.

TABLE 28-2	*Recommended Calcium Intake Levels*
Age Levels	**Calcium Intake (mg/day)**

Age Levels	Calcium Intake (mg/day)
Infants	
Birth-6 mo	210
7 mo-1 yr	280
Children and Adolescents	
1-3 yr	500
4-8 yr	800
9-18 yr	1300
Adults	
19-50	1000
19-51	1200
>70	1200
Pregnancy and Lactation	
<18	1300
19-50	1000

National Academy of Science. (1999). *Dietary reference intakes for calcium, magnesium, phosphorus, vitamin D, and fluoride.*, Washington, DC: Food and Nutrition Board, Institute of Medicine. National Academy Press.

BOX 28-4	*Calcium Equivalents of Dietary Sources (300 mg)*

1 cup of milk
1 carton of low-fat yogurt with fruit
1¼ cup frozen yogurt
1 cup vanilla pudding
1 cup baked egg custard
1 oz Swiss cheese
1 slice cheese pizza
½ cup ricotta cheese, part skim
1½ oz cheddar cheese
2¼ cup cottage cheese
11 dried figs
4 cups broccoli
7 oz baked wall-eyed pike fillet
¾ cup whole dried almonds

Prepared by Patricia T. Packard, R.D., C.N., Creighton University Osteoporosis Research Center, Omaha, NE.

loss. *Hormone replacement therapy* (HRT) is considered for women who are perimenopausal (see later discussion). Cigarette and alcohol cessation is advised.

Preventing Loss of Bone Mass. Osteoporosis is preventable. Strategies for prevention are most effective when they are started in childhood to maximize peak bone mass and to establish lifelong bone-healthy behaviors. Several interventions that maximize and preserve bone mass have general health benefits, including adequate intake of calcium and vitamin D, regular weight-bearing exercise, and avoidance of tobacco and alcohol abuse.

Calcium and Vitamin D Intake. A well-balanced diet containing the recommended level of calcium is an important component of bone health (Table 28-2). The major sources of dietary calcium are dairy products. Calcium can also be obtained from the wide range of calcium-fortified foods that are available (Box 28-4). National surveys of dietary intake indicate that many Americans are not consuming enough calcium. Most women consume less than half of the recommended daily levels. As early as age 10, the calcium intake of girls is considerably below that needed for optimal bone health.

People who have difficulty digesting milk because of a lack of the enzyme lactase, which breaks down the milk sugar lactose, may be able to tolerate acidophilus milk, yogurt, and hard cheeses; in addition, milk products may be tolerated if taken in small amounts. Skim milk and low-fat yogurt can be recommended for persons who are trying to maintain low-cholesterol diets. Diets high in dairy foods do not cause obesity. In fact, considerable research supports the role of dietary calcium in decreasing the risk of obesity. Dietary calcium is the preferred approach, but calcium supplements should be used when an adequate dietary intake cannot be achieved. All calcium supplements should be taken with food to enhance absorbability. Chewable supplements are preferred over those that are swallowed. Although a high dietary calcium intake is thought to increase the risk of renal calculi (stones), research findings suggest that high-calcium diets actually protect against stone formation.

Vitamin D plays a major role in both calcium absorption and bone metabolism. Vitamin D is made in the skin in the presence of sunlight, or it may be obtained from food sources, primarily vitamin D–fortified milk. Although exposure to sunlight is necessary for cutaneous synthesis of vitamin D, prolonged exposure to sunlight does not necessarily increase the amount that is synthesized. An average of 15 minutes a day of sunlight exposure to hands, face, arms, and legs probably meets the requirements for most people during the summer or below the 40th latitude. Although the use of sunscreen remains important to reduce photoaging and the risk of skin cancer, when sunscreen is applied the skin receives no sunlight and vitamin D is not synthesized in the skin. Vitamin D supplementation (400 to 800 international units/day) is recommended for institutionalized older people, for persons living in high northern or southern latitudes, and for people who have limited sun exposure.

COMPLEMENTARY AND ALTERNATIVE THERAPY

Oral Vitamin D₃ and Osteoporosis

A total of 2037 men and 649 women (mean age, 75 years) were eligible and agreed to participate in this British study of doctors and clients from a general practice. Clients were randomly assigned to receive vitamin D_3 (100,000 international units, equivalent to 800 international units/day) or placebo every 4 months for 5 years. The average calcium intakes were similar between the two groups. The 5-year overall, age-adjusted fracture risk was lower for clients receiving vitamin D_3 (relative risk [RR] = 0.78) versus placebo (NNT = 44 for 5 years). Fractures were also significantly lower for the hip, wrist, forearm, or vertebrae (RR = 0.67) with vitamin D_3 versus placebo. Women had a larger reduction in fracture risk at any site (RR = 0.68). The difference for men was not statistically significant, but the study may not have included enough men to find a difference. There was no significant difference between the vitamin D_3 and placebo group in self-reported health and falls or in the mortality rates from cardiovascular disease, cancer, or all causes. This intervention is safe and cheap because the average cost is less than $2 per year.

Reference

Trivedi, D., Doll, R., & Khaw, K. (2003). Effect of four monthly oral vitamin D3 (cholecalciferol) supplementation on fractures and mortality in men and women living in the community: A randomized, double-blind controlled trial. *British Medical Journal, 326,* 469–472.

NNT, Number needed to treat.

(See the Complementary and Alternative Therapy feature on Oral Vitamin D₃ and Osteoporosis, below.)

High dietary intake of sodium increases loss of calcium in the urine, and people who take in large amounts of sodium should increase their calcium intake accordingly. Although caffeine modestly increases calcium excretion in the urine, the loss is negligible compared with the effects of protein and sodium. The effect of caffeine can be offset by adding 40 mg of calcium to the diet for each cup of coffee. Phosphorus intake, such as that from drinking carbonated beverages, does not significantly affect calcium balance; however, people who drink a large number of carbonated beverages may not be consuming adequate calcium in the form of milk.

Low protein intake appears to play a distinct detrimental role in the causes and complications of hip fracture. Many older adults have an inadequate protein intake. The clinical outcome after hip fracture is significantly improved with the use of daily oral nutritional supplements or a calcium phosphate pill, which normalize protein intake. Protein supplementation also reduces further bone loss in older clients who have sustained a hip fracture.

Exercise. Weight-bearing exercise, such as walking and running, is necessary for maintaining bone mass because disuse results in bone loss. Swimming and biking have not been found effective in maintaining bone mass, probably because they do not adequately load the bones. The inactivity of older people increases the rate of bone loss and the risk of hip fracture. It has been suggested that regular exercise by older people would reduce the risk of hip fracture by at least half. In addition to maintaining bone mass by loading the bones, exercise leads to improved physical fitness, which is associated with improved muscle strength, stability, reaction time, balance, and coordination.

All these factors help to decrease the risk of falling and of subsequent fractures. Exercise regimens and weight training increase muscle strength even in persons older than 90 years of age. In light of the positive effects of exercise on bone and on health in general, nurses should recommend regular exercise for all clients. Previously sedentary clients who wish to start a more rigorous exercise program should undergo a physical evaluation before starting.

At least 30 minutes of any physical activity should be incorporated into daily schedules. Even activities such as walking, hiking, gardening, biking, and housework or yard work increase daily energy expenditure and help to promote muscular strength, flexibility, coordination, and endurance, which ultimately may decrease the number and severity of falls.

Alcohol and Tobacco. Alcohol abuse and smoking cigarettes increase the risk of osteoporosis. Current smokers have 2.1 times the risk of hip fractures as nonsmokers. If a woman quits smoking, she reduces her risk of hip fracture by 40%. Excessive alcohol intake reduces bone density and increases the risk of falls. Moderate alcohol intake has no known negative effect on BMD.

Pharmaceutical Prevention and Treatment of Osteoporosis. Medications approved by the FDA to prevent and treat osteoporosis include hormone replacement therapy (HRT), alendronate, raloxifene, risedronate, calcitonin, and teriparatide. Clients receiving drug therapy for osteoporosis should be taught about the importance of dietary intake and activity as part of any treatment regimen. Treatment should not be limited to persons who have had a fragility fracture but should include clients at high risk for osteoporotic fracture. See the Evidence-Based Practice in Action feature on Using Hormone Replacement Therapy for Osteoporosis, below.

Nonpharmaceutical Prevention of Osteoporosis. People who are at high risk of fracture and falling should be considered for hip protectors (Figure 28-12). These undergarments have protective shields or pads sewn into the area over the greater trochanter on each side. These shields are anatomically designed to shunt the energy of an impact away from the greater trochanter to the soft tissues. Large studies have shown that the rate of hip fracture per fall is 84% lower when hip protectors are worn. The design of the hip protectors is such that the garment is comfortable to wear and is not visibly apparent under slacks or a skirt. The garment has been modified with Velcro fasteners for nursing home clients. The cost of hip protectors is slightly more than the cost of one month of anti-resorptive medication.

Promoting Healing after Fracture. The goals of treatment after fracture are to manage pain, regain mobility and strength, promote healing, reduce bone loss, and

EVIDENCE-BASED PRACTICE IN ACTION

Using Hormone Replacement Therapy for Osteoporosis

Although HRT has been widely used in prevention and treatment of osteoporosis, new evidence about its benefits and risks requires consideration of its use for bone health. The Women's Health Initiative (WHI), a large randomized primary prevention trial of estrogen and estrogen plus progesterone, recently found that Prempro (combined estrogen and progesterone) reduced the risk of clinical vertebral fractures and hip fractures by 34%; however, Prempro also increased risks of probable dementia, coronary heart disease, stroke, thromboembolic disorders, breast cancer, and cholecystitis. It is important to note that the WHI used only one type of estrogen preparation at one dose and that a study arm that used estrogen *without* progesterone was not terminated. This raises the question of whether estrogen without progesterone involves fewer risks. Furthermore, the risks of lower doses of estrogen, which have been found to have bone health benefits, were not addressed in the WHI. Based on these findings, when use of HRT is considered solely for prevention of osteoporosis, approved non-estrogen therapies should first be considered. Currently, HRT is recommended for relief of menopausal manifestations and not for long-term prevention of osteoporosis. HRT prevents the estrogen-related bone loss that occurs during the perimenopausal period; however, this bone loss will occur when the HRT is stopped. The skeletal effects of estrogen are obtained with both oral and transdermal preparations.

Marketed as Evista, raloxifene is a member of a class of drugs called *selective estrogen receptor modulators* (SERMs). SERMs provide the benefits of estrogen but avoid the risks. They prevent bone loss and reduce the incidence of osteoporotic fracture. Their cardioprotective effects are under investigation.

SERMs do not increase the risk of breast or uterine cancer. In fact, Evista has been found to decrease the incidence of breast cancer. Evista increases the risk of DVT in a manner similar to that of ERT. Evista also increases hot flashes and is thus not effective in relieving menopausal manifestations.

Drugs that inhibit bone resorption are also prescribed. Alendronate and risedronate are bisphosphonates and are available as Fosamax and Actonel, respectively. These drugs must be taken after a prolonged fast (overnight) with 8 ounces of water, at least 30 minutes before eating or drinking. Clients should remain upright during this 30-minute interval. Calcitonin, a hormone that slows bone resorption, is available as Miacalcin and is delivered as a single daily dose of nasal spray. Calcitonin is less effective than Evista or Fosamax in maintenance of bone mass. Interestingly, calcitonin has analgesic effects, which may help to relieve pain associated with fractures.

Parathyroid hormone (PTH, Forteo) has recently been approved by the FDA for treatment of osteoporosis in postmenopausal women. It is an anabolic (bone-building) agent that is administered daily by subcutaneous injection. Forteo has few side effects, but some clients experience leg cramps and dizziness. The safety and efficacy of Forteo have not been demonstrated beyond 2 years of therapy.

Reference
Writing Group for the Women's Health Initiative Investigators. (2002). Risks and benefits of estrogen plus progestin in healthy postmenopausal women: principal results from the Women's Health Initiative randomized controlled trial, *Journal of the American Medical Association, 288,* 321-333.

FIGURE 28-12 Safehip. (Courtesy of Tytex Group, Woonsocket, RI.)

prevent further fracture. Furthermore, treatment is directed toward limiting the disability associated with existing fractures.

Managing Pain. One of the most important interventions in the care of the client with an osteoporotic fracture is pain management. Often clients present with back pain resulting from vertebral crush fracture syndrome. Strict bed rest for 5 to 7 days is most effective in relieving pain and shortening the course of pain. The client should lie supine or in a side-lying position. After 5 to 7 days of bed rest, the client is instructed to increase activity gradually.

Non-opioid analgesics may be needed for 1 to 2 weeks to aid in pain reduction. If NSAIDs are used, protect the client from gastric ulceration by administering medications with food or antacids.

Flexible corsets with adjustable self-fastening tape (Velcro) may help to relieve back pain and fatigue; however, these corsets cannot correct the underlying problem of bone loss and spinal deformity. Corsets may be worn in bed but are most helpful if worn when the person is in the upright position.

Physical therapy is of utmost importance in the long-term treatment of back pain. Often chronic back pain is associated with decreased ROM, weakness, muscle spasm, postural change, muscle tenderness, and decreased endurance. Physical therapy should be started during the period of bed rest with ROM exercises and mild resistive exercises of the extremities in bed. Heat or ice, ultrasound, and TENS may be used for pain reduction.

Regaining Mobility and Strength. After acute pain subsides, clients should carry out exercises specifically prescribed for them, such as stretching and strengthening. Water aerobics may be initiated early in the treatment before the client can tolerate weight-bearing exercise. A long-term physical activity program should include weight-bearing and aerobic exercise in addition to strengthening and flexibility exercise. Because osteoporotic clients are at risk for subsequent fractures, they should be taught how to move safely while maintaining or increasing physical activity. See the Management and Delegation feature on Assisting with Mobility and the Use of Splints on p. 605.

Promoting Healing. Good general nutrition should be encouraged after fractures to promote healing. Optimal calcium and vitamin D intake continue to be important, and special attention should be given to adequate protein in the diet, especially in older clients. Calcium phosphate supplements should be considered for persons with low protein intake.

Preventing Further Fractures. Medications and treatments used to prevent osteoporosis are continued after a fracture to maintain and improve bone mass in existing bone.

■ Nursing Management of the Medical Client

Nursing management for the client with osteoporosis is detailed in the Care Plan feature on The Client with Osteoporosis on the website.

■ Self-Care

Assess clients at high risk for fracture for activity level and dietary adequacy, and perform appropriate teaching to prevent fractures. In addition, assess these clients' risk of falling. Assessment includes visual acuity, medications that may cause dizziness or postural hypotension, and difficulties with balance or coordination as well as the home environment for potential safety hazards. Evaluation of the home setting is performed via the admission assessment, discussions with the client, consultation with a specialist in social services, and home safety evaluation by a visiting nurse.

Discussion about fall prevention strategies is imperative. Instruct clients who are prone to dizziness to get up slowly from a lying position, first sitting on the side of the bed. Eyeglass prescription may need to be updated to improve vision. An aid to ambulation, such as a cane or walker, may also be indicated to prevent falling. Alterations to the home may be recommended. Handrails in the bathroom, removal of scatter rugs, and increased lighting are some of the modifications that may be necessary.

Specific resources in the community that may be helpful to clients with osteoporosis include support groups and exercise programs. The National Osteoporosis Foundation (www.nof.org) is an excellent source of educational resources.

PAGET'S DISEASE

Paget's disease (osteitis deformans) is defined as an idiopathic bone disorder characterized by abnormal and accelerated bone resorption and formation in one or more bones. The normal bone is replaced by abnormal, structurally weaker bone that is prone to fractures. Paget's disease most frequently produces painful deformities of the femur, tibia, lower spine, pelvis, and cranium.

Although the cause of Paget's disease is unknown, it is thought to be of viral origin. Laboratory data suggest involvement of the measles virus, respiratory syncytial

virus (RSV), or canine distemper viruses, but these findings have not been confirmed. A genetic etiology of Paget's disease is probable because 15% to 30% of clients have a positive family history of the disorder.

Paget's disease increases in frequency with age in Western countries and is more prevalent in men than in women. It is seen infrequently in Africa and Asia. Epidemiologic studies suggest that Paget's disease is decreasing in both severity at diagnosis and in prevalence.

In many instances Paget's disease is diagnosed because the client has experienced trauma and x-rays demonstrate the characteristic changes of the disease; 10% to 20% of persons with the disease are asymptomatic. Before clinical manifestations occur, x-ray films show increased bone expansion and density. After clinical manifestations have developed, the bone shows a characteristic mosaic appearance (Figure 28-13). Bone scans are the most efficient means of identifying pagetic bone. Laboratory tests include indices of bone turnover such as serum alkaline phosphatase and urinary and serum deoxypyridinoline, N-telopeptide, and C-telopeptide.

In symptomatic Paget's disease, the most common presenting complaints include one or more of the following: deep, aching bone pain; skeletal deformity, such as a barrel-shaped chest, bowing of the tibia or femur, or kyphosis; changes in skin temperature; pathologic fractures through diseased bone; and manifestations related to nerve compression. Diseased bone pressing on the cranial nerves may result in vertigo, hearing loss with tinnitus, and blindness. Rheumatoid arthritis, ankylosing spondylitis, and gout are commonly associated with Paget's disease.

The NSAIDs, such as ibuprofen, and newer COX-2 inhibitors can often control bone pain. Pain may also be relieved with heat therapy, massage, and bracing. Further orthopedic treatment may be indicated for severe disabling arthritis, severe bowing deformities of the femur or tibia, and pathologic fractures.

Currently, five bisphosphonates are used for the treatment of Paget's disease. These include pamidronate (Aredia), alendronate (Fosamax), risedronate (Actonel), etidronate (Didronel), and tiludronate (Skelid). After a

FIGURE 28-13 A pagetoid bone demonstrating the characteristic mosaic pattern seen on x-ray examination. (From Merkow, R.L., & Lane, J.M. [1990]. Paget's disease of bone. *Orthopaedic Clinics of North America, 21*[1], 173.)

course of treatment, bone turnover indices such as alkaline phosphatase return to normal in 60% to 70% of clients, reflecting suppression of abnormal bone turnover. Existing data suggest that effective disease suppression will likely reduce future disabling problems. Unfortunately, deformity and hearing loss are not corrected with these medications. Re-treatment is indicated if bone turnover markers exceed the upper limit of normal (once they had decreased to within normal limits).

OSTEOMALACIA

Etiology and Pathophysiology

Osteomalacia is a disease in which the bone becomes abnormally soft because of a disturbed calcium and phosphorus balance secondary to vitamin D deficiency. Osteomalacia is characterized by widespread decalcification and softening of bones, especially in the spine, pelvis, and lower extremities. Bones become bent and flattened as they soften, leading to marked deformities of the weight-bearing bones and to pathologic fractures.

Osteomalacia mainly affects women, and it is endemic in Asia. It is also seen in Moslem women living in Western countries. Their style of dress prevents them from obtaining adequate vitamin D from sunlight exposure. Some causes are the following:

- Chronic use of anticonvulsants
- Strict vegetarianism
- Very-low-fat diets
- Renal osteodystrophy
- Hyperthyroid-induced osteopenia
- Fibrous dysplasia

Women who have had multiple pregnancies and who have breast-fed their children have a higher rate of the disease. Osteomalacia is similar to rickets, which occurs in children, and the condition is called *adult rickets.*

Clients generally report easy fatigability, malaise, and bone pain, which is diffuse, poorly localized, and accompanied by a general bony tenderness. Muscular weakness is often seen in severe cases. Serum calcium and phosphorus levels are reduced, and the alkaline phosphatase level is moderately elevated. Radiographs indicate generalized demineralization with trabecular bone loss. Pseudofractures (Milkman's syndrome) and cyst formation are common. Bone biopsy is frequently necessary for diagnosis.

Intervention for clients with osteomalacia includes daily vitamin D until signs of healing take place, at which time a daily low maintenance dose is continued. Adequate intake of calcium and phosphorus as well as protein should be ensured.

GOUT AND GOUTY ARTHRITIS

Gout is a metabolic bone disorder in which purine (protein) metabolism is altered and the by-product, uric acid, accumulates. Gout is classified as primary or secondary.

Primary gout is caused by an inherited defect of purine metabolism, leading to increased or decreased renal excretion. It accounts for 85% of all cases, of which 95% affect men. The initial attack of gout occurs in the third or fourth decade of life.

Secondary gout is an acquired condition that occurs following hematopoietic (multiple myeloma, polycythemia vera, and leukemia) or renal disorders. In hematopoietic disorders, cell turnover and uric acid production increase. In addition, gout may develop from the rapid induction of chemotherapy or radiation therapy when there is massive destruction of cells. Renal disorders that decrease the excretion of uric acid also may lead to gout. Hyperuricemia may also result from use of aspirin, thiazide, and mercurial diuretics, and some antituberculosis medications. Alcohol intoxication and starvation increase serum urate levels by inhibiting renal excretion as a result of lactic acidosis and ketosis, respectively. In addition, alcohol ingestion increases urate production by stimulating purine breakdown. Prolonged use of diuretics and other medications (levodopa, nicotinic acid, low-dose salicylates) also reduce the excretion of uric acid and precipitate gout.

In the body, uric acid is made by the enzymatic breakdown of tissue and dietary purines. Hyperuricemia develops because of underexcretion or overproduction of uric acid. In addition to accumulation in the blood, uric acid is concentrated in the synovial fluid, myocardium, kidneys, and ears. When uric acid levels reach a certain level, they crystallize, and the crystals (tophi) are deposited in connective tissue. Because the crystals are deposited in connective tissue, gout is classified as a form of arthritis (Figure 28-14).

Clinical manifestations of gout develop in stages (Table 28-3). The diagnosis of gout is confirmed by the presence of persistent hyperuricemia (>7 mg/dl) in addition to the clinical manifestations. The presence of uric acid in an aspirated sample of synovial fluid confirms the diagnosis.

Outcome Management

The management of the client with gout has two components: (1) management of the *acute* attack and (2) *long-term* management of hyperuricemia.

Management of the acute attack includes the use of colchicine and NSAIDs to reduce pain and inflammation. Colchicine reduces the migration of leukocytes to the synovial fluids. The initial dose of colchicine is 0.6 to 1 mg, followed by 0.5 mg/hr until pain is relieved or manifestations of toxicity develop. Use caution when giving colchicine because the therapeutic dose is close to the toxic dose. Manifestations of toxicity include nausea, vomiting, and diarrhea. Other NSAIDs can be used, such as indomethacin or naproxen. In resistant cases of gout, adrenocorticotropic hormone (ACTH) or steroids may be required. Ice over the inflamed joints may also relieve pain.

Medications to lower uric acid include allopurinol, which blocks formation of uric acid, and probenecid, which promotes resorption of uric acid deposits and excretion of uric acid. Long-term medication is advised in clients who have more than two attacks of gout a year, secondary forms of gout, or persistent hyperuricemia.

TABLE 28-3	*Manifestations of Gout by Stage*
Stage	**Manifestations**
Stage I	Asymptomatic hyperuricemia.
Stage II	Asymptomatic hyperuricemia again; laboratory and x-ray findings are unchanged from stage II.
Stage III	Acute attack is accompanied by redness, swelling, and exquisite tenderness in one joint (toes, fingers, wrists, ankles, knees, or other joints). The great toe is the most common site. This first attack develops quickly, often overnight. Fever, tachycardia, malaise, and anorexia may be noted. The acute episode usually subsides within a week. As the edema subsides, pruritus and local desquamation (tissue loss) may be noted. After the initial attack, the affected joint returns to normal and the client may be asymptomatic for years. Eventually, other attacks occur.
Stage IV	Permanent changes in multiple joints with restrictions in movement. Tophi may be detected on the ears, hands, elbows, feet, and knees. Renal and cardiac disorders may also develop. The client may have uric acid renal stones, renal colic, and hypertension. Atherosclerosis occurs in about 50% of all clients.

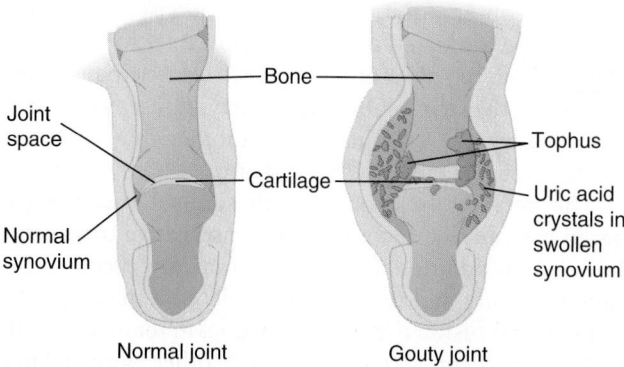

FIGURE 28-14 Comparison of a gouty joint and a normal joint.

Salicylates (aspirin) antagonize the action of uricosuric agents and must not be used concurrently.

Opinions differ regarding dietary treatment for gout. In the past, a low-purine intake was used to eliminate many proteins from the diet. Some physicians have prescribed a decrease in red and organ meats; others prescribe no dietary changes at all. Encourage ample fluid intake (2000 to 3000 ml/day) to promote excretion of uric acid. A moderate intake of distilled forms of alcohol does not seem to precipitate gouty attacks; beer, ale, and wine may precipitate them. Excessive alcohol in any form should be avoided.

Gradual weight loss is encouraged after the initial attack. Weight loss alone may reduce the incidence of attacks and uric acid levels; however, a sudden loss of weight may precipitate an attack because of the destruction of cells, which release uric acid.

Clients who can recognize early manifestations of gout may be able to avert the attack by the prompt use of colchicine or indomethacin. Long-term side effects (alopecia, bone marrow suppression, hepatic damage) from these agents, although rare, should be explained to the client.

Nursing management of the client with gout includes pain control. The client is usually placed at bed rest until pain subsides. Once ambulating, the client's need for crutches or a walker should be considered until gait is stable. Explain dietary restrictions, fluid requirements, and long-term self-management.

SPINAL COLUMN DEFORMITIES

The characteristic S curve of the lateral spine develops during fetal life and early childhood. Because other abnormal curves can occur because of defects in the bone, muscles, or nerves, every spinal problem must be considered from both an orthopedic and a neurologic viewpoint.

SCOLIOSIS

In the coronal plane, the spine should appear completely straight. Scoliosis is lateral curvature of the spine in any area—cervical, thoracic, thoracolumbar, or lumbar. It is important to distinguish curvature of *structural* origin from that of *nonstructural* origin. A structural curvature does not correct itself on forced bending against the curvature, and vertebral rotation can be demonstrated. A nonstructural curvature is easily corrected on forced bending or in the supine position, and rotation of the vertebral bodies is not demonstrated.

Idiopathic scoliosis is the most common form, appearing in growing children with no other apparent health problems. Scoliosis occurs most often in preadolescents and adolescents. It was once believed to be primarily a problem in girls, but school screening studies have shown small degrees of abnormal spinal curvature in equal numbers of boys and girls. Both boys and girls should be observed until it is proven that a curve is not progressive. Continued curve progression is possible even after skeletal maturity if the curvature is greater than 40 or 45 degrees, and excessive curvature can lead to cardiopulmonary problems and pain that prompt the client to seek medical care. The client may also seek help because of cosmetic deformity and loss in height. Skeletally mature clients with a curve less than 20 degrees do not require treatment. Skeletally immature clients with a curve between 20 and 40 degrees require brace management, whereas clients with curves greater than 45 degrees need surgical intervention.

Etiology

The cause of scoliosis can be congenital or neuromuscular. *Congenital scoliosis* results from a malformation of the bony vertebral segment of the spine, either because of failure of (1) formation (the absence of a portion of a vertebra) or (2) segmentation (the absence of normal separations between vertebrae). Neuromuscular conditions associated with spinal deformities include cerebral palsy, syringomyelia, polio, myelomeningocele, spinal muscle atrophy, spinal cord tumors, trauma, and myopathic conditions such as muscular dystrophy.

Clinical Manifestations

Clinical manifestations and a family history of spinal deformity are significant, but diagnosis is confirmed by upright posteroanterior and lateral radiographs that reveal a curvature of 10 degrees or more (Figure 28-15, *A*). X-rays are the only exact tool for monitoring changes in spinal deformity, but excessive radiation exposure is inappropriate in children. Two other noninvasive diagnostic techniques—Moire topography and the integrated shape-imaging system (ISIS)—produce images on the back surface shape that can be correlated to underlying spinal deformities.

Outcome Management

Nonsurgical treatments for clients with spinal deformity consist of observation, bracing, and exercise. Each client needs to be evaluated individually, not only for the medical problem but also for willingness to participate in any suggested therapies. One client may refuse to wear a brace under any circumstances; another may insist on treatment for even a slight curvature.

The decision to proceed with surgical treatment is based not only on the failure of conservative treatments but also on additional factors, such as the client's emotional stability and readiness to undergo a major procedure. Spinal fusion is the ultimate goal in many cases, attaching adjacent vertebrae to each other with a bone graft to prohibit motion between them. The surgical approach can be posterior or anterior, depending on the lo-

FIGURE 28-15 **A,** Scoliosis. **B,** Postoperative x-ray after correction with Cotrel-Dubousset instrumentation. (From Maher, A.B., Salmond, S.W., & Pellino, T.A. [Eds.]. [2002]. *Orthopedic nursing* [3rd ed.]. Philadelphia: W.B. Saunders.)

cation of the deformity. A combined anterior-posterior approach has become increasingly popular for adults with severe thoracolumbar scoliosis.

Various types of instruments can be used to stabilize the spine and correct deformity. The choice of instrumentation is based on the diagnosis, the magnitude of the curvature and the flexibility of the curve, the client's age and inherent bone strength, and the client's ability to wear a postoperative immobilization device. The Cotrel-Dubousset (CD), Texas Scottish Rite Hospital (TSRH), Moss-Miami, and Luque systems are commonly used for a posterior approach (see Figure 28-15, *B*). The Harrington rod system, developed in the 1960s, is still in use because of its availability and because many surgeons are familiar with it. The most common types of instrumentation for an anterior approach are the Zielke and Harris systems.

Complications

Possible complications following scoliosis surgery include neurologic compromise, infection, respiratory problems, spinal fluid leakage, phlebitis, excessive blood loss, implant problems, and pseudarthrosis. The most devastating complications are paralysis and death.

Postoperative Care

Postoperative nursing management focuses on the usual postoperative care (see Chapter 16). Assessment of motor and sensory function in the lower extremities is important because the nerves and muscles may have been stretched in surgery. Other postoperative care is discussed in the section on lumbar fusion in Chapter 73.

KYPHOSIS

Also called "humpback" or "dowager's hump," the term *kyphosis* describes a posterior rounding of the thoracic spine. Whereas a certain degree of kyphosis is considered normal, curvatures greater than 45 degrees are believed to be excessive and require additional evaluation as to the cause. Kyphosis is identified as *postural* if the client can voluntarily hyperextend the spine to correct the curvature and if there is no radiographic evidence of structural change. Kyphosis is common in metabolic disorders such as osteoporosis and osteomalacia, but it can also accompany neuromuscular diseases such as cerebral palsy and muscular dystrophy. Severe curvature can affect cardiopulmonary and gastrointestinal function, making intervention essential.

Kyphosis is most often treated with bracing or corsets to straighten the spine. Exercises to strengthen muscles and ligaments may also be encouraged. Spinal fusion with or without instrumentation may be required if response to other interventions is inadequate.

LORDOSIS

Lordosis is an excessive inward curvature of the lumbar spine that is sometimes seen in pregnant or obese clients or in people with large abdominal tumors. Extreme lordosis may lead to *swayback*, in which the lumbosacral spine curves sharply and the thoracolumbar spine exhibits kyphosis. Lordosis is often associated with sagging shoulders, an exaggerated pelvic angle, and medial rotation of the legs. If necessary, treatment may consist of bracing, spinal fusion, or osteotomy. Hyperlordosis in young children and prepubertal girls is a self-correcting problem thought to be related to rapid skeletal growth without corresponding soft tissue growth.

BONE INFECTIONS

Musculoskeletal system contamination can result either as infection spreads from other sites in the body or from external insults (e.g., puncture, surgery). Infections are often severe and difficult to treat because the bones are relatively inaccessible to protective macrophages and antibodies. Even a small number of microorganisms can be enough to establish a serious infection that can lead to loss of function or even death. For this reason, nurses should be diligent in wound care and alert to any manifestations that suggest infection.

OSTEOMYELITIS

Overview

Osteomyelitis is a severe pyogenic infection of bone and surrounding tissues. Although generally bacterial in origin, osteomyelitis can also be caused by a virus or fungus. *Staphylococcus aureus* is the most common infecting organism, but *Escherichia coli, Pseudomonas, Klebsiella, Salmonella,* and *Proteus* organisms may also be found. Because osteomyelitis can be extraordinarily difficult to cure even with long-term antibiotics, prompt recognition is crucial. Delayed identification or inadequate treatment can result in a chronic infection accompanied by continuing pain, chronically draining sinuses, loss of function, amputation, or death.

Osteomyelitis occurs most frequently in the femur, tibia, sacrum and heels. Males are affected more often than females, often as a result of trauma. Susceptibility to infection increases with IV drug use, diabetes, immunocompromising diseases, or a history of bloodstream infections. Osteomyelitis also develops in pressure ulcers and other chronic open wounds. Limiting the spread of osteomyelitis may also be more difficult in clients with a disorder such as malnutrition, alcoholism, or liver failure.

Clinical manifestations may vary slightly according to the site of involvement. Infection in the long bones is accompanied by acute localized pain and redness or drainage, often with a history of recent trauma or newly acquired prostheses. Fever and malaise may be present, but adults do not always appear acutely ill with other systemic manifestations. Infection in the vertebrae usually brings pain and mobility difficulties. The client with vertebral osteomyelitis often reports a history of genitourinary infection or drug abuse. Osteomyelitis in the foot is most commonly associated with vascular insufficiency. Older adults may become confused or disoriented.

Laboratory studies and x-rays or bone scans are important in the definitive diagnosis of osteomyelitis. Elevated WBC and ESR, along with clinical manifestations, usually allow initial diagnosis and early treatment while the physician waits for further evidence from blood cultures or needle aspirate analysis. Radiographic changes related to osteomyelitis are generally evident within 7 to 10 days, but in some cases the diagnosis is not confirmed radiographically until 3 to 4 weeks after infection develops. Early acute osteomyelitis can be identified more efficiently by radionuclide bone scans, which can detect lesions within 24 to 72 hours after the onset of infection. Because of its ability to distinguish between soft tissue

and bone marrow, MRI is also being used increasingly for definitive diagnosis of osteomyelitis.

Outcome Management

Elimination of the infecting organism, both locally from the bone and systemically from the body, is the major treatment goal for acute osteomyelitis. Prompt treatment also prevents further bone deformity and injury, increases client comfort, and avoids complications of impaired mobility. Surgery is initially performed on the adult client with osteomyelitis to ensure effective debridement and drainage, elimination of dead space, and adequate soft tissue coverage. Antibiotics alone rarely resolve infection in adults, but they do work more effectively after surgical preparation of the treatment area. High doses of parenteral antibiotics are frequently administered for 4 to 8 weeks to achieve a bactericidal level in the bone tissue. Oral antibiotics are continued for another 4 to 8 weeks, with serial bone scans and ESR measurements performed to evaluate the effectiveness of drug therapy. Open, draining wounds are packed with gauze to promote drainage. If initial treatment is delayed or inadequate, the necrotic bone separates from the living bone to form *sequestra,* which serve as a medium for additional microorganism growth. Chronic osteomyelitis can result.

SEPTIC ARTHRITIS

Overview

Septic arthritis (also known as pyogenic arthritis, infectious arthritis, septic joint disease, bacterial arthritis, and suppurative arthritis) is a closed-space infection caused by invasion of the synovial membrane by pus-forming bacteria or other pathogens. Joints most commonly affected in adult clients are the knee, hip, shoulder, wrist, and ankle.

A variety of microorganisms may infect the joint, but *Neisseria gonorrhoeae* is the most common causative pathogen in adults under 30 years of age. A significant percentage of staphylococci, the second most common causative organism in adults, is methicillin resistant. *S. aureus* invades the joint through hematogenous spread, as an extension of adjacent soft tissue infection, or from direct inoculation following trauma or an invasive procedure.

Hematogenous spread, in which organisms reach the joint from a remote site, is the most common etiologic mechanism. Because the synovial membrane is very vascular, any microorganism that is circulating in the blood may be easily trapped in the synovial space. Upper respiratory infection, otitis media, furuncle, or impetigo may seed a susceptible site such as a previously traumatized or diseased knee joint.

The presence of septic arthritis typically reflects the failure of multiple defense mechanisms. In the early stages of infection, the synovial membrane swells and becomes infiltrated with neutrophils. A purulent effusion distends the joint as the neutrophils release lysosomal proteolytic enzymes that destroy the articular cartilage, subchondral bone, and joint capsule. Enzymatic cartilage destruction can actually occur in 3 to 24 hours, creating a medical emergency that requires prompt treatment to avoid permanent joint damage.

The client often presents with complaints of pain, swelling, warmth, and tenderness in a single joint and also generally experiences an acute systemic reaction. The adult client is more likely than the child to experience only a low-grade fever and malaise; however, high temperatures and shaking chills are generally present in the client who has positive blood cultures.

Assessment focuses on the presence of factors that may predispose the client to joint infection, such as recent surgery or injury, diagnostic procedures, IV drug abuse, or systemic disease. Because effective treatment requires accurate identification of the causative agent, initial laboratory studies attempt to differentiate septic arthritis from autoimmune diseases with joint involvement (such as rheumatoid arthritis). Complete blood cell count (CBC), ESR, the antinuclear antibody (ANA) test, and rheumatoid factor (RF) measurements are often among the studies that are ordered. In addition, joint fluid is aspirated for analysis, and a synovial biopsy is performed. Radioisotope scanning techniques may also be helpful in the early detection of infection.

Outcome Management

Antibiotic therapy is a critical part of effective treatment of septic arthritis and must be promptly initiated to prevent permanent joint damage. Penicillin G, a bactericidal agent, is often administered initially because many common causative organisms are susceptible to the drug. After the specific organism and its sensitivities have been identified from synovial fluid cultures, the antibiotic therapy may be altered. Treatment time varies according to the duration of clinical manifestations, the causative organism, and the status of the client's immune system. For most clients, parenteral antibiotics are administered for 2 to 3 weeks and oral antibiotics continue for another 1 or 2 weeks. Older clients or those with more complex presentations may require parenteral therapy lasting 4 to 6 weeks. Decompression of the infected joint is also necessary, although controversy exists about the best methods. Open synovectomy and debridement or repeated joint aspirations and irrigations may be performed. Arthroscopic drainage and debridement have also been successful.

Effective nursing management requires scrupulous attention to the client's joint position, exercise, and rehabilitation. In the acute phase of septic arthritis, the client is likely to hold the joint in slight to moderate flexion as a position of comfort. Because this can lead to flexion deformities, slings, immobilizers, or splints may be used temporarily to hold the joint in an optimal position. As inflammation begins to resolve, passive ROM exercises are initiated to preserve joint function. CPM has also been used with some success. Active motion and weight-bearing may not be initiated until clinical manifestations and inflammation have almost totally disappeared. Pain management is also important for the client with septic arthritis to provide comfort and to allow greater ease in exercise participation.

BONE TUMORS

A bone tumor *(neoplasm)* may be benign or malignant (Table 28-4 and Figure 28-16). Benign bone tumors may remain undiagnosed because they often cause no pain. They may be noted as an incidental x-ray finding when the client is being evaluated for another complaint, such as fracture through a bone cyst; however, benign tumors that grow aggressively can cause bone pain, weakness, and destruction.

MALIGNANT BONE TUMORS

Primary malignant tumors originate in bone cells or form within the bone. Each year about 2500 new cases of primary bone tumors are diagnosed, including osteosarcoma, chondrosarcoma, and Ewing's sarcoma. Clients typically present with a mass or lesion or a pathologic fracture. They may also report weight loss, fever, chills, or pulmonary manifestations.

The exact cause of primary bone tumors remains largely unknown, but several factors are believed to play a role in their development. Past trauma has been associated with tumor development, as has exposure to carcinogens such as asbestos, dioxin, and radium. Bone tumors may also develop from benign medical conditions (enchondromatosis, neurofibromatosis) or from metabolic conditions (Paget's disease). Fewer than 5% of clients with malignancies have a hereditary predilection to cancer.

Metastatic bone tumors, which are more prevalent than sarcomas, spread to the bone from primary carcinomas in sites such as the breast, prostate, lung, and kidney. Thyroid, bladder, uterine, colorectal, and vaginal cancers can also metastasize to bone. Cancer cells may spread directly within a body cavity, or they may metastasize by hematogenous or lymphatic spread.

Laboratory studies such as CBC, blood and urine calcium levels, and ESR assist in client evaluation, but they are not diagnostic themselves. Other laboratory tests, however, are used as tumor markers. An elevated serum AP level may be noted with osteoblastic tumors, for example, and lactate dehydrogenase (LDH) may mark

Type	Description
Benign Cartilage-Forming Tumor	
Enchondroma	Lesion in mature cartilage but lacking histologic characteristic of chondrosarcoma; found in hands, feet, humerus, ribs, femur; age range, 20-40 yr
Osteochondroma	Most common bone tumor; cartilage-capped bony projection on external bone surface; metaphyses of long bone, especially proximal tibia and distal femur; age range, 0-30 yr
Benign Bone-Forming Tumor	
Osteoid osteoma	Small osteoblastic lesion (less than 1 cm) with demarcated outline and reactive bone formation; femur and tibia; age range 10-20 yr
Osteoblastoma	Similar to osteoid osteoma but larger (>2 cm); spine, long bones, hand
Giant cell tumor (osteoclastoma)	Aggressive benign bone tumor with richly vascularized tissue consisting of plump spindle-shaped cells and numerous giant cells; distal femur, proximal tibia, distal radius, proximal humerus; age range, 20-40 yr
Malignant Bone-Forming Tumor	
Osteosarcoma	Most common primary malignant bone tumor; formation of bone or osteoid by tumor cell; metaphyses, especially of distal femur, proximal tibia, and proximal humerus; intramedullary region involved; age range, 10-30 yr
Ewing's sarcoma	Composed of densely packed small cells with round nuclei; often confused with osteomyelitis because it presents with fever, anemia, leukocytosis, increased ESR; diaphyseal regions of long and flat bones; age range, 5-15 yr
Fibrosarcoma	Formation of spindle-shaped tumor cells of interlacing bundles of collagen fibers, absence of other types of histologic differentiation; femur, tibia; age range, 5-80 yr
Malignant Cartilage-Forming Tumor	
Chondrosarcoma	Formation of cartilage by tumor cells; higher cellularity and greater pleomorphism than in chondromas; femur, pelvis, ribs, scapula; age range, 30-60 yr

Data from Haynes, K.K. (2001). In D. C. Schoen (Ed.). *NAON* core curriculum for orthopaedic nursing (4th ed.). Pitman, NJ: National Association of Orthopaedic Nurses.

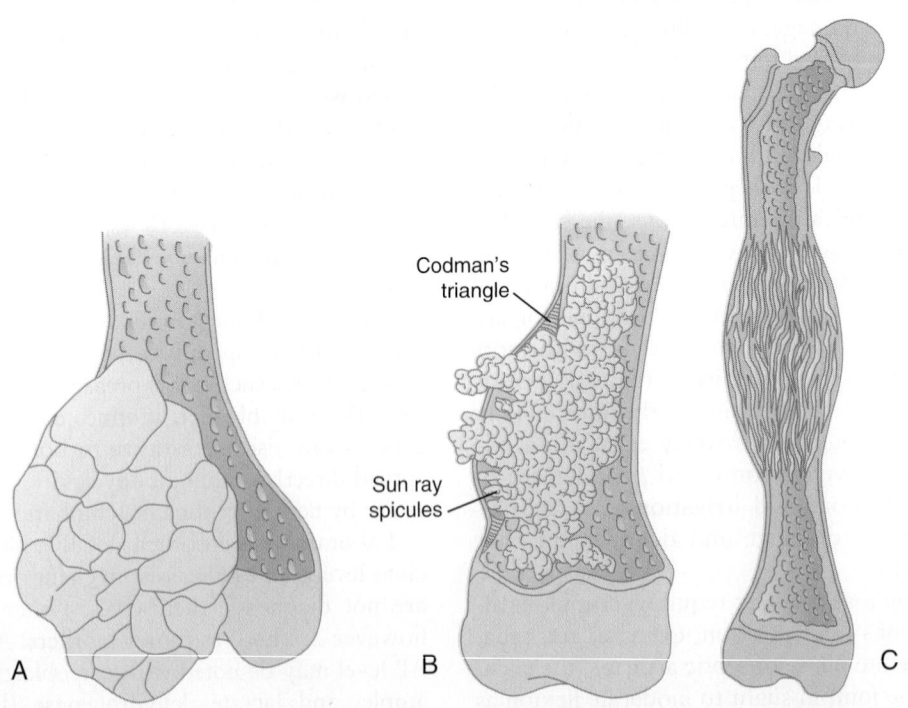

FIGURE 28-16 Bone tumors. **A,** A giant cell tumor. **B,** An osteogenic sarcoma. **C,** A malignant endothelioma (Ewing's sarcoma). (After Hughes, S. [1983]. *A short textbook of orthopedics and traumatology* [3rd ed.]. New York: ARCO.)

tumor progression for Ewing's sarcoma. A plain radiograph in anterior and posterior views may provide an initial diagnosis, but other studies—such as a CT scan, MRI, or bone scan—are also commonly performed. A bone biopsy is needed for definitive diagnosis of metastatic bone disease.

Outcome Management

The treatment goal for the client with a primary tumor is to eradicate the tumor completely and to promote long-term survival. *Chemotherapy* has dramatically increased the survival of clients diagnosed with primary bone tumors. *Radiation therapy* has become safer because of an increased understanding of cancer and radiobiology; it is also now better tolerated through the use of radiation machines that reduce skin sensitivity. *Surgery* may be performed to eradicate the disease, either through excision of the tumor and a wide zone of surrounding normal tissue or through amputation. If the tumor is excised, the resulting defect is repaired by using a joint prosthesis or bone graft with internal fixation. The bone graft can be taken from the client at another anatomic site, or an allograft (cadaver) bone may be used.

Pain management following surgery is a major focus. Opioids are often delivered by PCA pumps or via epidural catheter. Pain should be addressed aggressively and medication effectiveness assessed regularly. Frequent position changes and stimulation of non-tumor areas through heat, cold, or massage may be beneficial. Non-pharmacologic strategies, such as music therapy, imagery, and relaxation techniques, may provide powerful adjuncts to opioid administration. Postoperative nursing care also addresses the possible complications related to orthopedic surgery, including infection, DVT, and non-union of grafted bone.

For the client with metastatic disease, treatment goals include (1) palliation, (2) remission, and (3) extension of life. Pain management requires a collaborative effort of the client, family, and all members of the health care team. Because metastatic tumors can cause severe pain and have the potential to fracture, lesions in the long bones are commonly managed with excision, followed by insertion of intramedullary rods to stabilize the weakened bone. Radiation therapy may also be used to decrease tumor size, improve bone strength, and help in pain management.

Pharmacologic treatment of pain often includes morphine. Oral administration facilitates home care management for the client with metastatic tumors, but IV or transdermal medications may be indicated for the client with gastric problems. Other analgesics, such as acetaminophen and anti-inflammatory medications, may also be used because they act on the peripheral pain mechanism. Adjuvant medications, including antidepressants and anticonvulsants, are frequently used to increase the effectiveness of conventional analgesics.

The key to pain management is to administer all analgesics on an around-the-clock (ATC) rather than on a PRN basis. Nonpharmacologic measures should also be employed to maximize pain management.

As with postoperative treatment of the client with a primary tumor, pain should be addressed aggressively and medication effectiveness assessed regularly. Attempts at pain management for the client with a metastatic bone tumor may ultimately lead to a palliative neurosurgical procedure, such as a chordotomy, in which the anterolateral spinal cord tracts are severed to provide relief in the affected areas.

DISORDERS OF THE FOOT
HALLUX VALGUS (BUNIONS)

Bunions, a common foot deformity that involves the first metatarsal and the great toe (hallux), occur nine times more often in women than in men. Bunions may occur as a congenital disorder, or they may be acquired during periods of rapid growth, such as adolescence. They may also occur as a result of local irritation related to restrictive footwear. They result from a pronation abnormality and from hypermobility of the first metatarsal, phalanx, and cuneiform joints. The client typically complains of pain as the bony prominence of the metatarsal head becomes irritated from pushing against the inside of a shoe. *Calluses* under the second and third metatarsal heads occur from a shift in weight-bearing and may also cause pain. Standard anteroposterior and lateral x-rays show exostosis of the first metatarsal head with subluxation or dislocation.

To decrease pressure over the bunion and minimize the likelihood of bursitis, the client may try conservative treatment, consisting entirely of wearing shoes with a larger toe box to allow more space for the forefoot. If a change in footwear does not provide enough relief, orthoses may be ordered or steroid injections administered for acute inflammation. Surgery may be considered if conservative treatment fails, if the client desires cosmetic correction of the deformity, or if functioning of the lateral four toes is also affected. The procedure is designed to realign the great toe through osteotomy of the hallux or through fusion of the metatarsophalangeal joint (Figure 28-17). In addition to routine care, the client who has undergone bunionectomy may use open-toed flat shoes for ambulation.

MORTON'S NEUROMA (PLANTAR NEUROMA)

Athletes commonly experience Morton's neuroma because of excessive pressure placed on the branch of the medial plantar nerve between the third and fourth toes. The pressure causes a *neuroma,* or swelling of the nerve, that leads the client to complain of pain in the ball of the foot. Depending on the extent of the compression, pain may radiate into the toes and be accompanied by numbness. Pain may be increased if the client wears tight-fitting or high-heeled shoes. Hyperextension of the metatarsophalangeal joints or repetitive impact on the forefoot may also increase pain.

The usual treatment involves changing the type of shoe to one with a larger toe box that provides more room for the forefoot. Anti-inflammatory medications are often prescribed. If these are ineffective, steroid injections may be administered. Surgery to remove the neuroma may be considered if other treatments do not produce long-term relief.

HAMMER TOE

Hammer toe is a deformity caused by a flexion contracture of the proximal interphalangeal joint (PIP) with extension or slight hyperextension of the DIP (Figure 28-18). This deformity often accompanies hallux valgus and may occur in clients with a family history of hammer toe, RA, and clawfeet. Hammer toe leads to improper fit of footwear, creating pain with walking and a change in gait patterns. Corns and calluses on pressure areas of the foot may need to be removed.

Treatment centers on choosing footwear with a wide toe box. Pads and inserts can help relieve pressure, but they can also cause previously unaffected areas of the foot to rub against the shoe. Osteotomy of the toe and

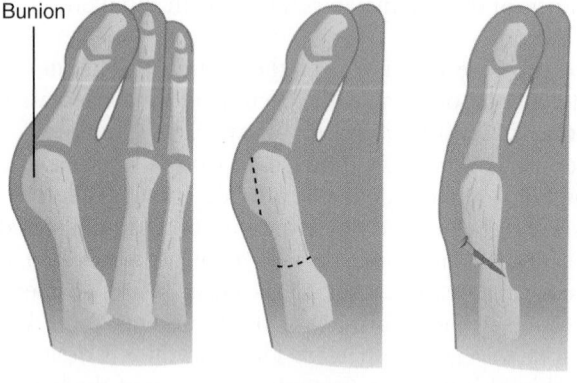

FIGURE 28-17 Bunions and their surgical correction.

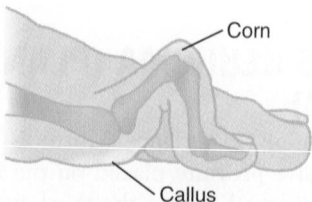

FIGURE 28-18 Hammer toe with characteristic joint deformity and soft tissue involvement.

resection of the proximal phalanx may be required for symptom relief.

MUSCULAR DISORDERS
MUSCULAR DYSTROPHY

Muscular dystrophy (MD) is a term that generally designates a group of genetic disorders involving gradual degeneration of muscle fibers. (For information on an

GENETICS LINKS
Myotonic Dystrophy

Description
Myotonic dystrophy is an autosomal-dominant disorder that affects skeletal muscle and smooth muscle as well as other body tissues, including the eyes, heart, endocrine system, and CNS. There are three forms of myotonic dystrophy (DM): mild, classical, and congenital. Mild DM presents with cataracts and mild myotonia; life span is normal. Classical DM is characterized by muscle weakness and wasting, myotonia, cataracts, and cardiac dysrhythmias; adults may be physically disabled and have a shortened life span. Congenital DM is associated with hypotonia and severe generalized weakness at birth, often with respiratory insufficiency, mental retardation, and early death. DM is considered the most common muscular dystrophy that affects adults, occurring in approximately 1 in 8000 people.

Genetics
DM is caused by an unstable inherited mutation in the myotonic dystrophy protein kinase gene (DMPK gene) located on chromosome 19. The disease mutation is an expanded CTG trinucleotide repeat that lies in the DMPK gene. The number of CTG repeats is strongly correlated with disease severity. Unaffected normal people can have from 5 to 37 CTG repeats. CTG repeat length exceeding 37 repeats is abnormal. The number of repeats often increases through successive generations, accompanied by increasing severity of the disorder and earlier age of onset (a tendency known as *anticipation*). Offspring of an affected individual have a 50% chance of inheriting the disease-causing mutation.

Diagnosis/Testing
Diagnosis is based on family history and clinical findings and is confirmed by the detection of an expansion of the CTG trinucleotide repeat in the DMPK gene. DNA-based testing is essentially 100% sensitive and is clinically available.

Management
No specific treatment for the progressive weakness of DM exists. Treatment can be offered to manage certain manifestations associated with the disease (e.g., medications to counter the effects of myotonia, surgery for cataracts, close monitoring of cardiac status).

TABLE 28-5	*Clinical Features in Muscular Dystrophy (MD)*		
	Duchenne's MD	**Becker's MD**	**Limb Girdle MD**
Incidence	Most common type of MD	Less common than Duchenne's MD	Less common than Duchenne's or Becker's MD
Age at onset	Usually <3 yr	Usually 5-15 yr	Usually by second decade
Inheritance	Sex-linked recessive gene, autosomal <10%	Sex-linked recessive gene	Usually autosomal recessive
Pattern of muscle involvement	Onset: Selected symmetrical weakness of proximal pelvic muscles, 3-5 yr Later: shoulder girdle muscle involvement	Similar to Duchenne's MD	Proximal shoulder and pelvic girdle
Late muscle involvement	Affects all muscles, including facial, oculopharyngeal, and respiratory	Face spared	Peripheral brachioradialis, hand, and calf
Pseudohypertrophy	Calf muscles	Calf muscles	Occurs in fewer than one third of cases
Contractural deformities	Common	Less common	Occurs in late disease; milder than Duchenne's MD
Scoliosis/kyphoscoliosis	Common in late disease	Not severe	Mild in late disease
Heart involvement	Yes	Uncommon in late disease	Rare
IQ	Decreased	Normal	Normal
Course	Steady progression	Slow progression	Slow progression, with greater variation among clients

Data from Mason K.J. (2001). Pediatric and congenital disorders. In D. C. Schoen (Ed.), *NAON core curriculum for orthopedic nursing* (4th ed.). Pitman, NJ: National Association of Orthopaedic Nurses.
IQ, Intelligence quotient.

autosomal-dominant disorder that affects skeletal muscle and smooth muscle as well as other body tissues, see the Genetic Links feature on Myotonic Dystrophy on p. 614.) The client experiences progressive weakness and skeletal muscle wasting accompanied by disability and deformity. The various forms of MD are differentiated by the affected muscle groups, the client's age at onset of the disease, the rate of progression, and the inheritance mode (Table 28-5). *Pseudohypertrophic MD (Duchenne's MD)* is the most common and severe form of the disease. A sex-linked recessive disorder that affects males almost exclusively, it has been linked to an abnormality of the Xp21 gene locus. The client experiences wheelchair dependency in early adolescence. Respiratory muscles are eventually involved, and myocardial degeneration leads to cardiomegaly and tachycardia.

Diagnosis of MD is accomplished through use of multiple modalities in an attempt to differentiate the disease from other disorders, such as myasthenia gravis and polymyositis. The most valuable laboratory test is serum creatine kinase analysis; levels are elevated in clients with MD because of an abnormality of striated muscle function. Enzyme levels do decrease, however, as muscle mass decreases. Muscle biopsy is essential to diagnosis of a neuromuscular disease such as

Duchenne's MD. Muscle shows degeneration, with fibers replaced by connective tissue and fat in later stages of the disease.

Treatment is largely symptomatic and supportive because there is currently no cure for MD. Care is aimed at increasing the comfort and functional ability through corrective surgery for related deformities or use of braces for the spine or lower extremities. Breathing exercises may also be initiated for respiratory decompensation. More than 60% of clients with MD live to age 21 years, but survival beyond age 30 is unusual.[6] Death generally results from respiratory or cardiac failure.

CONCLUSIONS

The focus of this chapter has been musculoskeletal disorders, including metabolic bone diseases such as osteoporosis. Osteoarthritis is a common degenerative disorder that is often treated with joint replacement surgery. Special nursing care is required after such surgery to maximize the client's outcome. Benign and metastatic bone tumors, common foot disorders, and MD, a hereditary neuromuscular disorder, have also been discussed. An understanding of these disorders is essential for the nurse who provides care for affected clients.

THINKING CRITICALLY *evolve*

1. You meet an older woman in the total joint class who is considering joint replacement surgery but has not yet scheduled the procedure with her orthopedist. She has osteoarthritis and, because of increasing pain in her hips, she now uses a wheelchair when she goes out in public. She tells you she also has diabetes mellitus. What would you discuss with her to help her prepare appropriately for surgery?

Factors to Consider. What would be the benefit of increased upper arm strength for this client? Is she maintaining tight control of the diabetes? Is weight loss an issue before surgery?

2. A middle-aged client is concerned about bone loss resulting from osteoporosis. She tells you that her mother has severe osteoporosis, and she realizes her lifestyle and family history are predisposing factors. She asks you to suggest a lifestyle program for her and her daughters. How should you proceed?

Factors to Consider. What focused assessment should you complete? How should you complete teaching for the client and her daughters?

3. An older woman tells you her physician wants her to eat a diet high in calcium. He wants her to consume 1500 mg of calcium without taking enriched antacids or calcium supplements. This woman is lactose intolerant and has a hiatal hernia. She lives alone on a limited income. What problems might impair her compliance with the prescribed treatment regimen?

Factors to Consider. What dietary sources of calcium are appropriate for the lactose-intolerant client? How does the presence of a hiatal hernia affect dietary intake?

Discussions for these questions can be found on the website and the CD-ROM.

BIBLIOGRAPHY

1. Alternatives for arthritis: Do unconventional treatments offer new options for an old scourge? (2000). *Consumer Reports on Health*, 12 (1), 6-9.

EB 2. American College of Rheumatology (ACR) Subcommittee on Osteoarthritis Guidelines (2000). Recommendations for the medical management of osteoarthritis of the hip and knee: 2000 update. *Arthritis and Rheumatology*, 43, 1905-1915.

EB 3. American Pain Society. (2002). American pain society releases new clinical guideline for treatment of arthritis pain. Available: http://www.ampainsoci.org/pub/principles.htm.

4. Anesthesiologists warn: If you're taking herbal products, tell your doctor before surgery (2000). ASA Public Education. Available: http://www.asahq.org/PublicEducation/herbal.html.

5. Burks, K. (2002). Health concerns of men with osteoarthritis of the knee. *Orthopaedic Nursing*, 21 (4), 28-34. **EB**

6. Burrage, R.L., & Sutter, C.A. (1999). Arthritis. In J.T. Stone, J.F. Wyman, & S.A. Salisbury (Eds.), *Clinical gerontological nursing: A guide to advanced practice*. Philadelphia: W.B. Saunders.

7. Carek, P.J., Dickerson, L.M., & Sack, J.L. (2001). Diagnosis and management of osteomyelitis. *American Family Physician, 63* (12), 2413-2420.

8. Cerrato, P.L. (1998). Alternatives. Complementary therapies: Can these compounds curb arthritis? *RN, 6*(4), 57-58, 67.

9. Childs, S.G. (2001). Nursing care for hand and wrist problems. In D.C. Schoen (Ed.), *NAON core curriculum for orthopaedic nursing* (4th ed.). Pitman, NJ: National Association of Orthopaedic Nurses.

10. Childs, S.G. (2002). Anatomy and physiology of the musculoskeletal system. In A.B. Maher, S.W. Salmond, & T.A. Pellino (Eds.), *Orthopaedic nursing* (4th ed.). Philadelphia: W.B. Saunders.

11. Crescimbeni, J.A. (1997). From bed to chair: Transferring the non–weight-bearing client. *Orthopaedic Nursing*, 16(2), 47-50.

12. Consensus Development Conference Statement. (2000). Osteoporosis prevention, diagnosis, and therapy. Available: http://consensus.nih.gov/cons/111/111-intro.htm. **EB**

13. Cummings, S., Eckert, S., & Krueger, K. (1999). Raloxifene reduced the incidence of breast cancer in postmenopausal women with osteoporosis. *Journal of the American Medical Association* 16, 2189-2197. **EB**

14. Davis. J.P., & Abbate, N. (2001). The knee. In D.C. Schoen (Ed.), *NAON core curriculum for orthopaedic nursing* (4th ed.). Pitman, NJ: National Association of Orthopaedic Nurses.

15. Fitzpatrick, L., & Heaney, R. (2003) Got soda? *Journal of British Medical Research*, 18, 1570-1573.

16. Fondaparinux: A new synthetic pentasaccharide for thrombosis prevention. (2002). *The Lancet, 359*, 1710-1711.

17. Geier, K.A., et al. (2002). Viscosupplementation: A new treatment option for osteoarthritis. *Orthopaedic Nursing*, 21 (5), 25-32.

18. Haynes, K.K. (2001). Tumors of the musculoskeletal system. In D.C. Schoen (Ed.), *NAON core curriculum for orthopaedic nursing* (4th ed.). Pitman, NJ: National Association of Orthopaedic Nurses.

19. Haynes, K. (2002). Neoplasms of the musculoskeletal system. In A.B. Maher, S.W. Salmond, & T.A. Pellino (Eds.), *Orthopaedic nursing* (4th ed.). Philadelphia: W.B. Saunders.

20. Hicks, M. (2001). The spine. In D.C. Schoen (Ed.), *NAON core curriculum for orthopaedic nursing* (4th ed.). Pitman, NJ: National Association of Orthopaedic Nurses.

21. Horstman. J. (2000a). Explorations: SAM-e. *Arthritis Today, 14* (1), 52-54.

22. Horstman, J. (2000b). Glucosamine goes legit. *Arthritis Today, 14* (2), 44-47.

evolve **Did you remember to check out the bonus material on the Evolve website and the CD-ROM, including free self-assessment exercises?**

http://evolve.elsevier.com/Black/medsurg/

23. Horstman, J. (1999). The Arthritis Foundation's guide to alternative therapies. Atlanta: Arthritis Foundation.

 24. Kannus, P., et al. (2000) Prevention of hip fracture in elderly people with use of a hip protector. *New England Journal of Medicine 343*, 1506-1513.

25. Labeling changes for arthritis drug. (2002). *FDA Consumer, 36* (5).

26. Lappe, J.M. (2001) Pathophysiology of osteoporosis and fracture. In L. Pachucki-Hyde, B. McClung, and M. Jennings (Eds.), *Nursing Clinics of North America*, vol. 36. Philadelphia: W.B. Saunders.

27. Lappe, J.M., et al (2003). Girls on a high calcium diet gain weight at the same rate as girls on a normal diet: A pilot study. *Journal of the American Dietetic Association (in press)*.

28. Maher, A.B. (2002). Assessment of the musculoskeletal system. In A.B. Maher, S.W. Salmond, & T.A. Pellino (Eds.), *Orthopaedic-nursing* (3rd ed.). Philadelphia: W.B. Saunders.

29. Mason, K.J. (2001). Pediatric and congenital disorders. In D.C. Schoen (Ed.), *NAON core curriculum for orthopaedic nursing* (4th ed.). Pitman, NJ: National Association of Orthopaedic Nurses.

30. Mauer, K.A., et al. (2002). National practice patterns for the care of the client with total joint replacement. *Orthopaedic Nursing, 21* (3), 37-46.

31. Morris, N.S. (1999). Complications associated with orthopaedic surgery. In *An introduction to orthopaedic nursing* (2nd ed.). Pitman, NJ: National Association of Orthopaedic Nurses.

32. Morris. N.S. (2001). Complications. In D.C. Schoen (Ed.), *NAON core curriculum for orthopaedic nursing* (4th ed.). Pitman, NJ: National Association of Orthopaedic Nurses.

33. Mosher, C.M. (1999). Total hip and knee replacement. In *An introduction to orthopaedic nursing* (2nd ed.). Pitman, NJ: National Association of Orthopaedic Nurses.

34. O'Koon, M. (1999). Shopping for a "cure." *Arthritis Today.* Available: http://www.arthritis.org/ReadArthritisToday/1999-03-04.shopping.asp.

35. Osteotomy and unicompartmental knee arthroplasty. (2002). AAOS Online Service Fact Sheet. Available: http://orthoinfo.aaos.org/fact/thr-report.cfm?Thread-ID=283&topcategory=Knee.

36. Pellino, T.A., et al. (2002). Complication of orthopaedic disorders and orthopaedic surgery. In A.B. Maher, S.W. Salmond, & T.A. Pellino (Eds.), *Orthopaedic nursing* (3rd ed.). Philadelphia: W.B. Saunders.

37. National Osteoporosis Foundation. (2003). Physician's guide to prevention and treatment of osteoporosis. Washington, D.C.: National Osteoporosis Foundation.

38. Recker, R., et al. (2000) Characterization of perimenopausal bone loss: A prospective study. *Journal of Bone and Mineral Research 15*, 1965-1973.

39. Roberts, D. (2001). Arthritis and connective tissue disorders. In D.C. Schoen (Ed.), *NAON core curriculum for orthopaedic nursing* (4th ed.). Pitman, NJ: National Association of Orthopaedic Nurses.

40. Roberts, D. (2002). Degenerative disorders. In A.B. Maher, S.W. Salmond, & T.A. Pellino (Eds.), *Orthopaedic nursing* (3rd ed.). Philadelphia: W.B. Saunders.

41. Rodts, M.F. (2002). Disorders of the spine. In A.B. Maher, S.W. Salmond, & T.A. Pellino (Eds.), *Orthopaedic nursing* (3rd ed.). Philadelphia: W.B. Saunders.

42. Salmond, S.W., & Fine, C. (2002). Infections of the musculoskeletal system. In A.B. Maher, S.W. Salmond, & T.A. Pellino (Eds.), *Orthopaedic nursing* (3rd ed.). Philadelphia: W.B. Saunders.

43. Schmitt, M. (2001). The foot and ankle. In D.C. Schoen (Ed.), *NAON core curriculum for orthopaedic nursing* (4th ed.). Pitman, NJ: National Association of Orthopaedic Nurses.

44. Simon, L.S. (1999). Arthritis: New agents herald more effective symptom management. *Geriatrics, 54* (6), 37-44.

45. Stein, R.R. (1999). An overview of the lumbar spine. In *An introduction to orthopaedic nursing* (2nd ed.). Pitman, NJ: National Association of Orthopaedic Nurses.

46. Theis, L.M. (2001). The hip, femur, and pelvis. In D.C. Schoen (Ed.), *NAON core curriculum for orthopaedic nursing* (4th ed.). Pitman, NJ: National Association of Orthopaedic Nurses.

47. Warner, C. (2002). The use of the orthopaedic perioperative autotransfusion (OrthoPAT) system in total joint replacement surgery. *Orthopaedic Nursing, 20* (6), 29-32.

48. Writing Group for the Women's Health Initiative Investigators. (2002). Risks and benefits of estrogen plus progestin in healthy postmenopausal women: principal results from the Women's Health Initiative randomized controlled trial. *Journal of the American Medical Association, 288*, 321-333.

49. Zemel, M. (2003) Mechanisms of dairy modulation of adiposity. *Journal of Nutrition, 133*, 252S-256S.

50. Zorn, K.E. (2001). Infection. In D.C. Schoen (Ed.), *NAON core curriculum for orthopaedic nursing* (4th ed.). Pitman, NJ: National Association of Orthopaedic Nurses.

Management of Clients with Musculoskeletal Trauma or Overuse

Dottie Roberts

---

evolve

Web Enhancements

http://evolve.elsevier.com/Black/medsurg/

Care Plan
The Client in Traction
The Client Following Hip Fracture and ORIF
Case Management
Hip Fracture

Appendix C
Laboratory Values of Clinical Importance in Medical-Surgical Nursing

---

Anyone who has experienced a broken bone or a ligament strain can appreciate the challenges facing a client who is recovering from musculoskeletal trauma or overuse. Activity restrictions and assistive devices both complicate and facilitate the healing process. Types of fractures and common soft tissue injuries and their medical and nursing management are discussed in this chapter.

FRACTURES

Trauma is the leading cause of death in the United States for those under the age of 45 and the fifth leading cause of death for all age groups. Nearly 60 million Americans suffer accidental injury each year.[25] Fractures account for a high percentage of traumatic injuries. They can create significant changes in one's quality of life by causing activity restrictions, disability, and economic loss.

A *fracture* is any disruption in the normal continuity of a bone. When fracture occurs, surrounding soft tissue is often damaged as well. A radiograph (x-ray) may confirm the bone injury, but it does not show evidence of the torn muscles or ligaments, severed nerves, or ruptured blood vessels that can complicate the client's recovery. To care appropriately for the client with a fracture, the nurse needs a concise and accurate description of the injury.

Etiology and Risk Factors

Fracture results from mechanical overload of the bone, when more stress is placed on the bone than it can absorb. The actual amount of force necessary to cause a fracture may vary greatly, depending in part on the characteristics of the bone itself. A client with a metabolic bone disease such as osteoporosis, for example, may experience fracture with even minor trauma because the bone is weakened by the pre-existing disorder. Fracture may result from direct force, as when a moving object strikes the body area over the bone. Force may also be applied indirectly, as when a powerful muscle contraction pulls against the bone. In addition, stress or fatigue can lead to fracture because of the bone's decreased ability to withstand mechanical force.

The two types of bone also respond differently to mechanical load. *Cortical* bone, the compact outer layer, is porous and can tolerate more stress along its axis (longitudinally) than across the bone. *Cancellous,* or *spongy,*

Nursing Outcomes Classification
for Nursing Diagnoses—Clients with Musculoskeletal Trauma or Overuse

Acute Pain
  Comfort Level
Imbalanced Nutrition: Less Than Body Requirements
  Nutritional Status: Food and Fluid Intake
  Nutritional Status: Energy
  Nutritional Status: Nutrient Intake
  Nutritional Status: Biochemical Measures
  Nutritional Status: Body Mass
Impaired Physical Mobility
  Ambulation: Walking
  Joint Movement: Active
  Mobility Level

Pain Control
Pain: Disruptive Effects
Risk for Constipation
  Bowel Elimination
  Hydration
  Knowledge: Medication, Medication Response
  Mobility Level
  Self-Care: Nonparenteral Medication
Risk for Impaired Skin Integrity
  Immobility Consequences: Physiological
  Tissue Integrity: Skin and Mucous Membranes

Risk for Infection
  Tissue Integrity: Skin and Mucous Membranes
  Treatment Behavior: Illness or Injury
Risk for Peripheral Neurovascular Dysfunction
  Joint Movement: Active
  Mobility Level
  Tissue Perfusion: Peripheral
Self-Care Deficit
  Self-Care: Activities of Daily Living (ADL)
  Self-Care: Bathing
  Self-Care: Dressing
  Self-Care: Grooming
  Self-Care: Hygiene

bone is the dense inner bone material. It contains web-like formations and spaces filled with red marrow that make it better able to absorb force than can cortical bone. Bony projections, called *trabeculae*, separate the spaces and are arranged along lines of stress, making cancellous bone even stronger.

Predisposition to fracture results from biologic conditions such as osteopenia (e.g., caused by steroid use or Cushing's syndrome) or osteogenesis imperfecta, which alters the strength and composition of the bone. Neoplasms can also weaken bone and contribute to fracture. Postmenopausal estrogen loss and protein malnutrition lead to decreased bone mass and increased risk for fracture. For persons with healthy bones, fractures can result from high-risk recreation or employment-related activities (e.g., skateboarding, rock climbing). Victims of domestic violence are also among people treated for traumatic injuries.

Pathophysiology

When fracture occurs, muscles that were attached to the ends of the bone are disrupted. The muscles can undergo spasm and pull the fracture fragments out of position. Large muscle groups can create massive spasms that displace even large bones, such as the femur. Although the proximal portion of the fractured bone remains in place, the distal portion can become displaced in response to both the causative force and the spasm in the associated muscles. Fracture fragments may be displaced sideways, at an angle (angulated), or as overriding bone segments. They may also be rotated or offset.

In addition, the periosteum and blood vessels in the cortex and marrow of the fractured bone are disrupted. Soft tissue damage frequently occurs. Bleeding occurs from both the soft tissue and from the damaged ends of the bone. In the medullary canal, a hematoma forms be-

tween the fracture fragments and beneath the periosteum. Bone tissue surrounding the fracture site dies, creating an intense inflammatory response. Vasodilation, edema, pain, loss of function, exudation of plasma and leukocytes, and infiltration of other white blood cells result. These processes serve as the initial step in bone healing.

Bone Healing

Unlike other specialized body tissues, bone heals uniquely through tissue regeneration rather than through scar tissue formation. Fracture repair occurs by the same mechanism as bone formation during normal growth and maintenance, with organized mineralization of newly synthesized bone matrix followed by remodeling to form mature bone. Adequate circulation to the fracture site and adequate fragment immobilization are crucial for effective bone healing. Factors such as the presence of systemic or bone diseases, the age and general health of the client, the type of fracture, and the treatment also can affect the speed and success of healing. For example, an impacted fracture may heal within several weeks, but a displaced fracture may take months or even years to heal. A radial or ulnar fracture may heal in 3 months, but fractures in the tibia or femur may require 6 months or longer to heal. A fracture in an infant may heal in only 4 to 6 weeks, but the same fracture in an adolescent may require 6 to 10 weeks to heal. The rate of fracture healing is not significantly decreased in older adults unless the client also has a metabolic disorder such as osteoporosis.

Fracture healing occurs in five stages (Table 29-1). These stages do not occur independently but tend to overlap as bone healing progresses. They are sometimes combined into a three-stage process.

TABLE 29-1	*Stages of Bone Healing*
Stage	**Description**
Stage I: Hematoma stage or inflammatory stage Time: 1-3 days	Immediate formation of a hematoma at the site of the fracture. The amount of damage to the bone and to the surrounding soft tissue and blood vessels determines the size of the hematoma. The blood forms a clot among the fracture fragments, providing a small amount of stabilization. Necrosis of adjacent bone occurs in direct relation to the loss of blood supply to the affected region and will extend to the area where collateral circulation begins. Vascular dilation occurs in response to the accumulation of dead cells and debris at the fracture site, and exudation of fibrin-rich plasma initiates the migration of phagocytic cells to the area of injury. If the vascular supply to the fracture site is inadequate, stage I healing will be greatly impaired.
Stage II: Fibrocartilage formation Time: 3 days to 2 weeks	Fibroblasts, osteoblasts, and chondroblasts migrate to the fracture site as a result of the acute inflammation and form fibrocartilage. Organization of the hematoma then offers the foundation for stage II bone and tissue healing. Osteoblastic activity is stimulated by periosteal trauma, and bone formation occurs quickly. The periosteum is elevated away from the bone, and within a few days the combination of periosteal elevation and granulation tissue formation creates a collar around the end of each fracture fragment. As the collars advance, they form a bridge across the fracture site. This early formation of fibrous tissue is sometimes called the *primary callus,* and it results in gradually increasing stability for the fracture.
Stage III: Callus formation Time: 2-6 weeks	Granulation tissue matures into a provisional callus (procallus) as newly formed cartilage and bone matrix disperse through the primary callus. The procallus is large and loosely woven. It is generally wider than the normal diameter of the injured bone. The procallus secures the bone fragments, extending some distance beyond the fracture site to serve as a temporary splint, but it does not provide strength. If cells are distant from the blood supply and oxygen tensions are relatively low, cartilage is formed. When calcium is deposited in the collagen network of the granulation tissue, fibrous bone forms. Proper bone alignment is essential during stage III. This stage may be the most important in determining successful healing; if it is slowed or interrupted, the final two stages cannot occur. Delayed union or non-union can then result.
Stage IV: Ossification Time: 3 weeks to 6 months	A permanent callus of rigid bone crosses the fracture gap between the periosteum and the cortex to join the fragments. In addition, medullary callus formation occurs internally to establish continuity between the marrow cavities. Trabecular bone gradually replaces the callus along stress lines. Bone union, which can be confirmed by x-ray, is said to have occurred when there is no motion with gentle stress and no tenderness with direct pressure at the fracture site. Weight-bearing in lower extremity fractures is also pain free after bone union.
Stage V: Consolidation and remodeling Time: 6 weeks to 1 year	Unnecessary callus is resorbed or chiseled away from the healing bone. The process of bone resorption and deposition along stress lines allows bone to withstand the loads applied to it. The actual amount and timing of remodeling depends on the stresses imposed on the bone by muscles, weight-bearing, and age.

Factors Affecting Bone Healing

If fracture healing is altered in any of the five stages, problems with bone union can result. Factors that affect bone healing are summarized in Box 29-1.

Most fractures heal adequately without any problems, but biologic interventions may be employed to stimulate fracture healing. For example, autogenous or allogeneic bone grafts can be used to stimulate bone growth. Injection or implantation of autogenous bone marrow is another intervention that is the subject of current research in fracture healing. A three-dimensional implant or graft can also be used as an aid to bone healing by supporting the attachment, spreading, division, and differentiation of bone cells. Osteoinduction involves the use of substances such as platelet-derived growth factor to stimulate bone healing.

BOX 29-1 *Factors Affecting Bone Healing*

Favorable

Location
- Good blood supply at bone ends
- Flat bones

Minimal damage to soft tissue
Anatomic reduction possible
Effective immobilization
Weight-bearing on long bones

Unfavorable

Fragments widely separated
Fragments distracted by traction
Severely comminuted fracture
Severe damage to soft tissue
Bone loss from injury or surgical excision
Motion/rotation at fracture site as a result of inadequate fixation
Infection
Impaired blood supply to one or more bone fragments
Location
- Decreased blood supply
- Midshaft

Health behaviors such as smoking, alcohol use

Clinical Manifestations

Fracture diagnosis is based on the client's clinical manifestations and history, physical examination, and radiographic findings. Some fractures are immediately obvious; others are detected only on x-ray. Use of the correct radiologic view is essential for adequate evaluation of the suspected fracture. Two views (e.g., anteroposterior and lateral) taken at right angles are generally considered the minimal number needed for evaluation, and they should include the joints above and below the suspected fracture to identify additional dislocations or subluxations. Abnormal x-ray findings include soft tissue edema or displacement of air in relation to a shift of the bone after injury. Radiographs of the fractured bone show an alteration in its normal contour and a disruption of the normal joint relationship. The fracture line itself demonstrates increased radiolucency (Figure 29-1). Radiographs are commonly taken before fracture reduction, after reduction, and then periodically during bone healing.

Physical assessment may reveal any of the following clinical manifestations:

- *Deformity.* Swelling from local hemorrhage may cause deformity at the fracture site. Muscle spasms can cause limb shortening, a rotational deformity, or angulation. Compared with the uninjured side, the fracture site may also have altered curves.

A   B

FIGURE 29-1 A, Fracture of the supracondylar femur. (Note the radiolucency of the fracture line.) **B,** Reduction of the fracture with traction. The fracture was eventually pinned.

- *Swelling.* Edema may appear quickly as a result of accumulation of serous fluid at the fracture site and extravasation of blood into surrounding tissues.
- *Bruising* (ecchymosis). Bruising results from subcutaneous bleeding at the fracture site.
- *Muscle spasm.* Frequently accompanying fractures, involuntary muscle spasm actually serves as a natural splint to decrease further motion of fracture fragments.
- *Pain.* If the client is neurologically intact, pain always accompanies fracture; the intensity and severity of the pain differ from client to client. Pain is usually continuous, increasing in severity until the fracture is immobilized. It results from muscle spasm, overriding of fracture fragments, or damage to adjacent structures.
- *Tenderness.* Tenderness over the fracture site is caused by underlying injuries.

- *Loss of function.* Any loss of function results either from pain caused by the fracture or from loss of the lever-arm function in an affected extremity. Paralysis may be caused by nerve damage.
- *Abnormal mobility and crepitus.* These manifestations are caused by motion in the middle of a bone or by fracture fragments rubbing together to create grating sensations or sounds.
- *Neurovascular changes.* Neurovascular injury results from damage to peripheral nerves or to the associated vascular structures. The client may complain of numbness and tingling or have no palpable pulse distal to the fracture.
- *Shock.* Bony fragments may lacerate blood vessels. Frank or occult hemorrhage can lead to shock.

Fracture Classification

More than 150 types of fractures have been identified according to various classification methods. See Table 29-2 for common descriptors.

The simplest classification method is based on whether the fracture is *closed* or *open* to the environment. A *closed fracture* has intact skin over the site of injury, whereas the *open fracture* is characterized by a break in the skin over the bone injury. Tissue damage can be extensive with open fractures, which are graded according to their severity:

- *Grade I.* The wound is smaller than 1 cm; contamination is minimal.
- *Grade II.* The wound is larger than 1 cm; contamination is moderate.
- *Grade III.* The wound exceeds 6 to 8 cm; there is extensive damage to soft tissue, nerve, and tendon; and there is a high degree of contamination.

Because the wound communicates with the external environment, the risk of infection must be promptly recognized and addressed.

Outcome Management
■ Medical Management

The goals of medical management include prompt and thorough assessment of the client to discover all injuries, reduction and stabilization of the fracture with immobilization, monitoring for complications, and eventual remobilization and rehabilitation.

Thorough Initial Assessment

Basic principles of trauma care must be followed during emergency management of fractures. Assessment and treatment are performed simultaneously as the rescuer addresses the general condition of the injured client. During primary assessment, the rescuer focuses on airway management, bleeding, and manifestations of shock. Any potentially life-threatening injuries must be stabilized immediately and emergency assistance summoned to transport the client to a medical facility for additional intervention. An injured client should not be moved unless the current location is not safe.

Because most fractures do not pose a serious threat to life, their management becomes a secondary priority in trauma care. Suspected injuries to extremities should be carefully splinted and moved as little as possible because multiple fractures frequently occur in the same limb. If the client complains of muscle spasm after a cervical spine or head injury, a fracture or dislocation is presumed to be present until radiographs can be performed and interpreted. The rescuer must stabilize the affected area and help the client remain still. An unconscious client should receive emergency management while the rescuer carefully notes any spontaneous movement as well as the client's position, head, and extremities. The rescuer performs a neurologic assessment that is based on the type of known or suspected injury. Any soft tissue damage must also be assessed because the injury may indicate a fracture site. Open fractures should be covered with sterile dressings and remain covered to prevent additional contamination until a thorough examination can occur in the nearest hospital.

When the client reaches the emergency department, the neurologic condition and vital signs are closely monitored, and food and fluids are withheld (*nil per os*, nothing by mouth, or NPO) in case surgery is indicated. Health care providers carefully examine the injured area and obtain the client's history. Details of the injury are helpful in determining the probable type of fracture and associated injuries. If the client was in a motor-vehicle accident, for example, was he or she sitting in the back or front seat? Was the client wearing a seat belt? What was the angle of impact? Was the client pulled from the car after a major collision? Or did the injury occur as a result of a fall on a hip or an outstretched arm?

Arterial damage is a possible early complication after fracture. The arteries may have been contused or lacerated, or they may have been constricted by tightly applied bandages or casts. With a displaced fracture, a hematoma may develop in the soft tissue as a result of damage to large blood vessels. Other indications of arterial damage include a variable pulse or absence of a pulse, poor capillary return, swelling, pallor or patchy cyanosis distal to the injury, pain, paresthesias, or coolness of an extremity as a result of poorly filled veins. Blood loss may be considerable, particularly with femur or pelvic fractures, and hypovolemic shock may become another complication. Extensive bleeding can occur even with closed fractures, and emergency surgery may become necessary; loss of blood supply to the fracture can result in areas of bone necrosis. Soft tissue infection can easily follow open fracture, and for optimal effectiveness, antibiotic therapy should begin as soon as possible after the injury.

TABLE 29-2	*Common Types of Fractures*			
Description	**Illustration**	**Description**	**Illustration**	

Appearance

Description	Illustration	Description	Illustration
Burst: Characterized by multiple pieces of bone; often occurs at bone ends or in vertebrae		Longitudinal: Fracture line extends in the direction of the bone's longitudinal axis	
Comminuted: More than one fracture line; more than two bone fragments; fragments may be splintered or crushed		Nondisplaced: Fragments aligned at fracture site	
Complete: Break across the entire section of bone, dividing it into distinct fragments; often displaced		Oblique: Fracture line occurs at approximately 45-degree angle across the longitudinal axis of the bone	
Displaced: Fragments out of normal position at fracture site	Torsion	Spiral: Fracture line results from twisting force; forms a spiral encircling the bone	
Incomplete: Fracture occurs through only one cortex of the bone; usually nondisplaced		Stellate: Fracture lines radiate from one central point	
Linear: Fracture line is intact; fracture is caused by minor to moderate force applied directly to the bone		Transverse: Fracture line occurs at a 90-degree angle to longitudinal axis of bone	

TABLE 29-2	*Common Types of Fractures—cont'd*			
Description		**Illustration**	**Description**	**Illustration**

General Description

Avulsion: Bone fragments are torn away from the body of the bone at the site of attachment of a ligament or tendon

Compression: Bone buckles and eventually cracks as the result of unusual loading force applied to its longitudinal axis

Greenstick: Incomplete fracture in which one side of the cortex is broken and the other side is flexed but intact

Impacted: Telescoped fracture, with one fragment driven into another

Anatomic Location

Colles': Fracture within the last inch of the distal radius; distal fragment is displaced in a position of dorsal and medial deviation

Pott's: Fracture of the distal fibula, seriously disrupting the tibiofibular articulation; a piece of the medial malleolus may be chipped off as a result of rupture of the internal lateral ligament

Reducing Fractures

The first step in management of a displaced fracture is *reduction*: the manipulation of the fracture to restore alignment, position, and length by bringing the fragments into close approximation. Reduction, which is also called *bone setting*, alleviates compression or stretching of nerves and blood vessels. Because reduction is generally painful, sedation or local or general anesthesia may be needed.

Not all fractures require reduction. Fragments of a nondisplaced fracture, for example, are already in proper alignment. Splinting or casting allows the alignment to be maintained as the fracture heals. A few other fractures cannot be adequately splinted and instead are treated simply by resting the affected area until healing occurs (e.g., distal phalangeal fractures).

When a fracture of an extremity divides a bone into two fragments, the fragments are referred to as *proximal* (nearer the trunk) and *distal* (farther from the trunk). Because of its muscle attachment and location, the proximal fragment cannot be manipulated or moved when the fractured bone is being set. Instead, the distal fragment is moved to realign it with the proximal bone segment. Reduction methods can be used alone or in combination.

FIGURE 29-2 Closed reduction to realign a supracondylar fracture.

Closed Reduction. To perform closed reduction, a health care provider applies manual traction to move the fracture fragments and restore bone alignment (Figure 29-2). Closed reduction should be performed as soon as possible after injury to decrease the client's risk for loss of function, to prevent or delay joint degeneration (traumatic arthritis), and to minimize the possible deforming effects of the injury. Fracture reduction is not an emergency procedure, however, and the client's life should never be jeopardized by attempting early reduction.

Manual reduction is accomplished through four maneuvers, beginning with a longitudinal pull on the distal end of the fracture or extremity. Because it reverses the mechanism of injury, this pull overcomes any initial muscle spasm, any effects on limb length, and the overriding of bone fragments. Second, the bone ends of the fracture must be disengaged from each other. This is sometimes accomplished by rotating the distal portion of the fracture. In the third maneuver, the fracture fragments are realigned. This is a complex step because forces from various muscle groups have held the fragments in their new positions. Finally, the distraction force is released while alignment is maintained.

Because gravity, weight-bearing, and muscle contraction can again move the fragments, an immobilization device must be applied after x-ray studies have confirmed bone alignment. The immobilizer most commonly used after closed reduction is a *cast*, a temporary device made of synthetic materials such as fiberglass or thermoplastic polymer or of plaster of Paris (anhydrous calcium sulfate). Casts are used for several purposes in addition to immobilization: prevention or correction of deformity; maintenance, support, and protection of realigned bone; and promotion of healing to allow early weight-bearing for ambulation. Casts may be applied in a hospital emergency department, in the operating room, or at the client's bedside in the hospital. They are also commonly applied in a physician's office or clinic.

Synthetic materials are used to construct a strong, light-weight cast that sets in about 5 minutes. They also come in a variety of colors and patterns that can enhance self-esteem in both young and older clients after injury. Synthetic casts maintain their shape and firmness even if they become wet, but they must be dried thoroughly to prevent skin maceration. If there is no incision under the cast, synthetic materials can be dried with a hair blow dryer on a low setting; however, several hours are needed for the cast to dry thoroughly.

Plaster of Paris bandages are individual rolls of precut crinoline impregnated with plaster. They come in various sizes, and the body part to be put in a cast determines the amount of plaster to be used. Plaster casts take at least 24 hours longer than synthetic casts to dry, and they lose their shape if they are allowed to get wet again.

Open Reduction and Internal Fixation. To perform open reduction, the surgeon makes an incision and realigns the fracture fragments under direct visualization. Open reduction is the treatment of choice for compound fractures that are comminuted or accompanied by severe neurovascular injury; it is also required if fracture fragments are widely separated or if soft tissue is interposed between pieces of bone.

Open reduction is usually performed in combination with internal fixation for femoral and joint fractures. Screws, plates, pins, wires, or nails may be used to maintain alignment of the fracture fragments (Figure 29-3). Rods may also be placed through the fragments or fixed to the side of the bone, or they may be inserted directly into the bone's medullary cavity. Internal fixation provides essential immobilization and helps to prevent deformity, but it is not a substitute for bone healing. If proper healing fails to occur, the internal fixation device may actually loosen or break as a result of stress.

External Fixation. Depending on the client's condition and the physician's judgment, external fixation devices may be used for fracture fragment immobilization (Figure 29-4). If, for example, soft tissue damage precludes the use of a cast, external fixation would be indicated for fracture immobilization. External fixation devices maintain position for unstable fractures and for weakened muscles, and they support areas with tissue or bone infection. They allow the client to use contiguous joints while the affected area remains immobilized. External fixation may also be indicated for bony non-union if fracture healing has not been successful after a certain time. Common sites for external fixation include the face and jaw, extremities, pelvis, ribs, fingers, and toes. Pins used in external fixation vary in number, length, and thickness on the basis of the treatment area.

FIGURE 29-3 Examples of different types of internal fixation devices. **A,** Tension band wiring with Kirschner wires for a fracture of the phalanx. **B,** Compression plate and screws in the lateral aspect of the femur. **C,** Sliding hip screw.

Client selection is critical to the successful use of external fixation. Any potential problems with compliance should be discussed thoroughly with the client and family, including the effects of external fixation on the client's lifestyle. Noncompliance with the medical regimen can lead to pin loosening, loss of fracture stabilization, and infection. Specific activity orders are written after the application of an external fixator, with special attention to weight-bearing status when the pelvis or a lower extremity is involved.

Traction. Traction has been used to treat fractures since prehistoric times, and its principles were well known to Hippocrates. Traction is the application of a pulling force to an injured body part or extremity while a countertraction pulls in the opposite direction. The pulling force can be achieved through the use of hands (manual traction) or, more commonly, the application of weights. The purposes of traction are shown in Box 29-2. With improved surgical technique and the development of femoral prostheses and intramedullary rods, traction is not as prevalent as it once was in the treatment of orthopedic injuries. Lower extremity traction, such as Buck or Russell traction, currently has limited application in the preoperative management of a client with a fractured hip, for example. Skeletal traction, however, continues to be an option for multiple trauma clients who are not immediate candidates for open reduction and internal fixation of orthopedic injuries. Various types of traction may also be treatment options before and after surgical reduction of injuries such as cervical fractures and for chronic conditions such as low back pain.

Skin traction involves the application of a pulling force directly to the skin through the use of skin strips, boots, or foam splints. Cervical halters and pelvic belts allow traction to be applied to the neck or pelvis. Skin traction bears a low longitudinal force load (5 to 7 pounds), which gives it minimal effectiveness. Because of the risk of skin breakdown, this type of traction should be used only temporarily.

Skeletal traction uses pins to apply force to the bone. With skeletal traction, a direct force can be applied after the physician aseptically inserts stainless steel pins through the bone itself. The most common sites for pin insertion are the distal femur, the proximal tibia, and the proximal ulna. Skeletal traction can be tolerated for longer periods than can skin traction. Weights may reach 15 pounds, although 7 to 10 pounds are more commonly used.

In addition to the mode of application, traction can be categorized as *static* (continuous) or *dynamic* (intermittent). Suspension may also be *running* or *straight* (exerting a direct pull on the affected part) or *balanced* (exerting a pull on the affected part and also supporting the extremity in a splint). Table 29-3 describes major types of traction.

Major disadvantages include the potential need for prolonged bed rest and the resulting effects of extended immobility. Long-term hospitalization is not always indicated if the client in traction can qualify for home care nursing services or, depending on the type of traction, receive additional treatment as an outpatient.

Complications After Fracture

Continuously assess the client with orthopedic trauma for potential complications and then intervene quickly to minimize effects. Certain client characteristics increase the likelihood of complications, particularly after

FIGURE 29-4 External fixation to provide immobilization of a tibial fracture. (From Stryker Howmedica Osteonics, Mahwah, NJ.)

BOX 29-2   *Purposes of Traction*

- Reduce, realign, and promote healing of fractured bones
- Decrease muscle spasms that may accompany fractures or follow surgical reduction
- Prevent soft tissue damage through immobilization
- Prevent or treat deformities
- Rest an inflamed, diseased, or painful joint
- Reduce and treat dislocations and subluxations
- Prevent the development of contractures
- Reduce muscle spasms associated with low back pain or cervical whiplash
- Expand a joint space during arthroscopy or before major joint reconstruction

From Ceccio, C.M. (1999). Key concepts in the care of patients in traction. In *An introduction to orthopaedic nursing* (2nd ed.). Pitman, NJ: National Association of Orthopaedic Nurses.

TABLE 29-3	*Major Types of Traction*		
Traction	**Type**	**Common Conditions Treated**	**Duration**
Cervical			
Chin halter	Skin	Severe strains or sprains; cervical trauma nerve root compression; torticollis	Intermittent
Skeletal tongs: Gardner-Wells, Crutchfield, Vinke	Skeletal	Fractures or dislocations of cervical or high thoracic vertebrae	Continuous
Halo traction	Skeletal	Fractures or dislocations of cervical or high thoracic vertebrae	Continuous
Upper Extremity			
Side-arm	Skin or skeletal	Vertical suspension to forearm	Continuous
Overhead/90-90	Skin or skeletal	Vertical traction to humerus; horizontal suspension to forearm	Continuous
Lower Back			
Pelvic belt or sling	Skin	Low back pain	Intermittent or continuous
Lower Extremity			
Buck	Skin	Hip and knee contracture; preoperative immobilization and muscle spasm relief for hip fractures	Continuous
Balanced suspension: Thomas ring and Pearson and Brady attachment	Skeletal	Used mainly with skeletal pins for supracondylar femur fracture; hip and knee contracture; postoperative positioning and immobilization	Continuous

Modified from Redermann, S. (2002). Modalities for immobilization. In A. B. Maher, S. W. Salmond, & T. A. Pellino (Eds.), *Orthopaedic nursing* (3rd ed.). Philadelphia: W. B. Saunders; and from Ceccio, C. M. (1999). Key concepts in the care of patients in traction. In *An introduction to orthopaedic nursing* (2nd ed.), Pitman, NJ: National Association of Orthopaedic Nurses.

surgical repair of fractures. These include the type of injury, the client's age, the presence of other health problems (co-morbidities), and the client's use of medications that affect bleeding, such as warfarin, corticosteroids, and nonsteroidal anti-inflammatory drugs (NSAIDs).

Nerve Injury. Bone fragments and tissue edema associated with the injury can cause nerve damage. Be alert for pallor and coolness of the client's affected extremity, changes in the client's ability to move the digits or the extremity, paresthesia, or complaints of increasing pain.

Compartment Syndrome. Muscle compartments in the upper and lower extremities are enclosed by tough, inelastic fascial tissue that does not expand if the muscle swells (Figure 29-5). Edema that occurs in response to a fracture can lead to an increase in compartment pressure that reduces capillary blood perfusion. When the local blood supply is unable to meet the tissue's metabolic demands, ischemia begins. *Compartment syndrome* is a condition of compromised circulation related to progressively increased pressure in a confined space. It is caused by anything that decreases the compartment size, including external compression forces such as a tight cast or internal factors such as bleeding or edema. Continued ischemia results in histamine release by the affected muscles, leading to even greater edema and a further decrease in perfusion. An increase in lactic acid production causes more anaerobic metabolism and a subsequent increase in blood flow that, in turn, increases the tissue pressure. This leads to a cycle of increasing compartment pressure. Compartment syndrome can occur anywhere in the body but occurs most often in the lower leg and forearm. If it goes unrecognized or untreated, the client can lose nerve and muscle function. Infection, myoglobinuria, and renal failure may follow, and amputation may become necessary.

Intracompartmental pressures can be measured by various monitors currently on the market. Normal compartment pressure is considered to be 0 to 8 mm Hg. Although co-morbid conditions such as shock or compensatory hypertension can affect the client's response, compartment pressures ranging from 30 to 45 mm Hg historically have been considered high enough to cause tissue necrosis if treatment is not initiated. According to more recent medical consensus, imminent surgical intervention is not required for pressures greater than 40 mm Hg if the client's diastolic blood pressure remains high enough to perfuse the muscle compartment.

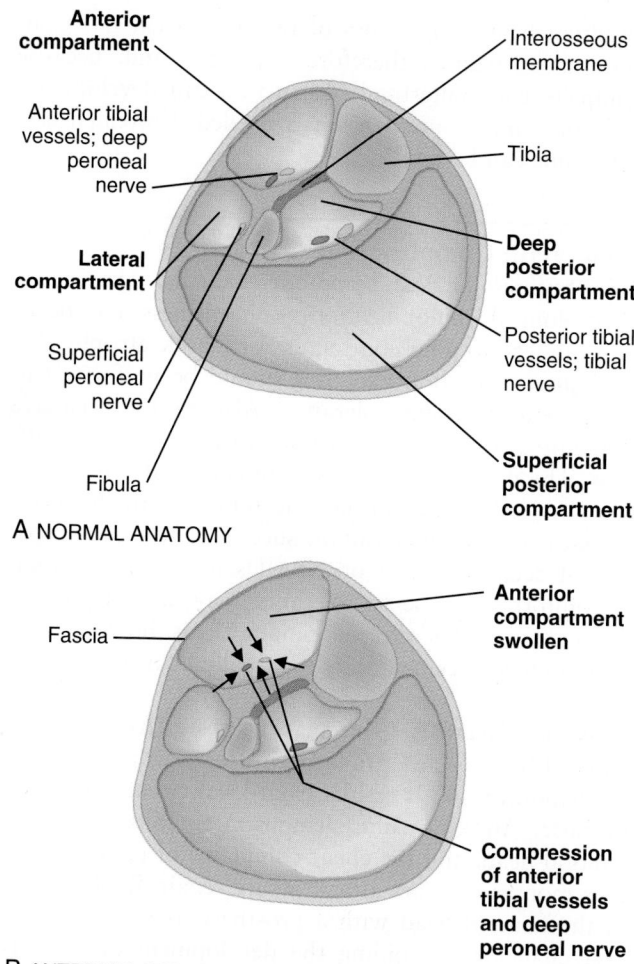

A NORMAL ANATOMY

B ANTERIOR COMPARTMENT SYNDROME

FIGURE 29-5 A, Dompartments of the proximal third of the lower leg. The four compartments are (1) anterior, (2) lateral, (3) deep posterior, and (4) superficial posterior. **B,** When swelling occurs in response to injury, the compartment is contained by the inelastic fascia that covers it. Unrelieved pressure compromises nerves and vessels within the compartment.

The primary treatment of compartment syndrome is relief of the source of pressure. To accomplish this, the physician may order a constrictive bandage to be removed or a cast to be bivalved (see Care of the Client in a Cast later in this chapter). The affected extremity should be kept at heart level because elevation above the heart actually decreases local arterial perfusion, further compromising blood flow. Cold applications should be avoided with suspected compartment syndrome because they lead to vasoconstriction, which can further compromise circulation. Adequate hydration is important for maintaining the client's mean arterial blood pressure. Pain should be managed to decrease the vasoconstrictive effects of the sympathetic nervous system.

If relief of external pressure is not enough to keep compartment pressures from rising, a fasciotomy may be necessary. An incision through the skin into the fascia of the muscle compartment allows tissue expansion and restores blood flow by relieving pressure on the microcirculation. The incision typically is left open until the swelling decreases; the area is then loosely wrapped and the wrapping is left on for several days. The wound is closed by tertiary intention when edema has subsided.

Volkmann's Contracture. *Volkmann's contracture* is a limb deformity that results from unrelieved compartment syndrome. As prolonged pressure causes ischemia, muscle is gradually replaced by fibrous tissue that traps tendons and nerves. Tibial fractures have been linked to the development of this condition, which can lead to deformities such as cavus of the foot, equinus, and adduction of the forefoot with varus of the hindfoot. In the upper extremities, Volkmann's contracture most commonly occurs after fractures of the elbow and forearm or after crushing injuries of the forearm, or it is caused by tight bandages or casts. It can lead to a permanently stiff, claw-like deformity of the hand and arm. Contractures may be avoided through prompt recognition of manifestations of compartment syndrome, followed by limb splinting and compartment decompression as indicated.

Fat Embolism Syndrome. Fat embolism syndrome (FES) is a major cause of delayed recovery and mortality after fracture. The mechanical theory of FES origin describes the release of fat globules from the bone marrow into the venous circulation after fracture, particularly fractures of the long bones, pelvis, ribs, sternum, vertebrae, and clavicle. A biochemical or metabolic theory suggests that trauma leads to the release of fatty acids and neutral fats. Platelet aggregation and fat globule formation then occur. In reality, the pathophysiologic process of FES is unknown; it may include parts of both theories or reflect an entirely different, unknown etiology.

The deposit of embolic fat in the pulmonary circulation can lead to the rapid onset of a disorder similar to adult (acute) respiratory distress syndrome (ARDS). Perfusion pressure increases, and pulmonary vessels become engorged. As the lung becomes more rigid, the workload of the right side of the heart increases. The fat globules occluding the pulmonary circulation are hydrolyzed into free fatty acids that increase capillary permeability and activate lung surfactant. Hemorrhagic pulmonary edema and patchy alveolar collapse occur, leading to severe hypoxia. Diagnosis of FES is not made on the basis of a single manifestation, laboratory test, or radiologic study. Instead, the client's presentation must be reviewed system by system.

The highest incidence of FES occurs following fractures of long bones, such as the femur, tibia, ribs, fibula, and pelvis. Up to 90% of clients with multiple traumas may develop FES.[27] Total joint arthroplasty also places the client at risk for FES, and the incidence increases after bilateral procedures. Primary manifestations typically occur within 24 to 72 hours after injury, but a fulminant form of FES can occur within just a few hours of injury and may progress rapidly to death.

Prevention of FES begins with prudent treatment of long bone fractures, including careful handling, appropriate splinting, and avoidance of unnecessary manipulation of the injured area. Prompt surgical fixation after injury (within 24 to 48 hours) is critical. Early aggressive resuscitation to prevent hypovolemic shock, adequate pain management, blood transfusion through a 20-μm filter, and prevention of sepsis are also considered standard preventive care.

If FES does occur, supportive treatment is directed at preserving the client's respiratory function. Oxygen is administered; intubation and continuous positive airway pressure are sometimes necessary. Steroids use is controversial but may be considered in overt and subclinical forms of FES in an attempt to decrease the inflammatory effects of the fatty acids on the alveolocapillary membrane. Fluid volume replacement is important to prevent circulatory instability.

Deep Vein Thrombosis and Pulmonary Embolism. The client with orthopedic injuries is at high risk for thromboembolic conditions such as deep vein thrombosis (DVT) and pulmonary embolism (PE). DVT results from the formation of a blood clot (thrombus) in a deep vein in the lower extremity. If the thrombus travels into the pulmonary circulation, it is termed a *pulmonary embolus.*

Prevention of DVT is a primary goal. Clot prophylaxis is recommended through the use of pharmacologic agents such as an oral anticoagulant or subcutaneous low-molecular-weight (LMW) heparin (fixed dose or weight adjusted). For appropriately selected clients, physical-mechanical measures such as intermittent pneumatic compression devices or elastic stockings may also have a role in DVT prevention. DVT is discussed fully in Chapter 55.

Infection. Infection continues to be a cause of morbidity among clients who have open or surgically repaired fractures. Pathogens can contaminate an open fracture or may be introduced at the time of surgery. Surgical wound infection during the postoperative period usually results from *Staphylococcus aureus* or *Staphylococcus epidermidis.* Osteomyelitis, a severe infection of the bone itself, can also result (see Chapter 28).

Cast Syndrome. Cast syndrome (superior mesenteric artery syndrome) occurs only with body spica casts. The duodenum is compressed between the superior mesenteric artery anteriorly and the aorta and vertebral bodies posteriorly, causing a decreased blood supply that can lead to hemorrhage and necrosis of the bowel. Cast syndrome can develop days to weeks after immobilization resulting from weight loss of retroperitoneal fat. Constant assessment is therefore a priority and, because complete gastrointestinal obstruction can develop, immediate nursing intervention is needed. Untreated cast syndrome can be fatal.

Long-Term Complications of Fractures

Joint Stiffness or Post-Traumatic Arthritis. After injury or prolonged immobilization, joint stiffness may occur and can lead to joint contracture or muscle atrophy. Active range-of-motion exercises should be performed to the extent of client tolerance. Also perform passive range-of-motion exercises to decrease the risk for stiffness. The occurrence of post-traumatic arthritis, which can also lead to joint stiffness, is influenced by the severity of the initial injury and the success of bone reduction. Use of acetaminophen or NSAIDs may decrease joint discomfort. Exercise to tolerance may also ameliorate the manifestations of developing arthritis; however, surgical joint replacement may eventually be needed.

Avascular Necrosis. Avascular necrosis (AVN) of the femoral head occurs primarily in fractures proximal to the femoral neck. It results from local circulatory compromise. An x-ray film demonstrates collapse of the femoral head, and the client complains of pain that occurs months to years after fracture repair. Replacement of the femoral head with a prosthesis is required. The best chance for avoiding the development of AVN is prompt surgical repair after fracture diagnosis.

Nonfunctional Union After a Fracture. Several types of problems can result in regard to proper bony union.

Malunion. Malunion results when fracture fragments heal in improper alignment as a result of unequal muscle pull and gravity. It can occur if the client bears weight on the affected extremity against medical advice or when an ambulatory device is applied before adequate healing has begun at the fracture site. The primary manifestation is external deformity of the involved extremity. Malunion is diagnosed by radiography. If it is identified early in the course of fracture healing, malunion can be corrected with adjustment of traction or remobilization. Malunion that is diagnosed after healing is complete must be surgically corrected. Prevention is accomplished by adequate fracture reduction and immobilization and by ensuring that the client understands the importance of any activity or position restrictions.

Delayed Union. Suspect delayed union if the client complains of continuation or increase in bone pain and tenderness beyond the healing period expected on the basis of the degree of trauma (3 months to 1 year). Healing is slowed but not completely stopped, possibly as a result of distraction of the fracture fragments or a systemic cause such as infection. If the cause can be identified and corrected early, the fracture usually heals.

Non-Union. Non-union is identified when fracture healing has not occurred 4 to 6 months after the initial injury and when spontaneous healing is unlikely to occur. It is generally caused by insufficient blood supply and uncontrolled repetitive stress on the fracture site, possibly as a result of the presence of muscle, tendon, or soft tissue between fracture fragments. Non-union can also result from prolonged or excessive traction; insufficient or inadequate immobilization that allows movement at the fracture site; inadequate internal fixation; or wound infection after internal fixation. On radiograph, non-union is characterized by a relatively narrow gap between fracture fragments. A soft tissue bridge of fibrocartilage and fibrous tissue spans the gap.

Once diagnosed, non-union is treated by bone grafting, internal or external fixation, electric bone stimulation, or a combination of these methods. Client education is especially important before the use of electric bone stimulation because weight-bearing on the affected extremity is contraindicated for 6 to 8 weeks. Weight-bearing on an unstable fracture prolongs healing time.

Fibrous Union. Fibrous tissue is interposed in a wide gap between fracture fragments. Loss of bone through surgery or injury predisposes the client to this type of fracture union. Additional surgical fixation may be required.

Complex Regional Pain Syndrome. Formerly known as *reflex sympathetic dystrophy*, this condition is a painful dysfunction and disuse syndrome that is characterized by abnormal pain and swelling of the affected extremity. It is usually precipitated by relatively minor trauma and generally is believed to be related to the sympathetic nervous system. The origin may be the client's pain, fear, or anxiety. Manifestations may include disproportionate pain at the site of injury, edema, muscle spasm or vasospasm, stiffness and decreased joint mobility, increased sweating, atrophy, contractions, and loss of bone mass. Some treatment success has been experienced with sympathetic nerve blocks, especially in early stages of the syndrome. Drug therapies typically involve use of analgesics, muscle relaxants, and antidepressants. Physical therapy and transcutaneous electric nerve stimulation may also be ordered. Psychological counseling is often suggested for the client living with this chronic condition.

■ Nursing Management of the Medical Client

Care of the Client in a Cast

Closed reduction of fractures is followed by immobilization to relieve or reduce pain and to prevent rotation and shearing at the fracture site. Immobilization is most often accomplished through the use of a cast or splint (Fig-ure 29-6). Before application of a cast, the nurse's role may entail preparation of the client for casting, including a detailed explanation of the procedure. Skin preparation involves thorough cleansing and assessment of any lesions. The presence of unremovable dirt or foreign particles should be reported to the physician. After the skin preparation, padding or a web roll is applied to the extremity surrounding the fracture site. Additional padding made be indicated over bony prominences, but too much padding can actually increase pressure. Stockinette is applied over the padding and is cut several inches longer than the expected finished cast length so that excess portions can be pulled over exposed cast ends to protect the client's skin. Make sure that these coverings fit smoothly and without wrinkles, which could produce pressure areas on underlying tissues.

Rolls of casting materials, whether plaster or synthetic, are individually submerged in clean water in a bucket. Excess water is squeezed from the roll, and then the bandage is applied to encircle the injured body part. Assist during cast application by supporting the extremity from underneath, using only the palms of your hands to avoid applying pressure to any one area. Fingertips should not be pressed into the cast, and the cast should not be allowed to rest on a hard or sharp surface; these actions might cause flattening or indentations in the cast, which could create pressure. As soon as the casting procedure is complete, the client's skin must be cleansed of excess casting material. Plaster-laden water should never be emptied into an ordinary sink because the plaster sediment solidifies and plugs the plumbing. If a sink with a plaster trap is not available, wait for sediment to settle to the bottom of the bucket, and then drain off the water from the top. The remaining plaster sediment can be scraped from the bottom of the bucket and placed into the garbage container.

Drying a Cast. As the water from a newly applied cast eventually evaporates, a mature cast of full strength develops. Synthetic casts dry to the touch in a few minutes, but they take about 30 minutes to set completely and allow weight-bearing. Plaster casts set quickly but take hours to days to dry completely; a lower extremity plaster cast may not be totally dry for up to 48 hours, and larger casts can take even longer. Because both plaster and synthetic casts generate heat while drying, the client should be instructed to expect the sensation of heat. The cast should not be covered with a blanket or towel while it is drying because the retained heat can burn the client. Several towels may be placed under the cast on the pillow to absorb dampness. While the cast is still damp, the client may feel cold and may experience a decrease in body temperature. Adequate covering is provided for the client while dry, warm air is allowed to circulate around the damp cast. To avoid excessive chilling for the client who is in a large cast, sections of the cast should be exposed for brief periods alternately. Unless it is

FIGURE 29-6 Common types of casts and possible pressure points.

contraindicated, the client should also be turned regularly to expose more of the new cast to air. Rapid drying through use of a blow dryer is not advised because it can burn the client's skin under the cast and crack the cast.

A wet plaster cast smells musty and is dull on percussion, gray, and cold to the touch. When dry, the plaster cast is odorless, resonant, and white, and it feels close to room temperature when touched. Wet fiberglass casts feel hot and sticky to the touch. A wet fiberglass cast should not be placed over drainage-containing pads,

such as incontinence pads, because paper and plaster adhere and the paper will become a permanent part of the cast. Once the cast is completely dry, it can safely be placed on a hard surface (e.g., a casted arm can rest on a table), but the client is usually more comfortable in continuing to rest the casted area on pillows.

Windowing or Bivalving a Cast. *Bivalving* a cast means cutting the cast along both sides and then splitting it to decrease pressure on underlying tissue. Windows may also be cut into the cast to allow the physician or nurse to visualize wounds under the cast or remove drains. In addition, windows may be cut to allow pulse assessment or to prevent cast syndrome. Bivalving also allows removal of half of the cast for wound care or x-rays. The remaining half of a bivalved cast is often used as an intermittent splint that can be removed and reapplied as the client adjusts to being without a cast. When reapplying a bivalved cast, take care not to pinch the client's skin between the cast halves. When the cast halves are properly fitted, secure them with an elastic wrap.

Neurovascular Assessment. Although casts are protective and therapeutic, they can also cause serious complications. Careful nursing assessment and prompt intervention are necessary to minimize the client's risk for detrimental effects. Be aware of the client's neurovascular status by assessing the following in a casted extremity:

- Color, warmth, pulses distal to the cast, capillary refill (circulatory function)
- Movement of distal fingers or toes, awareness of light touch distal to the cast, changes in sensation (nerve function)

The deep and superficial peroneal nerves and the tibial nerve are most at risk for injury with lower extremity fractures, whereas radial and ulnar nerve function must be assessed with upper extremity injuries. Encourage the client to report any numbness or tingling, although neither may be present even with nerve compression. Pulse, color, and warmth of the injured extremity should also be assessed by comparison with the unaffected extremity. Neurovascular assessment should be performed every 30 minutes for 4 hours after cast or splint application and then every 3 to 4 hours. Table 29-4 describes the technique used for assessment and expected findings.

Assessment of Pain. Careful assessment of pain must be completed regularly, and the client must be encouraged to verbalize the degree of pain. Inadequate analgesic effects should be reported promptly to the surgeon because an increased dosage or change in medication may be indicated. Unrelieved pain is also a classic manifestation of compartment syndrome; therefore any complaint of pain should be given your full attention. Be especially alert to complaints of progressive pain or pain out of proportion to the injury or treatment.

Assessment of the Cast. The skin around the cast edges should be observed for damage or swelling. Also assess the cast itself. "Hot spots"—areas of the cast that feel warmer than other sections—may indicate tissue necrosis or infection under the cast. "Wet spots" may indicate drainage under the cast or a need for additional drying. Stains can indicate wound drainage or bleeding, and any stained areas should be carefully measured and documented. Also be aware of possible pressure points on underlying structures, such as the lateral malleolus under a short leg cast or the epicondyle under a short arm cast. Closely inspect areas of the cast that are known to cover wounds with the understanding that drainage on the surface of synthetic casts may not wick outward but may go to a dependent area determined by cast position (e.g., beneath the cast if it is flat, posterior and superior if the limb is elevated).

An older cast may develop a sour smell because of perspiration or normal sloughing of outer skin layers. Musty, offensive odors under the cast, however, may indicate tissue necrosis or infection. If the odor of mildew is present, the synthetic cast may have not been thoroughly dried after it became wet; notify the physician because the cast needs to be changed.

Assessment for Complications

Compartment Syndrome. Any client with an extremity fracture should be assessed regularly for compartment syndrome for the first week after injury. Traumatic injury and treatment such as closed reduction usually produces swelling, which progresses for the first 12 to 24 hours after injury. The greatest swelling is likely to be evident in the first 24 to 48 hours. Mild swelling is expected; however, moderate or severe swelling associated with pain or discoloration is abnormal. Excessive swelling constricts the enclosed soft tissues and introduces the risk for compartment syndrome.

The affected extremity should be compared regularly with the uninjured extremity, and current findings should also be compared with baseline assessment data. Manifestations of compartment syndrome can begin as early as 30 minutes after ischemic injury. The primary manifestation is increasing pain or pain that is out of proportion to the injury. Specifically, pain with passive stretching of the muscles in an affected compartment is one of the earliest indicators. Assess for the presence of tingling or paresthesia in the affected extremity; muscle strength and motion; and circulation, including the presence and quality of pulses distal to the injury, capillary refill, skin color, and temperature. Increased tenseness and erythema of the skin also suggest increasing compartment pressures. If the intracompartmental pressure increases to a level above the client's systolic blood pressure, pulses are absent, capillary refill is delayed, and pallor results. Paralysis is a very late sign of compartment syndrome. If compartment syndrome goes unrecognized and tissue pressures are not relieved, muscle damage becomes irreversible after 4 to 6 hours of ischemia; nerve damage becomes irreversible after 12 to 24 hours.[8] The physician must be notified immediately of assessment findings that suggest the development of compartment syndrome (see the Critical Monitoring feature on The Client in a Cast on p. 634).

Fat Emboli. Be alert to manifestations of hypoxemia, such as apprehension, anxiety, agitation, or acute

TABLE 29-4 Neurovascular Assessments (CMS)

Parameter Being Assessed	Technique	Expected Finding
Circulation		
Color of affected extremity	Inspect the color of affected leg, foot, arm, or hand; compare to opposite side	Color should be the same; it is normal to have some paleness (pallor) in injured tissues; if incisions are present, some redness (erythema) may be noted along incision lines
Capillary refill in nail beds	Compress nail bed and measure time needed for refill (return of color)	Should be 2-3 sec; slowing to 4-6 sec should be reported
Edema	Inspect for edema in both extremities	No edema should be present; if edema is noted in affected extremity, consider whether it is caused by the trauma or surgery or thrombophlebitis; if present in both extremities, consider causes such as heart disease
Pedal pulses	Palpate for pedal pulses on dorsum of foot (dorsalis pedis) or adjacent to medial malleolus (posterior tibialis)	Pulses should be present bilaterally; if dorsal pulse is absent, may be normal variation; absent pulses could also signal compression of vessels from edema
Temperature of affected extremity	Use dorsum (back) of your hand to assess temperature	Temperature should be the same in each extremity; report any coolness or heat in the extremity
Movement		
Movement of affected extremity	Ask client to "move your toes/fingers"	Movement should be the same on each side; if decreased movement is noted, determine whether extremity normally moves (e.g., if the client has had a stroke, limited movement may have been present before); if client had surgery on toes or fingers, expect decreased movement as a result of pain and edema; look for even slight movement in the area
Sensation		
Sensation of affected extremity	Ask clients which digits they feel you touching; ask specifically if they have a "pins and needles" sensation or if the extremity feels as if it is "asleep"	Sensation should be the same on each side; any alterations in sensation should be reported
Pain	Ask clients to rate pain on scale of 0-10 (0 being no pain and 10 being the worst pain they have ever felt)	Pain is common in injured extremities; if no pain is reported, client may have recently had pain medication; uncontrollable pain may signal compartment syndrome and should be reported immediately

CRITICAL MONITORING

The Client in a Cast

Compartment Syndrome

Diminished or absent pulses; slow nail bed capillary refill (longer than 3 seconds)

Skin pallor, blanching, cyanosis, or coolness

Increasing pain, swelling, painful edema peripheral to cast, pain on passive motion

Paresthesias (tingling, prickling), heightened sensitivity, numbness; hypesthesia (diminished sensitivity to touch); anesthesia (numbness)

Motor paralysis of previously functioning muscles

Infection

Musty, unpleasant odor over cast or at ends of cast

Drainage through cast or cast opening

Sudden unexplained body temperature elevation

"Hot spot" felt on cast over lesion

New pain or increased pain

Cast Syndrome

Bloated feeling

Prolonged nausea; repeated vomiting

Abdominal distention; vague abdominal pain

Shortness of breath

confusion. The client with FES also exhibits fever (>103° F), dyspnea, tachypnea, and tachycardia. Diffuse rales and rhonchi may occur as late signs of FES. In 50% to 60% of clients, petechiae are noted on the chest, axillae, flanks, abdomen, clavicular fossae, and soft palate.[34]

Deep Vein Thrombosis. The typical manifestations of DVT are unilateral edema, at or below the site of thrombosis, that results from venous inflammation or obstruction. Affected clients often complain of pain and tenderness at the site, which may also be red and warm. Homans' sign (in which dorsiflexion of the foot causes discomfort in the upper calf) is present in fewer than one third of symptomatic clients with DVT. Because Homans' sign is present in more than 50% of symptomatic clients who do not have DVT, it is not considered specific or sensitive to the condition. Venous ultrasonography is a sensitive, accurate, noninvasive examination that has become the standard for diagnosis of DVT.

Pulmonary embolism results if a thromboembolism lodges in the pulmonary circulation, leading to decreased or absent blood flow distal to the clot. Because manifestations of PE can be nonspecific and vary greatly, PE is often undetected or misdiagnosed. The most common clinical manifestations are sudden unexplained dyspnea and pleuritic chest pain. In the event of a massive PE, diagnosis and successful treatment may be extremely difficult because of the extensive loss of gas exchange area and the severe strain placed on the right chambers of the heart by pulmonary hypertension. Although pulmonary angiography is still considered the standard for diagnosis, with a 98% sensitivity, the ventilation/perfusion ($\dot{V}/\dot{Q}$) scan is commonly ordered because it has a high sensitivity in ruling out PE. A chest radiograph can also be helpful in ruling out other pulmonary perfusion problems. (DVT is discussed more fully in Chapter 55, and PE is discussed in Chapter 63.)

Infection. The client may describe new pain or an increased level of pain and feelings of increased warmth under a bandage or cast. Assessment may reveal fever or chills, an odor from the area of injury, erythema and warmth around the wound, purulent drainage, and poor wound healing.

Cast Syndrome. If the client is in a body cast, closely attend to any complaints of nausea, abdominal pressure, vague abdominal pain, feelings of bloating or tightness, or inability to take a deep breath. These may be clinical manifestation of cast syndrome, a serious complication that can follow prolonged supine positioning, spinal surgery, or use of a body cast.

Management of suspected cast syndrome includes cutting a window or bivalving the cast to relieve pressure. Nasogastric intubation may be indicated to de-

compress the intestine, intravenous fluids may be ordered, and the client may be placed on NPO status. Antiemetics should be given sparingly to any client in a body cast because they can mask the manifestations of cast syndrome. The client who is discharged in a body cast should receive careful instruction about the clinical manifestations of cast syndrome and should be encouraged to report any complaints promptly to the surgeon.

Interventions for Clients in Casts. To prevent or relieve swelling, elevate the entire casted extremity higher than the client's heart for the first 24 to 48 hours. Place the affected extremity on pillows. A casted arm may also be elevated in a sling attached to an intravenous (IV) pole. The entire arm, including the elbow, wrist, and hand, must be supported, and the fingers must be kept higher than the elbow to minimize swelling. Also apply ice bags around the cast, and exercise the client's fingers or toes to encourage circulation. Relieve pressure at the cast edges by petaling the cast or loosely padding an uncomfortable area. To prevent footdrop in a cylinder-casted leg, splint or support the client's foot with the ankle in 90 degrees of flexion.

For the client in a hip spica or body cast, the buttocks should be exposed to prevent soiling or dampening of clothing during elimination and to provide adequate skin care. To prevent soiling, incontinence pads can be tucked into the edge of the cast before the client uses a fracture bedpan. Slightly raising the head of the bed facilitates elimination and also prevents excrement from running under the cast; this position is usually allowed unless the client is in shock, is hemorrhaging, or has a spinal injury. Dampness causes skin irritation and may increase the risk of infection if an open wound is present; therefore thorough perineal care must be completed after elimination.

Position changes at least every 2 hours are needed to help prevent complications of immobility, and a turning schedule is useful for ensuring that the client does not remain in one position too long. Give instructions on turning to encourage client activity, but also provide assistance with bed mobility as needed. When mobility assistance is needed, always have adequate staff help to reposition a casted client. Three or four people may be needed to turn a client in a body or hip spica cast, for example. Roller boards or mechanical lifts may also be useful.

Depending on the nature of the injury and the physician's orders, clients in casts can often bear weight as soon as the cast is dry. Be aware of the client's weight-bearing status when attempting a transfer. For client safety, also use a transfer belt when getting the client out of bed. Weak, older, or debilitated clients may have difficulty with the weight of the cast and may tire rapidly with initial activity. The client should be instructed about the likelihood of increased pain when a casted leg is lowered to a dependent position with initial attempts at ambulation. Help the client lower the leg, encouraging him or her about the decrease in pain as the leg becomes accustomed to the increased blood flow.

To ensure client cooperation, provide thorough instruction on pain management strategies. Ensure that the client understands the availability of analgesics for treatment of pain and is allowed to voice any concerns about their use, such as fears of addiction. Initiate an honest discussion about any barriers to analgesic use if the client seems hesitant about taking or asking for medication. Administer analgesics as prescribed, and promptly inform the surgeon of inadequate effects. Client instruction should also include alternative methods of pain management, such as distraction, visualization, or massage, that might help the client relax.

Care of the Client in External Fixation

Assessment. Because external fixation is commonly used following extensive soft tissue injury, the potential for neurovascular deficit or compartment syndrome is high. Even though the external fixator may be used for treatment of an open fracture, compartment syndrome can nonetheless develop in another compartment of the same extremity. Ongoing assessment of neurovascular status is critical. Current findings should be compared with baseline data, and the affected extremity should be compared with the unaffected extremity. Instruct the client to report any changes, and address any complaints promptly.

As with the client in a cast, careful assessment of pain must be completed regularly. Analgesia should be assessed, and inadequate effects should be reported promptly to the surgeon because an increased dosage or change in medication may be indicated. Unrelieved pain should raise suspicion of compartment syndrome, and any complaint of pain should be given full attention. Be especially alert to complaints of progressive pain or pain out of proportion to the injury or treatment.

Pin sites and wounds must be constantly assessed for signs of infection, and pins should be checked for loosening. A small amount of bleeding immediately after pin insertion is expected and can be controlled with small pressures dressings; however, bleeding that continues for more than 24 hours should be brought to the surgeon's attention. The progress of wound healing must be assessed, and changes must be carefully documented. The movement of adipose tissue at the pin sites may produce fatty drainage that looks a great deal like pus. Be alert to more specific signs of infection, such as pin instability, drainage with odor or color, and skin tension or puckering at the insertion site (tenting). If tenting occurs, the surgeon should be notified so that the wound can be extended.

The client's nutritional status greatly affects bone and wound healing; pay attention to the adequacy of food intake as well as the client's ability to eat and swallow. Be aware of complaints of nausea or vomiting. Any abnormal laboratory values should also be assessed as possible evidence of poor nutrition.

Interventions. Antibiotics may need to be administered prophylactically for 48 to 72 hours after application of an external fixator. Later, wound care may involve the application of wet-to-dry dressings. Because pin care methods still remain somewhat controversial, follow the surgeon's orders or institutional standards. Loose pins must be reported promptly to the surgeon; they will be removed to prevent osteomyelitis.

The client's sense of balance can be altered by the weight of a fixator frame on the lower extremity. Because the client often also has a prescribed weight-bearing limitation after application of a lower extremity external fixator, be scrupulous in assessing adherence to any weight-bearing restrictions and correct use of ambulatory aids. If the surgeon determines that the frame itself can be used to reposition the affected extremity, the client should be instructed to move the extremity and the external fixator as a unit to avoid stress on the fracture site. The amount of support needed from the nurse is determined by the client's ability to control the extremity during movement.

Nausea or vomiting should be addressed aggressively with an antiemetic agent, as ordered, to decrease the risk for nutritional deficits or aspiration. Dietary supplements may be used as needed. Client and family education is critical for achieving a successful outcome with use of external fixation. By the time of discharge, the client should have begun to accept the change in body image that accompanies the use of external fixation. The client should also understand his or her responsibility for pin and wound care. He or she should be knowledgeable about manifestations of infection and should be aware of the significance of neurovascular or integumentary changes. The client must also receive instruction on use of analgesics and antibiotics as ordered by the surgeon. Instruction should include alternative methods of pain management, such as distraction, visualization, or massage, that may help the client relax.

Before discharge, teach the client how to meet hygiene needs and discuss any resumption of sexual activity. Clothing may need to be modified with snaps or self-fastening (Velcro) closures before discharge to fit over fixators. Advise the client with a pelvic fixator to reduce intake of gas-producing foods, which can lead to abdominal distention. Once the affected bone is healed, the fixator is removed.

Care of the Client in Traction

Assessment. As with the other modalities for immobilization, the client in traction must be assessed for neurovascular compromise, pain, skin breakdown, nutrition deficit, and signs of infection. Pin tract infection and development of osteomyelitis are risks for the client in skeletal traction. Other complications of immobility, such as constipation or respiratory compromise, can also occur, especially in older clients and in clients with long-term traction use.

The client's position in relation to the traction device requires constant vigilance. Regular bedside rounds ensure proper positioning and alignment, especially if the client is active, confused, or noncompliant. Traction ropes and knots must be intact and secure. Ropes should move easily over pulleys and weights, which hang freely at the end or side of the bed. Traction mechanics should be checked at the beginning of each shift and after each application or position change; all clamps on the traction frame must be tight, and rope ends should not be frayed. A photograph or sketch of the correct traction setup may be useful for nursing staff.

Interventions. If the client's nutritional status becomes a concern, dietary supplements may be ordered. Small, frequent meals may be indicated for the client in a halo vest to avoid a feeling of excessive fullness. Bent straws and adapted utensils may be indicated for clients who have limitations on head elevation.

To provide client comfort with elimination, provide a fracture bedpan and ensure privacy when the client needs to use it. The client's diet should include ample fluids and fiber if there are no contraindications. Stool softeners or bulk-forming laxatives may be prescribed and should be administered regularly. Also determine whether the client has regular, effective personal strategies for maintenance of normal bowel elimination and incorporate those methods into the plan of care.

Encourage independence in client activities within the limitations of the traction. The client should be instructed on repositioning techniques, possibly using extended horizontal bars with roller traction to allow movement to a chair at the bedside. Unaffected joints should be exercised regularly through the use of free weights, foam balls, or elastic pull bands. A record book may be used to encourage the client to cross off the exercise session when it is completed.

Immediately after traction removal, the client is often weak and unsteady as a result of muscle atrophy or orthostatic hypotension. The client should be gradually assisted to a sitting position and then to a standing position later as tolerated. Movement of a previously bedridden client to a sitting or standing position may take several days, depending on the effects of previous immobility. Ensure adequate assistance and provide careful physical support when assisting the client with these position changes. An assistive device such as a walker or crutches may be needed for temporary support of weak muscles and stiff joints (see also the Care Plan feature on The Client in Traction on the website).

SPECIFIC FRACTURES
HIP FRACTURES

Hip fractures have become one of the leading causes of morbidity and mortality among the older population. An estimated 350,000 hospital admissions and 60,000 nursing home admissions occur annually as a result of hip fractures. More than 4% of those who sustain a hip fracture die during their initial hospitalization. Up to 24% die in the first year following injury, and 50% remain unable to walk without an assistive device.[2,3] In fact, up to 25% of previously independent clients remain in institutions for more than a year after a hip fracture.[6] Hip fractures also have a significant impact on health care costs; the annual expense of medical and nursing services is estimated to be $7 billion to $10 billion.

Etiology and Risk Factors

Numerous studies have associated low bone mass and increasing age with an increased risk of hip fracture. Women begin to lose bone about 1.5 years before the last menstrual period; the bone loss continues rapidly until about 1.5 years after the last menses. The rate of bone loss then slows, matching the rate of loss in men by age 65 or 70. The development of low bone mass is known to be influenced by genetic factors. For example, women tend to have lower bone mass if their mothers or fathers have experienced vertebral fractures. Additional factors that can lead to the development of low bone mass include (1) low body weight, (2) physical inactivity, (3) low dietary calcium intake, (4) inadequate levels of serum vitamin D, (5) cigarette smoking, and (6) consumption of alcohol.

More than 90% of hip fractures are caused by falling; however, attempts to decrease the risk of falling through controlled trials have generally been ineffective. Some researchers have concluded that it is the dynamic interaction between the client's physical environment and intrinsic risk factors that actually increases his or her vulnerability to fall and injury.

Other factors have been associated with occurrence of falls that lead to hip fractures. These include the client's orthostatic hypotension, impaired vision, lower limb dysfunction, and neurologic conditions as well as the use of barbiturates or long-acting benzodiazepines. Environmental hazards may also contribute to the older client's tendency to fall. These include loose carpeting or rugs, slippery floors, poor lighting, a slippery tub or shower, irregular pavement, and loose clothing or footwear (see the Evidence-Based Practice in Action feature on Assessing and Predicting Fall Risk on p. 638).

Pathophysiology

Fractures of the hip are either *intracapsular* (located within the joint capsule) or *extracapsular* (located outside the joint capsule). Fractures are also described on the basis of their location in one of the four anatomic areas of the

📖 EVIDENCE-BASED PRACTICE IN ACTION

Assessing and Predicting Fall Risk

Client falls are a difficult clinical problem that can result in substantial personal, financial, and emotional costs for everyone involved. Accurate fall risk assessment based on research can allow use of appropriate interventions to decrease occurrences in acutely ill populations.

In one study about predicting client falls, an interdisciplinary falls team developed and evaluated the Conley Scale for assessment of the risk of fall on the admission of hospitalized individuals.[1] Key predictors of fall were identified in the literature and in the at-risk population. Among those considered for inclusion in the scale were orientation/confusion, history of falls, medications, behavior/agitation, general weakness, immobility, sensory impairment, frequency of incontinence, intravenous lines, diagnoses, alcohol abuse, use of ambulatory aids, postoperative status, language barrier, orthostatic manifestations, and age. The team's literature review suggested that manifestations associated with increasing age (impaired mobility, vision deficits, impairments related to chronic disease) were more statistically predictive than was actual age of the client.

A preliminary assessment scale of the risk of fall was developed that included 10 indicators divided into four categories: history of falls, altered elimination, immobility, and cognitive impairment. Definitions of each category provided clarification of the indicators. During the first phase of scale implementation, 59 of 1168 assessed clients fell during their hospital stay. In the analysis of the occurrences, researchers noted that neither age nor gender was significantly associated with the client's fall. History of falls, incontinence on the way to the bathroom, disorientation, agitation, and impaired judgment were all significantly associated with the occurrence.

Based on this analysis and the clinical expertise of falls team members, the Conley scale was subsequently revised to include history of falls, impaired judgment or lack of safety awareness, agitation, impaired mobility, and incontinence on the way to the bathroom. Dizziness or vertigo was added based on input from staff in cardiology units that had experienced increased falls in the previous year. Items were assigned a weight based on their influence on fall risk. Authors suggested continued evaluation of the scale's predictability to support its use as an evidence-based fall prevention strategy.

Other researchers also confirmed that the first step in fall prevention is to identify the characteristics of at-risk clients.[2] They developed an instrument that included the following criteria: disturbed balance; intake of certain drugs (sedative, neuroleptic, hypnotic, diuretic); laxative use (motility-stimulating); disturbed gait, need for walking aids; need for human assistance with walking; dizziness; disturbed sleep at night; aggressiveness; confusion; and earlier falls within a 3-month period. Whereas admission assessment is important, the authors also noted that a plan of care should be developed based on the client's identified risk factors.

Staff seminars were held to discussion fall prevention strategies, including risk assessment, care planning, and appropriate interventions. Following staff education, records of 332 clients admitted during 1 year (study group) were reviewed and compared with a control group from the previous year. According to data in the study group, significantly more falls and fall incidents occurred in clients with a higher sum of risk factors. A standard care plan was believed to give basic information on the interventions that led to a positive result. Authors concluded that at-risk clients can be reliably identified using assessment tools and preventive strategies implemented.

Other authors also suggest that successful strategies to reduce fall rates include risk assessment plus implementation of effective nursing care protocols.[3] They indicate that enhanced staff awareness of fall risk factors, along with increased institutional attention to decreasing falls, plays a major part in preventing falls or diminishing their severity.

References

1. Conley, D. (1999). The challenge of predicting patients at risk for falling: Development of the Conley Scale. *MEDSURG Nursing, 8* (6), 348-354.
2. Udén, G., Ehnfors, M., & Sjöström, K. (1999). Use of initial risk assessment and recording the main nursing intervention in identifying risk of falls. *Journal of Advanced Nursing, 29* (1), 145-152.
3. Rutledge, D.N., Donaldson, N.E., & Pravikoff, D.S. (1998). Fall risk assessment and prevention in healthcare facilities. Available: www.cinahl.com/cgi-bin/ojcishowdoc.cgi?vol01.htm.

---

proximal hip (Figure 29-7). Femoral neck fractures are more common in frail older persons, especially women, and are often associated with osteoporosis. They generally result from relatively mild trauma. *Intertrochanteric fractures* (between the femoral neck and the greater trochanter) and *subtrochanteric fractures* are more often seen in males and in vigorous older persons; they are likely to be associated with greater traumatic force.

Because blood flow to the hip is an important influence on fracture healing, delayed healing or non-union may occur in areas of the hip where circulation is impaired after injury. Healing of femoral head fractures, for example, is unlikely if AVN develops after local circulatory compromise.

Clinical Manifestations

Hip fracture is often caused by a fall at home that involves only a moderate amount of trauma, such as slipping out of a chair onto the floor. Immediately after the fall, the client is unable to bear weight on the affected leg. Objective findings include a shortened leg and an externally rotated hip. Deformity may also be evident in the lateral hip if the fracture is displaced. Ecchymosis at the hip is most likely to occur with subtrochanteric fractures. Location of pain depends on the specific fracture site (see Figure 29-7, *A, C, E, G*). A femoral neck fracture, for example, is characterized by groin and hip pain that increases with hip movement. Intertrochanteric fractures are accompanied by severe pain over the greater trochanter of the femur, whereas subtrochanteric fractures typically produce pain over the proximal thigh. Additional tissue trauma such as head or hand lacerations may also be evident.

Diagnosis of hip fracture is based on the client's clinical manifestations, history of trauma, and radiologic findings. The presence of a fracture is often confirmed by anteroposterior radiograph, although in some instances additional studies may be ordered. Computed tomographic (CT) scans, bone scans, fluoroscopy, myelograms, or magnetic resonance imaging (MRI) may be necessary to identify the fracture site.

Outcome Management
■ Medical Management

For a relatively few clients, nonoperative treatment is the best option following hip fracture. A client who cannot tolerate anesthesia or who was nonambulatory before the fracture may be treated with skeletal traction or spica casting. While the client remains in traction (approximately 8 to 12 weeks), develop a plan of care that will decrease the effects of immobility. For example, excellent skin care must be provided to reduce the risk of pressure ulcer development. Because older clients are at increased risk for skin impairment even before immobilization, a pressure-reducing mattress and heel elevation are essential. Perform careful daily assessment of bony prominences such as the heels, sacrum, scapulae, and vertebrae. In addition, instruct the client about leg exercises that will decrease the probability of thromboembolism; pneumatic compression devices or anticoagulant medications may also be used to lessen the likelihood of clot development.

■ Surgical Management

Extensive blood loss can occur after hip fracture, particularly in older clients with other medical conditions. Additional deterioration can occur rapidly if the client is left on bed rest; therefore prompt surgical intervention and early mobilization are keys to successful rehabilitation. The goal of surgical treatment is to achieve a stable reduction and internal fixation of the fracture segments to support early ambulation.

Anatomic regions

A
Intertrochanteric fracture

B
Repair of an intertrochanteric fracture with an endoprosthesis

C
Intracapsular fracture

D
Repair of an intracapsular fracture with compression screws

E
Femoral neck fracture

F
Repair of a femoral neck fracture with compression screws

G
Subtrochanteric fracture

H
Repair of a subtrochanteric fracture with compression screws

FIGURE 29-7 Anatomic regions of the proximal femur and blood supply; **A-H,** Fracture patterns of the hip and surgical repairs.

Open Reduction and Internal Fixation

Postoperative treatment goals include the following:

- Complete union of the fracture (4 to 8 months)
- Prevention of deformity and contractures to the hip, knee, or foot
- Restoration of weight-bearing ambulation, with the use of assistive devices if needed
- Relief of pain and fear; prevention of complications
- Maintenance of optimal physiologic function

Fixation may be accomplished through the use of screws, plates, intramedullary pins or implants (see Figure 29-7, *B, D, F, H*). The term *open reduction* indicates that a surgical incision was made to expose the bone, in contrast to a closed reduction of a fracture (see Reducing Fractures earlier in this chapter). *Internal fixation* indicates that devices such as pins or plates were used to hold the bones in alignment during healing. Perfect anatomic reduction and fixation may be difficult to achieve if the client has decreased bone density as a result of osteoporosis. If the fracture is highly comminuted or the head of the femur has been destroyed, use of an endoprosthesis to replace the entire head of the femur may be necessary. For the client who has an accompanying acetabular fracture, total hip arthroplasty may be indicated (see Chapter 28).

■ Nursing Management of the Surgical Client

Preoperative Care

Clients who require surgical reduction and fixation of hip fractures most often go directly from the emergency department to the operating room. Delay in repair not only places an older client at risk for additional effects of immobility but also increases the likelihood that AVN will develop as a result of inadequate blood supply to the fracture fragments. Assess routine blood work and the client's baseline weight preoperatively. A bed scale should be used to minimize client discomfort with this procedure. Do not accept a stated weight from the client or family member because accurate comparison with postoperative changes will be impossible.

Occasionally, a client may require stabilization of medical conditions before being cleared for surgery. Underlying disorders such as heart failure or malnutrition, for example, must be evaluated and controlled. In such cases, skin traction through use of a Buck's boot may be applied to decrease painful muscle spasms surrounding the hip joint.

Routine preoperative assessment is performed (see Chapter 16). For the client who has experienced a hip fracture, preoperative assessment also includes determination of the preinjury level of functioning. Data should clearly address usual activities, ability to walk independently, and history of previous falls. Under the best of circumstances, the preoperative level of functioning is the level that the client can optimistically expect to achieve after surgery. Unfortunately, some loss of function is likely after fracture repair.

One significant factor in successful rehabilitation is the client's previous social functioning. The client who was previously independent and active and who enjoyed multiple social contacts is more likely to experience a full recovery than is the client who had restricted activity before injury.

Postoperative Assessments

After open-reduction, internal fixation (ORIF), the same basic nursing assessments are required as for any other surgical client (see Chapter 16). Additional assessment includes a comparison of the quality of peripheral pulses in the affected extremity with that in the unaffected extremity. Prompt recognition of abnormal data allows for early intervention for any neurovascular compromise (see the Care Plan on The Client Following Hip Fracture and ORIF on the website for additional interventions). As the client progresses into rehabilitation, collaborate with physical and occupational therapists in assessing the client's mobility and self-care needs.

Possible complications after hip fracture repair include fat emboli and infection (see Complications After Fracture earlier in this chapter). Other complications specific to or of high incidence in clients with hip fractures are discussed here.

Deep Vein Thrombosis. Prevention of DVT is a primary goal for the client after ORIF of a hip fracture. Pharmacologic agents such as LMW heparin or warfarin are prescribed for clot prophylaxis. Physical-mechanical measures such as intermittent pneumatic compression devices or elastic stockings may also have a role in DVT prevention. DVT is discussed more fully in Chapter 55.

Pressure Ulcers. A *pressure ulcer* is tissue damage that results from unrelieved pressure, usually over a bony prominence. Its development may have begun as the injured client lay on a hard floor at home, on hard surfaces in an ambulance or in the emergency department, on a table for radiographs or surgery, or in the bed after surgery. Pressure ulcer development is compounded because the client is unable to turn independently after injury or surgery. Without assistance, the client remains supine or in a semi-Fowler position for most of the hospitalization.

A turning schedule is essential for eliminating sustained pressure over bony prominences on the head, scapulae, vertebrae, coccyx, and heels. Other areas such as the elbows, ankles, and medial surfaces of the knees may also be affected by pressure that lasts as little as 15 minutes. Bony areas should be cushioned and supported with each position change. Heels should be elevated with calf pillows or foam boots. Prevention of ischemia can also be accomplished through the use of pressure-reduction bed overlays. An "egg-crate" mattress may contribute to client comfort in the bed, but it does not relieve pressure. Specialty mattresses or air beds are the only appropriate alternatives to assist in pressure reduction. The client who is using a specialty bed must still be turned on a regular schedule. Identification of the client's risk for skin impairment can be accomplished through the use of an assessment tool such as the Braden scale, presented in Chapter 51.

Acute Confusion. Confusion (delirium) is characterized by an abrupt onset of numerous global, transient changes in a client's attention, cognition, psychomotor activity, or sleep-wake cycle or in several of these. The client may appear forgetful, inattentive, disoriented, or fearful. Daytime sleepiness and nighttime insomnia may be noticed. In the hospitalized client, confusion creates concerns about safety and dependence on others for self-care needs and can greatly affect the emotional status of the client and family. It can also lead to prolonged hospitalization, possibly contributing to placement in a long-term care facility and definitely increasing costs. Some degree of confusion has been identified in up to 60% of hospitalized older clients.[29] The incidence of confusion after hip surgery may be as high as 42%.[29] Most affected clients have no history of confusion or mental impairment.

Consistent predictors of, or risk factors for, acute confusion have been difficult to identify clearly. The risk for development of confusion may in fact be a cumulative function of the client's biopsychosocial integrity, the level of illness and functional impairment, and the timing and magnitude of added stressors. Known contributors to confusion may be an unfamiliar environment; sensory overstimulation or deprivation; the client's loss of control and uncertain future; a disrupted routine; immobility and pain; and a disrupted elimination pattern. Because use of medications with anticholinergic effects has also been linked to client confusion, carefully monitor all medications.

Careful assessment of the client's attention, memory, orientation, psychomotor behavior, and sleep-wake cycle is needed. The risk for confusion may also be decreased by maintaining appropriate hydration, perfusion, and oxygenation in the client. Attention must be given to managing pain, meeting nutritional requirements, and correcting metabolic imbalances. The client must have easy access to glasses, hearing aids, and other functional devices. Also address environmental factors by reorienting the confused client in a consistent way and minimizing disruption to the usual diurnal rhythms. Companionship of family members or volunteers is helpful, as is the use of calendars, clocks, and newspapers to provide a time reference for the client. Follow institutional guidelines for the use of restraints.

Diagnosis, Outcomes, Interventions

Diagnosis: Acute Pain. Acute pain is expected after ORIF of the hip. The client may also have contusions or abrasions caused by the fall that led to hip fracture. The nursing diagnosis can be written as *Acute Pain related to local tissue trauma from surgical incision or other injuries.*

Outcomes. The client will demonstrate comfort after surgery, as evidenced by movement without grimacing, by requesting analgesics no more frequently than ordered, and by statements that the pain is tolerable and not interfering with rest or physical therapy.

Interventions. In the immediate postoperative period, the client may experience intense pain and require injectable analgesics to attain acceptable control. Common interventions include patient-controlled analgesia (PCA) or epidural analgesia. Ice application over the dressed surgical wound may also increase the client's comfort (see the Management and Delegation feature on the Application of Heat and Cold on p. 642). Within 24 to 48 hours, the client should be tolerating fluids and able to take oral analgesics. Because pain is intensified with movement, the client may attempt to limit activity. Medicate the client before physical therapy or activities such as transferring to the chair, and reinforce the importance of ambulation in decreasing the risk for postoperative complications. Use of non-opioid analgesics can also help with acute pain management, muscle spasms, and other chronic medical problems such as arthritis.

Concerns about becoming addicted to opioids should be addressed openly. Many older persons fear that they will become addicted quickly, and they may delay their recovery by tolerating unnecessary pain. Opioid addiction is rare, but the fear is quite intense.

Regularly assess for side effects of opioid analgesics. Confusion and sedation may be seen in the older adult. Respiratory depression is more likely to occur with PCA or epidural analgesia than with oral opioids. Pulse oximetry and regular measurement of vital signs help to assess for hypoxemia that results from shallow or slow breathing. Stimulating the client to deep breathe will raise oximetry values. Naloxone is seldom needed to reverse opioid analgesia.

Constipation can occur after hip fracture and repair as a result of the client's impaired mobility, opioid analgesic use, and progression to a regular diet. Encourage the client's intake of fluids and dietary fiber. In addition, stool softeners or laxatives may be indicated. If the client uses a bulk-forming laxative or other strategy to maintain bowel regularity at home, assist in continuing that program in the hospital. Regular assessment and implementation of a proactive bowel program are important for minimizing clients' concerns about bowel elimination.

MANAGEMENT AND DELEGATION

Application of Heat and Cold

Any equipment used to apply heat or cold may injure the client. Injury may result if the client is unable to perceive discomfort because of decreased peripheral circulation, decreased feeling, decreased sensorium, sedation, or agitation. The client may also be at risk if he or she cannot be left alone safely or if the client alters the controls of the heating pad or cooling device.

The application of heat or cold to an inflamed or painful area that is closed may be delegated to unlicensed assistive personnel. Before delegating the application of heat or cold, consider the following:

- What is the indication for the application of heat or cold? Check the physician's order. The order and indication may be sufficient to tell you whether you can delegate this task or not.
- What is the condition of the affected site? Assess for any areas of redness, swelling, breakdown, or scar tissue. It is important to know the baseline condition of the site before the application of heat or cold. There may be an indication to withhold this treatment or to confer with the physician about the order. You will also need to assess the condition of the site on completion of the treatment.
- What is the client's diagnosis? Is there any history of diabetes mellitus or impairment in sensorium or mentation? This may be an indication for you to perform this treatment yourself. If there is impairment of the client's mental or sensory status, it may be necessary for the unlicensed assistive personnel to remain with the client throughout the treatment.
- What is the competency level of the unlicensed assistive personnel who might perform this task?

Instruct the unlicensed assistive personnel providing the heat or cold application to do the following:

- Wash their hands.

- Assemble the necessary equipment. Advise them as to which method of applying heat or cold is ordered.
- When using ice cubes, they should be placed in an ice bag with a scoop through a funnel; the ice cubes should not be touched with bare hands.
- Check the temperature of the heat or cold device before applying it to the client's skin. A safe range for heat applications is 115° to 125° F for adults.
- Wrap any heat or cold application with a protective cover, such as a towel or a flannel sleeve.
- If using a heating pad, start with the device on the lowest setting to initiate treatment.
- Instruct the client not to adjust the heat setting.
- Check the client's response immediately. If the device is too hot or cold, an adjustment is necessary. Double the protective layer between the device and the skin or allow the temperature of the device to moderate slightly.
- Check the client's skin after 5 minutes. If it is tolerated, leave the heat or cold in place for 20 minutes. If it is not tolerated, the heat or cold should be removed immediately, and you should be made aware of this. Assess the situation and notify the physician as appropriate.
- Remove the heat or cold application at 20 minutes and to inform you that the treatment is complete.

You are responsible for examining the affected area and reassessing the client's skin at completion of this treatment. You should document your findings and the client's response to treatment in the medical record. The unlicensed assistive personnel should immediately report any difficulty encountered during the course of treatment.

Diagnosis: Impaired Physical Mobility. The client's degree of immobility after ORIF of the hip is affected by pain and fear of movement as well as any limitations in other joints. If previous mobility limitations contributed to the fall, the client may have even greater problems with mobilization after surgery. The nursing diagnosis can be written as *Impaired Physical Mobility related to pain or fear of movement.*

Outcomes. The client will demonstrate improved physical mobility, as evidenced by the need for less assistance in transfers (bed to chair, bed to standing), by safe use of a walker or crutches, and by the ability to ambulate a functional distance (150 feet). For the client with previous mobility limitations, outcomes may focus on bed mobility only.

Interventions. Moving the client after ORIF of the hip can create a great deal of anxiety for both the client and the nursing staff. First be aware of any weight-bearing limitations ordered for the client before transferring him or her (see Table 29-5 for a description of weight-bearing limitations). Non–weight-bearing orders are often received after hip fracture repair, and these must be strictly followed to avoid disruption of bone healing. If the client is not allowed to bear full weight, pay careful attention to the operative extremity while a transfer is made to ensure that the client avoids passing any weight through the leg. Record the amount of assistance that the client requires for safe transfer. This information provides the benchmark that will determine whether the goal for increased mobility is being met. For example, the client may have needed the assistance of two staff

TABLE 29-5	*Weight-Bearing Status*
Non–weight-bearing	The client does not bear weight on the affected extremity; the affected extremity should not touch the floor
Touch-down weight-bearing or toe-touch weight-bearing	The client's foot of the affected extremity may rest on the floor for balance, but no weight is distributed through that extremity
Partial weight-bearing	The client bears 30%-50% of weight on the affected extremity
Weight-bearing as tolerated	The client bears as much weight as he or she can tolerate on the affected extremity without undue strain or pain
Full weight-bearing	The client can bear weight fully on the affected extremity

members on the morning after surgery; by the next afternoon, increased mobility was demonstrated when only one nurse was needed to assist with transfer.

In addition to postoperative limitations, the client may suffer from arthritis in other joints or may have residual effects from a previous stroke. These conditions can increase pain and affect the ability to transfer from the bed to the chair. When the client stands and transfers for the first time, the assistance of at least two staff members will be needed. Use appropriate technique to ensure a safe transfer for the client and also to minimize the risk of injury to your lower back (see Chapter 28 for additional information on requirements for appropriate mobility assistance).

Diagnosis: Self-Care Deficit.

After hip fracture and surgical repair, the client is likely to experience some degree of self-care deficit in hygiene and dressing. Limited mobility may decrease independence in self-care, and assistive devices may be required. The diagnostic statement may read *Self-Care Deficit: Bathing/hygiene, dressing/grooming related to mobility impairment following hip fracture.*

Outcomes. The client will resume pre-injury level of independence in meeting self-care needs.

Interventions. After ORIF of the hip, the client will receive assistance from both physical and occupational therapists. Physical therapists help with ambulation and muscle strengthening. They offer instruction on climbing stairs and on getting in and out of a car. They also provide assistive devices that help in functional independ-

ence, including an elevated toilet seat and a walker. Occupational therapists instruct the client on bathing and dressing techniques. They may suggest use of a tub bench or a long-handled sponge. They may also provide long-handled reachers or sock aids to help the client dress with minimal assistance from others. Nursing staff will reinforce the use of techniques and assistive devices to encourage the client's optimal recovery.

Diagnosis: Risk for Impaired Skin Integrity.

If the client has fallen while alone and experienced an extended time on the floor before help arrived, even early assessment may show the development of pressure ulcers over bony prominences. After surgery, the client's mobility limitations and pain increase the risk for skin impairment. Malnutrition and dehydration, which may have existed before injury and could be exacerbated postoperatively, may also contribute. Older clients and clients receiving long-term corticosteroid therapy may have especially thin skin that is even more prone to breakdown and tears. The type of tape used to secure postoperative dressings, along with the method and direction of tape application, can also contribute to the development of skin blisters. An appropriate diagnostic statement may be *Risk for Impaired Skin Integrity related to mobility limitations or to the application of tape with dressing changes.*

Outcomes. The client will demonstrate intact skin, as evidenced by the absence of ulcers over bony prominences and heels and absence of epidermal stripping beneath tape used to secure postoperative dressings.

Interventions. After ORIF of the hip, the client should be assisted with position changes at least every 2 hours. The client can be turned to either side but is usually more comfortable on the nonoperative side with a pillow to support the operative leg. Carefully assess the skin over bony prominences such as the sacrum, coccyx, scapulae, elbows, and heels. If areas of skin breakdown are noted, measure and describe them thoroughly. Treat the ulcer using institutional protocols or see Chapter 51.

In addition to using a regular turning schedule, place a pressure-reducing mattress on the client's bed. Heels should be "floated" from the bed by placing a pillow under the calves. Pressure on the heels also can be relieved by placement of a towel roll for brief periods under the Achilles tendon. Specific skin care products are available to be rubbed gently into affected areas at the first sign of redness. Direct massage of stage I pressure ulcers is contraindicated.

Avoid epidermal stripping by placing postoperative dressings over a skin sealant that is applied wherever the tape would touch the skin. Elastic tape should be placed vertically (superior to inferior) without tension to allow for stretching that is related to postoperative edema. Any redness, blistering, or epidermal stripping should be evaluated, and an enterostomal nurse specialist should be consulted about the client's care as appropriate. Clients with thin skin should have gauze wraps rather than tape on their skin. Treatment of skin tears is discussed in Chapter 51.

Diagnosis: Risk for Infection.

Bone infection is a serious threat and can lead to loss of joint function. Pre-existent poor health also contributes to risk. State this nursing diagnosis as *Risk for Infection related to loss of primary defenses (skin) and malnutrition.*

Outcomes. The client will remain free of manifestations of infection, as evidenced by (1) white blood cell (WBC) count within normal limits, (2) an afebrile state, (3) absence of purulent wound drainage, (4) absence of increasing pain in wound, and (5) no inflammation in wound after 72 hours.

Interventions. Clients often receive prophylactic antibiotics during surgery and in the immediate postoperative period. After ORIF, the physician may prefer to perform the initial dressing change. Use strict aseptic technique in performing subsequent dressing changes, carefully assessing the wound each time for signs of healing or infection.

Diagnosis: Risk for Peripheral Neurovascular Dysfunction.

Be aware of the risk for peripheral nerve or vascular impairment after surgery on any joint. Edema or extremity positioning can place pressure on adjacent nerves. The nursing diagnosis can be written as *Risk for Peripheral Neurovascular Dysfunction related to lower extremity edema or positioning.*

Outcomes. The client will demonstrate normal neurovascular function, as evidenced by adequate peripheral pulses with capillary refill time of 3 seconds or less and by the absence of sensory impairments or motor weakness in the operative extremity.

Interventions. Assess the neurovascular function of the operative extremity at least every 4 hours or as directed by the surgeon, and then compare findings to the unaffected extremity. More frequent monitoring may be needed if indicated by the client's condition. Assessment includes the presence and quality of bilateral pedal pulses, skin color and temperature of the extremity, capillary refill in the toes, sensation and movement of the toes, and the client's ability to perform dorsoplantar flexion of the foot. Any pallor or coolness, numbness or tingling, or inability to move the extremity should be reported promptly to the surgeon.

Diagnosis: Risk for Constipation.

Impaired mobility and the use of opioid analgesics can lead to constipation. The risk is increased in older clients who have a pre-existing dependence on laxatives. The nursing diagnosis could be written as *Risk for Constipation related to impaired physical mobility and side effects of opioids.*

Outcomes. The client will maintain a pattern of regular bowel elimination by consuming adequate fluids and high-fiber foods and by having a bowel movement at least every 2 to 3 days.

Interventions. The client's diet should include ample fluids and fiber if not contraindicated. Stool softeners are often prescribed and should be administered regularly. Also, determine whether the client has regular, effective personal strategies for treating constipation and, if so, use those methods to assist with elimination. The client should be assisted to transfer to a bedside commode or ambulate to the bathroom whenever possible to meet elimination needs. To assist the bedridden client with bowel elimination, offer a fracture bedpan and ensure privacy when the client needs to use it.

Diagnosis: Risk for Imbalanced Nutrition: Less Than Body Requirements.

After surgery, the client may experience nausea that delays the progression to a regular diet. Decreased activity may also lead to poor appetite. If the client has experienced blood loss, a nutritional deficit may also occur. Remember that the presence of obesity does not ensure that the client is well nourished. This nursing diagnosis may be stated as *Risk for Imbalanced Nutrition: Less Than Body Requirements related to nausea or poor appetite following hip fracture.*

Outcomes. The client will maintain adequate dietary intake, as evidenced by energy for participation in physical therapy and by appropriate wound and bone healing.

Interventions. Stress the importance of a high-carbohydrate and high-protein diet for adequate healing, and then assist the client in making food choices as necessary. If the client's appetite remains poor, offer small, frequent meals. Encourage the client to eat at least some of every food at every meal to achieve balanced intake. After blood loss, increased dietary iron or iron supplements may be required. Encourage the client to eat foods high in iron, and administer a supplement as ordered. Inform the client that stool may appear black or tarry as a result of the iron supplement.

Evaluation

Clinical pathways or care maps are now often used to determine which outcomes have been met for the client with a hip fracture; they often suggest a time frame for each goal. Pain should decrease fairly soon after surgery. Injectable opioid analgesics are not typically required after 24 to 36 hours. The client should advance to oral analgesics as soon as nausea is controlled and liquids are being taken freely. A regular diet should be offered by the first or second day after surgery, again on the assumption that nausea is controlled. Early feeding primes the gastrointestinal tract, helping the client to avoid postoperative ileus. Adequate diet also contributes greatly to the client's physical stamina and to wound healing. If an indwelling urinary catheter has been used, remove it as soon as the client can transfer to a bedside commode to decrease any risk for urinary tract infection (see the Case Management feature on Hip Fracture on the website).

A clinical pathway also often describes the involvement of a case manager or social worker in planning the client's discharge. In collaboration with the staff nurse and the physician, the case manager assesses the client's discharge needs on the basis of information about the home environment and social support. An extended-care facility or rehabilitation unit may be one possible destination after acute care hospitalization. The client who can move from bed to chair with minimal or no assistance may go instead directly home with possible visits from a home health aide or nurse to meet other skilled needs, such as hygiene and mobility assistance. When the client is discharged directly to home, the nurse must ensure that the family can safely assist the client with mobility needs and activities of daily living. The case manager assists the client in obtaining any durable medical equipment that may be needed, such as a walker or crutches, and finalizes discharge transportation if necessary (see the Bridge to Home Health Care feature on Managing the Immobile Client, below).

CONDYLAR FRACTURES

The condyles are bony prominences at the distal end of the femur. Condylar fractures occur most often with high-energy injuries in young clients. They may be among several injuries sustained in a motor-vehicle accident, for example, when the client's flexed knee strikes the dashboard. Less severe condylar fractures are treated with knee immobilizers or casting. For more severe injury, ORIF is indicated. Bone grafting is used for comminuted fractures. Loss of knee mobility is a common outcome, and surgical revision may be needed to improve bony alignment. If the client develops severe pain and disability, *arthrodesis* (fusion) or *arthroplasty* (joint replacement) may be required.

BRIDGE TO HOME HEALTH CARE
Managing the Immobile Client

To prevent skin breakdown and manage other physical and emotional effects of immobility, the multidisciplinary team must collaborate with clients, their family members, and their informal caregivers. The core team members are a nurse, a physical therapist, a social worker, and an occupational therapist.

If the person is expected to spend much time in a chair or wheelchair, good seat cushions can be purchased from most pharmacies and vendors. Heavy foam (4 inches thick) provides pressure reduction for clients with wheelchairs that have sling seats. Cushions of air can be inflated to reduce pressure and prevent posture problems. Pillows or gel should not be used; a pillow allows too much hip adduction and internal rotation and becomes uncomfortable, and gel is expensive and heavy, breaks down, and makes it harder to move a wheelchair.

Evaluate how clients sit and use cushions. Inspect every cushion frequently for signs of wear. Avoid folds, wrinkles, or pockets on surfaces. The proper sitting position includes 90 degrees of flexion at the hips and knees. Clients should sit erect in chairs on their buttocks, not on the sacrum. Place pillows behind a client's back to promote more erect posture.

Teach clients to protect tissue, toughen skin, and avoid massaging lotion over bony prominences; massage makes skin soft and susceptible to breakdown or shearing. Minimize friction; avoid having tissue squeezed between two hard surfaces such as bedding and bony prominences. Teach clients, especially those with paraplegia, to use a mirror to check for friction or pressure. Clients may need assistance with repositioning at least every 2 hours. A footboard, a thoroughly padded plastic crate, or a box can be used to prevent feet from being forced into extreme plantar flexion. The clients' heels, ankles, trochanters, sacrum, scapulae, elbows, and ears need to be checked at least daily. Pillows, blanket or towel rolls, balloons, foam, or rolled-up clothing are useful for padding and positioning. Sheepskin, elbow and heel protectors, and egg-crate cushions provide little protection; thick foam is better. Even though good-quality alternating pressure pads are best, there are other options, including waterbeds, silicon bead beds, and air mattresses. When alternating pads are used, watch the skin for several days to ensure that the client is getting enough tissue off loading (see Chapter 51).

Daily exercise is essential. Passive exercise only increases flexibility, whereas active exercise increases circulation and air exchange, maintains joint lubrication and mobility, and helps prevent contractures. If you feel uncertain about whether to continue the exercise, request assistance from a physical therapist.

After clients progress through the acute stage, they need to consider long-term issues and dramatic lifestyle changes. Provide information about alternative housing options, transportation, yard and housekeeping services, financial assistance, recreation, and stores that deliver prescriptions. Mental health and sexuality issues are important, too. Clients also need to consider and make decisions about nutrition, clothing, informal caregivers, and health care services.

PELVIC FRACTURES

The pelvis is a ring-like structure composed mostly of cancellous bone and has a thin cortex. This structure provides great strength, allowing the pelvis to offer structural support and also to serve as a shock absorber that protects the abdominal organs. Pelvic fractures have become more common as a result of an increase in high-energy trauma, such as motor-vehicle accidents and gunshot wounds. Most pelvic fractures occur as a result of traffic accidents; pedestrians are injured more often than are the occupants of involved vehicles.

Because fractures of the pelvic ring can vary in stability, their management depends on the severity of the injury. Most cases can be diagnosed correctly with an anteroposterior radiograph. If there is any indication of an unstable fracture, a urethrogram or intravenous pyelogram is used to assess for possible damage to the kidneys and lower urinary tract. Pelvic fractures also often result in hemorrhage, and the pelvis can hold as much as 4 L of blood. Unstable fractures have been treated aggressively since the mid-1990s with internal fixation in which plates and screws are used to achieve an intact pelvic ring. External fixation is also still used. Less severe pelvic fractures may be treated with bed rest alone. The client needs adequate pain management as well as assessment for neurovascular compromise or the development of complications such as thrombophlebitis or fat embolism.

PATELLAR FRACTURES

Fracture of the patella (kneecap) often results from a direct blow to the area. Some separation or splitting of the patella invariably occurs, and the client is unable to extend the knee fully because of pain and related damage to extensor mechanisms. Patellar fractures are usually more evident on a lateral radiograph than on other views. A stellate fracture (cracked patella without fragment displacement) can be managed conservatively by placing the client in a long leg cast for several weeks and then beginning mobilization. Indirect trauma, such as a forced flexion injury sustained in a fall, can result in a transverse fracture. ORIF is often necessary to minimize the potential for later problems with knee motion or chondromalacia. After a comminuted fracture, fragments may be difficult to reduce accurately, and removal of the patella may be best. Surgical repair of extensors such as the quadriceps tendon and the patellar tendon may also be needed.

TIBIAL AND FIBULAR FRACTURES

The fibula can be fractured alone in several ways: from direct trauma to the outer surface of the leg, producing a transverse or comminuted fracture; through twisting injuries, which produce a spiral fracture; or from repeated stress as in long-distance running, which can cause a fatigue fracture usually just above the inferior tibiofibular ligament. Fatigue fractures require immobilization; for other nondisplaced fibular fractures, a cast may be needed to immobilize the ankle.

The tibia can also be broken, leaving the fibula intact. Fracture can result from direct trauma. Repeated stress can lead to a fatigue fracture at the junction of the middle and upper thirds of the tibia. This injury is commonly seen in long-distance runners, hurdlers, and ballet dancers who jump excessively. Twisting injuries rarely result in a lone tibial fracture. Tibial fractures are reduced and treated through cast immobilization, internal fixation, or external fixation. Although it may seem helpful to have the fibula intact, the undamaged bone actually holds the ends of the tibia apart, and it may be necessary to cut the fibula to attain satisfactory alignment of the tibia.

Fractures of both the tibia and fibula result commonly from motor-vehicle accidents and sports injuries. Treatment concerns include possible problems with fracture union, vascular and soft tissue damage, skin loss, and the development of compartment syndrome. As with lone tibial fractures, fragments may be held in the reduced position through casting from groin to toe. Alternatively, internal fixation would be the treatment of choice for clients with unstable or multiple fractures. External fixation would be necessary if the wound is dirty or if there is skin loss.

If the knee is struck violently on the lateral surface, a tibial plateau fracture may result. Four fracture patterns can occur: the lateral tibial plateau may be split vertically; part of the tibial plateau may be thrust downward into the tibia to produce a depressed fracture; both of these can occur together; or the whole plateau may be depressed. Because the full extent of injury may not be apparent on radiographs, CT scanning or MRI may be needed to determine the fracture anatomy. Any large fragment split off the tibia must be secured back in place with screws to restore the contour of the bone. Large depressed fragments can be elevated to reconstitute the bone's surface, but the cavity that results below the fracture must be filled with a cancellous bone graft. If only a slight depression occurred in the tibial plateau, more conservative treatment with early mobilization may be appropriate.

FOOT FRACTURES

Because it provides a contact point with the ground and protrudes forward from the body, the foot is especially susceptible to injury. Fracture most often is caused by falls or jumps from great heights, running or twisting, motor-vehicle accidents, or objects dropped on the foot. As with any other injury, the client with open fractures should be taken to the operating room for surgical debridement and repair. Closed fractures of the foot, however, can generally be treated conservatively through cast or brace immobilization or through the use of walking shoes. Weight-bearing is progressively resumed as tolerated.

UPPER EXTREMITY FRACTURES

Fracture of the proximal humerus is a common traumatic injury in older clients, often caused by a fall on an outstretched arm. A fall need not be serious to produce a humeral fracture in an osteoporotic client. Injury to the dominant arm of an older client can lead to dependence and immobility. The risk of falling also increases because the sense of balance is impaired as a result of loss of use of the arm. If the fracture is nondisplaced or minimally displaced, the extremity is usually immobilized with a sling. Gentle range-of-motion exercises can be started when shoulder discomfort subsides, usually within 2 or 3 weeks after injury. A displaced fracture is treated by ORIF. Prosthetic replacement is occasionally indicated for an intra-articular fracture or one that is severely comminuted. Prompt, appropriate treatment reduces the risk that AVN of the humeral head will develop.

Fractures of the humeral shaft usually result from a direct blow to the arm, a motor-vehicle accident, a gunshot injury, or a crush injury. Humeral fractures can also result from indirect injuries such as a fall on an outstretched hand or on the elbow. Most humeral shaft fractures can be treated by initial immobilization with a U-shaped splint. Once the swelling has subsided, a commercially available humeral fracture brace may be used in conjunction with an arm sling. Heavy hanging arm casts should be avoided because they may contribute to fracture non-union. Surgery is indicated for debridement of an open fracture. Surgical stabilization is also required for any fracture associated with a vascular injury.

Intra-articular injuries of the elbow include condylar, olecranon, and radial head or neck fracture. These injuries frequently result from falls on or direct blows to the elbow. Because associated injuries to the three major peripheral nerves (radial, median, and ulnar) are possible, careful neurovascular assessment is critical. A high potential for compartment syndrome also exists after intra-articular fractures of the elbow. Most nondisplaced fractures can be treated with immobilization, followed by early range-of-motion exercises once acute discomfort has diminished (usually after 1 week). A posterior long arm splint may be used with a shoulder sling. Displaced fractures, especially supracondylar fractures, often require ORIF. Repair of the brachial artery may also be necessary after traumatic injury. After surgery, immobilization can be accomplished with a posterior elbow splint, a cast, or traction.

Fractures of the shafts of the radius and ulna usually result from a direct blow to the forearm, a motor-vehicle accident, or a fall on an outstretched arm. Associated injuries to the nerves (median, ulnar, and radial) and arteries (radial and ulnar) are possible. A sugar-tong splint can be used to provide initial immobilization of forearm frac-

tures. Circumferential cast immobilization is generally not recommended in early treatment because fracture swelling in association with the constriction provided by the cast may lead to a compartment syndrome. Immobilization must include the wrist and the elbow to control rotation of the forearm. In adult clients, surgical treatment may be indicated for displaced or open fractures.

As with proximal humeral fractures, fractures of the distal radius are common injuries in older persons. Many older clients have a good outcome even with a residual deformity because their routine activities may not demand full use of the limb; however, deformity and possible resulting arthritic changes in younger clients may lead to inability to perform their current jobs. Colles' fracture is a common injury in which the distal radius fragment is displaced dorsally and proximally. Fracture reduction is greatly enhanced by the use of a nerve block such as the Bier block. This fracture may be treated with 2 weeks of splinting followed by 3 weeks in a short arm cast. Comminuted fractures may require external fixation or ORIF with bone grafting.

Most fractures of the metacarpals and phalanges are work related. A delay in seeking evaluation and diagnosis can make fracture reduction difficult because fractures in the hand form early callus within 7 to 10 days and become difficult to manipulate. Treatment involves accurate fracture reduction, movement of the uninvolved fingers to prevent stiffness, and elevation of the extremity to decrease edema. Simple measures such as "buddy taping" or splinting are usually sufficient treatment for stable fractures. Comminuted fractures and those requiring open reduction take longer to consolidate and are not ready for mobilization as quickly. Client motivation plays a critical role in rehabilitation after hand injury and often can be enhanced by a brief course of physical therapy. Motion typically can be started about 21 days after injury for clients with closed, nondisplaced fractures.

Neurovascular assessment is critical for all clients with upper extremity fractures. Carefully compare the color, warmth, movement, sensation, and capillary refill of the affected extremity with those of the unaffected extremity. Elevation of the injured extremity is typically indicated. At night, the client should be observed frequently to be certain that the arm does not move into a dependent position. If a cast or splint has been applied, the client and family should receive careful instruction about cast care and about the clinical manifestations of compartment syndrome.

DISLOCATIONS AND SUBLUXATIONS

Dislocation and subluxation both describe changes in joint relationships. In a dislocation, the opposing joint surfaces are no longer in contact. In subluxation, the joint surfaces are in partial contact, but their relationship is abnormal. Both injuries are caused by acute deforming forces applied to ligaments or tendons from a fall, a blow, or a strong muscle contraction. For example, the client who tries to break a fall down the stairs by holding on to the handrail may dislocate a shoulder. The nurse must identify the mechanism of injury that produced the dislocation so the action is not reproduced during the client's treatment.

Like fractures, dislocations are described in terms of the relationship of the distal bone to the proximal bone. In a posterior dislocation of the knee, for example, the tibia lies posterior to the femur. Although almost any joint can dislocate, some joints are more likely to become dislocated than others. Anterior dislocation of the humerus in the shoulder joint occurs commonly in adults. Anterior dislocation of the knee is the most common lower extremity dislocation. Its occurrence is a medical emergency because of related neurovascular injuries. The adult hip is usually stable, and its dislocation is often associated with severe trauma.

After dislocation, the client often complains of severe pain that increases with attempted movement. Swelling around or below the joint is likely, along with complete or nearly complete loss of function and a visible deformity that may alter the length of the extremity. Fracture of the joint surface often accompanies dislocation. Neurovascular status of the affected extremity must be assessed carefully because the displaced bone may tear blood vessels and impede circulation, damage nerves, and rupture ligaments or muscle attachments. Immediate reduction is preferred before inflammation and spasm can become significant. If immediate reduction is not possible, analgesics and muscle relaxants must be given before any later attempt to reduce the dislocation. A splint, a harness, or padding should be used for 4 to 8 weeks after acute dislocation or until pain is significantly reduced and muscle function provides adequate support in cases of recurrent dislocation.

After subluxation the client experiences variable pain and the feeling that the joint was out of position briefly. The joint typically feels weak, and pain increases with attempted movement. Because radiographs are often normal with subluxations, the physician must rule out other possible injuries such as sprain, strain, muscle tear, and fracture. Muscle-strengthening exercises can help the client avoid future subluxations. Joint restrictive supports such as a shoulder harness may also be useful.

SPORTS INJURIES
OVERUSE SYNDROMES

Overuse syndromes are common sports-related problems. They begin insidiously as the result of microtraumas that often do not completely stop the affected person's activity. The client must understand that the manifestations of pain, tenderness, and swelling result

from repeated stress on musculoskeletal structures. Eventual failure is likely because of fatigue or erosion if the client continues to exercise. Nonoperative treatment of stress injuries always includes relative rest. For example, the runner may be restricted from impact-loading activities but still allowed to cycle or run in the buoyancy of a swimming pool. Ice, compression (when swelling occurs), and NSAIDs are used routinely to reduce inflammation related to the injury. A supervised, stepped rehabilitation program is also helpful if the client plans to return to the athletic activity.

People who are at greatest risk for overuse include competitive athletes, first-time athletes, "born again" athletes (those who were once very active and now seek a return to athletics after a decade or longer of sedentary living), and those recovering from injury. Other factors can contribute to an increased risk for injury (Box 29-3) and should be shared with clients who exercise regularly or are considering involvement in an exercise program. The risk for developing an overuse syndrome decreases if the client avoids the following:

- Training errors, such as progressing too fast or allowing inadequate time for conditioning
- Improper technique based on the individual activity (e.g., elbow problems from poor tennis technique)
- Improper equipment, such as incorrect shoes for the sport
- Unsafe environment, such as exercising on a slippery surface or experiencing repeated impact on a hard surface

Prevention, the key to overuse injuries, is enhanced by pre-participation assessment and client teaching. Rather than trying to ensure that the client is in optimal health, a pre-participation assessment allows recognition of potential problems that can occur as the client progresses in a sport. Client teaching should emphasize the importance of stretching to maintain joint flexibility and range of motion. Stretching exercises

---

BOX 29-3 *Factors That May Increase Risk for Sports Injury*

- Age over 40 years
- Current inactive lifestyle
- Overweight by 20 lb or more
- Family history of cardiac disease
- Any past experience of pain or pressure in chest, arm, or throat
- Taking medications on a regular basis
- Documented high cholesterol level
- Smokes or has history of pulmonary disease
- History of diabetes or other chronic disorders
- History of joint disease

should be static (i.e., holding muscles in a stretched position for a few moments rather than repeatedly stretching and relaxing them). Static stretching reduces the danger of overstretching and tissue damage, causes less muscle soreness than a bouncing stretch, and relieves muscle soreness when it occurs. Box 29-4 presents additional information about injury prevention in fitness programs. (See the Complementary and Alternative Therapy feature in Oral Creatine Supplements to Improve Strength on page 650.)

Overuse syndromes are classified according to the severity of the injury. Intervention generally depends on the severity more than on the specific type of injury (Table 29-6).

BOX 29-4 *Preventing Injuries in Fitness Programs*

Lack of fitness is one of the main causes of sport injury.

Warm-up and Stretching

Always warm up for 5-10 minutes before strenuous exercises. Stretching may improve muscle flexibility, especially among older people.

Pacing

Build up an exercise program gradually. It takes at least 6 to 8 weeks to get into strong condition. Add small, gradual increments of exercise. Proceed gradually and do not overdo. Tired muscles are prone to injury.

Intensity

When preparing for a specific event, plan training programs accordingly (e.g., a marathon demands a more intensive training program than does a 10-km race).

Capacity Level

Exercise to the capacity of physiologic limits; monitor pulse rate.

Strength

Build strength gradually to gain greater endurance, speed, and power.

Motivation

Success depends on the individual's desire to exercise consistently.

Relaxation

Relaxation exercises relieve fatigue and tension.

Routine

Regular exercise is more valuable and less likely to lead to injury than bursts of activity followed by long periods of inactivity.

TABLE 29-6 *Grades of Overuse Injuries*

	Grade I	Grade II	Grade III	Grade IV
Assessment				
History	Hurts after, not during, activity	Hurts after and sometimes during activity	Hurts during and after activity	Hurts all the time
Physical examination	Generalized tenderness	Generalized tenderness over area	More localized tenderness	Localized tenderness
X-rays	Negative	Negative	Usually negative	May be positive
Bone scan	Negative	Negative	May be positive	Usually positive
Type of Tissue Injured	Soft tissue	Soft tissue	Soft, hard, or bony tissue	Hard or bony tissue
Management	Ice Treat underlying problem	Ice Correct underlying problem Anti-inflammatory medication (e.g., aspirin) Decrease exercise 25%-33%	Ice Correct underlying problem Anti-inflammatory medication (e.g., aspirin, NSAIDs); possibly prednisone Decrease exercise 50%-75%	Ice Correct underlying problem Anti-inflammatory medication (e.g., aspirin, NSAIDs); possibly prednisone Stop exercising altogether

Modified from The athlete's leg (1985). *Emergency Medicine, 17,* 83.
NSAIDs, Nonsteroidal anti-inflammatory drugs.

COMPLEMENTARY AND ALTERNATIVE THERAPY

Oral Creatine Supplemenation to Improve Strength

Oral creatine supplements may be the most widely used nutritional supplements among athletes. Therefore a meta-analysis was recently conducted on past studies of these supplements. Researchers found 16 studies for inclusion into their analysis. The summary difference in the maximum weight lifted was 6.85 kg greater after creatine supplements versus placebo for bench press and 9.76 kg greater for squats, but there was no difference for arm curls. In 7 of 10 studies evaluating maximal weight lifted, subjects were younger than 36 years of age and engaged in resistance training. The researchers concluded that oral creatine supplements combined with resistance training increase the maximal weight lifted in young men. There was no evidence of improved performance in older people or women or for other types of strength and power exercises. In addition, the safety of creatine supplements is unknown (one study reported gastrointestinal upset, rash, or headache in subjects taking creatine and no side effects in the three placebo group.) Therefore these supplements cannot be generally recommended until more trials are concluded.

Reference

Dempsey, R., Mazzone, M., & Meurer, L. (2002). Does oral creatine supplementation improve strength? A meta-analysis. *Journal of Family Practice, 51*, 945-951.

Lower Extremities

Common overuse injuries of the lower extremities include the following.

Stress Fracture

Stress fractures occur after usual activities, when there is no evidence of trauma to explain the fracture, and manifest with pain and swelling. The most common stress fracture occurs in the foot, particularly in the tarsal bones, as a result of fatigue from repetitive use or loading. Tarsal navicular stress fractures are fairly common in jumping athletes, but their recognition is frequently delayed. Once diagnosed, bone grafting and screw fixation may be necessary to obtain healing.

Plantar Fasciitis

Plantar fasciitis is one of the most common overuse syndromes of the foot experienced by people in running and jumping sports. It results from repetitive strain to the plantar fascia, the fibrous tissue that provides important support for the longitudinal arches of the feet. It attaches to the plantar surface (sole) of the calcaneus (heel bone), and its fibers fan out to attach to the forefoot. A bone spur may be seen occasionally on radiographs at the plantar origin of the fascia when new bone forms as a result of repeated tearing of the fascia. Diagnosis must rule out calcaneal stress fracture, tarsal tunnel syndrome, and other possible causes of heel pain.

Athletes with plantar fasciitis typically experience severe foot pain aggravated by weight-bearing with the first steps of the morning. The pain then gradually subsides with activity. These clients usually describe a deep ache or bruise at the anteromedial portion of the calcaneus on the plantar surface of the foot. Although more than 90% of athletes ultimately respond to conservative treatment, the prolonged duration of manifestations affects their ability to participate in sports.[34] Exercises may strengthen the major muscle groups in the lower leg to improve walking and running form. Ice is a mainstay of anti-inflammatory treatment. Ice baths of up to 10 minutes after activity and at the end of the day often help. NSAIDs are prescribed primarily for short-term pain relief. Corticosteroid injection is reserved for athletes who want more rapid pain relief or a quicker return to their sport. Little evidence supports the value of repeated injections. Orthoses, such as heel cups and night splints, can provide substantial pain relief. (See the Complementary and Alternative Therapy features on Magnet Therapy for Plantar Heel Pain and on Ionized Wrist Bracelets for Musculoskeletal Pain on p. 651.) Return to training is often recommended at 60% of the pre-injury level during rehabilitation, with the training load increasing no more than 10% per week.[34]

Shin Splints

A medial tibial stress syndrome results from excessive strain of the posterior tibial muscle origin. Shin splints are characterized by pain with activity and residual tenderness at the muscle origins for days after running or other repetitive activity. Shin splints are best treated by strengthening the involved muscles and by using orthotics to correct misalignment of the feet and reduce strain on injured muscles. Prevention begins with adequate stretching after working out to help tense muscles return to a more relaxed state.[38]

Patellar Tendinopathy

Also known as *jumper's knee,* patellar tendinopathy results from repetitive loads placed on the knee's extensor mechanism through sports that require jumping, such as basketball and volleyball. The client complains of pain, tenderness, and sometimes swelling at either pole of the patella. The pain is aggravated by additional jumping. Patellar tendinopathy is usually unilateral and rarely progresses to complete rupture. Treatment has histori-

COMPLEMENTARY AND ALTERNATIVE THERAPY

Magnet Therapy for Plantar Heel Pain

A randomized, double-blind, placebo-controlled trial of 101 adults with a diagnosis of plantar heel pain for at least 30 days was conducted, and daily pain diaries were kept for a total of 2 months. Cushioned insoles with either active bipolar magnets or sham magnets (placebo) were worn daily by the participants for 2 months. No significant differences were found between the two treatment groups.

Reference
Winemiller, M., et al. (2003). Effect of magnetic vs. sham-magnetic insoles on plantar heel pain: A randomized controlled trial. *Journal of the American Medical Association, 290,* 1474-1478.

COMPLEMENTARY AND ALTERNATIVE THERAPY

Ionized Wrist Bracelets for Musculoskeletal Pain

Researchers found that numerous advertisements support the use of an ionized bracelet to relieve musculoskeletal pain. Therefore they decided to study 610 adults with pain in at least 1 of 12 locations (from the neck to the feet). The mean age of the individuals was 48 years (74.2% female and 87.8% Caucasian.) Approximately 80% of the participants believed that the ionized bracelet would work. Participants were randomly assigned to wear either the ionized wrist bracelet or an identical placebo bracelet for 4 weeks. All 610 clients completed the study.

There was no significant difference between the two groups for either endpoint of the study (change in pain score or the sum total of pain scores for all locations). The baseline pain score for all body locations for both groups was between 4.2 and 5.8 out of a possible 10; at a 4-week follow-up the scores had decreased 1.3 to 2.6 points. Approximately 77% of the participants in both groups reported an improvement in their maximum pain score, and a similar number had an improved sum of pain scores. Therefore the bracelet did not work better than the placebo.

Reference
Bratton, R., et al. (2002). Effect of "ionized" wrist bracelets on musculoskeletal pain: A randomized, double-blind, placebo-controlled trial. *Mayo Clinic Proceedings, 77,* 1164-1168.

cally included NSAIDs, although this overuse condition has been shown to have a non-inflammatory pathology and NSAIDs do not provide significant long-term benefit.[19] Recommendations should include reducing the irritating activity as well as improving the flexibility of the hamstrings and rectus femoris to improve the efficiency of knee flexion and extension.

Upper Extremities

Overuse injuries that occur in the upper extremities may involve the shoulder, the elbow, and the wrist.

Impingement Syndrome

Impingement syndrome is one of the most common problems encountered by the athlete involved in repetitive above-the-shoulder activity (e.g., baseball pitchers); however, the disorder can also result from acromioclavicular arthritis, calcium deposits in the supraspinatus tendon, or a subluxation of the shoulder. Manifestations include pain and weakness associated with forward flexion or abduction of the shoulder above 90 degrees.[14] The subacromial bursa, long head of the biceps muscle, and the rotator cuff are the most frequently affected structures in the "painful arc." Initial conservative treatment involves rest with possible sport or job modifications. A sling is not used because adhesive capsulitis can result from shoulder immobilization. NSAIDs and ice applications may relieve pain. A subacromial injection of anesthetic and cortisone may be useful as a therapy and also as an aid to differentiating impingement syndrome from other shoulder problems. Physical therapy may be initiated once acute pain has subsided. Internal rotation, external rotation, and abduction exercises are emphasized for strengthening to prevent additional future injury. The client's return to activity should be slow and progressive.

Tennis Elbow

Despite the common term *tennis elbow,* lateral humeral epicondylitis is seen not only in tennis players but in anyone involved in activities that require repetitive use of the wrist extensors or flexors. Most clients are treated conservatively. Nonoperative treatment to reduce inflammation may include the use of iontophoresis, a modality that uses low-voltage electrical current to drive ions of anti-inflammatory medication into the affected area. A careful rehabilitation program includes gradual stretching and isometric exercises. As the client returns to full activity, a counter-force brace can be worn to inhibit full muscle expansion and decrease tension on the injured tissue.

Golfer's Elbow

The etiology and treatment of medial humeral epicondylitis are similar to those of tennis elbow.

Tendinitis and Tenosynovitis

Tendinitis and tenosynovitis involving the hand and wrist are quite common but are usually transitory. When they persist, they may impair the client's ability to work. People at risk include those who engage in activities that require gripping, pinching, pulling, or lifting with repetitive wrist motion. Radiographs are obtained to rule out foreign bodies, arthritis, calcification, fractures, and other abnormalities.

STRAINS

Strains result from trauma to a muscle body or to the attachment of a tendon from overstretching, overextension, or misuse. They often arise from twisting or wrenching movements and may occur in any body part that contains muscles and tendons. Strains can occur *acutely* during unaccustomed vigorous exercise. They may also be *chronic*, developing after repetitive muscle overuse.

Strains are characterized by muscle spasm and discomfort; severity of clinical manifestations is related to the degree of injury. With more severe strains, ecchymosis and edema may be evident, and range of motion may be quite limited. Radiographs are necessary to rule out the possibility of fracture.

Acute strains require rest and, if possible, splinting. The injured part should be elevated and ice should be applied for the first 24 to 48 hours to decrease swelling. Heat may be prescribed for comfort after 72 hours; it also hastens reabsorption of blood and fluid and promotes healing. Surgical repair may be needed if a rupture is present at the tendon-bone interface. During healing after strain (4 to 6 weeks), movement of the injured part should be minimized. Activity should never progress to the point that manifestations such as pain or swelling result. After mature scar tissue has formed, the injured part can be gradually and progressively exercised. Overactivity must absolutely be avoided during rehabilitation.

SPRAINS

A sprain is a ligamentous injury resulting from overstress that damages ligament fibers or their attachment to a bone. The ankle joint is most frequently injured during sports participation. An ankle sprain most often occurs when the foot is forced inward, stretching or tearing the ligaments that hold the joint in place. The greater the stress and the longer it is applied to the ankle, the more severe the sprain. The severity of the swelling depends on the extent of tissue injury; however, ecchymosis does not always reliably indicate either the severity or the site of the injury. To plan treatment, it is important to determine the number of ligaments affected and the severity of injury to them.

Sprains may be *mild* (first degree), *moderate* (second degree), or *severe* (third degree) (Figure 29-8). In a first-degree sprain, only a few ligament fibers are torn, with no loss of function and no weakening of the ligament. With a second-degree sprain, a portion of the ligament is torn and some loss of function results. In a

third-degree sprain, a ligament is completely torn, either from its attachment or within the body of the ligament itself. Treatment recommendations now call for early mobilization of mild and moderate sprains (first or second degree). The first phase of treatment includes *r*est, *i*ce, *c*ompression, and *e*levation (RICE) with protected weight-bearing as needed. The second phase of treatment begins when the client can place some weight on the injured extremity. Exercises focus on restoring strength, ankle motion, and proprioception. The third phase of rehabilitation includes activity-specific drills before the client is allowed to return to full sports participation.

If surgical repair is required for a complete ligament rupture, cast or brace immobilization is needed for 4 to 6 weeks after the injury. Once the conventional immobilizer is removed, the injured ankle may be placed in an air cast to allow dorsiflexion and plantar flexion of the foot while restricting lateral movements of the ankle. At this point, gentle range-of-motion and strengthening exercises can be initiated.

A

B

C

FIGURE 29-8 Various types of sprains (with the ankle as an example). **A,** Mild (first-degree) sprain is a small hematoma in a localized area. **B,** Moderate (second-degree) sprain is more severe, with more than half of the fibers torn. **C,** Severe (third-degree) sprains tear completely through the ligament.

Client education following an ankle sprain is extremely important. Explain all phases of recovery, and offer strategies to prevent future injury to the ankle.

ROTATOR CUFF TEARS

Most shoulder injuries involve the soft tissues, and many result directly from repetitive activities such as throwing or overhead motion within the shoulder girdle. The shoulder girdle includes the sternoclavicular joint, the acromioclavicular joint, the glenohumeral joint, the subacromial space, and the scapulothoracic space. Movement at all these articulations allows for the complexity of a pitcher's throwing motion. Four muscles also contribute to the shoulder's varied movements and form the rotator cuff: (1) the subscapularis (anterior), (2) the supraspinatus, (3) the infraspinatus, and (4) the teres minor (posterior).

Normal shoulder movement is a smooth, pain-free activity of the rotator cuff muscles; however, excessive joint activity can lead to repetitive trauma, or muscles can be injured by an external force. Careful history and appropriate examination by the physician often lead to a diagnosis of the extent of injury. If the rotator cuff is torn, the client is not able to perform abduction and external rotation. Activity at the glenohumeral joint is also painfully impaired. Confirmation can be gained through use of radiography, arthrography, CT scans, MRI, or arthroscopy.

Treatment of rotator-cuff injury often begins conservatively with rest and sling support for the shoulder. NSAIDs may relieve discomfort. Some physicians also advocate intra-articular injection of analgesics or steroids. When acute manifestations subside, the client should begin active exercises that address range of motion and strengthen the rotator cuff muscles. Any elastic graded equipment (e.g., TheraBand) can be used in a daily program of progressive gentle exercises. Exercise may be preceded by application of heat and followed by ice if discomfort occurs.

Surgery may be necessary to repair a tear in the rotator cuff. Repair will probably be performed on an outpatient basis, although the client may be hospitalized briefly if pain or nausea becomes problematic. Postoperative management includes instruction on the use of a shoulder immobilizer and introduction of a program of gentle exercises such as the pendulum shoulder movement. The neurovascular status of the affected arm should be assessed at regular intervals, and findings should be compared with the nonoperative arm. Pain management should also be a focus of postoperative care.

ANTERIOR CRUCIATE LIGAMENT INJURIES

More than 250,000 anterior cruciate ligament (ACL) injuries occur each year in the United States[10] (Figure 29-9). Most injuries occur during involvement in athletics, but falls and motor vehicle accidents also contribute to the number of ACL problems. Most injuries occur in people 15 to 44 years of age. Injury rates are two to eight times higher in females than in males, possibly related to anatomic differences or to ligamentous laxity that results from hormonal influences.[10]

The ACL is usually injured as part of a complex mechanism of hyperextension, internal rotation, extremes of external rotation, and deceleration. The ligament may actually be torn from the femur or tibia. More commonly, however, the tear occurs in the midportion of the ACL. The injured client often describes hearing a loud pop. Severe swelling can occur in the first few hours after injury. The knee feels unstable ("gives way"), particularly in rotation, and full extension is difficult.

The physician may attempt to determine knee stability during examination by using the Lachman test, the most sensitive test for ACL insufficiency. The client rests in a relaxed supine position with the injured knee flexed at 20 to 30 degrees. Placing one hand around the client's distal thigh and the other around the client's proximal tibia, the health care provider attempts anterior-

Medial collateral ligament tear

Medial meniscus tear

Anterior cruciate ligament tear

FIGURE 29-9 Common knee injuries: Medial collateral ligament tear, commonly caused by inversion and twisting. Anterior cruciate ligament injury, commonly caused by twisting a hyperextended knee. Medial meniscal injury, commonly caused by twisting an everted knee.

posterior translation. The test result is positive when anterior-posterior sliding occurs. The anterior drawer test is an alternative diagnostic maneuver. The health care provider grasps the tibia just below the joint line and pulls forward with both hands while assessing the amount of tibial displacement. An intact ACL allows the tibia to move forward only a few millimeters before stopping abruptly. An injured ACL allows greater movement and gives a mushy feel to joint mobility. Routine radiographs may also be used for diagnosis of ACL injury, but the MRI is especially sensitive and specific for difficult cases. Arthroscopy, the most important advance in the diagnosis of knee disorders, can enable the physician to confirm the degree of ACL damage and determine the extent of associated intra-articular injuries. Arthroscopy is also the surgical treatment of choice for ACL reconstruction.

Initial treatment focuses on decreasing pain and swelling and on protecting the joint from further injury by immobilization. ACL reconstruction can be accomplished within several weeks of injury and still allow a return of joint function and stability. Repair is often accomplished with the use of a portion of the client's patellar tendon. After ACL reconstruction, the surgeon often orders the use of a continuous passive motion (CPM) machine to help the client achieve rapid, satisfactory knee mobility. The CPM machine is generally applied in the recovery area and should be used at least 8 hours a day or until full range of motion is achieved. Some surgeons advocate the use of a long leg brace with fixed knee flexion, either alone or in combination with the CPM machine. After ACL reconstruction, the client receives instructions on performance of isometric exercises such as quadriceps setting, bent-knee leg exercises, and foot exercises. The exercise program is progressed over the next 4 to 6 weeks.

MENISCAL INJURIES

The meniscus is the fibrous cartilage that lies on top of the tibia, between the tibia and the femur, and acts as the shock absorber of the knee. It is torn less frequently than the ACL, but most longitudinal tears of the meniscus occur in conjunction with ACL or medial collateral ligament injuries (see Figure 29-9). Because the meniscus has little blood supply, it heals slowly, if at all, after injury.

Meniscal injuries often result from fixed-foot rotation in weight-bearing with the knee flexed. A combination of compression and rotational forces are thus exerted on the meniscus. Mild swelling may be evident, and the client may complain of joint-line pain. Popping, slipping, catching, or buckling of the knee can also occur, particularly if a piece of the cartilage is torn and floating within the knee capsule.

The McMurray test is the most widely used maneuver for assessing meniscal injury. The client is supine with the injured knee flexed to 90 degrees. The health care provider holds the client's foot with one hand and places the fingers of the other hand at the medial joint line. While applying a varus stress at the knee to compress the medial meniscus, the health care provider externally rotates the lower leg, ankle, and foot as a unit. The knee is then extended while the health care provider palpates the medial joint line. The test is considered positive if the client complains of pain localized to the medial or lateral joint line or if a palpable or audible click is produced.

Radiographs are usually normal, although some spurring may be evident if the tear has been present for a long time. Arthrography enables the physician to diagnose posterior tears, but MRI is a more sensitive and specific procedure for reliable diagnosis. Arthroscopy has an additional advantage as both a diagnostic and treatment option. After surgery, the leg is elevated and ice is applied. Effective pain management is an initial priority. An exercise program includes quadriceps strengthening and range of motion for the knee.

▌ REMOBILIZATION AFTER TRAUMATIC INJURY

Strategies for remobilization include therapeutic exercise, use of CPM machines, passive and active range-of-motion exercises, and active resistive range-of-motion exercises. Therapeutic exercise programs are developed to improve joint range of motion, muscle strength, and cardiovascular endurance. Before beginning an exercise program, the client must be aware of limiting factors such as pain and the inability to relax. Exercise should progress at a pace that allows the client to experience no more than a little muscle soreness. Pain in the exercising client may be caused by chronic compartment syndrome and should receive immediate attention.

Passive range-of-motion (PROM) exercises can be performed with the assistance of a therapist or a nurse or with equipment such as a CPM machine. This type of exercise helps to prevent joint contractures and maintain joint range of motion (ROM). If a CPM machine is ordered, make sure that the device properly fits the client. If, for example, the client is too short for the machine settings, the device may be too tight in the groin. Because the client must be supine when using the machine, assess the skin over pressure points such as the sacrum, scapulae, and heels for signs of impairment. The client should be taught the purpose of the CPM machine and how to stop and start it. He or she should also be encouraged to report any manifestations of pressure or irritation.

Active range of motion (AROM) results from the active contraction of the muscle against gravity. AROM exercises are part of a program that increases muscle strength and endurance. Examples include straight leg raises or knee flexion and extension when the client is in a sitting position. In active assistive range of motion, the therapist, a mechanical device, or the opposite extremity provides an external force to the affected extremity during joint motion. This type of exercise is often a second step in rehabilitation. It includes isotonic exercise, such as weight lifting, or isokinetic exercise through use of equipment such as Cybex machines.

Difficulties with ambulation can occur as a result of disorders of the musculoskeletal, nervous, and cardiovascular systems. Cognitive awareness, balance, and coordination are also important for safe walking. After an orthopedic injury, the client should ambulate as soon as possible. The client who has been bedridden even for brief periods may exhibit muscle atrophy and weakness, decreased endurance and cardiovascular fitness, and decreased joint flexibility. Orthostatic hypotension is also common after bed rest. A gradual progression of exercise is needed to remobilize the client. Bed exercises may be the first intervention. If the client has been on extended bed rest, a tilt table can be used to assist him or her to an upright position.

Be aware of the client's weight-bearing status before attempting to assist with ambulation. The degree of protected weight-bearing is determined by the physician on the basis of the client's injury and any surgical procedure. Ambulatory assistive devices such as canes, a walker, or crutches can be used as needed.

CONCLUSIONS

Musculoskeletal trauma ranges from simple strains or sprains to complex, life-threatening injuries. Your role is to promote early mobility, prevent possible complications, and teach the client how to prevent further injury.

THINKING CRITICALLY evolve

1. A young college student arrives in the emergency department holding his arm close to his body. His wrist is obviously misshapen, but swelling is minimal. He tells you he was playing basketball with friends and hit the gym wall after running toward the goal to attempt a lay-up shot. He complains of pain with attempted flexion or rotation of the wrist. A radiograph confirms a wrist fracture, and cast application is planned. What intervention should receive priority? What teaching about cast care should be completed?

Factors to Consider. How should you relieve the client's pain? What is involved in the healing process for a fracture? What complications might the client face because of the cast?

2. Friends of a 22-year-old woman assist her into the doctor's office. She twisted her knee on the pitcher's mound during a competitive softball game and says she heard a popping sound. Swelling over her knee is significant. The client states that her knee buckled when she attempted to walk off the field. What is your priority for care? What will be the long-range care goals?

Factors to Consider. What is the initial treatment for this type of injury? What postoperative treatments will be ordered?

3. An 80-year-old woman is brought to the nursing unit to await surgical repair of a femoral neck fracture. She is mildly confused. A neighbor says he found her on her kitchen floor after an apparent fall. What assessment should be performed on an ongoing basis? What will be the treatment goals after an ORIF of the fracture?

Factors to Consider. What possible complications could result after a hip fracture? How can they be prevented?

Discussions for these questions can be found on the website and the CD-ROM.

BIBLIOGRAPHY

1. Adamo, S.M. (2002). Modalities for mobilization. In A.B. Maher, S.W. Salmond, & T.A. Pellino (Eds.), *Orthopaedic nursing* (3rd ed., pp. 324-350). Philadelphia: W.B. Saunders.
2. Agency for Healthcare Research and Quality (AHRQ). (2001). Hip fracture study calls for assessing patients' risks of both functional impairment and death. Available: http://www.ahcpr.gov/news/press/pr2001/siupr.htm.
3. American Academy of Orthopaedic Surgeons (AAOS). (1999). Position statement: Hip fracture in seniors: A call for health system reform. Available: http://www.aaos.org/wordhtml/papers/position/1144.htm.
4. Austermuehle, P.D. (2001). Common knee injuries in primary care. *Nurse Practitioner, 26* (10), 26-45.
5. Bagwell-Crum, C. (2001). The shoulder. In D.C. Schoen (Ed.), *NAON Core curriculum for orthopaedic nursing* (4th ed., pp. 419-440). Pitman, NJ: National Association of Orthopaedic Nurses.
6. Buddenberg, L.A., & Schkade, J.K. (1998). Special feature: A comparison of occupational therapy intervention approaches for older patients after hip fracture. *Topics in Geriatric Rehabilitation, 13*(4), 52-68.
7. Ceccio, C.M. (1999). Key concepts in the care of patients in traction. In *An introduction to orthopaedic nursing* (2nd ed., pp. 45-60). Pitman, NJ: National Association of Orthopaedic Nurses.
8. Childs, S.G. (2001). Nursing care for hand and wrist problems. In D.C. Schoen (Ed.). *NAON Core curriculum for orthopaedic nursing* (4th ed., pp. 441-462). Pitman, NJ: National Association of Orthopaedic Nurses.

9. Childs, S.G. (2002) Athletic performance and injury. In A.B. Maher, S.W. Salmond, & T.A. Pellino (Eds.), *Orthopaedic nursing* (3rd ed., pp. 674-701). Philadelphia: W.B. Saunders.

10. Childs, S.G. (2002). Pathogenesis of anterior cruciate ligament injury. *Orthopaedic Nursing, 21*(4), 35-40.

11. Clarke, J. (2001). Organizing the approach to musculoskeletal misuse syndrome. *Nurse Practitioner, 26*(7), 11-25.

12. Demirtas, R.N., & Oner, C. (1998). The treatment of lateral epicondylitis by iontophoresis of sodium salicylate and sodium diclofenac. *Clinical Rehabilitation, 12*(1), 23-29.

13. Eckhouse-Ekeberg, D.R. (1999). Care of the patient with an external ambulatory device. In *An introduction to orthopaedic nursing* (2nd ed., pp. 31-43). Pitman, NJ: National Association of Orthopaedic Nurses.

14. Fongamie, A.E., Buss, D.D. & Rolnick, S.J. (1998). Management of shoulder impingement syndrome and rotator cuff tears. *American Family Physician, 57*(4), 667-674.

15. Gordon, D.B., & Pellino, T.A. (2002). Assessment and management of pain. In A.B. Maher, S.W. Salmond, & T.A. Pellino (Eds.), *Orthopaedic nursing* (3rd ed., pp. 129-151). Philadelphia: W.B. Saunders.

16. Hager, C.A., & Brncick, N. (1998). Fat embolism syndrome: A complication of orthopaedic trauma. *Orthopaedic Nursing, 17*(2), 41-46, 58.

EB 17. Healthy People 2010: Leading health indicators. (2000). Available: http://www.healthypeople.gov/LHI/.

18. Iero, J. (2001). Chronic or overuse injuries in sports. National Center for Sports Safety. Available: http://www.sportssafety.net/home.cfm?action=for-kids.

19. Khan, K.M., et al. (2002). Time to abandon the "tendonitis" myth. (2002). *British Medical Journal, 324,* 626-627.

EB 20. Koval, K.J., et al. (1998). Predictors of functional recovery after hip fracture in the elderly. *Clinical Orthopaedics and Related Research, 348,* 22-28.

21. Kunkler, C.E. (2002). Fractures. In A.B. Maher, S.W. Salmond, & T.A. Pellino (Eds.). *Orthopaedic nursing* (3rd ed., pp. 609-649). Philadelphia: W.B. Saunders.

22. Kunkler, C.E. (2001). Therapeutic modalities. In D. C. Schoen (Ed.). *NAON Core curriculum for orthopaedic nursing* (4th ed., pp. 205-234). Pitman, NJ: National Association of Orthopaedic Nurses.

23. Lappe, J.M. (1998). Prevention of hip fractures: A nursing imperative. *Orthopaedic Nursing, 17*(3), 15-23.

24. Loveridge, N. (2002). Lateral ankle sprains. *Emergency Nurse, 10* (2), 29-33.

25. Maher, A.B. (2001). Trauma. In D.C. Schoen (Ed.) *NAON Core curriculum for orthopaedic nursing* (4th ed., pp. 361-393). Pitman, NJ: National Association of Orthopaedic Nurses.

26. Morris, N.S. (1999). Complications associated with orthopaedic surgery. In *An introduction to orthopaedic nursing* (2nd ed., pp. 123-145). Pitman, NJ: National Association of Orthopaedic Nurses.

27. Morris, N.S. (2001). Complications. In D.C. Schoen (Ed.). *NAON Core curriculum for orthopaedic nursing* (4th ed., pp. 161-188). Pitman, NJ: National Association of Orthopaedic Nurses.

28. Murrell, G.A.C., & Walton, J.R. (2001). Diagnosis of rotator cuff tears. *The Lancet, 357,* 769-770.

29. National Center for Sports Safety. (2001). Injury facts. Available: http://sportssafety.org/home.cfm?action=injury-facts.

30. Redemann, S. (2002). Modalities for immobilization. In A.B. Maher, S.W. Salmond, & T.A. Pellino (Eds.). *Orthopaedic nursing* (3rd ed., pp. 302-323). Philadelphia: W.B. Saunders.

31. Roberts, D. (1999). Introduction to bone: Structure and function, fractures, and osteoporosis. In *An introduction to orthopaedic nursing* (2nd ed., pp. 3-16). Pitman, NJ: National Association of Orthopedic Nurses.

32. Sandor, R., & Brone, S. (2002). Rehabilitating ankle sprains. *The Physician and Sports Medicine, 30*(8), 48-50.

33. Schmitt, M. (2001). The foot and ankle. In D.C. Schoen (Ed.). *NAON Core curriculum for orthopaedic nursing* (4th ed., pp. 525-546). Pitman, NJ: National Association of Orthopaedic Nurses.

34. Shea, M., & Fields, K.B. (2002). Plantar fasciitis. *The Physician and Sportsmedicine, 30*(7), 21-28.

35. Slauenwhite, C.A., & Simpson, P. (1998). Patient and family per- spectives on early discharge and care of the older adult undergoing fractured hip rehabilitation. *Orthopaedic Nursing, 17*(1), 30-36.

36. Taggart, H.M. (1999). Caring for the elderly hip fracture patient. In *An introduction to orthopaedic nursing* (2nd ed., pp. 113-122). Pitman, NJ: National Association of Orthopedic Nurses.

37. Theis, L.M. (2001). The hip, femur, and pelvis. In D.C. Schoen (Ed.). *NAON Core curriculum for orthopaedic nursing* (4th ed., pp. 484-506). Pitman, NJ: National Association of Orthopaedic Nurses.

38. To stretch or not to stretch before exercising? (Dec. 2000). *Tufts University Health & Nutrition Letter,* 6.

39. Zorn, K.E. (2001). Infections. In D.C. Schoen (Ed.). *NAON Core curriculum for orthopaedic nursing* (4th ed., pp. 189-204). Pitman, NJ: National Association of Orthopaedic Nurses.

Nutritional Disorders

Anatomy and Physiology Review

The Nutritional (Gastrointestinal) System

Robert G. Carroll

The nutritional or gastrointestinal (GI) system is a long, hollow tube that passes through the body providing an isolated environment for digestion and absorption of the nutrients. Ingested contents pass sequentially through the mouth, esophagus, stomach, small intestine (duodenum, jejunum, and ileum), and large intestine (colon) before exiting the body at the anus.

GI tract function is regulated by a complex series of neural, hormonal, and local control systems. The enteric nervous system integrates motor and secretory activities along the GI tract. Ganglia have sensory neurons that respond to temperature, chemical agents, and mechanical deformation. Ganglia also have effector neurons to smooth muscle, secretory cells, endocrine cells, and autocrine cells. GI secretion and motility are enhanced by parasympathetic activity and inhibited by sympathetic activity.

GI hormones, which control and integrate both motility and secretion, are distributed in the stomach and small intestine. GI hormones are also important trophic factors, stimulating proliferation of the GI tract to enhance absorptive capacity.

Finally, the GI tract has an extensive immune system. Gut-associated lymphoid tissue (GALT) may account for up to 80% of the immunoglobulin-producing cells in the body. These cells are important because of the intimate association of the GU system and the "outside environment," the chyme in the lumen of the GI tract.

STRUCTURE OF THE GASTROINTESTINAL TRACT

In cross-section, the GI tract generally has four distinct layers (Figure U7-1). The innermost layer is the *mucosa*, where epithelial cells contact ingested food. The mucosa

FIGURE U7-1 Typical cross-section of the gastrointestinal tract. *Inset* shows enlargement of a cross-section of the small intestine. Microvilli of the mucosa enhance absorption of the diet, and smooth muscle orientation promotes mixing (circular) and peristalsis (longitudinal).

often has microvilli to increase the surface area available for absorption. Beneath the mucosa is the *submucosa (lamina propria)*, containing glands, blood vessels, and lymph nodules. Next is a *muscular layer,* with smooth muscle oriented either circularly or longitudinally. The outermost layer is the *connective tissue serosa layer.*

The entrance (mouth, upper esophagus) and exit (external anal sphincter) of the GI tract contain GI-associated skeletal muscle, which is partially under voluntary control. The remainder of the GI tract (Figure U7-2) has smooth muscle, which is under involuntary control. GI smooth muscle is electrically connected by gap junctions, allowing a wave of depolarization and contraction to spread along the tract (see Motility later in this chapter).

Food is chewed *(masticated)*, mixed with saliva in the mouth, and swallowed. It passes through the pharynx and into the *esophagus.* The upper third of esophagus has striated (voluntary) muscle, the middle third has both types of muscle, and the lower third has only smooth muscle. The vagus nerve innervates both the smooth and skeletal muscle of the esophagus. Sphincters isolate the esophagus from the remainder of the GI tract. The upper esophageal sphincter prevents entry of tracheal air and the lower esophageal sphincter prevents reflux of gastric contents *(aspiration).* Acute failure of the lower esophageal sphincter causes *esophagitis* (heartburn), and chronic gastric reflux causes digestion of the esophagus. The opposite problem, *achalasia,* occurs if the lower esophageal sphincter does not relax sufficiently to allow food to pass into the stomach.

The stomach is divided into the *fundus, body,* and *antrum.* The fundus and body are highly distensible and act as reservoir ingested meal. Food can be stored unmixed in the fundus and body for up to 1 hour. During

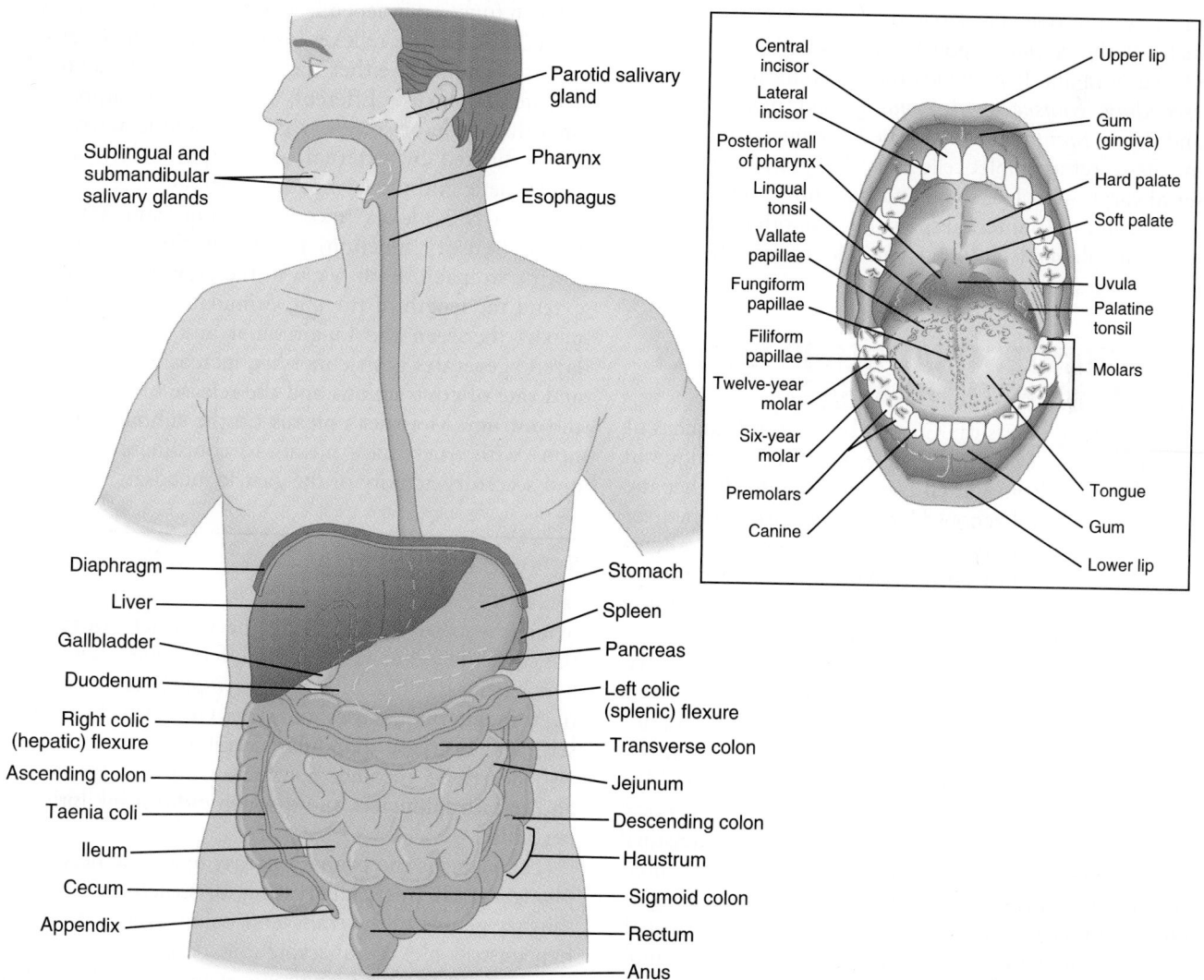

FIGURE U7-2 The digestive system. Ingested food passes through the mouth, esophagus, stomach, and small and large intestine before exiting at the anus. Liver, gallbladder, and pancreas assist the digestion and absorption of the diet. *Inset* shows the important structures of the oral cavity.

this time, there may be a separation due to density, because fats float to the top and liquids accumulate on the bottom. Thus liquids are the first to leave the stomach and be absorbed through the intestine. Gastric contents empty from the antrum through the pylorus into the duodenum. The gastroduodenal junction sequesters acid in the stomach and bile in the duodenum.

The small intestine is divided into *duodenum* (25 cm), *jejunum* (2.5 m), and *ileum* (3.6 m). The duodenum and jejunum are the major sites of digestion and absorption. Pancreatic and biliary ducts carry digestive enzymes, bicarbonate, and bile to the lumen of the duodenum. The continuous epithelial cell lining of the small intestine separates luminal contents from the body and provides a barrier across which nutrients must be absorbed. Epithelial cells reproduce rapidly and are lost (exfoliated) at the tip of the microvilli.

Chyme, the nonabsorbed component of the diet, passes through the *ileocecal valve* (a sphincter) to enter the large intestine. The large intestine (~1.5 m in length) includes the *cecum* (a pouch where small and large intestines join and from which the appendix projects); the *ascending, transverse, descending,* and *sigmoid colon*; and the *rectum* (anal canal). The large intestine contains mucus-secreting goblet cells and cells specialized for water absorption; it lacks villi and does not produce digestive enzymes. An internal sphincter (smooth muscle) and external sphincter (voluntary muscle) govern the expulsion of feces (defecation).

GASTROINTESTINAL BLOOD SUPPLY AND LYMPHATIC DRAINAGE

Arterial blood enters the GI tract by various branches of major arteries. Venous drainage, however, is unique in that the veins from the GI tract empty into the hepatic portal vein. Portal venous blood passes through the liver before entering the vena cava. This arrangement allows the liver to begin processing and detoxifying compounds absorbed across the stomach and intestines before those compounds enter the general circulation.

The esophageal arteries, the inferior thyroid artery, and the left gastric artery provide the esophagus with its arterial blood supply. The left gastric and inferior phrenic arteries supply the gastroesophageal area. Venous blood is returned via the azygos, thyroid, and left gastric veins. Lymphatic drainage from the cervical esophagus and from the tracheal and postmediastinal nodes flows to the internal jugular vein, whereas intercostal nodes drain the thoracic esophagus. The lymphatic drainage of the lower esophagus occurs through the diaphragmatic, intracardiac, and left gastric lymph nodes.

The arterial blood supply to the stomach is derived from the celiac artery, which branches off the lesser and greater curvatures. Gastric arteries, from the splenic ar-

tery, supply the fundus. The portal vein provides the venous drainage of the stomach. The right and left gastroepiploic veins drain the greater curvature; the right gastric and coronary veins drain the lesser curvature. Lymph nodes of the stomach arise in the submucosa and drain into the thoracic duct.

Except in the duodenum, arterial blood supply to the small intestine is derived from the superior mesenteric artery. Arterial blood from the hepatic artery supplies the duodenum. Venous drainage is via the superior mesenteric vein, which unites with the inferior mesenteric, splenic, and gastric veins and then empties into the portal system.

NEURAL REGULATION

Enteric Nervous System

The enteric system regulates motility and secretion along the entire length of the GI tract. The enteric nervous system can function independent of the central nervous system (CNS). Enteric reflexes, originating from GI sensory nerves, synapse in either the submucosal plexus or the myenteric plexus. Efferent nerves then supply the smooth muscle or secretory glands. Enteric activity can be modulated by external inputs, particularly by the sympathetic and parasympathetic nerves.

Auerbach's plexus (motor function) and *Meissner's plexus* (sensory function) provide intrinsic innervation for the stomach. Both begin in the esophageal wall and extend the length of the gut. Stimulation of Auerbach's plexus (between the longitudinal and circular muscle layers) generates gastric motility, increasing the intensity and rate of contractions and the release of gastrin from the antrum. Meissner's plexus (in the submucosa) functions with Auerbach's plexus to coordinate the motor and secretory activity of the gastric mucosa.

Sympathetic and Parasympathetic Nervous Systems

Sympathetic nerves supplying the GI tract originate in the celiac, superior mesenteric, inferior mesenteric, and hypogastric ganglia. In general, *sympathetics* inhibit activity in enteric plexuses, constrict GI system blood vessels, and decrease glandular secretions. GI motility is also decreased through contraction of circular muscle and certain sphincters and through indirect inhibition of peristalsis.

The vagus is the primary parasympathetic nerve supplying the GI tract, innervating all structures from the salivary glands to the transverse colon. Nerves from the hypogastric plexus innervate the remainder of colon. Parasympathetic postganglionic neurons are located in intramural plexus. In general, *parasympathetics* stimulate motor activity, stimulate secretory activity, and stimulate endocrine secretions.

FUNCTION OF THE GASTROINTESTINAL SYSTEM

The GI system isolates ingested food and provides an environment for digestion and absorption of nutrients. The major functions of the GI tract are (1) motility, (2) secretion, (3) digestion, and (4) absorption.

MOTILITY

Smooth Muscle

Smooth muscle of the GI tract is electrically connected by gap junctions, allowing a wave of depolarization and contraction to spread along the tract. Pacemakers along the length of the GI tract set the slow-wave contraction frequency. Nerves and hormones alter this rate and, therefore, GI motility.

GI smooth muscle produces long, strong contractions. Muscle basal tone provides some tension even at rest, and is influenced by neurotransmitters, hormones, and drugs. Stretch of GI system increases action potential frequency *(stress activation),* followed by a decrease back toward the original tension *(stress relaxation).* Contraction of GI smooth muscle defines a sphincter, or a region of higher tone, which may not have any anatomic features.

Peristalsis is an organized wave of contraction of the longitudinal muscle layer that propels contents aborally (away from the mouth). Distention of a segment of intestine elicits a reflex contraction. The smooth muscle aboral to the contraction relaxes, and the contents move. This sequence repeats, moving contents for a short distance before the wave diminishes and disappears. A descending wave of peristalsis initiates sphincter relaxation, mediated by vasoactive intestinal peptide (VIP) neurotransmitter in vagal nerves. Decreased vagal cholinergic activity also contributes to relaxation.

Intrinsic motility regulation uses interneurons to coordinate activity. The enteric nervous system has neuromodulators, similar to those in the brain. Intrinsic plexuses inhibit basal activity, and action potentials are thus elicited by less than half of the slow waves.

Contractions of the various layers of smooth muscle propel and mix luminal contents. Peristaltic contraction of the longitudinal muscle layer accomplish aboral movement. Contraction of circular muscle mixes luminal contents and increases contact with microvilli.

Mouth Through Esophagus

The process of moving food from the mouth into the esophagus is illustrated in Figure U7-3. The esophageal phase of swallowing is involuntary. Contraction of the upper esophageal sphincter isolates the pharynx from the esophagus. A primary peristatic wave, controlled by the swallowing center in the brain, moves food through the esophagus in 10 seconds. Secondary peristalsis is initiated by esophageal distention (enteric nervous system); it propels any food still remaining in the esophagus into the stomach.

Stomach

Gastric contractions after feeding occur at a rate of three per minute. They begin in the middle of body of the stomach, and increase in force and velocity as they approach the antrum. The antrum has strong contractions that fragment the food into smaller particles and mix the food with gastric secretions to initiate digestion. The rate of contractions is increased by gastrin and decreased by secretin. Sensory afferents from the stomach play a role in satiety. Increased intragastric pressure, gastric distention, gastric acidity, and pain all lessen the desire to eat food.

Gastroduodenal Junction

Gastric contents empty into the duodenal bulb at a controlled rate. The pylorus and terminal end of antrum contract almost simultaneously (systolic contraction), allowing only a small amount of antral content to enter duodenum. The remainder of antral contraction moves antral contents backward (retropulsion), causing further mixing. The rate of gastric emptying must match the duodenal buffering ability, or else acid may damage duodenal mucosa and cause duodenal ulcers. The pylorus prevents regurgitation of duodenal contents into stomach, or else bile may damage stomach mucosa, causing gastric ulcers.

Duodenal acidity (pH <3.5) decreases the rate of gastric emptying. A neural reflex causes secretin release, which increases bicarbonate buffer secretion from pancreas and liver. Chyme becomes more hypertonic as digestion progresses. Duodenal hypertonicity also decreases the rate of gastric emptying by a neural reflex. Fat content in the duodenal chyme also decreases the rate of gastric emptying. Cholecystokinin (CCK) released from duodenum and jejunum contracts the pyloric sphincter, and glucose-dependent insulinopeptide (GIP) may also have a role. Fatty acids (especially long chain and unsaturated) decrease the rate of gastric emptying. Monoglycerides increase contractility of pyloric sphincter. Amino acids (tryptophan) and peptides in duodenum slow gastric emptying by promoting gastrin release, which constricts the pylorus.

Small Intestine

Peristalsis moves chyme aborally an average of 10 cm per contraction, and chyme takes 2 to 4 hours to move 6 meters. Segmentation, the most frequent type of intestinal contraction, can be rhythmic, with adjacent sites

1.

ORAL PHASE (VOLUNTARY)

- Bolus of food
- Hard palate
- Tongue
- Vocal cords
- Larynx
- Posterior nares
- Soft palate
- Pharynx
- Epiglottis
- Esophagus

2.

PHARYNGEAL PHASE (INVOLUNTARY)

Early   Middle   Late

3.

ESOPHAGEAL PHASE (INVOLUNTARY)

- Bolus of food in esophagus
- Contracted muscle
- Bolus of food in esophagus
- Peristalsis
- Relaxed muscle

FIGURE U7-3 Swallowing occurs in three phases: (1) *Voluntary* or *oral* phase. The tongue presses food against the hard palate, forcing it toward the pharynx. (2) *Involuntary, pharyngeal* phase. *Early:* Wave of peristalsis forces bolus between tonsillar pillars. *Middle:* Soft palate draws upward to close posterior nares, and respirations cease momentarily. *Late:* vocal cords approximate and larynx pulls upward, covering the airway and stretching the esophagus open. (3) *Involuntary, esophageal* phase. Relaxation of the upper esophageal (hypopharyngeal) sphincter allows a peristaltic wave to move the bolus down the esophagus.

alternating contraction and relaxation. Eating slows ab-oral movement of chyme. The enteric nervous system controls the frequency of segmentation and peristalsis. An intrinsic rate of 11 to 13 contractions per minute exists in the duodenum, which decreases to eight to nine per minute in the terminal ileum. This rate is modified by extrinsic neural and hormonal inputs.

Migrating Myoelectric Complex

The migrating myoelectric complex generates periods of intense electrical activity, followed by long quiescent periods. The resulting contractions, initiated in stomach, traverse the entire small intestine. There is evidence for both vagal and hormonal (motilin) roles in initiation, and the enteric nervous system is required for propagation. This process sweeps the intestines clean and inhibits the retrograde movement of bacteria from the colon into the small intestine.

Large Intestine

Although chyme may move through the small intestine in 2 to 4 hours, it takes 1 to 3 days to complete its passage through the large intestine. Here sodium and water are absorbed. Bacteria consume more nutrients and release some vitamins (e.g., vitamin K). Solid wastes (sloughed epithelial cells, bile pigments, unabsorbed food) are prepared for elimination as feces. Abnormally fast movement of chyme through the large intestine results in diarrhea; abnormally slow movement results in constipation. Inflammation of the appendix (appendicitis) can lead to peritonitis and other complications.

Vomiting

Vomiting expels gastric (and sometimes duodenal) contents by mouth. Retching, wherein gastric contents are forced into the esophagus but not the pharynx, precedes vomiting. The vomiting reflex follows a set pattern:

1. Reverse peristalsis is initiated in middle of small intestine.
2. Pyloric sphincter and stomach relax to receive duodenal contents.
3. Forced inspiration against a closed glottis decreases intrathoracic pressure.
4. Forceful contraction of abdominal muscles increases intra-abdominal pressure.
5. Lower esophageal sphincter relaxes; pylorus and antrum contract.
6. Gastric contents enter esophagus.
7. Retching occurs when the upper esophageal sphincter remains closed.
8. Vomiting occurs when the upper esophageal sphincter opens.
9. Trachea closes as in normal swallowing to prevent aspiration.

The medulla has a separate vomiting center and retching center that normally interact. Afferent inputs include stomach and duodenal distention, and pain in genitourinary system. Dizziness or tickling the back of throat can also induce vomiting. Emetics are used to induce vomiting by stimulating receptors in the stomach and duodenum (ipecac) or by activating a chemoreceptive trigger zone (CTZ) in the area postrema (morphine).

SECRETIONS

Most ingested food cannot be absorbed directly. GI secretions digest foods into absorbable components, assist absorption, and help prevent autodigestion (Table U7-1). GI secretions are regulated by a series of hormonal and neural feedback mechanisms. Secretions include lubricants, ions, absorption facilitators, and bile.

Lubricants

Chewing of foods (mastication) is the initial step in digestion. Chewing mixes the food with salivary mucus, subdivides food, and exposes starches to salivary amylase. Chewing facilitates the mechanical breakdown of food, but chewing is not an essential component of digestion.

Saliva, with both watery and mucous secretions, helps lubricate food as it enters the GI tract. Mucus-secreting cells are located along the entire GI tract, but digestive secretions are limited to the prejejunal GI tract. Salivary glands contribute about 1.5 L/day to the GI tract. The stomach secretes about 2 L/day, and the pancreas secretes 1.5 L/day, helping to liquify the chyme. The small intestine secretes 1.5 L/day, and the large intestine secretes 400 ml/day. In addition, 0.25 to 1.5 L/day of hepatic secretions enter the duodenum.

Gastric secretions begin protein digestion and protect the gastric epithelium. After a meal, there are three distinct phases of gastric acid secretion. (1) The *cephalic phase* is due to a neural reflex initiated by the sight, smell, or taste of food. The decrease in antral pH acts directly on the parietal calls to attenuate the cephalic phase. (2) The *gastric phase* is due to gastric distention caused by food in the stomach. (3) The *intestinal phase* is initiated by chyme entry into duodenum.

Secretion of HCl from the gastric parietal cells involves the interplay of acetylcholine, gastrin, histamine, and a second cell type, the enterochromaffin cell. A powerful synergistic interaction between these stimuli causes difficulty in diminishing acid secretion by blocking only one pathway. HCl secretion can be blocked by atropine (acetylcholine) or cimetidine (H_2 histamine), but a blocker for gastrin is not yet available. Ranitidine, which is used to treat duodenal ulcers, is more effective and has fewer side effects. Gastric ulcers, although associated with increased HCl secretion, involve a gram-negative bacterium, *Helicobacter pylori*, which damages the gastric mucosa. Other agents, such as aspirin and

TABLE U7-1	*Gastrointestinal-Associated Secretions*	
Location	**Secretion**	**Role**
Lubricants		
Entire GI tract	Mucus	Lubricant
Salivary gland	Water	Lubricant and solvent
Pancreas	Water	Lubricant
Small intestine	Water	Lubricant
Digestive Enzymes		
Salivary glands	Amylase	Digest starch
	Lingual lipase	Digest triglycerides
Stomach	Pepsin (pepsinogen)	Digest proteins
	Gastric lipase	Digest triglycerides
Pancreas	Amylase	Digest starch
	Lipase	Digest triglycerides
	Colipase	Digest triglycerides
	Phospholipase	Digest phospholipids
	Trypsin	Digest peptides
	Chymotrypsin	Digest peptides
	Nucleases	DNA and RNA
Intestinal epithelium	Disaccharidases	Disaccharides
	Peptidases	Peptides
Hormones and Neurotransmitters		
Stomach	Gastrin	HCl secretion
Pancreas	Somatostatin	Inhibit insulin, glucagon release
Small intestine	Cholecystokinin	Pancreatic enzyme secretion
	Secretin	Pancreatic bicarbonate secretion
	Glucose-dependent insulinotropic peptide (GIP)	Pancreatic insulin release
	Motilin	GI smooth muscle contraction
	Enteroglucagons	Pancreatic insulin release
Enteric neurons	Vasoactive intestinal peptide (VIP)	GI smooth muscle relaxation
		Pancreatic secretion
	Bombesin	Gastrin release
Ionic Secretions		
Salivary glands	$NaHCO_3$	At high salivary flow rates
	KCl	At low salivary flow rates
Stomach		
Parietal cells	HCl	Activate pepsin
Mucous cells	K^+ and HCO_3	Protect stomach from acid
Pancreas	$NaHCO_3$	Neutralize gastric secretion
Absorption Facilitators		
Stomach	Intrinsic factor	Ileal absorption of vitamin B_{12}
Liver	Bile acids	Small intestine lipid absorption

DNA, Deoxyribonucleic acid; *GI*, gastrointestinal; *HCl*, hydrochloric acid; *KCl*, potassium chloride; *NaHCO₃*, sodium bicarbonate; *RNA*, ribonucleic acid.

nonsteroidal anti-inflammatory drugs (NSAIDs), can damage the gastric mucosa and cause gastric ulcers.

Absorption Facilitators and Ions

Pancreatic enzymes are essential for the normal absorption of lipids, proteins, and carbohydrates. Table U7-1 lists the important enzymes and ionic pancreatic secretions, and their function.

Bile and the Enterohepatic Circulation

Bile acids are secreted by liver as bile, stored in the gallbladder, and released into the duodenum after a meal. Bile acids are reabsorbed by both diffusion and active transport in the terminal ileum and are returned to liver by hepatic portal vein. The liver then actively extracts bile acids from the portal venous blood and secretes the reabsorbed bile acids into bile, thus beginning the process anew. Only about 15% to 35% of the bile acid pool is lost in feces each day and is replaced by new synthesis of bile acids.

Bile acids are normally secreted conjugated to glycine or taurine. At the neutral pH of the small intestine, bile is in the salt form.

With the sphincter of Oddi at the junction of the bile duct and duodenum normally contracted, bile is diverted to and stored in gallbladder between meals. The gallbladder extracts sodium ions (Na^+) actively, anions via electroneutrality, and water osmotically, thus concentrating bile. CCK is the primary stimulus for the gallbladder to contract (expel contents) into the duodenum. Vagal nerves also contract the gall bladder and relax the sphincter of Oddi, and sympathetics and VIP inhibit gallbladder emptying.

Disorders of bile secretions lead to crystal (stone) formation. Gallstones primarily are cholesterol crystals surrounding a bilirubin crystal core. Bile pigment stones, a calcium salt of unconjugated bilirubin, can also form. If cholesterol content exceeds the dissolving capability of the micelles, cholesterol crystals form and act as a nucleus for gallstones.

DIGESTION AND ABSORPTION

Complex carbohydrates are broken down to absorbable monoglycerides. Poorly absorbed large proteins are broken down into monopeptides, dipeptides, and tripeptides. Pancreatic lipases digest lipids to components, which are absorbed primarily as bile acid micelles.

Carbohydrates

Digestion and absorption of carbohydrates occurs primarily in the duodenum and the jejunum. The ability to absorb carbohydrates greatly exceeds normal dietary intake. Occasionally, an inability to absorb carbohydrate occurs because of deficiency of digestive enzymes or transport proteins. Microflora metabolize any carbohydrates that pass through to the colon, producing gas, in-creased motility, and diarrhea. Diagnosis of malabsorption is confirmed by exposure to a specific carbohydrate, such as an oral glucose tolerance test (GTT) or a biopsy of jejunal epithelial cells. Treatment involves dietary restriction or supplemental enzyme ingestion.

One common disorder, lactose malabsorption syndrome (lactose intolerance), is a genetic lactase deficiency that develops in 50% of adults. This syndrome is almost universal in people with Asian ancestry, it is common in native Africans and people from Mediterranean areas, but it is infrequent in people of Northern European descent.

Proteins

A protein intake of 0.5 g/kg/day is necessary for normal balance, and a higher intake is required for growth. Dietary intake varies among cultures. Separate from ingestion, the body recycles some protein from the intestines, mostly from digestive secretions (20 g/day) and desquamated epithelial cells (20 g/day). The little protein that is present in the feces is due mostly to colonic bacteria, desquamated cells, and proteins in colonic mucous secretion.

Digestion occurs in the stomach and small intestine, and absorption occurs primarily in the duodenum and jejunum. Large proteins are poorly absorbed. L-isomers and single amino acids as well as dipeptides and tripeptides are absorbed by a sodium-coupled process. Genetic malabsorption and intolerance affects intestinal and renal transport proteins. Hartnup's disease is a rare genetic defect in neutral amino acid transporter and prolinuria is a rare defect in proline transport.

Lipids

Triglycerides are the major component of dietary lipids. Other components include sterols, sterol esters, and phospholipids. Lipids are hydrophobic and separate from remainder of chyme as an oily phase in the stomach. In the duodenum, lipids are emulsified by bile acids and digested to form micelles with bile acids. The micelles are absorbed at the intestinal brush border.

Some digestion occurs in the intestine and stomach, but the duodenum, as a result of pancreatic lipases, is the major site of lipid digestion.

Micelles are essential to increase surface contact area for absorption in the duodenum and jejunum. Lipophilic cholesterol, fatty acids, and lysophosphatides diffuse across the cell membrane. The lipids accumulate in smooth endoplasmic reticulum and are resynthesized to triglycerides, phospholipids, and cholesterol esters. They are then packaged in chylomicrons and extruded by exocytosis. After entering the lacteals, chylomicrons pass through the lymphatics to enter venous circulation at the thoracic duct.

Fat lost in feces comes primarily from colonic microflora and desquamated cells. Malabsorption of lipids is tied to impaired digestion or absorption. Complete bile deficiency reduces fatty acids absorption by 50% and impairs absorption of other lipids. Complete absence of pancreatic lipases impairs absorption of all classes of lipids. Impaired absorption can also result from epithelial cell damage, such as intestinal mucosal atrophy, tropical sprue, and gluten enteropathy. The addition of nonabsorbable lipids (e.g., Olestra) and lipid absorption inhibitors also impairs the absorption of fat-soluble vitamins (A, D, E, and K).

Water and Electrolytes

The GI tract absorbs 99% of ingested water. Absorption is greatest in the jejunum and least in the colon as a result of the tightness of the "tight junctions" on the epithelial cells. The GI tract receives 2 L/day from ingestion and 7 L/day from GI secretions, and loses only 50 to 100 ml/day in feces. The colon absorbs 400 ml/day against an apparent osmotic gradient.

The jejunum is also the primary site of Na^+ absorption, secondary to amino acid and carbohydrate transport. The colon has an active Na^+ absorption. Potassium (K) is reabsorbed in jejunum and ileum, but net potassium balance is determined in the colon. The colon reabsorbs K^+ if the luminal K^+ concentration is high and secretes K if the luminal K^+ concentration is low. A significant K^+ loss accompanies water loss from diarrhea.

Intestinal chloride load is from ingestion and pancreatic secretions. Chloride is reabsorbed in jejunum, ileum, and colon. Bicarbonate intestinal load is from pancreatic secretions. It is absorbed in jejunum and may be secreted in the ileum and colon by HCO_3^-/Cl^- exchange. There is a net secretion if HCO_3^- levels are high (*alkalosis*) and a net reabsorption if HCO_3^- levels are low (*acidosis*).

Intestinal Ion and Water Balance

Sympathetic activity enhances water and sodium chloride (NaCl) absorption, and parasympathetic activity decreases water and NaCl absorption. Aldosterone provides the major hormonal control of absorption, causing Na^+ and water reabsorption and colonic and K^+ loss. Enkephalin (opioid peptides) enhances NaCl and water absorption, and somatostatin enhances colonic NaCl and water absorption.

Excessive GI secretions are a clinically important problem. Na^+, Cl^-, and water secretion in crypts in the small intestine can exceed the absorptive capacity of the remainder of the GI tract. Cholera toxin stimulates crypt cell secretion, as do other cyclic adenosine monophosphate (cAMP) stimulators such as VIP and prostaglandins. Pancreatic cholera results from a pancreatic tumor that secretes VIP.

Impaired nutrient absorption causes an excessive osmotic load and causes water and potassium loss in diarrhea. Carbohydrate malabsorption syndromes and fat malabsorption cause water loss in feces if colon absorptive capacity is exceeded.

Calcium absorption in the duodenum and jejunum is stimulated by vitamin D. Dietary iron is also reabsorbed primarily in the duodenum and jejunum, based on the bound state of iron. Approximately 5% to 10% of ingested heme iron is normally absorbed, but heme iron is better absorbed (20% of ingested). Epithelial cells secrete transferrin, which binds iron and is absorbed through receptor-mediated endocytosis. Approximately 50% of ingested magnesium is absorbed along the length of intestine. Phosphate is absorbed along the length of the intestine, possibly by active transport.

Flora

The small intestine flora are predominantly gram-positive lactobacilli, streptococci, and staphylococci. *Aerobacter aerogenes*, *Bacteroides*, *Candida albicans*, *Escherichia coli*, *Proteus*, *Pseudomonas*, and *Streptococcus faecalis* are also found. Bile acids and gastric acid may inhibit bacterial proliferation in the intestine.

Vitamins

Vitamins are essential amino acids that must be absorbed from a dietary source. Water-soluble vitamins can be absorbed by membrane transport proteins. Folic acid and nicotinic acid are absorbed by diffusion or facilitated diffusion. Diffusion causes absorption of pyridoxine and riboflavin. Secondary active transport absorbs vitamin C in the ileum, biotin in duodenum and ileum, and folic acid and thiamine in jejunum. Vitamin B_{12} absorption across the ileum requires intrinsic factor, a gastric secretion. Lipid-soluble vitamins are absorbed in micelles. These include vitamins A, D, E, and K. Compounds that diminish or impair fat absorption also impair absorption of fat-soluble vitamins.

EFFECTS OF AGING

Physiologic changes in the gastrointestinal tract are known to occur with aging. In the mouth, teeth may loosen from loss of supporting gums and bone. Circulation in the gums is reduced, and aging teeth darken and may become uneven and fracture. Decreased output of the salivary glands leads to dryness of mucous membranes and increased susceptibility to breakdown. This decrease can cause difficulty in swallowing and decreased stimulation of taste buds.

Secretion of digestive enzymes and bile also decreases. In the stomach, atrophy of gastric mucosa leads to a decreased secretion of HCl. A decrease in HCl reduces the absorption of iron and vitamin B_{12}, leading to development of anemia. A resulting proliferation of bacteria in the gut can lead to diarrhea and infection. With a decrease in bile secretion, absorption of fats and fat-soluble vitamins becomes impaired. This decreased absorption of fat can lead to weight loss, and the decrease in fat-soluble vitamins can lead to a variety of problems such as altered calcium metabolism and bleeding from the decrease of vitamin K, which is needed to synthesize prothrombin.

CONCLUSIONS

A thorough knowledge of the structure and function of the gastrointestinal system helps the nurse provide knowledgeable care to clients. Medical disorders are related to the four major functions of the GI system: digestion absorption, motility, and secretion. To provide effective interventions, the nurse must understand the normal physiology of this system and the digestive organs.

BIBLIOGRAPHY

1. Berne, R., et al. (2004). *Physiology* (5th ed.). St. Louis: Mosby.
2. Guyton, A.C., & Hall, J. (2001). *Textbook of medical physiology* (10th ed.). Philadelphia: W. B. Saunders.
3. Kierszenbaum, A.L. (2002). *Histology and cell biology: An introduction to pathology.* St. Louis: Mosby.
4. Silverthorn, D. (2001). *Human physiology* (2nd ed.). Upper Saddle River, NJ: Prentice-Hall.

Chapter 30

Assessment of Nutrition and the Digestive System

Vicki M. Ross

Adequate and appropriate nutrition underlies the success of all medical therapies. Nutritional health requires a functional gut that can receive, transport, absorb, and metabolize nutrients. Similarly, adequate and appropriate nutrition is necessary for the gut to function properly. Because of this interdependence, assessment of the gastrointestinal (GI) tract and nutritional status occurs simultaneously or in close succession. A systematic and thorough assessment of the client's nutritional status and upper GI tract can detect a wide range of actual or potential health problems.

This chapter focuses on assessment of nutritional status and the upper GI tract, which includes the mouth, esophagus, stomach, and small intestine. Assessments of the large intestine (colon), rectum, and accessory organs (liver, pancreas, and gallbladder) are presented in Chapters 34 and 44.

SCREENING AND ASSESSMENT OF NUTRITIONAL HEALTH

Nutritional Health

Nutritional health results when the body's nutrient requirements are consistently met.[12] To meet the body's nutrient requirements, adequate and appropriate nutrition must be delivered to, transported by, and absorbed by the GI tract. Furthermore, absorbed nutrients must be metabolized and used at the cellular level. Because of wide variation in factors affecting nutrient requirements, such as age, size, gender, metabolism, and activity level, it is difficult, if not impossible, to determine exact nutrient amounts required for individual clients. However, comparing individual characteristics to published standards or reference groups allows estimation of a client's nutrient requirements.

evolve *Be sure to check out the bonus material on the Evolve website and the CD-ROM, including free self-assessment exercises.*
http://evolve.elsevier.com/Black/medsurg/

To determine whether a client is receiving adequate nutrition, begin by collecting information about dietary intake. Ask the client to list the amounts and types of foods and beverages consumed over the past 24 hours and ask whether this is a typical daily intake. If it is not, ask the client to describe a typical day of food and beverage intake. Twenty-four–hour dietary recalls are quick and relatively easy to obtain; however, the accuracy of the information depends on the client's recall ability. Asking the client to maintain a food diary listing all foods and beverages consumed for 1 to 3 days is a prospective method for collecting diet information. In addition to listing all food and drinks consumed for a specific time period, food diaries should include the amount of each food or drink consumed, how the food or drink was prepared (fried, baked in butter, broiled, steamed), and the time of day the food or drink was consumed.

After obtaining information about dietary intake, assess the adequacy of the client's nutrient intake by comparing it to standard references such as the *Food Guide Pyramid* or the *Dietary Reference Intakes (DRI)*. Published by the United States Department of Agriculture, the Food Guide Pyramid is a graphic representation of the categories and servings of foods recommended for average, healthy persons (see Chapter 2). To use the Food Guide Pyramid, compare the number of servings and types of food (fruit, bread, dairy) consumed with the recommended number of servings from each food group. Clients who consistently omit one or more of the food groups are at nutritional risk, as are clients who consistently eat a disproportionate number of servings from one or more of the food groups.[11]

The DRI, formerly referenced as the Recommended Dietary Allowance (RDA), provides more detailed information about specific nutrients. The DRI may contain information and recommendations for adequate intake (AI), estimated average requirement (EAR), recommended dietary allowance (RDA), and tolerable upper intake level (UIL). For some nutrients, the AI is not available; in those cases, the RDA should be used. In consultation with a registered dietitian, determine the amounts of nutrients consumed by the client and compare them with the DRI.[9] For example, an adult who consumes less than 75 mg/day of vitamin C (the recommended amount for adults) is at risk for developing manifestations of scurvy. Table 30-1 contains the AI or RDA range for nonpregnant adults for selected nutrients.

In consultation with a dietitian, calculate the amount of calories and protein consumed by the client in a typical day. In general, the average, healthy person requires about 30 to 35 calories per kilogram and 0.8 to 1.2 g of protein per kilogram of body weight. For example, a woman weighing 55 kg (120 pounds) requires 1650 to 1925 calories and 44 to 46 g of protein. The Food Guide Pyramid and the DRI are based on average, healthy pop-

ulations and may need to be altered for clients who are ill or outside the average height or weight range. For example, fever increases caloric requirements 7% for each degree Fahrenheit of temperature increase. Some specialty groups such as the American Society of Parenteral and Enteral Nutrition publish nutritional recommendations for clients with specific diseases or conditions.[1] In general, protein requirements decrease and nonprotein calorie requirements increase when kidney or liver function is impaired. Dietary fats are restricted for pancreatic exocrine dysfunction and carbohydrates are restricted for pancreatic endocrine dysfunction.

The National Health and Nutrition Examination Survey, the National Food Consumption Survey, and the Continuing Survey of Food Intakes by Individuals are population-based surveys that provide information about dietary intake, nutritional status, or health outcomes related to nutrition. Information from these studies can be used to assess similar client populations. For example, analyses from population surveys indicate that an increasing percentage of Americans are overweight or obese. Furthermore, obesity is positively associated with increased caloric intake, sedentary lifestyle, and the risk of developing diseases such as diabetes and heart disease.[12] Therefore it is important to ask questions about the client's physical activity and the presence of diabetes or heart disease when assessing nutritional adequacy (see Chapter 31 for additional information about obesity).

Malnutrition

When nutrient availability is consistently inadequate or excessive, malnutrition occurs. Malnourished clients may suffer from starvation or obesity.

Starvation, or the inadequate delivery of nutrients to the body, can be primary or secondary:

- *Primary* malnutrition occurs when adequate nutrition is not delivered to the upper GI tract over an extended period (famine, anorexia, mechanical obstructions of the GI tract, fad diets).
- *Secondary* malnutrition occurs when the upper GI tract fails to absorb, metabolize, or use nutrients (ischemic bowel or Crohn's disease).

When inadequate amounts of proteins or calories are ingested or absorbed by the gut over an extended period, marasmus, kwashiorkor, or mixed-type malnutrition results. Table 30-2 contains information about the clinical presentation and laboratory findings for marasmus, kwashiorkor, and mixed-type malnutrition.[12]

Micronutrient malnutrition occurs when vitamins, minerals, or trace elements are not delivered, absorbed, or used by the body. Because most foods contain more than one micronutrient, inadequate food consumption rarely causes single micronutrient deficits. Instead, clients typically present with multiple nutrient deficits. Although laboratory tests are available to measure specific micronutrients, most are not specific or sensitive

TABLE 30-1	Recommendations for Daily Intake of Vitamin and Trace Micronutrients		
Micronutrient RDA or AI for Nonpregnant Adults	Foods High in Micronutrient	Manifestations of Deficit	Manifestations of Excess
Vitamin A 700-900 μg RE	Dark green, leafy or yellow-orange vegetables, milk fat, egg yolks, beef liver	Loss of appetite and taste; night blindness; bumpy or scaly skin	Dry lips, eyes, nasal mucosa, and skin; gingivitis; bone pain; hair loss; liver disease
Vitamin B₁ (thiamine) 1.1-1.4 mg	Lean meats, egg yolks, legumes, enriched or whole grain cereals, breads	Paresthesias; peripheral neuropathies; mental confusion; heart failure; edema	Dysrhythmias; wheezing; hypotension
Vitamin B₆ (pyridoxine) 1.3-1.7 mg	Yeast, wheat germ, pork, liver, whole grain cereals, legumes	Sore, reddened tongue; seborrheic-like dermatitis; paresthesias	Sensory ataxia; impairment of position and vibratory sense
Vitamin B₁₂ (cobalamin) 2.4 μg	Beef, fish, milk, eggs, cheese	Sore, reddened mouth; atrophy of the tongue; megaloblastic anemia; paresthesias	None known
Vitamin C (ascorbic acid) 75-90 mg	Oranges, lemons, strawberries, tomatoes, cabbage, green peppers	Gingivitis; dry mouth; alopecia; pruritus; ecchymotic lesions on the skin	Gastrointestinal upset; diarrhea
Calcium AI: 1000-1200 mg	Dairy products, sardines, salmon, dark green, leafy vegetables	Osteoporosis, osteomalacia	Calcification of soft tissue; hypercalcemia; constipation; impaired absorption of iron, zinc, or manganese
Copper 900 μg	Organ meats, legumes, chocolate, nuts	Decreased absorption of iron; anemia; neutropenia; leukopenia	Liver disease; Kayser-Fleischer rings (brown or green ring near corneal limbus and sunflower cataract)
Vitamin D (calciferol) AI: 5-15 μg	Fish and fish oil, fortified dairy products	Softening of the bones; joint pain; fatigue; muscle tetany	Calcification of soft tissue or tympanic membrane leading to deafness; anorexia; hypotonia
Vitamin E (tocopherol) 15 mg α-tocopherol equivalent	Sunflower, corn, or soybean oil, wheat germ oils	Lipid absorption or transport abnormalities	Pulmonary deterioration; thrombocytopenia; liver and kidney failure
Folate (folic acid) 400 μg	Legumes, liver, dark green or leafy vegetables, lean beef, potatoes	Sore, reddened tongue and mouth; glossitis; megaloblastic anemia	May decrease availability of zinc
Iron 8-18 mg	Organ meats, shellfish, poultry, legumes, blackstrap molasses, fortified cereals	Hypochromic, microcytic anemia	Vomiting; upper abdominal pain; pallor; cyanosis; shock
Iodine 150 μg	Seafood, iodized salt	Enlargement of the thyroid gland	Goiter; myxedema
Vitamin K AI: 90-120 μg	Broccoli, cabbage, turnip greens, green tea	Ecchymotic lesions; bruising	Hemolytic anemia; severe jaundice in infants
Manganese 2-5 μg	Whole grains, legumes, nuts, and tea	Magenta tongue; dermatitis	Manifestations of Parkinson's or Wilson's disease
Niacin 14-16 mg niacin equivalents	Organ meats, brewer's yeast, peanuts, fish, poultry, whole grains, beans	Sore, reddened mouth; atrophy of the tongue; angular stomatitis; dermatitis	Histamine release; liver toxicity
Riboflavin 1.1-1.3 mg	Liver, milk, cheddar cheese, cottage cheese, yogurt, brewer's yeast	Sore, reddened tongue and mouth; angular stomatitis; seborrhea-like dermatitis	None known
Zinc 12-15 mg	Oysters, wheat germ, beef, cheese	Angular stomatitis; seborrhea-like dermatitis; alopecia	Vomiting; diarrhea; impaired copper absorption

AI, Average intake; *RDA,* recommended dietary allowance; *RE,* retinol equivalents.

TABLE 30-2	*Types of Malnutrition Associated with Protein and Calorie Deficit*		
Type of Malnutrition	**Clinical History**	**Clinical Manifestations**	**Laboratory Results**
Kwashiorkor	Inadequate protein intake with adequate calorie intake	Body weight at or above ideal range, edema may be present	Visceral proteins (albumin, prealbumin, transferrin) below normal
Marasmus	Inadequate calorie/protein intake	Cachectic appearance, body weight and anthropometric measurements below normal	Visceral proteins within normal range
Mixed-type	Inadequate calorie/protein intake with increased nutritional requirements	Cachectic appearance, body weight and anthropometric measurements below normal	Visceral proteins below normal

enough to accurately determine whether the measured amount is adequate for a specific client.[12] The best method to identify whether an actual or potential micronutrient deficit exists is a thorough history and meticulous physical examination. Table 30-1 lists clinical manifestations of micronutrient deficits and foods high in specific micronutrients.

In addition to protein or calorie malnutrition, the client with chronic pancreatitis, short-bowel syndrome, pressure ulcers, cancer, acquired immunodeficiency syndrome (AIDS), or prior gastric surgery is at risk for developing micronutrient deficiencies. Chronic pancreatitis can lead to fat malabsorption and decreased absorption of fat-soluble vitamins. The decreased transit times through the gut in clients with short-bowel syndrome decreases the time for micronutrient absorption. Increased requirements of micronutrients such as vitamin C and zinc can result in micronutrient deficits for clients with pressure ulcers. Some drug therapies, especially those for cancer and AIDS, decrease the absorption or use of vitamins and minerals such as folate, potassium, and magnesium. Gastric surgery can impair absorption and use of vitamin B_{12}. If dietary intake is inadequate or if the client presents with a clinical history such as these, suspect and assess for micronutrient malnutrition.

Although not commonly regarded as a type of malnutrition, *obesity* results from nutrient delivery that exceeds the client's nutrient requirements. In the United States, the incidence and prevalence of obesity are reaching epidemic proportions. Chapter 31 contains additional information about obesity.

Nutrition Screen or Assessment?

Nutrition screening and nutrition assessment are not the same. Nutrition screening is a method of categorizing clients at high or low risk for malnutrition. In general, nutritional screening takes place within the first few days of the client's encounter with the health care system and includes general questions about nutritional status and upper GI function. When the nutritional screen indicates that a client is at risk for malnutrition, an in-depth nutrition and upper GI assessment are performed. Nutritional and upper GI assessments are client-centered and

include in-depth histories, physical examinations, and diagnostic testing to determine actual or potential problems involving the upper GI tract, nutritional status, or both. Table 30-3 compares characteristics of nutrition screens and nutrition assessments.

HISTORY

Assessment of nutritional status and the upper GI tract begins with collection of health history data. The historical account determines the direction and focus of the physical examination and the required diagnostic testing. Historical data include (1) biographical and demographic data, (2) current health, (3) past health history, (4) family health, (5) psychosocial factors, and (6) a review of systems.

Biographical and Demographic Data

Analyze the client's demographic information (gender, age, religious affiliation, and marital status) as it relates to his or her nutritional status and upper GI function. For example, women are at risk for calcium deficiency. Therefore specific and detailed questions about calcium intake should be incorporated into women's health histories. Because older people living alone are at increased risk for inadequate food intake, be sure to include questions about social and financial support as it relates to obtaining and preparing food.[8] The risks of GI conditions vary for different ages. For example, adolescents and clients in their teens are at increased risk of duodenal ulcers or gastric cancers, whereas older clients have an increased risk for developing gastric ulcers and colon cancers.[4] Culture and ethnic origin also affect the type, amount, and frequency of dietary consumption (see the Diversity in Health Care feature on Cultural Influences on Nutrition on the website).

Current Health

Chief Complaint

Clients often present with chief complaints that are related to nutrition or upper GI function. These complaints include nausea and vomiting, indigestion, abdominal pain, diarrhea, and changes in weight or

TABLE 30-3	Comparison of Nutrition Screen and Nutrition Assessment	
Characteristic	**Nutrition Screen**	**Nutrition Assessment**
Goal	Rapid identification of actual or potential malnutrition	Identification of specific causes and treatments of malnutrition
Question types	General and related to risk factors for malnutrition ("Have you noticed any recent changes in your weight? Do you live alone? Do you have any medical conditions?")	Detailed nutrition-related questions ("How much weight have you lost and over what period of time? Who buys and prepares your food? Do you eat alone? Do you have diabetes?")
Assessment techniques	Brief health history using standardized set of nutrition-related questions and readily available equipment such as scales for weight; many nutrition screening tools available	Client-centered and based on health history responses; may include sophisticated tests such as laboratory testing, endoscopy, radiologic or computerized body scanning
Health care professionals	Nurse or dietitian	Multidisciplinary health care team including nurse, dietitian, physician, pharmacist, social worker

appetite. When a client presents with these complaints, conduct an in-depth symptom analysis.

Symptom Analysis

Include the questions listed in the following sections.

Nausea and Vomiting. When does nausea or vomiting occur? How long does it last? Is it related to food intake? Does food relieve or worsen the manifestations? Does the vomitus contain undigested food or bile? What does it look like? What is the quantity vomited? Is pain associated with the onset of nausea and vomiting?

Indigestion. Have the client describe the indigestion. Is it a "burping" or burning sensation? Are the manifestations of indigestion related to food intake? Which foods worsen and which foods relieve the manifestations? Does the client take any medications or antacids for indigestion?

Abdominal Pain. Was the pain rapid or gradual in onset? What is the intensity of the pain? Has the pain increased in intensity over the past few hours, days, or weeks? Does the pain radiate? Does the pain worsen or improve with movement? Does food exacerbate or alleviate the pain? What specific foods alter the pain? Abdominal pain is a common presenting manifestation that may be associated with life-threatening conditions. It is important to differentiate abdominal pain caused by life-threatening conditions from pain associated with non–life-threatening conditions. Table 30-4 describes the etiology and associated characteristics of three life-threatening conditions associated with abdominal pain.

Diarrhea. How many stools are expelled per day? How much stool is expelled? Do feces fill the toilet or is the

amount small? Are stools liquid or solid? What color are the stools? Are the stools black or bloody? Do the stools sink or float? Is there pain with defecation? Does abdominal bloating or cramping accompany the diarrhea? Does diarrhea occur during the day, the night, or both day and night? Is fecal incontinence among the manifestations? How many days or weeks has the diarrhea persisted? Does diarrhea decrease at certain times during the month (indicating a hormonal influence)? Does physical activity change the diarrhea manifestations?

Ask specifically about the relationship of stool output and dietary intake. Bloating and diarrhea that occur after a diet containing dairy products may indicate lactose intolerance (see Allergies later in this chapter). High-fat diets that result in floating, greasy stools may indicate fat malabsorption. If vomiting or diarrhea persist, assess for fluid and electrolyte deficits (see Chapters 13, 14, and 15).

Nonspecific GI problems, such as nausea, vomiting, and diarrhea, can result from food-borne poisoning. Table 30-5 lists common sources and manifestations of food-borne poisoning. When clients present with these manifestations, ask about the type of food consumed over the past 2 or 3 days, how the food was prepared, and whether anyone else who ate the same food became ill.

Appetite and Weight Change. Have the client describe his or her appetite. Is it little, normal, ravenous? Has there been any change in appetite? Has the usual diet been modified, and, if so, why?

If the client has noticed a change in appetite, ask about associated factors such as changes in taste or smell, activity level, or mood states. Ask specific questions about the client's usual weight. Ask whether the client has lost or gained weight and, if so, ask over what period of time this occurred. Was the weight gain or loss intentional? If the weight loss was intentional, ask about the diet plan. Does a specific weight loss organization or

TABLE 30-4	*Etiology and Characteristics of Abdominal Pain*
Etiology	**Associated Characteristics**
Bowel obstruction	Intermittent or colicky pain. Pain near umbilicus associated with small bowel. Lumbar pain associated with colon. Distended abdomen with no flatus or bowel movement. As bowel fatigues, bowel sounds may progress from high pitched to absent.
Peritoneal inflammation (perforated ulcer, ruptured spleen, ruptured appendix)	Steady, aching pain directly over area of inflammation. Pain increases with motion. Intensity of pain varies with source of inflammation. Gastric acid may produce more pain than alkaline content of small bowel. May be associated with manifestations of shock.
Vascular catastrophe (aortic aneurysm or mesenteric infarction)	May be preceded by 2 to 3 days of mild to moderate pain and hyperperistalsis followed by severe abdominal pain and manifestations of shock. Back and flank pain are common with aortic aneurysms.

From Dang, C., et al. (2002). Acute abdominal pain. Four classifications can guide assessment and management. *Geriatrics 57*, 30-42.

TABLE 30-5	*Food-Borne Poisoning: Sources and Manifestations*	
Organism	**Associated Food**	**Clinical Manifestations**
Bacillus cereus (preformed enterotoxin)	Improperly refrigerated fried rice	Sudden onset of nausea and vomiting; possibly diarrhea within 1 to 6 hours of ingestion
Campylobacter jejuni	Raw or undercooked poultry, unpasteurized milk, untreated water	Fever, headache, myalgias progressing to abdominal pain, cramping, and possibly bloody diarrhea over 2 to 10 days
Clostridium botulinum (preformed toxin)	Improper canning of fruits and vegetables; foods held in warm ovens or potatoes held in aluminum foil	Mild to severe manifestations occur within 12 to 72 hours; nausea/vomiting with no fever; cranial nerve involvement results in ptosis, diplopia, dysarthria, and dysphagia
Enterohemorrhagic *Escherichia coli* (including *E coli 157*)	Undercooked beef, unpasteurized milk and juice, raw fruits, contaminated water	1- to 2-day incubation followed by bloody diarrhea, abdominal cramps; fever uncommon
Norwalk-like viruses	Ready-to-eat sandwich fillings touched by infected persons	Nausea, vomiting, large volume diarrhea within 24 to 48 hours; fever is rare
Salmonella (non-typhoidal salmonellosis)	Contaminated raw eggs, unpasteurized dairy products	24- to 72-hour incubation followed by nausea, vomiting, abdominal cramps, or fever
Staphylococcus aureus (preformed enterotoxin)	Unrefrigerated ham, poultry, potatoes, egg salad, mayonnaise, cream pastries	Nausea, vomiting, watery diarrhea, or fever within hours of consuming contaminated food
Trichinella spiralis	Undercooked meat, usually pork or wild game	Mild to severe abdominal pain, nausea, vomiting, diarrhea during first week and progressing over next 3 to 4 weeks; edema; rash; muscle weakness
Vibrio parahaemolyticus	Shellfish	Cramping and inflammatory diarrhea greater than 6 hours after consuming affected food

From U.S. Department of Health and Human Services. (2001). Diagnosis and management of foodborne illnesses: A primer for physicians. *MMWR, 50,* RR2.

health club sanction the client's diet? Does the client take diet pills, such as appetite stimulants or suppressants?

Unintentional changes in weight may stem from psychological, physiologic, or metabolic causes. Ask the following:

- Does the client feel sad or depressed?
- Has there been a change in activity level?

- Has the client experienced early satiety, anorexia, or any changes in the taste of food?
- Does the client have trouble chewing or swallowing or problems with teeth or gums? If the client wears dentures, ask about the fit of the dentures. Ill-fitting dentures can decrease appetite and lead to weight loss.

Past Health History

Major Illnesses and Hospitalizations

The client's history of illnesses or hospitalizations can provide important clues about nutritional status and gut function. For example, a client with a history of bleeding is at increased risk for iron deficiency anemia. A client with liver disease is at increased risk for protein malnutrition. Ask whether the client has been evaluated by a health care provider or been hospitalized for any of the following: peptic ulcer disease, vomiting blood (hematemesis), anemia, jaundice, gallbladder disease, pancreatitis, cancer, a change in bowel habits, tarry stools, or unexplained weight loss or gain. Has the client had diagnostic tests of the upper GI system, such as a barium swallow, upper GI studies, endoscopic examinations of the upper GI tract, or computed tomography (CT)? If so, ask when and where the tests were performed and the results of each test.

Past surgical procedures also provide information about nutritional status and the structure and function of the upper GI tract. Ask specifically about previous surgeries of the mouth, throat, stomach, liver, pancreas, gallbladder, or abdomen. Include dates and results of all tests, procedures, and operations performed.

Medications and Dietary Supplements

Because there are many potential drug-nutrient interactions, it is important to obtain information about the client's drug use. In addition, older clients who take multiple medications are at increased risk for malnutrition.[5] Obtain detailed information about current or previously prescribed and over-the-counter medications taken by the client. Table 30-6 contains a list of drug classes and possible drug-nutrient interactions.

Does the client use aspirin, aspirin compounds, or nonsteroidal anti-inflammatory drugs that may contribute to gastritis or bleeding? Does the client take antacids? If so, note the type and the frequency. Does the client use laxatives or stool softeners?

Dietary supplements sold over the counter are often viewed as harmless. However, taken in excess or with other drugs or supplements, dietary supplements can be harmful. Therefore it is important to determine the brand, amount, and frequency of use for all dietary supplements consumed by the client. Dietary supplements include vitamins, minerals, herbs used for medicinal purposes, amino acids, and meal supplements or replacements.

Vitamins are the most common supplement consumed by Americans.[13] Ask whether the client takes a vitamin supplement and, if so, determine the amount of specific vitamins, minerals, or trace elements contained in each dose. Because vitamin supplements differ in content and dose, it is important to compare the client's dietary requirements with the amount of each micronutrient (vitamins, minerals, trace elements) contained in the supplement. Taken in excess, some vitamins have toxic side effects. For example, a client taking calcium supplements may exceed the DRI upper limit of 2500 mg of calcium per day and experience manifestations of constipation or calcifications of soft tissue. Table 30-1 contains information about manifestations of vitamin and mineral excess.

There is little regulation in the production and distribution of medicinal herbs in the United States and relatively little is known about the safety and efficacy of these dietary supplements. Because clients who consume prescribed medications may also take herbal supplements, there is a growing concern about the interaction between prescription drugs and herbal supplements. Ask whether the client consumes any herbs or special products for his or her health. The herbs may be consumed as a tea or in

TABLE 30-6	*Drug-Nutrient Interactions*
Drug Class	**Possible Nutrient Interactions**
Antacids	Decreased absorption of calcium, iron, magnesium, zinc
Antibiotics	Cephalosporins: Increased vitamin K depletion
Anticoagulants	Vitamin K antagonist
Anticonvulsants	Decreased folate and biotin
Antituberculosis drugs	Interfere with metabolism of vitamins B_6 and B_{12}
Cathartics	Nonrenal losses of calcium, potassium, water
Cholesterol-reducing drugs	Inhibition of fat digestion and absorption
	Simvastatin: grapefruit juice may increase drug level
Diuretics	Increased renal loss of potassium, calcium, magnesium, and zinc
H_2 Blockers	Decreased vitamin B_{12} absorption
Monoamine oxidase inhibitors	Interact with tyramine-containing foods (cheese, smoked fish, wine, yeast)

From Skidmore-Roth, L. (2003). *Mosby's nursing drug reference.* St. Louis: Mosby.

pill, capsule, liquid, or powder form. It is important to note the brand and amount of herbal preparation consumed. Table 30-7 lists common herbal supplements, the associated common names, purported indications, potential side effects, and reported interactions with prescribed medications (see also Chapter 5).

Various forms of amino acids, hormones, and meal supplements are sold as over-the-counter health aids. Ask clients whether they consume preparations such as glucosamine, melatonin, or dehydroepiandrosterone (DHEA). Meal supplements or replacements are usually purchased in a liquid or wafer form and provide a convenient method of increasing nutritional intake. Because of the wide variation in nutritional content and the potential for consuming inadequate or excessive amounts of specific micronutrients, it is important to ask questions about the brand and amount of meal supplement the client consumes each day. See Chapter 31 for additional information about meal supplements.

Allergies

Inquire about the client's food intolerances to help differentiate food allergies from food intolerances. Food allergies typically result in systemic manifestations such as hives or dyspnea, whereas food intolerances are associated with GI manifestations such as abdominal cramping, flatulence, or diarrhea. Ask the client to describe the manifestations and determine whether these are associated with specific foods. Although less common than food intolerances, food allergies have been associated with foods such as nuts, shellfish, cow's milk, and food additives such as sulfites.[11]

Food intolerances are common and lactose is one of the most common causes of food intolerance, especially in adults of Asian, Hispanic, or African-American descent. When *lactase* (an enzyme necessary for the breakdown of lactose in the small bowel) is inadequate, large lactose molecules draw fluid into the small bowel

TABLE 30-7	*Common Herbal Supplements*		
Latin Name	**Common Name**	**Purported Uses**	**Manifestations of Toxicity/ Possible Drug Interactions**
Allium sativum	Garlic	Hypercholesterolemia; atherosclerosis; hypertension; anticlotting agent; increased peristalsis of GI tract	Heartburn; flatulence; rare allergic reaction; may potentiate action of antiplatelet drugs (aspirin or anticoagulants)
Echinacea angustifolia, E. purpurea, E. pallidus	Echinacea, purple coneflower, narrow-leaved Echinacea	Immunostimulant, anti-infective, topical wound therapy	Potential for allergic reactions
Ephedra sinica Stapf, *E. equisetina* Bunge	Ephedra, ma huang, ephedrine	Nasal decongestant, central nervous system stimulant, bronchodilator	Increased likelihood of hypertension, tachycardia, and cardiac irregularities when taken with antihypertensives, cardiac glycosides, or beta-blockers
Ginkgo biloba L.	Ginkgo	Dementia and intermittent claudication	Headache, GI upset, dizziness, nausea/vomiting, diarrhea; may potentiate effect of antiplatelet drugs
Hypericum performatum L.	St. John's wort, Klamath weed, amber touch-and-heel, goatweed, rosin rose	Treatment of depression, anxiety, bedwetting; diuretic, hemorrhoids; topical treatment for burns	Fatigue, allergic reactions, photosensitivity; synergistic effect for alcohol, barbiturates, benzodiazepines
Panax ginseng C.A. Mey (Orient) *P. quinquefolium* L. (American)	Ginseng	Strengthen body functions, increase vitality, aphrodisiac	Nervousness, excitation, diarrhea, skin eruptions; avoid use with hypertension; may increase headaches and tremors when taken with monoamine oxidase inhibitors or caffeine; may potentiate effect of corticosteroids

Data from Bartels, C., & Miller, S. (1998). Herbal and related remedies. *Nutrition and Clinical Practice, 13,* 5-19; Ernst, E., & Pittler, M. (2002). Herbal medicine. *Medical Clinics of North America, 86,* 149-161; and Kuhn, M. (2002). Herbal remedies: Drug-herb interactions. *Critical Care Nurse, 22,* 22-32.

resulting in abdominal cramping and diarrhea. Eliminating milk from the diet or taking a lactase replacement (Lactaid, Lactase, or Surelac) before eating dairy products eases or eliminates the manifestations of lactose intolerance. Lactose-free milk and ice-cream products are also available. Because dairy products are high in calcium, it is important to ask the lactose-intolerant client about calcium intake. Has the client eliminated all dairy products from the diet and, if so, is a calcium supplement taken? How much calcium is taken each day?

Family Health History

 Genetics and family environment may increase the client's risk of developing certain GI problems. Many diseases, such as ulcerative colitis and Crohn's disease, seem to have a familial component. Similarly, alcoholism and the associated liver disease also seem to have a strong familial link. Inquire about the health status of family members. Is there a family history of cancer, GI ulcers, or colitis? Is there a family history of diabetes, anemia, jaundice, alcoholism, hepatitis, pancreatitis, obesity, peptic ulcers, or irritable bowel syndrome?

Psychosocial History

Occupation

Exposure to environmental toxins and pathogens while at work or traveling increases the client's risk for developing diseases of the GI tract. Ask about the client's occupation and whether toxic substances such as arsenic, lead, mercury, or carbon tetrachloride are present in the workplace? Ask whether the client has recently traveled outside the country. Traveling abroad may increase the client's risk of contracting GI diseases caused by pathogenic bacteria, protozoa, helminths, or other parasites. Such clients usually present with GI manifestations such as nausea, vomiting, or diarrhea.

Diet

The type, amount, method, and timing of food intake are heavily influenced by psychosocial factors, such as ethnic origin, religion, and family structure (see the Diversity in Health Care feature on Cultural Influences on Nutrition on the website). When assessing the client's nutritional status, determine the client's cultural preferences. Ask the client to describe a typical meal. Ask about food preferences. Are food preferences associated with a specific cultural group (Hispanic, Chinese, American fast food)? Is the client a member of a specific religion that requires dietary fasting or prohibition of specific foods? Is food an important part of their family's tradition? Who purchases and prepares the meal?[13] Who usually dines with the client? Does the client consume alcohol? If so, ask how much, what type, and how frequently it is consumed.

Review of Systems

Inquire about the condition of the client's mouth, including the presence of dental caries, number and condition of teeth, condition of the gingivae, and use of dentures:

- Has the client noticed any oral lesions, halitosis, excessive salivation, or mouth dryness?
- How often does the client floss and brush?
- Is the client's water supply fluoridated?
- When was the last visit to the dentist for teeth cleaning?
- Has the client been treated for periodontal disease?
- Does the client have trouble tasting, chewing, or swallowing?
- If pain is reported with eating, is it related to specific foods or associated events?

Also see Chapter 44 for questions related to the hepatic and biliary systems.

PHYSICAL EXAMINATION

Anthropometric Measures

Anthropometric measures provide an assessment of body mass or body compartments. Height, weight, body mass index, frame size, and circumferential measurements are examples of anthropometric measures.

Height and Weight

Use a telescoping ruler and balance scale to measure height and weight. If the client cannot bear weight, consider using a calibrated sling or wheelchair scale. Clothing and shoes affect the obtained height and weight; describe any clothing and accessories (light clothing, shoes with or without heels, orthopedic casts, braces) worn by the client while obtaining the height and weight.

If the client cannot stand, use an arm span measurement to approximate height. To do so, extend the client's arms laterally and measure from the tip of the middle finger on one hand to the tip of the middle finger on the other hand.

Compare the client's current weight to the reported usual weight. Unintentional weight changes of less than 90% or more than 110% of the client's usual weight are considered significant. For example, a weight change of ±11 pounds for a client who usually weighs 100 pounds (current weight <90 pounds or >110 pounds) is considered significant and the cause of this significant weight change should be determined. To calculate the difference as a percentage of usual weight, divide the client's current weight by the usual weight and multiply by 100:

$$\% \text{ Usual weight} = (\text{Current weight}/\text{Usual weight}) \times 100$$

Body Mass Index

Past methods of determining ideal body weights for individuals have included mathematical formulas or comparison of heights and weights to life insurance tables. Based on numerous independent studies, body mass index (BMI) is gaining favor as the accepted standard for determining desirable body weight. The BMI standardizes weight for height. A desirable BMI range associated with good health is between 19 and 24.9. Table 30-8 contains the BMI for different heights and weights. To use the table, find the client's height in the left hand column, follow the row over to the client's weight, and then up to determine the BMI. Calculate the BMI by dividing the client's weight in pounds by the height in inches, then dividing by the height in inches again and multiplying by 703.

For example, a 64-inch tall woman weighing 140 pounds has a BMI of 24.

$$BMI = ([140 \div 64] \div 64) \times 703 = 24$$

A BMI of less than 18.5 is categorized underweight or less than desirable weight for height. A BMI between 25 and less than 30 is considered overweight, and a BMI of 30 or greater is considered obese.

Calculations for BMI are the same for males and females. Muscle mass and bone weigh more than fat and, for a few clients, the BMI may indicate they are overweight or obese when they are not. Therefore clients suspected of having a large frame size or muscle mass (weight lifters, football players) should be assessed for frame size and muscle mass.[12]

Frame Size

An estimation of frame size can be obtained by assessing the client's wrist circumference or elbow breadth (Box 30-1). Clients who have very small or very large frames may have a BMI at the low or high end of the desirable BMI range, respectively.

Circumferential Measurements

Circumference measurements are used to assess the proportion and distribution of muscle mass and body fat. Midarm muscle circumference (MAMC) and waist-to-hip ratio are examples of circumferential measurements.

To obtain a client's MAMC, measure the triceps skinfold thickness and midarm circumference and calculate the MAMC. Compare these measurements and calculated results with published standards for the client's gender and age (Figure 30-1).

Determine waist-to-hip proportions by dividing the waist measurement at its smallest circumference by the hip measurement at its largest circumference. Waist-to-hip proportions greater than 0.8 for women and 1 for

TABLE 30-8	*Body Mass Index (BMI)*																
BMI	**19**	**20**	**21**	**22**	**23**	**24**	**25**	**26**	**27**	**28**	**29**	**30**	**31**	**32**	**33**	**34**	**35**
Height							*Weight (in pounds)*										
4'10" (58")	91	96	100	105	110	115	119	124	129	134	138	143	148	153	158	162	167
4'11" (59")	94	99	104	109	114	119	124	128	133	138	143	148	153	158	163	168	173
5' (60")	97	102	107	112	118	123	128	133	138	143	148	153	158	163	168	174	179
5'1" (61")	100	106	111	116	122	127	132	137	143	148	153	158	164	169	174	180	185
5'2" (62")	104	109	115	120	126	131	136	142	147	153	158	164	169	175	180	186	191
5'3" (63")	107	113	118	124	130	135	141	146	152	158	163	169	175	180	186	191	197
5'4" (64")	110	116	122	128	134	140	145	151	157	163	169	174	180	186	192	197	204
5'5" (65")	114	120	126	132	138	144	150	156	162	168	174	180	186	192	198	204	210
5'6" (66")	118	124	130	136	142	148	155	161	167	173	179	186	192	198	204	210	216
5'7" (67")	121	127	134	140	146	153	159	166	172	178	185	191	198	204	211	217	223
5'8" (68")	125	131	138	144	151	158	164	171	177	184	190	197	203	210	216	223	230
5'9" (69")	128	135	142	149	155	162	169	176	182	189	196	203	209	216	223	230	236
5'10" (70")	132	139	146	153	160	167	174	181	188	195	202	209	216	222	229	236	243
5'11" (71")	136	143	150	157	165	172	179	186	193	200	208	215	222	229	236	243	250
6' (72")	140	147	154	162	169	177	184	191	199	206	213	221	228	235	242	250	258
6'1" (73")	144	151	159	166	174	182	189	197	204	212	219	227	235	242	250	257	265
6'2" (74")	148	155	163	171	179	186	194	202	210	218	225	233	241	249	256	264	272
6'3" (75")	152	160	168	176	184	192	200	208	216	224	232	240	248	256	264	272	279

From Evidence Report of Clinical Guidelines on the Identification, Evaluation, and Treatment of Overweight and Obesity in Adults, 1998. NIH/National Heart, Lung, and Blood Institute (NHLBI), Bethesda, MD.

BOX 30-1 *Calculating Body Frame Size*

Wrist Circumference Method

1. Measure the client's right wrist (in centimeters) at the point of the smallest circumference, just distal to the styloid process of the radius and ulna.

2. Obtain the client's height (in centimeters) without shoes.
3. Divide the client's wrist circumference into the client's height to obtain the *r* value:

$$r = \frac{\text{Height (in cm)}}{\text{Wrist circumference (in cm)}}$$

4. Use the chart below to determine the client's body frame size based on the calculated $r =$ value and sex:

	Men	*Women*
Small frame	$r > 10.4$	$r > 10.9$
Medium frame	$r = 9.6 - 10.4$	$r = 9.9 - 10.9$
Large frame	$r < 9.6$	$r < 9.9$

Elbow Breadth Method*

1. Instruct the client to extend his or her right arm, then bend the forearm to a 90-degree angle with the fingers pointing straight up.
2. Measure the width of the client's right elbow (in inches) across the greatest breadth of the joint between the bony prominences of the lateral and medial epicondyles of the humerus. To measure, either use calipers or place your thumb and index finger on the epicondyles and measure the distance between the thumb and finger.
3. Use the chart below to determine the client's body frame size based on the client's elbow breadth, gender, and height in 1-inch heels. The values shown are for a medium body frame. Measurements less than the values shown indicate a small frame; greater values indicate a large frame.

Height	Elbow Breadth
Men	
5'2"-5'3"	2 ½"-2 ⅞"
5'4"-5'7"	2 ⅝"-2 ⅞"
5'8"-5'11"	2 ¾"-3"
6'0"-6'3"	2 ¾"-3 ⅛"
6'4"	2 ⅞"-3 ¼"
Women	
4'10"-4'11"	2 ¼"-2 ½"
5'0"-5'3"	2 ¼"-2 ½"
5'4"-5'7"	2 ⅜"-2 ⅝"
5'8"-5'11"	2 ⅜"-2 ⅝"
6'0"	2 ½"-2 ¾"

Courtesy of Metropolitan Life Insurance Company.

men indicate fat distributions associated with negative health outcomes such as cardiovascular disease and diabetes.

Mouth

Assessment of the oral cavity includes inspection and palpation. Good illumination is essential. A headlamp provides direct illumination, and a head mirror provides indirect lighting; both items keep your hands free for the physical examination. A penlight and tongue blade may also be used. Always remember to wear gloves and use a gauze pad when palpating the oral cavity and handling

the tongue. Although discussed separately, inspection and palpation of the oral cavity usually proceed simultaneously.

Inspection

Begin assessment of the client's mouth by inspecting the lips for symmetry, color, hydration, lesions, or nodules. Put on clean gloves, and instruct the client to open the lips while clenching the teeth. Inspect the position of the upper and lower teeth for malocclusion or missing teeth. If dentures are worn, ask the client to remove them.

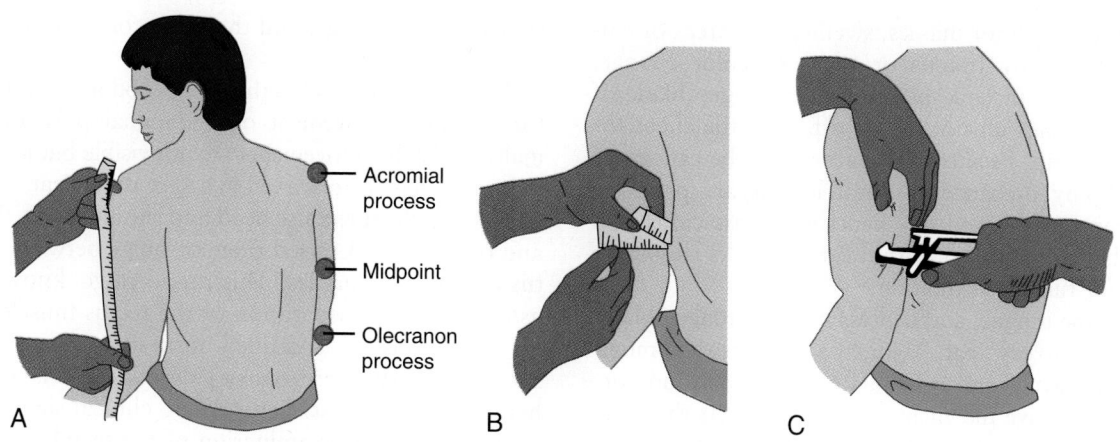

Calculate the midarm muscle circumference (MAMC) using the following formula:
MAMC (in cm) = [MAC in cm] − [(0.314) × (TSF in mm)]

MEASUREMENT		STANDARD	90%	60%
Midarm circumference (MAC)	Men	29.3 cm	26.4 cm	17.6 cm
	Women	28.5 cm	25.7 cm	17.1 cm
Triceps skinfold (TSF)	Men	12.5 mm	11.3 mm	7.5 mm
	Women	16.5 mm	14.9 mm	9.9 mm
Midarm muscle circumference (MAMC)	Men	25.3 cm	22.8 cm	15.2 cm
	Women	23.2 cm	20.9 cm	13.9 cm

D

FIGURE 30-1 Measuring adipose and skeletal muscle tissue to estimate the client's reserves of protein and calories. **A,** Locate the *midpoint* of the client's relaxed, nondominant upper arm by palpating the acromial and olecranon processes and measuring the distance between the two points with a tape measure. Mark the posterior aspect of the arm at the midpoint with a pen. **B,** Measure *midarm circumference* (MAC) at the midpoint, keeping the tape measure level. **C,** Just above the midpoint at the posterior aspect of the arm, grasp the client's skin and subcutaneous tissue between thumb and index finger, freeing it from the underlying muscle mass. Place the calipers at the midpoint just below the fold of grasped tissue. Squeeze the calipers until they are equilibrated at the "measure" markings. Read the measurement to the nearest millimeter. Repeat the readings two more times, allowing a rest period of 3 seconds between readings. Calculate the average of the three readings for the *triceps skinfold thickness* (TSF). **D,** Compare the client's values for MAC, TSF, and *midarm muscle circumference* (MAMC) to the following standards to determine nutritional risk status. *Undernutrition* is indicated by a measurement less than 90% of the standard. *Protein-calorie malnutrition* is indicated by a measurement of less than 60% of the standard, especially for MAMC. *Obesity* is indicated by a TSF measurement of at least 120% greater than the standard.

Note the symmetry of facial movements and the fit of the dentures as the appliance is removed.

Next, ask the client to open and close the mouth and note the symmetry and strength of movement. Ask the client to open the mouth wide, and inspect the structures inside (see Figure U-7-2). Start at the left side of the mouth and continue in a clockwise fashion. Note any evidence of dental caries, missing or broken teeth, and receding gums. Note the color of the mucosa and gums. Inspect for red lesions (erythroplakia), white lesions (leukoplakia), swelling, bleeding, or ulcers. Survey the pharynx for abnormalities of the tonsils, such as redness, swelling, lesions, ulcers, uvular deviations, drainage, or unusual mouth odor.

Inspect the tongue for symmetry, color, and moisture. Note any areas of atrophy, abnormal coatings, swelling, or lesions. Next, ask the client to stick out the tongue and move it from side to side, upward, and downward. Observe for symmetry of movement and voluntary or involuntary movement. Abnormal tongue movement may result from infiltration of the muscle by tumor or nerve entrapment.[6]

Palpation

Palpate the client's lips, gingivae, and buccal mucosa. Check for loose teeth, masses, swellings, or areas of tenderness. Note the location, size, color, consistency, and presence or absence of tenderness in any lesions.

Gently grasp, extend, and lift the tongue with a gauze pad while inspecting and palpating the underside and the floor of the mouth. Palpate all areas of the tongue and floor of the mouth for masses, swellings, or areas of tenderness. Note any lesions or areas of color change. Scrape all areas of leukoplakia with a tongue blade; if the white patches do not scrape off, refer the client for further work-up, because these areas may be cancerous lesions. Many precancerous oral lesions are pain-free and asymptomatic, and all clients with suspicious oral lesions that do not clear within 2 to 3 weeks should be referred for further evaluation.[10]

Release the tongue, and depress it with a tongue blade. Ask the client to say "aah." Note the symmetry and movement of the uvula and soft palate. If there are no contraindications, give the client a sip of water. As the client swallows, observe for manifestations of difficulty in swallowing (*dysphagia*). Clients who exhibit difficulty with swallowing or asymmetrical movement of oral cavity structures should be evaluated for dysphagia and risk for aspiration. Oral-pharyngeal dysphagia typically presents as difficulty moving solid foods to the back of the mouth and indicates further assessment and evaluation to rule out cranial nerve involvement (see Chapter 69). Esophageal dysphagia presents as difficulty swallowing solids or liquids and indicates motor disease or obstruction of the esophagus. Both oral pharyngeal and esophageal dysphagia should be referred for further evaluation.

Abdomen

Because a full bladder can interfere with abdominal assessment, ask the client to void before examining the abdomen. Place the client in a supine position with arms at sides. Place a small pillow under the client's knees to relax the abdominal muscles. Because percussion and palpation can alter intestinal activity, assess the abdomen in the following sequence: inspection, auscultation, percussion, and palpation. Visualize the underlying organs as you assess, and describe the abdomen by anatomic regions or quadrants (Figure 30-2).

Inspection

Stand at the client's right side and begin inspecting the abdomen by noting the condition of the skin and the abdominal contour. The skin should be smooth and intact, with varying amounts of hair. The contour should be flat, concave, or rounded, depending on the client's body type. Note any areas of distention or irregular contour, which may suggest obstruction, hernia, tumor, or previous surgery. Bulging flanks and glistening, taut skin are abnormal findings and suggest ascites (see Chapters 4 and 44).

Inspect the abdomen for rashes, discoloration, scars, petechiae, striae (stretch marks), and dilated veins. Scars on the abdomen should correlate with the client's history of past surgical procedures, and striae, an indication of changes in weight, should correlate with reported changes in weight. Note the shape, position, color, and presence of any discharge at the umbilicus. The umbilicus should be concave, located at the midline, with no evidence of drainage, and the same color as the abdominal skin.[14]

Next, sit at eye level to the client's abdomen and observe for peristaltic movement or abdominal pulsation. Normally, peristaltic movements are not visible but abdominal pulsations may be observed in a very thin client.

Ask the client to raise head and shoulders off the table and observe for a raised ridge or bulge between the rectus abdominal muscles. This raised ridge, known as *diastasis recti,* is a separation of the rectus muscle caused by conditions of sustained intra-abdominal pressure such as obesity or pregnancy. *Diastasis recti* is not a true hernia and, for most clients, of no clinical significance.[2]

Inspection and examination of the rectal area occurs after the abdominal examination (see Chapter 34).

Auscultation

Using the diaphragm of your stethoscope, begin auscultating the client's abdomen. Press the diaphragm lightly to the abdominal wall, beginning in the right lower quadrant at the area of the ileocecal valve. Continue in a clockwise fashion, auscultating each quadrant or region. As air and fluid move through the GI tract, soft clicks and gurgles can be heard every 5 to 15 seconds. Note the frequency and character of bowel sounds. Normal bowel sounds occur irregularly at a rate of 5 to 35 per minute.[2] Loud, high-pitched bowel sounds *(borborygmi)* represent hyperactivity of the GI tract. Borborygmi may be present in clients who are hungry or who have gastroenteritis, or they may be present in early intestinal obstruction.

Hypoactive bowel sounds occur at a rate of one or fewer every minute. To determine the absence of bowel sounds, listen for a total of 5 minutes or at least 1 minute per quadrant. If you do not hear bowel sounds, note the time allotted for auscultation of bowel sounds in the assessment record. Absence of bowel sounds does not mean absence of bowel peristalsis. Hypoactive or absent bowel sounds indicate the need for further assessment of bowel function. Hospitalized clients with nondistended abdomens and no complaints of nausea or vomiting may eat even though bowel sounds are not auscultated. Conversely, clients who have bowel sounds and nausea, vomiting, or abdominal distention should not be fed enterally.

Next, use the bell of your stethoscope to auscultate the abdomen for vascular sounds. A bruit, a venous hum, and a friction rub are examples of abnormal sounds that may be auscultated during the abdominal examination. Bruits auscultated over major blood vessels indicate turbulent blood flow, such as an aneurysm or partial obstruction of a vessel. A continuous venous hum heard in the periumbilical area indicates engorged liver circulation. Friction rubs sound like two pieces of leather rubbing together and suggest a hepatic tumor when heard loudest over the lower right rib cage or splenic inflammation when heard loudest over the lower ribcage in the anterior axillary line.[14]

QUADRANTS OF THE ABDOMEN
AND THEIR UNDERLYING ORGANS∗

Right Upper Quadrant (RUQ)
Adrenal gland (right)
Colon (hepatic flexure
    and portions
    of ascending and
    transverse)
Duodenum
Kidney (portion of
    right)
Liver (right lobe)
Gallbladder
Pancreas (head)
Pylorus

Left Upper Quadrant (LUQ)
Adrenal gland (left)
Colon (splenic flexure
    and portions
    of transverse and
    descending)
Kidney (portion of left)
Liver (left lobe)
Pancreas (body)
Spleen
Stomach

Right Lower Quadrant (RLQ)
Appendix
Bladder (if distended)
Cecum
Colon (portion of
    ascending)
Kidney (lower pole of
    right)
Ovary (right)
Salpinx (uterine tube;
    right)
Spermatic cord (right)
Ureter (right)
Uterus (if enlarged)

Left Lower Quadrant (LLQ)
Bladder (if distended)
Colon (sigmoid and
    portion of
    descending)
Kidney (lower pole of
    left)
Ovary (left)
Salpinx (uterine tube;
    left)
Spermatic cord (left)
Ureter (left)
Uterus (if enlarged)

∗ Small intestine loops in all quadrants.

ANATOMIC REGIONS OF THE ABDOMEN
AND THEIR UNDERLYING ORGANS

Right hypochondriac
Right lobe of
    liver
Gallbladder
Portion of
    duodenum
Hepatic
    flexure of
    colon
Portion of right
    kidney
Adrenal gland
    (right)

Epigastric
Pyloric end of
    stomach
Duodenum
Pancreas
Portion of
    liver

Left hypochondriac
Stomach
Spleen
Tail of
    pancreas
Splenic flexure
    of colon
Upper pole of
    left kidney
Adrenal gland
    (left)

Right lumbar
Ascending
    colon
Lower half of
    right kidney
Portion of
    duodenum
    and jejunum

Umbilical
Omentum
Mesentery
Lower
    duodenum
Jejunum and
    ileum

Left lumbar
Descending
    colon
Lower half of
    left kidney
Portions of
    jejunum and
    ileum

Right inguinal
Cecum
Appendix
Ileum (lower
    end)
Right ureter
Right
    spermatic
    cord
Right ovary

Suprapubic
Ileum
Bladder
Uterus (in
    pregnancy)

Left inguinal
Sigmoid colon
Left ureter
Left spermatic
    cord
Left ovary

FIGURE 30-2 Quadrants and anatomic regions of the abdomen and their underlying organs.

Percussion

Percuss the abdomen to determine the size and location of abdominal organs and to detect fluid, air, or masses. Percuss all quadrants or regions, and compare the sounds to expected findings. Normally when percussing over the abdomen, high-pitched, loud, or "musical" (tympanic) sounds are heard over gaseous areas and dull (thud-like) sounds are heard over fluid or solid organs. Percussion can be used to determine the size and position of the liver and spleen (see Chapter 44) and to assess the level of a distended bladder (see Chapter 34). Do not percuss the abdomen if you suspect an abdominal aneurysm or if the client has undergone abdominal organ transplantation.

Palpation

Palpate the abdomen in a systematic, quadrant-to-quadrant or region-to-region manner, beginning with nontender areas and progressing to painful ones. Start with light palpation, depressing the abdomen 1 to 2 cm. Palpate for masses or areas of tenderness. Note any areas of involuntary abdominal rigidity or guarding. McBurney's point is located in the right lower quadrant midway between the umbilicus and the anterior iliac crest. Localization of pain in this area suggests appendicitis.

After lightly palpating all areas, use deep palpation to determine the size and shape of abdominal organs and masses. Use caution when examining any tender areas. Rebound tenderness suggests peritoneal inflammation. To elicit rebound tenderness, depress the abdomen deeply over the area of tenderness and then quickly release it. If rebound tenderness is present, the client feels an increase in pain and tenderness upon release.

Palpation of organs such as the kidney, liver, and spleen is discussed in Chapters 34 and 44, and techniques are described in Chapter 4. The Physical Assessment Findings in the Healthy Adult feature on The Gastrointestinal System at right is an example of a recording for a normal abdominal physical examination.

DIAGNOSTIC TESTS

Diagnostic tests provide information about the nature and severity of upper GI tract or nutritional problems. Laboratory tests, radiography, ultrasonography, endoscopy, cytology, gastric analysis, and other tests are commonly used.

Laboratory Tests

Nutritional Anemias

Iron deficiency anemia is the most common cause of anemia in the world. In addition to iron, normal hematologic function requires adequate intake, absorption, use, and storage of nutrients, such as protein, vitamin B_{12}, and copper. Assessment of red blood cell function and iron stores is crucial to nutritional assessment. Chapters 76 and 77 describe assessment for hematologic disorders and anemias.

Serum Proteins

Serum proteins are important for maintaining intravascular oncotic pressure and as carrier molecules. Tests for serum proteins include albumin, prealbumin, retinol-binding protein, and transferrin. Measurement of serum proteins requires a venous blood sample with the client

---

PHYSICAL ASSESSMENT FINDINGS IN THE HEALTHY ADULT
The Gastrointestinal System

Inspection

Mouth. Lips symmetrical, pink, moist, without lesions. Buccal mucosa and gingivae pink, moist, intact, without lesions. Hard and soft palates pink, intact. Tonsils behind pillars, without inflammation. Posterior pharynx pink, without exudate. Uvula rises midline with phonation. Tongue midline, mobile, without deviation or fasciculations.

Abdomen. Flat, symmetrical, with umbilicus inverted, centered, and midline. No scars, lesions, dilated veins, visible peristalsis or pulsations, or separation of rectus muscles at rest or with straining.

Anus and Rectum. Perianal area free of lesions, inflammation, fissures, bulges, or external hemorrhoids.

Auscultation

Abdomen. Bowel sounds present in all four quadrants.

Percussion*

Abdomen. General tympany throughout, with liver and splenic dullness. Liver span 10 cm at right midclavicular line.

Palpation*

Abdomen. Liver and spleen nonpalpable. Abdomen soft, nontender, no masses or rebound tenderness; muscle tone firm, relaxed.

Anus and Rectum. Anus and rectum without tenderness, masses, hemorrhoids, or prolapse. Rectal mucosa smooth. Stool negative for blood.

*In assessment of the abdomen, palpation is performed after auscultation so that the bowel is not stimulated.

---

in a fasting or nonfasting state. Obtaining blood samples for laboratory tests are discussed in Chapter 4.

Table 30-9 lists serum proteins, normal values, half-lives, and conditions associated with abnormal values. In general, serum proteins with long half-lives (albumin) tend to be global indicators of nutritional status, and serum proteins with shorter half-lives (prealbumin and transferrin) suggest acute changes in nutritional status.

Total Lymphocyte Count

Immune function and nutritional status are closely related. Consequently, total lymphocyte count (TLC), an indicator of immune function, provides a gross measure of nutritional status. To determine TLC, obtain a white blood cell (WBC) count with differential from the client's venous blood sample. Next, multiply the per-

TABLE 30-9	Serum Proteins		
Protein	**Normal Range**	**Half-Life**	**Effect of Associated Conditions**
Albumin	3.5-5 g/dl	14-20 days	Increased with dehydration Decreased with malnutrition, overhydration, trauma, protein loss, liver disease
Prealbumin	20-40 mg/dl	3-5 days	Increased with nutrition intake and renal failure Decreased with poor dietary intake
Retinol-binding protein	3-6 mg/L	8-12 hours	Decreased with overhydration, liver disease, zinc and vitamin A deficit
Transferrin	200-400 mg/dl	8-10 hours	Increased with pregnancy, iron deficiency Decreased with chronic infection, cirrhosis

centage of lymphocytes by the total WBC count. For example, a client with a WBC count of 7000/mm³ and 30% lymphocytes has a TLC of 2100/mm³.

TLCs less than 1800/mm³ suggest malnutrition. Because the TLC is a gross indicator of immune function and nutritional status, normally nourished clients may have a low TLC after chemotherapy. Alternatively, an elevated TLC may be found in malnourished clients with sepsis.

D-Xylose Absorption Test

D-Xylose, a monosaccharide, is absorbed in the small intestine and is used to assess malabsorption. The client receives nothing by mouth (NPO) for 10 to 12 hours before the test. A blood sample and first-voided morning urine specimen are collected. After oral administration of a known quantity of D-xylose mixed in water, blood and urine levels of D-xylose are measured. Blood is drawn 2 hours after D-xylose is given, and all urine is collected for a specified time. Instruct the client to remain in bed during the test because activity alters the results. Decreased values of absorbed D-xylose in blood and urine indicate possible malabsorption in the small intestine.

Nitrogen Balance

Nitrogen balance is a measure of one's anabolic or catabolic state. To determine nitrogen balance, simultaneously record the amount and type of food consumed in a 24-hour period and obtain a 24-hour urine collection. The start and stop times for the food intake record and the 24-hour urine collection must be the same. Instruct the client about the procedure and about the importance of recording all food intake and saving all urine for 24 hours.

The 24-hour urine collection begins with discarding the first voided specimen, then collecting all urine for the next 24 hours in an iced, preservative-free container. After completing the 24-hour urine collection, send the urine to the laboratory for measurement of the urine urea nitrogen (UUN). Urine creatinine, sodium, and

potassium may also be measured to determine the adequacy of the urine collection. Consult a registered dietitian to calculate the client's 24-hour protein intake from the food intake record. If the client received tube feedings or parenteral nutrition during the 24-hour test period, the amount of protein from these sources must be included in the calculation.

Protein is approximately 16% nitrogen. To determine the amount of nitrogen consumed over the 24 hours, multiply the amount of protein consumed (in grams) by 0.16. UUN is the major source of nitrogen excretion. Subtract the UUN (in grams) from the amount of nitrogen consumed. Because nitrogen is also lost through the skin, stool, and the GI tract, subtract a correction factor of 3 from the nitrogen consumed, as follows:

Nitrogen balance = (Nitrogen consumed [in grams] – UUN [in grams]) – 3

Normal nitrogen balance is positive and ranges from 4 to 6 g. Negative nitrogen balance suggests a catabolic state indicating more protein is broken down than is consumed.

Fecal Analysis

Fecal content is an indicator of the absorptive capacity of the gut. Chapter 34 presents laboratory tests for fecal lipids and stool cultures.

Radiography

General principles for the following radiographic tests are explained in Chapter 4.

Flat Plate of the Abdomen

A flat plate of the abdomen is an x-ray (radiograph) of the abdominal organs. This test can help identify abnormalities, such as tumors, obstructions, abnormal gas or fluid collections, and strictures. The client may be required to lie flat or sit in the upright position for the x-ray.

Upper Gastrointestinal Series

An upper GI series, also known as a *barium swallow,* permits radiologic visualization of the esophagus, stomach, duodenum, and jejunum. It can aid in the detection of strictures, ulcers, tumors, polyps, hiatal hernias, or motility problems. The client drinks a radiopaque contrast medium (barium) while standing in front of a fluoroscopy tube. The client may also be asked to assume other positions, such as lying on the x-ray table and turning left or right. To prevent the swallowed barium from interfering with tests such as barium enemas and gallbladder radiographs, a barium swallow is usually done last.

Preprocedure Care

The client cannot have food or fluids for 6 to 8 hours before the test. Instruct the client about the procedure and about the barium preparation. Barium has a thick consistency and a chalky taste. It may be necessary to drink up to 16 ounces of barium for the procedure. The test lasts about 45 minutes.

Postprocedure Care

A laxative is given to help expel the barium and to prevent a fecal impaction. Assess the abdomen for distention, and observe the stool to determine whether the barium has been eliminated. Initially, the stool is white, but it should return to its normal brown color within 72 hours. A distended abdomen and constipation may indicate a barium impaction. Clients with ostomies should be closely monitored for retained barium.

Because the barium swallow is commonly performed on an outpatient basis, inform the client that the stool may be white for up to 72 hours after the procedure. Instruct the client to contact the physician immediately if constipation and abdominal distention occur.

Modified Barium Swallow

A modified barium swallow, also known as *videofluoroscopy* or an oropharyngeal motility study, is performed to assess swallowing and the risk of aspiration. While sitting in a chair equipped with videofluoroscopy, the client is asked to swallow a small amount of barium mixed in liquids and foods of various textures. During the procedure, a speech therapist or radiologist observes the client for difficulty with swallowing.

Clients are maintained on NPO status before the procedure. Maintain hydration with intravenous fluids if the client is expected to remain NPO for an extended period. After the procedure, nothing should be ingested by mouth until the speech therapist, radiologist, or physician has evaluated the test results. If diet alterations are required, consult a registered dietitian, speech therapist, or both to collaboratively develop an appropriate and adequate nutrition plan.

Computed Tomography

CT scanning is used to identify masses, such as neoplasms, cysts, focal inflammatory lesions, and abscesses of the liver, pancreas, and pelvic areas (Figure 30-3). CT also aids in evaluating local tumor spread, especially if barium studies suggest tumor growth beyond the bowel wall.[7] To distinguish normal bowel from abnormal intraperitoneal masses, dilute oral barium or other contrast media may be administered. The client is placed supine on the examination table and asked to lie still and hold his or her breath when instructed.

The client receives nothing by mouth for 6 to 12 hours before the procedure. Report any history of allergies to iodine to the radiologist. Non-iodine contrast medium may be used when the client is allergic to iodine. No follow-up care is needed. Chapter 4 covers the general preparation and care of the client undergoing CT scanning.

Ultrasonography

Ultrasonography of the GI system helps to identify pathophysiologic processes in the pancreas, liver, gallbladder, spleen, and retroperitoneal tissues. Ultrasound

FIGURE 30-3 Normal computed tomography (CT) scan of the stomach. The CT scan is through the body of the stomach *(B)* at a level just below the spleen. The lateral segment of the left lobe of the liver *(LS),* head of the pancreas *(P),* and splenic flexure of the colon *(C)* are adjacent structures. A, Aorta; D, duodenum; V, inferior vena cava. *Solid arrow* represents the superior mesenteric artery, and *open arrow* represents the vein. The rugae *(curved arrows)* are well visualized. (From Moss, A., Gamsu, G., & Genant, H.K. [1992]. *Computed tomography of the body: With magnetic resonance imaging* [Vol. 3, 2nd ed.]. Philadelphia: W.B. Saunders.)

studies can be used to identify fluid, masses (such as tumors), adipose tissue, abscesses, and hematomas. Physical examination is enhanced by ultrasound techniques because palpable masses and areas of tenderness can be correlated with anatomic structures while the client is on the examining table (see Chapter 4).

Because gas may interfere with the procedure, the client may take nothing by mouth for 8 to 12 hours beforehand. Reassure the client that the test is painless and safe. There are no specific postprocedure precautions or observations related to ultrasound.

Endoscopy

Endoscopy is the direct visualization of the GI system by means of a lighted, flexible tube. It is more accurate than radiologic examination because sources of bleeding, surface lesions, or healing tissues can be directly observed.

Procedure

Upper GI tract endoscopy includes esophagoscopy, gastroscopy, and esophagogastroduodenoscopy (Figure 30-4). These procedures are useful for examining clients who have acute or chronic GI bleeding, pernicious anemia, esophageal injury, masses, strictures, dysphagia, substernal pain, epigastric discomfort, or inflammatory bowel disease. Conscious sedation with a sedative, opioid, or tranquilizer may be given before or during the procedure. Anticholinergic medications may be given to decrease oropharyngeal secretions and to prevent reflex bradycardia.

When the client is sedated, a local anesthetic is sprayed on the posterior pharynx to ease discomfort and prevent gagging during insertion of the endoscope. The anesthetic often tastes unpleasant and makes the tongue feel swollen. To reduce the risk of aspiration, the client is placed in the left lateral decubitus (Sims) position to allow saliva to drain from the side of the mouth.

After the client is positioned, sedated, and anesthetized, a flexible fiberoptic tube is passed orally into the esophagus, stomach, pylorus, and duodenum. Some endoscopes are equipped with a camera that allows the physician to obtain color photographs. If cancer is suspected, cells or tissue can be collected for cytologic examination. Small, single polyps may be removed.

During the procedure, monitor for cardiac and respiratory complications. Assess the client's heart rate, blood pressure, respiratory rate, and pulse oximetry frequently. Specific antagonists to benzodiazepines and opioids should be available for emergency reversal of drug effects. Upper GI endoscopy should not be performed in clients with severe cardiovascular disease.

Preprocedure Care

Clients undergoing endoscopic procedures require a signed consent. If the client is going home within 24 hours after the procedure, someone should be available to drive. For clients with a history of cardiac valve disease or replacement, antibiotic prophylaxis may be required. To prevent aspiration of stomach contents into the lungs, keep the client NPO for 8 to 12 hours before the procedure. Assess the oral cavity, and report any loose teeth or lesions to the gastroenterologist. Remove the client's dentures and any removable bridges.

Even with anesthesia, the client may experience some discomfort, nausea, or pressure. Tell the client to breathe through the nose during the procedure. Explain that the room will be cool and dark and that he or she will not be able to talk while the endoscope is in place.

Postprocedure Care

To prevent aspiration, place the client in the Sims position until the sedation and local anesthesia wear off. Withhold fluids and solids for 2 to 4 hours after the procedure or until the gag reflex returns. Test for return of the gag reflex by stroking the back of the client's throat with a tongue blade to determine whether gagging occurs. Once the gag reflex returns, the physician may order anesthetic throat lozenges or normal saline gargles to ease throat irritation or hoarseness.

Monitor for bradycardia or other dysrhythmias that may occur as a result of sedatives or anesthetics. Assess for signs of esophageal or gastric perforation. Esophageal perforation may cause crepitus (crackling) in the neck (from air leakage), fever, bleeding, or pain. Neck and throat pain, aggravated by swallowing or moving, may also occur. Midesophageal perforation results in referred substernal or epigastric pain. Distal esophageal perforation results in shoulder pain, dyspnea, or manifestations similar to those of perforated ulcers. If you suspect perforation, an x-ray study should be obtained to confirm the presence of free air.[3]

Endoscopic examination of the lower GI tract is discussed in Chapter 34.

FIGURE 30-4 An endoscopic view of the esophagus showing an esophageal ulcer (*arrow*).

Exfoliative Cytologic Analysis

Exfoliative cytologic analysis, developed by George Papanicolaou, is a study of cells that have sloughed off from a tissue. The examination is performed to distinguish benign from malignant lesions. Malignant cells exfoliate more readily than normal cells. Specific areas of the GI tract are lavaged, and cells are collected and sent to the laboratory for analysis. Cells of the esophagus, stomach, small intestine, and colon can be examined. Stomach contents are examined for the presence of *Helicobacter pylori,* a bacterium that can cause gastritis and peptic ulcer disease.

In this procedure, a nasogastric tube is placed and cells are obtained by saline lavage through the tube. Explain the procedure to the client and, if required, obtain a written consent. Keep the client NPO before the procedure. Afterward, the client rests and may resume eating.

Gastric Analysis

Gastric analysis is performed to measure secretions of hydrochloric acid (HCl) and pepsin in the stomach. Analysis of gastric contents can aid in the diagnosis of duodenal ulcer, Zollinger-Ellison syndrome, gastric carcinoma, and pernicious anemia. Gastric analysis consists of (1) the basal cell secretion test and (2) the gastric acid stimulation test.

Procedure

For the *basal cell secretion test,* a nasogastric tube is inserted and attached to suction. Stomach contents are collected every 15 minutes for 1 hour. Label specimens carefully with time, volume, and client identification. The specimens are analyzed. If abnormal gastric secretion is suggested, a gastric acid stimulation test is performed.

The *gastric acid stimulation test* measures the amount of gastric acid for 1 hour after subcutaneous injection of a drug that stimulates its secretion (pentagastrin and betazole). If results are abnormal, radiographic studies or endoscopy may be done to determine the cause. A markedly increased level of gastric secretion may indicate Zollinger-Ellison syndrome, whereas a moderately increased level suggests a duodenal ulcer. Decreased levels of gastric secretion may indicate gastric ulcer or carcinoma.

Preprocedure Care

The client ingests nothing orally for 12 hours before the test. Insert a nasogastric tube, and remove any contents left in the stomach. Do not administer drugs that interfere with gastric acid levels, such as cholinergics, histamine blockers, or antacids. If a client requires coronary vasodilator therapy, change the oral form to an ointment or sublingual preparation during the procedure.

Postprocedure Care

If the nasogastric tube is left in place, attach it to low intermittent suction. Record the amount and color of the drainage.

Acid Perfusion Test

The acid perfusion test, also known as the *Bernstein test,* determines whether a client's chest pain is related to acid perfusion across the esophageal mucosa. A nasogastric tube is inserted, and gastric contents are aspirated. Normal saline solution (0.9%) and 0.1% HCl are alternately instilled into the lower esophagus. If the client does not experience pain, the test is considered normal. If pain occurs, normal saline is administered until pain ceases. To ensure that the pain is caused by acid perfusion, 0.1% HCl is readministered. After the test, the nasogastric tube is withdrawn.

Keep the client NPO the night before the test. Instruction about the procedure includes preparing the client for insertion of the nasogastric tube. After the procedure, the client may receive an antacid.

Esophageal Manometry

Manometry is used to assess esophageal motor function and can be used to assess and diagnose dysphagia, esophageal reflux, spasm, motility disorders, and hiatal hernia. A special enteric tube with fused small-caliber catheters is inserted into the esophagus. The tube is designed to measure simultaneous pressures of the esophagus and lower esophageal sphincter by infusion of water into the catheters. The client is asked to swallow small amounts of water, and esophageal pressures are recorded during muscular relaxation and contraction.

Instruct the client about the procedure and maintain the client in an NPO status for 6 to 8 hours before the procedure. The test takes about 15 to 20 minutes. After the test, remove the enteric tube. The physician may recommend medications or diet alterations based on the results.

Ambulatory Esophageal pH Monitoring

Ambulatory esophageal pH monitoring is used to distinguish chest pain caused by gastric acid reflux from chest pain caused by angina or myocardial infarction. Location of the lower esophageal sphincter (LES) is determined by esophageal manometry, and a nasoenteric tube with a pH sensor is inserted 5 cm above the LES. The enteric tube is secured to the client's face and attached to a battery-operated recorder. The client is then instructed to push a button on the recorder at the start and end of specific activities, such as eating, sleeping, and smoking. Tell the client to note when chest pain or indigestion starts and ends.

Because the location of the LES must be determined, inform the client that esophageal manometry may be performed first after which a second enteric tube may be placed for the pH monitoring. You may need to stop giving the client drugs that affect the GI tract (H$_2$ histamine blockers and motility drugs) before the procedure. Instruct the client about the importance of recording activities and manifestations. The tube must remain securely taped. Tell the client to avoid bumping or pulling the tube when dressing or during face washing. After the procedure, remove the tube and advise the client that normal activities may be resumed.

CONCLUSIONS

Nutritional health and a functional upper GI tract are basic to good health. Systematic assessment of the client's nutritional status and upper GI tract can lead to early detection, diagnosis, and treatment of nutrition-related problems and optimal nutrition outcomes.

BIBLIOGRAPHY

1. A.S.P.E.N Board of Directors. (2002). Guidelines for the use of parenteral and enteral nutrition in adult and pediatric patients. *Journal of Parenteral and Enteral Nutrition, 26,* 1S-138S.
2. Barkauskas, V.H., Baumann, L.C., & Darling-Fisher, C.S. (Eds.). (2001). *Health and physical assessment* (3rd ed.). St. Louis: Mosby.
3. Barkin, J., & O'Phelan, C.A. (Eds.). (1994). *Advanced therapeutic endoscopy* (2nd ed.). New York: Raven Press.
4. Elliot, D. (2002). The treatment of peptic ulcers. *Nursing Standard, 16*(22), 37-42.
5. Ennis, B.W., Saffel-Shrier, S., & Verson, H. (2001). Diagnosing malnutrition in the elderly. *The Nurse Practitioner, 26,* 52-65.
6. Estes, M.E. (Ed.). (2002). *Health assessment and physical examination* (2nd ed.). Australia: Delmar Thomson Learning.
7. Haubrich, W.S., Schaffner, F., & Berk, J.E. (Eds.). (1995). *Bockus gastroenterology* (5th ed.). Philadelphia: W. B. Saunders.
8. Holmes, S. (2000). Nutritional screening and older adults. *Nursing Standard, 15*(2), 42-44.
9. Institute of Medicine-National Academy of Sciences, Food and Nutrition Board. (2001). *DRI: Applications in dietary assessment.* Washington DC: National Academy Press.
10. Jarvis, C. (2000). *Physical examination and health assessment* (3rd ed.). Philadelphia: W. B. Saunders.
11. Mahan, L., & Escott-Stump, S. (Eds.). (2000). *Krause's food, nutrition, and diet therapy* (10th ed.). Philadelphia: W. B. Saunders.
12. Shils, E., et al. (Eds.). (1999). *Modern nutrition in health and disease* (9th ed.). Baltimore: Williams & Wilkins.
13. Stanhope, M. & Knollmueller, R.N. (2001). *Handbook of public and community health nursing practice. A health promotion guide.* St. Louis: Mosby.
14. Wilson, S.F., & Giddens, J.F. (2001). *Health assessment for nursing practice* (2nd ed.). St. Louis: Mosby.

Management of Clients with Malnutrition

Nancy Evans Stoner
Candace Cantwell
Charlene Compher

evolve

Web Enhancements

http://evolve.elsevier.com/Black/medsurg/

Ethical Issues in Nursing
How Can Nurses Ensure That Clients Have Given Their Informed Consent?

Appendix C
Laboratory Values of Clinical Importance in Medical-Surgical Nursing

---

Malnutrition can develop as a result of acute or chronic diseases and treatments that affect the ability to ingest or digest foods. In turn, it can cause such problems as delayed wound healing, impaired immune function, and a decreased functional status. Obesity, anorexia nervosa, and bulimia nervosa are eating disorders that reflect altered nutritional health. Nursing diagnoses pertinent to malnutrition include *Imbalanced Nutrition: More (or Less) Than Body Requirements,* and *Feeding Self-Care Deficit.*

PROTEIN-ENERGY MALNUTRITION

Malnutrition broadly describes *undernutrition* or *overnutrition* related to deficient or excess energy or nitrogen stores, possibly due to altered dietary intake. Protein-energy malnutrition (PEM) results when the body's need for protein or energy is not supplied in adequate quantity by dietary intake. Prolonged deficiencies in energy and protein can result in any of the following clinical syndromes of malnutrition:

- Kwashiorkor, which reflects primarily a chronic deficiency in protein
- Marasmus, which reflects primarily a prolonged deficit in caloric supply
- Marasmic kwashiorkor, which reflects both an energy and a protein deficit
- "Kwashiorkor-like malnutrition," which has been coined to describe the abnormally low serum protein concentrations observed in previously well-nourished clients during or after injury or operation

PEM can be classified as *primary* when the deficits result simply from poor food intake. Primary PEM is seen most commonly in developing nations or following natural disasters or war, where food supply is disrupted. The prevalence of primary PEM is greatest in developing countries, particularly where famine occurs.[41] Worldwide, 800 million people from developing countries are undernourished, a figure that includes 193 million (36%) underweight, 230 million (43%) stunted in growth, and 50 million (9%) wasted children younger than age 5 years.[41] The prevalence of underweight children is 36% in all developing countries with a range

---

evolve *Be sure to check out the bonus material on the Evolve website and the CD-ROM, including free self-assessment exercises.*
http://evolve.elsevier.com/Black/medsurg/

Nursing Outcomes Classification
for Nursing Diagnoses—Clients with Malnutrition

Chronic Low Self-Esteem	**Nutritional Status: Food and Fluid Intake**	**Nutritional Status: Food and Fluid Intake**
Self-Esteem	Self-Care: Eating	**Nutritional Status: Nutrient Intake**
Disturbed Body Image	Swallowing Status	Weight Control
Body Image	**Imbalanced Nutrition: More (or Less)**	**Impaired Swallowing**
Feeding Self-Care Deficit	**Than Body Requirements**	Swallowing Status
Nutritional Status	Nutritional Status	

from 11% in Latin America to 60% in South Asia.[42] The percentage of infants born small (<2500 g) for date is 19% in all developing countries, with a range of 11% in Latin America and East Asia to 34% in South Asia.[42] Although the overall percentage of malnourished children has been reduced in countries with economic and political stability, the actual number is unchanged because of burgeoning population growth. When a natural disaster, such as drought, flood, earthquake, or famine, occurs, the prevalence of PEM in a developing country may be increased. Similarly, when man-made disasters, such as war, political upheaval, or economic crisis, occur, malnutrition prevalence in the population is exacerbated.[41]

The age-groups at greatest risk for PEM are those with increased nutritional needs for growth, reproduction, or milk production—infants, pregnant or lactating women[41,42]—and older adults.[15] Maternal malnutrition peri-pregnancy is a key factor in the birth of an underweight newborn and that infant's development into a child with PEM.[41] Even though marasmic malnutrition (wasting) is most common in children younger than 1 year, weaning from breast milk later on is associated with kwashiorkor malnutrition when the available diet contains much lower protein content than milk. Older adults are particularly susceptible to PEM when their medical or socioeconomic status limits their ability to obtain and ingest nutritionally adequate diets.[15,32,40,41]

Secondary PEM refers to malnutrition associated with acute or chronic disease that causes one or more of the following: (1) decreased food intake, (2) decreased nutrient absorption, (3) increased nutrient losses, or (4) increased nutrient requirements. Secondary PEM is more common than primary PEM in developed nations. A relatively recent observation in developing countries is that obesity is increasing concurrently with prevalent PEM. Obesity occurs when caloric supply is adequate to promote chronic diseases (obesity, diabetes, hypertension, and cancer) but the nutrient content of the diet is poor.[12,15,16,34,40]

Severe marasmus, kwashiorkor, and marasmus-kwashiorkor are seen in Western health care facilities, particularly in very ill, older clients. The more usual pattern, however, in the general population is in clients with normal weight to overweight or obesity before hospital admission. Weight loss during the hospitalization is common, as is rapid development of severely depleted serum protein

levels in response to injury, infection, surgical or medical treatments, and prolonged limited intake of protein.[34,40]

PEM is a significant problem in adult medical and surgical clients in both hospital and home settings. Initial studies of malnutrition found PEM in up to 40% of hospitalized medical-surgical clients.[9,10] More recent studies have found similar rates of documented malnutrition on admission to the hospital in general medical clients (46%), clients with respiratory disease (45%), and older clients (43%).[12,15,16]

Malnutrition was documented in 10% of 441 clients who lived at home with cancer and chronic disease.[13,16] The older adult population is at particular risk for malnutrition; in one study of nursing home residents, 85% of those assessed had significant nutritional deficits.[13,16] Among community-dwelling older adults, the prevalence of PEM may be 5% to 10%. Decreases in functional capacity, mobility, and independence, which are common in older adults, can result from malnutrition or may contribute to its development.[32,34,40] The most important changes in body composition associated with aging are a loss of lean body mass and a gain in body fat. The loss of lean body mass is an important factor in the impairment of pulmonary function, immune function, and strength.[13,16,34] (See the Complementary and Alternative Therapy feature on Oral Protein and Energy Supplements to Reduce Mortality in Older Adults on p. 711.)

The cost of treating malnutrition varies greatly, depending on the level of nutritional care. For example, simply providing food snacks requires minimal cost; supplemental formulas typically cost $4 to $5 per six-pack. More sophisticated nutritional support therapies used to treat and prevent malnutrition are more expensive. *Enteral tube feedings* may cost up to $30 to $40 per day, and *parenteral nutrition* typically costs $250 to $350 per day. These costs are small relative to the complications associated with malnutrition, such as increased length of stay, delayed wound healing, and prolonged infection.

Etiology and Risk Factors

The etiology of PEM is multifactorial and is usually associated with the presence of acute or chronic disease. PEM can be related to socioeconomic factors, physiologic changes in nutrient absorption or nutrient requirements, or medical therapies used to treat disease. Socioeconomic factors that have a negative effect on nutritional status include the following:

- Social isolation
- Limited access to food
- Emotional depression
- Substance abuse
- Poverty

Physiologic factors leading to malnutrition usually result from other diseases that can cause compromised food intake, decreased absorption of nutrients, or increased demand for nutrients. Changes in nutrient intake can result from the disease or from its treatment.

Inadequate food intake is common in hospitals and can lead to malnutrition if diminished intake is prolonged or severe. Many disease processes affect the client's swallowing function and are common reasons for decreased food intake (see Chapter 32). Inadequate absorption of nutrients is the result of various disorders of the gastrointestinal (GI) tract, such as inflammatory bowel disease (see Chapters 33 and 35). In addition, the demand for nutrients increases in response to critical illness and to chronic and infectious diseases.

In your role of preventing and restoring nutritional status, you should take a multidisciplinary approach. Health *promotion* interventions include activities that support the client's knowledge of normal nutrition and provide nutritional information to maintain optimal health and prevent disease. Such strategies might include diet information related to decreasing cancer risk or identifying support for an older client who cannot prepare meals independently. Health *maintenance* interventions include targeting specialized diet therapy for a client with an illness (such as diet instruction for a client with Crohn's disease). Health *restoration* activities can include retraining a client to swallow after a stroke or administering total parenteral nutrition (TPN) to a malnourished client with severe inflammatory bowel disease.

Pathophysiology

PEM can develop gradually over weeks to months, or it can develop more quickly when coupled with severe stress and illness. When the total supply of nutrients is less than the body's requirement, malnutrition occurs. When the primary deficit is in energy balance, the result is, first, the depletion of adipose tissue or fat stores, with eventual loss of lean body tissue (muscle mass) and fatigue. This deficit is reflected in weight loss. An unintentional weight loss of 5% in 1 month or 10% in 6 months suggests that the client is at significant risk for malnutrition.[34,40] **EB**

When the nutrient deficit is primarily in protein, skeletal muscle is catabolized to meet the body's needs for glucose (in response to hormonal messages), and the liver's synthesis of proteins is altered. The production of serum proteins, such as albumin, transferrin, and prealbumin, is reduced during acute inflammatory conditions, postoperatively, and during significant infections. Rates of protein breakdown are also increased, and serum proteins may shift out of the vascular compartment, resulting overall in low serum protein concentrations.[12] Adequate protein intake is extremely important during these periods of clinical stress, to enable the production of these serum proteins at adequate levels during the recovery phase. Starvation related to severe stress affects organ function at the cellular level by impairing specific biochemical functions, which increases the risk of mortality and morbidity.[12,13]

Clinical Manifestations

Table 31-1 presents the pathophysiology and related clinical manifestations of malnutrition. You may also notice hair loss or hair that is dull and dry. The client's

TABLE 31-1	*Consequences of Malnutrition*	
Organ System	**Pathophysiology**	**Clinical Manifestations**
Cardiac	Decreased cardiac muscle mass	Postural hypotension Diminished venous return
Pulmonary	Decreased diaphragm strength Decreased respiratory strength Decreased endurance	Inability to clear secretions Decreased exercise tolerance Inability to wean from ventilator
Immune function	Decreased cell-mediated immunity Delayed cutaneous hypersensitivity	Increased incidence and severity of infection
Wound healing	Decreased collagen synthesis	Delayed wound healing
Skeletal muscle strength	Altered muscle contractions Relaxation response Decreased muscle endurance	Fatigue Inability to perform activities of daily living Risk of falling
Gastrointestinal function	Impaired intestinal absorption of lipids Decreased rate of glucose absorption Decreased gastric, pancreatic, and bile production	Diarrhea

EB EVIDENCE-BASED PRACTICE IN ACTION

Nutrition and Wound Healing

Adequate protein and calories are important to support the body while attempting to heal open wounds. Although this belief is fairly well accepted, research findings are beginning to clarify how much feeding should be done and when feeding should begin after injury.

Several studies indicate that protein is important in healing acute surgical wounds and chronic wounds such as pressure ulcers. Large open wounds not only need protein to heal but also continue to seep protein from the large open areas. Protein has traditionally been prescribed at 1.2 to 1.5 mg/kg/day. Two studies showed that pressure ulcers healed more rapidly when 1.8 mg/kg of protein was given by tube feeding[7] and when the diet contained 24% protein, an increase of 10% from usual dietary intake.[1,2,6] However, there was no increase in body weight or serum protein levels (e.g., serum albumin). There seemed to be an upper limit to increasing the protein intake because dehydration developed.

Vitamin C and zinc are also thought to be helpful in healing. However, data have shown no increase in the rate of healing by adding these supplements. Clients who are deficient in vitamin and minerals may benefit nutritionally from vitamin and mineral supplementation but data do not support their use in clients who are not deficient, and neither group (vitamin C or zinc) showed improved rates of wound healing.[1,8,12,13]

Enteral feeding after a major surgery or trauma has often been held until manifestations of GI function are present (i.e., bowel sounds, passing flatus, soft abdomen), which may be 2 to 3 days. However, data from multiple studies indicate that nutritional support should begin as soon as possible once hemodynamic stability is reached. After 3 days of not eating, the villa of the intestine atrophy, which reduces the capacity for nutrient absorption and also lowers immunoglobulin production in the gut. The loss of these immunoglobulins may increase the risk of infection.[5,9,10,11,14]

Tube feeding as a route to provide nutrition is a common method of providing nutrients. Three studies of more than 800 clients over 6 months showed that tube feeding was not associated with healing of pre-existing pressure ulcers or with prevention of new pressure ulcers. Reasons for these outcomes may be that the client is positioned at 30 degrees or more of elevation of the head of the bed, increasing friction and shearing of the sacrum, and that diarrhea may develop from the tube feeding.[3,4,15]

within hours of surgery. The general use of vitamins and minerals is also not effective to promote healing, except in those clients who are deprived of these supplements.

References

1. Agrawal, S., et al.(2003). Nutritional and vitamin status of non-healing wounds in patients attending a tertiary hospital in India. *The Journal of Dermatology, 30*(2), 98-103.
2. Avenell, A., & Handoll, H. (2003). Nutritional supplementation for hip fracture aftercare in the elderly. *The Cochrane Library, CD001880,* 1464-1780X.
3. Berlowitz, D., et al. (1996). Rating long-term care facilities on pressure ulcer development: Importance of case-mix adjustment. *Annals of Internal Medicine, 124,* 557-563.
4. Berlowitz, D., et al. (1997). Predictors of pressure ulcer healing among long-term care residents. *Journal of the American Geriatric Society, 45,* 30-34.
5. Braga, M., et al. (2002). Feeding the gut early after digestive surgery: Results of a nine-year experience. *Clinical Nutrition, 21*(1), 59-65.
6. Breslow, R., et al. (1993). The importance of dietary protein in healing pressure ulcers. *Journal of the American Geriatrics Society, 41,* 357-362.
7. Chernoff, R., Milton, K., & Lipschitz, D. (1990). The effect of very high protein liquid formula on decubitus ulcer healing in long-term tube fed institutionalized patients. *Journal of the American Dietetic Association, 90*(9), 1-130.
8. Costello, R., & Grumpstrup-Scott, J. (2000). Zinc: What role might supplements play? *Journal of the American Dietetic Association, 100,* 371-375.
9. Grant, J. (1994). Nutritional support in critically ill patients. *Annals of Surgery, 220,* 610-616.
10. Johnson Casto, C., Krammer, J., & Drake, J. (2000). Postoperative feeding: A clinical review. *Obstetrics and Gynecologic Surgery, 55*(9), 571-573.
11. Lewis, S., et al. (2001). Early enteral feeding versus "nil by mouth" after gastrointestinal surgery: Systematic review and meta-analysis of controlled trials. *British Medical Journal, 323*(7316), 773-776.
12. Long, C., et al. (2003). Ascorbic acid dynamics in the seriously ill and injured. *The Journal of Surgical Research, 109*(2), 144-148.
13. Racket, S., Rothe, M., & Grant-Kels, J. (1993). Diet and dermatology: The role of dietary manipulation in the prevention and treatment of cutaneous disorders. *American Academy of Dermatology, 29,* 447-461.
14. Sing, G., Ram, R., & Khanna, S. (1998). Early postoperative enteral feeding in patients with nontraumatic intestinal perforation and peritonitis. *Journal of the American College of Surgeons, 187*(2), 142-146.
15. Thomas, D. (2001). Improving outcome of pressure ulcers with nutritional interventions: A review of the evidence. *Nutrition, 17*(2), 121-125.

Implications

Adequate intake of protein is important to promote healing and may be underprescribed and withheld for too long. However, some studies indicate that when protein is given by tube feeding, the complications may outweigh the benefits, especially if the client develops diarrhea from the formula or remains positioned on the sacrum. Other studies support the use of enteral feeding to maintain immunocompetence and bowel function skin may be dry and bruised. Nails are brittle. Periodontal disease and bleeding gums as well as cheilosis may be present. Many malnourished clients are also anemic. With severe nutritional deficiencies, clients may experience decreased neurologic reflexes, weakness, edema, increased sensitivity to cold, amenorrhea, impotence, atrophied breasts, and delayed wound healing. (See the Evidence-Based Practice in Action feature on Nutrition and Wound Healing on p. 692.)

Abnormal laboratory values that may indicate malnutrition include decreased hemoglobin, blood urea nitrogen (BUN, also known as urea nitrogen), creatinine, albumin, total protein, transferrin, prealbumin (PAB), and lymphocyte proliferation. All of these findings are related primarily to a protein deficit. PAB is the most sensitive indicator of protein deficiency because of its short half-life of 2 days. It can be used to assess improvement in nutritional status with refeeding, and levels can increase by 1 mg/dl/day with adequate nutritional support.

Outcome Management
■ Medical Management

Management of PEM starts with identification of clients who are malnourished as well as clients at risk for malnutrition. All clients should be screened for nutritional problems. First-level screening can be done through admission forms or simple questionnaires. Nutritional screening generally focuses on a few key data points (such as a weight change, a change in dietary habits, and GI manifestations) to identify clients that require a more comprehensive nutritional assessment.

A comprehensive nutritional assessment includes a review of the medical history, weight and diet history, anthropometric measures, biochemical profiles, and physical examination (see Chapter 30 for an in-depth review of nutritional assessment).

Define Nutrient Outcomes. The outcomes for weight and fat stores and protein stores define the nutrient goals for each client. Weight maintenance is appropriate for clients within 90% to 120% of a reference weight, whereas depletion of fat stores and weight loss is appropriate for obese clients (>120% of reference weight). Clients with severely depleted fat stores and more than 10% weight loss need calories sufficient to replete these stores and to gain weight.

Define Nutrient Requirements Needed to Achieve Desired Outcomes. The energy needs of most clients can be determined with formulas that estimate the basal energy expenditure (BEE). Even though the studies occurred in the early 1900s, the Harris-Benedict equations for basal energy expenditure (BEE) are still the most commonly used formulas:

$$\text{BEE (men)} = 66 + (13.7 \times \text{Weight in kg})$$
$$+ (5 \times \text{Height in cm}) - (6.8 \times \text{Age})$$

$$\text{BEE (women)} = 655 + (9.6 \times \text{Weight in kg})$$
$$+ (1.7 \times \text{Height in cm}) - (4.7 \times \text{Age})$$

The BEE represents the basal metabolic rate and is multiplied by a factor that accounts for stress and activity. Table 31-2 outlines targets for daily energy requirements using predictive equations. These equations are most useful in mildly stressed clients and may overestimate or underestimate energy needs during critical illness. Indirect calorimetry can be used for severely stressed clients for a precise measurement of energy expenditure.

Alternatively, an estimate of 25 kcal/kg body weight is often used when weight maintenance is desired. If weight gain is needed, the caloric goal can be increased to 35 kcal/kg, or an additional 500 kcal/day (to promote a safe rate of weight gain of 1 pound per week) can be added to the caloric estimate for weight maintenance.

The protein needs of a hospitalized client may be nearly twice those of normal needs. The Recommended Daily Allowance (RDA) for protein in healthy people is 0.8 g/kg/day. Protein requirements for the metabolically stressed client range from 1.5 g of protein per kilogram (kg) to as much as 2 g of protein per kg of body weight.

Determine Route of Feeding. The goals to meet nutrient needs must be translated into a practical, safe, and medically appropriate nutritional plan of care. To prevent or correct existing malnutrition through oral dietary manipulation, a registered dietitian can assist in meal planning or can recommend diet modification to increase oral intake. Supplements to boost the oral intake of calories and protein are available in a variety of forms, such as liquid milk-like drinks, clear juice-like drinks, nutrient bars, and puddings (Table 31-3).

When the client is unable to eat or when oral intake is contraindicated, an alternative means of nutritional support is necessary, such as enteral or parenteral feedings. If the GI tract is functional, enteral feedings should be used. If the GI tract is not functional, however, the client is a candidate for parenteral nutrition. Figure 31-1 presents an algorithm for determining the appro-

TABLE 31-2	*Determining Daily Energy Requirements*	
Goal for Fat Stores	**kcal (in Hospital)**	**Requirement (kcal/kg/day)**
Replete	BEE × 1.5	30-35
Maintain	BEE × 1.3	25-30
Reduce	<BEE	20-25

From Evans Stoner, N. (1997). Nutritional assessment. *Nursing Clinics of North America, 32*(4), 648.
BEE, Basal energy expenditure.

TABLE 31-3	*Oral Nutritional Supplements*		
Type of Product	**Calories Per Serving**	**Protein (g Per Serving)**	**Features**
Milk-Based			
Nutra Shake (4 oz)	200	8	High-calorie/protein, lower-volume supplement
Carnation Instant Breakfast (8 oz) made with 2% milk	250	12	Widely available, economical, high-calorie/protein supplement
Ensure Pudding (5 oz)	250	6.8	Thicker consistency, low-volume supplement with added vitamins and minerals
Lactose-Free			
Boost Plus (8 oz)	360	14.6	High-calorie/protein supplement with added vitamins and minerals
Probalance (8 oz)	300	13.5	High calorie/protein, fiber-containing supplement with added vitamins and minerals
Disease-Specific			
Nepro (8 oz)	475	16.6	Specialized for clients with renal failure who are receiving dialysis; low in electrolytes and volume
Resource Diabetic (8 oz)	250	15	High-calorie/protein, low-carbohydrate supplement, lactose-free
Nutritional Bars			
Boost Bar (44 g)	190	4	Candy bar appeal, convenient, with added vitamins and minerals; various flavors
Powerbar Essentials (65 g)	180	10	High-protein, low-fat supplement with added vitamins and minerals; various flavors

priate route of feeding. Clients may need to alternate between oral, enteral, and parenteral feedings during the course of a hospital admission.

■ Nursing Management of the Medical Client

Assessment

Nurses play a vital role in identifying clients with nutritional problems. Of all the various health care providers who clients see, nurses are typically the first to assess clients as they enter a health system. Nurses also have the most constant contact during a hospitalization, and they are the last health professionals to see clients before they leave. Thus your continued monitoring of a given client's nutritional status is key.

Nursing admission forms should include questions regarding weight history, weight change, diet history, and food intolerance. Daily flow sheets or nursing records must include a section on nutrition, including weight measures and tolerance to nutritional therapy. Box 31-1 is an example of an admission nutrition screening tool that can be used to determine a client's nutritional risk.

Nursing Diagnosis, Outcomes, Interventions

Diagnosis: Feeding Self-Care Deficit. The nursing diagnosis most appropriate for the intervention of feeding is *Feeding Self-Care Deficit related to impaired mo-* *tor function, impaired cognitive function, sensory-perceptual alterations, or decreased appetite.* Neuromuscular impairments, such as Parkinson's disease, muscular dystrophy, myasthenia gravis, muscular weakness, and central nervous system tumors, are contributing factors. Visual disorders can occur with glaucoma, cataracts, or a stroke. A situational factor may include immobility, trauma, or the placement of external fixating devices that restrict arm movement. Older clients may have decreased visual and motor abilities, increased muscle weakness, and altered taste and appetite.

Outcomes. The client will maintain body weight or will gain 1 to 2 pounds per week to return to an ideal body weight by overcoming decreased appetite or motor, sensory-perceptual, or cognitive impairments.

Interventions

Improve Nutritional Intake. General strategies to improve nutritional intake relate to choices of menu items and the accessibility of dietitians and food service personnel who can evaluate client food preferences and assist in meal planning. Clients should be able to choose from a menu to avoid food monotony. Dietitians should be accessible during mealtimes to help assess individual preferences. Kitchen facilities and supplies should be available at the unit level to increase client choices. Ded-

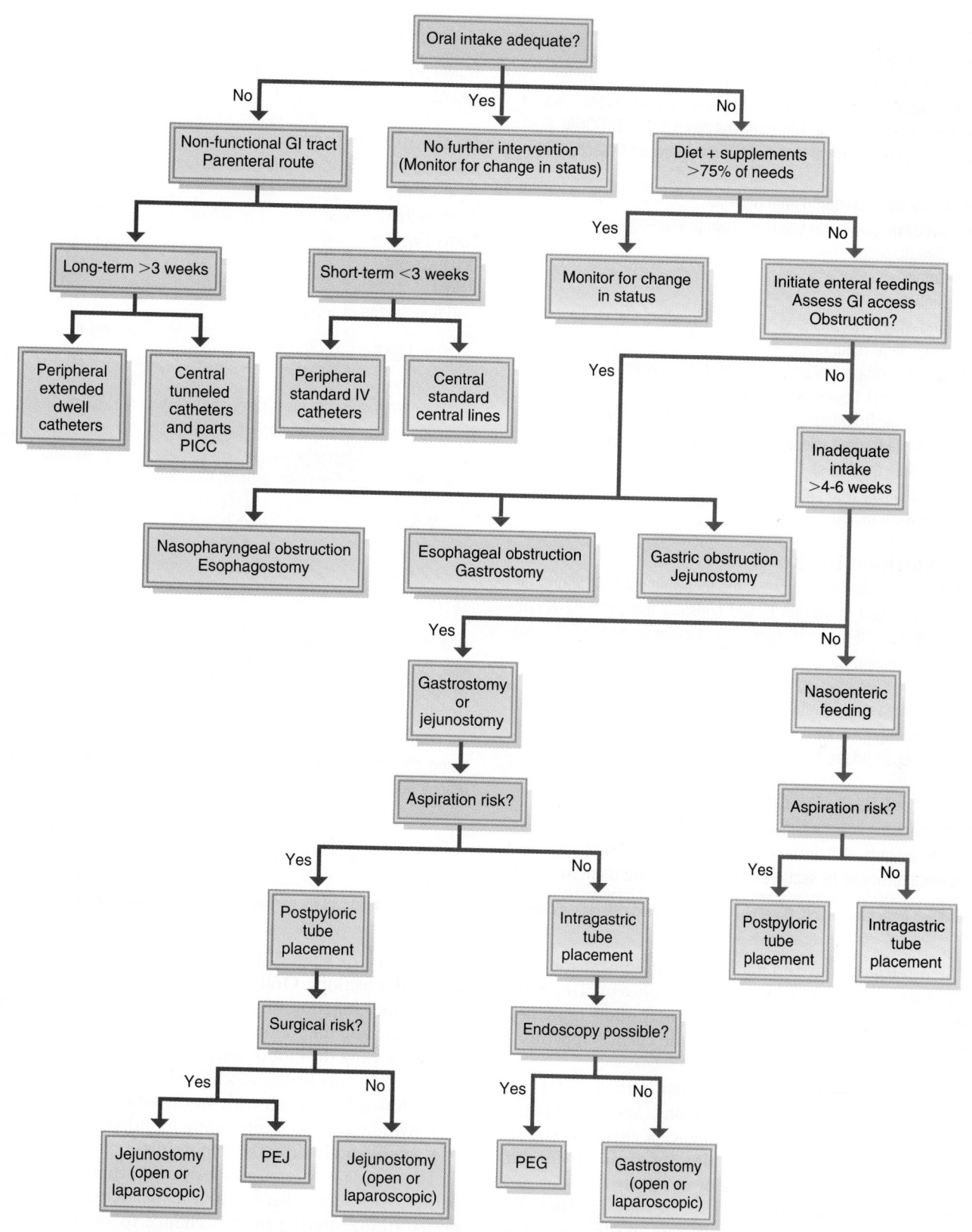

FIGURE 31-1 Algorithm to determine appropriate route of feeding. *PICC*, Peripherally inserted central catheter; *PEG*, percutaneous endoscopic gastrostomy; *PEJ*, percutaneous endoscopic jejunostomy. (Data from Mahan, L.K., & Escott-Stump, S.E. [2000]. *Krause's food, nutrition, & diet therapy* [10th ed., p. 467]. Philadelphia: W.B. Saunders; modified and adapted from Gorman R.C., Morris, J.B. [1997]. Minimally invasive access to the gastrointestinal tract. In J.L. Rombeau & R.H. Rolandelli [Eds.], *Clinical nutrition: Enteral and tube feeding* [p. 174]. Philadelphia: W.B. Saunders.)

BOX 31-1   *Features of the Admission Nutrition Screening Tool*

A. Diagnosis

If the client has one or more of the following conditions, circle it, proceed to section E, and consider the client AT NUTRITIONAL RISK. If the client has none of these conditions, proceed to section B.

- Anorexia nervosa/bulimia nervosa
- Cachexia (temporal wasting, muscle wasting, cancer, cardiac disease)
- Coma
- Diabetes
- End-stage liver disease
- End-stage renal disease
- Malabsorption (celiac sprue, ulcerative colitis, Crohn's disease, short-bowel syndrome)
- Major gastrointestinal surgery within the past year
- Multiple trauma (closed-head injury, penetrating trauma, multiple fractures)
- Nonhealing wounds
- Pressure ulcers

B. Nutrition Intake History

If the client has one or more of the following manifestations, circle it, proceed to section E, and consider the client AT NUTRITIONAL RISK. If the client has none of these manifestations, proceed to section C.

- Diarrhea (>500 ml for 2 days)
- Vomiting (> 5 days)
- Reduced intake (<½ normal intake for more than 5 days)

C. Ideal Body Weight Standards

Compare the client's current weight for height to a chart of ideal body weights. If the client weighs less than 80% of ideal body weight, proceed to section E and consider the client AT NUTRITIONAL RISK. If the client weighs more than 80% of ideal body weight, proceed to section D.

D. Weight History

Any recent unplanned weight loss? No _____ Yes _____
    Amount _____ (lb or kg)
If yes, within the past _____ weeks or _____ months
Current weight _____
Usual weight _____
Height _____
Find percentage of weight loss:

$$\frac{\text{Usual wt} - \text{Current wt}}{\text{Usual wt}} \times 100 = \underline{\hspace{1cm}}\% \text{ wt loss}$$

Compare the percentage of weight lost with the values on the following chart; circle the applicable value.

Length of Time	Significant (%)	Severe (%)
1 wk	1-2	>2
2-3 wk	2-3	>3
1 mo	4-5	>5
3 mo	7-8	>8
5+ mo	10	>10

If the client has experienced a significant or severe weight loss, proceed to section E and consider the client AT NUTRITIONAL RISK.

E. Nurse Assessment

Using the above criteria, what is this client's nutritional risk? (check one)

_____ LOW NUTRITIONAL RISK
_____ AT NUTRITIONAL RISK

Modified from Kovacevich, D., et al. (1997). Nutrition risk classification: A reproducible and valid tool for nurses. *Nutrition in Clinical Practice, 12,* 22.

icated refrigeration and microwave equipment for client and family use may encourage the families to bring foods that are appealing to the client and may allow more flexible mealtimes that coincide with the client's appetite.

Increase Appetite. Appetite is often impaired in a hospital setting for a variety of reasons. Several strategies can be used to maximize or enhance a client's desire for food. First, you can create a pleasant environment during mealtime. Clear the area of unsightly bedpans, urinals, suctioning equipment, and dressing supplies. Ensure adequate pain reduction before meals, and avoid invasive procedures or pulmonary treatments just before a meal. Increased activity through regular exercise may also increase the client's appetite.

Appetite can be enhanced by stimulation of the senses of taste, smell, and sight. Taste alterations can occur from injury or surgery to the oral cavity, medications, and oral infections. Oral hygiene is important to support the optimal function of taste buds. Routine mouth care should include the following:

- Cleansing the mouth after each meal and at bedtime
- Using a soft-bristle toothbrush
- Rinsing the mouth with warm saline (salt water)
- Avoiding alcohol-containing mouthwash
- Avoiding glycerin and lemon juice

The aroma of prepared foods may stimulate the appetite. Although clients cannot participate in food preparation, offering them a chance to smell food before a meal may be helpful. On the other hand, noxious odors may negatively affect appetite, and should be avoided.

Let the client see the food to help stimulate appetite, position the food to make it visible, and describe the different foods. Your description is especially important for clients with visual impairment.

Increase Social Interaction. Eating is ordinarily a time for social interaction, yet clients are usually given meals in their own rooms. Creating social contact by feeding clients in a central area or encouraging family and friends to visit during mealtimes may be an option. Client care assignments should be designed so that clients requiring feeding can be assigned to the same caregiver as much as possible. As the client and caregiver develop a therapeutic relationship, the feeding becomes a more pleasurable and successful experience for both.

Minimize Sensory-Perceptual Deficits. Clients with sensory-perceptual deficits require specific nursing actions to ensure adequate food intake. Make sure the client is wearing corrective lenses, if needed, and that they fit properly. If needed, describe the food and its location on the tray. The use of different-colored trays and dishes is helpful to clients with these deficits. Arranging the food in a clock-face pattern is an easy way to orient the client to the position of various foods on the tray. Describing the position of foods is imperative for clients with visual field disturbances. Do not place foods on the client's blind side.

Minimize the Impact of Neuromuscular Impairments. Various neuromuscular impairments can make the seemingly simple task of eating difficult or impossible. The occupational therapy staff can help in planning the feeding intervention and teaching the correct use of assistive devices. For a client with physical impairment, ensure privacy, allow adequate time for eating, position the client at a 90-degree angle with the meal tray at elbow height, and provide assistive devices, such as plate guards and built-up spoons.

Minimize the Impact of Cognitive Impairments. Cognitive impairments can result in the client's misunderstanding the task of eating or being unable to complete the task because of a short attention span. If so, the client requires frequent cues and close supervision. The following nursing actions are useful steps in feeding clients with cognitive impairments:

- Create a quiet, unhurried environment.
- Explain the procedure.
- Orient the client to the purpose of feeding equipment.
- Provide frequent cues to the client (e.g., "Mrs. S, pick up the toast" or "Mr. S, chew the food in your mouth").
- Provide several small meals for clients with short attention spans.

Minimize Fatigue. Another physical factor that can affect a person's ability to feed oneself is endurance. The client may be able to start the task but becomes quickly fatigued and cannot complete it. The client's ability to maintain a level of performance is related to cardiovascular, respiratory, neurologic, and musculoskeletal function.

For a client with reduced endurance, plan rest periods before mealtimes, especially when the meal follows an activity, such as physical therapy or ambulation. Help the client conserve energy for eating by helping with meal setup, opening packages, and cutting food.

Diagnosis: Impaired Swallowing. Chewing and swallowing dysfunction are frequent additional reasons for difficulties in eating. The client may experience malnutrition because of problems with swallowing. In this case, an appropriate nursing diagnosis is *Impaired Swallowing related to neuromuscular impairment (decreased or absent gag reflex), mechanical obstruction (edema, tracheostomy tube, tumor), fatigue, or limited awareness.*

Outcomes. The client will be able to freely swallow solids or liquids and will not experience any aspiration problems.

Interventions

Use a Team Approach. A team approach has been successful in the management of clients with swallowing impairments. Physicians, physical and occupational therapists, and speech pathologists can be helpful in addition to nurses in localizing the impairment and suggesting useful strategies. You must also understand the complexity of normal swallowing mechanisms in order to plan appropriate interventions.

Assess Swallowing. Take the following four steps before feeding a client to assess his or her readiness:

- Assess level of consciousness; the client must be alert.
- Assess the client's gag reflex by tickling the back of the throat.
- Have the client produce an audible cough.
- Have the client produce a voluntary swallow.

Implement Swallowing Techniques. Feeding should take place in a calm, adequately supervised environment. Place the client in a normal eating position with the feeder clearly visible. Some clients may have trouble moving the food bolus from the front to the back of the mouth. Food should be placed in the unaffected side of the mouth. If the tongue is damaged or impaired, assistive devices, such as adapted feeding syringes, can move food toward the pharynx, where the swallowing reflex (if intact) takes over.

Once the food bolus arrives at the pharynx, the client should tilt his or her chin down to decrease the risk of aspiration. Massaging the throat on the affected side helps stimulate the tactile areas that initiate the swal-

BRIDGE TO HOME HEALTH CARE
Managing Swallowing Difficulties

Swallowing difficulty (dysphagia) can vary in severity and duration. It can be mild to severe, short term (acute), or long term (chronic).

When you feed clients who have dysphagia, use good observational skills and plenty of communication and patience. Observe their responses to what you are doing. They may frown, spit, clamp their jaws together, or cough when food choices are not appealing. Try to adapt meals to their tastes. For example, if a client enjoys bananas, then dice, mash, or blend them into a shake, or even freeze them to offer variety; select the consistency that your client tolerates best.

Promote use of the sense organs during mealtime. Encourage your clients to think or talk about their favorite foods before meals to stimulate saliva flow and to aid in chewing. Ask clients to close their eyes and to visualize tasting and chewing these foods. Provide mouth care before and after the client eats meals and swallows medications to keep the mouth and breath fresh and facilitate saliva production. If your clients find it pleasurable, have them watch the food being prepared, smell the food cooking, and participate in the meal preparation as much as possible. Use an activity such as folding napkins to begin involvement. Play the client's favorite music tapes during mealtime.

The home health nurse should schedule shared visits periodically with the speech or occupational therapist to promote continuity of care. Discuss strategies related to mealtime and food preparation. Work with the therapists to help clients strengthen their mouth muscles by practicing pushing their lips or "puckering," humming, or whistling. Demonstrate the techniques you are trying to teach; hold a mirror so that clients can see their own mouth.

A high Fowler's position with 90-degree flexion of the hips is usually the best position for mealtime. Position your client with shoulders back and torso erect. Slightly flexing the client's head forward may aid in swallowing. Placing a pillow at the lower back and a towel roll behind the neck can facilitate a smooth flow of food from the mouth into the stomach. Observe your clients closely to see which position makes them most comfortable. Cushions, pillows, or bedrolls are used to support any dependent limbs or "weak" sides. Increasing physical comfort decreases distraction and allows more focus on eating.

Maintaining the high Fowler's position, with at least 75- to 80-degree flexion at the hips for at least 30 minutes after a meal, helps reduce reflux and aspiration. Check your client's mouth carefully for lingering food pockets that may become dislodged and cause aspiration long after the meal. For your safety, never place your unprotected fingers in the client's mouth when teeth or dentures are in place.

Close observation, good communication, and a sense of humor will keep mealtime pleasurable for your client and you.

---

lowing reflex. If the client has difficulty coordinating chewing, breathing, and swallowing, instruct the client to hold his or her head forward and to hold breath before swallowing.

Watch the thyroid cartilage to see whether the client has swallowed, and inspect his or her mouth before placing more food in the oral cavity. Allowing sufficient time between each mouthful helps ensure that the client adequately chews and swallows the food. Stay alert for signs that the client is becoming fatigued, restless, or agitated. Keep suction equipment available in case of an emergency. Also, know how to perform the Heimlich maneuver to prevent choking.

See the Bridge to Home Health Care feature on Managing Swallowing Difficulties, above.

■ Medical Management of the Client Receiving Enteral Nutrition

Enteral Nutrition. Total enteral nutrition (TEN) or tube feeding refers to a method of infusing nutrient solutions or formulas directly into the GI tract through tubes that enter through the nose, mouth, or abdominal wall. Enteral nutrition is indicated when the client has impaired ingestion but normal intestinal absorption.

Common indications for enteral nutrition are listed in Box 31-2. Enteral feeding is contraindicated in clients with complete intestinal obstruction, severe ileus or pseudo-obstruction, severe diarrhea, intestinal ischemia, severe acute pancreatitis, or malabsorption syndrome. In clients with impairments of the proximal GI tract, from fistulae or tumor, enteral feeding may be used if the tip of the tube is positioned distal to the impairment.

In clients with adequate GI tract function, *enteral* rather than *parenteral* nutrition should be used. One of the most important benefits of enteral nutrition relates to the importance of using the GI tract to maintain and support gut integrity and function and prevent atrophy of the gut mucosa. The protection offered by using the GI tract can result in a reduction of infectious complications.[2,13,14,21] Other factors that make enteral therapy desirable include reduced cost and safer administration.

The enteral feeding prescription is guided by the nutritional assessment and the definition of nutrient goals for calories and protein. The selection of an enteral for-

Modified from Guenter, P., et al. (1997). Delivery systems and administration of enteral nutrition. In J. Rombeau & R. Rolandelli (Eds.), *Clinical nutrition: Enteral and tube feeding* (3rd ed., p. 240). Philadelphia: W.B. Saunders.

BOX 31-2   *Indications for Enteral Feeding*

Neurologic and Psychiatric

Anorexia nervosa
Stroke
Demyelinating disease
Failure to thrive
Inflammation
Cancer
Severe depression
Trauma

Oropharyngeal and Esophageal

Inflammation
Cancer
Trauma

Gastrointestinal

Fistula (not mid-gut)
Mild inflammatory bowel disease
Mild malabsorption
Mild pancreatitis
Preoperative bowel preparation
Short-bowel syndrome (later stages)

Miscellaneous

Acquired immunodeficiency syndrome (AIDS)
Burns
Chemotherapy
Organ transplantation
Radiation therapy

mula is based on the client's nutrient needs, the absorptive function of the GI tract, the fluid status, and the level of stress. More than 100 enteral formulas are available; most can be placed into one of the following three classifications:

- *Standard formula:* contains intact (nonhydrolyzed) protein; provides 1 to 2 kcal/ml, variable protein, electrolyte, and fiber content.
- *Predigested semi-elemental formula:* contains hydrolyzed protein in the form of dipeptides, tripeptides, or amino acids. These products are designed for clients with limited digestive function.
- *Disease-specific formula:* enhances specific organ function (e.g., kidneys, liver, pulmonary system, or immune system) for clients with organ failure.

Table 31-4 outlines the classification of enteral products and includes brief descriptions of formula characteristics. Standard formulas, which contain 1 kcal/ml, are used most often. Concentrated calorie-dense formulas, which contain 1.5 to 2 kcal/ml, are helpful for clients who are fluid-restricted or unable to tolerate high volumes of formula. High-protein formulas contain more than 50 g/L of protein and are useful for critically ill clients who are hypercatabolic and have a proportionally lower calorie and fluid need with high protein requirements. The addition of fiber to standard formulas can help regulate bowel function and prevent diarrhea and constipation.

Enteral formulas provide the RDA of vitamins and trace elements based on an intake of 1500 to 2000 calories/day. Clients receiving lower-calorie regimens may require supplemental vitamins during extended enteral nutrition.

The daily fluid needs of the client receiving enteral nutrition must be calculated to avoid overhydration or underhydration. The most vulnerable client is the one receiving a calorie-dense or concentrated formula, which contains less free water than that in a standard formula. Such a client may require additional water delivered as an intermittent flush or bolus throughout the day to meet fluid needs. A client with excessive GI losses may also require supplemental water to maintain hydration.

Enteral Access. Enteral feeding requires the administration of a liquid solution through a tube into the GI tract. Enteral nutrients can be delivered into the stomach (intragastrically) or into the small intestine (duodenally or jejunally). Selection of the type of enteral access device depends on the functional status of the GI tract, the risk for aspiration, and the estimated length of therapy. Figure 31-2 depicts the various types of enteral access placements.

The functional status of the client's GI tract often defines the site of feeding. Resections, obstructions, motility disorders, or fistulae of the upper GI tract necessitate that the client be fed into the small bowel, distal to the impairment. A client who has aspirated or is at risk for aspiration may benefit from postpyloric feeding. The duration of enteral therapy defines the type of tube placed: temporary tubes for short-term therapy (<4 to 6 weeks) and permanent tubes for long-term therapy (>4 to 6 weeks).

For short-term feeding, nasogastric or nasoenteric tubes are preferred. Tubes varying in length and ranging in size from 5F to 16F are placed into the stomach or small intestine at the bedside, and the tip position is then verified with an abdominal radiograph. The smaller diameter tubes (<10F), however, are susceptible to blockage with formula and medication administration, and require frequent flushing and feeding pump administration of formula. If postpyloric feeding is indicated, the tip of the tube can be advanced under fluoroscopy, or via endoscopy, client positioning, or the administration of prokinetic agents (e.g., cisapride, metoclopramide, or erythromycin). Small-bore enteral feeding tubes are made of

TABLE 31-4   *Classification of Enteral Nutrition Products*

Classification	Formula Characteristics	Sample Products
Intact protein blenderized	Isotonic; nutritionally complete; containing fiber; lactose and lactose-free	Compleat Modified Formula Compleat Regular Formula, Vitaneed,
Low-residue standard protein	Isotonic; nutritionally complete; lactose-free	Entrition 1.0, Isocal, Isolan, Isosource, Osmolite, Resource
Intermediate, high-protein	Isotonic; nutritionally complete; lactose-free	Entrition 1.0, Isocal HN, Isosource HN, Osmolite HN
Concentrated	Calorically dense (1.5-2.0 cal/ml); lactose-free; nutritionally complete; hyperosmolar	Isocal HCN, Magnacal, TwoCal HN, Nutren 2.0
Fiber-supplemented	Isotonic; nutritionally complete; lactose-free; fiber range, 5-14 g/L; standard to intermediate protein	Fibersource, Jevity, Fiberlan, Ultracal
Disease-specific renal (pre-dialysis)	Low protein and standard protein; low-mineral, vitamin A, and vitamin D content; lactose-free; calorically dense; hyperosmolar	Suplena
Glucose-intolerant	Low-carbohydrate, high-fat; lactose-free; isotonic; containing fiber; nutritionally complete	Glucerna
Pulmonary	Low-carbohydrate, high-fat; lactose-free; nutritionally complete; hyperosmolar; calorically dense	Nutrivent, Pulmocare, Respalor
Trauma/stress	High-protein; isotonic to hyperosmolar; lactose-free; nutritionally complete; some containing fiber, hydrolyzed protein, supplemental amino acids (BCAA, arginine, glutamine), and β-carotene; low-fat	AlitraQ, Impact, Impact w/Fiber, Immun-Aid, Isotein HN, Promote, Replete, Replete w/Fiber, TraumaCal
Hydrolyzed protein, very-low-fat	Nutritionally complete; lactose-free, fewer than 10% of calories from fat; hyperosmolar, varying in peptide length; containing amino acids	Accupep HPF, Criticare HN, Vital High Nitrogen
Low-fat	Nutritionally complete; lactose-free, 11%-30% of calories from fat; hyperosmolar; varying in peptide length; containing amino acids	Travasorb HN, Travasorb STD
Moderate-fat	Nutritionally complete; lactose-free, 30%-35% of calories from fat (high MCT); hyperosmolar, varying in peptide length; containing amino acids	Peptamen, Reabilan
Disease-specific; trauma	Nutritionally complete; lactose-free, intermediate to high in protein content; 25%-35% of calories from fat (high MCT); varying in peptide length; containing amino acids; sometimes containing supplemental arginine and β-carotene	Perative, Reabilan HN
Crystalline amino acids	Nutritionally complete; lactose-free, low-fat (1%-3% of total calories); low protein to standard protein content; hyperosmolar	Tolerex, Vivonex T.E.N.
Disease-specific; hepatic failure	High BCAA; nutritionally incomplete; lactose-free; low-fat	NutriHep
Renal failure (with dialysis)	Essential and nonessential amino acids; nutritionally incomplete but containing water-soluble vitamins; hyperosmolar; lactose-free; low-fat	Nepro

Modified from Hopkins, B. (1994). Enteral nutrition products. In G. Zaloga (Ed.), *Nutrition in critical care*. St. Louis: Mosby.
MCT, Medium-chain triglyceride; *BCAA*, branched-chain amino acid.

Nasoenteric Routes
───── Nasogastric
─ ─ ─ Nasoduodenal
●●●●● Nasojejunal

Nasogastric tube

Cervical pharyngostomy or esophagostomy

PEG (percutaneous endoscopic gastrostomy); PEG button gastrostomy

Jejunostomy; PEJ (percutaneous endoscopic jejunostomy)

FIGURE 31-2 Placements for enteral access. (From Mahan, L.K., & Escott-Stump, S.E. [2000]. *Krause's food, nutrition, & diet therapy* [10th ed., p. 468]. Philadelphia: W.B. Saunders.)

polyurethane or silicone plastic and are thus softer and more flexible than a standard nasogastric tube used for decompression.

For long-term enteral feeding, gastrostomy and jejunostomy tubes are indicated. These tubes can be placed surgically, endoscopically, or radiologically. Surgically placed devices (gastrostomy or jejunostomy tubes) are used most commonly in clients undergoing a laparotomy, and general anesthesia is required. More recently, the percutaneous endoscopic gastrostomy (PEG) or jejunostomy (PEJ) approach has become the most common method of placing a permanent long-term feeding device. This nonsurgical approach avoids the need for general anesthesia and can be performed on an outpatient basis.

Table 31-5 describes various enteral feeding devices and their indications. Various GI tubes and their placement and management are discussed in Chapters 32 and 33.

Methods of Administration. Enteral feeding can be administered by either an *intermittent* or *continuous* drip. The method of delivery is determined by (1) the location of the tube tip and (2) the client's tolerance. When the tube tip is located in the small intestine, continuous feeding is the desired choice. For gastric feedings, the type of administration can be (1) bolus, (2) intermittent, or (3) continuous.

In *intermittent* or *bolus* feedings, 300 to 500 ml of enteral formula is delivered several times per day. Bolus feedings are usually delivered in 60-ml increments via a syringe over 10 to 15 minutes.

In *intermittent* feeding, formula is placed into a gravity bag and dripped in over 30 to 60 minutes. An infusion pump may also be used. Intermittent feeding is a more common method than bolus feeding to deliver periodic feedings into the stomach in the acute care setting because of improved tolerance.

Continuous feedings are administered via an infusion pump to more closely control the rate of infusion. The feedings are generally infused over 24 hours at rates ranging from 50 to 150 ml. As clients are switched to cycled nocturnal feedings in preparation for discharge, they often require and can tolerate continuous rates slightly greater than 150 ml/hr. However, clients usually cannot tolerate continuous feeding into the small intestine at rates greater than 200 ml/hr.

Continuous feeding into the stomach has been associated with less gastric distention and aspiration compared with bolus or intermittent feeding into the stomach.[14,17,21,30,39] In addition, continuous gastric feedings may reduce metabolic complications and protect against stress ulcers more effectively compared with intermittent gastric feedings.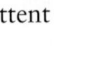

■ Nursing Management of the Client Receiving Enteral Nutrition
Assessment

In addition to the nutritional assessment measures described earlier, you should review the type of formula being used; the time, frequency, and amount of feeding; the client's specific indications; and the placement and patency of the tube. Monitor the client for aspiration of tube feeding or GI contents.

See the Bridge to Home Health Care feature on Managing Tube Feedings on p. 703.

Diagnosis, Outcomes, Interventions

Diagnosis: Imbalanced Nutrition: Less Than Body Requirements. The nursing diagnosis most appropriate for the client receiving enteral feeding is *Imbalanced Nutrition: Less Than Body Requirements related to difficulty swallowing, esophageal or gastric resection or ob-*

TABLE 31-5 *Enteral Access Devices*

Enteral Access	Tube Size and Length	Indications	Advantages	Disadvantages
Nasogastric (small-bore feeding tube)	8-12F, 17-36 inches	Functional stomach; Upper gastrointestinal tract obstruction; Dysphagia to solids; Not at risk for aspiration	Placed at bedside; Low morbidity; Easily inserted; Continued use of GI tract	Client discomfort; Risk of aspiration
Nasoduodenal	14-18F, 35-45 inches	Gastric atony; Risk of aspiration	Decreased risk of aspiration; Continued use of GI tract	Client discomfort; Difficult placement; Easily malpositioned
Nasojejunal	14-18F, 36-45 inches	High risk for pulmonary aspiration of gastric contents; Functional small bowel	Decreased risk of aspiration; Continued use of GI tract	Increased cost of tube and skilled professional to place tube; Easily malpositioned
Gastrostomy, surgical	14-30F	Inability to use percutaneous placement; GI surgery; Long-term feeding	Continued use of GI tract; Can be placed in clients with esophageal or pharyngeal cancers; Used in obese clients when unable to transilluminate abdominal wall for PEG placement	General anesthesia; Tube migration; Easily obstructed; Local stoma site complications
Gastrostomy, percutaneous	14-22F	Long-term feeding tube; No history of aspiration	No surgical procedure needed; Placement without general anesthesia; Continued use of GI tract	Potential for aspiration; Cannot be used in obese clients
Low-profile gastrostomy device (G-Button)	18-28F	Long-term feeding; Ambulatory patients; Disoriented patients who pull at gastrostomy tube	Increased mobility; Decreased cost over time because of device longevity; Decreased nursing time compared with time needed for replacement tube change; Continued use of GI tract	Skilled professional needed for placement; Increased trauma to client compared with replacement tube; Increased cost compared with cost of gastrostomy tube change; Second procedure required after gastrostomy tube placement
Jejunostomy, temporary	5F; Jejunostomy kit, 14F	Short-term enteral nutrition; Usually ≤2 weeks	Continued use of GI tract	Surgical placement; Tube easily obstructed; Costly
Jejunostomy, permanent	Whistle tip, 14-18F	Long-term jejunal feeding	Silicone plastic; Continued use of GI tract; Easily replaced when fistulous tract is formed; Larger-bore; Location proximal jejunum, thus elemental products not required	Continuous or slow intermittent tube feeding required via a pump
Combination tubes for gastric decompression	Gastric port, 16-30F; Jejunal feeding port, 9F	Long-term feeding; Dysfunctional stomach; Functional small bowel; Short-term postoperative care	Can decompress a dysfunctional stomach and prevent regurgitation of gastric contents during small intestine feeding; Continued use of GI tract	Skilled professional needed for placement; Expensive process; Jejunal feeding needed; Can be dislodged from original position; Placed during surgery

Modified from Shuster, M., & Mancino, J. (1994). Ensuring successful home tube feeding in the geriatric population. *Geriatric Nursing, 15*, 67-82.

BRIDGE TO HOME HEALTH CARE

Managing Tube Feedings

Home health agency nutrition support teams usually consist of a nurse, a registered dietitian, and a pharmacist. When these professionals regularly visit a client who has a new feeding tube, the chances for successfully managing the client and the tube feedings at home are greatly increased. In addition to providing direct care, the team provides instructions to the client and family, communicates with the client's physician, prevents problems if possible, and monitors any problems that develop.

Consistently flushing the tube with water before and after each feeding enhances the longevity of the tube. Although flushing the tube with carbonated beverages has been suggested, studies indicate few or no benefits over flushing with water. Flush all types of feeding tubes with a 50-ml syringe; smaller syringes can create pressure high enough to rupture a tube.

Teach the client and family to secure a nasogastric tube firmly to the nose and to either side of the face or to another position of comfort. To secure the tube, use tape, a transparent occlusive dressing, or a commercial tube holder with a hydrocolloid backing with a self-fastening tape (Velcro) closure.

When the client has a percutaneous endoscopic gastrostomy (PEG) or a percutaneous endoscopic jejunostomy (PEJ), observe daily for tube dislodgment, leaking, skin irritation, and clinical manifestations of infection. Clean the site daily with mild soap and water. Slide the external bridge away for cleaning, then reposition. No dressing is required. Good hand-washing technique is essential for all personnel.

Management of tube feedings varies with the type of infusion: continuous infusion with a pump, bolus infusion, or infusion by gravity. Numerous commercial products are available to meet the client's nutritional needs. The physician and the registered dietitian are responsible for assessing the type of feeding and method of infusion. However, the client may tolerate one formula better than another. Positioning clients at a 45-degree angle or greater helps them tolerate the feeding. Changing the rate and frequency of infusion may decrease or eliminate nausea, diarrhea, or tube displacement. Successful tube feeding begins in the hospital and continues at home as the client, family, home care nurse, registered dietitian, pharmacist, and physician work together as a team.

---

struction, or inability to ingest adequate calories and nutrients.

Outcomes. The client will maintain ideal body weight or will gain 1 to 2 pounds per week until ideal body weight is attained.

Interventions

Prevent Contamination of Formula and Delivery System. You are primarily responsible for administering and monitoring enteral feeding. The care and handling of the feeding formula and equipment is a key factor in the success of enteral feeding. To prevent contamination of the enteral formula, you must adhere to strict hand-washing before handling the feeding formula and equipment. *Open delivery systems,* which use cans, syringes, and bags, are the most vulnerable to contamination because of the great degree of manipulation. Formulas administered via an open system should hang for only 4 hours before being changed and the tubing flushed or rinsed. The equipment should be changed every 24 hours. *Closed delivery systems,* which use a prefilled container with sterile contents, minimize the preparation required by nurses before; thus the chance of formula contamination is reduced and the hang time is extended (24 to 48 hours).

Assess Tube Location. Before administering an enteral feeding, ensure that the tube is positioned properly. If a nasoenteric tube is being used to feed a client for the first time, make sure that an abdominal radiograph has verified that the tip is located in the GI tract.

Routinely evaluate the position of the enteral feeding device, and be alert for the possibility of tube migration or dislodgment. Nasoenteric tubes can be marked to indicate the position so that it will be evident if the tube has moved. Nasoenteric tubes can easily migrate when the client coughs or vomits, but more often the tubes are dislodged when a confused or agitated client inadvertently removes the tube.

In addition to determining whether the tube has migrated, you may need to evaluate the location of the tube tip. Is the tube tip in the stomach, small intestine, or respiratory tract? Four methods can be used to evaluate tip location:

- *Auscultation:* injecting air into the feeding tube and listening with a stethoscope for the sound
- *Aspiration:* observing the fluid that is removed through the feeding tube
- *pH paper testing:* checking the pH of the fluid removed from the feeding tube
- *Radiography:* checking the abdominal x-ray film for tube position

Auscultation is the least reliable method and should not be used to evaluate the tube tip position. Observing the aspirated fluid and checking its pH are more useful. However, aspiration should not replace a radiographic evaluation after the initial placement or when tube migration is suspected.

An enterostomy (e.g., gastrostomy, jejunostomy) tube can migrate in or out if it is not properly secured at the exit site with sutures or a tube attachment device. Enteral feeding tubes that are not well secured at the exit site can pivot, causing an accumulation of granulation tissue and a widening of the tract. If the tract becomes widened, formula and digestive enzymes can come up through it and excoriate the skin on the abdomen.

Administer Feedings. Starter regimens for enteral feedings differ according to tube tip location and the client's clinical status. Continuous feedings into the small intestine are usually started at 30 to 40 ml/hr and advanced as tolerated every 12 to 24 hours until the daily goal is reached. Intermittent feedings into the stomach are initiated at 100 to 120 ml every 4 hours and advanced every 12 to 24 hours as tolerated.

Prevent Aspiration. Preventing aspiration during enteral feeding is crucial. The use of postpyloric or small bowel feeding is recommended for a client with a high risk of aspiration. Proper administration and delivery techniques are especially important during gastric feedings. The head of the bed must be elevated 45 degrees for 1 hour before, during, and 1 hour after gastric feeding. Continuous gastric feedings require that the head of the client's bed remain elevated. Gastric residuals can be monitored every 4 hours initially and then as needed to assess gastric emptying and to prevent aspiration. A significant gastric residual is approximately 150 ml, but the volume can be more or less depending on the volumes and rates infused. Feeding into the jejunum theoretically reduces the risk of aspirating enteral formula, particularly for clients with any gastric resection. However, the head of the bed should still be elevated about 30 degrees during continuous jejunal feeding. The addition of blue dye to the enteral feeding should be discouraged. Recent case reports have documented systemic absorption of the dye in critically ill clients.[27]

Maintain Enteral Access. Maintenance of enteral access consists of caring for the external site, maintaining tube patency, and maintaining the correct tube position. Nasoenteric tubes most often exit the nose and are secured to the nose or cheek with tape or an adhesive attachment device. The nasoenteric tube should exit the nose, hang straight down, and then be gently looped up and secured to the cheek. Tubes that are sharply angled as they exit the nostril can cause necrosis or obstruct the flow of enteral formula through the tube. With any method of securing, the tube should be repositioned and resecured at least every other day to prevent skin irritation.

For tubes that exit the abdominal wall (e.g., PEG, gastrostomy, and jejunostomy tubes), a dressing is required for the first 24 hours after placement. The site care con-

sists of a daily cleaning with mild soap and rinsing with warm water. Dressings are optional for healed enterostomy sites, but a light nonocclusive dressing may help secure the tube as well as contain mucus that commonly drains from the tube tract.

Maintaining the patency of the enteral feeding tube is a critical nursing intervention for the client receiving enteral feeding. Enteral feeding tubes clog for a variety of reasons, the most common of which is the improper administration of medications through the tube. Medication administration via enteral feeding tubes is probably the most poorly understood part of working with enteral feeding devices and thus is highly susceptible to error. Medications should be given through an enteral access device only when there is an absolute contraindication to taking them by mouth. Problems that can result from incorrect medication administration via an enteral feeding tube include tube clogging, altered drug availability, and diarrhea. If a client has two tubes in place, such as a gastric tube for decompression and a jejunal or duodenal tube for feeding, consider whether medications could be delivered via the larger gastric tube, as long as the client can tolerate ½ hour of postmedication tube clamping. Box 31-3 lists steps to follow for safe administration of medications via an enteral feeding tube.

Tubes of any diameter clog without strict adherence to a flushing protocol. The most effective irrigant for flushing an enteral feeding tube is water. Flush the tube with at least 30 ml of warm water every 4 hours during continuous feedings and before and after each intermittent feeding or medication. Acidic flushing solutions, such as cranberry juice, may precipitate with protein and **EB** obstruct the tube; thus they are not recommended.[13]

See the Management and Delegation feature on Care of Nasogastric Tubes, Small-Bore Feeding Tubes, and Gastrostomy and Jejunostomy Tubes on p. 705.

BOX 31-3 *Guidelines for the Administration of Medications via an Enteral Feeding Tube*

- If possible, administer the medication by mouth.
- Use a liquid form of the medication if available.
- If the medication can be crushed, crush it to a fine powder and dissolve it in 30 ml of water.
- Do not crush enteric-coated or time-released tablets or capsules.
- Flush the tube with 30 ml of water before and after giving each medication.
- Do not mix multiple medications or give them together.
- Do not deliver a medication into the small intestine if it must be absorbed in the stomach, such as sucralfate (Carafate) or antacids.
- Hold feedings 1 to 2 hours before and after giving a medication that might have drug-nutrient interactions, such as phenytoin (Dilantin).

■ Medical Management of the Client Receiving Parenteral Nutrition

Parenteral Nutrition (PN). PN is indicated to maintain nutritional status and prevent malnutrition when the client has inadequate intestinal function or cannot be fed orally or by tube feeding. Box 31-4 outlines common indications for the use of parenteral nutrition.

The PN prescription is guided by the nutritional assessment and the definition of nutrient goals for calories and protein. The PN solution contains carbohydrates as glucose, fat as triglyceride, and protein as amino acids at

MANAGEMENT AND DELEGATION

Care of Nasogastric Tubes, Small-Bore Feeding Tubes, and Gastrostomy and Jejunostomy Tubes

Nasogastric Tubes

Decompression relieves stomach pressure by removing gas and fluids from the stomach. It can be used to prevent nausea, vomiting, and gastric distention when gastrointestinal (GI) motility is delayed or absent, or when the client has a distal obstruction or recent GI tract surgery. Nasogastric tubes may also be used to initiate enteral feedings upon resumption of bowel motility.

The detailed assessment and potential risks associated with nasogastric tube insertion, maintenance, and removal prevent delegation of these procedures to unlicensed personnel. You may delegate the gathering of equipment and the measurement, recording, and testing of nasogastric drainage to assistive personnel. Delegation of short-term disconnection of nasogastric tubes (for the purposes of toileting or ambulation) may be appropriate under the supervision of a registered nurse (RN). Reconnection of the nasogastric tube to suction requires the RN to verify pressure settings. You may delegate skin care of the client's nose and oral hygiene to unlicensed personnel.

Nasogastric Tubes: Mouth and Nose Care

Instruct assistive personnel to:
1. Wash hands and don gloves.
2. For nasal care:
   a. Gently clean and lubricate the client's external nares to prevent buildup of crusted secretions and skin breakdown.
   b. Use a clean cotton-tipped swab and a water-soluble lubricant to clean the client's nostril.
   c. Make sure that the skin on the client's nose is clean and dry.
   d. Apply tincture of benzoin or other skin adhesive on the tip of the client's nose and allow to dry.
   e. Secure tube with hypoallergenic tape, taking care to avoid pressure on nares.
3. For mouth care:
   a. Offer or administer frequent oral hygiene with non–alcohol-containing solutions to remove debris, increase comfort, and maintain a healthy oral cavity.
   b. Brush client's teeth or assist client in doing so.

Small-Bore Feeding Tubes and Gastrostomy and Jejunostomy Tubes

The most desirable and appropriate method of providing nutrition is via the oral route. For clients who are unable to meet their nutritional needs orally, enteral tube feedings may be an option. Tube-feedings may be delivered through large-bore or small-bore gastric tubes that may be inserted by the RN with a physician's order, through gastrostomy tubes, or through jejunostomy tubes. A gastrostomy tube is large and is surgically or endoscopically placed directly into the stomach, exiting through an incision in the left upper quadrant of the abdomen. A jejunostomy tube is also placed surgically (directly into the jejunum for small bowel feedings), or endoscopically (into the gastrostomy tube and passed through to the jejunum).

A physician's order is required for placement of a small-bore nasogastric or nasointestinal feeding tube. Accuracy of feeding tube placement is confirmed by abdominal radiograph. Insertion of nasogastric tubes and verification of placement of nasogastric, gastrostomy, and jejunostomy tubes require problem-solving and knowledge application unique to the professional nurse. For this reason, delegation of these skills is inappropriate. You may delegate skin care of the exit site of the tube to unlicensed personnel.

Gastrostomy and Jejunostomy Exit Site Care

Exit site care is performed 24 hours after feeding tube insertion. Instruct assistive personnel to:
1. Wash hands and don gloves.
2. Remove the old dressing.
3. Clean around the tube insertion site with normal saline and mild soap to remove exudate or dried blood.
4. Do not use hydrogen peroxide or any antiseptic cream unless specifically ordered by the physician.
5. Rinse the tube insertion site with clean water and dry thoroughly.
6. Apply a new split drain sponge dressing if needed.

Describe findings that are immediately reportable to you for assistive personnel, including redness, swelling, abnormal drainage (thick, foul-smelling, yellow or green color), or pain at the tube's insertion site. Have assistive personnel report any complaints of abdominal pain, bloating, cramping, or diarrhea. Verify the competence of assistive personnel in performing these tasks during orientation and annually thereafter.

BOX 31-4   *Clinical Indications for Total Parenteral Nutrition*

Malabsorptive syndromes
- Severe short-bowel syndrome
- Severe, prolonged radiation enteritis
- High-output fistulae that cannot be bypassed with small bowel enteral feeding

Motility disorders
- Persistent postoperative or disease-related ileus
- Intestinal pseudo-obstruction
- Severe persistent vomiting (as in hyperemesis gravidarum)

Intestinal obstruction
Perioperative nutrition for severe malnutrition
Critically ill client when enteral therapy is contraindicated
Low-flow state

Data from Shils, M., & Brown, R. (1999). Parenteral nutrition. In M. Shils, et al. (Eds.), *Modern nutrition in health and disease* (p. 1658). Baltimore: Williams & Wilkins.

TABLE 31-6   *Daily Electrolyte Recommendations*

Sodium	80-150 mEq	Diuretic therapy	↑
		Renal failure	↓
		Fluid overload	↓
Chloride	80-150 mEq	Gastric losses	↑
Potassium	80-100 mEq	Aggressive refeeding	↑
		Diuretic therapy	↑
		Gastrointestinal losses	↑
		Renal failure	↓
Calcium	10-20 mEq	Blood transfusions	↑
Magnesium	8-30 mEq	Aggressive refeeding	↑
		Gastrointestinal losses	↑
		Renal failure	↓
Phosphorus	15-45 mmol	Aggressive refeeding	↑
		Excessive antacid administration	↑
		Renal failure	↓
Acetate	0-60 mEq	Metabolic acidosis	↑
		Metabolic alkalosis	↓
		Sepsis	↑

From Evans, N. (1994). The role of total parenteral nutrition in critical illness: Guidelines and recommendations. In M. Ackerman, K. Puntillo, & J. Clochesy (Eds.), *Clinical issues in critical care nursing*, Philadelphia: J.B. Lippincott.
↑, Increased requirement; ↓, decreased requirement.

levels designed to meet the caloric and protein needs of the client.

Carbohydrates. Glucose usually accounts for 50% to 70% of the caloric supply. At least 100 or 150 g of glucose (350 to 500 kcal) should be given daily to prevent catabolism of muscle and to provide glucose for the brain.

Fat Emulsions. Lipid or fat emulsions generally provide about 10% to 30% of the daily caloric need. Fat emulsions (1) provide a calorie-dense (9 kcal/g fat) isotonic energy source and (2) supply fatty acids to prevent essential fatty acid deficiency.

Amino Acids. Crystalline amino acids of differing composition and a concentration varying from 3% to 15% are the source of protein in parenteral solutions. The standard commercially available solutions are a mix of essential and nonessential amino acids. Some amino acid solutions have been developed to target specific clinical problems, such as renal failure and liver failure. However, the increase in efficacy over the general amino acid solution is not conclusive, and the cost is considerably greater than for standard formulations.

Fluids, Electrolytes, Vitamins, and Trace Elements. Fluids, electrolytes, vitamins, and trace elements are all equally important in the parenteral nutrient solution. The daily electrolyte regimen should be individualized and should reflect the client's clinical condition (including any ongoing losses) and the function of major organ systems. Table 31-6 outlines recommendations for daily electrolyte requirements and situations that can result in an increased or decreased need.

Vitamins and trace elements are needed to promote optimal nutritional repletion, and they support a variety of important metabolic pathways. Multivitamin preparations contain both water-soluble and fat-soluble vitamins for daily use (Table 31-7). Vitamin K, a fat-soluble vitamin, is not contained in all of these commercial preparations and may be added to the TPN formula weekly (10 mg) or daily (1 mg). Other vitamins are sometimes added to the standard vitamin preparation, such as vitamin C to promote wound healing and vitamin B_{12}, thiamine, and folic acid to correct deficiencies commonly associated with alcohol abuse.

Guidelines for the administration of trace elements have been outlined by the American Medical Association's Nutritional Advisory Group (Table 31-8). Supplemental zinc may be indicated for clients with high-output fistulae, large wounds, or extreme catabolism.

Combination Systems. A *total nutrient admixture* (TNA) is a single-bag TPN delivery system that contains glucose, lipids, amino acids, electrolytes, vitamins, and trace elements. The main advantages of the TNA are decreased contamination from fewer manipulations of the IV delivery system, slow continuous infusion of all nutrients supplied, and the need for a single pump for de-

Vitamin	Amount Supplied
A	1 mg/3300 international units
D	5 μg/200 international units
E	10 mg/10 international units (as dl-α-tocopherol acetate)
B_1	3 mg
B_2	3.6 mg
B_3	40 mg
B_5	15 mg
B_6	4 mg
B_{12}	5 μg
C	100 mg
Biotin	60 μg
Folic acid	0.4 mg

TABLE 31-7 *Parenteral Multivitamin Supplementation**

From Galica, L. (1997). Parenteral nutrition. *Nursing Clinics of North America, 32*(4), 711.

*Roche and Astra products. Amounts of vitamins reflect the 1979 Nutritional Advisory Group recommendations of the American Medical Association.

livery. The main disadvantage is that it is more difficult to detect crystalline precipitates through the TNA and an inline filter is recommended.

Vascular Access. PN is most commonly infused into the central venous circulation, where the rapid flow of blood rapidly dilutes the concentration of the solution. In contrast, nutrient solutions infused into a peripheral vein are known as *peripheral parenteral nutrition.* Peripheral nutrition may result in caloric and nitrogen underfeeding. To avoid phlebitis of peripheral veins, it is necessary to keep the osmolarity of the solution less than 900 mOsm/kg, which may require either reduction in glucose and amino acid content or prohibitive fluid administration. Clients who have difficult peripheral venous access, particularly older adults, or those who require parenteral support for more than 5 days should not be treated with peripheral parenteral nutrition. In clients who have excessive caloric or nitrogen needs because of their illness, central access for PN is recommended.

In central vascular access, the tip of the catheter must be positioned in a high-flow vein, such as the superior or inferior vena cava. Access to this central system can be achieved through several veins, such as a peripheral vein, the jugular vein, the subclavian vein, or the femoral vein. Temporary central venous catheters are percutaneous nontunneled catheters that are best used in an acute care setting for a short time.

More recently, the peripherally inserted central venous catheter (PICC) (see Figure 19-2, C) has offered an option for long-term use. For extended therapy (>3 months), external tunneled central venous catheters or totally implanted ports are the best option (see Figures 19-2, *A* and *B*).

■ Nursing Management of the Client Receiving Parenteral Nutrition
Assessment

In addition to the nutritional assessment measures outlined earlier, you must check the infusion bag for correct ingredients and appearance of the solution, assess the condition of the venous access site, monitor blood glucose levels and the rate of infusion, and observe the client for untoward reactions to the solution.

Diagnosis, Outcomes, Interventions

Diagnosis: Imbalanced Nutrition: Less Than Body Requirements. The nursing diagnosis most appropriate for the client receiving TPN is *Imbalanced Nutrition: Less Than Body Requirements related to the need for IV delivery of nutrients, fluids, and electrolytes to maintain nutritional status secondary to malabsorption problems of the GI tract, gastric cancer, cancer cachexia, anorexia nervosa, excessive metabolic needs (as in extensive burns or draining wounds), or the need to rest the gut to promote healing (as in severe pancreatitis).*

Outcomes. The client will maintain ideal body weight or will gain 1 to 2 pounds per week until ideal body weight is attained.

TABLE 31-8 *Daily Parenteral Trace Element Supplementation*

Trace Element	AMA Guidelines	M.T.E.-4	M.T.E.-5	M.T.E.-5 Concentrate
Zinc	2.5-4.0 mg	1 mg	1 mg	5 mg
Copper	0.5-1.5 mg	0.4 mg	0.4 mg	1 mg
Manganese	0.15-0.8 mg	0.1 mg	0.1 mg	0.5 mg
Chromium	10-15 μg	4 μg	4 μg	10 μg
Selenium	20 μg	—	20 μg	60 μg

From Galica, L. (1997). Parenteral nutrition. *Nursing Clinics of North America, 32 (4)*, 711.
AMA, American Medical Association; *M.T.E.,* multiple trace elements.

Interventions

Administer PN. You are responsible for safely administering and monitoring the infusion of PN. Just before delivery, check every solution for its expiration date, the correct ingredients (glucose, fat, protein, and electrolytes), leaks or tears in the bag, and the appearance of the solution (separating or cracking of the solution). PN must be delivered using a peristaltic pump to accurately control the infusion rate and prevent the possibility of a bolus. PN solutions are typically infused over 24 hours in the acute care setting. In the home, clients often receive PN while sleeping.

Monitor Blood Glucose Levels. The first time PN is administered, blood glucose levels should be monitored every 6 hours to assess the client's response to glucose. If blood glucose is within the normal range for 24 hours, monitoring can be changed to daily. Persistent elevations of blood glucose are managed by delivering regular insulin in the PN solution after the daily requirement for insulin is determined. If the client's clinical status is unstable, the insulin dose cannot be stabilized over a 24-hour period, or both, the insulin should be delivered outside of the PN as an insulin drip or intermittent subcutaneous injections. Most clients can tolerate an acute discontinuation of PN and therefore do not need to be weaned from PN gradually.

Observe for Allergy to PN Components. Although rare, allergic reactions to lipid preparations or multivitamins have been reported and usually present within 30 minutes. A clinical manifestation of reactions can be any of the following: fever, shaking chills, shortness of breath, chest pain, back pain, or full anaphylaxis. If the client complains of any of these manifestations, stop the PN infusion immediately and inform the health care team of the manifestations to determine appropriate further treatment. If it is not necessary to rechallenge the client with PN, the risk of a more severe allergic reaction with rechallenge should be avoided.

Maintain Vascular Access. You play a pivotal role in ensuring the proper functioning of the vascular access system and preventing catheter-related infection. Maintain catheter patency by following a routine heparin flush protocol. Table 31-9 outlines the suggested protocols for central catheters that deliver TPN.

Prevent Infection. Prevention of catheter-related infection is key to the successful use of parenteral nutrition. Most infections that do occur result from contamination of the exit site or catheter hub.[6,26,35] You must follow strict guidelines or protocols for the care of the vascular access device before, during, and after its insertion. Although catheter site care is somewhat varied and is con-

TABLE 31-9 *Central Venous Catheter Maintenance*		
Catheter Type	**Site Care**	**Flushing**
Nontunneled central venous catheter	*Dressing:* Transparent or gauze Transparent dressing enhances catheter stability Performed as a sterile dressing Skin antisepsis protocols include one or a combination of the following: 70% alcohol (3 swabs), 10% povidone-iodine (3 swabs), chlorhexidine	*Internal volume:* 0.1-0.53 ml *Flush volume:* 1-2 ml *Frequency:* Usually daily
Tunneled, cuffed central venous catheter	*Dressing:* Transparent or gauze until incision healed Dressing commonly discontinued when incision healed and suture removed Performed as an aseptic dressing (skin antisepsis as above) Hydrogen peroxide may be used to remove crusting at the site	*Internal volume:* 0.15-1.8 ml *Flush volume:* 3-4 ml *Frequency:* Usually daily *Groshong catheters:* 5 ml 0.9% normal saline solution weekly
Peripherally inserted central catheter	*Dressing:* Transparent preferred to enhance catheter stability Performed as a sterile dressing (skin antisepsis as above) Dressings required as long as catheter is in place	*Internal volume:* 0.04-1.2 ml *Flush volume:* 2-3 ml *Frequency:* Daily
Ports	*Dressing:* Transparent when port is accessed to stabilize needle Sterile gauze may be placed between needle and skin Huber needle changed at least every 7 days Sterile approach needle insertion and dressing recommended (skin antisepsis as above before needle placement) Dressing remains until healed (several days postoperatively)	*Internal volume:* 0.5-1.5 ml *Flush volume:* At least 3 ml *Frequency:* Every 4 weeks

From Krzywada, E., & Edmiston, C. (1998). Parenteral access/equipment. *The ASPEN nutrition support practice manual.* Silver Spring, MD: ASPEN Board of Directors, with permission.

troversial, strict adherence to hand-washing and aseptic technique is clearly the most important way to prevent infection. Dedicate (and mark) one lumen of a multilumen catheter to the infusion of PN to minimize manipulations of the IV system. The most recent recommendations from the Centers for Disease Control and Prevention (CDC) are to change the tubing for PN solutions every 24 hours.[26,35]

Provide Dressing Changes. The dressing change protocol for central venous access devices continues to be controversial. Various protocols exist for skin cleaning and the type and frequency of dressing change. The catheter exit site should be cleaned with an antiseptic agent, such as 70% alcohol and 10% povidone-iodine. A preferred product that has shown positive results in preventing catheter-related infections is chlorhexidine.[35] Antibiotic ointments should not be applied to the catheter exit site.

The type of dressing applied over the catheter exit site should be either a sterile gauze or a transparent dressing. Frequency of dressing changes depends on client needs (e.g., more frequent changes are needed for a diaphoretic client) and the type of dressing. Gauze dressings typically are changed every 48 hours, transparent dressings every 3 to 7 days. The most important concept is that the dressing must remain adherent to be effective. Therefore any dressing must be changed immediately if it becomes damp, soiled, or loose. Follow your agency's policy regarding dressing change protocols.

Evaluation of Nutritional Interventions

When caring for a client receiving enteral or parenteral feedings, you must regularly evaluate the client's response to therapy. Assessing the client's tolerance to the nutrient regimen includes evaluation of the fluid status (intake and output data and weights) and a thorough assessment of the GI system. Evaluation also includes monitoring vital signs, reviewing laboratory tests, and assessing the function of the nutritional access device. Together with a nutritional support team, you will be collecting pertinent data, such as weight, intestinal tolerance, and pertinent laboratory values, to assess the success of the nutrient prescription.

Table 31-10 outlines common parameters used to monitor clients receiving enteral or parenteral nutrition. Comprehensive and routine monitoring can prevent complications related to nutritional support therapies.

■ Self-Care

Nutritional support therapies, such as enteral and parenteral feedings, are routinely administered in the home setting. Nurses play a pivotal role in determining appropriate candidates for home nutrition support by helping determine the plan of care and providing client and family education.

The nursing assessment includes a comprehensive review of the client and family or caregivers. The physical and cognitive abilities of the client or caregiver must be evaluated so that you can be sure of their ability to carry out complex procedures. Manual dexterity and eyesight are particularly important when care involves programming pumps for infusion and drawing up medication in syringes. The client's home environment must be evaluated to ensure that it is safe for home therapy. The client or caregiver education process should ideally start in the hospital and be reinforced after discharge. Clients receiving either enteral tube feedings or parenteral nutrition need to learn a wide range of related skills (Box 31-5).

■ EATING DISORDERS
OBESITY

Obesity is characterized by an excess accumulation of fat and reflects, on the most basic level, an overall positive balance between energy intake and expenditure. The causes of obesity are not fully understood, but are recognized as complex and pervasive.

TABLE 31-10	*Suggested Nutrition Monitoring Protocol*
Parameter	**Frequency of Assessment**
Biochemical Measures	
Electrolytes	Daily
Magnesium, calcium, phosphorus	Daily
Glucose	Every 6 hours for 48 hours, then daily
Albumin, prealbumin, transferrin	Weekly
Triglyceride	Pre-infusion, post-infusion, then daily
Liver function tests	Pre-infusion, then weekly
Complete blood count, prothrombin time, partial thromboplastin time	Weekly
Nursing Assessment	
Weight	Daily
Intake/output	Hourly/every 8 hours
Infusion rate	Every 4 hours
Temperature	Every 8 hours
Nutritional Monitoring	
24-hour urine collection for urinary urea nitrogen	Weekly
Measured resting energy expenditure	Weekly

BOX 31-5 *Teaching Topics for Clients Who Need Enteral or Parenteral Feedings at Home*

Care of the Nutritional Access Device
Flushing the venous access or feeding tube
Changing the dressing
Observing for evidence of infection

Formula Preparation
Adding medication to the TPN formula
Placing enteral formula in the feeding bag
Setting up the enteral or parenteral feeding pump or bag
Obtaining formula for TPN and related supplies

Monitoring for Complications
Assessing temperature
Monitoring weight

TPN, Total parenteral nutrition.

Definition

Obesity is defined worldwide by the body mass index (BMI):

$$BMI = Weight\ (kg)/Height\ (m^2).$$

Because BMI greater than 25 kg/m² is associated with increased prevalence of hypertension and type 2 diabetes, this level of BMI has been designated as overweight. The prevalence of chronic disease co-morbidities is increased [EB] further with BMI greater than 30 kg/m², which is defined as obesity. BMI greater than 40 kg/m² is accepted as severe obesity.[11] Obesity is a worldwide problem, and by the year 2010 obesity-associated chronic diseases, such as cardiovascular disease, type 2 diabetes, sleep apnea, and hypertension, will lead the causes of death in developing countries, far outpacing the current realities of starvation and infectious diseases.

According to the National Health and Nutrition Examination Survey's (NHANES) 2000 data, 61% of Americans are either overweight or obese, 30% are obese, and 5% are severely obese. African-American and Hispanic American women are particularly affected, out [EB] of proportion to their Caucasian counterparts. Obesity in children in the United States is also growing rampantly, with 15% of all children older than age 5 years being overweight or obese, and greater proportions of minority children than Caucasians being overweight.[36]

Etiology and Risk Factors

The etiology of obesity is multifactorial, making effective prevention and treatment a challenge. Environmental, biologic, and socioeconomic factors are currently seen as key:

1. *Environmental.* Both in the United States and by the evaluation of the World Health Organization, the environment is accepted as a key component of the burgeoning obesity epidemic. The environment impacts both the energy expenditure and the energy intake sides of the energy balance equation.

   As cultures become progressively more developed, individuals spend more time sitting (watching television, working with computers) than moving (sports, walking).[23] When the school budgets are tightened, priority is given to electronic resources such as computers and television, and sports programs are eliminated.

   Concurrently, the portion sizes of servings of food in restaurants and movie theaters have increased markedly over time, with minimal increment in cost. The end result of the combined effects of reduced energy expenditure and increased energy intake has been termed the "toxic environment," a combination that insidiously promotes weight gain.

2. *Genetic Tendency.* The broad prevalence of obesity in American culture suggests that genetic factors may be less important than previously thought. There are similarities in obesity prevalence within family units, but environment is also a common factor. Many obesity genes have been identified, but none have yet explained the broad prevalence of obesity, even in individuals with severe obesity.

   The Pima Indians of Arizona and Mexico have been used historically as an example of a group who may have a thrifty genotype. Severe obesity and type 2 diabetes are prevalent in the population of Pimas who live in Arizona, who are exposed to an inexpensive, high-calorie food supply. By contrast, those who live in Mexico, with a more traditional diet that is considerably lower in caloric content and which requires considerable expenditure of energy to produce, have much lower prevalence of obesity. These two groups have identical genetic make-up, suggesting that genetic influences may be less important than environmental influences.[33]

3. *Socioeconomic Factors.* Particularly in the United States, obesity is more prevalent in populations with lower socioeconomic status. This trend may reflect a more toxic environment in terms of energy-dense but nutrient-poor food supply and excess television watching. In poorer neighborhoods, outdoor physical activity is limited by concerns for physical safety and some efforts are underway to provide safe exercise environments in poor neighborhoods.

4. *Ethnic Disparities.* In the United States, Hispanic and African-American women are affected by obesity at greater rates than their Caucasian counterparts or men of the same ethnicity. The reasons for this phenomenon are not clear, necessitating particular sensitivity in dealing with obesity across

COMPLEMENTARY AND ALTERNATIVE THERAPY

Oral Protein and Energy Supplements to Reduce Mortality in Older Adults

An analysis of studies conducted since 1966 attempted to determine if oral protein and energy supplements could reduce all-cause mortality in older adults. A total of 31 randomized controlled trials met the inclusion criteria. In this meta-analysis, researchers found that oral protein and energy supplements were effective for reducing all-cause mortality in hospitalized or community-dwelling older adults. These supplements reduced mortality and length of hospital stay (3.4 days shorter) when a small (1.3 kg) but consistent increase in client weight occurred.

Most of these studies included clients who were not malnourished; therefore the benefit could have been more profound if supplementation had been given to malnourished older individuals (mini-nutritional assessment score <17). However, exactly which components of nutritional supplements (calories, protein, vitamins, and minerals) were responsible for the observed benefit could not be determined in this meta-analysis. A large clinical trial would be needed to answer this question. Regardless, health professionals should attempt to diagnose and treat poor nutritional status in older clients as much as they pursue abnormal blood tests or physical examination results.

References
Miline, A., Potter, J., & Avenell, A. (2002). Protein and energy supplementation in elderly people at risk for malnutrition. *Cochrane Database System Retreived CD003288 (3).*

COMPLEMENTARY AND ALTERNATIVE THERAPY

Intentional Weight Loss and Mortality

Researchers attempted to determine the effect of intention to lose weight, weight loss, and all-cause mortality. The study was a prospective cohort investigation from the United States. A total of 6391 overweight and obese individuals (body mass index of 25 or more) who were at least 35 years of age were studied and followed for 9 years. Compared with individuals not attempting to lose weight and reporting no weight change, those reporting intentional weight change had a 24% lower mortality rate, and those with unintentional weight loss had a 31% higher mortality rate. Interestingly, mortality rates were lower in individuals who reported trying to lose weight than in those not trying to lose weight, independent of an actual weight change. Attempted weight loss was associated with a lower all-cause or total mortality, independent of weight change. Therefore just the attempt to lose weight—regardless if any weight loss occurs—seems to provide a survival advantage versus individuals of the same weight who make no attempt to lose weight.

References
Gregg, E., et al. (2003). Intentional weight loss and death in overweight and obese U.S. adults 35 years of age and older. *Annals of Internal Medicine, 138,* 383-389.

---

cultures and possibly requiring different approaches toward prevention.

Pathophysiology and Clinical Manifestations

Obesity is a serious health risk and has been associated with increased risk of mortality and morbidity. Obesity is associated with a series of medical co-morbidities, including type 2 diabetes, cardiovascular disease, hypertension, hyperlipidemias, stroke, sleep apnea, obesity hypoventilation syndrome, arthritis, and some cancers.* Cancers, such as colorectal, breast, and prostate cancer, have been linked to obesity. However, whether this link between cancer and obesity is simply due to the excess weight, to specific dietary factors, or to difficulty in early diagnosis as a result of body build is unclear.

The mechanisms behind the obesity co-morbidities are not completely understood. It is clear, however, that the insulin resistance that is typical of truncal obesity is associated with type 2 diabetes and hypertriglyc-

eridemia. The sleep and respiratory problems seen with obesity are due to excess fat deposits in the airways and neck. Tendencies toward thrombosis may in part be due to reduced physical activity combined with venous stasis.

With loss of 5% to 10% of body weight, significant improvement in co-morbid conditions occurs (see the Complementary and Alternative Therapy feature on Intentional Weight Loss and Mortality, above). Blood pressure and cholesterol levels decrease with resultant reductions in medications. Type 2 diabetes improves greatly with weight loss and the sleep disturbances improve markedly.

Outcome Management
■ Medical Management

When a client has severe obesity, the quality of nursing care provided is key to client and caregiver safety. Oversized equipment may be indicated for safe transfer, transport, and skin management. Clients may require scales calibrated for accuracy at a higher range of body weight, larger blood pressure cuffs and tracheostomies, and oversized gowns for them to be cared for comfortably during a hospital admission or at home. Skin and wound problems are more prevalent in clients with severe obesity and require particular nursing attention for assessment and management.[19]

---

*References 11, 19, 23, 25, 33, 34, 36, 37.

The medical management of obesity should include a combination of diet, behavior modification, exercise, and occasionally medication. A team, including a psychologist with behavior modification skills and a registered dietitian, can provide the optimal intervention to encourage weight loss. A balanced deficit diet that supplies 500 to 1000 kcal less than total daily energy expenditure should promote the loss of 1 to 2 pounds per week. To prevent weight regain, it is also necessary to teach clients better diet management skills even if they use meal replacement formulas or very low-calorie diet regimens to begin weight loss. More severe calorie restrictions are difficult to maintain for longer periods and require vitamin and mineral supplementation. Clients on low-calorie diets should consume about 60 g/day of protein (~25% of total calories).

An exercise program should be part of the overall care of the obese client. Exercise is an important way to increase the energy expenditure and to facilitate weight loss. The inclusion of exercise into daily activities (e.g., taking the stairs rather than elevators, parking the car far away from the entrance at work), termed *lifestyle modification*, shows promise. Diet restriction in combination with an exercise program, compared with diet restriction alone, is a more successful way to lose weight and maintain the weight loss.

Commercial weight loss programs have been recommended for weight management but their efficacy has rarely been evaluated. A recent study conducted over 2 years in a multicenter, randomized trial determined that a structured commercial weight loss program provided more weight loss than self-help alone.[22]

The role of medications in promoting weight loss is an area of current research. At present, two drugs are approved by the Food and Drug Administration for the treatment of obesity. Orlistat (Xenical) is an intestinal lipase inhibitor, which acts by preventing the breakdown of dietary fat for absorption. The drug itself is not absorbed and has limited side effects unless a very high fat intake is taken, in which case steatorrhea may result. Clinical trials have documented a 30% reduction in dietary fat absorption, 9% versus 6% weight loss over 2 years, and a significant reduction in weight regain with orlistat use.[5]

Sibutramine (Meridia) is a serotonin, norepinephrine and dopamine reuptake inhibitor, and appetite suppressant. Sibutramine may also increase energy expenditure slightly in some individuals. The addition of sibutramine to a weight loss program induced significantly more weight loss than did a weight loss program and placebo.[5,8] Greater weight losses are sustained when the drug therapy is combined with dietary interventions and a comprehensive behavioral program.[5,8] The side effects of sibutramine, however, include sustained increase in blood pressure, as well as constipation, dry mouth, headache, and insomnia. Sibutramine is not recommended for clients with cardiovascular disease or uncontrolled hypertension, or in those taking monoamine oxidase inhibitors, serotonin reuptake inhibitors, or St. John's wort.

The use of a hypocaloric diet and zonisamide (Zonegran), an antiepileptic drug with serotonergic and dopaminergic activity, resulted in more weight loss than placebo and hypocaloric diet in the treatment of obesity.[18]

Although various drugs have been effective in promoting weight loss, any prescribed drug therapy regimen should be under the strict supervision of a qualified health care team to prevent potentially life-threatening complications.

■ Surgical Management

Surgical treatment of obesity is recommended by the National Heart, Lung, and Blood Institute (NHLBI) for clients who have BMI greater than 40 kg/m² or greater than 35 kg/m² with co-morbid complications (see http://www.nhlbi.nih.gov/guidelines/obesity/ob-exsum.pdf). These clients generally have been unsuccessful with multiple diet modifications, behavioral therapy, and drug therapy, and they are so obese that aggressive physical activity is not feasible.[37] Two surgical approaches are currently in use: (1) gastric restrictive and (2) restrictive plus malabsorptive.[1,11,33,37] An earlier procedure, the jejunoileal bypass, is no longer performed because of metabolic complications from the extreme malabsorption induced by the procedure.

Gastric Restrictive Procedure. The size of the stomach is reduced to a 2-ounce capacity by the placement of a line of staples from the esophageal-gastric sphincter to the gastroduodenal sphincter, just above which a Silastic ring is placed to prevent large food boluses from passing. This surgical approach, termed the vertical-banded gastroplasty, is associated with limited complications but lesser weight loss than the gastric bypass. Diet instruction must be part of the postoperative care of these clients, focusing on the increased frequency and decreased size of low-calorie meals. In addition, clients are instructed to take a chewable or liquid multivitamin every day.

Malabsorptive Procedure. In addition to the gastric stapling outlined above, the gastric bypass procedure bypasses a segment of duodenum from the food stream, thus inducing the malabsorption of nutrients and dumping manifestations when concentrated sugars are ingested. This gastric bypass procedure is most commonly performed in the United States when substantial weight loss is desired and the client has minimal surgical risk. Approximately 30% of the client's presenting weight is lost in the first year and maintenance of most of the lost weight has been documented for more than 14 years. The diet instruction for gastric bypass is similar to that for gastroplasty alone, but the importance of avoiding sweets to control manifestations of dumping syndrome is emphasized.

ANOREXIA NERVOSA AND BULIMIA NERVOSA

Anorexia nervosa is a condition of self-generated weight loss, usually seen in adolescent girls and young women, but also in middle-aged women or men.[7,24,33,44] The criteria for diagnosis of anorexia nervosa include a preoccupation with personal body weight and appearance, behaviors directed at thinness (excess activity and inadequate caloric intake), and the physical results of these behaviors (including extreme weight loss, amenorrhea, osteoporosis, and malnutrition). The psychopathologic presentation dictates the need for psychiatric intervention. A multidisciplinary team approach focused on consistency in addressing the behaviors characteristic of the disease has the greatest success with overall treatment.

Bulimia nervosa is a less serious and entirely separate illness. Clients with bulimia nervosa tend to maintain a relatively normal weight, but go through periods of eating excessively (bingeing) and vomiting (purging) gastric contents to prevent weight gain. It has been suggested that bulimia nervosa is a form of depressive illness.

Etiology and Risk Factors

Anorexia nervosa affects approximately 0.2% to 0.5% of young women.[44] Bulimia nervosa affects 2% to 3% of the same group.[44] Women are 10 times more likely to be affected by an eating disorder than men. These disorders are more prevalent in Western cultures, although their occurrence is increasing in Asian cultures.[44]

Although the cause of eating disorders is not certain, several factors are likely to contribute to development of the disorders. Sociocultural and environmental factors including media and peer influences, family factors including parental discord, and biologic factors including genetics, neurotransmitter regulation, and hormonal functioning have been implicated.[44] Negative affect, low self-esteem, and dieting behavior commonly predate the onset of an eating disorder.

Pathophysiology

The pathophysiologic changes associated with anorexia nervosa are similar to those seen in starvation. When caloric intake is severely limited, the body adapts by using the body's fat stores and sparing nitrogen stores. With prolonged starvation, significant shifts in fluid and electrolyte balance can occur and can be life-threatening. Alterations in the metabolism of insulin, thyroid hormone, and catecholamines explain common clinical manifestations, including decreases in pulse, respiratory rate, blood pressure, cardiac output, and gut motility.[7,24,33,44] The hypothalamus responds to the lack of nu-

trient intake with changes in pituitary function, resulting in amenorrhea and infertility. Clients with bulimia nervosa may or may not develop these changes. The extent of malnutrition will determine the pathophysiologic changes observed.

Clinical Manifestations

Clients with anorexia nervosa are usually first introduced to the health care system when the disordered eating behavior results in obvious weight loss. Clients may limit themselves to 200 to 500 kcal/day—only 60% to 70% of the amount needed for ideal body weight. Physical manifestations include dry skin, pallor, bradycardia, hypotension, intolerance to cold, constipation, and amenorrhea (Figure 31-3).

Clinical manifestations of bulimia nervosa include episodes of binge eating followed by self-induced vomit-

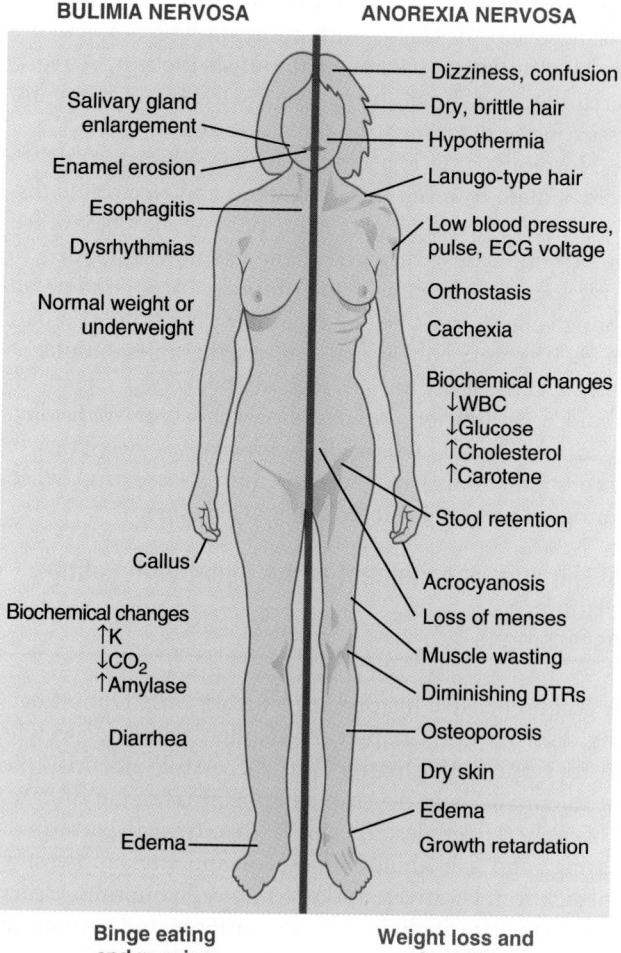

FIGURE 31-3 Physical manifestations of anorexia nervosa and bulimia nervosa. CO_2, Carbon dioxide; *DTRs*, deep tendon reflexes, *ECG*, electrocardiographic; *K*, potassium; *WBC*, white blood cell. (From Mahan, L.K., & Escott-Stump, S.E. [2000]. *Krause's food, nutrition, & diet therapy* [10th ed., p. 521]. Philadelphia: W.B. Saunders.)

ing. The eating and vomiting episodes occur most often in the late afternoon and evening and are done in secret. Some clients may abuse laxatives and diuretics as well. Personality characteristics typical of clients with bulimia are related to depression. Physical manifestations may not be as obvious, because the client with bulimia may be of normal weight without any depletion of fat stores. Less obvious clinical manifestations are erosion of tooth enamel from frequent vomiting and esophageal and throat irritation.

Outcome Management
■ Medical Management

The medical management of eating disorders must include psychological as well as nutritional components. Psychotherapy should focus on the underlying problems causing the disordered eating behavior. The physical rehabilitation of nutritional status targets ways to normalize the client's eating pattern and to help the client begin regaining weight, if needed. Excessive caloric intakes are not necessary in clients with anorexia and can actually be harmful in the severely malnourished client. A registered dietitian should be part of the treatment team and assist in the determination of caloric goals.

Hospitalization is necessary when malnutrition is severe enough to result in serious fluid and electrolyte disturbances. Enteral or parenteral therapy may be needed in extreme cases when the client has not responded to strategies to encourage and improve oral intake, although clients must be taught good eating skills as a part of the therapy. Nutritional support therapies should be introduced slowly in severely malnourished clients to avoid complications of refeeding syndrome. Refeeding syndrome is characterized by precipitous decreases in serum potassium, magnesium, and phosphorus when nutrients are administered to depleted clients.

■ Nursing Management of the Client with Eating Disorders
Assessment

A comprehensive history helps identify the type of eating disorder (see Chapter 30). Collect details of weight history and eating patterns to successfully identify the problem and help develop an appropriate plan of care. Have the client describe his or her typical pattern of eating, and ask about the use of appetite-suppressing medication, laxatives, and self-induced vomiting. Other pertinent data include exercise patterns and menstrual history.

Diagnosis, Outcomes, Interventions

Diagnosis: Imbalanced Nutrition: Less Than Body Requirements. The client with anorexia nervosa often experiences *Imbalanced Nutrition: Less Than Body Re-*

quirements related to inadequate food intake (anorexia nervosa).

Outcomes. The client will be able to resume normal eating behaviors. In clients with severe nutritional depletion, the client will be able to regain weight at a safe rate (1 to 2 pounds/week).

Interventions. When caring for a client with anorexia nervosa, help the client select foods from the Food Guide Pyramid for a nutritionally balanced diet. The client is usually allowed to refuse a specific number of foods (such as two or three) so that some sense of control is felt. Observe the client during mealtimes. Be supportive during mealtimes and, if needed, stay with the client after he or she eats to prevent him or her from purging. Education related to nutrition must include the client's family, caregivers, or co-residents. An accurate calorie count and regular monitoring of weight are other important interventions. Parenteral or enteral nutrition may be needed for refractory clients with extreme malnutrition.

Diagnosis: Imbalanced Nutrition: More Than Body Requirements. The client with bulimia nervosa or obesity often experience *Imbalanced Nutrition: More Than Body Requirements related to increased food intake.*

Outcomes. The client will lose 1 to 2 pounds per week until ideal body weight is achieved and maintain ideal body weight thereafter.

Interventions. Teach the client how to use the Food Guide Pyramid to select a healthy diet with portions of appropriate size. Encourage the client to eat slowly and develop a regular exercise pattern. Encourage the client to approach food, eating, and self-image in a new way. Provide emotional support and supervision for the client to overcome stressful periods and break the binge-and-purge cycle.

Diagnosis: Disturbed Body Image and Chronic Low Self-Esteem. The client with an eating disorder often has a *Disturbed Body Image and Chronic Low Self-Esteem related to misconception of body size or negative feelings (all disorders).*

Outcomes. The client will develop a more normal image of self, as evidenced by statements concerning increased self-esteem and by the client's ability to overcome the eating disorder.

Interventions. Recognize that clients suffering from eating disorders typically have low self-esteem. These clients see the regulation of food and exercise of self-control in eating patterns and amounts as ways to prove themselves successful. It is important that the client's significant others help the client find other areas of self-regard.

Evaluation

It is expected that the client will overcome the eating disorder with consistent and continued treatment and that weight will return to normal.

CONCLUSIONS

The nutritional care of the adult medical-surgical client is an important part of a comprehensive treatment plan. Preventing and treating malnutrition is just one way to facilitate recovery from acute and chronic illness. As a nurse, you have a vital role in nutritional assessment as well as in the prevention and treatment of malnutrition. Clients with eating disorders, such as obesity, anorexia nervosa, and bulimia nervosa may require medical, surgical, or psychological intervention.

THINKING CRITICALLY *evolve*

1. You are caring for a 62-year-old client in a nursing home. She has had a stroke and is paralyzed, sometimes confused, and incontinent. She refuses to eat and drink after many episodes of coughing and choking at mealtimes. A small-bore feeding tube has been inserted. When you check the tube for aspirate to confirm patency, you are unable to obtain any return aspirate. What nursing measures should be instituted to determine the problem? What is the priority nursing intervention?

Factors to Consider. What conditions contribute to the lack of aspirate return? What is your decision if the tube remains occluded?

2. You are assigned to care for two clients. One is an older man with a 6-month history of difficulty in swallowing and a weight loss of 25 pounds. The other client, a woman in her mid-30s, has Crohn's disease and has been admitted with an exacerbation of the disease. How should nutritional needs be addressed for each client?

Factors to Consider. How should nutritional needs be met for the client with an upper gastrointestinal tract disorder? With a lower gastrointestinal tract disorder?

3. D.A. is a 20-year-old white woman who is a sophomore in college and living away from home. She is 5 feet 1 inch tall. She has been steadily losing weight, although she participates in the campus meal plan

and takes her meals in the dormitory cafeteria. She plays on the college volleyball and basketball teams. Most of the students are excited about Thanksgiving holiday plans, but the dormitory counselor noticed that D.A. has not voiced any plans. She is found unconscious on the floor in the dormitory communal bathroom. She is taken by ambulance to the community hospital. Her college physical health record states that she weighed 98 pounds in June and had no known medical problems. On admission to the hospital, she weighs 79 pounds. What is her percentage of weight loss? What additional data need to be collected?

Factors to Consider. What interventions can be used to increase D.A.'s food intake? Is it feasible for a nurse on a busy medical-surgical unit to stay with D.A. during and after her meals? What alternatives might be used?

Discussions for these questions can be found on the website and the CD-ROM.

BIBLIOGRAPHY

1. Al-Saif, O., Gallagher, S., Banasiak, M., et al. (2003). Who should be doing laparoscopic bariatric surgery? *Obesity Surgery, 13*(1), 82-88.
2. ASPEN. (2002). Board of directors and the clinical guidelines task force: Guidelines for the use of parenteral and enteral nutrition in adult and pediatric patients. *Journal of the Parenteral Nutrition, 26*, 1SA.
3. ASPEN Publications. (2002). *ASPEN's set of guidelines and standards.* Silver Spring, MD: Author.
4. ASPEN Publications. (2002). *Clinical guidelines pocket guide.* Silver Spring, MD: Author.
5. Aronne, L. (2002). Current pharmacologic treatments for obesity. In C. Fairburn & K. Brownell (Eds.), *Eating disorders and obesity* (2nd ed.). New York: Guilford Press.
6. Barber, J., Miller, S., & Sacks., G. (2001). Parenteral feeding formulations. In M. Gottschlich (Ed.). *The science and practice of nutrition support: A case based core curriculum* (pp. 251-268). Dubuque, IA: Kendell/Hunt.
7. Beumont P. (2002). Clinical presentation of anorexia nervosa and bulimia nervosa. In C. Fairburn & K. Brownell (Eds.), *Eating disorders and obesity* (2nd ed.). New York: Guilford Press.
8. Berkowitz, R., et al. (2003). Behavior therapy and sibutramine for the treatment of adolescent obesity: A randomized control trial. *Journal of the American Medical Association, 289*(14), 1805-1812.
9. Bistrian, B., et al. (1974). Protein status of general surgical patients. *Journal of the American Medical Association, 230*, 858-860.
10. Bistrian, B., et al. (1976). Prevalence of malnutrition in general medical patients. *Journal of the American Medical Association, 235*, 1567-1570.

evolve **Did you remember to check out the bonus material on the** Evolve website and the CD-ROM, including free self-assessment exercises?

11. Blackwell, J. (2002). Identification, evaluation, and treatment of overweight and obese adults. *Journal of the American Academy of Nurse Practitioners, 14*(5), 196-199.

12. Bond, E., & Heitkemper, M. (2003). Protein calorie malnutrition. In V. Carrieri-Kohlman, A. Lindsay, & C. West (Eds.), *Pathophysiological phenomena in nursing: Human responses to Illness* (3rd ed.). Philadelphia: W. B. Saunders.

13. Bowers, S. (1999). Nutrition support for malnourished acutely ill adults. *MEDSURG Nursing, 8*(3), 145-161.

14. Charney, P. (2001). Enteral nutrition: Indications, options, and formulations. In M. Gottschlich (Ed.). *The science and practice of nutrition support: A case based core curriculum* (pp. 141-166). Dubuque, IA: Kendell/Hunt.

15. Covinsky, K., et al. (1999). The relationship between clinical assessments of nutritional status and adverse outcomes in older hospitalized medical patients. *Journal of the American Geriatric Society, 47*, 532-538.

16. Edington, J., Kon, P., & Martyn, C. (1996). Prevalence of malnutrition in patients in general practice. *Clinical Nutrition, 15*, 60-63.

17. Furhman, M. (2003). Nutrition support: Enteral and parenteral nutrition. In S. Williams & E. Schlenker (Eds.), *Essentials of nutrition and diet therapy* (8th ed., pp. 407-431). St. Louis: Mosby.

18. Gadde, K., Franciscy, D., Wagner, H., & Krishnan, K. (2003). Zonisamide for weight loss in obese adults: A randomized controlled trial. *Journal of the American Medical Association, 289*(14), 1820-1825.

19. Gallagher, S. (2002). Obesity and the skin in the critical care setting. *Critical Care Quarterly, 25*(1), 69-76.

20. Gottschlich, M. (2001). *The science and practice of nutrition support: A case based core curriculum.* Dubuque, IA: Kendell/Hunt.

21. Guenter, P., & Silkroski, M. (2001). Tube feeding: Practical guidelines and nursing protocols. Silver Spring, MD: ASPEN.

22. Heshka, S., et al., (2003). Weight loss with self-help compared with a structured commercial program: A randomized trial. *Journal of the American Medical Association, 289*(14), 1792-1798.

23. Hu, F., et al. (2003). Television watching and other sedentary behaviors in relation to risk of obesity and type 2 diabetes mellitus in women. *Journal of the American Medical Association, 289*(14), 1785-1791.

24. Huse, D., & Lucas, A. (1999). Behavioral disorders affecting food intake: Anorexia nervosa, bulimia nervosa and other psychiatric conditions. In M. Shils, et al. (Eds.), *Modern nutrition in health and disease* (9th ed., pp. 1513-1522). Baltimore: Williams & Wilkins.

25. Kannel, W., & Gordon, T. (1979). Physiologic and medical concomitants of obesity: The Framingham Study. In G. Bray (Ed.), *Obesity in America*. National Institutes of Health, Pub. No. 79. Washington, DC: Department of Health, Education, and Welfare.

26. Krzywda, E., et al. (2001). Parenteral access devices. In M. Gottschlich (Ed.), *The science and practice of nutrition support: A case based core curriculum* (pp. 225-250). Dubuque, IA: Kendell/Hunt.

27. Maloney, J., et al. (2000). Systemic absorption of food dye with sepsis. *New England Journal of Medicine, 343*(14), 1047-1048.

28. Matarese, L. (2001). Metabolic complications of parenteral nutrition therapy. In M. Gottschlich (Ed.), *The science and practice of nutrition support: A case based core curriculum* (pp. 269-286). Dubuque, IA: Kendell/Hunt.

29. Metheny N., et al. (1999). pH and concentration of bilirubin in feeding tube aspirates as predictors of tube placement. *Nursing Research, 48*(4), 189-197.

30. Minard, G., & Lysen, L. (2001). Enteral access devices. In M. Gottschlich (Ed.), *The science and practice of nutrition support: A case based core curriculum* (pp. 167-188). Dubuque, IA: Kendell/Hunt.

31. Mirtallo, J. (2001). Introduction to parenteral nutrition. In M. Gottschlich (Ed.), *The science and practice of nutrition support: A case based core curriculum* (pp. 211-224). Dubuque, IA: Kendell/Hunt.

32. Mitchell, M. (2003). Aging and older adults. In M. Mitchell (Ed.), *Nutrition across the lifespan* (2nd ed., pp 429-470). Philadelphia: W. B. Saunders.

33. Mitchell, M. (2003). Eating dilemmas: Dietary restraint, binging, purging, excessive consumption, and excessive exercise. In M. Mitchell (Ed.), *Nutrition across the lifespan* (2nd ed., pp 473-512). Philadelphia: W. B. Saunders.

34. Mitchell, M. (2003). Nutrition screening and assessment. In M. Mitchell (Ed.), *Nutrition across the lifespan* (2nd ed., pp 43-78). Philadelphia: W. B. Saunders.

35. O'Grady, A., et al. (2002). Guidelines for the prevention of intravascular catheter-related infections. *Morbidity and Mortality Weekly Report, CDC 51,* (RR-10), 1-31.

36. Ogden, C., et al. (2002). Prevalence and trends in overweight among U.S. children and adolescents, 1999-2000. *Journal of the American Medical Association, 288*(14), 1728-1732.

37. Rasheid, S., et al. (2003). Gastric bypass is an effective treatment of obstructive sleep apnea in patients with clinically significant obesity. *Obesity Surgery, 13*(1), 58-62.

38. Rombeau, J.L., & Rolandelli, R.H. (2001). *Clinical nutrition: Parenteral nutrition* (3rd ed.). Philadelphia: W. B. Saunders.

39. Russell, M., Cromer, M., & Grant, J. (2001). Complications of enteral nutrition. In M. Gottschlich (Ed.), *The science and practice of nutrition support: A case based core curriculum* (pp. 189-210). Dubuque, IA: Kendell/Hunt.

40. Shopbell, J., Hopkins, B., & Shronts, E. (2001). Nutrition screening and assessment. In M. Gottschlich (Ed.), *The science and practice of nutrition support: A case based core curriculum* (pp. 107-140). Dubuque, IA: Kendell/Hunt.

41. Torun, B., & Chew, F. (1999). Protein-energy malnutrition. In M. Shils, et al. (Eds.), *Modern nutrition in health and disease* (9th ed., pp. 963-988). Baltimore: Williams & Wilkins.

42. Victora, C., et al. (1999). Potential interventions for the prevention of childhood pneumonia in developing countries: Improving nutrition. *American Journal of Clinical Nutrition, 70*, 309-320.

43. Williams, S., & Schlenker, E. (2003). *Essentials of nutrition and diet therapy* (8th ed.). St. Louis: Mosby.

44. Wolfe, B., & Gimby, L. (2003). Caring for the hospitalized patient with an eating disorder. *Nursing Clinics of North America, 38*(1), 75-99.

Management of Clients with Ingestive Disorders

Elizabeth A. Murphy-Blake
Jane Hokanson Hawks

---

evolve

Web Enhancements

http://evolve.elsevier.com/Black/medsurg/

Appendix C
Laboratory Values of Clinical Importance in Medical-Surgical Nursing

---

The client with an ingestive disorder, regardless of the cause, may have a problem in the oral cavity or esophagus that indicates common nursing diagnoses, such as *Impaired Oral Mucous Membrane; Pain; Imbalanced Nutrition: Less Than Body Requirements; Impaired Verbal Communication;* or *Impaired Swallowing.* Usually, the client first experiences pain in the mouth or esophagus, or delay in passage of food, which is evidenced by difficulty with swallowing. Shortly thereafter, oral communication and nutritional intake may be compromised. These complications may also result in the development of personal and family coping problems as well as a lack of knowledge related to the treatment required for the disorder.

DENTAL DISORDERS

A person must have healthy teeth and gums for good general health. Health care providers strive to preserve their clients' healthy gums and natural teeth for as long as possible for the following reasons:

- Natural teeth are almost always more functional in masticating food than are dental prostheses.

- Effective mastication of food helps promote efficient digestion.
- Efficient digestion of food results in healthy gastrointestinal (GI) function and maintenance of general health.

The most common causes of tooth loss are dental decay and periodontal disease. Plaque is the major cause of both caries (decay) and periodontal disease. Tobacco use may also lead to tooth loss. *The best treatment for dental caries is prevention.* Early in childhood clients are encouraged to brush and floss frequently and regularly, eat a diet low in simple carbohydrates, use fluoride, and schedule regular visits (biannually) to the dentist for examination, cleaning, and treatment of dental caries.

Increasing the resistance of the enamel helps prevent caries. The resistance of enamel increases with the ingestion of fluoridated water during tooth formation and the continued use of fluoride throughout life. The daily use of fluoride rinses produces a more acid-resistant structure, enhances tooth mineralization, and interferes with bacterial growth. In addition, the dentist may apply topical fluoride to the teeth during biannual examinations.

Treatment of dental caries may include drilling out cavities and filling the tooth with material to restore the

---

evolve *Be sure to check out the bonus material on the Evolve website and the CD-ROM, including free self-assessment exercises.*

http://evolve.elsevier.com/Black/medsurg/

Nursing Outcomes Classification (NOC)
for Nursing Diagnoses—Clients with Ingestive Disorders

Acute Pain and Chronic Pain
 Comfort Level
 Acute and Chronic Pain: Disruptive
  Effects
Deficient Knowledge
 Knowledge: Illness Care
 Knowledge: Treatment Procedure
 Knowledge: Treatment Regimen
**Imbalanced Nutrition: Less Than Body
Requirements**
 Nutritional Status
 Nutritional Status: Food and Fluid
  Intake
 Nutritional Status: Nutrient Intake

Impaired Oral Mucous Membrane
 Oral Health
 Tissue Integrity: Skin and Mucous
  Membrane
Impaired Swallowing
 Swallowing Status
 Swallowing Status: Esophageal Phase
 Swallowing Status: Oral Phase
 Swallowing Status: Pharyngeal Phase
Impaired Verbal Communication
 Communication
 Communication: Expressive
Risk for Impaired Skin Integrity
 Nutritional Status

**Nutritional Status: Biochemical
 Measures**
Tissue Integrity: Skin and Mucous
 Membranes
Wound Healing: Secondary Intention
Risk for Ineffective Coping
 Coping
 Decision Making
 Information Processing
 Role Performance
 Social Support
Risk for Injury
 Risk Control
 Risk Detection

tooth, extraction (removal) of the entire tooth, and preservation of the tooth by *root canal therapy* (pulpectomy) followed by proper restoration. Any number of teeth can be removed because of tooth or gum disease. Teeth are usually replaced with some type of dental prosthesis (crowns, dentures, dental implants). If only one tooth or a few teeth are removed, local anesthesia is usually used. Removing several teeth or having a full mouth extraction may require sedation or general anesthesia. Potential complications include hemorrhage and abscess formation.

During root canal therapy, the entire pulp of the tooth is removed. The canal space within the roots is filled aseptically and sealed to prevent infection. The tooth remains rooted in the gingiva and can still be used. Subsequent restoration of the tooth is essential to retain the tooth in a normal functional relationship with the rest of the teeth.

Periodontal disease, caused by plaque formation and bacterial colonization, results in gingival inflammation if the plaque is not removed by proper brushing and flossing. Eventually, inflammation destroys the underlying tissues and separates the gingiva from the tooth. In periodontitis, the inflammation extends from the gums into the alveolar bone and periodontal ligament, destroying the supporting structures of the teeth. As a result, the teeth loosen and fall out or extraction may be required as a result of the severity of the periodontal disease.

Postoperative care of a tooth extraction includes assessing the oral cavity for bleeding and monitoring vital signs (if the client stays in an inpatient facility or recovery area). A gauze pad is usually placed over the extraction site, and the client is instructed to bite down gently on the pad to maintain pressure. Ice may be applied to the jaw over the site to decrease the blood flow and edema. Small amounts of bleeding may be normal; however, the dentist

or physician should be notified (or instruct the client to do so) if bleeding lasts longer than 1 hour.

The client usually requires analgesics to control pain. Instruct the client to eat soft foods and to avoid hot or cold foods for several days. The client should gently rinse the mouth with normal saline, but should avoid brushing any remaining teeth for about 24 hours. It is important for the client to maintain fluid intake to avoid dehydration, especially with full mouth extractions.

ORAL DISORDERS
STOMATITIS

Stomatitis, an inflammation of the oral cavity, may be of infectious origin or a manifestation of a systemic condition. It may be caused by *mechanical* trauma, such as injury, or *chemical* trauma, such as drugs used in the treatment of cancer. Jagged teeth, cheek-biting, and mouth-breathing may result in mechanical trauma. Certain foods and drinks as well as sensitivity to mouthwashes or toothpaste may produce chemical trauma. The inflammatory sloughing of tissue allows organisms to multiply, which may lead to infection by viruses, bacteria, yeasts, or fungus.

Stomatitis is classified as primary or secondary, depending on the cause. Primary stomatitis includes aphthous stomatitis (canker sore), herpes simplex, and Vincent's angina. Secondary stomatitis results when a client's lowered resistance allows an opportunistic infection to develop. Secondary stomatitis can be caused by a local or systemic disorder. Systemic disorders that can affect the oral mucous membranes include (1) allergies, (2) bone marrow disorders, (3) nutritional disorders, (4) immunodeficiency disorders, and (5) chemotherapy, radiation therapy, or immunosuppressive therapy.

Aphthous Stomatitis

The lesions caused by aphthous stomatitis, commonly known as *canker sores,* are recurrent, small, and ulcerated. The lesions develop in the soft tissues of the mouth, including the lips, tongue, and insides of the cheeks (Figure 32-1). Canker sores affect people of all age groups, although young adult women are more frequently affected. This is the most common oral ulcerative lesion. The cause of canker sores is unknown, but may be related to emotional stress, trauma, vitamin deficiency, food and drug allergies, endocrine imbalances, and viral infections. Prevention is almost impossible because the exact cause is unknown.

These lesions start as small, reddened areas that undergo central necrosis and ulceration. The lesions are not infectious, but are simply inflammatory. Lesions heal within 1 to 3 weeks without treatment. Assessment usually reveals a well-circumscribed erythematous macule that undergoes necrosis, creating a well-defined pseudomembranous ulcer with an erythematous border.

Medical treatment involves topical application of amlexanox (Aphthasol) to the ulcer. Topical or systemic steroids may shorten the healing time. In addition, to suppress recurrence, teach clients susceptible to allergic reactions to avoid tomatoes, chocolate, eggs, shellfish, milk products, nuts, and citrus fruits.

Herpes Simplex

Herpes simplex stomatitis is a form of inflammation and ulceration caused by the herpes simplex virus (HSV). By age 5 years, 90% of the population has been infected with *primary* herpes simplex. When the client is first infected with the primary herpes virus, lesions appear in the oral cavity. These vesicles, which can appear throughout the oral cavity, rupture to form ulcerated areas that resemble canker sores and heal within several weeks. The client's tongue has a characteristic heavy white coating. The client may have manifestations of generalized infection as well.

Secondary herpes is a recurrent infection that appears to lie dormant after the primary herpes infection. Secondary herpes takes the form of herpes labialis (fever blister, cold sore) and is often seen in clients receiving immunosuppressants and in those with human immunodeficiency virus (HIV) infection or acquired immunodeficiency syndrome (AIDS). Any infection, especially upper respiratory infections, fever, stress, or even sunlight, can reactivate the virus.

Assessment reveals clear, vesicular lesions, most often appearing at the mucocutaneous junction of the lips (Figure 32-2) and face. The lesions are contagious, last about 1 week, and heal without scarring. Later in the course of the infection, the tongue may appear coated and the client may complain of a foul breath odor.

General pain caused by herpes simplex may be treated with analgesics. Local or topical ointments and anesthetics may soothe the lesions. Clients who are immunocompromised are started on intravenous (IV) acyclovir (Zovirax). Clients with competent immune systems may be given acyclovir in oral or topical forms or penciclovir (Denavir) topical cream. Unless the ulcer is secondarily infected, antimicrobial treatment does not affect the progress of the ulcer.

Vincent's Angina

Vincent's angina (necrotizing ulcerative gingivitis, trench mouth) is an acute bacterial infection of the gingivae caused by resident flora in the mouth, fusiform bacteria, and spirochetes. Precipitating factors include poor oral hygiene, increased age, nutritional deficiencies, lack of rest and sleep, local tissue damage, and debilitating diseases, such as infectious mononucleosis, nonspecific viral infections, bacterial infections, blood dyscrasias, and diabetes mellitus. Most of these factors are unavoidable and therefore unpreventable. This condition is not contagious.

Vincent's angina has a sudden onset, causes erythema and ulceration of the gingivae, and affects the entire

FIGURE 32-1 Major aphthous ulcer (canker sore). (From Feldman, M., Friedman, L., & Sleisenger, M. [Eds.]). [2002]. *Sleisenger and Fordtran's gastrointestinal and liver disease: Pathophysiology/diagnosis/management* [7th ed.]. Philadelphia: W.B. Saunders.)

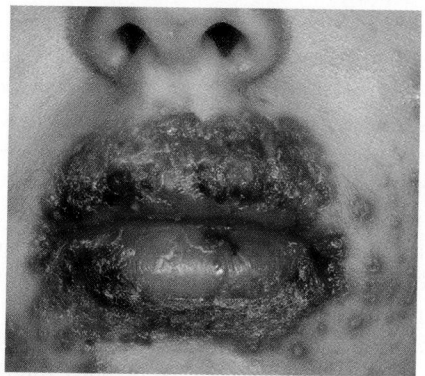

FIGURE 32-2 Herpes simplex of the lip. (From Habif, T.P. [2004]. *Clinical dermatology: Color guide to diagnosis and therapy* [4th ed.]. St. Louis: Mosby.

oropharynx. Once the tonsils are removed, this disorder rarely recurs. Assessment reveals ulcers covered with a pseudomembrane. A smear from an ulcer exudate identifies the causative organisms. Clients often have an elevated white blood cell (WBC) count. The client may complain of a foul taste, pain, a choking sensation, fever, thick secretions, anorexia, and, occasionally, local lymphadenopathy.

Management consists of removing the devitalized tissue and correcting the underlying cause with rest, improved oral hygiene, a bland diet, and vitamins. Pain medications as well as saline mouth rinses promote comfort.

CANDIDIASIS

Candidiasis (moniliasis, thrush) is caused by the organism *Candida albicans*, a yeast-like fungus that is part of the normal flora of the oral cavity. Candidiasis of the oral cavity is commonly seen in immunosuppressed clients, such as those receiving chemotherapy or those with HIV infection or AIDS. The incidence is also increased in clients with diabetes mellitus and those who are pregnant, under stress, receiving high-dose or long-term antibiotic therapy, or receiving long-term tube feeding. Clients with HIV have significantly lowered oral epithelial cells, whereas individuals with healthy oral mucosa resist oral candidiasis infections, which suggests an innate resistance.

Etiology and Risk Factors

When the client is in a state of immunosuppression or has decreased levels of some normal oral flora, an overgrowth of the normal flora *Candida* can occur. Candidiasis commonly occurs in critically ill clients with prolonged intubation. The major risk factors are immunosuppression and prolonged use of antibiotics that disrupts the normal flora. Clients with either risk factor should be monitored closely. Prophylactic treatment is often started for these high-risk clients.

Pathophysiology

Candidiasis is a secondary infection resulting from either an immunodeficiency or prolonged use of antibiotics. When the normal flora is disrupted, an overgrowth of the *Candida* organism may occur.

Clinical Manifestations

Assessment reveals white patches on the tongue, palate, and buccal mucosa (Figure 32-3). These lesions adhere firmly to the tissues and are difficult to remove. The lesions are often referred to as "milk curds" because of their appearance. Clients describe the lesions as dry and hot. Clients who have recurrent candidiasis infections should be examined for a possible systemic cause.

FIGURE 32-3 Oral candidiasis. Note white patches on the tongue and upper palate. (Courtesy of The Centers for Disease Control and Prevention, Atlanta, GA.)

Outcome Management
■ Medical Management

Medical management includes topical antifungal agents as well as other topical agents to alleviate the infection and provide pain reduction. Analgesics, such as acetaminophen or aspirin, may also be administered to promote pain reduction. Mouthwashes of warm saline (or water) are often ordered as part of an oral hygiene regimen. A bland liquid or pureed diet may be necessary. Prophylactic use of antifungal agents is indicated for high-risk clients. Oral pharyngeal cultures should be taken if infection is suspected. Fluconazole has become an integral part of the management of clients who are immunosuppressed.

■ Nursing Management of the Medical Client
Assessment

Clients with the risk factors of immunosuppression or prolonged antibiotic use should be monitored closely. Assess whether the client has pain, tenderness, or bleeding in any part of the oral cavity or has had any febrile episodes. Ask about a history of previous infection elsewhere in the body and the use of any medications, especially antibiotics. Ask the client about a history of treatment with radiation or chemotherapy because both can affect the oral mucosa. Prophylactic treatment for these high-risk clients may have been instituted.

To perform the oral assessment, use a tongue blade and bright lighting, and wear gloves. Inspect the oral cavity, noting any areas of inflammation, vesicular eruptions, ulcers, white patches, or erythema of the gingivae.

Diagnosis, Outcomes, Interventions

Diagnosis: Acute Pain and Impaired Oral Mucous Membrane. A common nursing diagnosis for the client with candidiasis is *Acute Pain related to impaired oral mucous membrane and ulcerations* or *Impaired Oral Mucous Membrane related to ulcerations.*

Outcomes. The client's oral mucous membranes will begin to heal, and pain will be relieved or controlled, as evidenced by expressions of pain reduction and demonstration of the ability to maintain normal nutrition.

Interventions

Minimize Pain. Assess for oral pain using a pain scale, and administer analgesics, such as aspirin or acetaminophen, as ordered. Topical agents and topical mouth rinses often provide pain reduction. Antifungal agents to rinse or swish and swallow are used to alleviate the infection. A change in diet to liquid or pureed foods often eases the discomfort of eating. The client should avoid spicy foods, citrus juices, and hot liquids.

Provide Oral Care. Clients with painful lesions cannot tolerate commercial mouthwashes because of the high alcohol level in these products. A solution of warm saline (or water) or mouthwash formulas specific to many institutions are better tolerated and may promote healing. If painful oral lesions are present, suggest modifications in the client's oral hygiene regimen. Gauze or sponge pads may replace toothbrushes, and oral rinses may be needed to clean the area of debris and promote healing.

Promote Self-Care. Give the client oral and written instructions regarding a dental hygiene regimen, diet, medications, and manifestations of complications. The client should demonstrate proper techniques of dental hygiene. Minimal home health care preparation is required unless the client requires alternative feeding routes. If the client is receiving tube feedings, referral to a home health agency may be appropriate. If home care is not affordable, teach the client or significant other how to perform the tube feedings (see Chapter 31 and later in this chapter). The client should be scheduled for medical follow-up to assess for recurrence.

Evaluation

The infection should clear up within a few days to a week in most clients. Assess the client for other risk factors if there is a reoccurrence. Educate the client about the clinical manifestations of infection to report to the health care practitioner.

TUMORS OF THE ORAL CAVITY

Benign Tumors of the Oral Cavity

The most common benign tumors of the mouth are fibromas, lipomas, neurofibromas, and hemangiomas. As with benign tumors in other parts of the body, oral tumors cause problems, primarily by occupying space and causing pressure. Benign tumors are usually excised if the mass causes functional or cosmetic problems.

Premalignant Tumors of the Oral Cavity

Leukoplakia

Leukoplakia, a potentially precancerous, yellow-white or gray-white lesion, may occur in any region of the mouth. The size and shape of lesions vary, but are usually elevated and have a roughened or leathery surface and clearly defined borders (Figure 32-4). Leukoplakia is a common disorder of the oral mucous membranes, usually seen in people in their 30s and 40s. Men are affected twice as often as women; however, the incidence in women is increasing because of the increasing number of women who smoke.

Leukoplakia results from chronic irritation of the mucosa by physical, chemical, or thermal factors. Physical factors include poorly fitting dentures, broken teeth, cheek nibbling, and occlusion problems. Chemical and thermal factors arise from the use of tobacco products, both inhaled and chewing products as well as pipe smoking. Ingestion of excessively hot food and beverages also places the person at risk. This condition may also develop from systemic factors such as poor nutrition or syphilis. A recent study suggests that both topical calcipotriol and topical tretinoin are equally effective therapy when treating oral leukoplakia.[13] Another study reported that surgical excision of the lesion prevented subsequent development of carcinoma in 1 of 75 subjects. No comparison studies between topical and surgical excision of the lesions were found.

Erythroplakia

Erythroplakia is a red, velvety appearing patch that commonly indicates early squamous cell carcinoma. It occurs most frequently in people ages 50 to 60, with men and women being equally affected. Risk factors are the same as those for squamous cell carcinoma.

FIGURE 32-4 Leukoplakia of the lateral edge of the tongue. (Courtesy of The Centers for Disease Control and Prevention, Atlanta, GA.)

Malignant Tumors of the Oral Cavity

Cancers of the oral cavity account for fewer than 3% of total cases of body malignancies. Cancers in this area are most frequently seen in people in their 40s and 50s and are seen in men more frequently than in women. Cancers of the oral cavity are most often associated with long-term alcohol consumption and tobacco use. Because of the increased use of tobacco by younger people, especially the use of smokeless (chewing) tobacco, and by women, the age and gender ratios are changing.

Health promotion actions include teaching clients to avoid excessive use of tobacco, alcohol, and very hot beverages and foods. Encourage clients to maintain meticulous oral hygiene, to eat a well-balanced diet, and to use sunscreen during exposure to sunlight. Health maintenance activities involve oral screening of smokers, tobacco chewers, and drinkers of alcohol and teaching these high-risk individuals to observe for early manifestations of oral cancer. Health restoration interventions include the management of chemotherapy and radiation for clients after tumor excision and providing nutritional support as needed.

Basal Cell Carcinoma

Basal cell carcinoma of the oral cavity, the second most common oral cancer, occurs primarily on the lips. It starts as a small scab that develops into an ulcer with a characteristic pearly border. Basal cell carcinoma primarily occurs as a result of excessive exposure to sunlight, tending to occur more commonly in fair-skinned individuals who are exposed to sunlight.

Squamous Cell Carcinoma

Squamous cell carcinoma is a malignant growth arising from tiny flat squamous cells that line mucous membranes. Squamous cell carcinoma is the leading type of oral cancer. Most tumors occur in clients older than age 45. Common sites include the lower lip and tongue. About 95% of cancers found on the tongue are squamous cell carcinomas. Malignancies of the tongue represent 1% to 1.5% of all malignancies in the United States.[1]

The primary cause of squamous cell carcinoma is chronic irritation of the mucous lining of the mouth and oral cavity. Overuse of alcohol and tobacco (both smoking and chewing) is the primary cause of oral irritation. In combination, tobacco and alcohol are extremely destructive to the oral mucosa.

Squamous cell carcinoma develops from tiny cells that line the oral cavity. It can occur on the lips, buccal mucosa, tongue (Figure 32-5), floor of the mouth, and tonsils. It is usually well differentiated, and the rate of metastasis is less than 10%. Cells metastasize by direct

FIGURE 32-5 Oral squamous cell carcinoma. This is an ulcerated lesion with surrounding leukoplakia on the posterior lateral and ventral portions of the tongue. (From Neville, B.W., et al. [2002]. *Oral and maxillofacial pathology* [2nd ed]. Philadelphia: W.B. Saunders.)

infiltration of local lymph nodes and can extend into the buccal fat and even to the mandible.

Manifestations may include a sore or lesion in the oral cavity that does not heal. Red-appearing (erythroplakia) squamous cell carcinomas may not be well delineated and often bleed easily. Because squamous cell carcinomas usually grow slowly, the lesion may be large before manifestations are detected. Other manifestations can include a mild irritation of the tongue, sore throat, trouble with wearing dentures, or pain in the tongue or ear.

Only a biopsy of lesions positively confirms a diagnosis of oral cancer. Cytologic examination of mucosa thought to be malignant, while valuable in screening, is not used widely enough to reduce the mortality rate. To be a valuable diagnostic aid, cytologic examination must be followed by biopsy when questionable cells are found. Biopsies may be performed with local or general anesthesia. To diagnose carcinoma at the base of the tongue, a laryngoscopic examination must be performed.

Outcome Management
■ Medical Management

Inhibit Tumor Growth. The survival rate of clients with oral cancer depends on the site and staging of the tumor. The tumor-node-metastasis (TNM) staging system (see Chapter 19) is used to stage oral cancers. Of the oral cancers, cancer of the lip carries one of the highest cure rates. Squamous cell carcinoma of the tongue carries the poorest prognosis because of the tongue's extensive vascular and lymphatic supply. Management of oral cancers includes surgery, radiation therapy, and chemotherapy, depending on the site and staging of the tumor.

Radiation Therapy. Oral cancers can be treated with *external beam therapy* or *interstitial radiation therapy* *(brachytherapy).* The external beam passes through the skin or mucous membrane to the tumor. Interstitial radiation involves implanting radioactive seeds into the tissue for a prescribed period of time. Because interstitial radiation affects local tissue, it is used for small lesions that have not infiltrated the surrounding tissue. The client undergoing interstitial radiation is hospitalized and placed on radiation precautions (see Chapter 19) while the materials are active.

Chemotherapy. The effectiveness of chemotherapy for the treatment of oral cancers is unknown. Several drugs are used to treat head and neck cancers. These drugs include bleomycin (Blenoxane), cisplatin (Platinol), cyclophosphamide (Cytoxan), doxorubicin (Adriamycin), 5-fluorouracil (5-FU), hydroxyurea (Hydrea), methotrexate (Folex), and vincristine (Oncovin). See Chapter 19 for discussion on chemotherapy.

■ Nursing Management of the Medical Client

Assessment

Carefully question the client about manifestations. A common finding is that of a painful ulcer. Assess the client for difficulty in swallowing, white or red patches on the oral mucosa, bleeding in the mouth, lumps in the neck, pain referred to the ear, foul odor, and hoarseness. Ask about the use of alcohol and tobacco, oral hygiene habits, and sun exposure. Assess the client's rehabilitative needs. Surgery can cause disfigurement and may alter speech; the client may experience depression from a change in body image and the diagnosis of cancer.

Diagnosis, Outcomes, Interventions

Diagnosis: Impaired Oral Mucous Membrane.
A common nursing diagnosis for the client who has oral cancer or who is at risk for oral cancer is *Impaired Oral Mucous Membrane related to irritants such as alcohol or tobacco, chemotherapy, radiation therapy, ill-fitting dentures, poor nutrition, and knowledge deficit of prevention and treatment of oral lesions.*

Outcomes. The client will understand and comply with measures to maintain the oral mucosa, as evidenced by statements of understanding of the substances and activities to avoid. The client will also be able to discuss the treatment regimen.

Interventions
Avoid Oral Irritants. Teach the client about the disease and treatment protocols. Advise the client to avoid chemical, physical, and thermal oral trauma; to perform careful, frequent oral hygiene, preferably three times daily; to see a dentist about ill-fitting dentures; and see a

practitioner about any mouth lesion that does not heal in 2 to 3 weeks.

Promote Comfort. If the client is receiving radiation therapy or chemotherapy, discuss possible side effects of these forms of treatment. Provide the client with comfort measures to minimize side effects, such as frequent oral hygiene and antiemetics to prevent nausea and vomiting.

Diagnosis: Imbalanced Nutrition: Less Than Body Requirements.
Clients with oral cancers often have nutritional difficulties, and a usual nursing diagnosis is *Imbalanced Nutrition: Less Than Body Requirements related to oral pain and difficulty eating and swallowing.*

Outcomes. The client will maintain weight or show weight gain before surgery, as evidenced by an increase in intake, maintenance of weight, or a weight gain of 1 pound per week until stable.

Interventions
Promote Nutrition. The location and size of a tumor, and the pain it causes, commonly interfere with a client's ability to eat. Small, frequent feedings can promote intake. Giving an analgesic 30 to 45 minutes before a meal can decrease the pain associated with eating. Provide oral care before and after meals to remove debris and minimize oral odors. Give the client with poor nutrition guidelines for improving the diet. Supply pamphlets outlining the basic nutrients for good health, and refer the client to a dietitian as needed.

Relieve Mouth Dryness. Treatments such as radiation alter salivation and taste perception. Xerostomia (dryness of the mouth) usually lessens with the use of pilocarpine and artificial saliva. Suggest that the client chew sugarless gum or suck on sugar-free hard candy to increase moisture. The client should perform frequent oral rinses with cool water to reduce dryness.

Evaluation

The best outcome is for the client to stop high-risk behaviors for oral cancer, undergo successful treatment, and promote and maintain nutritional status.

■ Surgical Management
Surgical management of oral cancers can range from local excision of small tumors to extensive surgery for invasive tumors. Small tumors can be treated in outpatient facilities by local excision, radiation, or laser therapy. Small tumors of the floor of the mouth can be locally excised with or without removing a portion of the mandible. Small tumors in the anterior floor of the mouth can be excised, and the area can be reconstructed with the use of a split-thickness skin graft.

A thin layer of skin, usually from the anterior thigh, can line the surgical site, allowing the client to maintain good mobility and function of the tongue. Xeroform gauze is usually placed over the skin graft and sutured into place. Both the graft and the gauze can restrict tongue movement, causing aspiration of secretions. Because of this packing and as a result of postoperative edema, a tracheostomy tube (see Chapter 62) is usually placed until edema subsides and the oral airway is patent. The client receives nothing by mouth (NPO) for 7 to 10 days after surgery to allow for healing. A nasogastric (NG) feeding tube, gastrostomy, or percutaneous endoscopic gastrostomy (PEG) is used to provide nutrition until the client can resume oral feedings (see Chapter 31).

Clients with invasive tumors require extensive surgical excision, usually involving removal of associated lymph nodes. Depending on the location, glossectomy (removal of the tongue), mandibulectomy (removal of the mandible), hemiglossectomy (removal of part of the tongue), or radical neck dissection may be performed. A radical neck dissection is an extensive procedure that involves removal of all tissue under the skin, from the jaw down to the clavicle, and from the anterior border of the trapezius muscle to the midline. To remove the cervical lymph nodes in this procedure, the surgeon must remove the sternocleidomastoid muscle, the spinal accessory nerve, and the jugular vein. A modified radical neck dissection involves removal of the lymph nodes only and is preferred when the disease is confined to mobile lymph nodes (see Chapter 62 for surgical management of cancer of the larynx). The Commando procedure is an extensive oral operation in which part of the mandible is excised along with the oral lesion. This procedure is often combined with a radical neck dissection. Any of these extensive surgical procedures require extensive preparation of the client for surgery.

■ Nursing Management of the Surgical Client
Assessment

Assessment of the surgical client is similar to assessment of the medical client. Complete routine preoperative and postoperative assessments, and ensure that the client understands the implications of the selected surgical approach and the associated postoperative assessments and treatments. Assessment of rehabilitative needs, such as speech therapy, coping with disfigurement, and depression may also be required.

Diagnosis, Outcomes, Interventions

Diagnosis: Risk for Injury. Surgery for oral cancer involves many potential risks. *Risk for Injury related to surgical procedure (including hemorrhage, ineffective airway clearance, impaired gas exchange, and risk for infection)* is an appropriate nursing diagnosis.

Outcomes. The client will remain free from injury, as evidenced by absence of excessive bleeding, maintenance of a patent airway and gas exchange, and wound healing without manifestations of infection.

Interventions

Maintain Airway. The most critical postoperative intervention is to maintain a patent airway. If the surgical procedure has been extensive, a tracheostomy is usually in place to help prevent respiratory difficulty from edema of the oral and pharyngeal structures. Clients at risk for ineffective airway clearance or impaired gas exchange should be in a semi-Fowler to a high Fowler position after surgery to promote venous lymphatic drainage. The client may have a dusky appearance about the face from venous congestion. Pulse oximeter readings also should be used to determine whether the client is sufficiently oxygenated.

The client with a tracheostomy may exhibit blood-tinged mucus in tracheal secretions for the first 48 hours after surgery. Bright red bleeding from the tracheostomy tube or site is a manifestation of hemorrhage. Notify the practitioner immediately if this occurs.

Provide Wound Care. The amount of nursing care required by the client after surgery depends on the extent of the procedure. After local excisions, teach the client how to perform hygiene gently. If a dressing and packing are in place, monitor the amount of drainage. After the dressing and packing are removed, the client should rinse the oral cavity with a water or saline solution every 4 hours to remove debris and promote healing. With more extensive surgery, the suture lines must be protected from trauma. Oral hygiene and oral suctioning are usually not implemented until healing has begun and the physician decides that this type of cleaning can be performed without damage to the sutured or incisional area.

Monitor for Bleeding. Hemorrhage may occur at any time after surgery, especially with extensive resection of the tongue. Hemorrhage can be massive because of the large vessels that supply the mouth and oral area. If bleeding occurs, apply pressure on the site until the bleeding stops spontaneously or stops with medical or surgical intervention. Surgical repair may be required to stop the bleeding. If an extensive resection is performed requiring skin grafts, monitor the site every 2 to 4 hours for drainage and manifestations of infection.

Diagnosis: Imbalanced Nutrition: Less Than Body Requirements. After surgical intervention for oral cancers, the client often continues to have difficulties with nutrition. *Imbalanced Nutrition: Less Than Body Requirements related to altered oral mucosa and surgical procedure* is an appropriate nursing diagnosis.

Outcomes. The client will maintain or gain weight after surgery, as evidenced by stabilization of weight and a weight gain of 1 pound per week until weight is stable.

Interventions

Administer Supplemental Nutrition. Immediately after surgery, monitor IV hydration. Assess bowel sounds every shift. The return of bowel sounds is often an indication to begin tube feedings. Assess the client for proper tube placement and measure retention of stomach contents every 4 hours or as ordered. Administer nutritional supplements by pump or bolus feedings as ordered. In addition, the practitioner may order total parenteral nutrition (TPN) as the first line of nutritional management (see Chapter 31 and discussion of achalasia later in this chapter).

Discuss Eating Modifications. Once the edema has subsided, healing has occurred, and the tracheostomy tube has been removed, the client may resume oral feedings. Caution the client about a decrease in sensation in the oral cavity after surgery. Assess swallowing carefully before eating begins. Instruct the client to avoid putting food directly on the surgical resection site. After meals, the client should always perform oral hygiene to remove any particles that remain and that may cause problems with the incision.

Diagnosis: Impaired Verbal Communication. When
the client has a tracheostomy after surgery, a common diagnosis is *Impaired Verbal Communication related to the presence of tracheostomy.*

Outcomes. The client will demonstrate the use of alternative forms of communication to communicate with staff and significant others.

Interventions

Promote Alternate Forms of Communication. Assess the client's literacy, and provide paper and pencil, magic slate, chalkboard, a marker board, or laptop computer for the client to write on as a substitute for talking. An alternative is to provide the client with a picture board to use for communicating any needs. Ideally, the assessment and instruction are completed preoperatively. The client should be allowed to communicate by gestures or written notes if this approach puts the client at ease. Most important, the nurse's manner should communicate acceptance, compassion, and caring. It is common to treat clients who cannot talk as though they cannot hear or understand. Be alert to any tendency to treat clients as if they are mentally incompetent or deaf. Help the client avoid social isolation by taking the client for walks and meeting others. Friendly social encounters and physical activity can help alleviate depression.

Relieve Anxiety. Help clients who cannot speak to express needs, concerns, and feelings. Check on the client frequently to reduce anxiety and loneliness. Place the call light within easy reach, and respond to the light promptly. If an intercom is used, it should be appropriately labeled regarding the client's limited ability to speak.

Evaluation

The most favorable outcome is that the client heals within 6 weeks to 3 months, according to the extent of the radical surgery, and without complications. Provide the name of the individual for the client to call or contact in case complications develop. Evaluate the client's ability to maintain intake of nutrients. If the client can self-feed via a tube until healing occurs and then gradually increase oral intake, then nutritional status should remain adequate. All clients need tremendous emotional support with this type of surgical intervention and need to be evaluated for possible complications related to lack of support from family or significant others.

■ Self-Care

On discharge, supply the client and family with complete instructions regarding diet, medications, manifestations of complications, and any treatments, such as care of the wound or tracheostomy. Explain how and when to contact health care practitioners. The client needs to be seen by the physician after discharge to ensure complete healing of any extensive surgical wounds. If the client has a tracheostomy, it may be permanent or may be closed at a later date. Clients who have undergone extensive surgery may need a referral to a home health agency for possible assistance with respiratory support (home oxygen), suctioning, nutritional support, and wound and tracheostomy care.

■ DISORDERS OF THE SALIVARY GLANDS

INFLAMMATION

Parotitis ("surgical mumps") is an inflammation of the parotid glands. It is the most common inflammatory condition affecting the salivary glands and probably results from inactivity of the glands caused by certain medications (such as diuretics), prolonged NG intubation, and lack of oral intake, such as that seen in postoperative clients. As secretions of the salivary gland diminish, oral bacteria have an opportunity to invade the gland and multiply. Interventions involve the following:

- Administering frequent oral hygiene to keep the bacterial count of the mouth low
- Keeping the client well hydrated

• Suggesting that the client use sugarless hard candies or chew sugarless gum to stimulate secretion of saliva

CALCULI

Stones, or calculi, form in the salivary glands when the glands are inactive and a metabolic condition favors the precipitation of salts. A nidus, or focus of origin, is necessary for stimulating salt precipitation. Assessment reveals that irritation from the stones causes local inflammation, swelling, and pain when the gland is stimulated to secrete, as during chewing. Intervention requires local excision by a physician. Stones occur most commonly in the submaxillary glands, probably because of the longer length of the duct and production of viscous alkaline secretions.

TUMORS

Most tumors in the salivary glands are benign. The most frequently seen malignant tumor is adenocarcinoma. Both benign and malignant tumors are characterized by enlargement of the gland. Pain occurs when expansion within the capsule of the gland creates pressure on sensory nerves. The treatment of choice for both benign and malignant tumors is usually surgical excision. If the tumor has recurred or is highly malignant, radiation therapy may also be used.

▌DISORDERS OF THE ESOPHAGUS

The most common manifestation of an esophageal disorder is dysphagia (difficulty with swallowing). Other manifestations include regurgitation, pain (which is probably linked with spasm), and heartburn or pyrosis.

DYSPHAGIA

Dysphagia can be caused by any esophageal disorder. Specific causes include neuromotor malfunction, mechanical obstruction, cardiovascular abnormalities, and neurologic diseases.

Dysphagia Caused by Mechanical Obstructions

Mechanical obstructions causing dysphagia include congenital defects, cancer, and acquired conditions such as a hiatal hernia. When an obstruction narrows the esophageal lumen, clients first experience dysphagia only with solid foods. Later, dysphagia becomes associated with semisolid foods and liquids. Finally, clients are unable to swallow their own saliva. Obstructive disorders, particularly esophageal cancer, may be accompanied by weight loss and cachexia.

Dysphagia Caused by Cardiovascular Abnormalities

Dysphagia may result from cardiovascular abnormalities, particularly in older people. Specific conditions causing vascular dysphagia include an enlarged heart, an

aortic aneurysm, and calcification of the descending aorta (review the anatomy of the heart and great arteries to the esophagus).

Dysphagia Caused by Neurologic Diseases

Dysphagia also may be caused by certain neurologic diseases, such as stroke, multiple sclerosis, poliomyelitis, and amyotrophic lateral sclerosis (ALS). Stroke is the most frequent cause of dysphagia.

Dysphagia from Other Causes

Dysphagia may be experienced after swallowing, if food gets caught in the esophagus. Clients may obtain relief by drinking liquids to force the impacted bolus through the narrow segment or by retching to dislodge the food. If vomiting does not succeed, endoscopy may be used to remove food lodged in the esophagus.

REGURGITATION

Regurgitation is the ejection of small amounts of chyme or gastric juice from the mouth without antecedent nausea. It is usually caused by an incompetent lower esophageal sphincter (LES). Regurgitation occurring immediately after swallowing results from structural or motor abnormality in the LES. Contributing factors include abnormal motor activity, increased abdominal pressure, and sphincter abnormality. Regurgitation occurs with achalasia, pylorospasm, lesions proximal to the cardia, hiatal hernia, reflux esophagitis, and esophageal ulcer or cancer. Stooping or lying down facilitates the flow of gastric contents into the esophagus, thus exacerbating regurgitation.

ACUTE PAIN

Pain, which may be constant or may occur only with swallowing, suggests diffuse esophageal spasm. Pain may result from alterations of the mucosa from reflux disease, radiation, or viral infection. Pain that affects the esophageal mucosa and occurs with swallowing is called *odynophagia*. The client usually describes the pain as sharp, constricting, sticking, crushing, stabbing, or knife-like. Odynophagia is usually severe, quite distressing, and often associated with a deep and long-lasting pain. The pain, located substernally, may radiate to the neck, back, and shoulder. Pain may occur throughout the day and can be confused with angina. Odynophagia can be triggered by a cold or carbonated beverage or by solid food passing through the esophagus. The most common cause is the reflux of gastric contents into the esophagus.

HEARTBURN OR PYROSIS

Heartburn or pyrosis, also known as (indigestion, or dyspepsia), is another common manifestation of esophageal disease. Generally, it is a painful sensation of warmth and burning in the lower retrosternal midline. Because clients may use the word "heartburn" to describe very different sensations, it is essential to find out exactly what this term means to the client using it. Heartburn usually means substernal, midline burning that tends to radiate, generally in waves, upward to the neck, resulting from abnormalities of the LES. Clients often describe this discomfort as *cramping* or *knotting*.

EB Heartburn is commonly experienced with obesity, postural changes (such as bending, stooping, and lifting), gulping of food or liquids, during pregnancy, or ingestion of alcohol. Manifestations often are relieved by standing or eructating. Heartburn also arises in the presence of refluxed gastric or duodenal contents. Disorders most commonly associated with heartburn are reflux esophagitis, hiatal hernia, achalasia, and gastric stasis. Heartburn is common in individuals with pyloric or duodenal ulcers and LES disorders.

ACHALASIA

Achalasia is a disorder characterized by progressively increasing dysphagia, with the client eventually having great difficulty swallowing and expressing the feeling that "something is stuck in the throat." Achalasia commonly occurs in individuals in their 20s and 30s and appears equally often in men and women.

Etiology and Risk Factors

Achalasia is a chronic, progressive disease of unknown cause. Occasionally, the client can relate the onset to an episode of acute dysphagia, but usually the onset is obscure. The disease is noticed only when dysphagia becomes severe. Because achalasia is idiopathic, there are no identified risk factors. There may be a familial component.

Pathophysiology

EB Achalasia is characterized by impaired motility of the lower two thirds of the esophagus. The LES fails to relax normally with swallowing. Inadequate functioning occurs because nerve impulses cannot pass through the esophagus or sympathetic receptors are absent from the LES. There may be degeneration of the ganglion cells or impairment of impulses from Auerbach's plexus. Impaired propulsion and a constricted LES result in accumulation of food and fluid within the lower esophagus. When hydrostatic pressure exceeds the force of resistance of the LES, the contents pass into the stomach. Reflux esophagitis with resultant ulceration (Figure 32-6) is a possible complication (see Gastroesophageal Reflux Disease later in this chapter). Aspiration of regurgitated esophageal contents may result in atelectasis and other pulmonary problems.

Clinical Manifestations

The initial manifestation of achalasia is dysphagia. It is difficult for food and fluid to pass through the LES. In the early stages of achalasia, the client may have substernal pain because of spasms of the esophagus or may

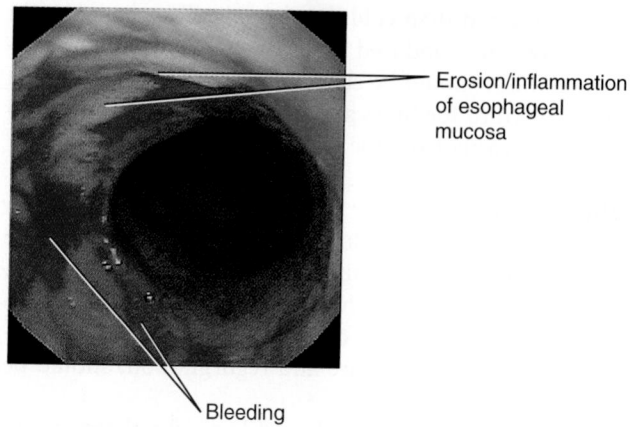

Erosion/inflammation of esophageal mucosa

Bleeding

FIGURE 32-6 Endoscopic view of severe esophagitis. Note arrows depicting erosion or inflammation of esophageal mucosa and bleeding.

be unable to eructate (belch). The client may regurgitate undigested food eaten many hours earlier as well as large amounts of mucus that have been stimulated by esophageal irritation. As achalasia progresses, manifestations increase in frequency and severity. Upper respiratory infections, emotional disturbances, overeating, obesity, and pregnancy may exacerbate the problem.

Diagnostic tests used to determine the presence of achalasia include barium swallow, endoscopy, and manometry. The barium swallow is considered positive for achalasia, if it reveals nonpropulsive waves and esophageal dilation. Barium may also be retained in the esophagus. Endoscopy helps determine the status of the LES, the amount of dilation, and the presence of food. Manometry (measurement of pressure in the esophagus) confirms the diagnosis with elevated resting pressures in the LES or slow, low-amplitude, or absent peristalsis.

Outcome Management
■ Medical Management

Relieve Manifestations. Treatment of achalasia is aimed at relieving clinical manifestations. Management usually begins with medical treatment on an outpatient basis. Often, as the problem progresses, hospitalization is required for surgical procedures or for placement of a gastrostomy, PEG, or percutaneous endoscopic jejunostomy (PEJ) tube for nutritional support.

Administer Medications. Medications that relax the LES or lower esophageal pressures (such as anticholinergic drugs, nitrates, gastrointestinal hormones, and calcium-channel blockers) have been studied, but none of them have proved to be of consistent value or effectiveness. Pain is managed with antacids, H_2 receptor antagonists, and proton pump inhibitors.

Modify Diet. Changes in diet may ease the pressure and reflux in the client with achalasia. Small, frequent feedings ease the passage of food, and semisoft, warm foods are better tolerated than cold, hard foods. The client should avoid hot, spicy, and iced foods as well as alcohol and tobacco. Foods should be chewed thoroughly to add saliva to the mixture for lubrication and to allow the bolus to pass more easily from the esophagus to the stomach.

Alternate Positions. The client should experiment with different positions to reduce pressure while eating. Some clients benefit from arching the back while swallowing. After eating, the client should remain upright by standing or sitting. Restrictive or tight clothing, which may increase esophageal pressure and regurgitation, should be avoided.

To prevent nocturnal reflux of food, the client should sleep with the head of the bed elevated. Place the client in a semi-Fowler position, using a wedge pillow to keep the head higher than the LES, or elevate the head of the bed on 4- to 6-inch blocks.

■ Nursing Management of the Medical Client
Assessment

Obtain a history, noting the manifestations the client is experiencing, onset and duration of aggravating factors, and any methods the client uses for relief. Assess respiratory manifestations because reflux or regurgitation can affect the respiratory tract. Assess the client's nutritional status, noting any weight changes and the effects of esophageal manifestations on dietary habits.

Diagnosis, Outcomes, Interventions

Diagnosis: Imbalanced Nutrition: Less Than Body Requirements. The client with achalasia experiences a great deal of difficulty swallowing, leading to the nursing diagnosis of *Imbalanced Nutrition: Less Than Body Requirements related to dysphagia.*

Outcomes. The client will maintain an adequate nutritional intake, as evidenced by maintenance of ideal body weight or regaining any weight lost at a rate of 1 pound per week.

Interventions. Consult with the client concerning dietary habits and daily intake of nutrients. Obtain a baseline weight and daily weights. Teach the client about changes in dietary habits that may relieve manifestations, as discussed under Medical Management. A gastrostomy tube, PEG tube, or PEJ tube may be used to provide adequate nutritional support if dysphagia continues to be a problem. Nursing management of tube feedings is discussed in Chapter 31 and later in this chapter under Nursing Management of the Surgical Client.

Diagnosis: Acute Pain. When the client experiences gastric reflux, the acid in the esophagus causes *Acute*

Pain related to episodes of gastric reflux, making this an appropriate nursing diagnosis.

Outcomes. The client will experience a decrease in pain or an absence of pain, as evidenced by verbalizing a reduction in or an absence of pain and an ability to maintain oral intake.

Interventions. Pain can be decreased or relieved through the use of medications (such as antacids, histamine H_2 receptor antagonists, and proton pump inhibitors), dietary changes, and repositioning. Assess the client every shift to determine whether medications, changes in diet, and repositioning are effective in controlling or relieving pain.

Evaluation

The most appropriate outcome is that the achalasia is controlled with medical treatment and the client's nutritional status is maintained. If the client's manifestations cannot be controlled with medical treatment, surgical intervention may be necessary.

■ Surgical Management
Surgical management of achalasia may involve dilating the LES (esophageal dilation) or enlarging the sphincter (esophagomyotomy). Esophageal dilation (bougienage) forcefully dilates the LES (Figure 32-7). This procedure, which is usually done on an outpatient basis, is used to

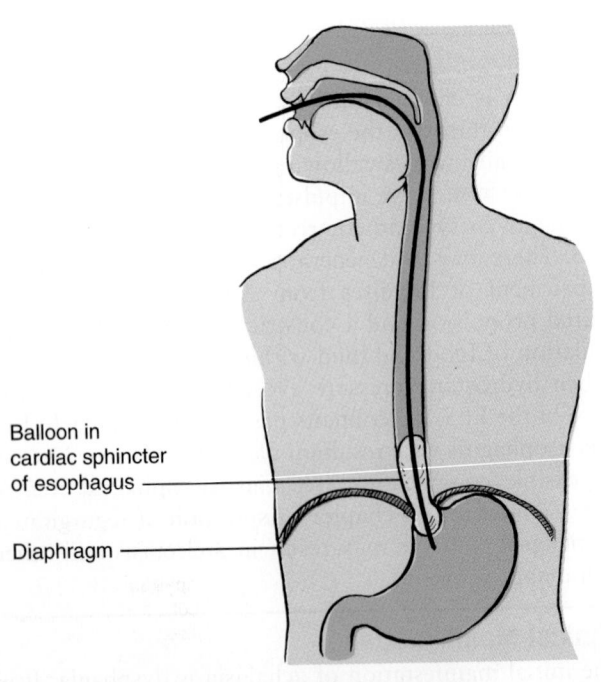

Balloon in
cardiac sphincter
of esophagus —

Diaphragm —

FIGURE 32-7 Bougienage (passage of a bougie) relieves dysphagia by dilating the lower esophageal sphincter.

help correct not only achalasia, but also esophageal spasms and strictures. Vigorous dilation is associated with a 75% success rate. Local anesthesia is used under radiologic guidance.

In the more complex procedure, esophagomyotomy (Heller's procedure), the surgeon enlarges the vestibule by incising the circular muscle fibers down to the mucosa (Figure 32-8). Complications may include reflux esophagitis and restenosis.

If a client cannot swallow for long periods, a gastrostomy tube, PEG, or PEJ may be inserted. The tubes may be inserted surgically, laparoscopically, or via percutaneous endoscopy.

For the laparoscopic or surgical method, the physician makes an incision in the wall of the abdomen and sutures the tube to the gastric wall. Usually these procedures are tolerated well by the client.

For a percutaneous endoscopic approach, the physician uses local anesthesia and inserts a cannula into the stomach through a small abdominal incision. A suture is threaded through the cannula. A second physician uses an endoscope to pull the suture through the client's mouth. The PEG tube is attached and advanced down the esophagus, through the abdominal incision, where crossbars (Figure 32-9) secure it internally and externally. Some tubes contain an internal balloon instead of an internal crossbar, whereas other tubes contain internal and external crossbars and an internal balloon. Skin care around the percutaneous site is necessary postoperatively. In the PEJ procedure, the tube is inserted into the jejunum instead of the stomach. See Chapter 31 for a comparison of enteral feeding routes.

■ Nursing Management of the Surgical Client

Preoperative Care
Assessment

Obtain a history, noting the onset and duration of manifestations the client is experiencing, aggravating factors, and any methods the client uses for relief. Assess the client's respiratory status and nutritional status in addition to the routine preoperative assessments.

Diagnosis, Outcomes, Interventions

Diagnosis: Deficient Knowledge. To prepare the client for surgery, consider the nursing diagnosis *Deficient Knowledge related to preoperative preparation and postoperative care.*

Outcomes. The client will understand and be prepared for surgery, as evidenced by asking questions and expressing statements of understanding.

Interventions

Teach about Esophageal Dilation. If the client is to undergo esophageal dilation, explain that the client will be awake during the procedure. A local anesthetic solution is sprayed on the throat, and an analgesic or tranquilizer may be given. The client should take long, slow breaths during passage of the bougies. As the bag is inflated, the client may feel brief discomfort. Weighted bougies with increasing weight can also be used for dilation. Esophageal dilation is often performed on an outpatient basis.

FIGURE 32-8 A and **B,** Esophagomyotomy (Heller's procedure) is the surgical procedure of choice when a segment of esophagus narrows and causes functional obstruction.

A — Line of incision into constricted section of muscle

B — Esophageal mucosa pouches through incision in muscle

FIGURE 32-9 Percutaneous endoscopic gastrostomy tube.

Tubing clamp · Plug-in adapter · External circle clamp · External cross bar · Abdominal wall · Stomach wall · Internal cross bar · Catheter tip

Explain Esophagomyotomy. Esophagomyotomy is a more complex procedure. The client requires a general anesthetic and remains hospitalized for more than 24 hours. Instruct the client undergoing an esophageal procedure about the usual preoperative procedures, such as remaining in an NPO status after midnight and administration of IV fluids and preoperative medications. Discuss pain control, drains, surgical dressings, and the presence of an NG tube, a gastrostomy tube, a PEG tube, or a PEJ tube. The possibility of a thoracotomy approach being used to reach the esophagus requires instruction concerning chest tubes. Discuss manifestations of respiratory complications related to esophageal reflux and aspiration.

Instruct clients who have undergone an esophagomyotomy to sleep with the head of the bed elevated and to recognize manifestations of respiratory complications. Explain the manifestations of infection and esophageal perforation; urge the client to notify the physician if any of these problems occur.

Postoperative Care
Assessment

Routine postoperative assessments, such as monitoring vital signs, pain, and drainage tubes placed during surgery, are required. In addition, monitor the client's respiratory and nutritional status and the site of the feeding tube (if placed).

Diagnosis, Outcomes, Interventions

Diagnosis: Imbalanced Nutrition: Less Than Body Requirements.
For the client experiencing dysphagia, the nursing diagnosis *Imbalanced Nutrition: Less Than Body Requirements related to dysphagia and placement of a gastrostomy, PEG, or PEJ tube* is appropriate.

Outcomes. The client will maintain an adequate nutritional intake, as evidenced by maintaining ideal body weight or gaining weight at a rate of 1 pound per week to replace previous weight loss.

Interventions. A baseline weight and daily weight measurement should be obtained. Evaluate the need for increased protein in the diet to promote wound healing.

Maintain Feeding Tube. Follow institutional policy regarding care for the client with a gastrostomy, PEG, or PEJ tube. Typically, the client is on NPO status for at least 24 hours before continuous or bolus tube feedings begin. Nursing interventions include checking tube placement via measurement of the tube and checking pH of stomach contents and residual amounts every 4 hours. (Do not assess this via aspiration if the tube is placed in the jejunum, because these tubes are flushed, not aspi-

rated.) If the gastric return is more than 150 ml or twice the hourly rate, hold the feeding for 1 hour and repeat aspiration before continuing the feeding. After checking placement and administering bolus feedings or medications, flush the tube with 50 to 100 ml of normal saline or water. Keep the head of the bed elevated at least 30 degrees at all times for continuous feedings or for 1 hour after completion of intermittent bolus feedings. Change the enteral feeding bag and tubing every 24 hours if an open delivery system is used, and rinse them with water every 4 hours or after each intermittent feeding to decrease the risk of bacterial contamination. If a closed delivery system is used, the bottle and tubing should be changed every 24 hours. (See Chapter 31 for additional information about enteral feedings.)

Diagnosis: Risk for Impaired Skin Integrity.
When a feeding tube has been placed, the nursing diagnosis *Risk for Impaired Skin Integrity related to placement of a gastrostomy, PEG, or PEJ tube* identifies a potential problem.

Outcomes. The client will maintain or regain normal skin integrity, as evidenced by the absence of exudate, swelling, excoriation, or erythema at the tube insertion site.

Interventions
Provide Feeding Tube Care. Follow your facility's policy regarding routine care. Usually, about 12 to 24 hours after the tube has been surgically placed, the initial dressing may be removed and the skin around the insertion site may be washed with soap and water. A dressing may be applied as needed. Manifestations of infection should be reported to the physician. Teach the client or significant other home care management. (See the Bridge to Home Health Care feature on Managing Tube Feedings in Chapter 31.)

Diagnosis: Risk for Injury.
A possible problem in the postoperative client is *Risk for Injury: Pneumothorax related to surgical procedure and presence of chest tubes.*

Outcomes. Injury will be prevented, as evidenced by absence of hemorrhage, absence of manifestations of perforation, normal temperature, and absence of problems associated with chest tubes, such as respiratory distress.

Interventions
Monitor for Complications. After esophageal dilation, monitor the client for manifestations of perforation, such as elevated temperature, chest or shoulder pain, and subcutaneous emphysema. If any of these manifestations are noted, notify the physician immediately. The client will require an x-ray study to determine whether air is in the mediastinum, indicating perforation.

Maintain Chest Tubes. After an esophagomyotomy, a thoracotomy incision and chest tubes are in place. Maintain chest tube drainage and the NG or gastric drainage system, and manage the client's pain. See Chapter 64 for care of the client with chest tubes.

Evaluation

An appropriate outcome is that the client will maintain adequate nutrition and that the condition will be reversed with surgery. The esophagus must heal completely before the client may return to eating the usual foods. An acceptable evaluation is that the client or significant others have been able to continue tube feedings for at least 6 weeks after surgery.

■ Modifications for Older Clients

An attempt is made to treat older clients with more local measures (pain medications, positioning, and dietary modification) and possibly esophageal dilation. The older adult is less likely to tolerate the more complicated procedures and, therefore, more likely to experience complications.

■ Self-Care

The client or significant others will require teaching if the feedings are required after discharge. Initially, home visits by a nurse may be necessary to assist the client with any home care needs related to tube feedings, diet, medications, and wound care and to provide an ongoing evaluation of the client's condition. A referral to a social worker may be needed to assist the client with financial assistance, community resources, counseling, and specialized equipment (see Chapter 31).

GASTROESOPHAGEAL REFLUX DISEASE

Esophageal reflux is a backward flow of gastric contents into the esophagus. Gastroesophageal reflux disease (GERD) refers to a syndrome resulting from esophageal reflux. Reflux exposes the esophageal mucosa to the gastric contents, which gradually breaks down the esophageal mucosa. This condition, sometimes called *reflux esophagitis,* is often associated with a sliding hiatal hernia. However, complications causing reflux may occur without a hiatal hernia, and individuals with a hiatal hernia may not have manifestations of reflux.

GERD can occur in any age group. About 10% of the population have daily manifestations of GERD, and as much as one third of the population have monthly manifestations. Manifestations are often overlooked and attributed to stress.

Etiology and Risk Factors

The cause of GERD seems to be an inappropriate relaxation of the LES (Figure 32-10). The exact cause of the relaxation is unknown, but reflux occurs with the following:

- An alteration in the innervation of the pressure zone in the region of the gastroesophageal sphincter
- Displacement of the angle of the gastroesophageal junction
- An incompetent LES

Risk factors as well as health promotion and maintenance behaviors are important teaching topics. These factors include obesity and weight gain, pregnancy, chewing tobacco, smoking, high-fat foods, theophylline, caffeine, chocolate, and high levels of estrogen and pro-

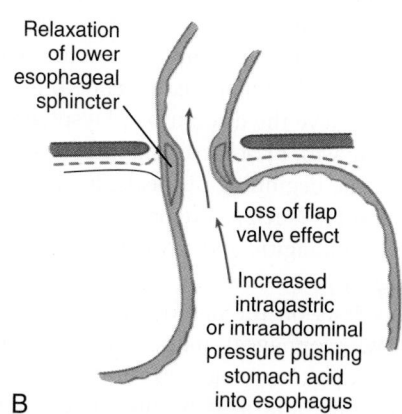

FIGURE 32-10 A, Normal mechanisms preventing esophageal reflux: contraction of lower esophageal sphincter (LES) creating high-pressure zone at the LES, acute gastroesophageal angle causing a flap valve effect, and phrenoesophageal ligament causing a pinchcock valve effect. **B,** Loss of normal mechanisms creating gastroesophageal reflux disease (GERD): relaxed LES and displaced angle of the gastroesophageal junction allowing increased intragastric or intra-abdominal pressure and resulting in gastric contents leaking into the lower esophagus. (**A** from Price, S.A., & Wilson, L.M. [2003]. *Pathophysiology: Clinical concepts of disease processes* [6th ed.]. St. Louis: Mosby.)

gesterone. Teaching clients to limit smoking, caffeine, chocolate, and high-fat foods helps prevent GERD. Eating small meals and increasing dietary protein also helps. Losing weight, elevating the head of the bed for sleeping, and avoiding lifting, straining, bending, and tight or constrictive clothing can further help prevent the problem. Once GERD has developed, a health restoration action is to instruct the client on taking prescribed medications.

Pathophysiology

Normally, a high-pressure zone exists in the region of the gastroesophageal sphincter. High pressure prevents reflux, but permits the passage of food and liquids. When there is an alteration in this region, reflux occurs.

Reflux esophagitis may occur with gastric or duodenal ulcer, after esophageal or gastric surgery, after prolonged vomiting, or after prolonged gastrointestinal intubation. The reflux most often consists of hydrochloric acid or gastric and duodenal contents containing bile acid and pancreatic juice. Frequent or prolonged reflux results in inflammation of the esophageal mucosa (esophagitis). The degree of reflux esophagitis present depends on (1) frequency of the reflux, (2) contents of the reflux, (3) buffering ability of the saliva and mucous secretion, and (4) rate of gastric emptying.

Clinical Manifestations

GERD may begin suddenly or gradually. The client may complain of heartburn, odynophagia, dysphagia, acid regurgitation, water brash (the release of salty secretions in the mouth), or eructation. Pain in GERD is typically described as a burning sensation that moves up and down. If the condition is severe, the pain may radiate to the back, neck, or jaw. Pain usually occurs after meals and is relieved with antacids or fluids. Discomfort sometimes accompanies activities that increase intra-abdominal pressure, such as lifting or straining. The client may state that discomfort occurs when lying supine or when the stomach is distended. Standing and walking may relieve the discomfort. Dysphagia resulting from edema, spasm, or a narrowed lumen is intermittent and worse at the beginning of meals. Responses to pain-relieving measures (such as nitroglycerin) help differentiate between esophagitis and problems of cardiac origin (such as angina pectoris).

Diagnosis rests on the demonstration of reflux. Barium swallow, esophageal manometry, esophagoscopy, esophageal biopsy, cytologic examination, analysis of gastric secretions, and acid perfusion tests confirm the diagnosis of GERD (see Chapter 30).

Outcome Management
■ Medical Management

Decrease Reflux with Medications. See the Integrating Pharmacology feature on Medications for GERD at right. For people receiving long-term therapy with non-steroidal anti-inflammatory drugs (NSAIDs), misopros-

tol (Cytotec) is useful for preventing gastric ulcer formation and, in some instances, GERD manifestations. Anticholinergic drugs, calcium-channel blockers, bisphosphonates, and theophylline should be avoided if possible because these drugs appear to decrease LES pressure, delay gastric emptying, or irritate the esophagus.

Decrease Reflux with Lifestyle and Diet Changes. In mild GERD, diet and lifestyle changes may be sufficient to relieve manifestations. Instruct the client to do the following:

- Restrict the diet to small, frequent feedings (four to six per day) to decrease the amount of food in the stomach.
- Drink adequate fluids at meals to assist food passage.

INTEGRATING PHARMACOLOGY
Medications for GERD

A variety of medications including antacids, histamine receptor antagonists, cholinergics, gastrointestinal stimulants, and proton pump inhibitors may be used for treatment of GERD.

Drug therapy for GERD often starts with an antacid, which commonly provides prompt relief (about 30 minutes). Typically, the client takes 30 ml of antacid 1 hour before and 2 to 3 hours after each meal to buffer or neutralize gastric acid secretions and soothe mucosal lining. Clients typically tolerate combination products such as calcium carbonate–magnesium carbonate (Mylanta) or magnesium hydroxide–aluminum hydroxide (Maalox). Aluminum hydroxide–magnesium carbonate (Gaviscon) is another excellent antacid because of its foaming action.

If manifestations are severe or persist, the client may be prescribed histamine receptor antagonists such as ranitidine (Zantac) or famotidine (Pepcid). These medications inhibit histamine at H_2-receptor sites in parietal cells, which decreases gastric acid secretions. If histamine receptor antagonists are used, they should be given an hour before or after antacids.

Bethanechol (Urecholine) may be added for clients with severe manifestations because it increases LES pressure and prevents reflux. Because bethanechol is a cholinergic drug, it is usually given with antacids and a histamine receptor antagonist because it can increase the secretion of gastric acid. It should be taken before meals.

Metoclopramide (Reglan), an antiemetic and cholinergic drug, may be prescribed because it increases LES pressure by stimulating the smooth muscle of the GI tract and increases the rate of gastric emptying (GI stimulant). This medication is taken 30 to 60 minutes before meals.

Lansoprazole (Prevacid) or esomeprazole (Nexium) are proton pump inhibitors that suppress gastric secretion by inhibiting the hydrogen and potassium ATPase enzyme system in the gastric parietal cell. They should be given at least 30 minutes before meals.

- Eat slowly and chew thoroughly to add saliva to the food.
- Avoid extremely hot or cold foods, spices, fats, alcohol, coffee, chocolate, and citrus juices to decrease acid.
- Avoid eating and drinking for 3 hours before retiring to prevent the common problem of nocturnal reflux.
- Elevate the head of the bed 6 to 8 inches to prevent nocturnal reflux.
- Lose weight, if overweight, to decrease the gastroesophageal pressure gradient.
- Avoid tobacco, salicylates, and phenylbutazone, which may exacerbate esophagitis.

Endoluminal Gastroplication. Endoluminal gastroplication is a medical therapy developed for the treatment of symptomatic GERD. The procedure works by creating plications, or pleats, at the LES. The EndoCinch System, like a tiny sewing machine, is attached to the end of a standard flexible endoscope, which allows the physician to place a suture (stitch) near the LES. Two stitches can be placed and tied together to create a pleat near the LES. Only mild sedation is required for this outpatient procedure and clients can resume normal activities the following day.

■ Nursing Management of the Medical Client

Assess Manifestations. Identify specific manifestations the client has been experiencing. Document onset of manifestations, the frequency and severity, and the relationship of manifestations to food and various food products. Assist in maintaining the client's general appearance and nutritional status. Assist the client to identify risk factors for GERD, and instruct the client concerning lifestyle changes to reduce risk factors.

Provide Teaching. Instruct the client in the prescribed diet regimen, and evaluate both the client's understand-ing of treatment and effectiveness. Administer medications ordered for pain, and document medication effectiveness. Instruct the client in the prescribed medication regimen, and evaluate the client's understanding of the treatment. Teaching to prepare the client for the endoluminal gastroplication is the same as teaching for a client undergoing endoscopic examination of the esophagus.

■ Surgical Management and Nursing Management of the Surgical Client

Clients who do not respond to medical management may undergo one of the surgical procedures discussed under Surgical Management for hiatal hernia.

HIATAL HERNIA

A hiatal hernia (diaphragmatic hernia) is a condition in which the cardiac sphincter becomes enlarged, allowing a part of the stomach to pass into the thoracic cavity. There are two major types of hernias: *sliding* hernias (type I) and *rolling* or *paraesophageal* hernias (type II). With a sliding hiatal hernia, the upper stomach and the gastroesophageal junction are displaced upward into the thorax (Figure 32-11, *A*). Sliding hiatal hernias account for about 90% of the total cases of esophageal hiatal hernias. With a rolling hiatal hernia, the gastroesophageal junction stays below the diaphragm but, all or part of the stomach pushes through into the thorax (see Figure 32-11, *B*).

The incidence of hiatal hernia is estimated as 5 per 1000 in the general population and may be as high as 60% in clients older than age 60 years. Women tend to be affected more often than men, and the incidence increases significantly with age.

Etiology and Risk Factors

Hiatal hernias are related to muscle weakness in the esophageal hiatus, which loosens the esophageal supports and allows the lower portion of the stomach to rise into the thorax. As with other hernias, the muscle weak-

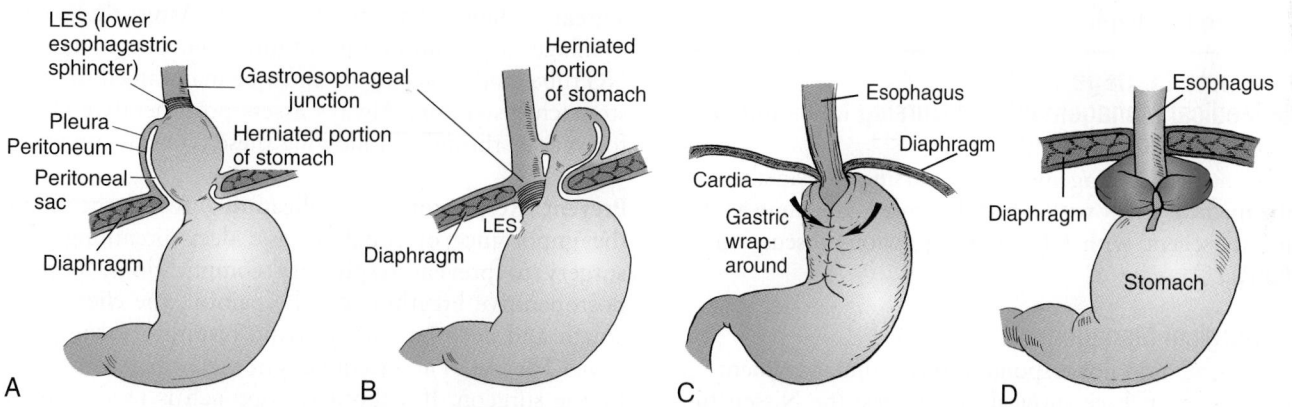

FIGURE 32-11 **A,** A sliding hiatal hernia. **B,** A rolling hiatal hernia. **C,** Nissen fundoplication for hiatal hernia. The gastric fundus is wrapped around the distal esophagus and sutured to itself. **D,** Angelchick antireflux prosthesis in place.

ness is caused by a variety of conditions, such as aging, trauma, congenital muscle weakness, surgery, or anything that increases intra-abdominal pressure such as lifting, coughing, pregnancy, and obesity.

Risk factors are those that weaken the diaphragm and increase intra-abdominal pressure. Pressure may be increased by conditions such as obesity, pregnancy, or ascites.

Health promotion behaviors to prevent or at least delay a hiatal hernia include avoiding any activities that increase intra-abdominal pressure. These activities include heavy lifting and wearing tight constrictive clothing, especially around the waist. Other than these measures, hiatal hernias are not preventable.

Pathophysiology

A hiatal hernia involves protrusion of part of the stomach through a weakness in the diaphragm. The resulting regurgitation and motor dysfunction cause the manifestations associated with hiatal hernia. The major problem with a sliding hiatal hernia is reflux (GERD), which appears to be caused by the exposure of the LES to the low pressure in the thorax.

With a rolling hiatal hernia, the LES remains below the diaphragm and reflux is not a problem. Complications of a rolling hiatal hernia include obstruction, strangulation, and the development of a volvulus.

Clinical Manifestations

Manifestations of hiatal hernia vary in kind and severity. In sliding hiatal hernias, the client may experience heartburn 30 to 60 minutes after meals. Reflux may also result in substernal pain.

The client with a rolling hiatal hernia does not have manifestations of reflux. The client may complain of a feeling of fullness after eating or may have difficulty breathing. Some clients experience chest pain similar to that of angina. Pain is usually worse when the client lies down.

A barium swallow with fluoroscopy can reveal a hiatal hernia by showing the position of the stomach in relation to the diaphragm.

Outcome Management
■ Medical Management and Nursing Management of the Medical Client

The medical management and nursing management of the medical client with a hiatal hernia is the same as that for the client with GERD. See previous discussion on GERD.

■ Surgical Management

Clients who do not respond to medical management undergo one of three surgical procedures: the Nissen fundoplication, the Hill operation, or the Belsey operation. The surgeon may use an open surgical approach or a lap-

aroscopic approach to complete these procedures. Recovery is usually faster with the laparoscopic approach.

The *Nissen fundoplication* is most common and involves suturing the fundus around the esophagus (Figure 32-11, C). An abdominal approach is usually used. An increase in pressure or volume in the stomach closes the cardia and blocks reflux into the esophagus. The surgeon creates a valve-like substitute sphincter with inherent contractility.

The *Hill operation* narrows the esophageal opening and anchors the stomach and distal esophagus to the median arcuate ligament (posterior gastropexy). This procedure reinforces the sphincter and recreates the gastroesophageal valve. A partial wraparound (180 degrees) of the stomach around the esophagus is created via an abdominal approach.

The *Belsey (Mark IV) repair* consists of plication of the anterior and lateral aspects of the stomach onto the distal esophagus. The surgeon creates the esophagogastric angle without opening the esophagus or the diaphragm. A 280-degree esophageal wraparound is created via a thoracic approach.

In clients with severe reflux, an Angelchick prosthesis may be inserted. A laparotomy is performed, and a synthetic C-shaped silicone prosthesis is tied around the distal esophagus (Figure 32-11, D). The prosthesis anchors the LES in the abdomen and reinforces sphincter pressure. The success of this procedure is variable, depending on the severity of the problem. In clients with severe reflux, this procedure may be unsuccessful.

Clients undergoing a surgical procedure are encouraged to follow the GERD antireflux medical regimen (medications, diet changes, lifestyle changes) because the recurrence rate is significant.

■ Nursing Management of the Surgical Client
Postoperative Assessments. The surgical client requires the same assessments as the medical client, as well as routine preoperative and postoperative assessments. If chest tubes are placed postoperatively, monitor the client for respiratory distress. An abdominal incision results in a greater chance of a wound infection. Assess the wound drainage for manifestations of infection. Clients have an NG tube, and tube patency must be maintained to avoid stomach distention. Always assess postoperative clients for venous thrombus following these types of surgery.

Prevent Respiratory Complications. Teach the client the importance of coughing and deep breathing after surgery to prevent respiratory complications. Because postoperative breathing can be painful, the client must cough and deep breathe to avoid respiratory complications. The use of an incentive spirometer may be ordered by the surgeon. If a thoracic approach is used, explain the purpose of the chest tubes and the care needed (see Chapter 64).

Prevent Gas-Bloat Syndrome. Fluids are usually resumed after 24 hours, and the diet is progressively advanced as tolerated when peristalsis returns. Small, frequent meals are provided to avoid overloading the stomach. After fundoplication, the client may experience gas-bloat syndrome if the wrap of the fundus is too tight, causing bloating and an inability to eructate. Clients should avoid carbonated beverages and gas-producing foods. Ambulating can assist peristalsis in removing air from the GI tract. The condition is usually temporary. Instruct clients to report dysphagia, epigastric fullness, bloating, or excessive borborygmi to physician or practitioner.

DIVERTICULA

An esophageal diverticulum is a sac-like outpouching in one or more layers of the esophagus. As food is ingested, it becomes trapped in a diverticulum and can later be regurgitated. The most common type of esophageal diverticulum is esophageal pulsion (Zenker's) diverticulum (Figure 32-12). Esophageal diverticula are considered rare. Zenker's diverticula occur three times more often in men as in women.

Etiology and Risk Factors

The cause of esophageal weakness may be a congenital defect, esophageal trauma, scar tissue, or inflammation. There are two categories of diverticula: traction and pulsion. With a *traction* diverticulum, the esophageal mucosa has pulled outward from the esophagus. Traction diverticula are most commonly found in the middle esophagus. With a *pulsion* diverticulum, the esophageal mucosa has pushed outward through a defect in the esophageal musculature. Pulsion diverticula are most commonly found in the upper esophagus. There is no means of prevention.

Pathophysiology

Diverticula in the esophagus often develop in areas of muscle weakness that arise from esophageal trauma, congenital weakness of the esophageal wall, or scar tissue that forms from chronic inflammation of the esophagus. When food becomes trapped in a diverticulum, it may cause a local abscess. Infected diverticula place the client at risk for esophageal perforation because the mucosa is without the protection of the normal esophageal muscle layer.

Clinical Manifestations

Initially, the client usually complains of difficulty swallowing. Other manifestations may include eructation, regurgitation of undigested food, halitosis, and a sour taste in the mouth. Coughing also may occur because of irritation of the trachea from regurgitated food.

A barium swallow is performed to locate the diverticulum. Endoscopy is usually contraindicated because the diverticulum may be perforated by the endoscope.

Outcome Management
■ Medical Management

Medical management of esophageal diverticula includes dietary management and positioning. Small, frequent meals of semisoft foods often facilitate passage of food. The client should note which foods ease or worsen the manifestations.

To prevent reflux of food, the caregiver should raise the head of the bed for 2 hours after meals. Sleeping with the head of the bed elevated can often prevent nocturnal reflux. The client also should avoid constrictive clothes and vigorous exercise after eating.

■ Nursing Management of the Medical Client

Obtain a history from the client, noting the onset and duration of manifestations and whether they occur at mealtimes or at night. Assess the client's respiratory status because regurgitation can cause respiratory complications.

Teach the client how changes in diet and positioning can control manifestations. Encourage the client to try various foods and various positions to evaluate which are most effective.

■ Surgical Management

When manifestations become severe, surgery may be indicated. A cervical approach is used for Zenker's diverticulum, whereas a thoracic approach is used for diverticula located lower in the esophagus. In both procedures, the diverticulum is excised and the esophageal mucosa is reanastomosed.

FIGURE 32-12 Endoscopic view of Zenker's diverticulum. Note how difficult it is to distinguish the true lumen of the esophagus from that of the Zenker's diverticulum. (From Feldman, M., Friedman, L., & Sleisenger, M. [Eds.]. [2002]. *Sleisenger and Fordtran's gastrointestinal and liver disease: Pathophysiology/diagnosis/management* [7th ed.]. Philadelphia: W.B. Saunders; Courtesy of D. Langdon, MD.)

■ Nursing Management of the Surgical Client
Assessment

Obtain a history, noting the onset and duration of manifestations, aggravating factors, and any methods the client uses for relief. In addition, routine preoperative and postoperative assessments are required.

Diagnosis, Outcomes, Interventions

Diagnosis: Risk for Injury. When an esophageal diverticulum is treated surgically, the nursing diagnosis *Risk for Injury related to surgical procedure and presence of chest tubes* is appropriate.

Outcomes. Injury will be prevented, as evidenced by a normal temperature and an absence of hemorrhage, infection, and problems associated with the chest tubes, such as respiratory distress.

Interventions

Provide Teaching. Discuss the normal preoperative routines. Explain that the client will be taking nothing by mouth after surgery and that an NG tube will be present until healing occurs. If a thoracic approach is used, preoperative and postoperative nursing care is similar to that for clients having thoracic surgery and chest tubes (see Chapter 64).

Maintain the Nasogastric Tube. After surgery, the client's NG tube is attached to low intermittent suction to avoid trauma to the stomach lining. Assess the amount and color of drainage during each shift. Check for continued bloody NG drainage as well as for external bleeding. Do not irrigate or reposition the NG tube unless told to do so by the physician. Moving the NG tube can perforate the esophagus or stomach (see Chapter 33 on irrigation of tubes if ordered by the surgeon). Assess the client for manifestations of esophageal perforation, such as chest pain, fever, and subcutaneous emphysema. The client receives IV fluids until tube feedings begin. Once fluids and supplemental feedings begin, record the client's response.

After surgery, the client may be discharged with an NG or a gastrostomy tube in place to allow for esophageal healing. Give the client written and verbal instructions about tube feedings, diet, and positioning. A visiting nurse should see the client at home to ensure that tube feedings are being tolerated well and should continue visits until the feeding tube is removed.

Promote Comfort. Assess the client's pain, and administer and evaluate prescribed analgesics. After surgery, the head of the bed should be elevated 30 degrees to reduce edema around the neck and upper chest. Frequent oral hygiene increases the client's comfort.

Evaluation

An appropriate outcome for the client with a diverticulum is that the altered diet will control the problem. If surgery is required, the client's nutritional intake should return to normal after healing occurs.

■ Modifications for Older Clients

Older adults are treated more conservatively, with an emphasis on diet and positioning rather than surgery. Surgery may entail too much risk for older clients.

ESOPHAGEAL CANCER

Cancer of the esophagus takes the form of either squamous cell carcinoma or adenocarcinoma of the esophageal mucosa (Figure 32-13). An estimated 13,900 new cases of esophageal cancer are projected to be diagnosed in 2003 in the United States.[1] The incidence is three times as high in men as in women, and it is higher in African-American and Asian men than in white men. Adenocarcinoma of the esophagus occurs less often than squamous cell carcinoma and develops primarily in the distal esophagus.

Etiology and Risk Factors

The cause of esophageal cancer is unknown, but researchers are studying environmental differences between locations with a low and a high incidence. In the Western world, evidence points to heavy smoking, nutritional deficiencies, and habitual ingestion of alcohol, hot foods, and hot drinks as underlying etiologic factors.

In other parts of the world, contaminants in the soil and food, high levels of nitrosamines, smoking opium, and nutritional deficiencies (especially of fruits and vegetables) have been linked to the condition. Chronic irritation from other esophageal problems, such as achalasia, hiatal hernia, and stricture, plays a minor role in the development of esophageal cancer.

FIGURE 32-13 Squamous cell carcinoma of the esophagus. (From Wilcox CM. [1995]. *Atlas of clinical gastrointestinal endoscopy.* Philadelphia: W.B. Saunders.)

These are preventable causes. Prevention should be targeted particularly toward the African-American population because their risk is higher. Risk factors include smoking tobacco or opium, nutritional deficiencies, ingestion of hot foods and beverages, habitual ingestion of alcohol, ingestion of smoked meats or meats cooked over very high heat, irritation from GERD, hiatal hernia, or achalasia. Health promotion and maintenance behaviors involve limiting or stopping smoking and avoiding chronic ingestion of alcohol, hot foods, and hot beverages. Restorative behaviors include advising the client to follow the appropriate medical or surgical regimen for treatment of the specific condition.

Pathophysiology

Cancer of the esophagus begins as slow-growing benign tissue changes. Most of these cancers are squamous epidermoid tumors that are commonly found in the middle or upper third of the esophagus. Because the esophagus has no serosal layer to limit its extension, esophageal tumors expand locally and rapidly. Early spread to the lymph nodes is common. The rich lymphatic supply to the mucosa provides an excellent means for the cancer to metastasize widely and quickly. The cancers are typically intraluminal, ulcerating lesions that encircle the esophageal wall and extend upward and downward.

The disease is progressive and almost always fatal. As it progresses, most clients experience some pulmonary complications because of the formation of tracheoesophageal fistulae that result in aspiration. If the condition is not treated, total esophageal obstruction is the inevitable outcome of the disease. Infiltration into blood vessels may predispose the client to hemorrhage. Metastasis is common because of the large supply of lymph channels in the area.

Clinical Manifestations

Typically, the first manifestations are dysphagia or odynophagia. Manifestations are usually not apparent until the cancer involves the circumference of the esophagus. By the time the client becomes aware of a swallowing problem and seeks medical care, the cancer frequently has invaded the deeper layers of the esophagus and, sometimes, adjacent structures such as the bronchus and mediastinum.

At first, dysphagia is usually mild and intermittent, occurring only after ingestion of solid food (especially meat). Soon, dysphagia becomes constant and manifestations of esophageal obstruction appear. These manifestations include an increase in salivation and mucus in the throat, nocturnal aspiration, regurgitation, and an inability to swallow even liquids.

Barium swallow, endoscopy, cytologic examination, and direct biopsy confirm the diagnosis. Computed tomography (CT) scans provide an excellent definition of the size of the primary lesion and reveal the extent of nodal involvement.

Outcome Management
■ Medical Management

Inhibit Tumor Growth. Treatment of esophageal cancer depends on the tumor's location and size, metastases, and the condition of the client. If the cancer is found in an early stage, treatment is directed toward cure; however, it is usually detected in the late stages, when treatment becomes palliative, aimed specifically at allowing the client to continue eating and live longer.

Radiation Therapy. Radiation therapy can be used alone or before or after surgery. It provides palliation by reducing tumor size and slowing tumor growth. Because high-dose radiation therapy may cause stenosis of the esophagus, treatments are usually administered over 6 to 8 weeks to minimize this effect.

Chemotherapy. Chemotherapy, combining several drugs, provides symptomatic relief. Neoadjuvant chemotherapy with cisplatin, (Platinol) and 5-fluorouracil (5-FU) before surgery can facilitate surgical resection by decreasing tumor size and invasiveness of the disease in about 50% of clients treated. Chemotherapy, combined with radiation and followed by surgery, shows promising early results.

Photodynamic Therapy. Photodynamic therapy is a relatively new therapy for treatment of esophageal cancer in clients who are not surgical candidates. The client receives an injection of a light-sensitive drug (Photofrin), which is followed 2 days later with a special fiberoptic probe with a light-bearing tip placed in the esophagus. The light activates the Photofrin and kills only cancer cells. This outpatient procedure uses conscious sedation, takes about 13 minutes to perform, and enables about 1 inch of tumor to be removed. Clients return home the same day and resume their usual activities the next day.

Maintain Nutrition. Maintaining nutrition is a major goal for the client with esophageal cancer. Early in the disease, the client may be able to tolerate small, frequent feedings of soft or semisoft foods. As the disease progresses, feeding tubes may be needed. If necessary, a feeding gastrostomy or jejunostomy may be created. Short-term TPN may be used to improve the client's nutritional status before surgery. Proper positioning after meals is necessary if the client is experiencing frequent regurgitation. The head of the bed should always be elevated 30 degrees.

■ Nursing Management of the Medical Client

Assessment

Obtain data concerning the client's nutritional status. Most clients complain of dysphagia that is both persistent and progressive. The client initially may have difficulty swallowing solid foods and then may have difficulty swallowing soft foods and liquids.

A careful assessment of dysphagia is important. Other manifestations, such as odynophagia, regurgitation, chronic cough, increased secretions, and hoarseness (from involvement of the larynx), also are important to assess.

Diagnosis, Outcomes, Interventions

Diagnosis: Imbalanced Nutrition: Less Than Body Requirements. Because of the progressively worsening dysphagia, the client with esophageal cancer exhibits the nursing diagnosis *Imbalanced Nutrition: Less Than Body Requirements related to the client's inability to swallow.*

Outcomes. The client will maintain an adequate nutritional status, as evidenced by maintenance of stable body weight or slowed weight loss.

Interventions. Monitor the client's nutritional status throughout treatment, including measurement of daily weight, intake and output, and calories consumed. In the beginning, teach the client about diet changes that can make eating easier. See the Evidence-Based Practice in Action feature on Quality of Life after Treatment for Esophageal Cancer, below.

As the disease progresses, tube feedings may need to be provided. Assess the skin around the feeding tube for impairment of skin integrity caused by leakage of gastric juices. Wash the skin around the opening with a gentle soap and dry thoroughly twice daily or as needed. Apply a protective ointment, such as zinc oxide or karaya gum, to the skin for further protection if needed.

Diagnosis: Impaired Swallowing. The client with esophageal cancer experiences increasing dysphagia that may lead to the nursing diagnosis *Impaired Swallowing related to esophageal obstruction from tumor.*

Outcomes. The client will not suffer from impaired swallowing, as evidenced by an absence of choking, the ability to consume oral intake, and the maintenance of a patent airway.

📖 EVIDENCE-BASED PRACTICE IN ACTION

Quality of Life After Treatment for Esophageal Cancer

The outcomes of treatment for gastroesophageal cancer surgery is important to the client's post-treatment experience and quality of life. Treatment may involve photodynamic therapy for Barrett's esophagus and high-grade dysplasia to complete esophagectomy.[1-4] Dysphagia is the most common manifestation reported after photodynamic treatment[1] and esophagectomy.[4] Other problems reported included hoarseness, reflux, weight loss, diarrhea, fatigue, and loss of physical strength, socialization, and happiness.[1,3,4] These clients reported that these manifestations affected their quality of life by decreasing their ability to perform usual activities of daily living. Clients who had a total gastrectomy reported a better quality of life than clients who had an esophagogastrectomy or esophogectomy.[3] Clients also reported not receiving enough information before treatment regarding the treatment details, side effects, cure, and prognosis.[1]

Implications

Nurses need to be aware of the client-reported problems related to treatment. Some clients reported that they would have refused treatment if they knew what the recovery period would entail. The clients asked for more dietary teaching related to eating smaller meals and eating more slowly, and ways to reduce reflux of food.

Nurses must develop teaching plans to fit individualized client's identified needs, especially those related to nutrition, fatigue, and socialization. A nutritional assessment should be performed and a plan developed to facilitate nutrition that includes increased protein for wound and tissue healing and increased energy. Additionally, clients may benefit from a support group to help with meeting socialization needs.

References

1. Hemminger, L., & Wolfsen, H. (2002). Photodynamic therapy for Barrett's esophagus and high grade dysplasia: Results of a patient satisfaction survey. *Gastroenterology Nursing, 25*(4), 139-141.
2. Mills, M., & Sullivan, K. (2000). Patients with operable oesophageal cancer: Their experience of information-giving in a regional thoracic unit. *Journal of Clinical Nursing, 9*(2), 236-246.
3. Spector, N., Hicks, F., & Pickleman, J. (2002). Quality of life and symptoms after surgery for gastroesophageal cancer. *Gastroenterology Nursing, 23*(3), 120-125.
4. Sweed, M., Schiech, L., Barsevick, A., et al. (2002). Quality of life after esophagectomy for cancer. *Oncology Nursing Forum, 29*(7), 1127-1131.

Interventions. Many problems arise when the client is unable to swallow. The client can easily choke on saliva and mucous secretions and must spit frequently or drool. Constant wiping of saliva from the lips can cause irritation, cracking of the skin, and open lesions. Because it is impractical to collect this quantity of secretions in tissues, the client should carry a receptacle to receive the saliva. While hospitalized, clients are often taught to do self-suctioning. To prevent oral lesions and oral infections, and to provide comfort, administer or assist with frequent oral care.

Diagnosis: Risk for Ineffective Coping.
The client with cancer of the esophagus has many problems associated with both the disease and its treatment. This can lead to a nursing diagnosis of *Risk for Ineffective Coping related to changes in body image and potentially terminal prognosis.*

Outcomes. The client will effectively cope with the alterations in body image and potentially terminal prognosis, as evidenced by maintenance of activities and continued social interaction.

Interventions. In addition to meeting the client's physical needs, you must provide emotional support. The gastrostomy tube may cause an alteration in body image and increased dependency. The constant drooling or need to spit may cause the client a great deal of emotional distress. The poor prognosis of esophageal cancer necessitates psychological support and interventions aimed at helping the client and significant others prepare for the client's death (see Chapters 19 and 23).

Evaluation

Successful control of manifestations and prevention of excessive weight loss, and supporting the client to a peaceful death, may be the desired outcomes. Few clients survive for 5 years.

◼ Surgical Management
Esophageal dilation may be necessary throughout the course of the disease to treat strictures and obstruction caused by the tumor. The physician should perform the treatment as often as needed to relieve dysphagia.

In advanced disease, a prosthesis may be inserted to bypass the tumor or to prevent aspiration in clients with fistulae. The prosthesis can maintain esophageal patency, but can perforate the esophagus if it becomes dislodged or the tumor increases in size.

Surgery may be performed for prophylaxis, cure, or palliation, depending on the extent of the disease. For high-risk clients with Barrett's esophagus (a premalignant healing process that occurs in association with GERD), the lower third of the esophagus is removed

prophylactically. One of three surgical procedures can be performed:

1. An *esophagectomy* consists of the removal of all or part of the esophagus. The resected esophagus is replaced with a polyester (Dacron) graft. This procedure is usually performed via a thoracotomy, but it may be performed transhiatally, which eliminates the need for a thoracotomy.
2. An *esophagogastrostomy* involves resection of the lower portion of the esophagus and anastomosis of the remainder to the stomach, brought up into the thorax.
3. In an *esophagoenterostomy* (colon interposition), the esophagus is resected and replaced with a segment of the descending colon.

◼ Nursing Management of the Surgical Client
Assessment

Obtain data about the client's nutritional status, ability to swallow, respiratory status, and ability to cope with the diagnosis. In addition, routine preoperative and postoperative assessments are required.

Diagnosis, Outcomes, Interventions

Diagnosis: Risk for Injury.
Surgery to treat esophageal cancer is often extensive, necessitating a thoracic approach and leading to the nursing diagnosis *Risk for Injury related to surgical procedure.*

Outcomes. Injury will be prevented, as evidenced by an absence of atelectasis, fever, wound infection, or problems associated with chest tubes.

Interventions
Improve Nutritional Status Before Surgery. Before surgery, clients usually require 2 to 3 weeks of nutritional support. Often, this support includes tube feedings or TPN. The client's weight and fluid and electrolyte status are monitored closely.

Provide Preoperative Teaching. Provide extensive instruction on postoperative respiratory care, including turning, coughing, deep breathing, and chest physiotherapy. Teach the client about all incisions, wound drainage tubes, feeding tubes, and chest tubes that may be present after surgery. Oral care should be performed four times a day to help prevent infection postoperatively. If an esophagoenterostomy is performed, a complete bowel preparation is performed before surgery.

Maintain Airway. After surgery, respiratory care is a high priority. The client may be placed on a ventilator in a critical care unit (see Chapter 65 for care of a client receiving mechanical ventilation). Otherwise, the client must turn, cough, and deep breathe every hour. Carefully assess the client's respiratory status, report any manifestations of atelectasis or pneumonia, and administer supplemental oxygen. Administer pain medication frequently, and assist the client in splinting the incision while coughing. Place the client in a semi-Fowler position to prevent reflux. Continually monitor the chest tube drainage for amount, color, and patency.

Maintain Fluid and Electrolyte Balance. Assess the client's fluid and electrolyte status. Monitor drainage from the NG, gastric, and all drainage tubes at least every shift. The client is NPO for 4 to 5 days until peristalsis returns. During the first 24 hours after surgery, NG or gastric drainage is bloody, but should then change to a greenish yellow color. If bloody drainage continues, it may indicate bleeding at the suture line and should be reported.

Leakage at the site of anastomosis may appear about 5 to 7 days after surgery. Assess the client for early manifestations of shock as well as for fever, fluid accumulation at the wound site, and inflammation. Check all dressings for bleeding, drainage, or separation of the suture lines.

Advance Diet as Tolerated. The client should be started on small sips of water. If this intake is tolerated, the quantity is slowly increased. Supervise the client, making sure the client stays in an upright position, and monitor for manifestations of leakage at the anastomosis site. If this is tolerated, the client gradually progresses to pureed and semisolid foods. Explain the importance of small, frequent feedings, and advise the client to sit upright at meals and for 1 hour after meals to prevent overdistention of the stomach and reflux.

Evaluation

The poor prognosis associated with the diagnosis of cancer of the esophagus means that successful control of manifestations and prevention of extensive weight loss may be the only reasonable outcomes for these clients. Few clients survive for 5 years. Provide support for the client during the process of dying.

■ Self-Care

Upon discharge, give the client and family written and oral instructions concerning wound healing, nutritional support, respiratory care, and medications. Teach the client about possible wound and respiratory complications, manifestations that should be reported immediately, and how to contact appropriate members of the health care team.

Make appropriate referrals to community agencies. Most clients need a great amount of assistance at home. Provide information about services offered by the American Cancer Society and palliative care (see Chapters 19 and 23) if it becomes apparent that end-of-life care is necessary.

VASCULAR DISORDERS

The principal vascular disorder of the esophagus is varices. Because esophageal varices result from portal hypertension, this condition is discussed with liver disorders in Chapter 49.

TRAUMA

Major traumatic conditions of the esophagus include chemical burns, the presence of foreign bodies, and injuries from external forces, such as endoscopic equipment. Chemical burns result from the ingestion of acids or alkalis and sometimes from highly spiced foods. Thermal burns can occur after drinking extremely hot liquids, accidentally ingesting foreign bodies that lodge in the natural narrow spots of the esophagus, and self-mutilating related to suicide attempts. Trauma can cause esophageal perforation, with resultant contamination of the mediastinum and stricture formation as complications of the healing process. Treatment of esophageal strictures involves dilation of the esophagus or surgical excision of the diseased portion and reanastomosis or interposition of a piece of gut from the stomach or colon (see Esophageal Cancer earlier in this chapter).

CONCLUSIONS

Disorders of the mouth and esophagus range from fairly simple problems, such as dental caries, to complex and potentially lethal problems, such as cancer of the esophagus. No matter how minor, disorders throughout the oral-esophageal area can interfere with the client's nutritional intake. Always keep this fact in mind when assessing and caring for clients with these disorders.

THINKING CRITICALLY *evolve*

1. The client is a 72-year-old retired schoolteacher who lives with her 70-year-old sister. She is being evaluated for complaints of chest pain, which have become increasingly more frequent. Yesterday, while she was lifting flats of bedding plants to prepare for planting, she became dyspneic and collapsed. Her sister called the ambulance, and the client was admitted to a medical-surgical unit. This morning, she underwent an abdominal ultrasound before an upper GI series. An electrocardiogram (ECG) followed the tests. When the nurse last checked, the client was sleeping soundly. Now the client's call light is on. When the nurse enters the room, the client is gasping, clutching at her chest,

and attempting to get out of bed, saying, "Please help me! I can't catch my breath!" What is your first priority?

Factors to Consider. Is the client experiencing manifestations of a cardiovascular problem or a gastrointestinal one? How can the nurse tell the difference?

2. A 61-year-old woman is being treated as an outpatient for gastroesophageal reflux disease. She tells the nurse that the doctor told her to take Maalox but did not tell her how else to treat her condition. What would the nurse teach this client?

Factors to Consider. What lifestyle changes might help the client manage her condition?

3. An 18-year-old man is seen at a dental clinic following the blow of a soccer ball to the head. Several teeth were loosened by the impact. During the oral examination, the nurse notes that the gums are reddened and tender and bleed easily when probed with a tongue blade. The area under the left premolar is swollen, tender, and abscessed. The client pulls away and tells the nurse to stop because it hurts too much to touch that tooth and states, "It's been hurting for the past several weeks." When questioned, the client states that he brushes his teeth once a day or every other day, has never flossed, and usually eats several candy bars a day. What nursing interventions are appropriate? Why?

Factors to Consider. What might be the problem with the client's tooth? What could be the cause of his gingival problems?

Discussions for these questions can be found on the website and the CD-ROM.

BIBLIOGRAPHY

1. American Cancer Society. (2003). *Cancer facts and figures*. Atlanta: Author.
2. American Medical Association. (2002). *New considerations in the evaluation and management of gastroesophageal reflux disease*. Chicago: Author.
3. Axford, S., et al. (2001). Cell biology of laryngeal epithelial defenses in health and disease: Preliminary studies. *Annuals of Otology, Rhinology and Laryngology, 110*(12), 1099-1108.
4. Aronson, B., et al. (2001). Care of the laparoscopic Nissen fundoplication patient. *Gastroenterology Nursing, 24*(5), 231-236.
5. Birek, C. (2000). Herpes virus-induced diseases: Oral manifestations and current treatment options. *Journal of California Dental Association, 28*(12), 911-921.
6. Castell, D.O. et al. (2002). Esomeprazole (40 mg) compared with lansoprazole (30 mg) in the treatment of erosive gastritis. *American Journal of Gastroenterology, 97*(3), 575-583.
7. Cooper, J., et al. (1999). Chemoradiotherapy of locally advanced esophageal cancer. *Journal of the American Medical Association, 281*(17), 1623-1627.
8. Copstead, L. (2000). *Pathophysiology: Biological and behavioral perspectives* (2nd ed.). Philadelphia: W.B. Saunders.
9. Cremonesse, G., Bryden, G., & Bottcher, C. (2000). A multidisciplinary team approach to preservation of quality of life for patients following oral cancer surgery. *Oral Head and Neck Nursing, 18*(2), 6-11.
10. Durkin, S. (1999). Photodynamic therapy: A cancer treatment for the 21st century. *Gastroenterology Nursing, 22*(3), 115-120.
11. Farup, C., et al. (2001). The impact of nocturnal symptoms associated with gastroesophageal reflux disease on health-related quality of life. *Archives of Internal Medicine, 161*(8), 43-52.
12. Feldman, M., Friedman, L., & Sleisinger, M. (2002). *Sleisenger & Fordtran's gastrointestinal and liver disease: Pathophysiology, diagnosis, management* (7th ed.). Philadelphia: Saunders.
13. Femiano, F., et. al. (2001). Oral leukoplakia: Open trial of topical therapy with calcipotriol compared with tretinoin. *International Journal of Oral Maxillofacial Surgery, 30*(5), 402-406.
14. Finley, R.J., et al. (2001). Laparoscopic Heller myotomy improves esophageal emptying and the symptoms of achalasia. *Archives of Surgery, 136*(8), 892-896.
15. Gislason, T., et al. (2002). Respiratory symptoms and nocturnal gastroesophageal reflux. A population-based study of young adults in three European countries. *Chest, 121*, 158-163.
16. Glenn, T. (2001). Esophageal cancer facts, figures and screening. *Gastroenterology Nursing, 24*(6), 271-275.
17. Goldsmith, H., & Herman, L. (2002). Endoluminal gastroplication. A new therapeutic endoscopic procedure for gastroesophageal reflux disease. *Gastroenterology Nursing, 25*(1), 115-119.
18. Inour, H. (2001). Treatment of esophageal and gastric tumors. *Endoscopy, 33*(2), 119-125.
19. Jailwala, J.A., & Shaker, R. (2000). Gastroesophageal reflux disease, Series #6: Reflux laryngitis. *Practical Gastroenterology, 24*(3), 15-47.
20. Johnson, M. (2001). *Primary Care: Gastroenterology, 28*(3), 459-486.
21. Katz, P. (2000). Gastroesophageal reflux disease, Series # 7: Pulmonary manifestations of gastroesophageal reflux disease. *Practical Gastroenterology, 24*(4), 27-50.
22. Lehne, R. (2001). *Pharmacology for nursing care* (4th ed.). Philadelphia: W.B. Saunders.
23. Luketick, J.D., et al. (2001). Outcomes after minimally invasive esophagomyotomy. *Annuals of Thoracic Surgery, 72*(6), 1909-1912.
24. Metheny, N., et al. (1999). pH and concentration of bilirubin feeding tube aspirates as predictors of tube placement. *Nursing Research, 48*(4), 189-197.

25. Moody, F. (1999). *Atlas of ambulatory surgery.* Philadelphia: W. B. Saunders.

 26. Pehl, C., et al. (1999). Effect of low and high fat meals on lower esophageal sphincter motility and gastroesophageal reflux in healthy subjects. *American Journal of Gastroenterology, 94*(5), 1190-1196.

27. Price, S., & Wilson, L. (2003). *Pathophysiology: Clinical concepts of disease processes* (6th ed.). St. Louis: Mosby.

28 Quinn, K.L., & Reedy, A. (1999). Esophageal cancer: Therapeutic approaches and nursing care. *Seminars in Oncology Nursing, 15*(1), 17-25.

29. Reeves, A. (2000). Endoscopic mucosal resection. *Gastroenterology Nursing, 23*(5), 215-220.

 30. Rice, D., et al. (2000). Surgical and interventional palliative treatment of upper gastrointestinal malignancies. *European Journal of Gastroenterology and Hepatology, 12*(40), 403-408.

31. Rockey, A. (2002). What you need to know about Barrett's esophagus. *Gastroenterology Nursing, 25*(6), 237-240.

32. Ryan, W. (2001). Herpes simplex virus: Clinical presentation and treatment. *Dentistry Today, 20*(5), 64-67.

 33. Saito, T., et al. (2001). Development of squamous cell carcinoma from pre-existent oral leukoplakia: With respect to treatment modality. *International Journal of Oral Maxillofacial Surgery, 30*(1), 49-53.

34. Shashy, R.G., & Ridley, M.B. (2000). Aphthous ulcers: A difficult clinical entity. *American Journal of Otolaryngology, 21*(6), 389-393.

35. Sial, S.H., & Catalano, M.F. (2001). Gastrointestinal tract cancer in the elderly. *Gastroenterology Clinics of North America, 30*(2), 565-590.

36. Spector, N., Hicks, F., & Pickelman, J. (2002). Quality of life and symptoms after surgery for gastroesophageal cancer. *Gastroenterology Nursing, 25*(3), 120-125.

37. Steele, C., et al. (2000). Growth inhibition of *Candida* by human oral epithelial cells. *Infectious Disease, 182*(5), 1479-1485.

38. Stein, H.J., et al. (2000). Multidisciplinary approach to esophageal and gastric cancer. *Surgical Clinics of North America, 80*(2), 659-682.

39. Terry, M., et. al. (2001). Outcomes of laparoscopic fundoplication for gastroesophageal reflux disease and paraesophageal hernia. *Surgical Endoscopy, 15*(7), 691-699.

40. Townsend, C. (2001). *Sabiston's textbook of surgery: The biological basis of modern surgical practice* (16th ed.). Philadelphia: W.B. Saunders.

41. Wong, R. (2000). Gastroesophageal reflux, Series #8: Barrett's esophagus. *Practical Gastroenterology, 24*(5), 15-59.

42. Vazquez, J.A. (2000). Therapeutic options for the management of oropharyngeal or esophageal candidiasis in HIV/AIDS patients. *HIV Clinical Trails 2000, 1*(1), 47-49.

Management of Clients with Digestive Disorders

Elizabeth A. Murphy-Blake
Jane Hokanson Hawks

---

evolve

Web Enhancements

http://evolve.elsevier.com/Black/medsurg/

Case Study
Perforated Ulcer Managed Surgically
Client Education Guide
Diet for Dumping Syndrome (English Version and Spanish Translation)

Clinical Pathway
Gastrointestinal Hemorrhage
Appendix C
Laboratory Values of Clinical Importance in Medical-Surgical Nursing

---

The client with a gastric disorder usually has a problem with nutritional intake. As a result, the most common nursing diagnoses are *Imbalanced Nutrition: Less Than Body Requirements*. Additional nursing diagnoses may include (e.g., *Acute Pain, Ineffective Therapeutic Regimen Management [Individual] related to dietary changes and pharmacologic management, Fear,* and *Risk for Injury related to complications*).

GENERAL CLINICAL MANIFESTATIONS OF GASTROINTESTINAL DISORDERS

Manifestations of gastrointestinal (GI) tract dysfunction are caused by excessive gastric secretions that can erode stomach mucosa, increase motility, and result in retention of gastric contents. The most prominent clinical manifestations are acute pain, acid reflux, anorexia, belching, flatulence, nausea, vomiting, bleeding, indigestion, and diarrhea.

Pain

Acute pain is the most characteristic clinical manifestation; it usually results from chemical irritation of nerve endings. Nerve irritation occurs when acid comes into contact with the eroded stomach mucosa. It also results from stretching and contracting of the stomach, caused in turn by increased motility and increased smooth muscle tension, as found in an obstruction.

Anorexia

Anorexia, or loss of appetite, is often experienced by clients with malignancy or various other disorders. Hunger is normally caused by several stimuli, including contraction of the empty stomach. When the stomach empties slowly or when gastric stasis occurs because of a gastric disorder, anorexia can result.

Nausea and Vomiting

Nausea is a result of conditions that increase tension on the walls of the stomach, duodenum, or lower end of the esophagus. Unpleasant stimuli, distention, gastritis, and carcinoma of the stomach can produce nausea. Vomiting may follow nausea or occur without it. Vomiting is caused by stimulation of the emetic center:

1. The chemoreceptor trigger zone (CTZ) in the fourth ventricle. The CTZ is stimulated by various drugs and body toxins. Conversely, medications of

---

evolve *Be sure to check out the bonus material on the Evolve website and the CD-ROM, including free self-assessment exercises.*
http://evolve.elsevier.com/Black/medsurg/

Nursing Outcomes Classification (NOC)
for Nursing Diagnoses—Clients with Digestive Disorders

Acute Pain or Chronic Pain
  Comfort Level
  Pain Control
  Pain: Disruptive Effects
  Pain Level
Fear
  Fear Control
  Anxiety Control
  Coping
Imbalanced Nutrition: Less Than Body Requirements
  Knowledge: Diet

Nutritional Status
Nutritional Status: Food and Fluid Intake
Nutritional Status: Nutrient Intake
Ineffective Therapeutic Regimen Management (Individual)
  Compliance Behavior
  Knowledge: Treatment Regimen
  Participation: Health Care Decisions
  Treatment Behavior: Illness or Injury

Risk for Injury: Postoperative Complications
  Circulation Status
  Risk Control
  Risk Detection
  Safety Status: Physical Injury
  Symptom Control
  Tissue Perfusion: Abdominal Organs
  Tissue Perfusion: Peripheral
  Vital Signs Status

the phenothiazine derivative groups, such as chlorpromazine (Thorazine) and prochlorperazine (Compazine), depress vomiting caused by chemoreceptor stimulation. Serotonin antagonists, such as ondansetron (Zofran), block serotonin receptors in the vagus nerve and CTZ.

2. Nerve impulses, which can be excited by
   a. Direct mechanical stimuli, as in increased intracranial pressure.
   b. Chemical stimuli from blood-borne metabolites or toxic substances.
   c. Sympathetic and parasympathetic afferent nerve impulses through the vagus, glossopharyngeal, vestibular, and splanchnic nerves (the most sensitive receptors are located in the proximal duodenum).
3. Unpleasant odors, subjects, and sights that stimulate higher center impulses.
4. Distention of stomach or duodenum.
5. Decreased gastric motility.
6. Pain, because the pain centers are close to the vomiting centers in the medulla.
7. Increased intracranial pressure.

Bleeding

Bleeding results from local trauma or irritations that cause erosion or ulceration of the GI tract mucosa. The disorders involved include stomach neoplasms, gastric ulcer, gastritis, anastomotic (marginal) ulcers, and duodenal ulcers. Duodenitis can also cause bleeding. Although bleeding may have numerous causes, up to 75% of all cases of upper GI tract bleeding result from esophagogastric varices (venous), hemorrhagic gastritis (capillary), or peptic ulcer. Ulcers account for 80% of all upper GI tract hemorrhage.

Diarrhea

Diarrhea can be caused by increased peristalsis resulting from an increased gastrocolic reflex or from the effort of the stomach and intestines to eliminate a local irritant.

Belching and Flatulence

Swallowed air causes most belching and flatulence. It is easy to swallow air during eating and drinking, especially when food is ingested rapidly. Frequently, clients attempt to belch to relieve a vague feeling of distress in the stomach caused by swallowed air. Attempting to belch with the mouth closed sometimes adds more air to the stomach than it removes.

Indigestion

Indigestion or dyspepsia can be caused by such factors as strong emotions, GI tract disease, eating too rapidly, chewing inadequately, gas-forming foods (e.g., beans and cabbage), and food allergy. Eating very large meals and lying down directly after eating can also cause indigestion.

GASTROINTESTINAL INTUBATION

Gastric and intestinal tubes are inserted for several purposes: (1) decompression, (2) lavage, (3) gastric analysis, and (4) tube feedings.

Decompression relieves the pressure caused by contents and gases that remain in the stomach or bowel because of some obstruction. Long intestinal tubes are sometimes used to dilate the lumen or to release an obstruction. Postoperative decompression removes secretions that cannot pass through the GI tract because of edema and decreased gastric motility. The placement of a tube (intubation) helps prevent vomiting, distention, and obstruction.

Lavage is the irrigation or washing out of an organ. Gastric lavage washes out the stomach. It is used most frequently as an emergency treatment in poisoning. Lavage is also used for exfoliative cytology to determine the presence of abnormal cells.

Tube feeding or *gavage feeding,* referred to as *enteral nutrition,* is a method of giving clients fluids and nutrients via a tube when oral intake is inadequate or impossible.

Types of Tubes

Three types of tubes are used for decompression: (1) *short* nasogastric (NG) tubes are used for the stomach, (2) *medium* tubes extend into the duodenum or jejunum, and (3) *long* tubes are used for the rest of the GI tract (Table 33-1).

Short Tubes

Short tubes include the Levin and Salem sump tubes. Short tubes are long enough to extend into the stomach but not into the bowel. These tubes are usually attached to suction. Occasionally, these may be used for short-term enteral feedings over a brief period. However, nasoduodenal tubes are preferred for feedings because of **EB** the high rate of aspiration pneumonia associated with NG tube feedings.

Levin Tube. The Levin tube is a single-lumen tube used to remove fluid or gas or to obtain a specimen of gastric contents. Because the tube has only one lumen, low in-**EB** termittent suction is required to minimize the irritation of the gastric mucosa. Levin tubes may be made out of plastic, rubber-like silicone (Silastic), or rubber.

Salem Sump Tube. The Salem sump tube is a double-lumen tube used to empty and decompress the stomach. Low, continuous suction is used because the "pigtail" lumen on the Salem sump tube vents the tube and protects gastric mucosa from being sucked against the tube. The pigtail lumen should not be clamped or irrigated and **EB** should be kept higher than the client's stomach to prevent drainage.

Medium Tubes

Medium tubes include a variety of nasoduodenal (e.g., Dobhoff) tubes that extend into the duodenum and are **EB** designed for short-term feeding. They are less likely to cause aspiration pneumonia because of their small size **EB** and weighted tip. Placement is verified by abdominal x-ray study (radiography).

Long Tubes

The long tubes extend into the small bowel, sometimes for its entire length. These tubes are between 1.8 and 3 m (6 and 10 feet) long and are used to prevent gas and fluid accumulation in the intestine, which is usually caused by intestinal obstruction. Use of long tubes has decreased substantially in the last several years. The more common long tubes are the Miller-Abbott, Cantor, and Harris tubes.

Miller-Abbott Tube. The Miller-Abbott tube is a double-lumen tube, 3 m (10 feet) long. One lumen is used to introduce mercury or to inflate the balloon at the end of the tube, and the other is used for aspiration. Markings on the tube indicate the distance the tube has been passed. Initial placement of the tube is completed by a physician. The nurse is responsible for advancing the tube as ordered.

Cantor Tube. The Cantor tube is used for aspirating intestinal contents and has only one lumen. It is 3 m (10 feet) long and is larger than the other tubes. This tube has 4 to 5 ml of mercury in a bag at the end, which is wrapped about the tube before insertion. For intestinal intubation, the tube is threaded through the nose into the stomach and then through the pylorus, where peristaltic activity of the bowel carries it to the desired intestinal area.

Harris Tube. The Harris tube is a single-lumen, mercury-weighted tube, 1.8 m (6 feet) long. A metal tip is introduced into the nostril after it is lubricated. The weight of the mercury carries the tube by gravity. This tube is used for suction and irrigation.

Sometimes it is difficult to get intestinal tubes to pass through the pylorus. The client is instructed to lie on the

TABLE 33-1	*Gastric and Intestinal Tubes*			
	Length	**Size (French)**	**Lumen**	**Other Characteristics**
Short Tubes				
Levin type (plastic or rubber)	125 cm (50 inches)	12, 16, 18	Single	
Salem sump	120 cm (48 inches)	12, 14, 16, 18	Double	Sump-type suction
Medium Tubes				
Dobhoff (nasoduodenal or nasojejunal)	160-175 cm (60-66 inches)	8, 10, 12	Single	Radiopaque, tungsten weighted
Long Tubes				
Cantor	300 cm (10 feet)	16	Single	Mercury weighted
Harris	180 cm (6 feet)	14, 16	Single	Mercury weighted
Miller-Abbott	300 cm (10 feet)	12, 14, 16, 18	Double	Mercury weighted

right side to facilitate passage. When the tube has passed into the duodenum, it is advanced, as ordered, an additional 4.8 to 9.6 cm (2 to 4 inches) every hour or half hour. When the tube has reached the desired location, tape it securely to the client's face to prevent further advancement.

Other Tubes

Long-term enteral feedings, gastrostomy tubes (GTs or G tubes) or jejunostomy tubes (JTs or J tubes) are often placed surgically. The GT and JT (see Chapter 31) can be inserted surgically or laparoscopically. The percutaneous endoscopic gastrostomy (PEG), which is the most common, and the percutaneous endoscopic jejunostomy (PEJ) have been discussed in Chapter 31.

Inserting Gastrointestinal Tubes

GI tubes are generally inserted through the nose into the stomach or small intestine. These tubes are rarely inserted through the mouth. Explain each step of the intubation procedure at the client's level of understanding. Assist the client to assume a high Fowler's position, which makes intubation easier. Measure the distance on the tube from the tip of the nose to the ear lobe plus the distance from the ear lobe to the tip of the xiphoid process (the NEX measurement). This approximates the distance that the tube must be passed to reach the stomach. Mark this distance on the tubing with adhesive.

After measuring the tube, lubricate and gently insert the tube through the nares and posterior nasal pharynx and into the oropharynx. When the tube is in the oropharynx, instruct the client to swallow; sometimes the client is allowed to drink water at this point to help with tube passage. Having the client swallow is important, because the sphincter at the proximal end of the esophagus remains closed except during swallowing. The larynx rises during swallowing, stretching the cricopharyngeal muscle and causing it to relax, thus reducing resistance to the tube. Swallowing also enables the tube to enter the esophagus rather than the trachea. After the tube passes the sphincter, advance it into the stomach.

To verify placement, perform at least two of the following activities:

1. Aspirate gastric contents.
2. Measure the pH of the aspirant; the pH of the stomach is less than that of the lungs. (See the Evidence-Based Practice in Action feature on Assessing Gastrointestinal Tube Placement on p. 747.)

3. Check with an x-ray study for the radiopaque lines on the tube.

After confirming placement, secure the tube to the nose with hypoallergenic tape. (This procedure is used for short tubes only; medium tubes are checked with an x-ray and long tubes need to be able to advance.)

Suctioning Gastrointestinal Tubes

When suction is applied to a GI tube to remove accumulated gas and fluid, ensure that the GI mucosa is not traumatized. Excessive negative pressure causes the mucosa to be sucked into the openings on the tube, impairing suction and injuring the mucosa. Intermittent suction is used to avoid this problem unless a double-lumen tube, such as the Salem sump, is used. Mucus tends to plug the openings of these tubes, making it necessary to irrigate with saline as ordered to maintain or check tube patency (usually every 4 hours) or more frequently if the client complains of nausea.

■ Nursing Management of Clients with Gastrointestinal Tubes

Maintain the client's comfort while the tube is in place. Helpful nursing interventions include the following steps:

1. Clean and lubricate external nares. The nares may become sore because of crusted secretions around the tube. Always use a water-soluble lubricant to avoid the possibility of lipid pneumonia when using an oil-based lubricant.
2. Tape the tube in a manner that prevents irritation of the nares.
3. Administer frequent oral hygiene to remove debris, increase comfort, maintain a healthy oral cavity, and stimulate saliva secretion. The client's mouth is usually dry because the absence of chewing prevents the normal stimulus to salivary secretions and the presence of the tube causes mouth breathing.
4. Permit the client, if possible, to chew gum or suck on sour candies or ice chips to help stimulate salivation. Excessive use stimulates gastric secretions and causes electrolyte loss through the suction.
5. Brush the client's teeth or assist the client in brushing teeth.
6. Request an order for anesthetic mouth rinses or lozenges because the presence of the tube frequently causes sore throat.

Placement of the tube in the throat may result in cricoid chondritis (irritation of the cricoid cartilage of the larynx) and laryngeal injuries. Presenting clinical manifestations include the following:

- Localized odynophagia
- Pain radiating to the ears
- Sore throat
- Stridor
- Bloody sputum
- Mild hoarseness

Assess for these potential complications and report the findings immediately. An order for anesthetic lozenges or gargles to relieve manifestations may be needed. Frequent assessment of secretions for color,

EB EVIDENCE-BASED PRACTICE IN ACTION

Assessing Gastrointestinal Tube Placement

Norma Metheny is one nursing researcher who has been conducting nursing research related to assessment of gastrointestinal tubes for more than 15 years.[1-9] Placement errors can lead to aspiration pneumonia, vomiting, increased residuals, and other complications.[2,7,9] The greatest error with nasoduodenal feeding tubes is not placing the tubes into the duodenum.[3,8,9] When these tubes are placed in the stomach, the risk of pulmonary aspiration increases.

Traditionally, checking placement of gastrointestinal tubes was done by nurses who injected air and auscultated to detect proper placement. This method was designed for assessing large nasogastric tubes and has been proven the least effective method for checking placement. Radiologic verification of weighted tubes and aspiration of gastric or duodenal contents and pH testing (using pH paper or tubes with a built-in probe and pH meter) of those contents are the most accurate predictors of gastrointestinal tube placement.[4,5] In addition, the ability to determine pepsin and trypsin levels as well as pH at the bedside facilitates assessment of proper position.[6]

Residual volumes of nasogastric, gastric, and nasoduodenal tubes have been researched as well.[1] A common mistake is aspiration of jejunal feeding tubes. These should never be aspirated. In one study, nasogastric residuals of more than 200 ml and gastrostomy residuals of more than 100 ml were shown to be of concern,[1] but further research is needed before thresholds can be established.

Implications

Nurses are the health care providers primarily responsible for nasogastric and nasoduodenal tube feedings, and nurses monitor all other gastrointestinal tubes and feeding tubes. It is imperative that correct assessment for placement (using pH or enzyme presence) be incorporated into practice. Further research is warranted regarding residual amounts that indicate that a tube feeding should be slowed or discontinued for an hour or more.

References

1. Edwards, S., & Metheny, N. (2000). Research for practice: Measurement of gastric residual volume: A state of the science. *MEDSURG Nursing, 9*(3), 125-128.
2. Metheny, N., et al. (1990). Detection of inadvertent respiratory placement of small-bore feeding tubes. *Heart & Lung, 19*(6), 631-638.
3. Metheny, N., et al. (1998). Detection of improperly positioned feeding tubes. *Journal of Healthcare Risk Management, 18*(3), 37-48.
4. Metheny, N., et al. (1993). Effectiveness of pH measurements in predicting feeding tube placement: An update. *Nursing Research, 42*(6), 324-331.
5. Metheny, N., et al. (1999). pH and concentration of bilirubin in feeding tube aspirates as predictors of tube placement. *Nursing Research, 48*(4), 189-197.
6. Metheny, N., et al. (1997). pH and concentrations of pepsin and trypsin in feeding tube aspirates as predictors of tube placement. *Journal of Parenteral Nutrition, 21*(5), 279-285.
7. Metheny, N., et al. (1994). Visual characteristics of aspirates from feeding tubes as a method for predicting tube location. *Nursing Research, 43*(5), 282-287.
8. Metheny, N., & Stewart, B. (2002). Testing feeding tube placement during continuous tube feedings. *Nursing Research, 15*(4), 254-258.
9. Metheny, N., & Titler, M. (2001). Assessing placement of feeding tubes. *American Journal of Nursing, 101*(5), 36-46.

odor, and quantity is essential. Report any changes to the physician or health care provider. It may be necessary to send samples of these secretions to the laboratory for analysis. Measure the contents of the suction containers to maintain an accurate record of GI losses. Metabolic alkalosis may result from a major loss of water and electrolytes. Monitor potassium levels, because potassium is one of the major electrolytes lost through suctioning.

The irrigating solution instilled into a GI tube is counted as intake if it is not removed when contents are aspirated. Keep accurate records of the amount instilled and the amount aspirated from the tube during irrigations. Normal saline is the preferred irrigating solution because water, a hypotonic solution, increases electrolyte loss through osmotic action if the tube is irrigated frequently.

GASTRITIS
ACUTE GASTRITIS

Gastritis, an inflammation of the gastric mucosa, is classified as either acute or chronic. The incidence of gastritis is highest in the fifth and sixth decades of life; men are more frequently affected than women. The incidence is greater in clients who are heavy drinkers and smokers.

Etiology and Risk Factors

The acute form of gastritis may be seen with nausea and vomiting, epigastric discomfort, bleeding, malaise, and anorexia. It usually stems from ingestion of a corrosive, erosive, or infectious substance. Aspirin and other non-steroidal anti-inflammatory drugs (NSAIDs), digitalis, chemotherapeutic drugs, steroids, acute alcoholism, and food poisoning (typically caused by *Staphylococcus*

organisms) are common causes. In addition, food substances, including excessive amounts of tea, coffee, mustard, paprika, cloves, and pepper, can precipitate acute gastritis. Foods with a rough texture or those eaten at an extremely high temperature can also damage the stomach mucosa. Ingestion of corrosive agents, such as lye or drain cleaner, also causes acute gastritis with the damage/loss of the mucosal layer.

Disorders linked with acute gastritis include uremia, shock, central nervous system lesions, hepatic cirrhosis, portal hypertension, and prolonged emotional tension. Acute gastritis is usually of short duration unless the gastric mucosa has suffered extensive damage.

Health promotion behaviors include limited use of NSAIDs, alcohol, and caffeine and avoidance of nicotine products; both smoking and chewing. Health maintenance behaviors include use of enteric-coated aspirin, misoprostol (Cytotec) to protect against NSAIDs or use of COX-2 inhibitors, histamine-receptor antagonists to decrease gastric acidity, or proton pump inhibitors to block gastric acid production. Clients with medical disorders that may lead to gastritis should follow orders for prescribed medications to minimize stomach irritation.

Pathophysiology

The mucosal lining of the stomach normally protects it from the action of gastric acid. This mucosal barrier is composed of prostaglandins. If this barrier is penetrated, gastritis occurs, with resultant injury to the mucosa. When hydrochloric acid comes into contact with the mucosa, injury to small vessels occurs with edema, hemorrhage, and possible ulcer formation. The damage associated with acute gastritis is usually limited.

Clinical Manifestations

Assessment typically reveals epigastric discomfort, abdominal tenderness, cramping, belching, reflux, severe nausea and vomiting, and sometimes hematemesis. Sometimes GI bleeding is the only manifestation. When contaminated food is the cause of gastritis, diarrhea usually develops within 5 hours of ingestion of the offending substance.

Diagnosis is based on a detailed history of food intake, medications taken, and any disorders related to gastritis. The physician may also perform a gastroscopic examination with a biopsy.

Outcome Management
■ Medical Management

Intervention involves removing the cause and treating the manifestations. Vomiting frequently responds to medications of the phenothiazine group; pain responds to antacids or histamine (H_2) receptor antagonists (see the Integrating Pharmacology feature on Medications for Peptic Ulcer Disease at right). If ingestion of NSAIDs is a problem, a prostaglandin E_1 (PGE_1) analog may be

prescribed to protect the stomach mucosa and inhibit gastric acid secretion.

Initially, foods and fluids are withheld until nausea and vomiting subside. Once the client tolerates food, the diet includes decaffeinated tea, gelatin, toast, and simple, bland foods. The client should avoid spicy foods, caffeine, and large, heavy meals. In the continued absence of nausea, vomiting, and bloating, the client can slowly return to a normal diet.

■ Nursing Management of the Medical Client

Nursing management of the medical client with acute gastritis is described in the section on chronic gastritis.

CHRONIC GASTRITIS

This condition appears in three different forms:
- *Superficial gastritis,* which causes a reddened, edematous mucosa with small erosions and hemorrhages

---

INTEGRATING PHARMACOLOGY
Medications for Peptic Ulcer Disease

Because most peptic ulcers are caused by *H. pylori* bacteria, a triple therapy aimed at eliminating the bacteria and reducing gastric secretions is prescribed. Triple therapy consists of two anti-infective agents (clarithromycin [Biaxin] or amoxicillin and metronidazole [Flagyl]) and a proton pump inhibitor (lansoprazole [Prevacid], pantoprazole [Protonix], omeprazole [Prilosec]). These are usually given for 1 week but may be repeated if necessary. Sometimes a quadruple therapy consisting of a proton pump inhibitor, tetracycline, metronidazole, and a bismuth salt may be administered.

Other medications prescribed include hyposecretory agents that reduce or inhibit acid secretions. These agents include H_2-receptor antagonists (ranitidine [Zantac]; cimetidine [Tagamet]; famotidine [Pepcid], prostaglandin analogs (misoprostol [Cytotec]), proton pump inhibitors (omeprazole [Prilosec]), and antacids. H_2-receptor antagonists inhibit the action of histamine on the H_2 receptors that trigger parietal cell response to chemical stimulation, which results in reduced gastric acid output and concentration. Prostaglandin analogs, in addition to decreasing acid secretion, stimulate production of cytoprotective mucus. Proton pump inhibitors act by inhibiting the gastric enzyme H^+, K^+, and ATPase, which catalyses the final step of HCl production at the secretory surface of the gastric parietal cells. Antacids neutralize gastric acid for approximately 30 minutes.

Another medication for short-term treatment of peptic ulcers is known as a mucosal barrier fortifier (sucralfate [Carafate]. These drugs prevent hydrogen ion back-diffusion into the mucosa and stimulate mucus production, which results in accelerated peptic ulcer healing.

- *Atrophic gastritis,* which occurs in all layers of the stomach, develops frequently in association with gastric ulcer and gastric cancer, and is invariably present in pernicious anemia; it is characterized by a decreased number of parietal and chief cells
- *Hypertrophic gastritis,* which produces a dull and nodular mucosa with irregular, thickened, or nodular rugae; hemorrhages occur frequently

Etiology and Risk Factors

Peptic ulcer disease (PUD), infection with *Helicobacter pylori* bacteria, or gastric surgery may lead to chronic gastritis. Other risk factors are similar to those for acute gastritis. Chronic gastritis is associated with atrophy of the gastrin glands. After gastric resection with a gastrojejunostomy, bile and bile acids may reflux into the remaining stomach, causing gastritis. *H. pylori* infection can lead to chronic atrophic gastritis, which predisposes to the development of gastric cancer. Age is also a risk factor; chronic gastritis is more common in older adults.

Pathophysiology

The initial pathophysiologic changes associated with chronic gastritis are the same as with acute gastritis. The stomach lining first becomes thickened and erythematous and then becomes thin and atrophic. Continued deterioration and atrophy lead to loss of function of the parietal cells. When the acid secretion decreases, the source of intrinsic factor is lost. This loss results in inability to absorb vitamin B_{12} and the development of pernicious anemia.

In chronic gastritis, the mucosa usually heals without scarring, but ulcer formation and bleeding can occur. The atrophic changes eventually result in a minimal amount of acid being secreted into the stomach (achlorhydria), which is a major risk factor for the development of gastric cancer.

Clinical Manifestations

Manifestations are vague and may be absent (because the problem does not cause an increase in hydrochloric acid). Assessment may reveal anorexia, a feeling of fullness, dyspepsia, belching, vague epigastric pain, nausea, vomiting, and intolerance of spicy or fatty foods.

Complications of Gastritis

The clinical course of clients with chronic gastritis may include such complications as bleeding, pernicious anemia, and gastric cancer. Bleeding can be a complication of gastritis, especially when the stomach mucosa becomes denuded or erosive. Bleeding is common with use of alcohol, aspirin, or NSAIDs. The client should undergo an endoscopic examination to determine the source of the bleeding. Another possible complication of atrophic gastritis is diminished ability of the stomach to secrete intrinsic factor, resulting in malabsorption of vi-

tamin B_{12}, which is confirmed by Schilling's test. Gastric cancer may be suspected in a client whose gastritis does not heal with therapy. (See Gastric Cancer later in this chapter.)

Outcome Management
■ Medical Management

Intervention begins when the health care provider rules out cancer as a causative factor. Discomfort may lessen with a bland diet, small frequent meals, antacids, H_2 receptor antagonists, proton pump inhibitors, and avoidance of foods that cause manifestations. If *H. pylori* bacteria are present, antibiotics and other medications are administered to eliminate the bacteria (see the Integrating Pharmacology feature on Medications for Peptic Ulcer Disease on p. 748). If 1 week of this regimen does not succeed in eliminating the bacteria, the regimen may be repeated for an additional week. If pernicious anemia develops, intramuscular injections of vitamin B_{12} may be administered monthly for the remainder of the client's life.

■ Nursing Management of the Medical Client

When assessing the client with acute or chronic gastritis, carefully focus on risk factors. Consider the client's diet, eating patterns, use of prescription and over-the-counter drugs, and lifestyle, including alcohol consumption and cigarette smoking.

Reduce Pain. Focus on teaching the client about the causes of gastritis and foods that may worsen the disease. Help the client assess factors that increase manifestations, such as stress or fatigue, taking certain medications on an empty stomach, ingestion of foods and beverages, alcohol consumption, and smoking. Encourage the client to avoid these factors.

Aluminum hydroxide with magnesium trisilicate (Gaviscon), which produces a soothing foam, is the best antacid for gastritis). H_2-receptor antagonists, proton pump inhibitors antisecretory agents, and drugs that enhance mucosal defenses also provide pain reduction (see the Integrating Pharmacology feature on Medications for GERD in Chapter 32).

If the nausea and vomiting are severe, the client may be restricted to nothing by mouth (NPO) until these problems decrease in severity. When the pain and nausea associated with gastritis have subsided, the client is instructed to have a well-balanced diet and avoid irritating foods and beverages.

Promote Self-Care. Cases of acute and chronic gastritis are managed at home unless complications develop. Instruct the client with chronic gastritis to see the health care provider at regular intervals. This is particularly important if the diagnosis is *H. pylori* infection and atrophic gastritis, because these problems are closely related to gastric cancer. Teach the client to use medications correctly, to maintain adequate nutrition, and to control risk factors that contribute to gastritis.

■ Surgical Management

If conservative measures have not controlled bleeding, surgery may be necessary. Subtotal gastrectomy, pyloroplasty, vagotomy, or total gastrectomy may be indicated with severe erosive gastritis. These procedures are discussed in the following section on PUD.

PEPTIC ULCER DISEASE

PUD involves a break in continuity of the esophageal, gastric, or duodenal mucosa. An ulcer may occur in any part of the GI tract that comes into contact with gastric juices (hydrochloric acid and pepsin). The ulcer may be found in the esophagus, stomach, duodenum, or the jejunum after gastroenterostomy.

PUD occurs in approximately 10% of the population. Gastric ulcers are more likely to occur during the fifth and sixth decades of life; duodenal ulcers more commonly occur during the fourth and fifth decades for men. For women, the occurrence is about 10 years later in life. Men are more likely to have both gastric and duodenal ulcers.

Duodenal Ulcers

Duodenal ulcers have a higher incidence than gastric ulcers. These ulcers usually occur within 1.5 cm (0.6 inch) of the pylorus and are usually characterized by high gastric acid secretion. Some are associated with normal gastric secretion that is associated with rapid emptying of the stomach. Hypersecretion of acid is attributed to a greater mass of parietal cells. Stimuli for acid secretion include protein-rich meals, alcohol consumption, calcium, and vagal stimulation.

Clients with a duodenal ulcer experience low pH levels in the duodenum for longer periods. The stomach lining is more sensitive to gastrin and secretes excess gastrin.

Finally, clients with duodenal ulcers have more rapid gastric emptying. The combined effect of hypersecretion of acid and rapid emptying of food from the stomach reduces the buffering effect of food and results in a large acid load in the duodenum. Within the duodenum, inhibitory mechanisms and pancreatic secretion (an alkaline solution) may be insufficient to control the acid load.

Gastric Ulcers

Gastric ulcers, which tend to heal within a few weeks, form within 1 inch (2.5 cm) of the pylorus of the stomach in an area where gastritis is common. Gastric ulcers are probably caused by a break in the mucosal barrier. The barrier, which differs from the layer of glycoprotein mucus that overlies the gastric epithelium, normally allows hydrochloric acid to be secreted into the stomach without injury to the epithelial cells. An incompetent pylorus may decrease production of mucus, the usual gastric defense. The reflux of bile acids through an incompetent pylorus into the stomach may break the mucosal barrier. Decreased blood flow to the gastric mucosa may also alter the defensive barrier and may make the duodenum more susceptible to gastric acid and pepsin trauma. The recurrence rate of gastric ulcer is lower than that of duodenal ulcer.

Table 33-2 distinguishes gastric from duodenal ulcers.

TABLE 33-2	Classification of Peptic Ulcers	
Assessment Data	**Duodenal Ulcers**	**Gastric Ulcers**
Location of ulcer	¼ to 1 inch from pylorus	Junction of fundus and pylorus, some in antrum
Acid secretion	Increased	Normal to decreased
Serum pepsinogen I	Increased	Normal
Serum gastrin		
Fasting	Normal	Elevated
Postprandial	Elevated	
Blood group	Most frequently type O	No difference
Age at onset	25-50 years	Peaks at 45-54 years
Gender predominance	Men to women, 4:1	Men to women, 2:1
Associated gastritis	None	Common and increased
Pain	Occurs on empty stomach, 2-3 hr after meals or in middle of night; relieved by food and antacids	Variable pain pattern; may be made worse by food; antacids ineffective
Nutritional status	Usually well nourished	Probably malnourished
Malignancy potential	Rare, no increase in incidence	Occurs in approximately 10% of clients
Bleeding pattern	Melena more common than hematemesis	Hematemesis more common than melena
Recurrence	May occur as marginal ulcers after surgery	Recurrence unlikely after surgery

Stress-Induced and Drug-Induced Ulcers

Besides peptic ulcers, acute gastric erosion, frequently called *stress ulcers* or *stress erosive gastritis,* can occur after an acute medical crisis. Major assaults that give rise to gastroduodenal ulcerations include the following:

- Severe trauma or major illness
- Severe burns (may cause what is known as Curling's ulcers)
- Head injury or intracranial disease (frequently called Cushing's ulcers)
- Ingestion of a drug (e.g., aspirin, NSAIDs, steroids, and alcohol) that acts on the gastric mucosa (Figure 33-1)
- Shock
- Sepsis

Etiology and Risk Factors

The causal factor in more than 90% of all peptic ulcers has been attributed to *H. pylori.* Eradication of the organism usually results in resolution of gastritis and subsequent ulcer healing. Multiple studies support this finding, which calls into question earlier theories about the causes of PUD. A vaccine, HELIVAX, is being tested to prevent infection with *H. pylori* and as an alternative to antibiotics in those already infected with *H. pylori.*

The occurrence of PUD depends on the defensive resistance of the mucosa in relation to the aggressive force of secretory activity. The defensive resistance of the mucosa depends on mucosal integrity and regeneration, presence of a protective mucous barrier, adequate blood flow to the mucosa, ability of the duodenal inhibitory mechanism to regulate secretion, and the presence of adequate gastromucosal prostaglandins. The aggressive factors of PUD are related to the presence of *H. pylori* and the volume of hydrochloric and biliary acids. Ulceration occurs when aggressive factors exceed the defensive barrier. The aggressive nature of the gastric juice may be the result of hypersecretion of gastric juices, increased stimulation of the vagus nerve, decreased inhibition of gastric secretions, increased capacity or number of the parietal cells secreting hydrochloric acid, or increased response of the parietal cells to stimulation.

Risk factors that contribute to PUD include smoking (nicotine), chewing tobacco, steroids, aspirin, NSAIDs, caffeine, alcohol, and stress. Certain medical conditions, including Crohn's disease, Zollinger-Ellison syndrome, and hepatic and biliary disease, may also play a role.

Health promotion and health maintenance actions for clients with PUD are the same as those discussed for acute gastritis. Health restoration for clients involves treating medical disorders that cause secondary PUD. Ensure that the client complies with the prescribed medication regimen to minimize stomach irritation. Treat aggressively any disorders that result in the development of PUD, for example, long-term use of steroids, severe burns, and chronic renal failure.

Pathophysiology

In addition to *H. pylori* inflammation as the primary pathophysiologic change, two different mechanisms for the development of PUD have been proposed. In the stomach, it is thought that a breakdown of the normally protective epithelial lining causes gastric ulcers. Under normal circumstances, flow of hydrochloric acid from the lumen of the stomach is prevented by the presence of tight, nonpermeable junctions between the epithelial cells and by the slightly alkaline layer of mucus that coats the surface of the gastric epithelium.

In the formation of a gastric peptic ulcer, this diffusion barrier may be interrupted by the chronic presence of such injurious substances as aspirin, NSAIDs, cortisone, adrenocorticotropic hormone (ACTH), caffeine, alcohol, chemotherapeutic agents, and hypersecretory conditions. These substances may stimulate acid production, cause local mucosal damage, and suppress mucus secretion. The substances strip away surface mucus and cause degeneration of epithelial cell membranes with massive diffusion of acid back into the gastric epithelial wall.

The pathogenesis of duodenal peptic ulcers has a different proposed mechanism, because excess acid secretion is responsible for ulcer development. Activity of the vagus nerve is increased in people with duodenal ulcers, particularly during a fasting state and at night. The vagus nerve stimulates the pyloric antrum cells to release gastrin, which travels via the bloodstream and acts on the gastric parietal cells to stimulate the release of hydrochloric acid.

Another factor in PUD is emotional stress, which can cause an increase in gastric secretion, blood supply, and gastric motility by thalamic stimulation of the vagal nerves. Hormonal influence takes place via the hypothalamus through the pituitary adrenal route. In clients with stress reactions, the sympathetic nervous system

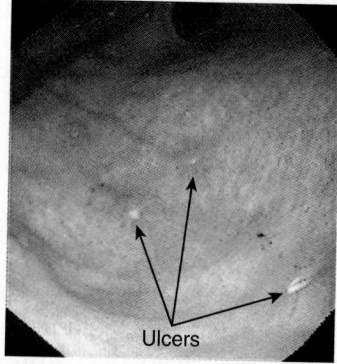

FIGURE 33-1 Gastric ulcerations caused by nonsteroidal anti-inflammatory drugs.

causes the blood vessels in the duodenum to constrict, which makes the mucosa more vulnerable to trauma from gastric acid and pepsin secretion. On activation of the adrenal cortex, mucus production decreases and gastric secretion increases. Together, these factors result in increased vulnerability to ulceration. Stress reactions thus upset the aggressive-defensive balance. Prolonged stress associated with burns, severe trauma, and other conditions can produce stress ulcers, or stress erosive gastritis, in the GI tract.

Zollinger-Ellison syndrome is characterized by abnormal secretion of gastrin by a rare islet cell tumor in the pancreas. Pathophysiologic changes associated with this syndrome include hypergastrinemia and diarrhea secondary to fat malabsorption resulting from decreased duodenum-inactivating pancreatic lipase or acid-induced injury of the villi. In addition to increased gastric secretion, hyperplasia of the gastric mucosa is induced by the trophic effects of gastrin. Treatment of the Zollinger-Ellison syndrome is aimed at suppression of acid secretion.

Treated ulcers usually heal without difficulty. Untreated ulcers or those that do not respond to treatment can result in perforation, hemorrhage, or obstruction, which may require surgical treatment. Some ulcers recur after healing, particularly if the risk factors associated with their development are not modified.

Critically ill clients are susceptible to *stress ulcers*. For example, gastric mucosal changes caused by stress develop within 72 hours in 78% of clients with greater than 35% burns on their body. Stress ulcers manifest with superficial gastric erosions, often accompanied by painless massive gastric hemorrhage. The client characteristically has multiple lesions, usually small and superficial, that do not extend through the muscularis mucosae. These lesions may appear to ooze blood. The mechanism causing stress ulcerations is unknown, but it probably involves ischemia. In the presence of acid, ischemia can produce erosive gastritis and ulcerations. Increased hydrogen ion back-diffusion and decreased mucosal perfusion may also contribute to stress ulcer formation. Low gastric pH (high acidity) is necessary for development of stress ulcers.

Researchers continue to seek the precise mechanism by which stress ulcers occur. Few manifestations accompany stress ulcer. These ulcerations are typically painless unless perforation occurs, which is rare. Upper GI tract hemorrhage is the major manifestation of stress ulcers. About 10% of clients experience dyspepsia before hemorrhage, but typically there are no warning manifestations. When stress ulcers cause profound hemorrhage, the mortality rate increases to about 50%.

Clinical Manifestations

Acute Pain
The principal manifestation of ulcers is an aching, burning, cramp-like, gnawing pain. The pain has a definite re-

lationship to eating. With gastric ulcers, food may cause the pain and vomiting may relieve it. Clients with duodenal ulcers have pain with an empty stomach, and discomfort may be relieved by ingestion of food or antacids. Clients usually describe the pain as circumscribed in an area 2 to 10 cm (0.8 to 4 inches) in diameter, between the xiphoid cartilage and the umbilicus. Gastric ulcer pain often occurs in the upper epigastrium, with localization to the left of the midline, whereas duodenal pain is in the right epigastrium. Ulcer pain also varies with the site, size, or penetration of the ulcer or the amount of surrounding fibrotic tissue.

In duodenal ulcers, steady pain near the midline of the back between the sixth and 10th thoracic vertebrae with radiation to the right upper quadrant may indicate perforation of the posterior duodenal wall. Fullness or hunger may also be present. Distention of the duodenal bulb produces epigastric pain, which may radiate to the back and thorax. Hydrochloric acid secretion may produce edema and inflammation, with resultant pain, or may activate motor changes with increased spasm, intragastric pressure, and increased motility, also with resultant pain. In addition, ulcer pain tends to occur in distinct periods (periodicity).

Nausea and Vomiting
Clients with a duodenal ulcer usually have a normal appetite unless pyloric obstruction is present. Carcinoma, gastric ulcers, or gastritis may be associated with anorexia, weight loss, and dysphagia. Vomiting occurs more often with gastric ulcer than with uncomplicated duodenal ulcer. It also occurs more frequently when the ulcer is in the pylorus or antrum of the stomach. Vomiting results from gastric stasis or pyloric obstruction, and the client typically vomits undigested food. Severe retching and vomiting may suggest an esophageal tear.

Bleeding
Clients with ulcers often bleed when the ulcer erodes through a blood vessel. Bleeding may occur as massive hemorrhage or may be occult, with slow oozing. Approximately 25% of clients with gastric ulcers may experience bleeding.

The diagnosis of ulcers is confirmed on the basis of manifestations, x-ray evidence, and endoscopy. The history and physical examination do not yield much significant information in a client with uncomplicated peptic ulcer. A complete blood count with decreased hematocrit and hemoglobin values may indicate bleeding. Stool testing for occult blood might also be positive if bleeding is present. Testing for the presence of *H. pylori* can be done via urea breath tests or identification of *H. pylori* serum antibodies in addition to esophagogastroduodenoscopy (EGD) with biopsy.

The major diagnostic tests include EGD and an upper GI tract x-ray series. The EGD has several advantages. It allows the physician to take tissue specimens and to treat the ulcer with either multipolar electrocoagulation (MPEC) or heater-probe therapy (see complications under Medical Management).

Outcome Management
■ Medical Management

The primary objective of intervention for peptic ulcer is to provide stomach rest. Approaches include neutralizing or buffering hydrochloric acid, inhibiting acid secretion, decreasing the activity of pepsin and hydrochloric acid, and eradicating *H. pylori* from the GI tract. Specific measures include medications (see the Integrating Pharmacology feature on Medications for Peptic Ulcer Disease on p. 748), physical and emotional rest, dietary management, and stress reduction. The vaccine HELIVAX, is being tested to prevent infection with *H. pylori* and could be added to the list of routine immunizations in children in the future. It is also being tested as an alternative to antibiotics in those already infected with *H. pylori*.

Response to the therapeutic program varies with clients' perception of their health status and the degree to which lifestyle influences the ulcer disease. The following list outlines the hallmarks of successful interventions:

- The client experiences a decrease in pain with eventual elimination of all ulcer pain and related manifestations.
- The client eats a nutritionally sound diet and reports increased tolerance of food.
- The client complies with the medication schedule.
- The client identifies stressors and develops ways to modify stress and make necessary lifestyle changes.

Modify Diet. For uncomplicated ulcer disease, few physicians or advanced practitioners favor strict dietary changes. There is scant evidence that diet treatment promotes or accelerates healing. Foods known to increase gastric acidity or cause discomfort should be avoided, such as coffee, alcohol, protein foods, and milk.

Prevent and Treat Complications. Hemorrhage, perforation, and obstruction are the main complications that develop after PUD.

Hemorrhage

Assess Bleeding. Hemorrhage varies in degree from minimal, manifested by the presence of occult blood in the stool (melena), to massive, manifested by vomitus containing bright red blood (hematemesis). The usual manifestation of GI tract bleeding is either vomiting of coffee ground–like material or passing of tarry stools. Acid digestion of blood in the stomach results in a granular dark emesis, whereas digestion in the duodenum or

below may result in a black stool. Hemorrhage tends to occur more often with gastric ulcers (Figure 33-2), especially in the older adult population. Although the onset of hemorrhage may be associated with fatigue, nervous tension, upper respiratory tract infection, dietary indiscretion, alcoholism, or irritating drugs, there may be no known precipitating factor.

Manifestations depend on the severity of the hemorrhage. With mild bleeding (<500 ml), the client may experience only slight weakness and diaphoresis. Severe loss of more than 1 L of blood per 24 hours may cause manifestations of shock (see Chapter 83). (See the Clinical Pathway feature on Gastrointestinal Hemorrhage on the website.)

Prevent Shock. Intervention for massive bleeding aims to treat hypovolemic shock, prevent dehydration and electrolyte imbalance, and stop the bleeding. The client, who should be fasting, receives intravenous fluids until the bleeding subsides. The nurse or the physician may insert an NG tube in the presence or absence of blood in the stomach to assess the rate of bleeding, prevent gastric dilation, and administer room temperature saline to remove blood from the stomach. The room temperature saline is cooler than the body temperature, which creates mild vasoconstriction. Gastric cooling may also be promoted by cool saline lavage, which, although controversial, further curtails hemorrhage through its vasoconstrictive effect. Iced saline is rarely used because it may lead to more mucosal damage by decreasing perfusion to the gastric mucosa and may cause a vagal response, decreasing systemic perfusion.

Replace Fluids. Blood volume depletion is a major problem for the client with severe hemorrhage. For those who have suffered a massive upper GI tract hemorrhage, a primary objective of intervention is to replace blood volume. Restlessness and tachycardia are the earliest manifestations of hypovolemia. The client has a greatly decreased urine output, which should be monitored with a Foley catheter and hourly urine measurement. This is important because fluids must be replaced to prevent damage to the kidneys. A urine output of less than 0.5 ml/kg/hr should be reported to the physician.

FIGURE 33-2 Bleeding ulcer on gastric mucosa.

Administer Vasopressin. Arterial administration of vasopressin (via an infusion pump) can also control acute hemorrhage. Vasopressin produces few complications if given intravenously for less than 36 hours to control bleeding.

Inject Artery with Emboli. Another approach to control bleeding is selective arterial embolization with angiography. The emboli may consist of autologous blood clots with or without an absorbable gelatin sponge. A modified clot may be made with a mixture of the client's own blood, aminocaproic acid, and platelets. Fibrin glue has also been used.

Maintain Rest. The client must have minimal activity for several days after bleeding has subsided. Rest decreases blood pressure and GI tract activity. When bleeding stops, the client is allowed bathroom privileges. If the client requires opioids, administer with caution. Morphine sulfate can cause nausea and vomiting; however, the drug may calm the client who is extremely restless and apprehensive. A better alternative is to manage anxiety with non-opioid alternatives.

Maintain High Gastric pH. During the first few days of hemorrhaging, gastric pH should be maintained between 5.5 and 7.0. To maintain the pH at this level, administer H_2-receptor antagonists intravenously for 4 days or as prescribed and advance to oral administration. Monitor gastric pH at least each shift. Anticholinergics are not recommended. Administer antacids for 1 week to complement the H_2-receptor antagonists. Give antacids 1 hour before or 2 hours after the H_2-receptor antagonists so that the antacids do not interfere with absorption of drugs. The client may require antacids every 30 minutes after starting intake of food or fluids.

Stop Bleeding Surgically. If bleeding continues beyond 48 hours, recurs, or is associated with perforation or obstruction, surgery may be indicated. Increased surgical risk is associated with prolonged bleeding, multiple transfusions, debilitation, electrolyte imbalances, and increased age. Surgical procedures include partial gastric resection, excision of the ulcer, and vagotomy and pyloroplasty.

Perform Multipolar Electrocoagulation or Heater-Probe Therapy. Two endoscopic procedures have been effective in treating bleeding ulcers: MPEC and heater-probe therapy. When using MPEC, a bipolar electric current cauterizes the bleeding lesion; with heater-probe therapy, direct heat cauterizes the lesion.

Perforation. Perforation is usually a surgical emergency. When the ulcer perforates, gastroduodenal contents escape through the anterior wall of the stomach into the peritoneal cavity, resulting in chemical peritonitis, bacterial septicemia, and hypovolemic shock. Peristalsis diminishes, and paralytic ileus develops. Posterior perforation is not as clear and often results in pancreatitis, because the pancreas plugs the perforation.

Assess Pain. Perforation occurs most frequently with duodenal ulcers (Figure 33-3). It occurs when the ulcer erodes through the tunica muscularis. The client experiences sudden, sharp, severe pain beginning in the midepigastrium. As peritonitis develops, the pain spreads over the entire abdomen, which becomes tender, hard, and rigid. (See discussion of peritonitis in Chapter 35.)

The degree of pain depends on the amount and type of contents that are spilled into the peritoneal cavity. The pain often causes the client to bend over or draw the knees up to the abdomen in an effort to decrease the tension on the abdominal muscles. If the perforation occurs on the posterior gastric wall, it may erode through to adjacent organs and become sealed, causing few manifestations. When a perforation erodes into the pancreas, manifestations of pancreatitis (see Chapter 48) develop.

Replace Fluids. If perforation occurs, the client needs immediate replacement of fluids, electrolytes, and blood as well as administration of antibiotics. Nasogastric suction should be instituted to drain gastric secretions and thus prevent further peritoneal spillage. A small perforation that closes immediately by adhering to adjacent tissues causes only a small loss of gastric contents.

Correct Perforation Surgically. When surgery is necessary, the surgeon evacuates the escaped gastric contents, cleans the peritoneal cavity by flushing it out with normal saline or an antibiotic or both, and closes the perforation by patching it with omentum. Vagotomy and hemigastrectomy or vagotomy and pyloroplasty provide definitive control of both the ulcer and the complications (see the Case Study feature on Perforated Ulcer Managed Surgically on p. 755). After surgery, antibiotics are given to combat peritonitis. The NG tube remains in the stomach until peristalsis returns. Postoperative complications include subphrenic abscess, hemorrhage, duodenal or gastric fistula, atelectasis, and pneumonia.

Obstruction. Long-standing ulcer disease causes scarring because of repeated ulcerations and healing. Scarring at the pylorus frequently causes pyloric obstruction,

FIGURE 33-3 Perforation of a duodenal ulcer.

manifested most often by pain at night, when the stomach cannot be emptied by peristalsis. Pyloric obstruction can also lead to vomiting. Surgery (pyloroplasty) is usually required to correct the problem.

■ Nursing Management of the Medical Client
Assessment

Nursing assessment involves gathering both psychosocial and pathophysiologic data concerning the client. To assess psychosocial aspects of ulcer disease, ask the client about a familial incidence of ulcer, ingestion of medications that cause gastric irritation, cigarette smoking, alcohol intake, stressors, and coping patterns. Questions about lifestyle, occupation, work, and leisure activities can yield valuable information.

Physical assessment includes accurately observing and immediately reporting manifestations that help pinpoint the diagnosis or that might indicate the presence of a complication. Manifestations include pain, vomiting, and, occasionally, bleeding and changes in appetite. Always obtain a complete history of previous ulcer attacks, including frequency, duration, manifestations, and response to intervention.

Monitor for the development of complications of ulcers, such as hemorrhage, perforation, or obstruction. Assessment also involves ascertaining a description of the bleeding, including hematemesis and melena. Note such factors as color, amount, consistency, and frequency. Bright red blood usually signifies new bleeding; dark red blood indicates old bleeding. If bleeding is severe, always maintain a current and accurate record of the client's hemoglobin, hematocrit, red blood cell count, and fluid intake and output. Monitor the client closely

for the development of manifestations of shock that might occur if bleeding is present.

Because of shock, the client may experience decreased renal blood flow, which causes a decrease in the glomerular filtration rate and in renal excretion. As the body absorbs the by-products of erythrocyte destruction and renal blood flow decreases, watch for an increase in blood urea nitrogen (BUN), creatinine, and ammonia levels. An elevated BUN may follow dehydration from vomiting.

Monitor the client for the development of perforation. Assess the abdomen for pain, tenderness, or rigidity. Report suspected perforation to the physician immediately, and prepare the client for possible surgery.

Monitor the client for the development of gastric obstruction. If the client vomits, record the frequency and the consistency (digested or undigested food or hematemesis) of the vomitus. If pyloric obstruction is present, nasogastric tube and intravenous fluids and electrolytes are needed until the problem is corrected surgically.

Diagnosis, Outcomes, Interventions

Diagnosis: Acute Pain or Chronic Pain. One of the most common nursing diagnoses for the client with a peptic ulcer is acute or chronic pain. *Acute Pain or Chronic Pain related to gastric mucosal injury.*

Outcomes. The client's pain will be relieved, as evidenced by healing of gastric or duodenal mucosal injury and the client's statement of decreased pain on a pain scale of 1 to 10 with the pain being less than 2 or 3.

Interventions

Administer Prescribed Medications. Administer medications as ordered to relieve the client's pain. The medications are discussed in the Integrating Pharmacology feature on Medications for Peptic Ulcer Disease on p. 748. Assess the effectiveness of the medications that the client is taking, and notify the physician if the pain is not relieved by the medications used in the treatment regimen.

Promote Rest and Relaxation. Avoidance of strenuous physical activity decreases gastric secretions and peristalsis. Help the client achieve rest, both physically and mentally. Be alert for factors that interfere with the client's rest. Arrange the environment to encourage relaxation. If certain visitors or telephone calls agitate the client, discourage these visits or calls until the client improves.

Encourage clients who attempt to carry on their normal work routine (despite prescribed rest) to schedule physical and mental relaxation. Explore with the client and significant others or co-workers ways to reduce work responsibilities temporarily.

CASE STUDY   *evolve*
Perforated Ulcer Managed Surgically

Mr. Fong is a 50-year-old, divorced, second-generation Asian-American and is the chief executive officer of a local telecommunications firm. He has a history of peptic ulcer disease. Mr. Fong has been taking clarithromycin (Biaxin) 250 mg bid, metronidazole (Flagyl) 250 mg bid, and omeprazole (Prilosec) 20 mg bid for 1 week. He reports that he has not been able to eat breakfast or lunch on a regular basis and has subsequently not taken sucralfate (Carafate) as ordered. He was taken to the emergency department today via rescue squad with complaints of a sudden onset of severe abdominal pain accompanied by emesis of bright red blood at his office. He is admitted to the hospital unit for preoperative diagnostic evaluation and preoperative preparation . . . *Case Study continued on the website and the CD-ROM with discussions, multiple-choice questions, and a nursing care plan.* *evolve*

Modify Diet. The diet must meet basic nutritional needs. Because an empty stomach stimulates gastric acid secretion, advise the client to eat small amounts at frequent, regular intervals. Discourage ingestion of alcohol, cola, tobacco, caffeine, milk, and foods that cause discomfort. The client may drink decaffeinated beverages.

During the acute phase, the client often requires a bland, nonirritating, low-fiber diet. Clients and their significant others need to learn the modifications in the diet. Have the dietitian review the home diet with the client or whoever will be cooking for the client.

Diagnosis: Ineffective Therapeutic Regimen Management (Individual).

For the client with an uncomplicated ulcer, most of the care must be done by the client at home. Write the nursing diagnosis as *Risk for Ineffective Therapeutic Regimen Management (Individual) related to lack of knowledge of cause of ulcer and measures to treat and prevent recurrence.*

Outcomes. The client will understand and be able to discuss the cause of the ulcer and the treatment and ways to prevent recurrence.

Interventions

Provide Teaching. Treatment of PUD places the responsibility for self-care on the client. To maintain self-care, the client must understand the process underlying ulcer development and the rationale underlying interventions. Help the client to do the following:

- Understand the pathogenesis of the ulcer and the significance of the pain
- Realize that healing takes place rapidly when the irritating effect is removed
- Understand what caused the condition to develop and what must be done to lessen the stimulation
- Discover which substances cause pain by stimulating secretion of gastric juices and eliminate the substances from the diet to promote ulcer healing
- Understand the importance of continuing the medical regimen, although the pain is gone, until healing is completed
- Recognize that once maintenance therapy stops, the ulcer may recur

Instruct the client to use acetaminophen instead of aspirin preparations when these medications are needed. Teach the client to examine the labels of all nonprescription medications, particularly cold remedies, for aspirin (acetylsalicylic acid), other salicylates, NSAIDs (ibuprofen), adrenocorticosteroids, and ACTH. These medications are ulcerogenic (ulcer causing), particularly used in combination. If any of these medications must be taken, advise the client to check with the physician first, to eat between meals, and to use H_2-receptor antagonists or antacids to protect the stomach lining.

Provide Support. Helping clients with PUD cope with psychosocial problems is a vital part of intervention. Encourage the client to learn about the stressors that may be causing the development of ulcers. Discussing coping and relaxation techniques may enable clients to better deal with problems.

Evaluation

Medical management usually controls PUD, often within a few weeks. Many clients must continue treatment to remain ulcer-free. The client must follow the therapeutic regimen and practice appropriate health maintenance and restoration behaviors to avoid complications and prevent future recurrence of PUD.

■ Surgical Management
Gastric Surgical Procedures

Indications. Various types of gastric surgery are performed to reduce the stomach's acid-secreting ability, to remove a malignant or potentially malignant lesion, to treat a surgical emergency that develops as a complication of PUD, or to treat clients who do not respond to medical intervention. Most chronic, recurring ulcers are eventually managed surgically. Many of the procedures described herein can be performed laparoscopically or with open surgical methods.

Surgery for prevention of ulcer recurrence is performed to do the following:

- Facilitate enterogastric regurgitation of mucus secretions, bile, and pancreatic juice
- Decrease the secretory capacity of the stomach by removing parietal cells
- Remove stimuli for hydrochloric acid secretion by cutting the vagus nerve
- Eliminate the gastrin hormone mechanisms by antrectomy

Contraindications. Most contraindications to gastric surgery involve the client's age and physical condition. Any life-threatening disease process, such as chronic obstructive pulmonary disease (COPD) or heart failure, may be a contraindication to surgery.

Complications. Complications are discussed in the section following the types of surgeries.

Outcomes. The outcomes desired from the various surgeries are that the client will survive and recover from the surgery without further injury related to surgery. After most procedures, the client will return home in 7 days or less and resume the previous lifestyle within 6 to 12 weeks. It may take 3 months to a year before the client can eat normally.

Types of Operations

Vagotomy. Vagotomy is performed to eliminate the acid-secreting stimulus to gastric cells. There are three types of vagotomy (Figure 33-4):

1. *Truncal vagotomy.* Each vagus nerve is completely cut.
2. *Selective vagotomy.* The surgeon partially severs the nerves to preserve the hepatic and celiac branches.
3. *Proximal vagotomy.* Partial cutting is performed, but only the parietal cell mass is denervated; innervation of both the antrum and the pyloric sphincter is preserved.

Cutting the vagal nerve fibers selectively avoids the problems of impaired emptying and diarrhea that follow the truncal vagotomy. It also eliminates the necessity for a drainage anastomosis to offset gastric stasis. Proximal vagotomy also reduces acid secretion and preserves the function of the antrum.

Vagotomy with Pyloroplasty. Vagotomy with pyloroplasty involves cutting the right and left vagus nerves and widening the existing exit of the stomach at the pylorus. This procedure prevents stasis and enhances emptying, thereby preventing belching, weight loss, and feelings of fullness (see Figure 33-4, *B*).

Gastroenterostomy. A simple gastroenterostomy (Figure 33-4, *C*) permits regurgitation of alkaline duodenal contents, thereby neutralizing gastric acid. A drain is made in the bottom of the stomach and sewn to an opening made in the jejunum. Because this neutraliza-tion interferes with the inhibition of gastrin release, a net increase in acid secretion may result. If the gastroenterostomy drains the stomach, it reduces motor activity in the pyloroduodenal area. Drainage also diverts acid away from the ulcerative area, which facilitates healing. A gastroenterostomy does not reduce the secretory capacity of the parietal cell mass, and the gastrin mechanism continues to function. Gastroenterostomy should be combined with vagotomy to reduce vagal influences.

Antrectomy. Antrectomy is performed to reduce the acid-secreting portions of the stomach. The procedure removes the entire antrum of the stomach; thus the cells that secrete gastrin are excised. This delays or eliminates the gastric phase of digestion by withdrawing the source of stimulation for acid release and slows the direct response to protein. The surgeon then anastomoses the remaining portion of the stomach to the duodenum.

Antrectomy is often accompanied by vagotomy; thus the cephalic and gastric phases of gastric secretion are eliminated and GI tract motor activity is decreased. This surgical procedure usually prevents recurrence and is probably superior to more extensive operations.

Subtotal Gastrectomy. Subtotal gastrectomy, a generic term referring to any surgery that involves partial removal of the stomach, may be accomplished by either a Billroth I or Billroth II procedure (Figure 33-5). In a *Billroth I* procedure, the surgeon removes part of the distal portion of the stomach, including the antrum. The remainder of the stomach is anastomosed to the duodenum. This combined procedure is more properly called *gastroduodenostomy*. It

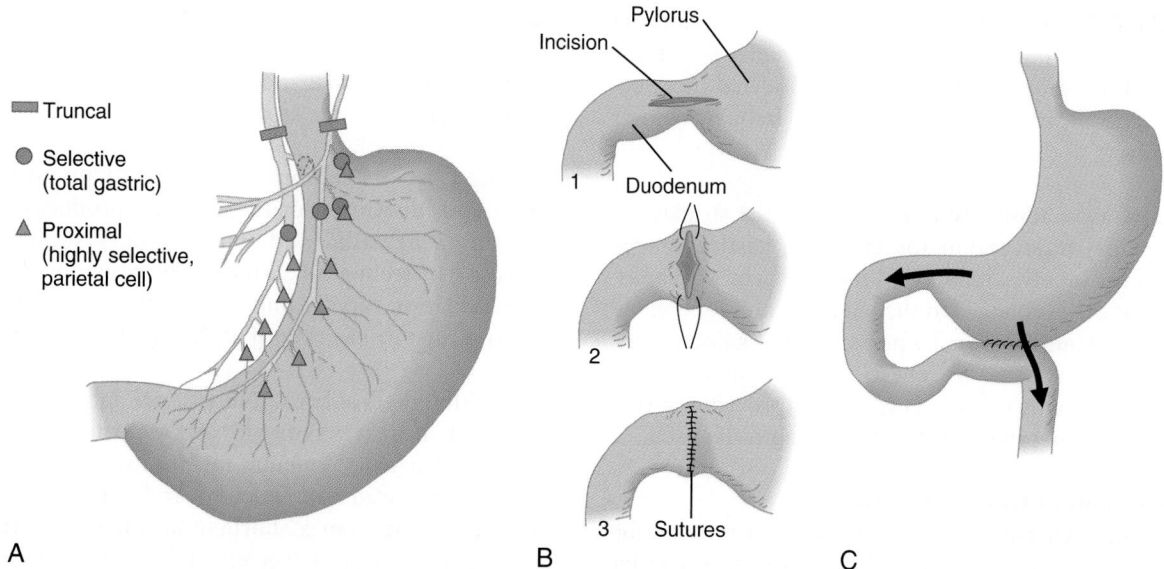

FIGURE 33-4 Vagotomy and drainage. **A,** Sites at which the three types of vagotomy are performed. **B,** Pyloroplasty provides a larger opening from stomach to duodenum to enhance emptying after vagotomy. **C,** Gastroenterostomy, another associated surgical procedure, creates a passage between the body of the stomach and the jejunum.

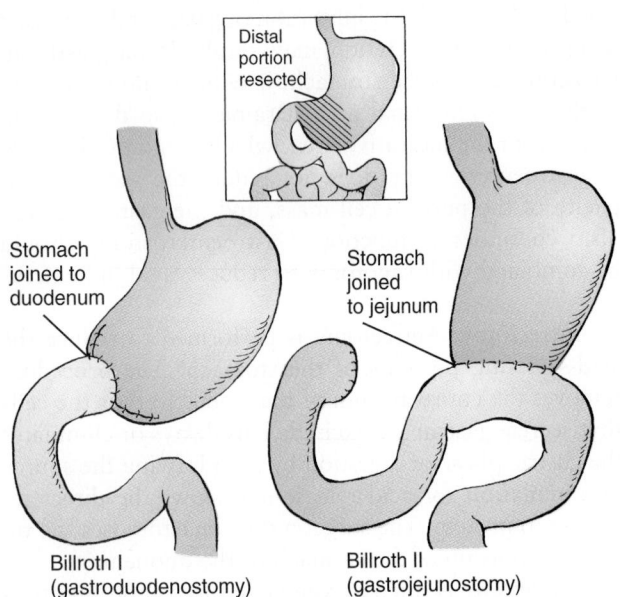

FIGURE 33-5 Subtotal gastrectomy removes acid-secreting portions of the stomach. After removing the distal stomach (*inset*), a surgeon sutures the remaining portion of the stomach to the duodenum (Billroth I procedure) or to the proximal jejunum (Billroth II procedure). The proximal duodenum is left with the Billroth II to allow bile and pancreatic secretions to flow into the duodenum to aid digestion and neutralize acid from stomach.

decreases the incidence of dumping syndrome that often occurs after a Billroth II procedure.

A *Billroth II* resection involves reanastomosis of the proximal remnant of the stomach to the proximal jejunum. Pancreatic secretions and bile continue to be secreted into the duodenum, even after gastrectomy. Because these secretions are necessary for digestion, a route to the intestine must be preserved. Surgeons prefer the Billroth II technique for treatment of duodenal ulcer because recurrent ulceration develops less frequently after this surgery.

Total Gastrectomy. Total resection of the stomach is the principal intervention for extensive gastric cancer. This surgery involves removal of the stomach, with anastomosis of the esophagus to the jejunum, an esophagojejunostomy (Figure 33-6). To perform total gastrectomy, the surgeon may enter the chest; thus the client returns from surgery with chest tubes. Newer procedures that eliminate opening the chest are beginning to be used.

Complications of Gastric Surgeries

Marginal Ulcers. A marginal ulcer can develop where gastric acids come in contact with the operative site, either at the site of the anastomosis or in the jejunum. Ulceration may cause scarring and obstruction. Hemorrhage and perforation can also occur at the surgical site.

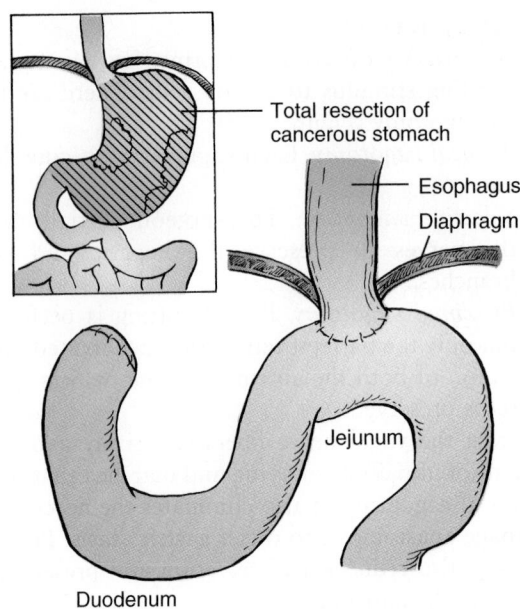

FIGURE 33-6 Total gastrectomy (*inset*) with anastomosis of esophagus to jejunum (esophagojejunostomy), which is the principal intervention for extensive gastric cancer.

Hemorrhage. The reported incidence of hemorrhage after gastric surgery is 1% to 3%. Bleeding is usually caused by a splenic injury or slippage of a ligature. Assess the client postoperatively for manifestations of bleeding and intraperitoneal hemorrhage.

Alkaline Reflux Gastritis. Alkaline reflux gastritis caused by duodenal contents occurs after gastric surgery in which the pylorus has been bypassed or removed. It also occurs after pyloroplasty and gastrojejunostomy. Usually, an associated vagotomy has been performed, which decreases gastric motility, allowing reflux of duodenal contents into the stomach.

Acute Gastric Dilation. In the immediate postoperative period, distention of the stomach produces epigastric pain, tachycardia, and hypotension. The client complains of a feeling of fullness, hiccups, or gagging. Gastric dilation rapidly improves after insertion of a nasogastric tube or clearing of a plugged nasogastric tube.

Nutritional Problems. Nutritional problems common after stomach removal include vitamin B_{12} and folic acid deficiency, calcium metabolism disorders, and reduced absorption of calcium and vitamin D. Such problems result from a shortage of intrinsic factor and inadequate absorption because of rapid entry of food into the bowel. With the Billroth II gastric resection, pancreatic juice and bile secretion are reduced because the usual stimulus of food passing through the duodenum is missing.

Dumping Syndrome. This postprandial problem occurs after gastrojejunostomy because ingested food rapidly enters the jejunum without proper mixing and without the normal duodenal digestive processing. It usually subsides in 6 to 12 months. Early manifestations, which occur 5 to 30 minutes after eating, involve the vasomotor disturbances of vertigo, tachycardia, syncope, sweating, pallor, palpitation, diarrhea, and nausea with a desire to lie down. The client's blood pressure and pulse may either rise or fall.

Dumping syndrome is most common after the Billroth II procedure. Intestinal manifestations include epigastric fullness, distention, abdominal discomfort, abdominal cramping, nausea (with only occasional vomiting), and borborygmi (rumbling sounds in the bowel). The client may experience tenesmus (ineffectual and painful straining to defecate). Pain is not present.

Early manifestations are probably caused by rapid movement of extracellular fluids into the bowel to convert the rapidly entering hypertonic bolus into an isotonic mixture. This rapid fluid shift decreases the circulating blood volume. A jejunum distended with food and fluid increases intestinal peristalsis and motility. Late manifestations, which occur 2 to 3 hours after eating, are a result of rapid entry of high-carbohydrate food into the jejunum, an increase in blood glucose level, and excessive insulin levels.

Management involves decreasing the amount of food taken at one time and maintaining a high-protein, high-fat, low-carbohydrate, dry diet. Gastric emptying can be delayed by eating in a recumbent or semi-recumbent position, lying down after meals, increasing the fat content in the diet, and avoiding fluids 1 hour before, with, or 2 hours after meals. (See the Client Education Guide feature on Diet for Dumping Syndrome on the website.)

The client may also be given sedatives and antispasmodic agents to delay gastric emptying. When manifestations persist, surgical intervention may include reducing the size of the gastroenterostomy or converting a Billroth II resection to a Billroth I by inserting a short segment of jejunum between the duodenal stump and the stomach.

Gastrojejunocolic Fistula. This postoperative complication follows recurrent PUD. The fistulae arise from perforation of a recurrent ulceration at the gastrojejunal anastomosis site. The perforation forms a fistula between the ulcer and adjacent bowel. Manifestations are variable but include fecal vomiting, diarrhea, weight loss, and anorexia. Belching of gas that has a fecal odor may also occur. The manifestations are caused by bacterial overgrowth in the small intestine.

Pyloric Obstruction. Pyloric obstruction, manifested by vomiting, occurs at the pylorus and is caused by scarring, edema, inflammation, or a combination of these conditions. When vomiting persists, alkalosis tends to develop because large quantities of acid gastric juice are vomited. A client who vomits persistently is usually hospitalized to receive intravenous fluids with electrolytes added.

Pyloroduodenal obstruction can cause gastric dilation, gastritis, and gastric stasis. These mechanisms create manifestations that gradually make it more difficult for the stomach to empty. Assess the client for feelings of fullness, distention, or nausea after eating, with loss of appetite and weight loss.

Management of obstruction focuses on restoring fluid and electrolytes and decompressing the dilated stomach; if necessary, surgical intervention is instituted.

■ Nursing Management of the Surgical Client

Preoperative Care
Provide Support. Surgical intervention for gastric and duodenal conditions may be either a planned procedure or an emergency. When emergency surgery is required (e.g., for acute obstruction, perforation, or hemorrhage), the client is very ill and is usually frightened. Provide calm, efficient, knowledgeable care, and explain what is being done. Note and respond to the client's nonverbal behavior. Help significant others provide the client with empathy and emotional support.

When cancer is suspected, the client may want to talk about fears and concerns. Listen to the client carefully, respond to cues, and offer support and understanding. The client may wish to attend to personal matters before surgery (e.g., review a will, see a member of the clergy).

When elective surgery is done, the client has an extensive series of preoperative tests, such as a GI tract x-ray series, endoscopy, and perhaps acid secretion studies (see Chapter 30).

Provide Teaching. Preoperative teaching should include an explanation of the surgery. Explain that the client will have either an NG tube or a gastrostomy tube with suction. An intravenous infusion line is placed in the client's hand or arm for fluids until the surgical site heals. Thoroughly demonstrate and discuss the importance of deep-breathing exercises or use of an incentive spirometer or both. Warn clients that the high abdominal incision makes deep breathing uncomfortable and that the high incision increases the risk of respiratory complications.

Postoperative Care
Assessment

Assess the client with surgical management of PUD in the same way as for the client being managed medically. In addition, perform routine preoperative and postoperative assessments (see Chapter 16).

Diagnosis, Outcomes, Interventions

Diagnosis: Risk for Injury. After surgery, the client is susceptible to postoperative complications. The nursing diagnosis is *Risk for Injury: Postoperative complications (immediate and delayed) related to bleeding, distention, and atelectasis.*

Outcomes. The client will not suffer injury related to postoperative complications (immediate and delayed) as evidenced by decreasing bloody drainage from the NG tube, absence of abdominal distention, and normal breath sounds.

Interventions. Nursing care after gastric surgery is the same as postoperative care for any client recovering from major abdominal surgery.

Maintain Nasogastric Tube. In addition to general postoperative care, perform the following functions:

- Assess drainage from the NG tube and document
- Maintain NG tube patency with saline irrigations, as ordered
- Ensure that the NG tube is attached to suction, and maintained on low suction as ordered
- Assess the operative site for excessive drainage; too much fluid in the remaining gastric stump may cause increased pressure and injury
- Assess the color and consistency of drainage from the operative site, and report or document bleeding or hemorrhaging

After surgery, the client has an NG or gastrostomy tube to prevent retention of gastric secretions. Carefully assess for abdominal distention. Do not reposition the NG or gastrostomy tube after gastric surgery because it may be placed directly over the suture line. Gently irrigate with saline *only* if specifically ordered to do so by the physician.

The color of the drainage in the NG tube may be bright red during the early hours after surgery, but it should become dark red by the end of 24 hours. The drainage has the appearance of coffee grounds for several days after surgery.

Monitor for Complications. Immediate complications after gastric surgery include hemorrhage, gastric distention, obstruction, and disruption of the suture line. Assess for general surgical complications, such as shock, hemorrhage, pulmonary problems, thrombosis, infection (peritonitis), evisceration, and paralytic ileus. Nausea and vomiting should not occur if the nasogastric tube is patent. Carefully measure and document intake (oral and intravenous) and output (urine, suction, and wound drainage).

Promote Comfort. Keep the client comfortable with liberal administration of pain medications; this helps the client to cooperate more fully during deep-breathing and coughing exercises. Give fluids by intravenous infusion, as ordered, until edema and swelling have diminished enough to allow fluids to pass the operative area (seen as a decrease in the gastric tube output and return of bowel sounds).

Diagnosis: Imbalanced Nutrition: Less Than Body Requirements. After surgery the client is at risk for *Imbalanced Nutrition: Less Than Body Requirements related to decreased nutrient absorption secondary to dumping syndrome.*

Outcomes. The client will maintain adequate nutrition, as exhibited by maintaining weight and with no evidence of dumping syndrome.

Interventions. When healing has occurred, clamp the NG or gastrostomy tube and begin oral intake by giving the client clear water, usually 30 ml at a time. Aspirate the tube after 1 hour to determine whether the fluid has been retained. When GI function has returned (e.g., active bowel sounds, passage of flatus) and the client tolerates clear water, the NG tube is usually removed and the diet progresses to soft foods; eventually, a regular diet of five or six small meals a day is given. The diet should not begin too early or progress too rapidly. At first, the client may experience discomfort if too much food is taken at one time.

Evaluation

Postoperatively, some clients need help to reduce the number of stressors in their lives. Strategies for altering lifestyle may be an important part of the rehabilitation and recovery plan. Clients need to know that convalescence after gastric surgery tends to be slow. It may be 3 months before clients regain strength and even partially begin to eat in a more normal manner. It may take a year or so before clients can eat three normal meals a day, and they may need to eat five times per day to accommodate changes in the anatomic structures. When complications such as dumping syndrome occur, clients may feel disappointed. Many clients expect a rapid recovery and may be unprepared when complications develop. Most clients can learn to control manifestations and lead a fairly normal life.

GASTRIC CANCER

Gastric cancer refers to the malignant neoplasms found in the stomach, usually adenocarcinoma, although there may be malignant lymphomas. The incidence of stomach cancer in the United States has diminished steadily since 1960.

The American Cancer Society estimated that 21,500 new cases of gastric cancer would be diagnosed in 2003, with 13,000 deaths attributed to gastric cancer.[1] Stomach cancer is twice as common in men as in women, more common in whites in the United States, and more frequent in clients who have pernicious anemia.

Etiology and Risk Factors

Although no specific cause of gastric cancer has been identified, several factors are associated with the development of the disease. The latest research indicates that the presence of *H. pylori* in the stomach increases the incidence of gastric cancer. Gastric cancer often develops in conjunction with chronic atrophic gastritis and affects individuals who live in urban areas, have a low socioeconomic status, eat smoked fish or meats, and have a history of exposure to background radiation or trace metals in soil. The changes in the mucosa may lead to an increase in absorption of carcinogens from the diet, such as pickled foods, salted fish, and nitrates. Other etiologic factors include achlorhydria, pernicious anemia, and smoking. There may also be a genetic factor because the disease seems to run in families. Metal crafts workers, coal miners, bakers, and those working in dusty, smoky, and sulfur dioxide–containing environments are at increased risk. Wood or tobacco smoke, nitrite food preservatives, and overheated fat products may predispose clients to gastric cancer.

Avoidance of the carcinogenic agents is important, especially in clients with other risk factors, such as chronic gastritis, *H. pylori* infection, and pernicious anemia. Cessation of smoking is an excellent health promotion behavior. The American Cancer Society recommends screening for cag A strain of *H. pylori* bacteria in people with a family history of gastric cancer.

Pathophysiology

Gastric cancer most often arises from the mucous lining of the stomach. Most of these cancers occur in the lesser curvature of the stomach in the pyloric and antral regions. Prognosis is best for stomach cancer involving polypoid lesions; it is poor for ulcerating cancers and poorest for infiltrating forms. Stomach cancer spreads by direct extension into the pancreas, via the lymphatics, and by hematogenous infiltration of the liver, lungs, and bones. The particular route depends on the location and the type of tumor. Some tumors penetrate, some ulcerate, and some spread along the tissue planes.

Gastric cancer is staged using the tumor, node, and metastasis (TNM) classification with stages I to IV (see Chapter 19). The cancer is resectable in early stages before it has invaded the wall of the stomach. The 5-year survival rate is about 90% for local disease and goes below 10% for stage III disease. In advanced gastric cancer, the survival rate is almost zero.

Clinical Manifestations

Because clinical manifestations occur late in the course of the disease, stomach cancer is seldom detected in an early stage. Unless hemorrhage or perforation occurs, manifestations are vague and indefinite. The presence of a palpable mass, ascites, or bone pain caused by metastasis may be the first manifestation. Manifestations vary, depending on the location of the tumor in the stomach. If the cancer grows near the cardia, the client may experience dysphagia because of early involvement of the esophagus. If the cancer is near the pylorus, manifestations may result from obstruction.

Assessment reveals weight loss, vague indigestion, anorexia, or a feeling of fullness or mild discomfort so insidious that the client does not recognize it as abnormal or seek medical assistance. Discomfort may be brought on by or relieved by eating. Anemia from blood loss commonly occurs, and occult blood may be present in the stool. The presence of lactic acid and a high lactate dehydrogenase (LDH) level in the gastric juice suggests carcinoma.

The diagnosis of gastric cancer is confirmed by upper GI tract x-ray examination and gastroscopy. Gastroscopy allows direct visualization and permits cytologic brushing or biopsies to facilitate retrieval of cells for cytologic examination.

Outcome Management
■ Medical Management

Little effective medical treatment is available for gastric cancer. Clients may receive chemotherapy and radiation therapy, but the primary treatment is surgical resection. At present, best results are achieved with multiple drug combinations. Drugs giving the best results are 5-fluorouracil, mitomycin C, cisplatin, etoposide, leucovorin, and doxorubicin (Adriamycin). A combination of radiation and chemotherapy after surgery may be used. Total parenteral nutrition (TPN) (see Chapter 31) is a method for providing nutrition to the client intravenously, bypassing the GI tract.

■ Surgical Management

Surgery is the only intervention that effectively treats stomach cancer. Unfortunately, because the diagnosis is usually late, surgery is more often palliative than curative. Gastrectomy, either partial (with Billroth I or II reconstruction) or complete depending on tumor location, is the usual procedure. Ideally, the surgeon removes all local growth and associated lymph nodes. When an extensive tumor makes resection impractical or impossible and the pylorus is obstructed, the surgeon may perform a palliative gastroenterostomy (surgical creation of a passage between the stomach and small intestine).

■ Nursing Management of the Surgical Client
Assessment

Clients may present with manifestations similar to those of PUD, but frequently manifestations are not present until the tumor is advanced. While assessing the client, note any history of risk factors predisposing to the development of gastric cancer. These include a history of chronic gastritis, pernicious anemia, previous gastric surgery, presence of *H. pylori* infection, or smoking. Ask the client if there is a history of ingestion of large amounts of nitrates, smoked fish, salty foods, or pickled foods.

Diagnosis, Outcomes, Interventions

Diagnosis: Acute Pain.
Both before and after surgery, a primary nursing diagnosis for the client is *Acute Pain related to gastric erosion and postoperative pain related to high surgical incision.*

Outcomes. The client will have pain controlled or experience a reduction in pain, as evidenced by the client's use of a pain scale of 1 to 10 and stating a pain score of less than a 2 or 3.

Interventions. It is important that the client experience pain reduction. Pain that is not controlled can interfere with sleep and eating and contributes to overall physical and mental deterioration. (Chapter 22 describes pain control in detail.) The client should have verbal and written instructions regarding medications, treatments, and follow-up care.

Diagnosis: Imbalanced Nutrition: Less Than Body Requirements.
An important nursing diagnosis for the client with gastric cancer is *Imbalanced Nutrition: Less Than Body Requirements related to decreased appetite, pain, possible gastric obstruction, and nausea and vomiting.*

Outcomes. The client will maintain nutritional intake to meet metabolic requirements, as evidenced by maintenance of normal body weight.

Interventions. Nutritional therapy is an important aspect of management of the client with gastric cancer. TPN or jejunostomy tube feedings may be used postoperatively (or for clients with inoperable disease) to maintain the nutritional status (see Chapter 31).

Diagnosis: Fear.
Because of the uncertainty of the disease, an appropriate nursing diagnosis for the client with gastric cancer is *Fear related to knowledge deficit, body image changes, treatment, and life-threatening illness.*

Outcomes. The client will have reduced or controlled fear, as evidenced by the client's ability to understand and discuss disease and treatment options.

Interventions. The client needs an explanation of the disease and all treatment options. Reinforce information

to the client as needed. The client also needs information concerning operative procedures and postoperative interventions (NPO status, NG tubes, other drains, intravenous infusions). This information helps decrease the client's fear.

Postoperative complications include hemorrhage, obstruction, anemia, nutritional deficiency, dumping syndrome, duodenal stump leakage, gastric dilation, and delayed gastric emptying. A home health care referral can assist the client with emotional support and treatments and provide an ongoing assessment of the client's condition. Referring the client to a dietitian, member of the clergy, and hospice team may also be necessary. Various community support groups are also available (e.g., I Can Cope). For terminal cancer care, see Chapters 19 and 23.

Evaluation

The prognosis for clients with gastric surgery for cancer is poor. Generally, surgery is performed to provide a palliative means of assisting the client to be more comfortable, rather than a cure of the stomach cancer. Therefore the only appropriate outcome may be as good a quality of life as possible and adequate control of manifestations.

CONCLUSIONS

Gastric disorders are common; unless treated promptly and completely, gastric disorders can continue to cause problems throughout the client's life. Assist clients to learn a new way to achieve and maintain health and to make necessary lifestyle changes. This may be a difficult task; however, unless the client is willing to modify behaviors, many of the gastric disorders recur. The foci of nursing interventions are education and modifications of the client's behavior to promote a healthier lifestyle pattern.

THINKING CRITICALLY *evolve*

1. A young female executive comes to the health clinic with complaints of epigastric pain and malaise. She works under stress and smokes heavily. She is in a hurry and wants quick action. The physician or advanced health practitioner recommends ranitidine (Zantac) for pain reduction and an upper gastrointestinal x-ray film to rule out a duodenal ulcer. What further nursing assessment is required? What nursing interventions should be planned?
Factors to Consider. What places the client at risk for a duodenal ulcer? What teaching is required for medication and dietary management? How should changes in lifestyle be addressed?

2. A 43-year-old male client is being evaluated for intractable peptic ulcer disease (PUD). He has a history

of recurrent duodenal ulcers. Last night he awakened at 2:00 AM and requested an antacid. This morning after breakfast, he passed a large, dark, liquid stool that tests positive for occult blood. Just before his 11:00 AM H_2-receptor antagonist, he turns on his call light. When the nurse enters the room, he is lying on his side with his knees drawn up, moaning and holding his pillow against his abdomen. He is diaphoretic, pale, and breathing rapidly and shallowly. The client states, "It's never hurt like this before. I feel as though I've been stabbed." What should the nurse's first actions be? What has probably happened to this client? Will he need surgery?

Factors to Consider. If surgery is needed, what type of surgery may need to be performed? What are the expected nursing assessments postoperatively? Is he at risk for complications? What discharge teaching will be needed to enhance his health maintenance and prevent future recurrence of PUD?

3. A 52-year-old man who had a subtotal gastrectomy for stage III gastric cancer 10 weeks ago is having difficulty maintaining his body weight. His usual body weight is 190 pounds; he currently weighs 165 pounds. His wife reports that her husband is depressed, will not eat, and sleeps all day in his chair. She states, "I don't know what to do anymore! I think he just wants to die." She then starts crying. What should the nurse say to the client's wife? Whom should the nurse contact to assist the family?

Factors to Consider. Why is the client at nutritional risk? What is his percentage of weight loss? What measures might be initiated to facilitate nutrition?

Discussions for these questions can be found on the website and the CD-ROM.

BIBLIOGRAPHY

1. American Cancer Society. (2003). *Cancer facts and figures.* Atlanta: Author.
2. Barrison, A., et al. (2001). Patterns of proton pump inhibitors in clinical practice. *American Journal of Medicine, 111*(6), 469-473.
3. Bookbinder, M., & Kiss, M. (2001). Death and society. In M.L. Matzo & D.W. Sherman (Eds.), *Palliative care nursing: Quality care to the end of life* (pp. 89-117). New York: Springer.
4. Braga, M., et al. (2002). Feeding the gut early after digestive surgery: Results of a nine-year experience. *Clinical Nutrition, 21*(1), 59-65.
5. Callahan, C., et al. (2000). Outcomes of percutaneous endoscopic gastrostomy among older adults in a community setting. *American Journal of Geriatric Society, 48,* 1048-1054.
6. Carswell, C., & Goa, K. (2001). Rabeprazole: An update of its use in acid-related disorders. *Drugs, 61*(15), 2327-2356.
7. Ciociola, A., Pappa, K., & Sirgo, M. (2001). Nonprescription doses of ranitidine are effective in the relief of episodic heartburn. *American Journal of Therapeutics, 8*(6), 399-408.
8. Copstead, L. (2000). *Pathophysiology: Biological and behavioral perspectives* (2nd ed). Philadelphia: W.B. Saunders.
9. Dempsey, D., et al. (2001). Descriptive study of nurses' compliance with postprocedural vital sign measurement in a gastrointestinal investigation unit. *Gastroenterology Nursing, 25*(5), 181-187.
10. Gene, E., et al. (2003). Triple vs. quadruple therapy for treating *H. pylori* infection: A meta analysis. *Alimentary Pharmacology and Therapeutics, 17*(9), 1137-1143.
11. Giese, L. (2000). A study of alternative health care use for gastrointestinal disorders. *Gastroenterology Nursing, 23*(1), 19-27.
12. Griffin-Sobel, J., & Suozzo, S. (2002). Nursing research priorities for the care of the client with a gastrointestinal disorder. *Gastroenterology Nursing, 25*(5), 188-191.
13. Hayes, A., & Buffum, M. (2001). Educating patients after conscious sedation for gastrointestinal procedures. *Gastroenterology Nursing, 24*(2), 54-57.
14. Heiser, M., & Malaty, H. (2001). Balloon-type versus non-balloon type placement of percutaneous endoscopic gastrostomy: Which is better? *Gastroenterology Nursing, 24*(2), 58-63.
15. Inoue, H. (2001). Endoscopic mucosal resection for the entire gastrointestinal mucosal lesions. *Gastrointestinal Endoscopic Clinics of North American, 11*(3), 459-478.
16. Lehne, R. (2001). *Pharmacology for nursing care* (4th ed.). Philadelphia: W.B. Saunders.
17. Marzio, L., Cellini, L., & Angelucci, D. (2003). Triple therapy for 7 days vs. triple therapy for 7 days plus omeprazole for 21 days in treatment of active duodenal ulcer with *H. pylori* infection: A double blind placebo controlled study. *Digestive and Liver Disease, 35*(1), 20-23.
18. Metheny, N., & Titler, M. (2001). Assessing placement of feeding tubes. *American Journal of Nursing, 101*(5), 36-46.
19. Nardone, G., et al. (1999). Effect of *Helicobacter pylori* infection and its eradication on cell proliferation, DNA status, oncogene expression in patients with chronic gastritis. *Gut, 44*(6), 789-799.
20. Otto, S. (2001). *Oncology nursing* (4th ed.). St. Louis: Mosby.
21. Powell, D. (2000). Gastrointestinal diseases. In Goldman, L. (Eds.). *Cecil textbook of medicine* (21st ed., pp. 643-766). Philadelphia: W.B. Saunders.
22. Pratt, B., & Greene, F. (2000). Role of laparoscopy in the staging of malignant disease. *Surgical Clinics of North America, 80*(4), 1111-1126.
23. Rajan, E., & Gostout, C. (2001). Widespread endoscopic mucosal resection. *Gastrointestinal Endoscopic Clinics of North of American, 11*(3), 489-497.
24. Raudonis, B. (2003). Palliative care update for gastroenterology nurses. *Gastroenterology Nursing, 26*(1), 26-30.
25. Robinson, M., et al. (2002). Control of nocturnal gastric acidity: A role for low dose bedtime ranitidine to supplement daily omeprazole. *Digestive Disease and Sciences, 47*(2), 265-273.

26. Soetikno, R.M., Inoue, H., & Chang, K.J. (2000). Endoscopic mucosal resection. Current concepts. *Gastrointestinal Endoscopic Clinics of North America, 10*(4), 595-617.

27. Stein, H., et al. (2000). Multidisciplinary approach to esophageal and gastric cancer. *Surgical Clinics of North America, 80*(2), 659-686.

28. Townsend, C. (2001). *Sabiston textbook of surgery: The biological basis of modern surgical practice* (16th ed.). Philadelphia: W.B. Saunders.

29. Ulmer, H., Beckerling, A., & Gatz, G. (2003). Recent use of proton pump inhibitor-based triple therapies for the eradication of *H. pylori*: A broad data review. *Helicobacter, 8*(2), 95-104.

Unit 8

Elimination Disorders

Anatomy and Physiology Review

The Elimination Systems

Robert G. Carroll

The urinary tract is composed of the following four structures:
- Kidneys
- Ureters
- Bladder
- Urethra

The kidneys balance the urinary excretion of substances against the accumulation within the body through ingestion or production. Consequently, they are a major controller of fluid and electrolyte homeostasis. The kidneys also have several non-excretory metabolic and endocrine functions, including blood pressure regulation, erythropoietin production, insulin degradation, prostaglandin synthesis, calcium and phosphorus regulation, and vitamin D metabolism.

Filtration at the renal glomerulus is the first step in urine formation. Normally, a volume equal to plasma volume is filtered every 45 minutes, and a volume equal to total body water is filtered every 6 hours. *Glomerular filtrate* is similar to plasma but lacks cells and large-molecular-weight proteins. The glomerular filtrate is modified by active transport, diffusion, and osmosis as it passes through the renal tubules. *Reabsorption* of filtrate components enhances conservation of glucose, peptides, and electrolytes. *Secretion* of plasma components enhances elimination of organic acids and bases (and some drugs). The remnants of the glomerular filtrate exit the kidney through the ureters.

The *ureters* conduct urine from the kidneys to the bladder by peristaltic contraction. The *bladder* is a distensible chamber that stores urine until it is eliminated. The *urethra* is the exit passageway from the bladder, and it carries urine for elimination from the body.

STRUCTURE OF THE ELIMINATION SYSTEM
KIDNEYS

The kidneys are located retroperitoneally, in the posterior aspect of the abdomen, on either side of the vertebral column (Figure U8-1). They lie between the twelfth thoracic and the third lumbar vertebrae. The left kidney is usually positioned slightly higher than the right. Adult kidneys average 11 cm in length, 5 to 7.5 cm in width, and 2.5 cm in thickness. Affixing the kidneys in position behind the parietal peritoneum is a mass of perirenal fat (adipose capsule) and connective tissue called *Gerota's* (subserosa) *fascia*. A fibrous capsule (renal capsule) forms the external covering of the kidney itself, except the hilum. The kidney is further protected by layers of muscle of the back, flank, and abdomen as well as by layers of fat, subcutaneous tissue, and skin.

The kidney has a characteristic curved shape, with the convex distal edge and a concave medial boundary. In the innermost part of the concave section is the hilus, through which pass the renal artery, renal vein, lymphatics, nerves, and the renal pelvis (the natural upper extension of the ureter). A fibrous capsule surrounds and adheres to the renal parenchyma. Each kidney is divided into three major areas: (1) cortex, (2) medulla, and (3) pelvis (Figure U8-2).

The cortex of the kidney lies just under the fibrous capsule, and portions of it extend down into the medullary layer to form the renal columns (columns of Bertin) or cortical tissue that separates the pyramids. The medulla is divided into 8 to 18 cone-shaped masses of collecting ducts called *renal pyramids*. The bases of the pyramids are positioned on the corticomedullary boundary. Their apices extend toward the renal pelvis, forming *papillae*. The papillae each have 10 to 25 openings on the surface, through which the urine empties into the renal pelvis (see Figure U8-2, *inset*). Eight or more groups of papillae are present in each pyramid; each empties into a minor calix, and several minor calices join to form a major calix. The two to three major calices are outpouchings of the renal pelvis. They channel the urine from the pyramids to the renal pelvis. The renal pelvis cavity is lined with transitional epithelium. The combined volume of the pelvis and calices is about 8 ml. Volumes in excess of this amount damage the renal parenchymal tissue. The renal pelvis narrows as it reaches the hilus and becomes the proximal end of the ureter.

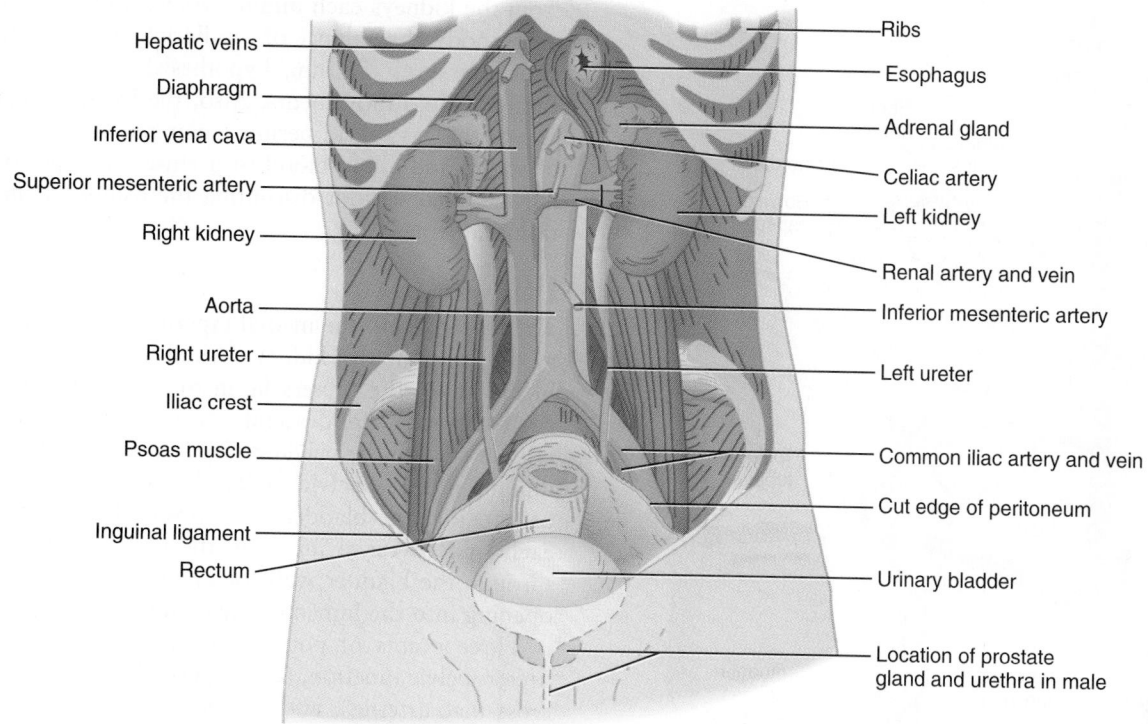

FIGURE U8-1 Anatomic relationship of the kidneys and related structures.

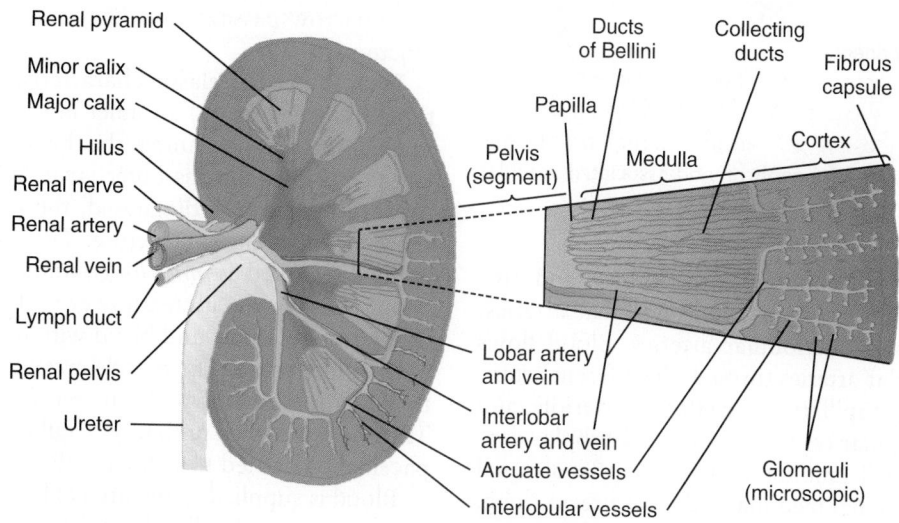

FIGURE U8-2 Anatomy of the kidney. *Inset,* Enlargement of a segment of the kidney.

Within the cortex lies the nephron, the functional unit of the kidney, which consists of both vascular and tubular elements (Figure U8-3). Filtration begins at the renal glomerulus. The glomerular tuft (glomerulus) contains capillaries and the beginning of the tubule system, called *Bowman's capsule.* Filtrate from the glomerulus enters Bowman's capsule and then passes through a series of tubule segments that modify the filtrate as it passes through the renal cortex and medulla and finally flows into the renal calyces. A second capillary bed, the peritubular capillaries, carries the reabsorbed water and solute back toward the vena cava.

Renal Blood Flow and Glomerular Filtration

The kidneys receive 20% to 25% of the cardiac output under resting conditions, averaging more than 1 L of arterial blood per minute. The renal arteries (see Figure U8-2) branch from the abdominal aorta at the level of

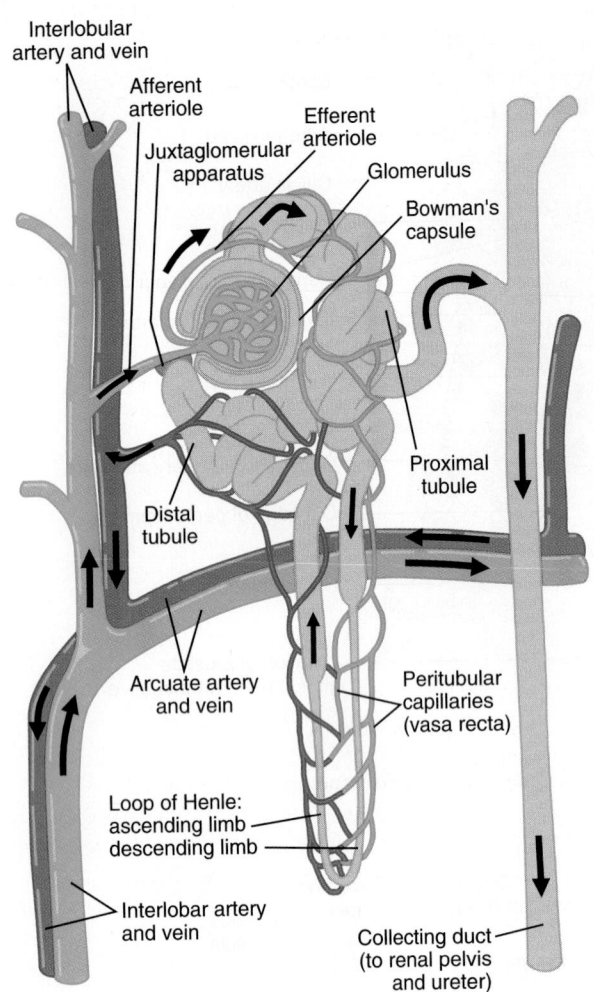

FIGURE U8-3 Diagram of a nephron and associated vascular structures.

Labels on figure:
- Interlobular artery and vein
- Afferent arteriole
- Juxtaglomerular apparatus
- Efferent arteriole
- Glomerulus
- Bowman's capsule
- Proximal tubule
- Distal tubule
- Arcuate artery and vein
- Peritubular capillaries (vasa recta)
- Loop of Henle: ascending limb descending limb
- Interlobar artery and vein
- Collecting duct (to renal pelvis and ureter)

from the kidneys each minute. As with other capillaries in the body, the balance of capillary hydrostatic and oncotic pressures (Starling hypothesis) determines transcapillary fluid movements. Also, the long, straight vessels of the vasa recta permit a countercurrent exchange of solute and allow blood to perfuse the hypertonic renal medulla without disrupting the osmotic concentration gradient.

URETERS

The ureters form the medial tapering of the renal pelvis at the hilus of the kidney. Usually 25 to 35 cm long in the adult, the ureters lie in the extraperitoneal connective tissue and descend vertically along the psoas muscle toward the pelvic cavity (see Figure U8-1). After dipping into the pelvic cavity, the ureters course anteriorly to join the bladder in its posterolateral aspect. At each ureterovesical junction, the ureter runs obliquely through the bladder wall for about 1.5 to 2 cm before opening into the lumen of the bladder.

Three points of potential obstruction exist: (1) the ureteropelvic junction, (2) the pelvic brim (where ureters cross iliac arteries), and (3) the ureterovesical junction. The ureter is much narrower at these points. This anatomic arrangement usually functions as a valve that prevents the backward flow (reflux) of urine into the kidney. Because it is difficult for calculi (stones) to traverse these narrow passageways, they typically lodge at these junctions.

Each ureter has elastic characteristics and is made of three tissue layers: (1) an inner mucosa (transitional epithelial membrane) lining the lumen, (2) a muscular layer, and (3) a fibrous outer layer. When cancer of the bladder or ureter is diagnosed, the potential for recurrence exists in either structure. The musculature is generally designated as *inner longitudinal* and *outer circular*. Along most of the ureter, however, the muscle fibers actually run obliquely and blend with one another to form a mesh-like tissue. The muscle arrangement allows urine to be propelled down the ureter by peristaltic action. This peristalsis is probably regulated by a myogenic pacemaker located near the renal calices.

Blood is supplied to the ureters by one or more vessels that run longitudinally along the tube. The number and assortment of arteries anastomosing with the ureteric vessels vary with each individual. Because the ureters travel through several anatomic areas, the ureteral vessels are fed by several of the following arteries: (1) renal (frequently), (2) testicular or ovarian, (3) aorta and common iliac, (4) internal iliac (frequently), (5) vesical, (6) umbilical, and (7) uterine.

The innervation of the ureter comes from the eleventh thoracic to the first lumbar nerves. The network of nerves becomes progressively more dense toward the terminal end of the ureters.

the second lumbar vertebra, enter the kidney, and progressively branch into *lobar arteries,* interlobar arteries, *arcuate arteries,* and interlobular arteries. Blood flows from the interlobular arteries through the afferent arteriole, the glomerular capillaries, the efferent arteriole, and the peritubular capillaries. Some of the peritubular capillaries carry a small amount of blood (~5% of renal blood flow) to the renal medulla in the vasa recta (long, straight blood vessels) before entering the venous drainage. The blood leaves the kidney in a venous system that closely corresponds to the arterial system: interlobular veins, arcuate veins, interlobar veins, and the renal vein. The renal circulation then empties into the inferior vena cava.

The arrangement of the two capillary beds in series in the nephron allows most of the large volume of filtrate at the glomerular capillaries to be reabsorbed by the peritubular capillaries. Normal glomerular filtration rate is 125 ml/min, but because of filtrate reabsorption at the peritubular capillaries, only about 1 ml of urine flows

BLADDER

The urinary bladder is a hollow organ located in the anterior half of the pelvis behind the symphysis pubis. (See the Unit 9 Anatomy and Physiology Review and Figures U9-1, *B*, and U9-4 for a discussion of anatomic structures.) The space between the bladder and the symphysis pubis is filled with a loose connective tissue that allows the bladder to stretch cranially as it fills. The peritoneum covers the top border of the bladder, and the base is held loosely in place by the true ligaments. The bladder is also enveloped by a loose fascia.

The bladder wall has several tissue layers. The internal lining of the vesical wall is transitional epithelium with some mucus-secreting glands. Then there are three ill-defined muscle layers: the inner and outer layers (longitudinal) and middle layer (circular). The fibers from these layers interweave to form a mesh-like muscle layer called the *detrusor muscle*. This arrangement allows the bladder wall to be elastic while maintaining strength. Bundles of these smooth-muscle layers come together at the base of the bladder to form the *internal sphincter*, or opening into the urethra. The *trigone* describes the triangular area formed by the ureterovesical junctions and the internal sphincter.

The superior and lateral aspects of the bladder are served by the superior vesical artery, which branches from the umbilical artery and internal iliac artery. The inferior vesical artery, which supplies the underside of the bladder, may arise independently or in common with the middle rectal artery. The veins draining the bladder pass to the internal iliac trunk.

Innervation for the bladder comes from the hypogastric sympathetic, pelvic parasympathetic, and pudendal somatic nerves. Ganglia are most commonly found in the bladder base and around the urethral orifice. These areas tend to act in continuity with each other, and their functions seem to be coordinated by both the sympathetic and parasympathetic nervous systems (Figure U8-4).

URETHRA AND MEATUS

The urethra is a tube that extends from the base of the bladder to the surface of the body. The female and male urethras differ greatly.

Female Urethra

The female urethra is about 4 cm long and curves slightly forward as it reaches the external opening, or *meatus*, located between the clitoris and the vaginal orifice. The urethra is lined with epithelium, which contains some mucus-secreting glands. The longitudinal muscle layer is a continuation of longitudinal layer of bladder muscle. The circular muscle fibers encompass the urethra and meet with the circular bladder muscle. This muscle thins out near the meatus. As the urethra passes through

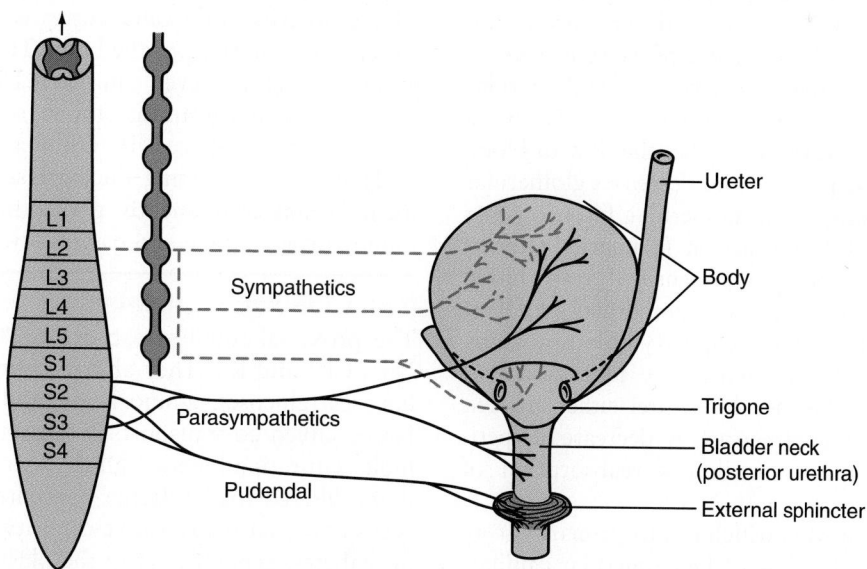

FIGURE U8-4 Innervation of the urinary bladder and associated structures involved in the micturition reflex. Bladder-wall stretch receptors send afferent projections along sensory nerves to the spinal cord. In the spinal cord, the sensory nerves stimulate parasympathetic activity and inhibit sympathetic activity. The resultant bladder contraction further increases pressure in the bladder. Decreased activity of the pudendal nerve relaxes the external sphincter, allowing expulsion of urine. (From Guyton, A.C., & Hall, J. [2001]. *Textbook of medical physiology* [10th ed.]. Philadelphia: W.B. Saunders.)

the urogenital diaphragm, the circular muscle fibers form the external sphincter.

Male Urethra

In males, the urethra is a common outlet for the reproductive system and urinary elimination. The prostate gland, although not a direct part of the urinary system, is a major cause of urinary dysfunction in men. Located below the bladder neck, the prostate completely surrounds the urethra. Normally, this relationship causes no problem, but if the prostate enlarges it constricts the urethra and obstructs the outflow of urine.

The male urethra is about 20 cm long and is divided into three main sections. The prostatic urethra extends about 3 cm below the bladder neck, through the prostate gland, to the pelvic floor. The ejaculatory ducts of the reproductive system empty into its posterior wall. The membranous urethra is about 1 to 2 cm long and ends where the muscle layer forms the external sphincter. The distal portion is the cavernous, or penile, urethra. About 15 cm long, it travels through the penis to the urethral orifice at the tip of the penis. It is also lined with epithelial cells.

FUNCTION OF THE ELIMINATION SYSTEM
TRANSCAPILLARY FLUID EXCHANGE

Fluid movement at each capillary bed depends on the balance of fluid pressures and osmotic pressures. Glomerular capillary blood pressure reflects resistance to flow at afferent and efferent arterioles. Preglomerular contraction (primarily afferent arteriole), such as caused by renal sympathetic nerves, decreases the flow of blood into the glomerular capillaries and decreases glomerular capillary blood pressure and glomerular filtration rate (GFR). Postglomerular contraction (primarily efferent arteriole), such as caused by angiotensin II, traps blood in the glomerulus and increases glomerular capillary pressure and GFR. Peritubular capillary blood pressure, because the peritubular capillaries are located downstream of the glomerulus, decreases after either afferent or efferent arteriolar contraction. A decrease in peritubular capillary pressure facilitates reabsorption of glomerular filtrate.

Plasma oncotic pressure, which results primarily from albumin, attenuates filtration at the glomerular capillaries. If the glomerular barrier is damaged, the permeability of the glomerular capillary to protein decreases the normal oncotic reabsorptive forces, and so GFR is increased. The primary barrier to protein filtration is the negatively charged endothelium and basement membrane of the glomerular capillaries. A loss of this negative charge, such as occurs in diabetes, allows some proteins to pass into the urine (*proteinuria*).

TUBULAR MECHANISMS FOR SECRETION AND REABSORPTION

The renal tubules are lined with epithelial cells that selectively secrete or reabsorb compounds (Table U8-1). This blind-ended tubular segment originates at the glomerulus. Transport proteins and tightness of tight junctions help to define functionally the segments of the tubules. Because the renal tubules and urinary tract are lined with epithelial cells, tubular fluid is functionally outside of the body (similar to the gastrointestinal [GI] tract).

Modification of ultrafiltrate occurs by diffusion and selective transport in tubules. Diffusion is quantitatively the most important process. Some compounds are absorbed by carrier mediated transport, such as sodium-coupled glucose transport.

Glomerular filtrate travels progressively through Bowman's capsule, the proximal tubules, loop of Henle, distal tubules, connecting segment, and the collecting duct; it then enters renal medullary space, passes into ureter, and is stored in the bladder before exiting body as urine. The tubule segments are anatomically adjacent to the vascular supply for that nephron. The juxtaglomerular apparatus consists of the glomerulus and the distal tubule that originated from that glomerulus. This arrangement allows negative feedback control of glomerular filtrate formation at the individual nephron level.

Water reabsorption is driven by osmotic gradients. The osmolarity of the renal cortex is 300 mOsm, similar to that in most areas of the body. The osmolarity of the renal medulla, however, can reach 1500 mOsm because of the high concentrations of urea, sodium, and chloride in the interstitial spaces. Two tubular segments, the loop of Henle and collecting ducts, pass through the renal medulla and consequently play a major role in determining urine volume and osmolarity.

Renal Tubular Segments

The proximal tubules reabsorb 65% of filtered water, Na^+, Cl^-, and K^+. They also reabsorb 100% of filtered hexoses (glucose), amino acids, and small peptides by Na^+ coupled co-transport. Because this mechanism exhibits saturation kinetics, glucose can pass into the urine if the filtered load (plasma concentration × GFR) exceeds the renal reabsorptive capacity (T_{max}). This occurs in diabetes, generally when the plasma glucose concentration exceeds 300 mg/dl.

The descending thin limb of the loop of Henle is water permeable, allowing water to exit the tubule as the filtrate passes into the osmotically concentrated renal medulla. Sodium chloride (NaCl) and urea, the osmotic particles of the medulla, can also enter the tubule in this segment. The thick ascending limb of the loop of Henle is water impermeable, as are the remaining segments of

TABLE U8-1 *Kidney Reabsorption and Secretion*

Compound	Mechanism	Blocker
Proximal Tubule Reabsorbed		
Na^+	Facilitated diffusion	Amiloride
HCO_3^-	Na^+/H^+ antiport	Carbonic anhydrase inhibitors
Cl^-	Electrical charge	
K^+	Diffusion	
Water	Osmosis	
Glucose	Na-coupled transport	
Amino acids	Na-coupled transport	
Urea		
Urate		
Proximal Tubule Secreted		
Penicillin	Active transport	Probenecid
PAH (para-aminohippuric acid)		
Quinine, choline, thiamine, others		
Creatinine		
H^+		
Thick Ascending Limb of the Loop of Henle Reabsorbed		
Na^+	Na/K/2Cl transporter	Furosemide and bumetanide
K^+	Na/K/2Cl transporter	Furosemide and bumetanide
Cl^-	Na/K/2Cl transporter	Furosemide and bumetanide
Mg^{2+}		
NH_4^+	Na/K/2Cl transporter	Furosemide and bumetanide
Thick Ascending Limb of the Loop of Henle Secreted		
H^+	H^+ ATPase	
Distal Tubule Reabsorption		
Na^+/Cl^-	NaCl symport	Thiazides
Na^+	Electrogenic (aldosterone)	Amiloride, spironolactone
H^+ or HCO_3^-	Intercalated cells	Carbonic anhydrase inhibitors
Distal Tubule Secretion		
K^+	Aldosterone Na reabsorption	Amiloride, spironolactone
H^+	H^+ ATPase	
Collecting Duct Reabsorption		
Urea	Transporters (ADH control)	
Water	Osmosis (ADH control)	
NaCl	NaCl symport	Thiazides

the urinary system, in the absence of antidiuretic hormone. In the ascending loop, the Na/K/2Cl transporter reabsorbs electrolytes, and this solute transport without water movement results in hypotonic filtrate (100 mOsm); so this tubule segment is sometimes called the *diluting segment.*

Transport in the distal tubule and collecting duct represent the final chance to modify the tubular fluid before it is lost as urine. Aldosterone promotes K secretion in the distal tubule, and antidiuretic hormone (ADH) increases water reabsorption in the collecting duct. The filtrate that flows from the collecting duct into the ureter is

the final excretory product: urine. The bladder stores urine for elimination, but it does not further modify urine composition.

Renal Mechanisms in Acid-Base Balance

Renal acid/base excretion complements pulmonary carbon dioxide (CO_2) elimination to regulate body acid-base status. Renal acids are hydrogen (H^+), ammonium (NH_3), phosphate and sulfate buffers. The renal base is predominantly HCO_3^-. Because of the high HCO_3^- filtered load, reabsorption of bicarbonate is the primary task of the tubule segments. This is accomplished in the proximal and distal tubules by H^+ secretion and carbonic anhydrase–mediated CO_2 formation. Ultimately, urinary acid secretion is determined by plasma CO_2 levels.

Ammonium (NH_4^+) formation in the proximal tubule augments acid secretion, particularly in chronic acidosis. The proximal tubule cells metabolize glutamine to form ammonia (NH_3). NH_3 is uncharged and diffuses into tubular lumen, where it combines with secreted H^+ to form NH_4^+. Ionic NH_4^+ does not freely diffuse, and it remains in the lumen in a process called *ammonia trapping*.

Distal nephron pH is regulated by intercalated cells. There are two populations of intercalated cells. One is oriented for HCO_3^- secretion, and the other is oriented for H^+ secretion. Increased plasma CO_2 causes net $NaHCO_3$ reabsorption, correcting the acidosis. Decreased plasma CO_2 promotes net HCl reabsorption, correcting the alkalosis.

Clearance

The clearance principle assumes that the substance being cleared has been completely removed from a hypothetical amount of plasma. The minimum flow of plasma required to deliver that substance to the kidney is defined as the clearance. Clearance is calculated as follows:

$$C_x = \frac{U_x \, [V]}{P_x}$$

$$\text{Clearance} = \frac{\text{Urine flow rate} \times \text{Urine concentration}}{\text{Plasma concentration}}$$

where U_x is urine concentration and $[V]$ is urine minute volume.

Clearance of inulin or creatinine provides a noninvasive measurement of GFR, and clearance of para-aminohippuric acid (PAH) or Diodrast provides an estimate of renal plasma flow.

Free water clearance is the rate of solute-free plasma (water) added to or subtracted from urine flow necessary to make the urine isosmotic to plasma. It provides a measure of water balance. A client may be in positive free water clearance if urine osmolarity is less than plasma osmolarity or in negative free water clearance if urine osmolarity is greater than plasma osmolarity.

Urinary Concentration and Dilution

Urine osmolarity reflects the balance of water and solute reabsorption rates. It is determined by the medullary osmolarity and the amount of antidiuretic hormone (ADH) acting on the collecting ducts. Glomerular filtrate is isosmotic with plasma (300 mOsm), and the filtrate osmolarity remains unchanged in the proximal tubule. Osmolarity increases in the descending loop of Henle. The ascending loop of Henle, where the Na/K/2Cl transporter removes ions, but not water, causes the filtrate osmolarity to drop to 100 mOsm. This value is close to the lower limit of urine osmolarity. ADH acts on the distal tubule and collecting duct to increase water and urea permeability, allowing the filtrate to become isosmotic with the cortex (300 mOsm); if a large amount of ADH is present, it becomes isosmotic with the inner medulla (1500 mOsm). The inner medulla osmolarity represents the upper limit on urine osmolarity.

REGULATION OF URINE FORMATION

Renal perfusion pressure is the dominant long-term regulator of glomerular filtrate formation and urine production (pressure diuresis and pressure natriuresis). Other mechanisms also alter the rate of filtrate formation and the efficiency of filtrate reabsorption.

Tubuloglomerular feedback at the juxtaglomerular apparatus provides negative feedback control of GFR. The juxtaglomerular apparatus is formed by the junction of the glomerular afferent arteriole and the macula densa of the distal convoluted tubule. A decrease in distal tubule NaCl delivery causes a reflex increase in GFR, both by afferent arteriolar dilation and an angiotensin II–mediated efferent arteriolar constriction. Blockade of angiotensin II formation reduces the effectiveness of this system and may cause a drop in GFR.

Neural regulation by the sympathetic nervous system also controls urine formation. Sympathetic contraction of afferent arterioles reduces filtrate formation and enhances salt and water conservation. Renal sympathetics are activated in response to hypotension sensed by arterial baroreceptors and in response to hypovolemia sensed by cardiopulmonary volume receptors.

RENAL ENDOCRINE AND METABOLIC ACTIONS

Most endocrine actions of the kidney are tied to the cardiovascular system. The kidneys synthesize and secrete erythropoietin, the hormone that increases blood cell synthesis in the bone marrow. Renin release from the afferent arteriole ultimately leads to the formation of vasoconstrictor angiotensin II and the release of aldosterone. Intrarenal prostaglandin production assists the regional distribution of renal blood flow. One exception to the renal-cardiovascular connection is vitamin D. Vitamin D_3 activated to 1,25 dihydroxycholecalciferol by renal proximal tubules to enhance Ca^{2+} absorption.

Second only to the liver, the kidney has a powerful gluconeogenesis capacity. Urine represents a possible loss pathway for nutrients, especially in disease. Proteinuria may cause a greater loss of protein than may be offset by ingestion. The glucosuria of diabetes may also represent a significant loss of potential calories.

MICTURITION

Urine production by the kidneys is relatively constant (~1 ml/min), but it can vary from 0.5 to 20 ml/min. The flow through ureters is intermittent and is controlled by the rate of peristaltic wave generation. The peristalsis that forces the urine into the bladder for storage occurs every 10 to 150 seconds. Parasympathetic activation increases frequency of peristalsis, and sympathetic stimulation decreases frequency. Afferent (pain) nerves initiate the ureterorenal reflex. This reflex, activated by obstruction, causes ureter constriction and also causes afferent arteriolar constriction to decrease urine production. Lodging of kidney stones in the ureter is a major cause of this response.

Both sensory and motor components of the pelvic nerves supply the bladder. Activation of the parasympathetic nerves causes a contraction of the detrusor muscle (bladder). The internal sphincter at neck of bladder is normally contracted, but it is relaxed when the bladder muscle contracts. The external sphincter is skeletal muscle under voluntary control, innervated by pudendal nerves. These nerves are tonically active, but activity can be decreased when controlled from higher central nervous system (CNS) centers.

The micturition reflex is initiated when bladder filling increases wall tension above a threshold point. Sensory nerves transmit tension information to the spinal cord, where an increase in parasympathetic activity causes contraction of the detrusor muscle. This contraction further increases wall tension, increasing reflex parasympathetic activity and enhancing the contraction. The process repeats until (1) tension plateaus (for a minute or so), (2) the reflex fatigues, or (3) the external sphincter is relaxed and the bladder empties. If emptying does not occur, the process will begin again after a few minutes.

Urination is facilitated by abdominal contraction, which compresses the bladder and increases wall tension, initiating the reflex. The micturition reflex is modulated by descending inputs from higher CNS structures. The pons has both strong facilitatory and inhibitory centers. The cerebral cortex also can modulate the reflex, allowing voluntary control of the timing of urination.

EFFECTS OF NUTRITION AND AGING
Aging causes shrinking of the kidneys and a progressive loss of renal function. This change is usually not critical because the kidneys have an excess function capacity. Damage or loss of one kidney, however, may allow the age-related changes to impair renal function in the remaining kidney. The increased capillary hydrostatic pressure caused by hypertension or protein ingestion causes progressive damage to glomeruli and accelerates the age related decrease in renal function. Low-protein diets attenuate the age related decrease in renal function and are recommended for clients with damaged kidneys.

The aging process also affects the act of micturition. The bladder becomes funnel shaped as a result of alterations in the connective tissue and weakening of the pelvic floor muscles. Irritability of the bladder wall often increases, adding more urgency to the normal desire to void. Finally, impairment of the detrusor muscle's ability to elongate results in decreased bladder capacity. Because of these changes, older people may have problems with incontinence, frequency, urine retention, or dysuria.

Dietary components can alter renal function at the glomerulus and tubule levels. Ingestion of a protein-rich meal dilates the afferent arteriole, and increases renal blood flow. The increase in glomerular capillary pressure increases GFR. These responses are termed *postprandial renal hyperemia*.

LARGE INTESTINE
COLON (LARGE INTESTINE)
Anatomically, the colon is divided into the cecum and the ascending, transverse, and descending colon. The cecum comprises the first 2 to 3 inches of the large intestine. It connects with the ileum at the ileocecal valve. Relaxation of the cecum allows ileal contents to enter the cecum. The distal end of the cecum forms a blind pouch to which is attached the vermiform appendix. The appendix is located in the lower right quadrant of the abdomen.

The anal canal is about 1 inch long. At the level of the crypts lies the dentate or pectinate line. This important landmark divides the (1) squamous epithelium (below) and columnar epithelium (above) and (2) the somatic nerve supply (below) and autonomic supply (above). The line also marks the division between internal and external hemorrhoids. Lymphatic drainage below the pectinate line goes largely to the inguinal nodes, and lymphatic drainage above this line goes to the pararectal and lateral pelvic (obturator) plexuses.

Colonic Blood Supply and Lymphatic Drainage
The cecum and colon receive their arterial blood supply from branches of the superior and inferior mesenteric arteries. The rectum and anal canal receive arterial blood from the superior, middle, and inferior rectal arteries. The superior and inferior mesenteric veins carry venous blood from the large intestine to the hepatic portal vein and then to the liver.

Neural Regulation
The enteric system regulates motility and secretion along the entire length of the GI tract. The enteric nervous system can function independently of the CNS. Sympathetic nerves that supply the GI tract originate in the celiac, superior mesenteric, inferior mesenteric, and hypogastric ganglia. In general, sympathetics inhibit activity in enteric plexuses, constrict GI system blood vessels, and decrease glandular secretions. GI motility is also decreased through contraction of circular muscle and certain sphincters and indirect inhibition of peristalsis.

The vagus is the primary parasympathetic nerve supplying the GI tract, innervating all structures from the salivary glands to the transverse colon. Nerves from the hypogastric plexus innervate the remainder of colon. Parasympathetic postganglionic neurons are located in intramural plexus. In general, parasympathetics stimulate motor activity, stimulate secretory activity, and stimulate endocrine secretions.

Motility

The colon reabsorbs water and salts as 1500 ml/day enters from the small intestine, and only 50 to 100 ml/day is excreted in feces. Segmental contraction divides colon into numerous haustra. Mass movements occurring three times each day are the most effective propulsion mechanisms. Enteric nerves primarily inhibit smooth-muscle contraction in the colon. Hirschsprung's disease has congenital absence of enteric nerves, and the colon is obstructed by a tonic contraction.

The final segments of the large intestine, the rectum and the anus, extend from the sigmoid colon to the anus. Two sphincter muscles (internal and external) control the opening of the anus. The distal portions of the rectal walls form longitudinal folds, called *rectal* and *anal columns*. These folds terminate about 12 inches from the anus and are connected to one another by transverse folds of tissue called *valves*. Pockets formed by the valves are called *sinuses* or *crypts*. Because the external portion of the anal opening is lined with skin that changes at this point to mucosa, this area is sometimes called the *mucocutaneous border*. The venous drainage and nerve supply also change at this point. Above this line, venous drainage is into the portal system. Below this line, drainage is into the vena cava. The autonomic nervous system supplies innervation above the line, and the somatic nervous system supplies innervation below it.

DEFECATION

The rectum is usually nearly empty. Following mass movement, the rectum fills, the internal sphincter relaxes, and the external sphincter reflexly contracts. This promotes an urge to defecate. The anal canal is normally closed. Voluntary relaxation of external sphincter allows defecation to proceed, facilitated by increased abdominal pressure.

REGULATION OF INTESTINAL ION AND WATER BALANCE

Sympathetic activity enhances water and NaCl absorption, and parasympathetic activity decreases water and NaCl absorption. Aldosterone provides the major hormonal control of absorption, causing Na^+ and water reabsorption colonic and K^+ loss. Enkephalin (opioid peptides) enhances NaCl and water absorption, and somatostatin enhances colonic NaCl and water absorption.

FLORA

The alkaline reaction of the large intestine permits the growth of organisms whose main functions are to putrefy and break down remaining proteins and indigestible residue. These organisms include *Escherichia coli, Enterobacter aerogenes, Clostridium perfringens,* and *Lactobacillus.*

Intestinal bacteria convert urea to ammonium salts and ammonia. Bacterial action in the large bowel causes the formation of gases, which provide bulk and help propel the feces. This action also synthesizes nutritional factors such as vitamin K, thiamine, riboflavin, vitamin B_{12}, folic acid, biotin, and nicotinic acid.

CHANGES WITH AGING

In the large intestine, peristalsis decreases and nerve impulses are dulled. In addition, the muscular tone of the intestinal wall and abdominal muscle strength are reduced. These changes can result in a decreased sensation to defecate and an increased incidence of constipation.

BIBLIOGRAPHY

1. Berne, R., et al. (2004). *Physiology* (5th ed.). St. Louis: Mosby.
2. Guyton, A.C., & Hall, J. (2001). *Textbook of medical physiology* (10th ed.). Philadelphia: W.B. Saunders.
3. Kierszenbaum, A.L. (2002). *Histology and cell biology: An introduction to pathology.* St. Louis, Mosby.
4. Nielsen, S., et al. (2002). Aquaporins in the kidney: From molecules to medicine. *Physiology Review* 82:205-244.
5. Silverthorn, D. (2001). *Human physiology* (2nd ed.). Upper Saddle River, NJ: Prentice-Hall.

Assessment of Elimination

Roberta A. Jorgensen
Karen A. Hanson

---

evolve

Web Enhancements

http://evolve.elsevier.com/Black/medsurg/

Assessment Terms
English and Spanish
Appendix A
Religious Beliefs and Practices Affecting Health Care

Appendix B
A Health History Format That Integrates the Assessment of Functional Health Patterns
Appendix C
Laboratory Values of Clinical Importance in Medical-Surgical Nursing

---

Despite advanced technology for diagnosing problems of elimination, every diagnostic evaluation is guided by an accurate, thorough, and documented assessment. Assessment of elimination is fundamental to the evaluation of the client.

Taking a health history requires exceptional skills in speaking, listening, observing, and interpreting the client's communication because anxiety and embarrassment often accompany the discussion of bowel, urinary, or genital problems. Language and semantic barriers can interfere with communication, especially with the variety of terms used to describe bowel and urinary elimination. Differences in educational background can result in fear and poor communication when the client has difficulty understanding medical terminology. A calm, caring, and accepting atmosphere during the interview promotes communication. The client may wish to have a family member present to assist with describing the details of the problem or health history.

BOWEL ELIMINATION
HISTORY

Assessment of the lower gastrointestinal (GI) system begins with the health history, followed by physical examination of the abdomen, anus, and rectum and diagnostic studies. Review previous hospitalizations, surgery, recent exposure to infection, recent travel, current medications, habits, and family history. Explore family risk factors for lower GI disorders, such as a history of colon cancer. Determine whether the client has regular screening for colon cancer.

Biographical and Demographic Data

A thorough review of biographical and demographic characteristics helps to elicit data related to the disorders that are most likely to occur. Many lower GI disorders are associated with age and gender. For example, colorectal cancer is predominantly a disease of older adults, peaking in the seventh decade, with a higher incidence in males than females.[23] Ulcerative colitis occurs typically between the second and fourth decades of life and more frequently in whites and in those of Jewish descent. Diverticular disease is most common in people who live in developed countries whose diets consist primarily of refined foods. Although the exact incidence of diverticular disease is not known, it is endemic in older populations of developed countries.[19]

Current Health

A simple, open-ended question, such as "How are you feeling?" can elicit concerns about conditions that

---

evolve
Be sure to check out the bonus material on the Evolve website and the CD-ROM, including free self-assessment exercises.
http://evolve.elsevier.com/Black/medsurg/

contribute to the current health problem. Explore potentially relevant areas such as the client's social situations, life events, and difficulties surrounding the health problem. Many lower GI manifestations are vague and have various causes.

Chief Complaint

Allow clients to describe the chief complaint in their own words. Elicit information about and learn to recognize a wide variety of manifestations that are potentially associated with a specific GI disorder. Colon pathology can result in diarrhea, constipation, obstipation, change in the caliber of stools, hematochezia, melena, rectal pain, or tenesmus. Manifestations may be influenced by socioeconomic status and culture. Objective findings, such as ascites and rebound tenderness, may be observed on physical examination. For any lower GI disorder, some manifestations may occur together. With experience, you will learn to recognize these as they relate to a specific GI disorder.

Symptom Analysis

Obtain more specific information about the problem by means of a symptom analysis (see Chapter 4). Include the information in the following sections.

Timing. When was the problem first noticed? How long did it last? Was the onset abrupt or insidious? Where was the client when it occurred? Has the problem been present since that time? Abrupt onset of abdominal pain could indicate emergent conditions such as appendicitis, volvulus, or bowel obstruction. Pain of gradual onset may be related to acute inflammation of the colon or diverticula, severe gastroenteritis, or constipation and gas. Is the problem related to food intake? If diarrhea is present, ask about nighttime manifestations, which may indicate inflammatory bowel disease (IBD) rather than irritable bowel syndrome (IBS).[16]

Quality and Quantity. Ask the client to describe the problem in detail. If the complaint is lower abdominal pain, determine whether it is sharp, dull, aching, burning, intermittent, or spasmodic. If the pain is deep, dull, and diffuse, it is probably visceral in origin, that is, the result of localized inflammation or ischemia. Pain that is sharp and more localized may be parietal or peritoneal pain that might be the result of generalized inflammation. If the client has noticed bloody stools, ask whether bleeding occurs with every bowel movement or only occasionally. Ask whether the blood is mixed in with the stool or present only on the surface.

Location. Assist the client in defining and locating abdominal pain. Does the pain radiate? The location of

pain provides clues to common causes. Right upper quadrant pain may be hepatic in origin, resulting from disorders such as hepatitis, liver abscess, or perihepatitis. Right lower quadrant pain may indicate appendicitis. Left upper quadrant pain may result from splenic rupture, infarct, or abscess. Pain in the left lower quadrant suggests a left colon origin and may indicate diverticulitis or ischemic colitis. Generalized abdominal pain suggests a number of possible causes, such as appendicitis, intestinal obstruction, IBD, or generalized peritonitis.

Precipitating Factors. Can specific events be identified that occur in relation to or before onset of the problem, such as stress, specific foods, medications, or activity? Does the problem occur at a certain time of the day? In cases of suspected gastroenteritis, has the client's source of drinking water changed recently, or has the client eaten unusual foods such as wild mushrooms or improperly handled food?

Aggravating and Relieving Factors. Do certain situations worsen the problem? Do particular medications or actions provide relief? What has the client done to make the situation better? Abdominal pain relieved by defecation is a hallmark of IBS.[16]

Associated Manifestations. Has the client noticed other recent manifestations? Disturbances in lower GI elimination may affect appetite, energy level, and weight. In addition to or in association with the problem, are there other GI manifestations such as nausea, vomiting, early satiety, anorexia, eructation (belching), flatulence, diarrhea, constipation, abdominal distention, heartburn, or indigestion? Does the client have food intolerances, abdominal cramping, weight gain or loss, hematemesis (vomiting of blood), melena (black, tarry stools), rectal pain, or anal pruritus? Other lower GI manifestations related to hepatic, biliary, or pancreatic disorders include jaundice, ascites, fatty stools, and colicky, abdominal pain. (Metabolic system assessment is discussed in Chapter 44.)

Abdominal pain that accompanies diarrhea is frequently associated with infectious gastroenteritis, IBD, diverticulitis, and early intestinal obstruction. Constipation preceding abdominal pain by several days may be associated with diseases of the colon or rectum.

Explore all manifestations because a health problem related to the GI system rarely occurs in the absence of other manifestations or etiologic events. Clients may be aware of other relevant manifestations. Review the client's health status and discuss general health, diet, lifestyle, and health risk factors. It is an opportune time to assess the client's health awareness and implement health promotion teaching. (See Chapters 4 and 30 for discussions of diet history and nutritional assessment and this chapter for assessment of elimination patterns.)

Past Health History

The past health history includes information about the general state of health, past illnesses, immunizations, injuries, hospitalizations, surgeries, current medications, and allergies.

Childhood and Infectious Diseases

Inquire about both childhood and adult diseases. In addition to common childhood infectious diseases, question the client about hepatitis, intestinal infections, encephalitis, sexually transmitted diseases, and human immunodeficiency virus (HIV) infection.

Immunizations

Record the immunization history. Ask whether the client has received routine childhood immunizations including *Haemophilus influenzae* type b (Hib) conjugate. Everyone should be immunized against hepatitis B, particularly people whose lifestyles put them at risk. Inquire about hepatitis A vaccination, which is indicated for international travelers or people employed in day care settings. Ask whether immunizations are current, and note dates of the last tetanus booster and influenza vaccination.

Major Illnesses and Hospitalizations

Note all hospitalizations and major illnesses. Has the client been hospitalized or treated for abdominal pain, anemia, GI bleeding, changes in bowel habits, colitis, unexplained weight loss, or colon cancer? What was the plan of care, and what was found? Ask for a summary of the hospitalization experience, including laboratory tests, diagnostic procedures, and their results. Ask about previous operations, particularly those involving the GI tract or accessory organs.

Try to determine what was found as a result of hospitalization. A discharge summary may be beneficial in treating the current health problem. How has the client been since having an operation performed? If the colon was resected, as for cases of severe chronic ulcerative colitis, the client may be functioning and feeling much improved.

Medications

Note all current medications and how they are taken. Ask about over-the-counter medications, such as vitamins, antacids, laxatives, enemas, pain relievers, herbal remedies, and nutraceuticals (health food supplements). Often clients consider these medications and natural remedies not worth mentioning. Be aware of potential relationships between what is taken and the client's cur-

rent GI manifestations. For example, nonsteroidal anti-inflammatory drugs (NSAIDs) can contribute to epigastric pain, gastric ulcers, and bleeding. Constipation can result from morphine, codeine, atropine, aluminum-containing antacids, calcium supplements, and bile acid binders such as cholestyramine. Medications known to cause diarrhea include antibiotics, lactulose, and magnesium-containing antacids and laxatives. Soluble fiber products such as oat bran, dried beans, and psyllium reduce fat absorption and have a laxative effect.

Herbal medicine is used with increasing frequency for GI disorders.[6] Be aware of potential GI-related adverse effects from herbal medicine. Poke root (*Phytolacca americana*) can cause abdominal pain; senega (*Acaia Senegal*), aloes (*Aloe vera*), senna (*Senna alexandrina*), Shavegrass (*Equisetum arvense*), and yellow dock (*Rumex crispus*) can cause diarrhea; Mormon tea (*Ephedra sinica*) has been associated with constipation.[13] Examples of herbs that can cause liver toxicity include comfrey (*Symphytum officinale*) and chaparral (*Larrea divaricata*).[6] Herbal medicine has been used as treatment for nausea and vomiting, constipation, peptic ulcers, diarrhea, and IBS. Chinese herbal medicine has been found to improve the manifestations of IBS.[1] Other remedies used for IBS but as yet unsubstantiated include St. John's wort (*Hypericum perforatum*) and peppermint oil (*Mentha x piperita*). Ginger (*Zingiber officinale*) is commonly used for nausea; celandine (*Chelidonium majus*), aloe vera, and psyllium (*Plantago psyllium*) have been used for constipation.[13] Numerous herbal remedies, including ginseng (*Panax quinquefolius*), garlic (*Allium sativum*), gingko (*gingko biloba*), Echinacea (*Echinacea angustifolia*), capsaicin (*Capsicum frutescens*), tamarind (*Tamarindus indica*), psyllium, and licorice (*Glycyrrhiza glabra*) can interact with conventional drugs of relevance to gastroenterology.[13]

Allergies

Ask about allergies related to the environment, food, or drugs. Seek specific details to determine the client's allergic response. Be careful to distinguish between foods that are merely difficult to tolerate and those that induce an actual allergic reaction. Ask what types of lower GI problems occur when the client ingests a particular food. Note allergic manifestations such as abdominal cramping, belching, or diarrhea.

Family Health History

A number of GI disorders have a familial association. Inquire whether any family members have been diagnosed with Crohn's disease, chronic ulcerative colitis, intestinal polyps, or colon cancer. Information about family incidence of other GI-related disorders such as jaundice, hepatitis or other liver disease, bleeding ulcers, or IBS is also relevant.

Psychosocial History

The psychosocial history includes information on occupation, current environment, life experiences, personal relationships, and lifestyle habits. Determine the client's knowledge about the manifestations and illness. Has the client lost time from work because of illness? Does the client have insight into the manifestations? Have environmental or psychosocial factors changed recently in the client's situation?

Occupation and Environment

Explore the client's occupational and environmental history to determine whether exposure to disease-provoking substances or environments has occurred. Ask about occupational exposure to substances that may be toxic if ingested or absorbed. If travel is a regular part of the client's job, has there been potential exposure to unusual or improperly handled foods or contaminated water? Does the client have any hobbies that involve possibly hazardous materials? Has there been increased stress in the workplace?

Geographical Location

Has the client recently traveled abroad and been exposed to contaminated food or water? The enteropathogens most commonly responsible for traveler's diarrhea are usually transmitted through fecally contaminated food and water. The most frequent causes are bacterial pathogens, of which enterotoxigenic *Escherichia coli* is the most common, occurring in 30% to 70% of cases.[7] Other causes include viruses and protozoa. Relatively few cases of travelers' diarrhea are caused by *Entamoeba histolytica* or *Giardia lamblia*.[7]

Exercise

Ask whether the client has a regular exercise program and whether physical activity is part of the daily routine. A sedentary lifestyle can be a causative factor in certain types of lower GI disorders, particularly constipation, **EB** and may play a role in IBS.[14]

Nutrition

Thorough assessment of dietary habits is essential when evaluating GI elimination disorders. The diet may be a causative factor, or it may have been altered to help ameliorate the manifestations. GI disorders may cause significant impairment of normal digestive function. In addition, nutritive factors may be related to GI disease, as exemplified by the relationship between a diet high in **EB** animal fat and the development of colorectal cancer.[24]

Fatty or gas-producing foods and foods containing lactose, fructose, or sorbitol tend to exacerbate IBS.[2]

When assessing the diet, ask the client to describe what was eaten the previous day because this is usually easiest to recall. Ask about consumption of high-fiber foods such as fruits and vegetables, whole grains, breads and cereals, red meats, and saturated fats. Are most of the meals eaten at home or at a restaurant, where there is a greater likelihood of high fat and high sodium content? Assess the client's knowledge of what constitutes a healthy diet. Could certain dietary modifications improve the client's nutritional intake?

What fluids are consumed in a day and in what amounts? Ask about water, coffee, cola, and alcohol intake in a 24-hour period. Many GI manifestations attributed to IBS may be related to excess alcohol and caffeine intake.

Assess the relationships between dietary intake and resultant GI manifestations. Excessive ingestion of synthetic, nonabsorbable sugars such as sorbitol may cause diarrhea. Lactose intolerance occurs when the intestine does not produce enough lactase to digest lactose (milk sugar), resulting in abdominal bloating and cramping. Other causes include bile acid malabsorption, pancreatic or biliary disease, and fluids or medications with high osmolality. Chapter 30 discusses nutritional assessment.

Habits

Certain lifestyle habits may contribute to GI manifestations. Lack of a regular bowel elimination routine in the daily schedule can lead to chronic constipation. Excessive alcohol consumption, if not curtailed, can lead to gastritis and eventual hepatic damage.

Inquire whether the client is experiencing increased stress either at home or at work. Altered stress levels can bring about GI-related manifestations such as epigastric pain, ulcers, and diarrhea.

Review of Systems

Review possible GI manifestations, and check each system to uncover additional manifestations of "unrelated" illness. Does the client have problems chewing or swallowing food? Ask about the condition of the teeth or whether dentures (if worn) fit properly. Are there sores in the mouth or on the tongue, or has there been difficulty with mouth dryness and odor?

Determine whether there has been a change in appetite, either excessive hunger or anorexia, and whether the client is having problems with indigestion such as excessive belching or heartburn. Has the client experienced abdominal pain, nausea, or vomiting? If vomiting has occurred, what was the character of the vomitus? Has there been a change in bowel movements, such as change in color, consistency, or caliber? Has there been rectal bleeding or black, tarry stools? Does the client experience rectal pain or pruritus? Determine whether there have been manifestations related to the accessory organs of digestion, such as the development of jaundice, ascites, peripheral edema, generalized intractable pruritus, clay-colored stools, or dark urine.

PHYSICAL EXAMINATION

Physical examination of the lower GI tract includes the abdomen, anus, and rectum. Discussions of upper GI tract, liver, pancreas, and spleen assessment appear in Chapters 30 and 44. An example of an abdominal assessment recording is given in Chapter 30.

Abdomen

Lower GI tract assessment begins with the abdomen. The abdomen is divided into either four quadrants or nine regions for descriptive purposes. Be familiar with the abdominal structures located in each of these areas (see Chapter 30).

The equipment for the examination of the abdomen and rectum includes a stethoscope, gloves, lubricant, tissues, materials for occult blood testing, and reagent. The client should be supine, with the abdomen fully exposed from the sternum to the knees (see Chapter 4). Place a sheet or towel over the genitalia. The arms should be at the sides and the legs extended. A pillow under the knees aids in relaxing the abdominal muscles. Stand at the client's right side. If the current problem is one of abdominal pain, examine the area of pain last to avoid stimulating tightening of the abdominal muscles (guarding). Proceed as follows: inspection, auscultation, percussion, palpation, and rectal examination.

Inspection

Inspect the abdominal contour and note whether it is flat, rounded, protuberant, or scaphoid. Look for evidence of distention, masses, asymmetry, or visible peristaltic waves, which are abnormal and should be reported. Note scars, striae, petechiae, and the presence of dilated veins. Note the shape, position, and color of the umbilicus. A protruding umbilicus may indicate ascites, mass, or an umbilical hernia.

Assess for inguinal, umbilical, and femoral hernias by asking the client to cough. A sudden bulge may indicate a hernia. Coughing may also elicit localized pain. Lastly, ask the client to perform the Valsalva maneuver (if not contraindicated) or attempt a stomach curl. Look for a separation of the rectus muscles at the midline *(diastasis recti)*, which may be accompanied by a bulge. This condition results from obesity, pregnancy, or problems in which sustained elevated intra-abdominal pressure weakens the muscles.

Auscultation

Auscultation of bowel sounds provides information about the motion of liquid and air through the intestinal tract. It is useful in assessing bowel motility and abdominal complaints. Perform auscultation before percussion and palpation. Palpation and percussion may affect intestinal motility and therefore may alter bowel sounds.

While the client is supine, place the diaphragm of the stethoscope gently over the mid-abdomen. Normal bowel sounds are high pitched and heard every 5 to 10 seconds. If no sounds are heard after listening for at least 2 minutes, bowel sounds are considered absent. Listening in one area of the abdomen, such as the lower right quadrant, is usually sufficient because bowel sounds are widely transmitted. The absence of bowel sounds suggests a paralytic ileus that may be related to diffuse peritoneal irritation. Rushes of rapid, high-pitched bowel sounds, or *borborygmi,* are associated with hyperperistalsis and may be present in gastroenteritis or early intestinal obstruction.

Auscultation helps to determine whether an abdominal bruit is present. Place the diaphragm of the stethoscope in the midline of the abdomen 2 inches above the umbilicus, and listen carefully for an aortic bruit. Next listen at a point 2 inches above the umbilicus and 1 to 2 inches laterally on both sides of midline for a renal bruit. A renal bruit may indicate renal artery stenosis. Bruit is discussed further in Chapter 53.

A *peritoneal friction rub,* like a pleural or pericardial rub, indicates inflammation. During respiration, a friction rub may be heard in the right or left upper quadrant, suggesting hepatic or splenic pathology. A rub is described further in Chapter 4.

Percussion

Percussion is used to detect the presence of fluid, gaseous distention, or solid masses and to determine the location and size of abdominal organs, primarily the liver and spleen. At times, it may be preferable to palpate before percussion, especially if the client is complaining of abdominal pain.

The client should be supine. Percuss the abdomen lightly in all four quadrants. The most common percussion note heard in the abdomen is *tympany* (high pitched, loud, or musical), which is due to the presence of gas in the stomach, small bowel, and colon. The presence of feces and fluid can cause areas of dullness. Observe any areas of dullness that might indicate mass or an enlarged organ such as a distended bladder, ovarian tumor, or enlarged liver or spleen. This observation will guide the palpation. If the bladder is full, the suprapubic area may sound *dull* (thud-like sounds over fluid or solid organs) when percussed (see the discussion of bladder percussion later in this chapter). Percussion of the liver and spleen is discussed in Chapter 44.

If ascites is suspected, a special percussion test for *shifting dullness* may be performed by nurses who have advanced assessment skills. Ascitic fluid sinks to the lower abdomen as a result of gravity (when standing), shifts to the side of the abdomen (when lying on one's side), and bulges in the flanks (when supine). While the client is supine, the borders between the areas of tympany and dullness are percussed. The area of tympany is due to gas in the bowel present above the ascites and is located above the area of dullness. The client is then asked to turn on the side, and the nurse again percusses the abdomen. If ascites is present, the area around the umbilicus that was initially tympanic becomes dull because the ascites has shifted to the more dependent position (see Figure 44-3). Ascites may also be detected by determining the presence of a *fluid wave*. This advanced assessment technique is discussed in Chapter 44 and is seen in Figure 44-3.

Palpation

Abdominal palpation usually proceeds from light to deep and then to the liver, spleen, and kidneys. The client is supine, and the examination begins with the area of the abdomen that is farthest from the area of pain, if pain is present.

Light palpation is used to detect masses, areas of muscular spasm or rigidity, and areas of direct tenderness. Deep palpation is used to determine the size and shape of abdominal organs and masses. Palpable findings are correlated with those found on percussion. Deep palpation

is used primarily by nurses in advanced practice areas. Palpation techniques are discussed in detail in Chapter 4.

Identify areas of tenderness or increased resistance. If resistance is present, distinguish voluntary guarding from involuntary muscle spasm by feeling for the relaxation of abdominal muscles on exhalation or by asking the client to breathe through the mouth. If these maneuvers do not decrease voluntary guarding or rigidity, peritoneal inflammation may be present.

Perform a test for *rebound tenderness* if the client has abdominal pain. Palpate slowly and deeply away from the area of suspected inflammation, and then quickly withdraw the palpating hand. The feeling of pain on the side of the inflammation that occurs when the palpating hand is withdrawn is *called rebound tenderness*. Because this maneuver may induce generalized pain, perform the test at the end of the abdominal examination.

Palpation of the liver and spleen is discussed in Chapter 44, and palpation of the kidneys is discussed later in this chapter.

Anus and Rectum

The abdominal examination concludes with examination of the anus and rectum. Maintain a calm, matter-of-fact approach because it is often embarrassing for the client.

Most nurses perform only a visual inspection of the perianal area, but advanced practice nurses can perform a complete digital examination of the rectum. Be familiar with rectal anatomy and expected physical findings. This information is necessary during digital assessment for rectal impaction or administering rectal medications (Figure 34-1).

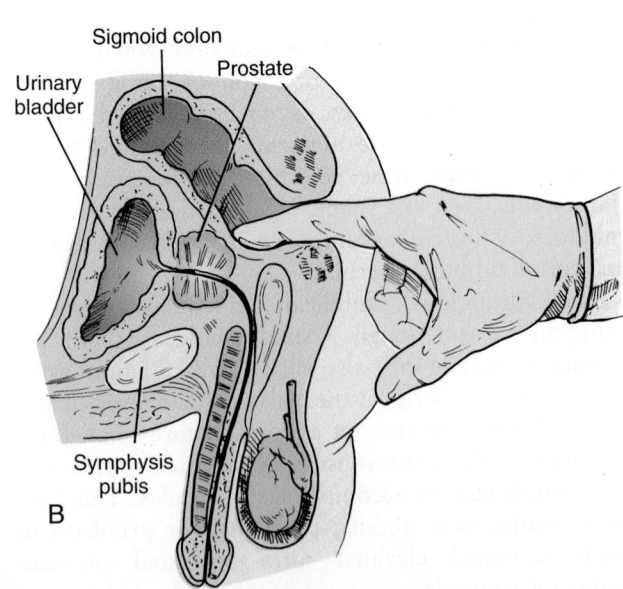

FIGURE 34-1 Palpation of the rectum in female clients (**A**) and in male (**B**) clients.

Inspection

Perform the rectal examination with female clients in the lithotomy position immediately after the pelvic examination. Sims' or dorsal recumbent are positions that can be used as alternatives (see Chapter 4). Male clients may be examined either in the Sims' position or while standing and leaning across the examination table, which makes examination of the prostate gland easier. Spread the buttocks apart with the gloved, nondominant hand, and examine the anus and surrounding tissue.

Inspect perianal skin for manifestations of inflammation, rashes, nodules, ulceration, fissures (cracks), fistulous openings, and hemorrhoids (dilated veins seen as reddened skin protrusions). Normally, the anus looks moist and hairless with coarse, folded skin that is more darkly pigmented than the perianal skin. The anal opening should be tightly closed. No lesions should be present. Inspect the sacrococcygeal area, which is normally smooth and even. Ask the client to strain while you look for evidence of rectal prolapse (protrusion of rectal mucosa through the anal opening), internal hemorrhoids, polyps, or fissures. There should be no break in the skin integrity or protrusion through the anal opening.

Palpation

Inform the client that a rectal examination will be performed. Tell the client that there will be the sensation of a cool lubricant and a feeling as if having a bowel movement.

Use the gloved nondominant hand to spread the buttocks apart, and place the lubricated index finger of the dominant hand on the anus. Apply gentle pressure over the anus, thereby relaxing the sphincter. Instruct the client to take a deep breath as the index finger is inserted into the anal canal. The anal sphincter should close completely around the examining finger, at which time sphincter tone may be assessed. Advance the examining finger approximately 6 to 10 cm (2 to 4 inches) into the rectum in the direction of the umbilicus. The rectal mucosa should feel smooth and should be nontender. Note irregularities such as polyps, masses, or undue tenderness, and describe their location and characteristics. Once the index finger is fully inserted, instruct the client to bear down again and feel for a mass descending from above against the palpating finger. No mass should be present.

In a female client, the cervix of the uterus may be felt through the rectovaginal wall along the anterior rectum (see Chapter 39). The rectovaginal wall is firm, smooth, and resilient. In a male client, the prostate gland may be palpated through the anterior rectal wall. This part of the examination is discussed in Chapter 39.

Note the color of the fecal material present on the glove when you withdraw your finger. Mucus, blood, or tan, gray, or black tarry stool is abnormal. Test the fecal material for occult blood (described later in this chapter). If a sexually transmitted disease is suspected, obtain a rectal culture (see the discussion later in this chapter). Wipe the perianal area clean, and inform the client that the examination is completed.

DIAGNOSTIC TESTS

Diagnostic tests are performed to determine the nature of the lower GI disorder. The general methods of diagnosis include laboratory tests (Table 34-1), radiographic studies, ultrasonography, and endoscopy. Hematologic studies and electrolyte determinations offer additional information; however, these reflect primarily general health status.

Laboratory Tests

Carcinoembryonic Antigen

Carcinoembryonic antigen (CEA) is a glycoprotein secreted on the glycocalyx surface of cells lining the GI tract and is normally produced during the first or second trimester of fetal life. High CEA levels are characteristic of various malignant conditions such as cancer of the colon, lung, or breast and of certain nonmalignant conditions such as liver disease, cirrhosis, alcoholic pancreatitis, heavy smoking, and IBD.

Although CEA levels cannot be used as a general indicator of cancer, they are useful for preoperative staging of colorectal cancer and assessing the adequacy of surgical resection. Often called a tumor marker, CEA is used to monitor the effectiveness of colorectal cancer therapy. Serum levels usually return to normal within 6 weeks if cancer treatment is successful.

Perform venipuncture and collect the sample in a 7-ml red-topped tube. Handle the sample gently to prevent hemolysis, which may alter test results. There is no postprocedure care.

Fecal Analysis

Fecal analysis aids in the evaluation of digestive efficiency and the integrity of the stomach and intestines. Analysis begins with gross examination of stool color, consistency, odor, and other characteristics and concludes with microscopic, chemical, or bacterial analysis.

If the colon is partially obstructed or loses its elasticity, stool in transit may cause bleeding. Blood in the stool also may result from hemorrhoids. A black, tarry stool can result from upper GI bleeding. A large, bulky, foul-smelling stool that floats in the toilet may indicate fat malabsorption. Diarrhea is a result of too rapid transit of food in the GI tract, often caused by a viral infection. Mucus or pus in the stool may be a result of rectal abscesses or ulcerative colitis. A stool specimen is often required for diagnosis of infectious diseases, GI bleeding, and other GI tract disorders. Because stool specimens

TABLE 34-1	*Laboratory Tests Used to Assess Lower Gastrointestinal (GI) Function*	
Test	**Normal Findings**	**Abnormal Findings**
Complete Blood Count		
Red blood cells	4.2-5.4 million/mm^3 (women)	Decreased values may indicate anemia or hemorrhage
	4.5-6.2 million/mm^3 (men)	Increased values indicate possible hemoconcentration, caused by dehydration
Hemoglobin	12-16 g/dl (women)	
	14-18 g/dl (men)	
Hematocrit	38%-46% (women)	
	42%-54% (men)	
Electrolytes		
Potassium	3.5-5.0 mEq/L	Decreased values indicate possible GI suction, diarrhea, vomiting, intestinal fistulas
Calcium	8.0-10.5 mg/dl	Decreased values indicate possible malabsorption
Sodium	135-145 mEq/L	Decreased values indicate possible malabsorption and diarrhea
CEA	<5 ng/ml (nonsmokers)	Increased values indicate possible colorectal cancer and inflammatory bowel disease
Fecal Analysis		
Stool for occult blood	Negative	Presence indicates possible peptic ulcer, cancer of the colon, ulcerative colitis
Stool for ova and parasites	Negative	Presence of *Entamoeba histolytica* (amebiases) or *Giardia lamblia*
Stool cultures	No unusual growth	Presence of *Salmonella typhi* (typhoid fever), *Shigella* (dysentery) *Escherichia coli* (gastroenteritis), *Staphylococcus aureus* (food poisoning), *Clostridium botulinum* (food poisoning), or *Aeromonas*
Stool for lipids	2-6 g/24 hr (normal diet)	Steatorrhea (increased values) can result from intestinal malabsorption or pancreatic insufficiency

cannot be obtained on demand, close cooperation is necessary to secure a suitable specimen.

Fecal Occult Blood Tests

A fecal occult blood test is the most frequently performed screening test for colorectal cancer in the United States and is the only test demonstrated through randomized, controlled trials to reduce risk of death from colorectal cancer.[17] The Hemoccult II test is the most widely used fecal occult blood test.[18] It is based on the change in the color of a guaiac-based colorless dye to blue caused by the peroxidase activity of hemoglobin. If any of the tests for fecal occult blood is positive, an evaluation of the whole colon is usually recommended. Annual fecal occult blood testing is recommended for persons of average risk 50 years of age or older by the American Cancer Society.[20]

The fecal occult blood test can be performed immediately after the rectal examination or on stool specimens collected over 3 days. Two samples from each of the consecutive stools are tested to avoid false-positives. A wooden applicator is used to apply stool to one side of guaiac-treated paper. Developing solution is applied, and

the result is immediately noted. Blue indicates a positive reaction and should be reported.

The client should abstain from rare meat and peroxidase-rich foods such as raw fruits and vegetables for 3 days before the test. Aspirin and NSAIDs, which may increase GI bleeding, should be withheld, although clients with painful arthritis may find this difficult. There is no postprocedure care.

Stool Examination for Ova and Parasites

Examination of a stool specimen can detect intestinal infection caused by several types of parasites and their ova (eggs). Wear gloves and collect the stool specimen directly in the container. Note the date and time of the collection, the consistency of the specimen, pertinent dietary history, and recent or current antimicrobial therapy. Send the specimen to the laboratory within 30 minutes of passage or refrigerate it if it will not be examined immediately.

Instruct the client to avoid treatments with castor oil or mineral oil, bismuth, magnesium or antidiarrheal compounds, barium enemas, and antibiotics for 7 to 10 days before the test. Three specimens should be tested by collection of a stool every other day or every third day. There is no postprocedure care.

Stool Cultures

Bacteriologic examination of the stool identifies pathogens that may cause overt GI disease. Identifying these organisms is necessary to treat the client and thereby prevent potentially serious complications. A sensitivity test may follow isolation of the pathogen. Some viruses may also cause GI manifestations but can be detected only by immunoassay or electron microscopy.

A stool specimen is collected on 3 consecutive days. Wear gloves and collect the specimen directly in the container. Stool may also be collected by means of a rectal swab inserted past the anal sphincter, rotated gently, and withdrawn. Place the swab in the appropriate container, and send it immediately to the laboratory. Note the dietary history, recent antimicrobial therapy, and any recent travel that might indicate endemic infection or infestation. There is no postprocedure care.

Fecal Lipids

Dietary lipids, emulsified by bile, are almost completely absorbed in the small intestine, provided biliary and pancreatic secretions are adequate; however, both digestive and absorptive disorders may cause *steatorrhea* (excessive secretions of fecal lipids). A quantitative test performed on stool collected over a 72-hour period confirms the presence of steatorrhea. Collect the stool in a non-wax container and keep it refrigerated.

Instruct the client to abstain from alcohol and to consume a high-fat diet (100 g daily) for 3 days before the test and during the collection period. Drugs that may affect test results, such as mineral oil, potassium chloride, and neomycin, should be withheld. There is no postprocedure care.

Radiography

Flat Plate of the Abdomen

A flat plate of the abdomen is an x-ray film of the abdominal organs. It is used to help identify tumors, obstructions, abnormal gas collections, and strictures.

Lower Gastrointestinal Series (Barium Enema)

Procedure

A barium enema is administered for the radiographic examination (with or without fluoroscopy) of the large intestine. Barium sulfate (single-contrast technique) or barium sulfate and air (double-contrast technique) are instilled rectally. The test is indicated for clients with a history of altered bowel habits; lower abdominal pain; or passage of blood, mucus, or pus in the stools. The test helps to detect tumors, diverticula, stenoses, obstructions, inflammation, ulcerative colitis, and polyps.

Preprocedure Care

Adequate preparation is essential and varies among agencies. Typical preparation includes a low-residue or clear liquid diet for 2 days before the test to reduce feces volume. The client usually receives a potent laxative and an oral liquid preparation for cleaning the bowel the day before the test and has nothing by mouth (*nil per os,* NPO) after midnight. The morning of the examination, a suppository or cleansing enema may be administered. If the client has active bleeding or an ileostomy, different bowel preparations may be needed. If ultrasonography, abdominal scan, or colonoscopy is also indicated, it should be performed first because barium interferes with these tests. The procedure is uncomfortable and takes 60 to 90 minutes.

Postprocedure Care

Barium impaction is a serious complication after a lower GI series if the barium is not evacuated. A laxative or cleansing enema is often given after the test to empty the large bowel. Stools are white for 24 to 72 hours after the examination. Encourage the client to increase liquid intake to prevent fecal impaction. Instruct the client to report any pain, bloating, absence of stool, or bleeding.

Computed Tomography

Computed tomography (CT) is a complementary test in assessing acute diverticulitis and abscess formation, diagnosing colorectal cancer, and staging rectal tumors. CT is a useful alternative to barium enema for clients who are unable to retain barium. CT is used primarily to identify masses such as neoplasms, cysts, focal inflammatory lesions, and abscesses of the liver, pancreas, and pelvic areas (see Chapter 4).

Ultrasonography

Ultrasonography is used to identify pathophysiologic processes in the pancreas, liver, gallbladder, spleen, and retroperitoneal tissues. Gas in the abdomen can interfere with the ultrasound waves (see Chapter 4).

Endoscopy

Endoscopy is the direct visualization of the GI system by means of a lighted, flexible tube. The physician can directly observe sources of bleeding and surface lesions and determine the status of healing tissues.

Proctosigmoidoscopy

Procedure

Proctosigmoidoscopy is the endoscopic examination of the lining of the distal sigmoid colon, the rectum, and the anal canal using two instruments: a proctoscope and a sigmoidoscope. Indications include a recent change in bowel habits, lower abdominal and perineal pain, prolapse on defecation, anal pruritus, and passage of mucus, blood, or pus in the stool. Sigmoidoscopy is not as thorough as colonoscopy because only half of the colon is visualized; however it is considered safer. If performed for cancer screening, it should be performed every 5 years in people at average risk at least 50 years of age.[20] The procedure involves three steps: a digital examination, sigmoidoscopy, and proctoscopy.

During digital examination, the anal sphincters are dilated to detect any obstruction that might hinder the passage of the endoscope. During sigmoidoscopy, a 25- to 30-cm (10- to 12-inch) rigid sigmoidoscope is inserted into the anus to allow visualization of the distal sigmoid colon and rectum. The flexible sigmoidoscope also permits visualization of the descending colon. During proctoscopy, a 7-cm (2-inch) rigid proctoscope is inserted into the anus to aid examination of the lower rectum and anal canal. Specimens may be obtained by biopsy, lavage, cytology brush, or culture swab at any point during the procedure from the mucosal areas under suspicion.

Preprocedure Care

Explain to the client that proctosigmoidoscopy allows visual examination of the lining of the distal sigmoid colon, the rectum, and the anal canal. Describe the preparation for the procedure and the position assumed (knee-chest or left lateral). Also explain that colicky, abdominal pain may result from passage of the instrument and introduction of air into the intestines. Reassure the client that there will be adequate draping to avoid embarrassment during the procedure. Obtain consent.

Agencies may specify various dietary and bowel preparations for this procedure. Clients are usually required to maintain a clear liquid diet for 24 to 48 hours before the test and to fast on the morning of the procedure. If a special bowel preparation is ordered, explain that this clears the intestine to provide a better view. A warm tap water or Fleet enema may be administered as ordered on the morning before the procedure.

Postprocedure Care

Observe closely for manifestations of bowel perforation (malaise, rectal bleeding, abdominal distention and pain, mucopurulent drainage, and fever) and for vasovagal attack related to emotional stress (depressed blood pressure, pallor, diaphoresis, and bradycardia). If the knee-chest position was used, instruct the client to rest supine for several minutes before standing to avoid postural hypotension. As ordered, the client is NPO and vital signs are monitored every 30 minutes until alert.

Colonoscopy

Procedure

Colonoscopy is the visual examination of the lining of the entire colon with a flexible fiberoptic endoscope. The procedure is indicated for clients with a history of constipation and diarrhea, persistent rectal bleeding, or lower abdominal pain when results of proctosigmoidoscopy and a barium enema are negative or inconclusive. Colonoscopy is also used to screen clients at high risk for colon cancer. Colonoscopy every 10 years is recommended for persons 50 years of age or older at average risk for colorectal cancer.[20]

Preprocedure Care

The client is sedated and placed on the left side. After the colonoscope is inserted through the anus, a small amount of air is insufflated to locate the bowel lumen. The scope is advanced through the rectum into the sigmoid colon under direct visualization. When the instrument reaches the descending sigmoid junction, the client may be assisted to the supine position to aid the scope's advance past the splenic flexure. After the scope has passed the splenic flexure, it is advanced through the transverse colon and past the hepatic flexure into the ascending colon and cecum. Abdominal palpation or fluoroscopy may help to guide the colonoscope through the large intestine.

Postprocedure Care

Observe the client closely for manifestations of bowel perforation (malaise, rectal bleeding, abdominal pain and distention, fever, and mucopurulent drainage). Monitor vital signs as ordered until they are stable.

■ URINARY ELIMINATION HISTORY

Urologic assessment includes the assessment of elimination as well as sexual and reproductive function. This chapter describes urologic assessment, and Chapter 39 describes reproductive assessment.

Biographical and Demographic Data

Biographical and demographic data, such as age, gender, marital status, race, occupation, and geographical location, provide the framework for the health history. Gather specific information regarding sexual preference or practices to assess the client's risk of venereal disease or HIV infection. Certain diseases and health states are more common in specific groups of people. For example, urinary incontinence affects approximately 13 million Americans, with the highest prevalence in the older population. It is more common in women than in men (10% to 30% versus 1.5% to 5%) and often affects older multiparous women (those who have had multiple pregnancies) in the form of stress incontinence.

Benign prostate hyperplasia (BPH) often occurs in men older than 40 years. BPH is usually the cause of irritative and obstructive voiding manifestations in older adult men. Prostatitis can mimic some of the manifestations of BPH but is more likely to be the diagnosis if the client is younger than 40 years of age.

Prostate cancer is the leading cancer diagnosis in the United States. Sixty percent of newly diagnosed and 80% of deaths from prostate cancer occur in men older than 70 years.[15] Risks include age, black race living in the United States, and family history. Testicular cancers most often occur in young men between ages 25 and 35. Bladder cancer occurs more often in men than women and in white than black or Hispanic males. The incidence rates are highest in industrialized countries and rise dramatically with age. Risk factors include cigarette smoking and exposure to arylamines.[15]

Current Health

Clients with urologic complaints may find it embarrassing to discuss their problems. Establish a private and relaxed atmosphere when obtaining the history. Continually assess verbal and nonverbal feedback, evaluate objectively, and provide information using language and diagrams that the client understands.

Chief Complaint

On identifying the chief complaint, ask specific questions about common urologic manifestations. Clients who have a urologic chief complaint describe problems in the categories of disturbances of voiding, alterations in urine characteristics, pain or referred pain, and systemic or GI manifestations. More than one manifestation may be present. Explore each one.

Symptom Analysis

Disturbances in Urination. Disturbances in urination include changes in urinary volume, irritative or obstructive manifestations, and urinary incontinence. Normal adult bladder capacity is about 300 to 500 ml. Adults normally void five or six times per 24 hours, more during the day than at night. Total daily urine output ranges between 800 and 1800 ml. This amount varies with changes in the amount and type of fluid intake, amount of perspiration, environmental or ambient temperature, and the presence of vomiting or diarrhea. It may also be affected by pathologic changes in the urinary system.

Changes in Urinary Volume. *Anuria* refers to a total urine output of less than 100 ml/24 hr, and *oliguria* refers to a total urine output of 100 to 400 ml/24 hr. Older clients may experience oliguria with up to 600 ml urine in 24 hours. Anuria and oliguria are associated with acute or chronic renal failure secondary to systemic events (shock, dehydration, reduced cardiac output), renal injury (glomerulonephritis, acute interstitial nephritis, renal artery aneurysms or emboli), or postrenal obstruction (ureteral, bladder outlet, or urethral). *Polyuria* (voiding in unusually large daily amounts) may be associated with systemic disease (diabetes mellitus or diabetes insipidus, adrenal insufficiency), diuretic medication, or chronic renal disease resulting in electrolyte imbalance.

Review the client's health history to determine any known precipitating medical causes of urine volume changes. Inquire about the onset and duration of the urinary volume change to establish whether it is acute or chronic or reflects an acute exacerbation of a chronic disease. Assess fluid intake, noting the amount and timing of consumption, especially of caffeinated and alcoholic beverages.

Irritative and Obstructive Manifestations. Irritative voiding manifestations of urgency, frequency, nocturia, and dysuria can occur with infection, inflammation, calculus, cancer, obstruction, or neurogenic dysfunction of the lower urinary tract (bladder, prostate, and urethra). Urgency and frequency often are present in combination.

Urinary frequency, voiding more often than every 2 hours, is common. It can occur because of changes in urine volume, decreased bladder capacity (such as with prostatic enlargement or detrusor instability), increased postvoid residual urine, inflammatory irritability of the bladder mucosa, and psychological disorders.

Urgency is a sudden strong desire to void that can usually be controlled. Urgency is caused by irritation of the lower urinary tract secondary to inflammation, calculus, bladder cancer, or neurogenic dysfunction.

Nocturia is excessive urination during the night (awakening with the need to urinate more than twice nightly). Nocturia may be related to the same urinary conditions listed for urinary frequency. It may also occur in clients who have circulatory problems that result in dependent edema during the day. The recumbent position helps to mobilize the sequestered fluids, resulting in increased venous return to the circulatory system and subsequent increased renal perfusion.

Dysuria, described as a burning sensation on initiation of, during, or at the end of urination, is usually

	Not at all	Less than 1 time in 5	Less than half the time	About half of the time	More than half the time	Almost always	Your score
Incomplete emptying Over the past month, how often have you had a sensation of not emptying your bladder completely after you finish urinating?	0	1	2	3	4	5	
Frequency Over the past month, how often have you had to urinate again less than two hours after you finished urinating?	0	1	2	3	4	5	
Intermittency Over the past month, how often have you found you stopped and started again several times when you urinated?	0	1	2	3	4	5	
Urgency Over the last month, how difficult have you found it to postpone urination?	0	1	2	3	4	5	
Weak stream Over the past month, how often have you had a weak urinary stream?	0	1	2	3	4	5	
Straining Over the past month, how often have you had to push or strain to begin urination?	0	1	2	3	4	5	

	None	1 time	2 times	3 times	4 times	5 times or more	Your score
Nocturia Over the past month, how many times did you most typically get up to urinate from the time you went to bed until the time you got up in the morning?	0	1	2	3	4	5	
Total IPSS score							

	Delighted	Pleased	Mostly satisfied	Mixed—about equally satisfied and dissatisfied	Mostly dissatisfied	Unhappy	Terrible
Quality of life due to urinary symptoms							
If you were to spend the rest of your life with your urinary condition the way it is now, how would you feel about that?	0	1	2	3	4	5	6

Total score: 0-7 Mildly symptomatic; 8-19 moderately symptomatic; 20-35 severely symptomatic.

FIGURE 34-2 International Prostate Symptom Score (IPSS) for assessment of the effects of benign prostate hyperplasia. (From Cockett, A.T.K., et al. [1994] The Second International Consultation on Benign Prostatic Hyperplasia [BPH]. In Cockett, A.T.K., et al. [Eds.]. The Second International Consultation on Benign Prostatic Hyperplasia [BPH]. Paris, Scientific Communication International.)

associated with infection, inflammation, or, rarely, cancer of the bladder or urethra. It is usually accompanied by urgency and frequency.

Irritative manifestations may be accompanied by obstructive manifestations such as hesitancy, straining to begin urination, intermittency, decreased force and caliber of the urinary stream, high postvoid residual, and urine retention. The cause is usually bladder outlet obstruction secondary to prostatic enlargement (in men), congenital urethral valves, urethral meatal stenosis, or urethral stricture. Baseline manifestations of bladder outlet obstruction in men can be assessed with the standardized International Prostate Symptom Score (IPSS), which is similar to the American Urologic Association (AUA) symptom index (Figure 34-2) but also contains an additional question about quality of life. Neurologic diseases may affect the striated or smooth muscles of the bladder and external sphincter and impair the bladder's ability to contract effectively.

Hesitancy refers to at least a 10-second delay in the initiation of urination. It is not associated with "bashful bladder," which can occur when urinating in a public restroom. It often leads to straining or pushing, which voluntarily increases intra-abdominal pressure to start the urinary stream. With prostatic obstruction or urethral stricture, straining is rarely helpful in initiating the stream.

When the client presents with obstructive manifestations, ask for a description of the urinary stream. Note whether (1) there is decreased force and caliber, (2) the stream is intermittent or interrupted (bladder stones or impaired bladder contractility), and (3) the stream is bifurcated or spraying (commonly seen with urethral stricture or meatal stenosis).

Clients who have significant amounts of *postvoid residual* urine or *urinary retention*, usually greater than 100 ml, may describe a sense of incomplete bladder emptying. This is noted either as bladder fullness after urinating or more commonly as "double voiding," a second urination necessary within 5 to 15 minutes after the initial void. Long-standing high-residual urine volumes, sometimes more than 1000 ml, is considered *chronic urinary retention*. Clients experience little or no pain but may demonstrate other obstructive manifestations. Continual overflow incontinence is common because the bladder remains full to capacity at all times.

Acute urinary retention is a sudden inability to void, accompanied by severe suprapubic pain (which distinguishes it from anuria) and urgency. It may occur postoperatively or postpartum (after delivery), with use of certain medications, or with worsening of bladder outlet obstruction. It is a medical emergency requiring immediate intervention (urethral or suprapubic catheterization).

Urinary Incontinence. *Urinary incontinence* refers to involuntary loss of urine. The social stigma and embarrassment of urinary incontinence result in loss of self-esteem and decreased ability to maintain an independent lifestyle. Decreased social interactions and decreased sexual activity are commonly reported. Considering the impact on one's quality of life, thoroughly investigate any mention of urinary incontinence by the client.

Urinary incontinence can be divided into several types: urge, reflex, stress, mixed, overflow, and functional.

Urge urinary incontinence is the involuntary loss of urine associated with a strong desire to void. It is present with detrusor instability (DI) and normal bladder sensation.

Urge urinary incontinence resulting from DI that is present without normal bladder sensation is considered *reflex urinary incontinence.* Diseases of the spinal cord above the sacral micturition center (S_{2-4}) produce reflex incontinence. DI with a neurologic cause is commonly referred to as *detrusor hyperreflexia.* It may also be accompanied by poor detrusor contractility and thus may contribute to difficulty emptying the bladder completely. Ask, "Are you able to feel when your bladder is full?" "Are you aware of urinary leakage when it happens?" "Do you still feel fullness in the bladder after you urinate?"

Stress urinary incontinence is the leakage of urine with physical exertion or with an increase in intra-abdominal pressure but without actual detrusor contraction. Stress incontinence in women is most often due to urethral hypermobility associated with the pelvic descent that occurs after childbearing. In both genders, it may be due to intrinsic urethral sphincter deficiency (ISD), congenital or acquired, in which the sphincter cannot create enough resistance to retain urine. Ask when the urine loss occurs. Is it with coughing, sneezing, laughing, or other physical activity?

A combination of stress and urge incontinence, or *mixed urinary incontinence,* typically occurs in older women. Urge urinary incontinence is more distressing for the client, probably because there is less control in social situations.

Overflow urinary incontinence is associated with chronic overdistention of the bladder secondary to impaired bladder contractility or bladder outlet obstruction. Clients present with frequent or constant dribbling or may have stress or urge urinary incontinence.

Functional urinary incontinence is associated with cognitive or physical impairments outside the lower urinary tract and is often seen in nursing home clients. It can often be remedied, even when it coexists with other types of incontinence, by changes in medications, improvements in hydration status, and removal of environmental barriers to toileting.

A careful interview and health history are instrumental to differentiate the types of incontinence so that the appropriate diagnostic evaluation can be performed.

Alterations in Urine Characteristics. When evaluating urine characteristics, ask the client to describe (1) the color, (2) the clarity, and (3) the odor of the urine.

Normal urine color is pale yellow to amber. Urine *color* is affected by blood, changes in hydration status, certain diseases, and ingestion of certain foods or medications (Table 34-2). Color can be clinically significant, especially if the client reports even a single episode of "bloody urine" *(hematuria),* which can be pink, red, tea colored, dark brown, or maroon, and may or may not be accompanied by blood clots. Gross hematuria is often the only presenting manifestation of bladder cancer. Further define the hematuria by asking at which point during voiding it occurs. *Initial* hematuria indicates a urethral, prostatic, or seminal vesicle origin. *Terminal* hematuria indicates bleeding from the bladder neck, trigone, or posterior urethra. Hematuria throughout the stream may indicate glomerulonephritis. *Total* hematuria indicates profuse bladder, ureteral, or kidney hemorrhage. Rule out menstrual contamination in female clients. Urinary tract infection is a common cause of hematuria in women.

Urine *clarity* is affected by infection or inflammation of the urinary tract that results in bacteriuria and *pyuria* (white blood cells in the urine). Most typically, cloudy urine is due to amorphous phosphates in alkaline urine. Other causes of hazy or cloudy urine are epithelial cells from the lower urinary tract, external contamination, yeast, crystals, mucus, or fecal material. Milky urine results from prostatic fluid or semen, lipids, lymphatic fluid (chyle), or blood. Microscopic urinalysis determines the cause of the cloudiness. Figure 34-3 depicts examples of urine casts and crystals.

Normal urine has a faint aromatic *odor.* Strong-smelling or foul-smelling urine may indicate infection or dehydration. Specific odors can be present with disease and are listed in Table 34-3. A strong ammonia odor may occur if the urine is left standing too long. Asparagus can affect urine odor.

Pneumaturia is the presence of gas in the urine during voiding. Pneumaturia suggests fistula formation between the bladder and bowel, recent bladder instrumentation, or the presence of a urea-splitting organism in the urine.

Pain or Referred Pain. Urinary tract disease does not always cause pain. When pain is present, ask the client to describe the location, intensity, onset, and duration to define the etiologic mechanism further. What seems to alleviate or worsen the pain? Is the pain affected by bladder fullness or urination? Is it better or worse with position change, ejaculation, or bowel movement?

Pain in the upper urinary tract (kidney and ureter) is frequently felt locally as a dull, constant ache in the costovertebral angle just lateral to the sacrospinal muscle and beneath the twelfth rib posteriorly. Sudden distention of the renal capsule secondary to acute

TABLE 34-2 *Causes of Urine Discoloration*

Color	Disease Etiology	Medication, Dyes, Dietary
Colorless	Chronic glomerulonephritis Diabetes mellitus Diabetes insipidus	Excessive fluid intake, alcohol, diuretics
Cloudy white	Phosphate in alkaline urine Epithelial cells Bacteria, pus, chyle	
Yellow	Concentrated urine	Tetracycline, rifampin
Dark yellow	Urobilinogen	Santonin, phenindione, rhubarb (in acid urine), nitrofurantoin, sulfasalazine, docusate calcium, thiamine (multivitamins)
Pink or red	Red blood cells Hemoglobin Urate excretion Myoglobin *Serratia marcescens* Menstrual contamination	Beet ingestion, vegetable dyes, phenolphthalein laxatives (in alkaline urine), cascara (in alkaline urine), senna (X-Prep, Senokot), rhubarb (in alkaline urine)
Brown	Highly concentrated urine Red blood cells	Metronidazole (left standing), porphyrin
Dark brown or black	Highly concentrated urine Bilirubin Melanin Red blood cells (old)	Porphyrin (after standing), tyrosine, phenacetin, quinine, senna, methyldopa
Blue-green	Bilirubin *Pseudomonas*	Methylene blue, indigo carmine, thymol, phenol, amitriptyline

pyelonephritis or ureteral obstruction is typically the cause of renal pain. Renal distention may refer pain to the epigastric area as well as to the subcostal area toward the umbilicus and lower abdominal quadrant. Ask when the pain occurs. Costovertebral pain caused by mechanical back pain and radiculitis differs from renal pain in that it becomes worse with heavy physical work and position changes of the spine.

If the pain is colicky, the ureter is probably involved. Ureteral colic may radiate to the bladder, scrotum, and testicle in a male and to the vulva in a female. Colicky pain can be continuous, spasmodic, severe, and unbearable. If ureteral stones are suspected, ask the client to identify the site of referred pain to help identify the location of the stone. Upper ureteral stones result in pain referred to the testicles, midureteral stones cause pain re-

FIGURE 34-3 Urine clarity can be affected by casts and stones. A, Cellular cast with cells trapped in cellular matrix. B, Red blood cell cast. C, Old leukocytes and staghorn calculus with *Proteus* infection. (From Walsh, P.C., et al. [Eds.]. [2002]. *Campbell's urology* [8th ed.]. Philadelphia: W.B. Saunders.)

TABLE 34-3	*Changes in Urine Odor Related to Chemicals or Disease Process*
Odor Characteristic	**Chemical or Disease Process**
Sulfur	Cystinuria and homocystinuria
Musty, mousy	Phenylketonuria
Cabbage, fishy	Tyrosinuria
Sweaty feet	Butyric/hexanoic academia
Brewery (yeast, hops)	Oasthouse urine

ferred to the intestine, and stones near the ureteral orifices in the bladder cause irritative bladder manifestations. Manifestations tend to be localized in adults but are more generalized in children, who often present with only GI manifestations of abdominal pain, nausea, and vomiting.

Bladder pain is usually associated with acute overdistention, infection, or irritation of the bladder wall. Acute urinary retention causes agonizing suprapubic pain and sometimes bladder spasms, which are experienced as intermittent, cramping, severe pain in the bladder. Bladder spasms also result from irritation of the bladder wall by a foreign body, such as an indwelling urinary catheter, infection, or bladder tumors. With bladder infections there may be only pain referred to the distal urethra, causing dysuria while voiding.

In the absence of a bacterial infection, manifestations of urgency and frequency can be caused by *interstitial cystitis,* a chronic inflammatory disorder that affects up to 500,000 men and women in the United States.[8] Pain in the spine or bony structure of the pelvis or pain that radiates down one or both legs may be related to metastasis of prostate, kidney, or bladder cancer.

Prostate pain is not common. Men with acute prostatitis may feel fullness in the rectum or perineum, have irritative voiding manifestations, and have postejaculatory pain. Testicular pain secondary to orchitis, trauma, or torsion of the spermatic cord is usually localized and severe and may radiate along the spermatic cord to the lower abdomen. Pain may be referred to the testicle from an inguinal hernia or upper ureteral stone.

Epididymal pain results from acute infection and initially occurs as local pain and swelling in the scrotum. The pain can progress to an exquisitely painful mass involving the entire hemiscrotum, possibly radiating to the groin and lower abdomen. Epididymal pain is reduced by elevating the scrotum (Prehn's sign).

Pain in the urethra is localized and results from inflammation and irritation of the urethral mucosa. It occurs with urethral stricture, urethritis, or urethral cancer. Urethral pain may be more apparent before and after voiding.

Systemic Manifestations. Fever and chills are usually associated with acute, not chronic, infectious processes in the urinary tract such as cystitis, pyelonephritis, prostatitis, and epididymitis. GI manifestations such as nausea, vomiting and diarrhea, abdominal distention, and pain commonly occur with many urinary tract disorders. With "silent" urologic disease, GI manifestations may be the only presenting complaint.

Renal pathology causes GI manifestations for several reasons. The renointestinal reflexes, which arise from common autonomic and sensory innervations of the urinary and GI tract, can trigger pylorospasm or changes in the smooth muscle of the GI tract when there is distention of the renal capsule. The kidneys are anatomically related to the colon, duodenum, liver, spleen, pancreas, diaphragm, and psoas muscle; inflammation of the kidney can create manifestations in any of these intraperitoneal or retroperitoneal organs. Anteriorly, the kidneys are covered by the peritoneum; thus renal inflammation may provoke muscle rigidity and rebound tenderness.

Clients with acute renal failure may have pre-existing systemic manifestations of hypovolemia, hypotension, sepsis, renal, hepatic or cardiac dysfunction, diabetes mellitus, or exposure to drug nephrotoxins. With elevated blood urea nitrogen and creatinine in chronic renal failure, observe for fatigue, anorexia, nausea, vomiting, pruritus, and neurologic changes. Observe for manifestations of end-stage renal failure, such as edema, confusion, lethargy, weakness, and muscle twitching or cramps. Weight loss, bone pain, and lethargy can occur with advanced stages of urinary cancer.

Past Health History

When obtaining the past health history, inquire about coexisting systemic disease. Many disorders affect urinary function. Because urinary tract infection, retention, urinary calculi, or incontinence can be chronic or recurrent, explore any history of these disorders, including their treatments and outcomes.

Childhood and Infectious Diseases

Congenital anomalies of the urinary tract are common but range in severity from being incidental radiologic findings to being incompatible with life. The kidney may be absent *(renal agenesis),* dysplastic or atrophic, ectopic (located outside the flank position), or fused (joined, as in "horseshoe" kidney). Note when a client has a solitary kidney because treatment must be tailored to preserve optimal renal function. Children with ectopic or fused kidneys are likely to have other genitourinary, skeletal, GI, or cardiovascular anomalies. When ectopia or fusion occurs alone, it is often asymptomatic. Ureters can be ectopic, incomplete, or absent *(agenesis);* duplicated; or markedly dilated *(megaureter).* Bladder extrophy, persistent urachus, and epispadias are congenital anomalies that require reconstructive surgery and potentially lead to long-term problems with urinary incontinence.

Malformations of the spinal cord, such as meningomyelocele and spina bifida, can cause neuropathic voiding disorders. Childhood streptococcal infections, mononucleosis, mumps, measles, and cytomegalovirus infections can result in acute glomerulonephritis.

Trauma

Is there a history of a motor-vehicle accident, falls, straddle injury, penetrating abdominal injury, or contact sports injury? Assess the injury, how long ago it occurred, and the medical or surgical management that followed. The most frequent renal injury is blunt trauma, which is often managed conservatively, whereas penetrating trauma is usually explored surgically. Assessment of blunt or penetrating renal injury involves observing for a flank mass, tenderness, or bruising, especially when there is visible evidence of abdominal trauma. Long-term complications are rare with early intervention and careful follow-up.

Injury to the ureters is rare and most often occurs after penetrating wounds or complicated pelvic surgery. If ureteral injury is promptly corrected surgically, long-term complications are rare. When treatment is delayed, the client may experience flank or abdominal pain, peritonitis, paralytic ileus, fever, and possibly fistulae. Delayed diagnosis increases the risk of renal damage secondary to infection, hydronephrosis, abscess formation, and ureteral stricture.

Bladder trauma is related to the amount of urine in the bladder at the time of the injury; the bony pelvis protects the empty bladder. Suspect trauma anytime a pelvic fracture has occurred. If the bladder wall is ruptured by a penetrating or blunt injury to the lower abdomen, urine may extravasate into the peritoneal cavity and cause an acute abdomen or peritonitis if the urine is contaminated. Typically, the client has suprapubic pain or is unable to void. Gross hematuria is usually present. Complications of bladder injury are rare if it is treated promptly but can include temporary incontinence.

Urethral injuries are more common in males than in females and can occur with instrumentation such as endoscopy or catheterization, straddle injury of the anterior urethra (distal to the urogenital diaphragm), or pelvic fracture in the posterior urethra (proximal to the urogenital diaphragm). In females, urethral injury is sometimes seen after traumatic intercourse, childbirth, or vaginal surgery. Assess for blood at the meatus, urinary retention, and bladder distention. Partial or complete disruption of the urethra may lead to urethral stricture, which can restrict urinary flow and predispose to urinary tract infections.

Major Illnesses and Hospitalizations

Ask about recent illnesses, including diarrhea, vomiting, trauma (abdominal, pelvic, or vascular), and associated manifestations such as visual disturbances or excessive thirst. Include chronic diseases that can affect urinary function. Hypertension, diabetes, electrolyte imbalance, coronary artery disease, heart failure, and anemia worsen renal disease. Diabetes mellitus and multiple sclerosis can impair urinary and erectile function by interfering with autonomic function of the bladder.

A history of tuberculosis is significant when a client reports manifestations of renal insufficiency or failure, ureteral obstruction, or chronic urinary tract inflammation. Genitourinary tuberculosis is the most common nonpulmonary tuberculosis infection after lymphadenopathy. Members of the *Mycobacterium tuberculosis* complex as well as the vaccine bacille Calmette-Guérin (BCG) can cause genitourinary disease. Mani-festations mimic urinary tract infection but can be differentiated by sterile pyuria. Clients with a history of sickle cell anemia are at risk for papillary necrosis of the kidney and erectile dysfunction secondary to recurrent priapism. If renal neoplasm is suspected, inquire whether the client has von Hippel-Lindau syndrome, an autosomal dominant disorder that causes angiomatous cerebellar cysts, angiomatosis of the retina, and tumors of the pancreas; it is associated with cysts or adenocarcinoma of the kidneys. Disorders of the central and peripheral nervous system can also affect innervation of the bladder. Disorders leading to hypercalcemia, such as hyperparathyroidism, or hyperoxaluria, such as Crohn's disease, or small bowel resections as well as limited mobility, dehydration, and dietary excess of calcium, sodium, oxalate, purines or refined carbohydrates can predispose to renal stones. External beam radiation therapy for bladder or prostate cancer can cause radiation cystitis. Immunocompromised clients such as those with HIV or acquired immunodeficiency syndrome (AIDS), and those on immunosuppressive therapy are susceptible to fungal infections of the urinary tract.

Scleroderma, an autoimmune disorder characterized by massive deposits of collagen, may involve the kidneys. Erythema multiforme, an inflammatory disorder of the skin associated with allergic or toxic reactions to drugs or microorganisms such as *Mycoplasma pneumoniae* and herpes simplex virus, can involve the kidneys of young adults and children in its most severe form (Stevens-Johnson syndrome). Systemic lupus erythematosus can lead to glomerulonephritis with hypertension and nephrotic syndrome.

Operations

Previous abdominopelvic or genitourinary procedures can affect urinary function through accidental trauma to the ureters and bladder. Document all invasive procedures, especially if the client might need surgery again. Ask about previous surgery for urinary cancer, calculus, obstruction, or incontinence. Surgical management of urologic cancers includes radical, partial, or simple nephrectomy, transurethral resection and fulguration of bladder tumors, radical cystectomy with urinary diversion through an ileal conduit or neobladder, radical prostatectomy with pelvic lymphadenectomy, and cryoablation of prostate tumors. Stones may be fragmented or extracted from the ureter with a transurethral ureteroscopy and from the kidney with a percutaneous nephrolithotomy. BPH may be treated with transurethral resection or less invasively with needle ablation or thermotherapy. Surgeries for incontinence include pubovaginal slings, periurethral collagen injections, colposuspension, anterior colporrhaphy, colpourethropexy, and retropubic urethropexy or pubococcygeal repair. Has the client had a hysterectomy? Has the client had other operations that could interfere with the innervation of the urinary tract, including neurosurgical and orthopedic procedures of the spine? Colon and rectal surgery can lead to a neurogenic bladder or erectile dysfunction.

Medications

Many medications can affect urinary function. Obtain a complete history of prescription and nonprescription medications, including herbs and nutraceuticals. Medications that can worsen some urinary conditions may be helpful in others. For example, anticholinergics and alpha-sympathomimetics can relieve urinary incontinence in some clients but can lead to urinary retention in others. If the client presents with urinary calculi, inquire about antihypertensives, diuretics, or silica antacids. Heavy consumption of acetaminophen has been associated with an increased risk renal cancer.[11] NSAIDs may cause interstitial nephritis. Herbal supplements used for prostate health include saw palmetto (Serenoa repens), pygeum (Pygeum africanum), pumpkin (Curcurbita pepo), and nettle root (Urtica dioica).[4] Nutraceuticals used for prostate cancer prevention include vitamin E, lycopene, and selenium.

Megadose vitamins (40,000 units of vitamin A, 100 mg of vitamin B_6, 2000 mg of vitamin C, 400 units of vitamin E, and 90 mg of zinc) were shown in one small study to have secondary prevention benefits over RDA vitamins in clients with bladder cancer.[22] Determine the medication, dose, dosage changes, length of time taken, type, and frequency to ascertain a possible relationship to the onset of the chief complaint. Medications known to alter urinary function are listed in Table 34-4.

Allergies

Document allergies to antibiotics. Nitrofurantoins, sulfonamides, and quinolones are often used in the treatment of urinary tract infections. Inquire about allergies to radiographic contrast dyes as well as to iodine because iodine dyes are used in some of the radiologic diagnostic tests routinely performed in a urologic evaluation. Clients with known contrast dye allergies can be given methylprednisolone before the procedure.

Family Health History

Ask about a family history of urinary calculi and renal or sickle cell disease when clients present with pain or hematuria or both. The client who has stones is twice as likely as one who does not have a first-degree relative with renal stones. Certain other diseases, such as prostate or testicular cancer and BPH, tend to be familial. Hypertension and diabetes are often inherited and can have a significant effect on renal function. Well-known genetic urinary disorders include adult polycystic kidney disease, tuberous sclerosis, von Hippel-Lindau disease, renal tubular acidosis, and cystinuria.

Psychosocial History

Psychosocial assessment is ongoing throughout the interview. Observe and assess for impairments in vision,

TABLE 34-4	Medications That Affect Urinary Elimination
Medication Type	**Effect on Urination**
Anticholinergics	Decreased detrusor contractility (oxybutynin, methantheline), urinary retention, hesitancy
Antispasmodics	Decreased detrusor contractility (dicyclomine), belladonna), urinary retention, urinary hesitancy
Tricyclic antidepressants	Decreased detrusor contractility (imipramine), urinary retention, less incontinence
Cholinergics	Increased detrusor contractility (bethanechol chloride), incontinence, urgency
Alpha-sympathomimetics	Increased sphincter resistance (pseudoephedrine), urinary retention, dysuria
Alpha-blockers	Reduced sphincter resistance (prazosin, terazosin), frequency, incontinence
Estrogens (women)	Increased urethral muscle tone (progestin, estriol), reduced incontinence
Antiandrogens (men)	Improved urinary flow (flutamide, bicalutamide)
Sedatives-hypnotics	Urinary incontinence
Nonsteroidal anti-inflammatories	Renal papillary necrosis (long term)
Diuretics	Polyuria, urinary incontinence (hydrochlorothiazide)
Aminoglycoside antibiotics	Nephrotoxicity (gentamicin, amikacin)
Calcium channel blockers	Urinary retention (diltiazem, verapamil)
Alcohol	Polyuria, frequency, urgency

hearing, or speech. Assess the level of mobility and social factors of living and work environment, caregivers, social contacts, and family. For clients who report (or you suspect have) involuntary incontinence, evidenced as wetness of clothing or odor, assess access to toilets and overall hygiene. Ask about positive or negative childhood experiences with toilet training that may have had a long-term effect on urination patterns. Assess the client's knowledge of variables in daily life at home and at work that may contribute to the urinary problem. Is the client anxious about urinating in a public place? Anxiety and stress can stimulate or inhibit urination and provoke urgency and frequency. Establish how the client recognizes and manages stress, particularly when the presenting manifestation is worsened by anxiety and stress. Clients may be unaware of lifestyle changes that they might make to improve their urinary problem.

Ascertain the client's knowledge and anxiety about a potential cancer diagnosis. Provide information and feedback according to the client's educational and emotional needs. Some clients have misconceptions or fears regarding their problem and the available treatments. Address fear of surgery and changes in body functions, which can seriously alter body image, so that support can be provided throughout the treatment process.

Occupation

Occupation can play a role in urinary function. Prolonged exposure to aromatic amines has been shown to increase risk of bladder cancer.[9] Diesel exhaust may also increase the risk of bladder cancer.[3] Assess the accessibility of toilets in the workplace, especially for clients who have urgency and urge incontinence. Prolonged exposure to heat or cold can affect urination.

Geographical Location

Hot climates can lead to chronic dehydration if fluid intake is inadequate. This, along with increased exposure to sunlight, can increase the risk of urinary calculi. People who live in warm climates are at increased risk for infection in larva-infested water used for swimming, bathing, and farming. Larvae may cause the disease schistosomiasis, which predisposes to urinary obstruction and bladder cancer.

Exercise

The positive effects of regular exercise on physical and psychological well-being cannot be overstated. What type of exercise does the client participate in regularly? How strenuous is the exercise? Does exercise affect the urinary problem in any way, or does the urinary problem prohibit participation? Does the client rehydrate as needed after heavy physical exertion? Long-distance runners sometimes have hematuria, which may originate from the kidney or bladder or may be a manifestation of underlying glomerular disease. Long-distance bikers may develop urethral and vulvar trauma or pudendal neuropathy, which can cause perineal pain and erectile dysfunction in men.[21]

Nutrition

Nutritional status can have a significant impact on urinary elimination. Diets rich in saturated and unsaturated fats, animal protein, and sugar and deficient in vegetable protein and unrefined carbohydrates (as seen in more affluent countries) can increase the risk of renal stone formation. Ask about dietary habits that could increase the risk for urinary stones, such as dairy products; purine in meats, fish, and poultry; and oxalate in tea, chocolate, and nuts.

Ingestion of caffeine can exacerbate conditions such as interstitial cystitis (Table 34-5). For the client who complains of nocturia, assess when and what type of fluid is consumed during the evening. Coffee, tea, and caffeinated sodas can have a diuretic effect on the urinary tract. Obesity has been linked to renal cell carcinoma. High-fat diets may increase the risk of prostate cancer.[12]

Habits

Obtain a history of tobacco, alcohol, and recreational drug use. Cigarette smoking has been consistently shown to be a risk factor for urothelial cancers. Smoking can also lead to peripheral vascular disease and to subsequent erectile dysfunction. The risk associated with cigarette smoking declines significantly with years of smoking cessation.

TABLE 34-5	Dietary Irritants of the Urinary Tract	
Irritant*	**Possible Substitutes**
Alcohol	Late harvest dessert wines
Apples, apple juice	Apricot or pear nectar, papaya juice
Coffee, tea	Kava, cold brewed coffee, herbal tea
Chocolate	Carob
Carbonated beverages	
Chilies, spicy foods	
Aspartame (NutraSweet)	Fructose
Strawberries, cranberries	
Grapes, guava, cantaloupe	
Peaches, pineapples, plums	
Tomatoes, onions	
Vinegar	

*Not all irritants have a corresponding substitute.

Alcohol can irritate the bladder and increase urine output. Chronic alcoholism can lead to autonomic and peripheral neuropathy that impairs urinary and sexual function and to decreased serum testosterone, testicular atrophy, and decreased libido. If the client is scheduled for surgery, heavy tobacco and alcohol use can increase the risk of perioperative complications significantly. (See Chapter 16 for a discussion of the effects of tobacco and alcohol on perioperative outcomes.)

Review of Systems

Ask about manifestations such as GI complaints, blood pressure changes, weight loss or gain, edema, fatigue, lethargy, headaches, blurred vision, changes in mentation, numbness or tingling of the extremities, pruritus, bleeding tendencies, exposure to infectious disease, and allergies that may be associated with urologic disorders. See the website for this textbook for additional questions to include in the review of systems.

PHYSICAL EXAMINATION

The urologic physical examination typically includes the following:

- Temperature, pulse, blood pressure, height, and weight
- General inspection of the skin for integrity, color, and peripheral edema
- Examination of the abdomen, pelvis, genitalia, and rectum

The examination may be tailored to the client's specific complaint or condition. Instruct the client to empty the bladder before the examination. When the physical examination is completed, document findings using the Physical Assessment Findings in the Healthy Adult feature on The Urinary System at right as a guide.

Abdomen

Inspection

Have the client lie supine with arms at the sides and knees slightly flexed to relax the abdominal muscles. If the client has complained of abdominal, back, or flank pain, note whether there is guarding or restlessness in this position. Inspect the abdomen for symmetry and contour. Asymmetry or a mass in the upper quadrants may indicate a renal tumor or hydronephrosis, although only a very large renal or adrenal mass in a very thin client would potentially be visible. Fullness in the suprapubic area may indicate a distended bladder.

Note any surgical or traumatic scarring that may have affected the urinary or GI tract or caused adhesions, especially if the client presents with abdominal complaints. Also note any herniation, either at the site of surgical scarring, around a stoma, or in the ventral area (epigastric or umbilical region), particularly with straining (see earlier discussion of lower GI tract physical examination).

For clients who have had previous urologic surgery, note the presence of a stoma, the type, whether it is a continent urinary diversion, and appearance of the stoma and surrounding skin. Observe the size and contour of the stoma, and note the color of the mucosa. Observe for abnormal findings such as retracted or prolapsed stomal mucosa, lesions, inflammation, or macerated skin. Document the type of ostomy appliance or stomal covering, if used. Also note the presence of an indwelling urethral or suprapubic catheter, its patency, and color and odor of the urine. Document the presence of sediment in the drainage collection system. Evaluate the drainage system for cleanliness and closed system integrity.

Auscultation

Auscultation is performed before palpation to avoid disruption of vascular murmurs and bowel sounds. Renal artery bruits are most commonly heard just above and slightly left of the umbilicus and can indicate renal artery stenosis or aneurysm or arteriovenous malformation. If a bruit is heard, avoid deep palpation. Evaluate bowel sounds in all four quadrants for frequency, intensity, and pitch, especially in the presence of GI manifestations (see earlier discussion of lower GI tract physical examination).

Percussion

Percussion is valuable in identifying a bladder containing at least 150 ml of urine. The percussion sound changes from tympanic to dull over a full bladder. Blunt percussion can also be valuable if performed anteriorly and

---

PHYSICAL ASSESSMENT FINDINGS IN THE HEALTHY ADULT
The Urinary System

Inspection
Lower abdomen flat, nondistended. External urethral orifice pink without discharge.

Auscultation
No renal bruit noted anteriorly or posteriorly over the right or left costovertebral angle.

Percussion
Flat note over symphysis pubis and tympany over lower abdomen. No tenderness posteriorly over the right or left costovertebral angle.

Palpation
Lower pole of right kidney palpable, smooth, nontender. Left kidney nonpalpable.

posteriorly to identify renal masses or tenderness when renal trauma and hemorrhage prevent deep palpation. Place one hand over the costovertebral angle on the left side and strike the hand lightly with the opposite fisted hand. The effect is perceived as a dull thud in a normal kidney but as sharp pain or tenderness in a distended kidney. Repeat for the right kidney. Figure 34-4 illustrates this maneuver, and Chapter 4 describes the blunt percussion technique.

Palpation

Begin palpation with a light touch, depressing the skin no deeper than 1 to 2 cm, to assess tenderness and muscle resistance or guarding, which might be a sign of peritoneal irritation. *Light palpation* allows examination of tender abdominal areas with minimal production of pain. Such pain may cause voluntary muscle rigidity and reduce the effectiveness of deep palpation.

Examine each of the four quadrants, noting areas of muscle resistance, which may indicate a superficial or large pelvic mass, either infectious or neoplastic, or bladder distention if it is in the suprapubic area. Involuntary muscle rigidity is usually unilateral, whereas voluntary rigidity is symmetrical. To differentiate between a rigid muscle and a mass, note whether the area of resistance follows an abdominal muscle or is lobular shaped.

Last, palpate any region under suspicion on the basis of the health history and previous inspection.

Deep palpation follows light palpation and is used primarily to detect renal enlargement or masses. The technique is similar to that of light palpation, but the depth is 4 to 5 cm. Reinforced *(bimanual)* palpation is used in cases of more resistant muscle tone. (See Chapter 4 for a discussion of bimanual palpation.)

Describe the identified masses in terms of location, size, consistency, surface characteristics, tenderness, mobility, and pulsation. Assess rebound tenderness to determine the presence of peritoneal inflammation. Deep palpation should never be used in cases of known renal trauma, polycystic kidneys, abdominal aortic aneurysm, kidney transplantation, or appendicitis.

The kidneys are normally well protected by the diaphragm and lower ribs and cannot be palpated easily. The right kidney is slightly lower than the left because of the presence of the liver. In a thin client, the lower pole of the right kidney can sometimes be detected with deep palpation. Palpate the kidney bimanually, with one hand on the costovertebral angle posteriorly and the other hand pushing firmly and deeply under the costal margin anteriorly, while instructing the client to inhale deeply. As the client inhales, the right kidney descends and may be felt by the anterior hand as it slides between the hands. A normal kidney feels smooth, firm, and rounded (Figure 34-5). The left kidney is usually not palpable because it lies higher under the rib cage. In older adults, the kidneys may be palpated more readily because of loss of abdominal muscle firmness.

An empty bladder cannot be palpated. In acute or chronic urinary retention, the bladder rises up out of the pelvis at the midline toward the umbilicus. It can be seen and usually felt. When chronic urinary retention is present, the bladder is atonic and difficult to palpate.

Genitalia

Use inspection and palpation to examine the genitalia. Clients tend to be more anxious about examination of the genitalia. Therefore remain straightforward and pro-

FIGURE 34-4 Blunt percussion over the costovertebral angle to assess renal tenderness. The client may be either sitting or prone.

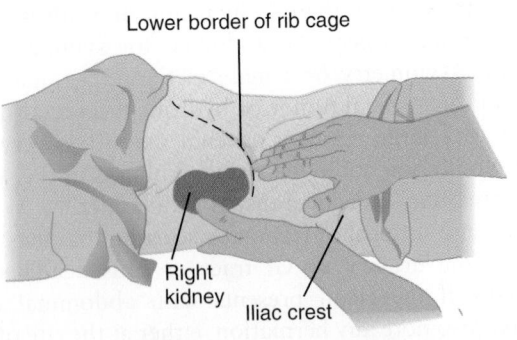

FIGURE 34-5 Palpating the kidneys.

fessional and perform this part of the examination after establishing rapport.

Male Clients

While the male client lies supine, inspect the perineum and groin area for manifestations of skin irritation or excoriation, especially if he has reported urinary incontinence. Examine the glans meatus. Circumcised males have a dry glans, whereas uncircumcised males have a relatively moist and pink glans. Examine the urethral meatus after carefully retracting the foreskin (in uncircumcised males). The foreskin should retract easily. Normally, the meatus is located centrally on the glans and the mucosa is pink and moist, readily separating when the glans is pressed between the thumb and forefinger.

A meatus opening dorsally on the glans, penile shaft, or penoscrotal junction indicates *epispadias*. *Hypospadias* is an anomaly in which the urethra opens on the ventral aspect of the glans, penile shaft, or penoscrotal junction. Malposition of the urethral meatus can interfere with normal voiding and can be associated with curvature of the penis that is called *chordee*. Note the presence of any urethral discharge or reddened edematous meatal edges that indicate urethritis. Difficulty exposing the distal meatal mucosa (fossa navicularis) may indicate stenosis. Next palpate the penile shaft ventrally along the urethra for tenderness, swelling, or mass. (Chapter 39 covers the examination of the genitalia.)

Female Clients

Urologic examination of the female genitalia includes examination of the external genitalia and in some cases a complete pelvic examination (see also Chapter 39). For an examination of the external genitalia, position the client in a supine recumbent position with knees and feet apart and knees flexed. Examine the urethral meatus for eversion or redness, which may indicate urethritis.

Palpate the urethra by inserting a gloved index finger into the vagina and palpating the anterior vaginal wall for induration or mass from the bladder to the meatus. Inspect for the presence of urethral discharge indicative of infection.

Ask the client to cough or strain, and note any bulging of the vaginal walls. Bulging of the anterior vaginal wall can indicate a *cystocele* and that of the posterior wall a *rectocele*. Cystocele is seen with relaxation of the pelvic floor musculature and may be the source of irritative voiding manifestations and stress incontinence.

Rectum

Male Clients

The urologic digital rectal examination of the male client is done to evaluate the prostate gland. Although the prostate is primarily a reproductive organ, disorders of the gland can affect urination. Disorders include BPH, prostatitis, prostatodynia, and prostate adenocarcinoma. Examination of the prostate is discussed in Chapter 39.

Depending on the skill of the examiner, the bulbocavernosal reflex can be assessed for neurologic abnormalities. Evaluate the reflex by gently compressing the glans penis with the thumb and forefinger of the opposite hand while the index finger remains in the rectum. When the reflex arc is intact, the sphincter contracts.

Female Clients

In the female client, the examiner can duplicate the evaluation performed for the male client by gently flicking the clitoris during the rectal examination. A rectal examination of the female urologic client is done primarily to assess sphincter tone and the bulbocavernosal reflex (see the earlier discussion of the rectal examination). It can also be done to evaluate for rectocele or enterocele.

Lymph Nodes

Inspect and palpate the supraclavicular and inguinal groups of lymph nodes if metastatic cancer of the prostate or testis is suspected. Chapters 39 and 76 describe examination of inguinal lymph nodes.

Related Body Systems

Assess pertinent information about other body systems, such as blood pressure, temperature, fluid balance, evidence of peripheral edema, and neurologic or vascular changes that affect the lower extremities. Document your findings because they may be related to disorders of the urinary tract.

DIAGNOSTIC TESTS

An overview of common urine and blood tests, imaging studies, voiding, and endoscopic procedures performed in urologic clients is given next (see also Chapter 4).

Laboratory Tests

Laboratory tests for the urinary system consist primarily of urine and blood studies.

Urine Studies

Urinalysis. Clients who present with urinary tract manifestations typically undergo a urinalysis. Urinalysis performed by dipstick provides information about color, odor, specific gravity, osmolality, pH, protein, glucose, ketones, bilirubin, urobilinogen, nitrites, leukocyte esterase, and blood or hemoglobin. Microscopic urinalysis quantifies white and red blood cells and indicates the presence of casts, crystals, bacteria, or epithelial cells (see Figure 34-3).

Microscopic urinalysis should always follow a report of red urine. Microscopic urinalysis differentiates between discoloration related to ingested substances and extracellular hemoglobin in the urine. The presence of erythrocyte casts indicates a renal origin of the blood. Gross hematuria and microscopic hematuria, defined as more than three red blood cells per high-power field (HPF), can indicate trauma, infectious processes, toxicity, calculus, and benign and malignant neoplasms (Table 34-6). Clients with asymptomatic microscopic hematuria who are at risk for urothelial cancer should undergo further evaluation.[10]

Specific gravity indicates the concentration of urine and reflects the client's hydration status as well as renal function. For example, clients who have diabetes insipidus consistently have specific gravity values less than 1.010. Clients with extensive tubular damage or endocrine disease involving antidiuretic hormone (ADH) insufficiency have specific gravity fixed at 1.010, the level of the plasma.

Osmolality is a measure of the concentrating ability of the kidney. Osmolality increases in hypernatremia, acidosis, and shock. It decreases in diabetes insipidus, hypercalcemia, excessive hydration, and renal tubular acidosis.

Urine pH is a measure of free hydrogen ion in the urine and indicates the renal tubules' ability to maintain normal hydrogen concentration in the plasma and extracellular fluid; 7.0 is the point of neutrality. Urine pH is helpful in determining systemic metabolic or respiratory acid-base disorders. It is also important in managing urinary conditions that require maintenance of alkaline or acidic urine (renal calculi, antibiotic therapy, and salicylate intoxication). The pH is affected by hydration, sleep, infections, medications, and diet.

Proteinuria, or persistent elevation of protein in the urine, may be glomerular, tubular, or overflow in origin. Glomerular proteinuria occurs with immunoglobulin A nephropathy or diabetes mellitus. Tubular proteinuria results from failure to resorb immunoglobulins because of defective tubular function. Overflow proteinuria is due to an increase in abnormal immunoglobulins and is often seen with multiple myeloma. Prolonged fever and excessive physical exertion can cause a transient elevation of urinary protein levels. Orthostatic proteinuria occurs occasionally when the client has been standing for several hours. A false-positive result for urine protein may be obtained when the urine is concentrated or contains white blood cells or vaginal secretions. Persistent proteinuria of

---

TABLE 34-6	*Understanding Urinalysis*	
Variable	**Normal Values**	**Causes of Abnormal Values**
Specific gravity	1.001-1.035	Decreased: increased fluid intake, diuretics, decreased renal concentration, diabetes insipidus
		Increased: dehydration, diabetes mellitus, increased ADH secretion, iodine contrast
Osmolality	50-1200 mOsm/L	Varies with hydration
pH	5.5-6.5	<5.5: metabolic or respiratory acidosis, renal tubular acidosis type II
		>7.5: presence of urea-splitting organism *(Proteus)*, renal tubular acidosis type I
Blood	None	Carcinoma, renal lithiasis
Protein	<20 mg/dl	Glomerular disease, nephropathy, interstitial disease, strenuous exercise, multiple myeloma
Glucose	Negative	Diabetes mellitus
Ketones	Negative	Diabetic ketoacidosis
Bilirubin	Negative	Intrinsic hepatic disease, bile duct obstruction
Urobilinogen	Trace	Hemolysis, hepatocellular disease
Nitrites	Negative	Bacteriuria
Leukocyte esterase	Negative	Bacteriuria
Red blood cells	<3 RBCs/HPF	Urinary tract cancer, IgA nephropathy, lithiasis, prostate enlargement, menstrual contamination, infection, papillary necrosis, renal artery embolism or thrombosis
White blood cells	0-5 WBCs/HPF	Infection
Bacteria	None	Urinary tract infection
Casts	0-4 hyaline/HPF	Red blood cell casts: glomerular bleeding
		White blood cell casts: glomerulonephritis
		Fatty casts: nephrotic syndrome
Crystals	Varies	Significant in renal lithiasis

ADH, Antidiuretic hormone; *HPF,* high-power field; *IgA,* immunoglobulin A; *LPF,* low-power field; *RBC,* red blood cell; *WBC,* white blood cell.

more than trace should be followed with a 24-hour urine evaluation.[5]

Glucosuria (glucose in the urine) occurs most often in clients with diabetes mellitus, which may result in renal papillary necrosis and recurrent urinary tract infections. Glucosuria occurs when the blood glucose level exceeds the resorptive capacity of the kidneys, a level of 180 mg/dl. Glucosuria in the absence of hyperglycemia indicates renal tubular, central nervous system, or thyroid disorders. *Ketonuria* (ketones in the urine) occurs when body fat is metabolized for energy, as in cases of diabetic ketoacidosis, fasting, pregnancy, vomiting, and diarrhea.

Direct bilirubin is made in the hepatocyte and appears in the urine as an early manifestation of extrahepatic biliary tract obstruction or intrinsic hepatic disease. *Urobilinogen* is the end product of conjugated bilirubin metabolism, and a small amount, 1 to 4 mg daily, is excreted in the urine. Increased levels indicate liver disease or hemolytic disorders. Absence represents obstruction of the biliary tract.

Leukocyte esterase indicates white blood cells in the urine. *Nitrites* in the urine strongly suggest bacteriuria. *Epithelial cells* are often present in urinary sediment. Renal tubular cells are least often seen but are indicative of renal disease.

Casts are formed in the distal tubules and collecting ducts of the kidneys; they signify renal disease when found in the urine. Red blood cell casts indicate glomerulitis or vasculitis. White blood cell casts indicate bacterial infection but are often difficult to distinguish from epithelial casts. Granular casts often represent disintegrated epithelial cells, leukocytes, or protein associated with renal tubular disease. Hyaline casts represent a mixture of mucus and globulin from the tubules and are not significant in small numbers.

Depending on the test ordered, urinalysis may be performed on a clean-catch specimen, midstream specimen, fresh urine specimen, first morning specimen, 12- or 24-hour collection, multiple bottle voidings (serial urine collections), or a specimen obtained with a catheter. First-voided morning specimens are helpful in evaluating renal function. Ideally, the urine should be obtained several hours after eating because postprandial specimens may contain lysed blood cells and disintegrated casts. Clean catch continues to be the standard method for obtaining urine specimens.

Instruct female clients to separate the labia and uncircumcised males to retract the foreskin. For a catheterized client, collect urine from the port on the tubing, not the urinary drainage bag, because this urine may be contaminated. Use a drip method to collect urine from a urostomy. Approximately 10 ml is required. In some situations, catheterization for a urine sample is required. In these cases, follow standard precautions and maintain sterile technique (see Chapter 4 for additional discussion of urinalysis). Refer to a nursing fundamentals textbook for specific information about the techniques for collecting urine specimens (random, clean catch, catheterized, timed, and from a urostomy). Always follow protocol for specimen collection and handling.

Urine Culture. When urinary tract infection is suspected from the client's history or the presence of bacteria or significant white blood cells on urinalysis, a urine culture is necessary. This test identifies the offending organism and quantifies the amount of colonization. Generally, the presence of organisms in a concentration greater than 100,000 colony-forming units (CFUs) per milliliter indicates infection, although treatment is recommended for 10,000 to 100,000 CFU per milliliter if manifestations of infection are also present.

Collection technique is as for midstream clean-catch or catheter specimens for urinalysis. Determining the sensitivity of the organism to specific antibiotics is not usually necessary because *E. coli,* known to cause 85% of routine infections, is sensitive to most oral antibiotics. Identifying the drugs to which the bacteria are sensitive is done in cases with recurrent or persistent manifestations of urinary tract infection.

Urine Cytology. When urothelial carcinoma or inflammatory disease of the bladder, renal pelvis, ureters, or urethra is known or suspected, urine cytologic evaluation is performed. This test is also helpful in diagnosing cytomegalovirus or other viral disease. The specimen may be clean voided or a bladder washing obtained either by catheterization or cystoscopically. Transitional cell carcinoma of the bladder typically sheds cells into the urine more than upper tract carcinomas, but the amount of cells retrieved for study depends on the adequacy of the specimen and the grade and volume of the tumor.

Flow Cytometry. Flow cytometry measures the DNA of the tumor cells. DNA diploid tumors have a favorable prognosis, whereas triploid to tetraploid tumors have a poor prognosis. This test is more accurate in identifying high-grade cancers.

Quantitative Fluorescent Image Analysis. This technique uses a computerized fluorescent microscopy to scan the nucleus of cells on a slide. The computer quantitates the amount of emitted fluorescence that is proportional to the nucleic acid content of the call and can identify abnormal amounts of DNA. Image analysis is more sensitive than standard cytology or flow cytometry.[22]

Quantitative Urine Studies. Urine creatinine clearance is most often part of quantitative urine studies. Creatinine determines the glomerular filtration rate and tubular excretion ability of the kidney. Creatinine is a byproduct of muscle energy metabolism and is excreted in the urine at a fairly constant rate. Creatinine level in the urine is equivalent to the glomerular filtration rate, and it may be diminished in renal disorders. Excretion rates of other urinary components and the completeness of the collection can be interpreted when measured with creatinine clearance. Other 24-hour urine studies are listed in Table 34-7.

For a creatinine clearance or other quantitative urine studies, collect the urine specimen for 12 or 24 hours as ordered (see Chapter 4). A blood sample is drawn at any point during the collection period in a 7-ml red-topped tube for creatinine clearance studies. There is no postprocedure care.

Concentration and Dilution Studies. Loss of ability to concentrate and dilute urine indicates significant renal tubular damage. Several tests can be performed to evaluate the ability of the kidneys to concentrate and dilute the urine. Many of these tests can be risky for clients who have compromised renal or cardiac function because of the severe fluid loading or fluid deprivation that is part of the procedure. Carefully assess and monitor the client's fluid balance and cardiovascular status (pulse, blood pressure, lung sounds) during urine concentration and dilution testing.

Urine Bence-Jones Protein. Urine Bence-Jones proteins are low-molecular-weight monoclonal immunoglobulin light-chain proteins. They may be present in the urine in multiple myeloma, lymphoma, macroglobulinemia, leukemia, osteogenic sarcoma, and amyloidosis. When present in urine, perform a urine test and serum electrophoresis. Collect a random urine sample as ordered (see Chapter 4).

Blood Studies

Blood Urea Nitrogen. Blood urea nitrogen (BUN) is a measure of renal function because urea is the primary end product of protein metabolism and is excreted by the kidneys. An elevated BUN level may indicate impaired renal function, although it is not specific for the kidneys. BUN may be elevated because of systemic factors such as sepsis, excess protein consumption, starvation, dehydration, and cardiac failure.

Serum Creatinine. Serum creatinine is more specific for renal function because it is not affected by dietary intake or hydration status. It can be elevated in cases of glomerulonephritis, pyelonephritis, acute tubular necrosis, nephrotoxicity, renal insufficiency, and renal failure.

TABLE 34-7	Quantitative (24-Hour) Urine Studies	
Substance	**Normal Values**	**Cause of Abnormal Values**
Calcium	100-300 mg/24 hr	Increased intestinal absorption, bone resorption, or loss of renal tubular resorption
Chloride	140-250 mEq/24 hr	Electrolyte imbalance
Creatinine	<0.8-1.8 g/24 hr (males) 0.6-1.6 g/24 hr (females)	Endocrine disorders, myopathies, renal disease, leukemia
Cystine	<38 mg/24 hr	Elevated with inherited impairment of renal tubular resorption of cystine
Magnesium	12-199 mg/24 hr	Intestinal malabsorption, alcoholism, Bartter's syndrome
Oxalate	7-44 mg/24 hr (males) 4-31 mg/24 hr (females)	Intestinal resections, increased vitamin C, ethylene glycol intoxication, renal failure
Potassium	25-125 mEq/24 hr	Renal, adrenal, water, or acid base imbalance
Sodium	40-220 mEq/24 hr	Renal, adrenal, water, or acid base imbalance
Uric acid	250-750 mg/24 hr	Increased in excess dietary intake of purines or endogenous uric acid production
Urine 5-hydroxyindoleacetic acid (5-HIAA)	3-15 mg/24 hr	Elevated in carcinoid tumors
Urine vanillylmandelic acid (VMA) and catecholamines	2-7 mg/24 hr (VMA) <100 μg/24 hr total <20 μg/24 hr epinephrine 15-80 μg/24 hr norepinephrine 65-400 μg/24 hr dopamine	Elevated with pheochromocytoma

Elevations are also seen in clients who have renal failure secondary to outlet obstruction. Elevated serum creatinine levels can occur with systemic disease such as hypertension or diabetes. The normal ratio of BUN to creatinine is 10:1.

Radiography

Kidney-Ureter-Bladder X-Ray Study

The kidney-ureter-bladder (KUB) x-ray study provides an anteroposterior film of the kidneys, ureters, and pelvis taken without contrast medium. It is used to evaluate suspected radiopaque urinary calculi or masses and as a preliminary study for other radiologic tests of the abdomen.

Client preparation includes bowel preparation if the KUB study is done as a preliminary evaluation test. Advise the client that the x-ray procedure is painless.

Intravenous Pyelography or Excretory Urography

Intravenous pyelography (IVP) or excretory urography (EXU) is a study in which a series of radiologic films are obtained after intravenous injection of radiopaque contrast medium. IVP or EXU provides information about the entire urinary tract because films are taken at regular intervals as the contrast medium moves through the tract. The final film is taken after the client voids to evaluate the ability of the bladder to empty. Applying pressure across the client's lower abdomen to compress the ureters enhances the renal pelvis and proximal ureters. This test is used to evaluate renal stones, masses, hematuria, obstructive uropathy, congenital anomalies, infection, and renal function.

Preprocedure Care

Client preparation includes careful screening for potential allergies or sensitivity to contrast medium and iodine. A steroid may be given before injection of contrast medium in cases of sensitivities. Instruct clients about the necessary bowel preparation. This includes a liquid meal before 6:00 PM the preceding evening, followed by a laxative such as senna extract (X-Prep). Fluids are withheld after 10:00 PM the evening before the procedure to promote greater concentration of the contrast medium in the kidneys.

Explain that there may be a sensation of flushing and warmth, an unpleasant or salty taste in the mouth, or nausea when the contrast dye is administered. Instruct the client to take deep, full breaths if this occurs. Assess for allergic reactions (urticaria, itching, diaphoresis, and respiratory distress or failure). Because reactions happen immediately after injection of the contrast medium, antihistamines, steroids, and an emergency cart must be readily available. Contraindications for IVP or EXU include renal insufficiency or failure, hypersensitivity or allergy to contrast dye, multiple myeloma, advanced pulmonary tuberculosis, current drug therapy for chronic obstructive pulmonary disease, asthma or emphysema, heart failure, pheochromocytoma, sickle cell anemia, and diabetes. Known allergies may necessitate premedication with methylprednisolone.

Postprocedure Care

Monitor hydration status after IVP or EXU to reduce the risk of renal failure in susceptible clients. Unless there is a contraindication, force fluids to promote renal clearance of the contrast medium. Monitor output. Observe for mild reactions to iodine, such as hives, nausea, or parotid swelling.

Retrograde Urography

Retrograde studies are performed in conjunction with cystoscopy in a surgical setting under local anesthesia, although sedation or general anesthesia may be required. For clients in whom IVP is contraindicated or insufficient, a *retrograde pyelogram* can be obtained (Figure 34-6). Contrast medium is administered directly into the urinary tract (rather than intravenously) during endoscopic visualization via cystoscopy. (Cystoscopy is

FIGURE 34-6 Normal retrograde pyelogram demonstrating pyelocalyceal system and ureters. (From Walsh, P.C., et al. [Eds.]. [2002]. *Campbell's urology* [8th ed.]. Philadelphia: W.B. Saunders.)

discussed later in this chapter.) A retrograde pyelogram details the ureter, ureteropelvic junction, renal pelvis, and calices.

A *cystogram* is obtained after instillation of contrast medium directly into the bladder via a catheter. Cystographic studies are used to evaluate recurrent urinary tract infections, vesicoureteral reflux, hematuria, trauma, postsurgical healing, and stress urinary incontinence.

A *voiding cystourethrogram* is similar to a cystogram except films are taken of the bladder and urethra while the client is voiding (see later discussion). A *retrograde urethrogram* is indicated when there is suspicion of urethral stricture, fistula, trauma, diverticulum, or tumor. Oblique x-ray films are taken after instillation of 15 to 30 ml of contrast medium into the urethra via a catheter or a catheter-tip syringe.

Urinary tract infection should be ruled out before any of these procedures are performed. Clients should remain NPO after midnight before the procedure. Instruct clients to watch for and report manifestations of infection, which may occur for up to 24 to 48 hours after the procedure (flank pain, dysuria, chills, fever). Encourage consumption of fluids. Transient flank pain, bladder, or urethral discomfort may occur but should resolve in 24 to 48 hours.

Computed Tomography

Computed tomography is used in urology to evaluate the kidneys, major renal vessels, ureters, and bladder as well as the abdominal and pelvic contents for malignant masses, metastases, or lymphadenopathy. It is used primarily for tumor staging and identifying abscesses. Other uses for CT are to evaluate a nonfunctioning kidney, urinary tract trauma, a transplanted kidney, renal calculi, and infections. CT urography combines CT of the abdomen and pelvis with IVP in a single study. Clients should fast for 4 hours before the procedure. (See Chapter 4 for general care of the client having a CT scan.)

Magnetic Resonance Imaging

Magnetic resonance imaging (MRI) is used to visualize the kidneys, retroperitoneum, bladder, prostate, testes, and penis. It is very sensitive in differentiating between cysts and neoplasms in the kidney and creates a vascular map of arteries and vessels when used preoperatively. MRI is better able to stage bladder and prostate cancers than other modalities. Use of phased-array pelvic and endorectal coils allows enhancement of the urethra and periurethral tissues. Gadolinium is a chelate-bound metal that is non-nephrotoxic and hypoallergenic and thus allows safe use in clients with renal insufficiency or allergies to contrast dye.[22] (See Chapter 4 for general care of the client undergoing MRI.)

Renal Angiography

Angiography is the visualization of blood vessels by the use of radiopaque contrast media, and it is usually used for therapeutic interventions. This modality visualizes renal and pelvic arteries and is usually part of the evaluation for renal vascular hypertension. Renal arteriography is also used to evaluate for arterial and venous thromboses, to obtain vascular maps preoperatively, or to evaluate potential kidney donors. Three-dimensional angiography combines CT, magnetic resonance angiography (MRA), or ultrasound with angiography. (Chapter 4 describes general care of the client undergoing angiography.)

Ultrasonography

Ultrasonography is used in urology to evaluate the kidneys, ureters, bladder, prostate, testes, and penis. In a renal scan, the client's abdomen and back are scanned in the longitudinal and transverse planes. The kidneys can be evaluated for size, hydronephrosis, calculi, solid tumors, and cysts. Renal ultrasonography is used to differentiate simple cysts from other types of mass lesions in the kidney. Other uses include localizing and mapping the kidneys before biopsy and evaluating transplanted kidneys.

The bladder can be scanned for residual urine volume, bladder wall thickness, bladder calculi, tumors, and diverticula with an ultrasound probe over the suprapubic area. Prostate ultrasonography is performed transrectally with a transducer probe inserted 4 to 5 inches into the rectum. Images are obtained in the anterior-posterior (AP), coronal, and sagittal planes to approximate size with an ellipsoid volume equation:

$$\text{Volume} = \text{AP} \times \text{Coronal} \times \text{Sagittal} \times 0.5236$$

Prostate ultrasonography is used to evaluate the size, volume, shape, and echogenicity of the prostate and seminal vesicles. (Chapter 39 describes ultrasonography of the testes and penis and further discusses prostate ultrasound.)

Reassure clients that ultrasonography is painless and not invasive. An exception is transrectal ultrasonography, which can cause discomfort and pressure when the anus and rectum are dilated. For prostate ultrasonography, instruct the client to evacuate the rectum by administering a Fleet enema about 45 minutes before the procedure. No colon or proctologic examinations should be performed on the same day.

Radionuclide Studies

Nuclear medicine studies are performed in urology to evaluate renal perfusion and function. Clients receive an intravenous injection of a technetium-based radioisotope followed by a nuclear scan 3 hours later, when the radioactive tracer has concentrated in the target organ.

Bone scintigraphy (radionuclide bone scan) is used to detect bone metastases in prostate cancer. A newer modality in which an intravenous infusion of a monoclonal antibody to prostate-specific membrane antigen (PSMA) before scintigraphy may identify prostate cancer cells in regional soft tissue and distant soft tissue and bone sites to aid in staging of prostate cancer.[22] Immediate and delayed images are taken. Encourage clients to force fluids before the scan. (See Chapter 4 for a general discussion of radionuclide studies.)

Endoscopy

Cystourethroscopy and Urethroscopy

Endoscopy (see Chapter 4) is utilized in urology, most commonly in *cystourethroscopy*. This endoscopic study is used to evaluate the anterior and prostatic urethra, bladder urothelium and trigone, and the ureteral orifices in the bladder of clients with hematuria, recurrent or persistent urinary tract infection, irritative or obstructive voiding manifestations, and bladder tumors. The procedure is performed transurethrally by either a rigid or flexible cystoscope (Figure 34-7). Cystoscopy allows diagnostic inspection of the urinary tract for evidence of urinary calculi, infection, vesicoureteral reflux, prostatic obstruction, bladder tumor, and urethral stricture. A variation of cystourethroscopy is *urethroscopy*, in which only the urethra is visualized.

Preprocedure Care

Before the procedure, a urine culture or Gram stain must be negative because an active urinary tract infection is a contraindication to the test. The procedure is usually performed with the client in the lithotomy position, and the urethra is prepared with a water-soluble lubricant containing 2% lidocaine. The external genitalia are prepped with an antiseptic solution such as povidone/iodine. A spinal or general anesthetic is administered if the cystoscopy is done before a surgical procedure such as transurethral resection of the prostate or bladder tumor. Instruct the client in the preoperative protocol for spinal or general anesthesia and obtain consent (see Chapter 16). Clients who have artificial joints, cardiac valvular disease, or valve replacement require prophylactic antibiotic therapy before the procedure to prevent the development of subacute bacterial endocarditis.

Postprocedure Care

Hematuria (red or pink-tinged urine) is expected after cystoscopy. Instruct the client to force fluids and to report any frank bleeding or clots in the urine or manifestations of urinary tract, gram-negative shock, or systemic infection (tachycardia, back pain, hypotension, dysuria, fever, or chills). Warm baths and NSAIDs may relieve dysuria. If acute urinary retention occurs after cystoscopy, intermittent bladder catheterization is required. Belladonna and opium suppositories or antispasmodics, may relieve bladder spasms. Antibiotics may be prescribed to prevent postprocedure infection.

Ureteroscopy, Ureteropyeloscopy, and Nephroscopy

Endoscopic procedures for the upper urinary tracts (see Chapter 36) include the following:

- *Ureteroscopy*, performed for diagnostic as well as therapeutic purposes, is used to evaluate radiologic filling defects, gross hematuria, and malignant cytology as well as to survey the ureters after conservative therapy for malignant tumors. Additional information regarding the grade and extent of malignant tumors can be obtained with ureteroscopic biopsy. Ureteroscopy has been performed safely in pregnancy.[22]
- *Flexible ureteropyeloscopy* allows visualization, diagnosis, and treatment of the ureteral as well as intrarenal collecting system pathology in a large number of clients.[22]
- *Nephroscopy* is performed with a flexible ureteroscope through a percutaneous nephrostomy tract. It is usually used during percutaneous nephrolithotomy, although it can be used as a second-look procedure to remove residual renal calculi and to diagnose upper urinary tract pathology and monitor treatment. It is useful in clients with conduit urinary diversions.

These procedures allow direct visualization of the ureter and kidney. The client is placed in a Trendelenburg

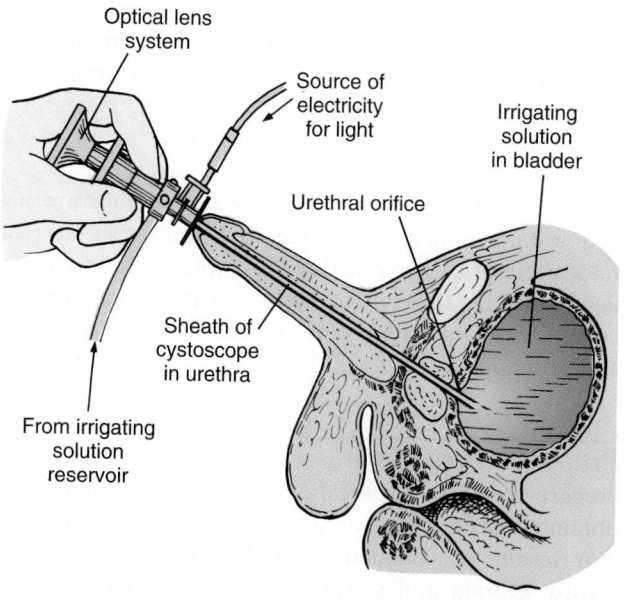

FIGURE 34-7 Cystoscope in the male bladder.

Labels in figure:
Optical lens system
Source of electricity for light
Irrigating solution in bladder
Urethral orifice
Sheath of cystoscope in urethra
From irrigating solution reservoir

position, and general or regional anesthesia or intravenous sedation is administered. Manipulation of the lower urinary tract, especially dilation of the ureteral orifice, can cause discomfort.

Preprocedure Care

Client preparation includes ensuring sterile urine, administering a perioperative broad-spectrum antibiotic, giving the client nothing by mouth, and obtaining consent. A history of previous radical surgery or ureteral manipulation should be known before ureteroscopic examination because it may make the procedure more difficult or impossible to complete successfully.

Postprocedure Care

Complications, including perforation, avulsion, submucosal dissection, and thermal injury, can occur, although most are recognized at the time of the procedure. Stricture may be a late complication. Observe for abdominal pain as well as infection, ureteral colic, and bleeding. A ureteral stent or temporary diversion catheter is left in place for at least 48 hours and up to 6 weeks if injury is known or suspected. Encourage the client to force fluids, and continue prophylactic antibiotics as ordered after the procedure.

Biopsy

Biopsies for malignancy in the urinary tract can be done transurethrally (kidney, ureter, bladder, and urethra) and transrectally (prostate). Biopsy of the kidney can be performed by either a percutaneous or an open surgical approach.

Transurethral Biopsy

Biopsy of a suspicious lesion in the bladder that is discovered during cystourethroscopy is done with the client under regional or general anesthesia. Biopsy specimens of surrounding bladder tissue are also taken randomly to evaluate the rest of the bladder. Care of the client is the same as for the client undergoing endoscopy but also involves preparation for anesthesia (see Chapter 16).

Intervention includes assisting the client in anesthesia recovery as well as using comfort measures for urethral pain, bladder spasms, flank pain, and dysuria, which are commonly experienced after biopsy. Instruct the client to watch for manifestations of urinary tract infection or infection of the puncture site and to report these promptly after the procedure.

Transrectal Prostate Biopsy

Biopsy of the prostate gland is performed via a rectal approach. The biopsy specimen usually is obtained with a multiple-core biopsy needle guided by ultrasonography.

The procedure is done in an outpatient setting when preliminary tests indicate the presence of prostate cancer. Before the procedure, instruct the client to avoid aspirin for 10 days and NSAIDs (excluding cyclooxygenase-2 [COX-2] inhibitors) for 48 hours. Clients taking warfarin (Coumadin) need to be off the medication for several days or long enough to obtain an International Normalized Ratio (INR) less than 1.5. Conversion to low-molecular-weight heparin in the periprocedure period may be necessary if discontinuation of warfarin (Coumadin) is too risky. A urine specimen is obtained for culture to ensure sterile urine. Prophylactic antibiotics are given for 1 to 3 days.

Observe for vasovagal reactions during or immediately following biopsy. Instruct clients that they may experience dysuria, hematuria, hematospermia, or rectal bleeding. Urinary retention or fever, chills, and manifestations of bacterial sepsis should be reported. (See Chapter 39 for additional discussion of prostate biopsy.)

Percutaneous Renal Biopsy

Percutaneous biopsy of the renal pelvis is used to diagnose benign and malignant masses, establish a prognosis, and follow progression and response to treatment. Renal biopsy is contraindicated for clients who have a solitary kidney, malignant tumors, hydronephrosis, infection or abscess, serious hypertension, or coagulation disorders. Small-gauge (21- to 25-gauge) needles are used for cytologic examination, and larger-gauge automated (14- to 20-gauge) needles are used to obtain tissue cores for histopathologic examination (Figure 34-8). Guided imaging such as fluoroscopy, ultrasonography, CT scanning, or MRI is used to help avoid large blood vessels. The physician inserts the biopsy needle as the client inspires deeply, and the client must be able to cooperate. Complications after biopsy include hemorrhage, pneumothorax, infection, and laceration or perforation of the kidney. Hematuria occurs in most clients but should resolve in 48 to 72 hours.

Brush biopsies of lesions of the upper tract urothelium are performed with a steel or nylon brush inserted via a ureteral catheter with endoscopic guidance. Biopsies of the renal pelvis, calices, and ureter can be obtained with this approach (see earlier discussion of ureteroscopy).

Preprocedure Care

Prepare the client for local anesthesia (see Chapter 16), obtain consent, and give nothing by mouth. Determine that results of coagulation studies are in the client's record. Obtain and record baseline vital signs. Clients are often managed in an outpatient setting with conscious sedation.

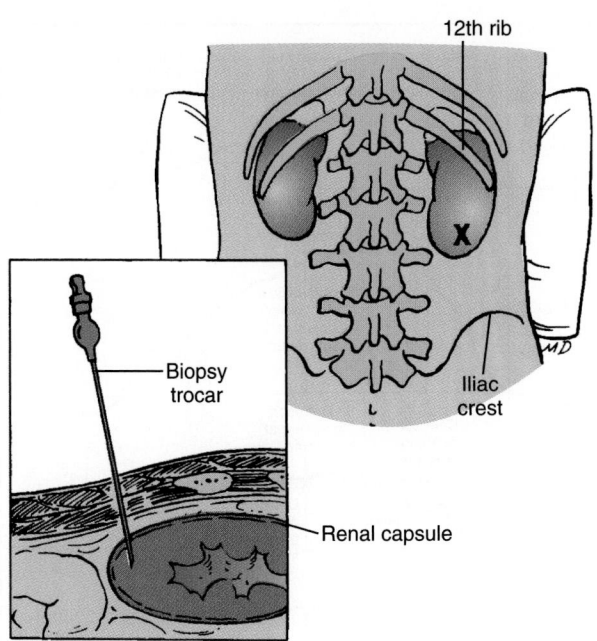

FIGURE 34-8 Percutaneous renal biopsy showing location of the trocar.

Postprocedure Care

Immediately after the biopsy, apply pressure to the puncture site for 20 minutes. Apply a sterile dressing. Pressure may be maintained by having the client lie on a sandbag placed against the biopsy site. Check the puncture site for bleeding and monitor vital signs. Force fluids to promote urination and to prevent clot formation, which can lead to urine obstruction.

Observe each voiding for hematuria; protocol may require checking each specimen with a dipstick for microscopic blood. Postbiopsy hematocrit levels are usually monitored.

The time for bed rest varies; clients may be discharged between 4 and 24 hours after biopsy. Encourage limited activity for the first 24 hours to prevent bleeding.

Complications after renal biopsy include gross hematuria, pain, infection, decreased hematocrit, and hypotension indicative of hemorrhage. Instruct the client to report immediately fever, increasing pain levels (back, flank, or shoulder), bleeding from the puncture site, weakness, dizziness, grossly bloody urine, or dysuria. Activity should be restricted if blood is seen in the urine. Advise the client to avoid strenuous lifting, physical exertion, or trauma to the biopsy site for up to 2 weeks after discharge.

Open Renal Biopsy

Open renal biopsy is indicated for tissue diagnosis and evaluation of the severity of renal disease; it is also used for evaluation of renal function in clients who are candidates for reconstructive surgery. It is preferred over percutaneous biopsy for clients with solitary kidney or co-

agulopathy and provides more tissue for analysis. The client requires preparation for local or general anesthesia (see Chapter 16) as well as renal function and coagulation studies. The procedure requires an extraperitoneal flank incision to permit direct visualization of the kidney.

After surgery, monitor vital signs, fluid balance, wound hemostasis, urine color, and pain levels. Complications and client management are similar to those for percutaneous renal biopsy (see earlier discussion) and general anesthesia.

Urodynamic Studies

Urodynamic studies are used to evaluate manifestations of voiding dysfunction related to pathology of the lower urinary tract (bladder and urethra). Studies include uroflowmetry, cystometry, pressure flow study, electromyography (EMG), leak point pressure (LPP), and urethral pressure profile. These studies can be performed with video or fluoroscopic capabilities.

Uroflowmetry

Urine flow rate is a measure of interaction between detrusor measure and urethral resistance. *Uroflowmetry* is a simple noninvasive procedure to measure the peak flow rate of urine in milliliters per second by having the client void into a special funnel device with a spinning disk at the base. A computerized module attached to the device digitally calculates a graph of the voiding episode. The graph yields information about peak and mean urine flow rates, duration of voiding, and the volume voided (Figure 34-9). It is indicated in clients with suspected bladder outlet obstruction. If impaired detrusor contractility is suspected, concomitant measurement of detrusor activity is recommended because uroflowmetry alone cannot distinguish between urethral obstruction and impaired detrusor contraction. Bladder outlet obstruction will diminish peak urine flow rates, although high detrusor pressures can compensate, resulting in a normal value. Peak urine flow rates are better at establishing clients with BPH than average flow rates. Peak flow rates greater than 15 ml/sec appear to have poorer treatment outcomes after prostate surgery.[22]

Instruct the client to prepare for the test by having a full bladder. Accuracy of the measurement depends on a voided volume of at least 125 ml, although clients should avoid overfilling the bladder. Complications or risks associated with this test are minimal. The bladder may be further evaluated for postvoid residual volume with ultrasonography (see earlier discussion of ultrasonography of the bladder).

Cystometry

Cystometry is a graph that shows vesical pressure as a function of volume and assesses detrusor activity, sensation, capacity, and compliance. The bladder is filled

FIGURE 34-9 Diagram of a normal uroflow curve showing frequently measured variables. *Shaded area* shows voided volume. *Dotted lines* show how voided volume is divided into time and flow rate. **A,** *Qura,* urine flow rate; **B,** *Qvol,* voided volume. (From Walsh, P.C., et al. [Eds.]. [2002]. *Campbell's urology* [8th ed.]. Philadelphia: W.B. Saunders.)

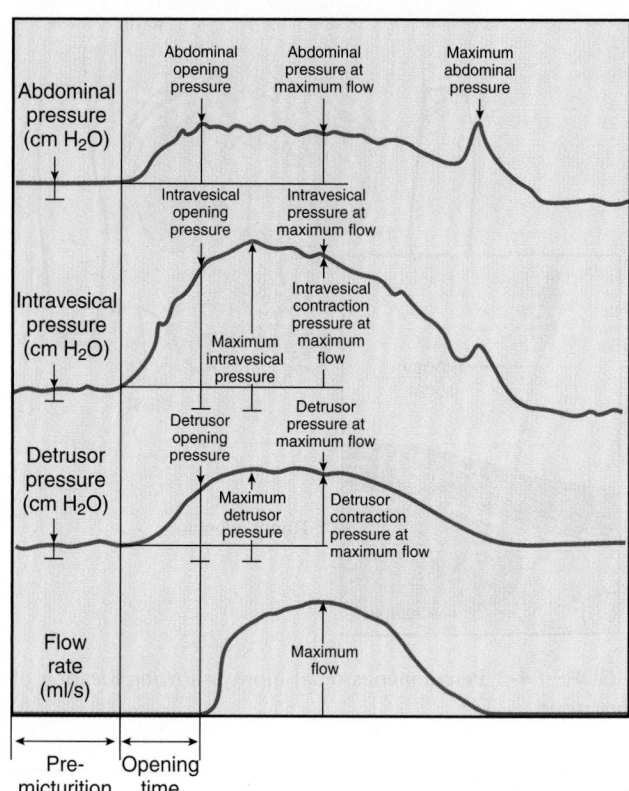

FIGURE 34-10 Diagram of a pressure flow graph with recommended terminology. (From Walsh, P.C., et al. [Eds.]. [2002]. *Campbell's urology* [8th ed.]. Philadelphia: W.B. Saunders.)

through a urethral catheter at a rate between 10 and 100 ml/min. A second catheter in the rectum or vagina measures intra-abdominal pressure, which is then subtracted from the vesical pressure measurement to obtain an accurate representation of the detrusor and bladder wall smooth muscle activity during filling and voiding. Cystometry is indicated for evaluating bladder outlet obstruction and urinary incontinence.

Pressure Flow Study

The pressure flow study is a combination of cystometry and urine flow rate. It can help to distinguish between poor detrusor contractility and bladder outlet obstruction (Figure 34-10).

Sphincter Electromyography

Electromyography is a measurement of electrical activity in the striated muscles of the urethral or anal sphincter or perineal floor muscles, and is often performed with cystometry. EMG evaluates for detrusor or sphincter dyssynergia, which occurs when the sphincter cannot relax or becomes overactive during detrusor contraction with voiding. This disorder can cause elevated postvoid residual volumes, urinary tract infection, or urinary retention, and it occurs in neurologic disorders.

Patch, wire, or needle electrodes are positioned on the perineum to monitor the response of the pelvic floor muscles to bladder filling and voiding. The patch and wire electrodes are painless but are prone to recording artifact. The needle electrodes provide detailed information but can cause discomfort and limit mobility. The sacral arc may be tested by eliciting the bulbocavernosal reflex during EMG (see earlier discussion of assessment of this reflex).

Leak Point Pressure

Leak point pressure is useful for clients with stress urinary incontinence or low urethral compliance. For clients with low compliance, it is measured during cystometry and determines the degree of vesical pressure present when there is leakage from the urethra without provocative maneuvers. High detrusor LPP >40 cm H_2O may result in hydronephrosis over time. Valsalva LPP measures sphincter function to determine the type of stress incontinence. The bladder is filled to capacity and the client is asked to perform a gradual Valsalva maneuver, increasing the vesical pressure until urinary leakage occurs. Cystometry measurements are taken of vesical and abdominal pressures during Valsalva, and

LPP is defined as the lowest pressure at which leakage occurs.

Urethral Pressure Profile

The urethral pressure profile measures sphincter closure pressure and evaluates urethral incompetence. The urethral length and continuous urethral response to filling, voiding, and provocative measures, such as coughing, may be assessed. A specialized catheter, either a membrane catheter or a catheter mounted with microtransducers, is withdrawn slowly through the urethra while recording pressure readings at every level. This test can be done in cases of sphincter dysfunction, urinary incontinence, or detrusor or sphincter dyssynergia.

Voiding Cystourethrogram

Voiding cystourethrogram allows radiographic visualization of the lower urinary tract during bladder filling and voiding to determine the source of bladder outlet obstruction, integrity of the bladder sphincter, and presence of vesicoureteral reflux as well as bladder wall abnormalities. It may be performed after other urodynamic studies.

Multichannel Fluoroscopic Urodynamics

This study is performed by filling the bladder with radiographic contrast to perform urodynamics. It has advantages over urodynamic studies and voiding cystourethrogram in that synchronous measures of abdominal pressure, urethral pressure, uroflow, and EMG measurements together with radiographic guidance allows evaluation of the complex interplay between all urodynamic variables. Results can be recorded on videotape for later evaluation.

Preprocedure Care

All urodynamic testing except uroflowmetry requires a negative Gram stain or urine culture. Advise clients to force fluids and to abstain from voiding approximately 1 to 2 hours before the procedure if possible. Clients may be advised to discontinue any medications that might affect urinary function before the study. The study should not be performed after recent cystoscopy or prostate biopsy. Clients who have artificial joints or cardiac valvular disease, valve replacements, and aortic grafts should have appropriate prophylactic antibiotics.

Explain how the procedure is performed, the catheters and equipment used, the client's role, and what the client can expect to feel during and after the study. If multichannel fluoroscopic urodynamics are measured, explain the need to have two or three people in the room (the nurse or technician performing the study, a radiologic technician, and possibly a urologist). Reassure the client that every effort will be made to preserve privacy.

Postprocedure Care

Teach the client to watch for and report manifestations of urinary tract infection, urgency, and frequency persisting after 24 hours. Encourage the client to drink at least two 8-ounce glasses of water each hour for 4 hours after the procedure. A warm bath or washcloth applied to the perineum may help alleviate the urethral irritation that is common after the procedure.

CONCLUSIONS

A thorough knowledge of the potential causes of elimination disorders is essential to obtain a pertinent health history and to perform an accurate physical assessment. Careful assessment facilitates formulation of accurate nursing and medical diagnoses and planning for the optimal treatment of the client. Knowledge of diagnostic testing is necessary to prepare the client for the tests and to facilitate the diagnostic process.

BIBLIOGRAPHY

1. Bensoussan, A., et al. (1998). Treatment of irritable bowel syndrome with Chinese herbal medicine: A randomized controlled trial. *Journal of the American Medical Association, 280*(18), 1585-1589.
2. Blackington, E. (2000). Irritable bowel syndrome: An update on treatment options. *Advance for Nurse Practitioners, 8*(10), 32-40.
3. Boffetta, P., & Silverman, D.F. (2001). A meta-analysis of bladder cancer and diesel exhaust exposure. *Epidemiology, 12*(1), 125-130.
4. Dvorkin, L., & Song, K. (2002). Herbs for benign prostatic hyperplasia. *Annals of Pharmacotherapy, 36*(9), 1443-1452.
5. Fischbach, F. (2000). *Manual of laboratory studies and diagnostic tests* (6th ed). Philadelphia: Lippincott Williams & Wilkins.
6. Giese, L.A. (2000). A study of alternative health care use for gastrointestinal disorders. *Gastroenterology Nursing, 23*(1), 19-27.
7. Goldman, L., & Bennett, J.C. (2000). *Cecil textbook of medicine* (21st ed.). Philadelphia: W.B. Saunders.
8. Gray, M., Albo, M., & Huffstutler, S. (2002). Interstitial cystitis: A guide to recognition, evaluation and management for nurse practitioners. *Journal of Wound, Ostomy and Continence Nursing, 29*(2), 93-102.

9. Greenberg, R.S., et al. (2001). A meta-analysis of cohort studies describing mortality and cancer incidence among chemical workers in the United States and Western Europe. *Epidemiology, 12*(6), 727-740.

 10. Grossfeld, G.D., et al. (2001). Asymptomatic microscopic hematuria in adults: Summary of the American Urologic Association best practice policy recommendations. *American Family Physician, 63*(6), 1145-1154.

 11. Kaye, J.A., Wald Myers, M., & Jick, H. (2001). Acetaminophen and the risk of renal and bladder cancer in the general practice research database. *Epidemiology, 12*(6), 690-694.

 12. Kolonel, L.N. (1999). Dietary fat and prostate cancer: Current status. *Journal of the National Cancer Institute, 91*(5), 414-428.

13. Langmead, L., & Rampton, D.S. (2001). Review article: Herbal treatment in gastrointestinal and liver disease—benefits and dangers. *Alimentary Pharmacologic Therapy, 15,* 1239-1252.

 14. Lustyk, M.K., et al. (2001). Does a physically active lifestyle improve symptoms in women with irritable bowel syndrome? *Gastroenterology Nursing, 24*(3), 129-137.

 15. Miller, B.A., et al. (1996). Racial/ethnic patterns of cancer in the United States 1988-1992. NCI, NIH Publication No. 96-4104, Bethesda, MD.

16. Olden, K.W. (2002). Diagnosis of irritable bowel syndrome. *Gastroenterology, 122,* 1701-1714.

17. Pignone M., et al. (2002). Screening for colorectal cancer in adults at average risk: A summary of the evidence for the U.S. Preventive Services Task Force. *Annals of Internal Medicine, 137*(2), 132-141.

18. Ransohoff, D.F., & Sandler, R.S. (2002). Screening for colorectal cancer. *The New England Journal of Medicine, 346*(1), 40-44.

19. Simpson, J., Scholefield, J.H., & Spiller, R.C. (2002). Pathogenesis of colonic diverticula. *British Journal of Surgery, 89*(5), 546-554.

20. Smith, R.A., et al. (2002). American Cancer Society guidelines for the early detection of cancer. *Ca: A Cancer Journal for Clinicians, 52*(1), 8-22.

21. Thompson, M.J., & Rivara, F.P. (2001). Bicycle related injuries. *American Family Physician, 63*(10), 2007-2014.

22. Walsh, P.C., et al. (2002). *Campbell's urology* (8th ed.). Philadelphia: W.B. Saunders.

23. Wu, X.C., et al. (2001). Subsite-specific incidence rate and stage of disease in colorectal cancer by race, gender, and age group in the United States, 1992-1997. *Cancer, 92*(10), 2547-2554.

24. Zhang, B., et al. (2002). A case-control study on risk of changing food consumption for colorectal cancer. *Cancer Investigation, 20*(4), 458-463.

Management of Clients with Intestinal Disorders

Helen Murdock Rogers

The client with an intestinal disorder usually has a problem with bowel elimination. Hence the most common nursing diagnoses are *Constipation, Bowel Incontinence,* and *Diarrhea.* Additional nursing diagnoses are *Acute Pain, Chronic Pain, Imbalanced Nutrition: Less Than Body Requirements, Deficient Fluid Volume,* and *Disturbed Body Image.*

GENERAL CLINICAL MANIFESTATIONS

Disorders of the intestine disrupt one or more of its functions. They can slow, obstruct, or accelerate the movement of intestinal contents *(chyme)* through the intestine, or they can disrupt the secretion, motility, and absorption of intestinal contents. Disorders occur in response to inflammation, tumors, infections, obstructions, and changes in the structure of the intestine. Manifestations of intestinal disorders vary according to which function (motility, digestion, or absorption) is disturbed. The major manifestations of dysfunction are hemorrhage, pain, nausea and vomiting, distention, constipation, diarrhea, and abnormal fecal contents.

Hemorrhage

Bleeding can be caused by trauma, ulceration, inflammation, or a growth that erodes through a blood vessel. The usual manifestation is blood in the stool *(hematochezia)* rather than in vomitus *(hematemesis)*. The amount of bleeding varies from a minute quantity that is invisible except by testing *(occult blood)* to large quantities that cause stools to be bright red to tarry black *(melena)*. The stool color is affected by (1) the digestive processes acting on the blood and (2) the rapidity with which chyme passes through the bowel. For instance, slow bleeding from the duodenum may not increase peristalsis and may produce a tarry stool. If the rate of bleeding or peristalsis increases, subsequent stools may become brighter red.

Pain

Pain may be acute or chronic. Mechanical, inflammatory, or ischemic changes cause pain by stimulating the nerve endings in the muscular or submucosal layers of bowel wall. Mechanical factors cause pain by stretching and distending the bowel; these actions then activate

Nursing Outcomes Classification (NOC)
for Nursing Diagnoses—Clients with Intestinal Disorders

Acute Pain and Chronic Pain
  Comfort Level
  Pain: Disruptive Effects
Bowel Incontinence
  Bowel Elimination
  Bowel Continence
  Tissue Integrity
Constipation
  Bowel Elimination
  Hydration
Deficient Fluid Volume
  Bowel Elimination
  Fluid Balance
  Hydration
Deficient Knowledge
  Knowledge: Treatment Procedures

Diarrhea
  Fluid Balance
  Hydration
  Symptom Severity
Disturbed Body Image
  Grief Resolution
  Psychosocial Adjustment: Life Change
  Self-Esteem
Effective Therapeutic Regimen Management
  Health Beliefs: Perceived Ability to Perform
  Knowledge: Treatment Regimen
  Participation: Health Care Decisions
Imbalanced Nutrition: Less Than Body Requirements
  Nutritional Status

Ineffective Coping
  Coping
  Decision-Making
  Role Performance
  Social Support
Risk for Infection
  Risk Detection
Risk for Injury
  Risk Control
  Safety Status: Physical Injury
Risk for Sexual Dysfunction
  Sexual Functioning
  Body Image
  Self-Esteem

---

nerve endings. For example, edema and vascular congestion cause painful stretching. Biochemical mediators that are released during the inflammatory process cause pain by stimulating nerve endings.

Obstruction of blood supply to the intestine *(ischemia)* also can cause pain. Acute or partial occlusion of the mesenteric artery causes intermittent pain during digestion because of the greater need for blood at that time. Occlusion can occur in the major artery or one of the smaller branches.

Discomfort occurs in various places and is characterized as three types:

- *Visceral pain* arises from a stimulus acting on the involved portion of the bowel. It results in a diffuse, poorly localized pain that clients describe as gnawing, burning, or cramping.
- *Somatic pain* arises from the parietal peritoneum and is more localized and intense than visceral pain.
- *Referred pain* is visceral pain felt at a distance from an affected organ.

Nausea and Vomiting

In intestinal disorders, nausea results from distention of the duodenum. Vomiting occurs from changes in the integrity of the intestinal wall (as in gastroenteritis) or from changes in the motility of the bowel (such as caused by an obstruction). Vomitus that contains fecal matter usually indicates a distal obstruction in the small intestine.

Distention

Distention is caused by excessive gas in the intestines. It may be due to the inability to digest adequately a specific nutrient, such as lactose, or it may result from a defect in intestinal motility. *Flatus* (passing of bowel gas) may be another clinical manifestation.

Diarrhea

Diarrhea is defined as an increase in the frequency, volume, and fluid content of stool. Rapid propulsion of intestinal contents through the small bowel results in diarrhea and may lead to a serious fluid volume deficit. Common causes are infections, malabsorption syndromes, medications, allergies, and systemic diseases.

Constipation

Constipation is the infrequent or difficult passage of stools or the passage of hard or pellet stools. It is a common manifestation that can be caused by inadequate fluid or bulk, mechanical blockage of the passage of intestinal contents (by a tumor), or slow peristalsis.

Abnormalities in Fecal Content

The presence of fats or other abnormal constituents, normally absorbed from the stool, indicates malabsorption. Other fecal abnormalities that can aid in diagnosis are bacteria, parasites, pus, blood, and abnormal quantities of mucus from the colon.

INFLAMMATORY DISORDERS

Inflammation can occur in any portion of the bowel and can be caused by organisms, toxins produced by organisms, infiltration of the bowel wall by granulomatous processes, trauma, medications, and injury from radiation.

VIRAL AND BACTERIAL INFECTIONS: GASTROENTERITIS

Gastroenteritis is an inflammation of the stomach and intestinal tract that primarily affects the small bowel. The major clinical manifestations are diarrhea of varying degrees and abdominal pain and cramping. Associated clinical manifestations are nausea, vomiting, fever, anorexia, distention, *tenesmus* (straining on defecation), and *borborygmi* (hyperactive bowel sounds).

Gastroenteritis occurs throughout the world, often in epidemic outbreaks. Contaminated food and water are major sources of these diseases and cause thousands of deaths yearly. The incidence of infections caused by food-borne diseases is rising. These diseases cost society billions of dollars each year. According to the Centers for Disease Control and Prevention (CDC), 33,000,000 cases of food-borne diseases occur annually in the United States, about 1 of every 10 Americans; about 9000 die. *Salmonella* and related strains cause an estimated four million cases of food-borne illnesses each year and, *Campylobacter* causes an estimated 2 million illnesses each year. Another bacteria, *Escherichia coli 0157:H7*, causes an estimated 30,000 infections and 250 deaths annually.

Infection with *Clostridium difficile (C. difficile),* also known as pseudomembranous colitis, is a bacterial dysentery commonly seen in clients who have been receiving large doses of antibiotics or who have taken antibiotics for longer than 7 days. Other medications that may predispose individuals to *C. difficile* are H$_2$ blockers, preoperative bowel preparations, and chemotherapy. *C. difficile* occurs most often in clients 65 years of age and older; in immunocompromised clients; in clients with chronic lung disease or chronic renal failure; in clients undergoing gastrointestinal (GI) procedures; and clients who use enemas, stool softeners, and GI stimulants. It is also more common in clients who undergo prolonged hospital stays, especially in intensive care units (ICUs), in clients transferred from small hospitals to tertiary care centers, and in clients placed in semiprivate rooms or wards. The condition is the most common cause of nosocomial infections in hospitalized clients, especially those undergoing surgical procedures.

Etiology and Risk Factors

Pathogens that cause GI disease are transmitted by the fecal-oral route, from person to person, and through ingestion of fecally contaminated food and water. GI infections are often referred to as "food poisoning" because food is frequently the vehicle for transmission of actively growing microbes or their toxins. Common bacterial sources of contaminated foods are eggs *(Salmonella),* raw or undercooked meat *(E. coli),* and chicken *(Campylobacter jejuni).* Outbreaks of food-borne viral infections are almost entirely caused by fecally contaminated shellfish. Unpasteurized milk, apple juice, ice

cream, and mayonnaise are also sources of food-borne infection. A multinational outbreak of food poisoning occurred from contaminated alfalfa sprouts *(Salmonella),* and also an outbreak in the United States of the food-related illness listeriosis was caused by the bacteria *Listeria.* Other causative organisms are *Vibrio cholerae* (cholera), *Shigella* bacilli (dysentery), and *Staphylococcus aureus* (staphylococcal food poisoning). The incubation period for all viral and bacterial infections ranges from 6 hours to 4 or 5 days.

Health-promotion actions for avoiding such GI infections involve instructing clients about (1) good hand-washing technique after defecation and before handling food and (2) obtaining available vaccinations against bacterial and viral gastroenteritis. Encourage cleanliness and sanitation as well as proper food handling, preparation and storage techniques, such as cooking meats to 150° F, cooking chicken to 170° F, and not allowing food to sit at room temperature for long periods. Warn clients not to eat food containing raw eggs and to refrain from buying cans, boxes, or jars that are damaged. Advise clients to avoid the use of antibiotics over a long time. Teach travelers going to developing countries about safe food practices, such as avoiding tap water, ice cubes, milk products, raw meat or seafood, salads, and foods that cannot be cooked or peeled.

Health maintenance activities include the assessment of clients who are receiving high or continued doses of antibiotics for manifestations of *C. difficile* infection and other manifestations of GI infection secondary to antibiotic use. Health-restoration interventions involve client self-management of manifestations. Instruct clients to follow their medication regimen and to call their health care provider if (1) manifestations continue for several days, (2) they might be dehydrated, or (3) body temperature is higher than 100° F. Promote bowel rest and replacement of fluids and electrolytes as needed.

Pathophysiology

Normally, human intestinal flora protects the bowel from colonization of pathogens; however, the intestinal flora can be (1) disrupted by harmful bacteria and viruses that cause tissue damage and inflammation or (2) depressed by antibiotic therapy, administered either orally or parenterally. Antibiotics most often implicated in the depression of normal flora are clindamycin, penicillins, cephalosporins, and aminoglycosides.

Pathogens cause tissue damage and inflammation by releasing endotoxins that stimulate the mucosal lining of the intestine, resulting in greater secretion of water and electrolytes into the intestinal lumen. The active secretion of chloride and bicarbonate ions in the small bowel leads to inhibition of sodium reabsorption. To balance the excess sodium, large amounts of protein-rich fluids are secreted in the bowel, overwhelming the large bowel's ability to reabsorb the fluid and leading to diarrhea. Pathogens also cause damage and inflammation by invading and destroying the mucosal lining of the bowel, resulting in bleeding and ulceration. When the integrity of the GI tract is impaired, its ability to carry out digestive and absorptive functions can be affected. See Figure 35-1 for pathophysiology of *C. difficile*-associated diarrhea (CDAD).

FIGURE 35-1 How *Clostridium difficile*–associated diarrhea (CDAD) develops. **A,** *C. difficile* bacteria attach to intestinal lining and begin to secrete toxins A and B. **B,** Toxin A, an enterotoxin, causes hemorrhaging and fluid leakage into the gut. Toxin B, a potent cytotoxin, decreases cellular protein synthesis. A third substance secreted by toxins A and B inhibits gut motility. (From Sheff, B. [1999]. Minimizing the threat of *C. difficile*. *Nursing 99,* 33-39.)

Clinical Manifestations

The universal manifestation of gastroenteritis is diarrhea, which occurs in varying intensity, depending on the organism involved and the health status of the individual client. The diarrhea may be mild (two to three stools per day) or intense (more than 10 watery stools per day). Nausea, vomiting, and anorexia may occur from abdominal distention caused by increased fluid content and undigested food. Abdominal pain, cramping, and borborygmi may occur from gas released from undigested food, irritation of bowel mucosa, and distention of the intestines. The client may have a fever, depending on the causative organism. The stool may test positive for leukocytes and may contain the causative organism as well as mucus and varying amounts of blood. The "gold standard" for *C. difficile* is the cytoxin neutralization test that confirms the presence of toxins in the stool. Other stool tests for confirming the diagnosis of *C. difficile* are the latex agglutination test, which is less sensitive than the previous test, and the newest test, enzyme-linked immunosorbent assay (ELISA), which is rapid and reliable. An endoscopic examination will reveal a bowel mucosa that is inflamed, edematous, and containing numerous plaques. Diagnosis can be confirmed by biopsy of the intestine.

Prognosis

Most cases of gastroenteritis are temporarily disabling and self-limiting, with resolution in 1 to 5 days; however, gastroenteritis can be fatal in debilitated, older, or very young people. Early detection and treatment with fluids and electrolytes are critical to prevent death or disability in such cases. Up to 16% of clients infected with *E. coli 0157:H7* develop hemolytic uremic syndrome (HUS), which causes death in 3% to 5% of the people it affects. Of the clients who survive HUS, 10% to 50% develop chronic sequelae that include chronic renal failure, cardiomyopathy, pulmonary problems, chronic hypertension, and encephalopathy. HUS is the major cause of renal failure in children.

PARASITIC INFECTIONS

More than two million cases of parasitic illnesses are recorded annually in the United States. An increasing number of people in the United States are being exposed to parasitic diseases because of increased international travel, international food trade, and consumption of raw and undercooked foods. Currently more than 100 parasites are known to cause food-borne disease, and many have only recently been identified.

Protozoa

Protozoa organisms are parasites that replicate in the intestines of infected hosts and are excreted in the feces. They are transmitted in the same way as bacterial and viral pathogens; however, fewer numbers or organisms are needed to produce clinical manifestations. Enteric protozoa are the leading cause of water-borne disease and are becoming more frequently implicated as causes of food-borne infections. Several new protozoa have been identified, for example, *Cyclospora*, which has been linked to contaminated raspberries. Some protozoa are becoming resistant to methods used to eliminate them, such as chlorination.

Giardiasis, the most common protozoal diarrheal illness in the United States, is caused by the protozoan *Giardia lamblia*. It generally spreads through spoiled food or surfaces contaminated with feces from infected animals or humans. It can also be spread by swallowing contaminated recreational water found in swimming pools, hot tubs, Jacuzzis, and lakes. Most infected people are asymptomatic; however, those with manifestations may present several weeks after exposure with nausea, vomiting, excessive foul flatulence, and malabsorption, which results in weight loss and copious, foul-smelling, greasy stools. Organisms infect the small intestine mucosa and submucosa and are found in the stool. The medications used for treatment include metronidazole (Flagyl), quinacrine (Atabrine), and furazolidone (Furoxone). A new vaccine may be available in the near future; however, at present no agent is effective in preventing giardiasis.

Cryptosporidium is associated with water-borne and food-borne outbreaks in nursing homes and day care centers. It is spread by drinking contaminated water or swimming in infected lakes or swimming pools. The organism attaches itself to the intestinal epithelium, causing surface damage, inflammation, and watery diarrhea.

Amebiasis produces diarrhea when a protozoan *(Entamoeba histolytica)* invades the lining of the colon. Manifestations include rectal inflammation as well as blood, pus, and amebae in the stool. Metronidazole (Flagyl) is the drug of choice for treatment.

Helminths

The intestinal tract may be infested with any of several species of helminths or parasitic worms, including *Ascaris* (roundworms), *Enterobius* (pinworms), *Trichinella spiralis* (which causes trichinosis), and various species of *Cestoda* (tapeworms). These parasites are found worldwide. Worm infestations, contracted through the skin or from ingesting contaminated food or water, can cause serious, even fatal disease, if the parasites are not eradicated from the intestinal tract. Worms also may cause urinary tract infections or pruritus ani. Fortunately, most of these parasites are susceptible to medications such as mebendazole and pyrantel pamoate. Piperazine and quinacrine hydrochloride also may be used, but they have more side effects. Treatment of all household members may reduce reinfection.

Schistosomiasis is caused by a blood fluke (a parasitic flatworm). The infection is prevalent worldwide, occurring in about 1 in 30 people. The cercariae (larvae) of the parasite penetrate the skin, migrate to the liver via the lungs, and remain in intrahepatic portal venules until the worm matures. The mature worm, which does not multiply within humans, then moves into its final habitat. Depending on the species involved, the worm may settle in the veins of the large bowel, small bowel, or bladder, where it lays eggs. These eggs, which form pseudotubercles (small, nobby prominences), have been found in every system of the body. Schistosomiasis may have mild or severe manifestations, depending on the species of worms involved and the number present. Laboratory studies to identify the species are completed before pharmacologic treatment with oxamniquine, metrifonate, praziquantel, or niridazole is started.

Outcome Management for Viral, Bacterial, and Parasitic Infections
■ Medical Management

Treatment for food-borne illnesses is usually supportive as most infections are self-limiting. Most infected clients do not benefit from antibiotics. An exception to this is traveler's diarrhea that is usually caused by *E. coli*, rotavirus, or salmonella. Treatment with a fluoroquinolone has proven to be effective.

Rest the Bowel. Rest, with nothing by mouth (NPO [from the Latin *nil per os*]) until the vomiting has stopped, is the best intervention.

Decrease Diarrhea. When diarrhea is severe and does not resolve within 2 to 3 days, the infecting organism needs to be identified from stool specimens and blood samples. Medications to decrease intestinal motility are usually not administered because the infecting agents need to be eliminated, particularly *C. difficile* infection, because the bacteria multiply if GI motility is slowed and the bacteria are retained. For severe cases of *C. difficile* infection, the client is placed on metronidazole orally or intravenously. Vancomycin is used if this proves to be ineffective.

Restore Fluids and Electrolytes. The client is started on small amounts of clear liquids as tolerated. An electrolyte replacement beverage may be given. The diet is advanced after 24 hours as tolerated. If the client has a severe fluid depletion, an intravenous (IV) agent such as 0.45% sodium chloride may be required. A potassium supplement may be ordered if the client's serum potassium level is low.

■ Nursing Management of the Medical Client

Most clients present with an acute onset of diarrhea. Carefully note a description of the diarrhea, including (1) onset; (2) number, color, and consistency of stools;

and (3) accompanying manifestations, such as nausea and vomiting. Ask the client about recent foreign travel and antibiotic use. Obtain a diet history that includes all foods the client has eaten in the past 5 days. Ask especially about foods known to be at high risk for causing infection.

Assess the client's abdomen. Examination may reveal hyperactive bowel sounds, distention, and tenderness. Dehydration and electrolyte imbalance may be present, depending on the amount of fluids and electrolytes lost. Assess muscle weakness and fatigue that are due to hypokalemia. Metabolic alkalosis from bicarbonate loss is also a potential problem. Carefully examine all stools for blood and mucus, and record intake and output. Examine the client's anal area for irritation. After cleaning the area, apply a protective moisture barrier product for clients with irritation. Be especially cautious in caring for a client with a colostomy or ileostomy.

Administer anti-infective medications, such as antibiotic and antiparasitic agents, to treat the specific cause of the diarrhea if appropriate. Antidiarrheals may be ordered if the diarrhea is uncontrollable. If manifestations of fluid and electrolyte imbalance are noted, start IV fluids until oral fluids are tolerated. Begin clear liquids with electrolytes in small amounts until the client can tolerate toast and crackers. Advance the diet as tolerated.

Prevent spread of the disease to others. Remind the client to wash hands and maintain absolute cleanliness. If the client is hospitalized, transfer him or her to a private room and initiate contact isolation precautions. Follow the facility's protocol. Spores from *C. difficile* live for months on environmental surfaces, for example, toilets, bedpans, and floors. Therefore ensure meticulous cleaning of the environment and use dedicated equipment when possible. Follow the facility's guidelines for the disposal of contaminated equipment. Never use an electronic rectal thermometer because of the potential for spreading bacteria. Provide written and oral instructions regarding medications, diet, and rest as well as about when and how to report any continued problems. Teach family and visitors about precautions and how to follow procedures. Ensure them that their chance of becoming infected is remote.

Relapses and reinfection are common. Therefore the client should be closely monitored for any clinical manifestations of recurring disease.

APPENDICITIS

Appendicitis is an inflammation of the vermiform appendix that develops most commonly in adolescents and young adults (Figure 35-2). It can occur at any age but is rare in clients younger than 2 years and reaches a peak incidence in clients between 20 and 30 years. It is not common in older adults; however, when it does occur in such clients, rupture of the appendix is more common. Appendicitis affects 7% to 12% of the population.

FIGURE 35-2 Appendicitis. This appendix is inflamed and distended with yellowish pus. (From Price, S.A., & Wilson, L.M. [2003]. *Pathophysiology: Clinical concepts of disease process* [6th ed.]. St. Louis: Mosby. Courtesy Gerald D. Abrams, MD, Department of Pathology, University of Michigan—Ann Arbor.)

Etiology and Risk Factors

Appendicitis can be caused by the following:

- A fecalith (a fecal calculus, or stone) that occludes the lumen of the appendix
- Kinking of the appendix
- Swelling of the bowel wall
- Fibrous conditions in the bowel wall
- External occlusion of the bowel by adhesions

No particular risk factors for appendicitis have been identified. Because it is not preventable, early detection of the condition is important.

Pathophysiology

When the appendix becomes obstructed, the intraluminal pressure increases, leading to decreased venous drainage, thrombosis, edema, and bacterial invasion of the bowel wall. After the initial obstruction, the appendix becomes increasingly hyperemic, warm, and covered with exudate, progressing to gangrene and perforation.

Clinical Manifestations

The classic manifestations of appendicitis begin with acute abdominal pain that comes in waves. At first, the pain may be perceived merely as discomfort that makes the client feel that passing flatus or having a bowel movement will bring relief. Unfortunately, many clients take a laxative during this period, which may lead to rupture of the appendix and peritonitis.

The pain typically starts in the epigastrium or periumbilical region. It then shifts to the right lower quadrant as the inflammatory process spreads to involve the serosal layers of the bowel, thereby bringing the inflammatory process into contact with the peritoneum. The pain becomes steady rather than intermittent, and the client often *guards* or protects the area by lying still and drawing the legs up to relieve tension on the abdominal muscles.

Assessment also may reveal vomiting that begins after the pain starts, loss of appetite, low-grade fever, coated tongue, and bad breath. Mild leukocytosis is usually present, with the white blood cell (WBC) count between 10,000 and 15,000/mm³. Pain at McBurney's point, which lies midway between the right anterior superior iliac crest and the umbilicus, confirms the diagnosis.

Outcome Management
■ Surgical Management

Appendectomy

There is no medical treatment for appendicitis. Preoperatively, IV fluids and antibiotics are administered. Pain medication is withheld until the diagnosis is confirmed.

Indications. Surgical intervention involves removal of the appendix *(appendectomy)* within 24 to 48 hours of onset of the manifestations. The surgery can be performed through a small open incision or a laparoscope (a lighted scope used to visualize and remove the appendix). When the operation is performed in time, the mortality rate is less than 0.5%. Delay usually causes rupture of the organ and resultant peritonitis (see Peritonitis).

Complications. Perforation of the bowel is the most common complication. Antibiotics and surgical drainage are required if perforation occurs. Peritonitis may develop after perforation.

Outcomes. Following a laparoscopic procedure, the client is usually discharged in 24 to 48 hours. Another day of hospitalization may be indicated after an open surgical procedure. Lifting is restricted for 2 to 4 weeks. The client can resume all activities 4 to 6 weeks after surgery.

■ Nursing Management of the Surgical Client
Assessment

The client is usually admitted with severe abdominal pain. Carefully assess the pain, especially to determine its location. Also assess the client for rebound tenderness (sharp pain when pressure is released on abdomen after deep palpation) and the presence of peritonitis (see Peritonitis). Carefully assess the client's vital signs, fluid and electrolyte status, and laboratory data. The client with appendicitis should fast preoperatively.

Diagnosis, Outcomes, Interventions

Diagnosis: Acute Pain. One of the most appropriate nursing diagnoses for the client with acute appendicitis is *Acute Pain related to inflammation.*

Outcomes. The client describes decreased postoperative pain.

Interventions. An abrupt change in the character of the pain preoperatively may indicate perforation. Postoperatively, pain control, as described in Chapters 16 and 22, should be practiced. Sometimes pain medication is not given until the client is actually ready for surgery. Never give an enema or a laxative or apply heat to the abdomen of the client with appendicitis because any one of these actions may lead to bowel perforation.

Diagnosis: Risk for Deficient Fluid Volume. Another appropriate nursing diagnosis for the client with acute appendicitis is *Risk for Deficient Fluid Volume related to vomiting.*

Outcomes. The client maintains fluid and electrolyte balance, as evidenced by balanced intake and output and electrolyte levels within normal limits.

Interventions. As soon as the client is admitted, IV fluids are started to maintain fluid balance, with electrolytes added as needed. If the client is vomiting, a nasogastric (NG) tube may be inserted. Carefully measure intake and output.

Diagnosis: Risk for Infection. The diagnosis *Risk for Infection related to rupture of appendix* is common.

Outcomes. An infection will not develop, or rupture will be diagnosed early, as evidenced by (1) removal of the appendix before rupture or (2) prompt treatment of the rupture.

Interventions. Check the client's vital signs regularly, monitoring closely for an increase in temperature and a change in pulse and blood pressure, which may signify a ruptured appendix. Preoperative antibiotics are usually administered to reduce the infection. Monitor pain closely. If the pain becomes generalized throughout the abdomen and the abdomen becomes rigid and board-like, the appendix may have ruptured.

After surgery, monitor vital signs, urine output, level of consciousness, and IV therapy; also assess the client's respiratory status and the surgical wound. The client may have a drain, and if the appendix ruptured, packing may be present. Assess the dressings, provide wound care, reposition the client approximately every 2 hours, and adequately manage the client's pain.

The client who has had a ruptured appendix with an infected wound needs to be taught the proper way to care for the wound. Wound care usually involves irrigation of the wound with sterile saline and application of a sterile dressing at least several times a day. Assess the client's ability to function at home and to care for the wound. A home health care referral may be needed to assist the client with physical needs and to ensure that the wound is healing properly.

Evaluation

The usual outcome after an uncomplicated appendectomy is healing within a few weeks. If the appendix has ruptured, however, healing takes longer. With a ruptured appendix, healing cannot occur until the infection has cleared and the wound is clean. A secondary closure may be required after the wound is clean. Some incisions are left open to heal through granulation *(regeneration)* of tissue.

PERITONITIS

Peritonitis is inflammation of the peritoneal membrane. The *peritoneum* is a semipermeable two-layered sac filled with about 1500 ml of fluid. This sac covers all the organs in the abdominal cavity. Because it is well supplied with somatic nerves, stimulation of the parietal peritoneum that lines the abdominal and pelvic cavities causes sharp, well-localized pain. The visceral peritoneum is relatively insensitive.

Etiology and Risk Factors

Peritonitis can be primary or secondary. Major sources of inflammation are from the GI tract, from the external environment, and through the bloodstream. Normal flora of the intestine becomes a source of infection when they enter the sterile peritoneal cavity. The most common organism is *E. coli,* although streptococci, staphylococci, and pneumococci also may be involved. The peritoneum may produce an inflammatory reaction and wall off (prevent the spread of) a localized process to combat an infection if the stimulus is not too massive and if the source of infection does not continue.

There are no risk factors for peritonitis because the condition is a result of another problem. Causes include ruptured or gangrenous gallbladder, perforated peptic ulcer, perforated stomach or intestine secondary to cancer or inflammatory bowel disorders, bowel obstruction, penetrating wounds, and other conditions (such as acute pancreatitis and mesenteric thrombosis). The major preventive measures are early diagnosis of clients at risk for peritonitis and initiation of early treatment help to prevent spread of the infection.

Pathophysiology

Peritonitis produces severe systemic effects. Circulatory alterations, fluid shifts, and respiratory problems can cause critical fluid and electrolyte imbalances. The inflammatory response shunts (diverts) extra blood to the inflamed area of the bowel to combat the infection. Peristaltic activity of the bowel ceases. Fluids and air are retained within its lumen, raising pressure and increasing fluid secretion into the bowel. Thus circulating blood volume diminishes. The inflammatory process increases oxygen requirements at a time when the client has difficulty ventilating (breathing) because of abdominal pain and increased abdominal pressure, which elevates the diaphragm.

Clinical Manifestations

Manifestations of peritonitis vary according to the cause. Pain may be localized or generalized. Well-localized pain that causes rigidity of abdominal muscles and pain that increases with any pressure or motion of the abdomen are characteristic of peritonitis. Also, the client usually experiences nausea, vomiting, and, possibly, a low-grade fever. Assessment reveals absence of bowel sounds and shallow respirations because the client is trying to avoid the pain caused by body movement.

The client with peritonitis commonly has an elevated WBC count ($20,000/mm^3$) with a high neutrophil count. Abdominal x-ray studies are performed, which may show dilation and edema of the intestines or free air or fluid in the abdominal cavity. If the client is vomiting, manifestations of imbalanced fluid and electrolyte balance also may be present.

Outcome Management
■ Medical Management

Maintain Fluid and Electrolyte Balance. If peritonitis is advanced and if surgery is contraindicated by shock and circulatory failure, oral fluids are prohibited. IV fluids are necessary for the replacement of electrolyte and protein losses. An NG tube or a long intestinal tube may be inserted to reduce pressure within the bowel. See Chapter 33 for nursing care of a client with an NG or intestinal tube.

Control Infection. Once the infection has been walled off and the client's condition improves, surgical drainage and repair can be attempted. The other major treatment of peritonitis is IV antibiotic therapy with potent broad-spectrum agents.

■ Surgical Management

Surgery may be performed to prevent peritonitis, such as an appendectomy for an inflamed appendix or a colon resection (surgical removal) for inflamed diverticulum. If the perforation is not prevented, the major surgical intervention is incision and drainage of the abscess once it is walled off.

■ Nursing Management of the Surgical Client

Preoperatively, obtain a thorough history, including specific information about the client's pain. Assess the abdomen, noting the presence or absence of bowel sounds. Palpate the abdomen, noting whether the abdomen is firm, distended, or rigid. Note areas of rebound tenderness.

Clients with peritonitis are acutely ill and are given broad-spectrum antibiotics immediately. The perforated organs are usually repaired as soon as the client is stable enough to withstand the stress of surgery. During surgery, any leakage can be sampled for culture so that specific antibiotic therapy can be implemented. The peritoneal cavity is irrigated with an antibiotic solution to reduce the bacterial count. Often the wound is packed open or drains are placed so that infection can be treated.

Postoperatively, carefully monitor clients for the development of postoperative complications, such as adult respiratory stress syndrome (ARDS), sepsis, and shock. Closely monitor the client's fluid balance by assessing vital signs, bowel sounds, urine output, skin turgor, mucous membranes, and weight. Immediately report any manifestations of sepsis, such as a drop or rise in temperature or a drop in blood pressure. IV fluids are administered along with antibiotic therapy. On discharge, provide the client with oral or written instructions regarding wound care, medications, activity restrictions, and follow-up visits.

INFLAMMATORY BOWEL DISEASE

Inflammatory bowel disease (IBD) consists of two chronic inflammatory disorders: Crohn's disease (regional enteritis) and ulcerative colitis. About one million Americans suffer from Crohn's disease and one million suffer from ulcerative colitis. Each year, 30,000 people learn that they have a moderate to severe form of IBD. It is estimated that IBD costs between $1.8 and 2.6 billion annually in lost wages and disability and health care payments.

These chronic, recurrent diseases can occur in people at any age but usually are diagnosed in young adults between 15 and 30 years of age. A definitive diagnosis is hard to make because the manifestations mimic other conditions and because there may be long periods of remission. There is no known cure. Treatment is symptomatic. Responses are often unpredictable and clients with IBD frequently require surgery to remove diseased sections of the bowel and to repair holes in the intestine. Because of the similarities between Crohn's disease and ulcerative colitis, the two conditions are compared throughout the following discussion and in Table 35-1.

Etiology and Risk Factors
The cause of IBD remains unclear, but it probably involves a combination of genetic predisposition, environmental conditions, and defects in immune regulation. Chromosome 16 recently was strongly linked to Crohn's disease, but not ulcerative colitis.[34] Some believe that the disease is of bacterial origin because many clients have a history of bacterial infection before the onset of the condition. It is believed that any one of these factors weakens the intestinal wall, allowing it to become more sus-

ceptible to inflammation and tissue breakdown when in contact with disease producing organisms. Other theories suggest that destructive enzymes and a lack of protective substances in the bowel wall cause the inflammatory process. An emotional disturbance can precipitate an exacerbation or prolong an attack, but it is not the primary cause. The only risk factors identified for IBD are genetic. There are no preventative measures.

Relatives of clients with IBD are more likely to experience IBD than the general population. A 20-fold to 50-fold increase in occurrence among siblings and a 50-fold to 100-fold increase in children have been noted in families of clients with IBD. The chance of having IBD is estimated at 2% to 10% if a first-degree relative (children, siblings, parents) is affected; about 10% of clients with IBD have a positive family history of the disease

Crohn's Disease
Crohn's disease is a chronic relapsing disease that can develop discontinuously (without sequence and skipping sections) in any segment of the alimentary tract. The most common locations are the terminal ileum and colon. Half of clients experience perianal involvement. Crohn's disease more characteristically involves the entire thickness of the bowel wall *(transmural)*, particularly the submucosa. The mortality rate is not high, but recurrences and complications can result in disability. The client feels well between attacks; however, each bout leaves the intestine more scarred and less able to absorb nutrients.

Ulcerative Colitis
Ulcerative colitis is a disease that spans the entire length of the colon and involves only the mucosa and submucosa. The disease usually starts in the rectum and distal colon, spreading upward beyond the rectosigmoid valve to involve most of the sigmoid and descending colon. The disease extends in a contiguous manner with distinct demarcations between normal and unhealthy areas. Ulcerative colitis causes inflammation, thickening, congestion, edema, and minute lacerations that ooze blood and eventually develop into abscesses. The edema can lead to extreme friability of the mucosa, and bleeding can thus occur from any minor trauma. It occurs at all ages, but the incidence is higher among young adults, women, and Jews.

Pathophysiology

Crohn's Disease
Lesions typically develop in several separated segments of bowel. They are visible on gross examination (without aid of a microscope), and their color differs dramatically from that of normal tissue (Figure 35-3). Examination of

TABLE 35-1	Differentiation Between Crohn's Disease and Ulcerative Colitis	
Characteristic	**Regional Enteritis (Crohn's Disease)**	**Ulcerative Colitis**
General Description		
Age at onset	Young	Young to middle age
Pathology and Anatomy		
Depth of involvement	Transmural (all layers of submucosa)	Mucosa and submucosa
Rectal involvement	50%	95%
Right colon involvement	Frequent	Occasional
Small bowel involvement	Involved, ileum narrow	Usually normal
Distribution of disease	Segmental	Continuous
Inflammatory mass	Chronic and extensive	Rare (crypt abscess)
Cobblestone-like mucosa and granuloma	Common	Absent
Mesentery lymph involvement	Edema and hyperplasia	Not involved
Toxic megacolon	Occasional	Occasional
Steatorrhea	Frequent	Absent
Malignancy results	Rare	After 10 years
Fibrous stricture	Common	Absent
Clinical Characteristics		
Course of disease	Slowly progressive	Remissions and relapses
Rectal bleeding	Occasional	Common (90%-100%)
Abdominal pain	Colicky (45%)	Predefecation (60%-70%)
Hematochezia	Unusual or absent	Almost always present
Diarrhea	Present (65%-85%)	Early and frequent (80%-95%)
Vomiting	Present (35%)	Present (15%)
Nutritional deficit	Common	Common
Weight loss	Present (60%-70%)	Present (10%)
Fever	Present (35%)	Present (10%)
Anal abscess	Common (75%)	Occasional (10%)
Fistula and anorectal fissure fistula	Common (80%)	Rare (10%-20%)
Systemic Manifestations		
Arthritis	20%	Uncommon (10%)
Peripheral sacroiliitis	18%	18%-20%
Hepatobiliary involvement	Uncommon	15% cholestatic dysfunction
		19%-38% fatty liver
		30%-50% pericholangitis
Skin: erythema nodosum, pyoderma gangrenosum	Common	Present (5%-10%)
Nephrolithiasis	Occasional	Rare

FIGURE 35-3 Endoscopic appearance of Crohn's disease. **A,** Typical aphthous ulcers consisting of a central white depression surrounded by a slightly elevated, erythematous rim only a few millimeters in diameter. **B,** Findings more typical of advanced disease, with erythema, edema, and a cobblestone appearance. (From Feldman, M., Friedman, L.S., & Sleisenger, M.H. [2002]. *Sleisenger and Fortran's gastrointestinal and liver disease* [7th ed.] [Vol. 2]. Philadelphia: W.B. Saunders.)

A   B

the bowel tissue by endoscopy reveals edematous, heavy, reddish purple areas. Granular spots also may be present. Enlarged lymph nodes appear in the submucosa, and Peyer's patches are seen in the intestinal mucous membrane. These areas undergo small superficial ulcerations with granulomas and fissures. Fissures may completely penetrate the bowel wall, leading to fistulas and abscesses. Fistulas, in turn, release toxic substances from the intestine into the bloodstream, the abdominal cavity, and other organs. Collections of lymphocytes throughout the mucosa, submucosa, and serosa are the only microscopic features of Crohn's disease. The small bowel wall becomes congested and thickened, narrowing the lumen.

Extraintestinal complications include malabsorption; kidney stones; hydronephrosis; stomatitis; peripheral arthritis; and pyoderma gangrenosum, an inflammatory, ulcerative condition of the skin. Gallstones occur in 13% to 34% of clients. Anorectal problems include internal fistulae and abscesses. Anal fissure (see later discussion) is common and is directly related to the severity of the diarrhea, which produces ulceration of the perianal skin. Pain is aggravated by walking, sitting, and defecation.

Ulcerative Colitis

The appearance of the colon depends on the stage, activity, and severity of the disease (Figure 35-4). The most characteristic lesion of ulcerative colitis is an inflammatory infiltrate called a *crypt abscess*. This abscess consists of polymorphonuclear leukocytes, lymphocytes, red blood cells, and cellular debris appearing at the base of the crypts of Lieberkühn. Secretions from crypt abscesses result in purulent discharge from the bowel mucosa. Abscesses may become necrotic and may ulcerate.

Infections secondary to ulcerative colitis produce further inflammatory reactions in the mucosa and submucosa. When the inflammatory lesions heal, scarring and fibrosis, with narrowing, thickening, and shortening of the colon, and loss of haustral folds, may follow.

Cancer of the colon is more common among clients with ulcerative colitis than in the general population. The incidence is greatly increased when ulcerative colitis develops before the client is 16 years of age and in clients who have had the condition for more than 20 years.

Toxic megacolon is an extreme dilation of a segment of the diseased colon (often the transverse segment) that results in complete obstruction. Toxic megacolon usually occurs during an acute exacerbation of ulcerative colitis, and it may follow hypokalemia, a barium enema, or the use of anticholinergics, opioids, corticosteroids, or antibiotics. Bacterial overgrowth contributes to this complication. Perforation and peritonitis may complicate the condition.

Clinical Manifestations

Crohn's disease and ulcerative colitis produce similar manifestations. Clients suffer from abdominal pain, diarrhea, fluid imbalances, and weight loss. Severe diarrhea or vomiting may cause metabolic acidosis. Remis-

FIGURE 35-4 Spectrum of severity of ulcerative colitis. **A,** Colonoscopy in mild ulcerative colitis demonstrated by edema, loss of vascularity, and patchy subepithelial hemorrhage. **B,** Colonoscopy in severe ulcerative colitis with loss of vascularity, hemorrhage, and mucopus. (From Feldman, M., Friedman, L.S., & Sleisenger, M.H. [2002]. *Sleisenger and Fortran's gastrointestinal and liver disease* [7th ed.] [Vol. 2]. Philadelphia: W.B. Saunders.)

sions are followed by exacerbations of acute disease. When the disease is acute, the client has a fever. The general appearance of clients with IBD varies from reasonably healthy to wasted, drawn, and malnourished, with varying degrees of pallor. Clients usually report a steady and progressive weight loss. Inspection reveals a flat or concave shape to the abdomen, with visible peristaltic activity. Palpation of the abdomen reveals tenderness over the area of inflamed bowel. Increased bowel sounds are heard on auscultation. Hemorrhoids and, in Crohn's disease, perianal abscess, fistula, and ulcers may be apparent.

Hematocrit and hemoglobin values are usually decreased. A barium enema study with air contrast is often performed to differentiate ulcerative colitis from Crohn's disease. The client with suspected IBD routinely undergoes colonoscopy. Biopsy and cytologic studies also help to distinguish among carcinoma, ulcerative colitis, and Crohn's disease. The clinical manifestations of Crohn's disease and ulcerative colitis are compared in Table 35-1.

Crohn's Disease

Diarrhea in Crohn's disease is usually less severe than that in ulcerative colitis. Stool consistency is typically soft or semiliquid. Urgency to expel stools may awaken the person at night. The client rarely passes gross blood unless ulceration is present. Malabsorption, associated with steatorrhea, may develop. If so, stools may be foul smelling and fatty.

The client with severe steatorrhea, diarrhea, or long-standing enteritis may have associated nutritional deficits, weight loss, anorexia, pain, anemia, debility, fatigue, and metabolic disturbances. Nutritional deficits arise from (1) a reduction in the intestinal absorptive surface; (2) malabsorption of protein and carbohydrates; and (3) impaired absorption of fat, folic acid, iron, calcium, and vitamins A, B_{12}, C, D, E, and K. Alterations in bile salt and vitamin metabolism may result from surgery or mucosal defects. Metabolic requirements increase because of the inflammatory process and infection, the decrease in food intake, and the loss of nutrients in the feces because of rapid GI transit time. Electrolytes lost from diarrhea include sodium, potassium, chloride, the trace elements (magnesium, zinc, copper), and minerals. Nitrogen excretion remains normal if there is no loss of protein from the inflammatory exudate. The consequences of malnutrition include the following:

- Loss of immunocompetence
- Decreased resistance to infection
- Diminished wound healing
- Reduced pancreatic enzyme output
- Impaired healing (fistula and surgical wounds)
- Decreased iron-binding capacity resulting from chronic infection or blood loss

Ulcerative Colitis

The predominant manifestation of ulcerative colitis is rectal bleeding. Clients often experience diarrhea, possibly 20 or more stools per day. The severity and frequency of diarrhea depend on the extent of involved colon. Severe diarrhea can cause a loss of 500 to 17,000 ml of water in 24 hours. Liquid stools occur with tenesmus and may contain blood, mucus, and pus. A sense of urgency and cramping abdominal pain may occur with the diarrhea. The client typically experiences colicky pain in the lower left quadrant.

Nausea, vomiting, anorexia, fever, weight loss, and decreased serum potassium concentration may occur with severe disease. In addition, the client loses plasma proteins, prothrombin, and fluids. Anemia may develop with severe blood loss and decreased dietary iron intake.

Physical findings include tenderness in the lower left quadrant, guarding, and (in severe ulcerative colitis) abdominal distention. Following remissions, ulcerative colitis may recur after bouts of emotional stress, dietary indiscretion, or the ingestion of irritants such as laxatives and antibiotics. Physical exertion, respiratory infections, and fatigue also may cause an attack.

Prognosis

Remissions and exacerbations characterize both types of IBD. The only known cure for ulcerative colitis is surgical removal of the colon. Surgical procedures and medication therapy can control the manifestations in Crohn's disease, but currently there is no known cure.

Outcome Management
■ Medical Management

Decrease Diarrhea. Medical treatments, which aim primarily to control the manifestations, are similar for ulcerative colitis and Crohn's disease. Because the inflammatory process in Crohn's disease involves deeper layers of the bowel wall and is more chronic, healing may occur more slowly than in ulcerative colitis. Thus anti-inflammatory therapy, including steroids, is required for longer periods in Crohn's disease than in ulcerative colitis.

Fluids, electrolytes, and blood are replaced as needed to maintain the client's homeostasis. Physical activity should be kept to a minimum during an acute attack to decrease intestinal motility. The client with a mild attack can work but will need extra rest. The client with fever, toxemia, frequent bowel movements, bleeding, or pain requires bed rest. Failure of the inflamed colonic mucosa to reabsorb water and electrolytes, bile salts, and lactose interferes with the control of diarrhea. The extent of large bowel involved by the disease influences the severity of diarrhea. The client should keep a record of the number of stools, their consistency and color, and the presence or absence of blood.

Bowel rest and parenteral hyperalimentation may result in restored immunocompetence, greater resistance to infection, correction of nutritional deficiencies, and relief of edema and bowel inflammation.

Pharmacologic Agents. Once inflammatory bowel disease has been diagnosed, the client is started on pharmacological agents with the hope of bringing the disease into remission. A variety of pharmacologic agents are used to control diarrhea, reduce inflammation, and treat pain. See the Integrating Pharmacology feature on Medications for Inflammatory Bowel Disease, below, for a discussion of specific medications.

Increase Nutritional Intake. Nutritional deficiencies are the most common complications of IBD. These deficits derive from decreased intake, increased losses, greater nutritional requirements, and side effects of certain medications. Diarrhea leads to fluid and electrolyte losses with resultant muscle wasting and edema. Malabsorption resulting from bacterial overgrowth or mucosal involvement of the bowel may cause further problems. Deficiencies of fat-soluble vitamins (A, D, E, and K) and folate may develop. Vitamin K deficiency causes bleeding tendencies.

Diet and Supplements. A diet high in protein and calories is given in an attempt to restore normal nutri-

INTEGRATING PHARMACOLOGY

Medications for Inflammatory Bowel Disease

Medications that target the inflammatory process are usually effective in controlling active IBD in most clients and sustaining remission for prolonged periods in many. Most health care providers used a stepped approach to therapy in which more potent agents are added to the regimen if less active drugs fail to achieve an adequate response.

The 5-aminosalicylate-based compounds have remained the mainstays of treatment for clients with mild to moderate active ulcerative colitis and Crohn's disease. These drugs block the production of prostaglandins and leukotrienes to decrease the inflammatory process. Examples include sulfasalazine (Azulfidine), mesalamine (5-ASA, Asacol, Rowasa), and olsalazine (Dipentum). Oral formulations should be used for more proximal disease in the small bowel or ileum while suppositories and enemas should be used for distal colonic disease.

Clients whose IBD fails to respond to the salicylates may require corticosteroid medications. These may be administered orally or rectally as well as intravenously. They should only be taken during remissions and not continually. Antacids or histamine receptor antagonists should be given during steroid therapy to prevent gastric ulceration. Steroids reduce adrenal function and may impair resistance, causing defective healing of abscesses and fistulas. Steroids do not cure IBD, but they modify its course. Clients should be tapered off steroids as soon as possible to prevent long-term complications.

A new, nonsystemic steroid, budesonide (Entocort), has been shown to be effective in treating active Crohn's disease, but it is not effective in preventing remissions of the disease. Budesonide has fewer systemic side effects than other steroids and can be administered topically as an enema and orally in a controlled release form.

When salicylates and corticosteroids are not successful, management of the disease with more toxic, secondary-line agents

becomes crucial. These immunosuppressive and immunoregulatory agents include 6-mercaptopurine (Purinethol), methotrexate (Folex), and azathioprine (Imuran). These drugs have many toxic side effects, however, including blood dyscrasias, infection, pancreatitis, and digestive intolerance. Cyclosporine (Sandimmune) is another effective agent but is also associated with much toxicity. Infliximab (Remicade) is a drug for Crohn's disease that blocks the action of tumor necrosis factor-alpha, a natural protein that causes intestinal inflammation. It is the only drug used specifically for Crohn's disease and is given by a single IV infusion that may be repeated every 2 to 3 months. The newest immune medication used for IBD is natalizumab (Antegren), which attaches to immune cells and stops them from leaving the bloodstream and going to the site of inflammation.

Several new drugs currently in clinical trials are the selective cytokine-inhibiting drug CDC 801 (SelCID) and successor compounds to SelCID called inflammation modulator imidazoles (IMIDs). Interleukin 11 and 12 are also being investigated as treatment options for Crohn's disease. Human growth hormone is another experimental drug that repairs the intestines and strengthens the intestinal wall. Recent research studies indicate that this drug has few side effects and is safe and effective for long-term treatment of Crohn's disease.

Other medications that may be given during acute exacerbations include anticholinergic and antidiarrheal medications to relieve abdominal cramps and help control diarrhea. Anticholinergic, antidiarrheal, and antispasmodic agents allow the colon to rest. Antibiotics may be used to prevent or control infections and to treat anal fistulas and perianal disease. The sulfonamides and antibiotics such as metronidazole (Flagyl) and ciprofloxacin (Cipro) are the medications of choice.

tional levels but is not always well tolerated. Liquid supplements are residue free, low in fat, and digested mainly in the upper jejunum.

Anemia and vitamin deficiencies should be corrected nutritionally or with supplements. Folate deficiency, which may be due to the therapeutic use of sulfasalazine, may be prevented by (1) increasing dietary intake of folate, (2) having the client take sulfasalazine between meals, or (3) supplementing the intervention regimen with folic acid.

Total Parenteral Nutrition. Total parenteral nutrition (TPN) is indicated when a client has not responded to medical intervention, is being prepared for surgery, or has undergone intestinal resection. TPN provides bowel rest by removing all stimulation of secretion and by decreasing fecal bulk. Weight gain, positive nitrogen balance, and a temporary remission of manifestations can occur. TPN appears to be more useful in Crohn's disease than in ulcerative colitis.

When oral food and fluids are resumed, they should be chemically and mechanically nonirritating and high in calories, protein, and minerals. The client should avoid cocoa, chocolate, citrus juices, cold or carbonated drinks, nuts, seeds, popcorn, and alcohol.

■ Nursing Management of the Medical Client Assessment

Assess the client's bowel elimination pattern, noting the number of stools, their color and consistency, and the presence or absence of blood or steatorrhea. Also assess the client's abdomen. Note bowel sounds and the location of pain. Complete a nutritional assessment, as directed in Chapter 30.

Diagnosis, Outcomes, Interventions

Diagnosis: Diarrhea. Diarrhea is the most common manifestation of IBD, and so the primary nursing diagnosis is *Diarrhea related to inflamed intestinal mucosa.*

Outcomes. The client will experience a decrease in diarrhea, as evidenced by a decrease in number and a more solid consistency of stools.

Interventions. Antidiarrheal medications may be administered to control the client's diarrhea. Perianal excoriation often occurs with diarrhea. After every bowel movement, gently clean the skin with warm water and apply a protective moisture barrier product. (See the Management and Delegation feature on the Application and Care of Rectal Pouches and Rectal Tubes on p. 821.)

Diagnosis: Imbalanced Nutrition: Less Than Body Requirements. The client with inflammatory bowel disease has many difficulties with nutrition, making *Imbalanced Nutrition: Less Than Body Requirements related to diarrhea and malabsorption* a common nursing diagnosis.

Outcomes. The client will increase nutritional intake to meet metabolic requirements as evidenced by weight stabilization and possibly weight gain.

Interventions. Monitor the client's nutritional intake. The type of diet ordered depends on the client's condition. If the client can tolerate a diet, encourage intake of fluids and food. Because eating stimulates the gastrocolic reflex and the urge to defecate, many people are afraid to eat; small servings may enable the client to avoid this problem. Foods should be easily digested to promote absorption during the short time the food remains in the bowel.

Clients with Crohn's disease are often receiving home TPN because as a result of disease exacerbation they cannot tolerate foods for long periods (see Chapter 31). These clients also may have undergone multiple bowel resections, resulting in short-bowel syndrome and problems of malabsorption.

Diagnosis: Acute Pain. Another common nursing diagnosis for the client with inflammatory bowel disease is *Acute Pain related to inflamed mucosa.*

Outcomes. The client will experience a relief in abdominal pain as evidenced by the client's statement that pain has been relieved.

Interventions. Assess the client's pain, and give pain medications as ordered. Note any changes in the client's complaints of pain because they may indicate the development of complications. Opioids are generally used sparingly so that they do not mask manifestations.

Diagnosis: Risk for Ineffective Coping. Stress is associated with IBD and clients frequently report a poor quality of life. Write the nursing diagnosis as *Risk for Ineffective Coping related to stress of disease and exacerbations related to stress.*

Outcomes. The client will cope effectively with the disease as evidenced by fewer exacerbations and an improved coping style. The client will report an improved quality of life. (See the Evidence-Based Practice in Action feature on Quality of Life with Inflammatory Bowel Disease on p. 822.)

Interventions. Although emotional factors may not contribute to the cause of the disease, they do influence its course. Prolonged stress often precedes the onset of IBD and exacerbations. Recommend that the client schedule a follow-up physical examination and colonoscopy every 1 to 2 years. Refer clients with IBD to the Crohn's

MANAGEMENT AND DELEGATION

Application and Care of Rectal Pouches and Rectal Tubes

Diarrhea is the rapid movement of fecal matter through the gastrointestinal (GI) tract, resulting in poor absorption of nutrients, water, and electrolytes. Because of this rapid transit, the client experiences frequent evacuation of watery, liquid, or unformed stools. The stool in diarrhea is usually alkaline because it contains digestive enzymes. Skin breakdown results if there is prolonged or frequent cutaneous contact. A rectal pouch may be applied to collect feces, to protect the skin from prolonged contact with fecal material, and to prevent subsequent skin breakdown.

You can delegate the application and care of rectal pouches to unlicensed assistive personnel.

Application of Rectal Pouches

Instruct assistive personnel to:
- Wash hands and don gloves.
- Provide privacy for the client.
- Wash and dry the rectal area thoroughly with soap and water.
- Assist the client to a side-lying position, with upper knee drawn to the chest to expose the perineal area.
- Remove the rectal pouch from packaging, and enlarge the opening in the skin barrier with scissors if necessary.
- Remove paper backing from the skin barrier.
- Spread the client's buttocks, and then apply the adhesive backing to the perineal area; apply firm, gentle pressure to ensure adherence.
- Release the buttocks, allowing them to assume a relaxed position.
- Assist the client to a comfortable position, returning the bed to its lowest position.
- Remove gloves and wash hands.

Emptying the Collection Bag
- Wash hands and don gloves.
- Empty the collection bag by opening the cap on the drain and by directing stool into a collection container or bedpan.
- Remove gloves and wash hands.
- Record stool volume per physician's order.

Removing the Rectal Pouch
- Wash hands and don gloves.
- Empty and reseal the collector bag.

- Gently ease the skin barrier away from the client's skin.
- Discard the pouch into an appropriate receptacle.
- Wash and dry the perineal area thoroughly with soap and water.
- Assist the client to a comfortable position, returning the bed to its lowest position.
- Remove gloves and wash hands.

Rectal Tubes

Flatulence (presence of abnormal amounts of gas in the GI tract) may occur anytime peristalsis is decreased or absent. Excess gas may lead to a bloated feeling, abdominal distention, and cramping pain. A rectal tube may be inserted and left in place for 20 to 30 minutes to facilitate the client's passage of excessive flatus. You may delegate the skin care and positioning of a client with a rectal tube to unlicensed assistive personnel.

Skin Care and Positioning of a Client with a Rectal Tube
- Wash hands and don gloves.
- Provide privacy for the client.
- Wash the client's rectal area with soap and water.
- Place a waterproof pad under the client's hips and buttocks.
- Assist the client to a left Sims position.
- Assist the registered nurse with insertion of the rectal tube as needed.
- Instruct the client to remain in a side-lying position to prevent dislodgment of the tube.
- Wash hands and don gloves before assisting with removal of the rectal tube after 20 to 30 minutes.
- Wash and dry the perineal area thoroughly with soap and water if needed.
- Assist the client to a comfortable position, returning the bed to its lowest position.
- Remove gloves and wash hands.
- Describe findings that are immediately reportable to you for assistive personnel, including any difficulty with application of the rectal pouch, continued complaints of abdominal pain or discomfort by the client, and any areas of skin breakdown.
- Verify the competence of assistive personnel in performing these tasks during orientation and annually thereafter.

and Colitis Foundation of America (386 Park Ave. S., New York, NY 10016-8804) to learn about the condition and about meetings of local support groups. Instruct the client to call the physician at the first manifestation of IBD recurrence.

Evaluation

It is hoped that the client's disease will respond to medical management and that the client will achieve remission, improved coping, and adequate nutritional

EB EVIDENCE-BASED PRACTICE IN ACTION

Quality of Life with Inflammatory Bowel Disease

Inflammatory Bowel Disease (IBD) is a chronic disorder with no known cure. It is characterized by remissions and exacerbations. Clients with IBD suffer from physical and psychological symptoms and must live with the uncertainty of the disease course. As a result, many clients report a poor quality of life.

Recently, some nursing and medical research studies, both quantitative and qualitative, have assessed the quality of life in clients with IBD. Research participants included clients in an outpatient clinic,[5] parents with IBD,[4] and young adults with the disease.[2] In addition, one experimental research study examined the effects of nursing led counseling sessions to help clients cope with the disease.[5] Data were collected by means of questionnaires[1] and interviews.

Findings from these studies were that clients have maladaptive coping skills and suffer from life-disrupting challenges that profoundly affect their peers, families, and individuals in their social support systems. One study found that parents with IBD have difficulty with parenting and suffer from guilt, worry, and depression in regard to effective parenting. Participants in this study reported that their children became angry, anxious, and frustrated when their social activities were interrupted because of the disease. On a positive note, parents with IBD reported closer relationships with their children as a result of the disease and children who were caring and understanding.[4]

Recommendations from the studies were that any comorbid psychiatric illnesses be treated and that risk factors for psychological distress be identified early.[3] Those at particularly high risk for psychological distress are those who lack family support, those with severe symptoms, and those with young children. Nurses should strive to understand the disease from each client's perception.[2] Clients need help with problem-solving coping strategies, stress reduction, assistance with dealing with uncertainty, and assistance with gaining personal control.[3] They need social support and education about the disease for both them and individuals in their support system.

Implications

Clients with IBD often suffer from poor qualities of life due to the chronic nature of the disease and its clinical manifestations. Learning how to manage the disease and gain personal control is essential to a good quality of life. Nurses are in an ideal situation to help these clients achieve good qualities of life through education, counseling, and support.

References

1. Casellas, F., et al. (2001). Influence of inflammatory bowel disease on different dimensions of quality of life. *European Journal of Gastroenterology and Hepatology, 13*(5), 567-572.
2. Daniel, J. (2002). Young adults' perceptions of living with chronic inflammatory bowel disease. *Gastroenterology Nursing, 25*(3), 83-94.
3. Dudley-Brown, S. (2002). Prevention of psychological distress in persons with inflammatory bowel disease. *Issues in Mental Health Nursing, 23*(4), 403-422.
4. Mukherjee, S., et al. (2002).An insight into the experiences of parents with inflammatory bowel disease. *Journal of Advanced Nursing, 37*(4), 355-363.
5. Smith, G. et al. (2002). Impact of a nurse-led counseling service on quality of life in patients with inflammatory bowel disease. *Journal of Advanced Nursing, 38*(2), 152-160.

intake. If the client's IBD does not respond to medical management, surgical intervention may be required.

■ Surgical Management

Surgery, the only cure for ulcerative colitis, is usually indicated when medical management fails and the condition is intractable. Of clients with ulcerative colitis, 25% to 40% must undergo surgical removal of the colon with a permanent ileostomy or a continent ileostomy such as an ileal pouch–anal anastomosis or a Kock pouch. Surgery is not indicated in Crohn's disease except to treat complications. Surgery may be indicated in either or both conditions, however, for complications such as perforation, hemorrhage, obstruction, toxic megacolon, abscess, fistula, and disease intractability.

Total Proctocolectomy

In a total proctocolectomy, the colon and rectum are removed and the anus is closed. The terminal ileum is brought out through the abdominal wall, and a permanent ileostomy is formed.

Kock Pouch

Indications. A Kock pouch is a procedure in which a reservoir or pouch is constructed from the distal 45 cm of the ileum. This allows stool to be stored intra-abdominally until it is drained through a nipple valve made from an intussuscepted portion of ileum (prolapse of one part of intestine into an adjacent section) (Figure 35-5). The client has a flat stoma on the right side of the abdomen. Advantages of the continent ileostomy are (1)

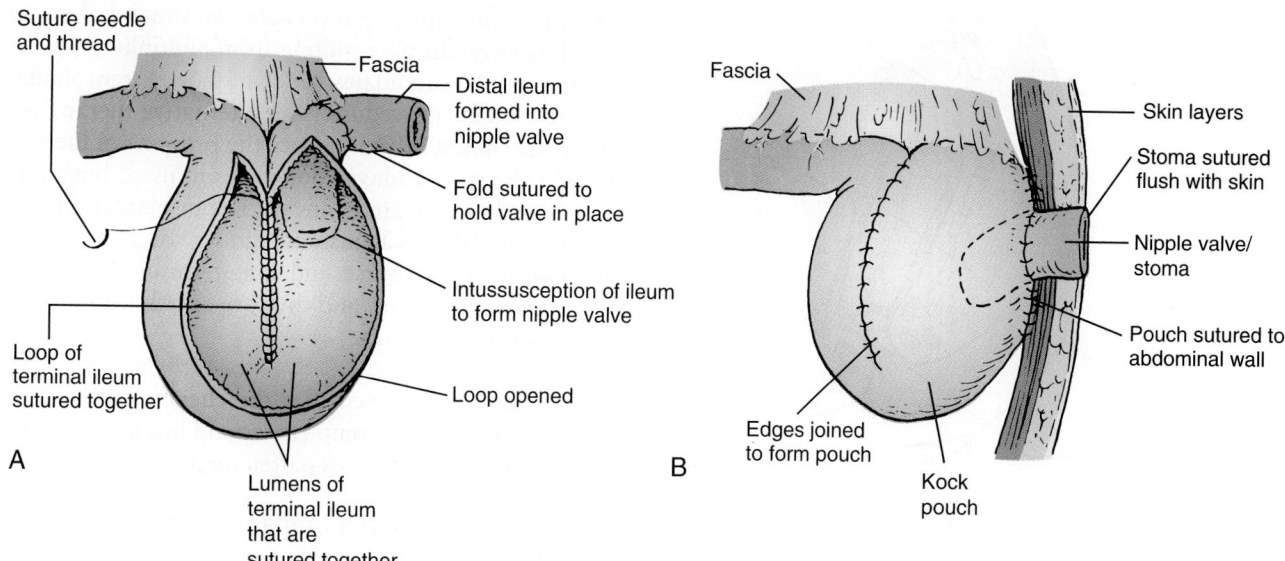

FIGURE 35-5 Continent ileostomy (Kock pouch). **A,** Loop of terminal ileum is sutured together and cut open. Using forceps, the surgeon intussuscepts the distal ileum to form a nipple valve. **B,** Free edges are sutured together to form the reservoir, the stoma is sutured flush with the skin, and the pouch is sutured to the abdominal wall.

no need to wear an external pouch, (2) minimal skin problems, and (3) usually, no flatus or leakage of stool. The client drains the pouch several times a day by intubation with a catheter through the nipple valve, usually in response to a feeling of fullness.

Contraindications. A Kock pouch should not be performed for Crohn's disease because of the likelihood of recurrent disease in the ileal pouch. If the client has malnutrition, TPN may be required to improve the outcome of surgery and promote wound healing.

Complications. After the formation of the Kock pouch, suture line leakage with local or generalized peritonitis may occur in the early postoperative period. The client may be unable to intubate the pouch because of slippage of the nipple valve. Other complications that may occur later in the recovery period include pouchitis, fistula formation, and obstruction by food residue.

Outcomes. The client resumes usual activities within 4 to 6 weeks. Nutritional status also improves. The client experiences improved quality of life without the necessity of frequent trips to the bathroom.

Ileal Pouch–Anal Anastomosis

Indications. Ileal pouch–anal anastomosis is the preferred surgical procedure for clients with ulcerative coli-

tis. Several surgical procedures result in the creation of a pelvic pouch, an internal reservoir created from the distal ileum, and sutured into the anorectal canal. The most common procedure is the J pouch. Clients who choose this procedure avoid an ostomy.

Surgery is usually performed in two steps. During the first step, the rectal mucosa is excised and the colon removed. An ileoanal reservoir (pouch) is then created in the anal canal, and a temporary loop ileostomy is formed to divert fecal contents until the pouch heals. After healing has taken place, usually in 2 to 3 months, the ileostomy is reversed so that stool drains into the reservoir, which is created by suturing two loops of bowel together (Figure 35-6). Some surgeons are completing this procedure in one surgery so that a temporary ileostomy is not required.

Contraindications. This anastomosis should not be performed for Crohn's disease. If malnutrition is a problem, TPN may be needed to improve the outcome of surgery and promote wound healing.

Complications. Complications include anastomotic leakage, pouchitis (inflammation of the pouch), and bowel obstruction.

Outcomes. The client resumes regular activities in 4 to 6 weeks after the second procedure or after the first procedure if a temporary ileostomy has not been performed. Nutritional status improves, and the client ex-

J-pouch

Anal sphincter

FIGURE 35-6 Ileal J pouch–anal anastomosis. The two-loop ileal pouch is simple to construct, provides adequate storage capacity, and is evacuated spontaneously and fully.

periences improved quality of life with nearly normal bowel movements and fewer trips to the bathroom.

Surgical Resection of the Small Bowel

Indications. In Crohn's disease, surgery is used only to treat the complications because even when the diseased portion is removed, the incidence of recurrence is 50%. The physician may prescribe antibiotics to control infection. During surgical resection for Crohn's disease, attempts are made to preserve as much of the small intestine as possible. Two thirds of the small intestine may be removed with no ill effects if the remaining portion is normal.

Contraindications. Clients may be too malnourished to undergo surgery. TPN is needed to prepare the client for surgery and to improve wound healing.

Complications. With resection of the distal ileum, the client cannot absorb vitamin B_{12} and removal of more than 6 to 8 feet results in impaired absorption of glucose, fat, and protein. If the colon is diseased, an ileotransverse colectomy (right colon and ileum), segmental colectomy, or total colectomy may be performed. A total colectomy with ileorectal anastomosis may be the surgery of choice.

For 1 to 3 weeks after extensive small bowel resection, the client may be unable to tolerate oral intake and may experience further losses in body protein or lean body mass. TPN is given until oral intake can be resumed. Diarrhea usually occurs during the first 6 weeks after surgery. Anemia (from iron deficiency, steatorrhea, or decreased protein absorption) also may ensue. Paralytic ileus (see later) is another possible complication.

Clients with either irreversible intestinal failure or short-bowel syndrome resulting from multiple bowel resection, may be candidates for small bowel transplantation (SBT). This procedure is an alternative therapy for clients who might otherwise face the prospect of lifelong TPN. In the past, cadaver donors were used, but more recently a living-related intestinal transplantation has been accomplished. Clients undergoing SBT have a difficult postoperative course and long-term complications of immunosuppression, and they are at risk for graft rejection (see Chapter 82).

Outcomes. It is hoped that the client can return to regular activities with complete wound healing and adequate nutrition 4 to 6 weeks after surgery.

■ Nursing Management of the Surgical Client
Assessment

Assessment of the surgical client is similar to assessment of the medical client; however, routine preoperative and postoperative assessments as discussed in Chapter 16 are also necessary. If the client is malnourished, TPN may be required preoperatively to improve nutritional status.

Diagnosis, Outcomes, Interventions

Preoperative Care
Diagnosis: Deficient Knowledge. The client who is to undergo surgical resection for IBD has many learning needs. The nursing diagnosis is *Deficient Knowledge related to surgical procedure and possible ileostomy or other bowel resection.*

Outcomes. The client will understand the surgical procedure and implications of bowel resection as evidenced by the ability to describe the procedure and perform a demonstration of ileostomy care.

Interventions. Describe the anticipated postoperative course, including the types of tubes that will be in place. Ostomy care must be fully explained to the client scheduled for ileostomy surgery. A preoperative visit from a member of any ostomy association may be helpful. An enterostomal therapy nurse should assist with the preoperative preparation. Before surgery, the site of the ileostomy is selected, with consideration being given to the location of the disease, body contours, convenience, and type of clothing the client wears. The client may wear the pouch for 1 to 2 days before surgery to ensure comfort with the site selected. To provide assistance and support, assess the client's body image as well as feelings about loss of a major body part and wearing a pouch for a lifetime.

If the client is having a continence-sparing surgery, extensive teaching is still required. The client needs to understand the type of bowel resection to be performed and the implications of the surgery. With some procedures, a temporary ileostomy (ileal pouch–anal anastomosis) may be necessary; with other procedures (e.g., the Kock pouch), the client's method of waste elimination is imbalanced permanently.

Postoperative Care
Diagnosis: Risk for Injury: Postoperative Complications (Stomal Necrosis, Retraction, Prolapse, Stenosis, Obstruction).
The client undergoing stoma formation is prone to complications. The nursing diagnosis is *Risk for Injury related to postoperative complications of stomal necrosis, retraction, prolapse, stenosis, or obstruction.*

Outcomes. The client will not suffer injury, as evidenced by minimal distention, rapid return of normal peristalsis, and absence of fluid and electrolyte imbalance.

Interventions
Monitor Stoma. Monitor the stoma after surgery. Ensure that there is no pressure on the stoma that could interfere with circulation. Assess the color of the stoma frequently (see Figure 35-13 for appearance of a normal stoma). If the stoma becomes pale, dusky, or cyanotic, notify the physician immediately. When blood supply to the stoma is compromised, surgical revision is required.

Advance Diet. An NG tube is in place for several days after surgery to remove gases and fluids that would increase intestinal distention and put pressure on the suture line. The drainage must be accurately noted. The passage of flatus indicates return of peristalsis. As bowel sounds return, clamp the tube as prescribed, and give the client ice chips and water. When the client has tolerated ice chips and water for a minimum of 24 hours, the tube is usually removed, and clear liquids are given.

Monitor for Complications. Although the postoperative course for most clients with ileostomy is uneventful, several complications can occur. The most common is an intestinal obstruction, which may be caused by obstruction of the lumen, adhesions, food, or stomal edema. Early manifestations of obstruction are (1) anorexia; (2) abdominal cramps; (3) absence of ileostomy drainage or a foul, brown, watery discharge in the pouch; and (4) visible peristalsis. Other early postoperative complications are hemorrhage, hypoxia, and fluid and electrolyte imbalance. If severe or prolonged problems with absorption occur, parenteral nutrition may be necessary.

Diagnosis: Risk for Disturbed Body Image.
The client with an ostomy has to face alterations in self-concept and body image. Write the nursing diagnosis as *Risk for*

Disturbed Body Image related to alteration of lifestyle secondary to ostomy.

Outcomes. The client experiences a positive body image and self-concept as evidenced by the client's statements and the ability to care for the ostomy without embarrassment.

Interventions. A few days after surgery, the client needs to begin to (1) confront the stoma and (2) integrate its function and appearance into his or her body image. Help the client to look at and touch the stoma as soon as possible. Always use proper terms for the stoma and equipment.

Because clothing can be a concern for the client with an ostomy, clothing options should be discussed. Discourage the client from wearing a tight waistband, which might rub on the stoma. Encourage the client to try on various outfits to ensure that the stoma and pouch are not visible. A visit from another person with an ostomy, usually available through the local chapter of the American Cancer Society, often helps the client realize that the ostomy can be easily hidden beneath clothing.

Encourage the client to verbalize feelings about the stoma and its appearance. The client may be accepting of the stoma because the illness (ulcerative colitis) is now gone and his or her life can be more normal and productive than it had been with the disease. Young men and unmarried women may express the greatest concern about body image. Find out how family or significant others now view the client. Their response might be positive because the client may have been chronically ill before surgery and now appears much healthier.

Diagnosis: Effective Therapeutic Regimen Management.
The client with a new stoma has much to learn about self-care. The nursing diagnosis is *Effective Therapeutic Regimen Management related to ileostomy care, care following ileorectal anastomosis, care of an ileal pouch–anal anastomosis, or care of a continent ileostomy.*

Outcomes. The client will understand proper care of the chosen surgical procedure as evidenced by (1) the ability to apply the appliance correctly, without leakage, and to empty the pouch appropriately; and (2) absence of perianal breakdown.

Interventions
Ileostomy
Teach Ostomy Care. The client must master the skills needed to provide self-care. Stoma care is the area of greatest concern to the client with an ileostomy. Consultation with an enterostomal therapy nurse, if available, may enhance teaching and care (see the Management and Delegation feature on Stoma Care and

MANAGEMENT AND DELEGATION

Stoma Care and Application of Ostomy Appliances

The care of a mature stoma and the application of an ostomy appliance may be delegated to unlicensed assistive personnel. The assessment and care of a newly created ostomy, however, should be performed only by a registered nurse. Before delegating stoma care and applying an ostomy appliance, consider the following:

The age of the ostomy. Is this a postsurgical client with a new ostomy or a client with an ostomy that is several weeks, months, or years old? For the client with a new ostomy, you or a trained ostomy nurse should provide care. For the client with a long-standing ostomy, assess the ostomy to ensure that the client is caring for it properly and that the stoma and surrounding skin are intact before you delegate ostomy care to assistive personnel.

The client's need to learn self-care of the stoma and ostomy. You or a trained ostomy nurse should provide this instruction for a client needing to learn self-care.

The client's acceptance of the ostomy, altered appearance, and bowel function. Clients having difficulty accepting their altered body image would benefit from having you or an ostomy nurse help them increase the acceptance and their ability to cope with the new ostomy.

The competency level of the unlicensed assistive personnel who will potentially perform this task.

The assistive personnel providing stoma care and applying ostomy appliances should be instructed to:

- Provide privacy for the client.
- Place a waterproof pad around the ostomy or under the client to protect the skin and bed linens.
- Empty the contents of the ostomy bag before removing the bag, noting the consistency, color, volume, and odor of the feces.
- Gently remove the skin barrier and bag while supporting the client's skin. An adhesive remover may be applied if necessary to remove adhesive residue from peristomal skin. This should be avoided if there is evidence of skin irritation or excoriation.
- Place a gauze pad or tissues over the exposed stoma to avoid soiling from leakage.
- Wash the skin around the stoma with warm water and a mild soap, and wash the stoma with clear water.
- Thoroughly rinse the area with water and pat it dry.
- Note the color, moisture, and protrusion of the stoma and the condition of the surrounding skin.
- Create a circle $1/8$ to $1/4$ inches larger than the size of the stoma on the back of the appliance. A stoma-measuring guide may be helpful for this procedure. The appliance wafer may have to be cut in an irregular shape to accommodate a noncircular stoma.
- Prepare the wafer and appliance as a unit.
- Smooth the wafer to remove all air bubbles.
- Fill in irregular stoma borders with skin paste applied around the opening in the wafer before applying it to the skin.
- Apply the unit, appliance, wafer, and bag around the stoma. Position the bag to hang in a dependent position. If the client is ambulatory, remember to position the bag for optimal drainage while the client is upright.
- Dispose of the soiled bag and appliance properly. Do this outside the client's room to prevent embarrassment about any odors.

Assistive personnel should report immediately to you if they find black, tarry stools or overt signs of blood in the bag or bleeding from the stoma. Reddened, inflamed skin surrounding the stoma should also be brought to your attention. Information pertaining to the care and condition of the stoma should be recorded.

Application of Ostomy Appliances, above). Initially, the client can simply observe care of the stoma. Begin by telling the client what the stoma looks like; that it extends $1/2$ to $3/4$ inches beyond the abdominal wall, is 1 to $1\frac{1}{2}$ inches in diameter, and is red and swollen at first. Assure the client that permanent changes in stoma size occur within the first 3 months after surgery as the swelling subsides.

The frequency with which the ileal pouch needs to be emptied varies with each client. It should be emptied whenever it is approximately one third to one half full. Instruct the client to empty the pouch during times of low output, usually before meals, at bedtime, and on arising in the morning. It is best to change the pouch when the ileostomy is the least active, usually first thing in the morning. Coating the pouch with drops of vegetable oil before using it prevents the contents from sticking to the sides and helps it to slide out easily.

When changing the pouch, have all equipment ready before removing the old pouch. Remove the old pouch carefully using a moist cloth. A piece of gauze may be held over the stoma until the new pouch is attached. Encourage the client to inspect and touch the stoma at this time. Remind the client who has a new ileostomy to take ostomy supplies along when traveling. The client may want to keep supplies handy in a shaving or cosmetic case instead of a suitcase. Many different types of pouches are available (Figure 35-7). Clients should try to find the best pouch for their needs.

FIGURE 35-7 Natura brand ostomy products. (Courtesy of ConvaTec, Bristol-Myers Squibb, Skillman, NJ.)

Teach Stoma Assessment. When changing the pouch, the client should learn to check the size and color of the stoma, assess the odor of the drainage, and observe for manifestations of irritation. When the ileostomy begins to function, the output is minimal. As the client takes in more food, the drainage becomes thicker and has a weak odor. Because an ileostomy may drain continuously (drainage is related to eating patterns), a pouch must be worn continuously, and the stoma must be covered with gauze when the pouch is being changed.

Prevent Skin Irritation. The pouch should be cut to fit the stoma, allowing only $\frac{1}{16}$ inch of room around the stoma. If the pouch does not fit well, severe skin irritation can occur because of the alkalinity of the effluent. Skin irritation can vary from redness to weeping dermatitis or ulceration. Irritation also can result from adhesives or frequent removal of the appliance. Any hair around the stoma should be cut with small scissors or shaved with an electric razor following the grain of hair. This helps prevent folliculitis and soreness. The skin should be washed and rinsed thoroughly between removing one pouch and applying another. Some appliance companies suggest using an adhesive remover wipe each time the pouch is changed, followed by washing with a mild soap and thoroughly rinsing with water. Then towel- or air-dry. With a two-piece setup, a pouch is snapped onto the faceplate, which is applied to the skin. This arrangement allows easy emptying of the pouch. The faceplate usually remains adherent to the skin for 5 to 7 days but may need to be changed sooner if it becomes loose or if leakage occurs.

Treat Skin Problems. If skin irritation occurs, first check the fit of the pouch. The best initial treatment for this problem would be to reapply the ostomy appliance, en-

suring a proper fit and seal. The skin barrier of the appliance is usually sufficient to protect and heal the skin. If this method does not work, other barriers must be used. A wide variety of skin care products are available. If the problems continue, consult an enterostomal therapy nurse for further assistance.

Skin infection also can occur. *Candida* is the most common cause. The peristomal skin takes on a rash-like appearance. An antifungal powder should be rubbed onto the affected skin area. The barrier can then be applied over the powder.

Reduce Odor. Foods such as eggs, fish, onions, cabbage, and some greens cause stool odor; therefore deodorizing solutions and tablets may be placed in the pouch. Spinach, parsley, yogurt, and buttermilk reduce drainage odor.

Discuss Medications. The client also needs special instructions regarding prescription and over-the-counter medications. Enteric-coated tablets, such as iron preparations, vitamins, hormones, multilayer tablets, timed-release capsules, and gelatin capsules may not be absorbed in the small intestine. The client should note whether any medications are obvious in pouch drainage; if so, the physician must prescribe different medications or different forms of medication.

Emphasize Fluid Intake. The client who has had an ileostomy needs to pay close attention to fluid intake. It is easy for such a client to become dehydrated. The approximate output from an ileostomy is 1200 to 1500 ml/day. The client must monitor this output for any increase that could lead to severe fluid and electrolyte imbalance.

Explain Dietary Recommendations. A low-residue diet that is high in protein, carbohydrates, and calories is recommended after ileostomy surgery. Supplemental vitamins A, D, E, K, and B_{12} may be needed. Berries, whole-grain cereals, and raw fruits and vegetables can cause problems for the client with an ileostomy. Any foods that cause discomfort or diarrhea should be omitted. Ingested foods pass through the ileostomy within 4 to 6 hours. It is not advisable to eat a large meal close to bedtime.

The client with an ileostomy must learn to chew food well (20 to 25 chews for each bite) because the shortened bowel transit time would cause poorly chewed food to be passed undigested. High-fiber and high-cellulose foods may absorb excessive moisture, leading to swelling and possibly constipation or even obstruction. Foods that should be avoided or limited, at least initially, include popcorn, peanuts, tough fibrous meats, vegetables with skins, rice, bran, and coconuts.

Clients may find that the postoperative diet is less restrictive than the diet they followed before the surgery.

The diet required by the presence of the disease was often restricted because so many foods increased the diarrhea and other manifestations. Clients with ileostomies often gain weight after surgery, sometimes to the point of having to restrict caloric intake.

Prevent Urolithiasis. Some clients with ileostomies tend to have calcium oxalate, uric acid, or urinary calculi because greater amounts of fluid are lost through the ileostomy, leading to decreased urine output. Uric acid stones tend to form when urine volume is low and the urine is persistently acidic. Ingestion of sodium bicarbonate or potassium citrate alkalinizes the urine. Allopurinol may be used if uric acid levels remain elevated. Fluid intake should be at least 2000 ml daily.

Ileal Pouch–Anal Anastomosis. The client with an ileal pouch–anal anastomosis has no need to learn about stoma or pouch care unless a temporary ileostomy was created. The client will learn to prevent leakage by responding to the sensation to defecate. After the bowel adapts to the surgical alteration, the stool becomes more formed, although it will always be loose. Most clients have between two and eight stools per day. Kegel exercises, to strengthen the tone of the anal sphincter muscles, will facilitate continence. Teach the client to tighten the anal sphincter muscles as if stopping a bowel movement. Hold for a count of 10 while squeezing tightly and then relax for a count of 10. These exercises should only be carried out when approved by the surgeon. Perianal skin irritation is likely to occur as a result of seepage and the enzyme content of liquid stool. The client should be taught to gently wipe the perianal area after each bowel movement. A moisture-barrier ointment such as Desitin can provide comfort. Pouchitis occurs in about 30% of clients. Clinical manifestations are an increase in number of stools, malaise, bleeding, and fever. Pouchitis is treated with metronidazole (Flagyl); ciprofloxacin, mesalamine, or steroids are used for severe cases. The client should maintain an adequate fluid intake.

Kock Pouch (Continent Ileostomy)
Maintain Ileal Drainage. During surgical formation of the Kock pouch, an evacuation catheter is inserted. A skin barrier and special gauze dressing are then applied. These hold the catheter in an upright position to avoid stress on a healing nipple valve. It is imperative to avoid distention of the ileostomy reservoir in the early postoperative period because of the pressure it would put on the suture line. Thus the reservoir is attached to straight drainage for several days after surgery. Then it is emptied every 2 hours for about 2 weeks.

Carefully observe for the start of ileal drainage, which usually begins 3 or 4 days postoperatively. About 2 weeks after surgery, the catheter is removed from the pouch. The catheter may then be used to drain the pouch. The intervals between drainings are gradually in-

creased each week until the ileostomy is emptied four to six times per day and once or not at all at night.

Teach Reservoir Catheterization. Explain the following procedure for emptying the reservoir, which should be performed with the client sitting on the toilet:
1. Lubricate the catheter with a water-soluble lubricant, and insert it into the stoma through the valve.
2. Allow the contents to drain by gravity through the catheter into the bathroom toilet; drainage should be complete in 3 to 5 minutes.
3. Apply a small gauze dressing over the stoma.
4. Clean the equipment with mild soap, and rinse it; the equipment can be carried in a plastic case.

The reservoir volume continues to increase to a maximum of around 600 ml in 6 months.

Explain Dietary Recommendations. The client needs an oral intake of at least eight 8-ounce glasses of fluid per day. Foods that could cause a blockage of the valve and the stoma, including mushrooms and nuts, may need to be avoided. All foods need to be chewed thoroughly because partly digested food may occlude the stoma.

Diagnosis: Risk for Sexual Dysfunction.
In the client with an ileostomy, there are no physiologic reasons for sexual dysfunction; however, after J-pouch surgery, both men and women may experience alterations in sexual function due to injury to nerves in the pelvic region. Men might experience impotence or retrograde ejaculation. Women may experience vaginal dryness and painful intercourse. Psychological reasons may also lead to dysfunction. Therefore the nursing diagnosis is *Risk for Sexual Dysfunction related to concern about ileostomy and disturbed body image and self-concept.*

Outcomes. The client will not have sexual dysfunction as evidenced by the ability to resume presurgery sexual functioning and role.

Interventions. The client with an ileostomy or pouch may be concerned about sexual activity and pregnancy. Encourage the client to express any such concerns and to discuss them with the sexual partner. Clients can be taught activities to lessen the intrusiveness of the pouch during intercourse, such as emptying the pouch before intercourse, wearing a soft flannel pouch cover, and being open to using different positions for intercourse. If problems arise, a sexual therapist should be consulted for further information and assistance. Impotence is uncommon; psychological reasons should be explored if it does occur.

Pregnancy and normal vaginal delivery are possible for a client with an ileostomy. The United Ostomy Association has a wide variety of booklets available for clients with an ostomy. Titles include *Sex, Pregnancy and the Female Ostomate; Sex, Courtship and the Single*

Ostomate; *Sex and the Male Ostomate*; and *Insight into the Emotional Aspects of Ileostomies and Colostomies*. Similar resources are available from the American Cancer Society.

Evaluation

If teaching is adequate, the client should be able to care for the ostomy and to handle the altered elimination. Preoperative activities can usually be resumed within 6 weeks.

■ Self-Care

Postoperative care and care of the stoma or diversion should be reinforced before the client is discharged. The client with an ileostomy should be encouraged to join the United Ostomy Association. This organization often helps clients regain self-esteem and improve self-concept and body image. The successful rehabilitation of others helps clients believe that they, too, can return to a normal lifestyle.

See the Client Education Guide on Ostomy Supplies on the website for the equipment needed to care for an ileostomy. The client should be aware of the nearest ostomy supply center so that equipment will be easy to obtain. If the client experiences difficulty with self-care, a visiting nursing or enterostomal therapy nurse should visit the client at home to follow up on learning needs. Clients with J pouches can find information on the Internet at http://www.ccfa.org.

No long-term restrictions are placed on physical activities. Tell the client to wear a medical alert identification bracelet and to carry a brief description of the pouch and drainage procedure in case of an emergency.

■ NEOPLASTIC DISORDERS
BENIGN TUMORS OF THE BOWEL

Various types of benign tumors are found in the bowel. Polyps, lesions that project into the lumen of the bowel, are the most commonly found benign tumor (Figure 35-8). Some polyps have stems *(pedunculated)*, whereas others do not *(sessile)*. Polyps are usually benign lesions, but some types are precursors of cancer (i.e., premalignant tumors). Polyps are dangerous because (1) they can mask the presence of a malignant tumor, and (2) they may serve as the focus for bowel obstruction or intussusception. Benign bowel tumors have clinical manifestations similar to those of malignant tumors. Some benign tumors bleed profusely and cause abdominal discomfort. Bleeding benign tumors are usually removed surgically.

CANCER OF THE SMALL BOWEL

Fewer than 5% of all GI cancers involve tumors of the small bowel. It was estimated that, in 2003, about 4700 people would have had cancer of the small bowel

FIGURE 35-8 Colonic polyps. (From Copstead, L.C., & Banasik, J.L. [2000]. *Pathophysiology: Biological and behavioral perspectives* [2nd ed.]. Philadelphia: W.B. Saunders. Courtesy of L.E. Copstead.)

and 1200 will have died of it. The average age of onset is 53 to 58 years. Most tumors are in the ileum, with the remainder almost equally divided between the duodenum and jejunum. Manifestations are vague and nonspecific; they include weight loss, pain, anemia, nausea, vomiting, obstruction, a palpable mass, and hemorrhage.

Surgery is the only intervention that offers hope of cure. Unfortunately, even with early diagnosis and bowel resection, only about 20% of clients with small bowel cancer survive 5 years. With late diagnosis, the 5-year survival rate decreases to about 5%.

COLORECTAL CANCER

Colon and rectal (colorectal) cancer is the most common GI cancer in the United States. It occurs equally in men and women, is the third most common cancer, and is the second leading cause of death from cancer in the United States. Colon cancer is three times more common than rectal cancer. It is estimated that about 135,000 new cases of colorectal cancer are diagnosed each year and that about 56,000 people die of it. The probability of developing colorectal cancer at some point in one's lifetime is roughly 6%, or 1 of 17 people. The incidence rates have been declining in the last 20 years, a trend most likely attributable to increases in screening and polyp removal. Likewise, mortality rates have also been declining, most likely a reflection of the falling incidence rates and rising survival rates from early diagnosis and treatment.

Most tumors are found in the distal portion of the large bowel. Survival following diagnosis correlates with the stage of tumor invasion (Figure 35-9). The 5-year survival rate for colorectal cancer is 91% when disease is diagnosed and treated in the early stage. Once the can-

cer has spread to regional organs, the 5-year survival rate decreases to 60%. For clients with metastasis to distant organs, the 5-year survival rate is 6%.

Etiology and Risk Factors

The cause of colorectal cancer is not definitely known. It occurs equally in men and women and occurs in all ethnic groups; however, the highest prevalence and mortality rates occur in those of African-American descent. It may be related to low-residue, high-fat diets and highly refined foods with an inadequate intake of fruits and vegetables (see the Complementary and Alternative Therapy feature on Trans-Fatty Acids and Colon Cancer on p. 852). There is a higher incidence in cities and industrialized countries. Two types of hereditary forms of colorectal cancer are caused by genetic mutations (see the Genetic Links feature on Hereditary Colorectal Cancer on p. 831). Gene mutations found in people with hereditary nonpolyposis colorectal cancer (HNPCC) suggest a predisposition for the development of colon cancer to be 90%, with the typical age of onset occurring in the 40s. Those with a genetic disposition to familial adenomatous polyposis (FAP) also have a higher risk of developing colorectal cancer. Only about 5% to 10% of clients with colorectal cancer have a hereditary basis for the disease, however. The risk of cancer increases sharply with age, with 90% of colorectal cancers developing after 50 years of age. Other risk factors are a history of breast, ovarian, or endometrial cancer; or

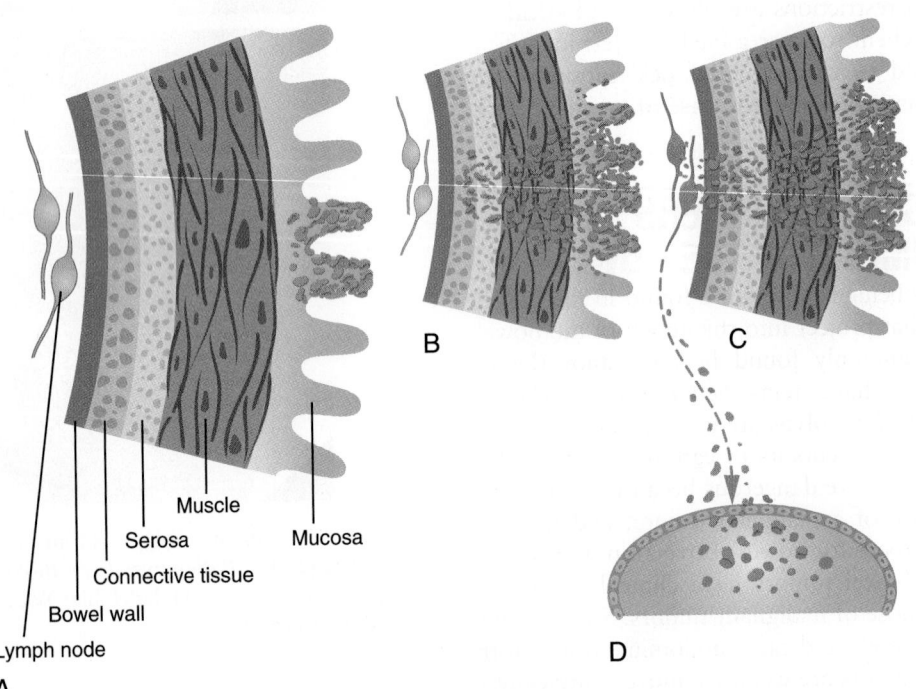

FIGURE 35-9 Stages of colon cancer, tumor (T), node (N), metastasis (M) system. **A,** Dukes' A or TNM I. Cancer is confined to bowel mucosa. **B,** Dukes' B or TNM II. Cancer extends into muscle, serosa, and connective tissue or adheres to or invades adjacent organs. **C,** Dukes' C or TNM III. Cancer penetrates the bowel wall and adheres to or invades adjacent organs; lymph nodes are positive. **D,** Cancer metastasizes to distant organs.

IBD, especially ulcerative colitis. (See the Complementary and Alternative Therapy feature on Iron Deficiency and Gastrointestinal Cancer on p. 852.)

Epidemiologic studies indicate that diet may be a major factor in the development of cancer of the large bowel. Studies on bulk in stool and the rate of transit of fecal matter have so far given mixed results. Some researchers propose that metabolic and bacterial end products are carcinogenic and that constipation allows a longer contact with the bowel wall, thus raising the probability that cancer will develop. Increasing fiber in the diet may reduce exposure to carcinogens by speeding stool transit through the intestines (see the Complementary and Alternative Therapy feature on Low-Fat, High-Fiber, and Fruit and Vegetable Diet to Reduce Rectal Mucosal Proliferation on p. 852). Folate, calcium, and selenium have been found possibly to prevent colon cancer.

Some studies have indicated that hormone replacement therapy and regular use of nonsteroidal anti-inflammatory drugs (NSAIDs) may reduce the risk of colon cancer (see the Complementary and Alternative Therapy feature on Chemoprevention of Colorectal Cancer on p. 852). Aspirin has been show to decrease the incidence of polyps. Uses of these agents are health-promotion actions, such as the dietary inclusion of fiber; fruits; and vegetables, especially cruciferous vegetables such as cauliflower, broccoli, brussels sprouts, and cabbage. Recent studies suggest that regular physical exercise may be protective against colon but not rectal cancer.

Health maintenance activities include yearly screening with fecal occult blood test (FOBT) and digital rectal examination (DRE) for people at average risk for colorectal cancer who are 50 years of age and older. A flexible sigmoidoscopy, colonoscopy, or double-contrast barium enema study should be performed every 5 to 10 years in clients with normal screening results and more frequently in clients from whom polyps have been removed. Several tests have become available. The stool gene test looks for abnormal genetic material in the stool that is shed from colorectal cancer cells. A positive test indicates the presence of early cancer cells or precancerous polyps. The virtual colonoscopy is a new

GENETICS LINKS

Hereditary Colorectal Cancer

Currently there are two well-described hereditary colorectal cancer syndromes.

Hereditary Nonpolyposis Colon Cancer (HNPCC)

Description. Colorectal cancer associated with HNPCC typically develops in a single colonic lesion, with most occurring in the proximal (right side) colon. Affected persons are also at risk for extracolonic malignancies including carcinoma of the endometrium, ovary, stomach, small bowel, pancreas, upper renal tract, and the hepatobiliary tract. Mean age of onset is 45 years of age.

Incidence. About 1% to 6% of all colorectal cancer is thought to be due to HNPCC.

Genetics. Autosomal dominant pattern of inheritance; each offspring of an affected parent has a 50% chance of inheriting the HNPCC genetic mutation. HNPCC results from a germ-line mutation in one of several DNA mismatch repair genes (*MLH1, MSH2, MSH6, PMS1,* and *PMS2*).

Diagnosis/Genetic Testing. A hallmark of HNPCC colorectal tumors is microsatellite instability (MSI). The presence of MSI in the tumor suggests the presence of a germline mutation. Testing generally begins with MSI testing of tumor tissue, followed by mutation analysis of the five genes if the tumor is positive for microsatellite instability. Mutations in *MSH1* and *MLH1* account for 95% of mutations found in HNPCC families.

Management. Close surveillance with annual colonoscopy is recommended for clients with strong clinical evidence of HNPCC or those with a known germline mutation. Annual screening for extracolonic malignancies is recommended, including transvaginal ultrasonography and endometrial aspiration for pathologic assessment beginning at age 30 years.

Familial Adenomatous Polyposis (FAP)

Description. FAP is a heritable colon cancer syndrome in which hundreds, if not thousands, of precancerous colonic polyps begin to develop from 7 to 36 years of age. Without a total colectomy, the risk of cancer is almost 100%. Extracolonic manifestations include polyps of the gastric and duodenum, osteomas, dental anomalies, congenital hypertrophy of the retinal pigment epithelium (CHRPE), soft tissue tumors, desmoid tumors, and associated cancers. A milder variant known as *attenuated FAP* has been described in which fewer polyps develop at a later age (around 50 to 55 years of age).

Incidence. Estimated to be responsible for 1% of all colorectal cancer.

Genetics. FAP is inherited in an autosomal dominant manner. About 75% to 80% of clients with FAP have an affected parent. Offspring of an affected parent have a 50% risk of inheriting the altered *APC* gene.

Diagnosis/Testing. FAP is caused by mutation in the APC gene, but the diagnosis primarily relies on clinical findings by colonoscopy. Molecular genetic testing is clinically available and detects about 95% of the disease-causing mutations.

Management. Management involves close surveillance of clients who carry an *APC* mutation or clients who are at risk but whose genetic status has not yet been determined. Recommended treatment for individuals with classic FAP is often colectomy.

FIGURE 35-10 Carcinomas of the cecum seen at colonoscopy. Carcinomas of the proximal colon are often large and bulky polypoid lesions (**A, B**) involve the ileocecal valve (**C**) and may outgrow their blood supply and become necrotic (**D**). (From Feldman, M., Friedman, L.S., & Sleisenger, M.H. [2002]. *Sleisenger and Fortran's gastrointestinal and liver disease* [7th ed.] [Vol. 2]. Philadelphia: W.B. Saunders.)

technique that uses a computerized imaging scanning machine to produce a three-dimensional image of the colon. The colon is scanned after the bowel is filled with fluid. It is less costly and less invasive than a colonoscopy; however, polyps cannot be removed or biopsies performed. Magnetic resonance colonography is an alternative to colonoscopy. It detects endoluminal masses and lesions and is used to screen clients who are at high risk for colon cancer. Finally, the pill camera is a large pill containing a tiny camera that the client swallows. It takes pictures of the bowel lining every few seconds and is most effective in filming the small bowel.

Clients who have a family or personal history of colorectal cancer, polyps, or IBD or genetic indicators for colorectal cancer should begin colorectal cancer screening at a younger age and should undergo screening more frequently. It is vital to explain to all clients the necessity for early detection and the importance of reporting manifestations such as rectal bleeding and a change in bowel habits to a health care provider.

Pathophysiology

More than 95% of colorectal cancers develop from adenomatous polyps (adenomas). The three types of adenomas are tubular, tubulovillous, and villous. The last type

has the highest risk of becoming cancerous. The polyps glow slowly, and most take 5 to 10 years or longer to become malignant. As a polyp becomes malignant, it increases in size within the lumen and begins to invade the bowel wall (Figure 35-10). Tumors in the right intestine tend to be bulky and to cause necrosis and ulceration. Tumors in the left intestine start as small, button-like masses that cause ulceration of the blood supply. Clients with FAP develop hundreds to thousands of polyps in their colons at an early age and have an almost 100% chance of developing cancer by the age of 40. As a result, some elect to have a prophylactic colectomy as a preventative measure.

Colon cancer is staged using the TNM (tumor-node-metastasis) or Dukes' classification system. The TNM system is described in Chapter 19. Figure 35-9 compares the TNM system with the Dukes system, the system most commonly used for colon cancer. Dukes' classifications (A, B, C, D) correlate with the TNM stage groupings (I, II, III, IV).

Malignant bowel tumors spread by (1) direct extension to a nearby organ, such as to the stomach from the transverse colon; (2) lymphatic and hematogenous channels, usually to the liver; and (3) seeding of, or implanting of cells into, the peritoneal cavity. The urinary bladder, ureters, and reproductive organs are frequently involved by direct extension. Blood-borne metastasis extends most commonly to the liver but also may involve the lungs, kidneys, and bones.

Clinical Manifestations

Manifestations of colon cancer include rectal bleeding, changed bowel habits, abdominal pain, weight loss, anemia, and anorexia. In general, tumors in the small bowel and right colon are more likely to cause abdominal pain and cramping, nausea, and vomiting. Because the large intestine distends, cancer located there has fewer early manifestations. At this location, lesions often ulcerate, resulting in anemia and dark, reddish brown stools. Anorexia, weight loss, weakness, debility, and a palpable mass in the right lower quadrant may be present at the time of diagnosis. Lesions of the ascending colon and transverse colon often manifest as progressive obstruction.

Tumors in the descending colon and rectum frequently cause obstructive manifestations, ribbon-like stools containing bright red blood and mucus, altered bowel habits, and tenesmus, but not weight loss, anemia, or dyspepsia. Bleeding is the manifestation that often prompts the client to seek health care.

One third of malignant tumors of the distal colon and rectum can be felt with an examining finger, which makes DRE one of the most important diagnostic methods. A stool guaiac test is performed to check for gastrointestinal bleeding. Serum carcinoembryonic antigen (CEA) and cancer antigen (CA) 19-9 are markers (indicators) that may be elevated in colorectal cancer and may aid in determining the progress of the disease. X-ray studies of the colon may show either a filling defect or a stricture. Ultrasound and computed tomography (CT), which help establish tumor size and metastasis, identify more than half of colorectal tumors. Flexible fiberoptic colonoscopes permit better visualization into the right colon, extend the diagnostic capabilities of the procedure, and enable collection of biopsy specimens (see Chapter 34). A new screening test that detects DNA shed from precancerous colon polyps and early stage colon cancer in the stool is in the developmental stages.

Prognosis

The prognosis in colorectal cancer depends on (1) the health of the client, (2) how early the disease is diagnosed, and (3) how effective the treatment is. The 5-year survival rates, listed according to Dukes' classification, are as follows: Dukes' A, 80% to 90%; Dukes' B, about 60%; Dukes' C, 25% to 40%; Dukes' D, less than 5%. Overall, 51% of clients with a diagnosis of colorectal cancer survive for 10 years. Early diagnosis and treatment are essential for a good outcome; however, only 37% of colorectal cancers are identified in the early stages.

Outcome Management
■ Medical Management

Decrease Tumor Growth. The primary treatment for colon cancer is surgery; however, medical treatment is used as an adjunct to improve survival in tumors that cannot be completely removed. Electrocoagulation may be used to destroy small tumors. Radiation therapy and chemotherapy are given alone or together. The combination can increase the survival of clients with rectal cancer; there is less evidence that the combination increases survival of clients with colon cancer. A vaccine called OncoVAX, manufactured from a person's own colon cancer cells, has shown promise in decreasing the rate or recurrence in clients with stage 2 cancer and increasing the survival rates.

Radiation Therapy. Radiation therapy is often used before surgery to reduce the size of the tumor and make it more resectable. Local interventions at the tumor site after surgery include implantation of radioactive isotopes into the tumor area. Isotopes used include radium, cesium, and cobalt. Iridium has been used in the rectum. Postoperatively, radiation therapy is used for clients classified with Dukes' B or C tumors. It may also be used for clients with Dukes' D cancer. Radiation therapy is not begun until surgical healing has taken place.

Chemotherapy. Chemotherapy may be used to reduce metastasis and control its manifestations; however, drug resistance limits the effectiveness of chemotherapy in colorectal cancer. Entire classes of cytotoxic drugs are rendered ineffective. There are effective drugs that are not influenced by these multi-drug resistance mechanisms. For example, the combination of oral levamisole (Ergamisol) and IV 5-fluorouracil (5-FU) has improved survival in Dukes' C tumors. Leucovorin (folinic acid) also may be given with 5-FU, with or without levamisole, to increase its effects. Recent studies demon- strated that adding irinotecan (Camptosar) to the first-line therapy has been effective in treating metastatic cancer. The combination of irinotecan, 5-FU, and leu- covorin is known as IFL, or the Saltz regimen. Toxic effects (nausea, vomiting, diarrhea) are more frequent with IFL. Bevacizumab (Avastin), which blocks angio- genesis, is the newest chemotherapy agent for treatment of colorectal cancer and has been shown to increase life expectancy.

■ Nursing Management of the Medical Client

Care of the client undergoing medical treatment for colon cancer revolves around care of a client undergoing chemotherapy and, occasionally, radiation therapy. See Chapter 19 for further information about the care of these clients.

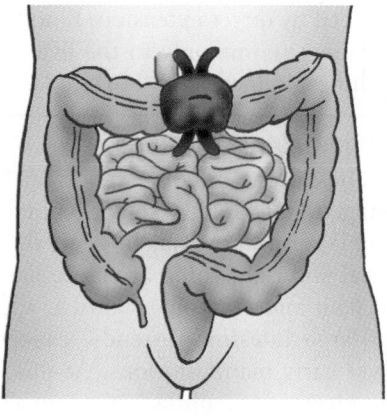

Single-barrel   Double-barrel   Loop

FIGURE 35-11 Types of colostomies. Single-barreled colostomies are usually permanent. Double-barrel colostomies are usually temporary, and stomas may be adjacent or several inches apart. Loop colostomies are temporary and are formed by bringing a loop of colon through the abdominal wall and supporting it with a plastic brace.

■ Surgical Management

About three of four clients undergo surgery and about 60% are cured. Intervention depends on the type of tumor, its location and stage, and the client's general condition. The basic goal of surgery is to remove the tumor with proximal and distal margins of the normal bowel tissue that contain blood vessels, lymph nodes, and the lymphatics. Poor margins associated with rectal cancer make the procedure difficult. As a result, there is a higher rate of recurrence with rectal cancer than with colon cancer.

A variety of surgical procedures are performed to treat colorectal cancer (Figures 35-11 and 35-12). Early colorectal cancers can be excised and removed through a colonoscope; however, most procedures entail colon resection, which can be completed laparoscopically or through an open surgical procedure. The tumor is removed with several inches of colon on either side of the tumor. An end-to-end anastomosis is performed, if possible. A sleeve resection may be performed for clients with advanced disease; it is a less involved procedure in which segments of the intestine are resected to relieve obstruction and bleeding.

Several different procedures are used for rectal cancer, depending on tumor location. It may be possible to preserve sphincter function by resecting tumors located in the proximal area. It may not be possible, however, to preserve sphincter function if tumors are less than 8 cm from the anal opening.

Colostomy

Indications. A colostomy may need to be performed for colorectal cancers. This procedure involves creating an opening between the colon and abdominal wall, from which fecal contents will pass. Because the main func-

tion of the large bowel is to absorb water, the colostomy is easier to manage nearer the sigmoid colon because the stool is more formed here than in the transverse or right colon. A colostomy can be located in the ascending, transverse, descending, or sigmoid colon and can be permanent or temporary.

A temporary colostomy allows the bowel to rest and later may be reanastomosed. The temporary colostomy also can be used to treat inoperable bowel cancer, with the ostomy placed proximal to the cancer. A temporary colostomy is made most commonly at the midpoint of the left colon or transverse colon, whereas a permanent colostomy is usually placed in the sigmoid colon. When creating a temporary loop colostomy, the surgeon brings a loop of bowel out through a wound that is separate from the surgical incision. To keep the loop from slipping back into the abdominal cavity, the surgeon places a rod or bridge beneath it. Although the bowel is usually opened with a cautery in surgery, the surgeon may wait 2 or 3 days postoperatively to open the bowel. Because there are no sensory nerve endings in the bowel wall, this procedure is essentially painless, except for some cramping. The surgeon usually indicates which is the proximal loop and which is the distal loop.

A colostomy may also be single-barreled or double-barreled. When only one loop end of bowel is opened onto the abdominal surface, the result is called an *end* or *single-barreled colostomy;* the client has only one stoma. An end colostomy is permanent if the bowel distal to it has been resected. A *double-barreled colostomy* is one in which both loops, distal and proximal, are open onto the abdominal wall. It may be closed later, depending on the disease present. A double-barreled colostomy can be two separate stomas, a loop with one stoma and two openings, or one stoma and a mucus fistula. The fistula expels mucus and is covered with a gauze dressing or pouch.

A   B   C

FIGURE 35-12 Resecting malignant tumors in the rectosigmoid segment of the bowel. **A,** Anterior resection with primary anastomosis is used for cancer at any point in the bowel except the terminal rectum. Associated lymph nodes are resected. **B,** Abdominoperineal (anteroposterior) resection with formation of permanent colostomy (Miles' operation) for cancer involving the anus and terminal portion of the rectum. **C,** Proctosigmoidectomy with pull-through and preservation of external sphincter muscles is appropriate when the tumor is in the proximal rectum and unlikely to metastasize further.

Contraindications. Any health condition that makes the client a poor surgical risk is a contraindication to a colostomy procedure.

Complications. Suture line leakage with local or generalized peritonitis may occur in the early postoperative period. Other complications are hemorrhage and stomal necrosis, retraction, prolapse, and stenosis. Stomal complications may require additional surgery to revise the stoma.

Outcomes. The client resumes usual activities within 4 to 6 weeks and is able to perform self-care of the stoma. If needed, radiation therapy and chemotherapy are initiated.

Abdominal-Perineal Resection

Rectal tumors may require an abdominal-perineal resection, with the formation of a permanent or end colostomy. The affected colon and entire rectum are excised, and the anus is closed. The colon is removed through an abdominal incision, and the rectum through a perineal incision. Newer surgical techniques allow removal of low sigmoid tumors while leaving the rectal sphincter intact; normal bowel elimination is maintained.

■ Nursing Management of the Surgical Client

Preoperative Care

The client often presents with weight loss and a change in bowel habits. Obtain accurate descriptions of manifestations as well as an assessment of major risk factors,

such as a family history of colon cancer, ulcerative colitis, or familial polyposis. Assess the abdomen, noting any abnormalities, such as pain, distention, and masses.

Preoperatively, a diet high in calories, protein, and carbohydrates but low in residue may be given to provide nutrition and reduce peristalsis. TPN may be necessary to provide nutrients and vitamins the client requires.

The bacteria level in the bowel must be lowered preoperatively to decrease the risk of infection. Clients needing a bowel resection must undergo a bowel preparation to minimize bacterial growth in the bowel and postoperative wound infection. This preparation usually involves the following:

- A low-residue or liquid diet to reduce the fecal contents of the bowel
- Oral administration of cathartics, such as polyethylene glycol–electrolyte solution (GoLYTELY) or a preprocedure bowel evacuator (Fleet Prep Kit), which is started at least 12 to 24 hours preoperatively
- Administration of antibiotics, such as sulfonamides and possibly neomycin and cephalexin, usually by mouth, for 12 to 48 hours preoperatively
- Administration of enemas to clean the bowel (the inside of the bowel lumen should be as clean and as bacteria free as possible)
- Blood transfusions to correct severe anemia and enhance wound healing

Identify the client's level of anxiety and provide supportive efforts. Explain all treatments and procedures fully. Clarify and reinforce the information provided by the physician. Encourage clients to ventilate their feelings and meet with health team members to discuss treatments and prognosis. The client also needs to know how treatment decisions will be made when the results of pathologic study are available and what to expect after the operation, such as placement of tubes and measures to prevent postoperative complications.

If a colostomy is necessary, an enterostomal therapy nurse should be asked to educate the client about the ostomy, answer questions, and advise about the optimal placement of the stoma. If an enterostomal therapy nurse is not available, assume the responsibility for teaching the client about the stoma. The risk of sexual dysfunction should be explained to the client in a supportive atmosphere.

Postoperative Care
Assessment

Immediate postoperative assessments are as discussed in Chapter 16. Assess for the return of peristalsis; indications are passage of flatus and return of bowel sounds, heard during auscultation of the abdomen. Gastric suction may be continued until peristalsis returns. Make sure the NG tube is patent.

Additionally, if a colostomy was created, monitor the colostomy output, and use special care to keep fecal contents from the colostomy (which contain bacteria) away from the surgical incision. Assess the client's stoma closely for the presence of stomal ischemia. The stoma should be red and moist. If it becomes dark or dusky, report this change to the surgeon immediately.

If an abdominoperineal resection with creation of an end colostomy is performed, assess both the abdominal and perineal wounds. The incision may be sutured completely closed; however, sometimes drains are left in the incision and may be attached to a suction device such as a Hemovac. When suction is not used, a Penrose drain can be placed in the wound. Change the dressing frequently or as ordered. A large amount of serous drainage can be expected from the perineal wound. It often takes several weeks to months for the wound to heal completely because of its size.

Diagnosis, Outcomes, Interventions

Diagnosis: Risk for Injury. The postoperative client is at risk for the development of postoperative complications. The nursing diagnosis is *Risk for Injury related to postoperative complications, including infection, hemorrhage, wound disruption, thrombophlebitis, and abnormal stomal function.*

Outcomes. The client does not experience an injury as evidenced by absence of manifestations of infection, bleeding, and evidence of wound disruption, thrombophlebitis, stomal ischemia, and bowel spillage.

Interventions

Monitor Vital Signs. Immediate postoperative interventions are the same as those used for any major abdominal procedure; they involve monitoring vital signs for manifestations of infection and shock.

Advance Diet as Tolerated. An NG tube is usually in place until peristalsis returns. It is usually several days before the NG tube is discontinued and the client begins to consume fluids and food. As the client tolerates food, he or she is slowly advanced to a regular diet.

Decrease Cramping. Abdominal cramps commonly occur after surgery, as does distention of the bowel. Distention is uncomfortable and may put pressure on suture lines. The insertion of a rectal tube for 20 to 30 minutes per physician order will help if the rectum contains gas. Early ambulation helps to relieve distention and promotes peristalsis.

Apply Rectal Dressing. Prepare the client to wear a rectal dressing throughout the healing period. The character, volume, and odor of the drainage should be assessed. If the drainage in any way suggests a developing infection, arrange for a culture of the wound to identify the organism.

Occasionally, in the immediate postoperative period, sump drainage is placed in the perineal wound. This is also indicated if the wound becomes infected. The sump tube is attached to suction, allowing the wound to heal from its deepest portion without forming an abscess.

Reduce Pain. The perineal wound can be very painful, and the client should receive sufficient medication to control the pain. Once the packing is removed, the wound is irrigated, and the client should take a sitz bath three or four times a day. The client will find a side-lying position in bed most comfortable.

Monitor Stoma Drainage. There may be a colostomy pouch over the stoma. Make sure that this pouch is not applying pressure to the stoma, which would interfere with its blood supply. When changing or emptying the pouch, prevent contamination of the surgical wound by fecal discharges. Monitor the return of bowel function by observing the type and quantity of discharges from the stoma.

Prevent Thrombophlebitis. The high lithotomy position associated with the abdominoperineal resection is associated with an increased risk of development of postoperative phlebitis. To prevent this problem, subcutaneous injections of heparin, usually 5000 units every 12 hours after surgery, are often prescribed. Sequential pressure stockings or thigh-high antiembolic hose also must be worn. The client must perform leg exercises before and after surgery. Monitor the client for manifestations of thrombophlebitis.

Diagnosis: Risk for Disturbed Body Image.

The client with an ostomy must face alterations in self-concept and body image. Write the nursing diagnosis as *Risk for Disturbed Body Image related to colostomy and lifestyle changes.*

Outcomes. The client adjusts to changes in body image as evidenced by the ability to identify and use effective coping methods in dealing with the disease and losses experienced.

Interventions. Give emotional support while the client begins the process of adjusting to the colostomy. It is also important to provide extensive teaching about how to care for the colostomy. The client's significant others also must adjust to the colostomy; help them by listening to their reactions and explaining the client's problems to them.

A client's reactions to a new colostomy may range from apparently easy acceptance to total withdrawal from social contacts. How well clients adjust depends partly on their attitudes toward excretory functions, previous knowledge about colostomies, and general ability to adjust to stressful situations.

Some clients refuse to look at the stoma and find it difficult to accept its presence, whereas others begin to participate in stoma care almost immediately. Your reactions to and manner toward the client and the care required can affect the client's adjustment. For some clients, the colostomy represents a "cure"; for others, it is palliation when the cancer has spread.

Continuing sexual relationships is a major concern for the client with a colostomy and the significant other. There is no physical reason that a client cannot enjoy normal sexual relations, although a small number of men become impotent after a radical perineal dissection. If this complication occurs, the physician may recommend a urology consultation to discuss treatment options for impotence (see Chapter 40). Psychological barriers may cause problems. With love, patience, understanding, and good hygienic practices, there should be no problem; however, it may be several months after surgery before a couple manages to reestablish a satisfactory sexual relationship. Referral to a social worker, counselor, psychiatric liaison, sex therapist, or registered nurse with a counseling background may be beneficial.

Diagnosis: Effective Therapeutic Regimen Management.

The client with a colostomy needs to learn about self-care. The nursing diagnosis is *Effective Therapeutic Regimen Management related to colostomy care, irrigation, and possible complications associated with colostomies.*

Outcomes. The client understands care of the colostomy, as evidenced by the ability to (1) apply the pouch; (2) care for peristomal skin; (3) irrigate the colostomy, if applicable; and (4) prevent or treat any associated problems.

Interventions.

Carefully assess the client's physical condition and emotional and mental attitudes toward the colostomy before attempting to teach ostomy self-care. Pace the teaching to the client's level of acceptance of the colostomy and ability to manage it.

Teach Ostomy Care. Teach the client how to apply the pouch to the stoma correctly. The client first should be taught how to examine the stoma. A healthy stoma is red and slightly raised. (Figure 35-13 shows a colostomy during the application of an appliance.) The skin around the stoma *(peristomal skin)* should be clear, without evidence of irritation. The peristomal area should be cleaned well with a mild soap and water and dried well before the new pouch is applied. The skin should be treated with a skin barrier and the new pouch applied, cut about $\frac{1}{16}$ to $\frac{1}{8}$ inch larger than the stoma. The pouch should be changed every 4 to 5 days or when leakage occurs. If a two-piece system is used, the faceplate may stay in place for 7 days. Types of pouches are shown in Figure 35-7.

Teach the client to empty the pouch when it is about half full and how to clean out the pouch when emptying it. The client should demonstrate the ability to empty and change the pouch independently before being discharged. See the earlier discussion of ileostomy care for further information.

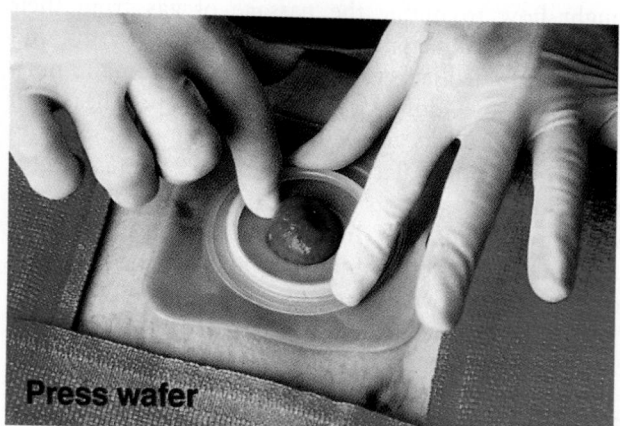

Press wafer

FIGURE 35-13 Healthy stoma during application of wafer. Note that the stoma is red, moist, and healthy looking. The nurse is pressing the wafer onto the skin. The temperature of the client's skin warms the wafer to help it adhere to the client. (Courtesy of ConvaTec, Bristol-Myers Squibb, Skillman, NJ.)

Teach Stoma Irrigation. Clients with end sigmoid colostomies can be taught to regulate the colostomy through regular irrigation. Clients who are physically, mentally, and emotionally capable should be encouraged to attempt irrigation and regulation. Some clients, despite irrigation, may never achieve regularity of elimination. If they have not achieved regularity within 6 months, they probably never will.

See the Client Education Guide on Colostomy Irrigation on the website for the steps involved in irrigation. The best time for irrigation is when the client formerly had a daily bowel movement because the bowel is already "trained" to evacuate at this time. If inserting the catheter proves difficult, let a little solution flow in and rotate the catheter. If the catheter will not go in, teach the client to apply gloves or a finger cot, lubricate the finger, and gently pass it into the stoma. This method often dislodges any feces that might be near the stoma. If the client cannot pass a catheter and no obstruction is felt digitally, the client should notify the health care provider.

If cramping occurs, the client should stop the solution temporarily, take a few deep breaths, and restart the solution slowly. The client should *never* (1) use more than 1000 ml, (2) irrigate the colostomy more than once a day, or (3) irrigate the colostomy if diarrhea is present.

If there is no return after irrigation, the client should ambulate, gently massage the abdomen, and try drinking some warm water. If there is still no return, the client should apply a pouch and try the irrigation again the next day. If there is no return the second day, the client should notify the health care provider.

Minimize Flatus. Flatus is an embarrassing problem because the client may have no control over its passage and no sensations to indicate when it is about to pass. Flatus can make clients avoid social situations. Clients can be taught how to muffle the passage of gas from their colostomies. Women may hold their purses or arms, and men their folded jackets or hats, over the stoma to muffle the noise. Odor-proof pouches and pouches with charcoal filter disks are available, but the most satisfactory way to control flatus is through diet. Because everyone is different, clients must learn by trial and error which foods cause gas. In general, nuts, corn, cabbage, sauerkraut, broccoli, cauliflower, and legumes are gas-forming foods. Swallowing air by eating too rapidly, chewing gum, and drinking carbonated beverages also cause intestinal gas.

Evaluation

The client should recover from surgery without complications and should resume usual activities within 6 weeks. When a colostomy has been performed, the client should be able to manage it within 2 months. If the client is unable to accomplish self-care, the need for further teaching should be explored.

■ Self-Care

In preparation for discharge, clients need support and knowledgeable advice as they learn to live with their colostomies. The client needs to know the nearest location for purchase of ostomy supplies (see the Client Education Guide on Ostomy Supplies on the website). Immediately after dismissal, home delivery of supplies may be necessary. The enterostomal therapy nurse can help the client learn to manage and accept the ostomy and to achieve a smooth transition from the health care facility to the home. Some cities have established ostomy rehabilitation clinics to help clients, and most large communities have an ostomy association that maintains contact with the American Cancer Society. These support groups are helpful because clients can share their ostomy concerns with others who have similar problems. A home health care referral can add to the client's peace of mind, identify problems that might not otherwise be known, and ensure necessary follow-up care. (See the Bridge to Home Health Care feature on Adjusting to Life with a Colostomy on p. 839.)

Before discharge, advise clients that it may take several weeks for them to regain their strength after major bowel surgery; further, when segments have been removed from the bowel, bowel habits may alter until the body adjusts to the situation. You may need to teach the client and his or her significant others how to change dressings at home because wounds may not be healed totally by the time the client is discharged. In general, teaching should cover (1) dressing changes, (2) dietary or activity restrictions, (3) colostomy care if applicable, and (4) manifestations of intestinal obstruction and perforation.

The client who is having a problem with the colostomy should see an enterostomal therapy nurse. The client with an abdominoperineal resection needs follow-up from the surgeon to ensure that the perineal wound is healing properly.

OTHER DISORDERS OF THE LARGE AND SMALL BOWEL

HERNIATIONS

A *hernia* is the abnormal protrusion of an organ, tissue, or part of an organ through the structure that normally contains it. Hernias most commonly occur in the abdominal cavity when a section of the bowel protrudes through as a result of a congenital or acquired weakness of abdominal musculature. Hernias can occur at any age and in either gender. About 700,000 inguinal herniorrhaphies are performed in the United States each year. Indirect inguinal hernias, the most common type, typically occur in men. Direct inguinal hernias are found

BRIDGE TO HOME HEALTH CARE

Adjusting to Life with a Colostomy

When you visit a client who has a new colostomy, assess the stoma and peristomal skin thoroughly before selecting a pouch. The stoma should be beefy red; a pale red or pale pink stoma indicates a limited blood supply. A healthy stoma is moist; dryness suggests dehydration. Note whether the outer edges are intact and attached to the peristomal skin. The stoma should be round and raised; it will shrink during the next 4 to 6 weeks. Assess the stoma when the pouch is off and the client is lying down; repeat when the client sits. Watch for (1) changes in stoma shape, (2) skin folds, (3) creases, and (4) dimpling of the peristomal skin.

Clients and caregivers are more likely to manage a colostomy independently if they understand and follow your instructions and participate in care. Demonstrate how to clean the stoma; request return demonstrations. Some bleeding is normal; applying pressure should stop the bleeding. Excessive bleeding is abnormal; if this happens, they should call a physician immediately. Tell the client and caregiver to expect output (effluent) daily. The effluent will by runny initially but will thicken within 2 to 4 weeks. Expect excessive flatulus (bowel gas) for 4 to 8 weeks. Teach clients and caregivers to watch for manifestations of intestinal obstruction that require immediate medical care, such as nausea or vomiting, body temperature exceeding 101° F, severe abdominal pain, distention, limited or no output, and decreased bowel sounds.

Leakage is a common problem. To minimize leakage, provide detailed instructions about pouch fit and care; the pouch should be changed twice a week. *Do not* assume that the appliance the client took home from the hospital will fit when the stoma shrinks. If the peristomal skin retracts, the client needs a pouch with a convex wafer, not a flat wafer. If the stoma is round, you may use a precut pouch; if it is not round, use a cut-to-fit pouch. Make and date a pattern of the stoma by tracing the outline of the stoma on a clear piece of rigid plastic with an indelible marker. Cut out the pattern and check it for proper fit against the stoma; it may not fit when the stoma shrinks. Use an ostomy belt that is snug but not tight to improve the bond between the pouch and peristomal skin. If the client is using a two-piece pouch system, make sure that there is a good seal between the pouch and the wafer.

To reinforce instructions between your visits, leave simple, step-by-step directions for pouch changing for clients and caregivers. Also leave written details about purchasing ostomy supplies locally or by mail order. Provide verbal and written diet and hydration information. Suggest that the client avoid foods high in fiber initially, such as corn, popcorn, mushrooms, peanuts, and Chinese foods; these foods can cause the bowel to swell and become obstructed. When the swelling decreases in 4 to 8 weeks, clients should be able to gradually resume eating a regular diet and to increase fluid consumption to prevent constipation at resumption of regular diet.

Refer clients with a colostomy and their family members to organizations that can help them cope with the colostomy diagnosis and changed body image, such as the United Ostomy Association (1-800-826-0826); the American Cancer Society (1-800-227-2345); and the National Wound, Ostomy, and Continence Nurses Association (1-888-224-9626). Nurse members of the last group can provide valuable information about resuming a normal lifestyle and can help manage complicated ostomies.

---

more commonly in older people. Incisional or ventral hernias occur most often in clients who had poor wound healing after surgery. Obese or pregnant clients are more likely to develop umbilical hernias.

Etiology and Risk Factors

Hernias develop when there is a defect in the integrity of the muscular wall accompanied by increased intra-abdominal pressure. Congenital muscle weakness is one risk factor, as are any factors that increase intra-abdominal pressure. The muscle weakness cannot be prevented, but exercises can be performed to strengthen weak muscles. Because obesity is one cause of increased intra-abdominal pressure, such an increase can be prevented by weight control. Avoiding heavy lifting and straining also reduces intra-abdominal pressure. Early diagnosis is important to prevent incarceration and strangulation of the herniated tissue.

Pathophysiology

Defects in the muscular wall may be congenital and due to weakened tissue or a wide space at the inguinal ligament or may be caused by trauma. Intra-abdominal pressure increases with pregnancy, obesity, heavy lifting, coughing, and traumatic injuries from blunt pressure. When two of these factors coexist with some tissue weakness, a hernia may occur. Increased pressure without a weakness is not likely to cause a hernia. Weakness, in addition to being present from birth, is acquired as part of the aging process. As clients age, muscular tissues become infiltrated and are replaced by adipose and connective tissues.

When the contents of the hernial sac can be replaced into the abdominal cavity by manipulation, the hernia is said to be *reducible. Irreducible* and *incarcerated* are terms that refer to a hernia in which the contents of the sac cannot be reduced or replaced by manipulation. When pressure from the hernial ring (the ring of muscular tissue through which the bowel protrudes) cuts off the blood supply to the herniated segment of bowel, the bowel becomes *strangulated*. Incarcerated hernias usually become strangulated. This situation is a surgical emergency because unless the bowel is released, it soon becomes gangrenous because of the lack of blood supply.

Hernias can penetrate through any defect in the abdominal wall, through the diaphragm, or through some internal structure within the abdominal cavity (Figure 35-14). This discussion covers only the more common types of hernias: inguinal (both indirect and direct), femoral, umbilical, and incisional. (Hiatal hernia is discussed in Chapter 32.)

Indirect Inguinal Hernia

An indirect inguinal herniation occurs through the inguinal ring and follows the spermatic cord through the inguinal canal. It is more common in males than females because of the space allowed for the testicles to descend. There is a high incidence of indirect inguinal hernia in young people. The incidence is also high among clients 50 to 60 years of age and then gradually decreases in older age groups. These hernias can become extremely large and often descend into the scrotum.

Direct Inguinal Hernia

In a direct inguinal hernia, bowel passes through the abdominal wall in an area of muscular weakness, not through a canal, as do indirect inguinal and femoral hernias. This type of hernia is more common in older clients. Direct inguinal hernia gradually develops in an area that is weak owing to a congenital deficiency in the number of fibers it contains.

Femoral Hernia

A femoral hernia occurs through the femoral ring and is more common in females than in males. It begins as a plug of fat in the femoral canal that enlarges and gradually pulls the peritoneum, and almost inevitably the urinary bladder, into the sac. There is a high incidence of incarceration and strangulation with this type of hernia.

Umbilical Hernia

Umbilical herniation in the adult is more common in women and is due to increased abdominal pressure. It usually occurs in obese clients and in multiparous women.

Incisional or Ventral Hernia

The incisional or ventral hernia occurs at the site of a previous surgical incision that has healed inadequately because of a postoperative problem, such as infection, inadequate nutrition, extreme distention, or obesity.

Outcome Management
■ Medical Management

Hernias that are not strangulated or incarcerated can be mechanically reduced. A truss, a firm pad held in place by a belt, also can be used to keep the hernia reduced. The pad is placed over the hernia after it has been reduced and is left in place to prevent the hernia from recurring. The client is taught to apply the truss daily before arising. The client should carefully inspect the skin under the truss for any manifestation of breakdown.

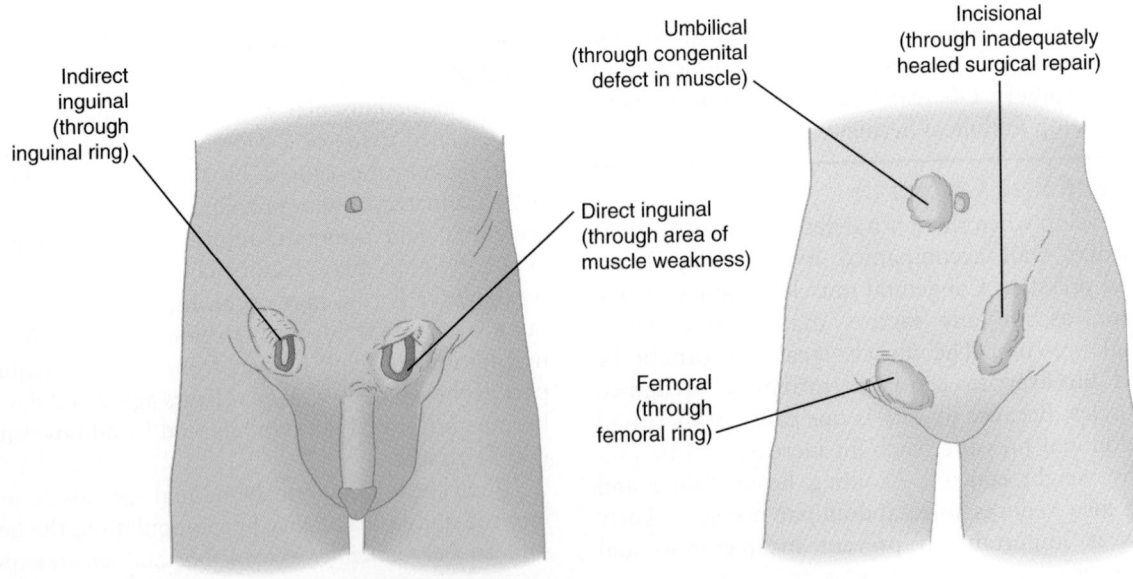

FIGURE 35-14 Common types of herniation.

■ Surgical Management

Inguinal hernia repairs (herniorrhaphies) are common, occurring in an estimated 28 of every 10,000 population in the United States. A hernia repair is performed using a small incision directly over the weakened area. The intestine is then returned to the perineal cavity, the hernia sac is excised, and the muscle is closed tightly over the area. Mesh may facilitate healing and prevent recurrence. Hernias in the inguinal region are usually repaired with the use of spinal or local anesthesia. Most hernia repairs are now performed as outpatient procedures. Laparoscopic extraperitoneal (LEP) herniorrhaphy is a newer technique that results in higher success rates with less recurrence, less pain, and shorter postoperative recovery periods.

Some repairs are difficult because there is insufficient muscle mass to keep the intestines in place. In this case, mesh grafts are used to reinforce the area of herniation. Clients with difficult repairs are usually hospitalized for 1 to 2 days to receive prophylactic antibiotics.

■ Nursing Management of the Surgical Client

Make certain the client voids after hernia surgery because urinary retention is a common problem, especially in males. Return the client to a general diet as soon as he

or she tolerates food. When general anesthesia is used, postoperative progress is slower. Assure the client that during the immediate postoperative period, the hernia will not recur. Some clients hesitate to become active because of this fear. The client should be told not to engage in any lifting for 4 to 6 weeks after surgery. Obese clients progress more slowly, heal more slowly, and may need more encouragement to participate in postoperative activities.

Following an inguinal hernia repair, an ice pack is usually applied to the incisional area to control pain and reduce swelling. In males, the scrotal area should be carefully assessed for swelling. An ice pack also can be applied to the scrotal area. To reduce scrotal swelling, position the client so as to elevate the scrotum and have the client wear a scrotal support when out of bed.

DIVERTICULAR DISEASE

Diverticular disease refers to two disorders: diverticulosis and diverticulitis. A *diverticulum* is a blind out-pouching or herniation of intestinal mucosa through the muscular coat of the large intestine, usually the sigmoid colon. *Diverticulosis* is the presence of noninflamed diverticula (Figure 35-15). *Diverticulitis* is inflammation of a diverticulum. Diverticulitis is common in obese clients and af-

A   B

FIGURE 35-15 A, A barium enema showing right-sided diverticulosis. **B,** Endoscopic appearance of a diverticulum in the right colon. (**A** courtesy of Mark Feldman, M.D. **B** from Feldman, M., Friedman, L.S., & Sleisenger, M.H. [2002]. *Sleisenger and Fortran's gastrointestinal and liver disease* [7th ed., vol. 2]. Philadelphia: W.B. Saunders.)

fects 5% to 10% of men and women over 45 years of age and 80% of those over 85 years of age. It is estimated, however, that only 20% of those with diverticulitis will develop manifestations of disease. Although diverticula may be found all through the bowel, 85% of diverticulitis arises in the sigmoid and descending colon.

Etiology and Risk Factors

Low-fiber diets have been implicated in the development of diverticula because such diets decrease bulk in the stool and predispose to constipation. The etiology of diverticular disease is related mainly to two factors: weakening of the bowel wall and increased intraluminal pressure. In the presence of muscle weakness in the bowel, this increase in intraluminal pressure can lead to the formation of diverticula. Diverticulitis occurs when undigested food blocks the diverticulum, leading to a decrease in blood supply to the area and predisposing the bowel to invasion of bacteria into the diverticulum.

Pathophysiology

Diverticula have a narrow neck like that of a flask that communicates with the bowel lumen. Weak points in the bowel musculature exist where branches of the blood vessels penetrate the colonic wall. These weak points create areas for bowel protrusion when there is increased intraluminal pressure. Diverticula frequently develop in the sigmoid colon because of the high pressures required in this area to move the stool into the rectum.

Diverticulitis may be acute or chronic. If the diverticulum is not infected, it causes few problems. When fecaliths do not liquefy and drain from the diverticulum, however, they may become trapped, causing irritation and inflammation (diverticulitis). The inflamed area becomes congested with blood and may bleed or perforate. Chronic diverticulitis results in increased scarring and eventual narrowing of the bowel lumen, potentially causing obstruction.

Diagnosis of acute diverticulitis can be confirmed by computed tomography (CT). Sigmoidoscopy is of little diagnostic value since the disease is usually extraluminal.

Clinical Manifestations

The manifestations of diverticulitis depend on the extent of the inflammation and the site of occurrence. Discomfort consists of dull, episodic, or steady left quadrant or midabdominal pain. Assessment also reveals alteration in bowel habits (constipation, diarrhea, or both), increased flatus, anorexia, and low-grade fever. Localized tenderness may occur in the left lower quadrant. The inflammatory process usually subsides within several weeks. If the infection penetrates the pelvic floor or retroperitoneal tissues, abscesses may result. Extension of the inflammation to adjacent organs can lead to fistulas of the bladder or vagina and peritonitis. Repeated inflammation can result in narrowing and obstruction of the bowel.

Trace blood may be found in the stools, but profuse bleeding is uncommon. Stools also may contain mucus. Urinary frequency can occur if the inflammation is in the proximity of the bladder. Straining, coughing, or lifting causes an increase in intra-abdominal pressure and manifestations such as diarrhea, constipation, pain, mucus, and flatus. The clinician may palpate a tender mass on digital rectal examinations.

Outcome Management
■ Medical Management

Asymptomatic diverticular disease requires no specific therapy other than diet modification. Mild disease can be treated by adherence to a high-fiber diet and prevention of constipation with bran and bulk laxatives (hydrophilic colloids). Advise clients to notify the physician of any change in bowel movement pattern (constipation or diarrhea) or character (the presence of mucus or blood) or if fever, abdominal pain, or urinary manifestations develop.

Diverticulitis may be treated conservatively with medical intervention by allowing the colon to rest. Clients with acute diverticulitis are assigned to NPO status, may have an NG tube, and receive parenteral fluids and antibiotics until pain, inflammation, and temperature decrease. If opioids are required for pain management, meperidine is the drug of choice. Morphine sulfate should be avoided because it has been shown to cause spasm of the colon. When the acute episode subsides, oral liquids and, later, a progressively more inclusive diet can be added. Nursing care involves the preceding interventions and teaching the client about diet changes.

■ Surgical Management

About 20% of clients with diverticulitis will require surgery. Surgery is indicated for diverticular disease with complications such as hemorrhage, obstruction, abscesses, and perforation. Surgical procedures usually involve ligation and removal of the sac or resection of involved bowel if complications develop. With abscess or obstruction, the surgeon performs a colon resection with a temporary colostomy, which is left in place until the client's condition improves. For some clients, the temporary colostomy alone allows the bowel to rest and heal. For nursing care, see the earlier discussion of bowel resection.

MECKEL'S DIVERTICULUM

Meckel's diverticulum, an outpouching of the bowel, is a vestige of embryonic development found on the ileum within 10 cm of the cecum. The pouch may be lined with gastric mucosa or may contain pancreatic tissue. The gastric mucosal lining sometimes ulcerates and bleeds or perforates. In addition, the diverticulum may become inflamed and may mimic appendicitis. Meckel's diverticulum is sometimes attached to the umbilicus by a fibrous band and may be the focus around which the bowel twists, causing obstruction. Treatment involves surgical excision of the diverticulum.

INTESTINAL OBSTRUCTION

Partial or complete impairment of the forward flow of intestinal contents is known as an *intestinal obstruction.* About 90% of bowel obstructions occur in the small bowel, especially in the ileum, which is the narrowest segment. Obstructions of the small intestine are a common surgical emergency. Large bowel obstructions usually occur in the sigmoid colon. The mortality rate for acute obstruction in the small bowel is 10% and in the large bowel, 30%. Obstruction produces nausea, vomiting, dehydration, and severe pain. Intestinal obstruction has a high mortality rate if it is not diagnosed and treated within 24 hours.

Etiology and Risk Factors

Obstruction of the small intestine may be caused by narrowing of the intestinal lumen as a result of inflammation, neoplasms, adhesions, hernia, volvulus, intussusception, food blockage, or compression from outside the intestine. Paralytic ileus (see later discussion), vascular problems such as mesenteric embolus and thrombus, and hypokalemia from diuretics or antihypertensive agents also may result in small bowel obstructions. Lobar pneumonia, peritonitis, and pancreatitis frequently produce an ileus (see later discussion) of infectious origin.

Cancer accounts for about 80% of obstructions of the large intestine, with most occurring in the sigmoid colon. Other causes are diverticulitis, ulcerative colitis, and previous abdominal surgery. Factors that cause intestinal obstructions may be mechanical, neurogenic, or vascular.

Mechanical Factors

Adhesions. Adhesions are probably the most common cause of obstruction in both the small and large intestines. Adhesions form after abdominal surgery, and for unknown reasons, some clients have massive adhesions. Irritants that remain in the abdomen following surgical procedures enhance the formation of adhesions. These fibrous bands of scar tissue can become looped over a portion of the bowel. The loops then can become either the focus around which the bowel can twist *(volvulus)* (Figure 35-16) or the band that mechanically obstructs the bowel by external pressure. The presence of multiple adhesions increases the risk of obstruction.

Hernia. An incarcerated hernia may or may not cause obstruction, depending on the size of the hernial ring; however, the potential for obstruction is always present in any hernia. A strangulated hernia is always obstructed because the bowel cannot function when its blood supply is cut off.

Volvulus. Volvulus is a twisting of the bowel that commonly occurs about a stationary focus (e.g., tumor or Meckel's diverticulum) in the abdominal cavity (see Figure 35-16). It can cause infarction of the bowel and can occur in either the large or small bowel. Volvulus sometimes can be corrected without surgical intervention. Successful decompression of the bowel with a long tube (Cantor or Miller-Abbott tube) releases pressure against the proximal end of the loop, thus allowing a small bowel volvulus to relax.

Intussusception. *Intussusception,* which sometimes complicates IBD, is a telescoping of the bowel (slipping of a section of bowel into an adjacent section) (Figure 35-17). The condition is often associated with tumor of the large bowel. Peristaltic action telescopes the proximal bowel into the bowel distal to it. Intramural lesions often cause intussusception.

Cancers. Cancer accounts for about 80% of mechanical obstructions in the large bowel and mostly affects the sigmoid colon. Carcinogenesis is slow and, because of the large lumen of the bowel, may become advanced before a fecal mass lodges at the constricted site and pre-

FIGURE 35-16 Volvulus. Intestine twists at least 180 degrees, causing obstruction and ischemia.

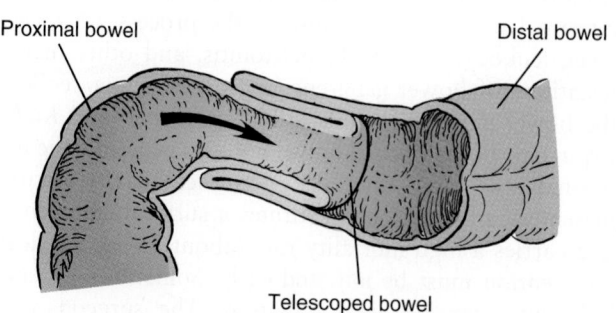

FIGURE 35-17 Intussusception. A portion of bowel telescopes into adjacent (usually distal) bowel.

cipitates an acute obstructive process. In the small bowel, obstructive manifestations are frequently the first indication of a tumor. Even though the lumen of the small bowel is smaller, manifestations do not appear early in the process because the intestinal contents are liquid.

Neurogenic Factors

Neurogenic factors are responsible for an adynamic (or functional) obstruction, the most common type of intestinal obstruction. An adynamic obstruction, also called *paralytic ileus*, is caused by lack of peristaltic activity and commonly occurs after abdominal surgery. The bowel ceases to function for longer than 72 hours as a result of the sympathetic nervous system's response to an insult to the peritoneum. Extensive surgical procedures in the bowel and in the retroperitoneal area may cause a postoperative neurogenic problem. Additional causes of adynamic ileus are trauma, hypokalemia, myocardial infarction, and vascular insufficiency. Treatment involves aspiration of secretions by NG suction until the bowel begins to function.

Vascular Factors

When the blood supply to any part of the body is interrupted, the part ceases to function and pain occurs. Blood is supplied to the bowel by way of the celiac and superior and inferior mesenteric arteries. These vessels have anastomotic intercommunications at the head of the pancreas and along the transverse bowel. Obstruction of blood flow can arise as a result of complete occlusion *(mesenteric infarction)* or partial occlusion *(abdominal angina)*.

Complete Occlusion (Mesenteric Infarction). Any occlusion of arterial blood supply to the bowel, as in mesenteric thrombosis, effectively stops bowel function. The usual cause is an embolus. An acute occlusion, at its onset, causes intense abdominal pain. Usually, there are no manifestations of advanced intestinal obstruction because the pain results from ischemic tissue rather than from obstruction. Ischemia is the most serious result of intestinal obstruction because as the process advances, fever, leukocytosis, shock, peritonitis, and other manifestations of bowel gangrene appear. Ischemia renders the bowel more permeable, allowing *E. coli* and *Klebsiella*, part of the normal bowel flora, to penetrate the intestinal wall and enter the peritoneal cavity. Acute mesenteric obstruction constitutes a surgical emergency and carries a high mortality rate (about 75%). Surgical intervention must be initiated early. Sometimes an embolectomy can restore circulation. The surgeon also must resect necrotic (dead) segments of the bowel.

Partial Occlusion (Abdominal Angina). Abdominal angina usually results from atherosclerosis of the mesenteric arteries, a common although often asymptomatic problem found in 33% of routine autopsies. Because there is a greater need for oxygenation during the digestive process, pain may develop 15 to 30 minutes after eating in a client with abdominal angina. Initially, pain may occur only after ingestion of a large meal. As the arterial process extends, however, it may occur even after a small meal, and eventually the pain becomes almost continuous.

Manifestations arise only when interruption of blood supply is sufficient to compromise bowel function. At this time, in addition to pain after eating, assessment reveals a change in bowel habits, nausea and vomiting, and weight loss as a result of the client's restriction of intake to avoid the discomfort of eating. Vascular or bypass grafts can sometimes improve the blood supply to the affected portion of the bowel.

Pathophysiology

Normally, the bowel secretes 7 to 8 L of electrolyte-rich fluid, and most of the fluid is reabsorbed. When the bowel is obstructed, this fluid is partially retained within the bowel and partially eliminated by vomiting, causing severe reduction in circulating blood volume, which results in hypotension, hypovolemic shock, and diminished renal and cerebral blood flow. Because fluid is lost but blood cells are not, hematocrit and hemoglobin values rise, thus increasing the potential for vascular occlusive disorders such as coronary, cerebral, and mesenteric thromboses.

For instance, with the onset of an obstruction, fluids and air collect proximal to the site of the problem, causing distention. Manifestations occur sooner and are more intense in a small bowel blockage because the small bowel is narrower and normally more active. The large volume of secretions from the small bowel adds to the distention. The only significant secretion from the large bowel is mucus.

Distention causes a temporary increase in peristalsis as the bowel attempts to force the material through the obstructed area. Within a few hours, the increased peristalsis ends and the bowel becomes flaccid, thus reducing pressure within the lumen and slowing the process caused by the obstruction. Greater pressure within the bowel reduces its absorptive ability, which increases the fluid retention still further. Soon the intraluminal pressure reduces venous return, increasing venous pressure, congestion, and vessel fragility. This process in turn raises capillary permeability and allows plasma to extravasate (escape) into the bowel lumen and the peritoneal cavity. The bowel wall becomes permeable to bacteria, and bowel organisms enter the peritoneal cavity. Rising pressure in the bowel wall soon slows arterial blood flow, causing necrosis and, in some cases, toxemia and peritonitis.

Strangulation of the bowel results in decreased arterial blood supply. Necrosis and perforation may force the intestinal contents into the peritoneal cavity, causing peritonitis. Bacteria proliferate in the strangulated bowel and may form endotoxins. When the endotoxins are released into the peritoneal cavity or systemic circulation, there is rapid circulatory collapse with endotoxic shock, accounting for the high mortality rate associated with this condition. These complications are especially likely to occur in older adults, who tend to have atherosclerotic narrowing of these vessels, making thrombosis more likely.

Clinical Manifestations

Manifestations of intestinal obstruction depend on the level and length of bowel involved, the extent to which the obstruction interferes with blood supply, the completeness of the obstruction, and the type of lesion producing the obstruction. Local changes in the bowel wall include congestion, fragility, reduced circulation, and increased pressure. Increased pressure leads to reverse peristalsis, producing vomiting that helps prevent overdistention of the bowel. These local effects result from (1) loss of fluids, electrolytes, and plasma; (2) bacterial proliferation; and (3) perforation. Systemic effects include a reduction in extracellular fluid and circulating blood volume, toxemia, and peritonitis.

The client with small bowel obstruction typically experiences abdominal pain in rhythmically recurring waves. The pain results from distention and the small intestine's peristaltic efforts to push its contents past the obstruction. Small intestinal pain is felt in the upper and midabdomen, whereas colonic pain is experienced in the lower abdomen. Soon after the small intestine becomes distended, the peristaltic waves are visible, accompanied by high-pitched tinkling sounds. The client usually becomes nauseated and vomits, bringing some relief from the pain if the obstruction is high or proximal to the ileum.

If the obstruction is distal to the ileum, vomiting fails to empty the bowel completely, allowing the accumulation of fluids, residue, and gases. As the muscles become atonic, loops of small bowel dilate, compounding the problem of distention. Eventually, severe distention may raise the diaphragm, thereby inhibiting respirations. Hypoxia (due to inadequate respirations, decreased circulating blood volume, and hypotension) often develops. Vomiting is more severe if the obstruction is located high in the small bowel. At first, vomitus is composed of semidigested food and chyme; later, it becomes watery and contains bile. Finally, the client vomits dark fecal material, the result of bacterial growth in the fluid that has stagnated in the obstructed bowel.

When the colon is obstructed, the competent ileocecal valve prevents regurgitation (and vomiting), and pressure within the lumen increases, resulting in distention. The cecum may perforate. Obstruction of the colon results in imbalanced bowel habits, lower abdominal pain, a desire to defecate, distention, and borborygmi. In the presence of an incompetent ileocecal valve, distention progresses to the small intestine. Vomiting that accompanies large intestine obstruction is a very late manifestation that occurs only from a distended small intestine.

Clients with vomiting may experience severe fluid and electrolyte imbalances. They lose not only water but also sodium, chloride, potassium, and bicarbonate. The result is an acute extracellular volume deficit (dehydration), which in turn lowers the circulating blood volume. Hydrogen ion imbalances frequently occur in intestinal obstructions, with metabolic acidosis being the most common problem.

Specific diagnostic tests for possible bowel obstruction consist of a plain x-ray film, which shows gas shadows, barium or radiopaque x-ray studies, and complete blood studies. Increased hemoglobin and hematocrit values may indicate dehydration. Leukocytosis may point to a strangulated bowel. A decrease in sodium, potassium, and chloride levels and a rise in nonprotein nitrogen and blood urea nitrogen (BUN) levels may indicate small bowel obstruction.

Outcome Management
■ Medical Management

Decompress the Bowel. The major treatment for an intestinal obstruction is the insertion of an intestinal tube (see Chapter 33). Often an intestinal tube both decompresses the bowel and breaks up the obstruction.

In adynamic ileus, the best intervention is bowel rest and prevention of distention by gastric suction. Medications are not effective in stimulating bowel activity. The bowel will respond when it recovers completely from the effects of obstruction.

■ Nursing Management of the Medical Client
Assessment

Obtain a complete history of the onset of manifestations, eating patterns, food tolerance, vomiting episodes, stools (number per day and appearance), distention, and factors that increase or decrease pain.

During physical assessment, note abdominal distention, the quality of bowel sounds, the presence and extent of dehydration, and manifestations of abdominal pain, such as muscle guarding. A lack of bowel sounds indicates peritoneal irritation or adynamic ileus. Usually, in the case of bowel obstruction, auscultation reveals high-pitched peristaltic rushes with high, metallic tinkling sounds.

Diagnosis, Outcomes, Interventions

Diagnosis: Deficient Fluid Volume. A priority nursing diagnosis for the client with an intestinal obstruction is *Deficient Fluid Volume related to vomiting, decreased intestinal reabsorption of fluid and decreased intestinal secretions.*

Outcomes. The client maintains fluid balance, as evidenced by balanced intake and output, no manifestations of dehydration, and blood pressure within the client's normal range.

Interventions

Maintain Fluid Balance. Maintain good fluid balance in the client with an obstruction by carefully replacing fluids and electrolytes. Administer parenteral fluids with sodium chloride, bicarbonate, and potassium added as ordered.

Decompress the Bowel. An intestinal tube is inserted and attached to suction to relieve the vomiting and distention. If the obstruction is not mechanical, an intestinal tube can achieve decompression. If the obstruction is due to adhesions, hernia, or tumors, the tube stops at the point of obstruction and keeps the bowel decompressed above the obstruction.

Note the progress of an intestinal tube, the amount and type of drainage, and whether or not relief of distention and nausea occurs. Assess and measure drainage from the intestinal tube; document color, odor, consistency, and volume. Inform the physician of blood levels of sodium, potassium, and bicarbonate, and the pH of the blood, all of which reflect fluid and electrolyte balance.

Provide Discharge Teaching. For dismissal following medical resolution of the obstruction, the client needs to learn ways to prevent recurrence and to maintain bowel elimination. The client must be seen by a primary health care provider at intervals after the obstruction is relieved to confirm that it has not recurred. The client's nutritional status also should be monitored to ensure that adequate nutrition is maintained.

Evaluation

Once the obstruction is relieved medically, bowel function should return to normal within a matter of days. If the obstruction cannot be relieved medically, surgery is required.

■ Surgical Management

If intestinal intubation does not relieve the obstruction, surgery is the only remaining option. The major objective in treating bowel obstruction is to relieve the cause and thus eliminate the problem; however, the cause is not always immediately obvious. Diagnosis of the cause of the acute abdominal condition may be difficult and commonly can be made only during surgery. Document specific observations to aid in the diagnosis.

In most vascular and mechanical obstructions, surgical excision of the cause is the only intervention. Surgery relieves the obstruction and removes any ischemic bowel. Relieving the obstruction should reestablish bowel patency. The type of surgery depends on the location and type of obstruction. The surgeon may perform bowel resection, colostomy, or a bypass procedure.

■ Nursing Management of the Surgical Client

Assessment of the surgical client is the same as assessment of the medical client. In addition, routine preoperative and postoperative assessments are required. Additional nursing interventions are the same as those discussed for other GI procedures.

IRRITABLE BOWEL SYNDROME

Irritable bowel syndrome (IBS) is a functional disorder of motility in the intestines. There is no organic disease or anatomic abnormality, nor are there any genetic markers. It is not life threatening, nor is it associated with development of cancer. Other descriptive names for this condition are spastic colon, irritable colon, nervous indigestion, spastic colitis, intestinal neurosis, and laxative or cathartic "colitis." IBS is the most common GI disorder in Western society, accounting for 50% of subspecialty referrals and the writing of more than five million prescriptions annually. In the United States, three of every four of those affected are women. It is most often diagnosed during middle age, although 50% of those affected report that they had clinical manifestations in childhood. It is estimated to affect 17% to 20% of the American population and is the second leading cause of missed workdays.

Etiology and Risk Factors

Clients at risk for IBS are those who consume diets high in fat, gas-producing foods, lactose, carbonated beverages, caffeine, and alcohol. Also at risk are clients who smoke, are lactose intolerant, have high stress in their lives, or complain of alterations in sleep and rest. Recent studies have suggested a relationship between childhood sexual abuse and IBS in women.

Health-promotion strategies are to instruct clients to consume a high-fiber, low-fat, well-balanced diet that avoids problematic foods and carbonated beverages. Also encourage clients to reduce stress, limit smoking and alcohol consumption, engage in regular exercise, and get 8 hours of sleep each night. To promote health maintenance, advise clients to stop smoking and to follow the diet and fluid recommendations previously described. Encourage clients to practice stress relaxation techniques. Health-restoration actions are to administer sedative and antispasmodic medications. Encourage clients to follow diet, exercise, and relaxation regimens and to increase fiber in their diets.

Pathophysiology

Four components appear to be involved in IBS: GI motility, visceral hypersensitivity, central nervous system processing, and autonomic nervous system (ANS) imbalance. Motility can be altered by any number of factors, including diet and emotional state. The most recent theory states that there is a hypersensitivity to bowel wall distention that results in disruption in the normal function of the muscles in the small and large bowel. The alteration in motility can cause diarrhea, constipation, or alternating diarrhea and constipation. The structure of the bowel mucosa is not changed, although the disease continues whenever the client is exposed to the causative agents. Causative agents vary among clients; however, most clients can clearly identify them. More recent in-

terest has focused on linking chemical mediators to IBS, specifically serotonin (5-hydroxytryptamine or 5-HT). It is believed that 5-HT may transmit pain to the gastrointestinal tract as a result of its role as an intermediary of bowel motility and visceral sensitivity (Figure 35-18).

Clinical Manifestations

The manifestations of IBS are thought to be related to abnormalities in bowel motility and visceral sensitivity caused by the action of 5-HT. The client with IBS usually has some combination of the following manifestations: crampy abdominal pain usually located in the lower abdomen, change in bowel function, constipation or diarrhea, hypersecretion of colonic mucus, dyspeptic manifestations (flatulence, nausea, anorexia), and some level of anxiety or depression. There is usually relief after defecation. Women report that manifestations are often worse around the time of menses. Manifestations vary in

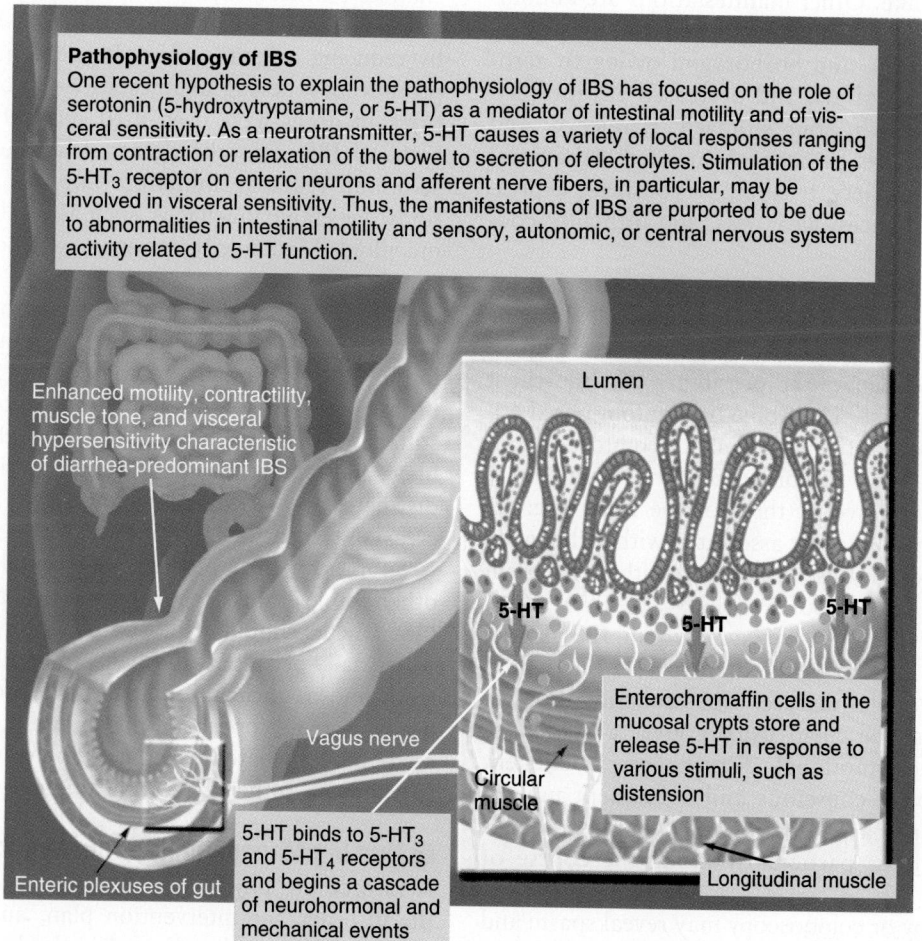

Pathophysiology of IBS
One recent hypothesis to explain the pathophysiology of IBS has focused on the role of serotonin (5-hydroxytryptamine, or 5-HT) as a mediator of intestinal motility and of visceral sensitivity. As a neurotransmitter, 5-HT causes a variety of local responses ranging from contraction or relaxation of the bowel to secretion of electrolytes. Stimulation of the 5-HT_3 receptor on enteric neurons and afferent nerve fibers, in particular, may be involved in visceral sensitivity. Thus, the manifestations of IBS are purported to be due to abnormalities in intestinal motility and sensory, autonomic, or central nervous system activity related to 5-HT function.

Enhanced motility, contractility, muscle tone, and visceral hypersensitivity characteristic of diarrhea-predominant IBS

Lumen

5-HT   5-HT   5-HT

Enterochromaffin cells in the mucosal crypts store and release 5-HT in response to various stimuli, such as distension

Vagus nerve

Circular muscle

Longitudinal muscle

5-HT binds to 5-HT_3 and 5-HT_4 receptors and begins a cascade of neurohormonal and mechanical events

Enteric plexuses of gut

FIGURE 35-18 Pathophysiology of irritable bowel syndrome (IBS). The manifestations of IBS are thought to be related to abnormalities in serotonin (5-hydroxytryptamine or 5-HT), which is a mediator of intestinal motility and visceral sensitivity. (From Heitkemper, M., & Jarrett, M. [2001]. It's not all in your head: Irritable bowel syndrome. *American Journal of Nursing, 101*[1], 26-33.)

intensity. Fiber, fruits, alcohol, caffeine, and fatigue may aggravate or precipitate manifestations. Clients complain about interference with activities of daily living and a poor quality of life.

Emotional disturbances affect the ANS and its innervation of the bowel. Disturbances of ANS function probably alter motor activity and bowel transit time. Manifestations may mimic various organic and systemic diseases. Pain may be steady or intermittent, and there may be a dull, deep discomfort with sharp cramps in the morning or after eating. The typical pattern consists of lower left quadrant abdominal pain and constipation or diarrhea. Tenderness over the sigmoid area also may be present.

Diarrhea tends to be the major problem but does not usually occur at night; nocturnal diarrhea tends to be associated with organic disease of the bowel. Examination of the stool reveals mucus but not blood. Eating may aggravate pain and defecation, and passing flatus or stool may provide temporary relief. Spastic contractions sometimes occur with stools that are small, dry, hard, and pellet-like. Other manifestations are abdominal disturbances such as nausea, distention, dyspepsia, eructation (belching), and borborygmi owing to aerophagia (swallowing of air) and decreased gas motility. Anorexia, foul breath, sour stomach, flatulence, and cramps also may be present. Associated behavioral disturbances are anxiety, tension, nervousness, depression, sleep disturbances, weakness, and difficulty concentrating.

Because there are no confirmatory diagnostic tests for or histologic features of IBS, diagnosis generally is made by excluding other diseases. Diagnostic techniques, therefore, must eliminate the possibility that the client has organic GI disease. The Rome II symptom-based criteria for IBS state that the abdominal discomfort or pain must last for at least 12 consecutive weeks within 12 months along with two of three of the following: relieved with defecation, onset associated with a change in frequency of stool, or onset associated with a change in form or appearance of stool.[22]

Clients older than 50 years in whom IBS is suspected must be carefully evaluated to rule out malignancy and diverticular disease. When functional bowel disease develops, the client usually gives a history of nervousness and emotional disturbance. The client also may be bowel conscious and a frequent user of cathartics and enemas. Palpation may demonstrate abdominal tenderness, particularly along the course of the colon.

Sigmoidoscopy or colonoscopy may reveal spasm and mucus in the colonic lumen. A barium enema study is usually performed. A complete blood count and stool examination are needed to rule out occult blood, ova, parasites, and pathogenic bacteria.

Outcome Management
■ Medical Management

Encourage Lifestyle Changes. Treatment is supportive. Advise the client to limit responsibilities, seek rest, and adopt measures to reduce stress, such as progressive relaxation, biofeedback, and a regular exercise routine. The client can control manifestations through diet, medication, and regular physical activity. The client must continue with routine follow-up assessment and care.

Administer Medications. No specific class of medications is universally effective, although new drugs that block or modulate 5-HT receptors are being developed. Tegaserod (Zelnorm), a 5HT4 receptor blocker, has been effective in the treatment of constipation in clients with IBS. Antidiarrheals may be used. Loperamide (Imodium) slows bowel transit, enhances water absorption, and strengthens anal sphincter tones resulting in fewer stools. Antispasmotics, especially anticholinergics, are commonly prescribed to relax smooth muscle. Calcium channel blockers have been proposed for the treatment of IBS because of their ability to relax GI smooth muscle by reducing calcium influx. Peppermint oil has shown promise in relieving manifestations in children. Antidepressant drugs have been used successfully in management of IBS. Tricyclic agents delay bowel transit and serotonin reuptake inhibitors improve pain manifesta- tions. Vegetable mucilages, such as psyllium hydrophilic mucilloid (Metamucil), can increase stool bulk.

Modify Diet. A high-fiber diet helps control IBS through the production of bulkier stools and reduction of tension in the walls of the sigmoid colon. Fiber helps to manage both constipation and diarrhea. In constipation, the softer, bulkier, and heavier stools produced by dietary fiber tend to decrease transit time. In diarrhea, the fiber diet helps absorb water, giving form to the stool and increasing transit time.

Sources of fiber include bran cereals, whole wheat, other whole grains such as brown rice, and fresh vegetables. Clients should drink six to eight 8-ounce glasses of water daily because water helps to regulate stool consistency and frequency. If diarrhea is a problem, the client needs to avoid foods that may cause it, such as carbonated and caffeinated beverages, and to drink liquids between meals rather than at mealtime.

■ Nursing Management of the Medical Client

Reinforce the physician's explanation of the nature of the disorder, the intervention plan, and the prognosis. Make it clear to the client that the bowel responds to stress, foods, and medications. Emphasize the importance of regular hours, nourishing meals, and adequate sleep, exercise, and recreation. Help the client to establish a regular bowel routine. Advise the client with diarrhea to limit foods that produce gas or irritate and to avoid (1) caffeinated and carbonated beverages, (2) alcohol, (3) foods containing nondigestible carbohydrates, such as beans, and (4) milk and milk products. Provide empathy and support.

CELIAC DISEASE

Celiac disease, also known as *nontropical sprue,* is a disorder that causes severe malabsorption. The disorder is characterized by marked atrophy of the villi in the proximal small intestine induced by ingestion of gluten-containing foods. *Gluten* is a high-molecular-weight protein found in rye, oats, barley, and wheat. It is found in bread, bread products, beer, and many other processed foods. Clients present with diarrhea, steatorrhea, and weakness, which is relieved when the client begins a gluten-free diet. Corticosteroids may be required if the gluten-free diet is not successful in relieving manifestations.

DISORDERS OF THE ANORECTAL AREA

The major function of the rectum is to store feces until evacuation. When feces enter the rectum, peristalsis occurs. Many disorders in the rectal area result from constipation or failure to empty the rectum when peristalsis occurs.

At the mucocutaneous border of the anal canal, the mucous membrane changes to skin that has cutaneous somatic nerve endings. Because of this anatomic structure, lesions of the external anal canal are very painful. The two most common manifestations are bleeding and pain. Drainage of mucus and fecal matter and irritation of the skin by organisms can cause intense itching.

Hemorrhoids and skin tags may protrude from the anal opening, and there may be drainage of pus from abscesses. Bright-red blood per rectum usually indicates a lesion of the left colon or anorectal region. Blood on the toilet paper alone usually indicates perianal disease, whereas blood on the surface of a formed stool may suggest a polyp or carcinoma of the left colon or rectum. Blood mixed with the stool suggests inflammatory bowel disease or carcinoma of the proximal colon. Blood in the toilet bowl after the passage of formed stool suggests hemorrhoidal bleeding, the most common source of bright-red blood in the stool. All rectal bleeding must be evaluated by a health care provider.

HEMORRHOIDS

Hemorrhoids are perianal varicose veins. They may be internal or external (Figure 35-19). Internal hemorrhoids are varicosities of the superior hemorrhoidal plexus occurring above the mucocutaneous border

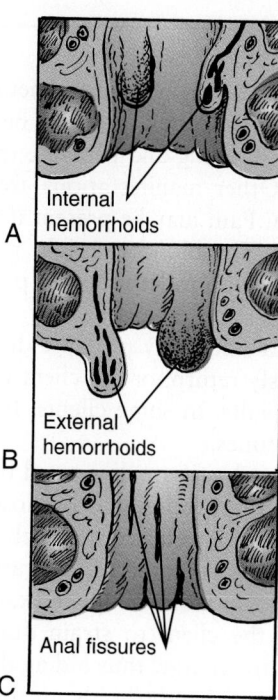

FIGURE 35-19 A, Internal hemorrhoids. **B,** External hemorrhoids. **C,** Anal fissures.

(pectinate line); they are covered by mucous membrane and are innervated by the autonomic nervous system. Hemorrhoids are a common disorder, affecting both men and women of any age, but the incidence is higher in people between 20 and 50 years of age.

Etiology and Risk Factors

By the age of 50, almost half of the population has hemorrhoids. Enlargement of hemorrhoids is caused by increased intra-abdominal pressure. Pregnancy, constipation with prolonged straining, obesity, heart failure, prolonged sitting or standing, and cirrhosis with portal hypertension also raise the incidence of hemorrhoids. Any condition that increases constipation, intra-abdominal pressure, or hemorrhoidal venous pressure raises the risk of development of hemorrhoids. Prevention of constipation through more fiber in the diet is an excellent measure to reduce the risk of hemorrhoids.

Pathophysiology

Tenesmus increases intra-abdominal and hemorrhoidal venous pressures, leading to distention of the hemorrhoidal veins. When the rectal ampulla (pouch) is filled with formed stool, venous obstruction is believed to occur. As a result of the repeated and prolonged increase in this pressure and the obstruction, hemorrhoidal veins become permanently dilated. As a result of the distention, thrombosis and bleeding also may occur.

Clinical Manifestations

The major manifestation of external hemorrhoids is an enlarged mass at the anus. Internal hemorrhoids are characterized by bleeding and prolapse (protrusion outside the anus). Other manifestations are rectal itching and constipation. Pain may be present if there is associated thrombosis. The blood is bright red and may be seen in the stool or on toilet tissue. A prolapse may occur in severe cases after exercise or after prolonged standing. Hemorrhoids may prolapse during defecation and spontaneously return, or the client may need to replace them manually. In some clients, hemorrhoids are prolapsed at all times.

External hemorrhoids are diagnosed by visual examination; internal hemorrhoids are diagnosed through history; digital palpation; anoscopy which is using a hollow, lighted tube to view the rectum; and proctoscopy, which is useful for a more complete examination of the rectum. Asking the client to strain during assessment causes the veins to enlarge, thus aiding diagnosis.

Complications of hemorrhoids are bleeding, thrombosis, and hemorrhoidal strangulation. Severe bleeding from prolonged trauma to the vein during defecation can cause iron deficiency anemia. Blood oozes or may even spurt out following a bowel movement. Thrombosis within the hemorrhoids can occur at any time and manifests as intense pain. Strangulated hemorrhoids, which are prolapsed hemorrhoids in which the blood supply is cut off by the anal sphincter, can result in thrombosis when blood within the hemorrhoid clots. Assessment reveals severe pain, extreme edema, and inflammation.

Outcome Management
■ Medical Management

Medical therapy is used for small, uncomplicated hemorrhoids with mild manifestations.

Prevent Constipation. Dietary changes used to treat constipation include increasing fluids and fiber in the diet. Constipation unrelieved by diet may require use of a stool softener (docusate sodium) or a hydrophilic psyllium preparation (e.g., Metamucil).

Relieve Pain. For pain, an initial application of cold packs, followed by warm sitz baths three or four times a day, should help. A topical anesthetic or steroid preparation, such as lidocaine (Xylocaine) or steroid cream, also reduces pain and itching.

■ Nursing Management of the Medical Client

Prevent Constipation. The client with hemorrhoids should take measures to avoid constipation. The anal area is very painful, and the client may avoid defecating, resulting in hard stool or fecal impaction. Encourage the client to take bulk laxatives, stool softeners, or mineral oil as prescribed to promote stool passage. Monitor the stool for consistency and blood.

Counsel the client to (1) eat fiber-containing foods and drink ample fluids to prevent straining and (2) avoid laxatives as much as possible. Remind the client not to sit on the toilet longer than necessary; this position impairs blood flow and puts added pressure on anal vessels.

Relieve Pain. Encourage 15-minute warm sitz baths three or four times per day for 15 minutes. Witch hazel compresses are soothing to the mucosa. Other over-the-counter preparations may temporarily relieve pain.

■ Surgical Management

Several surgical procedures are used to treat hemorrhoids. Most are performed as outpatient or clinic procedures. Botox injections into the internal sphincter of clients who have just undergone hemorrhoidectomy have been used to reduce pain postoperatively.

Sclerotherapy. Sclerotherapy is performed by the injection of a sclerosing agent (a substance that causes formation of scar tissue) between and around the veins. This produces an inflammatory reaction that leads to thrombosis and fibrosis. This procedure can be performed on an outpatient basis but requires one to four injections 5 to 7 days apart. The sclerosing agent can scar the anal canal.

Ligation. Ligation, a common procedure for internal hemorrhoids, is performed in the office setting. The client can usually resume normal activities immediately after the treatment. Unfortunately, the procedure cannot be used for external hemorrhoids and may be only temporarily effective. The surgeon inserts a ligator, a small, double-lumen cylinder with a small rubber band on the inner layer, through an anoscope. The hemorrhoid is then grasped with forceps and pulled through the ligator. The rubber band is placed around the neck of the hemorrhoid. Although bleeding can occur, the most common problem is some pain during ligation. The client takes a bulk laxative after the procedure to avoid local trauma from a hard fecal mass. In 8 to 10 days, the rubber band cuts through the neck of tissue, and the tissue sloughs.

Cryosurgery. Cryosurgery (freezing) of hemorrhoids is performed less commonly today. It is also an outpatient procedure. The freezing of the tissue leads to necrosis and sloughing of the hemorrhoids. The problems associated with this procedure are the prolonged periods of drainage, the amount of foul drainage, the presence of large residual skin tags, and possibly incomplete destruction of the hemorrhoids.

Laser. Laser removal of hemorrhoids also is performed on an outpatient basis. The hemorrhoid is burned off with the laser. There is minimal bleeding, although the procedure causes some pain.

Hemorrhoidectomy. With a hemorrhoidectomy, the vein is excised, and the area either is left open to heal by granulation or is closed with sutures. The open method is very painful but has a high rate of success. The suture method, although far less painful, is more likely to cause infection and result in poor healing. Complications include infection, stricture formation as the lesion heals, and hemorrhage. Hemorrhage may occur immediately after surgery or about 10 days later as a result of sloughing of tissue. Also, bleeding may not be evident because it can occur into the rectum without being passed immediately.

■ Nursing Management of the Surgical Client

Promote Healing. After the client has undergone a procedure to remove hemorrhoids, stress the importance of keeping the area clean and the stool soft but formed to help prevent strictures. Encourage the client to wash the area after defecation and to pat it dry. Local moist heat, applied with a washcloth or piece of cotton to the anal opening for a few minutes, cleans, soothes, and promotes healing. Never apply heat in the immediate postoperative period because of the increased risk of hemorrhage. Beginning 12 hours after surgery, sitz baths three or four times a day, as the client desires, and after each bowel movement are encouraged. A sanitary napkin is the most convenient perianal dressing if one is required.

Prevent Complications. Postoperative complications requiring nursing assessment include hemorrhage and urinary retention. The proximity of the bladder and tenderness in the area sometimes make urination difficult. Reestablishment of bowel habits is another potential postoperative problem. The client may need instruction on the relationship of proper diet and adequate fluid intake to bowel regularity, the physiology of defecation, and the importance of establishing a regular bowel routine.

Relieve Pain. Postoperative pain can be controlled with parenteral and then oral analgesics. Warn the client to avoid vigorous perianal wiping during the immediate postoperative period. The client is usually given a stool softener and mineral oil to soften and lubricate the first stool. Warn clients that fainting can occur, from pain and vagal stimulation, during the first postprocedure bowel movement.

ANAL FISSURE

An *anal fissure* is an ulceration or tear of the lining of the anal canal, usually the posterior wall that occurs as a result of excessive tissue stretching and possibly from passage of a hard or large stool. The skin tear is tender and tends to reopen at subsequent defecation.

Chronic fissures are usually secondary to infectious material retained in the anal crypts. Sharp pain accompanies defecation, followed by burning. Severe muscle spasm of the sphincter usually accompanies chronic conditions. The client may try to avoid defecation, aggravating the conditions.

If the acute lesion does not heal with local dilations, cleaning, and control of constipation, the tract can be excised surgically. A chronic fissure usually does not heal spontaneously and requires surgery.

Advise the client to (1) keep the stool soft with psyllium hydrophilic mucilloid (Metamucil), mineral oil, or docusate sodium, as prescribed; (2) have a bowel movement daily; and (3) clean the area after defecation, preferably with warm water. Sitz baths aid healing and may relieve pain. Suppositories with a local anesthetic may relieve constipation. Some colorectal surgeons are using Botox injections for treatment of chronic anal fissures.

ANAL FISTULA

A *fistula* is a sinus tract that develops between two body cavities or between a body cavity and the surface of the body. A rectal fistula is a tract that leads from the anal canal to the skin outside the anus or from an abscess to either the anal canal or the perianal area. It usually is preceded by an abscess. A fistula may heal over temporarily and then open and drain periodically.

Anal fistula is a chronic condition for which surgery is the only cure. The surgeon excises the tract and cleans the area, leaving it open to heal by granulation. It may heal very slowly and be very painful. Advise the client to keep the area clean, especially after a bowel movement.

ANORECTAL ABSCESS

Anorectal abscesses form in several locations. Most abscesses begin as cryptitis, with the formation of cysts that extend through the tubular ducts into the submucosal spaces. They also can originate from abrasions of the local tissues, with entry of a virulent organism. Anal intercourse may also cause a rectal abscess. Treatment involves drainage of the abscess and surgical excision of any associated fistulas. Two stages of surgery may be required to accomplish the needed resection.

CANCER

Carcinoma and melanoma can occur at the anus but are rare, constituting fewer than 5% of anorectal cancers. They spread by local extension into the perirectal spaces and then to the inguinal nodes. Cancer of the anal canal or lower rectum can coexist with other rectal conditions, and the client may falsely attribute bleeding to a hemorrhoid instead of carcinoma. Anal cancers are more common in African Americans, in clients who have had human papilloma virus or HIV, and in clients with pre-existing anal and perianal problems, such as fistulas.

COMPLEMENTARY AND ALTERNATIVE THERAPY

Trans-Fatty Acids and Colon Cancer

Trans-fatty acids are also known as "partially hydrogenated" fats or oils. These compounds are found in numerous food products because they tend to increase shelf life. However, these fatty acids tend to raise low-density lipoproteins, or LDL ("bad cholesterol"), and they tend to reduce high-density lipoproteins, or HDL ("good cholesterol"). Few studies have evaluated their impact on cancer risk.

One of the first studies to examine a potential relationship with cancer was a case-control study (1993 cases and 2410 controls) from Utah, Northern California, and Minnesota. Researchers found a higher risk for colon cancer with trans-fat intake, especially in older individuals ($\geq$67 years), in individuals who did not use nonsteroidal anti-inflammatory drugs (NSAIDs) regularly, and in women who were not taking hormone replacement therapy (HRT). As of 2003, the U.S. government requires that all foods sold in the United States report the exact amount of trans-fat in their product.

Reference
Slattery, M., et al. (2001). Trans-fatty acids and colon cancer. *Nutrition and Cancer 39*, 170-175.

COMPLEMENTARY AND ALTERNATIVE THERAPY

Iron Deficiency and Gastrointestinal Cancer

A cohort study with 2 years of follow-up was conducted in the United States. A total of 9024 civilian, non-institutionalized persons 25 to 74 years of age (60% women, 83% Caucasian) were included. Men and postmenopausal women (n = 6227) with iron deficiency alone (n = 223) and iron deficiency anemia (n = 51) had an increased risk for gastrointestinal malignancy (any malignancy of the esophagus, stomach, small intestine, colon, or rectum). Similar results were found for individuals 50 years of age or older (n = 4447) and in individuals 65 years of age or older (n = 2733). The researchers concluded that men and postmenopausal women with iron deficiency (with or without anemia) had an increased risk for gastrointestinal cancer within 2 years. One potential recommendation from this study is that any individual over 50 years of age who is found to have an iron deficiency should at least be encouraged to have a colonoscopy.

Reference
Ioannou, G., et al. (2002). Iron deficiency and gastrointestinal malignancy: A population-based cohort study. *American Journal of Medicine, 113*, 276-280.

COMPLEMENTARY AND ALTERNATIVE THERAPY

Chemoprevention of Colorectal Cancer

Consensus is forming on the potential drugs and supplements that have the most data for the prevention of polyps and/or colorectal cancer. These agents include aspirin, calcium and vitamin D, celecoxib (a COX-2 inhibitor), estrogen, exisulind (a sulfone metabolite of sulindac), and folic acid. Health professionals should continue to follow the data on these supplements and drugs.

Reference
Burke, C., Bauer, W., & Lashner, B. (2003). Chemoprevention of colorectal cancer: Slow, steady progress. *Cleveland Clinic Journal of Medicine 70(4)*, 346-350.

COMPLEMENTARY AND ALTERNATIVE THERAPY

Low-Fat, High Fiber, and Fruit and Vegetable Diet to Reduce Rectal Mucosal Proliferation

Researchers evaluated the effects of a 4-year, low-fat, high-fiber, fruit and vegetable–enriched dietary intervention on colorectal epithelial cell proliferation among 399 patients from the Polyp Prevention Trial. This trial is a randomized, multicenter trial with adenoma recurrence as the primary endpoint. Rectal biopsies were performed on clients at baseline, after 1 year, and after 4 years. No significant differences occurred between the dietary intervention group and control group. This observation is similar to the findings in the larger primary study, in which dietary intervention did not reduce the recurrence rates of adenoma.

Reference
Pfeiffer, R., et al. (2003). The effect of a low-fat, high-fiber, fruit and vegetable intervention on rectal mucosal proliferation. *Cancer, 98*, 1161-1168.

Bleeding, local pain and itching, and tenesmus are characteristic manifestations. The client is usually aware of a lump near the anus that has bled and that gradually becomes more and more painful, particularly during or just after a bowel movement. Many cancers are not diagnosed until they are large, and by then the prognosis is poor. Some tumors are treated with radiation and chemotherapy, whereas others may require surgical excision. Surgical intervention involves excision of the anus with an abdominoperineal resection.

BOWEL INCONTINENCE

Bowel incontinence may develop in clients as a result of aging, trauma, diabetes, rectal prolapse, or childbirth injuries or a neurogenic cause, such as spina bifida. Clients with cancer in the lower pelvic and rectal areas or with a history of radiation therapy to the rectal region are also at risk for bowel incontinence.

As an aid to promote continence, a device called an artificial rectal sphincter (ARS) has been used successfully to promote bowel continence in almost all clients except those who have a history of cancer or radiation and who would be unable to activate the pump. The device mimics the natural process of bowel control and elimination.

The ARS consists of three parts: (1) a cuff, placed under the skin to fit around the anal canal for an artificial rectal sphincter; (2) a pressure-regulating balloon placed in the abdominal wall and filled with liquid such as a contrast agent that can be seen on x-ray; and (3) a control pump placed in the scrotum or labia to inflate the cuff. The cuff inflates like a balloon to prevent the passage of stool and to promote continence. To evacuate the rectum, the client deflates the plastic ring and stool is able to pass. After a bowel movement, the cuff automatically inflates in 10 minutes.

General or spinal anesthesia is used for surgical implantation of the ARS, and the procedure takes about 1 hour. The bowel is cleaned with antibiotics, laxatives, and enemas.

Postoperatively the client is given IV antibiotics for several days to prevent infection. The nurse teaches the client how to deflate the cuff for bowel evacuation and monitors the client's bowel patterns as well as for complications such as mechanical failure, infection, and ulceration. If mechanical failure is suspected, manometry is used to measure the closing pressure of the ARS. Client satisfaction has been reported. (See also the Management and Delegation feature on Application and Care of Rectal Pouches and Rectal Tubes on p. 821 for clients with diarrhea.)

PILONIDAL CYST

A *pilonidal cyst* occurs at the base of the sacrum, usually contains hair, and becomes infected, forming an abscess and then a sinus tract. It is most common in young adults, especially men. It may result from hairs that penetrate the skin and cause sinus tracts to form. Constant irritation (e.g., from clothing and perspiration from activity) can cause hairs to become embedded and then infected. Acute pain and swelling result, followed by a discharge. Treatment involves surgical excision of the abscess. Healing is slow, and if the infectious process is not completely removed, the condition may recur. The client also may receive antibiotics.

BLUNT OR PENETRATING TRAUMA

Blunt or penetrating trauma to the abdomen refers to accidental or intentional trauma causing internal injuries. Most blunt abdominal trauma is caused by automobile steering wheel or pedestrian accidents, whereas most penetrating trauma is caused by gunshot wounds or stabbings.

Etiology and Risk Factors

Almost any kind of injury can cause blunt trauma to the abdomen. In automobile accidents, rapid, uncontrolled deceleration is the force that produces the trauma, when the client's body hits the steering wheel or some other object. Penetrating trauma commonly results from gunshot wounds, which cause a great deal of internal damage. Stabbings are the next most common cause of penetrating abdominal wounds, although the wounds are less traumatic.

Trauma is the leading cause of death in adults younger than 40 years and the fifth leading cause of death in all adults. Although not all cases of trauma involve abdominal trauma, abdominal injuries are common with motor vehicle accidents. One method of prevention is wearing seat belts, which could decrease abdominal trauma during accidents.

Pathophysiology

Blunt trauma to the abdomen can cause shearing, crushing, or compressing forces that rupture the bowel and other abdominal structures. Gunshot wounds can damage every structure in the abdomen. The bullets may perforate the stomach or bowel, causing peritonitis and sepsis.

Stab wounds produce fewer traumas to internal abdominal structures because the abdominal organs have more time to shift out of the way of the penetrating instrument.

Clinical Manifestations

Assessment of the client first involves obtaining a thorough history of the accident so that the extent of blunt trauma can be estimated. For penetrating trauma, careful assessment of the position of entry and possibly exit wounds is vital.

The client may show manifestations of an acute abdomen with either type of trauma. With both injuries, either internal or external hemorrhage may occur. If the bowel is ruptured, manifestations of peritonitis are present. All abdominal drainage is closely assessed for the presence of bowel contents.

Abdominal lavage is commonly used to assess the presence of bleeding in all abdominal wounds. This procedure involves instillation of a crystalloid solution into the peritoneal cavity followed by paracentesis (drainage of contents). Note and record the color and amount of the drainage.

A CT scan of the abdomen is now considered the base assessment of intra-abdominal injury. Angiography, intravenous pyelography (IVP), and other studies may be performed to assess different organs and the degree of trauma suffered.

Outcome Management
■ Medical Management

If minimal blunt trauma was sustained without severe injury to any abdominal organs, the client may simply be observed for problems once the diagnostic tests have been performed. Penetrating trauma always requires surgical intervention. The major complications of trauma are hemorrhage, shock, peritonitis, and sepsis.

The client's pain is treated conservatively until the severity of trauma has been determined. If the bowel has been ruptured, large doses of IV antibiotics are given to control infection. If hemorrhage and shock are present, IV fluids, colloids, and vasopressors may be used. The client is assigned to NPO status until the abdomen has been assessed and found to be intact.

■ Surgical Management

The treatment of choice for abdominal trauma with injury is an exploratory laparotomy. Depending on the injury, the surgery may be as simple as a closure of tears or as complex as a bowel resection and even a temporary colostomy.

■ Nursing Management of the Medical-Surgical Client

Careful assessment of the client's injury is vital. The client often must be prepared for immediate emergency surgery. Prepare the client as quickly as possible, knowing that postoperatively much more teaching and support will be required.

Usually, once the injuries and repair have had sufficient time to heal and the infection has been adequately treated, the client returns to the hospital so that the temporary ostomy may be closed and the bowel returned to normal.

Discharge Teaching. Before discharge, the client may need education regarding home health care, which may include ostomy care and extensive wound care. The client or his or her significant others may have to learn to change dressings and to care for an open, draining wound. Follow-up care from a visiting nurse may also be required for the administration of antibiotics at home, further ostomy teaching, or wound care for an open draining wound.

CONCLUSIONS

Intestinal disorders are common and may cause problems for the client throughout life if he or she is not treated promptly and completely. Even with early treatment, many clients require ostomies for treatment of large and small bowel disorders. The resultant body image changes are the focus of nursing interventions to educate the client and to facilitate behavior modifications that will promote health and adaptation to the changes.

THINKING CRITICALLY *evolve*

1. A young man is admitted with an exacerbation of inflammatory bowel disease. He reports frequent watery stools, general weakness, lack of appetite with a loss of 5 pounds in a week, and cramping abdominal pain. What nursing history and physical assessment are required? How will his exacerbation be treated?
Factors to Consider. What are the clinical manifestations of inflammatory bowel disease? What are priority nursing interventions?

2. An older client has undergone a bowel resection with placement of a temporary transverse colostomy for treatment of colon cancer. He lives with his wife of 25 years. She is very interested in learning how to help her spouse manage care for the stoma and how to change the colostomy bags. What is your priority assessment? What teaching methods should you use to teach the client and his wife?
Factors to Consider. What is the appearance of a healthy stoma and healthy skin around the stoma? What dietary management is important?

3. A woman in her 50s schedules an appointment with her health care provider because she has found blood in her stool and has noticed a change in bowel habits. She states that her father died of colon cancer and she has been afraid to see her health care provider because she fears she might also have colon cancer. What are priority nursing interventions? What teaching methods should be used for this woman?
Factors to Consider. What are the causes of colorectal cancer? What are its clinical manifestations? How is it treated?

Discussions for these questions can be found on the website and the CD-ROM.

BIBLIOGRAPHY

1. American Cancer Society. (2003). *Cancer facts and figures.* Atlanta: Author.

 2. Arroyo, A., et al. (2001). Randomized clinical trial comparing suture and mesh repair of umbilical hernia in adults. *British Journal of Surgery, 88*(10), 1321-1323.

3. Ball, E. (2000). Part Two. A teaching guide for continent ileostomy. *RN, 63*(12), 35-42.

4. Banks, N., & Razor, B. (2003). Preoperative stoma site assessment and marking. *American Journal of Nursing, 103*(3), 64A-64D.

5. Borum, M. (2001). Colorectal cancer screening. *Primary Care: Gastroenterology, 28*(3), 661-674.

6. Borum, M. (2001). Irritable bowel syndrome. *Primary Care: Gastroenterology, 28*(3), 523-533.

7. Bryant, D., & Fleischer, I. (2000). Changing an ostomy appliance. *Nursing 2000, 30*(11), 51-53.

8. Catassi, C., et al. (2002). Risk of non-Hodgkin lymphoma in celiac disease. *Journal of the American Medical Association, 287*(11), 1413-1419.

9. Cerrato, P. (1999). When food is the culprit. *RN, 62*(6), 52-59.

10. Chung, D., & Rustgi., L. (2003). HNPCC syndrome: Genetics and clinical implications. *Annals of Internal Medicine, 138*(7), 560-570.

11. Chutkan, R. (2001). Inflammatory bowel disease. *Primary Care: Gastroenterology, 28*(3), 539-555.

 12. Colorectal Cancer Collaborative Group. (2001). Adjuvant radiotherapy for rectal cancer: A systematic overview of 8507 patients from 22 randomized trials. *Lancet, 358*(9290), 1291-1304.

13. Crohn's & Colitis Foundation. (2002). *Crohn's disease and ulcerative colitis.* New York: Author.

14. Dest, V. (2000*).* Oncology today: New horizons, colorectal cancer. *RN, 63*(3), 53-63.

15. Fathi, J., Isler, J., & Billingham, R. (Eds.). (1999). Office management of common anorectal problems. *Primary Care, 26*(1), 1-187.

16. Giardiasis (On-line). (2003). Available: http://www.cdc.gov/ncidod/dpd/parasites/giardiasis/factsht.giardia.htm.

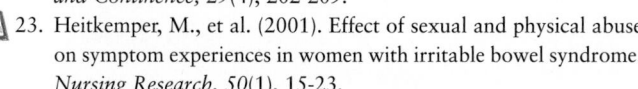 17. Giovannucci, E. (2003). Diet, body weight and colorectal cancer: A summary of epidemiologic incidence. *Journal of Women's Health, 12*(2), 173-182.

18. Glaser, E., & Grogan, L. (1999). Molecular genetics of gastrointestinal malignancies. *Seminars in Oncology Nursing, 15*(1), 3-9.

19. Goldman, L., & Bennett, J.C. (2000). *Cecil textbook of medicine* (21st ed.). Philadelphia: W.B. Saunders.

20. Guyton, A.C., & Hall, J.E. (2000). *Textbook of medical physiology* (10th ed.). Philadelphia: W.B. Saunders.

21. Heitkemper, M., & Jarrett, M. (2001). It's not all in your head: Irritable bowel syndrome. *American Journal of Nursing, 101*(1), 26-33.

22. Heitkemper, M., Jarrett, M., & Bond, E. (2002). Irritable bowel syndrome: More than a gut feeling. *Journal of Wound, Ostomy, and Continence, 29*(4), 202-209.

23. Heitkemper, M., et al. (2001). Effect of sexual and physical abuse on symptom experiences in women with irritable bowel syndrome. *Nursing Research, 50*(1), 15-23.

24. Hemorrhoids (On-line). (2003). Available: http://www.niddk.nih.gov/health/digest/pubs/hems/hemords.htm.

25. Khaitan, L., & Holzman, M. (2002). Laparoscopic advances in general surgery. *Journal of the American Medical Association, 287*(12), 1502-1505.

26. Klonowski, E., & Masoodi, J. (1999). The patient with Crohn's disease. *RN, 62*(3), 32-37.

27. Lerman, C., et al. (1999). Genetic testing in families with hereditary nonpolyposis colon cancer. *Journal of the American Medical Association, 281*(17), 1618-1622.

28. Levin, T., et al. (1999). Predicting advanced proximal colonic neoplasia with screening sigmoidoscopy. *Journal of the American Medical Association, 281*(17), 1611-1617.

29. Mackenzie, D. (1999). When E. coli turns deadly. *RN, 62*(7), 28-32.

 30. Mitka, M. (2003). Colon cancer screening guidelines stress initial test's importance. *Journal of the American Medical Association, 289*(9), 1089-1090.

31. Molbach, K., Mead, P., & Griffin, P. (2002). Antimicrobial therapy in patients with *E. coli* 0157:H7 infection. *Journal of the American Medical Association, 288*(8), 1014-1016.

32. Moody, F. (1999). *Atlas of ambulatory surgery.* Philadelphia: W.B. Saunders.

33. Otto, S. (2001). *Oncology nursing* (4th ed.). St. Louis: Mosby.

34. Podolsky, D. (2002). Inflammatory bowel disease. *New England Journal of Medicine, 347*(6), 417-429.

35. Price, S., & Wilson, L. (2003). *Pathophysiology: Clinical concepts of disease processes* (6th ed.). St. Louis: Mosby.

36. Rayhorn, N., & Rayhorn, D. (2002). An in-depth look at inflammatory bowel disease, *Nursing, 32*(7), 36-43.

37. Saddler, D., & Ellis, C. (1999). Colorectal cancer. *Seminars in Oncology Nursing, 15*(1), 58-69.

38. Sheff, B. (1999). Minimizing the threat of C. *difficile. Nursing, 99,* 33-39.

39. Shrag, D., et al. (2001). Age and adjuvant chemotherapy use after surgery for stage III colon cancer. *Journal of the National Cancer Institute, 93*(11), 850-857.

40. Steffen, R., et al. (1999). Epidemiology, etiology, and impact of traveler's diarrhea in Jamaica. *Journal of the American Medical Association, 281*(9), 811-817.

41. Swidsinski, A., et al. (2002). Mucosal flora in inflammatory bowel disease. *Gastroenterology, 122,*44-54.

42. Syngal, S., et. al. (1999). Interpretation of genetic test results for hereditary nonpolyposis colorectal cancer: Implications for clinical predisposition testing. *Journal of the American Medical Association, 282*(3), 247-253.

 43. Tang, T., et al. (2001). Randomized clinical trial of the effect of open versus laparoscopically assisted colectomy on systemic immunity in patients with colorectal cancer. *British Journal of Surgery, 88,* 801-807.

44. Thompson, J. (2000). Part One. A practical ostomy guide. *RN, 63(11),* 61-68.

45. Tilg, H., et al. (2002). Treatment of Crohn's disease with recombinant human interleukin 10 induces the proinflammatory cytokine interferon y. *Gut, 50,* 191-195.

46. Townsend, C. (Ed.). (2001). *Sabiston textbook of surgery: The biological basis of modern surgical practice* (16th ed.). Philadelphia: W.B. Saunders.

47. Walsh, J., & Terdiman, J. (2003). Colorectal cancer screening: Scientific review. *Journal of the American Medical Association, 289*(10), 1288-1296.

48. Weeks, J., et al. (2002). Short-term quality-of-life outcomes following laparoscopic-assisted colectomy vs open colectomy for colon cancer. *Journal of the American Medical Association, 287*(3), 321-328.

49. Whiteford, M., et al. (2002). The evolving treatment of anal cancer: How are we doing? *Archives of Surgery, 136,* 886-891.

Management of Clients with Urinary Disorders

Francie Bernier

Web Enhancements

http://evolve.elsevier.com/Black/medsurg/

Client Education Guide
Learning to Care for a Urinary Diversion (English Version and Spanish Translation)
Preventing Recurrence of Urinary Stones (English Version and Spanish Translation)
Complementary and Alternative Therapy
Inorganic Arsenic in Drinking Water and the Risk of Bladder Cancer

Ethical Issues in Nursing
What Can You Do to Prevent a Premature Hospital Discharge?
Table
Urologic Instruments Most Commonly Encountered in a Clinical Setting
Appendix C
Laboratory Values of Clinical Importance in Medical-Surgical Nursing

Nurses commonly provide the initial assessment, diagnosis, and outcome management of altered urinary elimination and related nursing diagnoses. *Impaired urinary elimination* is a nursing diagnosis used for dysfunction involving the urethra, bladder, or ureters. More specific nursing diagnoses include *Stress Urinary Incontinence, Reflex Urinary Incontinence, Urge Urinary Incontinence, Functional Urinary Incontinence, Total Urinary Incontinence,* and *Urinary Retention.* Several additional nursing diagnoses are discussed throughout the chapter.

Because of the personal nature of the urinary system, its proximity to the reproductive system in females, and the shared urinary and reproductive system of males, urinary disorders commonly lead to feelings of shame, isolation, and embarrassment. It is vital that nurses be sensitive to the psychosocial needs of any client with a urinary disorder.

It is also important to recognize that urinary diagnoses may signal that other medical conditions coexist. Long-term sequelae or conditions occurring as a consequence of altered urinary elimination may include such

problems as impaired kidney function, changes in fluid volume and electrolytes, skin breakdown, changes in quality of life, and other associated conditions.

INFECTIOUS AND INFLAMMATORY DISORDERS
CYSTITIS

The diagnosis of a *urinary tract infection* (UTI) is typically confirmed on the basis of a certain number of microorganisms in the urinary system (usually 10^5 organisms), although manifestations may begin with many fewer organisms. The infectious process usually affects the bladder, but the urethra, ureters, and kidneys may be involved. *Cystitis,* the most common type of UTI, is an inflammation of the bladder wall, usually caused by ascending bacteria or obstructive voiding patterns that lead to decreased flow or stasis of urine. *Urethritis,* inflammation of the urethra, may cause the same manifestations as cystitis.

Nursing Outcomes Classification (NOC)
for Nursing Diagnoses—Clients with Urinary Disorders

Acute Pain
 Comfort Level
 Pain Control
 Pain: Disruptive Effects
 Pain Level
Deficient Knowledge
 Knowledge: Disease Process
 Knowledge: Health Behaviors
 Knowledge: Health Resources
 Knowledge: Illness Care
 Knowledge: Medication
 Knowledge: Prescribed Activity
 Knowledge: Treatment Procedure
 Knowledge: Treatment Regimen
Effective Therapeutic Regimen Management
 Adherence Behavior
 Compliance Behavior
 Family Participation in Professional Care
 Knowledge: Treatment Regimen
 Participation: Health Care Decisions
 Risk Control
 Symptom Control
Functional Urinary Incontinence
 Urinary Continence
 Urinary Elimination

Impaired Urinary Elimination
 Urinary Continence
 Urinary Elimination
Powerlessness
 Depression Control
 Depression Level
 Family Participation in Professional Care
 Health Beliefs
 Health Beliefs: Perceived Ability to Perform
 Health Beliefs: Perceived Control
 Health Beliefs: Perceived Resources
 Participation: Health Care Decisions
Reflex Urinary Incontinence
 Neurologic Status: Autonomic
 Urinary Continence
 Urinary Elimination
Risk for Disturbed Body Image
 Body Image
 Grief Resolution
 Psychosocial Adjustment: Life Change
 Self-Esteem
Risk for Impaired Skin Integrity
 Nutritional Status
 Risk Detection
 Tissue Integrity: Skin and Mucous Membranes

Tissue Perfusion: Peripheral
 Wound Healing: Primary Intention
 Wound Healing: Secondary Intention
Risk for Injury
 Risk Control
 Risk Detection
 Symptom Control
Risk for Sexual Dysfunction
 Body Image
 Role Performance
 Self-Esteem
Stress Urinary Incontinence
 Urinary Continence
 Urinary Elimination
Total Urinary Incontinence
 Tissue Integrity: Skin and Mucous Membranes
 Urinary Continence
 Urinary Elimination
Urge Urinary Incontinence
 Tissue Integrity: Skin and Mucous Membranes
 Urinary Continence
 Urinary Elimination
Urinary Retention
 Urinary Continence
 Urinary Elimination

UTI is one of the most common infections treated by primary care providers. Untreated, it has the potential for serious consequences, such as pyelonephritis (inflammation of the kidney) (see Chapter 37) and bacteremia (bacteria in the blood). On rare occasions, complications of a UTI can lead to death.

The prevalence of UTIs is about eight times higher in women than in men, probably because the female urethra is shorter and lies closer to the anal and vaginal openings. This position increases the risk of bacterial contamination of the lower urinary tract. About 6 to 7 million young women see physicians for UTIs each year, second in frequency only to upper respiratory infections.[59] In 5% to 10% of cases, the UTI recurs after initial treatment.

UTIs rarely develop in men younger than 50 years because of the length of the male urethra and the antibacterial properties of prostatic fluid. The incidence of UTIs in men increases with age, as does the incidence of prostate disease. This medical problem leads to dysfunctional voiding patterns with incomplete emptying of the bladder. Stasis of urine in the bladder increases the risk of cystitis.

The incidence of UTIs increases during hospitalization, usually from catheterization procedures and possibly from inadequate catheter care. Nosocomial (hospital-acquired) UTIs occur in about 2% of inpatients. About 1% of nosocomial UTIs (5000 each year) become life-threatening. Catheter-associated urinary infections account for about 40% of all nosocomial infections and increase the duration of hospital stay, the cost, and mortality risk.[32]

Etiology and Risk Factors
The most common UTI-causing bacteria are gram-negative organisms found in the intestine. *Escherichia coli* probably causes about 80% of UTIs, and *Klebsiella* causes about 5% of reported UTIs. *Enterobacter* and *Proteus* are found in about 2% of reported cases.[59]

Women with vaginal *candidiasis* commonly complain of UTI manifestations. Other causative organisms, such as *Chlamydia trachomatis, Trichomonas vaginalis, Neisseria gonorrhoeae,* and herpes simplex, may be responsible for UTI manifestations as well. Therefore, ask female clients about any gynecologic manifestations when clients present with potential UTIs.

Besides the shorter urethra and its proximity to the vagina and anus, other risk factors for women may be **EB** related to sexual intercourse, pregnancy, poor hygiene, dysfunctional voiding patterns, or a history of female genital mutilation (see Chapter 41). Colonization of the vaginal opening and urethral meatus with *E. coli* is characteristic of women who have recurrent UTIs. Hormonal changes in pregnant and postmenopausal women alter **EB** the vaginal pH, change the vaginal flora, and may allow abnormal levels of normal bacteria to grow.

In addition, shrinkage of the mucosal layer of the lower urogenital system of postmenopausal women in- **EB** creases the risk of urethral irritation during intercourse. In fact, sexual intercourse may increase the risk of UTI in all women. The thrusting motion during coitus can push organisms up the urethra and into the bladder, which can lead to cystitis if the woman does not void after intercourse. The term "honeymoon cystitis" is frequently used to describe this phenomenon.

A poorly fitting contraceptive diaphragm or pessary **EB** may lead to recurrent UTI as well. Pressure against the urethra may obstruct the flow of urine, leading to irritation and incomplete emptying of the bladder. Spermicides are also associated with an increased number of UTIs. **EB** They seem to increase the vaginal pH, alter the normal vaginal flora, and increase colonization of *E. coli*.

In women, synthetic underwear and pantyhose, tight jeans, and wet bathing suits can also foster the develop- **EB** ment of cystitis. Allergens or irritants—feminine hygiene sprays, bubble baths, perfumed toilet paper, sanitary napkins, and soaps—contribute to the development of cystitis in some women.

Indwelling urethral catheters dramatically increase **EB** the occurrence of UTIs. Indeed, UTIs are the most common nosocomial infection. Among catheterized clients, the rates for UTIs in most hospitals are greater than 50%, with some rates reported as high as 100%. Indwelling catheters can introduce bacteria into the urinary tract, possibly from poor insertion technique, irritation and consequent inflammation of the urethra, and ascension of bacteria along the length of the catheter. The rate of infection increases significantly if the drainage system does not remain closed.

Diabetic clients are at increased risk for UTIs because increasing neuropathy can keep the bladder from emp- **EB** tying completely. Anything that interrupts the integrity of the bladder lining opens the way to possible infection. Loss of integrity of the mucosal lining may be caused by an indwelling catheter, calculus, tumor, or diminished estrogen levels. In addition, anything that contributes to urinary stasis significantly increases the risk of UTI.

In older men, obstructive uropathy, loss of the bacte- **EB** ricidal properties of prostatic secretions, poor bladder emptying, and other medical disorders contribute to the development of UTIs. The incidence of UTI in older men is about 15%.

Health promotion and health maintenance strategies are discussed under Nursing Management of the Medical Client.

Pathophysiology

The most common mechanism by which a UTI develops is via ascending and invading bacteria. The organism triggers an inflammatory response in the lining of the urinary tract. This irritation leads to pain, frequent voiding, and other clinical manifestations.

Clinical Manifestations

Any change in a client's voiding habits should be assessed as a possible UTI. The most common clinical manifestations of cystitis are burning pain on urination **EB** (dysuria), frequency, urgency, voiding in small amounts, an inability to void, incomplete emptying of the bladder, cloudy urine, and hematuria (blood in the urine). Lower back or suprapubic pain may be present as well. Other manifestations may include malaise and abdominal and flank pain related to upper tract infection. Manifestations of ureteral involvement may include abdominal distention, nausea, and diarrhea.

Asymptomatic bacteriuria (bacteria in urine) is seen in about 10% of cases, most often in older adults. The only reported manifestation of asymptomatic bacteriuria in an older client may be a change in the mental status with or without fever.

A urine culture is the most accurate diagnostic tool. Initially, a dipstick test for leukocyte esterase and nitrite activity may detect bacteriuria, allowing for immediate broad-spectrum antibiotic therapy to begin. However, the dipstick test should not be used as the exclusive diagnostic tool for a UTI. Some bacteria, such as enterococci, do not convert from nitrates to positive nitrites. Therefore, a urine culture is essential for all clients with evidence of cystitis or a positive dipstick test. Sensitivity **EB** testing can determine which antibiotics the bacteria will respond to. A urine specimen drawn by catheter yields a more accurate test than a voided specimen does.

An area of controversy arises in asymptomatic clients with indwelling urinary catheters and a high bacterial count. Some believe that the UTI should not be treated until the catheter is removed or manifestations develop. Others say that the infection should be treated when a culture is found to grow bacteria. However, most clinicians believe that specimens must be obtained for culture before antibiotics are started.

Traditionally, a bacterial count greater than 100,000/ml for voided specimens has been considered **EB** appropriate for antibiotic intervention. However, symptomatic clients may need treatment even with bacterial counts as low as 1000 to 10,000/ml.

Diagnostic testing, such as an intravenous pyelogram (IVP), voiding cystourethrogram (VCUG), retrograde pyelogram, or cystoscopy, may be used to evaluate clients

INTEGRATING PHARMACOLOGY

Medications for Urinary Tract Infection

The primary medication for the treatment of acute urinary tract infection is an antibiotic aimed at targeting the specific bacteria causing the infection. The specific bacteria should be cultured from a clean or sterile urine specimen. Each of the most commonly prescribed antibiotics and urinary antiseptics act in a specific method to inhibit bacterial growth. Commonly used pharmacologic agents include urinary antibiotics such as sulfonamides (trimethoprim-sulfamethoxazole [Bactrim]), fluoroquinolones (ciprofloxacin [Cipro], and nitrofurantoin (Macrobid). In addition, medications containing azo dyes, such as phenazopyridine (Pyridium), may also be prescribed to minimize the burning sensation often felt with cystitis. Pyridium turns urine bright orange and makes the client feel better after one dose. However, the client needs to understand that the complete course of the prescribed antibiotic must be taken to eradicate the bacteria.

Simple, acute bacterial cystitis may be treated with a single dose of fosfomycin (Monurol). This is a very expensive drug so many health care providers may prescribe a 3-day course of a cheaper antibiotic such as Bactrim or Macrobid.

If infection recurs, the preferred course of treatment is a 7- to 10-day antibiotic regimen. Some clients may be treated for 14 days if they are medically compromised, such as a hospitalized client with an indwelling catheter or a client with a history of diabetes or immunosuppression.

---

with recurrent UTIs or clients at risk for strictures from previous interventions that have been used to identify structural abnormalities, stones, tumors, or foreign bodies in the lower urologic tract. The VCUG detects obstructive voiding patterns, as from an enlarged prostate, that increase the client's risk for recurrent cystitis.

Outcome Management
■ Medical Management

Inhibit Bacterial Growth. To promote comfort and decrease complications, broad-spectrum antibiotics typically begin before the culture and sensitivity results are known. Later, on the basis of the sensitivity report, a more specific antibiotic may be prescribed. See the Integrating Pharmacology feature on Medications for Urinary Tract Infection, above.

A client who reports continued manifestations after completing an antibiotic course or who complains of recurrent UTIs should return for a follow-up culture after antibiotic therapy. If the urine is not yet sterile, antibiotic therapy may be continued with the same or another antibiotic, based on the sensitivity report of the repeated culture.

Chronic or recurrent infections are a frustrating problem. Each infection must be treated with antibiotics. Persistent infections may call for suppression to keep the urine sterile. This measure consists of a small dose of antibiotic taken once daily or several times a week. Clients should be educated to avoid self-diagnosis and self-treatment with over-the-counter products, such as phenazopyridine. Each infection necessitates culture and sensitivity testing with specific treatment. The primary caregiver either may prescribe continuous suppression therapy or may continue episodic administration of antibiotics when a UTI recurs.

There is a growing trend to provide self-care for medication administration in clients with chronic infections. For example, women who experience UTIs in relation to sexual activity may receive a prescription for an antibiotic and instructions to take the medication after coitus. Other clients with frequent recurrences are:

- Offered a prescription for medication
- Taught to recognize early manifestations of a UTI
- Instructed to begin antibiotic therapy at the first hint of infection
- Reminded to complete the full course of antibiotics even if the manifestations disappear

Treating the client with asymptomatic bacteriuria is yet another problem. Some clinicians suggest that an asymptomatic infection be treated only if intervention is certain to prevent further morbidity or if the client is medically compromised. Others suggest immediate antibiotic treatment to reduce the risk of damage to the upper urinary tract.

Modify Diet. Certain foods are known to irritate the bladder, such as caffeine, alcohol, tomatoes, spicy food, chocolate, and some berries. Clients should be encouraged to avoid bladder irritants during the acute phase of the UTI. **[EB]**

Cranberry juice and ascorbic acid (vitamin C) have been used to acidify the urine. The use of these various dietary measures is under investigation. The tannin (proanthocyanidins) is thought to block bacteria from attaching to the bladder wall, thus flushing it from the urinary system. See the Evidence-Based Practice in Action feature on Cranberry-Based Products in the Prevention/Treatment of Urinary Tract Infections on p. 861. **[EB]**

Increase Fluid Intake. To treat and prevent UTI, encourage increased fluid intake, especially water, if the client is not required to restrict fluids. The desired amount is 3 to 4 L/day. Research suggests that calculating 0.5 ounce of fluid per pound of body weight (or dividing body weight in half to find the ounces of fluid needed) is an easy way to individualize fluid intake. Increased fluids flush the urinary system and are important in preventing *urolithiasis* (urinary calculi, or stones) in clients treated with sulfa drugs. Fluids containing alcohol and caffeine should be avoided because they increase mucosal irritation. **[EB]**

EB EVIDENCE-BASED PRACTICE IN ACTION

Cranberry-Based Products in the Prevention/Treatment of Urinary Tract Infections

Urinary tract infections (UTIs) account for more than 11 million visits to physicians' offices annually. Additionally, UTIs have been noted to become increasingly resistant to first-line antibiotic therapy.[4] Recently, evidence has suggested that the ingestion of cranberry juice or cranberry products has been effective in the prevention of UTIs or to decrease the manifestations of UTIs.[1,2,5-8] Cranberry juice, a red tart juice, is available in juice concentrations of 10% to 25%. The pure cranberry juice is acidic and is often unpalatable to clients even when mixed with a sweetener. Although the berry when harvested before it is ripe produces a milder and clear juice, no studies have discussed the evaluation of red cranberry juice versus white cranberry juice in the treatment of UTIs.[3]

According to earlier studies, the active ingredient proanthocyanidins (condensed tannins) found in cranberries and blueberries acidify the urine, inhibiting certain urinary pathogens to adhere to the epithelial cells of the bladder. When the urinary pH goes to 4.5 to 5.0 and urine osmolarity is elevated, the proanthocyanidins affect the adherence of *Escherichia coli (E. coli)* to the bladder epithelial wall.[1,6] The evidence suggests that this phenomenon is most effective in the presence of *E. coli* and *Enterococci fecalis*. However, it has not been tested for other bacteria such as *Pseudomonas aeruginosa, Staphylococcus epidermidis,* or *Candida albicans.*

Kontiokari and colleagues compared cranberry and lingonberry juice with *Lactobacillus GG* drink and no intervention to determine which was most effective in preventing recurrent UTI in women.[5] Their findings indicated that cranberry and lingonberry juice prevented recurrence of UTIs in women, whereas *Lactobacillus* GG drink or no intervention did not prevent recurrence of UTIs.[5] Another study by Dignam and colleagues found a decrease in institutional UTI rates from 27.2 per month to 20 per month after all residents were given 4 ounces of cranberry juice per day.[2]

Additionally, cranberry tablets are available in strengths of 400 to 500 mg for dietary supplementation. The recommended dosing of cranberry tablets is from 1 to 2 tablets per day to 1 to 2 tablets with each meal.[3] McGuinness and colleagues conducted a study that used placebo and cranberry tablets containing 8000 mg of cranberry concentrate.[6] They found that UTIs developed in 32% of the placebo control group and in 34% of the cranberry tablet group.[6] The failure of the cranberry tablets was thought to be related to the inability to ensure that proanthocyanidins (the active ingredient in cranberries) were actually present in the cranberry tablets. They recommended that clients drink cranberry juice or eat cranberries. When studying the effects of cranberry

tablets, Stothers[8] found that both cranberry juice and cranberry tablets statistically reduced the number of UTIs compared to placebo, with tablets being cheaper ($624 for tablets versus $1400 for juice per year.[8] Use of the tablets and use of the juice both decreased the use of antibiotics during the year as well.

Implications

Recent evidence supports the use of cranberry products to prevent UTI. Evidence supports the use of cranberries or cranberry juice but is mixed with regard to cranberry tablets. Hence, additional research is warranted before conclusions regarding cranberry tablets can be made. Nurses should offer supplemental cranberry juice as a preventive measure for those who are at risk for UTIs, especially those in long-term care facilities. In addition, teaching clients with UTIs about the preventive properties of cranberry juice or cranberries is appropriate.

References
1. Chambers, S.T., et al. (1999). Inhibitors of bacterial growth in urine: What is the role of betaines? *International Journal of Antimicrobial Agents, 11,* 2933-2936.
2. Dignam, R., et al. (1998). The effect of cranberry juice on urinary tract infection rates in a long-term care facility. *Annals of Long-Term Care, 6*(5), 163-167.
3. Gray, M. (2002). Are cranberry juice or cranberry products effective in the prevention or management of urinary tract infection? *Journal of Wounds, Ostomy and Continence, 29,* 122-126.
4. Howell, A.B., & Foxman, B. (2002). Cranberry juice and adhesion of antibiotic-resistant uropathogens. *Journal of the American Medical Association, 287*(230), 3083-3084.
5. Kontiokari, T., et al. (2001). Randomized trial of cranberry-lingonberry juice and *Lactobacillus* GG drink for the prevention of urinary tract infection in women. *British Medical Journal, 322,* 1571-1573.
6. McGuinness, S., Krone, R., & Metz, L. (2002). A double-blind, randomized, placebo-controlled trial of cranberry supplements in multiple sclerosis. *Journal of Neuroscience Nursing, 34*(1), 4-7.
7. Robbins, B., & Bondi, S. (2003). Does cranberry juice prevent or treat urinary tract infection. *Journal of Family Practice, 52*(2), 154-156.
8. Stothers, L. (2002). A randomized trial to evaluate effectiveness and cost effectiveness of naturopathic cranberry products as prophylaxis against urinary tract infections in women. *Canadian Journal of Urology, 9*(3), 1558-1562.

Prevent Complications. Broad-spectrum antibiotic therapy may destroy normal flora in the body and allow an overgrowth of opportunistic organisms. On occasion, diarrhea, associated bowel problems, and vaginal candidiasis may develop. Some antibiotics may reduce the

effectiveness of oral contraceptives and estrogen, whereas sulfa drugs increase sensitivity to the effects of the sun.

Complications can also occur if the infection is not completely eradicated. An ascending infection can migrate from the bladder to the kidneys, resulting in pyelonephritis. Recurrent pyelonephritis can predispose the client to renal scarring and chronic renal failure if damage to the kidneys is severe enough. In clients with a history of recurrent or chronic infections, diagnostic testing is necessary to prevent complications associated with recurrent UTIs.

■ Nursing Management of the Medical Client Assessment

Direct the initial nursing assessment at the history and clinical manifestations, as described earlier, to determine whether the problem is acute or chronic. Also, take a gynecologic, sexually transmitted disease (STD), and contraceptive history from female clients. Question male clients about presenting manifestations and take an STD history.

A key nursing responsibility is to instruct the client about clean-catch urine collection to minimize contamination from surface organisms. Appropriate collection of a clean-catch urine specimen for a dipstick test and culture and sensitivity should be included in the assessment. The urine specimen should initially be checked for leukocytes, blood, and nitrites. Color, odor, and clarity should also be evaluated. The urine specimen should then be sent for culture and sensitivity testing. If a client presents with chronic manifestations, additional radiologic diagnostic testing may be ordered to locate the origin of the disease process.

Diagnosis, Outcomes, Interventions

Diagnosis: Impaired Urinary Elimination. The primary
nursing diagnosis when a client is experiencing problems related to cystitis is *Impaired Urinary Elimination related to irritation and inflammation of the bladder mucosa.*

Outcomes. The client will have return of normal voiding
habits within 3 days of starting antibiotic treatment as evidenced by an absence of fever, pain, burning, frequency, and urgency.

Interventions

Inhibit Bacterial Growth. Give adequate instructions to the client regarding antibiotic therapy and dietary and activity restrictions needed during antibiotic therapy. Make sure the client understands the drug, its side effects, whether to take it with or without food, and the importance of taking the full course of the drug even after manifestations disappear. Have the client restate the antibiotic instructions by asking questions to ensure that the instructions have been understood.

Modify Diet. Provide information about dietary changes needed to keep the urine acidic and to reduce

bladder irritation, such as avoiding alcohol and caffeinated beverages. Caffeine is found in coffee, tea, chocolate, some carbonated beverages, and some over-the-counter medications. Spicy foods and tomatoes are also associated with increased bladder irritation. Encourage clients with chronic UTIs to drink 10 oz of cranberry juice daily to acidify the urine and decrease the likelihood of bacterial attachment to the bladder wall.

Increase Fluid Intake. To control the urgency and frequency caused by a UTI, clients may limit rather than increase fluid intake. Instruct your client to eliminate fluids that increase urgency and frequency, such as caffeinated beverages, and to increase the intake of other fluids to 3 to 4 L/day to flush the urinary system. To treat infection and prevent recurrence, teach the client how to calculate an appropriate fluid intake: 0.5 ounce of fluid per pound of body weight per day unless this amount is contraindicated.

Prevent Complications. Tell the client about the increased manifestations that might result from infection of the upper urinary tract and what to do if those manifestations occur. You should maintain a closed urinary drainage system and provide meticulous perineal care with mild soap and water for clients with an indwelling catheter. Keep the catheter bag below the level of the bladder at all times.

Teach Health Promotion Strategies. Encourage the client to engage in health promotion activities to prevent UTIs. For example, encourage a fluid intake of at least 3 L/day, especially of water and acid-ash items to acidify the urine (such as cranberry juice). Advise clients to avoid caffeinated and alcoholic beverages or any of the foods that may irritate the bladder lining.

An important health promotion activity centers on client teaching to prevent recurrence of UTI. Female clients should learn the risks associated with chemical irritants such as spermicides, intercourse, poorly fitted vaginal devices, and the additional risk of lowered estrogen levels associated with menopause. A review of correct hygienic practices should also be included. Alert both male and female clients that STDs can cause manifestations similar to those of a UTI. Inform male clients about obstructive voiding problems caused by benign prostatic hypertrophy (BPH) that lead to urinary stasis.

Emphasize the importance of increased fluids and avoidance of foods and fluids that increase irritation. Also, remind the client to void every 2 to 4 hours during the day (unless the bladder program is planned otherwise) to keep the urinary system flushed. Pregnant women should be encouraged to void every 2 to 3 hours.

Encourage women to void before and after coitus. Suggest that sexually active women use positions that minimize pressure on the anterior vaginal wall during intercourse. Also emphasize the need to maintain good perineal hygiene. For example, instruct women to wipe the urinary meatus from front to back. Encourage women who experience frequent UTIs to shower rather than take tub baths, and urge them to avoid bubble baths, salts, and scented feminine hygiene products. Wearing cotton underpants, which are more absorbent and breathable or porous than synthetic undergarments, and avoiding pantyhose with slacks, a practice that can trap moisture in the perineal region, are additional ways to lower the risk of UTI in women.

The application of vaginal estrogen increases circulation to the lower urogenital system and increases the mucosal layer of atrophic tissues commonly seen in postmenopausal women. Because the lower urogenital system is heavily enriched with estrogen receptors and blood supply before menopause, women should be informed about the need for topical estrogen and systemic estrogen in the postmenopausal period. Using a vaginal lubricant during intercourse is helpful as well.

Health maintenance activities include (1) monitoring pregnant women and older male clients (especially those with BPH) for the presence of UTI, (2) teaching high-risk clients the clinical manifestations of infection, and (3) monitoring clients with an indwelling catheter for the presence of infection. Many postoperative clients receive prophylactic antibiotics while an indwelling catheter is in place.

Finally, clients with a UTI are managed with antibiotics and increased fluid intake. To restore health, clients should be taught ways to prevent recurrence and the importance of taking all antibiotics, followed with repeated cultures and sensitivity testing as ordered.

Diagnosis: Acute Pain. Another common nursing diagnosis for clients with cystitis is *Acute Pain related to irritation and inflammation of bladder and urethral mucosa.*

Outcomes. The client will be able to urinate with minimal or no discomfort within 24 hours after treatment begins and will return to normal voiding habits within 3 days, as evidenced by an absence of pain and burning on urination.

Interventions. Medications prescribed specifically to treat pain, such as phenazopyridine (Pyridium), should be administered. Other comfort measures include forcing fluids to dilute urine and taking a warm sitz bath to decrease urethral smooth muscle spasms. Some clients find a heating pad applied to the suprapubic area helpful in reducing bladder spasms and suprapubic pain.

Evaluation

After the first 24 hours of treatment, the client should be able to report a reduction in pain, burning, urgency, and frequency. Antibiotic therapy usually brings about complete resolution of irritation and pain within 3 days. If indicated, urine culture specimens should be negative after 1 week of treatment or after the course of antibiotics is completed.

■ Surgical Management

The need for surgery is rare; operations are performed only to address structural anomalies that cause repeated infections. Strictures of the bladder neck or urethra are the most common problems requiring surgical intervention. BPH may also be treated surgically (see Chapter 40). Correction of structural abnormalities or obstruction should resolve recurrent UTIs. Nursing care after surgery is discussed under the specific disorder. Chapter 40 describes nursing care of men after surgery for BPH.

■ Self-Care

Promotion of self-care for a client with a UTI includes recognition of lifestyle changes needed to decrease risk factors, the ability to restate the medication protocol, and return for follow-up urine cultures, if indicated. Explain risk factors for UTIs and health promotion strategies to prevent recurrence. These strategies include increased fluid intake, fluid and diet modifications, voiding every 2 hours, and lifestyle modifications, as previously discussed. Advise the client to seek care if manifestations recur.

■ Modifications for Older Clients

In older people, cystitis may occur more often than in younger people but for different reasons. Such a cause might be immobility, constipation, fecal and urinary incontinence, urinary retention (incomplete voiding), altered mental status, or systemic disease.

In older women, atrophic changes resulting from decreased estrogen affect the vagina and urethra. This alteration causes bladder dysfunction, which may predispose this population to infection.

In older men, BPH is one of the main risk factors for UTIs. BPH becomes more common with increased age. Management of recurrent UTIs in men involves treatment of BPH. Once BPH is treated, the infections should diminish.

When administering medications to older or compromised clients, you must consider their renal and hepatic status. Many drugs used to treat UTIs necessitate that the client have adequate renal and hepatic function, particularly with long-term administration. Also, consider any changes in cardiovascular status that might prevent an increase in fluid intake.

URETHRITIS

Urethritis, or inflammation of the urethra, is commonly associated with STDs or sexually transmitted infections (see Chapter 43) and is an associated manifestation of cystitis. The most common causes of urethritis are gonorrhea, chlamydial infection, and other bacterial infections. Among women, common causes also include feminine hygiene sprays, scented toilet paper, sanitary napkins, spermicidal jellies, UTIs, and changes in the vaginal mucosal lining. In short, any irritant that comes into contact with the urethra can cause urethritis.

Exposure to irritants causes the mucosal lining of the urethra to become inflamed. The mucosal lining becomes swollen, painful, red, and irritated. Pus may be produced. *Pyuria*, the presence of pus in the urine, is a common indication of urethritis. Manifestations are similar to those described for cystitis. Frequently, women reveal a history of chemical irritant exposure. Male clients frequently exhibit a urethral discharge.

The diagnosis is often confirmed on the basis of the client's history and clinical manifestations. Culture and sensitivity testing of the urine should be performed, and culture specimens should be obtained to exclude STDs if indicated.

Management of urethritis includes removing the etiologic mechanism. If a microorganism is the cause, administration of systemic and topical antibiotics is essential. Sitz baths and an increased fluid intake are also encouraged. Advise the client to avoid coitus until the manifestations subside or treatment of the STD is completed. The use of lubricants with intercourse decreases irritation in women who have had frequent episodes. Common medications are the same as those used to treat cystitis. The physician may also prescribe topical estrogens for a menopausal woman.

Prevention of urethritis by decreasing exposure to STDs is essential. Inform women about the increased risk of urethritis from spermicides and about the need to avoid feminine hygiene sprays, perfumed toilet paper, and scented sanitary napkins.

URETERITIS

Ureteritis, or inflammation of the ureter, is commonly associated with pyelonephritis (see Chapter 37). Once the kidney infection is treated, ureteral inflammation usually subsides. Chronic pyelonephritis can cause the ureter to become fibrotic and narrowed by strictures, which in turn can continue to foster this condition.

UROSEPSIS

Urosepsis is a gram-negative bacteremia originating in the genitourinary tract. It has become more prevalent among institutionalized clients, especially if the client has an underlying condition. The most common predisposing factors are an indwelling catheter or an untreated UTI in a medically compromised client. Two other primary risk factors for urosepsis are immunosuppression therapy and chemotherapy.

The most common organism responsible for gram-negative bacteremia is *E. coli*, which has the ability to develop resistant strains. Traditionally, gram-negative bacteria have always been recognized as the causative organism of urosepsis. However, there is increasing evidence to suggest that gram-positive bacteria, fungi, viruses, and parasites may also be responsible. Therefore, more research, better diagnostic testing, and better and more aggressive implementation of a therapeutic program directed at eliminating bloodstream invasion of the bacteria with correction and prevention of the pathophysiologic events that cause urosepsis is essential.

The pathophysiologic mechanisms of urosepsis are complex and not fully understood. The disorder can lead to septic shock and death if it is not treated immediately and aggressively (see Chapter 83). The cell wall of the gram-negative bacillus is composed of a lipid-carbohydrate complex. Bacteria release endotoxins, which damage cells. The cells release lysosomes, which further damage tissues and set off kinins and the complement cascade. Cellular metabolism becomes anaerobic, and lactic acidosis develops. Fever and altered mental status are the most common early manifestations. Additionally, research indicates that hyperventilation is often observed before fever begins in clients suffering from urosepsis.

To prevent sepsis and shock, treatment of urosepsis must be instituted right after specimen collection for culture and sensitivity testing. Initial treatment consists of intravenous (IV) aminoglycosides, beta-lactam antibiotics (such as aztreonam), or third-generation cephalosporins until culture results are available. As soon as culture and sensitivity results are available, the antibiotic may be changed if necessary. IV treatment is directed by the status of the client and continued for 3 to 5 days once the client becomes afebrile. Oral antibiotics are continued for the duration of therapy.

INTERSTITIAL CYSTITIS

Cystitis may be noninfectious or abacterial. One type, interstitial cystitis (IC), is also called painful bladder disease (PBD), Hunner's ulcer, urethral syndrome, pseudomembranous trigonitis, and other names. This greatly underdiagnosed condition involves urgency, frequency, and a painful bladder despite a lack of bacteria in the urine culture. The most severe forms of this disease involve ulcerations and hemorrhages in the bladder wall. The cause of these ulcers is unknown, but the ulcers may stem from a defect in the epithelial molecular layer of the bladder wall.

Etiology and Risk Factors

IC occurs mainly in young women (90% to 95% of all cases), usually white but occasionally African American. The disease is increasing significantly among Jewish women, which may be somehow related to the increase in inflammatory bowel disease associated with autoimmune disorders in this population.[56]

Pathophysiology

IC is a poorly understood disorder with an unclear pathophysiology. It may be a local autoimmune phenomenon. Despite clinical manifestations, the urine is usually sterile. The most current theory seems to be associated with a breakdown in the permeability of the glycosaminoglycan layer of the bladder mucosa, which is usually impermeable to urea and bacteria. This theory has been questioned in some studies, which suggest that the permeability of the bladder in clients with IC is no greater than that in normal people.[25,56]

Characteristic pathologic changes are found in more severe forms of IC, including nonspecific chronic inflammatory infiltrate, edema, vasodilation, and eventually fibrosis of the submucosa and detrusor layers of the bladder wall. The fibrosis of the submucosa seems to decrease the elasticity of the detrusor muscle, which decreases bladder capacity.

Mast cell infiltrates have been identified in the bladders of clients with IC, particularly in the detrusor layer. Because mast cells are associated with allergic reactions, it is worth noting that about half of clients with IC are reported to have allergies and 30% have inflammatory bowel disease. Finally, another hypothesis is that bacteria are found only in the mucosal wall of the bladder and not in the urine.[25,56]

Clinical Manifestations

The clinical manifestations of IC are tenderness in the area of the bladder trigone during anterior palpation during a vaginal examination, complaints of lower abdominal or pelvic pain, urinary urgency, and frequency (up to 60 times a day), *nocturia* (excessive urination at night), and, in some women, dyspareunia (painful intercourse). Presenting manifestations and their severity vary from client to client. Some women find the disorder debilitating. Manifestations may be present for years and treated as bacterial cystitis before an appropriate diagnosis is made.

The National Institute of Diabetes, Digestive, and Kidney Diseases recommends specific diagnostic criteria for identifying clients with clinical manifestations. These criteria include the following:

- A detailed client history with physical examination
- A completed bladder diary
- Urine cytology
- Urodynamic evaluation to determine bladder capacity and evaluate bladder function
- Cystoscopy with the client under anesthesia and with hydrodistention of the bladder
- Bladder biopsy

During cystoscopy and hydrodilation of the bladder, the presence of outpouches in the bladder wall, Hunner's ulcers, and a severely decreased bladder capacity is considered by many physicians to be the clinical diagnostic feature of IC. Others believe that IC may be present even without these findings.

Outcome Management
■ Medical Management

Reduce Pain. The treatment of IC is controversial, with no single accepted treatment. Anti-inflammatory, antispasmodic, antidepressant, and antihistamine medications and, occasionally, tranquilizers or opioids may be used.

Pentosan polysulfate sodium (Elmiron) is the newest oral medication of choice. This drug increases the bladder defense mechanism or detoxifies irritants in urine that might break down the bladder lining. The mechanism of action is like heparin, with anticoagulant and antifibrin effects. Relief of manifestations may take up to 3 months.

Other treatments include instillation of a variety of agents into the bladder to promote healing and pain reduction, such as sodium oxychlorosene (Clorpactin), silver nitrate, and dimethyl sulfoxide (DMSO). Heparin itself has been instilled in the bladder, initially daily for 3 to 4 months. Therapy is continued three times a week for 3 to 6 months. Some clients may not notice any improvement in manifestations until after the first 2 to 4 months of treatment.[25] All of these treatments are designed to decrease the permeability of the bladder mucosa so that the causative agent has more difficulty penetrating the lining.

Although the mechanism of action is unclear, bacille Calmette-Guérin (BCG) has been effective as an intravesical agent administered weekly. BCG instillations for 6 weeks have led to a decreased need for pain medications, a doubling of cystometric capacity, and sometimes a decrease in client discomfort.[25]

Referrals to centers providing conservative management programs with behavioral intervention, electrical stimulation, and biofeedback to the pelvic floor musculature may also alleviate manifestations of IC. Because of the chronic nature of the disorder, physicians are reluctant to offer opioids for pain reduction. During severe exacerbations, however, opioids may be appropriate.

Improve Coping. Many clients with IC complain of exhaustion and depression. The exhaustion usually stems from poor sleep patterns caused by nocturnal urgency, frequency, and pain. Depression can result from frustration, exhaustion, chronic pain, and difficulty in obtaining effective medical care.

During the acute phase, these clients may require medications to improve sleep as well as antidepressant therapy to increase coping ability. Referrals to social workers or other health care professionals to improve coping strategies and mental status may be needed. You also may need to refer the client to a center that specializes in treating IC.

■ Nursing Management of the Medical Client

Reduce Pain. Nurses provide a great deal of education about drug therapy. Many of the medications have a cumulative effect, making long-term therapy necessary for maximal results. You may need to continuously reinforce this point if the client grows frustrated with pharmacologic intervention. You also should counsel the client before opioid intervention. Because IC is a chronic problem, inform the client about risk factors associated with opioids.

Improve Coping. Your major responsibility is to support the client through diagnosis and treatment. Because the cause of IC is unclear, few nursing interventions are aimed at prevention. IC is a chronic disorder requiring long-term client support. Clients may need additional psychological counseling to help with stress-related coping strategies. Become familiar with national and local resources for clients with IC or painful bladder disease (Interstitial Cystitis Association), and refer clients as appropriate.

Bladder retraining with conservative management programs can help reduce clinical manifestations. Teaching clients to void by the clock rather than by urge gently and slowly increases bladder capacity. Biofeedback-directed pelvic floor exercises teach the client the urge suppression technique. This process decreases episodes of urgency and frequency and promotes control of manifestations. The additional use of transvaginal or transanal electrical stimulation may help override bladder spasms and can increase the quality of pelvic floor contractions.

■ Surgical Management

Surgery is rarely used to manage the client with IC. The traditional therapy is hydraulic distention of the bladder, with or without instillation of DMSO to increase the bladder's functional capacity. Clients with severely reduced bladder capacity and incapacitating manifestations may be candidates for a transurethral resection (TUR), laser surgical resection of the lesions, a partial or complete *cystectomy* (resection of the bladder), and *urinary diversion* (surgical rerouting of the normal urinary flow) (see Bladder Cancer, below).[25]

■ OBSTRUCTIVE DISORDERS
BLADDER CANCER

Most bladder cancers are transitional or papillary tumors in the bladder urothelium. These tumors may infiltrate the bladder wall. Bladder cancer is the most frequent neoplasm of the urinary tract, accounting for about 6% of all cancer cases in men and 2% in women.[1]

The American Cancer Society estimated 57,400 new cases of bladder cancer in 2003 and 12,500 associated deaths.[1] Bladder cancer is rarely seen in adults younger than 40 years of age and occurs most frequently in 50- to 60-year-old adults. Now the fourth most common cancer in men and the tenth most common cancer in women, it affects whites twice as often as blacks.[1]

Etiology and Risk Factors

The disease process has several possible causes. There is a strong correlation between cigarette smoking and bladder cancer. Hence, a health promotion and health maintenance strategy is to encourage smokers to stop smoking and to be screened regularly after age 50 years for hematuria and other manifestations of bladder can-

COMPLEMENTARY AND ALTERNATIVE THERAPY

Supplements to Reduce the Risk of Bladder Cancer

A large epidemiologic study found somewhat similar results to the Health Professionals Follow-up Study. Researchers investigated the association between individual vitamin C and vitamin E supplements and bladder cancer mortality among more than 991,000 U.S. adults in the Cancer Prevention Study II cohort. This data set covered 16 years of follow-up, and 1289 deaths (962 men and 327 women) from bladder cancer were recorded.

Regular vitamin C supplement use was not related to bladder cancer mortality during any follow-up period. However, regular vitamin E supplement use for 10 or more years (but not of shorter duration) was associated with a reduced risk of bladder cancer mortality (RR = 0.60). A reduction in bladder cancer mortality was found in adults who never smoked (RR = 0.84) and in ex-smokers (RR = 0.69), but the reduction was most evident in current smokers (RR = 0.31).

The authors of this study did not endorse the use of vitamin E supplements for smokers because of the large impact on overall disease risk in current smokers from other studies. The primary recommendation, which seems most appropriate, was to stop smoking completely to prevent both bladder cancer and early morbidity and mortality from other diseases. Thus the preliminary data so far indicates that current smokers may not benefit from individual vitamin C and vitamin E supplements in terms of overall disease morbidity and mortality reduction, but ex-smokers and those who have never smoked may derive some benefit (mostly from vitamin supplements), especially in regard to bladder cancer reduction.

Reference
Jacobs, E., et al. (2002). Vitamin C and vitamin E supplement use and bladder cancer mortality in a large cohort of U.S. men and women. *American Journal of Epidemiology 156*, 1002-1110.

RR, Relative risk.

cer. (See the Complementary and Alternative Therapy feature on Supplements to Reduce the Risk of Bladder Cancer on p. 866.)

Industrial exposure to certain substances, such as aniline dyes, asbestos, and aromatic amines (e.g., benzidine and 2-naphthylamine) may also result in bladder cancer. The latency period of industrial exposure can be as long as 18 to 45 years. Workers in this high-risk group should also be screened regularly after age 50 years for hematuria and other manifestations of bladder cancer.

Artificial sweeteners have been weakly linked to the development of bladder cancer. Attempts to connect coffee consumption and bladder cancer have produced contradictory findings because of the increased use of artificial sweeteners and cigarettes associated with coffee consumption. Other risk factors may be chronic cystitis, pelvic radiation, and the chemotherapeutic drug cyclophosphamide (Cytoxan). For more information, see the Complementary and Alternative Theapy features on Fluid Consumption to Reduce the Risk of Bladder Cancer, below, and on Fruits and Vegetables and the Risk of Bladder Cancer on p. 868. (See also the Complementary and Alternative Therapy feature on Inorganic Arsenic in Drinking Water and the Risk of Bladder Cancer on the website.)

Clients who have undergone transurethral resection or removal of superficial bladder cancer should return for regular cystoscopic follow-up as a health maintenance and restoration activity. Teaching clients to care for a urinary diversion is a health restoration activity provided by nurses.

Pathophysiology

Bladder cancer appears to result from exposure of the bladder wall to a *carcinogen* (a cancer-causing agent). Cigarette smoking or second-hand smoke may result in carcinogenic metabolites produced by abnormal tryptophan metabolism, with the metabolite excreted in the urine. Cigarette smoke also contains nitrosamines as well as 2-naphthylamine (both carcinogens), which are also excreted in the urine.

Premalignant proliferative changes are often found in the transitional cell layer. These changes are called *dysplasia* and refer to abnormal cell configuration found in several degrees of severity. The extent of dysplasia may be described as mild, moderate, or severe, leading to carcinoma in situ (localized).[67] Most bladder cancers start as papillary or transitional cell tumors and account for 70% of bladder tumors. These tumors are most commonly found in the trigone of the bladder and lateral wall of the bladder.

Staging of a tumor indicates the depth of penetration into the bladder wall and degree of *metastasis*. Staging must be done to determine the treatment modality. Clin-

---

COMPLEMENTARY AND ALTERNATIVE THERAPY

Fluid Consumption to Reduce the Risk of Bladder Cancer

Increased fluid consumption from numerous sources may reduce the risk of bladder cancer. The largest cohort study attempting to determine the relationship between fluid intake and bladder cancer risk was taken from the Health Professionals Follow-up Study. Approximately 48,000 male health professionals were followed for 10 years, with a total of 252 cases of bladder cancer found during this time period. Men in this study updated their diet and medical history every 2 years. Data on total fluid intake was taken from the reported intake frequency of 22 beverage types on a diet questionnaire.

Age and smoking were found to have a major relationship with bladder cancer risk. Total fluid consumption was inversely related with the risk of bladder cancer (RR = 0.51) for the highest quintile of intake (>2531 ml/day) versus the lowest (<1290 ml/day). Water intake was responsible for a significantly lower risk (*p* for trend = 0.001) when comparing 6 or more cups/day versus 1 cup (RR = 0.49). This risk decreased by 7% for each 240 ml daily increment of fluid consumption.

The baseline questionnaire used in this study could not provide insight regarding the source of water (tap and/or bottled) consumed on a regular basis. Thus the investigators in this study could not clearly comment on the effect of the water source and any potential risk. However, data from approximately one third of the cohort found that the majority of these men (78%) consumed municipal water. In addition, the inverse relationship for water and risk was consistently observed in all regions of the United States and were also observed for the individuals who reported drinking water from municipal sources.

This investigation suggests that a greater consumption of water could decrease the risk of bladder cancer by an average of 50%. No beverage except water demonstrated a significant inverse relationship with bladder cancer, but the consumption of all of other types of fluids, with the exception of fruit juice, was also related to a lower risk (RR = 0.63). Other fluids that reduced the risk included milk, sodas, lemonade, coffee, tea, and alcoholic beverages. Whether or not greater fluid intake affects risk remains to be determined, but if it does it may be a partial explanation of why certain regions of the world experience lower rates of bladder cancer despite a higher rate of smoking.

Reference
Michaud, D., et al. (1999). Fluid intake and the risk of bladder cancer in men. *New England Journal of Medicine, 340,* 1390-1397.

RR, Relative risk.

COMPLEMENTARY AND ALTERNATIVE THERAPY

Fruits and Vegetables and the Risk of Bladder Cancer

One of the largest prospective studies on fruit and vegetable consumption and the risk of bladder cancer derived data from the Health Professionals Follow-up Study, which included approximately 48,000 men. Over a 10-year period (1986-1996), 252 cases of bladder cancer were diagnosed. Each individual in this cohort completed a very detailed (131-item) dietary questionnaires in 1986 and again in 1990 and 1994. Age, smoking status, residence, total fluid intake, and caloric intake were adjusted for in this investigation.

An overall nonsignificant and minimal but inverse relationship was found between total fruit and vegetable consumption and the risk of bladder cancer. However, the consumption of cruciferous vegetables was significantly associated with a reduced risk when comparing the highest intakes versus the lowest intakes (RR = 0.49). The intake of other types of vegetables was not related to risk. All cruciferous vegetables (except coleslaw) were associated with a decreased risk, but only broccoli (RR = 0.61) and cabbage (RR = 0.56) were found to be statistically significant when comparing intakes of less than once a week versus one or more times per week.

The reduction in bladder cancer risk with the intake of cruciferous vegetables was observed to be strongest for individuals with no smoking history. Overall this study supports the possibility that a greater intake of cruciferous vegetables may reduce the risk of bladder cancer.

Reference

Michaud, D., et al. (1999). Fruit and vegetable intake and incidence of bladder cancer in a male prospective cohort. *Journal of the National Cancer Institute, 91,* 605-613.

RR, Relative risk.

ical staging includes the results and review of an excretory urogram, cystoscopy, biopsy, and bimanual examination with the client under anesthesia. For evaluation of specific areas of metastasis as well as for staging, chest radiography, lymphangiography, isotope bone scans, computed tomography (CT), and liver function analysis are needed. The most frequently used staging systems are the Jewett-Marshall-Strong System and the tumor-node-metastasis (TNM) classification. The stages refer to the depth of invading tumor found during biopsy (Figure 36-1).[60]

Metastasis to other organs begins once the invading cancer penetrates the submucosal and muscular layer of the bladder. The invasion progresses through pelvic lymph nodes and spreads to liver, bones, and lungs. As metastasis progresses, it can extend into the rectum, vagina, other pelvic soft tissues, and retroperitoneal structures. The prognostic "dividing line" lies between stages B1 and B2; stage C and D tumors portend a much poorer prognosis. Clients with superficial bladder tumors have a survival rate of 70% after 5 years. Other clients with muscle invasive disease experience tumor recurrence within 18 to 24 months of the diagnosis.[48]

Superficial tumors have a good chance of being eradicated or stabilized; however, recurrence is frequent. Therefore, it is crucial to do follow-up cystoscopic examinations every 3 months for 2 years, with additional cystoscopic examinations every 6 months for 2 years, then yearly. In a study of 114 clients, the interval between the original intervention and recurrence ranged from 3 months to 27 years. Nineteen percent involved a new tumor of a higher grade, and 22% of the tumors were of a more advanced stage. Most recurrences of superficial tumors represent lesions that can be controlled by transurethral resection.[48]

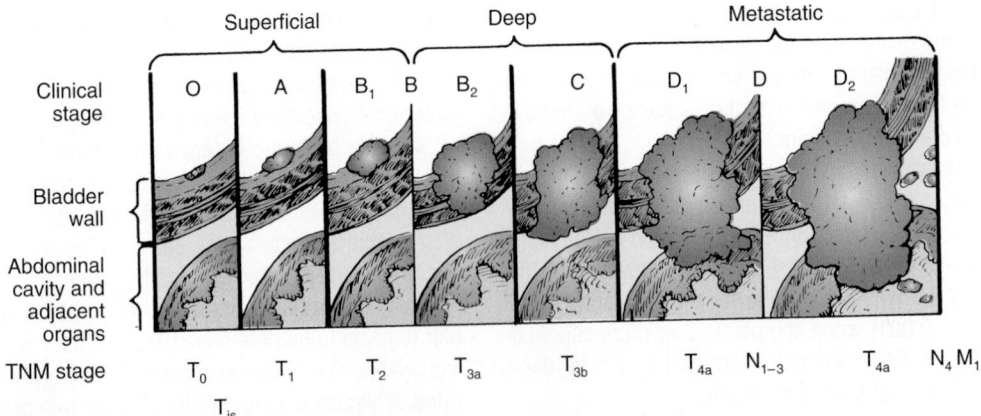

FIGURE 36-1 The Jewett-Marshall-Strong clinical staging of bladder cancer. The diagram shows the degree of tumor infiltration at each stage and compares it with the tumor, node, metastasis (TNM) system. (Modified from K. Karlowicz [Ed.]. [1995]. *Urologic nursing: Principles and practice.* Philadelphia: W.B. Saunders.)

Clinical Manifestations

Gross painless hematuria is most frequently the first manifestation of bladder cancer, occurring in 85% of all cases. Initially, the bleeding is usually intermittent, which may lead a client to delay seeking health care. As the disease becomes more invasive, the client may experience frequent bladder irritability with dysuria, frequency, and urgency. Frequently, gross hematuria or obstruction in voiding forces the client to seek help. The amount of hematuria does not correlate with stage of disease.

When gross or microscopic hematuria is identified without any known etiologic agent, an extensive evaluation is necessary. Cystoscopy is indicated to identify and visualize the tumor directly and to obtain a biopsy specimen of the lesion for cytologic study. Flow cytometry can be done to examine the deoxyribonucleic acid (DNA) content of the cells in the urine. Bladder washings during cystoscopy produce more accurate specimens compared with a voided specimen. The mechanical action resulting from saline washings enhances tumor shedding, with better quality specimens sent for cytologic study.

Numerous attempts have been made to identify other screening tests including the BTA (Bladder Tumor Antigen) test, NMP22 (nuclear matrix protein) test, and TRAP (telomeric repeat amplification protocol) assay, but all lack sufficient sensitivity. Newer techniques under investigation include assays designed to detect hyaluronic acid, hyaluronidase or survivin, a substance that inhibits cellular apoptosis.[23]

Another examination, IVP, is a dye-enhanced x-ray examination that allows one to evaluate not only the bladder but also the ureters and kidneys. CT, magnetic resonance imaging (MRI), and ultrasonography also may be done to assess the bladder and surrounding structures, such as the rectum or uterus, possible sites of spread. A tumor marker, serum carcinoembryonic antigen (CEA), which is present with adenocarcinomas of the bladder, can also be evaluated.

Outcome Management
■ Medical Management

The outcome desired with medical management is to eradicate the bladder of transitional or papillary cell carcinoma in situ in the early stages. This is best achieved with alkylating intravesical chemotherapy or BCG instillations, which are the first-line and most common therapies. Advanced cancer that has invaded muscle is usually treated surgically with a radical cystectomy. Radiation therapy is rarely used except in cases of advanced disease or as palliative treatment.

Chemotherapy Administration. Intravesical therapies can be administered for superficial tumors, such as transitional cell, papillary cell, or stage 0-A tumors. Intravesical BCG therapy appears to be successful in treating carcinoma in situ. The best results have been obtained with BCG as an intravesical agent for transitional cell tumors, although it has also been used for papillary tumors, adenocarcinoma, and squamous cell carcinoma.

Usually, BCG is instilled into the bladder through a urethral catheter. The catheter is clamped or removed. The client is directed to retain the fluid for 2 hours, with side-to-side position changes or supine-to-prone changes required every 15 to 30 minutes. Once the 2 hours have passed, the client voids in a sitting position or the catheter is unclamped to allow drainage. Finally, the client is instructed to drink two glasses of water to help flush the bladder. Steroids and ciprofloxacin (Cipro) have sometimes been given after intravesical BCG treatment to prevent recurrence. If two treatments of intravesical BCG have been ineffective, most urologists recommend a cystectomy. (See the Complementary and Alternative Therapy feature on Combination Mega-Dose Supplement and the Recurrence of Bladder Cancer, below.)

COMPLEMENTARY AND ALTERNATIVE THERAPY

Combination Mega-Dose Supplement and the Recurrence of Bladder Cancer

An older trial that has yet to be duplicated included 65 clients with transitional cell carcinoma (TCC) of the bladder and BCG (bacille Calmette-Guérin) immunotherapy. Clients were randomly assigned to a group that received by mouth either the recommended daily allowance (RDA) of several vitamins and a mineral or the RDA of several vitamins and a mineral plus 40,000 international units of vitamin A, 100 mg vitamin B_6, 2000 mg vitamin C, 400 international units of vitamin E, and 90 mg zinc.

No difference in the time to recurrence was noted in the first 10 months of the study, but significant differences occurred after that time period. The overall follow-up was a mean of 45 months (40 months for the RDA group and 49 months for the RDA-plus-other-vitamins group). The 5-year estimates (Kaplan-Meier interval) of recurrence were 91% in the RDA group ($n = 30$) and 41% in the RDA-plus-other vitamins group. This difference was statistically significant, and mild nausea was the most common side effect.

This study obviously requires a larger randomized trial to confirm its findings, but the initial result is interesting and should probably at least be discussed with clients undergoing a similar conventional treatment protocol. Some questions concerning the individual clients in this study were not addressed, such as nutritional or vitamin and mineral deficiency status and other lifestyle and genetic differences between the groups. These issues need to be addressed in future studies.

Reference

Lamm, D., et al. (1994). Megadose vitamins in bladder cancer: A double-blind clinical trial. *Journal of Urology, 151*, 21-26.

Intravesical instillation of an alkylating chemotherapeutic agent, another common practice, provides concentrated topical treatment with relatively little systemic absorption. Thiotepa, mitomycin, doxorubicin (Adriamycin), valrubicin (Valstar), and cyclophosphamide (Cytoxan) are all used for low-grade, superficial papillary tumors. Systemic chemotherapy drugs are used for more advanced disease, to treat the metastasis of the bladder tumor, and to prolong life. However, surgical removal of the bladder is the most common approach in advanced disease when tumor has invaded muscle.

The major side effects or complications of intravesical chemotherapy or BCG instillation include bladder irritation, frequency, urgency, and dysuria. These manifestations usually resolve within 1 or 2 days. Occasionally, hematuria, fever, malaise, nausea, chills, arthralgia (joint pain), and pruritus (itching) are reported. These manifestations are more representative of systemic reaction and should be reported to the physician.

Radiation Therapy. Radiation therapy alone is not as effective a treatment for bladder cancer as surgery and chemotherapy; the 5-year survival rate after radiation alone is less than 40%. Radiation therapy is rarely used except as palliation for advanced disease that cannot be eradicated by intravesical chemotherapy or radical surgery. Most bladder cancers are poorly radiosensitive, and high doses of radiation are necessary.

External supervoltage radiation, somewhat unsuccessful by itself, is effective when used in combination with surgery or chemotherapy. Hyperbaric radiation therapy increases the oxygen tension of the tumor cells and their radiosensitivity. Palliative radiation may be used to relieve pain, to prevent and relieve bowel obstruction, to control potential hemorrhage, and to alleviate leg edema secondary to venous or lymphatic obstruction.

The major side effects of radiation are hemorrhagic cystitis and bladder irritation. Local instillation of formalin may control bladder hemorrhaging resulting from the cancer or the treatments. Hemorrhagic cystitis may occur even as late as 10 years after pelvic radiation. Other complications include manifestations of cystitis and proctitis, such as dysuria, frequency, urgency, nocturia, and diarrhea. Delayed adverse effects, such as ileitis, colitis, persistent cystitis, bladder ulceration, and fistula formation, may occur as late as 6 to 12 months after radiation.

A *fistula* is an abnormal passage between two organs or between an organ and the skin. It allows for intercommunication of secretions and other substances. After radiation to the bladder, a vesicovaginal fistula may be found in women or a colovesical fistula may develop. A fistula is suspected when urine leaves the body from an unnatural site, such as the vagina, when fecal material or air appears in the urine, or when the client has recurrent UTIs. Diagnosis is confirmed by IVP, cystography, cystoscopy, or sigmoidoscopy. To further delineate the path of a fistula, a dye, such as Congo red or indigo carmine, is instilled into the bladder and all outlets are identified.

Before surgical repair of a fistula, the client must maintain a continuous flow of urine from the kidney through temporary urinary diversion, either externally or with a catheter. Surgical repair often requires a long and slow surgical procedure and may require several procedures. The primary goals are to excise the fistula and to reestablish tissue integrity.

■ Nursing Management of the Medical Client
Assessment

Begin your assessment of a client being evaluated for bladder cancer with a careful health, medical, and surgical history. Because this client will be undergoing extensive diagnostic evaluation, be sure to collect additional information about drug, chemical, and food allergies. Explain risk factors from exposure to known carcinogens. Ask the client about changes in urine or urination patterns, noting changes in color, frequency, and amount.

Diagnosis, Outcomes, Interventions

Diagnosis: Powerlessness. The client with bladder cancer may experience *Powerlessness related to lack of knowledge of disease process, options, treatment, and side effects of therapy; fear of the disease process and treatment; and loss of control following the diagnosis and decisions regarding treatment offered.*

Outcomes. The client will learn about the medical management of the disease process, with a full understanding of client responsibilities during the treatment. The client and family will be involved with decisions about therapies and care. The client will also be encouraged to help direct care with involved health care professionals.

Interventions

Provide Education. To increase knowledge, educate the client and family about the use, rationale, risks, side effects, and expected outcomes of intravesical chemotherapy, BCG instillation, radiation, and surgery. You play an important role in client education of treatment modalities and complications that may accompany them.

Encourage Decision Making. Encourage the client to discuss and make decisions about care. Provide opportunities for the client to express desires for care as well as time to discuss what the diagnosis and treatment mean personally.

Diagnosis: Impaired Urinary Elimination. *Impaired Urinary Elimination related to urgency, frequency, dysuria, and hematuria resulting from chemotherapy, radiation, or BCG instillation for treatment of bladder cancer.*

Outcomes. Normal voiding will resume by day 3 after removal of the catheter, and the client will not experience sequelae to BCG instillation, chemotherapy, or radiation therapy.

Interventions. Nursing management of intravesical chemotherapy includes client education, administration of the chemotherapy agent, care of the client throughout the procedure, and monitoring for complications after administration.

Provide Education. Preparation before BCG or chemotherapy bladder instillation requires fluid restriction for 4 hours before the procedure to decrease the need to void for 2 hours afterward. Tell the client that a catheter will be inserted before the instillation and that it will be necessary to rotate and change positions every 15 to 30 minutes during treatment. After the 2-hour instillation, fluids are encouraged to flush the urinary system. Explain that treatments are typically repeated weekly for 4 to 8 weeks and then monthly for varying periods. Follow-up cystoscopy is required to monitor tumor growth.

Promote Safety. Because of the toxicity of the intravesical chemotherapy or BCG instillation, it is important to provide a safe environment for health care workers who may come in contact with the chemotherapeutic agent. For 6 hours after treatment, all urine and the toilet bowl must be disinfected with bleach.

Promote Comfort. Dysuria or irritation while voiding may result from the side effects of chemotherapy, placement of an indwelling catheter, and the presence of the tumor, and it must be managed. Tumor pain is managed with analgesics. Irritative problems of dysuria, frequency, and urgency from the catheter will diminish when the catheter is removed. Irritation from the chemotherapy will decrease after about 2 days.

Reassure the client that dysuria, frequency, and urgency from catheter placement and intravesical treatment will diminish over 2 days. Discuss prescribed analgesics, antispasmodics, or anticholinergics, and explain how they should be taken.

Diagnosis: Risk for Injury. The client who undergoes chemotherapy, BCG instillation, or radiation therapy is at *Risk for Injury from side effects of these treatments.*

Outcomes. Complications resulting from these treatments will be minimized. The client will verbalize an un-

derstanding of risk and side effects following the selected treatment option.

Interventions. Explain expected and unexpected outcomes of BCG instillation, chemotherapy, or radiation therapy. Inform the client and family how and when to alert medical staff to potential complications. Interventions for side effects include administration of antispasmodics, increasing fluid intake, and administering urinary tract antiseptics or analgesics.

If a high temperature develops after BCG instillation, treatment with isoniazid or other medications used to treat tuberculosis may be indicated.

For radiation proctitis, the client requires a low-residue diet and drugs to decrease intestinal motility. For complete information on nursing care for clients receiving radiation therapy, see Chapter 19.

Urine from a client undergoing this intervention should be sent to the radioisotopes laboratory for monitoring. A client with radioactive implants is typically placed in a private room with limited visitation, but hospital policies may vary.

Evaluation

Complications that arise from medical treatment may be difficult to manage, but they typically resolve after the treatment has ended. Evaluation of the nursing management of radiation therapy and intravesical BCG and chemotherapy are based on the client's ability to restate personal responsibilities, to verbalize an understanding of the disease process, and to participate in care.

Because clients with bladder cancer require long-term follow-up care and continuous evaluation, they must understand the disease process and long-term follow-up responsibilities needed to maintain optimal health. If medical therapies are unsuccessful, surgical removal of the bladder may be required.

■ Surgical Management

Several surgical options may be used to treat bladder cancer that has not responded to medical therapies or that has invaded the bladder muscle. Surgical intervention ranges from local resection and fulguration of the tumor (destruction of tissue by electrical current through electrodes placed in direct contact with the growth) to total cystectomy, which requires diversion of normal urinary flow.

Transurethral Resection

The simplest procedure is transurethral resection of the bladder tumor and fulguration done for low-grade, superficial, isolated papillary tumors or, sometimes, for inoperable tumors for palliation. The bladder is accessed through a cystoscope, which has been inserted through the urethra (see Chapter 34). This procedure is commonly followed by intravesical BCG or chemotherapy to prevent recurrence from reattachment of loose bladder cancer cells. (See the Complementary and Alternative **EB** Therapy feature on Probiotic Agents to Reduce the Risk of Recurrence of Bladder Cancer, below.)

Partial Cystectomy

A segmental or partial cystectomy may be done if the client cannot tolerate a radical cystectomy and for an isolated tumor that cannot be treated by transurethral resection. Up to half the bladder can be removed. This procedure is appropriate for 10% to 15% of clients. The recurrence rate can be high.

COMPLEMENTARY AND ALTERNATIVE THERAPY

Probiotic Agents to Reduce the Risk of Recurrence of Bladder Cancer

Two randomized controlled/double-blind investigational trials were conducted in clients with superficial transitional cell cancer (TCC) of the bladder to determine the effect of oral *Lactobacillus casei* powder (biolactis powder [BLP], 3 g/day) on the recurrence post-transurethral resection. Study 1 included 48 clients ($n = 23$ BLP and $n = 25$ placebo), and study 2 included 125 clients ($n = 61$ BLP and n = 64 placebo).

The two groups in study 1 had similar clinical qualities, but their 50% recurrence-free interval after BLP treatment was 1.8 times longer ($p = 0.03$) versus the placebo arm (350 days versus 195 days). Study 2 referred clients to one of three subgroups according to their tumor status. Subgroup A consisted of multiple primary tumors, subgroup B consisted of single recurrent tumors, and subgroup C consisted of multiple recurrent bladder tumors. The 50% recurrence-free interval in subgroups A and B was longer with BLP versus the placebo (688 versus 543 days). No significant difference was recognized in subgroup C. Multivariate analysis showed that the result with BLP was significantly greater than with the placebo ($p = 0.01$). Mild diarrhea was the primary side effect in 4.6% of the individuals (3 clients) taking BLP, and they did not require treatment.

These preliminary observations suggest that BLP powder has a good short-term safety profile and may play a role in preventing or prolonging the recurrence of superficial bladder in some clients.

References
Aso, Y., Akaza, H., & the BLP Study Group. (1992). Prophylactic effect of a *Lactobacillus casei* preparation on the recurrence of superficial bladder cancer. *Urology International, 49*, 125-129.
Aso, Y., et al. (1995). Prevention effect of a *Lactobacillus casei* preparation on the recurrence of superficial bladder cancer in a double-blind trial. *European Urology, 27*, 104-109.

During the initial postoperative period, bladder capacity is markedly reduced. The postoperative bladder may be able to hold no more than 60 ml. Over several months, bladder tissue expands, increasing its capacity from 200 to 400 ml.

Radical Cystectomy and Urinary Diversion

A radical cystectomy with urinary diversion is the procedure of choice when potentially curable stage B disease is too advanced for transurethral resection or intravesical chemotherapy. The procedure may also be performed for treatment of the following:

- Neurogenic bladder (see later discussion)
- IC or radiation-induced cystitis with severely reduced bladder capacity
- Congenital anomalies of the lower urinary tract, such as bladder exstrophy

Radical cystectomy entails removal of the bladder, urethra, uterus, fallopian tubes, ovaries, and anterior segment of the vagina in women. In men, the bladder, urethra, and usually the prostate and seminal vesicles are removed. Cystectomy also involves removal of perivesical fat and dissection of the pelvic lymph nodes. This procedure is necessary when the tumor has invaded the bladder wall, involves the trigone, or cannot be treated adequately by less radical methods. When the bladder and urethra are removed, permanent urinary diversion is required. The entire surgical procedure is done in one step, with urinary diversion and cystectomy performed at the same time.

Ileal Conduit. An ileal conduit (also called ureteroileostomy, ileal bladder, or Bricker's procedure) is one type of urinary diversion. Using a segment of the intestine as a conduit, the surgeon constructs a system in which urine empties through an artificial opening in the skin called a *stoma* (Figure 36-2). Usually, a portion of the terminal ileum, which has the least reabsorptive power, is used for the conduit. After the continuity of the remaining intestine is reestablished with end-to-end anastomosis, the proximal end of the segment is closed. The distal end is brought out through a hole created in the abdominal wall, folded back, and sutured to the skin to form a stoma. The ureters are then implanted into the ileal segment. Urine flows into the conduit and is continually propelled out through the stoma by peristalsis. Mucous shreds are present in the urine because of the mucus produced by the lining of the bowel.

Indications. The client who has undergone an ileal conduit must wear an appliance over the stoma to collect the urine. This treatment is rarely selected for clients with a life expectancy of more than 1 to 2 years. The procedure involves less time, and the conduit is easier to construct compared with other diversion procedures, which makes it an excellent choice for older clients who are unable to tolerate a lengthy surgery because of other medical conditions. Because the ileal segment is not a reservoir, absorption of electrolytes and the frequency of other complications are minimal.

Contraindications. Clients who cannot maintain follow-up care or treatment because of physical limitations or mental impairment are not candidates for an ileal conduit; clients with chronic bowel disease or colon cancer may not be candidates either. Any medical condition that prevents a major surgical procedure is also a contraindication.

Complications. Several complications related to stoma management (e.g., skin irritation, stomal defects, and stomal pouching problems) may arise. Leakage at

FIGURE 36-2 Ileal conduit. A segment of the terminal ileum is used to create an artificial bladder to which the ureters are attached. Urine continually drains from the ileal conduit through a stoma and into an ostomy pouch.

the anastomosis site, stenosis, peristomal hernia, ulceration, and obstruction at the ureteroileal anastomosis may develop. Finally, clients who have undergone an ileal conduit procedure are at increased risk for pyelonephritis, hydronephrosis (distention of renal pelvis and calices with urine), and formation of calculi.

Outcomes. Eight weeks after surgery, it is expected that the client will adjust to the stoma and appliance, maintain stoma and appliance care, have a urine output of 0.5 ml/kg/hr, and return to most previously enjoyed activities.

Indiana Pouch. Other diversionary procedures are the Indiana pouch, Florida pouch, Kock pouch, and continent internal ileal reservoir. A reservoir is created from the ascending colon and terminal ileum. The Indiana pouch is an improved and larger version of the original Kock pouch (Figure 36-3). Other continent reservoir operations vary slightly regarding surgical technique and the portion of the colon and ileum used.

Once the reservoir has been created, the ureters are implanted into the side of the diversion. A special nipple valve is then constructed and used to attach the reservoir to the skin. Several weeks after surgery, the client is taught to use a catheter to drain the reservoir at 3- to 4-hour intervals. Internal storage of up to 800 ml of urine is possible, with a daytime continence rate of up to 96% and a nighttime continence rate of up to 86%.

Indications. Because this procedure involves no appliance for collecting urine, it is used for clients with a life expectancy of more than 2 years. Creation of the reservoir and nipple valve requires 1 to 3 more hours more surgical time compared with the time needed to construct an ileal conduit. The client's serum creatinine level should be 2.5 mg/dl or less. The client will need gross and fine motor coordination to catheterize the nipple valve and must be willing and able to participate in

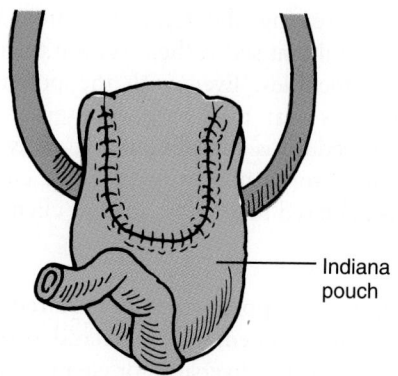

FIGURE 36-3 Indiana pouch procedure.

self-care. Electrolyte reabsorption is minimal with this diversion technique as long as the urine is drained regularly.

Contraindications. Clients with a history of significant bowel resection and malabsorption related to diarrhea, irritable bowel syndrome, ulcerative colitis, diverticular disease, bowel cancer, Crohn's disease, progressive neurologic disorders, morbid obesity, kidney disease (creatinine >2.5 mg/dl) and pelvic radiation are not candidates for an Indiana pouch.

Complications. Possible complications include incontinence, difficult catheterization, urinary reflux, anastomotic leaks, pyelonephritis, obstruction, bacteriuria, calculi, erectile dysfunction, electrolyte imbalances, and rupture of the reservoir.

Outcomes. About 8 to 10 weeks after surgery, the client will have urinary continence, will remain free of UTI, and will return to activities pursued before surgery. Self-catheterization should begin 3 weeks postoperatively.

Neobladder. Sometimes the urethra can be spared, allowing the creation of a *neobladder,* also known as an ileal W-bladder. This operation is the treatment of choice for a client with bladder cancer that has invaded the bladder muscle. Although this procedure differs from one in which the reservoir empties through an abdominal stoma, a neobladder empties via a pelvic outlet to the urethra. Maintaining continence can be a problem unless the lower portion of the bladder can be spared.

Some surgeons believe that the urethra should be removed because of the risk of tumor recurrence. If the urethra is resected, a reconstructed neourethra together with an artificial sphincter is created. This procedure is more successful in males because of the longer urethra.

Several weeks after surgery, the catheter is removed and the client empties the neobladder by relaxing the external sphincter and creating abdominal pressure. The client must learn intermittent self-catheterization to cope with any voiding difficulties. Even with the potential postoperative problems that may be encountered, acceptance of this procedure is high because it allows a more normal anatomy to be maintained for the client. Total continence is achieved in 84% to 96% of clients at 5 years.

Indications. Because an appliance is not required and normal anatomy is maintained, the neobladder technique is the preferred urinary diversion for clients with a life expectancy of more than 2 years and with no contraindications. Other indications are as described for an Indiana pouch.

Contraindications. In addition to the contraindications listed for an Indiana pouch, clients with bladder tumors in the trigone region of the bladder, diffuse carcinoma in situ, multifocal tumors, or bladder cancer involving the prostate are not candidates for this procedure.

Complications. Possible complications include pouch rupture from hypercontinence, inability to empty the bladder completely, incontinence, electrolyte imbalances, erectile dysfunction, and calculi. With resection of the ileum, possible metabolic changes include (1) malabsorption of bile salts; vitamin B_{12}; fat; fat-soluble vitamins A, D, E, and K and (2) increased risk of biliary and kidney stones and steatorrhea.

Outcomes. The client will go home 4 to 8 days after surgery with a catheter in place. The catheter will be removed about 4 weeks after surgery, and the client will be taught to "strain to void" (see later discussion on strain voiding or "Valsalva voiding" and self-catheterization). After 2 to 3 months, the client is expected to have urinary continence, to be able to empty the bladder completely, and to return to previously pursued activities.

Palliative Procedures

Percutaneous Nephrostomy or Pyelostomy. For the client with inoperable bladder cancer, a percutaneous nephrostomy or pyelostomy may be performed to prevent obstruction. A catheter is inserted into the renal pelvis by surgical incision or, more likely, a percutaneous puncture procedure. In the surgical approach, a balloon-tipped or mushroom-tipped catheter is connected to an external drainage system.

In the percutaneous nephrostomy procedure, a trocar is inserted under fluoroscopy by direct puncture into the renal pelvis or calyx. A flexible small-gauge needle is then used to instill contrast material to verify proper location. Using angiographic wire as a guide, the surgeon places the nephrostomy tube and connects it to a closed drainage system. The entire procedure is done with the client under local anesthesia. It is important to stabilize the tube to prevent dislodgment.

Ureterostomy. A ureterostomy may be performed as a palliative procedure if the ureters are obstructed by a tumor. During a cutaneous ureterostomy, the surgeon attaches the ureter to the surface of the abdomen where urine flows directly into a drainage appliance without an intermediary conduit. For clients with ureterostomies, infection, obstruction to urine flow secondary to strictures at the opening, and skin irritation are potential problems. This procedure includes several variations.

■ Nursing Management of the Preoperative Client Assessment

Preoperative nursing management of the client with bladder cancer is directed at educating the client and family. Assess the client and family's understanding of pending diagnostic testing, bladder cancer, and proposed surgical procedure. Evaluate the client's anxiety level by providing opportunities to talk about feelings and to ask questions about the upcoming surgery, potential for distorted body image, and support systems outside the hospital.

In addition to educating and counseling the client, obtain physical assessment findings. Check for (1) costovertebral tenderness and masses in the upper abdomen and flank, (2) distention before and after urination, (3) vaginal or rectal masses, and (4) manifestations of discharge in urethral meatus and perianal areas. Assessment of other body systems includes (1) monitoring vital signs, (2) measuring intake and output, (3) examining skin for color, bruises, petechiae, and hydration, and (4) auscultating heart and lung sounds.

Complete a self-care or functional assessment to determine whether the client can manage drains and indwelling catheters and is able to catheterize a continent stoma or urethra. Finally, determine whether a family member can provide care or whether home health care is available to the client.

Diagnosis, Outcomes, Interventions

Diagnosis: Deficient Knowledge. The most common nursing diagnosis preoperatively is *Deficient Knowledge related to bladder cancer and diagnostic testing, possible bowel preparation prior to surgical intervention, and surgical intervention with associated expected course of treatment.*

Outcomes. Preoperative education will bring about an increased awareness of the procedure and lowered anxiety preoperatively and postoperatively. The client will understand diagnostic tests, bowel preparation, surgical intervention, and the anticipated postoperative course, as evidenced by statements and demonstrations of self-care.

Interventions

Provide Preoperative Teaching. Assess the client's educational deficits surrounding bladder cancer, proposed treatment, and expected outcomes by encouraging discussion. Include the family in the discussion to review diagnostic evaluation, preoperative treatment, and postoperative expectations. Explain the purpose of various tubes, such as IV lines, the nasogastric (NG) tube, stents, drains, and catheters that will be present after surgery and when they will be discontinued. As needed, discuss support services available after discharge.

Discuss Bowel Preparation. If a diversion or pouch procedure has been chosen as the appropriate surgical intervention, discuss the preoperative bowel preparation ("bowel prep"). Because a segment of bowel will be used to create the conduit or reservoir, this measure relates to the segment of intestine to be used in the procedure.

Bowel preparation calls for a clear liquid diet for 1 to 3 days, laxatives and enemas to clear the bowel, and antibiotics to lower the bacterial count in the bowel. Because this step takes several days and includes enemas, dietary restrictions, and medications, it is extremely important to teach the client and family to strictly adhere to the directions.

Provide Enterostomal Nurse Visitation. If the client will have a pouch or diversion procedure, a visit from an enterostomal nurse may be reassuring for the client and family. This visit allows the client and family to interact and learn the expected postoperative course with a nurse with expertise in this field.

Before surgery, the enterostomal nurse selects and marks the best site for ostomy placement if the surgeon plans to construct a stoma. The main criterion for stomal placement is finding a site that allows the faceplate of the drainage appliance to bind securely to the surface of the abdomen.

The stoma must be clearly visible to the client. This means that the surgeon should avoid the umbilicus, rib margins, pubis, iliac crests, and pre-existing scars, wrinkles, or crevices. Placing the stoma directly on the client's waistline can cause excessive pressure from clothing.

The client is observed in the supine, standing, and sitting positions during the selection process. Stoma placement is usually on the right lower quadrant of the abdomen, in the abdominal rectus muscle, about 2 inches below the waist and 2 inches from the midline. Explain the proper way to care for the urinary diversion.

Diagnosis: Risk for Disturbed Body Image. The client is at *Risk for Disturbed Body Image related to surgery, possible stoma formation, possible sexual dysfunction, and potential change in urinary elimination.*

Outcomes. The client will not experience body image disturbance postoperatively, as evidenced by the ability to discuss concerns regarding altered body image, stoma placement, change in urination pattern, risk of sexual dysfunction, and verbalization of fears.

Interventions. Identify factors that reveal the client's difficulty in coping with anticipated changes in body image. If a diversion procedure is necessary, in addition to a preoperative visit from an enterostomal nurse, you may want to suggest a visit from a client with a similar diagnosis and procedure. These visits provide the client with a comfortable opportunity to ask questions, to experi-

ence a sense of comfort and support, and to receive information.

Preoperative teaching should include explanations of the expected anatomic and physiologic alterations and possible effects for the client. Because of the lifestyle changes that are required by diversion or pouch surgery, be sure to offer support and refer the client for additional counseling if indicated. Community associations, such as the United Ostomy Association and the American Cancer Society, provide tremendous help for clients undergoing urinary diversion.

Radical bladder surgery may cause a disturbance in sexual function. Because of the private and personal nature of this surgery, you should use this opportunity to discuss the risk for sexual dysfunction following radical surgery for bladder cancer. Although nerve-sparing procedures and vaginal reconstruction procedures can reduce sexual dysfunction, clients should be prepared to take advantage of available resources in case impotence or difficulty with intercourse develops after surgery.

Evaluation

It is expected that the client will be prepared for and will undergo the selected surgery successfully. The client should restate information about bladder cancer, diagnostic testing, bowel preparation, and surgical intervention. In addition, the client should voice concerns about body image disturbance and sexual dysfunction after surgery. The client should be aware of outside resources available following discharge.

■ Nursing Management of the Postoperative Client
Assessment

Routine postoperative evaluation and care involve the usual assessments for a client after major abdominal surgery. The stoma, if present, should be inspected hourly for 24 hours after surgery, then every 4 hours for 24 hours, then every 8 hours. The stoma should be red and moist at all times and is edematous just after surgery. The edema diminishes by 200% to 500% within a few weeks. Peristomal sutures may be seen adhering to the skin and mucosal bowel edge. Any sign that the stoma is becoming pale, dark, dusky, gray, or cyanotic may mean loss of vascular supply; this event must be corrected immediately to avoid necrosis.

Peristalsis in the intestinal tract is absent for several days because of the manipulation and resection of the bowel. The client continues to receive nothing by mouth (i.e., remains on NPO status) with IV lines and a nasogastric tube in place until peristalsis returns. Assessment of bowel sounds and nasogastric contents is required.

Urine flow never stops after surgery. Ureteral stents originating in the renal pelvis extend through the ureters and through the reservoir, conduit, or neobladder. The stents that exit through a stoma are contained in the pouch. With continent reservoirs, a catheter is placed through the nipple valve to drain the internal reservoir for 2 to 3 weeks until healing occurs. For a neobladder, a suprapubic catheter may be placed through the abdominal wall into the reservoir to keep it drained while another catheter is placed through the urethra and is used as a stent. This protects the anastomosis of the urethra and neobladder.

In some instances, ureteral stents or catheters may drain urine after neobladder or continent reservoir surgery. The stents and catheter are removed once adequate healing has occurred, usually in 3 to 4 weeks. The catheter is usually the last tube to be discontinued. Constantly monitor the tubes for patency and continuous drainage, usually in separate closed gravity systems. For the first 24 to 48 hours, hourly intake and output records may be required. Clients should be kept from manipulating tubes immediately after surgery.

Hematuria

Assess for hematuria, stenosis, and other complications after surgery. Hematuria, a common problem after transurethral resection, is controlled with a three-way indwelling catheter and, if necessary, bladder irrigation. The greatest potential problems after any diversion or pouch procedure are infection, wound dehiscence, skin irritation, ulceration, and stomal defects. Later complications are renal deterioration caused by reflux, stenosis of the stoma, strictures at the site of the anastomosis, hydronephrosis, calculi, and peristomal hernia.

Stenosis

Stenosis of the stoma may occur from scarring during stomal maturation. If the opening on the faceplate is too large, epithelial hyperplasia or thickening of the peristomal skin may contract the stoma. Clients with urinary diversion are also susceptible to uric acid and calcium stone disease. The onset of urinary stone development usually occurs at least 2 years postoperatively and sometimes as long as 5 to 10 years later. UTI is a perpetual threat because of the exposure of the urinary tract. Obstruction anywhere in the urinary tract may interfere with normal urine flow.

Other Complications

The potential complications of continent reservoirs or pouch procedures include incontinence, difficult catheterization, urinary reflux, and possible pyelonephritis, obstruction, bacteriuria, electrolyte imbalances, urolithiasis, or absorptive problems. The reservoir may rupture if the client does not comply with the self-catheterization protocol.

Monitor the client for other complications as well following a radical cystectomy. Cystectomy is a very invasive surgery that puts the client at risk for most of the usual postoperative complications, including shock and hemorrhage. The extensive pelvic dissection associated with this surgery can increase the risk of thrombophlebitis. Additionally, pelvic lymph node dissection can predispose the client to lymphedema in the lower limbs. You may need to assess calf circumference during each shift.

Diagnosis, Outcomes, Interventions

Diagnosis: Risk for Injury: Occlusion of Urinary Drainage.
A potential problem for the postoperative client is *Risk for Injury: Occlusion of urinary drainage device related to hematuria, clot formation, and swelling following the surgical procedure.*

Outcomes. Catheters and other drainage tubes will not become obstructed, and urine will flow freely.

Interventions. After transurethral resection of the bladder, the client usually has hematuria. A three-lumen, indwelling urethral catheter is attached to a continuous or intermittent closed bladder irrigation system to facilitate urine flow, minimize blood clots, and monitor for postoperative bleeding. Nursing care is similar to that after transurethral resection of the prostate (see Chapter 40). Bright red or pink urine fades to clear in about 3 days.

Nursing care after segmental bladder resection centers on maintaining constant urinary drainage to ensure that the remaining bladder does not become distended, putting strain on the suture line. The client usually has both urethral and suprapubic catheters. The client is discharged with the catheters in place, and they remain in place for about 2 weeks or until complete healing has occurred.

As with any major abdominal surgery, clients who undergo a radical cystectomy and urinary diversion are at an increased risk for hemorrhage. Monitor the client's vital signs, the incision, and the drainage tubes closely for early signs of excessive bleeding. If an ileal conduit is formed, the client has a pouch in place to collect urine from the ileal conduit or ureteral catheters or stents.

After a continent diversion, make sure that the catheter is draining urine freely. If any obstruction occurs, the newly created reservoir can become damaged and internal leakage along the suture line can occur. Monitor the catheter output closely, and perform irrigations at regular intervals as directed. Perform catheter irrigation gently in the immediate postoperative period, using about 60 ml of normal saline solution. Irrigation is necessary to prevent obstruction from clots or mucus.

After neobladder surgery, one or two catheters will be in place to prevent overdistention of the newly created bladder. These catheters are treated as closed drainage systems. Carefully monitor the neobladder for possible obstruction. Regular irrigation is needed to rid the neobladder of mucus.

When ureteral stents or catheters are placed, patency is important to prevent hydronephrosis and pyelonephritis. Because there is no mucus in urine from the kidney, irrigation is usually not required and is kept to a minimum to prevent pyelonephritis and hydronephrosis. Do not irrigate ureteral catheters unless you have a specific order to do so, and then only use 5 to 10 ml of sterile saline solution. Urine output from each ureteral catheter should be 0.25 ml/kg/hr or roughly half of the 0.5 ml/kg/hr normally expected from a urethral catheter. Ureteral catheters may drain into a pouch when a stoma is present (see the Critical Monitoring feature on Postoperative Monitoring After Urinary Diversion Procedures, below).

CRITICAL MONITORING

Postoperative Monitoring After Urinary Diversion Procedures

- Measure urine output every hour for the first 24 hours, and at least every 8 hours thereafter; report any amount less than 0.5 ml/kg/hr (~30 ml/hr) or no output for more than 15 minutes.
- Check the ostomy pouch for leaks and the skin under it for irritation every 4 hours initially, then every 8 hours.
- Inspect the stoma every hour for the first 24 hours after surgery. (This gives a baseline from which you can quickly detect deviations. The stoma should be red and moist.) If you find no problems, extend intervals to every 4 hours, then to every 8 hours.
- Note the size, shape, and color of the stoma. Expect it to be edematous in the immediate postoperative period. However, other changes may indicate complications, warranting action from the physician. A dusky or cyanotic stoma color may denote an insufficient blood supply and the onset of necrosis. This is an emergency. The reduced blood supply may result from surgical technique, from an appliance faceplate that is too small or improperly centered, or from peristomal protective materials that have been poorly applied. Other complications with the stoma include prolapse (protrusion from the skin) or retraction into the abdomen beneath the skin.
- Watch for manifestations of peritonitis, such as fever and abdominal pain and rigidity. Leakage at the site of the anastomosis or ureteral separation from the conduit may allow urine to seep into the peritoneal cavity, leading to peritonitis.
- Observe for bleeding. Although bleeding from the stoma may indicate a surgical defect, it is also common for the intestinal mucosa, which is fragile, to bleed during a change of appliance or because of a poorly fitted collection pouch.

If the client has a stoma, a temporary, clear urostomy pouch over the stoma is connected to a gravity drainage system. Sometimes ureteral catheters are used to splint the ureters while they heal. These catheters, usually removed before the client is discharged from the hospital, may extend through the stoma.

Label all catheters, stents, and drainage tubes to prevent errors in irrigation and output calculations. Secure all tubes. Use a separate closed gravity drainage system for each tube unless, as with an ileal conduit, ureteral catheters exit into the pouching system until they are discontinued. A separate system for each tube minimizes the risk and extent of bacterial infection.

Diagnosis: Effective Therapeutic Regimen Management.
Clients undergoing any type of urinary diversion need to learn new self-care strategies. The nursing diagnosis of *Effective Therapeutic Regimen Management related to complexity of therapeutic regimen* is applicable for this client.

Outcomes. The client will effectively manage the urinary diversion or neobladder, as evidenced by the ability to describe the regimen and to perform the required care successfully.

Interventions
Ileal Conduit. For a client with an ileal conduit, teach stoma care and skin care, promote self-care of the collection device, prevent odor, promote independence, and encourage follow-up.

Teach Stoma Care. The client needs to learn to care for the stoma and skin with proper application of a urinary pouch (see the Bridge to Home Health Care feature on Managing an Ileal Conduit, below). An opening must be cut in the skin barrier just large enough to fit over the stoma. The barrier is then applied to the skin before attaching the pouch or faceplate. A skin cement or adhesive disk may help the faceplate stick more securely to the skin. A non–water-soluble adhesive spray allows the

BRIDGE TO HOME HEALTH CARE
Managing an Ileal Conduit

When clients first come home from the hospital, they need your help to get organized and feel in control. Use a small plastic basket, such as one purchased at a discount store, to store small supplies, such as adhesive tape, stoma adhesive, a pen, and a small scissors. A wash basin, a small box, or a small organizer on wheels works well for the larger items, such as faceplate or wafers, skin barriers, pouches, and paper towels.

Typically, clients are taught about stoma care before discharge, but they may have been so overwhelmed that they did not hear or remember instructions. Once home, they may have many questions. While you change the appliance, have your clients lie down with a mirror positioned so they can become accustomed to seeing the stoma and can learn to care for the stoma without experiencing side effects such as faintness or dizziness. Eventually, the client should face the toilet while sitting comfortably on a stool or chair.

Before removing the original wafer, cut the new faceplate or wafer to size, snap it on the pouch, and make certain that everything is ready. Some clients may need a circular insert in the wafer to form a convex angle that makes a tighter seal around the small stoma. Once you take off the old appliance, cover the stoma; peristalsis causes urine to squirt out spontaneously.

Do not make your client laugh; pressure will cause urine to leak out. It is frustrating to repeatedly reclean the area. Use thick, absorbent paper towels to cover the stoma; they are also inexpensive and readily available.

Before cleaning the skin surface, make sure that the stoma is open and not becoming filled with mucus from the bowel. Use a small amount of lubricating jelly (e.g., K-Y) on your little finger,

and gently enter the stoma. Quickly cover the stoma with a paper towel to absorb urine. To keep the skin healthy, wash around the stoma with soap and water, and prepare the skin with a skin barrier. Cover the stoma, and allow the skin barrier to dry. Once you are ready to secure the appliance, remove the paper towel quickly and apply the wafer.

Place your warm hands on the faceplate or wafer for a few minutes to help it adhere to the skin. You may need to apply an extra piece of adhesive tape in the corner or side to prevent leaking. Assess skinfolds before applying the wafer; consider shifting the wafer to a diamond position to decrease the bend at the fold and the potential for leaking.

Leakage is one of the most distressing aspects of the ileal conduit. Instruct clients to attach an overnight Foley bag to the pouch at bedtime and to be sure that there are no kinks in the tubing. Back-pressure and overflow into the pouch cause the faceplate or wafer to pop off or leak. Until they feel confident, clients may decide to awaken about 2:00 AM to check the pouch. During the day, they need to empty the pouch often because the tension of a full pouch causes leakage. Clients should change the pouch every 3 to 4 days; the faceplate or wafer should be changed once a week to once every 10 days to avoid odor problems and to decrease the risk of a UTI. The pouch is made with a hard plastic ring that snaps onto the faceplate or wafer because frequent changes are necessary.

Clients may call on enterostomal nurses at local hospitals, the United Ostomy Association, and the American Cancer Society for help in adjusting to an ileal conduit.

client to go swimming. Most pouches come as two pieces, a faceplate or wafer and a removable pouch. Not having to remove the faceplate or wafer as frequently makes care much easier for many clients.

Teach Skin Care. Skin irritation or breakdown is a constant threat to a client with a urinary diversion. Advise the client to prevent urine from contacting the skin. This can be achieved in part when a well-fitted and properly attached appliance is used (Figure 36-4). The opening in the adhesive backing of the faceplate or wafer should be cut no more than 3 mm larger than the stoma. This opening should be remeasured after the edema in the stoma recedes.

Each time the faceplate or wafer is changed, the skin around the stoma should be cleaned with a mild, non-residue soap and water, and thoroughly dried. A gauze pad, absorbent paper towel, or tampon should be held

A

C

B

D

FIGURE 36-4 Applying a disposable ostomy pouch. **A,** Gently remove the old pouch, using warm water or an adhesive solvent around the seal if necessary. Place the gauze pad over the stoma to prevent leakage as you gently clean peristomal area with moist gauze. **B,** Measure the stoma with the stoma template. Trace the shape onto the skin barrier and adhesive, using the template. Cut openings no more than 3 mm larger than the stoma. **C,** Remove backing from the adhesive surface of the disposable ostomy pouch. **D,** Center a pouch opening over the stoma with the pouch drain pointing to floor or, if the client is bedridden, with the drain to the side. (If the client ambulates frequently, the pouch drain should point to the client's feet.) Make sure that the seal is complete.

over the stoma during cleaning to prevent urine from flowing out over the skin. Remove this pad or tampon just as the appliance is reapplied. The appliance should be changed early in the morning because urine production is slowest at this time.

Promote Self-Care of the Collection Device. Urine pouches have a valve in the bottom for intermittent urine drainage. Alternatively, the pouch may be drained by gravity into a leg or bedside bag, especially at night. The self-contained pouch drainage system allows the client to resume most, or all, former activities with little or no change in style of dress.

However, instruct clients to empty the pouch when it is one-third to one-half full. The weight of accumulating urine may pull the faceplate away from the skin and cause leakage. Advise clients to check the seal often if they are perspiring heavily.

Prevent Odor. Urine odor is a common problem with urinary stomas. Noxious odors result mostly from poor hygiene, alkaline urine, normal breakdown of urine (ammonia), concentrated urine from insufficient fluid intake, and the ingestion of certain foods, such as asparagus.

Because diluted urine has less odor, adequate fluid intake is helpful. Reusable appliances can be washed with soap and lukewarm water. The pouch can also be soaked in diluted white vinegar or in a commercial deodorant product for 20 to 30 minutes. Rinse the pouch, and allow it to dry. Deodorant tablets are available for placement in the pouch while it is being worn.

Promote Independence. Long-term nursing intervention aims to maintain a functional urinary system and prevent complications. It takes time for clients and significant others to adjust to a urinary diversion. Even though counseling may have been excellent during the preoperative period, the reality of the diversion commonly produces anxiety, depression, and anger. The client may need help at first to look at or even talk about the stoma. As soon as possible after surgery, the client must begin to help care for the stoma, peristomal skin, and drainage system, gradually assuming more responsibility until achieving independence (see the Client Education Guide feature on Learning to Care for a Urinary Diversion on the website).

Encourage Follow-Up. A client with bladder cancer must receive follow-up at regular intervals to assess for a recurrence of the cancer. The client should also continue to be seen by an enterostomal therapy nurse to check for problems with the ostomy.

Continent Diversion. Postoperative care for the client with an Indiana pouch is similar to that for any client with a urinary diversion, except there is no external pouch. The client has a 24F to 26F or Medina catheter in place to drain urine continuously until the pouch heals. The reservoir is irrigated through the catheter with about 50 to 60 ml of normal saline every 4 hours to wash out clots or mucus, which may cause obstruction.

Teach Reservoir Catheterization. After a radiographic study, remove the catheter at 3 to 4 weeks after surgery to make sure that the continent reservoir is functioning properly. The client must learn to empty and irrigate the reservoir at regular intervals. The principles of catheterization of a urinary reservoir are the same as for clean, intermittent urinary self-catheterization.

Using a 16 to 20F catheter with a generous amount of water-soluble lubricant, show the client how to insert the catheter into the nipple valve. Warn against forcing the catheter into the reservoir. If resistance occurs, tell the client to pause and apply only gentle pressure while slightly rotating the catheter. If this does not work, the client should call the physician. Advise the client to insert the catheter every 2 to 3 hours to drain the reservoir. Each week thereafter, the interval is increased by 1 hour, until finally catheterization is completed every 4 to 6 hours during the day.

Teach Reservoir Irrigation. Once the urine has stopped flowing, the client should take several deep breaths and move the catheter in and out 2 to 3 inches to be sure that the pouch is fully emptied. The catheter should be withdrawn slowly so additional urine can drain.

After urine has been drained from the reservoir, tell the client to leave the catheter in place and to use 50 to 60 ml of normal saline solution to irrigate the reservoir and to prevent excess mucus buildup, which may cause obstruction. The fluid can be either gently aspirated or allowed to drain from the catheter. Once the irrigant is drained, the catheter is removed and the end of the catheter is pinched before removal to prevent dripping. The irrigations may be repeated until the drainage returns free of mucus. If the mucus is viscous (thick), increasing fluid intake and drinking cranberry juice can decrease the viscosity. Usually, mucus production lessens over time.

Because the catheterization procedure can be unpredictable, advise clients to carry catheterization supplies with them. Most clients develop a sensation of abdominal pressure when catheterization is needed. Regular fluid intake and adherence to the catheterization schedule are important. A full reservoir puts pressure on the nipple valve, making catheterization much more difficult. Clients should be taught to practice these skills before discharge. They may need follow-up with a visiting nurse for additional help.

Teach Strain Voiding and Intermittent Self-Catheterization. With a neobladder, the client must learn how to *strain void,* relaxing the external sphincter and increasing ab-

dominal pressure to start the urine stream. Show the client how to perform clean self-catheterization in case the bladder cannot be emptied by regular voiding.

Encourage Follow-Up. Following urinary diversion, the client should be monitored at 3, 6, 9, and 12 months. The assessment includes electrolyte values, serum creatinine and blood urea nitrogen (BUN) values, renal function studies, vitamin B_{12} levels, and urine cultures. Renal damage may occur in noncompliant clients who neglect to empty the pouch and who then develop infection. These clients often experience severe kidney infections and damage, and an ileal conduit must be created to replace the neobladder or Indiana pouch so that urine will drain freely.

Diagnosis: Risk for Impaired Skin Integrity. If the client has an ileal conduit, the nursing diagnosis of *Risk for Impaired Skin Integrity related to irritation of peristomal skin* is a potential problem.

Outcomes. The client will not demonstrate altered skin integrity or irritation of peristomal skin, as evidenced by intact, clear skin.

Interventions. Begin interventions for any skin irritation promptly. Check the pH of a urine specimen because strongly alkaline urine irritates the skin and facilitates crystal formation. Encourage the client to drink cranberry juice to help acidify the urine. Any positive urine culture result necessitates treatment. Check appliances carefully to identify leakage and detect skin sensitivity.

Skin irritation may result from changing the pouch too frequently. A general recommendation is to leave the pouch in place as long as it is not leaking. During appliance changes, leave the skin open to the air as much as possible. Apply a pouch with a non-karaya (sterculia gum) skin barrier. Karaya cannot be used with urinary pouches because urine erodes karaya.

Skin irritation around the stoma commonly results from a yeast infection. Nystatin creams or powders are effective against topical yeast. Nystatin powder is applied directly over the irritated skin area and sealed to the skin with a liquid skin barrier.

Diagnosis: Risk for Sexual Dysfunction. Extensive surgical dissection may alter the reproductive anatomy, creating a *Risk for Sexual Dysfunction related to potential postoperative impotence in men or painful intercourse in women following a radical cystectomy and changes in body image affecting sexuality.*

Outcomes. The client will accept and adopt alternative methods of sexual expression and will obtain additional information about sexuality through questions and statements.

Interventions. Male clients have a risk of impotence after a radical cystectomy related to the resection. Offer counseling both before and after the surgery to help the client adjust to any alterations (see Chapter 40 for information about alterations in male sexuality). Sildenafil (Viagra), 50 to 100 mg three times weekly, is offered to most male clients immediately after the catheter is removed to maintain blood flow to the corpora cavernosa, so that when sexual intercourse can be resumed the client will have fewer problems with impotence. Other medications and devices are available to increase blood flow in the penis.

For women who have had a total abdominal hysterectomy, bilateral salpingo-oophorectomy, and anterior vaginal resection, the result can be shortening and tightening of the vagina, leading to painful intercourse. Alternative positions, lubricants, topical estrogen, and vaginal dilators may decrease the discomfort. Booklets discussing both female and male sexual dysfunction are available from the American Cancer Society.

For partners of any client, encourage holding, touching, kissing, and other activities to promote intimacy. Partners are often afraid to touch the client for fear of inflicting hurt; embarrassment may also be an issue. Encourage open discussions.

Evaluation

Carcinoma in situ is considered curable with a simple transurethral resection. Intravesical chemotherapy or BCG may be combined to decrease the risk of recurrence. If the postoperative care of the client has been successful, the client will be able to make the transition to self-care with minimal difficulty. Even with a radical cystectomy, however, the 5-year survival rate for clients with muscle invasive tumor (stage C or greater) is only 40% to 50%.

■ Self-Care

Motivation to promote preoperative self-care may influence the postoperative course. Direct the client toward self-care by improving knowledge, encouraging independence, and fostering participation in care and treatment. When the client increases self-care, the need for nursing care decreases and health promotion activities increase.

The client may need referrals to durable medical equipment companies for ostomy supplies or catheters for reservoir irrigation or intermittent self-catheterization. These items can be delivered to the client's home. If the client lives alone, it may be necessary to arrange home delivery of groceries and medications.

Housekeeping and lifting are limited for the first 6 to 8 weeks after surgery. Evaluate the client's ability to engage in self-care, and identify the need for additional care from home health nurses. If the client cannot pro-

vide care and if a family member is involved with care, respite services may be required. Also consider directing the client and family to local support groups.

■ Modifications for Older Clients

The major modification for older clients with urinary diversion stems from difficulties with self-care. Changing an appliance is one area of difficulty because some dexterity is required. Older clients commonly have arthritis and other disabilities, including decreased visual acuity, that may limit their ability to manipulate catheters and pouches. These concerns must be closely assessed and appropriate assistance offered.

URETERAL TUMORS

Primary tumors of the ureter are rare. In men, ureteral cancer occurs mainly during one's 50s and 60s. This form of cancer rarely affects women. Ureteral neoplasms usually extend from renal or bladder neoplasms or from tumors originating in the bowel, uterus, or ovary. Those primary neoplasms usually occur first as a papillary, transitional cell, or squamous cell carcinoma. These tumors are most frequently found in the lower third of the ureter. In later stages of ureteral cancer, the tumor extends outside the ureter to adjacent structures and regional lymph nodes or to distant sites. Common sites for metastasis include the lungs and liver.

Usually, the first manifestation of ureteral malignancy is gross hematuria. The tumor normally develops painlessly until obstruction occurs. At this point, the client may experience flank pain. Diagnosis is made through urine cytology, IVP, cystoscopy, ultrasonography, and CT scanning.

Treatment of ureteral cancer almost exclusively involves surgical excision and resection. Radiation may also be used in advanced cases with local extension. When the lesion is located in the middle or proximal third of the ureter, the surgical procedure usually involves nephroureterectomy, removal of the kidney, ureter, and attached segment of the bladder on the affected side. If the tumor is in the distal third of the ureter and noninvasive, a more conservative procedure may be used; in this case, just the distal portion of the ureter is resected with ureteral reimplantation.

Silicone rubber (Silastic), polytetrafluoroethylene (Teflon), polytetrafluorourethane, and bovine carotid heterograft are used to replace the resected ureter, facilitating reimplantation in the bladder. A ureter-ureter anastomosis also may be performed. Preoperative and postoperative intervention is similar to that for clients undergoing nephrectomy, ureteral reimplantation, or segmental resection of the bladder.

If the decision is made not to perform any of these procedures, some palliative measure may be needed to prevent or alleviate ureteral obstruction. Urinary diversion may be performed, as described previously, or a ureteral stent catheter may be placed into the ureter during cystoscopy to maintain its patency. The older catheter, a flanged, winged stent (Gibbon's stent), or the newer double J stent prevents migration up the ureter or dislodgment by ureteral peristaltic waves or gravity.

URINARY CALCULI

Urinary calculi *(urolithiasis)* are calcifications in the urinary system. Commonly called stones, calculi form primarily in the kidney *(nephrolithiasis)*, but they can form in or migrate to the lower urinary system. They are typically asymptomatic until they pass into the lower urinary tract. Stones are usually managed by a urologist. Primary bladder calculi are rare and usually develop from a history of urinary stasis from obstruction or chronic infection.

Up to 4% of the population in the United States have urolithiasis. About 12% of the male population have a renal stone by age 70 years. More than 200,000 Americans require hospitalization for treatment of stones each year. Many more people pass stones spontaneously with only minor manifestations that require no treatment, whereas others are treated in an ambulatory setting. The recurrence rate for calcium oxalate stones is about 50% within 5 years.[36,37]

Etiology and Risk Factors

The two primary causative factors are (1) urinary stasis and (2) supersaturation of urine with poorly soluble crystalloids. Increased solute concentration occurs because of fluid depletion or an increased solute load. This increased concentration leads to the precipitation of crystals, such as calcium, uric acid, and phosphate. Urinary pH influences the solubility of certain crystals, with some crystal types precipitating readily in acid urine and some in alkaline urine. Abnormal pH levels occur in renal tubular acidosis with the administration of carbonic anhydrase inhibitors, in the presence of urea-splitting bacteria, and in severe, chronic diarrhea. Stasis of urine from bladder neck obstruction, continent urinary diversion, and immobilization increases the risk for development of stones because the crystals in unmoving urine precipitate more readily.

Infection, foreign bodies, failure to empty the bladder completely, metabolic disorders, and obstruction in the urinary tract contribute to the formation of calculi as well. The presence of precipitators has been noted in the urine (such as protein matrix and bacteria or inflammatory elements).

Inhibitor substances, such as citrate and magnesium, appear to keep particles from aggregating and forming crystals; a lack of inhibitors increases risk of stone development. Not only does the deficiency of inhibitors predispose the client to calculi, but there may be "anti-inhibitors" in the urine, such as aluminum, iron, and silicone. Certain medications may induce calculus forma-

tion, such as acetazolamide, absorbable alkalis (e.g., calcium carbonate and sodium bicarbonate), and aluminum hydroxide. Massive doses of vitamin C increase urinary oxalate levels.

There is an increased risk of calculus formation in the southeast part of the United States—an area known as "the stone belt." Men between ages 30 and 50 years have three times the risk of calculi.[44] Stones are also more common among people of European or Asian descent. Once a client has had calculi, there is an increased risk of additional ones.

Urolithiasis results not from any single factor but from multiple phenomena. One unanswered question is "Why do some clients form calculi when others do not?" This problem is particularly important with recurrent "stone formers."

Risk factors for stone formation include anything that either causes stasis or supersaturation of the urine:

- Immobility and a sedentary lifestyle, which increase stasis
- Dehydration, which leads to supersaturation
- Metabolic disturbances that result in an increase in calcium or other ions in the urine
- Previous history of urinary calculi
- Living in stone-belt areas
- High mineral content in drinking water
- A diet high in purines, oxalates, calcium supplements, animal proteins
- UTIs
- Prolonged indwelling catheterization
- Neurogenic bladder
- History of female genital mutilation

Health promotion and health maintenance activities are discussed under Nursing Management of the Medical Client.

Pathophysiology

The exact mechanism of stone formation has not been clearly defined. Some researchers believe that a low dietary calcium intake contributes, whereas others contend that a high calcium intake contributes. Both groups agree on the role of supersaturation, however. Crystallization appears to be the primary factor in calculus development from the following[9]:

- Supersaturation of urine with increased solutes
- Matrix formation caused when mucoproteins bind to the mass of the stone
- Lack of inhibitors caused by increased or absent protectors against stone formation
- A combination of these conditions

In general, crystal growth involves *nucleation,* in which crystals are formed from supersaturated urine. Growth continues by aggregation to form larger particles. One of these particles may travel down the urinary tract until it is trapped at some narrow point where for stone formation occurs.

Inhibitor substances (e.g., citrate, pyrophosphate, and magnesium) have been identified as *chelating agents.* When present in adequate amounts, they act to keep crystals from aggregating and forming stones. When inhibitors are absent, stone formation following crystal aggregation is more likely. Also, a fibrous matrix of urinary organic material (mostly mucoproteins) may form in the kidney or bladder, producing a substance into which crystallites are deposited and trapped. This, then, becomes the nidus of the stone. The excessive production of this mucoprotein may, in part, account for a family history of urolithiasis in clients with calculi.

Types of Calculi

Stones may be of one crystal type or a combination of types.

Calcium. Calcium is the most common substance and is found in up to 90% of stones.[44] Calcium stones are usually composed of calcium phosphate or calcium oxalate. They may range from very small particles, often called "sand" or "gravel," to giant staghorn calculi, which may fill the entire renal pelvis and extend up into the calyces (Figure 36-5). The peak onset is during a person's 20s, and these stones affect primarily males.

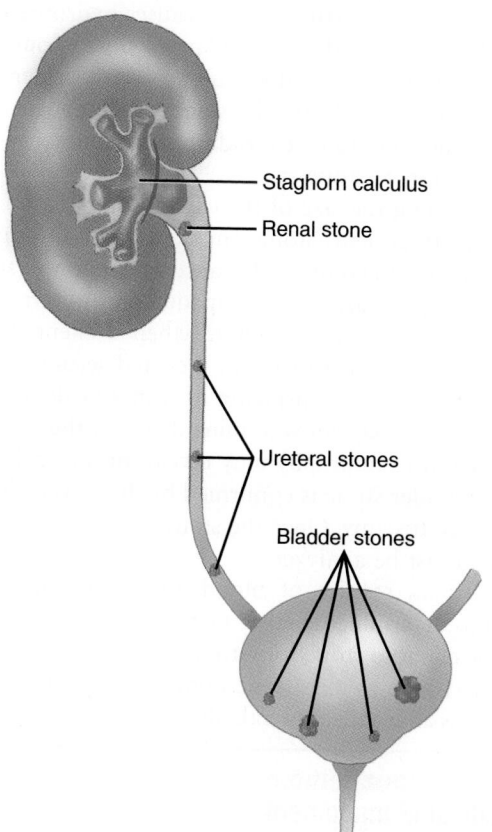

Hypercalciuria (an increased solute load of calcium in the urine), is caused by four main components:

- A high rate of bone reabsorption, which liberates calcium, as in Paget's disease, hyperparathyroidism, Cushing's disease, immobility, and osteolysis caused by malignant tumors of the breast, lung, and prostate
- Gut absorption of abnormally large amounts of calcium, as in milk-alkali syndrome, sarcoidosis, and excessive intake of vitamin D
- Impaired renal tubular absorption of filtered calcium, as in renal tubular acidosis
- Structural abnormalities, such as "sponge kidney"

About 35% of all clients with calcium stones do not have high serum levels of calcium and demonstrate no apparent cause of hypercalciuria.

There are two variants of hypercalciuria:

- The primary abnormality is increased intestinal absorption of calcium or increased bone reabsorption. The resulting higher serum calcium level triggers increased renal filtration of calcium and parathyroid hormone (PTH) suppression. This in turn decreases tubular reabsorption, thereby increasing the concentration of calcium in the urine.
- "Renal leak" of calcium, the other abnormality, is caused by a tubular defect. The resulting hypocalcemia stimulates PTH production, which increases intestinal absorption of calcium. This cycle fits into the previous one, causing an increased solute load of calcium. Clients with this problem are often called "calcium wasters."

Oxalate. The second most frequent stone is oxalate, which is relatively insoluble in urine. Its solubility is affected only slightly by changes in urinary pH. The mechanism of oxalate availability is unclear but may be closely related to diet. The disease is most common in areas where cereals are a major dietary component and least common in dairy farming regions.

An increased incidence of oxalate stones may be related to the following:

- Hyperabsorption of oxalate, seen with inflammatory bowel disease and a high intake of soy-based products
- Postileal resection or small bowel bypass surgery
- Overdose of ascorbic acid (vitamin C), which metabolizes to oxalate
- Familial oxaluria (oxalate in the urine)
- Concurrent fat malabsorption, which may cause calcium binding, thus freeing oxalate for absorption

Struvite. Struvite stones, also called triple phosphate, are composed of carbonate apatite and magnesium ammonium phosphate. Their cause is certain bacteria, usually *Proteus,* which contain the enzyme urease. This enzyme splits urea into two ammonia molecules, which

FIGURE 36-5 Staghorn calculus (stone) and other locations of calculi in the urinary tract.

Labels on figure: Staghorn calculus · Renal stone · Ureteral stones · Bladder stones increases the urine pH. Phosphate precipitates in alkaline urine. This action is responsible for the label "ureasplitter" characterizing these organisms.

Stones formed in this manner are staghorn calculi (see Figure 36-5). Abscess formation is common. Struvite stones are difficult to eliminate because the hard stone forms around a nucleus of bacteria, protecting them from antibiotic therapy. Any small fragment left after surgical removal of the stone begins the cycle again.

Uric Acid. Uric acid stones are caused by increased urate excretion, fluid depletion, and a low urinary pH. *Hyperuricuria* is the result of either increased uric acid production or the administration of uricosuric agents. Approximately 25% of people with primary gout and about 50% of persons with secondary gout develop uric acid stones. A high dietary intake of food rich in *purine* (a protein) may predispose clients to uric acid stone formation. Also, treating neoplastic disease with agents that cause rapid cell destruction may increase the urinary uric acid concentration. Moreover, a link between hyperuricuria and calcium stone formation may exist. It is hypothesized that uric acid crystals absorb some of the crystal inhibitors normally found in urine.

Cystine. Cystinuria is the result of a congenital metabolic error inherited as an autosomal recessive disorder. Cystine stones typically appear during childhood and adolescence; development in adults is very rare.

Xanthine. Xanthine stones occur as a result of a rare hereditary condition in which there is a xanthine oxidase deficiency. This crystal precipitates readily in acid urine.

Summary

Despite the type of stone that forms, the potential damage is essentially the same: (1) pain, spasm, or colic from peristalsis movements of the ureter contracting on the stone; (2) obstruction with possible hydronephrosis or hydroureter; (3) tissue trauma with secondary hemorrhage; and (4) infection.

Clinical Manifestations

The most characteristic manifestation of renal or ureteral calculi is a sharp, severe pain of sudden onset caused by movement of the calculus and consequent irritation. Depending on the site of the stone, this pain may be either *renal colic* or *ureteral colic*. Renal colic originates deep in the lumbar region and radiates around the side and down toward the testicle in the male and the bladder in the female. Ureteral colic radiates toward the genitalia and thigh.

When the pain is severe, the client usually has nausea, vomiting, pallor, grunting respirations, elevated blood pressure and pulse, diaphoresis, and anxiety. Visceral pain such as renal colic is mediated by the autonomic nervous system via celiac ganglia, which causes nausea, vomiting, decreased intestinal motility, and possibly paralytic ileus. Some people, especially those with bladder stones, experience manifestations of urgency, frequency, hematuria, and chronic cystitis. Pressure against the bladder neck during micturition (voiding) may cause a heavy feeling in the suprapubic region, obstruction in voiding, a decreased bladder capacity, and an intermittent urinary stream. If the stone enters the urethra, urine flow is obstructed. The pain lasts for minutes to days and can be somewhat resistant to opioid intervention.

Pain may be intermittent, which usually means that the stone has moved. Physicians hypothesize that the ureter dilates just proximal to the calculus, which allows urine to pass, relieving the ureteral distention. Then, as the stone moves into a new obstruction site, the pain returns. The pain subsides when the stone reaches the bladder.

Pain caused by renal stones is not always severe and colicky. It may be dull or aching or may be experienced as a heavy feeling. This is particularly true during the early stages of hydronephrosis. Sometimes, there may be no sensation, and the first clue the client has is seeing blood in the urine or hearing a "clink" against the toilet when the stone passes.

Other manifestations of calculi include infection with an elevated temperature and white blood cell (WBC) count and urine obstruction that causes hydroureter, hydronephrosis, or both. A flat plate of the abdomen and an x-ray study of the kidney, ureter, and bladder (commonly called a KUB) are the standard diagnostic tools. These studies should reveal radiopaque stones and aid in the evaluation of stone size.

Determining the size of the calculus is essential in selecting the treatment. Stones smaller than 4 or 5 mm can pass without intervention. Because some stones, such as uric acid stones, are not radiopaque and not visible on x-ray film, it is crucial to note when a client presents with manifestations of calculi. Elevated serum uric acid levels may confirm a suspicion of urinary calculi. In addition, an IVP may show a filling defect at the site of the stone or ultrasonography may reveal the stone. Diagnosis of a bladder stone is confirmed by direct visualization through cystoscopy. Once the stone is retrieved, its components must be analyzed.

Additional studies of blood and urine may be required to determine whether metabolic problems predispose the client to stone formation. Other possible disease processes, such as metastatic bone cancer, must be ruled out as possible causes of calculi.

Outcome Management
■ Medical Management

Conservative or medical management is appropriate if there is no obstruction, if the pain can be managed, if the client can be hydrated with oral fluids, and if the stone is less than 5 mm. Medical management is directed at relieving the acute manifestations while facilitating the passage of small stones. The desired outcomes of medical management are to increase fluids, reduce pain, and minimize calculus formation by implementing diet changes and administering medications. Most clients pass the stone naturally from the ureter and bladder. If the stone does not move, if it causes obstruction, or if x-ray studies suggest that the calculus is too large to pass safely to the urethra, more invasive treatment is necessary. After the acute phase, medical management is directed toward preventing recurrence of stone formation.

Increase Fluids.
The most effective management strategy is to increase fluid intake to facilitate passage of small stones and to prevent the development of new ones. Encourage clients to increase fluids to 3 to 4 L daily, unless contraindicated, to ensure a urine output of 2.5 to 3 L daily. The increased urine volume resulting from this high fluid intake decreases the concentration of solutes and alleviates urinary stasis. Increased fluids may also decrease pain, prevent an increase in stone size, and prevent infection. The kind of fluid the client drinks depends on dietary restrictions, but at least one half of the fluid should be water.

Reduce Pain.
Pain is most severe in the first 24 hours. In addition to pain control with increased fluids, the client usually requires treatment with opioids and antispasmodic agents. Opioids such as morphine sulfate are given intravenously or intramuscularly (IV or IM) to control moderate to severe pain. Nonsteroidal anti-inflammatory drugs (NSAIDs) may also be effective.

Antispasmodic agents, such as oxybutynin chloride (Ditropan), are very effective for relieving and controlling colic pain associated with spasms of the ureter. Clients with repeated stone formation may have a family member drive them to a clinic, ambulatory care center, or emergency department for administration of opioid analgesics and antispasmodic agents so that they can relax, go home, and pass the stone naturally. Other clients may require admission to an acute care setting for administration of these medications. For nausea and vomiting associated with colic, antiemetics may also be necessary.

Prevent Stone Recurrence.
Diet modifications and medications may be required to prevent further calculus formation in clients who return with repeated stones. Increased fluid intake is still the primary prevention measure. Results of a stone analysis are essential before these recommendations are implemented.

Implement Dietary Changes.
Some controversy exists over dietary restrictions because of their uncertain effectiveness and the problems clients experience in following the regimen. In the past, calcium stones and hypercalciuria may be controlled by limiting excessive calcium intake to 800 mg daily. However, more recent research has supported increasing the diet with calcium-rich foods. **EB** See the Evidence-Based Practice in Action feature on Calcium Intake and Its Relationship to Kidney Stone Formation on p. 886.

Clients with oxalate stones should avoid high-oxalate foods, such as tea, tomatoes, instant coffee, cola drinks, beer, rhubarb, green beans, asparagus, spinach, cabbage, celery, chocolate, citrus fruits, apples, grapes, cranberries, peanuts, and peanut butter. Megadoses of vitamin C increase oxalate excretion in the urine and should be avoided. If the stone is composed of uric acid, the client should follow a low-purine diet, which involves limiting such foods as aged cheeses, wine, bony fish, and organ meats. (See the Complementary and Alternative Therapy **EB** feature on Diet to Reduce the Risk of Calcium Oxalate Kidney Stones on p. 886.)

Administer Medications.
Following recurrent stone formation, analysis of the stone, or abnormal metabolic findings, medications may be required. For hypercalciuric clients, a thiazide diuretic such as hydrochlorothiazide (HydroDIURIL) promotes calcium resorption from the renal tubules, thereby preventing excess calcium loads in the urine. Potassium citrate is commonly added to the thiazide diuretic to replace potassium as needed.

For low urine citrate levels, potassium or sodium citrate may be ordered. Because these medications can be expensive, many urologists encourage the client to drink a quart of lemonade for both the increased fluid and citrate benefits.

Calcium oxalate stones may be treated with vitamin B_6 (pyridoxine), magnesium oxide, or cholestyramine. For clients with hyperuricosuria and calcium oxalate stones, allopurinol (Zyloprim) is prescribed only if a reduced purine diet fails and stones persist.

Uric acid stones are treated with drugs to lower uric acid, such as allopurinol. In addition, sodium bicarbonate or citrate may be indicated to raise urinary pH because uric acid stones form in acidic urine. This treatment is also effective for xanthine stones, which are inhibited in alkaline urine. Cystine stones are treated with tiopronin (Thiola) and D-penicillamine, which make cystine more soluble for excretion. Long-term antibiotics are used to control the infection that leads to struvite stone formation.

■ Nursing Management of the Medical Client
Assessment

Ask the client about any family history of calculi, previous UTIs, immobility, and recent dietary habits. For instance, a large intake of purines may be significant, as would be drinking a large amount of fruit juice or tea,

EB EVIDENCE-BASED PRACTICE IN ACTION

Calcium Intake and Its Relationship to Kidney Stone Formation

In the past, clients with a history of calcium-oxalate kidney stones have been advised to decrease their intake of calcium rich foods to 800 mg/day to reduce the recurrence of kidney stones. However, more recent literature contradicts these previous dietary instructions. New theories propose that calcium stone formation in the kidney may be linked to a diet high in protein. A high protein diet increases urinary calcium, oxalate, and uric acid secretion and increases the probability of stone formation in normal subjects.

Study findings by Curhan and colleagues questioned previous research findings and treatment of kidney stones.[2] Their results suggest that a higher intake of dietary calcium was strongly associated with a decreased risk of calcium-based renal stones.[2] Curhan et al. reported the incidence of kidney stones was lower by 50% in men with the highest calcium of up to 1326 mg/day compared with the incidence in those who took lower amounts of calcium of 516 mg/day.[2] The men who ingested up to two glasses of milk per day had half the risk of stone formation as those who drank less than one glass per month. Another study reported a similar diet of high-calcium, low protein, and low-sodium does reduces the risk of reoccurrence of kidney stones.[1]

In women, it has been reported that increased dietary intake of calcium was not associated with risk of kidney stone formation. However, the intake of supplemental calcium was related to an increased risk of kidney stones. Additionally, an increased intake of sucrose and sodium increased the risk of stone formation, whereas increased fluids or potassium decreased the incidence.[3]

Implications

Nurses should encourage clients who have had at least one calcium-oxalate kidney stone to increase fluids and dietary calcium intake and reduce protein and sodium intake. Intake of dietary calcium should be encouraged in all clients to prevent osteoporosis and to prevent calcium-oxalate kidney stones. Other dietary adjustments to lower oxalate intake may also be recommended.

References

1. Borghi, L., et al. (2002). Comparison of two diets for the prevention of recurrent stones in idiopathic hypercalciuria. *New England Journal of Medicine, 346,* 77-84.
2. Curhan, G.C., et al. (1993). Prospective study of dietary calcium and other nutrients and the risk of symptomatic kidney stones. *New England Journal of Medicine, 328,* 833-838.
3. Curhan, G.C., et al. (1997). Comparison of dietary calcium with supplemental calcium and other nutrients as factors affecting the risk of kidney stones in women. *Annals of Internal Medicine, 126,* 497-504.

COMPLEMENTARY AND ALTERNATIVE THERAPY

Diet to Reduce the Risk of Calcium Oxalate Kidney Stones

A large-scale, 5-year, randomized trial was recently conducted in Parma, Italy. This trial included a total of 120 men (mean age 45 years) who were diagnosed with idiopathic hypercalciuria (urinary calcium excretion >300 mg/day), on an unrestricted diet, experiencing recurrent formation of calcium oxalate stones, and undergoing no current treatment. A total of 103 men (86%) completed the trial (13 withdrew, 2 were lost to follow-up, and 2 died). A total of 60 men were placed on a normal-calcium (30 mmol/day), low–animal protein (52 g/day), low-salt (50 mmol/day) intervention diet. Another group of 60 men were placed on the low-calcium diet and were instructed to avoid milk, yogurt, and cheese so that calcium ingestion would be reduced to 10 mmol/day. Both groups were recommended to avoid large quantities of oxalate-rich foods (e.g., walnuts, spinach, chocolate) and to drink 2 to 3 L of water/day.

The primary outcome of the study was the first recurrence of a symptomatic renal stone or the presence of a radiographically identified stone. Kaplan-Meier analysis demonstrated that over 5 years, men that received the intervention diet (normal calcium, low protein, low salt) reduced their risk of a recurrent stone by 50% versus the control group (low-calcium diet). Health professionals should advocate this type of diet in clients who have a history of calcium oxalate stones.

Reference

Borghi, L., et al. (2002). Comparison of two diets for the prevention of recurrent stones in idiopathic hypercalciuria. *New England Journal of Medicine, 346,* 77-84.

which could cause oxalate precipitation. Also assess the amount, pattern, and types of fluids consumed.

Assess the client for the clinical manifestations described earlier. Use rating scales to measure the severity of pain. Many clients describe renal or ureteral colic as "the worst pain I've ever had." Vital signs should be monitored. A decreasing blood pressure may indicate severe pain and impending shock; increased pulse and temperature may result from infection. A sudden onset of little or no urine output suggests obstruction, which is an emergency that must be treated immediately to preserve kidney function. Frequency and dysuria commonly occur when a stone reaches the bladder.

All urine voided should be strained through several layers of gauze or through a commercial urine strainer. Carefully examine all debris caught by straining. Save any stone material so that the stone's composition can be analyzed as a basis for treatment and to show how much has passed through the urinary tract. A routine urinalysis, urine for culture and sensitivity testing, and a 24-hour urine specimen may be needed.

Diagnosis, Outcomes, Interventions

Diagnosis: Acute Pain.
The priority nursing diagnosis is *Acute Pain related to irritation and spasm from stone movement in the urinary tract.*

Outcomes. The client will report pain reduction or control.

Interventions. During the acute phase of treatment, offer pain medications, antispasmodics, and antiemetics, if necessary. For severe pain, give the medications on a regular schedule. Use a rating scale to help evaluate the client's pain.

Once pain is controlled, the client should force fluids and ambulate, which facilitates passage of the stone. Relaxation techniques, such as guided imagery or therapeutic or healing touch, can help relieve pain. Help the client find a comfortable position to alternate with ambulation.

Diagnosis: Effective Therapeutic Regimen Management.
More than half of clients with a urinary calculus experience another episode within 5 years. As a result, an important nursing diagnosis is *Effective Therapeutic Regimen Management related to prevention of recurrent calculi.*

Outcomes. The number of recurrences will be reduced, and the interval between stones will increase.

Interventions

Increase Fluids. Teach the client to drink 3 to 4 L of fluid daily to flush the urinary system. At least half the fluid consumed should be water. Intake should be as consistent as possible throughout the 24-hour period.

As a rule, encourage the client to drink a full glass of water every hour during the day and two large glasses just before going to bed. This schedule may create the need to void during the night, at which time the client should drink another glass of water.

Teach Stone Prevention Measures. Besides increased fluid intake, teach the client about other measures to prevent stone recurrence, such as diet modifications, medications if required, and avoidance of urinary stasis (see the Client Education Guide feature on Preventing Recurrence of Urinary Stones on the website). Prompt treatment of UTIs and early recognition of manifestations of stone recurrence are also important.

Health promotion activities include frequent turning and range of motion for immobilized clients, increased fluid intake, and decreased intake of stone-forming solutes in the diet, such as oxalates, purines, and animal proteins. Health maintenance interventions include monitoring high-risk clients with indwelling catheters or obstructions for calculi.

Evaluation

If medical management is successful, the client's pain is controlled, the stone passes unaided, and the client has no complications of obstruction or infection. The client is able to describe factors that increase the risk of developing stones and is able to identify self-care strategies to prevent stone recurrence.

■ Surgical Management
About 20% of stones require additional treatment with shock wave lithotripsy or endourologic or surgical procedures. Open surgery is used only for the small percentage of clients who cannot be successfully treated with lithotripsy or endourologic procedures.

Endourologic Procedures
Depending on the position of the calculus, cystoscopy may be done. Small stones may be removed transurethrally with a cystoscope, ureteroscope, or ureterorenoscope. Additionally, one or two ureteral catheters or stents may be inserted past the stone. From this point, several different interventions are appropriate. The catheters may be left in place for 24 hours or longer to drain urine trapped proximal to the stone and to dilate the ureter, which may prompt spontaneous movement of the calculus. Otherwise, the catheter may mechanically guide the stone downward as it is removed.

At times, a continuous chemical irrigation may be used to dissolve uric acid, struvite, and cystine stones.

Finally, an attempt may be made to manipulate or dislodge the stone with a variety of special catheters with loops and expanding baskets used to snare the stone. Care is the same as that following cystoscopy.

Larger stones may be crushed with an instrument called a *lithotrite* (stone crusher) to facilitate removal. *Cystolitholapaxy* is performed when a bladder stone is soft enough to be crushed. In cystoscopic lithotripsy, an ultrasonic lithotrite is placed to pulverize the stone, followed by extensive flushing of the bladder. Possible complications associated with this procedure include hemorrhage, urinary retention, infection, bladder perforation, and possibly retained stone fragments.

A flexible ureteroscope, passed through a cystoscope, is used to collect stones in the ureter. This procedure, called *ureteroscopy*, is used to retrieve 4- to 5-mm stones or, combined with ultrasonic lithotripsy, to remove fragments after treatment. Minimal sedation or anesthesia is necessary, and postoperative complications are usually few.

A flexible ureterorenoscope can be passed for access to the entire upper urinary tract, including the distal ureter and intrarenal collecting system so that stones or lesions in the lower pole or lateral calices can be reached.

A nephroscope may be inserted to retrieve free-lying renal stones. Figure 36-6, *A* shows a nephroscope in place. The stone may be removed with alligator forceps or a stone basket followed by irrigation. Electrohydraulic, laser, or ultrasound lithotripsy may be completed through the nephroscope. After this procedure, a nephrostomy tube remains in place for 1 to 5 days. The client can go home with it in place. Increased fluids are essential to achieve a urine output greater than 3000 ml (3 L). The tube is removed after diagnostic studies determine that all stone fragments have been removed.

Lithotripsy

Laser Lithotripsy. A newer treatment for calculi is laser lithotripsy. Lasers are used together with a ureteroscope to remove or loosen impacted stones. Constant water irrigation of the ureter is required to dissipate the heat. Complications resulting from this procedure are the same as those of any endourologic procedure.

Extracorporeal Shock Wave Lithotripsy. *Extracorporeal shock wave lithotripsy* (ESWL) is the use of sound waves applied externally to break up stones in the kidney or ureter (Figure 36-7). High-energy shock waves, aimed by fluoroscopy, are transmitted to the stone. The shock waves break the stones into small fragments, which are passed or retrieved endoscopically. The client may be strapped to a frame in a water bath or secured on a table, depending on the type of lithotripsy equipment used. The client is usually offered conscious sedation or general anesthesia.

The procedure lasts 30 to 50 minutes with administration of 500 to 1500 shock waves. Cardiac monitoring is required to synchronize shock waves with the R wave to prevent cardiac dysrhythmias. Complications of ESWL include ecchymosis on the affected flank, retained fragments, urosepsis, perinephric hematoma, and hemorrhage.

FIGURE 36-6 Surgical techniques for removal of kidney stones. **A,** Percutaneous nephroscopic removal of kidney stones. **B,** Pyelolithotomy—open surgical procedure to retrieve stones from renal pelvis. **C,** Nephrolithotomy—open surgical procedure to remove stones from renal calyx.

FIGURE 36-7 Water bath extracorporeal shock wave lithotripsy. Electrically generated shock waves fracture kidney stones.

Stone fragments may bunch up in the distal ureter, obstructing the kidney. To prevent this accumulation and obstruction, a double J stent is commonly placed via cystoscopy before ESWL for stones larger than 6 mm. The stent is removed during a follow-up visit.

After ESWL, the client may experience renal or ureteral colic that needs to be treated with antispasmodics. Early ambulation and increased fluid intake are important for flushing out stone fragments. The fragments may be passed for up to 3 months after the procedure.

Percutaneous Lithotripsy. Percutaneous lithotripsy involves the insertion of a guide percutaneously (through the skin) under fluoroscopy near the area of the stone. An ultrasonic wave is aimed at the stone to break it into fragments.

Open Surgical Procedures

If the stone is too large or if endourologic and lithotripsy procedures fail to remove it, an open surgical procedure is performed. Surgery is rarely needed because of the success of modern, less invasive options.

A *ureterolithotomy* is the surgical removal of a stone from the ureter through a flank incision for higher stones or an abdominal incision for lower ones. A Penrose drain and ureteral catheter are usually placed postoperatively for healing and drainage of urine.

Cystolithotomy, removal of bladder calculi through a suprapubic incision, is used only when stones cannot be crushed and removed transurethrally. Stricture (abnormal narrowing) is the most common postoperative complication. A stone is removed from the renal pelvis by *pyelolithotomy* and from the renal calyx by a *nephrolithotomy.* Figures 36-6, *B* and *C* illustrate these procedures.

Rarely, a partial or total *nephrectomy* (see Chapter 37) is necessary because of extensive kidney damage, overwhelming renal infection, or abnormal renal parenchyma, which can be responsible for stone formation.

■ Nursing Management of the Surgical Client
Assessment

Preoperative assessment includes the general condition of the client, including the presence of conditions that may present problems postoperatively. It is a priority to assess the client's understanding of the condition and the procedure to be performed. Other assessments are similar to those described under Nursing Management of the Medical Client.

Diagnosis, Outcomes, Interventions

Diagnosis: Risk for Injury. With any endourologic procedure, lithotripsy, or surgery, the client has a *Risk for Injury related to postoperative complications.*

Outcomes. The client will remain free from injury, as evidenced by absence of hemorrhage, by vital signs within preoperative limits, by normal WBC count and temperature, and by a total urine output of at least 0.5 ml/kg/hr from all sources.

Interventions

Increase Fluids. Increase the client's IV or oral fluids to 3 to 4 L daily as described earlier, unless contraindicated.

Monitor Urine Output. Maintain the client's urine output at 0.5 ml/kg/hr or more. Assess any indications of hemorrhage, stone retention, urinary retention, or infection. As needed, irrigate the client's bladder to wash out possible stone fragments. See Chapter 40 for discussion of continuous bladder irrigation (CBI). Continue to strain all urine.

Nursing care after a ureterolithotomy may involve care of a ureteral catheter. Output of at least 0.25 ml/kg/hr from the ureteral catheter should be expected and closely monitored. Because the renal pelvis holds only 5 ml, ureteral catheters must be kept patent (open) and are never clamped. Institute prompt intervention with any unexpected reduction in urine flow. Several conditions—such as mucus shreds, blood clots, and chemical sediment—can interfere with the flow of urine through these catheters. Plus, ureteral peristalsis occasionally pushes the catheters out of the ureter into the bladder.

Closely monitor the catheter output. Each ureteral, suprapubic, and urethral catheter should drain into its own collection bag so that the source of the reduced urine flow is noticed immediately. Each tube or bag should be labeled. Measure and record the output of each catheter every hour for the first 24 hours. Output from each catheter should be monitored every 4 to 8 hours until removal. Most of the urine will drain from the ureteral catheters for the first 48 to 72 hours postoperatively. As the inflammation decreases, urine flows around ureteral catheters and is drained by the urethral or suprapubic catheters. Report a total urine output of less than 0.5 ml/kg/hr or a lack of output from ureteral catheters for more than 15 minutes to the physician immediately.

If the physician orders ureteral catheter irrigation, use strict sterile technique. A maximum of 3 to 5 ml of irrigating solution, usually sterile saline solution, should be allowed to flow in by gravity. Very gentle force should be used. If you cannot confirm patency, notify the physician immediately. Use extreme care to ensure that the catheter is not dislodged. If it is not sutured in place, secure it carefully to the client's skin with tape.

Drainage from a nephrostomy tube should also be carefully monitored and cared for with interventions similar to those used for ureteral catheters. Irrigation amounts, if ordered, are no more than 3 to 5 ml. Because the tube goes directly into the kidney, maintain sterile technique to prevent infection.

Clients with any type of catheter must be taught how to care for them before returning home. They should learn how to clean around them, empty them, prevent kinking, and irrigate them if necessary. A home health nurse may be required to assist with these activities.

Prevent Complications. If the client has a flank incision, care is similar to that needed after nephrectomy (see Chapter 37). To prevent pneumonia, the client should cough and deep breathe 10 to 20 times each hour. To facilitate this, administer opioids regularly to control incisional pain. Other postoperative interventions are similar to those for a client with any major abdominal incision, such as monitoring bowel sounds, vital signs, and output from drains and nasogastric tube. Antibiotics may be given prophylactically or at the first sign of infection.

Evaluation

It is expected that surgical intervention for stone removal would be completed with the least invasive procedure possible and before renal damage occurs. In most instances, the client can go home the day of the procedure and does not need to be hospitalized. Clients may go home with catheters in place for about a week; they need to learn catheter care or have home health follow-up. For major surgical intervention, the client is dismissed 3 to 4 days after the procedure.

■ Self-Care

A client with urolithiasis is at risk for recurrence. You have a major role in helping the client develop and maintain an effective, individual regimen to prevent stone recurrence. The main components of prevention are (1) increased fluids, (2) dietary modifications, (3) medications as ordered, and (4) prompt treatment of UTIs. The client must understand that these are lifelong changes in lifestyle. If catheters are in place after surgical intervention, client management of the tubes is necessary before discharge from the hospital.

URINARY REFLUX

Urinary reflux is the backward flow of urine in the urinary tract. It usually begins at the vesicoureteral junction. Urine flows back into the ureter and upward into the renal pelvis. The severity of vesicoureteral reflux is stated as grade I, which is least severe, through grade V, which is most severe. There is an increase in the development of reflux in men older than 50 years of age because of chronic bladder neck obstruction from BPH. Reflux typically occurs in younger children or in young adults from congenital abnormalities of the vesicoureteral junction.

Etiology and Risk Factors

Reflux can be caused by a congenital abnormality, such as ectopic ureter, chronic bladder infections secondary to dysfunctional bladder, or outlet obstruction in the bladder neck. Urinary reflux is more frequently seen as a result of another condition. Reflux contributes to the increase of intravesical pressure (within the bladder) until it finally overwhelms the resistance of the intramural ureteral sphincters, allowing reflux to occur. Clients with obstructions must be evaluated to have the cause identified and treated to prevent and relieve intravesical pressure.

Pathophysiology

In bladder outlet obstruction, the main result is the continuous presence of residual urine, which leads to chronic UTIs. Continual overdistention of the bladder can also decrease detrusor tone, increasing the bladder's capacity and raising the threshold needed to start the micturition reflex.

Renal damage and pyelonephritis are the two primary problems resulting from vesicoureteral reflux. Because the capacity of the renal pelvis is only 5 ml, larger amounts of urine can cause renal parenchymal changes, hydronephrosis, or hydronephroureterosis if they result from ureteral obstruction or reflux. The increased hydrostatic pressure leads to renal cortical atrophy from ischemia and hypoxia and then to calicectasis (dilation of the renal calices). The destruction of kidney tissue, often asymptomatic and undetected, can progress to end-stage renal disease. The kidneys are usually protected from ascending infections by the intramural portion of the distal ureter. With reflux, however, any pathogens in the bladder are carried through the ureters to the kidney. This problem leads to recurrent pyelonephritis. Chronic pyelonephritis leads to renal failure.

Clinical Manifestations

The major manifestation of reflux in the bladder neck is pyelonephritis. When the obstruction is in the vesicoureteral junction or higher, renal failure may be clinically evident. The major diagnostic studies are (1) the VCUG to visualize the lower urinary system during voiding, (2) cystoscopy to evaluate manifestations of obstruction, (3) ureteroscopy to assess the vesicoureteral junction, (4) ultrasound to assess for hydronephrosis, and (5) IVP to evaluate the entire collecting system. Blood studies of BUN and creatinine levels are also done to assess renal function.

Outcome Management
■ Surgical Management

Because there are no medical regimens to prevent or treat reflux caused by ectopic ureter, the primary therapy is surgical. Renal damage from the reflux usually calls for surgical intervention. Surgery is also indicated for obstruction at the ureteropelvic junction, for intractable infection, and for a problem not resolved by maturation. Because the most common causes of reflux are ureteral defects, surgical procedures focus on reimplantation or other treatments for the ureter.

Postoperatively, a urethral or suprapubic catheter keeps the bladder empty to reduce tension on the suture line. A ureteral catheter is also inserted into the ureter involved in the surgical procedure. The tip of this tiny, semi-rigid catheter usually rests in the renal pelvis. The distal end extends through the bladder and out through the urethra or through an abdominal incision.

A ureteral catheter provides three benefits: it splints the ureter to facilitate healing, it prevents obstruction from edema after surgery or other trauma in the area, and it drains urine.

■ Nursing Management of the Surgical Client

Carefully assess any client with a high risk of obstruction for any manifestation of urinary reflux. The client being evaluated for urinary reflux requires support during this diagnostic process. Preoperative preparation for ureteral surgery is similar to that required by any client who needs surgery (see Chapter 16).

Postoperative care is similar to that discussed earlier for urinary calculi. Assess the color of the client's urine frequently. Expect it to progress from bright red to clear yellow over a matter of days. Discharge teaching depends on a variety of factors, including the cause of the reflux, the treatment or procedure done, and the amount of renal damage present. For the client with kidney damage, renal function must be monitored at regular intervals to evaluate any changes in status.

■ VOIDING DISORDERS
URINARY RETENTION

Urinary retention is the inability of the bladder to empty partially or completely during voiding. Treatment is directed at relieving the cause of the problem.

Etiology and Risk Factors

Detrusor failure is the most common cause of urinary retention in women. Failure of the bladder to contract, demonstrated on urodynamic evaluation, is often associated with neurologic conditions. In men, obstructive voiding due to an enlarged prostate is the frequent cause of retention. Other disorders, urethral strictures, medications, detrusor-sphincter dyssynergia, calculi, blood clots, tumors, bladder neck contractures, and history of female genital mutilation may also cause retention. Neuropathies affecting bladder function include diabetes, strokes, and spinal cord injuries. These long-term problems affect the neurologic status of the bladder and interfere with the

micturition reflex. Remember, urinary retention is a manifestation of another pathologic condition.

Retention may be caused by decreased sensory input to and from the bladder, muscle tension, anxiety, or other neurologic conditions affecting the bladder. Surgery has traditionally been a factor; spinal anesthesia causes retention more often than general anesthesia does. After surgery, 10% to 15% of clients who received general anesthesia require catheterization because of an inability to void, and 20% to 25% of those who received spinal anesthesia require a catheter.

In women, prolapse of the back wall of the vagina (rectocele or enterocele) increases the risk of retention by exerting pressure against the urethra. Also, a large cystocele may cause kinking of the bladder neck, decreasing the bladder's ability to empty.

More than half of men older than age 50 experience BPH, a common cause of retention. This is not a preventable problem, although the client with an enlarged prostate should be monitored closely for obstruction secondary to the enlargement. Neurologic injury or disease, such as diabetes mellitus, spinal cord injuries, or multiple sclerosis, may lead to urinary retention as well. Other risk factors are a history of structural abnormalities and use of certain medications, such as tricyclic antidepressants. In some clients, a psychogenic origin may be found.

Pathophysiology

Retention of urine is hazardous because the resulting urinary stasis contributes to UTIs, stone formation, and eventual complications of long-term structural damage to the bladder, ureters, or kidneys. Additionally, continued bladder distention leads to loss of bladder tone.

The pathologic process of retention produces a snowball effect. Retained urine increases hydrostatic pressure against the bladder wall, which results in hypertrophy of the detrusor muscle, formation of trabeculae (connective tissue in the bladder wall), or development of diverticula. At the same time, peristalsis in the ureteral musculature increases against the pressure of the accumulating urine. The ureter may gradually become elongated, tortuous, and fibrotic. Increasing pressure is also transmitted through the renal pelvis and calices into the renal parenchyma. The resulting hydronephrosis exerts pressure on the blood vessels, causing ischemia and increasing the renal damage. If the process is not interrupted, it can proceed to renal failure and death. Figure 36-8 demonstrates the sequence. Even after the retention is relieved, when the alterations caused by increased pressure reach the renal parenchyma, the damage may be permanent and irreversible.

Medications, such as opioids, tricyclic antidepressants, sedatives, antispasmodics, anti-Parkinson drugs, beta-adrenergic blockers, and psychotropic agents, can interfere with normal neurologic function and the mic-

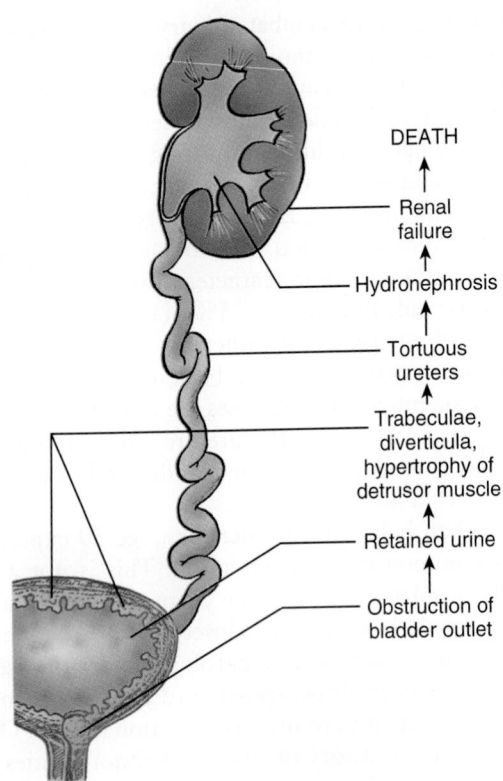

DEATH
↑
Renal
failure
↑
Hydronephrosis
↑
Tortuous
ureters
↑
Trabeculae,
diverticula,
hypertrophy of
detrusor muscle
↑
Retained urine
↑
Obstruction of
bladder outlet

FIGURE 36-8 Potential effects of urinary tract obstruction.

turition reflex. Diseases with neurologic effects, such as stroke, multiple sclerosis, diabetes mellitus, tabes dorsalis, and spinal cord lesions, also disrupt the micturition reflex.

Urinary retention may result in chronic UTI or a series of UTIs and dysfunctional voiding. Conversely, chronic UTIs and dysfunctional voiding may result in urinary retention. The detrusor muscle may become irritated and fail to function correctly, leading to incomplete bladder emptying. Irritation and scarring of the bladder neck or urethra may develop, thus placing these clients at greater risk for urinary retention.

A disorder of psychogenic origin, such as anxiety or fear of voiding in a public restroom, may lead to distention of the bladder and urinary retention. Inability to relax the urethra because of anxiety or neurologic deficit may lead to urinary retention as well.

Anorectal problems, such as hemorrhoids, abscess, fecal impaction, and vaginal prolapse, can be contributing factors, either from obstruction or from secondary spasms of the perineal musculature that interfere with the urethra during voiding.

Decreased oral or IV fluid intake reduces the glomerular filtration rate (GFR), which causes very slow urine production and overfilling of the bladder. The slow increase allows the detrusor muscle to accommodate the increased volume until the muscle's fibers are stretched beyond their ability to contract, hampering micturition.

Urinary retention with overflow incontinence results from the following events. As the bladder continues filling, the intravesical pressure increases. Eventually, this pressure overcomes the resistance of the sphincter. Urine flows out of the bladder until it reduces the intravesical pressure, but only to the level at which the external sphincter can again control the flow of urine. Most clients report that the bladder does not feel empty. It overfills again, and the cycle is repeated.

Prolonged obstruction leads to increased pressures in the urinary tract and may predispose the client to bladder diverticula. A *diverticulum* is a pouch or sac resulting from the herniation of the mucous membrane lining caused by weakness in the muscular wall of an organ. Bladder diverticula are most common in men. Many diverticula are asymptomatic and are usually discovered by chance during assessment of other conditions.

Bladder diverticula can cause two major problems: (1) UTIs, resulting from stasis of urine, and (2) malignancies, probably a result of chronic irritation by persistent infection. Intervention involves removing the obstruction and relieving the retention, followed by surgical excision of the pouch and reestablishment of normal patency of the urinary tract. Postoperatively, catheter drainage of urine is required to allow complete tissue healing. Clients who have had chronic or recurring infections usually require long-term antibiotic therapy after surgery.

Clinical Manifestations

The primary manifestation of urinary retention is a distended bladder or an inability to empty the bladder completely. Voided amounts of 25 to 50 ml one or more times an hour may indicate retention with overflow. The major diagnostic test is catheterization. A postvoid residual amount greater than 100 ml after an attempt to void signals retention. Other diagnostic measures, such as cystoscopy and urodynamic testing to include pressure voiding studies, help identify the cause of the retention.

Outcome Management
■ Medical Management

Identifying the cause of urinary retention is the first step in determining treatment. Finding the underlying neurologic problem or obstructive disorder is crucial in selecting a treatment plan.

Administer Medications. In some cases, cholinergic medications have been known to help stimulate bladder contractions. If a mechanical obstruction is present, however, cholinergic drug therapy should not be used. In this instance, intravesical pressure increases against an obstructed outlet, causing ureterovesical reflux or a ruptured bladder.

Although their effects are somewhat controversial, bethanechol (Urecholine) and neostigmine (Prostigmin) are commonly given. Bethanechol not only improves detrusor tone but also increases bladder outlet and urethral resistance. To counteract this, bethanechol is sometimes combined with phenoxybenzamine (Dibenzyline), prazosin (Minipress), and terazosin (Hytrin), which are potent alpha-adrenergic blockers.

Urethral Dilations. In some instances, urinary retention is relieved by dilation of the urethra by means of the placement of progressively larger urethral sounds (see the table on the website, Urologic Instruments Most Commonly Encountered in a Clinical Setting for examples of sounds). Local or sometimes general anesthesia is used for sedation during sound placement.

■ Nursing Management of the Medical Client

Interventions described next are appropriate for the nursing diagnosis *Urinary Retention.*

Assess Urine Output Patterns. It is important to distinguish retention from *oliguria* (diminished urinary secretion) and *anuria* (complete suppression of urinary secretion). In urinary retention, the kidneys are producing a normal amount of urine but the bladder does not function properly. It fills with urine and rises above the level of the pubic symphysis, sometimes being displaced to either side of midline. Percussion over the bladder produces a dull sound. The client may experience increasing discomfort and the need to urinate. The client also may complain of restlessness, sweating, anxiety, bladder pain, and feelings of bladder fullness. A bladder scan estimates urine amounts in the bladder accurately.

Implement Measures to Stimulate Independent Voiding. Nursing interventions may be used initially to treat retention. Provide privacy, and place the client in a normal sitting or standing position, using gravity and increased intra-abdominal pressure to help relieve an acute problem. Running the water or flushing the toilet within earshot of the client may encourage voiding. Tape-recorded aquatic sounds may be effective. A warm bath or pouring warm water over the perineum often promotes muscle relaxation. Immersing the client's hands in water sometimes works. Applying ice or gently stroking the inner thigh sometimes works as well. These measures may stimulate trigger points of the micturition reflex. If the client is tense and anxious, any measure that induces relaxation may aid in relieving the situation, even a back rub or soothing music.

Catheterize the Client. The client should not be catheterized unless urine amounts by bladder scan are greater than 300 ml or the client complains of discomfort. For clients with persistent urinary retention, a straight or retention catheter may be inserted through the external meatus, into the urethra beyond the internal

sphincter, and into the bladder. A straight catheter is removed after the bladder drains. An indwelling (Foley) catheter is usually inserted after two straight catheterizations. The catheter is kept in place for continuous or intermittent drainage by inflating a balloon near the catheter's tip. Strict sterile techniques are used for insertion except for clients on an intermittent self-catheterization program; these clients may use clean technique.

The indwelling catheter is attached to either a bedside drainage bag or a leg bag. A leg bag may be used for long-term catheterization, especially for a client going home with the catheter in place. A newer belly bag is also available for clients with long-term catheter placement. These devices allow the client more mobility and eliminates the embarrassment of carrying a drainage bag in public view.

Because of the bag's small capacity, the leg bag must be emptied frequently. A conventional drainage system is used at night to avoid the need to empty the leg bag at night. (The change in bags is not necessary with the belly bag.) Instruct the client to avoid attaching the rubber straps too tightly, because doing so may cause skin irritation, thrombophlebitis, and ulcer formation. Loose straps tend to tighten as the bag fills. Recent improvements have led to the use of nylon self-fastening tape (Velcro) leg straps for clients with circulatory problems, those with latex allergy, and those at high risk for skin breakdown. Meticulous skin care and periodic removal of the bag help prevent these problems. Cleanliness and odor control are managed by washing the apparatus with soap and water and soaking the bag in a 1% acetic acid (white vinegar) solution overnight.

Prevent Infection. Prolonged use of an indwelling catheter increases the risk of UTI and tissue trauma. More than 80% of people who develop nosocomial (hospital-acquired) UTIs have undergone urologic instrumentation. The risks of bacteriuria leading to urosepsis increases in direct relationship to duration of catheter placement; estimates of infection rates range from 4% (within 24 hours) to 95% (within 4 weeks). Organisms enter the catheter through any contamination or break in the system or intrude via the thin layer of fluid and exudate that forms around the outside of the catheter.

Catheter insertion should be avoided unless necessary to monitor urine output. Wash your hands thoroughly before and after handling a catheter or drainage system. In addition, do the following:

1. Maintain a closed drainage system.
2. Avoid backflow of urine.
3. Avoid unnecessary manipulation of the catheter during perineal cleaning.
4. Prevent microbial invasion and colonization in the urine collection bag.
5. Maintain patency of the catheter.
6. Encourage a high fluid intake.

On occasion, prophylactic antibiotics are given to clients with catheters in place. The practice is not routine, however, because of the threat of resistant organisms and possible adverse reactions.

Prevent Tissue Injury. Tissue trauma may occur during catheterization. Tissue irritation or necrosis may result from the following:

- Using an oversized catheter
- Continuous pressure and pulling of the catheter between the meatus and the site of taping on the leg or abdomen
- Friction caused by the continuous movement of the catheter, causing tissue breakdown and enhancing encrustation on the outside of the catheter
- Local or systemic allergic reactions to rubber in clients with a history of latex allergy; silicone catheters may be used in these clients

The subject of bladder decompression drainage is still misunderstood. In the past, it was incorrectly assumed that rapid emptying of a distended bladder through a catheter could result in bladder hemorrhage and hypotension. Consequently, the catheter was clamped after 1000 ml of urine had been drained, reopened after an hour to drain another 1000 ml, and clamped and reopened again until the bladder was decompressed. Cystometric studies have shown that this problem does not occur with retention. It is currently thought that any amount of urine can be drained. Drainage does not occur rapidly, because the usual size of a catheter does not allow rapid drainage.

■ Surgical Management
Surgical intervention is usually done when a structural defect is found. Intervention may include (1) removal of an enlarged prostate gland or urethral stricture or (2) correction of a structural abnormality.

Bladder Neck Repair. Surgical intervention is sometimes needed for obstructions below the bladder. If the bladder neck becomes rigid as a result of inflammation, cystoplasty may be done by insertion of an elastic wedge into the area. A transurethral incision of the bladder neck might also be done. Excision of urethral strictures, sometimes with a *urethroplasty* (plastic repair of the urethra), helps return proper functioning. Alternatively, a meatotomy may be performed to open the urethral meatus.

Suprapubic Cystotomy
Indications. Suprapubic catheterization is sometimes used to relieve urinary retention. Placement of the catheter allows postoperative clients to begin a bladder training program. The catheter is placed when urethral catheterization is difficult, as in clients with a severely enlarged prostate, urethral strictures, or quadriplegia.

Local anesthesia is used, although general anesthesia may be used if another surgical procedure is also performed. To facilitate proper placement of the catheter, the bladder must be distended with urine or water before insertion. If the bladder is insufficiently distended with urine, additional fluid is instilled through a catheter or cystoscope.

The suprapubic skin is prepared. Under sterile technique, the suprapubic catheter is inserted through a small surgical incision or by passing a trocar through the skin into the bladder. Once the trocar is in place, the pointed core of the cannula is removed. The catheter is threaded through the cannula and attached to a closed drainage system. The catheter is commonly sutured in place or secured with a commercially made retention seal. When the catheter is removed, the muscle layers of the bladder immediately contract over the puncture site and shrink the surface wound.

Contraindications. Short-term catheter placement may be a possible contraindication.

Complications. Potential complications of a suprapubic catheter include dislodgment of the catheter, hematuria (especially after the use of a large-bore catheter), bowel perforation during trocar insertion, and failure of the wound to close, which results in a urinary fistula.

Outcomes. When a suprapubic catheter is used instead of a urethral catheter, a lower rate of UTIs, increased comfort, and easier implementation of a bladder training protocol are expected.

■ Nursing Management of the Surgical Client
The client with a suprapubic catheter requires care similar to that needed for clients with a urethral catheter. The most frequent problem is catheter obstruction caused by (1) twisting or kinking or (2) sediment or clots. Disconnecting the catheter from the drainage tubing can disrupt the siphon drainage. When the catheter is removed, dressing changes may be needed to protect the skin from urinary leakage from the site. The suprapubic catheter site usually closes completely immediately or within 24 hours of removal.

■ Self-Care
The client who is discharged with an indwelling suprapubic or urethral catheter needs to know how to care for the catheter at home. The family and significant others should learn how to empty the drainage bag and how to prevent infection. They should also be taught the clinical manifestations of UTI and instructed to call the physician if they occur. When the client is discharged with a catheter in place, follow-up care is required. Removal of the catheter depends on the cause of the retention.

■ Modifications for Older Clients

Older clients are more susceptible to urinary retention because of a chronic decrease in bladder tone. Retention leading to infection may also be worse in older clients. Treatment, however, remains the same.

URINARY INCONTINENCE

Urinary incontinence has been defined by the International Continence Society (ICS) as "a condition in which involuntary loss of urine is a social or hygienic problem and is objectively demonstrable."[18] Some 13% to 56% of noninstitutionalized adults older than age 60 years and at least half of nursing home residents have problems related to incontinence.[51] The annual cost of incontinence exceeds $15 million.[51] Yet most people avoid seeking treatment because they feel shame and embarrassment, which means that the problem is severely underreported and underdiagnosed. Many health care providers do not understand the effects of urinary incontinence on quality of life. Affected people may forfeit their active lifestyles and turn to a reclusive existence because they fear embarrassment.

There are three major types of incontinence: (1) *stress urinary incontinence,* (2) *urge urinary incontinence,* and (3) *overflow urinary incontinence.* Under each of these types are many subtypes that may present in clients as an individual diagnosis or a combination of diagnoses.

Etiology and Risk Factors

Urinary incontinence commonly results from many factors, including anatomic defects and physical, physiologic, psychosocial, and pharmacologic factors. Anatomic and physiologic incontinence results from sphincter weakness or damage, urethral deformity, altered muscle tone at the urethrovesical junction, and detrusor instability.

Stress urinary incontinence is an involuntary loss of urine that occurs without detrusor (bladder) contraction when intravesical pressure exceeds urethral pressure.[18] It commonly results from obstetric or surgical trauma, the loss of estrogen associated with menopause, repeated straining, urogenital prolapse, and congenital weakness. After a suprapubic prostatectomy and transurethral prostatectomy, men may experience some exertional urine loss after the postoperative catheter is removed. Surgical interventions may cause bladder neck damage, with possibly permanent incontinence. A radical perineal or retropubic prostatectomy may cause permanent incontinence if the bladder neck is partially damaged during surgery.

Dysfunction of the urethrovesical junction (the area where the bladder meets the urethra) occurs mainly in women. Common causes include pregnancy, vaginal delivery, menopause, and surgical procedures that damage nerves leading to muscles of the pelvic floor. These in-

juries may lead to stress incontinence of varying degrees. A change in the angle of greater than 30 degrees from a horizontal plane during straining indicates hypermobility due to relaxation of the urethrovesical junction.

A simple diagnostic test for a hypermobile urethrovesical junction is a *Q-tip test.* A sterile, well-lubricated cotton applicator is placed in the urethra. The client is asked to strain as if to have a bowel movement. More than a 30-degree difference in a horizontal plane indicates a positive result or urethral hypermobility of the urethrovesical junction (Figure 36-9).

Detrusor instability has many possible causes, although in many cases the cause remains unknown. On occasion, the cause can be identified as a bladder lesion, lower or upper spinal cord lesion, complication of pelvic surgery, or neurologic deficit. The ICS offers two descriptions to characterize detrusor instability. In the first, the bladder contracts either spontaneously or with provocation while the client attempts to inhibit micturition. These contractions are seen during the filling phase of a cystometrogram in a neurologically intact client. In the second, detrusor overactivity results from disturbances of the nervous control mechanism. These clients have objective evidence of bladder dysfunction from a neurologic disorder. This type of detrusor instability, known as *detrusor hyperreflexia,* is commonly seen in the client with a history of a stroke or neurologic impairment.

Urge urinary incontinence occurs randomly when involuntary urination is preceded by the warning of a few seconds to a few minutes. It is caused by uncontrolled contraction or overactivity of the detrusor muscle seen with central nervous system disorders (Alzheimer's dis-

FIGURE 36-9 Diagnostic "Q-tip test" determines the descent of the normal urethrovesical junction contributing to stress incontinence in women. More than a 30-degree increase during exertional activities indicates a hypermobile urethrovesical junction.

ease, brain tumor, Parkinson's disease, multiple sclerosis), bladder disorders (interstitial cystitis, radiation effects, carcinoma in situ), and spinal cord interference with spinal inhibitory pathways (spondylosis, cancer growth in spinal cord).

Overflow urinary incontinence, as defined by ICS, is an involuntary urine loss associated with overdistention of the bladder.[18] The bladder is able to store urine but does not empty completely, causing urine loss as a result of diminishing resistant pressures.

Physical causes of incontinence independent of disorders of the urinary tract are often related to physical immobility, especially with older adults. These clients are often physically unable to get to the toilet independently because of stroke, fractures, or weakness. Failing vision and distances from the bathroom can also contribute to incontinence if the client cannot see the commode or bedpan.

Psychosocial causes of incontinence range from true psychological problems, such as dementia, to simple confusion. Clients may be unaware of the need to void or may be unable to respond appropriately when they feel the urge to empty the bladder. Other possible causes include regression, dependence, insecurity, sensory deprivation, and the disturbance of conditioned reflexes.

Drugs can also contribute to incontinence, especially overflow incontinence. Examples include the following:

- Opioids, tranquilizers, sedatives, and hypnotic agents, all of which may affect sensory perception
- Alcohol
- Rapid-acting diuretics
- Antihistamines
- Atropine and atropine-like substances
- Hypotensive agents
- Alpha-adrenergic blockers
- Beta-adrenergic agents
- Ganglionic blockers

Other causative factors include fecal impaction, bladder scarring, urethral adhesions, diabetes mellitus, and obesity. Frequent voiding by clients who fear "accidents" leads to decreased bladder capacity, increased detrusor tone, and thickening of the bladder wall, which only fosters the dysfunction.

Incontinence health promotion activities involve prevention of impaired mobility and UTIs, exercise to minimize muscle weakness, and assisting clients to the bathroom by the clock to prevent accidents. Health maintenance measures are to thoroughly assess clients who report incontinence and monitor high-risk clients for development of incontinence. Teaching clients to perform pelvic muscle exercises (Kegel exercises) to improve muscle tone, follow bladder training protocols, and decrease incontinence by regulating fluid intake (e.g., not drinking large amounts of fluid at bedtime) are examples of health restoration interventions.

Pathophysiology

Pathophysiologic changes associated with incontinence vary with the specific cause of the disorder. In *stress incontinence,* increased vesical pressure commonly stems from such activities as sneezing, coughing, laughing, and exertion. There may be some dysfunction of the urethral sphincter or, in women, changes in the urethrovesical junction caused by weakness of periurethral muscles. Muscle weakness from childbirth, menopause, or other problems loosens the pelvic floor. In addition to the loss of muscle tone supporting the urethrovesical junction, there is increased descent, with a funneling effect of the bladder neck during exertion. In men, the pathophysiologic change usually results from BPH, which causes retention, overflow, and stress incontinence.

Urge urinary incontinence is associated with several pathophysiologic changes. One problem is uninhibited detrusor contraction associated with motor disorders. Another cause is decreased mobility from an upper motor neuron spinal lesion combined with an inability to stop voiding once the impulse is felt.

Overflow urinary incontinence stems from overdistention of the bladder and eventual overflow of the excessive amount of urine. Usually, this problem results from obstruction at the bladder outlet, as with BPH.

If incontinence is not controlled, it can lead to both psychological and physical problems. The psychological consequences of incontinence are serious. Clients may isolate themselves, and the fear of embarrassment may lead to depression. Incontinence is also a leading cause of nursing home admissions. The physical complications of incontinence include infection, skin breakdown, and permanent voiding dysfunctions.

Clinical Manifestations

The major manifestation of urinary incontinence is involuntary urine loss. Manifestations vary from client to client. An excellent diagnostic tool, the *bladder diary,* reveals voiding frequency, fluid intake, patterns of urinary urgency, and number and severity of incontinent episodes. A 7-day diary reveals patterns of incontinence and may be helpful before a diagnostic evaluation.

Urodynamic evaluation provides the best diagnostic information in determining the precise cause of the client's incontinence. The purpose of urodynamics is to reproduce the manifestations. The information collected is used to determine and guide treatment. Additionally, an evaluation of pelvic floor prolapse in women can reveal other contributing factors of urogenital dysfunction.

The variety of urodynamic examinations, including cystometrography and electromyographic (EMG) monitoring, are described in Chapter 34. Urine flow rate studies help identify hypotonic detrusor or an obstructional or dysfunctional voiding mechanism. A urethral pressure profile helps determine whether there is pressure in the urethra, which may contribute to a severe type of stress incontinence *(intrinsic sphincter deficiency)* (see Bladder Neck Suspensions later in this chapter). Ultrasonography or catheterization of the bladder can detect elevated residual urine levels. Additionally, cystoscopy can be used to diagnose tumors, foreign bodies (such as stones or sutures), trabeculations, or structural abnormalities in the bladder and urethra.

Outcome Management

Successful management of urinary incontinence requires appropriate diagnostic testing. Treatments include pelvic floor behavioral interventions, drug therapy, and surgery. The least invasive treatment should be tried first.[51] Many therapies aimed at improving incontinence can be implemented without risk to the client. Success is based on motivation, competency, and willingness to add these changes to one's lifestyle. Surgery should be performed only when a structural or anatomic defect is found.

The goals of treatment for a client with urinary incontinence include the following:

- Careful evaluation
- Treatment decisions based on the specific abnormalities identified for each client
- Treatment modalities that coordinate with the client's personality, expectations, environment, and clinical status
- A treatment plan that includes ways to circumvent environmental constraints
- Ability of the client to make an informed choice among treatment options

■ Medical Management

Many noninvasive, behavior-based therapies may be effective in controlling some types of incontinence. The Agency for Health Care Policy and Research guidelines provide numerous algorithms that detail the diagnosis and treatment of various forms of incontinence.[18] Injectable agents such as Botox are being explored for medical treatment of incontinence.

Pelvic Muscle Exercises. Originally designed for postpartum women, these exercises—commonly known as Kegel exercises—have long been the technique of choice for reducing urinary incontinence. Reports of success range from 30% to 90%. New devices have improved the success rate by fostering the correct use of these exercises. See the Evidence-Based Practice in Action feature on Pelvic Muscle Exercise for Treatment of Urinary Incontinence on p. 898.

Pelvic Floor Reeducation. Biofeedback has been used for clients with incontinence to help them learn to reuse the pelvic floor musculature. Clients are educated to control incontinence by isolating and contracting the pelvic floor muscles. The use of biofeedback has been success-

ful in eliminating incontinence in about 54% to 77% of clients who try it.[13]

Biofeedback provides a "relay-like" system by which the client can visualize the isolation and contraction of the pelvic floor musculature. Either pressure manometry or EMG monitoring records the muscle strength or muscle activity.

Clients are taught to use the pelvic floor muscles to override the sense of urgency in an effort to retrain the bladder. They can also be taught to contract the correct muscle group to inhibit urine loss caused by exertion. Biofeedback can also be used to teach clients to relax the pelvic floor if they have problems with urinary retention.

Electrical Stimulation. Electrical stimulation of the pelvic floor can be used to inhibit the micturition reflex and to contract the pelvic floor muscles. Delivery of a weak electrical current helps to close the urethra more tightly by direct and reflexogenic contraction of the striated periurethral muscles. Electrical stimulation also helps increase bladder volume through bladder inhibition and stabilized detrusor activity.

The most common method of delivery is by insertion of a vaginal or anal sensor. The procedure can be done in a physician's office or at home. The client inserts the internal device, and the stimulation level is directed at maintaining a synchronous pelvic floor contraction during an on-and-off cycle. Figure 36-10 shows the computerized systems used for biofeedback and electrical stimulation.

Bladder Training and Behavioral Training. The client who uses bladder and behavioral training to address incontinence first voids at short intervals throughout the day—once an hour or less, if necessary. The client then tries to gradually lengthen the time between voiding up to 3 hours. Behavioral training with biofeedback or verbal feedback to teach pelvic floor muscle control showed a 63% to 69% improvement in continence in community-dwelling older women.[13]

Institutionalized clients can also use a form of bladder training. With these clients, health care workers encourage voiding at hourly intervals and give positive feedback. The time between voiding can then be gradually increased to 2 hours.

Medications. Drug therapy for incontinence is guided primarily by the following events. During the bladder filling phase, the detrusor relaxes because of beta-adrenergic activity. At the same time, the bladder outlet contracts in response to alpha-adrenergic stimulation. If these actions are insufficient to keep urine in the bladder, drugs can be prescribed to supplement or replace them. See the Integrating Pharmacology feature on Medications for the Treatment of Urinary Incontinence on p. 899.

EB EVIDENCE-BASED PRACTICE IN ACTION

Pelvic Muscle Exercises for Treatment of Urinary Incontinence

Kegel exercises, first introduce by Dr. Arnold Kegel in the 1940s, have been encouraged for clients as a method to treat urinary incontinence. Dr. Kegel reported symptomatic relief of stress and urge incontinence with a daily regimen of pelvic muscle exercise. Over the years, physicians have encouraged clients to perform pelvic muscle exercise as the first-line treatment of urinary incontinence. Over the past 15 years, many nurses have offered continence programs with biofeedback-directed pelvic muscle exercise programs. These instructional rehabilitation programs have repeatedly demonstrated cost-effective care while decreasing or eliminating the manifestations associated with urinary incontinence.

Although surgery and medications have been developed for those with incontinence, the cost and risk associated with surgery and the side effects associated with medications are not treatments chosen by clients. Pelvic muscle exercise has been recommended by the Agency for Health Care Policy and Research as the first-line treatment for urinary incontinence.[6] It provides improved continence with little risk. Studies have demonstrated that verbal instructions are not adequate in teaching clients correct performance of pelvic muscle exercise.[1-5,7] Continence nurses use biofeedback to help clients recognize the specific events that initiate incontinence episodes. Clients are then taught to contract the pelvic floor muscle quickly to eliminate the urgency, frequency, and urine loss associated with urge incontinence. The quick squeezes excite the inhibitory reflex to relax the bladder while the squeezes associated with stress incontinence close the urethra by increasing urethral pressure. During a stress incontinent episode, urine loss is experienced during increased abdominal pressure, for example, while sneezing, coughing, or laughing. To decrease these manifestations, clients are taught to squeeze before the specific exertional activities that precede the incontinent episode. Eventually, clients perform these pelvic muscle contractions automatically to control their incontinence manifestations. Additionally, these specifically educated continence nurses offer a well-rounded program consisting of emotional support, behavioral interventions, dietary changes, and individualized plans that are specific to each client's diagnosis and clinical manifestations.

References
1. Bump, R.C., et al. (1994). Assessment of Kegel pelvic performance after brief verbal instruction. *American Journal of Obstetric & Gynecology, 170*(2), 208-212.
2. Burgio, K., et al. (1998). Behavioral vs drug treatment for urge urinary incontinence in older women. *Journal of the American Medical Association, 280*(23), 1995-2000.
3. Burgio, K., et al. (2003). Behavioral training with and without biofeedback in the treatment of urge incontinence in older women: A randomized, controlled trial. *Journal of the American Medical Association, 288*(18), 2293-2299.
4. Burns, P. (1993). A comparison of effectiveness of biofeedback and pelvic muscle exercise treatment of stress incontinence in older community-dwelling women. *Journal of Gerontology, 48*(4), 167-174.
5. Dougherty, M., et al. (2002). A randomized trial of behavioral management for continence with rural older women, *Research in Nursing and Health, 25*(1), 3-13.
6. Urinary Incontinence Guideline Panel. (1992). *Urinary incontinence in adults: Clinical practice guideline.* AHCPR Publication No. 92-0038. Rockville, MD: Agency for Health Care Policy and Research, Public Health Service, U.S. Department of Health and Human Services.
7. Wyman, J., et al. (1998). Comparative efficacy of behavioral interventions in the management of female urinary incontinence. Continence Program for Women Research Group. *American Journal of Obstetrics and Gynecology, 179*(4), 999-1007.

Fluid Intake and Dietary Changes. The major nutritional aspect of management involves controlling fluid intake. Decreasing fluid intake, especially after dinner, may help decrease nocturia. For obese clients, weight reduction may help decrease stress incontinence by decreasing pressure against the bladder neck during exertion. The client should also avoid bladder irritants, such as alcohol, chocolate, and caffeinated drinks.

■ Nursing Management of the Medical Client

Multiple nursing diagnoses can be used, depending on the specific type of incontinence: *Stress Urinary Incontinence, Reflex Urinary Incontinence, Urge Urinary Incontinence,* and *Functional Urinary Incontinence.* All of the following interventions may be implemented as appropriate. Nurses often offer the first intervention for the client with urinary incontinence. The primary intervention is asking about bladder health with sensitivity. Many clients feel shame and embarrassment about incontinence, and they may be reluctant to acknowledge the existence of a bladder control problem that affects their quality of life.

Implement a Bladder Training Program. A successful bladder training program requires patience. The client must accept the program and be a willing and active participant. The first step is to discuss all procedures, expectations, and anticipated outcomes with the client. Do your best to inspire a sense of hope and a positive attitude when discussing the client's prognosis.

FIGURE 36-10 An electrical stimulation and biofeedback system can be used to treat men and women with incontinence. This system is called the InCare PRS 9500. (Courtesy Hollister Incorporated, Libertyville, IL.)

A bladder training program involves (1) adequate fluid intake, (2) accessibility to a toilet, (3) muscle-strengthening exercises, and (4) carefully scheduled voiding times. Implementing the program also requires well-organized teaching guidelines. The client also may need behavioral modification or intermittent catheterization.

Monitor Fluid Intake. Many clients with incontinence reduce their fluid intake to decrease urine production and increase control. Actually, adequate fluid intake and adequate urine production are necessary to stimulate the micturition reflex. Unless the client's physical status is a contraindication, encourage a daily fluid intake of 0.5 ounce of fluid for every pound of body weight. Carefully space these fluids throughout the day, limiting fluids in the evening to allow longer sleep periods at night. Fluids should be free of caffeine and alcohol, both of which may irritate the bladder.

Teach Kegel Exercises. Performed diligently, Kegel exercises strengthen the pubococcygeal muscle, help resolve stress incontinence, and decrease urgency and frequency. Instruct the client to contract the pelvic floor muscles as if to hold back intestinal gas. Do not ask the client to start and stop the urine stream as a way to isolate the correct muscle group. Stopping and starting the urine stream may cause dysfunction of the micturition reflex and may encourage urinary retention.

Once the client can isolate the correct muscle group, he or she should contract these muscles 10 times in sitting, standing, and lying positions, three times a day,

INTEGRATING PHARMACOLOGY

Medications for the Treatment of Urinary Incontinence

Medication is often the first treatment offered to clients with incontinence. These medications are diagnosis specific. Urge incontinence is treated with anticholinergic agents such as oxybutynin (Ditropan) and tolterodine (Detrol). Anticholinergics work by increasing the volume in the bladder that can be tolerated before an involuntary bladder contraction occurs, decreasing the strength of the involuntary bladder contraction, and increasing the total bladder capacity. Extended-release formulas of these drugs are available. Additionally, Ditropan has an antispasmodic action as well. It has an inhibitory effect on the smooth muscle of the bladder and has a local anesthetic effect. Tolterodine has an antimuscarinic property that has fewer side effects than other anticholinergics.

Tricyclic antidepressants such as imipramine (Tofranil) and amitriptyline (Elavil) are also often prescribed for urge incontinence as well as for interstitial cystitis. The tricyclics act by increasing the synaptic concentration of serotonin or norepinephrine in the central nervous system. This leads to bladder wall relaxation and increased bladder capacity.

A commonly used drug for stress incontinence is pseudoephedrine (Sudafed). The alpha-adrenergic properties of this drug can increase the closure mechanism within the urethra, decreasing the manifestations of stress incontinence in some clients. Because this medication stimulates the alpha-receptors in the body, clients with a history of high blood pressure should have their blood pressure checked regularly. New medications to treat stress incontinence are undergoing clinical studies.

Another commonly prescribed medication for incontinence in women is vaginal estrogen. Before the menopausal years, the urogenital system is enriched with estrogen receptors that bring an excellent blood supply to the vaginal mucosa. During the perimenopausal years and through the postmenopausal years, the decreasing circulating estrogens lead to atrophic changes of the vagina, urethra, and bladder trigone. As the mucosal layers atrophy, the tissues become less elastic as the urethra loses its ability to close properly. The application of vaginal estrogen increases the circulation, leading to improved function of the lower urogenital system.

working up to 10-second contractions. Then encourage the client to contract the pelvic floor muscles to learn the urge suppression technique or before any exertion that might cause incontinence. As with any exercise program, the program takes a conscious effort and may take months for the muscles to become adequately toned.

Develop a Voiding Schedule. At the same time that the client is strengthening pelvic floor muscles, the nurse should develop a voiding schedule with the client. Determine how often the client urinates during the day by asking him or her to maintain a voiding record. Depending on the voiding pattern, help the client to the toilet or commode every 30 minutes, increasing the time to 2 hours. As the program progresses, encourage the client to hold the urine longer. This increases voiding intervals, which increases bladder capacity.

Implement Biofeedback Techniques. Biofeedback and behavior modification may improve the outcome of the bladder-training program. Use biofeedback techniques to help the client regain control over the external urethral sphincter and pelvic floor musculature. An internal probe is placed to measure the pelvic floor muscle activity. As the client contracts the pelvic floor, a visual analog scale or video graphs (see Figure 36-10) indicate the activity, strength, and duration of the muscle contraction. The system gives immediate feedback of progress. The therapy can be offered in the practitioner's office or with the use of a home unit.

Use Behavior Modification. Behavior modification is a variation of the voiding schedule. This program conditions the bladder to empty when the client attempts to void. The client is encouraged to void by the clock rather than by urge. The initial time between voiding is based on a completed bladder diary before therapy is begun. The time between voiding may be as little as every 30 minutes, with weekly increases of 15 to 30 minutes between. The gradual increase in time between voiding helps to decrease urge incontinence and to increase bladder capacity.

Explore Obstructive Devices. Obstructive devices are sometimes used for women with stress incontinence and vaginal prolapse (Chapter 41). For example, certain types of vaginal pessaries can reduce incontinence by supporting the descending urogenital angle at the bladder neck. When a pessary is fit properly, the client should be able to void completely without urethral obstruction. Women using such devices should have the dexterity to remove the device for cleaning several times a week or when not in use. If the client is unable to remove the pessary, she should return to the clinic every 3 weeks to have the pessary removed, cleaned, and reinserted, and she should undergo a vaginal inspection for infection and irritation.

Recommend Counseling. A mental health consultation may help clients with depression that stems from incontinence. Talking to a counselor can help clients manage the fear of embarrassment, sense of increased dependence, and self-image problems accompanying incontinence. Avoid medications such as antidepressants because of the potential for more bladder dysfunction.

Use Other Incontinence Products

Disposable Pads. Sometimes none of the measures described are effective. Nursing interventions must then be aimed at protecting the client's skin, clothing, and bed linen. Adult-sized disposable pads or briefs help protect and increase the social mobility of clients with chronic incontinence. These commercially available undergarments have elastic legs and cellulose padding that draws fluid away from the skin by capillary action. Some brands include an odor-reducing agent.

Skin Care. If the skin becomes wet, it must be meticulously cleaned with a pH-balanced cleaner and dried to prevent serious rashes and skin breakdown from maceration and ammonia. The skin should then be carefully moisturized. Indwelling catheters to drain urine should be used only to avoid skin breakdown.

Condom Systems. External condom catheter drainage involves placing a thin rubber or plastic sheath over the penis and connecting it to either a leg bag or a bedside drainage bag. When the bladder releases urine, it runs down the tube into the collecting device. Problems include leakage (with or without detachment of the condom), twisting of the condom, and stasis of urine, which can macerate the penis.

Select the correct size of sheath, attaching it to stay in place without compromising circulation to the distal penis. Make sure that the sheath is not too tight, particularly at the ring. You may need to remove some of the client's pubic hair before preparing the skin. Wash the penis with soap and water and allow it to dry thoroughly to remove skin oils. If appropriate, apply an adhesive paste or commercial skin barrier.

Many commercially prepared condom systems contain a double-sided adhesive liner that is applied to the penis before the condom. Many newer devices are self-adhesive.

When rolling the condom sheath over the penis, allow at least 1.5 cm between the distal end of the penis and the internal end of the sheath. This reduces skin irritation. Make sure that the foreskin is over the glans.

Use only elastic tape to allow for expansion or erection. Apply this tape in a spiral only. To avoid impaired circulation, never encircle the penis completely with tape. Frequently monitor the patency of the system, and remove the condom daily to clean and dry the skin.

Encourage Follow-Up. The client should be seen at regular intervals to make sure that interventions are adequate and continence is improved. Referral to a continence clinic may sometimes be appropriate to ensure close follow-up of continuing problems. The National Association for Continence and the Simon Foundation for Continence both publish newsletters containing important information for the incontinent client and family (see the Management and Delegation feature on Helping Clients with Urinary Incontinence on p. 901).

MANAGEMENT AND DELEGATION

Helping Clients with Urinary Incontinence

Various underlying conditions can result in urinary incontinence. Although women are at greater risk than men, incontinence also affects men. You and the physician assess and evaluate the client to determine the appropriate interventions to manage incontinence, possibly using a bladder record or voiding diary to document patterns and trends. Pelvic muscle rehabilitation, behavior therapy, pharmacologic interventions, and surgical procedures are the recommended treatments. For many, incontinence is an acute problem; for others, it is a chronic one.

Bladder training, assistance with toileting, and providing good skin care are duties that may be delegated to unlicensed assistive personnel. These measures are necessary for improving continence and for keeping clients dry and clean to prevent complications associated with skin irritation and ulceration.

Helping the incontinent client who cannot get out of bed is crucial in preventing skin breakdown and pressure ulcers. Utilizing a bedpan, a bedside commode, or a raised toilet seat may be helpful at times. If the client uses a walking aid to ambulate, ensure that the wheelchair, walker, or cane is near the bed and that the pathway to the bathroom is well lit and clear. Indicate which modality is appropriate for each client.

Instruct unlicensed assistive personnel to:
- Respond promptly to all call lights in their assigned area.
- Closely measure and record urine output. Cloudy, foul-smelling, or dark urine should be reported immediately to you.
- Give each client plenty of time to void. Create privacy by closing the door or pulling the bedside curtain.
- Never scold a client who is wet. The client may be upset or feel ashamed about incontinence.

With bladder training instruction, direct unlicensed assistive personnel to:
- Assist or prompt the client to the bathroom on a scheduled interval, usually every 1 to 2 hours at the beginning of the training period.
- Increase the interval of time to assist or prompt the client to the bathroom as the client begins to achieve dryness.

Ask unlicensed assistive personnel to:
- Explain when the next bathroom time will be before they leave the room.
- Offer positive reinforcement to the client who can successfully void or asks for assistance to the bathroom to urinate, or has a dry absorbent pad.

- Assist clients with exercises to strengthen pelvic muscles to help minimize incontinence, reinforcing your previous instruction.

Direct unlicensed assistive personnel about which toileting methods to use:
- *Scheduled toileting:* Assist the client to the bathroom every 2 to 4 hours whether or not the client is wet or dry.
- *Prompted voiding:* Check whether the client is wet or dry; ask the client whether he or she needs to void, and help the client to the bathroom if the client answers "yes."
- *Habit training:* Once the client's voiding times each day are determined, help the client to the bathroom at the same times each day.

Maintaining clean, dry, and intact skin is necessary to prevent skin breakdown and unnecessary complications associated with wet skin. Instruct unlicensed assistive personnel to provide proper skin care and to identify any changes such as red, excoriated, or tender skin to you. The regimen may include:
- Cutting back on evening or night fluid intake to decrease voiding accidents during the night.
- Changing disposable wet pads or diapers every time the client is wet.
- Using ointments or creams to protect the skin and to serve as a barrier after cleaning the client.
- Applying absorbent pads or diapers that are not chafing to the skin.

Have unlicensed assistive personnel communicate and report (1) any changes in skin or urine, (2) the client's inability to follow the toileting plan, and (3) any other questions that arise. You are responsible for assessing, implementing, evaluating, and making all changes to the client's plan of care.

Bibliography

Agency for Health Care Policy and Research. (1996). *Clinical practice guideline: Urinary incontinence in adults: Acute and chronic management.* AHCPR Publication No. 96-0682. Rockville, MD: U.S. Department of Health and Human Services.

Agency for Health Care Policy and Research (1996). *Clinical practice guideline: Caregiver guide: Helping people with incontinence.* AHCPR Publication No. 96-0683. Rockville, MD: U.S. Department of Health and Human Services.

■ Surgical Management

Surgical procedures are performed only to correct or compensate for anatomic defects leading to incontinence. After an injury to the bladder neck, the surgeon can resuspend the bladder neck and attempt to recreate normal anatomy. Implantation of an artificial sphincter can bring about opening and closing of the urethra to allow voiding. Other procedures, such as collagen or fat injections, are used to fill or occlude a urethra that cannot close completely.

Bladder Neck Suspensions. Bladder neck suspensions restore the normal urethrovesical junction or lengthen and support the urethra. Resuspending the bladder neck allows the urethrovesical junction to function correctly.

The *Burch colposuspension* is a popular surgical procedure for women with stress incontinence. This surgical intervention is a modification of an older procedure known as the MMK (Marshall, Marchetti, Krantz). In the Burch procedure, a surgeon fixes the periurethral tissue to Cooper's ligament, whereas in the MMK procedure, the surgeon sutures the periurethral tissue to the symphysis pubis. After surgery, a suprapubic catheter must usually be in place for up to 14 days. The drainage system must remain patent because the pressure of a filling bladder can inhibit the healing process.

A *sling procedure* is used for intrinsic sphincter deficiency, a severe type of stress incontinence. Material is placed beneath the urethra to elevate it and to increase urethral compression. The sling material may be synthetic or autologous (from one's self), such as fascia from another part of the client's abdomen. There are many variations of the procedure; some present a significant risk of voiding dysfunction and others present risk of rejection of the synthetic material used for urethral support.

One type of *sling procedure* is called a *TVT*, or transvaginal tape. When a TVT procedure is placed in a woman, a synthetic material made of Prolene is loosely positioned under the urethra at the bladder neck. It supports the urethra and bladder neck during the activities that trigger a stress incontinent episode. The procedure is done as an outpatient surgery and the client is often discharged within several hours of completion of the TVT.

Other surgical procedures provide an intact, patent route for the transport of urine. Scar tissue that interferes with normal bladder neck function must be removed.

Implantation of an Artificial Urinary Sphincter. Implantation of an artificial urinary sphincter may help some clients achieve continence. This procedure usually is avoided until all other treatments have failed. Figure 36-11 shows a sphincter device, which consists of an inflatable cuff, a reservoir, and a control pump. The surgeon implants the cuff around the bladder neck or urethra, the deflation (or control) pump in the scrotum or labia, and the fluid reservoir in the abdomen.

The cuff keeps the urethra closed until the client manually squeezes the pump. This moves the fluid from the cuff to the reservoir. The bladder then drains. The cuff automatically refills after 3 to 5 minutes, again occluding the urethra.

Candidates for this treatment must not have an obstructed lower urinary tract, detrusor hyperreflexia, or progressive neurologic disease affecting bladder func-

tion. Clients must have adequate manual dexterity and motivation to manage the system. Failure of the device poses a long-term risk that the client will need more surgery. Clients must be absolutely compliant, or else the upper tracts of the urinary system can be damaged by obstruction.

■ Nursing Management of the Surgical Client

Nursing care of clients undergoing surgery focuses on maintaining adequate urinary drainage. With bladder suspension, preventing distention is a priority to help avoid excessive pressure on the healing surgical site. During the immediate postoperative period, a bladder training program is initiated to help the client regain detrusor muscle tone. Clamp the catheter for lengthening intervals while urine collects in the bladder, unclamping it periodically to empty the bladder. If the client reports severe pressure, the catheter should be unclamped immediately.

If a suprapubic catheter is used, the client should try to void every 2 to 3 hours. After voiding is attempted, the catheter is drained to measure the residual urine and determine the effectiveness of bladder emptying.

■ Self-Care

The expected outcome is that the client will resume control over bladder function. Many strategies to achieve continence may be tried, and the client selects what is most comfortable and best able to support preferred activities. Management options can be expensive, such as multiple biofeedback sessions. If continence is achieved

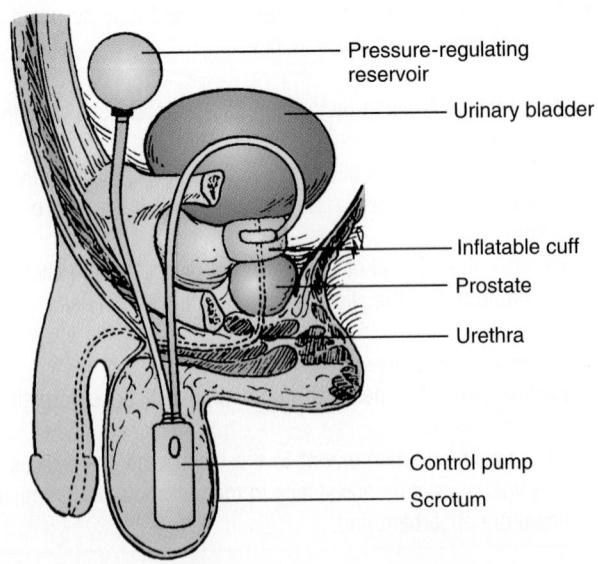

FIGURE 36-11 Artificial urinary sphincter. This surgically implanted urethral sphincter restores continence. To urinate, the client deflates the cuff around the bladder neck by squeezing the control pump within the scrotum. The cuff reinflates automatically.

with any of the described therapies, however, treatment to achieve continence is cheaper than the purchase of adult briefs for daily use; in addition, the client would be free to engage in desired activities. Teach the client about continence options, and help the client make decisions about treatment options.

■ Modifications for Older Clients

Incontinence is not a normal part of the aging process, but it is a common problem among older adults. Older clients can be treated with any of the previously mentioned treatments. Because older people are more sensitive to many medications, care should be used when drugs are administered.

NEUROGENIC BLADDER

The term *neurogenic bladder* refers to several bladder dysfunctions caused by lesions of the central or peripheral nervous systems (Figure 36-12). Their manifestations depend on the site of the lesion. A neurogenic bladder may involve a combination of one or more nervous system dysfunctions. There are five major types of neurogenic bladder dysfunction:

- Uninhibited
- Sensory paralytic (detrusor muscle hyperreflexia)
- Motor paralytic (detrusor muscle areflexia)
- Autonomous
- Reflex

Neurogenic bladder dysfunctions may also be classified according to the level of the lesion in the central nervous system.

Upper motor neuron lesions occur above the sacral segments of the spinal cord. They produce bladders that are spastic or characterized by exaggerated reflexes (hyperreflexia).

Lower motor neuron lesions occur at or below the sacral vertebrae. They produce bladders that are lacking reflexes (areflexic) or tone (atonic).

The incidence of neurogenic bladder dysfunction reflects the incidence and etiology of neurologic injuries or disorders. With certain disorders, a neurogenic bladder may develop in 100% of clients, as with transection of the spinal cord. Clients with conditions such as multiple sclerosis are affected with varying degrees of manifestations.

Etiology and Risk Factors

Risk factors for neurogenic bladder disorders include tumors, neurologic disorders, and trauma to the nervous system. Accidents are the only preventable cause of this problem.

Uninhibited

The uninhibited neurogenic bladder produces "infantile" or uninhibited voiding. The urge to void causes urine to flow. The primary cause is a lesion in the corticoregulatory tracts, as from a stroke or multiple sclerosis.

Sensory

A sensory paralytic bladder results from an interruption in the lateral spinal tracts, as occurs in tabes dorsalis, diabetic neuropathy, and pernicious anemia. Because of the sensory loss, the client cannot sense the bladder filling. This lack of perception leads to atonic bladder, retention with possible overflow incontinence, and upper tract involvement.

Motor

A motor paralytic bladder is the most uncommon type and is caused by lesions in the motor outflow from vertebrae S2 to S4. Disease processes causing this dysfunction include poliomyelitis, tumor, trauma, spina bifida,

FIGURE 36-12 Types of neurogenic bladder dysfunction.

and infection. This dysfunction may be temporary if a bacterial or viral infection is the cause. Although there is full sensation of bladder filling, even to the point of pain, the client cannot initiate micturition.

Autonomous

Clients with an autonomous neurogenic bladder cannot perceive bladder fullness, or they cannot start and maintain urination without some type of exertional pressure. Retention and incontinence are common problems. The autonomous type of dysfunction occurs after destruction of all nerve connections between the bladder and the central nervous system at vertebra S2, S3, or S4 following trauma, inflammatory processes, spinal anesthesia, or malignancy.

Reflex

Transection of the spinal cord above the sacral segments causes a reflex neurogenic bladder. There is no sensation, and the bladder contracts reflexively but does not empty completely.

Pathophysiology

Lesions at the lower motor neuron level of the spinal cord often directly interfere with the reflex arc leading to inappropriate interpretation of efferent and afferent impulses. When the bladder fills, the message is transmitted through afferent fibers to the brain cortex. The injury keeps these impulses from being correctly interpreted, leading to loss of the micturition reflex. A flaccid bladder with urinary retention is the result.

With upper motor neuron lesions, impulses are not transmitted to or from the lower spinal areas to the cortex. When the bladder distends, no sensation is transmitted. Because the lower cord is intact, activity of the reflex arc can occur. The client would have reflex incontinence as a result.

When the damage is to the cortical area itself, as with a stroke or trauma, the client cannot correctly interpret the impulses that are being transmitted. Unless the client is evaluated and treated appropriately, serious UTIs, skin breakdown associated with incontinence, and even renal failure due to chronic overdistention of the bladder are more likely to develop.

Clinical Manifestations

The major clinical manifestation of neurogenic bladder dysfunction is retention with or without incontinence. The client may or may not feel a need to void or feel a sense of bladder distention. The diagnosis is made from the location of neurologic dysfunction. Urodynamic studies, including EMG monitoring, should be done to determine the extent of neurologic involvement to guide an appropriate treatment plan.

Outcome Management
■ Medical Management

Bladder Training. If possible, some form of bladder training should be attempted for a client with neurogenic bladder dysfunction. This measure includes a bladder training program, medication, possible intermittent catheterization, and sometimes surgical intervention.

Medications. A number of medications are used to treat neurogenic bladder dysfunction. Antispasmodics and anticholinergics (such as Detrol, Ditropan, dicyclomine, propantheline, and flavoxate) are given to relieve uninhibited or reflex bladder contractions. Phenoxybenzamine and other alpha-adrenergic blockers may be used. Bethanechol may help stimulate an atonic bladder. Other medications described in the discussion of incontinence may be useful as well.

Preventing Complications. *Autonomic dysreflexia* is a serious, potentially life-threatening complication affecting clients who have spinal cord injuries. It may occur during bladder training programs if the urinary system or bowel becomes obstructed. The most frequent cause is bladder distention or feces in the rectum, although autonomic dysreflexia can be triggered by visceral distention or stimulation of pain receptors in the skin. This condition results from an excessive autonomic response to normal stimuli and affects primarily clients with upper motor neuron lesions.

The most common manifestations are severe hypertension, bradycardia, a throbbing headache, flushing, diaphoresis above the level of the lesion, blurred vision, nasal congestion, nausea, and pilomotor spasm ("goose bumps") above the lesion. If left untreated, this problem can lead to retinal hemorrhage, seizures, or stroke. It is important for the client to recognize the earliest manifestations and summon help immediately. Preventing bladder distention is one way to prevent this emergency. If stool is accumulating in the rectum, careful evacuation should be done to avoid either overdistention or overstimulation.

Medications such as diazoxide (Hyperstat), phenoxybenzamine (Dibenzyline), guanethidine monosulfate (Ismelin), propantheline bromide (Pro-Banthine), phentolamine mesylate (Regitine), and mecamylamine (Inversine) relieve both acute manifestations and the chronic recurrence of episodes.

■ Nursing Management of the Medical Client

Prevent Autonomic Dysreflexia. Always be prepared for the development of autonomic dysreflexia. If severe hypertension (sometimes 300/180 mm Hg), flushing, and a pounding headache suddenly develop, you must address the manifestations immediately.

Nursing interventions involve removal of the triggering stimuli by reestablishing urine flow or removing the fecal impaction. Remove any fecal impaction only after a topical anesthetic agent has been inserted into the rectum to avoid further stimulation. In addition, a catheter may be necessary; if one is already in place, restore its patency by irrigation or by removing kinks and obstructions. Monitor the client's vital signs every 5 minutes, and raise the head of the bed to the semi-Fowler's position. Administer medications as ordered.

Teach Methods to Stimulate Micturition. Neurogenic bladders are difficult to control, but you can teach many clients how to stimulate the micturition reflex and maintain urination. Assist the client by providing external pressure on the abdomen. The client can lean forward or press on the abdomen. Have the client breathe deeply to push the diaphragm downward. Wearing a corset or girdle can provide an extra source of external pressure. The Valsalva maneuver is another method of increasing intra-abdominal pressure on the urinary bladder.

Another method that helps the client learn to empty the bladder is the Credé maneuver. The client places the fingers over the bladder and presses downward slowly toward the symphysis pubis, as though "milking" the urine out of the urinary system. This should be done with great caution. If the client has sphincter dyssynergia (failure of muscle coordination) or if the sphincter does not readily relax, the Credé maneuver can lead to sphincter damage and may cause ureteral reflux if there is any obstruction of outflow. The Credé maneuver is often combined with intermittent self-catheterization.

The client can use several other methods to initiate and maintain micturition. Locate trigger points on the body (lower abdomen, inner thighs, and pubic area), and explain how to stimulate them by stroking, pinching, or applying ice. Stretching the anal sphincter also relaxes the reflexes of the external urethral sphincter because they are both innervated by the pudendal nerve. The client leans forward while sitting on the toilet and inserts two gloved fingers into the anus. The fingers are then either widened apart or pulled posteriorly. Men must be careful to avoid touching the glans penis, which stimulates the bulbocavernosus reflex, contracting the external sphincter.

Perform Intermittent Catheterization. For the treatment of long-term or short-term bladder atony (lack of tone), an intermittent catheterization program is an alternative to indwelling catheterization. A straight urethral catheter is inserted into the bladder at specified intervals, the urine is drained, and the catheter is removed. This may be done in a health care facility or in the client's home (see the Bridge to Home Health Care feature on Inserting Urinary Catheters on p. 906).

Teach Intermittent Self-Catheterization. Clients with bladder atony should be encouraged to learn self-catheterization because it increases independence and mo-

bility. The client or any other person who has been properly educated about the technique may insert the catheter.

Sterile technique is necessary in health care facilities because of the high risk of nosocomial infections. At home, *clean technique* can be used for catheterization without increasing the rate of UTIs. Clean technique is also easier and less expensive for the client. To reduce the risk of bacteriuria, urinary antiseptics and acidification or bladder irrigation with antibiotics and antiseptics are used with each catheterization.

There are several procedural differences between clean and sterile techniques. For clean technique:
1. Gloves are not worn. The client must perform thorough hand-washing before starting.
2. A clean (rather than a sterile) catheter is used.
3. The catheter can be washed and reused indefinitely.
4. Lubricant should be used because the urethra is susceptible to traumatic urethritis.

The catheter should be washed thoroughly after use with soap and water and stored in a clean sandwich-size plastic bag or other clean container.

During self-catheterization, the client may sit or stand. When a female client stands, she should separate her legs or place one leg on a toilet seat. After separating the labia, she can use a mirror to find the meatus.

Timing is important for successful catheterization programs. Catheterization should be carried out at specified intervals throughout the day until bedtime. The interval between catheterization is set according to the degree of continence. The average interval for adults is every 3 to 4 hours, but the client usually has to start at intervals of 2 to 3 hours. Clients should use the catheter to remove 350 to 400 ml of urine each time. A client who cannot follow a schedule is not an appropriate candidate for the program.

The amount of fluid intake allowed is under debate. Some programs allow fluid as desired; others restrict fluid intake to varying degrees. This aspect of the program requires systematic investigation. Clinicians generally recommend that the client drink about 250 ml of fluid at about 2-hour intervals. Ingestion of large amounts of fluid within a short period can cause bladder distention and reflux. Most clients are urged to drink up to 2 L of fluid daily at regular intervals.

A catheter-free bladder and absence of bacteriuria indicate a successful intermittent catheterization program. Controversy exists about the treatment of asymptomatic bacteriuria. A successful catheterization program may be due to several factors, including intermittent bladder distention, which causes stimulation of the normal micturition reflex and reactivation of the bladder's normal antibacterial properties. Other advantages include continence, independence, good hygiene, prevention of complications arising from urinary stasis or a retention catheter, decreased cost, and comfortable sexual relations.

BRIDGE TO HOME HEALTH CARE

Inserting Urinary Catheters

Indwelling catheters may be inserted to treat urinary incontinence. Indications include pressure ulcers or surgical wounds that do not heal, overflow incontinence associated with obstructions that cannot be removed, and decisions of the client or family that dryness and comfort outweigh the risks, especially in cases of serious or terminal illness.

Catheters affect the client's quality of life and self-esteem and are frequently accompanied by recurrent urinary tract infections (UTIs) that can lead to more serious complications and hospitalization. Therefore, you must evaluate whether a catheter is in the client's best interest and whether it will meet the particular client's needs. Catheters should be the last treatment option; consider a referral to a continence care nurse or continence clinic first. You are responsible for providing instructions about daily cleaning, adequate fluid intake, manifestations of UTI, and indications to call the nurse or physician.

Use the smallest French size catheter to meet the client's needs. A 14 to 16F catheter may be the best size for a woman; a 16 to 18F catheter may be best for a man. The balloon should hold 5 to 10 ml of fluid. A catheter that is too large or overinflated causes bladder spasms and urine to leak around the catheter. Men who have an enlarged prostate may need a coudé tip catheter.

Adequate lighting is often a challenge in the home. Consider using a flashlight or small lamp. It may be necessary to ask a family member or informal caregiver to help position the client and to hold the light.

When inserting a urinary catheter, place a female client in the supine position with her knees flexed and separated. Arrange pillows laterally under her knees to provide comfort and increase relaxation. Consider using the posterior approach if the client is obese or has severe lower extremity contractures; turn her on her side facing the other way.

Using sterile technique, check the catheter balloon for appropriate filling, deflate, and set aside on the sterile field. Cleanse the labia and meatal opening one side at a time, using downward stokes; discard the swabs after each stroke. The last swab may be left slightly inside the vagina as a marker.

Ask the client to breathe deeply, and insert the well-lubricated catheter into the meatal opening. When urine returns, insert the catheter another inch and inflate the balloon with the preattached saline syringe; gently pull back to seal the catheter. If no urine returns, gently insert the gloved little finger into the vagina to assess for slippage of the catheter into the vagina.

If a catheter is accidentally inserted into the vagina, leave it in place as a marker. Never reuse a catheter. Obtain a new catheter, and insert with sterile technique as before.

Place male clients in a supine position. Using sterile technique, check the balloon for appropriate filling, then deflate and set aside on the sterile field. Retract the foreskin, and hold the penis at a 60- to 90-degree angle. Clean the glans penis in circular motion, starting at the meatus and working outward. Using a rotating motion, insert the well-lubricated catheter into the meatus. Do not force the catheter if resistance is met, but maneuver it gently as the client breathes deeply, coughs, or bears down.

When urine returns, inflate the catheter balloon with the saline-filled syringe. If placement cannot be verified, notify the physician. Always hang the drainage bag below the bladder level. Many clients prefer to hang the drainage bag on a clean wastepaper can to prevent urine from leaking onto the floor.

Intermittent catheterization is not a panacea. The program requires the client to assume a great deal of personal responsibility. Some clients are not sufficiently motivated to fulfill the responsibilities involved in self-catheterization. Also, some problems can occur when the client is away from home.

Clients with high resting pressures in the bladder that are incontinent between catheterizations are likely to have difficulty with intermittent self-catheterization. All clients should be evaluated before starting the program. If urodynamic evaluation reveals high resting pressures, anticholinergic medications are administered.

■ Surgical Management

Surgery is not the primary treatment option for the client with neurogenic bladder. However, if conservative measures are ineffective in treating the neurogenic bladder, surgical intervention may be necessary. External sphincterotomy or incision of the bladder neck may restore normal bladder emptying. Interrupting innervation to the bladder reflex can aid an uninhibited bladder. Injection of alcohol into the subarachnoid space or rhizotomy (cutting) of the sacral nerves increases bladder capacity by inhibiting reflex bladder contractions, without interfering with normal sphincter function. Sometimes a temporary sacral nerve block is performed before surgery to evaluate the potential candidate. Electrodes may be implanted at thoracic or cervical levels of the spinal epidural space and attached to a percutaneous stimulator. As soon as the client learns to regulate the electrical stimulation properly, the device can be used to inhibit or interrupt reflex bladder contractions.

Continuous intrathecal baclofen administered through an implanted infusion pump is another method of treating a neurogenic bladder. Baclofen helps decrease spasms and detrusor sphincter dyssynergia. Clients report improvement in bladder compliance and capacity. Finally, if all else fails, urinary diversion may be performed to provide the client with a more manageable urinary system.

Nursing Management of the Surgical Client

Nursing care of the client undergoing surgery for a neurogenic bladder with either an external sphincterotomy or a revision of the bladder outlet is the same as for any client undergoing bladder surgery. Urine output maintenance is the priority of these clients. A suprapubic or urinary catheter may be needed until healing occurs.

As with the other surgical procedures, focus care on teaching the client self-care. The client needs to learn to regulate electrical stimulation appropriately to inhibit or interrupt the reflex bladder contractions.

Proper care of the implantable infusion pump is another important area of client education. Care of clients undergoing urinary diversion has been discussed under Bladder Cancer.

Self-Care

The focus of discharge teaching for the neurogenic bladder client is intermittent self-catheterization. Teach the client and significant others a bladder training program and, possibly, a catheterization program. Assess the client's ability to understand and perform self-care procedures, and ensure that the client understands the self-catheterization program. Written materials, teaching videos, and diagrams can be used to reinforce the teaching.

Clients need to be assessed in the home setting to make sure they can function as well as in the hospital. A visiting nurse may be included to help in the discharge planning of the self-catheterization or bladder training program. The client's urinary function should be monitored at regular intervals, including renal function tests and yearly renal ultrasound studies. Teach the client to call the health care provider if manifestations of a UTI develop.

Modifications for Older Clients

Older clients are more likely to have other medical problems, such as arthritis and visual changes, that can interfere with their ability to use the self-catheterization program. However, they may still be able to use this method if they have adequate help.

TRAUMATIC DISORDERS
BLADDER TRAUMA

Bladder trauma is defined as a blunt or penetrating injury to the bladder that may cause bladder rupture. Bladder trauma often results from automobile accidents, when the seat belt compresses the bladder. A bladder distended by urine can rupture with a direct blow to the lower abdomen. The bladder may also be punctured by a bullet, knife, bony splinter from a fractured pelvis, or internal medical instrumentation. When the bladder ruptures, urine spills into the peritoneal cavity. Complications of peritoneal urine accumulation from a ruptured bladder are peritonitis and pelvic cellulitis.

Clinical Manifestations

Bladder injuries usually produce hematuria and pain low in the abdomen or pain referred to a shoulder. The client also may have trouble voiding. Manifestations of peritonitis may develop as well. Fever is usually present as the peritonitis and pelvic cellulitis continue to develop. If the client has had an injury or blow to the abdomen, suspect bladder injury as the cause of the manifestations.

Diagnostic tests include an IVP with lateral views or a CT scan with the bladder full and empty, a cystogram, and a voiding cystourethrogram. If blood is flowing from the meatus, urethral disruption may be present. In this case, catheterization should be avoided until the urethra is evaluated. This allows assessment of both bladder integrity and the bladder's ability to empty.

Outcome Management
Medical Management

The first treatment for suspected bladder injury is insertion of an indwelling or suprapubic catheter to monitor for hematuria or urine production and to keep the bladder decompressed during healing. Any injury other than a simple contusion or very small perforation requires surgical repair.

Nursing Management of the Medical Client

Immediately assess for a suspected bladder injury if the client has had blunt trauma to the lower pelvis or abdomen. Closely monitor the client's urine output for both amount and the presence of hematuria. Report any decrease in urine output in relation to fluid intake to the physician immediately. Careful catheter insertion is necessary for the client with suspected bladder trauma.

Surgical Management

Clients with bladder injuries usually require surgical intervention. After a urethral or suprapubic catheter has been inserted, surgical repair of the damaged bladder wall is performed. The extravasated urine in the perivesical area is drained. It is important to maintain urinary drainage through a patent catheter to promote healing and to avoid the potential development of fistulae or leakage.

Nursing Management of the Surgical Client

Postoperatively, maintain urinary drainage to prevent tension on the sutures in the bladder. A Penrose drain is left in place to allow drainage of any urine remaining in the pelvis. This may necessitate dressing changes.

Because the client may be discharged with an indwelling or suprapubic catheter, teach catheter care to the client and significant others. Assess the client's self-care abilities to determine a possible need for assistance at home. If the client or significant others cannot care for the catheter, arrange for a home health visit.

Follow-up care is essential after discharge to assess healing. A cystogram may be done before the catheter is removed. If a suprapubic catheter has been placed, the client can begin bladder training before the catheter is removed. If the client has a urethral catheter, the catheter is removed before the client can attempt to void. If clients do not void within 4 to 6 hours after removal, the catheter should be reinserted.

URETHRAL TRAUMA

The urethra as well as the bladder may be injured in a pelvic fracture. Falling astride an object, such as the bar on a boy's bike, with sudden force to the groin may cause urethral contusion and laceration. Injury may also occur during medical or surgical interventions, may be self-inflicted, or may occur after female genital mutilation (see Chapter 41). Penetrating wounds also cause urethral damage.

Evaluation of urethral damage is indicated if the client cannot void, has an altered urine stream, or has visible blood at the meatus. Even if the client can pass some urine through the urethra, voiding causes urinary extravasation, resulting in swelling of the scrotum or inguinal areas, which can lead to sepsis and necrosis. Blood may appear at the external meatus and may also extravasate into the surrounding tissues, giving the area an ecchymotic appearance.

The two most common complications of urethral trauma are (1) development of urethral strictures and (2) risk of impotence in men. Impotence occurs because the corpora cavernosa of the penis, blood vessels, or nerves supplying this area are damaged.

Proper management of urethral injuries is controversial. Clinicians generally agree that urinary drainage must first be established with either a urethral or suprapubic catheter. Some physicians suggest an immediate primary surgical repair of the urethra. Others prefer to wait 2 to 3 weeks to see whether the urethra will heal around the urethral catheter without surgery. During any waiting period, the client must be monitored for developing infection and continuing extravasation of urine.

URETERAL TRAUMA

The ureters are located deep within the abdomen and are protected by the spine and surrounding musculature. Thus most ureteral trauma takes place accidentally during surgery. Perforation or tearing may occur during manipulation of intraureteral catheters or other instruments. The ureters may be occluded by ligating sutures or a misplaced clamp, or they may be transected during pelvic surgery. Many surgeons insert ureteral stents before pelvic procedures to easily identify the ureters and prevent trauma. Gunshot and stab wounds may also traumatize the ureters. On occasion, blunt trauma from a car accident can tear these structures.

Trauma is often not discovered until a clinical manifestation develops, such as hematuria, flank pain, or the presence of extravasated urine. As the urine seeps out into the tissues, pain may occur in the lower abdomen and flank. As extravasation continues, there may be sepsis, paralytic ileus, a palpable intraperitoneal mass, and the appearance of urine in an external wound. IVP and ultrasonography are the most definitive means of diagnosis.

Surgical intervention is used to repair the defect, preferably with end-to-end anastomosis. More radical procedures may be needed, such as cutaneous ureterostomy, transureteroureterostomy, and reimplantation. The surgeon may use prosthetic ureteral implants. A nephrectomy is performed if obstruction or sepsis causes severe renal damage. It is essential to treat sepsis aggressively. Significant extravasation of urine may necessitate that the surgeon open the abdomen and drain the urine.

CONGENITAL ANOMALIES

A congenital anomaly of the bladder is exstrophy of the bladder that develops when the symphysis pubis fails to close in utero. The lower anterior abdominal wall and anterior bladder wall are absent, allowing the bladder to protrude through the defective abdominal wall. These conditions are often treated with urinary diversion in childhood, but additional revisions may be needed as the child grows. Children who have had a diversion may be candidates for continent reservoir revisions.

Although congenital anomalies of the ureter are uncommon, several types are described:

1. *Ectopic ureter* occurs when a ureter follows an abnormal course or has an abnormal distal opening. It is the most common congenital ureteral anomaly. An ectopic ureter occurs as a result of the abnormal embryologic development of the ureter. During micturition, this anomaly often results in a back-flow of urine. Misplacement of the meatus (hypospadias and epispadias) is discussed in Chapter 40.

2. *Duplicate ureters,* arising from the same renal pelvis, may develop when the ureters on one side unite at some point; both may open in the normal portion of the trigone or both may open into the urethra or vagina. This anomaly is not usually recognized unless a radiographic study is done for another reason. Pyelonephritis develops, and an evaluation reveals the anomaly. Surgical intervention is usually not necessary unless complications occur.

3. *Abnormal dilation of the ureter (megaureter)* is characterized by dilation and pouching of the ureteral wall just adjacent to the vesicoureteral junction. Resulting manifestations are seen as reflux or obstructive effects, which predispose the client to recurrent UTIs.

4. *Congenital ureteropelvic obstruction* occurs at the junction of the renal pelvis and the ureter. This anomaly is usually bilateral. A mild obstruction may never cause manifestations of a urinary tract disorder. As long as the kidney produces urine at a rate less than 6 ml/min, the ureter can generally handle the flow; however, urine production greater than this rate causes urinary stasis in the kidney, which results in hydronephrosis. If the condition is symptomatic, treatment consists of surgical repair of the narrowed section at the ureteropelvic junction.

CONCLUSIONS

Urinary system disorders can be extremely problematic for clients. Nurses play a major role in the diagnosis, prevention, and treatment of these disorders. Many of the disorders of the urinary system are chronic or become chronic problems, leading to renal disease or incontinence. Some of the manifestations of these disorders can drastically alter the client's self-concept and lifestyle. Problems of the lower urinary tract may become life-threatening, and the nurse must ensure that the client receives prompt and adequate treatment of disorders within the lower urinary system.

THINKING CRITICALLY *evolve*

1. A 28-year-old newlywed woman has been experiencing pain and burning with urination for the past 24 hours. This is the third episode of urinary manifestations she has had in the past 3 months. What is the probable cause of the urinary manifestations? What further information do you need to assess her problem? What can you do to help her treat this problem and prevent further difficulties?

Factors to Consider. For what urinary tract problems does the client's status as a newlywed place her at risk? Which tests would help differentiate an infectious problem from a noninfectious one?

2. The client had a radical cystectomy with formation of an Indiana pouch 12 hours ago. He has a catheter in place, which has drained 10 ml in the last hour. The stoma is a very pale pink. His vital signs are elevated from their preoperative levels. His pulse rate is 100 beats/min, and his temperature is slightly increased. What actions would be appropriate at this point in the client's care?

Factors to Consider. Is the client's urine output within expected limits? What color should a fresh stoma normally be?

3. A 69-year-old man with diabetes is admitted with severe left flank pain, nausea, vomiting, and diarrhea. His abdomen is soft and only slightly tender. His urinalysis reveals increased red blood cells, and his KUB shows a large staghorn calculus in the left kidney with hydronephrosis of the left kidney. What would be a priority assessment for this client?

Factors to Consider. What other diagnostic tests should be done? What are the treatment options for large renal stones?

Discussions for these questions can be found on the website and the CD-ROM.

BIBLIOGRAPHY

1. American Cancer Society. (2003). *Cancer facts and figure*. Atlanta: Author.
2. Appell, R. (2002). Injection therapy for urinary incontinence. In P. Walsh, et al.(Eds.). *Campbell's urology* (8th ed., pp. 1172-1186). Philadelphia: W. B. Saunders.
3. Atala, A., & Keating, M. (2002). Vesicoureteral reflux and megaureter. In P. Walsh, et al.(Eds.). *Campbell's urology* (8th ed., pp. 2053-2116). Philadelphia, W. B. Saunders.
4. Bassi, P. (2002). BCG therapy of high-risk superficial bladder cancer. *Surgical Oncology, 11*(12), 77-83. **EB**
5. Bates, F. (2002). Assessment of the female patient with urinary incontinence. *Urologic Nursing, 22*(5), 305-314.
6. Baumgartner, R., et al. (2002). Causes of increased length of stay following radical cystectomy. *Urologic Nursing, 22*(5), 319-323. **EB**
7. Benson, M., & Olsson, C. (2002). Cutaneous urinary diversion. In P. Walsh, et al. (Eds.). *Campbell's urology* (8th ed., pp. 3789-3834). Philadelphia: W. B. Saunders.
8. Bernier, F., & Jenkins, P. (1997). The role of vaginal estrogen in the treatment of urogenital dysfunction in postmenopausal women. *Urologic Nursing, 17*(3), 92-95. **EB**
9. Bihl, G., & Meyers, A. (2001). Recurrent renal stone disease—advances in pathogenesis and clinical management. *The Lancet, 358*(9828), 651-656.
10. Blaivas, J. & Groutz, A. (2002). Urinary incontinence: Pathophysiology, evaluation, treatment overview, and nonsurgical management. In P. Walsh, et al. (Eds.). *Campbell's urology* (8th ed., pp. 1027-1043). Philadelphia: W. B. Saunders.

11. Blumenfeld, J., & Vaughn, E. (2002). Renal physiology and pathophysiology. In P. Walsh, et al. (Eds.). *Campbell's urology* (8th ed., pp. 169-227). Philadelphia: W. B. Saunders.

12. Boyd, L. (2003). Intravesical bacillus Calmette-Guérin for treating bladder cancer. *Urologic Nursing, 23*(3), 189-192, 199.

 13. Burgio, K., et al. (2002). Behavioral training with and without biofeedback in the treatment of urge incontinence in older women: A randomized controlled trial. *Journal of the American Medical Association, 288*(18), 2293-2299.

 14. Chambers, S.T., et al. (1999). Inhibitors of bacterial growth in urine: What is the role of betaines? *International Journal of Antimicrobial Agents,* 11, 2933-2936.

15. Chancellor, M.B., & Yoshimura, N. (2002). Physiology and pharmacology of the bladder and ureter. In P. Walsh, et al. (Eds.). *Campbell's urology* (8th ed., pp. 831-886). Philadelphia: W. B. Saunders.

16. Cunningham, E., & Marcason, W. (2002). Are there special dietary guidelines for interstitial cystitis? *Journal of the American Dietetic Association, 102*(3), 379.

17. Dusgupta, P., et al. (2001). Cimetidine in painful bladder syndrome: A histopathological study. *British Journal of Urology International, 88*(3), 183-186.

18. Fantl, J. A., et al. (1996). *Urinary incontinence in adults: Acute and chronic management.* AHCPR Publication No. 96-0682. Clinical Practice Guideline, No. 2 (update). Rockville, MD: Agency for Health Care Policy and Research, Public Health Service, U.S. Department of Health and Human Services.

19. Goldman E. L. (2002). Interstitial cystitis: "Evil twin of endometriosis." A 70%-90% concordance between the two. *Ob/Gyn News,* March 15.

20. Gray, M. (2002). Are cranberry juice or cranberry products effective in the prevention or management of urinary tract infection? *Journal of Wound, Ostomy & Continence Nursing,* 29, 122-126.

21. Gray, M. (2002). Continence nursing at the dawn of the 21st century: A futurist perspective. *Urologic Nursing, 22*(4), 233-236.

22. Gray, M., & Krissovich, M. (2003). Does fluid intake influence the risk for urinary incontinence, urinary tract infection, and bladder cancer? *Journal of Wound, Ostomy and Continence, 30*(3), 126-131.

23. Gray, M., & Moore, K. (2004). *Urologic disorders.* St. Louis: Mosby.

24. Greenburg, R., & Ignatoff, J. (2001). Intravesical therapy for refractory transitional cell carcinoma in situ. *Contemporary Urology, 13*(7), 19-21.

25. Hanno, P. (2002). Interstitial cystitis and related disorders. In P. Walsh, et al. (Eds.). *Campbell's urology* (8th ed., pp. 631-670). Philadelphia: W. B. Saunders.

26. Hanson, K. (2002). BCG installations for bladder cancer and latent tuberculosis infections. *Urologic Nursing, 22*(2), 132-134.

27. Herschorn S., & Carr, L.K. (2002). Vaginal reconstructive surgery for incontinence and prolapse. In P. Walsh, et al. (Eds.). *Campbell's urology* (8th ed., pp. 1092-1139). Philadelphia: W. B. Saunders.

28. Howell, A., & Foxman, B. (2002). Cranberry juice and adhesion of antibiotic-resistant uropathogens. *Journal of the American Medical Association, 287*(23), 3083-3084.

29. International Cystitis Association. (1999). Interstitial cystitis and cystoscopy and hydrodistention. *Urologic Nursing, 19*(1), 53-54.

30. Jiminez, V., & Marshall, F. (2002). Surgery of the bladder cancer. In P. Walsh, et al. (Eds.). *Campbell's urology* (8th ed., pp. 2809-2844). Philadelphia: W. B. Saunders.

31. Johnson, W.D., Johnson, C.W., & Lowe M.D. (2002). Tuberculosis and parasitic diseases of the genitourinary system. In P. Walsh, et al. (Eds.). *Campbell's urology* (8th ed., pp. 743-795). Philadelphia: W. B. Saunders.

32. Kunin, C.M. (2001). Nosocomial urinary tract infections and indwelling and indwelling catheter: What is new and what is true? *Chest, 120* (1), 10.

33. Lehmann, S., & Dietz, C. (2002). Double-J stents: They're not trouble free. *RN, 65*(1), 54-60.

34. Li-Ming, S. & Sosa, R.E. (2002). Ureteroscopy and retrograde ureteral access. In P. Walsh, et al. (Eds.). *Campbell's urology* (8th ed., pp. 3306-3318). Philadelphia: W. B. Saunders.

35. Lindberg J.S., & Sprague S. (2001). Nephrolithiasis: Causes and treatment. *Journal of Critical Illness, 16*(10), 446-452.

36. Lingeman, J., et al. (1999). Divergence between stone composition and urine supersaturation: Clinical and laboratory implications. *Journal of Urology, 161,* 1077-1081.

37. Lingeman, J.E., Lifschitz, D.A., & Evan, A.P. (2002). Surgical management of urinary lithiasis. In P. Walsh, et al. (Eds.). *Campbell's urology* (8th ed., pp. 3361-3451). Philadelphia: W. B. Saunders.

38. Lockman, A.R. (2002). What is the best diet to prevent reoccurrence calcium oxalate stones in patients with idiopathic hypercalciuria? (Patient-Orientated Evidence that Matters). *Journal of Family Practice, 5*(4), 305-307.

39. Malkowicz, S.B. (2002). Management of superficial bladder cancer. In P. Walsh, et al. (Eds.). *Campbell's urology* (8th ed., pp. 2785-2802). Philadelphia: W. B. Saunders.

40. Matthews, S.D., & Courts, N.F. (2001). Orthotopic neobladder surgery: Nursing care promotes independence in patients. *American Journal of Nursing, 101*(7), 24AA-24EE.

41. McDougall, E.M., et al. (2002). Percutaneous approaches to the upper urinary tract. In P. Walsh, et al. (Eds.). *Campbell's urology* (8th ed., pp. 3320-3360). Philadelphia: W. B. Saunders.

42. McGuire, E.J., & Clemens, J.Q. (2002). Pubovaginal slings. In P. Walsh, et al. (Eds.). *Campbell's urology* (8th ed., pp. 1151-1172). Philadelphia: W. B. Saunders.

43. McDougall, W. (2002). Use of intestinal segments and urinary diversion. In P. Walsh, et al. (Eds.). *Campbell's urology* (8th ed., pp. 3745-3788). Philadelphia: W. B. Saunders.

44. Menon, M., & Resnick, M.I. (2002). Urinary lithiasis: etiology, diagnosis, and medical management. In P. Walsh, A. Retik, E. Vaughan, & A. Wein (Eds.) *Campbell's urology* (8th ed., pp. 3229-3305). Philadelphia: W.B. Saunders.

45. Messing, E. (2002). Urothelial tumors of the urinary tract. In P. Walsh, A. Retik, E. Vaughan, & A. Wein (Eds.) *Campbell's urology* (8th ed., pp. 2732-2784). Philadelphia: W.B. Saunders.

46. Middelton, L., & Lessick, M. (2003). Inherited urologic malignant disorders: Nursing implications. *Urologic Nursing, 23*(1), 15-29.

47. Miller, A., & Bartsch, H. (2001). Hair dye use and bladder cancer. *International Journal of Cancer, 94*(6), 901-902.

48. Millikan, R. (2001). Chemo's used in bladder cancer must be individualized. *Urology Times, 29,* 4.

49. Moody, F. (Ed.). (1999). *Atlas of ambulatory surgery.* Philadelphia: W. B. Saunders.

50. Morris, R. (1999). Female genital mutilation: Perspectives, risks, and complications. *Urologic Nursing, 19*(1), 13-19.

51. Newman, D., & Palmer, M. (Eds.). (2003). The state of the science on urinary incontinence. *American Journal of Nursing, 3*(suppl.), 1-58.

52. Parsons, C.L. (2000). Interstitial cystitis: New concepts in pathogenesis, diagnosis, and management. *AUA News, 5*, 20-31.

53. Patient-initiated treatment of recurrent urinary tract infection in woman (summaries for patient). (2001). *Annals of Internal Medicine, 135*(1), S18-S24.

54. Payne, C.K. (2002). Urinary incontinence: Nonsurgical management. In P. Walsh, et al. (Eds.). *Campbell's urology* (8th ed., pp. 1069-1091). Philadelphia: W. B. Saunders.

55. Peeker, R., et al. (2000). Intravesical BCG and DMSO in the treatment of classic and nonulcer interstitial cystitis: A prospective randomized double-blind study. *Journal of Urology, 164*, 1912-1915.

56. Ratner, V., & Perilli, L. (2003). Interstitial cystitis: An updated overview. *Urologic Nursing, 23*(2), 107-111.

57. Rosser, M. (2002). Alarming rise in bladder cancer seen in UK: Incidence increased 34% in women vs. 8% men in 25 years, possibly because of smoking. *Urology Times, 5,*1.

58. Sasso, K. (2003). Case study: Challenges of pessary management. *Journal of Wound, Ostomy and Continence Nursing, 30*(3), 152-158.

59. Schaeffer, A. (2002). Infections and inflammations of the genitourinary tract. In P. Walsh, et al. (Eds.). *Campbell's urology* (8th ed., pp. 515-602). Philadelphia: W. B. Saunders.

60. Schoenberg, M. (2002). Management of invasive and metastatic bladder cancer. In P. Walsh, et al. (Eds.). *Campbell's urology* (8th ed., pp. 2803-2817). Philadelphia: W. B. Saunders.

61. Smith, J.J, & Barrett, D.M. (2002). Implantation of the artificial genitourinary sphincter in men and women. In P. Walsh, et al. (Eds.) *Campbell's urology* (8th ed., pp. 1187-1194). Philadelphia: W. B. Saunders.

62. Society of Urologic Nurses and Associates. (1997). *Scope and standards of urologic nursing practice.* Pitman, NJ.

63. Stein, J.P., & Skinner D. (2001). Orthotopic urinary diversion: The new gold standard? *Contemporary Urology, 13*(11), 26-37.

64. Stockert, P. (1999). Getting UTI clients back on track. *RN, 62*(3), 49-52.

65. Stone, J., Wyman, J., & Salisbury, S. (1999). *Clinical gerontological nursing: A guide to advanced practice* (2nd ed.). Philadelphia: W. B. Saunders.

66. Swibold, L. (1999). Maintenance therapy with bacillus Calmette-Guérin in clients with superficial bladder cancer. *Urologic Nursing, 19*(1), 38-41.

67. Urinary Incontinence Guideline Panel. (1992). *Urinary incontinence in adults: A client's guide.* AHCPR Publication No. 92-0040. Rockville, MD: Agency for Health Care Policy and Research, Public Health Service, U.S. Department of Health and Human Services.

68. Urinary Incontinence Guideline Panel. (1992). *Urinary incontinence in adults: Clinical practice guideline.* AHCPR Publication No. 92-0038. Rockville, MD: Agency for Health Care Policy and Research, Public Health Service, U.S. Department of Health and Human Services.

69. Urinary Incontinence Guideline Panel. (1992). *Urinary incontinence in adults: Quick reference guide for clinicians.* AHCPR Publication No. 92-0041. Rockville, MD: Agency for Health Care Policy and Research, Public Health Service, U.S. Department of Health and Human Services.

70. Webster, G., & Gurlnick M.L. (2002). Retropubic suspension surgery for female sphincteric incontinence. In P. Walsh, et al. (Eds.). *Campbell's urology* (8th ed., pp. 1140-1150). Philadelphia: W. B. Saunders.

71. Wein, A. (2002). Neuromuscular dysfunction of the lower urinary tract and its treatment. In P. Walsh, et al. (Eds.). *Campbell's urology* (8th ed., pp. 931-1026). Philadelphia: W.B. Saunders.

72. Wein, A. (2002). Pathophysiology and categorization of voiding dysfunction. In P. Walsh, et al. (Eds.). *Campbell's urology* (8th ed., pp. 887-899). Philadelphia: W.B. Saunders.

Management of Clients with Renal Disorders

Anita E. Molzahn

The kidneys regulate the body's fluid, electrolyte, and acid-base balances while removing toxic substances from the blood and excreting them in urine. The kidneys also play a significant role in erythropoietin and prostaglandin synthesis, in insulin degradation, and in the renin-angiotensin-aldosterone system.

This chapter identifies the common disease processes and injuries that can interfere with normal renal function. Although the effects of extrarenal influences on the kidneys are briefly described, the primary purpose of this chapter is to discuss specific renal pathologic processes. Some of these disorders can result in renal failure (see Chapter 38). Because of the potential seriousness of any renal problem, the client and his or her significant others have physical as well as psychological needs. You need to know about both aspects and should maintain a consistent awareness of the need for appropriate intervention.

EXTRARENAL CONDITIONS

Many conditions located primarily in other parts of the body affect the kidneys, such as diabetes mellitus, hypertension, and sepsis. This chapter provides a brief description of the renal implications of these extrarenal conditions. For further discussion, see Chapters 47, 54, and 83.

DIABETES MELLITUS

One of the most common extrarenal diseases affecting the kidney is diabetes mellitus. *Diabetic nephropathy*, a progressive process, commonly leads to renal failure. About 30% of clients with end-stage renal disease (ESRD) have diabetes mellitus. Researchers estimate that 25% to 50% of clients with insulin-dependent diabetes mellitus (IDDM, or type 1 diabetes) have ESRD within 10 to 20 years of beginning insulin therapy. Renal disease can also occur in the non–insulin-dependent diabetic client. The incidence of proteinuria is about 25% after 20 years of diabetes.

Several pathologic changes lead to renal failure in clients who have diabetes mellitus. The most common is a characteristic intercapillary *glomerulosclerosis*, or scarring of the capillary loops. Progressive microangiopathy, called *nephrosclerosis*, affects the afferent and efferent arterioles and eventually scars the glomerulus, tubules, and interstitium. *Pyelonephritis* (kidney infection) can scar the renal parenchyma and lead to ischemia. It may also lead to renal papillary necrosis and sloughing of the papillae. *Neurogenic bladder* dysfunction may contribute to renal failure. The high incidence of urinary tract infection or the increased pressure in the kidney caused by the backup of urine may also contribute to renal dysfunction.

evolve *Be sure to check out the bonus material on the Evolve website and the CD-ROM, including free self-assessment exercises.*
http://evolve.elsevier.com/Black/medsurg/

Nursing Outcomes Classification (NOC)
for Nursing Diagnoses—Clients with Renal Disorders

Acute Pain and Chronic Pain
  Comfort Level
  Pain Control
  Pain: Disruptive Effects
  Pain Level
Anxiety
  Anxiety Control
  Coping
Excess Fluid Volume
  Fluid Balance
  Hydration
Fatigue
  Activity Tolerance
  Endurance
  Energy Conservation
  Nutritional Status: Energy

Imbalanced Nutrition: Less Than Body Requirements
  Nutritional Status: Food and Fluid
    Intake
Readiness for Enhanced Therapeutic Regimen Management
  Health-Promoting Behavior
  Health-Seeking Behavior
  Knowledge: Health Behaviors
  Knowledge: Health Promotion
  Self-Direction of Care
Risk for Deficient Fluid Volume
  Bowel Elimination
  Fluid Balance
  Hydration
  Knowledge: Medication

  Knowledge: Treatment Regimen
  Urinary Elimination
Risk for Impaired Skin Integrity
  Nutritional Status
  Tissue Integrity: Skin and Mucous
    Membranes
  Tissue Perfusion: Peripheral
Risk for Infection
  Immune Status
  Risk Control
  Risk Detection
Risk for Injury
  Risk Control
  Risk Detection
  Symptom Control

Initially, the sclerotic, or hardening, process of glomerulosclerosis increases renal vascular resistance, contributing to systemic hypertension. This does not cause renal insufficiency. Indeed, the glomerular filtration rate (GFR) may increase as much as 20% to 50% above the normal GFR during this early "silent" phase. It is now recognized that microalbuminemia (measurable by assay) occurs quite some time before clinical proteinuria. If it is diagnosed, it may be a much earlier indicator of eventual renal failure. As more nephrons are destroyed, available functioning renal tissue decreases and the client begins to show clinical proteinuria (a key manifestation), hypertension, edema, and evidence of renal failure.

The kidney metabolizes 30% to 40% of insulin, and as renal function declines the degradation of insulin also decreases, resulting in a lower insulin requirement. Renal failure may be initially identified when the client is evaluated for recurrent insulin reactions. Researchers hope the sclerotic process can be slowed by the following:

- Carefully controlling hypertension
- Adjusting insulin therapy and carefully monitoring blood glucose to maintain euglycemia
- Restricting dietary protein (see the Evidence-Based Practice in Action feature on Managing Hypertension in Diabetics to Slow Progression of Renal Disease on p. 915 and the Complementary and Alternative Therapy feature on Slowing the Progression of Diabetic Nephropathy with a Unique Diet on p. 937).

Regardless of diabetic control, however, renal failure inevitably develops within 5 to 10 years after the appearance of significant proteinuria.

HYPERTENSION

Because the kidneys receive quite a large share of cardiac output, renal function can affect or be affected by cardiovascular changes. Renal blood flow determines the GFR, which directly affects renal function. Hypertension is one condition that can either cause or be affected by renal disease. For example, renovascular hypertension results from renal artery stenosis or renal infarction. The reduction in renal blood flow activates the renin-angiotensin-aldosterone system and increases systemic blood pressure.

Renal hypertension associated with parenchymal renal disease (e.g., glomerulonephritis, polycystic disease, pyelonephritis) usually results from the kidney's decreasing ability to excrete salt and water. Other causes include increased renin release from increased glomerular perfusion and inadequacy of renal vasodilating substances, as occurs with analgesic nephropathy. Among clients with renal failure, 80% to 85% of hypertension results from excess salt and water retention; renovascular hypertension accounts for up to 15% of all systemic hypertension.

On the other hand, sustained systemic high blood pressure adversely affects the kidneys. Researchers report that nephrosclerosis can be seen microscopically in clients who have had uncontrolled hypertension for more than 5 years, although all other renal diagnostic tests may be normal. Kidney damage is the direct result of degenerative changes in the arterioles and interlobular arteries caused by increased blood pressure.

There is a direct correlation between the duration and degree of elevated blood pressure and the severity of renal vascular disease. Progression of the disease usually can be halted or slowed by controlling blood pressure (see the Evidence-Based Practice in Action feature on

EB EVIDENCE-BASED PRACTICE IN ACTION

Managing Hypertension in Diabetics to Slow Progression of Renal Disease

Both diabetes mellitus and hypertension can result in renal failure. One third of hypertensive males lose renal function over 7 years. It has been estimated that 5% of hypertensive clients with elevated serum creatinine levels will require dialysis therapy.[1,3,4,8] Diabetic nephropathy may reduce glomerular filtration rate at a rate of 10 to 12 ml/min/yr if hypertension is untreated. It has been found that lowering blood pressure to less than 130/80 mm Hg in clients with chronic kidney disease slows renal disease progression.[1,4] People with proteinuria of greater than 1 g/24 hr benefit from even tighter control of blood pressure to levels of less than 125/75 mm Hg. Lowering blood pressure reduces mortality in those at risk for cardiovascular events, including diabetic clients.[1,2]

Despite this evidence, management of blood pressure in diabetic clients is less than optimal. Chronic disease management focusing on care processes and intermediate outcomes such as glycemic control found positive outcomes in type 2 diabetic clients. A recent randomized trial of a specialized clinic focusing on intensified multiple risk factor intervention showed improved microvascular disease and a trend toward improved macrovascular disease in diabetic clients within 4 years.[7] Similar benefits were seen in a before-and-after study of diabetic clients with more advanced chronic kidney disease.[9] Multidisciplinary clinics offering care by nurses and physicians and sometimes other professionals, have demonstrated improved outcomes.[5,6,8]

Implications

Control of blood pressure in diabetic clients and good disease management can improve outcomes and can slow progression of renal disease in diabetic clients. Nurses, in their roles as primary health care providers and as members of specialized disease management teams, can reduce the morbidity and complications associated with diabetes and hypertension. Further research should address the specific interventions and strategies that are most effective.

References

1. Chobanian, A. et al. (2003). The Seventh Report of the Joint National Committee on Prevention, Detection, Evaluation, and Treatment of High Blood Pressure: The JNC 7 Report. *Journal of the American Medical Association, 289*(19), 2560-2572.
2. Estacio, R.O., et al. (2000). Effect of blood pressure control on diabetic microvascular complications in patients with hypertension and type 2 diabetes. *Diabetes Care, 23 (suppl2)*, B54-B64.
3. Hajjar, I., & Kotchen, T. (2003). Trends in prevalence, awareness, treatment, and control of hypertension in the United States, 1988-2000. *Journal of the American Medical Association, 290*(2), 199-206.
4. Hansson, L., et al. for the HOT Study Group. (1998). Effects of intensive blood pressure lowering and low dose aspirin in patients with hypertension: Principal results of the Hypertension Optimal Treatment randomized trial. *Lancet, 351,* 1755-1782.
5. Norris, S.L., et al. (2002). The effectiveness of disease and case management for people with diabetes: A systematic review. *American Journal of Preventative Medicine, 22,* 15-38.
6. Sidorov, J., et al. (2002). Does diabetes disease management save money and improve outcomes? *Diabetes Care, 25,* 684-689.
7. UK Prospective Diabetes Study Group. (1998). Tight blood pressure control and risk of macrovascular and microvascular complications in type 2 diabetes. *British Medical Journal, 317,* 703-713.
8. Wagner, E.H., et al. (2001). Chronic care clinics for diabetes in primary care: A system wide randomized trial. *Diabetes Care, 24,* 695-700.
9. Walker, W.G., et al. (1992). Renal function change in hypertensive members of the Multiple Risk Factor Intervention Trial. *Journal of the American Medical Association, 268,* 3085-3091.

Managing Hypertension in Diabetics to Slow Progression of Renal Disease, above). Client teaching is vital to managing the hypertension and preventing renal failure.

HYPOTENSION

Cardiovascular shock, or hypotension, also affects renal function. Renal vasoconstriction reduces renal blood flow. Because of the autoregulation capabilities of the kidneys (see Chapters 13, 14, 34, and 83), however, GFR remains at a functional level until the advanced stages of systemic shock, at which time acute renal failure develops. Restoring systemic blood pressure usually reverses the renal vasoconstriction, and kidney function returns, typically within 2 to 8 weeks provided prolonged ischemia has not occurred. A period of polyuria (excessive urination) may follow the correction of hypovolemia, although the mechanisms for this are unclear.

Before renal function returns to normal, another oliguric period may occur, followed by a "mobilization phase" in which sequestered fluid is shifted into the intravascular space. This shift may cause some hypertension until the kidneys can remove the extra fluid. Careful assessment of the client's fluid status and meticulous fluid management are crucial during these recovery phases.

RHABDOMYOLYSIS

Rhabdomyolysis is a disorder usually associated with traumatic injury of skeletal muscle tissue, which releases myoglobin and intracellular substances into the blood. It can also occur after serious crush injuries, strenuous exercise, seizures, heat stroke, prolonged coma, and drug overdose. The resulting acute renal failure is usually reversible with treatment.

Clinical evidence of rhabdomyolysis includes fever, malaise, nausea, vomiting, muscular weakness, pain, and swelling. The release of substances from damaged muscles results in myoglobinemia, myoglobinuria (which can be seen as brown urine and confirmed through urinalysis), hyperkalemia, hyperphosphatemia, hyperuricemia, and elevated creatine kinase levels. Hypocalcemia occurs initially because of the precipitation of calcium with phosphate. Later, in the diuretic phase of acute renal failure, hypercalcemia can occur as calcium is mobilized.

Treatment is typically symptomatic, including bed rest to reduce muscle metabolism and steps to correct acidosis and electrolyte imbalances and maintain normal fluid volume. In severe cases, dialytic therapy may be necessary.

CARDIOVASCULAR DISEASE

Cardiac disease influences kidney function primarily through its effect on cardiac output and circulating blood volume. The hemodynamic and hormonal changes of cardiac disease may decrease the kidneys' ability to excrete sodium and water. This, in turn, increases intravascular congestion and edema and establishes a pathologic cycle.

Hemodynamic changes also occur with normal aging. Blood flow to the kidneys decreases by up to half by age 70 years, and GFR can decrease by 40% to 50% as well. Renal function deteriorates as glomeruli become sclerotic and atrophy.

PERIPHERAL VASCULAR DISEASE

Thromboembolic disease can affect the renal circulation and cause infarction of the tissue supplied by the affected blood vessel. In clients with sickle cell disease, the interstitial hypertonicity and low oxygen pressure found in the renal medulla seem to favor sickling of red blood cells in the kidney's juxtamedullary region. These cell masses cause gross hematuria as venules rupture, papillary necrosis, renal infarction, concentrating disturbances resulting from interference with the countercurrent mechanism, nephrotic syndrome, pyelonephritis, and, finally, renal failure.

In disseminated intravascular coagulation (DIC), in which diffuse clotting consumes clotting factors and causes hemorrhage in affected areas throughout the body, the kidney is the organ most affected.

SEPSIS

Extrarenal sepsis may affect kidney function either through its effect on systemic circulation or by stimulating the immune system. Renal reactions to septic shock are similar to those in hypotension. Immunologic injury can lead to glomerulonephritis (see Glomerulonephritis

later in this chapter). Occasionally, pathogens may break away from extrarenal foci of infection and travel to the kidney to establish additional sites.

PREGNANCY

Pregnancy has a definite influence on kidney function. During the first trimester, the collecting system dilates and the kidneys enlarge; this may persist 9 to 12 weeks after delivery. Renal blood flow and GFR increase by 30% to 50% during pregnancy, contributing to increased creatinine clearance and decreased uric acid excretion. These normal changes (such as lower serum creatinine) must be taken into account in interpreting laboratory findings for pregnant women. Pregnancy also increases the likelihood of proteinuria (usually transient), polyuria, and nocturia (excessive urination at night). These disorders may be caused by external bladder compression and alterations in antidiuretic hormone metabolism.

OTHER CAUSES

Kidney function is influenced by many other extrarenal disease processes, such as cancer, connective tissue disorders, and metabolic disturbances. Many systemic diseases produce clinical manifestations like those of glomerulonephritis, although they typically have other systemic features characteristic of the disease (see Glomerulonephritis). These diseases include systemic lupus erythematosus (SLE), systemic scleroderma, polyarteritis nodosa, thrombocytopenic purpura, Wegener's granulomatosis, hemolytic-uremic syndrome, gout, amyloidosis, and Henoch-Schönlein syndrome. Diagnosis can be confirmed by renal biopsy.

Renal disease has become an increasingly common complication for people infected with the human immunodeficiency virus (HIV). Among the several renal disorders associated with HIV and acquired immunodeficiency syndrome (AIDS) are renal tuberculosis and cytomegalovirus, such malignancies as lymphoma and Kaposi's sarcoma, and HIV-associated nephropathy, a focal glomerulosclerosis that is manifested by nephrotic syndrome (see Nephrotic Syndrome later in this chapter).

NEPHROTOXINS

Nephrotoxins have specific, destructive effects on renal cells. They can cause the following types of renal injury:
- Acute tubular necrosis
- Defects in the tubular transport system
- Interstitial nephritis
- Vasculitis
- Nephrotic syndrome

Nephrotoxic substances in the environment include heavy metals, such as mercurial compounds, lead, cadmium, bismuth, arsenic, copper, and phosphorus; carbon tetrachloride; ethylene glycol; trichloroethylene; carbon monoxide; and chlorinated hydrocarbons. Exposure to many of these substances occurs in industrial locations. Other environmental nephrotoxins include snake venom and certain mushrooms. Acute tubular necrosis is the most frequent injury resulting from exposure to nephrotoxins. Some nephrotoxins also cause tubular transport defects and nephrotic syndrome. Box 37-1 presents some common nephrotoxic substances.

All five types of kidney damage may result from nephrotoxic reactions to medications. Two types of medications well known to cause renal damage are antibiotics and certain analgesics. Because the kidneys are the major route of excretion for many antibiotics, renal tissue is directly exposed to these compounds. The longer the exposure, the higher the risk of renal toxic effects. Pre-existing renal disease, decreased renal blood flow, electrolyte imbalances, and concurrent use of other nephrotoxic medications enhance a medication's nephrotoxic effect.

High-risk antibiotics include cephalosporins, sulfonamides, polymyxins, aminoglycosides, and amphotericin B. Carefully monitor renal function tests to identify early nephrotoxic reactions so that causative medications can be discontinued or the dose decreased. Closely monitor drug levels to ensure that dosages stay in the therapeutic range. Besides using these medications as briefly as possible and at as low a dose as possible, maintaining a high fluid intake may help prevent nephrotoxic effects. A high urine output keeps the medication diluted in the kidney and helps prevent crystallization.

The risk of renal damage caused by excessive use of certain analgesics has been receiving more attention. Salicylates, acetaminophen, phenacetin, and nonsteroidal anti-inflammatory drugs (NSAIDs) are the most common nephrotoxic agents. Short-term overdose or long-term consistent use of these medications may cause acute tubular necrosis or chronic renal failure. Researchers estimate that 5% to 10% of clients with ESRD have analgesic nephropathy.

Anesthesia reduces the kidney's vasoconstrictive ability, which helps protect it against systemic blood pressure drops; thus the kidney is made more vulnerable to the effects of shock. In addition, certain anesthetics, particularly methoxyflurane, have a direct nephrotoxic effect. Administration of this general anesthetic agent can cause acute tubular necrosis and has been associated with fatal acute renal failure. Halothane may also adversely affect renal function.

Diuretics may have nephrotoxic effects as well and, when used aggressively, can cause hypovolemia. Other common medications that may have nephrotoxic effects include probenecid, phenytoin, low-molecular-weight dextran, rifampin, phenindione, lithium, and gold. You must know about the possible adverse effects of any medication a client takes so that you can assess and intervene appropriately.

Radioiodinated contrast agents used in radiographic and computed tomographic (CT) studies have been associated with acute tubular necrosis. Risk factors include:

- Age older than 60 years
- Pre-existing renal insufficiency, especially diabetic nephropathy
- Dehydration
- Low cardiac output with pre-existing renal disease
- Proteinuria
- Hypoalbuminemia
- Multiple myeloma
- Multiple contrast studies within a 24-hour period

Using non-dye studies whenever possible and keeping the client well hydrated throughout the test will reduce the risk of acute renal failure. Baseline renal function tests before the contrast study should be available to compare with post-test findings. Monitor the client's urine output carefully for several hours after the study is completed. (See the Complementary and Alternative Therapy feature on Oral Acetylcysteine Supplements for Preventing Acute Deterioration in Renal Function After Coronary Angiography in Moderate Renal Insufficiency on p. 937.)

ACQUIRED DISORDERS
NEPHROLITHIASIS

Although calculi (stones) can form anywhere in the urinary tract, the most frequent site is the kidney. These stones may travel down the urinary tract, lodge anywhere along the tract, and cause obstruction and tissue damage, or they may stay in the kidney. Urolithiasis is described in detail in Chapter 36.

BOX 37-1   *Nephrotoxins*

Antibiotics
Aminoglycosides
Tetracyclines
Amphotericin B
Cephalosporins
Sulfonamides
  (co-trimoxazole)
Bacitracin
Polymyxin
Colistin

Heavy Metals
Lead
Mercury
Arsenic
Copper
Gold
Lithium

Poisons
Mushrooms
Insecticides
Herbicides
Snake bites

Anesthetics

Contrast Dyes

Organic Solvents
Glycols
Gasoline
Kerosene
Turpentine
Tetrachloroethylene

Other Drugs
Acetaminophen
Nonsteroidal anti-
  inflammatory drugs
Salicylates
Heroin
Dextran
Mannitol
Interleukin-2
Cisplatin
Amphetamines

Treatment and nursing care of clients with renal calculi are similar to those of people with calculi lower in the urinary tract. Damage to the kidney caused by calculi can be permanent, however, and may require nephrectomy (described later).

PYELONEPHRITIS

Pyelonephritis is an inflammation of the renal pelvis and parenchyma caused by a bacterial infection. The cause may be an active infection in the kidney or the remnants of a previous infection. The two main types of pyelonephritis are acute and chronic. They differ primarily in their clinical picture and long-term effects.

Etiology and Risk Factors

Sometimes an infection may be a primary disease, as happens with reduced host resistance (e.g., calculi, malignancy, hydronephrosis, or trauma). Most kidney infections, however, are extensions of infectious processes located elsewhere, especially the bladder. Chapter 36 discusses the etiologic mechanism and pathogenesis of infections in the lower urinary tract.

The bacteria spread to the kidney primarily by ascending the ureter to the kidney. Blood and lymphatic circulation also provide channels for the organisms. Ureteral reflux, which allows infected urine back into the ureter, and obstruction, which causes urine to back into the ureter and allows organisms to multiply, are the most common causes of ascending urinary tract infections. *Escherichia coli* is the most common bacterial organism that causes pyelonephritis.

Health promotion is key to preventing the recurrence of infection and further renal damage. The nurse provides information to clients about health and lifestyle measures to prevent urinary tract infections, including (1) perineal hygiene measures such as wiping from front to back, (2) acidification of the urine (by drinking cranberry juice or taking ascorbic acid), and (3) ensuring adequate fluid intake. Early detection and adequate treatment of lower urinary tract infections greatly reduce the incidence of pyelonephritis.

After infection health maintenance includes education about the importance of completing the course of antibiotics. Follow-up cultures are important with recurrent pyelonephritis to ensure that the infection has been eradicated. Health restoration measures depend on the extent of renal damage and the cause of the disease. If obstruction precipitated the infection, the cause of the obstruction must be treated.

Acute Pyelonephritis

Acute pyelonephritis often occurs after bacterial contamination of the urethra or after introduction of an instrument, such as a catheter or a cystoscope.

Chronic Pyelonephritis

Chronic pyelonephritis is more likely to occur after chronic obstruction with reflux or chronic disorders. It is slowly progressive and usually is associated with recurrent acute attacks, although the client may not have a history of acute pyelonephritis.

Pathophysiology

Pyelonephritis occurs when bacteria enter the renal pelvis, causing an inflammatory response and an increase in white blood cells (WBCs). The inflammation leads to edema and swelling of the involved tissue, beginning at the papillae and sometimes spreading to the cortex. The infection can be either ascending, as occurs after cystitis or prostatitis, or descending, as from a streptococcal infection in the bloodstream.

As the infection is treated and the inflammation recedes, fibrosis and scar tissue may develop. The calices become blunted with scarring in the interstitial tissues. If the infection recurs, more scar tissue develops; fibrosis and altered tubular reabsorption and secretion lead to decreased renal function.

Acute Pyelonephritis

Acute pyelonephritis is associated with the development of renal abscesses, perinephric abscesses, emphysematous pyelonephritis, and chronic pyelonephritis, which can lead to renal failure.

Acute pyelonephritis is usually brief. It often recurs, however, either as a relapse of a previous infection not eradicated or as a new infection; 20% of these recurrences take place within 2 weeks after completion of therapy. A client must be treated adequately to prevent the development of chronic pyelonephritis. The infection may also progress to bacteremia.

Chronic Pyelonephritis

This disease is characterized by a combination of caliceal abnormalities and overlying cortical scarring. The kidney becomes contracted, and the number of functioning nephrons decreases as they are replaced by scar tissue. Renal failure may ensue, although uremia is less common than once thought.

Clinical Manifestations

Acute Pyelonephritis

Acute pyelonephritis is characterized by enlarged kidneys, focal parenchymal abscesses, and accumulation of polymorphonuclear lymphocytes around and in the renal tubules. Typically, the client seems to be in acute distress, although in some cases this disorder causes minimal or no manifestations.

Assessment usually reveals high fever, chills, nausea, flank pain on the affected side (costovertebral angle [CVA] tenderness), headache, muscle pain, and general prostration. The pain commonly radiates down the ureter or toward the epigastrium and may be colicky if the infection is complicated by calculi or sloughed renal papillae. Percussion or deep palpation over the CVA elicits marked tenderness. Commonly, the client has experienced dysuria, frequency, urgency, and other evidence of cystitis for several days. The urine may be cloudy or bloody, is foul smelling, and shows a marked increase in WBCs and casts. Chapter 34 describes the assessment of the renal system.

Urine culture and sensitivity studies, along with a physical examination, are the primary diagnostic tests. Studies may be done to detect calculi, especially with recurrent infections, because calculi may seed and cause reinfection, particularly with *Proteus*. X-ray studies, as of the kidney, ureter, and bladder (a KUB study), and intravenous pyelography (IVP) are commonly done. A cystourethrogram may be obtained, especially after an initial episode of pyelonephritis, to look for underlying defects, particularly any cause of reflux. Magnetic resonance imaging (MRI) or a CT scan may also be used to evaluate the kidney size or the presence of other problems.

Chronic Pyelonephritis

This disease has no specific manifestations of its own. Thus it is usually discovered incidentally when the client is being evaluated for hypertension or its complications. Hypertension itself is the most frequent manifestation of the disease.

Abnormal laboratory studies may show azotemia, pyuria, anemia, acidosis, and proteinuria. They may also demonstrate poor urine-concentrating ability.

Outcome Management
■ Medical Management

Acute Pyelonephritis

Ideal outcomes of medical management include the following:

- Elimination of the pathogenic organisms with appropriate antibiotics, as identified by urine culture and sensitivity studies
- Removal of any factor or disease contributing to decreased host resistance

If calculi or other obstructions are found to be the cause of recurrent infection, appropriate treatment must be instituted.

Inhibit Bacterial Growth. Antibiotic therapy is based on the results of urine culture and sensitivity tests. Typically, a broad-spectrum antibiotic is prescribed; it may be changed after the results of the culture are available. Sulfonamides or the combination of sulfamethoxazole and trimethoprim is commonly used as first-line therapy unless the client is allergic to one of these drugs. Typically, antibiotic therapy continues for 10 days to 2 weeks.

Antibiotics may be administered orally or by the single large-dose method described in Chapter 36. In severe cases of acute pyelonephritis, intravenous antibiotics may be administered. With oral therapy, the client must understand that completing the full course of antibiotic therapy is important to prevent recurrence of the infection. Recurrent infections are commonly treated with long-term prophylactic antibiotic therapy. Additional pharmacologic therapy may be needed to correct any predisposing factors.

Relieve Pain. Analgesic or urinary antiseptic medications can be prescribed to reduce discomfort. Antibiotics quickly reduce discomfort as well.

Chronic Pyelonephritis

The desired outcome of medical management is prevention of further renal damage. If bacteria are found, appropriate antibiotics are given, as in acute pyelonephritis. Chronic pyelonephritis tends to be less painful. Above all, hypertension must be controlled. Additional intervention depends on the degree of renal failure that has already occurred. Although high fluid intake may be advisable in acute pyelonephritis, it may be contraindicated in chronic pyelonephritis if the degree of renal dysfunction is significant.

Inhibit Bacterial Growth. Antibiotics specific to the bacteria present are given to treat chronic pyelonephritis (see Acute Pyelonephritis and Chapter 36).

Control Hypertension. Renal damage can cause hypertension, which can cause further renal damage. Thus it is important to control the client's blood pressure. Reduction of dietary sodium and pharmacologic therapy may be indicated. Management of hypertension is discussed in Chapter 54.

■ Nursing Management of the Medical Client
Assessment

Assessment of the client with pyelonephritis begins with a thorough history and physical examination, giving close attention to the presence of risk factors, previous urinary tract infections, hypertension, and CVA tenderness. Look for evidence of pyelonephritis.

Diagnosis, Outcomes, Interventions

Diagnosis: Risk for Deficient Fluid Volume. A common diagnosis is *Risk for Deficient Fluid Volume related to fever, nausea, vomiting, and possible diarrhea.*

Outcomes. The client will remain free of fluid volume deficiency as evidenced by balanced intake and output, maintenance of adequate hydration, and an absence of manifestations of dehydration.

Interventions. Prepare the client for the diagnostic tests and probable antibiotic therapy. Clients with severe nausea and vomiting may require intravenous fluids. Keep in mind that overhydration may dilute antimicrobials, diminishing their effectiveness. See Chapter 36 on the nursing care of the client with cystitis.

Diagnosis: Acute Pain. Another common nursing diagnosis is *Acute pain related to an inflammatory process in the kidney and possible colic.*

Outcomes. The client will report either no pain or that pain is controlled.

Interventions. Medications can be given to control pain caused by calculi. CVA tenderness should decrease as the antibiotics control the infection. Medication for nausea can be given as needed with antipyretics for high fevers. Adequate treatment of the infection quickly reverses the dysuria, pyuria, and frequency. Urinary analgesics (see Chapter 36) can also help the client with these problems. Fluid intake of 3 to 4 L daily is recommended. This fluid helps to dilute the urine and to reduce irritation and burning. The continual flow of urine serves to prevent stasis and discourage multiplication of bacteria in the urinary tract.

Diagnosis: Readiness for Enhanced Therapeutic Regimen Management. Client teaching is important to promote self-care and to prevent recurrent infections. Write the diagnosis *Readiness for Enhanced Therapeutic Regimen Management to prevent recurrent infections.*

Outcomes. The client will understand how to prevent recurrent infections as evidenced by the client's statements and no recurrence of infection.

Interventions. The preventive measures for acute and chronic pyelonephritis are similar to those for cystitis (see Chapter 36). It is important to prevent permanent renal damage. Ensure that the client can recognize the manifestations of a urinary tract infection and knows to seek prompt medical attention when these manifestations do occur.

When the acute infection subsides, instruct the client to continue follow-up care. This care includes completing the full course of antibiotic therapy and having repeated urine cultures. Also, teach ways to prevent further infections in the urinary tract, including ensuring a high fluid intake (see Chapter 36).

It is vital that the client return for follow-up urine cultures and possibly other diagnostic tests if the cause of the pyelonephritis is not clear. Emphasize that follow-up cultures are important because bacteriuria may be present without producing any manifestations. Advise the client to report any manifestations of recurrence immediately so that retreatment can begin.

Evaluation

The infection should subside with adequate antibiotic treatment. Successful management results in reduced pain and negative findings on follow-up urine cultures. The client must also be made aware of the cause of this infection and ways to prevent further infections (see Chapter 36).

■ Self-Care
The focus of client self-care is to maintain high levels of fluid intake and prevent recurrence of infection. If manifestations arise, the client must report them promptly and begin treatment to prevent further renal damage.

■ Modifications for Older Clients
In older clients, the kidneys may be less able to recover from a severe infection. Antibiotic therapy should be monitored closely because older adults often vary in their sensitivity and response to the medication. Older adults may also have altered blood levels of antibiotics because renal perfusion decreases with age, reducing the kidney's ability to excrete drugs.

OTHER INFECTIOUS PROCESSES
Bacteria cause most cases of pyelonephritis, but renal candidiasis, a fungal infection, is increasing. Renal tuberculosis and renal abscesses and perinephric abscesses are other less common infectious processes. They are briefly described in Table 37-1.

HYDRONEPHROSIS
Hydronephrosis is distention of the renal pelvis and calices caused by an obstruction of normal urine flow. Urine production continues, and the urine is trapped proximal to the obstruction. Causes of occlusion include calculus, tumor, scar tissue, congenital structural defects, and a kink in the ureter.

Whatever the cause, the accumulating urine exerts pressure on the renal pelvis wall. At low to moderate pressures, the kidney may dilate with no obvious loss of function. Over time, sustained or intermittent high pressure causes irreversible nephron destruction. In addition to pressure-related problems, pyelonephritis is always a risk because of urinary stasis.

Outcome Management
■ Medical Management
Treatment aims to relieve the obstruction and prevent infection. Depending on the location of the obstruction, it may involve placement of a ureteral catheter or stent

TABLE 37-1	*Less Common Renal Infectious Processes*			
Type of Infectious Process	**Clinical Manifestations**	**Diagnosis**		**Treatment**
Renal candidiasis	Ureteral obstruction Progressive oliguria Pyuria Progressive renal failure	Urine culture Presence of serum *Candida precipitans* Radiological findings of hydronephrosis, caliceal erosion, filling defects		Amphotericin B Flucytosine
Renal tuberculosis	Often nonspecific General malaise Weight loss Low-grade fever Night sweats Manifestations of cystitis Flank pain, hematuria Pyuria, epididymitis	Growth of *Mycobacterium tuberculosis* in culture		Anti-tubercular agents, usually several medications Possible total or partial nephrectomy Possible urinary diversion if severe strictures or bladder damage
Renal abscess or perinephric abscess	Fever, tenderness Flank or loin pain Manifestations of sepsis Weakness Anorexia Weight loss	Ultrasound findings		Aggressive antibiotic therapy Surgical incision and drainage

above the point of obstruction. Typically, surgery is required (see Chapter 36) to relieve the obstruction and restore adequate drainage of the urinary system.

Removal of the obstruction results in sudden release of the pressure on the renal parenchyma caused by the trapped urine, which leads to diuresis. Thus postobstructive diuresis occurs and can lead to fluid and electrolyte imbalances, including dehydration. The kidney gradually begins to concentrate urine appropriately.

■ Nursing Management of the Medical Client
Assessment

Assessment of a client with hydronephrosis includes monitoring for the presence, location, intensity, and character of pain. Monitor urine output, and report manifestations of renal failure (oliguria, anorexia, lethargy), hematuria, and dysuria. Reduced urine output could indicate obstruction. Palpate the client's bladder to assess for any manifestations of distention. The kidneys, if palpated, may be tender.

Diagnosis, Outcomes, Interventions

Diagnosis: Risk for Deficient Fluid Volume. *Risk for Deficient Fluid Volume related to increased urine output* is the most important nursing problem. Because of the

dangers involved in postobstruction diuresis, it is crucial to monitor the client closely after an obstruction is released.

Outcomes. The client will maintain a normal fluid volume, as evidenced by balanced intake and output, maintenance of adequate hydration, and no manifestations of dehydration.

Interventions. Make frequent assessments, including hourly outputs; daily weights; vital signs every 30 minutes for the first 4 hours and then every 2 hours; urine for specific gravity, albumin, and glucose; and edema. Also make periodic serum electrolyte and glucose determinations, and consider the expected presence of severe fatigue caused by urinary losses and the need for frequent observation. Fluid management during this period is crucial; hourly fluid replacement is based on the previous hour's output.

Evaluation

The client with hydronephrosis must understand the importance of fluid balance, the need to monitor urine output, and the need to report any changes in condition. Specific evaluation criteria will vary depending on the cause of obstruction.

■ Surgical Management

Surgery is commonly required to relieve the obstruction causing hydronephrosis. Management of the surgical client is discussed under urolithiasis in Chapter 36.

■ Self-Care

Clients who have had hydronephrosis should watch for manifestations of infection and obstruction, such as pain and reduced urine output. Avoiding urinary tract infections is important in preventing pyelonephritis and preserving renal function (see Chapter 36).

RENAL CANCER

Benign kidney tumors are rare. Classifications include lymphangioma, lipoma, medullary fibroma, adenoma, leiomyoma, and oncocytoma. When large benign tumors occur, it is relatively impossible to distinguish them from a malignant tumor by x-ray examination.

At least 85% of all renal tumors are malignant, and about 11,900 people die of kidney cancer each year. The tumors are most common in people 50 and 70 years of age. They affect men more often than women. About 31,900 new cases of renal cancer were expected to be diagnosed in the United States in 2003.[1]

Etiology and Risk Factors

The exact cause of renal tumors is unknown. Some links have been established between renal cancer and tobacco, lead, cadmium, and phosphates. A genetic link has also been postulated.

Because of the possible association between smoking and renal cancer, one means of avoiding renal cancer may be to quit or not to start smoking; avoiding exposure to chemicals such as lead, phosphate, and cadmium may also prevent some renal cancers. The cause of many renal cancers is not established, however, and prevention may not be possible.

After surgery, most people have difficulty in dealing with cancer and the risk of recurrence. If nephrectomy is required, clients are often concerned about living with only one kidney. Assure clients that one kidney can meet the body's needs but that care should be taken to protect that kidney. The care includes preventing injuries and infections; controlling blood pressure if necessary; and maintaining overall health and well-being through adequate nutrition, rest, and so on.

Pathophysiology

Renal cell carcinoma, or adenocarcinoma, is the most common tumor type; it accounts for 90% of all kidney neoplasms. Tumor growth begins in the renal cortex and usually continues for some time before it produces manifestations. The tumor can grow very large and tends to compress the adjacent renal parenchyma rather than infiltrate it. The tumor, usually avascular, tends to surround blood vessels and constrict them. The lungs and

mediastinum are the most frequent metastatic sites of occurrence. Liver, bone, skin, spleen, renal vein, and brain are other common sites of metastases.

Other types of renal cancer include (1) nephroblastoma, (2) sarcoma, and (3) epithelial tumors in the renal pelvis.

Nephroblastoma, or Wilms' tumor, is primarily a childhood disease, although it occasionally occurs in adults. The prognosis for adults is worse than for children, with some sources reporting only a 25% survival rate. Sarcoma is infrequent and typically arises in the renal capsule. Most tumors of the renal pelvis are primarily urothelial in origin and include three tissue types: transitional cell, squamous cell, and adenocarcinoma.

Spontaneous regression of renal adenocarcinoma reportedly occurs in fewer than 1% of all cases. Most of these regressions occur after nephrectomy and involve metastatic areas. Authorities consider these episodes as evidence that the disease is associated with immunologic or hormonal factors.

Clinical Manifestations

Manifestations of renal malignancies vary, and tumor growth may advance significantly before the disease is discovered. It is not uncommon for the client to have clinical manifestations apparently unrelated to renal disease. Frequently, a palpable abdominal mass found during a routine physical examination arouses the first suspicion. The average time between the onset of hematuria and the onset of pain is 9 months and that between initial pain and diagnosis is 14 months. Extrarenal manifestations are commonly found before a diagnosis of renal cancer is confirmed. Up to 35% of clients have metastasis when the final diagnosis of a renal neoplasm is made.

The common triad of manifestations consists of hematuria, flank pain, and a palpable abdominal or flank mass. The hematuria is usually gross and intermittent, which helps to explain the client's delay in seeking medical advice. The clinical picture also contains a combination of the following usual findings: fever, weight loss and cachexia, fatigue, hypertension, amyloidosis, thrombophlebitis, anemia, erythrocytosis, hypercalcemia, abnormal serum liver profile, and an elevated erythrocyte sedimentation rate (ESR). Less frequent findings include peripheral neuropathy, inferior vena cava obstruction, priapism, and varicocele. Hydronephrosis may occur if the tumor obstructs the ureteropelvic junction. The incidence of pulmonary embolus as a presenting manifestation may be higher than previously thought because of the high rate of vena cava and renal vein involvement. Plasma erythropoietin, renin, and chorionic gonadotropin levels are elevated, and prostaglandin production increases in renal cell carcinoma.

Several diagnostic tests help confirm a diagnosis of renal cancer. IVP is probably the most helpful in identifying a space-occupying lesion. Ultrasonography helps differentiate a cyst from a solid mass. Other noninvasive procedures include CT scan, nephrotomography, and radioisotope studies. Arteriography is used to evaluate the renal vascular system. Renal biopsy, usually done percutaneously, provides definitive data about the lesion.

Outcome Management

Staging of the tumor helps delineate the appropriate treatment and can suggest the client's prognosis (Figure 37-1). Five-year survival rates for stage 1 are about 65%; for stage 2, about 40%; 10-year rates drop to 40% and 35%, respectively. Five-year survivals are rare in stages 3 and 4.

■ Medical Management

Radiation Therapy. Radiation may be used as an adjunct with chemotherapy and surgery. Irradiation is most useful in preoperative preparation of the tumor. It is sometimes also used postoperatively to destroy residual or recurrent tumor cells, treat lymphatic involvement, and treat metastatic sites, such as bones, palliatively.

Chemotherapy. Clinical investigators continue to search for an effective chemotherapeutic regimen. Medroxyprogesterone and testosterone have been used as hormonal therapy, but their effectiveness has been limited. Vinblastine seems to be the most effective single agent, with response rates of 25%. Combination regimens seem to increase toxic effects without improving response rates. Many agents are being studied, but renal cancer cells seem insensitive to chemotherapeutic or hormonal agents, possibly because of their slow growth rate.

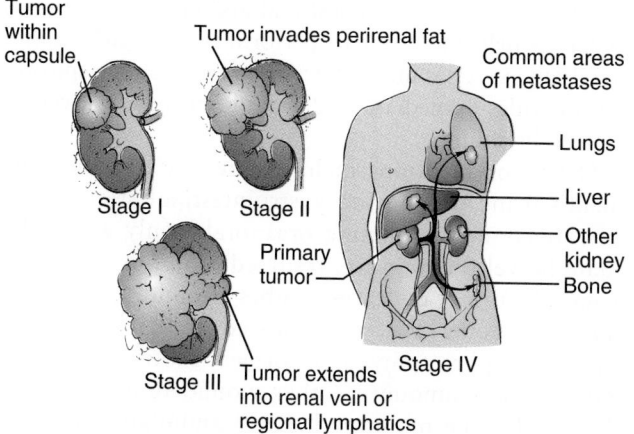

FIGURE 37-1 Staging system for renal carcinoma. Stage 1 tumor is confined within the renal capsule. Stage 2 tumor extends beyond the renal capsule to invade local perinephric fat but has no metastasis. Stage 3 tumor extends into the renal vein or involves local lymphatics. Stage 4 tumor has metastasized to other parts of the body.

Immunotherapy. Immunotherapy holds some promise in the treatment of renal cancer. Stimulants of the immune system have led to some positive results as long as the tumor is not too large and the immunosuppression is not too severe. There has also been some response to natural and recombinant interferon-alfa. Interleukin-2 has been approved by the Food and Drug Administration for treating renal carcinoma.

■ Nursing Management of the Medical Client

Nursing management of the client with renal cancer must include general aspects of care for any cancer (see Chapter 19).

■ Surgical Management

Nephrectomy. For renal cell carcinoma, the surgical procedure of choice is generally radical nephrectomy, which includes removal of the kidney, the adrenal gland, and perinephric fat with the retroperitoneal lymphatics. Several surgical approaches can be used to remove the diseased kidney. Transabdominal and thoracoabdominal approaches are preferred to secure the renal artery and vein and to prevent the spread of malignant cells.

A retroperitoneal approach is also possible. An incision of 6 to 10 inches is made, usually in the flank area; muscle layers are divided; and tissues are excised. The renal artery and vein are clamped and cut, and the ureter is dissected. When the tumor is in the renal pelvis, a nephroureterectomy is usually performed because of a tendency for transitional cell cancer to "seed" down the ureter into the bladder. With nephroureterectomy, a cuff of the adjacent bladder is removed.

Lymphadenectomy remains controversial. Even in advanced cases, when the prognosis is poor, nephrectomy is sometimes done to relieve pain and hematuria.

If the neoplastic disease is bilateral or if there is a solitary functioning kidney, a partial nephrectomy can be done on at least one kidney, leaving enough renal tissue to support life without long-term dialysis. If partial nephrectomy is not possible in either instance, the entire kidney is removed and the client undergoes dialysis. These clients may be candidates for renal transplantation, but they are usually maintained with dialysis for about a year to watch for recurrence of the disease.

Although open nephrectomy tends to be the procedure of choice for many urologists, laparoscopic nephrectomy is being performed in a number of centers with considerable success. Four small incisions are made through fewer muscle layers. A special laparoscope is inserted through one of the incisions, and laparoscopy instruments are placed in the others. Carbon dioxide is passed through a tube in one incision to inflate the abdominal cavity, which enables the surgeon to see the organs and provides room for manipulation of instruments. At the end of the procedure, the kidney is removed through a small 2- to 3-inch incision below the navel.

The laparoscopic surgical procedure tends to be longer (6.9 versus 2.2 hours), but clients who undergo the laparoscopic procedure require fewer analgesics, resume oral intake earlier, are discharged home earlier, and return to work sooner than those undergoing open surgery. Increasingly, removal of a kidney for organ donation is being performed laparoscopically.

Indications. Nephrectomy or heminephrectomy is indicated with tumors of the kidney. Other treatments are not successful.

Contraindications. As with any surgery, nephrectomy is contraindicated in clients with systemic or respiratory infections. General health must be satisfactory to withstand anesthesia, blood loss, and surgical stress. Any metabolic and systemic disorders should be stabilized before surgery.

Complications. Because the kidney is a very vascular organ, the risk of hemorrhage is high. Renal artery embolization of the affected kidney may be done to obstruct the tumor's blood supply and reduce its vascularity, thereby reducing the risk of hemorrhage. Embolization is usually accomplished by occluding the renal artery using an absorbable gelatin sponge (Gelfoam), metal coil, barium, subcutaneous fat, isobutyl-2-cyanoacrylate, absolute ethanol, or a balloon. This procedure may also be performed to control hemorrhage in an inoperable kidney. In addition, some researchers believe that embolization may stimulate an immune response against the dying cancer cells.

Other possible complications include those associated with any major surgery, such as atelectasis, pneumonia, thromboembolism, and infection of the surgical wound.

Outcomes. Nephrectomy reduces pain and hematuria caused by the tumor. The hospital stay is typically 4 to 6 days, with a return to work in 4 to 8 weeks. With laparoscopic nephrectomy, hospitalization is reduced and return to work after 2 to 4 weeks is not uncommon. Living with one kidney has few, if any, negative effects. Long-term outcomes, however, depend on the stage of the cancer.

■ Nursing Management of the Surgical Client

Preoperative Care

Preoperative preparation of the client having renal surgery includes the general guidelines described in Chapter 16. Increase fluid intake, if indicated, to ensure adequate excretion of waste products before surgery. Give emotional support because the client may be anxious, not only about the surgery but also about postoperative renal function and possible recurrence of the disease. If the remaining kidney functions adequately, assure the client that this kidney can fully meet the body's needs.

Postoperative Care
Assessment

Postoperatively, monitor the client's vital signs frequently and watch for any manifestations of bleeding or hemorrhage. Bleeding may be through the incision or internal.

Surgically induced or spontaneous pneumothorax occurs occasionally after nephrectomy; monitor for this complication by assessing for sudden shortness of breath and loss of breath sounds on the affected side.

Diagnosis, Outcomes, Interventions

Diagnosis: Risk for Injury: Postoperative Complications. The nursing diagnoses are likely to include *Risk for Injury: Postoperative complications related to surgical procedure.* Although postoperative care is similar to that for laparotomy, one of the greatest challenges is reestablishing effective breathing patterns. Deep breathing and coughing are difficult because the incision is very close to the diaphragm. Also, assuming the jackknife position on the surgical table increases pain and soreness in the thoracic region, limiting respiratory excursion. Paralytic ileus is a common problem. Urine output must be maintained.

Outcomes. The client will maintain normal respiratory excursion and have no additional breath sounds and no signs of atelectasis or infection. There will be normal bowel sounds within 2 to 3 days. Urine output will be at least 0.25 ml/kg/hr if one kidney is removed and 0.5 ml/kg/hr if a partial nephrectomy is performed.

Interventions. Liberal use of opioids (including patient-controlled analgesia) to reduce pain and external mechanical support of the chest and abdomen with pillows or hands help the client to perform deep-breathing and coughing exercises more effectively. An incentive spirometer provides immediate feedback about the effectiveness of deep breathing.

Other interventions include carefully assessing the client's urine output and gastrointestinal status postoperatively and beginning oral intake only after adequate bowel function has resumed. Total urine output from all urine collection tubes should total 0.25 ml/kg/hr if one kidney is removed or 0.5 ml/kg/hr if a partial nephrectomy is performed. Notify the physician of lesser amounts. Other wound drainage tubes also need to be monitored. Early ambulation is indicated.

Diagnosis: Acute Pain. A nursing diagnosis of *Acute Pain related to surgery* is common because the nephrectomy incision is extensive and causes significant discomfort. Muscle pain may develop from the prolonged position maintained during surgery.

Outcomes. Pain will be reduced, as indicated by the client's reports of reduced discomfort or of pain as tolerable, as well as by nonverbal indications of reduced discomfort, particularly during movement.

Interventions. The pain may be reduced by opioid analgesics (including the use of patient-controlled analgesia) and proper positioning. Epidural fentanyl or morphine sulfate can provide effective analgesia.

Diagnosis: Anxiety. Clients with cancer and clients undergoing surgery experience anxiety because of uncertainty about the future. A diagnosis of *Anxiety related to disease and surgery* is probable.

Outcomes. Ideally, the client will report having the information needed to reduce uncertainty and will report that the information reduced anxiety.

Interventions. To help reduce feelings of anxiety, continue to keep the client and his or her significant others informed about the progress made. Encourage them to express their concerns and to talk with one another. This need for support continues throughout the follow-up period.

Evaluation

The client should be able to resume regular activities within 6 to 8 weeks after surgery. Long-term survival is dependent on the stage of cancer diagnosed.

■ Self-Care

With shorter hospitalizations, clients who have undergone nephrectomy may require home care and support. Clients are weakened by surgery and possibly by other treatments. Activity should increase gradually; typically, 6 weeks must elapse before clients are ready to return to work or lift more than 10 pounds.

Concern about recurrence of the cancer is common. The American Cancer Society and other support groups may be helpful in the client's adjustment to cancer. People with one kidney can lead normal lives. There is, however, a need to protect the remaining kidney by prevention of infection and trauma.

TUBULOINTERSTITIAL DISEASE

Traditionally, the term *interstitial nephritis* has been applied to renal disease characterized by the presence of inflammatory cells in the spaces between the renal tubules. Not all disease processes included in this classification are inflammatory, however. Therefore the term *tubulointerstitial disease* is being advocated for this category of renal disorders.

Tubulointerstitial diseases are commonly classified as either acute or chronic. The acute form usually represents an allergic reaction and has a rapid onset. Assessment

findings are typically related to tubular injury. Manifestations often include fever, skin rash, eosinophilia, oliguric renal failure, and occasionally gross hematuria. The disease may progress along any of three courses:
- Complete recovery
- Rapid progression to renal failure and death
- Movement to the chronic form

Although corticosteroids are commonly prescribed, their value is unclear. Treatment is similar to that for acute renal failure.

Chronic tubulointerstitial disease is characterized by progressive interstitial fibrosis and usually chronic inflammatory cell infiltration with tubular atrophy. In the terminal stages, the altered renal vasculature and renal structure make the disease virtually indistinguishable from chronic pyelonephritis.

Morphologic findings in tubulointerstitial disease include interstitial edema, cellular infiltration of the interstitium, tubular cellular atrophy and flattening, and interstitial fibrosis. As the disease progresses, renal involvement extends beyond the tubules to progressive fibrosis of Bowman's capsule with secondary involvement of the glomeruli.

There are many potential causes of this pathologic process:
- Acute pyelonephritis
- Septicemia
- Analgesic abuse, especially with phenacetin, aspirin, and acetaminophen
- Immunologic mechanisms, for example, renal allograft, SLE, and Sjögren's syndrome
- Heavy metal toxicity
- Drug toxicity
- Hypercalcemia
- Hypocalcemia

In addition, several medication hypersensitivities can contribute. The medications involved include rifampin, penicillin and its analogs, sulfonamides, cephalosporins, allopurinol, captopril, cimetidine, azathioprine, phenytoin, thiazide, lithium, NSAIDs, and possibly furosemide.

An early manifestation of tubulointerstitial disease is a sudden, unexplained decrease in renal function that may be mild to severe. Specifically, there may be inability to concentrate urine, salt wasting, and poor acidification of the urine leading to metabolic acidosis. Finding a variety of urine sediment abnormalities is also common. Because glucose, uric acid, phosphates, amino acids, and bicarbonate are not effectively reabsorbed in the tubules, they appear in the urine. Severe bicarbonaturia is an indicator of renal tubular acidosis. Proteinuria is less severe than with other renal disease. Systemic hypertension is a common finding.

GLOMERULONEPHRITIS

Glomerulonephritis encompasses a variety of diseases, most of which are caused by an immunologic reaction that results in proliferative and inflammatory changes in glomerular structure. Glomerulonephritis can be acute or chronic. It is usually manifested by either a nephrotic syndrome or a nephritic syndrome. Percutaneous renal biopsy is typically used to identify the type of glomerulonephritis, and the findings assist in planning interventions and determining the prognosis.

NEPHROTIC SYNDROME

Nephrotic syndrome is a set of clinical manifestations caused by protein wasting secondary to diffuse glomerular damage. Manifestations include proteinuria (>3.5 g/day), hypoalbuminemia, and edema. Abnormal permeability of the glomerular basement membrane (especially to albumin) results in loss of protein in the urine. The resulting hypoalbuminemia alters oncotic pressure in the vascular tree, and fluid moves into the interstitial spaces, causing edema. This movement stimulates plasma renin activity and augments aldosterone production; as a result, the kidney retains sodium and water, thus adding to the accumulation of extracellular fluid.

Hyperlipidemia usually occurs also, probably because of increased hepatic lipoprotein synthesis in response to decreased serum albumin. Depending on the degree of renal failure, some level of normocytic anemia is common.

The causes of nephrotic syndrome are numerous. Besides glomerulonephritis, certain systemic disorders can cause it, such as diabetes mellitus, SLE, amyloidosis, hepatitis B, syphilis, carcinoma, leukemia, infectious disease, and preeclampsia. Other predisposing factors include the following:

- Allergic reactions
- Reactions to such drugs as penicillamine, anticonvulsants, probenecid, captopril, gold salts, heroin, and NSAIDs
- Renal vein thrombosis
- Sickle cell disease
- Heart failure

Potential complications of nephrotic syndrome include the effects of extracellular fluid accumulation and the progressive development of renal failure. The client may also experience severe hypovolemia, thromboembolism, secondary aldosteronism, abnormal thyroid function, osteomalacia, and increased susceptibility to infections.

Usually, edema is the client's chief problem. Although its onset may be insidious, it becomes massive. The client's skin typically takes on a characteristic waxy pallor resulting from the edema rather than anemia. Other manifestations include anorexia, malaise, irritability, and abnormal or absent menses. Large amounts of protein appear in the client's urine along with granular and epithelial cell casts and fat bodies; proteinuria may account for losses of 4 to 30 g/day. Some hematuria may be present. Serum albumin concentrations may drop as low as 1 to 2.5 g/dl.

The primary aim of treatment for nephrotic syndrome is to heal the leaking glomerular basement membrane, stop the loss of protein in the client's urine, and break the cycle of edema. Interventions typically include maintaining the client's fluid and electrolyte balance, reducing inflammation, preventing thrombosis, and minimizing protein loss.

Maintain Fluid and Electrolyte Balance. Unless the client is hyponatremic, fluids are not usually restricted. The client's fluid balance, however, should be carefully monitored via daily weights, girth measurements, and intake and output determinations. These data are important because weight loss may represent true tissue loss involving protein rather than fluid.

Loop diuretics (i.e., those that work on the loop of Henle), such as furosemide (Lasix), are typically prescribed. Plasma volume expanders, such as albumin, plasma, and dextran, may be administered to raise the oncotic pressure in the vascular tree. The increased pressure pulls fluid from the extracellular spaces, making it available for kidney filtration. Diuresis in older clients must be handled with particular caution because of their reduced ability to tolerate sudden shifts in intravascular volume.

Because the kidneys have a reduced capacity to excrete sodium, mild sodium restriction usually is instituted. The diet should be as palatable as possible, however, because the client must consume adequate protein and calories. Potassium may also be restricted as serum potassium levels rise.

Because edema disrupts cellular nutrition, the client is at increased risk for skin breakdown. Thus skin care is vital. Interventions include good hygiene, massage, position changes, and possibly special mattresses. Use research-based tools to assess the client's risk of breakdown (see Chapter 20).

Reduce Inflammation. Steroid therapy helps some clients, depending on the cause of disease. Cytotoxic agents such as cyclophosphamide and chlorambucil, indomethacin, anticoagulants, and antiplatelet agents may be used as well.

Prevent Thrombosis. Because clients with nephrotic syndrome are vulnerable to renal vein thrombosis, some are given long-term anticoagulation therapy. Teach such clients how to monitor for hemorrhage, and encourage them to carry identification that lists the drugs they take.

Minimize Protein Loss. For clients with nephrotic syndrome, most physicians recommend a protein intake of 1 to 1.5 g/kg/day with more than 35 kcal/kg/day to prevent further protein breakdown. Twenty-four-hour urine collections are used to measure urinary protein losses and monitor the success of treatment. Treatment to reduce inflammation ultimately reduces protein loss.

An important nursing role is to help the client with nephrotic syndrome maintain health and cope with the illness. Teach the client to take prescribed medications regularly, follow the prescribed diet, and report changes in health status, such as increasing edema, reduced urine output, weight gain, respiratory distress, and signs of infection. Explain that the amount of exercise allowed is based, at least in part, on the severity of the edema. Bed rest is imposed only during severe edema. As the fluid level moves toward normal, the client is allowed more activity. Other important areas of teaching include nutrition, prevention of infection, and methods of careful self-assessment.

NEPHRITIC SYNDROME

EB Nephritic syndrome refers to a set of clinical manifestations that includes hematuria and at least one of the following: oliguria (urine output <400 ml/24 hr), hypertension, elevated blood urea nitrogen (BUN), or decreased GFR. Nephritic syndrome is common with many types of glomerulonephritis, including immunoglobulin A (IgA) nephropathy and Henoch-Schönlein purpura. Treatment includes management of the underlying disease (usually through immunosuppressive drugs, as noted later) and symptomatic treatment of blood pressure and uremia.

TYPES OF GLOMERULONEPHRITIS

There are many types of glomerulonephritis, most of which involve either nephrotic syndrome or nephritic syndrome. The diagnosis of the specific type can be made by assessment of clinical manifestations and through renal biopsy. Box 37-2 presents a classification system based on etiology. Table 37-2 describes the onset, diagnostic findings, and prognosis for various types of glomerulonephritis.

Pathophysiology

EB Glomerulonephritis is an immunologic disorder that causes inflammation and increased cells in the glomerulus. Because the primary function of the glomerulus is to filter blood, most cases result when antigen-antibody complexes produced by an infection elsewhere in the body become trapped in the glomerulus. This entrapment causes inflammatory damage and impedes glomerular function, reducing the glomerular membrane's capacity for selective permeability. The source of the antigens may be either *exogenous* (e.g., after streptococcal infection) or *endogenous* (as in SLE). Evidence also indicates that some antigen-antibody complexes may form in the kidney itself.

Glomerulonephritis may also result from antibodies affixed to the glomerular basement membrane. For example, Goodpasture's syndrome involves pulmonary hemorrhage and glomerulonephritis.

The primary pathologic processes in glomerulonephritis, lipoid nephrosis, and focal glomerular scle-

---

BOX 37-2 Classification of Glomerulonephritis Based on Etiology

Primary Glomerulonephritis—Immune Response to Pathogens
- Acute glomerulonephritis
- Postinfectious glomerulonephritis
- Group A beta-hemolytic streptococcus
- Other infectious conditions such as cytomegalovirus infection, measles, mumps, staphylococcus, or pneumococcal bacteremia
- Infectious glomerulonephritis
- Membranoproliferative glomerulonephritis
- Rapidly progressive glomerulonephritis
- Idiopathic membranous glomerulonephritis
- Immunoglobulin A (IgA) nephropathy
- Chronic glomerulonephritis
- Lipoid nephrosis
- Focal glomerular sclerosis

Secondary Glomerulonephritis—Related to Systemic Disease
- Goodpasture's syndrome
- Hemolytic-uremic syndrome
- Henoch-Schönlein purpura
- Polyarteritis
- Progressive systemic sclerosis
- Systemic lupus erythematosus
- Wegener's granulomatosis
- Thrombocytopenic purpura
- Postpartum renal failure

---

rosis are proliferation and inflammation; however, lipoid nephrosis and focal glomerular sclerosis are characterized by degeneration. Figure 37-2 depicts the pathophysiologic mechanisms of glomerulonephritis.

Clinical Manifestations

Acute glomerulonephritis may develop insidiously or suddenly, varying considerably with the pathophysiology involved. Classic manifestations of sudden onset include hematuria with red blood cell casts and proteinuria. Fever, chills, weakness, pallor, anorexia, nausea, and vomiting may be present. Generalized edema, particularly facial and periorbital swelling, is a typical finding. The client may have ascites, pleural effusion, and heart failure.

The client is likely to have a headache and moderate to severe hypertension. Visual acuity may be reduced because of retinal edema. Abdominal or flank pain may develop, probably because of kidney edema and distention of the renal capsule. Oliguria, even anuria, may be present for several days; the longer it persists, the more irreversible the kidney damage. In contrast, the disease

TABLE 37-2 Types of Glomerulonephritis: Onset, Findings, and Prognosis

Type	Onset	Diagnostic Findings	Prognosis
Poststreptococcal glomerulonephritis	1 to 3 weeks after beta-hemolytic streptococcal infection of throat or skin Nephritic syndrome	Underlying infection Elevated antistreptolysin O titer Microscopic urinalysis, urine with many casts	Variable Complete recovery to end-stage renal disease
Membranoproliferative glomerulonephritis	Nephrotic syndrome sometimes preceded by a streptococcal infection	Proteinuria Hematuria (microscopic or gross)	Gradual progressive chronic renal failure
Rapidly progressive glomerulonephritis	Nephritic syndrome Sudden May follow antigen or infection Peak ages 40-60 yr	Hematuria Edema Hypertension Proteinuria Oliguria Acidosis	Progresses to renal failure within weeks or months
Idiopathic membranous glomerulonephritis	Insidious Peak ages 40-70 yr Unknown antigen	Asymptomatic proteinuria or nephrotic syndrome	Mixed: 25% have spontaneous remission, 25% have renal failure, 25% have persistent proteinuria, 25% have deteriorating renal function
Immunoglobulin A (IgA) nephropathy (also called Berger's disease)	Most common in young adults Nephritic syndrome	Hematuria Red blood cell casts on microscopic urinalysis	Usually progresses slowly over 10-20 yr; a small proportion progress to renal failure
Lipoid nephrosis (also called minimal change glomerulonephritis)	Nephrotic syndrome	Found on biopsy	Generally good May be relapses and spontaneous remission
Focal glomerular sclerosis	Peaks between ages 30 and 50 yr Nephrotic syndrome	Found on biopsy May be few symptoms	Poor, although rate of deterioration varies widely Recurs after transplantation
Membranous glomerulonephritis	Commonly secondary to drug therapy toxins or systemic autoimmune disease Nephrotic syndrome Insidious onset	Heavy proteinuria	Variable 30% have spontaneous remission
Hemolytic-uremic syndrome	Follows infection with *Escherichia coli* (01571 H7 serotype) History of eating undercooked hamburger Children and older adults particularly vulnerable	Hemorrhagic manifestations, such as bleeding and bruising Purpura manifestations, such as acute renal failure, hemolytic anemia, and thrombocytopenia	Recovery rate 95% but may leave residual renal damage

may be so mild that the client reports only vague weakness, anorexia, and lethargy.

Acute glomerulonephritis can become a fulminant process, proceeding quickly to uremia or chronic glomerulonephritis. Most clients, however, start to recover within 14 days. Most clinical manifestations disappear within several weeks, although hematuria and proteinuria may be present for longer periods. If complete recovery does not occur within 2 years, it probably will not occur at all.

Some clinicians use the term *subacute glomerulonephritis* to describe disease persisting longer than 6 to

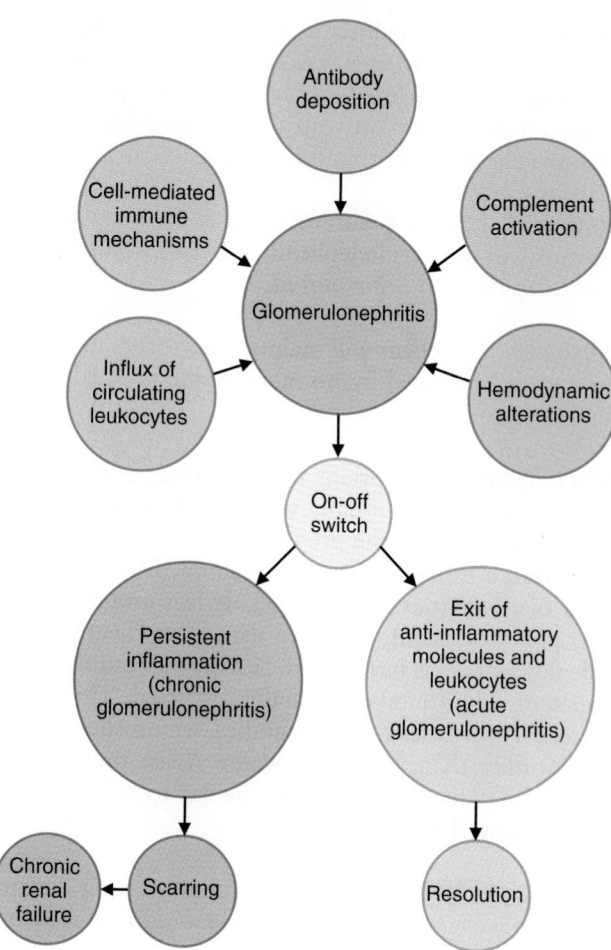

FIGURE 37-2 Pathophysiologic mechanisms of glomeru-lonephritis.

headache, dizziness, and digestive disturbances. As the disease progresses, these manifestations intensify, and the client may experience respiratory difficulty and angina.

The cardinal manifestation of this disease is hypertension. It is not uncommon for the client to experience such complications as nosebleed, manifestations of arteriosclerosis, cardiomegaly, and hemorrhage into the kidneys, lungs, retina, or cerebrum. Edema increases as heart failure becomes more severe and the serum albumin decreases. Examination of the eye grounds shows vascular changes and edema of the discs. Urinalysis shows a fixed specific gravity, small amounts of proteinuria except during exacerbation, casts, WBCs, renal tubular cells, and consistent hematuria. Anemia tends to be severe.

Examining the urine usually provides the information necessary for a diagnosis of glomerulonephritis (see Chapter 34). Gross hematuria and proteinuria are the cardinal findings. The client's urine, which may be scant, usually has a dark, smoky, cola-colored, or red-brown hue. The proteinuria produces a persistent and excessive foam. The urine may have a low pH and a specific gravity in the midnormal to high-normal range if there is enough renal damage to affect the kidneys' ability to concentrate.

Other studies may assist in the diagnosis as well. Serum urea nitrogen and creatinine levels may be elevated, and creatinine clearance rates may be decreased. C-reactive proteins and anti-streptolysin O titer are usually elevated in poststreptococcal glomerulonephritis, and the serum complement level is low in many forms of glomerulonephritis. Hematocrit and hemoglobin studies may indicate anemia, particularly if renal failure is imminent.

Outcome Management
■ Medical Management

Medical intervention aims to eliminate antigens, to alter the client's immune balance, and to inhibit or alleviate inflammation to prevent further renal damage and improve kidney function. Although some clients may require initial hospitalization, treatment is typically on an outpatient basis.

Reduce Inflammation. Plasmapheresis has been used in some research protocols to reduce the number of antigens in certain types of glomerulonephritis, including rapidly progressive glomerulonephritis. This interven- tion is usually administered in conjunction with corticosteroids and immunosuppressive agents (azathioprine, cyclophosphamide). The technique is designed to remove the specific circulating antibody or mediators of the inflammatory response. Large volumes of the client's plasma are cyclically removed and replaced with fresh frozen plasma through a continuous-flow blood cell separator.

8 weeks. Although most of the manifestations of the acute disease have disappeared, the client is still at high risk for exacerbation of glomerulonephritis. The term *latent glomerulonephritis* refers to an asymptomatic condition characterized by significant albumin levels and casts in the urine for more than 1 year after acute onset. These findings indicate continued but slow parenchymal changes.

Most types of glomerulonephritis can progress to a chronic state. Sometimes, glomerulonephritis is first seen as a chronic process. Chronic glomerulonephritis progresses over an extended period, often as long as 30 years. When it progresses to end-stage renal failure, dialysis must begin or the client will die.

As the glomeruli and tubules are destroyed by the pathologic process, the kidneys shrink and become severely contracted. Fibrous and scar tissue replaces functioning renal tissue. Sclerosis of renal blood vessels also occurs. The destruction rates vary.

Common manifestations include malaise, weight loss, edema, increasing irritability and mental cloudiness, a metallic taste in the mouth, polyuria and nocturia resulting from the kidney's inability to concentrate urine,

Antibiotic therapy (such as penicillin for streptococcal organisms) is used to treat poststreptococcal glomerulonephritis. It is also used prophylactically after streptococcal infections to prevent further damage.

Maintain Fluid and Electrolyte Balance. Volume overload and hypertension are treated with diuretics, antihypertensives, and restriction of dietary sodium and water. Common complications of fluid overload include heart failure with pulmonary edema and increased intracranial pressure. Renal failure may develop (see Chapter 38). Appropriate monitoring is essential and should include vital signs, intake and output, and weight. Recognizing complications early facilitates prompt medical intervention.

■ Nursing Management of the Medical Client
Assessment

For any client with suspected glomerulonephritis, take a comprehensive history that includes upper respiratory tract infection (such as strep throat), skin infections, scarlet fever, or a history of glomerulonephritis. Also question the client about systemic disorders that might be present, such as SLE, scleroderma, amyloidosis, and hypertension. Any recent invasive procedures should also be noted.

Physical examination may reveal ascites, pleural effusion, and manifestations of heart failure with pulmonary edema. Examine the urine closely for color, amount, and abnormal substances. In particular, microscopic analysis of the urine can be a valuable diagnostic tool with glomerulonephritis; urinary casts are commonly seen under high magnification (see Chapter 34). Check the client's vital signs closely, especially the blood pressure.

Diagnosis, Outcomes, Interventions

Diagnosis: Imbalanced Nutrition: Less Than Body Requirements. If the client has a reduced appetite or an aversion to food, the nursing diagnosis *Imbalanced Nutrition: Less than body requirements related to anorexia and increased metabolic demands* is appropriate.

Outcomes. The client will maintain adequate nutritional intake, as evidenced by no weight loss, an absence of a negative nitrogen balance, and normal electrolytes.

Interventions. It is important to protect the kidneys while they are recovering their function. The prescribed diet is likely to be high in calories and low in protein. This diet is designed to avoid protein catabolism and enables the kidney to rest because it handles fewer protein molecules and metabolites.

The degree to which protein is restricted depends on the amount excreted in the urine and the client's individual requirements. Sodium is also restricted, depending on the amount of edema present. Anorexia, nausea, and vomiting may interfere with adequate intake, requiring creative intervention on your part. A dietitian can help plan the client's diet around these restrictions.

Diagnosis: Excess Fluid Volume. A common nursing diagnosis in glomerulonephritis is *Excess Fluid Volume related to reduced urine output.*

Outcomes. The client will maintain balanced intake and output, as evidenced by no manifestations of edema or fluid overload.

Interventions. Appropriate fluid balance is important. Careful monitoring of daily weight and intake and output helps determine the progress of the edema and thus provides an estimate of renal function. Daily measurement of edematous parts (especially legs and abdomen) also provides useful, objective data. The client's allowable fluid intake is based on the intake and output measurements. Fluid intake is usually restricted. Thirst may be relieved by offering hard candies, lemon slices, or ice chips rather than a glass of water. Assist the client to "plan" fluid distribution during the day to make the best use of allowed fluids.

Diagnosis: Fatigue. Another common nursing diagnosis is *Fatigue related to increased metabolic demands and anemia.*

Outcomes. The client will have an adequate balance of rest and activity, as evidenced by absence of complaints of fatigue.

Interventions. Rest is essential—both physical and emotional. As mentioned, activity level correlates directly with the amount of hematuria and proteinuria. Exercise also increases catabolic activity. The allowable amount of activity depends on the results of serial urinalyses. Bed rest interspersed with periods of limited activity may continue for several weeks to months. Therefore the client may need help in arranging personal matters, such as family, home, job, finances, and community responsibilities.

Encourage the client to talk about any fears or concerns, and, if necessary, help the client deal with the emotional reactions expected during a long-term illness with a questionable prognosis. Only after handling these problems can the client rest emotionally. Appropriate diversionary activities may help the client cope with prolonged physical immobility.

Diagnosis: Risk for Impaired Skin Integrity. A typical nursing diagnosis is *Risk for Impaired Skin Integrity related to edema.*

Outcomes. The client will remain free of skin break-down as evidenced by continued intact skin.

Interventions. Edema interferes with cellular nutrition, which makes the client more susceptible to skin break-down. Take precautions to prevent this complication. Interventions include good hygiene, massage, and position changes as well as other prophylactic measures, such as mattress devices. Use research-based tools to assess the client's risk of breakdown (see Chapter 20).

Diagnosis: Risk for Infection. Another diagnosis after immunosuppressive therapy is *Risk for Infection related to altered immune response secondary to treatment.*

Outcomes. The client will remain free of infection as evidenced by normal temperature and an absence of local or systemic manifestations of infection.

Interventions. Glomerulonephritis markedly diminishes a client's natural defenses to infection, especially to streptococcal organisms. Immunosuppressives and corticosteroids further reduce host resistance. Although isolation is not necessary, take care to protect the client from people with obvious infectious processes. General supportive measures help boost the client's defense mechanisms. Client teaching should involve appropriate ways to avoid infections, especially respiratory and urinary tract infections.

Evaluation

The client must be able to understand the condition and the reasons for limitations, including dietary and fluid restrictions. Stress the importance of follow-up treatments to minimize the risk of recurrence.

■ Self-Care

Clients with glomerulonephritis are followed as outpatients, often for many years. Self-care activities should include regular follow-up, recommended medications and dietary restrictions, and monitoring for changes in condition. It is vital that blood pressure be controlled to prevent further renal damage; many clients learn to monitor their own blood pressure at home. Because the disease may progress to renal failure, there are numerous quality-of-life issues, as discussed in Chapter 38.

■ Modifications for Older Clients

The older client is at greater risk for renal damage because of the pre-existing effects of age on the kidneys. The older client is also more likely to have concurrent chronic diseases—such as hypertension and diabetes—that may have affected the kidneys, although treatment is the same.

RENAL TRAUMA

Serious kidney injury is relatively rare because of the protection afforded by the rib cage, the heavy muscles of the back, and the tough capsule surrounding the kidney. Traffic accidents and falls in which the client lands on the abdomen, flank, or back are the most common cause of injury, usually from blunt trauma. Kidney lacerations can result from fractures of the spine and ribs as well as penetrating injuries from bullets and knives.

Pathophysiology

Five categories of traumatic injury can affect the kidney:
- Contusion with intrarenal hemorrhage
- Minor laceration (rupture with subcapsular hemorrhage)
- Major laceration (rupture into the renal pelvis)
- "Fractured" kidney (shattered rupture)
- Vascular (pedicle) injury, which damages renal blood supply (Figure 37-3)

In a contusion a hematoma develops and remains confined within the renal parenchyma. Rupture of the kidney may cause hemorrhage between the capsular walls; bleeding may or may not reach into the renal pelvis. A shattered or fractured kidney causes hemorrhage throughout the renal tissue. The pedicle holds the renal artery and other vital circulatory and nervous sys-

Contusion   Minor laceration   Major laceration   "Fractured" kidney   Vascular injury

FIGURE 37-3 Categories of renal trauma.

tem connections to the kidney. Injury to the pedicle may jeopardize the life of the kidney and may occur with or without intrarenal hemorrhage.

Clinical Manifestations

The type of injury the client has suffered gives the first real key to identifying renal trauma. Commonly, the client has multiple serious injuries, and renal trauma may not be immediately apparent. Hematuria (gross or microscopic) is a cardinal manifestation and is found in about 80% of cases. However, serious renal injury can occur without hemorrhage, and clear urine does not automatically rule out renal trauma. Other findings include shock, flank pain, and a palpable mass in the affected flank area or over the 11th or 12th rib. Paralytic ileus may also occur. You may see bruises over the client's flank and lower back secondary to retroperitoneal hemorrhage, a development known as Grey Turner's sign. A KUB film, IVP, retrograde pyelography, renal scan, ultrasonography, CT scan, and renal arteriography all help confirm the type and degree of kidney injury.

Complications

In addition to the immediate problems of hemorrhage and loss of functioning renal tissue, kidney trauma makes the client highly susceptible to a number of other problems. Even in closed injuries, there is a high risk of sepsis leading to kidney and perinephric abscesses. Secondary hemorrhage is not uncommon. Other complications include hypertension resulting from fibrosis and ischemic kidney, renal artery thrombosis, arteriovenous aneurysms, fistula formation from extravasation of urine, urinomas, and pseudocysts.

Outcome Management

Whether conservative or surgical treatment should be used for renal trauma is controversial. Most physicians agree that kidney contusion calls for conservative treatment. Other minor injuries, such as small subcapsular hematomas and minor lacerations without extravasation, may also be better followed conservatively.

Clients with major injuries (e.g., renal fracture, parenchymal injury with major arterial occlusion, avulsion injuries, tears in the renal artery or vein, and parenchymal lacerations with extending perirenal hematomas or urinary extravasation) may require surgical exploration. Possible indications include continued moderate to severe hemorrhage and continued urinary extravasation. Urinary extravasation itself is not a definite reason for surgery because sterile urine usually resolves or is encapsulated spontaneously; however, it sometimes produces a severe tissue reaction and causes fistula formation. The pocket of extrarenal urine may also become obstructive.

Medical Management

Medical management, which primarily involves waiting and watching, is possible because the retroperitoneal space allows tamponade. In the absence of other injuries, a client with microscopic hematuria and normal findings on IVP may be observed on an ambulatory basis with careful instructions about activity restrictions and the need for adequate hydration. If there is gross hematuria, bed rest is required until the urine clears. Serial observations of the urine, hematocrit, and vital signs are made to watch the progress of the hemorrhage. Sequential urine specimens may be collected to compare current and previous urine color and turbidity.

Even if replacement fluids are not needed, a prophylactic intravenous line may be established, and a type and crossmatch for blood may be done. If a hematoma is present or IVP shows urine extravasation, the client may receive antibiotics to prevent sepsis. The physician prescribes blood transfusions if the hematocrit is low. After the urine clears, the client can be more active. After discharge, the client needs follow-up blood pressure checks and IVP studies to rule out secondary hypertension and anatomic changes in the renal system.

Nursing Management of the Medical Client

Nursing management of the client with renal trauma varies considerably, depending on extent of injury. The goals of nursing care are to prevent further bleeding and injury and to alleviate the client's anxiety.

Assessment

Assessment includes checking for tenderness at the CVA. Watch for bleeding, which may occur as hematuria or may be internal, depending on the nature of the injury. Assess the client's vital signs for evidence of shock. Make serial observations of urine, hematocrit, and vital signs to watch the progress of hemorrhage. Sequential urine specimens may be collected to compare current and previous urine color and turbidity.

Diagnosis, Outcomes, Interventions

Diagnosis: Risk for Injury: Hemorrhage. The goals of nursing after renal trauma are related to monitoring for shock and minimizing the risk of further bleeding. For this reason, the nursing diagnosis is *Risk for Injury: Hemorrhage related to blood loss, further injury, and hypovolemia.*

Outcomes. The client will not experience shock, and bleeding will stop, as evidenced by a decrease in hematuria, pain, or other bleeding.

Interventions. Nursing interventions during conservative treatment center on monitoring urinary elimination patterns and helping the client to cope and comply with the medical regimen. If there is gross hematuria, bed rest is required until the urine clears. Monitoring includes assessment of vital signs as well as intake and output. Notify the physician if urine output drops below 0.5 ml/kg/hr. Because bed rest can cause problems with bowel elimination and adequate fluid intake, circulation, and respiratory function, take appropriate measures to minimize the risk of these complications (passive exercise, for example). A client with microscopic hematuria and normal IVP results who is observed on an ambulatory basis should be given careful instructions about activity restrictions and the need for adequate hydration.

Diagnosis: Anxiety.

Renal trauma can cause considerable anxiety over the possible loss of renal function and possible shock. Hence a nursing diagnosis of *Anxiety related to injury* is highly likely.

Outcomes. The client will report less anxiety and will have the information needed to understand the situation and prognosis.

Interventions. Nursing care related to anxiety involves providing information about the plan of care, including activity restrictions. The client is concerned about the progress, and you may be in a position to facilitate communication between the client and other members of the health care team.

Evaluation

It is expected that the client will have no further bleeding or injury and that renal function will be maintained, whether monitoring is done on an outpatient basis or in an acute care setting. With limited activity, most clients can be managed at home unless surgical intervention is required.

■ Surgical Management

The greatest diversity of opinion concerns proper handling of the renal damage discovered during exploration. When the other kidney is functioning effectively, some physicians recommend free use of nephrectomy to avoid later sequelae, whereas others believe that the goal should be salvaging maximal renal function. The latter group advocates giving the conservative approach a fair trial and, if surgery is necessary, attempting to repair the kidney before deciding to remove it. With renal vascular injury, fewer than half of kidneys can be salvaged if the injury is 18 hours old; there is virtually no chance of renal recovery after 24 hours.

Renal hemorrhage may be controlled by injection of an autologous clot into the secondary arteries supplying the bleeding site. Blood is drawn from the client and allowed to clot. The clot is then injected angiographically. Because normal endothelium has a strong clot-lysing effect, the clot disappears from the normal adjacent vasculature after several hours and affects only the damaged portion.

If kidney repair is attempted rather than nephrectomy, the surgical procedure is designed to debride devitalized tissue, achieve hemostasis, establish a watertight seal of the collecting system, approximate the renal parenchymal edges, and drain the renal fossa.

Two surgical techniques improve the outcome of repair:

- *Extracorporeal,* or *bench, surgery* allows the kidney to be removed from the body for better visualization and manipulation of the organ during the repair process; the kidney is returned by autotransplantation. During its time outside the body, the kidney is maintained by hypothermia or by a perfusate mechanically pulsed through it.
- The *slush technique,* in which the kidney is immersed in iced saline slush, slows the metabolism and oxygen requirement of renal tissue, allowing longer intraoperative ischemic times. This technique causes some systemic hypothermia, but it is not significant. Pedicle vascular injury may also be repaired.

If either technique fails, nephrectomy is necessary.

■ Nursing Management of the Surgical Client

Nursing management of the client undergoing surgery for renal trauma is similar to that for other surgical procedures on the kidney (see Nephrectomy earlier in this chapter).

■ Self-Care

The client being observed on an ambulatory basis requires an appropriate teaching plan covering health maintenance activities and the need for a follow-up program. The client should promptly report any change in condition or recurrence of bleeding or pain to the physician. Strenuous activity should be avoided for several weeks or more, depending on the extent of the injury. The client must also maintain adequate hydration.

RENAL VASCULAR ABNORMALITIES

The kidneys depend on adequate blood circulation to nourish tissues and provide blood for filtration so that they can perform their intended functions. Anything that interferes with the normal circulatory flow significantly reduces renal function.

RENAL ARTERY DISEASE

Etiology and Risk Factors

Of all cases of renal artery disease, 90% are caused by atherosclerosis or fibromuscular dysplasia. Atherosclerosis affects males more often than females and usually involves the proximal third of the artery. Health promotion activities are the same as those for atherosclerosis as discussed with circulatory and cardiac disorders. Fibromuscular dysplasia is an alternating stenosis and dilation; arteriographic studies demonstrate a "string-of-beads" appearance of the artery. This condition affects females four to five times as often as males. Because the cause is unknown, there are no health promotion actions.

There are several other, less common, causes of renal artery disease. Cancer may obstruct the vessels. Embolism or thrombosis can cause acute obstruction. Trauma, as described earlier, can interrupt blood flow. The renal artery may be purposely occluded to produce a "medical nephrectomy" or total renal infarction; the occlusion may be done preoperatively in the case of renal adenocarcinoma or to control proteinuria or hypertension. Shredded Gelfoam can be used, or a liquid substance that polymerizes instantly when it comes in contact with blood may be injected into the renal artery. A dissecting aneurysm in the renal artery may also interrupt renal circulation.

Pathophysiology

The end result of any of these conditions, if severe enough, is reduced renal blood flow. The reduced flow causes renal parenchymal ischemia and, finally, renal atrophy. The role of renal artery disease in renovascular hypertension is also well documented, and hypertension alone may indicate treatment of the condition.

Clinical Manifestations

Because of the kidney's compensatory mechanisms, the gradual development of renal artery stenosis from atherosclerosis and cancer may give rise to few manifestations, at least until the resulting hypertension and decreasing renal function become evident. Acute obstruction makes itself known relatively quickly, however. Manifestations of this sudden episode include flank pain over the affected kidney or abdominal pain and fever. Atrial dysrhythmias are a frequent finding; however, because they commonly alternate with periods of normal sinus rhythm, this manifestation can be missed. Urinalysis may be normal, and blood chemistry profiles may show elevated aspartate aminotransferase and lactic dehydrogenase. IVP shows a nonfunctioning kidney, and a renal scan shows no arterial blood flow.

In response to reduced renal circulation, collateral circulation helps preserve the kidney if sufficient development takes place before total obstruction. Collateral circulation, in addition to a marked reduction in filtration, renal work, and oxygen requirements, allows the kidney to tolerate ischemic periods for up to several weeks. In acute total occlusion, a normal kidney can remain viable for about 2 hours before infarction and tissue necrosis begin.

Outcome Management
■ Surgical Management

Treatment of the ischemic kidney usually involves surgical revascularization. Arterial endarterectomy may be done with follow-up anticoagulant or antiplatelet therapy. In the technique known as *percutaneous transluminal renal angioplasty* (PTRA), the vessel is cleared with a balloon catheter. If it cannot be recanalized, a renal artery resection with end-to-end anastomosis or an aortorenal bypass graft procedure may be performed.

Percutaneous Transluminal Renal Angioplasty. In clients undergoing PTRA, a balloon-tipped catheter is inserted, usually through the femoral artery, and threaded under radiologic guidance to the obstructed renal artery. The physician inflates the balloon and pulls it through the obstructed area, stretching it and increasing the size of the arterial lumen. A stent may be placed at the site of occlusion to maintain the size of the lumen, prevent restenosis, and minimize the risk of abrupt vessel reclosure. If a stent is placed, antiplatelet agents or anticoagulants may be prescribed to minimize the risk of acute thrombosis.

Indications. Renal artery angioplasty is usually the first intervention for renovascular hypertension. If angioplasty is unsuccessful or if the condition recurs, more invasive surgical approaches are considered.

Contraindications. Angioplasty may be contraindicated if there is previous damage to the femoral artery or severely impaired circulation to the limb.

Complications. Renal artery angioplasty is considered a relatively safe procedure. The overall complication rate is about 10%. The most common complications include renal artery dissection, renal artery thrombosis or occlusion, segmental renal infarction, and hematoma formation or puncture trauma.

Outcomes. About one third of clients with renovascular hypertension do not respond to this therapy. A significant number are cured, and about half improve significantly. The treatment can be repeated if necessary. Clients usually return home in 24 to 48 hours.

■ Nursing Management of the Surgical Client

Preoperative Care

Because the length of stay is limited for most clients undergoing PTRA, it is a challenge to coordinate their care during the diagnostic and intervention phases of treatment. Typically, diagnostic tests such as angiograms and blood work are completed during the week before the procedure. Teaching about angioplasty and discharge instructions must be provided in a short period.

Postoperative Care

Care after PTRA is similar to other care after any angioplasty. Just after the procedure, vital signs are monitored every 15 minutes for 1 hour, every 30 minutes for 2 hours, hourly for 3 hours, and then regularly according to the established protocol. Check the dressing at these times for manifestations of bleeding or hematoma formation, and check peripheral pulses to assess circulation in the affected limb. Bed rest for up to 24 hours may be ordered.

In the longer term, the client's blood pressure should be monitored because hypertension can indicate recurrence of the lesion. Control of hypertension is crucial to preserving renal function.

After renal artery bypass graft surgery, nursing care is similar to other care after any kidney surgery, such as nephrectomy (discussed earlier in this chapter); however, in the postoperative period after an aortorenal bypass graft procedure, the client may experience an initial exacerbation of hypertension. Its cause is unclear, but it is thought to be related to systemic vasoconstriction secondary to general anesthesia and intraoperative hypothermia, severe pain, or transient renin secretion caused by clamping the aorta and manipulating the kidney. This episode usually lasts no more than 48 hours, but it can be significant and may require medical intervention. You must monitor blood pressure frequently.

RENAL VEIN DISEASE

The primary pathologic process involving the renal vein is thrombosis. Obstruction of venous drainage increases interstitial pressure, which reduces renal function. Findings include severe lumbar pain, renal enlargement, proteinuria, and hematuria. If the obstruction is bilateral, oliguria and azotemia occur. Contributing factors include diabetic nephropathy, chronic glomerulonephritis, and renal amyloidosis.

Kidney survival depends largely on the development of collateral circulation before the vessel is fully occluded. Embolectomy or ligation of the renal veins may be done, and anticoagulants may be prescribed. Intravenous streptokinase is used to lyse the occluding clot. If enough renal damage has occurred, nephrectomy is an option.

CONGENITAL DISORDERS

Renal congenital anomalies usually involve abnormalities in the number, position, form, size, or structure of the kidneys. Blood supply may be abnormal, although malformations that significantly affect renal function are rare. Anomalies of the ureteropelvic junction usually obstruct at that point and result in hydronephrosis. Typically, this situation is discovered and treated during childhood.

ANOMALIES INVOLVING KIDNEY NUMBER AND POSITION

Renal agenesis is the absence of one or both kidneys. Having only one kidney presents no difficulty if this kidney functions adequately. A client can live normally with one properly functioning kidney, as kidney donors aptly demonstrate. Bilateral agenesis, however, is fatal. Even in unilateral agenesis, the functioning kidney is at high risk for development of additional anomalies.

Supernumerary kidneys (more than two kidneys) are usually asymptomatic and are discovered during IVP. The extra ureter enters either the ipsilateral ureter or the bladder.

Ectopic, or malpositioned, kidneys are usually found in the pelvis, although thoracic kidneys have been documented. Problems associated with this anomaly include respiratory difficulties, pain caused by pressure on nerves or surrounding structures, and difficulty in childbirth.

Occasionally, one kidney may be across the midline so that both kidneys are on the same side. This condition usually remains undiscovered until infection or obstruction indicates a need for x-ray examination.

ANOMALIES INVOLVING KIDNEY FORM AND SIZE

Anomalies of kidney form and size include aplasia, hypoplasia, dysplasia, and *horseshoe kidney.* Aplastic kidneys are small and contracted and contain no functioning renal tissue. Renal hypoplasia produces miniature kidneys with some functioning tissue. Although clinically this condition may be asymptomatic, it may cause hypertension and recurrent urinary tract infection.

Horseshoe kidney results when two kidneys are joined into a single organ whose shape somewhat resembles that of a horseshoe (Figure 37-4). The kidneys are connected, usually at the lower poles, by an isthmus of tissue. Because the developmental error interferes with normal ascent and medial rotation, the kidney is usually located in the lower lumbar region with its pelvis facing anteriorly. Although clients with horseshoe kidney may be asymptomatic, they are susceptible to hy-

FIGURE 37-4 A horseshoe kidney is usually created by tissue joining the lower poles.

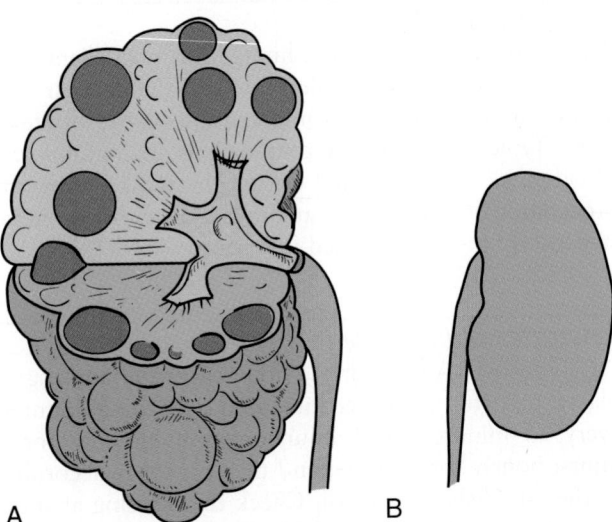

FIGURE 37-5 Polycystic kidney (**A**) filled with fluid or blood-filled cysts which alter the architecture of the kidney. Notice how much larger it is in size compared to a normal kidney (**B**).

dronephrosis, infection secondary to ureteropelvic junction obstruction, and calculus formation.

ANOMALIES INVOLVING CYSTIC DISEASE

Cystic disease in renal tissue can range from a simple, solitary fluid-filled mass to almost complete replacement of renal structures by cystic tissue. A simple renal cyst commonly originates superficially in the renal parenchyma. It grows slowly and usually produces no manifestations until adulthood, when it may cause heaviness and pain in the abdomen and become a palpable mass. Arriving at a diagnosis may be complicated because renal cysts closely resemble malignant tumors; naturally, differentiation between the two is vital. As long as a simple renal cyst remains asymptomatic, intervention is usually unnecessary. If intervention is necessary, the cyst may be aspirated with a needle, or a partial nephrectomy may be performed to remove it.

Polycystic Kidneys

Polycystic disease of the kidney is a hereditary disorder in which grape-like cysts containing serous fluid, blood, or urine replace normal kidney tissue (Figure 37-5). The condition may develop at any age.

Infantile polycystic kidney disease is inherited as an autosomal recessive trait, and both parents must have carried the gene. It is a rare disorder that affects both kidneys and often the liver. In an infant, the disease usually causes death within days. Milder forms of the disease do not appear until childhood.

Adult polycystic disease accounts for about 10% of the clients receiving dialysis or transplantation. It is inherited as an autosomal dominant trait (see the Genetic Links feature on Autosomal Dominant Polycystic Kidney Disease on p. 937). It usually appears after age 40 years, although it may begin as early as age 20 or as late as age 80. There are diverse manifestations; the most common are dull, aching lumbar or flank pain, which may be colicky, and hematuria. Other common findings are proteinuria, palpable kidney masses, pyuria, calculi, and uremia.

Early in the disease, the ability to concentrate urine decreases. Hypertension develops along with cardiac enlargement and heart failure.

Polycystic liver disease occurs in about one third of cases, and cystic lesions are sometimes found in the thyroid, lung, pancreas, spleen, ovary, testis, epididymis, uterus, and bladder. Cerebral aneurysms occur in about 2% of clients with polycystic kidney disease.

The cystic kidney can become so enlarged that it causes severe pressure on other organs, with production of additional extrarenal manifestations. The ultimate result of this disease is chronic renal failure (see Chapter 38). As the disease slowly progresses, renal nephrons are destroyed, renal function deteriorates, and uremia ultimately results. The mean duration of polycystic kidney disease from onset of manifestations to development of uremia varies a great deal and may be 15 to 30 years or longer.

Because there is no known way to arrest the progress of the destructive cysts, conservative medical treatment is designed to preserve kidney function. Urinary tract in-

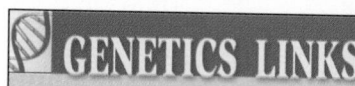

GENETICS LINKS

Autosomal Dominant Polycystic Kidney Disease (ADPKD)

Description

An adult-onset disorder characterized by progressive cyst development and bilaterally enlarged polycystic kidneys. Clinical features include renal function abnormalities, hypertension, pain, and renal insufficiency. About 50% of clients develop end-stage renal disease by about age 60. Cysts can also occur in other organs (e.g., liver, pancreas).

Genetics

ADPKD is caused by mutations in the *PKD1* gene (~85% of cases) located on chromosome 16 or the *PKD2* gene (~15% of cases) located on chromosome 4. Molecular genetic testing of the *PKD1* and *PKD2* genes is available clinically. As an autosomal dominant condition, offspring of an affected individual with ADPKD have a 50% chance of inheriting the disease-causing mutation. Most clients have a parent with ADPKD, but de novo mutations (new or spontaneous mutations) occur in about 10% of families.

Diagnosis/Testing

Diagnosis is established by imaging studies of the kidneys or molecular genetic testing of the *PKD1* gene and the *PKD2* gene.

Management

As yet there is no treatment specifically directed towards the disease. Current therapy is aimed at reducing morbidity and mortality from the renal and other complications of the disease.

COMPLEMENTARY AND ALTERNATIVE THERAPY

Slowing the Progression of Diabetic Nephropathy with a Unique Diet

In general, clients with end-stage renal disease are encouraged to follow a low-protein diet to slow the progression of their disease. However, a recent study challenged this notion by using a carbohydrate-restricted, low-iron, polyphenol-enriched diet. Foods rich in polyphenols include olive oil, cranberries, green tea, red wine, and grapes.

A total of 191 clients with type 2 diabetes and impending renal failure were included (men and women 49 to 62 years of age). Clients had a history of diabetes for 5 to 15 years and a glycosylated hemoglobin of 6.0% to 9.3%. Current medications for both hypertension and glucose control were continued. Clients were assigned to either the low carbohydrate diet or a conventional protein-restricted diet (0.8 g/kg). The main features of the low-carbohydrate diet were a 50% reduction of carbohydrates; replacement of iron-enriched meats with iron-poor meats and foods known to inhibit iron absorption; elimination of all liquids except tea, water, and red wine; and the use of olive oil for frying and dressings. Unfortunately, compliance was not assessed.

Clients were followed for an average of 3.9 years. No significant differences were seen in the baseline characteristics of the two groups. Serum creatinine doubled in 21% of the clients following the lower carbohydrate diet versus 39% of the control group ($p < 0.01$). Thus a polyphenol-enriched diet with 50% carbohydrate reduction and low iron availability was better than a conventional protein-restricted diet in slowing the progression of diabetic nephropathy. More studies are needed, but the results are interesting.

Reference

Facchini, F., & Saylor, K. (2003). A low-iron-available, polyphenol-enriched, carbohydrate-restricted diet to slow progression of diabetic nephropathy. *Diabetes 52,* 1204-1209.

COMPLEMENTARY AND ALTERNATIVE THERAPY

Oral Acetylcysteine Supplements for Preventing Acute Deterioration in Renal Function After Coronary Angiography in Moderate Renal Insufficiency

Acetylcysteine tablets already play several roles in medicine. For example, they seem to reduce hepatic damage from acetaminophen overdose and have a role in clearing lung function in cystic fibrosis. However, other roles for this supplement are being explored.

A randomized, blinded, placebo-controlled trial with a 7-day follow-up was recently conducted in a university hospital in Hong Kong. A total of 200 clients (mean age 68 years, 61.5% men, 100% Chinese) with moderate chronic renal insufficiency and upcoming elective coronary angiography were studied. Clients received either oral acetylcysteine (600 mg twice daily, n = 102) or a placebo (n = 98) both the day before and the day of angiography (total treatment duration of 2 days). All clients received a nonionic, low-osmolality contrast agent (iopamidol).

Researchers found that in clients with moderate chronic renal insufficiency, oral acetylcysteine was safe and effective in preventing acute deterioration in renal function after elective coronary angiography. In fact, acute contrast media–induced reduction in renal function was reduced by 68% in the supplement group compared to the placebo group (NNT = 12). Therefore this intervention should be considered for high-risk clients who have diabetes or chronic renal disease and are about to undergo coronary angiography.

Reference

Kay , J., et al. (2003). Acetylcysteine for prevention of acute deterioration of renal function following elective coronary angiography and intervention: A randomized controlled trial. *Journal of the American Medical Association, 289,* 553-558.

NNT, Number needed to treat.

fection is the most common complication because of the distorted renal architecture; chronic infection can occur if resistant bacteria develop. Aggressive control of hypertension is essential.

Unlike clients with decreasing creatinine clearance rates caused by other kidney diseases, those with polycystic kidney disease seem to waste rather than retain sodium. Thus they need increased sodium and water intake. When ESRD develops, dialysis or renal transplantation is required. Nursing interventions for clients with renal failure are discussed in Chapter 38.

Genetic counseling (see Chapter 17) is advisable because of the hereditary nature of the disease, especially if the disease is diagnosed during childbearing years. Because the disease typically appears after the childbearing period, however, the likelihood of transmitting the disease to another generation is high. Therefore counseling the extended family is essential when the disease has been identified.

Adult-Onset Medullary Cystic Disease

Adult-onset medullary cystic disease, sometimes called *uremic sponge kidney* or *medullary polycystic disease,* is also an autosomal dominant disorder. It is similar to polycystic disease in all aspects except that it progresses to uremia rapidly after its onset in the teenage years or in one's 20s. Hemodialysis and renal transplantation are likely to be required.

Medullary Sponge Kidney

Medullary sponge kidney is a cystic disorder in which spaces are produced at the apex of the renal pyramids. Onset peaks during adolescence or between ages 30 and 40 years. Infection, calculi, pain, and hematuria are potential complications. Renal function usually remains adequate unless the client has uncontrolled infection or calculi.

OTHER HEREDITARY RENAL DISORDERS

Other hereditary renal disorders include some types of chronic nephritis (such as Alport's disease), congenital nephrotic syndrome, distal renal tubular acidosis, idiopathic hypercalciuria, and nephrotic diabetes insipidus. Many of these conditions are fatal during childhood, but some persist into adulthood and are discussed in the appropriate parts of this text.

CONCLUSIONS

Renal disorders are highly complex. You must have a clear understanding of the structure and function of the renal system to care for clients with these conditions. The outcomes of successful treatment include preservation of renal function.

THINKING CRITICALLY *evolve*

1. A 35-year-old newlywed woman enters the emergency department with acute abdominal pain and a temperature of 101.8° F. Her abdomen is distended, and she has not had a bowel movement today, even though she is usually regular. The abdominal pain is diffuse and on the right side. She has no rebound tenderness and no pain at McBurney's point. Her WBC is 15,000/mm³. What problems other than appendicitis might she be experiencing? What other assessments should be made?

Factors to Consider. What type of renal problem might she be experiencing? What teaching would she need once the diagnosis is made? What medication might be prescribed and why? What follow-up is needed?

2. L.S. is a 22-year-old male college student with a diagnosis of acute glomerulonephritis. Three weeks ago, he received oral antibiotic therapy for strep throat. He is scheduled for a renal biopsy to confirm a diagnosis of acute poststreptococcal glomerulonephritis. What other diagnostic assessments should be made? What is the expected course of treatment?

Factors to Consider. What teaching does this client need when the diagnosis is confirmed? What medication might be prescribed, and how will it be delivered? What follow-up is needed?

3. C.H. is a 68-year-old retired mail carrier who lives with his wife. They spend 6 months living in their home state in the Midwest and spend the winter months in Arizona. The client is admitted with a diagnosis of suspected renal cell carcinoma. Diagnostic tests confirm the diagnosis. What surgical procedure will be scheduled? What nursing interventions are associated with this procedure?

Factors to Consider. What diagnostic tests were used to confirm the diagnosis of renal carcinoma? What tests will be used to determine whether radiation, chemotherapy, and immunotherapy are needed? Describe the postoperative assessments you should make for pain management, vital signs, surgical dressings, drainage tubes, and urine output. If Mr. and Mrs. H. plan to drive to Arizona a month after surgery, what should you discuss with them about their travel plans?

Discussions for these questions can be found on the website and the CD-ROM.

BIBLIOGRAPHY

1. American Cancer Society. (2003). *Cancer facts and figures.* Atlanta: Author.

2. Bevan, M. (2001). Assessing renal function in older people. *Nursing Older People, 13*(2), 27-28.

3. Brenner, B.M. (Ed.). (2000). *Brenner and Rector's the kidney* (6th ed.). Philadelphia: W.B. Saunders.

4. Chertow, G.M., et al. (2001). Guided medication dosing for inpatients with renal insufficiency. *Journal of the American Medical Association, 286*(22), 2839-2844.

5. Chmielewski, C. (2003). Renal anatomy and overview of nephron function. *Nephrology Nursing Journal, 30,* 185-192.

6. Chow, W., et al. (1999). Rising incidence of renal cell cancer in the United States. *Journal of the American Medical Association, 281*(17), 1628-1631.

7. Clark, P. (1999). 13-year experience with percutaneous management of upper tract transitional cell carcinoma. *Journal of Urology, 161,* 772-776.

8. Deedwania, P.C. (2000). Hypertension and diabetes: New therapeutic options. *Archives of Internal Medicine, 160*(11), 1585-1594, 1708-1709.

9. Diamond, G.L., & Zalups, R.K. (1998). Understanding renal toxicity of heavy metals. *Toxicology and Pathology, 26*(1), 92-103.

10. Fox, H.L., & Swann, D. (2001). Goodpasture syndrome: Pathophysiology, diagnosis, and management. *Nephrology Nursing Journal, 28,* 305-311.

11. Goldman, L., & Bennett, J.C. (Eds.). (2000). *Cecil textbook of medicine* (21st ed.). Philadelphia: W.B. Saunders.

12. Gonzalez, R.P., et al. (1999). Surgical management of renal trauma: Is vascular control necessary? *Journal of Trauma: Injury Infection and Critical Care 47,* 1039-1044.

13. Guyton, A.C., & Hall, J.E. (2000). *Textbook of medical physiology* (10th ed.). Philadelphia: W.B. Saunders.

14. Halperin, M.L., & Bohn, D. (2002). Clinical approach to disorders of salt and water balance: Emphasis on integrative physiology. *Critical Care Clinics, 18*(2), 249-272.

15. Hebert, L.A., Spetie, D.N., & Keane, W.F. (2001). The urgent call of albuminuria/proteinuria: Heeding its significance in early detection of kidney disease . . . second in a series. *Postgraduate Medicine, 110*(4), 79-82, 87-88, 93-94.

16. Holechek, M.J. (2003). Glomerular filtration: An overview. *Nephrology Nursing Journal, 30,* 285-292.

17. Hornstein, G. (2001). Short course: Pyelonephritis. *Office and Emergency Pediatrics, 14*(1), 8-13.

18. Howard, V.B., & Tasota, F.J. (2001). Eye on diagnostics: Assessing for rhabdomyolysis. *Nursing, 31*(9), 70.

19. Karnik, J., & Chertow, G.M. (2000). Analgesic-related renal disease: Causes, patients at risk, management. *Journal of Critical Illness, 15*(1): 49-51, 55-58.

20. Kelly, A.L. (1999). Acute pyelonephritis: altered physiology, diagnosis and management in the emergency department. *Australian Emergency Nursing Journal, 2*(3), 8-12.

21. Koeppen, B.M., & Stanton, B.A. (2000). *Renal physiology* (3rd ed.). St. Louis: Mosby.

22. Kumar, S., & Berl, T. (1999). NSAID-induced renal toxicity: When to suspect, what to do. *Consultant, 39*(1), 195-198, 201-202.

23. Lang, M.M., & Towers, C. (2001). Identifying poststreptococcal glomerulonephritis. *Nurse Practitioner: American Journal of Primary Health Care, 26*(8), 34, 37-38, 40-42.

24. Loeb, W.F. (1998). The measurement of renal injury. *Toxicology and Pathology, 26*(1), 26-28.

25. Lubkin, I.M., & Larsen, P.D. (2002). *Chronic illness: Impact and interventions* (5th ed.). Boston: Jones & Bartlett.

26. Massry, S.G., & Glassock, R.J. (Eds.). (2001). *Massry and Glassock's textbook of nephrology* (4th ed.). Philadelphia: Lippincott Williams & Wilkins.

27. Matthews, L.A., & Spirnak, J.P. (1995). The nonoperative approach to major blunt renal trauma. *Seminars in Urology, 13*(1), 77-82.

28. Meister, J., & Reddy, K. (2002). Rhabdomyolysis: An overview: this rare disease may be on the rise. *American Journal of Nursing, 102*(2), 75, 77, 79.

29. Melville, A., Richardson, R., & Lister-Sharp, D. (2000). Learning curve: Complications of type 2 diabetes: Renal disease and the promotion of patient self-management. *Nursing Times, 96*(17), 37-38.

30. Melville, A., Richardson, R., & Lister-Sharp, D. (2000). Type 2 diabetes. *Health Service Journal, 110*(5696), 32-33.

31. Miller, O., & Hemphill, R.R. (2001). Urinary tract infection and pyelonephritis. *Emergency Medicine Clinics of North America, 19*(3), 655-674.

32. Moody, F. (1999). *Atlas of ambulatory surgery.* Philadelphia: W.B. Saunders.

33. Morey, A.F., & McAninch, J.W.R. (1996). Renal trauma: Principles of evaluation and management. *Trauma Quarterly, 13*(1), 79-94.

34. Myhre, M.J. (2000). Herbal remedies, nephropathies, and renal disease. *Nephrology Nursing Journal, 27*(5), 473-480.

35. Nelson, D.B. (2003). Minimal change glomerulopathy in pregnancy. *Nephrology Nursing Journal, 30,* 45-57.

36. Palmieri, P.A. (2002). Obstructive nephropathy: Pathophysiology, diagnosis and collaborative management. *Nephrology Nursing Journal, 29,* 15-23.

37. Porrovecchio, S. (2000). RHABDO — what?! *Pulse, 37*(1), 15.

38. Raynovich, W. (2000). Crush syndrome: Indications & treatment options. *Journal of Emergency Medical Services 25*(1), 82-90, 92-93.

39. Rupert, S.A. (2002). Pathogenesis and treatment of rhabdomyolysis. *Journal of the American Academy of Nurse-Practitioners 14*(2), 82-87.

40. Russell, T.A. (2000). Acute renal failure related to rhabdomyolysis: pathophysiology, diagnosis, and collaborative management. *Nephrology Nursing Journal, 27,* 567-577.

41. Sarnak, M.J. (2002). How can the cardiac death rate be reduced in dialysis patients? *Seminars in Dialysis, 15*(1), 18-29.

42. Scholz, M. (2001). News watch: Pain clinic: Will long term analgesic use lead to kidney damage? *RN, 64*(11), 95.

43. Schneiderman, H., & Pazmino, P. (2001). What's your diagnosis? . . . nephrotic syndrome. *Consultant, 41*(7), 1017-1018, 1021-1022.

44. Schrier, R.W. (1999). *Atlas of diseases of the kidney.* Philadelphia: Blackwell Science.

45. Schrier, R.W. (2001). *Diseases of the kidney and urinary tract* (7th ed.). Philadelphia: Lippincott Williams & Wilkins.

46. Schrier, R.W. (2000). *Manual of nephrology* (5th ed.). Philadelphia: Lippincott Williams & Wilkins.

47. Schrier, R.W. (2002). *Renal and electrolyte disorders* (6th ed.). Philadelphia: Lippincott Williams & Wilkins.

48. Schrier, R.W., & Gottschalk, C.W. (Eds.). (2001). *Diseases of the kidney and urinary tract.* Philadelphia: Lippincott Williams & Wilkins.

49. Smith, D.M., Fortune-Faulkner E.M., & Spurbeck, B.L. (2000). Continuing education: Lupus nephritis: Pathophysiology, diagnosis, and collaborative management. *Nephrology Nursing Journal, 27*(2), 199-236.

50. Spitalewitz, S. (2000). In consultation: How to best control hypertension in patients with renal insufficiency. *Journal of Critical Illness, 15*(9), 468.

51. Staples, B.J. (2001). Primary IgA nephropathy: Pathophysiology, diagnosis, and clinical management. *Nephrology Nursing Journal, 28,* 151-158.

52. Stone, J., Wyman, J., & Salisbury, S. (1999). *Clinical gerontological nursing: A guide to advanced practice* (2nd ed.). Philadelphia: W.B. Saunders.

53. Tambimuttu, J. (2000). Crush injury and its management. *Australian Emergency Nursing Journal, 3*(1), 20-23.

54. Tanagho, E.A., & McAninich, J.W. (2000). *Smith's general urology* (15th ed.). Norwalk, CT: Lange Medical Books/McGraw-Hill.

55. Tran, M., & Rutecki, G.W. (2000). Renal disease: Tips on prevention and early recognition. *Consultant, 40*(2), 222-225, 228-229.

56. Vig, E.K., & Hu, H. (2000). Lead toxicity in older adults. *Journal of the American Geriatrics Society, 48*(11):1501-1506.

57. Walsh, P., & Retik, A.B. (2002). *Campbell's urology* (8th ed.). Philadelphia: W.B. Saunders.

58. Weir, M.R. (2001). Decision making in medicine: Hypertension in patients with type 2 diabetes . . . including commentary by Henrich W.L. *Hospital Practice, 36*(1), 41-42, 47-48, 51-52.

Management of Clients with Renal Failure

Anita E. Molzahn

A disruption in renal function impairs the body's ability to maintain fluid, electrolyte, and acid-base balance. Reduced renal function interferes with erythropoietin and prostaglandin synthesis. Insulin degradation and the renin-angiotensin-aldosterone system are also affected by decreased renal function.

The most common diseases and problems that cause renal failure are described in Chapter 37. This chapter identifies manifestations of acute and chronic renal failure and outlines treatments used to replace or restore renal function, such as dialysis and transplantation. For clients and families, psychosocial needs may arise from the physiologic problems caused by renal failure. You have a key role in helping promote quality of life and rehabilitation for these clients.

UREMIC SYNDROME

The terms uremia, uremic syndrome, and renal failure are used synonymously. *Uremia* literally means "urine in the blood." This term and the term *uremic syndrome* describe a set of manifestations that result from loss of renal function. This loss may be of sudden onset or may develop over a long period. It may be self-limiting or irreversible. Sudden loss of kidney function, as occurs with damage from trauma, shock, toxins, or acute glomerulonephritis, brings on uremia rapidly and usually causes severe deterioration of the client's condition. Gradual loss of kidney function over an extended period may occur with glomerulonephritis, hypertension, chronic pyelonephritis, and other diseases.

Because the kidneys perform a wide variety of functions, the effects of uremia occur not only in the kidneys but also in other organ systems. Because of the time involved, chronic renal failure (CRF) causes more degenerative changes throughout the body than acute uremia does. However, both types of renal failure have many of the same consequences. Unless the process can be halted or replacement therapy initiated, coma, seizures, and death result.

ACUTE RENAL FAILURE

Acute renal failure (ARF) refers to the abrupt loss of kidney function. Over a period of hours to a few days, the glomerular filtration rate (GFR) decreases. Serum creatinine and urea nitrogen or blood urea nitrogen (BUN) levels increase. A healthy adult who eats a normal diet needs a minimum urine output of about 400 ml over 24 hours to excrete the body's waste products through the

Nursing Outcomes Classification (NOC)
for Nursing Diagnoses—Clients with Renal Failure

Anxiety
  Anxiety Control
  Coping
Constipation
  Bowel Elimination
  Hydration
Deficient Fluid Volume
  Electrolyte and Acid-Base Balance
  Fluid Balance
  Hydration
Excess Fluid Volume
  Electrolyte and Acid-Base Balance
  Fluid Balance
  Hydration
Fatigue
  Activity Tolerance
  Endurance
  Energy Conservation
  Nutritional Status: Energy
Imbalanced Nutrition: Less Than Body Requirements
  Nutritional Status

Nutritional Status: Food and Fluid Intake
Risk for Compromised Family Coping
  Family Coping
  Family Normalization
Risk for Impaired Skin Integrity
  Dialysis Access Integrity
  Nutritional Status: Biochemical Measures
  Risk Control
  Risk Detection
  Self-Mutilation Restraint
  Tissue Integrity: Skin and Mucous Membranes
  Tissue Perfusion: Peripheral
Risk for Ineffective Breathing Pattern
  Respiratory Status: Ventilation
Risk for Ineffective Coping
  Coping
  Decision Making
  Role Performance

Risk for Ineffective Family Therapeutic Regimen Management
  Family Functioning
  Family Health Status
  Family Participation in Professional Care
Risk for Ineffective Individual Therapeutic Regimen Management
  Family Functioning
  Family Health Status
  Family Participation in Professional Care
Risk for Infection
  Dialysis Access Integrity
  Immune Status
  Risk Control
  Risk Detection
  Tissue Integrity: Skin and Mucous Membranes
Risk for Injury
  Risk Control
  Risk Detection
  Symptom Control

kidneys. Any lower amount indicates a decreased GFR. *Oliguria* refers to daily outputs of urine between 100 and 400 ml; *anuria* refers to urine output of less than 100 ml.

Etiology and Risk Factors
There are many possible causes of ARF, the most common of which are hypotension and prerenal hypovolemia. The etiologic mechanisms of these disorders are discussed in Chapter 37.

Classification
The numerous causes of ARF can be categorized into three major areas: prerenal, renal, and postrenal (Figure 38-1).

Prerenal Causes
Prerenal causes of ARF are those that interfere with renal perfusion. The kidneys depend on adequate delivery of blood to be filtered by the glomeruli. Therefore reduced renal blood flow lowers the GFR and can lead to ARF. Conditions that contribute to decreased renal blood flow include the following:
- Circulatory volume depletion, as may occur with diarrhea, vomiting, hemorrhage, excessive use of diuretics, burns, renal salt-wasting conditions, or glycosuria

- Volume shifts, as from third-space sequestration of fluid, vasodilation, or gram-negative sepsis
- Decreased cardiac output, as during cardiac pump failure, pericardial tamponade, or acute pulmonary embolism
- Decreased peripheral vascular resistance, as from spinal anesthesia, septic shock, or anaphylaxis
- Vascular obstruction, such as bilateral renal artery occlusion or dissecting aneurysm

Intrarenal Causes
Intrarenal (or renal) causes of ARF involve parenchymal changes caused by disease or nephrotoxic substances. Acute tubular necrosis is the most common intrarenal cause of ARF and accounts for about 75% of cases. This destruction of the tubular epithelial cells results from impaired renal perfusion or direct damage by nephrotoxins. In addition to the nephrotoxins described in Chapter 37, acute tubular necrosis may be caused by heme pigments, such as myoglobin and hemoglobin, which are liberated from damaged muscle tissue. This release may result from trauma (rhabdomyolysis), such as surgery, crush injury, and electric shock, or from nontraumatic conditions, such as severe muscle exertion, genetic conditions (such as diabetes mellitus or malignant hyperthermia), infectious disease,

PRERENAL
FAILURE

Shock
Circulating volume depletion
Volume shifts
Decreased cardiac output
Decreased peripheral
     vascular resistance
Renal artery obstruction

INTRARENAL
FAILURE

Acute tubular necrosis
Renal trauma
Severe muscle exertion
Genetic conditions
Infectious disease
Metabolic disorders
Glomerulonephritis
Renal artery lesions

POSTRENAL
FAILURE

Prostate disease
Obstruction
Spinal cord injury
Pelvic trauma

FIGURE 38-1 Causes of acute renal failure: prerenal, intrarenal, and postrenal.

metabolic conditions (such as hypokalemia, phosphatemia, or heat stroke), and rejection of a transplanted kidney.

Other intrarenal causes of ARF include glomerulonephritis; microvascular and large vascular lesions, as in hemolytic-uremic syndrome; thrombosis; vasculitis; scleroderma; trauma; atherosclerosis; tumor invasion; and cortical necrosis, which is caused by prolonged vasospasm of the cortical blood vessels.

Postrenal Causes

Postrenal causes of ARF arise from an obstruction in the urinary tract, anywhere from the tubules to the urethral meatus. Common sources of obstruction include prostatic hypertrophy, calculi, invading tumors, surgical accidents, ureteral or urethral strictures or stenosis, and retroperitoneal fibrosis. Spinal cord injury may lead to decreased bladder emptying and a functional obstruction.

General Considerations

In management of the client with ARF, it is important to determine whether the disorder originates from prerenal, intrarenal, or postrenal causes before intervention begins. Appropriate interventions require determining the cause of the disorder.

One health promotion strategy is to teach clients about the risks of nephrotoxic agents identified in Chapter 37. Other health promotion and health maintenance actions include monitoring of vital signs and urine output and early identification and reversal of hypotension and hypovolemia, the two causes of ARF associated with the highest mortality rates. Prevention of urinary obstruction is another health promotion and maintenance action.

Pathophysiology

The pathogenesis of ARF is not clear. One hypothesis is that the damaged tubules cannot conserve sodium normally, which activates the renin-angiotensin-aldosterone system. The effect is to redistribute the renal vascular supply by increasing the tone of both the afferent and efferent arterioles. The resulting ischemia may cause an increase in vasopressin, cellular swelling, inhibition of prostaglandin synthesis, and further stimulation of the renin-angiotensin system. The reduced blood flow decreases glomerular pressure, GFR, and tubular flow; thus oliguria occurs.

Another theory is that cellular and protein debris in the tubule obstruct the lumen, which raises the intratubular pressure. The increasing oncotic pressure opposes filtration pressure until glomerular filtration stops. A biochemical theory claims that decreased renal blood flow leads to decreased oxygen delivery to the proximal tubules; this causes a reduction in cellular adenosine triphosphate, which increases cytosolic and mitochondrial calcium concentrations. The result of this process is cell death and tubular necrosis. Vasomotor nephropathy, which causes spasms of peritubular capillaries, may result in tubular damage. Other possible pathogenic mechanisms include leakage of filtered urine through damaged tubules back into the peritubular capillaries and chemical or morphologic changes in the basement membrane of the glomerular capillary, which decrease nephron filtration. The reversibility of this mechanism depends on the level of destruction of the basement membrane.

Clinical Manifestations

The clinical course of ARF is marked by several phases. The onset (or initiating) phase covers the period from the precipitating event to the development of renal manifestations. Manifestations may begin immediately or up to a week after the precipitating event. The oliguric-anuric (or nonoliguric) phase lasts 1 to 8 weeks. The longer the oliguric-anuric phase, the poorer the prognosis. Dialysis may be required during the oliguric-anuric phase.

A gradual or abrupt return to glomerular filtration and leveling of the BUN signal the diuretic phase. Urine output may be 1000 to 2000 ml/day, which may lead to dehydration; 25% of the deaths from ARF occur during this phase.

The recovery phase lasts 3 to 12 months. During this time, the client commonly returns to an activity level similar to that before the onset of the illness. Mild tubular abnormalities, including glycosuria and decreased concentrating ability, may continue for years, and the client is continually at risk for fluid and electrolyte imbalance, especially during times of stress.

The effects of ARF are widespread. The major consequences include the following:

- Fluid and electrolyte imbalances (fluid overload or depletion, hyperkalemia, hyponatremia, hypocalcemia, and hypermagnesemia)
- Acidosis
- Increased susceptibility to secondary infections
- Anemia
- Platelet dysfunction
- Gastrointestinal complications (anorexia, nausea, vomiting, diarrhea or constipation, and stomatitis)
- Increased incidence of pericarditis
- Uremic encephalopathy characterized by apathy, defective recent memory, episodic obtundation, dysarthria, tremors, convulsions, and coma
- Impaired wound healing

Other manifestations are usually a result of these sequelae. The most common overall manifestation of ARF is alteration of the expected urine output. Usually, oliguria or anuria is found, but polyuric ARF accounts for 30% of the cases. There are two varieties of ARF: nonoliguric and oliguric.

Nonoliguric Renal Failure

Although nonoliguric, or polyuric, ARF is being recognized more often, its status remains controversial. It may be an independent entity or may be a phase of oliguric ARF.

Clients with nonoliguric renal failure may excrete as much as 2 L/day, and this must be recognized as a possible manifestation of ARF. The urine produced is dilute and nearly iso-osmolar, reflected in a low urine specific gravity indicating that not all nephrons have stopped filtering. Hypertension and tachypnea, with manifestations of fluid overload, are commonly found. The client may also demonstrate manifestations of extracellular fluid depletion, such as dry mucous membranes, poor skin turgor, and orthostatic hypotension. Nonoliguric renal failure is usually associated with less morbidity and mortality than the oliguric form, probably because of the lesser degree and shorter duration of azotemia.

Oliguric Renal Failure

In oliguric ARF, urine production is usually less than 400 ml/day. However, the aging kidney normally loses its concentrating ability, and renal function becomes more susceptible to insult. Therefore an older client may have had oliguria even at urine volumes of 600 to 700 ml/day.

The clinical manifestations of oliguric ARF depend on the cause. In prerenal failure, assessment findings are diverse, depending on the underlying condition. The client commonly has a history of a precipitating event, such as hemorrhage or cardiac insult. The urine has a high specific gravity and osmolarity, and there is little or no proteinuria. Urine sediment is usually normal, although it may contain a few hyaline and granular casts. There is little urinary sodium excretion. The BUN-creatinine ratio is significantly elevated, reaching levels between 10:1 and 40:1.

Systemic manifestations of intrinsic renal failure may include edema, weight gain, hemoptysis resulting from elevated left ventricular end-diastolic pressure, weakness from anemia, and hypertension. The urine has a fixed specific gravity, a high sodium concentration, and definite proteinuria. The client with glomerulonephritis has hematuria and red blood cell and hemoglobin casts. Acute tubular necrosis causes muddy brown granular casts. If there has been significant tissue damage, expect elevated levels of serum creatinine, phosphokinase, and potassium.

Urine produced in postrenal failure may have fixed specific gravity and elevated sodium concentration with little or no proteinuria. Urine sediment is generally normal. The most definitive manifestations are those indicating obstruction, as described with calculi and neoplasms. Wide fluctuations between anuria and polyuria may indicate intermittent urinary tract obstruction.

Urinalysis and determinations of urine specific gravity and sodium levels, serum creatinine, and urea nitrogen (BUN) are common diagnostic tests for ARF. The amount of urine in relation to intake is also important in formulating the diagnosis. To measure the exact urine output or to obtain a specimen for culture and sensitivity, the client may need to be catheterized one time only (with a straight catheter).

Prognosis

The mortality rate in ARF may be as high as 50%; the highest mortality rates occur when failure is caused by trauma or surgery. The lowest mortality rate is in ARF caused by nephrotoxic substances (see Chapter 37). When obstruction or glomerulonephritis is the cause, the mortality rate is low.

Outcome Management
■ Medical Management

Prevent Acute Renal Failure. The medical management of ARF is largely based on preventing and treating its effects. As with any disease process, prevention is the primary intervention. Attaining and maintaining adequate hydration and diuresis in high-risk clients is crucial, as is the prevention of contributing factors.

Once ARF has developed, prompt recognition and action facilitate restoration of optimal renal function. Correction of the underlying condition, such as hydration for a client with hypovolemic shock, may be all that is necessary in ARF caused by prerenal disorders. Postrenal causes must be rectified. In the meantime, the sequelae of ARF require specific intervention.

Maintain Fluid and Electrolyte Balance. In ARF, maintenance of fluid and electrolyte balance is key to survival. Imbalances are common and pose significant challenges to the clinician.

Fluid replacement must be done carefully to avoid fluid overload. Fluid replacement volumes are usually calculated on the basis of some fraction of the previous day's urine output plus an amount (commonly 400 ml) to account for the usual insensible losses that occur during a 24-hour period. Amounts lost in other ways, such as vomiting and diarrhea, are added to the daily allotment. Unless the client is receiving total parenteral nutrition (TPN), some physicians use a daily weight loss of 0.2 to 0.5 kg/day as a measure of the success of the fluid replacement program. This amount represents the usual daily weight loss through catabolism and loss of lean body mass.

Diuretic therapy may be used cautiously. Furosemide and mannitol are the drugs used most often, but furosemide can be nephrotoxic, increasing the risk of further renal damage. It is also important to avoid dehydration, and fluids should be replaced as needed to maintain adequate blood flow to the kidneys.

Electrolyte replacement is based primarily on urine and serum electrolyte concentrations. Hyperkalemia is probably the most dangerous imbalance because of its contribution to cardiac dysrhythmias and arrest. In addition to the kidney's inability to excrete potassium, this electrolyte is released in greater quantities from the body cells when acidosis is present and is further increased by rapid tissue catabolism.

Electrocardiographic monitors are commonly used to check for effects of hypokalemia or hyperkalemia. Treatment of hyperkalemia is described in the Integrating Pharmacology feature on Medications for Acute Renal Failure on p. 946. Hyponatremia usually results from dilution rather than true lack of sodium. Therefore intervention is a matter of proper fluid replacement (i.e., fluid restriction and self-correction).

Because magnesium is normally excreted by the kidneys, it can accumulate in renal failure. Dark green vegetables, unrefined grains, seeds, nuts, legumes, and antacids and osmotic laxatives containing magnesium should be avoided because they increase serum magnesium levels.

Metabolic acidosis usually results from the accumulation of acid waste products. Sodium bicarbonate, sodium lactate, or sodium acetate may be used in the short term to correct this condition. Dialysis is usually used for severe acidosis.

The Integrating Pharmacology feature highlights some of the common medications used in ARF.

Replace Renal Function. Dialysis (detailed later in the chapter) is frequently required for treatment of ARF. Indications for dialysis include the following:

- Significant volume overload
- Uncontrolled hyperkalemia or acidosis
- Progressive uremia, as evidenced by rising BUN and creatinine concentrations
- Altered central nervous system function
- Pericarditis

There are some special considerations for dialysis of clients with ARF. First, heparin is generally decreased to reduce the risk of bleeding. Because hypotension is common, clients must be carefully monitored and replacement fluids provided as appropriate.

For clients with ARF, continuous renal replacement therapy (CRRT) has benefits. There are several types of CRRT, including (1) continuous arteriovenous hemofiltration, (2) continuous venovenous hemofiltration, (3) continuous venovenous hemodialysis, (4) continuous arteriovenous ultrafiltration, and (5) slow continuous ultrafiltration (Box 38-1). In essence, these methods involve removal of plasma water and dissolved contents from the client's blood across a membrane. In contrast, in dialysis, particles are removed by diffusion. Slow continuous removal of waste products and water through CRRT is less stressful to the client than shorter, more efficient dialysis treatments.

Prevent Infections. Secondary infections are a significant cause of death in clients with ARF. The client must be monitored carefully for infectious processes; if these occur, they should be treated aggressively. Except to monitor urine output during ARF, indwelling urethral catheters are usually avoided because of their great potential for introducing infection. If a catheter is placed, meticulous catheter care is essential.

Monitor the Client. Treatment of ARF may take place in an intensive care unit or other critical care unit, depending on the cause. Much of the care consists of physiologic monitoring and assessment. In addition to monitoring fluid and electrolyte balance, you should monitor the progression of manifestations associated with renal failure. Pericarditis occurs in as many as 18% of clients with renal failure. Assessment findings include pleuritic

INTEGRATING PHARMACOLOGY

Medications for Acute Renal Failure

Treatment of acute renal failure (ASF) depends on the cause of the renal failure. For instance, in some autoimmune diseases, immunosuppressive agents may be prescribed. Generally, treatment is based on manifestations. Low doses (1 to 5 μg/kg/min) of dopamine hydrochloride (Intropin) may be given to activate dopamine receptors in the kidney. Dopamine, a sympathomimetic, can dilate renal blood vessels, which improves renal function, increases urine flow, and increases sodium excretion to improve renal function.

Metabolic acidosis is common and is typically treated with sodium bicarbonate. Hypertension is also a common manifestation of ARF. Where hypertension is a result of fluid volume excess, fluid removal through renal replacement therapy is generally preferable to the administration of antihypertensive medications. In other cases, hypertension is caused by an excess of renin production by the kidneys (starting the renin-angiotensin system); aggressive antihypertensive therapy is then needed to control blood pressure effectively. Diuretic therapy may be used cautiously. Furosemide and mannitol are the drugs used most often, but furosemide can be nephrotoxic, increasing the risk of further renal damage. Diuretics are typically not very effective in people with advanced renal failure.

Hyperkalemia is potentially life-threatening because of the risk of cardiac arrest; it should be treated immediately and aggressively. Treatment may include administration of calcium, which antagonizes membrane actions. Cation exchange resins may be administered orally or rectally to facilitate excretion of potassium through the gastrointestinal tract. Cation exchange resins (e.g., Kayexalate) that exchange potassium for other electrolytes can be administered orally or rectally. They start to act within 2 to 3 hours. Sorbitol, an osmotic cathartic, is given with cation exchange resins to induce a diarrhea to eliminate the potassium ions that were exchanged for sodium ions in the resins. Sorbitol can be given orally, as an enema, or by nasogastric tube. Potassium-containing foods and medications should be avoided. In an emergency, administration of 50% glucose and regular insulin, with sodium bicarbonate if necessary, can temporarily prevent cardiac arrest by moving potassium into the cells and reducing serum potassium levels. Insulin and glucose, beta-2-adrenergic agonists, and sodium bicarbonate force potassium into the cells; these three types of medications work within 30 to 60 minutes and last several hours.

Infection is one of the most frequent complications of ARF and occurs in as many as 70% of cases. Prophylactic use of antibiotics is sometimes indicated and treatment of infections is based on culture and sensitivity reports.

In ARF, particular care should be taken to avoid nephrotoxic agents to prevent further injury to the already damaged kidneys. The absorption, distribution, metabolism, and elimination of medications must be considered before medications are prescribed or administered. If the kidneys are not functioning, drugs that are normally excreted by the kidney can accumulate to toxic levels. Some drugs are removed by dialysis; others are not. All these factors should be considered when determining dosage, route, and time of administration. Also, drugs that are nephrotoxic (e.g., aminoglycosides, intravenous pyelogram [IVP] dye) may cause further damage to a dysfunctional organ and should be avoided.

---

pain (which may subside when the client assumes an upright position), pericardial friction rub, tachycardia, and fever. Treatment usually starts with steroids or nonsteroidal anti-inflammatory drugs (NSAIDs). Pericardiocentesis and pericardiectomy may be necessary if cardiac function is compromised.

Other problems call for relief of manifestations. The increasing BUN decreases the seizure threshold, resulting in an increase in the number of seizures. These seizures may be relieved by intravenous phenytoin or phenobarbital. Anemia is treated by transfusions or the use of recombinant erythropoietin. Erythropoietin is a hormone produced by the kidney that stimulates red blood cell production. Erythropoietin is used in CRF, but its use in ARF has not been studied extensively. Bleeding tendencies may be minimized by correcting vitamin K deficiencies as well as by reducing the serum BUN level, because BUN interferes with platelet aggregation.

Maintain Nutritional Status. Proper nutrition is crucial. A high-calorie, low-protein diet is usually prescribed. The diet may also be low in sodium, magnesium, phosphate, and potassium. The protein must be of high biologic value (complete), containing the essential amino acids to reduce nitrogenous waste products. Adequate carbohydrate intake reverses the process of gluconeogenesis. During the acute phases, intake should be 135 to 150 nonprotein kilocalories (kcal) for each 6.25 g of protein ingested; this ratio is considered adequate for preventing protein catabolism. Liquid supplements, low in potassium, may also be used. If oral intake is not sufficient to meet requirements, tube feedings or TPN, including lipids, may be instituted.

■ Nursing Management of the Medical Client

Assessment

Carefully monitor any client with risk factors for ARF. It is important to assess fluid balance in any hospitalized or seriously injured client. Because hypovolemia is a common cause, assess the client closely for this problem. When the diagnosis is ARF, carefully assess for such complications as

BOX 38-1 *Types of Renal Replacement Therapies*

Modalities of continuous renal replacement therapies (CRRT) are similar in that they slowly remove water from the body. However, they differ in the way they remove solutes.

Diffusion is the process where particles move from an area of high concentration through a semipermeable membrane to a solution of low concentration. *Convection* is the process whereby replacement fluid pulls waste through the semipermeable membrane. High flow rates of fluid (e.g., 1000 to 2000 ml/hr) drag more particles across the membrane than slower flow rates.

Ultrafiltration is a process of removal of fluid from the extracorporeal circuit by creating pressure across the membrane.

Continuous arteriovenous hemofiltration (CAVH) was the first slow renal replacement procedure. CAVH involved circulation of blood from an artery through a hemofilter and returned through a vein. It requires a blood pressure high enough to circulate the blood. More recently, other forms of CRRT use pumps to circulate blood and replacement fluids and dialysate and a double lumen catheter is inserted into a large vein rather than using both an artery and a vein.

Slow continuous ultrafiltration (SCUF) is used to remove fluid; it involves convection through a process called ultrafiltration. It is used when fluid removal is the prime therapeutic goal. While some urea is removed with plasma water, the rate of urea removal is low.

Continuous venovenous hemofiltration (CVVH) works by convection. Blood is removed and returned through venous access. Fluid is infused into the extracorporeal circuit and removed rapidly by the hemofilter. As a result, wastes and toxins are removed by convection.

Continuous venovenous hemodialysis (CVVHD) is a slow form of dialysis in which blood is removed and returned through a venous access. Diffusion is the process used to remove wastes and electrolytes. However, the flow rate of blood and dialysate is slower than in conventional hemodialysis.

Continuous venovenous hemodiafiltration (CVVHDF) uses both convection and diffusion to remove fluids, waste particles, inflammatory mediators, and other toxins. Like dialysis, a dialysate solution runs counter to the blood and particles are removed by diffusion. In addition, an electrolyte solution is pumped into the blood to promote convection. It has the best clearances but is more expensive and technically challenging.

Continuous arteriovenous ultrafiltration (CAVU) is a process of fluid removal from the blood whereby blood is removed from an artery, through an extracorporeal circuit where fluid is removed and then returned through a vein. Ultrafiltration is the process used to remove fluid.

---

pleural effusion, pericarditis, acidosis, and uremia. See the Case Study feature on Acute Renal Failure and Abdominal Aortic Aneurysm Reaction at right.

Diagnosis, Outcomes, Interventions

Diagnosis: Deficient Fluid Volume or Excess Fluid Volume. A common nursing diagnosis in ARF is *Deficient Fluid Volume related to fluid loss from a variety of causes.* Another common nursing diagnosis is *Excess Fluid Volume related to inability of the kidneys to produce urine secondary to ARF.*

Outcomes. The client will not have deficient fluid volume and ARF; if ARF does occur, fluid volume excess will not develop or it will be managed with dialysis or CRRT, as evidenced by a return to balanced intake and output.

Interventions. Careful monitoring of fluid balance indicators is crucial to the management of ARF. Accurate intake and output measurements guide the fluid replacement regimen. Compare these values and look for 24- to 48-hour trends. Check the client's vital signs (including postural blood pressures and apical pulses), skin turgor, and mucous membranes about every 4 hours, depending on the severity of the illness. Carefully obtain daily weight measurements using the same scale at the same time of day. Obtain blood pressure measurements via an arterial line, if one is in place.

CASE STUDY   *evolve*

Acute Renal Failure and Abdominal Aortic Aneurysm Resection

Mr. Carlson is a 70-year-old retired farmer who is brought in by squad to a small rural hospital. He complains of boring-type abdominal pain that radiates through to the back. A computed tomography scan of the abdomen reveals a dissecting abdominal aneurysm. Mr. Carlson is flown to an urban hospital for emergency resection of the aneurysm. Complications encountered in surgery require that the aorta be cross-clamped for a number of hours. Multiple blood products are administered to replace those lost through hemorrhage. Mr. Carlson is admitted to the surgical intensive care unit for postoperative care and monitoring. . . . *Case Study continued on the website and the CD-ROM with discussions, multiple-choice questions, and a nursing care plan.* *evolve*

Urine specific gravity, usually an indication of fluid balance, may not be useful with intrinsic renal disease. Abnormalities in heart sounds, breath sounds, and mental status may indicate the presence of fluid and electrolyte imbalances.

When the physician has determined the client's fluid allotment, make sure that intake amounts for each shift are followed. This means carefully monitoring fluid intake to ensure that the prescribed amount is taken. Often, this amount represents a significant fluid restriction for the client, which causes a problem with thirst. Help the client stay within the prescribed restriction with careful oral hygiene and judicious use of ice chips, lip ointments, and appropriate diversionary activities. Placing the allotted water in a spray bottle may help spread out the amount taken. Fluid from foods must be taken into account as well. To conserve fluids for the client, administer medications with meals, if possible.

Diagnosis: Imbalanced Nutrition: Less Than Body Requirements.

Another common nursing diagnosis for clients with this disorder is *Imbalanced Nutrition: Less Than Body Requirements related to anorexia and altered metabolic state secondary to renal failure.*

Outcomes. The client will maintain adequate nutrition, as evidenced by sufficient intake to prevent protein catabolism and laboratory values within safe levels.

Interventions. A client with renal failure commonly experiences anorexia, nausea, stomatitis, and taste changes. These, combined with a generally less palatable diet, make adequate nutrition a challenge for nurse and client. Work with the client to plan a diet that is most acceptable. The therapeutic dietitian is a good resource.

Provide a pleasant environment at mealtime. Preparing foods in an attractive manner and presenting them in small amounts may help. Medications to alleviate the discomfort of nausea and stomatitis may be useful. Enteral or parenteral nutrition may be instituted if the client's nutritional status cannot be maintained with oral intake.

Diagnosis: Risk for Impaired Skin Integrity.

You may need to use the diagnosis *Risk for Impaired Skin Integrity related to poor cellular nutrition and edema.*

Outcomes. The client will not develop impaired skin integrity, as evidenced by intact skin.

Interventions. The poor systemic nutrition and edema that accompany renal failure may cause skin breakdown. Meticulous skin care, frequent turning, and special mattresses are important. Range-of-motion exercises facilitate movement and increase circulation.

Diagnosis: Risk for Infection.

Acute or chronic renal failure makes clients more susceptible to infection, resulting in a nursing diagnosis of *Risk for Infection related to lowered resistance.*

Outcomes. The client will not develop infection, as evidenced by normal vital signs, a normal white blood cell count, and no outward manifestations of infection.

Interventions. The client with ARF is immunocompromised and susceptible to secondary infection, a stress that the kidneys cannot handle. Nursing intervention must be designed to prevent infection in the usual high-risk sites (e.g., respiratory tract, wounds, central catheters, and mouth). Urethral catheters are avoided if possible. If they must be used, provide meticulous catheter care. Also, be alert to early manifestations of infection so that aggressive medical treatment may be instituted.

Diagnosis: Anxiety.

Inevitably, the client experiences *Anxiety related to unknown outcome of disease process.*

Outcomes. The client will demonstrate an ability to manage the anxiety, as evidenced by calmness and an ability to focus on the disease and its outcome.

Interventions. Because the client's physical needs are obvious, it is easy to forget that the client as well as significant others will be anxious and frightened. Give frequent, careful explanations, and provide emotional and psychological support.

Evaluation

The client is expected to maintain fluid balance. If fluid volume excess develops, it is managed with dialysis or CRRT to reduce body weight and to achieve balanced intake and output. The client should also maintain intact skin, demonstrate normal vital signs and white blood cell count, appear to be less anxious, and show ability to focus on the information provided.

Although ARF manifestations may continue, most clients with ARF recover within 4 to 10 weeks of correction of the underlying problem. Results of renal function studies may continue to improve for up to 12 months after the onset of ARF. The client is particularly vulnerable to additional renal injury during this time.

■ Self-Care

It is important for the client to understand the implications of ARF and the importance of following the therapeutic regimen. The client and significant others have to understand which manifestations might indicate further renal damage or CRF. The client must be closely observed by a nephrologist for at least a year after ARF is reversed so that deterioration of renal function can be monitored. The client and significant others require knowledge of renal failure and an understanding of the possible need for ongoing treatment.

■ Modifications for Older Clients

Older clients are at increased risk for ARF because of reduced cardiac contractile function, vascular compliance, renal plasma flow, and renal mass. The older adult has more difficulty maintaining a homeostatic fluid balance. The ability to retain sodium declines with age, as does the ability to concentrate urine. Older clients are also more likely to have pre-existing renal damage from such diseases as hypertension, diabetes, and benign prostatic hypertrophy in men. Therefore dosages of medications that are nephrotoxic or excreted by the kidney may need to be adjusted.

CHRONIC RENAL FAILURE

Chronic, or irreversible, renal failure is a progressive reduction of functioning renal tissue such that the remaining kidney mass can no longer maintain the body's internal environment. CRF can develop insidiously over many years, or it may result from an episode of ARF from which the client has not recovered.

The incidence of CRF varies widely by state and country. In the United States, the incidence is 331 new cases per million people. According to the U.S. Renal Data System, at the end of 2001, a total of 378,862 people were being treated for end-stage renal disease (ESRD); of these, 24.7% had a functioning transplant, 64.5% received hemodialysis, and 6.1% were on a form of peritoneal dialysis (for some people, data were not available).[60]

Etiology and Risk Factors

The causes of CRF are numerous. Chapter 37 discusses various injuries and disease processes that may end in renal failure. Chronic glomerulonephritis, ARF, polycystic kidney disease, obstruction, repeated episodes of pyelonephritis, and nephrotoxins are examples of causes. Systemic diseases, such as diabetes mellitus, hypertension, lupus erythematosus, polyarteritis, sickle cell disease, and amyloidosis, may produce CRF. Diabetes is the leading cause and accounts for more than 30% of clients who receive dialysis. Hypertension is the second leading cause of CRF.

To reduce the risk of CRF, the client should be closely observed and should receive adequate treatment to control or slow the progress of these problems before they progress to ESRD. Some conditions, such as lupus and diabetes, can progress to renal failure despite close treatment.

Pathophysiology

The pathogenesis of CRF involves deterioration and destruction of nephrons with progressive loss of renal function. As the total GFR decreases and clearance is reduced, serum urea nitrogen and creatinine levels increase. Remaining functioning nephrons hypertrophy as they filter a larger load of solutes. A consequence is that the kidneys lose their ability to concentrate urine adequately. To continue excreting the solutes, a large volume of dilute urine may be passed, which makes the client susceptible to fluid depletion. The tubules gradually lose their ability to reabsorb electrolytes. Occasionally, the result is salt wasting, in which urine contains large amounts of sodium, which leads to more polyuria.

As renal damage advances and the number of functioning nephrons declines, the total GFR decreases further. Thus the body becomes unable to rid itself of excess water, salt, and other waste products through the kidneys. When the GFR is less than 10 to 20 ml/min, the effect of uremic toxins on the body becomes evident. If the disease is not treated by dialysis or transplantation, the outcome of CRF is uremia and death.

Clinical Manifestations

The clinical manifestations of the early stages of renal failure depend on the disease process and contributing factors. As nephron destruction progresses to ESRD, the manifestations become similar and are described as uremic syndrome. The clinical course of irreversible renal disease and uremic syndrome follows a pattern:

- *Reduced renal reserve* refers to the state in which BUN is high-normal but the client has no clinical manifestations. Normal functioning is evident as long as the client is not exposed to unusual physiologic or psychosocial stress.
- *Renal insufficiency* reflects a more advanced pathologic process with mild azotemia when the client is receiving a general diet. Impaired urine concentration, nocturia (excessive urination at night), and mild anemia are common findings. Renal function is easily impaired by stress.
- *Renal failure* is indicated by severe azotemia, acidosis, impaired urine dilution, severe anemia, and a number of electrolyte imbalances, such as hypernatremia, hyperkalemia, and hyperphosphatemia.
- *ESRD* is characterized by two groups of clinical manifestations: deranged excretory and regulatory mechanisms and a distinctive grouping of gastrointestinal, cardiovascular, neuromuscular, hematologic, integumentary, skeletal, and hormonal manifestations. The kidneys can no longer maintain homeostasis.

Recently, the National Kidney Foundation proposed a set of clinical practice guidelines outlining a uniform classification system for chronic kidney disease (CKD). (See Table 38-1 on p. 968 for a description of stages 1 to 5 CKD.) In coming years, this classification and stratification system will replace less precise terms such as "chronic renal insufficiency" and "chronic renal failure."

The clinical manifestations of CRF are present throughout the body. No organ system is spared. Renal alterations (described previously) include the inability of the kidney to concentrate urine and regulate electrolyte excretion. Polyuria progresses to anuria, and the client loses normal diurnal patterns of voiding. In addition, all normal functions of the kidney, such as regulation of acid-base balance, regulation of blood pressure, synthesis of 1,25-dihydroxycholecalciferol, biogenesis of erythropoietin, degradation of insulin, and synthesis of prostaglandins, become curtailed and are eventually lost.

See the Concept Map on Understanding Chronic Renal Failure and Its Treatment on pp. 950 and 951.

Understanding Chronic Renal Failure and Its Treatment

CONCEPT MAP—cont'd

evolve

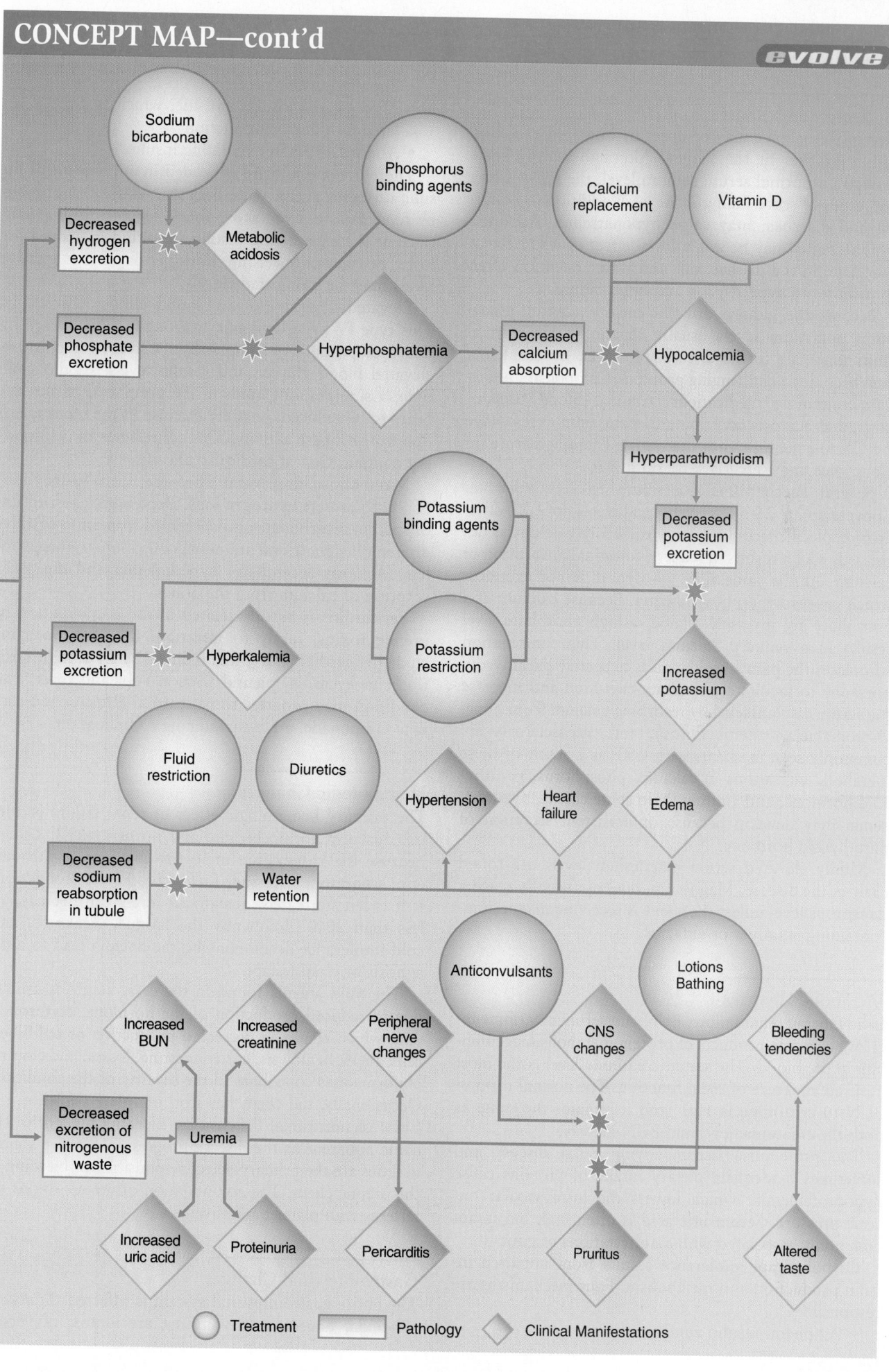

○ Treatment   ▭ Pathology   ◇ Clinical Manifestations

Electrolyte Imbalances

Electrolyte balance may be upset by impaired excretion and utilization in the kidney. Although many clients maintain a normal serum sodium level, the salt-wasting properties of some failing kidneys, in addition to vomiting and diarrhea, may cause hyponatremia. Apparent hyponatremia may be a dilutional effect of water retention. Late in the disease, salt and water retention often contributes to hypertension and heart failure.

Because the kidneys are efficient at excreting potassium, potassium levels usually remain within normal limits until late in the disease. However, hyperkalemia then becomes a challenging problem. Catabolism, potassium-containing medications, trauma, blood transfusions, and acidosis contribute to potassium excess. (See the Complementary and Alternative Therapy feature on Noni Juice and Renal Disease on p. 970.

Several mechanisms contribute to hypocalcemia. Conversion of 25-hydroxycholecalciferol to 1,25-dihydroxycholecalciferol (necessary to absorb calcium) is decreased, which results in reduced intestinal absorption of calcium. At the same time, phosphate is not excreted, which causes hyperphosphatemia. Because calcium and phosphate are inversely related, a high phosphate level results in a reduced calcium level. This combination stimulates the parathyroid glands to secrete parathyroid hormone to facilitate phosphate excretion and increase the serum calcium level by resorbing calcium from bone. Osteomalacia, osteitis fibrosa, and osteosclerosis are commonly seen in clients with CRF as a result of these metabolic alterations in calcium, phosphorus, parathyroid hormone, and vitamin D. In some clients, hypercalcemia may develop because of persistent secretion of parathyroid hormone.

Mildly elevated serum magnesium levels are found early in the disease. Magnesium does not usually reach a dangerous level unless the client is receiving magnesium-containing laxatives or antacids.

Metabolic Changes

In advancing renal failure, BUN and serum creatinine increase as waste products of protein metabolism accumulate in the blood. The serum creatinine level is the most accurate measure of renal function. The normal ratio of BUN to creatinine is 10:1, and it remains the same as both the creatinine level and BUN increase.

The proteinuria accompanying renal disease and sometimes inadequate dietary intake of proteins cause hypoproteinemia, which lowers the intravascular oncotic pressure. Serum uric acid is often high but is not commonly associated with manifestations of gout.

Carbohydrate intolerance results from impaired insulin production and metabolism. Four mechanisms are responsible:

- Peripheral insulin antagonism
- Impaired insulin secretion
- A prolonged insulin half-life, which is directly related to kidney malfunction
- Abnormalities in circulating insulin

Therefore special care is needed in adjustment of insulin doses for clients with diabetes mellitus complicated by renal failure. Even short-acting regular insulin functions as a longer-acting insulin, resulting in a need for lower dosages or fewer injections per day. Blood glucose levels must be monitored closely.

Elevated triglycerides are found almost universally. This type IV hyperlipidemia is thought to be caused by increased production of lipids by the liver in response to elevated blood glucose and insulin levels. At the same time, assimilation of lipids in the peripheral tissues appears to be reduced, possibly because of the blockage of lipoprotein lipase activity. This contributes to a secondary complication of cardiovascular disease.

Metabolic acidosis occurs because of the kidney's inability to excrete hydrogen ions. Decreased reabsorption of sodium bicarbonate and decreased formation of dihydrogen phosphate and ammonia contribute to this problem. Acidosis accentuates hyperkalemia and the reabsorption of calcium from the bones.

Pericarditis is usually related to the accumulation of uremic toxins, rarely to infection. Manifestations include pericardial pain (often reduced by an upright position), tachycardia, pleural friction rub, and fever. The condition may progress to pericardial effusion and cardiac tamponade, a life-threatening complication.

Hematologic Changes

The primary hematologic effect of renal failure is anemia, usually normochromic and normocytic. It occurs because the kidneys are unable to produce erythropoietin, a hormone necessary for red blood cell production. If it is left untreated, hematocrit levels can decrease to less than 20%. Frequently the fatigue, weakness, and cold intolerance accompanying the anemia lead to a diagnosis of renal failure.

The mild anemia found in the early stages is usually due to reduced production of the hormone, erythropoietin, which results in decreased production of red blood cells. Later, hemolysis, gastrointestinal losses, and clotting abnormalities contribute to the severity of the condition. Occasionally, the client has iron or folate depletion because of nutritional deficiencies. Bleeding tendencies become apparent as the disease progresses. Platelet abnormalities are the primary defect responsible for bleeding in the uremic client. The accumulation of uremic toxins interferes with platelet adhesiveness.

Gastrointestinal Changes

The entire gastrointestinal system is affected. Transient anorexia, nausea, and vomiting are almost universal.

Clients often experience a constant bitter, metallic, or salty taste, and their breath commonly smells fetid, fishy, or ammonia-like. Stomatitis, parotitis, and gingivitis are common problems because of poor oral hygiene and the formation of ammonia from salivary urea. Accumulations of gastrin (from increased secretion of gastric acid) may be a major cause of ulcer disease. Esophagitis, gastritis, colitis, gastrointestinal bleeding, and diarrhea may be present. Serum amylase levels may be increased, although they do not necessarily indicate pancreatitis.

Constipation is a common problem. It often results from phosphate-binding agents, restriction of fluids and high-fiber foods (many of which are rich in potassium and phosphorus), and decreased activity. Constipation is a particular challenge because many of the usual interventions to prevent it (i.e., adding fruits, vegetables, and grains to the diet) and to treat it (e.g., using magnesium-containing laxatives) are contraindicated for a client with renal failure.

Immunologic Changes

Impairment of the immune system makes the client more susceptible to infection. Several factors are involved, including depression of humoral antibody formation, suppression of delayed hypersensitivity, and decreased chemotactic function of the leukocytes. Immunosuppression is an important part of the medical management of renal diseases such as glomerulonephritis. Immunosuppression after transplantation is discussed later in this chapter.

Changes in Medication Metabolism

CRF has a serious effect on the metabolism of medications. The uremic client is at high risk for medication toxicity because of the effect of renal changes on the pharmacokinetics (absorption, distribution, metabolism, and excretion) of otherwise therapeutic medications. There are three main causes of this toxicity:

- A high plasma level of the medication caused by low serum albumin, decreased binding sites, impaired renal excretion, or impaired hepatic metabolism of the drug
- Increased sensitivity to the medication because of uremia-induced changes in the target organ
- A metabolic load due to administration of the medication; for example, hypoalbuminemia means less protein available for binding

Various tables and formulas are available to help guide dosage decisions. Medication dosages must be altered and the usual dosage ranges are not safe for a client with CRF. Assess the client carefully for toxic reactions. Keep in mind that many medications, particularly water-soluble ones, are removed by dialysis.

Cardiovascular Changes

Between 50% and 65% of deaths that occur during CRF result from cardiovascular complications. The most common clinical manifestation is hypertension (which may also be the cause of renal failure), produced through the following:

- Mechanisms of volume overload
- Stimulation of the renin-angiotensin system
- Sympathetically mediated vasoconstriction; for example, increased levels of dopamine β-hydroxylase
- Absence of prostaglandins

Any of the many systemic complications of prolonged high blood pressure may be found.

The effects of volume overload on the heart are seen, including left ventricular hypertrophy and heart failure. Heart failure may also result from anemia, vascular access, complications of coronary artery disease, electrolyte imbalance, acidosis, myocardial calcification, and thiamine depletion. Dysrhythmias may be caused by hyperkalemia, acidosis, hypermagnesemia, and decreased coronary perfusion.

Atherosclerosis is accelerated because of abnormal carbohydrate and lipid metabolism, impaired fibrinolysis (which leads to the development of microemboli), and hyperparathyroidism. Arterial calcifications have been identified, with the ankles being the most common early location. Other sites include the abdominal aorta, feet, pelvis, hands, and wrists. These vascular calcifications also occur within the heart, particularly at the mitral valve.

Respiratory Changes

Some of the respiratory effects, such as pulmonary edema, can be attributed to fluid overload. Pleuritis is a frequent finding, especially when pericarditis develops. A characteristic condition called *uremic lung* is a type of pneumonitis that responds well to fluid removal. Metabolic acidosis causes a compensatory increase in respiratory rate as the lungs work to eliminate excess hydrogen ions.

Musculoskeletal Changes

The musculoskeletal system is affected early in the disease process, and up to 90% of clients with CRF experience renal osteodystrophy. This condition develops insidiously and takes several forms: osteomalacia, osteitis fibrosa, osteoporosis, and osteosclerosis. The etiologic mechanism involves the kidney-bone-parathyroid and calcium-phosphate-vitamin D connections. As the GFR decreases, phosphate excretion decreases and calcium elimination increases. Abnormal levels of calcium and phosphate stimulate the release of parathyroid hormone, which mobilizes calcium from the bones and facilitates phosphate excretion.

As renal failure progresses, the kidney no longer converts vitamin D to its active form, 1,25-dihydroxycholecalciferol. The lack of this substance interferes with calcium absorption from the intestine and paradoxically facilitates phosphate retention. Thus mineralization of the bone with calcium and phosphate is impaired. Demineralization of the bone frees more calcium and phosphorus into the blood. As the disease progresses, the parathyroid gland may become unresponsive to the normal feedback system and continue to produce parathyroid hormone, accelerating renal osteodystrophy. Partial parathyroidectomy is the treatment of choice when hypercalcemia and high plasma levels of parathyroid hormone cannot be controlled with medication.

In addition to bone demineralization, this process leads to deposition of calcium in subcutaneous, vascular, and visceral tissues throughout the body. In advanced stages, joint pain is severe. The client may also report diffuse and generalized bone and muscle pain. Bone deformities and frequent fractures are common. In children, bones fail to calcify, causing growth retardation. Tissue calcifications may be lethal if they develop in vital tissues, such as cerebral, coronary, or pulmonary vessels.

Some clients complain of muscle cramps. These may result from osmolar changes in the body fluids or sometimes from hypocalcemia.

Integumentary Changes

Integumentary problems are particularly uncomfortable for some clients with CRF. The skin is also often very dry because of atrophy of the sweat glands. Severe and intractable pruritus may result from secondary hyperparathyroidism and calcium deposits in the skin. Pruritus can lead to excoriated skin caused by continued scratching.

Several color changes affecting the skin are found in clients with renal failure. A bleeding tendency often results in increased bruising, petechiae, and purpura. These do not usually cause problems themselves, but their presence may be alarming to the client. The pallor of anemia is evident. The cause of retained urochrome pigments, making the skin orange-green or gray in color, is not clear.

Hair is brittle and tends to fall out; nails are thin and brittle as well. Characteristic red bands that develop on the nails are called Muehrcke's lines. Another nail pattern that has been observed is a "half-and-half" nail, with the proximal half normally white and the distal portion brown.

Neurologic Changes

Although dialysis has reduced the incidence of neurologic changes, some clients experience these problems early in the disease process. Peripheral neuropathy causes many manifestations, such as burning feet, inability to find a comfortable position for the legs and feet (restless legs syndrome), gait changes, footdrop, and paraplegia. These manifestations move up the legs and may extend to include the arms. Initially, it is primarily a problem of the sensory system; however, if left untreated, it may progress to the motor system. Nerve conduction becomes slower, and deep tendon reflexes and vibratory sense are diminished.

Central nervous system involvement is demonstrated through forgetfulness, inability to concentrate, short attention span, impaired reasoning ability and judgment, impaired cognitive functioning, increased nervous irritability, nystagmus, twitching, dysarthria, seizures, central nervous system depression, and coma. Involvement of the cranial nerves may alter any of the senses. Hearing threshold levels show a high-frequency deficit early in the disease, and hearing progressively deteriorates. Uremic amaurosis is the sudden onset of bilateral blindness, which seems to be reversed in hours to days. The eyes often contain calcium salts, which give them an irritated appearance.

Reproductive Changes

Reproductive system changes can be alarming. Women commonly experience menstrual irregularities, particularly amenorrhea (absence of menstrual periods), and infertility. However, some women with CRF have conceived and had successful full-term pregnancies. Men commonly report impotence of both physiologic and psychological causes. They may also experience testicular atrophy, oligospermia (decreased sperm count), and reduced sperm motility. Both genders report decreased libido, possibly from both physiologic and psychological factors.

Endocrine Changes

CRF also affects the endocrine system, such as the insulin utilization and parathyroid function discussed already. Pituitary hormones, such as growth hormone and prolactin, may be increased in some people. The levels of luteinizing hormone and follicle-stimulating hormone vary greatly from client to client. Thyroid-stimulating hormone is usually normal, but it may show a blunted response to thyrotropin-releasing hormone; this commonly results in hypothyroidism.

Psychosocial Changes

Psychosocial changes probably result from both the physiologic alterations and the extreme stress experienced by a client who has a chronic, life-threatening disease. Common stressors include feelings of powerlessness and lack of control over the illness and treatment, intrusive therapy, restrictions imposed by the medical regimen, changes in body image, and changes in sexuality.

Clients commonly suffer from role reversal, loss or reduction of work, financial strain, and many lifestyle changes. Scheduling dialysis can create many difficulties. The client's self-concept and body image may be altered, leading to further problems with work and relationships.

People cope with these stressors in various ways, and not all coping strategies are positive. They can range from obtaining support from family and friends and seeking more information about the condition to depression and thoughts of suicide. Indeed, helping a client cope with psychosocial changes is one of the hardest nursing challenges you face.

Prognosis

The survival rate of people with CRF has improved with the advent and improvement of dialysis and transplantation. At 1 year after dialysis begins, the survival rate is about 79%. After 5 years, the rate decreases to 33%.[60]

Outcome Management
■ Medical Management

Conservative intervention does not cure CRF, but it may slow the progress of the disease. Eventually, most clients need renal replacement therapy. However, even successful dialysis and transplantation do not preclude the potential for death from complications of renal failure or its treatment.

After correcting contributing factors, control of blood pressure and fluid and dietary adjustments are the mainstays of conservative intervention for a client with CRF. The following are the five goals of medical management:

1. To preserve renal function
2. To delay the need for dialysis or transplantation as long as feasible
3. To alleviate extrarenal manifestations as much as possible
4. To improve body chemistry values
5. To provide an optimal quality of life for the client and significant others

Preserve Renal Function and Delay Dialysis. Preservation of renal function can delay the need for dialysis therapy. It can be accomplished by controlling the disease process (see Chapter 37), by controlling blood pressure, and by reducing dietary protein intake and catabolism.

CRF commonly causes hypertension, which accelerates kidney damage. Good blood pressure control helps to preserve renal function. Blood pressure can be controlled through diet, weight control, and medications (see Chapters 37 and 54).

Specific adjustments of dietary elements often depend on the results of the client's blood chemistry studies. Although there is some debate over whether and how to restrict proteins, keeping the daily intake of protein of high biologic value below 50 g may slow the progression of renal failure. Generally, recommendations range from no restriction other than avoiding high-protein fad diets to a restriction to 1 g/kg/day. This protein must be of high biologic value so that the essential amino acids can be used more efficiently with less nitrogenous waste. This restriction of proteins also limits accumulation of acid, potassium, and phosphate.

It is also important to provide adequate nonprotein calories to prevent or reduce catabolism. One recommendation is a carbohydrate and fat intake of 40 to 50 kcal/kg/day. As the renal disease progresses, the client's ability and willingness to take in adequate nutrition diminish and the challenge becomes not only to maintain appropriate intake of nonprotein calories but also to satisfy protein needs. In these instances, elemental diets, enteral feedings, or TPN may be used instead of or in addition to regular food intake.

Alleviate Extrarenal Manifestations. Pruritus can be annoying. Many interventions have been tried, including topical emollients and lotions, antihistamines, intravenous lidocaine, and ultraviolet B light, but relief has been inconsistent and usually temporary. Subtotal parathyroidectomy has sometimes helped, but there have been reports of recurrence. Effective dialysis seems to relieve the manifestations for many clients.

Neurologic manifestations require safety measures to protect the client from injury. Anticonvulsants and sedatives may be used. Phenothiazines are potentiated by uremia and should be avoided. The increase of uremic toxins causes a reduction in cognitive functioning, and patience is required in explaining things to the client.

The hematologic changes can also be treated medically. Therapy with epoetin alfa three times a week (or weekly as darbepoetin alfa) helps stimulate the production of red blood cells. Supplemental iron, vitamin B_{12}, and folic acid are usually administered as well.

Cardiovascular disease is the major cause of mortality in people with chronic renal failure. Increasingly, hyperlipidemia is being treated with statins to minimize the risk of myocardial infarction and stroke.

Improve Body Chemistry. The client's body chemistry can be improved through dialysis, medications, and diet. Dialysis removes excess water and nitrogenous wastes, reducing the manifestations of renal failure. Dialysis can be used temporarily if the client has ARF or as a permanent, life-sustaining treatment if the client has CRF. In the latter case, dialysis must continue for the rest of the client's life unless a successful kidney transplantation is performed.

Dialysis is also used to control uremia and to physically prepare the client to receive a transplanted kidney. Dialysis is usually necessary to keep the client alive until a suitable donor kidney is found. If the transplanted kidney does not immediately function adequately, dialysis may help prevent uremia until the kidney begins functioning sufficiently.

The following are the four basic goals of dialysis therapy:

1. To remove the end products of protein metabolism, such as urea and creatinine, from the blood
2. To maintain a safe concentration of serum electrolytes
3. To correct acidosis and replenish the bicarbonate levels of the blood
4. To remove excess fluid from the blood

Principles of ultrafiltration and diffusion are used to accomplish the goals of dialysis. *Ultrafiltration* refers to removal of fluid from the blood using either osmotic or hydrostatic pressure to produce the necessary gradient. *Diffusion* is the passage of particles (ions) from an area of high concentration to an area of low concentration. Both processes occur across a semipermeable membrane with pores large enough to allow certain particles (such as urea, creatinine, and electrolytes) to pass through but too small to allow the passage of larger particles (such as protein and red blood cells). When the two solutions are separated by a semipermeable membrane, solute particles move toward the solution of lower concentration. Simultaneously, water moves toward the solution of higher solute concentration.

Solute particles and water can move freely across the membrane in either direction between the blood and the dialysate. Thus if the blood has a higher concentration of urea, creatinine, and certain electrolytes than does the prepared dialysate solution, these particles move into the dialysate solution, lowering the level in the blood. If the blood is deficient in a substance, such as bicarbonate, the higher concentration of this substance in the dialysate causes it to move into the blood, raising the blood level.

There are two types of dialysis: *peritoneal dialysis* and *hemodialysis*. The semipermeable membrane in the dialyzer or "artificial kidney" used is either the peritoneal membrane (for peritoneal dialysis) or an artificial membrane (for hemodialysis). The blood and a specially prepared electrolyte solution, called the *dialysate*, are placed in compartments on opposite sides of the membrane. The tendency is always toward equalization of the concentrations of the two solutions.

Peritoneal Dialysis. Peritoneal dialysis involves repeated cycles of instilling dialysate into the peritoneal cavity, allowing time for substance exchange, and then removing the dialysate. The procedure is useful for both ARF and CRF and for fluid and electrolyte imbalances. It has been used to treat overdoses of drugs and toxins, but because its clearance is much slower than that with hemodialysis, it may not be satisfactory for this purpose.

One of the primary advantages of peritoneal dialysis is its relative ease, which allows it to be used in community health care facilities without the sophisticated equipment needed for hemodialysis. It can be easily managed at home and commonly allows the client more independence and mobility than hemodialysis does.

Peritoneal dialysis is typically used for clients with severe cardiovascular disease, especially those whose problems would be worsened by the rapid changes in urea, glucose, electrolytes, and fluid volume that occur during hemodialysis. Some physicians prescribe peritoneal dialysis for diabetic clients to reduce the risk of retinal hemorrhage associated with the heparin used during hemodialysis and because good blood glucose control can be achieved by adding insulin to the dialysate. Peritoneal dialysis is the dialysis treatment of choice for children because it seems to have less effect on growth.

Contraindications to peritoneal dialysis include hypercatabolism, in which peritoneal dialysis cannot adequately clear uremic toxins, and poor condition of the peritoneal membrane because of adhesions or scarring. Relative contraindications to peritoneal dialysis include obesity, a history of ruptured diverticula, abdominal disease, respiratory disease, recurrent episodes of peritonitis, abdominal malignancies, severe vascular disease, back problems (because the increased weight of fluid may increase back strain), and extensive abdominal surgery with drains or tubes that may increase the risk of infection.

Types of Peritoneal Dialysis. Several types of peritoneal dialysis are in use. The most common are continuous ambulatory and automated peritoneal dialysis.

Continuous Ambulatory Peritoneal Dialysis (CAPD). In the continuous type of peritoneal dialysis, 1.5 to 3 L of dialysate is instilled into the abdomen and left in place for a prescribed period of time. The empty dialysate bag is folded and carried in a pouch or pocket until it is time to drain the dialysate. The bag is then unfolded and placed lower than the insertion site so that the fluid drains by gravity flow. When full, the bag is changed and new dialysate is instilled into the abdomen as the process continues.

Another version of this procedure is the disconnect system. With this system, the client removes the empty dialysate bag after inflow and attaches a protective cap to the dialysis catheter. A new sterile bag is used for each drainage and infusion, which eliminates the need to wear the tubing and bag between exchanges.

CAPD usually uses four dialysis cycles every 24 hours, including an 8-hour dwell overnight. There are two major advantages. First, because there is no need for machinery, electricity, or a water source, the client can go about almost any desired activity during dialysis. Second, because the continuous exchange process closely resembles normal renal function, the body more easily maintains homeostasis, allowing fewer dietary and fluid restrictions. For management of diabetic clients, insulin can be added to the dialysate.

See the Bridge to Home Health Care feature on Living with Peritoneal Dialysis on the website.

Automated Peritoneal Dialysis. Automated peritoneal dialysis necessitates use of a peritoneal cycling machine. This method can be performed as continuous cyclic, intermittent, or nightly intermittent peritoneal dialysis.

Continuous Cyclic Peritoneal Dialysis. In this variation, there are usually three cycles at night and one cycle with an 8-hour dwell in the morning. The advantage of this procedure is that the peritoneal catheter is opened only for the on-and-off procedures, which reduces the risk of infection. Another advantage is that the client does not require exchanges at work or school.

Intermittent Peritoneal Dialysis. This is not a continuous dialysis procedure. Instead, dialysis is performed for 10 to 14 hours, three to four times a week, by the same peritoneal cycling machine as in continuous cyclic peritoneal dialysis. Hospitalized clients may be dialyzed for 24 to 48 hours at a time if they are catabolic and require additional dialysis time.

Nightly Intermittent Peritoneal Dialysis. Dialysis is performed for 8 to 12 hours each night with no daytime dwells.

Peritoneal Dialysis Procedures. Several steps are involved.

Peritoneal Catheter Insertion. For a client who needs peritoneal dialysis, one of several types of soft catheters is inserted through the abdominal wall and into the peritoneal cavity. Usually, the catheter is inserted in the operating room, with the client under local anesthesia, although it may be inserted at the client's bedside. The client is medicated before the procedure to provide relaxation and to reduce discomfort.

The preferred insertion site is 3 to 5 cm below the umbilicus, an area that is relatively avascular and has relatively low fascial resistance. Figure 38-2 illustrates three types of peritoneal catheters. The Tenckhoff catheter has two polyester (Dacron) felt cuffs bonded to the catheter. Over a period of 1 to 2 weeks, there is an ingrowth of fibroblasts and blood vessels into the cuffs, which fix the catheter in place and provide an effective barrier against dialysate leakage and bacterial invasion. Note in Figure 38-2 that a subcutaneous tunnel is created for the catheter to reduce direct bacterial invasion into the peritoneum. The other catheters illustrated have cuffs to provide stability.

Dialysate. The dialysate is usually allowed to run into the peritoneal cavity by gravity flow. It is warmed slightly to avoid chilling the client and to dilate the peritoneal blood vessels, thus facilitating substance exchange. In an adult, 2 L is usually instilled, although smaller amounts are generally used at first until the wound heals. Throughout the procedure, care must be taken to prevent air from entering the peritoneal cavity.

The *dwell time* is the period during which the dialysate is left in the peritoneal cavity. In intermittent peritoneal dialysis, equilibrium between the dialysate and the body fluids usually occurs within 15 to 30 minutes, with the maximum exchange occurring during the first 5 minutes. Therefore the solution is typically left in place 30 to 45 minutes for manual dialysis or 10 to 20 minutes when an automatic cycler is used. The fluid is then allowed to run out through the catheter by gravity. In continuous ambulatory and automated peritoneal dialysis procedures, the dwell time is prolonged to 4 to 8

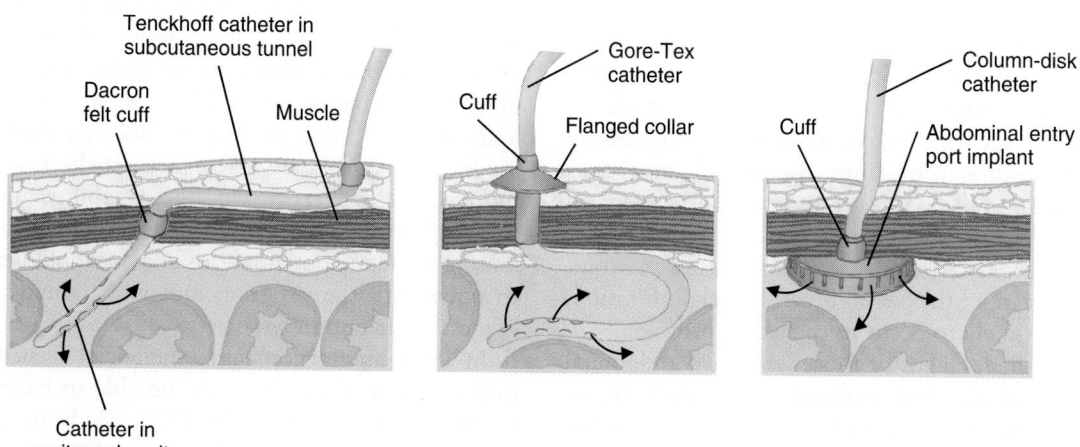

FIGURE 38-2 Three types of peritoneal dialysis catheters. The Tenckhoff catheter has two polyester (Dacron) felt cuffs that hold the catheter in place and prevent dialysate leakage and bacterial invasion; a subcutaneous tunnel also helps prevent infection. The Gore-Tex catheter has a Dacron cuff above a flanged collar. The column-disk catheter has a cuff and a large abdominal entry port implant.

hours with a solution that allows continuous exchange and better clearance of certain elements.

Cycles. The number of dialysis cycles depends on the normalization of body fluids and blood chemistries, as indicated by laboratory studies. Peritoneal clearance is influenced by several factors, including the size of the membrane area, blood flow to the peritoneum, and alterations in the permeability of the peritoneal membrane.

Complications of Peritoneal Dialysis. Although peritoneal dialysis is considered a safe procedure, a number of complications can be attributed to it.

Peritonitis. Peritonitis is the major concern; therefore meticulous aseptic technique must be maintained during handling of the catheter, tubing, and dialysate solution. Bacteria may enter the peritoneal cavity through contaminated dialysis fluid, a contaminated catheter lumen, or the catheter insertion site.

Clinical evidence of peritonitis includes fever, rebound abdominal tenderness, nausea, malaise, and a cloudy dialysate output. Laboratory tests routinely used to diagnose peritonitis include white blood cell counts with differential, culture, and sensitivity and Gram's stain of the peritoneal fluid. Peritonitis is the diagnosis when the dialysate white blood cell count exceeds 100/mm^3 and neutrophils are greater than 50%. The causative organism does not always grow in routine cultures, but Gram's stain is positive in up to 40% of the samples.

If peritonitis develops, appropriate antibiotics are added to the dialysate; in addition, systemic antibiotics may be used.

Catheter-Related Complications. Catheter problems include displacement and obstruction. Obstruction may be due to malposition, adherence of the catheter tip to the omentum, or infection. Constipation can reduce catheter flow, possibly because peristalsis facilitates outflow. A bisacodyl suppository may be used prophylactically even if the client is not constipated. Fluid leakage may indicate improper catheter function, incomplete healing of the insertion site, or excessive instillation.

Especially in the early stages, it is sometimes necessary to use small-volume instillations. Bloody effluent is usually insignificant and disappears spontaneously. Heparin may be added to the dialysate to prevent fibrin clot formation in a new catheter or after treatment for peritonitis. Also be aware of the possibility of bowel perforation, which is most likely to occur in cachectic (profoundly ill and malnourished) clients or those who have abdominal adhesions. Fecal material returned in the dialysate or massive diarrhea after instillation may also signal perforation. Bladder perforation can also occur if the bladder has not been emptied before catheter insertion.

Dialysis-Related Complications. Pain during dialysis may result from rapid instillation, incorrect dialysate pH or temperature, dialysate accumulation under the diaphragm, or excessive suction during outflow. Some pain

is expected in the early stages but should disappear after 1 to 2 weeks. Low back pain may develop with continuous dialysis procedures because the abdominal weight affects posture; appropriate exercises help relieve this problem. Hernia may occur. Systemic cardiovascular and neurologic effects are usually the result of fluid and electrolyte imbalances. Especially during small-volume exchanges, a significant amount of dialysate fluid may be absorbed by the body.

Hypotension may result from too rapid removal of fluid. Overhydration, from insufficient fluid removal, may be manifested as heart failure and pulmonary edema. Hypoalbuminemia leading to hypovolemia often occurs because the peritoneal membrane allows the passage of albumin, as much as 100 g/day if the client is infected. It is especially a problem if dietary intake of protein is poor, the client is infected, or dialysis treatment is used for several consecutive days. Hyperglycemia may occur in diabetic clients as a result of absorption of glucose from the dialysate and electrolyte changes. These clients require extra insulin. Respiratory difficulties may occur during dwell time because of pressure on the diaphragm. Weight gain may occur because of the high concentration of glucose in the dialysate.

Outcomes. Long-term outcomes associated with peritoneal dialysis are considered good. The treatment is usually effective for years. However, scarring of the peritoneum and repeated infections may require a change to hemodialysis.

Hemodialysis. Hemodialysis is used for clients with acute or irreversible renal failure and fluid and electrolyte imbalances. It is usually the treatment of choice when toxic agents, such as barbiturates after an overdose, need to be removed from the body quickly.

Historical Overview. The first artificial kidney was developed in 1943 in The Netherlands. In 1960, the first successful treatment of clients with CRF was reported. In the early years, although the technology was available, the exorbitant cost and lack of equipment required a stringent selection process in choosing clients for hemodialysis. Clients were screened on the basis of their motivation, intelligence, emotional stability, and rehabilitative potential. In essence, it had to be decided who among the many potential candidates would best be able to cope with the program and who would make the biggest contribution to society.

In 1972, an amendment to the Social Security Act required that anyone with CRF be able to have any lifesaving treatment needed. In 1973, Medicare took over the financial responsibility for many clients receiving hemodialysis. Thus availability of this treatment for clients with end-stage renal failure has become more prevalent. Generally, self-selection is the only criterion used now. As a result, the population receiving hemodialysis represents a wide cross-section of age, rehabilitative potential,

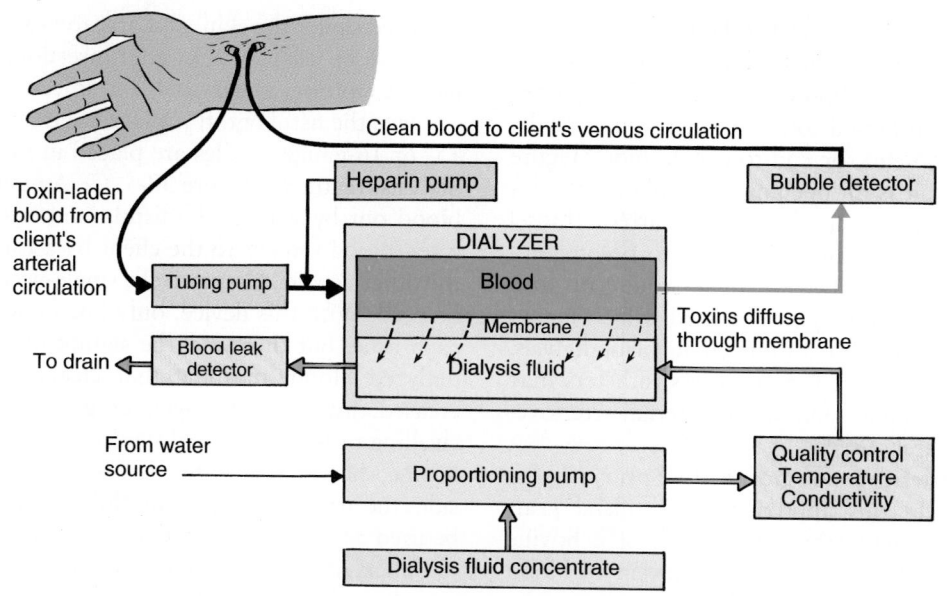

FIGURE 38-3 Typical hemodialysis system. Toxin-laden blood from the client diffuses across the membrane within the dialyzer into the dialysis fluid. Clean blood is returned to the client.

and socioeconomic status. There continue to be problems with selection of appropriate candidates, when to start, and when and how to stop. With the reduction in available health care dollars, the problems associated with selection criteria will only increase.

Hemodialysis Procedure. In hemodialysis, the client's toxin-laden blood is diverted into a dialyzer, cleaned, and then returned to the client (Figure 38-3). While the blood is in the dialyzer, a mechanical proportioning pump causes dialysis fluid to flow on the other side of the membrane (Figure 38-4). Toxins diffuse across the membrane from the blood to the dialysate. Strict asepsis must be maintained throughout the procedure.

One of the vital aspects of hemodialysis is the establishment and maintenance of adequate blood access. Without it, hemodialysis cannot be done. The major routes of access are external arteriovenous shunts and subclavian catheters for acute dialysis and internal arteriovenous fistulae and grafts for chronic dialysis.

The external arteriovenous shunt requires surgical placement of two rubber-like silicone (Silastic) cannulas into the forearm or leg. The two cannulas are connected to form a U shape. Blood flows from the client's artery through the shunt into the vein.

When the client is to be connected to the hemodialyzer, a tube leading to the membrane compartment is connected to the arterial cannula. Blood then fills the membrane compartment and flows back to the client by way of a tube connected to the venous cannula. When dialysis is completed, the arterial cannula is clamped. Once the blood in the membrane compartment has been returned to the body, the venous cannula

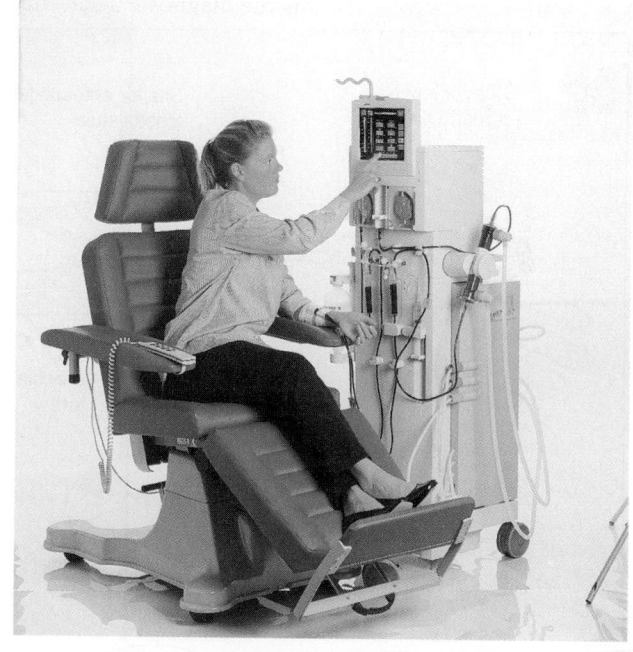

FIGURE 38-4 A client undergoing hemodialysis. (Courtesy of Althin Medical, Inc., Miami Lakes, FL.)

is clamped and the ends of the two cannulas are reattached to form their U. This access can be created quickly and thus is particularly suitable when dialysis must be started immediately.

Infection at the insertion site and clotting are complications that often necessitate moving the cannula sites. Other problems that occur with shunts are accidental dislodgment, hemorrhage, and skin erosion.

The internal arteriovenous fistula is the access of choice for clients receiving chronic dialysis. The fistula is created through a surgical procedure in which an artery in the arm is anastomosed to a vein in an end-to-side, side-to-side, side-to-end, or end-to-end fashion (Figure 38-5, A). The result is an opening or fistula between a large artery and a large vein. The flow of arterial blood into the venous system causes the veins to become engorged (Figure 38-5, B). These fistulae require up to 6 weeks to mature before they can be used, which makes this approach inappropriate for immediate hemodialysis. Peritoneal dialysis or large venous access catheters may be used while the fistula is maturing. External arteriovenous shunts are rarely used.

The internal arteriovenous graft is used primarily for chronic dialysis. In this approach, an artificial graft made of water-repellent fabric (Gore-Tex) or a bovine carotid artery is used to create an artificial vein for blood flow. The graft is used in clients who do not have adequate blood vessels for surgical creation of a fistula. One end of the artificial graft is anastomosed to an artery, tunneled under the skin, and anastomosed to a vein. The graft can be used 2 weeks after insertion. Complications include clotting, aneurysms, and infection.

Once the fistula graft is placed and ready for use, two 15- or 16-gauge needles are placed in the access at each dialysis treatment (Figure 38-5, C). A pump pulls arterial blood out by way of the fistula and into the hemodialyzer. Blood returns to the client by a tube connected to the other needle. Alternatively, single-needle dialysis may be used. With this device, only one puncture is required each time, but there may be significant recirculation of dialyzed blood, meaning that clearance rates are decreased. Internal arteriovenous grafts may cause hand swelling or ischemia (steal syndrome), carpal tunnel syndrome, hemorrhage, thrombosis, and aneurysms. Besides the arm, the subclavian, thigh, and ankle areas may be used as sites for hemodialysis access.

Subclavian, jugular, and femoral catheters can be inserted at the bedside for vascular access or surgically placed in the operating room. Double-lumen catheters are usually used to provide access for both removal and

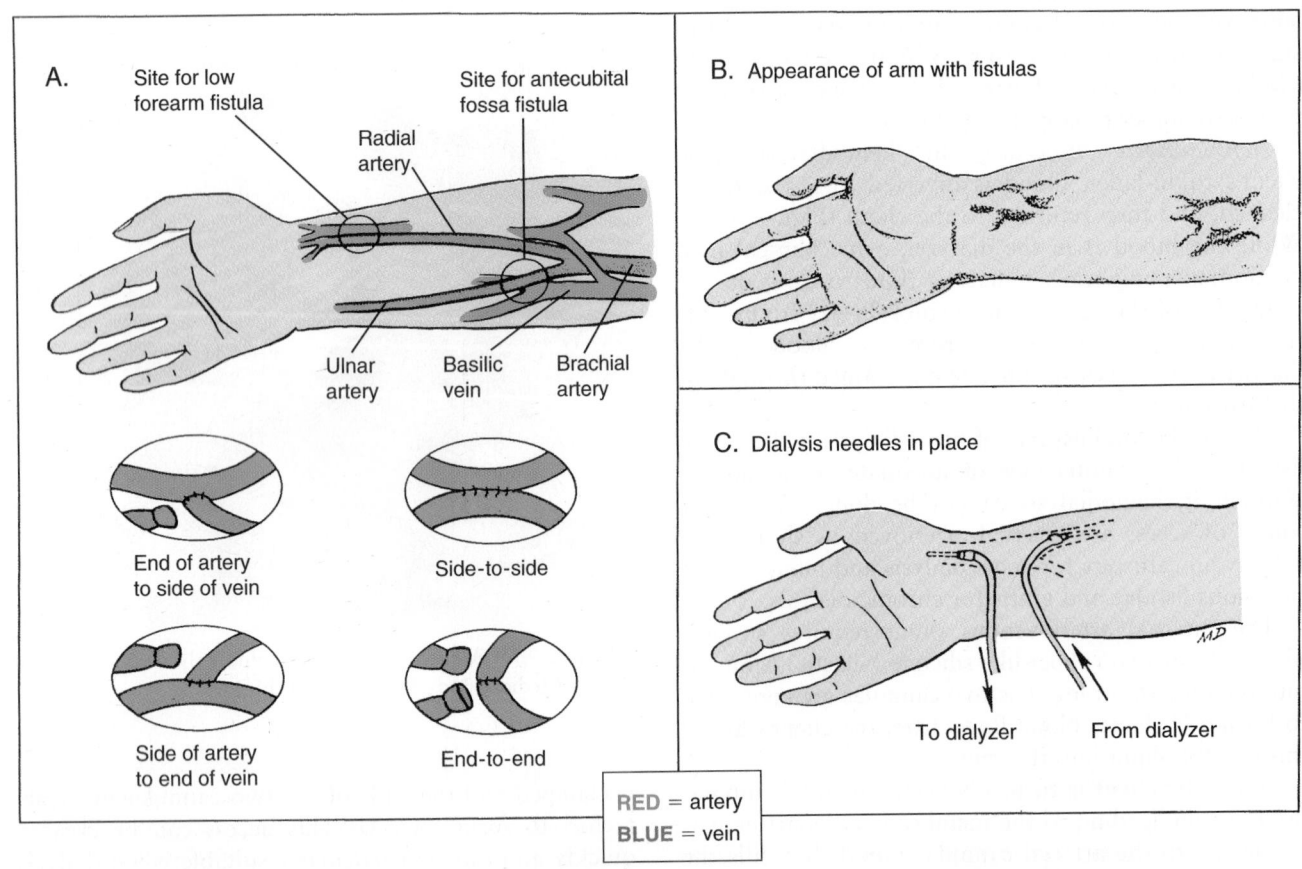

FIGURE 38-5 Internal arteriovenous fistula. Surgical creation of an arteriovenous anastomosis provides easy access to blood for hemodialysis. This method reduces the risk of infection and makes external shunts unnecessary except during hemodialysis. The internal fistula must be created 2 to 6 weeks before it can be used. **A,** Types of fistulae. **B,** Appearance of arm with fistulae. **C,** Dialysis needles in place.

return of blood. These catheters are usually a temporary source of vascular access and must be replaced frequently to prevent infection. Strict aseptic technique must be used during insertion, and dressing changes are usually performed by a limited number of trained nurses. Thrombosis and infection are the most common complications.

Dialyzers. Several types of dialyzers are available, including flat plate and hollow fiber mold devices. Choice of a particular system is mostly a matter of preference. There are differences in urea and creatinine clearance rates as well as ultrafiltration rates. Many centers that perform long-term dialysis now reprocess and disinfect the unit and reuse it for the same client to reduce costs. The dialysate solution is altered to fit the client's need.

Hemodialysis Schedules. Hemodialysis as a treatment for CRF must be continued intermittently for the client's lifetime unless successful kidney transplantation is performed. A typical schedule is 3 to 4 hours of treatment 3 days per week. This schedule varies with the size of the client, the type of dialyzer used, the rate of blood flow, the personal preference of the client, and other factors.

Therapeutic Effects of Hemodialysis. The overall therapeutic effects of hemodialysis are to (1) clear waste products from the body; (2) restore fluid, electrolyte, and acid-base balances; and (3) reverse some of the untoward manifestations of irreversible renal failure. Success is varied. Excess fluid, potassium, urea nitrogen, and acid ions are removed, but only temporarily; between dialyses, these elements build up again. Nutritionally, carbohydrate intolerance is usually reduced. Amino acids, protein, glucose, and water-soluble vitamins are lost. Anemia generally worsens because of blood loss associated with the therapy. The predialysis causative factors are still present, and additional losses occur during dialysis because of blood sampling, residual blood left in the dialyzer, and bleeding secondary to anticoagulation during dialysis. Serum iron stores are also further depleted.

Hyperlipidemia (elevated serum lipid levels) is more prevalent in people with chronic renal failure and is associated with accelerated atherosclerosis. Renal osteodystrophy usually improves with dialysis; this can be further enhanced by adding calcium to the dialysate. Pruritus may occur for reasons not yet understood. Men who have maintenance dialysis often have low testosterone levels and develop gynecomastia, which is usually transient. Many other sexual manifestations of uremia are reversed after a period of adaptation.

The usual effect of hemodialysis on serum concentration of medications is increased clearance, which is therapeutic in the case of overdose. Dosage schedules are altered to prevent, as much as possible, loss of medications through dialysis. Supplemental doses may be necessary to maintain therapeutic levels of certain medications.

Complications of Long-Term Hemodialysis. In addition to its therapeutic effects, chronic hemodialysis can cause a number of complications:

- Technical problems, such as blood leaks, overheating of the dialysate solution, insufficient loss of fluid, improper concentration of salts in the dialysate, and clotting
- Hypotension or hypertension
- Cardiac dysrhythmias from potassium imbalance
- Air embolus
- Hemorrhage resulting from heparinization with particular concern for subdural, retroperitoneal, pericardial, and intraocular bleeding
- Restless legs syndrome
- Pyrogenic reactions

Gastrointestinal ulcer disease is often complicated by hemorrhage. Muscle cramps may occur as a result of hyponatremia or hyposmolality and too rapid removal of fluid. Infection is a significant complication, with hepatitis B being a significant risk. Frequent infectious processes include local access infection, bacteremia, and infectious endocarditis.

Dialysis disequilibrium syndrome can occur, particularly during the client's first few dialysis episodes. It is characterized by mental confusion, deterioration of the level of consciousness, headache, and seizures. It may last for several days. Rapid solute removal from the blood probably causes a relative excess of solutes interstitially or intracellularly (an osmotic gradient). The excess causes cerebral edema, which leads to increased intracranial pressure. Many dialysis centers avoid this complication by first-time dialyzing for shorter times at a reduced blood flow rate.

Diet. Dietary adjustment is dictated by many components of CRF, including accumulation of nitrogenous waste products, impaired excretion of electrolytes, vitamin deficiencies, and continued catabolism. The wasting syndrome is a major problem. The client with renal failure constantly loses body weight, muscle mass, and adipose tissue.

Dietary intake of electrolytes may be encouraged or restricted. The regulation of sodium is a delicate matter. At times, the kidneys waste salt, and sodium intake must be encouraged to replace it. More frequently, however, the kidneys retain sodium. Some believe that there should be moderate restriction with careful monitoring of urinary sodium excretion as a guideline. Serial monitoring of fluid status also gives important information about sodium needs. Many regimens are used.

Potassium is frequently restricted. Clients must be reminded not to use salt substitutes because they contain potassium chloride. When hyperkalemia becomes evident, restriction of potassium in food and fluids is instituted. In an emergency situation, when the serum potassium is greater than 7 mEq/L, the client may require emergency treatment (see the Integrating Pharmacology feature on Medications for Acute Renal Failure on p. 946). Dialysis is also effective in removing potassium from the blood.

If serum calcium levels are low, adequate calcium intake is important. Dietary sources may be supplemented with calcium carbonate, calcium lactate, or calcium gluconate. If serum calcium levels are high, however, dietary restriction may be recommended. Phosphorus is restricted. In addition, calcium carbonate may be used to reduce phosphorus levels further. Finally, mild magnesium restriction may be imposed.

Medications. Medications commonly prescribed for people with chronic renal failure are described in the Integrating Pharmacology feature on Medications for Chronic Renal Failure, below.

Promote Quality of Life. Renal failure and its therapies significantly affect the quality of life of the client and family members. As noted earlier, there are numerous stressors and life changes. Much of the care required by clients receiving chronic peritoneal dialysis and hemodialysis and their significant others concerns the psychosocial aspects of dialysis.

Clients receiving maintenance dialysis often have ambivalent feelings. They realize that dialysis therapy is their tie to life, but the many restrictions and lifestyle changes it imposes make continuation of the program extremely difficult. Clients often report that they feel in limbo between the worlds of life and death.

The process of adaptation to loss is part of adjustment. It is not uncommon for clients to feel grateful and optimistic at the start of dialysis treatments. Usually, they have felt ill for some time, and they view the intervention as a route to survival and feeling well again. It takes a few days or weeks for them to realize fully the permanent place of dialysis in their lives. Depression

---

INTEGRATING PHARMACOLOGY

Medications for Chronic Renal Failure

People with chronic renal failure typically take numerous medications to manage manifestations of their illness. Many factors must be considered before administering these drugs, including absorption, distribution, metabolism, and elimination of the medication. Because the kidneys are not functioning, drugs that are normally excreted by the kidney can accumulate to toxic levels. Some drugs are removed by dialysis; others are not. All these factors should be considered when determining dosage, route, and time of administration. Also, drugs that are nephrotoxic (e.g., aminoglycosides, intravenous pyelogram [IVP] dye) may cause further damage to a dysfunctional organ and should be avoided.

All people with renal failure need vitamin supplements and folic acid, because water-soluble vitamins are dialyzed out, and because dietary restrictions may preclude adequate dietary intake. Also, in renal failure, there are significant disturbances in calcium and phosphorus balance. This is because vitamin D is normally activated in the kidney, and when kidneys are not functioning properly, calcium is not absorbed in sufficient quantities. Vitamin D analogs, such as calcitriol, help with the absorption of calcium. These drugs require close monitoring of serum calcium and phosphorous levels. Furthermore, many people with renal failure take calcium supplements. Calcium carbonate and calcium acetate are relatively inexpensive and are useful as both calcium supplements and as phosphate binders. Because phosphorus is not excreted normally, serum phosphorus level is high and serum calcium level tends to be low. This can result in severe bone disease, known as osteitis fibrosa. Phosphate binders lower serum phosphorus by binding with phosphates in the gut. However, they also tend to cause constipation. As a result, many people also take stool softeners or cathartics. Laxatives with magnesium should be avoided because of the risk of toxicity.

Hypertension is common in people with renal failure. In some cases, this is a result of fluid volume excess and in other cases it can be caused by an excess of renin production by the kidneys (starting the renin-angiotensin system). Fluid volume removal through dialysis is one strategy to manage hypertension, but many people need antihypertensives to control blood pressure effectively. There are many classifications of antihypertensives including angiotensin-converting enzyme inhibitors (e.g., captopril, enalapril, benazepril), beta-adrenergic blockers (e.g., propranolol, atenolol, metoprolol, labetalol), calcium channel blockers (e.g., nifedipine, verapamil), alpha-1 receptor blockers (e.g., prazosin), alpha-2 agonists (e.g., methyldopa, clonidine), and vasodilators. Each has a different mechanism of action, and, typically, considerable monitoring and adjustment of dosage and types of medication takes place before normotension is attained. Diuretics are typically not effective in people with chronic renal failure.

Erythropoietin is a hormone that is produced by the kidney and stimulates the production of red blood cells. A common manifestation of renal failure is anemia. Since 1989, this deficiency has been treated with epoetin alpha (EPO), a recombinant erythropoietin that increases hematocrit to near-normal levels. It can be administered intravenously, after hemodialysis, or subcutaneously. This results in significant improvements in the energy level and quality of life of people with the illness. If iron levels are low, oral or intravenous iron treatment should also be initiated to optimize treatment with EPO. Long-acting forms of EPO (e.g., Aranesp) have recently been made available.

during this period is expected. The suicide rate among clients receiving dialysis has been estimated as 100 times that of the general population.

Common psychosocial problems include changes in body image, dependence on technology, and uncertainty regarding the future. The client's own feelings of weakness and illness and the presence of the arteriovenous fistula and dialysis equipment are constant reminders that the client is no longer a "whole person." Relationships with relatives and friends, job, and community roles and responsibilities are probably altered. The client's normal need for independence is continually threatened by dependence on the dialysis equipment and care providers. This is especially true of adolescents and young adults. Other emotional problems include the need for identity, safety, control of the environment, love, esteem, and communication. The stress on marital relationships and significant others is extreme.

Research suggests that the quality of life of people with ESRD is influenced positively by transplantation, erythropoietin therapy, social support, a positive outlook on life, and the ability to function (including work and activities of daily living). (See the Evidence-Based Practice in Action feature on Quality of Life in End-Stage Renal Disease, below.) Providing an optimal quality of life involves a concerted effort by all members of the health care team with the client and family members as active partners. Many dialysis facilities have established active rehabilitation programs. Elements of these programs include education, exercise, encouragement, employment, and evaluation.[59]

■ Nursing Management of the Medical Client
Assessment

When a client is thought to have CRF, take a complete history and look closely for risk factors. Question the client about past and present medications, diet and weight changes, energy levels and unexplained fatigue, and the pattern of urinary elimination.

Assess the client for the multiple effects of CRF on all body systems, such as the presence of cardiovascular or

EB EVIDENCE-BASED PRACTICE IN ACTION
Quality of Life in End-Stage Renal Disease

Many aspects of renal replacement therapy have a negative impact on quality of life of people with end-stage kidney disease. Numerous manifestations, a restricted diet, and a demanding dialysis schedule prevent people from living normal lives. However, in recent years, there has been considerable research addressing factors to enhance quality of life in this population. It has been recognized that a positive outlook, social support, and higher subjective health status are related to quality of life.[4,5] It has also been noted that renal transplantation offers a higher quality of life than dialysis therapy.[4]

In recent years, there has been increasing emphasis on rehabilitation of people with end-stage renal disease. In a study of 226 people at approximately 60 days after the initiation of treatment, exercise activity was the most important predictor of quality of life.[3]

Qualitative research approaches have been used to explore why some people live long and live well on dialysis. In one study, 18 people who had been receiving dialysis therapy for more than 15 years were interviewed.[2] Life on dialysis was described as a transformation into comprehensive, active self-management of disease, its treatment and its manifestations. Participants in the study described affirmations such as self-preservation (i.e., I want to live), self-identity (i.e., I am still me), self-worth (i.e., I am still valuable), and self-efficacy (i.e., I am in control).[2] Management of their illness included selective manifestation report and management, vigilant oversight of care, proposal of treatment, confrontation of the system through active self-advocacy, and independent adoption of treatment and use of alternative therapies.[1]

Implications
Chronic renal failure and its treatment can severely compromise quality of life of people affected by the disease. Self-management is integral to ensuring a good quality of life. This requires considerable time and energy on the part of the client affected by the disease. Nurses can support self-management through education of clients, planning for exercise programs, and through supportive communication.

References
1. Curtin, R.B., & Mapes, D.L. (2001). Health care management strategies of long-term dialysis survivors. *Nephrology Nursing Journal, 28,* 385-394.
2. Curtin, R.B., et al. (2002). Long-term dialysis survivors: A transformational experience. *Qualitative Health Research, 12,* 609-624.
3. Kutner, N.G., Zhang, R., & McClellan, W.M. (2000). Patient reported quality of life early in dialysis treatment: Effects associated with usual exercise activity. *Nephrology Nursing Journal, 27,* 357-367.
4. Molzahn, A.E., Northcott, H.C., & Dossetor, J.B. (1997). Quality of life of individuals with end stage renal disease: Perceptions of patients, nurses, and physicians. *American Nephrology Nurses Association Journal, 24,* 325-333.
5. Molzahn, A.E., Northcott, H.C., & Hayduk, L. (1996). Quality of life of patients with end stage renal disease: A structural equation model. *Quality of Life Research, 5,* 426-432.

respiratory abnormalities, neurologic changes, gastrointestinal problems, or skin changes.

Assess the client's understanding of CRF, the diagnostic tests that will be done, and the possible treatment regimens. Evaluate the client's level of anxiety and ability to cope. Involve the family in the assessment to determine their ability to cope with the disease and treatments.

When a client has CRF, the client and significant others, the nephrologist, and the nephrology nurse discuss the use of dialysis and decide which type best meets the client's needs. If the client is to receive dialysis, assess the client's and significant others' understanding of the treatment regimen and the client's ability to cope with the treatment regimen. The family's ability to cope and their ability to support the client are also vital.

When the client begins peritoneal dialysis, the first assessment is for infection. Inspect the insertion site carefully for redness or other problems. Carefully assess the drained dialysate or effluent for cloudiness, fibrin streaks, or blood. Monitor the client's vital signs and weight closely.

If the client is undergoing hemodialysis, the first assessment is for the patency of the venous access site. In a patent arteriovenous fistula or graft, a "thrill" or vibrating sensation should be palpable and a bruit should be audible with a stethoscope. It is vital that this site be assessed for possible occlusion or, if it is an external site, for infection. Also ascertain the client's understanding of the access site and its care.

Diagnosis, Outcomes, Interventions

Diagnosis: Deficient Fluid Volume or Excess Fluid Volume. As with all renal disorders, a common nursing diagnosis is *Deficient Fluid Volume or Excess Fluid Volume related to impaired renal function, fluid shifts between dialysate and blood, and blood loss during hemodialysis.*

Outcomes. Neither a fluid volume deficit nor an excess will occur, as evidenced by the absence of edema or dehydration.

Interventions

Monitor Fluid Volume Status. A fluid volume deficit or overload is a serious problem. The current fluid status must be known and fluid intake carefully regulated in keeping with it. Monitor the client's fluid status by observing daily weights, orthostatic blood pressure, skin turgor, and mucous membrane moistness and by meticulous intake and output comparisons.

Give written instructions to outpatients that explain how to weigh themselves properly and how to interpret the relationship of daily weight loss or gain to their need for sodium and water. Help the client understand that vomiting, diarrhea, and working or playing in a hot environment may cause excessive fluid loss and must be

prevented or controlled. Teach the client how to take his or her blood pressure and record it daily.

Follow Fluid Restrictions. When the fluid allowance for the day has been determined, help the client follow the recommendation. Fluid restrictions are difficult for most clients. Offer suggestions about reducing thirst and moistening lips with lip balms, frequent oral hygiene, and taking ice chips or spray bottles rather than drinking. Spread out fluid intake over a longer period of time. If intravenous fluids are used, carefully attend to them to ensure proper administration rates. Water may be restricted so that the client can drink more nutritious liquids, such as apple juice, cranberry juice, or milk.

Monitor Fluid Status During Dialysis. During dialysis, carefully monitor the client's vital signs, including postural blood pressure, pulse, weight, and intake and output. Watch for hypovolemia and retention of dialysate. The amount of desired fluid loss may be ordered by the dialysis physician. Alternatively, a "dry" or "ideal" weight is established and you select appropriate solutions to remove additional fluid.

If fluid does not drain properly during peritoneal dialysis, check the system for kinks or other obstructions. Inform the physician about fluid accumulations that exceed the limit set in the dialysis orders. If the client is undergoing hemodialysis, hypotension and excess fluid removal are risks; monitor carefully.

Diagnosis: Imbalanced Nutrition: Less Than Body Requirements. Another common nursing diagnosis in CRF is *Imbalanced Nutrition: Less Than Body Requirements related to anorexia and nausea.*

Outcomes. The client will maintain adequate nutrition, as evidenced by maintenance of weight without loss of muscle mass.

Interventions. Dietary management is vital to the conservative management of CRF. Anorexia results from many of the manifestations of irreversible renal failure, emotional depression, and a frequently unpalatable diet. Thus a major nursing challenge is to help the client take in adequate nutrition while minimizing uremic toxicity. This problem grows as the disease progresses, and the client may develop an aversion to meat and other sources of protein.

To help stimulate the client's appetite, take measures to relieve nausea and vomiting, stomatitis, and other gastrointestinal manifestations. Diet counseling is essential. Teaching aids (such as those in Figure 38-6) may be helpful. Arrange for dietary consultation if possible. The client needs to know how to translate the dietary regimen into a palatable, understandable food program. Help the client select and prepare foods and learn where

CLIENT EDUCATION TIPS ON PROTEIN INTAKE

THERE ARE TWO DIFFERENT TYPES OF PROTEIN

One is called animal or high biological protein, which contains ALL essential amino acids.

The other type is vegetable or low biological protein, which contains SOME amino acids.

THE HEMODIALYSIS AND THE PERITONEAL MEMBRANE ARE NOT SELECTIVE, WHICH MEANS THAT VITAL AMINO ACIDS AND VITAMINS AS WELL AS UNWANTED WASTES ARE REMOVED

If you are on HEMODIALYSIS, you should aim for **1.2 grams of protein per kg of body weight**; e.g., if you weigh 65 kg (143 lb), your protein intake should be about 78 grams per day.

If you are on PERITONEAL DIALYSIS, you should aim for **1.3 grams of protein per kg of body weight**; e.g., if you weigh 70 kg (154 lb), your protein intake should be about 91 grams per day.

EXAMPLES OF PROTEIN SOURCES

3.5 oz. of extra lean ground beef has 24 grams of protein, whereas rib eye has 28 grams of protein.

Half of a chicken breast (3.5 oz.) has 29 grams of protein. Turkey white meat (3.5 oz) has 30 grams of protein.

One can of Ensure has 13 grams of protein, whereas 1 scoop of Promod has 5 grams, and one egg has 6 grams of protein.

15 large cooked shrimp have 17 grams of protein. A 3 oz. can of white tuna in water has 22 grams of protein.

One cup of milk has 8 grams of protein, whereas ½ cup of regular tofu has 10 grams, and one slice of white bread has 2 grams of protein.

One cup of cooked corn, peas, potato, pasta, or rice has about 4 grams of protein.

FIGURE 38-6 Renal teaching aids: tips on protein intake. (Modified from Darlene Michl, Sidney, British Columbia.)

to obtain special foods if necessary. Exercise may also improve appetite.

Diagnosis: Constipation.
The treatment of CRF leads to the predictable nursing diagnosis of *Constipation related to medications, fluid and dietary restrictions, and decreased activity level.*

Outcomes. The client will remain free of constipation, as evidenced by a bowel movement at least every other day.

Interventions. Constipation is a major problem for clients with CRF. Because of fluid restrictions, inability to eat most high-fiber foods, and limited activity, it is difficult to use customary measures for preventing constipation. Phosphate-binding agents contribute to the problem as well.

Bran, which is not rich in potassium or phosphorus, can be used. Stool softeners are often administered regularly, although care should be taken to avoid those that contain calcium and sodium. If necessary, bulk laxatives (such as psyllium hydrophilic mucilloid) may be given. The recommended amount of fluid should be taken with the powder and subtracted from the day's fluid allotment.

Stimulant and lubricant laxatives should be used only if necessary, especially compounds containing magnesium or phosphorus, such as sodium biphosphate–sodium phosphate (Fleet) enemas. If none of these measures is effective, small-volume, gentle stimulant enemas may be used sparingly, but large-volume enemas should be avoided because of possible fluid and saline absorption. Clients with renal failure are at risk for diverticular disease because of the constipation and straining.

Diagnosis: Fatigue.
Physiologic alterations can ensure a nursing diagnosis of *Fatigue related to anemia and altered metabolic state.*

Outcomes. The client will have a balance of rest and activity, as evidenced by the client's statement of decreased fatigue.

Interventions. Rest is important to any client whose body is under a great deal of stress. Encourage frequent naps. Insomnia is frequently a problem, and you may need to make suggestions about how to solve this problem (as by observing a presleep quiet time and establishing a presleep routine). Assessment in a sleep center may be helpful.

Hypnotics and sedatives must be used cautiously because they may alter mentation and may be metabolized differently by a client with renal failure. The client also needs to establish and maintain an appropriate exercise program. Anemia should be treated with iron and erythropoietin therapy to increase energy levels.

Diagnosis: Risk for Impaired Skin Integrity.
Edema and skin changes create a *Risk for Impaired Skin Integrity related to edema, dry skin, and pruritus.*

Outcomes. The client will not develop impaired skin integrity, as evidenced by intact skin.

Interventions. Dry skin is a common problem. Use of soap may need to be eliminated. Because of the increased risk of secondary infection, however, the client's skin still needs to be kept clean. Moisturizing oils in the bath water or applied directly to the skin help to correct dryness. Avoid any products that contain alcohol or perfumes; they increase dryness and pruritus. If edema is present, avoid sustained pressure on the area. The potential for skin breakdown is particularly acute in clients with diabetes. Observe for poor circulation and areas of breakdown or infection.

Diagnosis: Risk for Compromised Family and Ineffective Individual Coping.
An important diagnosis is *Risk for Compromised Family and Ineffective Individual Coping related to chronic illness, uncertain future for the client, role reversal, and effects of long-term dialysis.*

Outcomes. The client and family will cope with the client's chronic illness and future deterioration, as evidenced by acceptance of the client's problems and ability to support the client. The client and family will cope effectively with the effects of long-term dialysis, as evidenced by the client's level of activity, feelings of self-worth, and participation in dialysis treatment.

Interventions

Involve in Decision Making. Assistance for the client and significant others must begin before dialysis is started. A client with CRF faces a future of continued deterioration but with an unknown course and timetable. In addition, the disease itself produces behavioral manifestations that contribute to the client's susceptibility to stress.

Many such clients must make important decisions about the choice of treatment modes at a time when they do not feel well. It is often difficult for the client to voice concerns about discontinuing dialysis, and it may be difficult for care providers and families to accept the client's decision to stop treatment and choose death instead. For these reasons, you need to assess how the client handled change and stress before the illness began. The client and significant others need to be actively involved in the care planning process because they will be living with the disease for many years.

Provide Support. The client and significant others will have many questions about such issues as family functioning, job or school demands, dependence, and sex. The client may experience reduced self-esteem. Significant others commonly report a decline in their quality of life that correlates directly with changes in the client's quality of life. Encourage the client and significant others to discuss their feelings and concerns, together and individually, using therapeutic communication techniques. Support groups and peer counseling programs are often helpful.

Offer Home Dialysis. About 15% of all clients who receive dialysis do so at home. The cost of this type of program is less than that of in-center dialysis, and it usually improves the client's quality of life. Home dialysis offers the client more access to significant others and greater feelings of independence and control. However, this type of treatment also produces stress on personal relationships, especially on the person who becomes the "dialysis helper" during home hemodialysis. Some spouses have voiced concern about lack of free time and increased responsibility; others see it as an opportunity to give something back to their spouse or loved one. Some states have funding available to pay for a non-family member to serve as dialysis helper. In some instances, this may reduce tension and improve the quality of life for the family.

Clients for home dialysis programs must be selected carefully. Criteria might include stability of relationships, psychological stability, financial support, and lack of severe physical complications. A successful program requires care providers who are advocates of home dialysis, a good training program, and good support services, possibly including nursing, medical, and social services; provision of supplies; equipment maintenance; dietary counseling; home visits; and retraining as necessary.

Diagnosis: Risk for Ineffective Family and Individual Therapeutic Regimen Management.
There is *Risk for Ineffective Family and Individual Therapeutic Regimen Management related to lack of knowledge of the disease process and treatment.*

Outcomes. The client will understand the disease process and treatment regimen as evidenced by ability to describe the disease and treatment and participate in the treatment regimen.

Interventions

Provide Information. Teaching is a crucial part of the nursing management plan. Usually, the client is observed on an outpatient basis and is responsible for following the recommended treatment regimen. The client and significant others must know about normal renal function and how the disease has altered it, the details of the management protocol and how to follow it, a number of self-assessment skills as described earlier, and when to seek professional consultation for possible complications. Teaching aids are available from many sources, such as the National Kidney Foundation, the National Association of Patients on Hemodialysis and Transplantation, various corporations, and the Internet. The Life Options Rehabilitation Program offers an award-winning website known as Kidney School (see http://www.KidneySchool.org).

Explain Dialysis. The client and significant others need to know about dialysis and how to work with its ramifications. With peritoneal dialysis, most clients continue the treatment mode in their homes; hence, their knowledge needs to be complete and detailed. They participate in a complete training program so that they can handle the entire dialysis process independently.

Continuous monitoring during hemodialysis provides vital information about the progress of the treatment and allows early diagnosis of potential complications. There should be a well-organized plan for observing and recording vital signs, dialysate composition and temperature, and functioning of the entire dialysis system and blood flow. The client should also be alert to early manifestations of potential complications, as listed earlier. The nurse often serves as case manager and coordinates the services provided by the nephrology team, which includes the physician, nurses, social worker, and dietitian.

Reduce Anxiety. Although clients with renal disease must learn about their disorder, they may not always be ready to learn. Anxiety itself interferes with learning. In addition, the disease interferes with normal cognitive functioning; memory deficits and a short attention span may require simple presentations and frequent repetition of information. Retained learning must be continually evaluated.

Significant others may be especially frustrated during teaching sessions by the client's inability to grasp the concepts being presented. The client may seem out of touch with reality. Significant others need reassurance that this is an effect of the disease and that the client will become more capable of learning, especially after institution of dialysis.

Diagnosis: Risk for Infection.
Indwelling catheters carry a high *Risk for Infection related to the presence of an indwelling peritoneal catheter and instillation of dialysate or related to venipuncture and connection of tubing during hemodialysis.*

Outcomes. The client will remain free of infection, as evidenced by a normal white blood cell count, absence of fever, and clear dialysate.

Interventions. Because peritonitis is the main complication of peritoneal dialysis, strict aseptic technique must be used throughout the procedure. Masks are worn by the nurse and client when the peritoneal dialysis circuit is opened. Gloves are worn by anyone touching the catheter during all connection and disconnection procedures. The catheter is soaked before and after these procedures in a povidone-iodine or other disinfecting solution. Dressing changes around the catheter site are performed according to the specific unit protocol. Be sure dressings are kept dry at all times.

With hemodialysis, use strict aseptic technique during venipuncture and when attaching the tubing and solution.

Diagnosis: Risk for Ineffective Breathing Pattern.
Peritoneal dialysis also creates a *Risk for Ineffective Breathing Pattern related to pressure from dialysate.*

Outcomes. The client will have an effective breathing pattern, as evidenced by an absence of shortness of breath.

Interventions. Because dialysate presses on the diaphragm, its full excursion may be reduced and an immobilized client may be at risk for respiratory problems. Encourage the client to cough and deep-breathe regularly. Keep the client in the semi-Fowler position to ease breathing. Also, remind the client to stay alert for early manifestations of compromised respiratory function.

Diagnosis: Risk for Injury.
Trauma and complications associated with the vascular access for hemodialysis may occur, leading to the nursing diagnosis of *Risk for Injury related to trauma to hemodialysis vascular access site.*

Outcomes. The client will not experience injury to the vascular access site, as evidenced by continued patency of the site.

Interventions. Careful attention to the access site—to prevent infection and clotting—is important to the life expectancy of the access site. A dressing is used to protect cannulas and subclavian catheters from infection. The access site must also be protected from trauma that could cause clotting, bleeding, or physical disruption of the site. For example, warn the client against wearing tight sleeves or carrying a purse over the access site. The limb that contains the access site should not be used to take blood pressure or to draw blood.

Between dialysis periods, the skin over the fistula or graft requires only routine care with soap and water. The site of a fistula should be carefully assessed. To assess patency, palpate over the fistula for a thrill and auscultate for a bruit at regular intervals. The client must also learn to assess the access site for patency.

Evaluation

The client is expected to improve physically and mentally when dialysis begins. The client's weight and blood pressure should begin to stabilize if dietary and fluid restrictions are followed and as fluid balance stabilizes.

Normal electrolyte and albumin levels reflect adequate nutrition and compliance with diet. The client should report regular, normal bowel movements. The client should report less fatigue and increased energy and activity as hematocrit values approach normal levels. Skin should remain intact.

The client should understand and adapt to the treatment regimen and be successfully maintained with peritoneal dialysis or hemodialysis. Clients receiving peritoneal dialysis (and some receiving hemodialysis) should be able to demonstrate successful performance of the dialysis procedure and care of the vascular access site or peritoneal catheter. They should remain free from complications associated with dialysis. As long as venous or peritoneal access can be maintained, the client can be managed with dialysis until transplantation (if the client is a candidate) is completed, the client elects to stop dialysis, or other complications result in death.

Significant others should cope with the client's chronic illness and dialysis, show acceptance of problems, support the client, and report improved satisfaction with their own quality of life. The family and significant others should assist the client with treatment as needed.

■ Self-Care

Clients must comply with dietary and fluid intake modifications and take prescribed medications as ordered. They must monitor and record weight and blood pressure daily and care for the vascular access or peritoneal catheter as ordered. Noncompliance with the regimen leads to complications. The client or family must perform dialysis at home or keep scheduled dialysis appointments.

■ Modifications for Older Clients

The type of dialysis selected for older clients is based on an assessment that includes the presence of other chronic disorders that would preclude various treatment modalities. Older clients may have had multiple abdominal surgical procedures with the development of adhesions that limit the usefulness of peritoneal dialysis. They are more likely to have pre-existing cardiovascular problems that may limit the usefulness of many vascular access sites.

RENAL TRANSPLANTATION
■ Surgical Management

Indications. Renal transplantation is the surgical implantation of a human kidney from a compatible donor in a recipient. This procedure is performed as an intervention in irreversible kidney failure. The kidney is surgically placed extraperitoneally in the iliac fossa. The renal artery is anastomosed to the recipient's hypogastric internal or external iliac artery (occasionally the aorta) and the renal vein to the recipient's iliac vein (Figure 38-7). Usually, the kidney begins to function immediately.

Selection of a transplant recipient is based on careful evaluation of the client's medical, immunologic, and psychosocial status (see Chapter 82). Usually, a recipient is younger than age 70, has an estimated life expectancy of

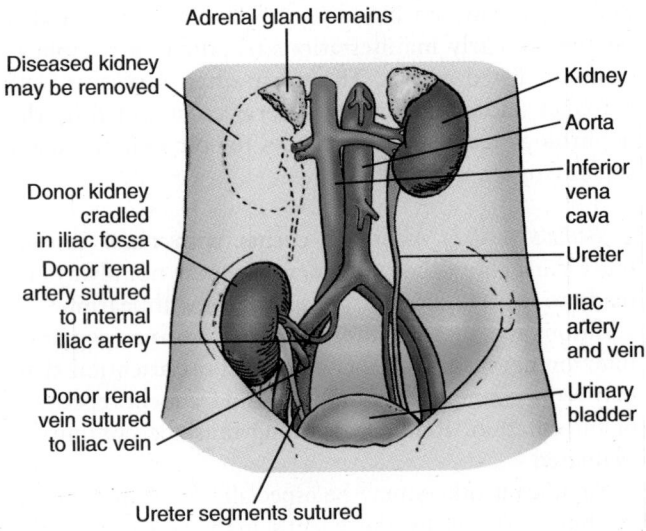

FIGURE 38-7 Transplanted kidney placement in the right iliac fossa.

TABLE 38-1	National Kidney Foundation Classification of Chronic Kidney Disease		
Stage	Description	Other Terms Used	GFR (ml/min/1.73m²)
1	Kidney damage with nomal glomerular filtration rate (GFR)	At risk	>90
2	Kidney damage with mild decrease in GFR	Chronic renal insufficiency (CRI)	60-89
3	Moderate decrease in GFR	CRI, chronic renal failure (CRF)	30-59
4	Severe decrease in GFR	CRF	15-29
5	Kidney failure	End-stage renal disease (ESRD)	<15

Modified from National Kidney Foundation: *K/DOQI (Kidney/Dialysis Outcomes Quality Initiative) Clinical Practice Guidelines for Chronic Kidney Disease: Evaluation, Classification and Stratification.* Accessed January 30, 2004: http://www.kidney.org/professionals/doqi/kdoqi/toc.htm.

2 years or more, and is expected to have an improved quality of life after transplantation. Conservative management and dialysis should have made the client's state as nontoxic as possible. Bilateral nephrectomy may be performed before the transplantation procedure for persistent or active bacterial pyelonephritis, uncontrolled renin-mediated hypertension, polycystic kidneys, or rapidly progressive glomerulonephritis.

Successful transplantation prolongs life and markedly improves its quality. The client is freed from the restrictions of dialysis and from the reversible manifestations of uremia.

Because graft survival rates are higher, the most desirable source of kidneys for transplantation is a living related donor who matches the client closely. Willing family members are evaluated for physical and mental health and screened for ABO blood group, tissue-specific antigen, and human leukocyte antigen histocompatibility (see Chapter 82). Consideration has been given to transplanting kidneys from emotionally related donors, such as friends or spouses. In recent years, the number of living donations is close to the number of cadaveric donations, because of the limited supply of the latter.

Contraindications. Infection and active malignancy are the only absolute contraindications to transplantation. Some physical conditions markedly increase the risk for the client, however, primarily because long-term immunosuppressive medications are necessary to avoid graft rejection. Clients with liver disease, psychological disorders, advanced atherosclerosis, hypertension, respiratory disease, and gastrointestinal bleeding need particular consideration. The primary factor limiting the number of transplantations done is the availability of kidneys.

Complications. Major complications of transplantation, such as graft rejection (and antirejection therapy), infection, skin and gastrointestinal problems, and other complications, are discussed in Chapter 82.

Graft Rejection. The manifestations of renal transplant rejection include fever, graft tenderness at the site of the transplanted kidney, anemia, and malaise.

Urinary Tract Complications. Several complications may occur in the urinary tract. Although it is rare, spontaneous rupture of the kidney may occur because of rejection or ischemic damage. Leaking of urine from the ureter-bladder anastomosis causes the development of a urinoma, which eventually puts pressure on the kidney and ureter, reducing renal function. Long-term uremia and steroid therapy may predispose the client to ureteral, bladder, or caliceal-cutaneous fistulae. Other urinary tract complications include ureteral, bladder, or pelvic leaks, as well as obstruction, reflux, and lymphoceles.

Cardiopulmonary Complications. Hypertension occurs in 50% to 60% of adult recipients and may be caused by renal artery stenosis, acute tubular necrosis, acute and chronic graft rejection, hydronephrosis, hyperaldosteronism, large-dose steroids, and cyclosporine. Cardiac dysrhythmias and heart failure may result from fluid and electrolyte imbalances.

Pneumonia caused by bacteria and fungi is the most frequent respiratory complication. Other respiratory problems include pulmonary edema, pulmonary emboli, and reactivated tuberculosis.

Other Complications. The reproductive problems associated with CRF commonly disappear after transplantation. The incidence of gynecologic malignancies is higher than in the general population, with cervical cancer dominating. Successful pregnancies have been completed after transplantation, although there is a risk for both the fetus and the mother with a transplanted kidney.

Outcomes. Over the years, both recipient and graft survival rates have greatly improved. One-year graft survival rates are 85% to 90% with transplants from living related donors and 75% to 80% with cadaver kidneys. The overall mortality rate 2 years after transplantation is about 10%. This represents a dramatic decrease; two decades ago, the 2-year survival rate was 40% to 50%.

In particular, the decrease in the death rate related to infection in the first 2 years after transplantation has been dramatic. Advances in immunosuppressive therapy and the treatment of infectious diseases have contributed to the overall improvement. Cardiovascular problems remain the leading cause of death in the late transplantation period. Myocardial infarction, stroke, and heart failure are the primary causes of death.

■ Nursing Management of the Surgical Client

Preoperative Care
Before kidney transplantation, assess the client's understanding of the procedure and follow-up regimen. Also, assess the client's ability to cope with a complex medication regimen after transplantation. The client needs to understand the transplantation and therapeutic regimen. Preoperative preparation of both the living donor and the recipient includes all aspects of general preoperative care as outlined in Chapter 16.

Postoperative Care
Assessment for renal transplant recipients is similar to that for most other postoperative clients (see Chapter 16), with the exception of the focus on renal function. Give particular attention to fluid balance, and carefully monitor intake and output (every 30 to 60 minutes) and weight (daily). To monitor renal function and maintain electrolyte balance, obtain serial laboratory determinations of hemoglobin, hematocrit, BUN (urea nitrogen), creatinine, electrolytes, white blood cell count, and platelets. Auscultate the kidney regularly to check for

COMPLEMENTARY AND ALTERNATIVE THERAPY

Noni Juice and Renal Disease

Noni juice (Morinda citrifolia) is a popular drink in some alternative medicine circles. It has been advertised by some as promoting health and as helping to cure many types of conditions. However, no good research studies have been completed to see if this is true. The general recommended dose for noni juice (as found on the Internet) is approximately 1 ounce/day, but some websites promote higher intakes. Individuals with kidney disease whose blood levels of potassium get too high may experience irregular heart rhythms or even a heart attack. Noni juice contains moderate levels of potassium in small doses. Therefore clients should be careful and find out the potassium level of their brand, or they should just play it safe and stay away from this alternative medicine until more studies are concluded.

Reference

Mueller, B., et al. (2000). Noni juice (Morinda citrifolia): Hidden potential for hyperkalemia? *American Journal of Kidney Disease, 35,* 310-312.

bruits, which might indicate stenosis. Monitoring of vital signs is key, because even a slight temperature increase may indicate an infection.

The function of the transplanted kidney is a primary concern after surgery. A kidney from a cadaver may not function immediately, and the client may be maintained with hemodialysis until it functions adequately. Postoperatively, manage intravenous fluids carefully; the amount of fluid infused is typically based on the previous hour's output. A high urine output is usually desired. The additional care required by the recipient is related to potential complications. Care of the client with a transplant is discussed in more detail in Chapter 82.

Psychologically, the client must be helped to incorporate the new kidney as a part of the whole being. Provide education and counseling to enhance changes in lifestyle that promote health-seeking behaviors and compliance with transplantation medications. If the graft fails, expect the client to feel anger, hostility, guilt, and a helplessness-hopelessness syndrome. Relatives and friends may mirror these feelings. Role changes that were well established during the chronic illness may lead to problems, as with the family member who no longer feels needed as the caregiver. Likewise, the client may have difficulty giving up the sick role.

◾ Self-Care

Failure to follow the prescribed regimen is a major problem after transplantation, and your knowledge and creativity are needed to help the client follow the recommended regimen. Many clients—particularly adolescents—miss doses of their immunosuppressive medications (see Chapter 82). This practice contributes to early loss of renal function and possible graft loss.

Clients may be reluctant to take medications for many reasons. For some, the side effects disrupt their lives. Others may believe that they no longer need the medications because their condition is stable. Economic concerns also need to be addressed. Work with the client to provide needed information and to develop strategies that fit the client's lifestyle.

Overall, transplantation offers clients with CRF a much better quality of life than does dialysis therapy. Renal function returns and many of the clinical manifestations of CRF disappear. Complications do occur, and care must be taken to prevent graft loss. Renal transplant recipients are monitored regularly at transplantation clinics. The visits become less frequent as renal function stabilizes and time passes. Blood tests are done regularly to monitor serum creatinine levels and cyclosporine levels. Every transplantation center has protocols for routine follow-up tests.

◾ Modifications for Older Clients

Fewer treatment options are available for older clients. Renal transplantation is not routinely done for older clients. Clients older than 60 years are evaluated on an individual basis; clients as old as 75 years of age have had successful transplantations. In older clients, a less effective immune system in conjunction with immunosuppressants can lead to further complications.

CONCLUSIONS

Caring for the client with renal failure involves many challenges. Numerous physical and psychosocial manifestations are associated with renal disease and its treatment. The nurse can significantly impact the client's quality of life through the provision of education, encouragement, promotion of exercise, and ongoing assessment of the client and family as well as evaluation of programs offering treatment for ESRD. The nurse, in collaboration with the multidisciplinary team, can facilitate positive outcomes.

THINKING CRITICALLY *evolve*

1. You are caring for a 74-year-old man 1 day after coronary artery bypass surgery. His urine output is about 15 ml/hr. He has a long history of hypertension (controlled), and his blood pressure usually ranges from 180 to 190 over 90 to 100 mm Hg. His blood pressure since surgery has ranged from 120 to 130 over 70 to 76 mm Hg. His serum sodium concentration is 145 mEq/L and potassium is 4.9 mEq/L. His

skin turgor is poor, and his mucous membranes are dry. What is your first assessment and action?

Factors to Consider. What has his intake been since surgery? What are the possible causes of his low blood pressure, increased electrolytes, and decreased urine output? If he has renal failure, what is the probable cause? What other assessments should you make?

2. You are caring for a 60-year-old woman with diabetes, hypertension, and chronic renal failure. She has had hemodialysis for over a year and has decided that she no longer wants to continue living this way. She has informed her physician and family that she no longer wishes to continue dialysis. Her family is trying to persuade her that she should go for her next treatment. She asks you your opinion, "Would you want to live this way?" How would you respond? How would you ensure that she is making the right decision?

Factors to Consider. What is the client's cognitive and emotional status? How have the client and her family members coped with the illness and its treatment? Given the information you have, what is her prognosis? Do people have the right to refuse life-sustaining therapy? Knowing that health care resources are finite, what is the best use of resources for all members of society?

Discussions for these questions can be found on the website and the CD-ROM.

BIBLIOGRAPHY

1. Abdeen, O., & Mehta, R.L. (2002). Dialysis modalities in the intensive care unit. *Critical Care Clinics, 18*(2), 223-248.
2. Abernethy, V.E., & Lieberthal, W. (2002). Acute renal failure in the critically ill patient. *Critical Care Clinics, 18*(2), 203-222.
3. Agrawal, M., & Swartz, R. (2000). Acute renal failure. *American Family Physician, 61*(7), 2077-2088, 1969-1972, 2266.
4. Ahee, P., & Crowe, A.V. (2000). The management of hyperkalemia in the emergency department. *Journal of Accident and Emergency, 17*(3), 188-191.
5. Astle, S.M. (2001). A new direction for dialysis. *RN, 64*(7), 56-60.
6. Bleyer, A.J., et al. (1999). An international study of patient compliance with hemodialysis. *Journal of the American Medical Association, 281*(13), 1211-1213.
7. Bliwise, D.L., et al. (2001). Survival by time of day of hemodialysis in an elderly cohort. *Journal of the American Medical Association, 286*(21), 2690-2694.
8. Borkan, S.C. (2002). Extracorporeal therapies for acute intoxications. *Critical Care Clinics, 18*(2), 393-420.
9. Brenner, B.M. (Ed.). (2000). *Brenner and Rector's the kidney* (6th ed.). Philadelphia: W. B. Saunders.
10. Bro, S. (2003). How abnormal calcium phosphate and parathyroid hormone relate to cardiovascular disease. *Nephrology Nursing Journal, 30,* 275-281.
11. Burrows-Hudson, S. (Ed.). (1999). *Standards and guidelines of clinical practice for nephrology nursing.* Pitman, NJ: American Nephrology Nurses Association.
12. Butterly D.W., & Schwab, S.J. (2001). Catheter access for hemodialysis: An overview. *Seminars in Dialysis, 14*(6), 411-415.
13. Chertow, G.M., et al. (2001). Guided medication dosing for inpatients with renal insufficiency. *Journal of the American Medical Association, 286*(22), 2839-2844.
14. Cliffe, M., Bloodworth, L.L.O., & Jibani, M.M. (2001). Can malnutrition in predialysis patients be prevented by dietetic intervention? *Journal of Renal Nutrition, 11*(3), 161-165.
15. Collins, A.J., et al. (2002). Dialyzing the elderly: Issues and concerns: Comparison and survival of hemodialysis and peritoneal dialysis in the elderly. *Seminars in Dialysis, 15*(2), 98.
16. Curtin, R.B., & Mapes, D.L. (2001). Health care management strategies of long-term dialysis survivors. *Nephrology Nursing Journal, 28,* 385-394.
17. Daugirdas, J.T., Blake, P.G., & Ing, T.S. (2001). *Handbook of dialysis* (3rd ed.). Philadelphia: Lippincott Williams & Wilkins.
18. Davison, S.N. (2001). Quality end-of-life care in dialysis units. *Seminars in Dialysis, 15*(1), 41-44.
19. Dember, L.M. (2002). Critical care issues in the patient with chronic renal failure. *Critical Care Clinics, 18*(2), 420-440.
20. Dirkes, S.M. (2000). Continuous renal replacement therapy: Dialytic therapy for acute renal failure in intensive care. *Nephrology Nursing Journal, 27,* 581-592.
21. Duncan, M.G. (1999). The effects of nutritional supplements on the treatment of depression, diabetes, and hypercholesterolemia in the renal patient. *Journal of Renal Nutrition, 9*(2), 58-62.
22. Fishbane, S., & Goldman, R. (2002). Quality outcomes and obstacles to their achievement in end-stage renal disease. *Seminars in Dialysis, 15*(1), 30-34.
23. Gauthier, P.M., & Szerlip, H.M. (2002). Metabolic acidosis in the intensive care unit. *Critical Care Clinics, 18*(2), 289-308.
24. Gennari, F.J. (2001). *Medical management of kidney and electrolyte disorders.* New York: Marcel Dekker.
25. Gennari, F.J. (2002). Disorders of potassium homeostasis: Hypokalemia and hyperkalemia. *Critical Care Clinics, 18*(2), 273-288.
26. Guyton, A., & Hall, J. (2000). *Textbook of medical physiology* (10th ed.). Philadelphia: W.B. Saunders.
27. King, B. (2000). CE: Meds and the dialysis patient. *RN, 63*(7), 54-60.
28. Klassen, P.S., et al. (2002). Association between pulse rate and mortality in patients undergoing maintenance hemodialysis. *Journal of the American Medical Association, 287*(12), 1548-1555.
29. Kosier, J., et al. Darbepoetin alfa (Aranesp) for treating anemia associated with chronic kidney disease. *Urologic Nursing, 23,* 77-79.
30. Krishnan, M., Lok, C.E., & Jassal, S.V. (2002). Dialyzing the elderly: Issues and concerns: Epidemiology and demographic aspects of treated end-stage renal disease in the elderly. *Seminars in Dialysis, 15*(2), 79.

31. Kutner, N.G., & Jassal, S.V. (2002). Dialyzing the elderly: Issues and concerns: Quality of life and rehabilitation of elderly dialysis patients. *Seminars in Dialysis, 15*(2), 107.

32. Lameire, N. & Mehta, R.L. (2000). *Complications of dialysis.* New York: Marcel Dekker.

33. Lancaster, L.E. (Ed.). (2001). *Core curriculum for nephrology nursing* (4th ed.). Pitman, NJ: American Nephrology Nurses Association.

34. Lawson, J.A., Lazarus, R., & Kelly, J.J. (2001). Prevalence and prognostic significance of malnutrition in chronic renal insufficiency. *Journal of Renal Nutrition, 11*(1), 16-22.

35. Lindqvist, R., Carlsson, M., & Sjoden, P.O. (2000). Perceived consequences of being a renal failure patient. *Nephrology Nursing Journal, 27,* 305-310.

36. Lowance, D.C. (2002). Dialyzing the elderly: Issues and concerns: Withholding and withdrawal of dialysis in the elderly. *Seminars in Dialysis, 15*(2), 88.

37. Lubkin, I., & Larsen, P.D. (2002). *Chronic illness: Impact and interventions* (5th ed.). Boston: Jones & Bartlett.

38. Madore, F. (2002). Plasmapheresis: Technical aspects and indications. *Critical Care Clinics, 18*(2), 375-392.

39. Massry, S.G., & Glassock, R.J. (Eds.). (2001). *Massry and Glassock's textbook of nephrology* (4th ed.). Baltimore: Lippincott Williams & Wilkins.

40. Mistiaen, P. (2001). Thirst, interdialytic weight gain, and thirst interactions in hemodialysis patients: A literature review. *Nephrology Nursing Journal, 28,* 601-615.

41. Myhre, M.J. (2000). Herbal remedies, nephropathies, and renal disease. *Nephrology Nursing Journal, 27*(5), 473-480.

42. Noortgate, N.V. de, et al. (2002). Dialyzing the elderly: Issues and concerns: The dialytic management of acute renal failure in the elderly. *Seminars in Dialysis, 15*(2), 127.

43. Parker, K.P., Bilwise, D.L., Rye, D.B. (2000). Hemodialysis disrupts basic sleep regulatory mechanisms: Building hypotheses. *Nursing Research, 49*(6), 327-332.

44. Polaschek, N. (2003). The experience of living on dialysis: A literature review. *Nephrology Nursing Journal, 30,* 303-309.

45. Owen, W.F. Jr., et al. (1998). Dose of hemodialysis and survival: Differences by race and sex. *Journal of the American Medical Association, 280*(20), 1764-1768.

46. Robert Wood Johnson Foundation. (2003). ESRD Workgroup Final Report Summary on End-of-Life Care: Recommendations to the field. *Nephrology Nursing Journal, 30,* 59-63.

47. Ross, C.A. (2000). Emergency: Dialysis disequilibrium syndrome. *American Journal of Nephrology, 100*(2), 53-54.

48. Russell, T.A. (2000). Acute renal failure related to rhabdomyolysis: Pathophysiology, diagnosis, and collaborative management. *Nephrology Nursing Journal, 27,* 567-577.

49. Sarnak, M.J. (2002). How can the cardiac death rate be reduced in dialysis patients? *Seminars in Dialysis, 15*(1), 18-29.

50. Schiffl, H. (2002). News: Patients in acute renal failure may be undertreated. *American Journal of Nephrology, 102*(5), 18.

51. Schiffl, H., & Innenstadt, M.K. (2002). Abstracts: Daily hemodialysis and the outcome of acute renal failure. *Journal of the American Medical Association, 287*(14), 1780.

52. Schrier, R.W. (Ed.). (2000). *Manual of nephrology* (5th ed.). Philadelphia: Lippincott Williams & Wilkins.

53. Schrier, R.W. (2002). *Renal and electrolyte disorders* (6th ed.). Boston, Little, Brown.

54. Schrier, R.W. (Ed.). (2001). *Diseases of the kidney and urinary tract* (6th ed.). Philadelphia: Lippincott Williams & Wilkins.

55. Singri, N., Ahya, S., & Levin, M. (2003). Acute renal failure. *Journal of the American Medical Association, 289*(6), 747-751.

56. Spitalewitz, S. (2000). In consultation: How to best control hypertension in patients with renal insufficiency. *Journal of Critical Illness, 15*(9), 468.

57. Stevens, L.M. (2001). Kidney failure. *Journal of the American Medical Association, 286*(22), 2898.

58. Stone, J., Wyman, J., & Salisbury, S. (1999). *Clinical gerontological nursing: A guide to advanced practice* (2nd ed.). Philadelphia: W. B. Saunders.

59. Tawney, K. (2000). Clinical consult: Developing a dialysis rehabilitation program. *Nephrology Nursing Journal, 27*(5), 524, 539.

60. U.S. Renal Data System. (2002). *Annual data report: Atlas of end-stage renal disease in the United States.* Bethesda, MD: National Institutes of Health, National Institute of Diabetes and Digestive and Kidney Diseases.

61. Welch, J.L., & Davis, J. (2000). Self-care strategies to reduce fluid intake and control thirst in hemodialysis patients. *Nephrology Nursing Journal, 27,* 393-395.

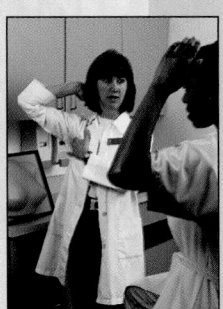

Unit 9

Sexuality and Reproductive Disorders

Anatomy and Physiology Review

The Reproductive Systems

Robert G. Carroll

The human reproductive system is specialized for the production and joining of *germ* cells—the ovum, or egg (female), and the sperm (male). The female reproductive system is also specialized to nurture and protect the fertilized ovum during the 9-month gestation period. Gonadal development begins in utero, but maturation of the reproductive system *(puberty)* is delayed until adolescence. At 45 to 60 years of age, fertility gradually decreases, ending at *menopause* (permanent cessation of menstruation) in women.

GONADAL DEVELOPMENT

The *gonads* are the sex glands of the female *(ovaries)* and male *(testes)*. Their primary function is to form germ cells, which have half the normal number of chromosomes. The ovaries produce ova; the testes produce spermatozoa (sperm).

Gonadal development begins during the 5th week of fetal life. Gonadal differentiation occurs in the 7th and 8th weeks of gestation. Human chorionic gonadotropin (HCG) is released from the placenta, stimulating the fetal ovaries to release estradiol and progesterone and the testes to release testosterone. In males, the wolffian ducts develop into the epididymis, vas deferens, and seminal vesicles, and the müllerian ducts regress. In females, the wolffian ducts regress and the müllerian ducts develop into fallopian tubes, uterus, and upper vagina. The external genitalia, the glans penis and scrotum, are complete in the male by 14 weeks of gestation from the stimulation of testosterone. The clitoris, labia majora, and labia minora are complete in the female by 11 weeks of gestation by the absence of testosterone.

FEMALE REPRODUCTIVE SYSTEM GENITAL STRUCTURES

External Structures

The female reproductive organs consist of both external and internal structures. The external structures, collectively termed the *vulva* or *pudendum,* play a role in sexual stimulation and provide a barrier to protect the body from foreign materials (Figure U9-1, *A*). External female genital structures consist of the mons pubis, labia majora, labia minora, clitoris, vestibule, and vestibular bulbs. The *perineum* is the area posterior to the vestibule, between the vestibule and the anus.

Internal Structures

The internal female genital structures produce and release the reproductive cell or ovum, transport ova to the potential site of fertilization, and provide an appropriate environment for the implantation, growth, and delivery of the fetus (Table U9-1).

Ovaries are the female gonads, producing the female germ cell (ovum) and hormones (estrogen and progesterone). Normally two ovaries are located in the pelvis, one on either side of the uterus and below the fallopian (uterine) tubes (Figure U9-1, *B*). The ovaries are contained in the posterior surfaces of the broad ligaments. They are also supported by the suspensory ligament (to the side of the pelvis) and by the utero-ovarian ligament (to the uterus). Each ovary is about the size, shape, and weight of an almond. In young females, ovaries are smooth; with age, they become pitted.

Ova, in various stages of development, together with their surrounding tissue, make up the *ovarian follicles.* Each follicle contains a developing ovum; it grows and matures in the stroma, close to an abundant blood and lymphatic supply. A mature follicle (a mature ovum and its surrounding tissues) is an endocrine gland secreting estrogen hormones (see Estrogens later in this chapter). At birth, several hundred thousand follicles, each containing an oocyte (endstage ovum), are present. They decrease in number as puberty approaches (the onset of function reproductive capability), and they gradually disappear around menopause.

The *corpus luteum* is a glandular body that produces the hormones progesterone and estrogen. It develops from a graafian follicle after ovulation (see Secretory [Luteal] Phase later in this chapter).

Two *fallopian tubes* connect the uterus to the ovaries and are the usual site of fertilization (Figure U9-1, *C*).

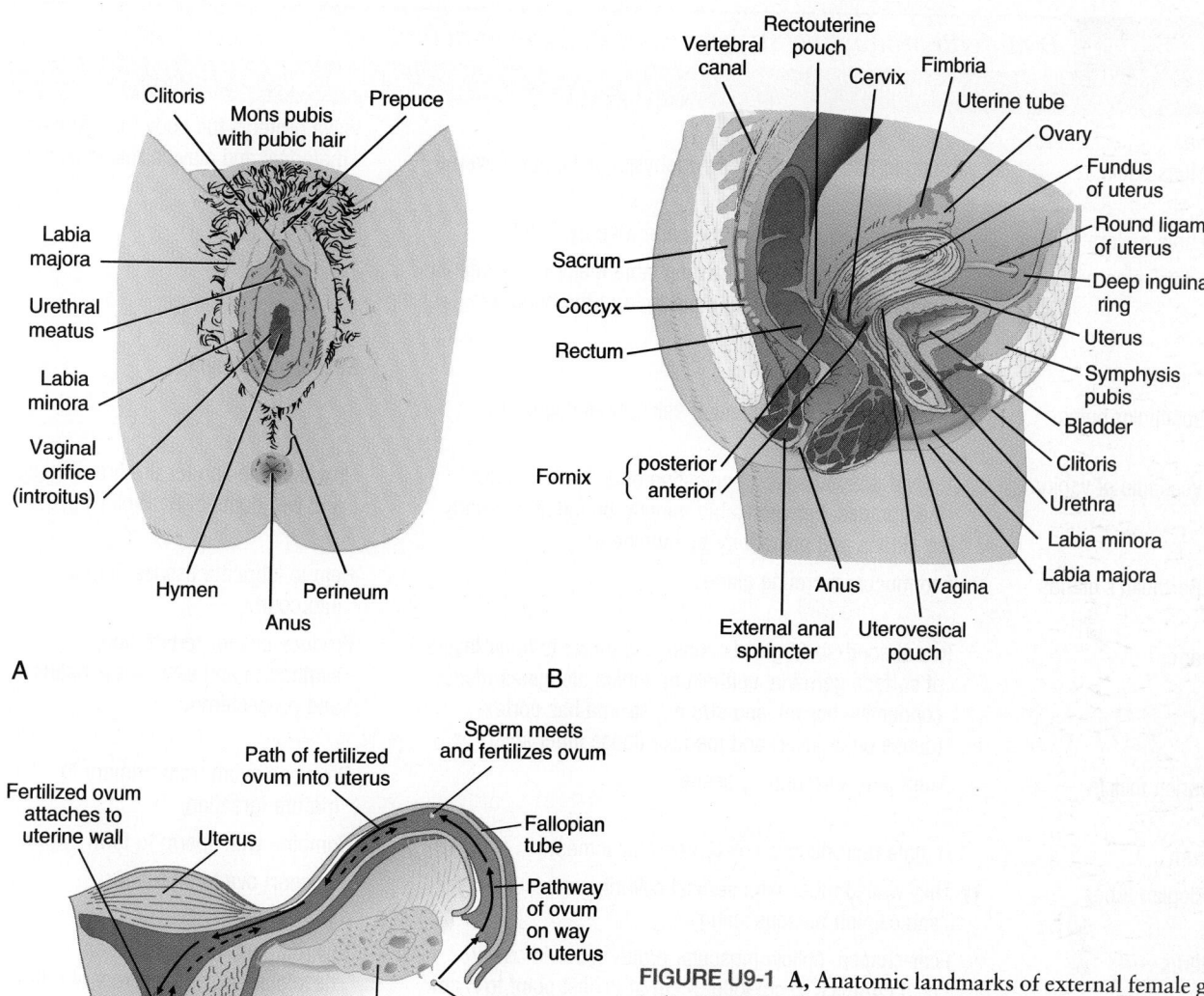

FIGURE U9-1 **A,** Anatomic landmarks of external female genitalia. **B,** Midsagittal section of the female pelvis. **C,** Pathways of sperm and ovum in the female reproductive organs.

They connect the ovum to the uterus. Each fallopian tube is about 10 cm long.

The *uterus* is located in the pelvic cavity slightly below and between the fallopian tubes, almost at a right angle to the vagina. The normal uterus is movable in all directions. However, it maintains a normal position in the body cavity through the action of various ligaments and the pelvic floor. The cardinal (lateral cervical) ligaments run between the pelvic wall and the cervix and vagina and provide the most support. Round ligaments extend from the external genitalia to the uterus, just below the fallopian tubes. If these ligaments

are weak, the uterus is likely to prolapse (drop) into the vagina.

The uterus has three functional layers: (1) the *parametrium,* the thin peritoneal and fascial covering of the uterus; (2) the *myometrium* (bulk of the uterus), a muscular layer composed of three layers, mainly of involuntary muscles; and (3) the *endometrium,* the mucous membrane lining the inner surface of the uterus. The superior two thirds of the endometrium responds cyclically to hormones. A fertilized ovum implants in the endometrium. When the ovum is not fertilized, the endometrial lining is shed (see Menstrual Cycle later in this chapter).

TABLE U9-1	Female Reproductive Structures and Their Functions	
Structure	**Description**	**Function**
Vulva		Vulva protects the body from foreign materials and plays a role in sexual stimulation
Mons pubis	Rounded pad of flesh over symphysis pubis; hair-covered after puberty	
Labia majora	Two elongated folds of tissue separated by a cleft	
Labia minora	Two thin folds of tissue between labia majora and vaginal opening; they divide and unite to form the hood-like prepuce of the clitoris	
Clitoris	Homologous to penis	Sexual stimulation
Vestibular bulbs	Two sacculated collections of veins; homologous to corpus spongiosum	
Vestibule of vagina	Almond-shaped space, consisting of delicate mucous membranes, between labia minora; bounded anteriorly by clitoris and posteriorly by fourchette	Provides opening for urethra, vagina, and two ducts of Bartholin's glands
Bartholin's glands	Two mucus-secreting glands	Help to lubricate tissues during intercourse
Ovaries	Two almond-sized glands consisting (outer to inner layers) of surface germinal epithelium, tunica albuginea (dense connective tissue), and stroma; stroma has cortex (dense outer layer) and medulla (loose inner layer)	Produce ova for fertilization; synthesize and secrete estrogens and progesterone
Ovarian follicle	Ovum plus surrounding tissue	Develops ovum from primary to mature (graafian)
Ovum	Female reproductive cell (23 chromosomes)	Combine with sperm to form zygote
Fallopian tubes	Thin-walled tubes with serosal covering, muscular layer, and ciliated mucous lining	Transport ova to uterus for implantation
Uterus	Pear-shaped, hollow muscular organ in pelvic cavity (2-5 cm thick, 5 cm long, 5 cm at widest point to 2 cm at narrowest point with opening to vagina (cervix)	Environment for implantation, development, and delivery of fetus; cervix allows entry of sperm for fertilization
Vagina	Canal between uterus and vestibule having three layers: epithelium, fibrous connective tissue, and muscular layer	Route of entry for sexual intercourse; exit for menstrual blood and birth canal
Breasts	Modified sebaceous glands and skin appendages lying within superficial fascia of anterior chest wall (vertically from second to sixth rib, horizontally from sternum to midaxillary line); parenchyma consists of ductular, lobular, and acinar epithelial structures; stroma is made of fibrous and fatty tissue	Produce milk to feed infants

The *vagina* is a musculomembranous canal connecting the uterus with the external genitalia. The mucosa of the inner surface of the vaginal wall folds over in small ridges (rugae) extending laterally upward. This rugal pattern adds to the elasticity of the vagina, making it very distensible. The rectum is posterior to the lower two thirds of the vagina. The smooth rugal pattern and elasticity of the vagina diminish with age during the menopausal and postmenopausal years. The vagina can easily become infected from urethral or rectal secretions.

Pelvic Blood Supply, Innervation, and Lymphatic Drainage

Blood Supply

The most important *blood supply* to the external genitalia comes from the internal iliac (hypogastric) artery. This artery branches to supply the pelvic floor, pelvic walls, and pelvic viscera. The principal vessels supplying the female pelvic genitalia are the *uterine arteries* from the internal iliac artery and the *ovarian arteries*, which stem directly from the aorta. The uterine artery provides a rich vascular bed to the uterus and anastomoses the arterial supply to the vagina (vaginal arteries). The ovarian artery supplies blood to the ovaries, fallopian tubes, and body of the uterus. Venous drainage roughly parallels the arterial supply.

Innervation

Both the sympathetic and parasympathetic autonomic nervous systems provide innervation to the pelvic structures. Sexual arousal is controlled by the parasympathetic dilatation of blood vessels in the vestibular bulbs and clitoris. The uterine myometrium is innervated only by the sympathetic nerve fibers. The perineum is supplied principally by the pudendal nerve.

Lymphatic Drainage

The pelvic *lymphatics* are a rich network of superficial and deep systems that roughly parallel the blood supply. The intermingling of the pelvic lymphatics and blood vessels is significant for the potential spread of cancer.

THE BREASTS

Breasts have an important role in modern culture. Because breasts are visible, their size and shape are often viewed as a measure of sexuality, femininity, and attractiveness. However, breasts are a secondary sex characteristic; that is, reproduction can occur without them. The physiologic function of female breasts is milk secretion to feed infants. An average nonlactating breast weighs between 150 and 250 g, and a lactating breast weighs 400 to 500 g.

The *parenchyma* of a breast consists of ductular, lobular, and acinar epithelial structures. The stroma of a breast is made of fibrous and fatty tissue. The upper lateral quadrant of the breast, which is mostly glandular, is the most common site of tumor occurrence. A breast consists of 12 to 20 *lobes,* subdivided into *lobules,* made up of acini. Breast lobes are arranged like the spokes of a wheel around the nipple. Each lobe is drained by a duct, 12 to 20 of which open independently on the surface of the nipple.

The *nipple,* located at the fourth intercostal space, is surrounded by a circular pigmented area, called the areola. Estrogen increases pigmentation of the areola at any age. The areolar epithelium contains some small hairs and sebaceous glands, sweat glands, and accessory mammary glands. The sebaceous glands (Montgomery's glands) enlarge to lubricate the nipple during pregnancy and lactation.

Blood Supply

The two main sources of the breast's blood supply are the lateral mammary artery and the lateral thoracic artery. These arteries form an extensive network of anastomoses. The main veins follow the arterial pattern.

Lymphatic Drainage

Lymphatic pathways, in general, follow the pathways of the veins. There are three types of lymphatic drainage of the breast (Figure U9-2):

- Cutaneous or superficial lymphatic drainage from the skin
- Areolar lymphatic drainage from the areola and nipple
- Glandular lymphatic drainage from deep glandular tissue

Lymphatic drainage pathways and lymph nodes are important in the prognosis and treatment of breast cancer (see Chapter 42). The nerve supply is derived from the anterior and lateral branches of the fourth to sixth intercostal nerves.

Functions of the Breast

The following physiologic changes affect the breast:

- Growth and development
- The menstrual cycle
- Pregnancy and lactation

Estrogen and progesterone act synergistically with the pituitary growth hormones prolactin and corticotropin to produce breast development and function. Breast development usually occurs between 9 and 16 years of age and takes 4 to 5 years. Estrogen is responsible for the growth of the breast and periductal stroma. Progesterone promotes the development of lobular and acinar structures.

After menopause, the ovaries stop producing estrogen and progesterone. Estrogen is then produced by the adrenals through stimulation from the anterior pituitary. During this life stage, there is a continuous involution of the breast with loss of glandular elements and tissue atrophy.

During pregnancy, estrogen, progesterone, and pituitary hormones increase, increasing breast vascularity and the permeability and dilation of breast lymphatics. When pregnancy ends, prolactin initiates lactation. Prolactin and corticotropin help maintain lactation. The "letting down" (flow) of milk is a complex response involving a mother's subjective response and the mechanical stimulation of suckling. Suckling releases the pituitary hormone oxytocin into the bloodstream, which causes the mammary acini to contract and release milk into the duct system.

FEMALE REPRODUCTION

Role of Hormones

Under control of the hypothalamic releasing factors and anterior pituitary follicle-stimulating hormone (FSH) and luteinizing hormone (LH), the ovaries manufacture

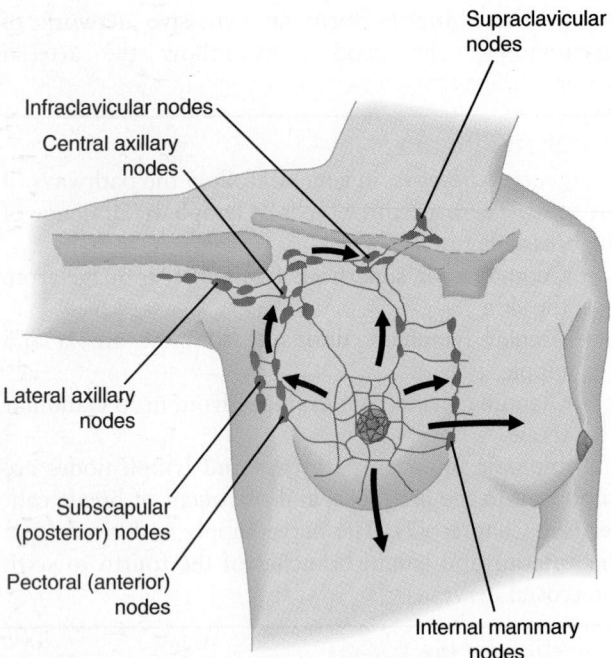

Supraclavicular
nodes

Infraclavicular nodes

Central axillary
nodes

Lateral axillary
nodes

Subscapular
(posterior) nodes

Pectoral (anterior)
nodes

Internal mammary
nodes

FIGURE U9-2 Routes of lymphatic drainage from the breast. These routes are important routes of spread of breast cancer.

estrogens and progestins. These hormones accomplish the following functions:

- Stimulate sexual desire
- Interact with the hypothalamic-pituitary unit and the uterus for (1) ovarian changes (follicular development, ovulation, corpus luteum formation), (2) pregnancy (implantation of a fertilized ovum), or (3) menstruation
- Exert additional effects elsewhere in the body

Estrogens

Estrogens (female sex hormones) produce cyclic changes in the uterine endothelium and vaginal epithelium. Estrogens are steroids secreted in both males and females by the adrenal cortex and in women by the ovary (main source) and placenta. Natural estrogens include estradiol, estrone, and estriol. Estrogens in low doses may be used therapeutically as a replacement hormone during menopause.

The main effects of estrogenic stimulation on the body occur at puberty and include breast growth (fatty tissue deposition, pigmentation), fat deposition in the vulva, pubic and axillary hair growth, bony pelvis growth and broadening, closure of the epiphyseal plates of long bones, vaginal epithelial changes, and general growth. The effects of hormones on menstruation are discussed later in this chapter.

It is not known precisely how the trophic actions of estrogen interact with other endocrine systems. Thus whether estrogen replacement should be given during

menopause is under investigation. Osteoporosis (increased bone porosity) is associated with estrogen deficiency in adult women.

Progesterone

Progesterone is a steroid hormone that helps prepare the endometrium to receive and implant the fertilized ovum; it also promotes development of the placenta (a spongy structure in the uterus that provides nourishment for a developing fetus) and the mammary glands.

Progesterone is used therapeutically to treat threatened abortion and such menstrual problems as dysmenorrhea or amenorrhea. It is secreted from the placenta and the corpus luteum under control of the anterior pituitary hormone LH. Progesterone plays a minor role in sodium and water balance. It also influences nitrogen balance, breast function, and body temperature during the menstrual cycle, raising body temperature by 1° F in the postovulatory phase of the cycle.

Menarche

The beginning of menstrual life (menarche) is a biologic, psychological, and social milestone. Psychosocial support, education about the physical changes that are happening, and knowledge about self-care are essential at this stage of life.

The average age for menarche in the United States is 12.8 years. Menarche is preceded by characteristic body changes (such as breast development) occurring between ages 9 and 16 years.

The age at which menarche occurs is affected by genetic factors. Menarche may be delayed by poor nutrition, high levels of exercise (athletes or dancers), and several medical conditions, such as diabetes mellitus, congenital heart disease, and ulcerative colitis. Early menarche can occur with other conditions, such as hypothyroidism, central nervous system (CNS) tumors, and head trauma. Girls usually show an increase in height of only 2 to 3 inches after the onset of regular menstruation.

Early menstrual cycles are often irregular and anovulatory (menstrual flow is not preceded by ovulation, production, and discharge of an ovum). Although regular menstrual cycles may not occur for several years, the woman is still potentially fertile.

Menstrual Cycle

The menstrual cycle is a complex set of recurrent changes in the uterus, ovaries, cervix, and vagina (Figure U9-3). The menstrual cycle consists of the following stages:

- Proliferation
- Secretion
- Premenstrual phase
- Menstruation

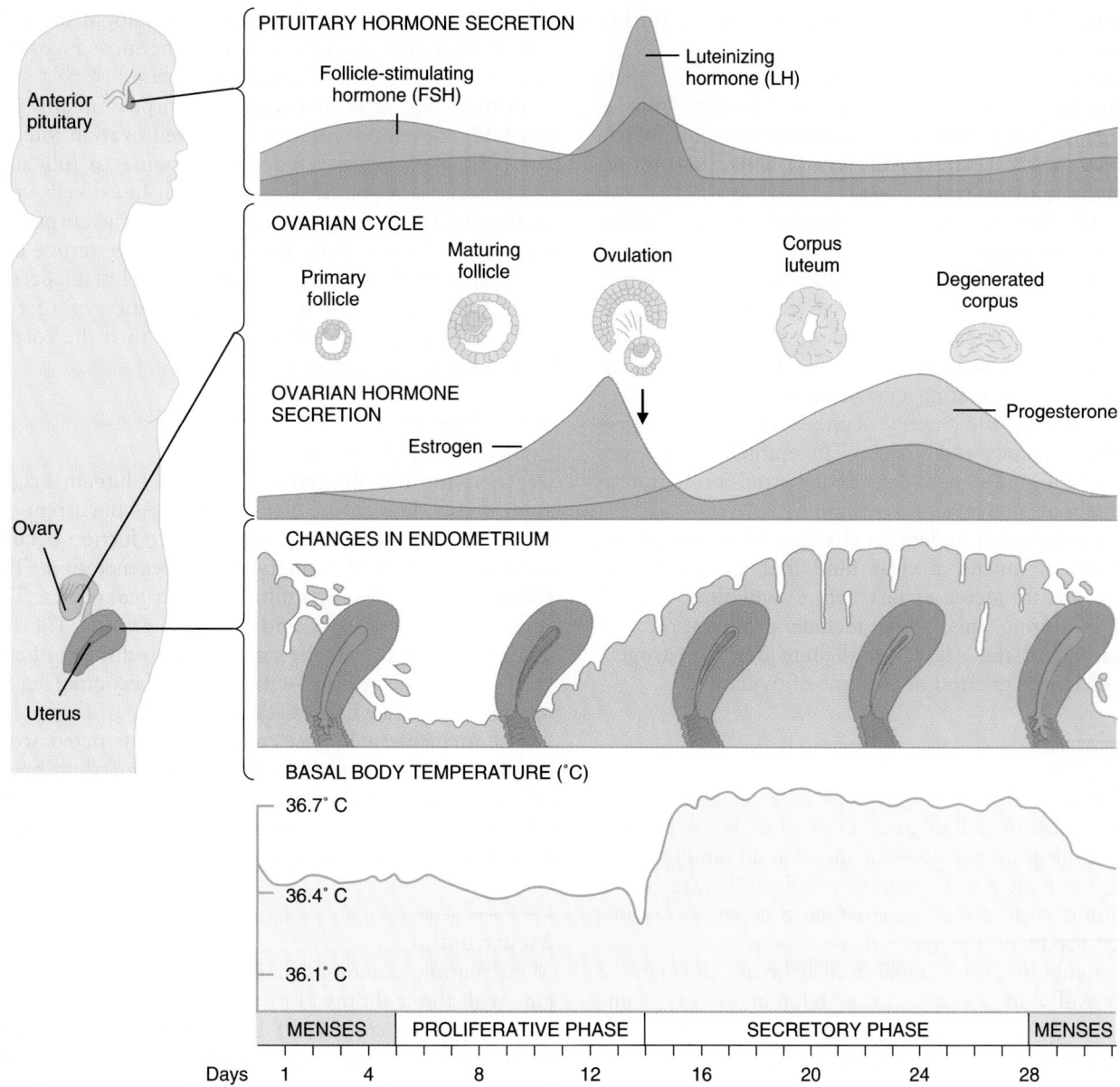

FIGURE U9-3 Menstrual (uterine) cycle. Note hormonal control of the menstrual cycle and the effects on ovaries (*center*) and endometrium (*bottom*).

Each phase is characterized by specific histologic changes in the endometrium. The length of the menstrual cycle is calculated from the first day of menstrual flow. The cycle generally runs 25 to 32 days but can vary from month to month.

The menstrual cycle depends on interactions between the CNS, anterior pituitary, ovaries, and uterus. Variations in the length of the proliferative phase (which ends with ovulation) typically cause a change in the length of the entire cycle. Environmental influences, climatic changes, emotionally traumatic experiences, stress, or acute or chronic illness also may affect the menstrual cycle.

Proliferative Phase

The proliferative phase of the menstrual cycle depends on the ratio of FSH to LH. In the ovary, after menstrual flow has begun, primary follicles (containing oocytes, or primitive ova) and follicular cells begin to develop under the influence of FSH from the anterior pituitary gland (see Figure U9-3). The thecal (stromal) cells surrounding ova produce estrogens. The increased level of estrogen signals the pituitary to inhibit FSH production and to stimulate secretion of LH. Acting together, the two pituitary hormones stimulate further estrogen production. Estrogens further inhibit FSH release from the anterior pituitary. LH becomes dominant, stimulating further maturation of the follicle.

About 2 days before ovulation, a graafian follicle reaches full maturity and the remaining primary follicles degenerate. Ovulation occurs when the graafian follicle migrates to the cortex of the ovary, where it ruptures through the ovary wall.

In the uterus, meanwhile, related changes occur, largely in response to increased estrogen from the developing follicle. At the end of a menstrual flow, the uterine endometrium (containing surface epithelium, glands, connective tissue, spaces, and blood vessels) is thin because much of it has sloughed off during menstrual flow. Estrogen begins creating a new endometrial surface layer and restoring the uterine epithelium. It stimulates growth of glands and stroma. The epithelium becomes thicker and more vascular. Endometrial proliferation peaks about 2 days before ovulation.

The cervix also undergoes changes. Most important, secretion of mucus, a clear fluid that is receptive to sperm, greatly increases just before ovulation. Vaginal changes during this phase include proliferation and thickening of the vaginal epithelium due to estrogen. This change is greatest at the time of ovulation.

Ovulation

Increasing levels of estrogen cause a decrease in FSH secretion, allowing a flood of LH to occur. Over a 24-hour period, this process causes the thecal and granulosa cells lining the follicle to hypertrophy and proliferate. When ovulation occurs, the ovarian follicle collapses and estrogen production temporarily decreases.

At ovulation, the graafian follicle breaks through the ovary wall and passes into the abdominal cavity. Some hemorrhage occurs into the center of the ruptured follicle, where a clot quickly forms. Ovulation may produce a transient abdominal pain (mittelschmerz).

Once in the abdominal cavity, the graafian follicle is usually picked up by the fimbriated ends of the fallopian tube and is slowly transported to the uterus. Unless it is fertilized, it eventually passes out of the body with the menstrual flow.

Ovulation occurs 12 to 15 days before the onset of the next menstrual period. It is almost impossible to determine exactly when ovulation will occur, even by counting from the first day of the preceding menstrual period.

Secretory (Luteal) Phase

During the secretory phase (lasting 10 to 14 days), progesterone and estrogen promote marked changes in the endometrium. Connective tissue hypertrophies. The arteries coil and become tortuous. The glands become larger and more tortuous, and abundantly secrete a substance containing glycogen. The endometrium becomes edematous, compact, and thickened. Development peaks 7 to 8 days after ovulation. This is the most favorable time for implantation of a fertilized ovum.

In the ovary after ovulation, the corpus luteum (yellow body) develops within the ruptured ovarian follicle. First, the clot that developed in response to follicular hemorrhage is replaced with yellowish luteal cells containing lipids. These cells eventually form the corpus luteum, an endocrine body that secretes progesterone and some estrogen. Full maturity of the corpus luteum occurs about 9 days after ovulation. If implantation of a fertilized ovum (pregnancy) does not occur, then the corpus luteum begins to degenerate.

Premenstrual (Ischemic) Phase

Degeneration (involution) of the corpus luteum occurs about 2 to 4 days before menstruation. A concurrent decrease in progesterone and estrogen production occurs, causing endometrial retraction and degeneration. The endometrium is heavily infiltrated with leukocytes. The coiled arteries constrict and ischemia results. The endometrium shrinks. At the same time, production of cervical mucus decreases, with mucus becoming more opaque and somewhat resistant to sperm.

The premenstrual phase ends as the constricted arteries open. Small patches of necrotic endometrium break off, and menstrual flow begins. The LH and FSH ratio changes; the pituitary is stimulated to increase its production of FSH; and the cycle begins again.

Menstruation

Menstruation, commonly called a *period* or *menses* begins with the withdrawal of estrogen and progesterone. Menstrual flow consists of blood, mucus, endometrial tissue fragments, and vaginal epithelial cells. Menstrual flow is usually dark red, has a characteristic odor, and contains 60 to 150 ml of fluid. Fifty percent to 75% of this fluid is blood, which usually does not clot, but some small clots are normal. Menstruation usually lasts about 4 to 5 days, but 1 to 10 days may be normal for some women.

Chapter 41 covers menstrual disorders, and methods of contraception (prevention of pregnancy) may be found in obstetrics nursing texts.

Menopause

Like menarche, menopause (permanent cessation of menstruation) is an important developmental event in a woman's life having physical, psychological, and social implications for the woman. Menopause is one event of a complex sequence of biologic aging events of the climacteric or perimenopausal period. This period lasts about 15 to 20 years from about age 40 to 60 years, during which time the body makes the transition from fertility to infertility. Menopause usually occurs between the ages of 48 and 54 years, but it may occur as early as age 35. The average age at menopause appears to be increasing in industrialized countries.

Menstrual cessation may be abrupt, but usually occurs over 1 to 2 years. Periodic menstrual flow gradually lessens and becomes irregular. Anovulatory cycles are common during this time, and occasional episodes of profuse bleeding may be interspersed with episodes of scant bleeding. Menopause is said to have occurred when there have been no menstrual periods for 12 consecutive months. Because unplanned pregnancy may occur during the premenopausal period, sexually active women should use contraception for at least 6 months after menses have ceased. Any spontaneous uterine bleeding after menopause is abnormal and should be investigated.

Although the cause of menopause is not known, certain predictable physiologic changes and experiences occur. During the climacteric period, a gradual decrease in the number of maturing ovarian follicles and a parallel decline in the production of ovarian estrogen occur. Over time, as the ovaries become unresponsive to pituitary hormones, and toward the end of the climacteric period, the ovaries atrophy. Other changes associated with menopause, such as hot flashes and vaginal atrophy, are related to decreased estrogen production.

Menopause is not a disease. Most women pass through menopause with minimal or no problems. The modern menopausal woman is younger-looking, more active, and has more positive attitude about menopause than in the past. The stereotype of the menopausal woman who is miserable and who seeks medical assistance for a wide range of symptoms has been disproved. Research shows that menopause itself does not cause poorer health or greater use of health care facilities. Menstrual variation (irregular menses, skipped periods, and occasional scanty or moderately heavy menses) usually do not warrant any intervention. However, some women do become distressed enough to require professional assistance.

Although further study of the psychosexual changes associated with the perimenopausal period is needed, any changes that occur are the result of the complex interaction of anatomic, physiologic, psychological, and social factors. Vaginal lubrication may be reduced in the perimenopausal years, and this dryness may cause discomfort or bleeding with intercourse. Estrogen or hormone replacement therapy (HRT) can usually relieve this discomfort. Some studies have reported lessened interest in sexual activity among menopausal women, but other authors claim freedom from pregnancy allows women to relax and enjoy intercourse more. With increased life expectancy, the typical woman can spend more than one third of her life in the postmenopausal years.

During the menopausal years, many women are faced with life situations that affect mood, such as growing older, adjusting to the children's leaving home, and ac-

cepting increased responsibility for aging parents. Nurses can help counter some misconceptions and negative connotations associated with menopause by stressing the normal and positive aspects of the experience, clarifying misconceptions about menopause, and differentiating the physiologic manifestations of menopause from midlife developmental changes.

MALE REPRODUCTIVE SYSTEM STRUCTURES

The male reproductive organs consist of paired *testicles* lying within the scrotum, epididymides, seminal ducts, spermatic cords, seminal vesicles, ejaculatory ducts, bulbourethral (Cowper's) glands, the prostate gland, and the penis (Table U9-2 and Figure U9-4). The penis and scrotum are external, visible genitalia, whereas the other structures are internal. The male perineum is the external area between the scrotum and the anus.

Penis and Related Structures

The *penis* is both a sexual organ (organ of copulation) and an organ for urination. This cylindrical, pendulous structure suspends from its attachment to the pubic arch. The skin of the penis is dark, hairless, thin, and loose (permitting considerable distention).

The portion of the penis between its end or head and its attachment to the pubic bone is the *shaft*. In males, the external opening of the urethra (*meatus* or orifice) is in the glans (*glans penis*), the cone-shaped end or head of the penis. The glans is the conical expansion of the corpus spongiosum. The expanded posterior border of the glans is the *corona*. At its junction with the shaft is the *coronal sulcus*. A flap of movable skin (*foreskin* or *prepuce*) covers the glans. *Smegma* is a cheesy, thick, odoriferous secretion of sloughed-off epithelial cells that collects under the prepuce. (In females, smegma is the secretion of the apocrine glands of the clitoris, together with epithelial cells.)

The penis is homologous to the female clitoris. Usually, the penis is flaccid. However, when stimulated (physically or during sexual excitement), it becomes rigid. An *erection* occurs when the corpora cavernosa fill with blood. The tissue becomes congested (hyperemic) with blood. Following *orgasm* (climax of sexual excitement) and *ejaculation* (emission of semen), the blood leaves. An erect penis may differ in size from a flaccid penis. Penis size, however, does not physically influence sexual pleasure. The secretion of the bulbourethral (Cowper's) glands forms part of the semen.

Scrotum and Testes

The *scrotum* is a double pouch hanging from the base of the penis. It is separated into halves internally by muscular contractile tissue (*tunica dartos*) and externally by a *raphe* (ridge) that runs over the scrotum from the base

TABLE U9-2 *Male Reproductive Structures and Their Functions*

Structure	Description	Function
Penis	Erectile tissue arranged in three columns, each enclosed in a fascial sheath (tunica albuginea): two lateral columns (corpora cavernosa) and a median column (corpus spongiosum) that contains the urethra; all are surrounded by a thick, fibrous envelope (Buck's fascia)	Ejects semen for fertilization; excretes urine
Bulbourethral (Cowper's) glands	Two small glands above the corpus spongiosum; homologous to Bartholin's glands	Enhances lubrication during intercourse
Scrotum	Double pouch of muscular contractile tissue between the root of the penis and the perineum; bisected by a ridge; each half contains a testicle and epididymis and part of a spermatic cord made up of nerves, testicular vessels (spermatic artery, vein, lymph vessels), and vas deferens	Provides protective environment for production of sperm
Testicles	Two smooth, solid, ovoid structures (4 cm × 2 to 2.5 cm) with outer coat of inelastic fibrous tunica albuginea; lobules in testicles contain tubules composed of germ cells (develop into sperm) and Sertoli cells (support spermatogenesis); between the tubules are Leydig cells (source of testosterone)	Produce testosterone and sperm
Sperm	Germ cell with flattened, broad, oval heal with a nucleus, protoplasmic middle piece or neck, and a hair-like tail (flagellum); has 23 chromosomes	Fertilizes ovum
Epididymis	Small oblong structure consisting of a convoluted tube 4 to 6 m long; attaches to upper end of testicle	Transports sperm
Vas deferens	Smooth muscle tube about 46 cm long	Stores and transmits sperm from testicles
Prostate gland	Partly muscular, partly glandular structure posterior to the symphysis pubis; urethra and ejaculatory ducts pass through it	Contributes to liquefaction of semen
Seminal vesicles	Two sac-like structures 5 cm long; they connect to the vas deferens	Secretions contribute to sperm nutrition and activation

of the penis to the anus. Each half of the scrotum contains (1) a testicle with its epididymis and (2) part of a spermatic cord held together by spermatic fascia.

The *vas deferens* (ductus deferens, seminal duct) is the excretory duct of the testicle. It is the continuation of the epididymis and conveys sperm from the testicle to the prostatic urethra (from the epididymis to the ejaculatory duct). The *ejaculatory duct* then conveys semen to the urethra.

The spermatic cord goes through the inguinal canal, and the vas deferens continues into the abdominal cavity. It passes behind the bladder, anterior to the rectum, to join the duct of the seminal vesicle, becoming the ejaculatory duct. The spermatic cord is movable for protection from trauma and facilitates optimal production of mature, functional sperm.

Testicles produce the male hormone *(testosterone)* and the male reproductive cells *(sperm)*. Many lobules,

separated by septa, divide a testicle. Each lobule contains one to three seminiferous tubules where sperm are produced. Each testicle contains 600 to 1200 seminiferous tubules (90% of the mature testis). Between the seminiferous tubules are interstitial cells called *Leydig cells*, the source of testosterone, the male hormone. The lobules of the testicles lead to straight ducts that join a plexus, from which efferent ducts lead to the epididymis.

The *epididymis* rests on and beside the posterior surface of the testicle. Its head caps the upper end of the testicle and its tail becomes continuous with the vas deferens, which joins other vessels to form the spermatic cord. The head of the epididymis contains 12 to 20 testicular efferent ducts.

Sperm

Sperm are mature male sex or germ cells that develop after puberty. Resembling tadpoles, sperm self-propel

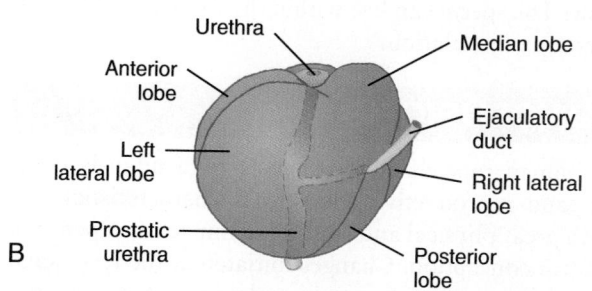

FIGURE U9-4 **A,** Midsagittal section of the male pelvis and external genitalia. **B,** Anatomy of the prostate gland.

themselves by hairlike tails like flagella. A normal sperm has a flattened, broad, oval head with a nucleus. A middle piece or protoplasmic neck connects to the tail. During fertilization, the sperm's head pierces an ovum. The sperm's tail is lost when fusion of two cells occurs. Sperm are produced in the seminiferous tubules of the testicles. Sperm develop in great quantities from spermatids (spermoblasts) and are stored in the vas deferens.

Prostate and Related Structures

The prostate gland surrounds the neck of the male urinary bladder and urethra. In children, the prostate is small, but during puberty, it grows to the size of a chestnut. The adult prostate gland (see Figure U9-4) lies like a flattened cone in the pelvis, about 2 cm posterior to the symphysis pubis. A normal adult male's prostate weighs 15 to 20 g and is 4 to 6 cm long. The prostate is inverted, so its apex is inferior, and is suspended by the urogenital diaphragm. The base of the prostate is superior and, at the bladder neck, anterior to the rectum. A firm, fibrous capsule containing smooth

muscle fibers in its inner layer encloses the prostate. The bladder overlies the basal surface of the prostate. The posterior surface of the prostate is in close contact with the rectal wall. This is the surface of the prostate available for digital examination.

The portion of the urethra that passes through the prostate is called the *prostatic urethra*. Prostatic muscle fibers encircle the urethra and separate the prostate's glandular tissue.

The seminal vesicles are sac-like structures whose secretion, a component of semen (seminal fluid or ejaculate), may contribute to sperm nutrition and activation. They lie behind the bladder. The seminal vesicles connect to the vas deferens on each side.

Male Breasts

The male breast is similar to that of a preadolescent girl. It contains a few ducts surrounded by connective tissue. Estrogen can cause a man's breast to enlarge (gynecomastia) (see Chapter 42). Accumulation of fat in obese men can also make the breasts appear large.

MALE SEXUAL DEVELOPMENT AND FUNCTION

Development of the male genitalia requires two hormones: (1) müllerian duct inhibitory factor, secreted by Sertoli cells, and (2) testosterone, secreted by Leydig cells (see Gonadal Development earlier in this chapter). Germ cells develop into spermatozoa, and Sertoli cells support spermatogenesis.

The hypothalamus and pituitary gland regulate testicular function. The hypothalamus secretes gonadotropin-releasing hormone (GnRH) in a pulsatile fashion. GnRH stimulates the anterior pituitary gland to produce LH and FSH. LH stimulates Leydig cells to produce testosterone, which modulates the secretion of GnRH and, therefore, LH through negative feedback to the hypothalamus and pituitary gland. FSH and testosterone stimulate Sertoli cells and germ cells to start and complete spermatogenesis. Inhibin, released from Sertoli cells, provides a negative feedback on FSH by the anterior pituitary.

Testosterone is the primary androgen secreted by the testis. The testis also secretes androstenedione and estradiol. Estradiol may be important for skeletal maturation in the male.

Spermatogenesis

Spermatogenesis is the process of sperm production and development that occurs within the seminiferous tubules during active sex life. This process begins at puberty as a result of stimulation by the gonadotropic hormones from the anterior pituitary.

Spermatogonia are the germinal epithelial cells found in the outer border of the tubular epithelium. These cells are continually formed to replenish themselves, while a portion continue to develop into sperm. During the first stage of spermatogenesis, the spermatogonia divide and migrate toward the Sertoli cells. The spermatogonia penetrate the membranes of Sertoli cells and become enveloped within the cytoplasm of these cells. The spermatogonia continue this close relationship with Sertoli cells throughout their development.

During the 24 days when it is in contact with Sertoli cells, the spermatogonium changes and enlarges to form a primary spermatocyte. After this development, the spermatocyte splits into two secondary spermatocytes, each with only 23 chromosomes. After 2 to 3 days, the spermatocytes undergo a second division to form four spermatids, each with 23 chromosomes, half the original number. The sperm that eventually fertilizes the female ovum contains half the genetic material, while the ovum contains the other half.

The period of spermatogenesis from germinal cell to sperm takes about 74 days. During this time, the spermatocytes lose some cytoplasm, the chromatin material of the head reorganizes to form a compact head, and the remaining cytoplasm and cell membranes collect at one end of the cell to form the tail of the sperm.

Role of Hormones

Testosterone is essential to the growth and division of the germinal cells that form the sperm. LH stimulates Leydig cells to secrete testosterone. FSH stimulates Sertoli cells, promoting spermatogenesis. Estrogens, formed from testosterone when Sertoli cells are stimulated by FSH, appears to be essential in spermatogenesis. Growth hormone promotes early division of spermatogonia.

Maturation in the Epididymis

After the sperm are formed in the seminiferous tubules, they spend several days passing through the epididymis. After the sperm have spent about 24 hours in the epididymis, they become motile and capable of fertilization (i.e., they are mature).

Sperm are stored in small amounts in the epididymis but are mainly stored in the vas deferens and the ampulla of the vas deferens. With low levels of sexual activity, the sperm can be stored there up to a month, maintaining their motility and fertility. When sexual activity is frequent, sperm may be stored only a few days.

Prostatic Fluid

The prostate gland secretes a milky fluid that forms part of the semen. This fluid aids the passage of sperm and helps keep them alive, supplying them with food, if needed. Prostatic secretion is manufactured in a network of branching glands embedded in muscle within the prostate. This muscle contracts during ejaculation, and prostatic secretions are ejected through the ejaculatory ducts into the urethra.

Semen

Semen is a viscid, thick, opalescent secretion discharged by males at the climax of sexual excitement or orgasm. It contains sperm and other secretions. About 10% of the semen is composed of sperm and fluid from the vas deferens, with about 60% made up of fluid from the seminal vesicles. The remaining 30% is composed of prostatic fluid and small amounts of mucoid secretion from the bulbourethral glands.

Semen is slightly alkaline, with a pH of about 7.5. The prostatic fluid contains a clotting enzyme, which causes the fibrinogen of the seminal vesicle fluid to form a weak coagulum. This coagulum holds the semen near the uterine cervix. The coagulum dissolves in about 15 to 30 minutes, at which time the sperm become highly motile. The sperm can live within the vagina for 24 to 48 hours after ejaculation.

CONCLUSIONS

The human reproductive system is tremendously complex, and reproductive and sexual characteristics can have a great physical and emotional impact on a person's life from conception. Changes initiated at the fetal stage cause differentiation between male and female. Sexual maturation, starting between the ages of 9 and 13 years, alters both external and internal structures. A thorough knowledge of the structure and function of the female and male reproductive systems is important so the nurse can provide safe, effective care for clients with associated problems. The nurse must be sensitive to the delicate nature of reproductive problems because many disorders affect sexuality.

BIBLIOGRAPHY

1. Berne, R., et al. (2004). *Physiology* (5th ed.). St. Louis: Mosby.
2. Guyton, A.C., & Hall, J. (2001). *Textbook of medical physiology* (10th ed.). Philadelphia: W. B. Saunders.
3. Kierszenbaum, A.L. (2002). *Histology and cell biology: An introduction to pathology.* St. Louis: Mosby.
4. Silverthorn, D. (2004). Human physiology (3rd ed.). Upper Saddle River, NJ: Prentice-Hall.

39

Assessment of the Reproductive System

Rhonda Holloway

evolve

Web Enhancements

Assessment Terms
English and Spanish
Appendix A
Religious Beliefs and Practices Affecting Health Care

http://evolve.elsevier.com/Black/medsurg/

Appendix B
A Health History Format That Integrates the Assessment of Functional Health Patterns
Appendix C
Laboratory Values of Clinical Importance in Medical-Surgical Nursing

Your ability to assess the reproductive system competently and compassionately is important to your clients on both physical and psychosocial levels. To perform this task well, you will need a combination of sound assessment skills and a nonjudgmental attitude that is both professional and empathic.

Because of the close association between the reproductive, urinary, and bowel elimination systems, you must be prepared for some overlap in their assessment (see also Chapter 34). You also must be prepared for some difficulty in discussing reproductive and elimination topics because many clients are uncomfortable talking about them. Language and semantic barriers may interfere with communication as well, in part because of the many words and slang terms used to describe reproductive anatomy, function, and problems. Educational or cultural barriers also can inhibit a client from discussing a problem. Remain sensitive and nonjudgmental, and do your best to put the client at ease.

Clients have the right to be informed and to participate actively in decisions about their health. A supportive, respectful attitude promotes comfort, cooperation, and participation in health care. Be alert to sexist attitudes in yourself and in the health care system, either of

which may lead to ignored health complaints, unnecessary or inappropriate prescriptions, and unneeded procedures. Be an advocate, and positively influence the client's perception of health care and the importance of health maintenance.

Especially when assessing the reproductive system, provide privacy and create an environment conducive to the expression of feelings. Encourage the client to voice concerns and ask questions. Assess the client's understanding of health care information, and explore what the client perceives as needs and problems. You may need to repeat information, especially if the client is anxious or feeling stressed, for example, during a pelvic or prostate examination. Provide a sensitive, humane orientation to reproductive health care. Teaching and counseling promote health maintenance.

Besides providing a history and physical examination, an adequate reproductive assessment should include an in-depth review of the client's lifestyle, health habits, self-perception, body image, and developmental stage, along with cultural, religious, socioeconomic, and educational factors. These factors influence the client's health and health-seeking behaviors. Throughout the assessment, you will find that a respect for others' values

---

evolve *Be sure to check out the bonus material on the Evolve website and the CD-ROM, including free self-assessment exercises.*

http://evolve.elsevier.com/Black/medsurg/

facilitates effective care. Cultural or ethnic background, socioeconomic status, and sexual preference should never limit a client's access to, or quality of, health care.

THE FEMALE REPRODUCTIVE SYSTEM

Many women receive most, if not all, of their primary health care from obstetric and gynecologic health care providers, not only for gynecologic conditions but also for general health. An annual gynecologic examination provides opportunity to discuss health maintenance activities. For example, during a client's health visit for a Papanicolaou (Pap) smear, take the opportunity to teach breast self-examination and discuss risk factors associated with gynecologic cancer and heart disease. Explain developmental changes (adolescence, menarche, or menopause) and menstrual hygiene and symptom management. Discuss lifestyle factors that affect health maintenance, such as diet, exercise, adequate sleep and rest, stress management, cessation of smoking, and general risk factor identification. If appropriate, provide information about protection against sexually transmitted diseases (STDs).

After establishing rapport, perform a comprehensive gynecologic nursing assessment appropriate to the situation. (For a review of a comprehensive history and psychosocial assessment, see Chapter 4.) Follow the health history with a systematic physical examination. Diagnostic tests may be ordered, some of which you will perform. The resulting data are the basis for nursing intervention.

HISTORY

The health history for the female reproductive system includes data related to the genitals, the reproductive system, the breasts, and the woman's overall health status. Conduct the interview in private while the woman is clothed to maintain her level of comfort.

Biographical and Demographic Data

Biographical and demographic data can help to establish the client's health risk status. The incidence of some gynecologic cancers is higher in certain age groups. For example, the risk of breast cancer rises with age. Ethnicity may also be a risk factor for certain gynecologic cancers, such as cancer of the cervix. Because controversy exists about the influence of environmental factors in the development of reproductive disorders, the client's living and working environments may prove important.

Current Health: The Chief Complaint

Ask the client to describe her reason for seeking gynecologic care. Be alert to the possible nature of the problem and the woman's level of understanding of the problem.

This information will direct the health history interview and your health teaching. If the client's visit is for a specific problem rather than for a routine examination, ask her to relate the history of the problem and conduct a symptom analysis (see Chapter 4).

Past Health History

To investigate the client's past health history, review her childhood and infectious diseases, major illnesses and hospitalizations, medications, and allergies.

Childhood and Infectious Diseases

The most serious childhood infectious disease that may affect a woman of childbearing age is rubella. Maternal rubella during the first trimester increases fetal risk for congenital disorders. Ask the client whether she has had rubella or has immunity to it. If she is contemplating pregnancy, suggest that a rubella titer be drawn to determine her immunity status. If the titer is negative, indicating that immunity is lacking, encourage the woman to be vaccinated. Advise the newly immunized woman to avoid pregnancy for at least 3 months. A pregnant woman should not be vaccinated.

Ask the client about her history of STDs and STD exposure. Some of these diseases, left unrecognized or untreated, can damage the reproductive system, particularly the fallopian tubes. The result may be problems with fertility and achieving pregnancy.

Major Illnesses and Hospitalizations

Ask about major illnesses. For instance, diabetes is associated with increased maternal and fetal morbidity and mortality. Pregnancy and oral contraceptive use are also linked with higher morbidity and mortality rates in women who have a history of cardiovascular disease, such as angina, hypertension, and thrombophlebitis. Anemia can result from menstrual disorders, such as dysfunctional uterine bleeding. Hypothyroidism and hyperthyroidism can affect the menstrual cycle, as can other endocrine disorders.

Urinary tract disorders can interfere with sexual function. Women who have migraine headaches or seizure disorders may need to avoid oral contraceptives because of the increased risk of migraines and seizures associated with their use. Oral contraceptives, pregnancy, dietary changes, or a high-fat diet may worsen cholecystitis. Hepatitis and other liver disorders may contraindicate some estrogen use because of its route of metabolism. Estrogens are usually contraindicated in women who have had breast cancer or cancers of the reproductive tract.

Ask about surgery involving the reproductive system. Specific surgical procedures include dilation and curettage (D&C), tubal ligation, cryosurgery or cryotherapy, cystocele and rectocele repair, hysterectomy, oophorectomy, salpingectomy, and salpingotomy. Inquire about interrupted pregnancies, including both elective and spontaneous abortions.

Medications

Collect a complete medication history, including prescription and over-the-counter medications, vitamin and mineral supplements, and recreational or illegal substances. Contraceptive medications can include oral contraceptive pills, medroxyprogesterone or estradiol cypionate/medroxyprogesterone injections, vaginal preparations, and uterine devices. Ask about episodic medications, such as those used for premenstrual dysphoric disorder (PMDD) and menstrual discomforts (diuretics and selective serotonin re-uptake inhibitors), and the use of herbal or other "natural" substances, such as the following:

- Black cohosh *(Cimicifuga racemosa)* for menstrual irregularity, PMDD, and menopausal problems
- Chamomile *(Matricaria recutita, Chamaemelum nobile)* for menstrual cramps
- Chaste tree *(Vitex agnuscastus)* for PMDD and menopausal problems and possibly for mastalgia
- Evening primrose *(Oenothera biennis)* for PMDD
- Feverfew *(Tanacetum parthenium)* for menstrual problems
- Sage *(Salvia officinalis)* for menstrual irregularity
- Soybeans and other legumes for their phytoestrogens, which may help to prevent breast cancer

Ask specifically about hormone replacement therapy (including estrogen, progesterone, thyroid hormones, and corticosteroids). Recreational or illegal substances, such as alcohol, amphetamines, barbiturates, marijuana, and hallucinogens, may affect sexual behavior and risk status for exposure to a STD, among other problems.

Allergies

Ask about all allergies, including allergic reactions. Antibiotics are used to treat genitourinary infections. Latex and rubber are used in contraceptive devices such as condoms, cervical caps, and diaphragms, some of which are used in conjunction with spermicides. Some intrauterine contraceptive devices contain copper. Allergies to these substances eliminate their use for contraception. Use vinyl gloves instead of latex while examining the client, if necessary.

Gynecologic History

A gynecologic history includes questions about breasts, menstruation, contraceptives, sexual practices, obstetric problems, genitourinary problems, and reproductive health practices. For a menopausal or older woman or a woman who has had a hysterectomy, ask only the appropriate questions.

Breast History

Ask the client about breast pain or tenderness and its occurrence in relation to the menstrual cycle. Many women experience breast tenderness before menstruation in relation to hormonal changes. Ask whether the woman has had in the past or currently has breast lumps or masses. If a lump is present, ask the woman to describe its location, onset, and size and whether it is painful. Determine whether the lump has changed shape, size, consistency, or the degree of tenderness since it was first noticed. Does the lump change during the menstrual cycle? Because the breasts become more firm and cystic during the luteal phase, the best time to perform breast palpation is 7 to 10 days after onset of menses.

Ask about any nipple discharge, which would be abnormal in women who are not pregnant or lactating. If discharge is present, determine the color, consistency, amount, and odor.

Ask whether the woman performs monthly breast self-examination (BSE) (see Figure 2-4). Ask about frequency of examination and the technique used so that you can decide whether the client needs a review of the procedure and supervised practice. Note whether the woman includes the axillary nodes in the BSE (see Figure 39-2).

Finally, ask whether there is a history of breast cancer in the client's blood-related female relatives, including mother, sisters, maternal grandmother, or maternal aunts. Breast cancer in these relatives indicates an increased risk of breast cancer for the client.

Menstrual History

Ask the woman at what age she started menstruating. Determine the first day of her last menstrual period. Ask the number of days per cycle and the regularity of cycles. Assessing the amount of menstrual flow is difficult. Knowing whether more than one pad or tampon per hour becomes saturated helps to determine whether the flow is unusually profuse. Are there clots in the flow? How long does the menstrual period last?

Does the woman experience pain during menstruation? If so, have her describe the pain, its duration, whether it occurs with every cycle, and what she uses for relief. Does she experience midcycle bleeding, spotting, or pain? Are there any moliminal (premenstrual discomfort) manifestations? Are there menopausal manifestations, including menstrual cycle changes?

Contraceptive History

Document the current contraceptive method (if any), satisfaction with the method, duration of use, any contraceptive problems, and any desire to change methods. Ask about previous contraceptive methods, problems

TABLE 39-1 *Sexual Health Assessment*

Sexual health assessment may include consideration of the client's current:

Knowledge about sexuality

Attitudes about sexuality and toward sexual partner(s)

Level of comfort and feelings of adequacy regarding own sexuality

Concerns about sexuality of significant others

Perception of own sex role and that of sexual partner(s)

Sexual self-concept as a female or male

Fears and anxiety about intimacy and other aspects of sexuality

Self-perception of own body (body image)

Ability to function sexually (to obtain an erection and control ejaculation, to please sexual partner, to achieve pain-free orgasm, to reproduce, to obtain adequate contraception, to obtain sufficient vaginal lubrication, to give and receive effective sexual stimulation and pleasure)

Typical sexual patterns and activities (partner choice [female, male, spouse, extramarital, multiple, single, same partner, different partners], frequency of sexual activity, type of sexual activity [vaginal, anal, oral, masturbation], partner satisfaction, self-satisfaction)

Level of interest in sexual activity (sex drive)

Level of satisfaction regarding current sexual opportunity and activity

Physical health problems affecting sexuality (menstrual problems, pregnancy, medication, surgery [colostomy, surgical amputation, recent heart surgery or brain surgery], paralysis, illness [hypertension, diabetes, recent myocardial infarction, stroke, injury [recent spinal cord injury, recent head injury, burns, traumatic amputations], sexually transmitted disease, genitourinary problems)

Sexual History

There is no single approach to taking a sexual health history. Information obtained may relate to historical (past) information about the following:

Both Females and Males

Pregnancies (information about unplanned pregnancies)

Fertility management

Genitourinary problems

Sexually transmitted disease

Sexual abuse (incest, rape, pedophilia, battering)

Relationship-partner history (number of sexual partners, sexual orientation [bisexual, homosexual, heterosexual])

First experience of sexual activity

Early sexual development and influences

Adolescent sexual experiences

Sexual technique used (masturbation, intercourse ([oral, vaginal, anal])

Role models for sexuality (peers, parents, guardians, famous people, advertising models)

Spiritual-philosophical models influencing the client's sexuality

Females

History specific to menstruation, abortion, pregnancy

Males

History specific to impotence, nocturnal emissions

---

encountered, and reason for discontinuation. Provide contraceptive information if appropriate. For a woman of reproductive age who is not sterilized and who is heterosexually active, determine whether she wants to become pregnant.

Sexual History

Obtain a sexual history using a direct approach and terms the woman understands. The purpose of a sexual history is to identify sexual problems and to give the woman an opportunity to ask questions or express concerns (Table 39-1). To help put the client at ease, explain why you are asking for this information, and assure her that it will be kept confidential.

Begin with general questions about whether the woman is satisfied and comfortable with her current sexual activity. A nonjudgmental approach is essential; make no assumptions about anything, including the gender or number of partners. Follow up on any concerns or issues she raises. Of particular importance are difficulties or concerns she may have. Be alert for any risk-taking behaviors, including those that put her at risk of STDs. See the website for this textbook for further information on sexuality assessment.

Obstetric History

If the woman is in her childbearing years, ask whether she thinks she could be pregnant. (Pregnancy may contraindicate mammography or other radiologic studies as well as certain medications.) If the woman has been pregnant, obtain information about each pregnancy, including the delivery and postpartum period. Document details of difficulties or complications (physical or psychosocial). Record spontaneous or planned abortions. If the woman has never been pregnant, ask whether children were or are desired. If the woman has relinquished a child for adoption, explore the circumstance and her feelings about it. See the website for this textbook for detailed questions to assess the obstetric history.

Genitourinary History

Ask about previous problems with genitourinary infections and vaginitis. Determine whether the woman has had a previous pelvic infection or STD, treatment, or complications. Determine whether the woman experiences urinary or fecal incontinence and the circumstances surrounding the incontinence. (Chapter 36 discusses urinary incontinence, and Chapter 35 discusses fecal incontinence.)

Reproductive Health Practices

Seek information about menstrual, sexual, and gynecologic hygiene, including douching. Ask about the frequency of gynecologic examinations. If appropriate, ask the client whether she uses protection against STDs and unwanted pregnancy.

Family Health History

A family history of diabetes, cardiovascular disease, or cancer of a reproductive organ may indicate a higher risk for development of those diseases. If the woman's mother received diethylstilbestrol (DES) while pregnant with the client, the woman might be at risk for reproductive tract cancer or structural and functional abnormalities.

Psychosocial History

Occupation and Environment

Ask the woman about any exposures to hazards encountered at work, including toxins or radiation. Many substances can affect overall health status generally and reproductive function specifically.

Habits

Ask whether the client smokes cigarettes. Smoking is associated with an increase in morbidity, especially when used in conjunction with oral contraceptives, and also may be related to an earlier than normal onset of menopause. Note the use of alcohol, recreational drugs, and habits that increase risk of acquiring STDs.

Domestic Violence

In private, ascertain whether the woman is a victim of domestic violence. Ask every client about violence in her life. Explain that the same question is asked of all women and that she is not being singled out. (She might assume that you ask the question because of her race, nationality, or socioeconomic status.) Clients frequently deny domestic violence many times before acknowledging it; consequently repeated questioning in a variety of ways may help determine whether the client is a victim. Be alert to physical and behavioral manifestations that are inconsistent with the explanation of their cause. Also be aware of an overprotective significant other. This is also a good time to educate women about available options if violence is or becomes a problem.

Psychosocial Factors

Because the genital organs and their reproductive capacity have symbolic significance for many women, problems in this area can affect a woman's sexuality and sense of femininity. Gynecologic problems may be associated with changes in self-concept, body image, personal identity, and role performance. Reproductive capabilities, the expression of sexuality, and sexual activities may be affected. In short, gynecologic disorders may result in psychological consequences. For this reason, psychological assessment is especially important. A woman's outward reaction to gynecologic problems does not necessarily correspond with either her inner experience or the seriousness of the condition.

Be sensitive when interviewing and examining a woman. Do not insist on obtaining information that she is hesitant to reveal. The woman herself may not understand her responses. Empathic listening is supportive and may lessen the stress the woman feels.

The woman may express fear because of a suspected unhealthy change in the genitals or of unwanted pregnancy. She may feel anxious and embarrassed before undergoing a pelvic examination. Many women consider the pelvic examination unpleasant despite its minimal risk of injury or physical pain. Other feelings that may be expressed include humiliation, guilt, or anger. Deep, powerful feelings may prevent women from seeking gynecologic care. Intrusive gynecologic procedures may evoke memories or strong reactions in women who have experienced sexual abuse or assault. The opportunity to express and discuss feelings with a nurse who is skilled in therapeutic communication may help these women cope more effectively and follow through with appropriate care. A therapeutic conversation can provide opportunities for clarifying a woman's misconceptions about her diagnosis, proposed treatment, and preventive care. Many women have never received accurate information about reproductive problems.

Review of Systems

Review the client's physical health history, proceeding from head to toe. Note especially (1) cardiovascular disorders (hypertension, angina [pain], myocardial infarction [MI], thrombophlebitis), (2) endocrine disorders (hypothyroidism, hyperthyroidism), (3) disorders of the pituitary gland, (4) liver disorders, and (5) cholecystitis. Ask about problems involving the urinary tract and reproductive system, such as urinary tract infection, urinary incontinence, vaginitis, and any bleeding disorders associated with menstruation (amenorrhea, dysmenorrhea, breakthrough bleeding, menorrhagia, or postcoital bleeding). Detailed questions for the review of systems *evolve* are found on the website for this textbook.

PHYSICAL EXAMINATION

Elements of a standard gynecologic examination can vary slightly but usually include the following physical assessment and laboratory data:

- Vital signs (temperature, pulse, respiration, and blood pressure)
- Height
- Weight
- Hematocrit (or complete blood count)
- Urinalysis
- Pelvic examination and Pap smear
- Physical assessment of skin, heart, lungs, breasts and axillae, thyroid, and abdomen
- Periodically, lipid profile and thyroid-stimulating hormone (TSH) level
- As appropriate for age and history, endoscopic procedures, including colonoscopy and colorectal sigmoidoscopy, fecal occult blood testing, and mammography

If unusual or abnormal findings are obtained during the gynecologic history or physical examination, additional data must be sought.

Breasts and Axillae

Examination of the breasts and axillae is an important part of the gynecologic examination. Good lighting is essential. Some examiners complete this portion of the examination before assessing the anterior lungs and heart. Because the breasts are sensitive and are closely associated with sexuality, some examiners delay this portion until there has been more hands-on interaction with the client during assessment of the lungs and heart. Others integrate assessments so that the client is sitting for those portions of the heart, lungs, breasts, and axillae examination before being helped to a supine position for the remaining portions. Any sequence is acceptable as long as you are thorough, you maintain the client's privacy, and the client can tolerate the position changes. Instruct the client in BSE while examining the breasts. (BSE is discussed in Chapter 2.)

Ask the client when her last menstrual period began. Breasts are usually tender the week before onset of menses and least tender the week after menses has ceased. If the client reports that one breast is tender, begin palpation with the opposite breast. Thorough examination requires exposure of both breasts for comparison.

Inspection

Begin breast inspection while the client is seated with her arms at her sides. Ask her to raise her hands over her head. Finally, ask her to press her hands firmly on her hips or together to tighten the pectoral muscles. Examine women who have large or pendulous breasts while they bend at the waist and face forward with the breast hanging down (Figure 39-1). In all positions, inspect the breasts for symmetry, size, shape, contour, and skin characteristics, including the vascular pattern.

Breasts are symmetrical, although it is not unusual for one breast to be slightly larger than the other. The breasts should hang evenly between the third and fourth ribs with the nipples about level with the fourth intercostal space when the client sits with her arms at her sides. With aging and loss of tissue elasticity, the breasts hang lower, especially after pregnancy and breast-feeding. The contour is even. Dimpling (retraction), masses, or surface flattening are abnormal. Skin color is the same as that of the abdomen. *Striae* (stretch marks from rapid skin stretching) may be present; recent striae are reddened and become paler with time. Venous patterns, if noticeable, should be symmetrical. Local areas of hyperpigmentation or edema should be absent.

Ask the client to raise her arms over her head while you examine the lateral and undersurfaces of each breast. Contraction of the pectoral muscles exaggerates manifestations of retraction or skin flattening. Note areas of redness or excoriation from poorly fitting brassieres. The breasts should elevate evenly so that the areolae remain at the same level. Ask the client to put her hands on her hips and press inward firmly while you repeat the inspection for masses, retraction, or skin flattening.

Inspect the areolae and nipples for size, shape, contour, symmetry, surface characteristics, and masses or lesions. Areolae are pink in fair-skinned women and darker in dark-skinned women. Slight asymmetry is common, but the nipples should point in symmetrical directions. Masses or lesions are abnormal. Montgomery's

FIGURE 39-1 Positions for breast examination. **A,** Arms at side. **B,** Hands raised over head. For tightening pectoral muscles, the examiner asks the client to press hands firmly on hips (**C**), or to press hands together (**D**). **E,** Breasts may also be examined with the woman leaning forward at the waist, allowing the breasts to hang down.

tubercles may be prominent around the nipple, which is normal. The nipples are round or oval, equal in size, of the same color, soft, and smooth. If one or both nipples are inverted, ask whether this is a recent occurrence or has been present for a while and how long. Recent nipple inversion is abnormal, and the client should be referred to an appropriate health care provider for follow-up. Rashes, crusts, or discharge should be absent unless the client is in the late stages of pregnancy, when colostrum (a yellowish fluid) may leak from the nipples.

Inspect the axillae for rashes, masses, and areas of unusual pigmentation, which should be absent. Axillary hair should be present unless the client removes it.

Palpation

Palpation of axillae is usually done while the client is seated; breast palpation is facilitated with the client supine. For clients who have large, pendulous breasts, who have a history of breast masses or cancer, or who are at increased risk for breast cancer, the breasts should be palpated in both positions.

Palpation of the axillae includes examination of five sets of lymph nodes (Figure 39-2). Encourage the client

to relax her arm; this relaxes the chest muscles and eases palpation. Begin by palpating the edge of the pectoralis major muscle along the anterior axillary line, using a bimanual technique if necessary, to examine the pectoral (anterior) nodes. Then reach high up into the axilla at the midaxillary line to palpate the midaxillary (central) nodes against the ribs and serratus anterior. Palpate the subscapular (posterior) nodes along the posterior axillary fold along the anterior edge of the latissimus dorsi. Palpate the brachial (lateral) nodes along the humerus in the upper inner arm.

Finally, palpate the infraclavicular area. The supraclavicular nodes, which also receive lymphatic drainage from the breasts, are usually examined with the neck nodes. All the nodes should be nonpalpable, although detection of one or two small, nontender, mobile central nodes is often a normal finding. Abnormal findings include firm, fixed nodes that may or may not be tender. If nodes are palpated, note the number of nodes felt, their location, size, shape, mobility, tenderness, and consistency.

Conduct breast palpation systematically to examine all breast tissue, including the tail of Spence in the upper outer quadrant. Any one of several approaches can be

FIGURE 39-2 Assessment of axillary lymph nodes. **A,** Location of the groups of nodes examined. **B,** Pectoral (anterior) nodes. **C,** Midaxillary (central) nodes. **D,** Subscapular (posterior nodes). **E,** Brachial (lateral) nodes. **F,** Infraclavicular (subclavicular) nodes. Axillary nodes are also palpated for male clients.

used as long as each portion of the breasts, areolae, and nipples is palpated. The breast and areola may be palpated in concentric circles, in a wheel-and-spokes pattern, or back and forth from superior to inferior. When the client is sitting, you may prefer to use a bimanual technique, especially if the breasts are large. When the client is supine, place a small folded towel under her shoulder to enhance breast flattening against the chest wall. Have her place her arm behind her head. Slide your fingers along the tissue using a rotary motion to press the breast against the chest wall. Your fingers remain in contact with the skin surface. The firm, curved ridge along the inferior breast is the inframammary ridge.

Breast consistency varies from firm and elastic in young women to stringy and nodular in older women. If the client reports a mass, begin palpation with the unaffected breast so that you have a basis for comparison. Pay particular attention to the upper outer quadrant and tail of Spence, where most of the glandular tissue is located and 50% of breast lesions are found. No masses or local areas of warmth should be present. If you feel a lump or mass, note its characteristics. Include the exact location (and the position the client is in for the palpation), using the areola as a reference point. Note the size, shape, contour, consistency, mobility, tenderness, and discreteness. Visualize the breast as having four quadrants plus the tail; the location of lesions can be diagrammed in the written record. For a recording example,

see the Physical Assessment Findings in the Healthy Adult feature on The Female Reproductive System on p. 993.

Palpate the areola and nipple gently. Compress the nipple between your thumb and index finger. There should be no discharge. Nipple erection and wrinkling with manipulation are normal.

Pelvis

Women often find pelvic examinations embarrassing, humiliating, and anxiety provoking, especially if they are performed roughly or in a perfunctory and hurried manner. Insensitive professional treatment produces fear, humiliation, submission, and low self-esteem. Meet the client, and interview her before she disrobes in the examining room. Memories of an uncomfortable or otherwise unpleasant pelvic examination may make women avoid future examinations and neglect gynecologic health care.

Put the woman at ease before and during the pelvic examination. Promote comfort by being nonjudgmental, relaxed, and competent. Explain your actions before proceeding. Avoid quick movements because they may cause the client to tense her muscles, which results in greater discomfort. Enhance comfort with gentleness, privacy, keeping the woman warm, warming hands and instruments, using a lubricant to ease insertion during invasive maneuvers, and cleaning the perineum after the

PHYSICAL ASSESSMENT FINDINGS IN THE HEALTHY ADULT

The Female Reproductive System

Inspection

Breasts and Axillae. Breasts symmetrical, full, rounded, smooth in all positions, without dimpling, retractions, or masses. Faint, even vascular pattern and striae are noted. Nipples everted, areolae even. Axillae even color, without masses or rash.

Genitalia. Pubic hair distribution varies with stage of sexual development; clean, coarse. Labia majora covered with pubic hair in adult women; may gape open slightly. Labia minora pink, smooth. Clitoris midline, smooth. Urethral meatus pink, discharge absent. Vaginal orifice clean, without bulges. Vaginal walls intact, pink, glistening, rugae present; discharge, bulges, and masses absent. Cervix round with os round or oval in nulliparous women and slit-like in parous women; discharge absent.

Palpation

Breasts and Axillae. Breasts firm without masses, lumps, local areas of warmth, or tenderness. Nipples without discharge. Axillae smooth, nodes nonpalpable.

Genitalia. Pelvic floor musculature firm. Skene's glands without discharge or tenderness. Bartholin's glands without masses or tenderness. No bulges in vaginal wall with straining. Uterus anteverted, firm, smooth, mobile, nontender, without masses. Ovaries oval, firm, movable, nontender.

examination. Protect the woman's dignity, and communicate with her before, during, and after the examination. Use a mirror during the examination to show the woman her anatomic structures, if she desires, to facilitate the learning process.

A pelvic examination will be less dreaded when a woman can participate and learn while retaining a sense of power and self-control. Encourage questions and expression of concerns, feelings, and wishes. Some women are afraid the examiner will detect their sexual "secrets" from a pelvic examination. Provide these clients with a sense of control over self-disclosure so that they do not feel you are prying or are able to "read their past."

Remain professional, and avoid actions or remarks that might be misconstrued by the client as demeaning or sexually provocative. For example, use a firm touch instead of gentle stroking. Be aware that the client may become sexually stimulated; alter the sequence of the examination, if necessary, but continue in a professional manner. Some facilities mandate that a female assistant be present when an examiner performs a pelvic examination both to comfort the client and to discourage accusations of sexual impropriety.

Preparation

Instruct the woman not to douche, have intercourse, or use any vaginal products for 2 to 3 days before a pelvic examination. If a Pap smear is to be obtained, the woman should not be menstruating. Just before the examination, ask the woman to empty her bladder and bowels to enhance comfort and accuracy. If necessary, collect a urine specimen at this time.

Ask the woman to remove enough clothing to allow examination of the abdomen and perineum. If a breast examination is planned, request that the woman disrobe completely and have her put on a gown. Ask about previous experiences with pelvic examinations, and acknowledge any feelings the woman may have. If this is the client's first examination, explain the procedure fully and show her how the speculum works. All women should be told which examinations are to be performed. Tell the woman when and where she will be touched to help her avoid tensing up, which produces discomfort.

Equipment

The following equipment is used during a pelvic examination:

- Vaginal speculum of an appropriate size
- Materials for obtaining smears and culture specimens for cytologic and microbiology tests, including sterile cotton-tipped swabs, vaginal spatulas (wooden or plastic) or cytology brush, glass slides and coverslips, cytology fixative, culture plates, and enzyme immunoassay kits for *Chlamydia* and gonorrhea screening
- Adequate, adjustable light source
- Water-soluble lubricant
- Appropriately sized examination gloves (vinyl if the client is latex-sensitive)

Long forceps and cotton balls may be used after smears and specimens have been obtained to clean the cervix or vaginal areas so that any suspected areas may be examined more easily. Have biopsy equipment available in case the examination reveals that a biopsy is necessary.

Position

Help the client to assume a dorsal recumbent or lithotomy position, and keep her draped until it is time for the examination. In the lithotomy position, the buttocks should be aligned with the end of the table. The client may not have to put her feet into stirrups if only the external genitalia are examined. Help the client to flex and abduct her hips and knees with her arms at her sides or crossed over the chest. Adjust the stirrups to accommodate the woman's height.

The lithotomy position, with the perineum exposed, may be uncomfortable and embarrassing. Do not keep a woman exposed any longer than necessary. Elevate the client's head on a small pillow to aid abdominal muscle relaxation and facilitate the examination. Low back pain or a hip deformity may contraindicate this position; an alternative position, such as Sims, might be necessary (see Chapter 4), or an assistant can help the client abduct one or both legs. There must be an adjustable light source. Wear nonsterile, disposable examining gloves (latex or vinyl).

External Genitalia

Inspect the external genitalia and perineum (see Figure U9-1, A for the anatomy of the female peritoneum and genitalia). Assess secondary sexual characteristics, such as pubic hair distribution and developmental stage of external genitalia, during examination of the external genitalia and rectum while these areas are uncovered. Before touching the client's perineum, place one hand on the client's thigh to avoid startling her.

The mons pubis is a mound of tissue superior to the labia. In adults, it is usually covered by pubic hair distributed as an inverse triangle over the mons, anterior perineum, and medial aspects of the upper thighs. Inspect the hair for nits and the skin for parasites, irritation, inflammation, edema, and lesions. An offensive odor should not be present. Any discharge should be scanty and clear to white.

Perineal skin is slightly darker than the rest of the body. The labia majora are symmetrical, rounded, and full. If the client has had a previous vaginal delivery, the labia majora gape slightly and the labia minora are evident. After menopause, the labia majora slowly atrophy. They should be free of edema, inflammation, and lesions. The labia minora are thinner than the labia majora, and one side may be larger than the other side. Gently separate the labia to inspect the vulva and remaining external structures. Place the thumb and index finger of your nondominant hand inside the labia minora, and retract the tissues laterally. Maintain a firm hold to avoid unnecessary manipulation of sensitive tissues.

Inspect the clitoris, urethral meatus, hymen (if present), and vaginal orifice (introitus); discharge, inflammation, edema, or lesions, should be absent. The clitoris is approximately 1 cm wide and 2 cm long, the same color as the rest of the vulva. It can be the site of syphilitic chancres (more likely in younger women), and the site of dry, scaly, nodular lesions that are malignant (more likely in older women). While examining the introitus, also inspect the hymen, which is just inside the introitus. The hymen may be prominent and may restrict the vaginal opening in a virgin, or it may be mostly absent in a sexually active client. Bartholin's glands are found near the base of the introitus and normally are not visualized

or palpable. If inflammation and edema are present near the posterior introitus, palpate each gland between your thumb and index finger. Insert your index finger into the introitus, and rotate it laterally and posteriorly (Figure 39-3, A). Palpate the gland against the thumb at the posterior aspect of the labia majora. Repeat the maneuver for the other side.

The urethral meatus, between the clitoris and introitus, can be difficult to locate, particularly in women who have had a vaginal delivery. It is a small slit just above the vaginal opening and is the same color as the sur-

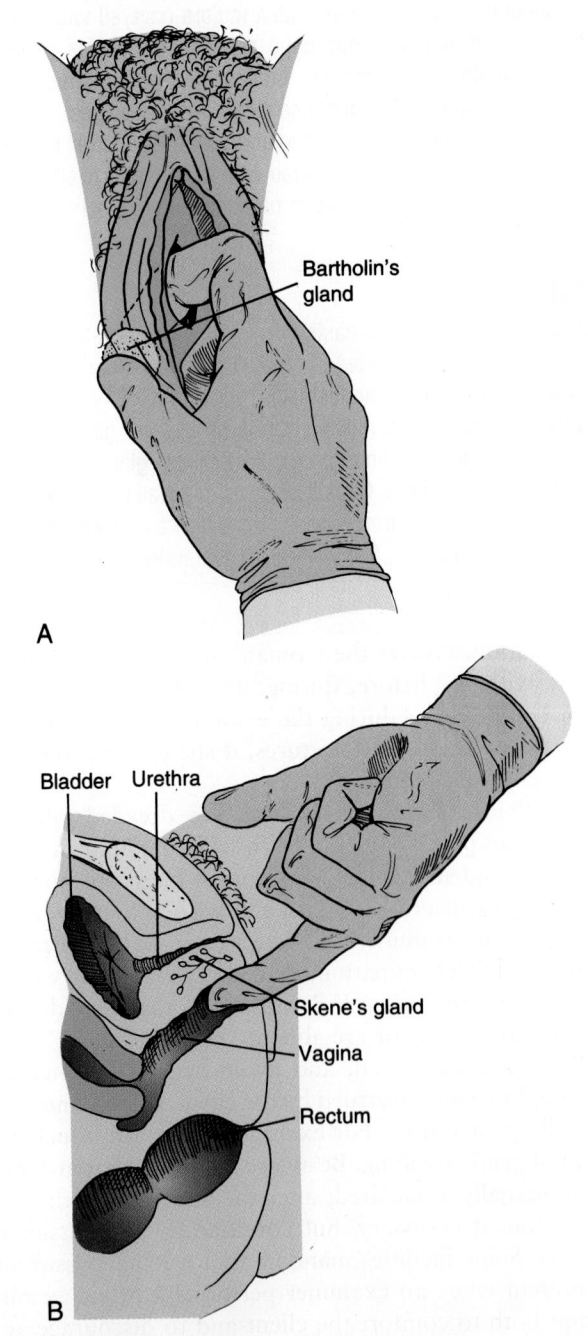

FIGURE 39-3 A, Palpation of Bartholin's glands. **B,** Palpation of Skene's glands.

rounding tissues. In women who have had several vaginal deliveries, the opening may be located just inside the vaginal orifice. The meatus should be free of discharge, inflammation, or swelling. If these manifestations are present, palpate Skene's glands (paraurethral glands), which are at both sides of the urethral meatus (Figure 39-3, *B*). They are usually not visualized or palpable. Insert a gloved index finger palm up into the introitus and about 1 inch (2.5 cm) into the vagina. Press gently upward to palpate the glands, and note their characteristics. Draw your index finger along the vaginal wall as you remove it from the vagina so that any discharge is "milked" from the glands into the urethra and out the meatus. If a discharge is present, collect a specimen for culture and change gloves before proceeding.

Vaginal Speculum Examination

Select a vaginal speculum of appropriate size; specula differ in width and length. Lubricants cannot be used because they interfere with various cytologic studies, such as the Pap smear. If a cervical smear is not needed, use a water-soluble lubricant. Wear gloves and insert the speculum, either rinsed in warm water or lubricated as indicated, gently into the vagina.

To do so, place the index and middle fingers of your nondominant hand in the vaginal orifice and gently pull posteriorly. Insert the closed speculum at a 45-degree angle, with the tip pointing downward into the vaginal orifice over your fingers (Figure 39-4, *A*). Withdraw your fingers while slowly rotating the speculum downward

FIGURE 39-4 Pelvic examination and insertion of the vaginal speculum. **A,** The speculum blades are turned obliquely, and any pressure is directed downward onto the perineum. **B,** After full insertion, the blades are rotated to a horizontal position. **C,** Squeezing the speculum handles opens the blades. **D,** A full view of the cervix and cervical os. **E,** The bimanual examination. The abdominal hand presses the pelvic organs to be palpated toward the intravaginal hand. **F,** Rectovaginal examination combines bimanual and rectal examination. The index finger is in the vagina and the middle finger is in the rectum.

into the vagina until the handle is in a vertical position and the blades are fully inserted (Figure 39-4, *B*). Open the blades to observe the vaginal walls and cervix (Figure 39-4, *C* and *D*). You may need to make several gentle attempts to correctly position the cervix between the blades of the speculum. Offer the woman a mirror if she wants to see her cervix.

Vaginal mucous membranes are moist and pink, without discharge. If a discharge is present, it should be thin and clear to white. Abnormal findings include dry or inflamed mucosa; a discharge that is thick, curdy, yellow, green, odorous, or profuse; ulcers; lesions; masses; and bulges of the vaginal wall (which could be from a cystocele or rectocele).

The cervical os (Figure 39-4, *D*) is usually round, but it may be a slit or irregularly shaped after vaginal delivery. It is pink and smooth. A discharge is usually present that varies from thin and clear to thick, white, and stringy, depending on the phase of the menstrual cycle. Abnormal findings include unusual color of the mucosa, abnormal consistency of discharge, ulcerations, growths, masses, nodules, inflammation, and bleeding. If an abnormal discharge is present, obtain a specimen for culture.

Before removing the speculum from the vagina, obtain cytologic and microbiologic specimens, if indicated, as discussed later in this chapter. To visualize the vaginal walls, leave the speculum blades open slightly as they are withdrawn. Rotate the blades obliquely, and remove the speculum slowly to assess the vaginal walls fully. Do not allow the blades to press on the urethra or the blades to close fully, which can cause extreme discomfort.

Bimanual Examination

Wear appropriate disposable examination gloves. Lubricate the glove and gently insert one or two fingers of your dominant hand into the vagina, palm up, and place the other hand on the client's lower abdomen (Figure 39-4, *E*). Palpate the pelvic contents between the fingers in the vagina and the hand on the abdomen. Locate and assess the cervix. Assess the size, shape, surface characteristics, consistency, position, mobility, and tenderness of the uterine body and fundus. Finally, palpate each of the adnexal areas (left and right). Normal ovaries may or may not be palpable, and normal fallopian tubes are not palpable. Postmenopausal ovaries should not be palpable.

A normal cervix can be gently moved from side to side without pain. The cervix should feel smooth and firm, located deep in the vagina, most often on the anterior wall. It usually points away from the fundus of the uterus. Abnormal findings include tenderness or pain with palpation, immobility, and an abnormal position.

The uterus is typically in an anterior position but may be retroverted or in midposition in 15% of women. It is normally firm, smooth, mobile, and nontender and is about 2⅛ to 3⅛ inches (5.5 to 8 cm) long. Abnormal findings include prolapse into the vagina, hard or soft consistency, being fixed in position, irregular contour, enlargement, or tenderness.

A normal ovary is 4 to 6 cm in diameter and feels smooth, firm, and oval. Slight tenderness on palpation is normal, but extreme tenderness, pain, and masses are not.

Withdraw your hand, palm up, halfway from the vaginal orifice, and assess the integrity of the pelvic floor musculature. Ask the client to contract her pelvic floor muscles as if trying to stop the flow of urine. The muscles will constrict around your fingers with more tone in a nulliparous client than in a client who has had a vaginal delivery. Next ask the client to bear down as if straining to void. Feel for bulging of the vaginal walls pressing down against the introitus. If the anterior wall of the vagina bulges, the client probably has a *cystocele* (prolapse of the urinary bladder). A posterior vaginal wall bulge is often the result of a *rectocele* (rectal wall prolapse). Both of these are common in multiparous or obese clients.

Rectovaginal Examination

Insert your lubricated middle finger into the rectum and the index finger into the vagina (Figure 39-4, *F*) to assess the rectal tissues for abnormalities, such as hemorrhoids (see Chapter 34). Ask the woman to bear down so as to ease insertion of your finger into the rectum. Rectal examination also confirms uterine position. If the uterus is retroverted, palpate the body and fundus. Reassess the adnexal areas, and palpate the rectovaginal septum and cul-de-sac. Normal pelvic organs can be palpated through the posterior cul-de-sac. Abnormal masses or normal ovaries are often felt in the cul-de-sac.

Assess the anal sphincter tone and the rectal wall, which should be smooth. Assess the rectovaginal wall, which should be smooth, firm, and resilient (see Chapter 34). If the uterus is retroverted, it may be felt through the rectovaginal wall. The cervix feels smooth, round, firm, and movable without tenderness. Do not mistake the cervix or a vaginal tampon (if one is left in place) for a rectal mass.

If a stool specimen is needed for occult blood testing, obtain it at this time (see Chapter 34). When the examination has been completed, help the client sit up and offer her tissues or wipes to clean the perineum.

If it has been well performed, a vaginal examination in women who have no pathologic conditions usually causes no or minimal discomfort. Some discomfort may occur during palpation of the ovaries during the bimanual and rectal examinations. Acknowledge this, and help the woman relax by asking her to bear down during the rectal examination and to breathe deeply through her mouth during palpation of the ovary. After completing the examination, give instructions and conduct appropriate health instruction.

Sometimes abnormal cervical or vaginal tissue, a mass, or other problem is discovered during a pelvic examination. Colposcopy or biopsy of the abnormal tissue may be performed. Further examination under anesthesia may be necessary for exploration of a mass or unexplained tenderness. A pelvic examination is conducted before various other gynecologic tests (such as colposcopy or hysterosalpingogram) and before surgery (such as laparoscopy or laparotomy).

DIAGNOSTIC TESTS

GYNECOLOGIC STUDIES

Laboratory Studies

The most common gynecologic laboratory studies are the Pap smear, wet smear, and cervical culture. The woman should not be menstruating at the time specimens are collected. Instruct her to avoid sexual intercourse, douching, or using vaginal hygiene sprays or deodorants for 2 to 3 days before a test.

Papanicolaou Smear

Cytology is examination of the structure, function, pathology, and chemistry of the cell (Figure 39-5). In gynecology, the most common cytologic test is the Pap smear, named after George Papanicolaou, the physician who devised it. The Pap smear identifies preinvasive and invasive cervical cancer. A newer technique that improves the quality of Pap smears is the ThinPrep Pap test. Cells are collected and processed in such a way that a thinner layer of cells can be examined on the slide. Clinical trials have demonstrated improved detection of precancerous cervical cells using the ThinPrep Pap test compared with the conventional Pap smear.

Procedure

The principle of the Pap test is based on the fact that both normal and abnormal cells are shed from the uterine and cervical linings and pass into their secretions. When a cytologic smear of these secretions is examined under a microscope, early cellular changes can be detected before disease becomes clinically apparent. Conventional Pap tests (slides) are about 78% accurate in the diagnosis of early cervical carcinoma provided that correct sampling and handling techniques are used. Liquid-based Pap tests are considered to be 93% to 94% accurate under the same conditions.[10] Pap tests are only about 40% accurate in detecting endometrial carcinoma.[5,8]

Specimens for the Pap test consist of a small amount of secretions taken from the endocervix and exocervix

(Figure 39-5, *B* and *C*). With the conventional Pap test, these secretions are smeared separately on clean, dry slides, or they may be placed on one slide divided into sections (Figure 39-5, *E*). The slides are marked with "C" for cervix and "E" for endocervix. Immediately after the smears are made on the slides, they are fixed with either a commercial spray or solution. The secretions must be fixed before they dry. Cells in the specimen may be distorted if they dry or are contaminated with lubricant, which makes accurate reading difficult or impossible. With the ThinPrep test, the collected secretions are placed in a small bottle of preservative.

A Pap smear is usually painless. The American Cancer Society (ACS) recommends that women who are or have been sexually active or who have reached age 18 years should have annual Pap tests and pelvic examinations. After a woman has had three or more consecutive normal annual examinations, the Pap smear may be performed less often at the discretion of the health care provider. Many health care providers, however, continue to recommend annual examinations. The Pap test should be continued after menopause. Vaginal smears are obtained for Pap smear in women who have had a hysterectomy with removal of the cervix (see Chapter 41). Secretions are obtained from the vaginal pool, located in the posterior fornix (Figure 39-5, *D*).

In the past, reported findings were classified numerically; however, descriptive reports are preferred because they are more useful in clinical decision-making. Reports either classify findings as normal or describe more fully the cellular changes seen. Specific infections may also be identified, and hormonal assessment may be done.

An abnormal Pap smear does not always mean malignancy. There is about a 6% to 22% false-positive or false-negative rate for the Pap test, and this rate is much higher if the specimen has been incorrectly collected or handled.[10] Having an abnormal Pap smear can be a frightening experience. Careful interpretation of cytologic findings is crucial. The woman needs an opportunity to ask questions, to discuss concerns and feelings, and to participate in follow-up care planning.

If the cervix appears abnormal to the naked eye during the examination, colposcopy may be done at that time if it is available (see later discussion). If the Pap smear result reveals a vaginal infection, the woman may be treated for vaginitis and the Pap test repeated later. If the Pap test result shows dysplasia or abnormal tissue, treatment will vary according to extent of the lesion, grade of the dysplasia, and preference of the woman and her health care provider. For more information on cervical cancer, see Chapter 41.

Postprocedure Care

Care is minimal following a Pap test. Help the client out of the stirrups, and tell her not to get up too rapidly, par-

A. SPECIMEN COLLECTION EQUIPMENT

B. ENDOCERVICAL SPECIMEN

Moisten swab with saline. Insert cotton-tipped end into cervical os. Rotate handle to obtain specimen.

C. EXOCERVICAL SPECIMEN

Insert Ayre spatula with longer tip in cervical os. Rotate end of spatula around cervical opening.

E. SLIDE PREPARATION

Smear specimen evenly on glass slide. Add drop of KOH or saline and cover with cover glass. Label with name, date, area of sample, identification number.

F. GONOCOCCAL CULTURE

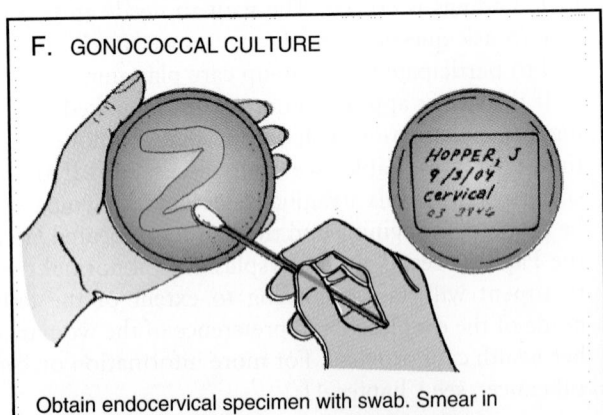

Obtain endocervical specimen with swab. Smear in Z pattern on agar plate. Cover and label as above.

D. CUL-DE-SAC   POOL SPECIMEN

Insert saline-moistened swab into cul-de-sac pool to obtain specimen.

FIGURE 39-5 **A-F,** Collection of cervical cytology specimens.

ticularly if she is older. Clean off any excess lubricant, or allow the client to do so. Ensure that the client understands how she will receive the results of her Pap test.

Wet Smear

The wet smear is used to detect vaginal infection with *Candida albicans, Trichomonas vaginalis,* or organisms that cause bacterial infections. A copious specimen of discharge from the vaginal vault is obtained with a cotton-tipped swab and placed in about 1 ml of warm normal saline to check for *T. vaginalis* and clue cells (indicative of bacterial vaginosis). A second specimen can be placed in about 1 ml of potassium hydroxide to check for *C. albicans.* Both specimens are mixed to produce a suspension and then placed on a glass slide with a coverslip for microscopic examination (Figure 39-5, *E*).

Cervical Culture

A cervical culture or antigen detection test can be done to detect infection with *Neisseria gonorrhoeae* or *Chlamydia trachomatis.* A cotton-tipped swab is rotated in the endocervical canal and placed in the appropriate Culturette tube or rolled in a **Z** pattern onto a culture medium, depending on the organism. The culture medium should be at room temperature before inoculation with the specimen (Figures 39-5, *B* and *F*). Because of the asymptomatic nature of these infections, sexually active women are often tested routinely during regular examinations.

Radiography

Computed tomography (CT) and magnetic resonance imaging (MRI) are modalities in which images of the pelvic organs are obtained in the assessment of reproductive and urologic disorders (see Chapters 4 and 34). There is no special preparation for CT scan or MRI unless a contrast agent (dye) is given. Pregnancy and morbid obesity contraindicate both tests. Ask the woman whether she has a copper-containing intrauterine device in place, the presence of which may contraindicate MRI.

Ultrasonography

Obtain informed consent. For a transabdominal scan, the client may be asked to arrive for the appointment with a full bladder (see Chapter 4).

When performed with a vaginal probe, an ultrasound examination enhances the view of the adnexae. This technique is used to evaluate ovarian cancer, cysts, and ovaries that have been stimulated with fertility-enhancing drugs. For this approach, the bladder is usually emptied. The woman inserts the vaginal probe (sheathed in a protective, lubricated cover). Once the probe is inserted, the technician maneuvers it to obtain the best images. Inform the woman to expect the technician to manipulate the probe.

Sonohysterography utilizes a saline infusion in conjunction with transvaginal ultrasound to enhance the endometrial imaging and aid in the diagnosis of uterine and endometrial abnormalities. Preparation for sonohysterography is the same as for ultrasonography.

Endoscopy

Endoscopic procedures for assessing the female reproductive system include colposcopy, hysteroscopy, and laparoscopy.

Colposcopy

Colposcopy involves the use of stereoscopic binocular microscope (colposcope) to examine the cervical epithelium, vagina, and vulva. It is indicated for all women whose Pap smears show dysplasia. It also may be used to examine suspected lesions in the lower genital tract.

Explain to the woman that the procedure is similar to a pelvic examination and that, when the speculum is in place, a special microscope is used to look at the cervix. Colposcopy increases diagnostic accuracy and reduces the need for biopsy. The procedure is safe and painless, and it can be performed in pregnant women.

Help the woman into the lithotomy position. The cervix is exposed with a vaginal speculum. A solution of 3% acetic acid (common household vinegar) is applied to the cervix to remove mucus and cellular debris and to slightly dehydrate the cells. The cervix and upper vagina are then inspected with the colposcope. Biopsy is usually performed at this time if a lesion is present and can be done easily without the use of anesthesia. Cervical biopsy is avoided on pregnant women. (See discussion of cervical biopsy later in this chapter.)

Hysteroscopy

During a hysteroscopic examination, the intrauterine cavity is viewed directly through an endoscope called a hysteroscope (Figure 39-6). Hysteroscopes have a fiberoptic lighting system and use 5% glucose in water, highly viscous dextran solutions or carbon dioxide as the uterine-distending medium. After an anesthetic agent is administered, the hysteroscope is passed into the uterus via the vagina. The uterine cavity is distended and may be rinsed to clear away blood and debris that would obstruct vision. In addition to direct visualization of the uterine cavity, directed biopsies and resections of endometrial abnormalities can be done. The hysteroscope can also be used to deliver a laser beam into the uterus for therapeutic procedures.

Hysteroscopy can be used for (1) ruling out organic causes in abnormal uterine or postmenopausal bleeding,

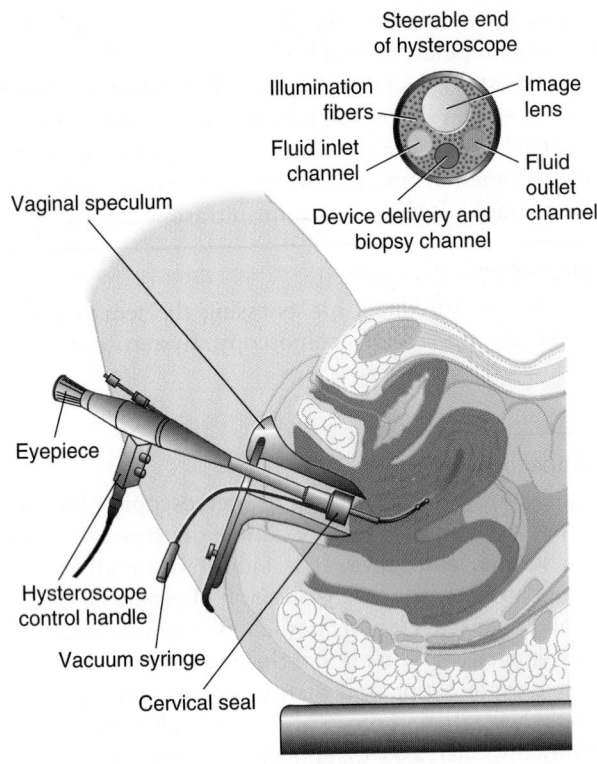

FIGURE 39-6 Hysteroscopy. An endometrial biopsy may be obtained during hysteroscopy.

(2) examining suspected leiomyomas or polyps, (3) removing an intrauterine device with a missing string, (4) evaluating infertility, and (5) performing surgical techniques for uterine abnormalities. It is contraindicated if the client has acute pelvic inflammatory disease, recurrent chronic upper genital tract infection, or recent uterine perforation. It also is contraindicated in pregnancy.

Explain the procedure and obtain informed consent. Position the client in the lithotomy position, as for a pelvic examination. Complications of the procedure may include bleeding, uterine perforation, infection, and, rarely, bowel injuries. The woman may have referred shoulder pain if carbon dioxide was introduced into the pelvic cavity during the procedure; it usually resolves within 24 hours. Monitor the client's vital signs, and assess pain levels and location carefully.

Laparoscopy

A laparoscope, a common diagnostic and therapeutic tool, is a telescope with an illuminated optical system. It is inserted into the abdomen through a small incision in or near the umbilicus to visualize abdominal and pelvic organs. Laparoscopy is a safe, convenient procedure that can be performed in hospitals, offices, or clinics equipped for outpatient surgery. The postprocedure recovery period is short, and the scar is small.

Laparoscopy may be performed diagnostically for conditions such as pelvic pain, pelvic masses, infertility, suspected ectopic pregnancy, and endometriosis. It also may be performed therapeutically for such procedures as tubal ligation, lysis of adhesions, treatment of endometriosis, drainage and removal of cysts, and for laparoscopy-assisted hysterectomy.

The main contraindication to laparoscopy is serious cardiac or pulmonary disease, although severe obesity may preclude its use. Previous lower abdominal surgery is not a contraindication, but it should be considered.

To prepare a client for laparoscopy, explain the procedure and inform the client how she can expect to feel afterward. Tell her to take nothing by mouth past midnight on the night before the procedure. Someone else should drive her to the health care facility because she should not drive after the procedure. Suggest that she wear loose-fitting clothes because it will be easier to dress after discharge. Typically, women who have laparoscopy in a same-day surgery setting can go home 2 to 4 hours after the procedure.

After laparoscopy, take the client's vital signs every 15 minutes for the first hour or until they are stable. If local anesthesia has been used, the woman can have fluids and a light snack as soon as she wants. After general anesthesia, the woman may have fluids and a light snack as soon as she is fully awake and has no nausea.

Explain that she may experience mild to moderate transient shoulder pain or a feeling of bloating as a result of the carbon dioxide or nitrous oxide that was used to distend the abdomen, separate the organs, and allow better visualization during the procedure. The discomfort usually lasts only a few hours and can be reduced by positioning or mild analgesics. The woman may also experience mild incisional pain or abdominal cramping for the first few hours or days after the procedure; these are usually reduced by rest.

If general anesthesia was used, the client might have a sore throat from intubation. Soreness should disappear within 48 hours.

Teach the client how to keep the incision clean and dry. After it heals, the scar will be barely noticeable. Sexual intercourse can be resumed within a week or less.

Biopsy

Cervical Biopsy

Cervical biopsy is performed to rule out malignancies. A specimen of the cervical lesion that has been identified with the naked eye or with colposcopic magnification is usually obtained in the outpatient setting with little or no anesthesia. A solution of 3% acetic acid can be applied to the cervix to identify areas suspected to be dysplastic, metaplastic, or malignant. These areas undergo a color change and appear white after acetic acid is applied.

View

Biopsy site

FIGURE 39-7 Cervical biopsy, if indicated, is performed following colposcopic examination.

When colposcopy cannot identify an abnormal lesion on the cervix or vagina, the Schiller's test may be performed. Lugol's iodine solution is applied to the vagina and cervix. Normal tissue takes up the stain and appears as a homogeneous mahogany-brown color. Usually, abnormal tissue does not take stain as well and may appear light yellow instead. This is a positive finding and can indicate areas needing biopsy. A biopsy may be done when a cervical lesion is first noted, or it may be delayed until about 1 week after the menstrual period, when the cervix is least vascular. Multiple biopsy specimens are usually obtained at specific sites with biopsy forceps (Figure 39-7). Hemostasis is achieved with topical application of Monsel's solution or silver nitrate. For ruling out disease in the endocervical canal, endocervical curettage may be performed.

Before a cervical biopsy, explain the purpose of the test and obtain the client's informed consent. The test is usually not done while the client is menstruating. The lithotomy position is assumed.

After a cervical biopsy, allow the client to rest for a short time before she goes home. Although she may note a small amount of blood-tinged vaginal discharge or the mustard and blackish discharge from the Monsel's solution, tell her to report any excessive bleeding immedi-

ately. Advise her to abstain from vaginal sexual activity and to avoid tampons and douching until the bleeding has completely stopped to achieve hemostasis, to lessen trauma, and to promote healing.

Endometrial Biopsy

An endometrial tissue sample is obtained for histologic study through the technique of endometrial biopsy. Tissue may be analyzed for endometrial cancer, dysfunctional uterine bleeding, and occasionally for infertility. The biopsy is performed after bimanual examination of the uterus. Because the biopsy procedure may result in cramping, the woman may receive a nonsteroidal anti-inflammatory drug, a paracervical block, or both to reduce the discomfort.

The cervix is dilated under sterile conditions, and a uterine sound is inserted to measure the depth of the uterine cavity. An aspirating instrument is passed into the uterus, and a small amount of tissue is removed from the endometrium for examination (see Figure 39-6).

Explain the purpose of the test and the procedure, including the use of an anesthetic block. Obtain an informed consent. Position the client as for a pelvic examination.

If cramping persists after the procedure, administer analgesics as ordered or apply heat to the lower abdomen.

BREAST STUDIES

Laboratory Studies

No reliable laboratory tests have been found for screening for breast cancer. Identifying a reliable biologic tumor marker for breast cancer could possibly aid in the detection or treatment of the disease.

Radiography

Various techniques have been tried to identify early stage breast cancer in women accurately and safely when assessment indicates breast lesions. Such techniques are also important in finding an effective method to screen women without clinically apparent manifestations. At present only mammography has been shown to be useful for widespread screening. Whereas ultrasonography is not specific enough to identify lesions suggestive of cancer, it can differentiate cystic from solid lesions. Other methods of testing are being investigated.

Mammography

A mammogram is a soft tissue radiographic breast examination used to detect small invasive and noninvasive tumors and benign lesions (Figure 39-8). Common ques-

A   B

FIGURE 39-8 **A,** Mammography, a technique for obtaining an x-ray image of the breast, is a reliable mechanical method of detecting a breast cancer before it can be felt. This technique is also used to help diagnose breast cancer. **B,** A normal mammogram of the left breast.

tions and possible answers about mammography include the following:

1. *How often should I have a screening mammogram?* Use the ACS or National Cancer Institute (NCI) guidelines for the age and risk group.
2. *What is the cost?* Prices vary. Inquire at the facility where the mammogram will be performed. Tell the client that although it is worthwhile to compare prices, ensure that the facility meets the necessary quality standards.
3. *How much time is involved?* About 15 to 30 minutes. Results are usually available within 1 to 21 days, depending on the facility.
4. *What preparation is required?* The woman should not wear any body powder, creams, or deodorant on the torso the day of the procedure.
5. *Is there pain?* Discomfort may be experienced because of the compression needed to obtain the best image. Some women find it helpful to schedule a mammogram for the week after the end of their menses, when the breasts are less tender. Women who have tender breasts may take a nonsteroidal anti-inflammatory drug, if not contraindicated, about 1 hour before the procedure.
6. *Is there a risk in the exposure to the radiation?* Mammography uses the smallest dose possible.

The long-term effects of an annual mammogram are considered to be harmless.

During a mammogram, the woman disrobes from the waist up and her gown is separated to expose one breast at a time. The breast is placed between an x-ray plate and a compression paddle that is adjusted so the breast is compressed between the two plates to obtain the best image possible (see Figure 39-8). Usually, two views of each breast are taken from different angles. Cranial-caudal and oblique views are most common.

Mammography can identify some breast cancers before they are palpable. The Breast Cancer Detection Demonstration Project included 280,000 participants who were followed up by mammogram for at least 5 years. Mammography alone detected 41.6% of the cancers—an impressively high rate in the diagnosis of small cancers.[12]

Indications for mammography include the following:
- Diagnosis of potentially curable cancer and follow-up after treatment
- Evaluation of questionable breast masses or other abnormal physical findings to help determine whether and where a biopsy should be performed
- Detection of breast cancer in a woman with metastatic cancer if the primary site is unknown
- Routine screening

Some controversy exists about the age at which to begin routine screening mammograms. The ACS recommends a baseline mammogram for all women by 40 years of age and mammography screening of asymptomatic women 40 to 49 years of age at intervals of 1 to 2 years and annually for women 50 years of age and older.[1] The NCI no longer recommends routine screening of women under age 50 years. Until there is further evidence, the decision of when to begin should be made on an individual basis, with the woman and her health care provider together evaluating her risk for breast cancer as well as the possible risks and benefits of the screening test. A woman who is at high risk for breast cancer should follow the recommendations of her health care provider.

Ultrasonography

An ultrasound study of the breast involves scanning with a hand-held real-time sector scanner. Ultrasonography is useful in determining the consistency of breast masses and differentiating cystic (fluid-filled) from solid lesions; however, it cannot differentiate solid benign from solid cancerous lesions (see Chapter 4). Ultrasound is useful in confirming the fluid consistency of cystic-appearing lesions seen on a mammogram. It is also useful in guiding fine-needle aspiration of cysts and other breast masses. No special preparation is needed, and the procedure is painless; no radiation risk is involved.

Biopsy

Biopsy is essential to the diagnosis of breast cancer. No treatment should be undertaken without an unequivocal histologic diagnosis of cancer. A core needle biopsy and a fine-needle aspiration (FNA) biopsy may be performed with local anesthesia during an office visit.

Core needle biopsy, a simple procedure, takes just a few minutes. After the site is cleaned and prepared with povidone-iodine, a small core of tissue is obtained with a special needle (Vim-Silverman). The core of tissue removed is placed in formalin and sent to the pathologist for histologic diagnosis. Occasionally a suture is needed to close the skin.

With an FNA *biopsy,* a needle and syringe are used to aspirate cells from a breast mass or fluid from a cyst. The cells are fixed on a slide (as in a Pap smear), and a cytologic diagnosis is made. Mammography is used to guide the needle for aspiration of nonpalpable lesions. The cytologic examination is useful for confirming the diagnosis of clinical and mammographic findings of fibroadenoma (a fibrocystic condition), intramammary lymph nodes, fat necrosis, subareolar papillomatosis, chronic subareolar abscess, and cancer. If the cytologic findings suggest that the specimen is acellular or that only blood and adipose cells are present, a biopsy or further evaluation is needed to rule out breast cancer.

Both FNA and core needle biopsy involve taking only a small amount of cells and tissue from a lesion. Because false-negative results are possible, an open biopsy still may be required.

Incisional or excisional open biopsies are usually performed in an operating room or a minor surgical suite with the use of local anesthetic or intravenous (IV) sedation. About 35% of clients who require an open biopsy for a breast lesion have a malignancy. *Excisional* biopsy involves removal of the entire palpable mass, *incisional* biopsy only a portion of the mass. In both cases, the tissue removed is sent to the pathologist for histologic assessment. The incision is closed with sutures, and a dressing (sometimes a pressure dressing) is placed over the site. Typically, the dressing is in place for 24 to 48 hours before it is removed.

Percutaneous needle localization determines the area for an open biopsy if a mass is very small, for example, those detected by a mammogram alone. The lesion is localized in the radiology department. A thin needle is passed into the area in question that has been identified by mammography. A second mammogram confirms the position of the lesion. The needle is secured in place with tape, and the woman is taken to the operating room, where an open biopsy is immediately performed. Frozen-section examination may be done for rapid diagnosis.

Before a breast biopsy, explain the purpose of the biopsy to the client and obtain her consent. Restrict food and fluids if IV sedation is to be used. Discuss the post-procedure self-care activities that the client should follow. Most women fear that the biopsy will result in a finding of cancer; some clients will ask about what will happen if cancer is found (see Chapter 42).

After the biopsy, instruct the woman to report any bleeding, swelling, or evidence of infection. After a needle biopsy, normal activity can be resumed as soon as it is comfortable to do so. Vigorous activity should be avoided for 1 to 2 weeks after an open biopsy. The woman may find it more comfortable to wear a supportive brassiere 24 hours a day until the site is healed so long as the wires and elastic do not rub on the incision.

THE MALE REPRODUCTIVE SYSTEM

Disorders of the male reproductive and urinary tract (which is closely associated with the reproductive tract) occur in men of all ages. Assessing these disorders requires expertise in conducting the health history interview and physical examination. Be sensitive and tactful because many men are uncomfortable discussing issues associated with these disorders. Discuss lifestyle factors that affect health maintenance, such as diet, exercise, adequate sleep and rest, stress management, smoking cessation, and identification of individual risk factors. If appropriate, provide information about protection against STDs. Explain what is involved in the physical examination, use easily understood terms, and discuss any diagnostic tests that may be indicated.

HISTORY

A complete health history, including sexual and reproductive systems, and physical examination are necessary for men experiencing reproductive disorders. History-taking provides an opportunity to achieve the following:

- Allow men to express sensitive concerns
- Identify and dispel myths and misinformation
- Teach health information
- Offer referrals
- Facilitate further communication

The following discussion addresses the major risk factors pertinent to men's reproductive health history.

Biographical and Demographic Data

Review the client's biographical and demographic data to determine his health risk status. Age, race, and occupation all have health risk implications. Men over 50 years of age may have benign prostatic hypertrophy (BPH), an enlargement of the prostate gland. Men younger than age 40 who have manifestations that resemble those of BPH are more likely to have prostatitis. African-American men and those over 40 years of age are at increased risk for adenocarcinoma of the prostate. Younger men, particularly those between ages 25 and 35, have a higher incidence of testicular cancer. Occupations and activities that involve prolonged, strenuous lifting or straining can provoke hernias. Exposure to some chemicals and pesticides may be linked to fertility and reproductive disorders.

Current Health: The Chief Complaint

The client may present with problems related to the genitourinary or reproductive system or to sexuality. A chief complaint may include the following areas:

- Systemic disturbances, such as weight loss, fever, and malaise
- Voiding disturbances, such as frequency, polyuria, oliguria, nocturia, pyuria, enuresis, dysuria, urgency, or incontinence
- Disturbances in urine characteristics, such as hematuria and pyuria
- Gastrointestinal disturbances, such as nausea, vomiting, anorexia, abdominal discomfort, constipation, or diarrhea
- Reproductive disturbances, infertility, history of STDs, genital lesions, or genital discharge in self and partner; genital trauma
- Sexual functioning (whether the client is sexually active or celibate), such as changes in libido;

changes in erectile ability; decreased ejaculatory ability; gynecomastia (breast enlargement); and the effects of disability, chronic disease, trauma, surgery, or treatment

For each reported manifestation, conduct a symptom analysis (see Chapter 4).

Past Health History

Significant health history for the male reproductive system includes childhood and infectious diseases, immunizations, major illnesses and hospitalizations, medications, and allergies.

Childhood and Infectious Diseases

The most significant childhood infectious disease to affect male fertility is mumps. Its occurrence in young men is associated with sterility. Ask whether the client has ever had mumps or been immunized against it. Question the client also about the presence of cryptorchidism at birth and the age at which the testicles descended or were brought down surgically.

Major Illnesses and Hospitalizations

Ask about major illnesses, such as diabetes, hypertension, stroke, and MI. Men who have diabetes commonly have problems with potency related to the accompanying neurologic and vascular changes. Hypertension and stroke can cause impotence related to physiological or psychological factors. Impotence may also occur in men who have had an MI because they fear having another episode as a result of sexual excitement and activity.

Urinary tract disorders can interfere with sexual functioning because of the close proximity of anatomic structures. Endocrine disorders can also affect sexual performance. Be alert to the man's concerns and fears, remain nonjudgmental, and offer the support of counseling and referral to peer groups established for this purpose.

Ask the client about any previous surgery involving the reproductive system, such as herniorrhaphy, vasectomy, prostatectomy, varicocelectomy, orchiopexy, and testicular torsion repair.

Medications

Obtain a complete medication history for prescription, over-the-counter, and recreational drugs; nutritional supplements; and herbal remedies. Some medications prescribed for hypertension (methyldopa, clonidine, guanethidine, and hydralazine) can cause impotence. Tranquilizers can interfere with sexual performance. Other medications can decrease sperm count and motility. Recreational drugs (marijuana and hallucinogens) that alter behavior can also affect physiologic reproductive function and may raise the risk of STDs. Herbs frequently used to treat reproductive disorders include saw palmetto *(Serenoa repens)* for BPH and yohimbe *(Pausinystalia yohimbe)* for erectile dysfunction and impotence.

Allergies
Ask the client about allergies to antibiotics, rubber, or latex. Male genitourinary disorders are often treated with antibiotics, and latex and rubber are found in condoms as well as in examination gloves commonly worn during the physical examination. If the man is allergic to latex, wear vinyl gloves.

Sexual and Reproductive History
A sexual and reproductive history includes questions about breasts, contraceptives, sexual practices, genitourinary problems, and reproductive health practices (see Chapter 4).

Breast History
Collect data about the breasts and axillae. Ask about breast pain, masses, skin changes, and nipple discharge. Ask whether the man has noticed any changes in breast tissue, such as enlargement. Gynecomastia can occur in obese or older men and as a side effect of some medications. Ask whether the client performs BSE, similar to the technique taught to women.

Contraceptive History
Document the man's current contraceptive method (if any), his satisfaction with the method, the effect of contraception on sexual function, and any desire to change methods. Has the man used contraceptive methods previously? If so, did any problems lead to their discontinuation?

Sexual History
Inquire about the client's patterns of sexual relationships. Can the man relate the total number of sexual partners he has had and the frequency of sexual activity? Multiple partners and contacts increase the client's risk of STDs. Does the man use condoms during sexual intercourse? Does he have homosexual or bisexual relationships, both of which increase the risk of human immunodeficiency virus (HIV) infection?

Does the client have any sexual concerns, such as an inability to attain or maintain an erection? If so, does this problem occur frequently or occasionally? Is the client able to discuss sexual concerns with his partner? Have he and his partner developed ways to cope with or adjust to disturbances in sexual function? If sexual dysfunction exists, does the client want a referral to, or consultation with, a sex counselor?

Throughout the interview, ask questions directly. Phrase questions in a neutral, nonjudgmental way. This interview technique helps preserve dignity and self-esteem instead of fostering guilt or shame. The website provides further information on sexuality assessment. *evolve*

Genitourinary History
Ask about past problems with genitourinary infections, such as prostatitis. Determine whether the client has had a previous pelvic examination. Does he have such problems as urinary incontinence, dribbling, hesitancy, a weak urinary stream, or other manifestations? Chapter 34 describes assessment of the urinary system.

Reproductive Health Practices
Inquire about sexual and reproductive hygiene. How often does the man examine his breasts (see Figures 2-4 and 39-2) and testes (Box 39-1)? Does he protect himself against STDs? Chapter 4 discusses health risk management.

Family Health History
Ask whether the client has a family history of infertility, diabetes, hypertension, strokes, or endocrine disorders. As with women whose mothers took DES during preg-

---

BOX 39-1   *Testicular Self-Examination*

Testicular self-examination (TSE) is a simple technique that men can use to assess for changes in their testicles that may signal testicular cancer. The risk is highest in adolescents and in men under age 35 years. As with BSE, the man should become familiar with the normal appearance and feel of his genitals to feel confident of his ability to perform TSE. Advise the man to schedule a regular time each month to assess his genitals. The best time is after bathing, because the warm water causes the scrotum to relax and makes the testicles easier to examine.

Teach the client to perform TSE as follows:
1. Hold the scrotum in the palms of your hands, and examine each testicle with the thumbs and fingers of both hands. The index and middle fingers should be on the underside of each testicle with the thumbs on the top.
2. The testicle is rolled between the thumb and fingers. A normal testicle is shaped like an egg and is about 4 cm (1⅗ inches) long. It feels firm but not hard (like an ear lobe) and should be smooth without lumps.
3. After examining the testicles, examine the epididymides (behind the testicles); they should be soft and may feel sponge-like.
4. Examine the spermatic cords, which ascend from the epididymides up into the body. They are normally firm, smooth tubular structures.

nancy, men who have been exposed to DES *in utero* are at increased risk for congenital anomalies, including structural defects of the genitourinary system and reduced semen quality.

Psychosocial History

Assess the client's occupation, environment, habits, and psychosocial factors.

Occupation and Environment

Determine the client's type of work and recreational activities to identify any exposure to chemicals, pesticides, heat, heavy metals, hormones, and radiation. These materials can directly affect the number and integrity of sperm and the quality of germinal tissue.

Habits

Assess the client's use of caffeine, alcohol, tobacco, and recreational drugs, including marijuana. These substances may affect the sperm count, contribute to impotence, decrease libido, or encourage risk-taking behaviors. Physical and recreational sports can put the client at risk for genital trauma if protective gear is not used.

Psychosocial Factors

Review the following subjects when conducting a health history interview with a man who has a reproductive disturbance. You may not be able to obtain detailed information in each of these areas, but the outline should help you to view each man and his significant others as individuals and to avoid stereotypical and possibly judgmental nursing care. Note the following:

1. *Self-concept.* How has the client's health affected how he feels about himself? How do his partner and significant others feel about him? What is his posture, dress, grooming? What is his emotional response? What is his mood? His tone?
2. *Role relationships.* Who are the important people in this client's life? Who accompanied him to the health care facility? Who is his most significant other? How is he able to carry out his various social roles (partner, husband, friend, father, worker)? How has his health affected his economic situation and his partner or significant others?
3. *Communication.* How does the client communicate, both verbally and nonverbally, with you and his significant others? Does he maintain eye contact? Does he use gestures or touch? How does he speak (volume, tone, vocabulary, repetition)?
4. *Value system.* What values, opinions, and beliefs does the client hold? What is his predominant lifestyle? What is his cultural or subcultural background?

5. *Coping and stress tolerance.* Who supports and nurtures the client? Does he experience intimacy with anyone? How connected is the client with significant others? What supports and resources does he have? How does he spend his leisure time? To what extent does he engage in physical activity or exercise?
6. *Cognitive-perceptual.* How does the client use words? Can he read? What is his level of comprehension? What is his major source of information about reproductive health?

Review of Systems

Ask about diabetes, hypertension, stroke, angina, MI, endocrine disorders, renal disorders, and urinary tract problems. Detailed questions for the review of systems may be found on the website for this textbook.

PHYSICAL EXAMINATION

Skillful history-taking helps to establish a therapeutic relationship that facilitates physical examination. Many men find physical examination of the reproductive system stressful and embarrassing. Some men may view the genitals as private or unclean.

Help the client become more comfortable by sharing normal findings while you proceed. Explain each step. Increase the client's comfort by maintaining eye contact, proceeding in an unhurried manner, and involving the client in self-examination. Occasionally, a man will have an erection during an examination. A kind, professional manner and a firm yet gentle touch lessen this possibility. If the man does have an erection, explain that this is normal and does not have sexual connotation.

The physical examination focuses on findings that may be associated with reproductive or sexual disorders. These may include the following disorders:

- Inflammatory, such as enlarged, tender, movable, or fixed lymph nodes in the inguinal region
- Endocrine and genetic, including indications of such conditions as Cushing's syndrome or acromegaly, hair distribution, and gynecomastia
- Neurologic, including a gross neurologic examination of the legs
- Vascular, including the femoral and pedal pulses
- Traumatic, such as a hernia

Follow an orderly sequence for the physical examination, and teach the client how to perform similar self-examinations regularly. The male breasts and axillae are included here as part of the reproductive system examination.

Breasts and Axillae

Examine the client's breasts and axillary nodes. Although the incidence of breast cancer in men is low, it can occur because men have glandular tissue beneath each nipple.

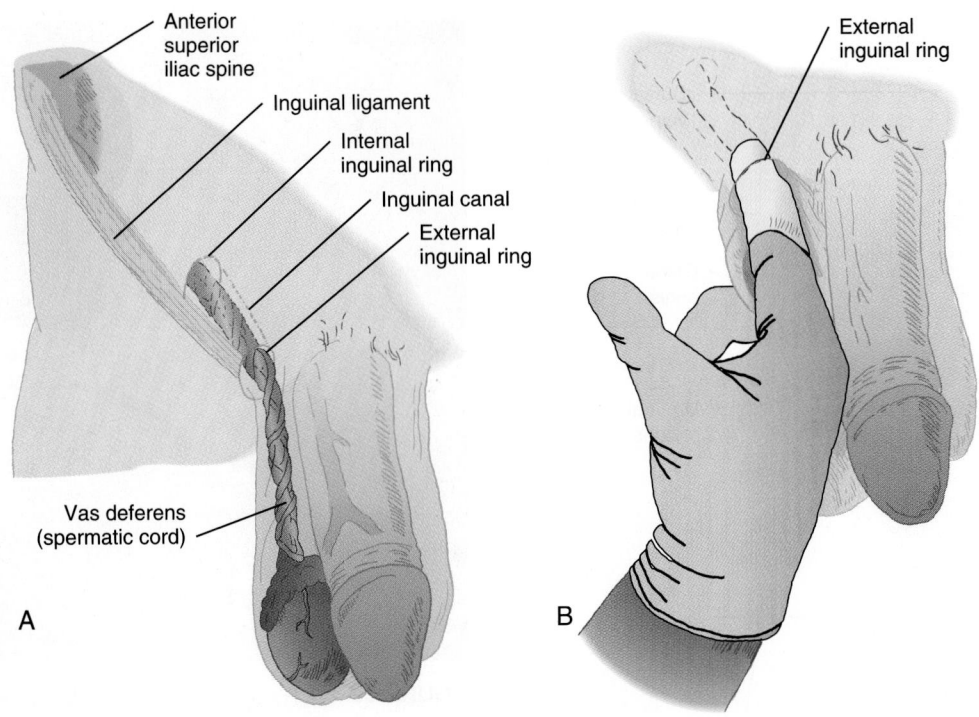

FIGURE 39-9 **A**, Anatomy of male inguinal structures. **B**, Palpation to detect an indirect hernia.

Inspect and palpate the breasts and axillae while the man is sitting, following the same guidelines as for the female breast examination. The male breast is flat and symmetrical, without nodules, edema, or ulceration. One-sided (unilateral) breast enlargement that persists beyond puberty is abnormal. Palpation reveals a small, flat disk of glandular tissue under the areola. No masses or discharge should be present. Axillary nodes should be nonpalpable (see Figure 39-2).

External Genitalia

The client's urinary bladder should be empty. The client may be supine or lying on his side with his legs spread slightly for the first portion of the genital examination; ask him to stand during the assessment for inguinal herniation. Alternatively, the client might stand for the entire examination of the genitals while you remain seated. Because the male urethra is the common conduit for both urine and semen, examination of the male reproductive tract also includes assessment of the urinary system. Wear nonsterile, disposable examining gloves.

Inspect the external genitalia and perineum (Figure U9-4, *A*), observing the pubic hair and skin. You must be familiar with normal growth and development of the male genitalia. Observe general appearance and body build. Note the hair distribution. Pubic hair distribution in men is triangular, with hair covering the symphysis pubis, base of the penis, and inner aspects of the thighs. Hair distribution may also spread toward the umbilicus in a diamond pattern. Inspect hair for nits and the skin for parasites, rashes, excoriation, and lesions. Masses, lesions, edema, and offensive odors should be absent. Scrotal skin is darker than other skin surfaces and is loose and wrinkled.

The penis includes the penile shaft, prepuce (foreskin), glans, and urethral meatus (Figure 39-9). Inspect and palpate these structures for lesions, nodules, swelling, inflammation, atrophy, and discharge. Penile skin in a flaccid penis is wrinkled. The foreskin, if present, covers the glans. The foreskin is absent in a circumcised client (Figure 39-10). Instruct the client to retract the foreskin to expose the glans, which is easily accomplished. You may see a small amount of cheesy, thick, white, odoriferous smegma between the glans and the foreskin; it is normal. If other discharge is noted, obtain a specimen for culture. The area between the glans and foreskin is a common site of venereal lesions. The area is normally free of lesions; if any are present, palpate them for tenderness, size, shape, and consistency, then change gloves before proceeding.

Next inspect the urethral meatus, located at the tip of the penis. It looks like a slit. Malposition of the meatus on either the underside of the penile shaft *(hypospadias)* or upper side *(epispadias)* is usually a congenital condition. The meatus is pink and without ulcers, scars, inflammation, or discharge. Gently compress the glans between your thumb and index finger to open the meatus, and inspect for discharge. If the client reports a urethral discharge, ask the client to compress the penis from base to tip between his thumb and fingers in an attempt to express

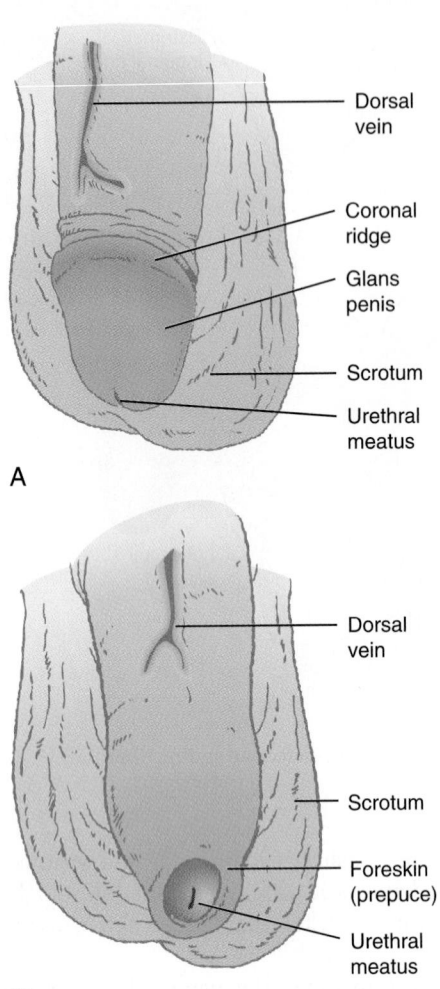

- Dorsal vein
- Coronal ridge
- Glans penis
- Scrotum
- Urethral meatus

A

- Dorsal vein
- Scrotum
- Foreskin (prepuce)
- Urethral meatus

B

FIGURE 39-10 Appearance of a circumcised (**A**) and an uncircumcised (**B**) penis.

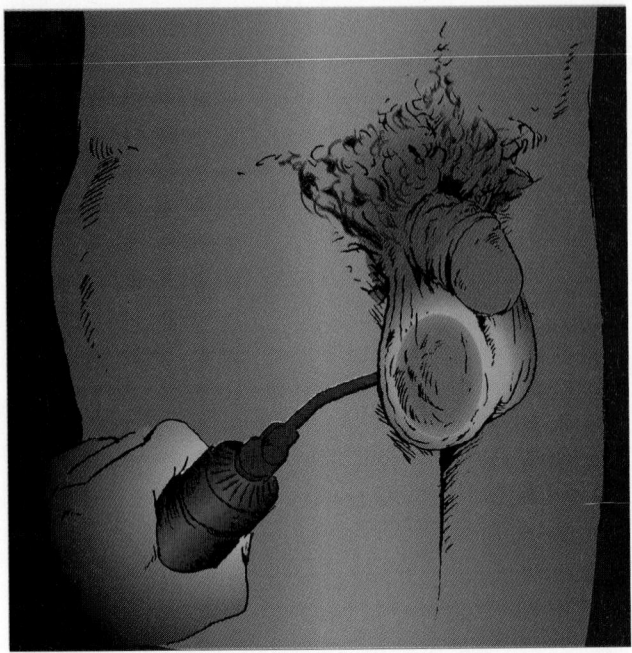

FIGURE 39-11 Transillumination of the scrotum. In a darkened room, place a strong, lighted flashlight or transilluminator next to the scrotum, as shown. Light normally passes through the scrotum (transillumination), but this does not occur with testicular tumor. A hydrocele shines red.

a discharge. If one appears, obtain a specimen for culture or microscopic examination. You may need to change gloves again before continuing with the examination.

Palpate the penile shaft gently between your thumb and first two fingers. It is smooth and semifirm, and the skin should move easily over underlying structures. The normal penis is free of nodules, thickened or hard areas, and tenderness.

Inspect the scrotum and palpate for symmetry, size, shape, and swelling. Size and shape vary from one individual to another. The scrotum has a right and a left half, each containing a testis, epididymis, and vas deferens. The left testis hangs lower than the right. Scrotal size varies with ambient temperature; cold results in contraction, warmth in relaxation. Ask the client to hold the penis to one side and then the other and to lift the scrotum up for inspection. The skin should be loose, without tension. The testes are ovoid, about $\frac{4}{5} \times 1\frac{3}{5}$ inches (2 × 4 cm). On palpation they are normally smooth, firm, and rubbery and without nodules, masses, or tenderness. Older clients have smaller, less firm testes.

In younger, adolescent males, note whether both testes are present in the scrotum. Testes may temporarily migrate from being touched during examination or being exposed to cold air. They may be palpable later in the examination, when the client is more relaxed. If a testis is not apparent, palpate the femoral and inguinal area. If the client has an undescended testis, refer him to an appropriate health care provider. A small (pea-sized), hard lump located on either the anterior or lateral aspect of a testis suggests a malignancy; again, refer the client for follow-up. Compare the testes bilaterally for similarity.

Palpate each epididymis between your thumb and index finger. The epididymis is located on the superior aspect of the testis and extends down the posterior surface. It feels soft, resilient, and tender. Swelling and hardness are abnormal. The vas deferens (spermatic cord) begins at the superior, lateral aspect of the testis. It is differentiated from the epididymis by its firmer, tubular feel. Compare findings bilaterally. Palpate the vas deferens along its length toward the inguinal canal. Note any thickening and asymmetry, which are abnormal.

If you find swelling, nodules, or other abnormalities during the scrotal examination, perform transillumination of the scrotum (Figure 39-11). Darken the room, and shine a flashlight through the scrotum from behind the mass. A scrotum filled with serous fluid will transilluminate as a red glow. More solid lesions, such as a hematoma or a mass, do not transilluminate and may be seen as a dark shadow. Record the characteristics of the abnormality, including whether it transilluminates.

While the client is standing, examine for an inguinal hernia (a prolapse or protrusion of a loop of intestine through the inguinal wall or canal). Inspect the inguinal areas for bulges while the client stands quietly and again after he bears down and strains as though attempting a bowel movement. Bulges should be absent.

A *direct* inguinal hernia enters the inguinal canal behind the external ring because of a weakened abdominal wall; it does not pass through the inguinal canal. Assess for a direct hernia by gently inserting an index finger into the loose scrotal skin over the external inguinal ring; the finger does not enter to the external ring. Use the left index finger to palpate the client's right side and the right finger for the client's left side while he faces you. Instruct the client to bear down while you feel for a bulge, which should be absent.

An *indirect* inguinal hernia enters the inguinal canal through the internal ring and can remain in the canal or pass down through the external ring and into the scrotum. To palpate for an indirect hernia, gently invaginate the scrotal skin with the index or little finger, following the vas deferens to where it passes into the external ring (Figure 39-9, *B*). Ask the client to flex the knee on that same side to help relax the muscles so that the finger can be inserted through the external ring and into the inguinal canal. Advance the palpating finger as far as possible, and instruct the client to bear down while you feel for a tissue mass touching the finger. The mass retreats up the canal when the client relaxes.

A *femoral* hernia, which is more common in women, occurs inferiorly and more laterally compared with an inguinal hernia; it often has the appearance of an enlarged inguinal lymph node. Palpate the inguinal area directly for a femoral hernia while the client is relaxed and again after instructing him to bear down. A palpable mass should be absent. Surgical repair of hernias is discussed in Chapter 35.

Prostate

After examining the anterior genitalia, assess the anus, rectum, and prostate gland. A rectal-prostatic examination should be performed annually in men over the age of 50 years (over 45 in high-risk clients) to look for manifestations of an STD, changes in the size and consistency of the prostate gland, and evidence of a tumor or acute or chronic infection. Emphasize the importance of regular examinations as the best way to detect prostatic cancer for effective treatment.

Just before the examination, ask the client to empty his bladder, and collect a urine specimen at this time if one is needed. Explain that an empty bladder makes the examination more comfortable and more accurate. Also explain that it is normal to experience sensations of having to urinate or defecate during the examination.

Two possible positions for the client during the rectal examination are the knee-chest position, with the buttocks elevated, or bending over from the hip, with elbows placed either on the knees or on the examining table. (Positions are discussed in Chapter 4, and the anal and rectal examination is discussed in Chapter 34.)

Wear gloves and apply water-soluble lubricant to the examining finger. Place your dominant hand on the client's hip to stabilize his position and to reassure him. Gently spread his buttocks with the nondominant hand. Observe the perineum and perianal areas for lesions, hemorrhoids, inflammation, or discoloration. Ask the client to bear down. Explain that this helps relax the anal sphincter and makes it easier to insert the examining finger.

Insert the ball of the finger toward the anterior wall of the rectum. The normal prostate is located 2 to 5 cm beyond the anal sphincter along the anterior wall of the rectum. It is normally about 4 cm long and 5 cm wide (Figure U9-4, *B*). The prostate is shaped like a doughnut wrapped around the neck of the urethra. Only the posterior and lateral lobes can be felt through the rectal wall (Figure 39-12, *A*). The lateral lobes should be symmetri-

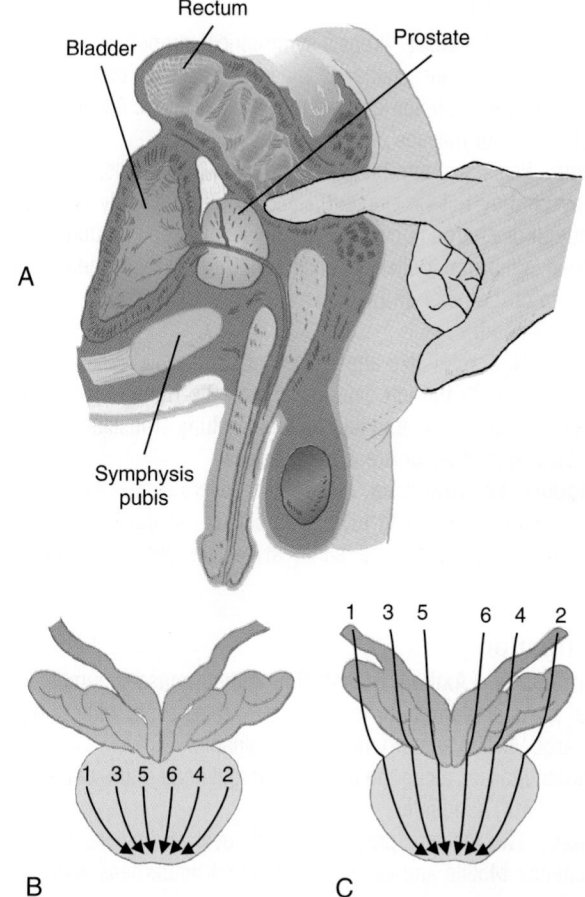

FIGURE 39-12 Rectal-prostatic assessment. **A,** Rectal examination. Insert a gloved index finger into the anus while the client is bearing down. Palpate all surfaces. **B,** Prostatic massage. Roll the pad of the index finger across the prostate, starting laterally and superiorly and moving toward the midline of the prostate. **C,** Seminal vesicles and prostatic massage. Use the same technique as for prostatic massage, but extend the finger over the area of the seminal vesicles.

cal. A normal prostate feels smooth, rubbery, and firm, somewhat like the base of the thumb. In a man with BPH, the prostate feels larger than normal, with a firmer consistency, like that of the chin. Tenderness and bogginess (like the cheek of the face) may indicate acute or chronic prostatitis. Carcinoma feels like a stone or hard nodule, that is, a circumscribed area of induration. Any induration is abnormal. The seminal vesicles (superior and lateral to the prostate) are normally nonpalpable.

Prostatic massage may be indicated even when the client is asymptomatic to aid in the detection of prostatitis. Roll the pad of your index finger across the prostate gland, starting laterally and superiorly and moving to-

---

PHYSICAL ASSESSMENT FINDINGS IN THE HEALTHY ADULT
The Male Reproductive System

Inspection
Breasts and Axillae. Breasts symmetrical, smooth in all positions, without retractions or masses. Vascular pattern and striae absent. Nipples everted and areolae even. Axillae even color, without masses or rash.

Penis. Penis size and shape vary among individuals. Foreskin may or may not be present. Head of penis slightly rounded without discharge (if client is circumcised). Smegma under the foreskin (normal if client is uncircumcised). Urinary meatus at the tip of the head of the penis, free of discharge or drainage. Shaft smooth.

Scrotum. Scrotal size and shape vary normally. Hangs below the penis with the left side lower than the right. Scrotal skin thin and rugose. Sparse hair on the scrotum. Transillumination shows no masses or areas of thickness.

Inguinal-Femoral Area. Coarse hair covers symphysis pubis, inner thighs, extending toward umbilicus. No bulges over the inguinal or femoral area either at rest or with coughing or straining.

Palpation
Breasts and Axillae. Breasts firm without masses, lumps, local areas of warmth, or tenderness. Nipples even, without discharge. Axillae smooth, nodes nonpalpable.

Penis. Masses along the penile shaft and head of the penis absent. Firm, nontender.

Testis. Two testicles present, smooth, oval, and similar in consistency. Mobile and equal in size. Slight tenderness with palpation.

Epididymis. Present at the posterior of the scrotum (found in the anterolateral or anterior area of the testis in a small percentage of men). No tenderness.

Vas Deferens. Cord-like, mobile, smooth, and nontender. No masses.

Inguinal Canal. No bulge or mass in inguinal canal either at rest or with straining.

---

ward the midline of the prostate (Figure 39-12, *B*). Then strip (or "milk") the area of the seminal vesicles, starting laterally and superiorly, toward the midline (Figure 39-12, *C*). Send the resulting meatal secretions for microscopic examination. A large number of pus cells suggests prostatitis. Staining may identify acid-fast organisms. Cultures may be needed to identify organisms such as gonococcal, chlamydial, or tuberculosis bacilli. If a culture is required, the glans of the penis must be cleaned and the bladder emptied to clear the urethra before prostatic massage. Collect meatal secretions in sterile culture media.

Withdraw your finger from the rectum, and observe for stool on the glove. Feces, if present, are normally brown. Mucus or blood and black, tarry, light tan, or gray stools are abnormal. Test the stool sample for occult (hidden) blood, which should be absent (see Chapter 34). If you suspect an STD, obtain a rectal swab for culture. Wipe the perianal area, and inform the client that the examination is complete. For an example of a recorded examination of the male reproductive tract, see the Physical Assessment Findings in the Healthy Adult feature on The Male Reproductive System at left.

DIAGNOSTIC TESTS

Various diagnostic tests are available to assess for disorders of the male reproductive system. Men and their significant others are often anxious about diagnostic tests. You can help to reduce anxiety by giving careful explanations before and during the tests. It is much less frightening if a client knows what to expect and what is included in the process. Sedation or pain reduction may be required before a test. An informed consent may be necessary. Physiologic preparations may be required, such as fasting or an enema. During the test, tell the client what is happening. Help him maintain the required positions. Observe him during and after the test for adverse reactions, such as pain, excessive anxiety, pallor, or nausea.

Laboratory Studies

Blood Studies
Prostate cancer screening has been revolutionized by the prostate-specific antigen (PSA) assay. PSA, a glycoprotein produced by the prostate gland and found in prostatic fluid, aids the liquefaction of semen. Normal PSA levels are less than 2.6 ng/ml.[6] The PSA level increases with age. PSA levels may also be elevated with BPH or prostatitis. When a PSA is 2.6 to 10 ng/ml, the likelihood of prostate cancer is judged as moderate, but values greater than 10 ng/ml indicate a high level of suspicion. Prostatic massage, urethral instrumentation (such as catheterization or cystoscopy), or rectal examination within 48 hours before the assay can cause elevated PSA levels.[6]

Several additional tests are available: (1) PSA *density* (PSAD), (2) PSA *velocity* (PSAV), and (3) fractionated PSA. PSA density relates PSA level to prostate size.[6] The

PSA density test is combined with transrectal ultrasonography (TRUS) to determine prostate volume. Scores are calculated by dividing the PSA by the prostate volume. Men who have PSA density levels less than 0.15 ng/ml are considered unlikely to have significant prostate cancer. As PSA levels rise, however, the presence of cancer cells is more likely. PSA velocity involves the rate of change in PSA level over time. Men who have a PSA velocity that rises more than 0.7 ng/ml per year or that increases 20% or more a year are considered at high risk of having prostate cancer. Fractionated PSA measures free versus protein-bound PSA in blood. Men with prostate cancer have a higher proportion of PSA bound to protein; the proportion of free PSA is higher in men with BPH. Other PSA testing methods are being investigated.[6]

Semen Examination

Semen testing is used to evaluate fertility. One to three samples of semen, collected at intervals of 2 to 4 weeks, are examined to accommodate for normal variations. To provide an adequate sample, the client should abstain from ejaculation for 2 to 5 days before the test. Prolonged abstinence may decrease sperm quality and motility, whereas more frequent ejaculations reduce sperm concentration and volume.

In the laboratory or office, the client masturbates into a clean, dry specimen container. Using ordinary condoms or coitus interruptus is not an appropriate method because contamination or loss of the specimen is likely. If the client must collect the specimen outside the laboratory or office, the specimen should be kept at room temperature and brought to the laboratory within 30 minutes of collection.

Semen analysis is used to assess infertility and to evaluate the effectiveness of a vasectomy. Tests for infertility include a sperm count, morphology, and motility along with semen pH, viscosity, appearance, and volume. If abnormalities are found, further analysis for the presence of antibodies can also be performed. If the test is being done to evaluate the effectiveness of a vasectomy, the presence or absence of sperm is sufficient.

Secretion Analysis

Secretions from the throat, penis, and anus or lesions from the oral, pharyngeal, and perineal areas may be examined for microorganisms. A sterile, cotton-tipped applicator is placed on or in the affected area, and the specimen is transferred to a sterile tube or slide. Be careful not to touch any other surface with the applicator.

Radiography

Both CT scanning and MRI are used to assess male reproductive and urologic disorders. Procedures include clinical staging of testicular and prostate cancers and imaging of pelvic organs for epididymitis, hydrocele, sper-

matocele, scrotal hernia, or testicular torsion and infarction. Chapter 4 covers these diagnostic procedures.

Ultrasonography

A transrectal approach is used in prostatic ultrasonography. The rectum must be free of feces. Help the client into a left lateral Sims position. After a rectal examination, a well-lubricated transducer is inserted. The probe is covered with a water-filled condom to enhance sound-wave transmission; a full bladder may also improve sound transmission. The examiner moves the probe along the prostate to complete the scan. Tell the client that some discomfort may be felt with probe insertion and manipulation. Once the probe has been removed, there should be no further discomfort.

Radionuclide Imaging

Radioisotope scans may be used to assess testicular abnormalities, such as torsion, epididymitis, abscess, tumors, hydroceles, varicoceles, and spermatoceles. A radioactive substance is administered intravenously, and several scans are taken. Before a scan is taken, ask the client whether he has a history of allergies.

Cystoscopy

Cystoscopy is indispensable for assessing and treating prostate and urologic problems. It is used to determine the cause of urinary manifestations, such as those related to prostatic hypertrophy, and to obtain specimens, such as in a transurethral prostatic biopsy. Cystoscopy can be done in a urologist's office or in an operating room before surgery. Inspection of the bladder interior includes looking for trabeculation, diverticula, and bladder neck contracture, and checking the size and contours of the prostatic lobes. Chapter 34 describes the procedure and client care in detail.

Urodynamic Assessment

Urodynamic studies measure pressure from the bladder or urethra, urinary flow, and striated muscle activity. Common tests include uroflowmetry, cystometry, electromyography, and a urethral pressure profile. They are useful in determining the cause of frequency and decreased urinary stream in men (as from prostatic obstruction). Chapter 34 describes urodynamic testing in detail.

Prostatic Biopsy

Areas of the prostate that suggest a problem are assessed by biopsy after abnormal findings in PSA level, TRUS, or digital rectal examination (DRE). Biopsy of the prostate allows cytologic examination for the presence of cancer. The tissue may be obtained by a transurethral, transrectal, or perineal approach. The client must understand the approach to be used, the preparation, and the procedure for it. Obtain an informed consent. Physical preparation often includes an enema for the transrectal or perineal approach. The client must void before the procedure.

For *the transurethral* approach, place the client in the lithotomy position. Local anesthesia is used. The biopsy tissue is removed through transurethral endoscopy. Even though direct visual guidance is used in this approach, malignant tissue may be missed. This is partly because prostate cancer commonly begins in the posterior lobe, making it more difficult to obtain a specimen by this approach.

For the *perineal* approach, the lithotomy position is usually used; a jackknife position is an alternative. After the perineal area is cleaned and anesthetized, one or more biopsies are taken. This approach allows direct access to the posterior lobe of the prostate. Direct pressure is applied to the area. If there is no bleeding, a sterile dressing is applied.

For a *transrectal* approach, place the client in Sims position. A rectal examination is performed to identify any hard nodules. The biopsy is performed with the examiner's finger as a guide. Some consider this approach to be inappropriate because malignant cells from the nodule may be seeded into the rectal mucosa.

After the procedure, monitor the client's vital signs at regular intervals to detect signs of hemorrhage. If a transurethral approach was used, some hematuria is normal, although frank bleeding should be reported. The client must be able to void after the procedure. With the perineal approach, carefully assess the dressing for blood. After a transrectal approach, monitor for bleeding or infection.

PREVENTION OF MALE REPRODUCTIVE PROBLEMS

Primary prevention (preventing a problem before it occurs) includes genetic counseling, immunization against infectious diseases, good nutrition, careful genital hygiene, the use of condoms to prevent STDs, knowing one's partner, avoiding multiple sex partners, and avoiding sexual intercourse (oral, anal, or genital) with a person who has genital lesions.

Secondary prevention (detecting and treating a problem early) includes screening activities, such as serum PSA levels in men over 50 years of age and testicular self-examination (TSE). See Chapter 2 for a discussion of BSE; TSE is discussed earlier in this chapter.

Tertiary prevention (avoiding complications and rehabilitation) is health care provided for clients experiencing acute and chronic disorders. For example, teaching perineal exercises after a prostatectomy helps men regain urinary control.

CONCLUSIONS

Assessment of the female and male reproductive systems requires knowledge of the physiologic and psychological implications associated with reproductive disorders. Exhibit a concerned, caring attitude when assessing any client with a reproductive disorder because these disorders are laden with psychosocial overtones. Assess the client in a thorough but matter-of-fact manner to put the client at ease and to expedite a complete assessment.

BIBLIOGRAPHY

1. American Cancer Society. (2003). *Cancer prevention and early detection.* Atlanta: Author.
2. American Cancer Society. (2003). *Cancer facts and figures.* Atlanta: Author.
3. Bast, R.C., et al. (2000). *Cancer medicine* (5th ed.). Hamilton, Ontario: B.C. Decker.
4. Bickley, L.S., Szilagyi, P.G., & Stackhouse, J.G. (2002). *Bates' guide to physical examination and history taking* (8th ed.). Philadelphia: Lippincott Williams & Wilkins.
5. Belinson, J., et al. (2001). Shanxi province cervical cancer screening study: A cross-sectional comparison trial of multiple techniques to detect cervical neoplasia. *Gynecologic Oncology, 83*(2), 439-444.
6. Gretzer, M., & Partin, A. (2003). *Campbell's urology updates: PSA and PSA molecular derivatives, 1*(1), 1-12.
7. Hutchinson, M.L., et al. (1999). Utility of liquid-based cytology for cervical carcinoma screening. *Cancer Cytopathology, 87*(2), 48-55.
8. Jarvis, C. (2000). *Physical examination and health assessment* (3rd ed.). Philadelphia: Elsevier.
9. Kee, J.L. (2001). *Laboratory and diagnostic tests with nursing implications* (6th ed.). Old Tappan, NJ: Prentice Hall.
10. Krane, J.F., et al. (2001). Papanicolaou smear sensitivity for the detection of adenocarcinoma of the cervix. *Cancer Cytopathology, 93*(1), 8-15.
11. Scott, J.R., Hammond, C., & Gordon, J. D. (2003). *Danforth's handbook of obstetrics and gynecology* (2nd ed.). Philadelphia: Lippincott Williams & Wilkins.
12. Seidman, H., et al. (1987). Survival experience in the breast cancer detection demonstration project. *CA: A Cancer Journal for Clinicians, 39*(5), 258-291.
13. Walsh, P.C., et al. (2002). *Campbell's urology* (8th ed.). Philadelphia: Elsevier.

Management of Men with Reproductive Disorders

Mikel Gray

Today men are more actively involved in health maintenance as evidenced by their increased interest in fitness and exercise, increased attainment of lifestyle factors related to fitness (such as smoking cessation), and increased participation in childbirth and parenting. With the recent emphasis on prostate health and prostate cancer, these interests have expanded to incorporate issues of reproductive and urinary health maintenance. Armed with knowledge about risk factors, preventive measures, and improvements in disease management, men are more likely to engage in preventive health-promoting behaviors and participate in health screening and early detection programs designed to avoid the morbidity and mortality associated with delayed diagnosis and management of common chronic diseases.

This increased attention to health promotion behaviors in adult males has provoked health care professionals, including nurses, to champion the concept of "men's health" services or clinics using similar strategies to those that have evolved in women's health services. Disorders of the genitourinary system are an important component of men's health. Nevertheless, men are often reluctant to ask for help because they regard such problems as a potential threat to their sexuality or identity as a man. Some men may also fear negative reactions from their health care providers because of their age or sexual preference.

Because of this reluctance to seek help, skillful therapeutic interaction is essential to help men express their concerns. Sensitivity to fear and embarrassment, respect for privacy and confidentiality, careful history taking, and addressing information needs help to put male clients at ease. When the client allows, partners should be brought into management plan discussions because most reproductive and genital disorders affect relationships.

Statements such as "Many men are concerned about how this problem will affect their sex lives," "It is common to worry about how your partner might feel about this problem," and "What are some of your concerns?" may help the client begin to talk about his concerns.

Giving men permission to express their feelings and their health-related concerns draws them and their significant others into the process of health care. Having topic-related brochures visible may provide the impetus for a man to ask questions.

evolve *Be sure to check out the bonus material on the Evolve website and the CD-ROM, including free self-assessment exercises.*
http://evolve.elsevier.com/Black/medsurg/

Nursing Outcomes Classification (NOC)
for Nursing Diagnoses—Men with Reproductive Disorders

Acute Pain
  Comfort Level
  Pain Control
  Pain: Disruptive Effects
  Pain Level
Impaired Urinary Elimination and Urinary Retention
  Urinary Continence
  Urinary Elimination

Ineffective Therapeutic Regimen Management
  Compliance Behavior
  Knowledge: Treatment Regimen
  Participation: Health Care Decisions
  Treatment Behavior: Illness or Injury
Risk for Injury: Postoperative Complications
  Circulation Status
  Electrolyte and Acid/Base Balance

Fluid Balance
Risk Control
Risk Detection
Safety Status: Physical Injury
Symptom Control
Tissue Perfusion: Abdominal Organs
Tissue Perfusion: Peripheral
Urinary Continence
Urinary Elimination
Vital Signs Status

PROSTATE DISORDERS
BENIGN PROSTATIC HYPERPLASIA

The prostate is the genital organ most commonly affected by benign and malignant neoplasms. Benign enlargement of the prostate gland is an extremely common process that occurs in nearly all men with functioning testes. The term *benign prostatic hyperplasia* or *hypertrophy* (BPH) is used to describe the disorder that occurs when the prostate growth sufficiently obstructs (blocks or encroaches upon) the urethral outlet resulting in bothersome lower urinary tract symptoms (LUTS), urinary tract infection (UTI), hematuria, or compromised upper urinary tract function. Histologic evidence of prostate enlargement begins about the third decade of life and in- creases proportionally with aging. Specifically, about 43% of men in their 40s will have evidence of BPH, as will 50% of men in their 50s, 75% to 88% in their 80s, and nearly 100% of men reaching the ninth decade of life. The prevalence of BPH of sufficient magnitude to produce moderate to severely bothersome LUTS is lower, however, varying from about 17% of men in their 50s, 27% of men in their 60s, and 35% of men in their 70s. European and African Americans have similar prevalence rates of BPH, but Asian Americans tend to have lower rates of BPH. The incidence of BPH is lowest among immigrants, however, and it increases with subsequent generations, suggesting environmental as well as possible racial differences.

Etiology and Risk Factors

The etiology of BPH is partly understood. Whereas prostate enlargement is nearly universal in men with functioning testes, it is arrested following bilateral orchiectomy. Although androgens, and particularly testosterone, are not direct causes of BPH, their presence is

The authors would like to thank Patricia McCallig Bates for her contribution to this chapter in the sixth edition of *Medical-Surgical Nursing* and for her review of this edition's chapter.

critical to the normal growth and development of the prostate as well as BPH. Within the prostate, testosterone is converted to dihydrotestosterone (DHT) under the influence of an enzyme called 5-alpha reductase. DHT is the locally active form of testosterone that supports prostate growth and development throughout life, and the prostate remains sensitive to androgen production throughout life to maintain both prostate size and function. As a man ages and prostate enlargement occurs, 5-alpha reductase and DHT levels remain similar to those seen in younger men, but recent evidence has shown that the balance between two forms of this enzyme may be compromised, contributing to prostatic enlargement. Additional factors associated with BPH include a defect in local substances that regulate the programmed cellular death *(apoptosis)* common to many tissues within the body, including the skin and gastrointestinal tract. Imbalances of local growth factors, local inflammation, and genetic factors are also thought to influence the risk of BPH and the timing of its onset.

Multiple possible risk factors for BPH have been studied. For example, dietary factors have been examined, and lycopene in cooked tomatoes, green and yellow vegetables, and other elements of a traditional Japanese diet appear to provide some protection against BPH. Obesity (particularly an increased abdominal girth) may increase the risk for BPH, but diabetes mellitus appears to exert only a modest affect on the incidence of BPH or its severity. Smoking has been hypothesized to exert a protective effect on BPH because it reduces serum testosterone levels, but epidemiologic studies have shown that it has only a slight effect on BPH risk compared with the well-documented and severe adverse health risks associated with cigarette use. Heavy alcohol use and cirrhosis of the liver impede prostate enlargement. Frequent use of alpha-adrenergic agonists commonly found in over-the- counter cold medications or diet pills increases the severity of bothersome LUTS associated with BPH and the risk for acute urinary retention.

Pathophysiology

Histologic evidence of prostate enlargement alone does not constitute a clinically relevant problem. Instead, the clinical disorders associated with BPH occur when this enlargement obstructs the bladder outlet, leading to bothersome LUTS, an increased risk of urinary infection, and compromised upper urinary tract function. Two processes produce this obstruction: hyperplasia and hypertrophy. Hyperplasia originates in the glandular (stromal) cells near the urethra, the *transitional zone*. On the microscopic level, prostatic hyperplasia is nodular, but the effect on palpation is a symmetrically enlarged gland free from the palpable nodes characteristic of prostate cancer. Obstruction occurs when this hyperplasia narrows the lumen of the segment of the prostate that courses through the prostate (the *prostatic urethra*), when it encroaches upon the bladder neck reducing its ability to funnel in response to micturition, and when growth of the so-called median lobe of the prostate extends into the proximal urethra. BPH is also influenced by the prostatic capsule (connective tissue covering the gland); in some men the capsule allows hyperplasia to expand outward, increasing the size of the prostate rather than the severity of urethral compression and urinary obstruction. Hypertrophy of the smooth muscle of the prostate also contributes to urethral obstruction via both active and passive forces. Hyperplasia of the prostate is accompanied by hypertrophy of the smooth muscle of the gland; this is the rationale for the alternative description of BPH as benign prostatic hypertrophy. Smooth muscle hypertrophy exacerbates urinary obstruction by increasing muscle tone at the bladder neck and proximal (prostatic) urethra and by mechanically adding to the tissue constricting the urethral lumen.

Our understanding of the lower urinary tract and urethral obstruction remains incomplete, but it has grown significantly over the past decade (Figure 40-1). The bladder's initial response to increasing urethral resistance to outflow is to amplify the strength of the detrusor contraction. This strategy is often initially successful, leading many men to report relief from bothersome LUTS that may persist for a period of months to years. Further growth of the prostate and exacerbation of urethral obstruction, however, ultimately overwhelms the detrusor muscle's ability to ensure effective bladder evacuation by micturition. As a result, the man may note a decline in the force of the urinary stream, and feelings of incomplete bladder emptying despite urination. In addition to these LUTS, men tend to note bothersome LUTS that affect bladder filling, including daytime voiding frequency, nocturia and urgency. These LUTS are often associated with overactive detrusor contractions that may lead to urge urinary incontinence in some cases. It is these manifestations that typically provoke men to seek help from a health care professional. If the man does not

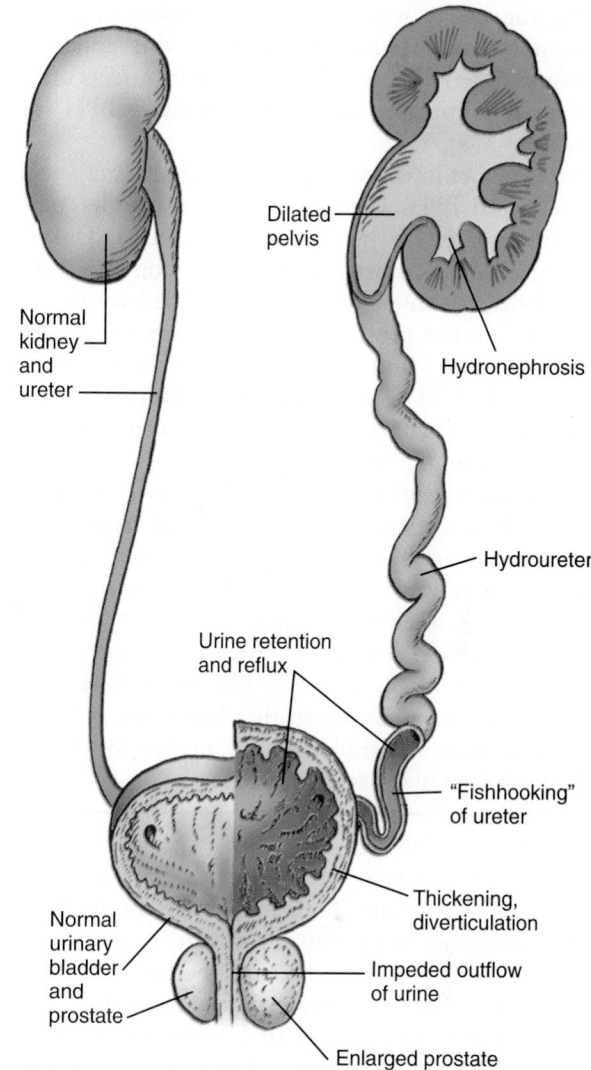

FIGURE 40-1 Complications of benign prostatic enlargement. *Left,* Normal kidney, ureter, bladder, and prostate. *Right,* Potential complications.

seek help for his bothersome LUTS and the process of prostatic enlargement continues, the detrusor eventually *decompensates,* leading to urinary residual volumes and, ultimately, to a weakened muscle contraction, even after relief from urethral obstruction. Alternatively, decompensation of the detrusor muscle may lead to an episode of *acute urinary retention,* defined as the complete inability to urinate. This condition is a medical emergency because uremia or bladder rupture and peritonitis will occur if the bladder is not relieved. In addition, acute urinary retention is associated with an increased risk of postoperative complications following surgical management of BPH.

A minority of men do not experience the bothersome LUTS described above, or they do not interpret these manifestations as indicating the need to seek care. When the obstruction associated with BPH is prolonged and severe, the client will experience compromised renal function or renal failure. Fortunately, this condition, sometimes referred to as *silent prostatism,* affects only a very small portion of men who experience BPH (i.e., fewer than 1%).

Urinary tract infection and hematuria also may be associated with BPH. Obstruction of the bladder outlet and urinary retention increase the risk of UTI. This risk is greatest when catheterization, cystoscopy, or transurethral surgery are performed that enable bacteria contained within the prostatic acini to reach the bladder. Urinary retention and obstruction also complicate the treatment of a UTI because incomplete bladder emptying compromises the complete evacuation of urine, bacteria, and toxins from the bladder.

The pathophysiology of hematuria caused by BPH is not entirely understood. It is known that *angiogenesis* (growth of blood vessels) is a part of hyperplasia and that these vessels may be prone to disruption and bleeding. Prolonged bleeding also may occur after catheterization, cystoscopy, or transurethral prostate surgery. The incidence of hematuria among men with BPH is unknown, but it has been noted that hematuria is the primary indication for transurethral surgery for BPH in 12% of all men diagnosed with BPH.

Clinical Manifestations

Bothersome LUTS provoke men with BPH and urethral obstruction to seek care. These manifestations usually develop slowly and may persist for months or years before the man defines them as sufficiently bothersome to seek help. Bothersome LUTS associated with bladder filling include *nocturia* (awakening from sleep because of the desire to urinate). Men younger than 65 years of age normally experience none or one episode of nocturia, and up to two episodes of nocturia is normal in men over age 65 years. In contrast, men with BPH often experience four or more episodes of nocturia per night that may lead to chronic sleep deprivation. Men with BPH also tend to report *daytime urinary frequency,* defined as urination more often than every 2 hours while awake and *urgency* (a sudden and severe desire to urinate). LUTS associated with micturition include hesitancy, a decline in the force of urinary stream, intermittent urinary stream, and feelings of incomplete bladder emptying. The severity of obstruction and bothersome LUTS caused by BPH is not related to the size of the enlargement. This lack of correlation occurs because physical assessment of prostate size is based on palpation of the exterior of the gland while the severity of obstruction and related BPH reflect a combination of active and passive factors.

Acute urinary retention is the complete inability to urinate. The client may report no urine output at all or dribbling leakage, called *overflow urinary incontinence.* Suprapubic discomfort and restlessness crescendo as the bladder fills beyond physiologic capacity (the volume at which a strong desire to urinate is perceived) and approaches anatomic capacity (the maximum volume the bladder can safely hold without imminent risk of rupture or other damage).

History-taking includes specific questions about daytime voiding frequency, nocturia, urgency, urinary incontinence, the force of the urine stream, hesitancy, need to strain, perception of bladder emptying, and prior episodes of acute urinary retention. The American Urological Association's International Prostate Symptom Score Index (IPSS) is a short questionnaire commonly used by urologists to assess the client's opinion about the severity of these manifestations (the IPSS appears in Figure 34-2). This instrument provides a reliable and valid description of bothersome LUTS associated with BPH, but it fails to differentiate LUTS caused by BPH from those caused by other, nonobstructive etiologies. It demonstrates good predictive validity (it accurately reflects the success of various treatments for the relief of bothersome LUTS).

A digital rectal examination (DRE) is performed to assess prostate size and to differentiate BPH from prostate enlargement owing to adenocarcinoma or infection. BPH reveals a symmetrically enlarged prostate with an obliterated central sulcus. Prostatic infection (prostatitis) is associated with symmetric enlargement, a boggy consistency, and discomfort on palpation. Adenocarcinoma of the prostate is associated with asymmetric enlargement, hardened nodules, or induration. Urinalysis and blood tests for kidney function (urea nitrogen or blood urea nitrogen [BUN] and creatinine) are routinely performed, and a urine culture or *prostate-specific antigen* (PSA) to assess for cancer are performed in selected cases. Chemistry panels, such as electrolyte, liver function, and blood coagulation studies, may be added if surgery is being considered.

Uroflowmetry may be completed to assess the voiding pattern and measure maximum and average flow rates. A man starts this test with a full bladder, voids into a specific toilet or container, and empties his bladder to the best of his ability. Residual urine is determined after the urine flow either by catheterization or by ultrasonography. A maximum urinary flow of 12 ml/sec or greater in a man aged 55 years or older greatly reduces the likelihood of urethral obstruction associated with BPH, but a voiding pressure flow study must be completed to measure definitively the severity of obstruction and to determine its cause. Depending on the severity of the client's manifestations and general medical condition, cystourethroscopy, intravenous pyelography (IVP), or urodynamic studies may be done (see Chapter 34).

Outcome Management
■ Medical Management

Medical management has become a common initial approach for BPH because it is noninvasive and effective in cases of mild to moderate obstruction. "Watchful waiting" is a relatively new approach to BPH, particularly for the client with mild LUTS assessed by IPSS. Ongoing assessment, including repeated measurement of a symptom score such as the IPSS, is necessary to determine whether the magnitude of bothersome LUTS increases or other complications (such as acute urinary retention) occur. An increase in IPSS score (reflecting exacerbation of voiding symptoms or high symptom score at baseline) indicates the need for more definitive treatment, as does the occurrence of a complication such as a UTI, hematuria, or episode of acute urinary retention. (See the Complementary and Alternative Therapy feature on Acupuncture Treatment for Benign Prostatic Hyperplasia on the website.)

Relax Prostate Muscle/Slow Prostate Growth. More aggressive medical treatment is aimed at reducing urethral obstruction by relaxing smooth muscle within the prostate, proximal urethra, and bladder neck or blocking the action of 5-alpha reductase, the enzyme that converts testosterone to DHT, allowing local growth of the prostatic stroma. See the Integrating Pharmacology feature on Medications for Benign Prostatic Hyperplasia at right.

In addition to the U.S. Food and Drug Administration (FDA)-approved drugs listed in the preceding section, a growing number of men use phytotherapeutic agents (use of herbs for healing purposes) to manage BPH. The most widely used agent is *Serenoa repens* (saw palmetto). Saw palmetto is derived from a dwarf palm tree that grows in the southwest United States; it contains a mixture of fatty acids, sterols (alcohol-based steroid), and flavonoids. Its principal action in relationship to BPH appears to be inhibition of 5-alpha reductase enzyme activities similar to the action of finasteride. (See the Complementary and Alternative Therapy feature on Saw Palmetto for Benign Prostatic Hyperplasia on the website.) Beta-sitosterol is extracted from *Hypoxis rooperi* (South African star grass) to form the primary active ingredient in Harzol and Azuprostat. Its actions on BPH are unknown, but it is hypothesized to inhibit one or more growth factors involved in prostatic hyperplasia. Nevertheless, at least two randomized, controlled trials show symptom relief among men taking these preparations compared with those taking placebo. Other agents purported to relieve bothersome LUTS associated with BPH include cough grass, pumpkin, pipsissewa, and pygeum (see the Complementary and Alternative Therapy feature on Pygeum Africanum Supplements for Benign Prostatic Hyperplasia on p. 1018.) Of these, pipsissewa is not recommended because dosages and its side effect profile have not been determined. Pumpkin has not been shown to be beneficial for managing BPH manifestations. The efficacy of pygeum compared with finasteride or saw palmetto has not been documented, and it should not be used in combination with other medica-

INTEGRATING PHARMACOLOGY
Medications for Benign Prostatic Hyperplasia

Medical management of benign prostatic hyperplasia (BPH) involves the use of medications that slow prostate growth or relax prostate muscle. Alpha-1-adrenergic blockers relax the smooth muscle of the prostate, bladder neck and proximal urethra. These drugs are often also used in the treatment of hypertension. Examples of medications in this category include terazosin (Hytrin), doxazosin (Cardura), and tamsulosin (Flomax). A 4-week treatment trial is needed to evaluate the maximum efficacy of these drugs. The medications are typically taken at bedtime because peak serum levels (and greatest risk for side effects) occur approximately 2 hours after administration. Orthostatic hypotension, dizziness, tachycardia, and nasal congestion are the most common side effects. A new drug, alfuzosin, soon to be released in the United States, has fewer side effects.

5-alpha-reductase inhibitors slow prostate growth by inhibiting the conversion of testosterone into dihydrotestosterone (DHT) in the prostate gland. Finasteride also lowers serum PSA levels and may mask the occurrence of prostate cancer. Examples of medication in this category include finasteride (Proscar) and dutasteride. These drugs must be taken for 6 to 12 months to assess maximum ability to relieve bothersome LUTS. Because 5-alpha-reductase also acts on hepatic tissue and finasteride is primarily metabolized by the liver, hepatic function tests are important before therapy is started. Side effects are mild and include a decrease in ejaculatory semen, decreased libido, and erectile dysfunction in about 1% to 5% of men taking this drug. These drugs can cause abnormal development of a male fetus. Hence, pregnant women should not handle the medication without gloves or come in contact with the semen of a man taking this drug.

Anti-androgens and LHRH antagonists, agents used to treat prostate cancer, have been tried in the treatment of BPH but the side effects outweigh the benefits for most men.

tions for BPH until studies assessing its safety in combination with these agents have been completed.

Relieve Retention. Acute urinary retention is initially managed by an indwelling catheter. It is usually left in place for 2 to 4 weeks to allow the bladder to recover from injury caused by the acute overdistension of the bladder wall associated with acute retention. Following this period, the client may be given a voiding trial. The bladder is filled with sterile water or saline, preferably heated to body temperature, and the catheter is removed. The client is then asked to urinate and the voided volume is compared with the infused volume to determine the efficiency of micturition. Alternatively, the

COMPLEMENTARY AND ALTERNATIVE THERAPY

Pygeum Africanum Supplements for Benign Prostatic Hyperplasia

Saw palmetto has the most evidence to date of any supplement for improving the manifestations of benign prostatic hyperplasia (BPH) or non-cancerous enlargement of the prostate. However, several other supplements may have some limited evidence. An analysis of all studies that included extracts of the African plum tree, or *Pygeum africanum,* was recently conducted. Researchers found that 18 studies met the selection criteria that included 1562 clients. However, only 5 trials ($n = 430$) provided information on a global assessment of improvement of clinical manifestations after treatment with this supplement, which was rated by physicians and not clients. In addition, most trials were short and did not compare this herbal product to standard prescription drugs. Therefore it is possible that this herb is providing nothing more than a placebo effect. Regardless, more men in the supplement versus placebo group had an overall improvement in manifestations rated by their physician. The increase in peak urine flow was 23% greater, and the reduction in residual urine volume was 24% greater in the *Pygeum africanum* versus placebo group. The groups did not differ in dropout rates and side effects. Thus very limited evidence suggests that *Pygeum africanum* extract is more effective than a placebo for improving clinical manifestations and urodynamic study results in men with BPH.

Reference
Wilt, T., et al. (2002). *Pygeum africanum* for benign prostatic hyperplasia. *Cochrane Database System Retrieval* (1): CD001044.

client may be taught to perform clean intermittent catheterization, particularly if long-term retention occurs (see the Bridge to Home Health Care feature on Intermittent Self-Catheterization for Men on p. 1019). Men who are not candidates for surgery or intermittent catheterization may require long-term indwelling catheterization.

■ Nursing Management of the Medical Client

Assessment

Ask the client to describe all urinary manifestations, including the pattern of urination, urgency, frequency, decreased or altered urinary stream, hesitancy, and nocturia. Ask about the presence of *hematuria* (blood in the urine).

Clients often consume herbal agents in the belief that they are safer than physician-prescribed medications. You should ask your clients whether they are taking saw palmetto, couch grass, pipsissewa, pumpkin, or pygeum or other preparations for BPH. Client teaching for the

man using phytotherapy includes information about the actions of these agents, their efficacy, and the safety of their use in combination with prescribed drugs.

Diagnosis, Outcomes, Interventions

Diagnosis: Ineffective Therapeutic Regimen Management. The nurse has a major teaching role to help the client avoid *Ineffective Therapeutic Regimen Management related to lack of understanding of disease, manifestations, and medical treatments.*

Outcomes. The client will understand disease, manifestations, and medical treatment, as evidenced by client statements, increased fluid intake, and ability to follow medication regimen.

Interventions

Provide Teaching About BPH. Men often have only a vague understanding of what an enlarged prostate is, much less where the gland lies. Many men fear they have prostate cancer or that BPH is a precursor of prostate cancer. Beliefs about treatment affecting their sexual functioning are also a concern. Show the client and significant other a picture of the reproductive organs and prostate, and explain the effects of enlargement on urine excretion.

Encourage Fluids. Many clients limit their fluid intake to combat the manifestations of BPH. Explain that concentrated urine acts as an irritant to the bladder. Caffeine and alcohol also can exacerbate bothersome LUTS, and their intake should be reduced or avoided. Clients increase their risk of UTI with limited fluid intake. Unless otherwise contraindicated, the client should maintain an intake of 30 ml/kg/day or ½ ounce per pound of body weight.

Explain Medications. If medications are being used to treat BPH, men need a thorough explanation of how the medications work, their side effects, and precautions. Warn the client to increase dosage only under the physician's orders because more medication may not help manifestations and may cause serious cardiovascular problems. Encourage clients to be patient because the effects of medication on the prostate may take time. Discourage clients from taking medications that contain alpha-adrenergic agonists (e.g., cold medicines and diet pills) because they can cause a man with BPH to experience acute urinary retention. Clients are also discouraged from taking over-the-counter cold remedies containing diphenhydramine (Benadryl), which has strong anticholinergic properties that may relax the decompensated detrusor muscle and precipitate acute urinary retention. Clients are counseled to inform all health care providers of their BPH because multiple medications (in-

BRIDGE TO HOME HEALTH CARE
Intermittent Self-Catheterization for Men

Intermittent self-catheterization is indicated for transient or persistent urinary retention. Retention occurs when clients are unable to empty their bladders completely as a result of neurologic conditions such as spinal cord injury, multiple sclerosis, or brain injury. An obstructive condition such as an enlarged prostate is another common cause of retention. The amount of residual urine that clients retain can vary greatly.

When intermittent self-catheterization is used to manage urinary retention, an indwelling catheter is not needed and the risk of infection is decreased. The procedure can be used as a temporary measure, for example, for the development of temporary bladder atony after bladder surgery. Before self-catheterization is selected for long-term management, a thorough assessment should be completed and noninvasive methods should have been attempted without success.

To use intermittent self-catheterization successfully, clients should have sufficient manual dexterity and cognitive ability, and they should follow guidelines. Because they must not overfill their bladders, it is essential that clients be motivated to catheterize four or five times daily. The goal is to obtain a quantity of urine that does not exceed 500 ml per catheterization. Most physicians recommend a moderate daily fluid intake. They tell clients to establish a consistent plan that includes the time and amount of their intake so that they do not overfill their bladders. It is also important that clients understand that poor or inconsistent technique increases the risk of complications. Infection is the most frequently occurring complication; persistent overfilling of the bladder can cause ureterovesical reflux with subsequent renal damage.

Clean self-catheterization is acceptable in the home setting. Using clean technique implies that clients do not wear gloves and do not need to use a sterile field or supplies. Clients should use a comfortable position; they may prefer to sit or stand. They need the following supplies: straight or curved-tip Tiemann (the Tiemann is most common and desired to navigate in the male urethra) catheter (12 or 14F) in a clean container or plastic bag, water-soluble lubricant (K-Y or Surgilube), washcloth prepared with soap and water, receptacle for urine, and receptacle for catheter. Clients should use the following procedure:

1. Wash hands and gather equipment. (Storing all equipment in one easy-to-carry container simplifies the procedure.)
2. Assume the desired position. If sitting on a bed, place plastic under a towel to protect bedding.
3. Retract the foreskin if present, and wash the tip of the penis thoroughly with soap and water.
4. Remove the catheter from the container and lubricate first 4 to 6 inches with lubricant; place other end over the receptacle or toilet to catch urine.
5. Hold the penis at right angles to the body, keeping the foreskin retracted.
6. Insert the catheter 7 to 10 inches into the penis or until urine flows; then insert one more inch.
7. Allow the catheter to drain while pressing down with abdominal muscles to promote complete emptying.
8. After drainage is complete, gently withdraw the catheter.
9. Wash and dry the area.
10. Wash the catheter in warm, soapy water, rinse with clear water, shake dry (to eliminate excess water in lumen), and dry outside with paper towel. Place in a plastic bag for storage. (Use catheters for 2 to 4 weeks; then discard.)
11. Wash hands.

cluding antimuscarinics, certain antidepressants, antipsychotics, and calcium channel blockers) may adversely affect bladder function and increase the risk for acute urinary retention.

Diagnosis: Impaired Urinary Elimination.
The client with BPH usually experiences manifestations such as frequency, urgency, hesitancy, change in stream, incontinence, retention, and nocturia. Write the nursing diagnosis as *Impaired Urinary Elimination related to increasing urethral occlusion.*

Outcomes. The client will remain free of manifestations of BPH or those manifestations will decrease with treatment, as evidenced by absence of frequency, urgency, hesitancy, change in stream, incontinence, retention, or nocturia.

Interventions

Catheterize. When the client has urinary difficulties, such as obstruction, urinary retention, or diminished renal function, some form of catheterization may be necessary. See the table on the website, Urologic Instruments **evolve** Most Commonly Encountered in a Clinical Setting, which shows various types of urethral catheters. (The Bridge to Home Health Care feature above explains intermittent self-catheterization for men.) Never force a urinary catheter. If it cannot be inserted with gentle pressure, notify the urologist, who may need special instruments to get the catheter past the obstruction. Bladder spasms are common with indwelling catheters. If bladder discomfort and leakage are significant, medications can be ordered to reduce them (see Chapter 36). Clean the meatus several times a day with water and mild soap.

Monitor Urine Output. If an indwelling catheter is placed for acute retention, observe the client for hourly urine output (should be at least 0.5 ml/kg/hr), hematuria, and shock caused by postobstructive diuresis. Hematuria can occur because of the sudden release of pressure on the blood vessels supplying the bladder or mild trauma owing to catheterization. *Postobstructive diuresis* means increased urine output caused by inability of the renal tubules to absorb water and electrolytes after prolonged urinary obstruction. It is usually self-limiting but can cause sodium depletion in some clients, which leads to vascular collapse and death if not detected and treated.

Evaluation

The client should be able to manage the manifestations of the disease and to take the medication appropriately. Clients should also continue follow-up so that the usefulness of the medical treatment can be assessed. Surgical intervention may be needed if medical management fails.

■ Surgical Management

Surgery is indicated in cases of high magnitude obstruction (particularly when complicated by an episode of acute urinary retention), severe LUTS, recurrent UTI, hematuria, bladder stones or upper urinary tract distress. The part of the gland causing the obstruction is removed in a procedure called a *prostatectomy.* The term *prostatectomy* is a misnomer because the procedure is actually removal of new tissue growth. Figure 40-2 illustrates various surgical approaches. The method used depends on the size of the prostate, the health of the client, and surgeon preference. Since 2002, robotic assistive devices have been used for laparoscopic prostatectomy procedures in major medical centers.

Regrowth of prostate tissue after prostatectomy for BPH occurs over a period of 1 to 15 years, and it occasionally requires a repeat procedure. In addition, prostate cancer may still develop because the total prostate is not removed. These clients need the same follow-up as other men who have not had prostate surgery.

Operative Technique

Transurethral Resection of the Prostate. Transurethral resection of the prostate (TURP) remains a widely used technique for managing BPH, and it continues to be the "gold standard" against which all other procedures are measured. A resectoscope is inserted through the urethra (Figure 40-2, *A*). The surgeon visualizes the inside of the bladder by inserting a cystoscope (telescopic lens) through the resectoscope. A movable loop is inserted through the resectoscope that cuts tissue and coagulates bleeding vessels with high-frequency electric current. (A cold-punch resectoscope that punches out tissue, piece by piece, with a circular knife blade is rarely used today.)

Irrigating fluid is infused into the bladder via the cystoscope, allowing visualization of the resection. Repeated irrigation and drainage of this fluid ensure that resected tissue and debris are removed from the bladder. Sterile irrigation fluid is used for transurethral surgery that allows the electrical conductance needed for resection and coagulation. An isotonic fluid is selected; however, normal saline is avoided because of its suboptimal conductivity properties. In addition, a hypotonic solution such as water must never be used because it will readily absorb into the bloodstream and creates a high risk for transurethral resection (TUR) syndrome. TUR syndrome is characterized by hyponatremia, hypervolemia, hemolysis, and acute renal failure. Clinical manifestations of TUR syndrome include agitation, acute delirium, bradycardia, tachypnea, and vomiting. Although unusual, it can occur even when isotonic solutions are used, particularly if resection involves surgical times longer than 60 to 90 minutes, allowing extensive absorption of irrigation into the vascular system. If manifestations of TUR syndrome occur, the physician is notified immediately and fluid and other supportive measures are initiated promptly. Bleeding is common after this procedure, and constant or intermittent irrigation is necessary.

Suprapubic Prostatectomy. Suprapubic prostatectomy is a surgical approach that involves a lower abdominal incision (Figure 40-2, *B*). It may be the operation of choice when (1) the prostate is too large to be resected transurethrally; (2) a large, pedunculated middle prostatic lobe or later lobes are present; (3) a bladder abnormality needs correction; or (4) an abdominal surgical exploration is necessary. An incision is made into the bladder, and the enlarged tissue is enucleated by blunt dissection. Both suprapubic and urethral catheters are inserted. Bladder abnormalities can be treated concurrently with this procedure, and complete tissue removal is facilitated; however, hemostasis can be difficult to achieve.

The client may experience more bladder spasms, urinary leakage into the abdominal wound around the suprapubic catheter, and a relatively prolonged and uncomfortable convalescence. Incontinence and *erectile dysfunction* (ED) *(impotence)* can occur after this procedure.

Retropubic Prostatectomy. In the retropubic prostatectomy (Figure 40-2, *C*), the surgeon approaches the prostate through a low abdominal incision without entry into the bladder. This is the operation of choice when the prostate is very large and a severe urethral stricture is present. Advantages include direct visualization of the prostate and direct hemostasis in the prostatic fossa. Disadvantages are that associated bladder problems cannot

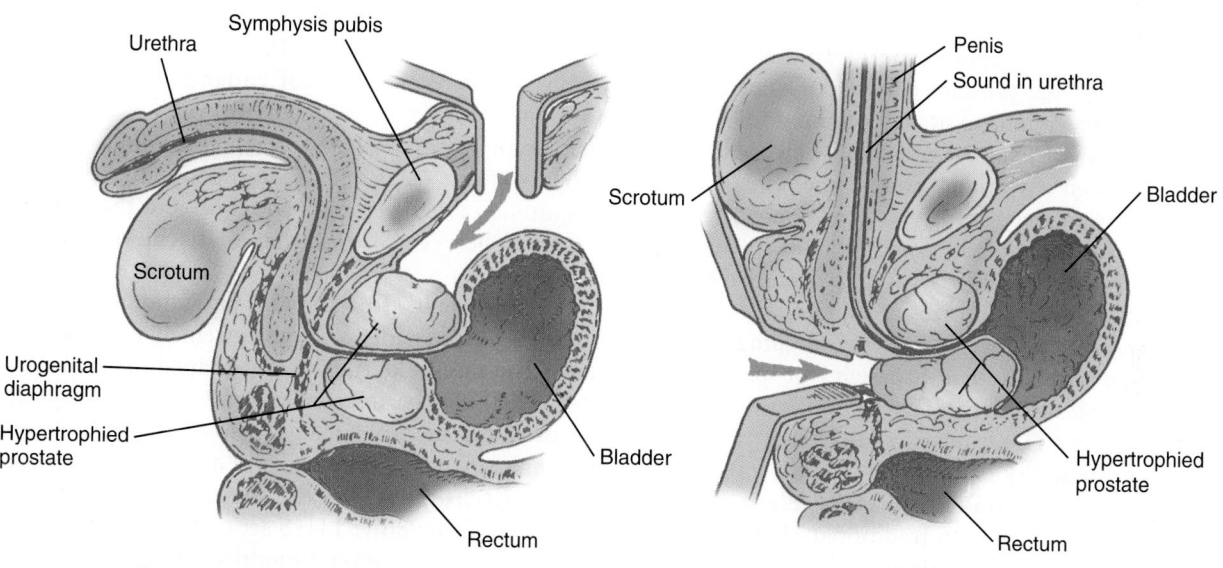

FIGURE 40-2 Surgical approaches to the prostate. **A,** Transurethral resection of the prostate (TURP) is a closed method of treatment; no incision is made, and the hyperplastic prostate tissue is removed through a resectoscope (like a cystoscope), which is inserted through the urethra. **B,** Suprapubic (transvesical) prostatectomy is an open method of treatment in which the hyperplastic prostatic tissue is enucleated through the anterior walls of the abdomen and bladder. **C,** Retropubic (extravesical) prostatectomy is an open method of treatment; a low abdominal incision is made between the pubic arch and the bladder. **D,** Perineal prostatectomy is an open method of treatment involving an incision between the anus and the scrotum.

be treated and osteitis pubis (pubic bone inflammation) may occur.

Perineal Prostatectomy. An incision is made into the perineum between the anus and the scrotum (see Figure 40-2, *D*). This operation is rarely used for treating BPH because of the great potential for ED. The client must be in a lithotomy position, which is contraindicated for people with severe arthritis or cardiopulmonary disease. Other complications include rectourethral fistula, UTI, epididymitis, and urinary retention.

Minimally Invasive Therapies. A number of newer procedures have been developed that offer potential advantages compared with open surgery or TURP. Collectively, these techniques have been termed *minimally invasive therapies.* Although the morbidity and need for hospitalization vary among these procedures, they are generally associated with less bleeding and minimal or no need for hospitalization compared with the gold standard for surgical management for BPH, the TURP.

Transurethral Incision of the Prostate. Transurethral incision of the prostate (TUIP) is an option for men with a small prostate that is causing outlet obstruction. Incisions are made into the prostatic tissue to enlarge the lumen of the prostatic urethra. This procedure is associated with relatively few postoperative complications and can be performed with local anesthesia for high-risk clients. High client satisfaction has also been reported with this procedure; many clients report no change in ejaculation, which makes this an excellent procedure for younger men with a small prostate gland.

Transurethral Electrovaporization. Transurethral electrovaporization of the prostate (the VaporTrode procedure) uses similar equipment as that required for TURP, with the exception of a specially designed ball or bar that is inserted through a working port of the resectoscope and attached to an electrocautery power source. Tissue vaporization requires electric power of 200 to 300 W, compared with the 80 to 150 W used to cauterize blood vessels during TURP. It vaporizes prostatic tissue and offers the potential advantage of reducing bleeding. It also destroys tissue samples that are sent for pathologic analysis following traditional TURP. Studies comparing the VaporTrode to TURP reveal similar short-term results, but the durability of these results may not be as good as those seen with traditional TURP. Electrovaporization may be combined with traditional TUR, particularly when prostate size is considerable or tissue protrudes into the proximal urethra.

Laser-Assisted Procedures. Transurethral ultrasound-guided laser incision of the prostate (TULIP) is a newer procedure in which a laser is used to make the incision into the prostate. It is associated with minimal blood loss, no irrigation is necessary, and the client does not always need a catheter after surgery. Visual laser ablation of the prostate (VLAP) has become more successful since the development of right-angle laser fibers. Neodymium-yttrium aluminum garnet (YAG) is the medium that produces the energy to destroy tissue through a special endoscope. Sloughing of tissue may be delayed, but blood loss is minimal. *Dysuria* (painful urination) and the need for longer catheterization have been noted.

Compared with TURP, each of these procedures is associated with reduced bleeding, and they may be completed in an outpatient (ambulatory surgery) setting. The magnitude of tissue destruction and the durability of results is less than that achieved with TURP, however.

Hyperthermia and Thermal Therapy. Hyperthermia and thermal therapies are new procedures. *Hyperthermia* refers to the administration of temperatures below 45° C; *thermal therapy* refers to administration of higher temperatures. Three techniques—microwaves, radiofrequency, or high-intensity ultrasound waves—may be used to heat prostate and destroy prostate tissue. Transurethral microwave thermotherapy requires passage of a catheter into the urethra that is used to deliver microwave energy. A temperature probe is placed in the rectum, and water is circulated through the system to prevent urethral or rectal heat injury. The transurethral needle ablation (TUNA) system uses radiofrequency energy to destroy prostatic tissue. Special needles are placed into the prostate, and radiofrequency energy is used to provoke tissue coagulation and necrosis. A shield is used to protect the urethra, and multiple treatments are usually required. Water-induced thermotherapy (WIT) uses heated water to destroy obstructive prostate tissue; it is delivered via a 20F catheter in a single 30- to 45-minute session.

Each of these therapies can be completed in an outpatient setting using local anesthesia only. The initial magnitude of relief from obstruction and the durability of results, however, are less than that achieved by TURP.

Prostatic Stent. Traditionally, prostatic stent insertion is indicated for clients who are extremely poor operative risks. The mesh-like tube (a coil-shaped device has also been used) can be inserted through an endoscope into the prostatic urethra, where it holds the urethra open mechanically. Over time, usually about 3 to 6 months, epithelial cells grow over the stent, which is permanent in most cases. Irritative LUTS are common, but they usually subside within several months. The stents have had to be removed when they migrate, become encrusted or infected, or cause persistent perineal discomfort. Removal may be difficult. To prevent complications, clients are cautioned to avoid catheterization through the stent for 3 months after placement.

Complications

Complications after treatment vary between treatments. They may include bleeding (particularly associated with TURP), infection, persisting obstruction (particularly seen with minimally invasive therapies), accidental displacement of the catheter, stenosis of the urethra or bladder neck, epididymitis, urinary incontinence, ED, or retrograde (backward) ejaculation. Urethral stricture or bladder neck contracture is usually treated with dilation, although urethroplasty may be required in severe or refractory cases. Persistent incontinence after TURP affects

1% to 2%. Clients with overactive detrusor contractions (overactive bladder), voiding frequency, and sensory urgency initially may note an increase in the frequency of urinary leakage or de novo incontinence. Pharmacotherapy, combined with pelvic muscle rehabilitation, fluid and dietary control may be required to control overactive bladder that has been "unmasked" by removal of obstructive prostatic tissue.

Erectile dysfunction occurs in 5% to 10% of clients and only when nerves are damaged during surgery for prostate resection. Of major concern to clients is the occurrence of retrograde ejaculation. Because the verumontanum is destroyed during most prostate surgery, antegrade (forward) ejaculation cannot occur. Instead, semen goes into the bladder during ejaculation and is voided with the next urination, creating cloudy urine. This effect is harmless, but sexual function may be impaired unless the client is advised of this anticipated effect and reassured that it is expected to alter fertility potential but not libido or erectile function.

Outcomes

It is expected that the client will achieve significant relief from bothersome LUTS without complications. In addition, objective measures of lower urinary tract function should reveal alleviation of obstruction and urinary retention.

■ Nursing Management of the Surgical Client

Preoperative Care

Assess the client's ability to empty his bladder. The bladder should be palpated for distention. If the client cannot void, a urethral catheter may have to be placed. Clients taking any drug or supplement with anticoagulant effects must discontinue these substances before surgery. The nurse should carefully review all prescription drugs, over-the-counter, and herbal agents for anticoagulant properties. This review also incorporates high-dose vitamin E or multivitamins because daily supplementation with vitamin E of 400 international units or higher exerts a dose-dependent anticoagulant effect. Preoperative assessment should also include attention to expectations about the procedure, such as anticipated changes in voiding and sexual function. You are often able to lessen the client's fear and anxiety during the nursing history by reinforcing preoperative teaching provided by the urologist and by ensuring that the client (and partner if possible) understands the anticipated outcomes of the procedure. Respond to the concerns of the client and significant others with empathic listening, accurate information, and ongoing support. Restating the explanations given by the surgeon and anesthetist when securing informed consent is particularly helpful because stressed clients frequently forget what they have been told.

Informed consent requires that the man understand the risks (e.g., possible sexual dysfunction, including ED; retrograde ejaculation; and infertility) and short-term and long-term benefits (e.g., relief of urinary manifestations and promotion of optimal renal function). It is important for the client to receive honest answers to questions concerning sexuality and reproduction.

Postoperative Care
Assessment

Immediately after surgery, your major task is to observe the vital signs and maintenance of urinary drainage. Indwelling catheters are used to facilitate urinary drainage after many types of prostate procedures. Document the urine color, including the presence of blood clots, each time urine output is recorded.

Various types of catheter irrigation systems may be used with these catheters. Closed irrigation, or *closed bladder irrigation* (CBI) (Figure 40-3), permits either constant or intermittent irrigation without the hazard of

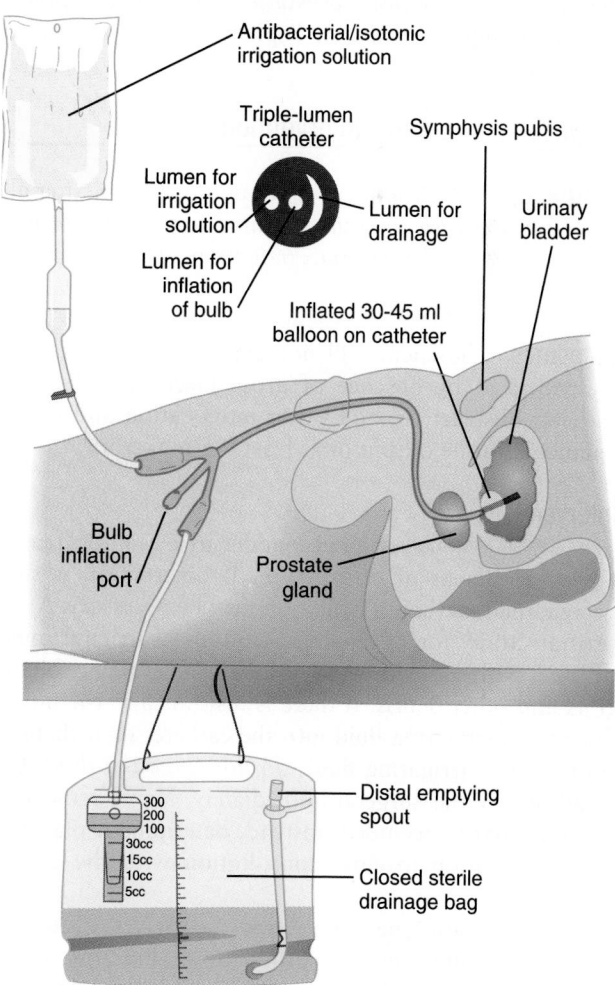

FIGURE 40-3 A closed bladder irrigation system.

violating aseptic technique. Isotonic fluid is used to maintain the outflow of clear or slightly pink urine. Pay close attention to the irrigation rate, and *never* reduce the rate until directed to do so because premature reduction of the irrigation rate will predispose the client to stasis of debris or blood leading to catheter blockage. Ensure that the catheter drainage bag is emptied regularly and when it is approximately three quarters filled to avoid stasis or interruption of urinary drainage.

Frequently assess the client's urine output. Documentation of output must include records of intake and output, and it should include the amount instilled with the irrigation. Differentiation of urine output versus output from the irrigation process is important because it is possible for the client to have a urine output of less than 0.5 ml/kg/hr that is easily missed if irrigation drainage is not subtracted to calculate true urine output.

Ensure catheter patency frequently to make sure the catheter is draining; blockage of an irrigated bladder rapidly leads to overdistention, secondary hemorrhage, and formation of blood clots or infection. Proper positioning of the catheter and drainage system is important to maintain good drainage and prevent obstruction of the system. Blood clots, prostatic debris, mucus plugs, kinked tubing, or catheter displacement may obstruct urinary flow.

Diagnosis, Outcomes, Interventions

Diagnosis: Risk for Injury.
A common problem after all procedures is *Risk for Injury related to presence of urinary catheters, hematuria, irrigation, or suprapubic drains.*

Outcomes. The client will not experience hemorrhage, as evidenced by absence of gross bleeding, infection, catheter obstruction, and water intoxication and maintenance of urine output of at least 0.5 ml/kg/hr.

Interventions

Maintain Irrigation. Closed bladder irrigation decreases the development of obstruction. If obstruction is suspected, manual (hand) irrigation may be necessary. After prostatectomy for BPH, at least 60 ml of irrigant must be used, with some force, to dislodge and evacuate blood clots and other debris. If there is resistance to the introduction of irrigating fluid into the catheter or if there is no return of irrigating fluid, *do not force the fluid.* Instead, notify the surgeon immediately. Never remove a catheter that is occluded; instead, determine a plan for recatheterization in close consultation with the physician.

Catheters and the procedures themselves cause increased urethral mucus production. Practice good **EB** meatal care. Keep the penis and meatal area clean by washing them with soap and water at least twice a day.

Antibacterial ointments were formerly used, but they are no more effective than cleansing. Antibacterial soaps or antiseptics may dry out skin.

Monitor for Bleeding. Some hematuria is usual for several days after surgery; however, frank bleeding, arterial or venous, may occur during the first day after surgery. Arterial blood is bright red, has numerous clots, and is viscous. Blood pressure may fall, and emergency surgical intervention may become necessary. Venous bleeding in the prostatic area may be controlled by increasing the pressure in the balloon end by adding to its retention balloon or by placing traction on the catheter. Traction is increased by pulling the catheter out by using firm but gentle pressure so that the balloon moves into the prostatic fossa. Traction is maintained by securing the catheter to the thigh with a Velcro catheter strap. Traction may be maintained for 24 hours or longer and is released by the physician when the bleeding has stopped. In selected cases, the surgeon may remove fluid slowly from the balloon as the bleeding decreases to partially decrease traction.

Prevent Catheter Dislodgment. The client may be confused immediately after surgery or may forget that he has a catheter and accidentally pull out the catheter. Show him how to get in and out of the bed or chair without pulling on the catheter. Remind the client that he has a tube in his bladder through his penis or abdomen (whichever it is), and instruct him not to touch it. A displaced or removed urinary catheter after prostatic surgery is painful and disrupts recovery. Securing the catheter with a Velcro catheter strap (holder) is strongly recommended. If the client does pull the catheter out, notify the surgeon immediately.

Prevent Infection. Observe the client carefully for local or systemic indications of infection. Handle catheters, drainage apparatus, and urine collection carefully to avoid introducing microorganisms into the urinary tract. Maintain a closed urinary drainage system unless manual irrigation is absolutely required. Encourage increased fluid intake, ambulation, and deep-breathing exercises.

Wound drains are usually removed earlier than suprapubic catheters. Keep skin around the drain and catheter sites clean, dry, and protected. Observe for redness, edema, or infection.

In some cases, a suprapubic catheter may remain in place until voiding function has returned. When the client is voiding well, the suprapubic catheter can be removed. Expect urinary leakage from the suprapubic catheter site, mostly on the day the catheter is removed, until the wound is completely healed. Frequent dressing changes are necessary at first. If a suprapubic catheter is removed before the client has returned to normal voiding, the wound may not heal properly, leading to fistula formation.

Monitor for Retention. The length of time urethral catheters are left in place varies according to the surgeon's judgment, the type of surgery, and the client's preoperative lower urinary tract function. Removal of the catheter is associated with a risk for urinary retention owing to changes in detrusor contractility, transient obstruction resulting from urethral edema or local discomfort, or urethral blockage due to clots or other debris. A voiding trial may be completed to evaluate voiding function after a TURP or similar procedure. Whereas this procedure assesses the client's immediate ability to urinate, it does not exclude the possibility of urinary retention occurring hours to 1 day following catheter removal. Therefore the client is informed of the possibility for delayed retention and instructed about management of this unanticipated outcome.

Manage Temporary Incontinence. Advise the client that irritative LUTS such as daytime voiding frequency, urgency, leakage, and dysuria are anticipated and will persist until complete healing occurs. Keep reminding him that these problems are temporary and may take some time to resolve. Be understanding of the man's feelings, and keep him dry without embarrassing him. Absorbency products may be needed temporarily. They vary in size, shape, and absorbency capacities. Pelvic muscle exercises may help to reduce this problem. Additional surgery is occasionally required for persistent incontinence.

Diagnosis: Acute Pain.
A common nursing diagnosis is *Acute Pain related to surgery and bladder spasms.*

Outcomes. The client's pain will be under control, as evidenced by the client's report.

Interventions. Pain control after surgery is discussed in Chapters 16 and 22. Bladder spasms frequently occur after prostate procedures, and incisional pain will occur if an open surgery (prostatectomy) is completed. Incisional pain is usually described as continuous, dull, boring pain of moderate to severe intensity; bladder spasms are typically described as periods of intense cramping discomfort or pressure. When bladder spasms are suspected, ensure that the drainage system is not blocked because obstruction as well as bladder irritation causes bladder spasms. Antispasmodic medications, such as belladonna and opium (B&O) suppositories, propantheline bromide (Pro-Banthine) or immediate release oxybutynin (Ditropan IR), may be prescribed to relieve bladder spasm. Side effects associated with these medications include dry mouth, drowsiness (especially with B&O suppositories), or acute confusion in the older clients. Be-

cause antispasmodic drugs can cause constipation, and straining at stool can precipitate bleeding from the operative site, stool softeners such as docusate sodium (Colace) are often given. Men with severe cardiac disease or narrow angle glaucoma should not receive these agents.

Evaluation

It is expected that the client will be discharged without complications and resume regular activities within 4 to 6 weeks. Depending on the procedure performed, some clients return home the same day. The client who has undergone TURP is usually discharged about 2 to 3 days after the operation. Clients who had open procedures are discharged after 4 to 6 days. Voiding of urine improves, and complications such as urgency, frequency, and dribbling end within 3 months.

■ Self-Care
Provide Teaching. In addition to teaching the client verbally, give him written materials to take home after discharge. If applicable, review catheter and wound management. Clients who go home with a catheter may have a leg bag for day use and a Foley bag for use at night.

Some activities are limited after prostatectomy. The surgeon's orders should be followed regarding heavy lifting, strenuous activity, prolonged sitting, sexual activity, and driving or riding in an automobile. Because prolonged sitting increases intra-abdominal pressure and may precipitate bleeding, the man should avoid sitting except during meals. Clients should avoid driving an automobile or taking prolonged automobile rides until at least 2 weeks after surgery, when the risk of bleeding lessens. Strenuous exercise is also contraindicated for 4 to 6 weeks.

Prevent Injury. Advise the client not to strain during defecation for at least 6 weeks after surgery because this can lead to bleeding from the operative site. Docusate sodium, prune juice, and milk of magnesia are usually satisfactory bowel stimulants during this time. Increasing the amount of fluids also helps to prevent constipation. The client should avoid or limit intake of alcohol and other bladder irritants such as caffeine. Smoking should be discouraged because coughing puts strain on the surgical area.

Teach Pelvic Muscle Rehabilitation. Activity-induced incontinence (stress urinary incontinence) is typically a transient problem, although 1% to 2% of men may have long-term UTI following prostate surgery. Transient urine loss may be managed by containment products such as a pad that inserts into the underclothing. Simultaneously, men should be taught the principles of pelvic floor muscle rehabilitation or referred to a nurse specialist or physical therapist that specializes in this type of treatment. Pelvic muscle rehabilitation comprises three components: (1) biofeedback to promote muscle identification and isolation; (2) muscle training to improve maximal strength, endurance, and function; and (3) neuromuscular reeducation to enable the client to contract the muscles strategically in a way that maximizes continence. Biofeedback methods are usually needed to help the client identify the pelvic muscles. Options include contracting the muscles during DRE, contraction while seated in a chair with a firm seat, or interruption of the urinary stream. If the latter strategy is used, it is critical to differentiate this *biofeedback* strategy from an exercise and instruct the man to practice this no more than once daily or every other day over a period of 1 to 3 days until effective muscle identification is learned. Muscle training consists of a graded exercise program of repeated pelvic muscle contractions. Teach the client to tighten the pelvic muscles for 6 to 10 seconds followed by a rest period of equal duration. Begin with 5 to 10 exercises daily and gradually increase to 25 to 35 daily exercises over a period of 6 to 12 weeks. Neuromuscular reeducation focuses on teaching the knack. Teach the client to contract his pelvic floor muscles consciously whenever he coughs, sneezes, or lifts a heavy object. Although this is a conscious effort initially, eventually it will be incorporated by most clients as a subconscious response to activities likely to provoke urinary leakage over time. Clients who are unable to identify the pelvic floor muscles or who do not respond to treatment after 4 to 6 weeks should be referred to a specialist for clinician-directed rehabilitation. (See the Evidence-Based Practice in Action feature on Pelvic Muscle Rehabilitation Following Prostatectomy, below.)

EB EVIDENCE-BASED PRACTICE IN ACTION

Pelvic Muscle Rehabilitation Following Prostatectomy

Urinary incontinence can be a complication of radical prostatectomy procedures. Despite improvements in surgical approaches, many men experience moderate to severe urinary incontinence postoperatively.[4,6] The treatment of this condition varies widely from medications or additional surgery to progressive therapy programs to increase the activity of the muscles of the pelvic floor and improve urinary leakage experienced by prostatectomy clients.[9]

Men with post-prostatectomy incontinence who practiced repeated pelvic muscle contractions with or without behavioral biofeedback (to assist with correct muscle identification) or electrical stimulation several times per day reported decreased incontinence following treatment in more than 75% of the cases.[1-3,5,8,9] By instituting biofeedback sessions with pelvic floor muscle exercises prior to radical prostatectomy even better outcomes were achieved.[7] Clients who received the sessions and performed the exercises before surgery had significantly better outcomes than clients who received the sessions and performed the exercises after the radical prostatectomy.

Implications

Nurses have an important role in providing teaching and interventions related to pelvic floor muscle strengthening exercises prior to radical prostatectomy procedures to improve client outcomes related to urinary continence following surgery. Completing the biofeedback sessions with pelvic floor muscle exercises before surgery increases the nurse's role in educating the prostatectomy client to achieve continence. It gives the client knowledge about exactly what is involved in doing the pelvic muscle exercises and what to expect after surgery. Additionally a rapport can be established between the nurse and client that can be carried through the postoperative period.[7]

References

1. Burgio, K., Stutzman, R., & Engle, B. (1989). Behavioral training for post-prostatectomy urinary incontinence. *Journal of Urology, 141*, 303-306.

2. Jackson, J., et al. (1996). Biofeedback: A noninvasive treatment for incontinence after radical prostatectomy. *Urologic Nursing, 16*(2), 50-54.

3. Moore, K., Griffiths, D., & Hughton, A. (1999). Urinary incontinence after radical prostatectomy: A randomized controlled trial comparing pelvic muscle exercises with or without electrical stimulation. *British Journal of Urology International, 83*, 57-65.

4. Moorhouse, D., et al. (2001). Behavioral treatments for post-prostatectomy incontinence. *Ostomy/Wound Management, 47*(12), 30-31, 33-38, 40.

5. Moul, J. (1999). Pelvic muscle rehabilitation in males following prostatectomy. *National Association for Continence, 17*(2), 1-3.

6. Shell, J. (2002). Evidence-based practice for symptom management in adults with cancer: Sexual dysfunction. *Oncology Nursing Forum, 29*(1), 53-69.

7. Sueppel, C., Kreder, K., & See, W. (2001). Improved continence outcomes with preoperative pelvic floor muscle strengthening exercises. *Urologic Nursing, 21*(3), 201-210.

8. Van Kampen, M., et al. (2000). Effect of pelvic floor reeducation on duration and degree of incontinence after radical prostatectomy: A randomized controlled trial. *The Lancet, 355*, 98-102.

9. Wisinski, C., Rolf-Carbaugh, L., & Bangs, K. (2001). Physical therapy treatment for urinary incontinence utilizing rectal weights following radical prostatectomy. *Journal of the Section on Women's Health, 25*(4), 9-11.

Treat Erectile Dysfunction. Erectile dysfunction is an uncommon complication of prostatectomy and the greatest risk is associated with open surgical procedures. Sildenafil (Viagra) may be given to postprostatectomy clients postoperatively in an attempt to maintain blood flow to the corpora cavernosa during the recovery period and prevent or reverse apoptosis (programmed cellular death) caused by prolonged disuse of the erectile mechanism. Research has shown that this strategy is beneficial for men undergoing radical prostatectomy, but its efficacy in men undergoing TURP or prostatectomy for BPH is not known.

Information and supportive care for the client and his partner are extremely important. The client needs to know that he can still please a partner and that love-making techniques other than intercourse may be necessary. The partner should be reassured that sexual intimacy will not harm the client. The couple may need information about alternatives to intercourse, such as cuddling, stroking, or manual or oral stimulation to orgasm. Vacuum erection devices, intracorporeal injections, and intraurethral or oral medications are also topics that sexual counselors can discuss. A penile implant may be considered in selected cases (see Erectile Dysfunction later in this chapter), and referral for sexual counseling is often helpful.

Arrange Follow-Up. Be sure the client knows when and where to reach the surgeon and how to get in touch with health care professionals if he has concerns. He should especially report any elevated temperature, unusual bleeding, manifestations of wound infection or UTI, and obstructed urinary flow. He should know the date and time of his follow-up appointment with the surgeon.

PROSTATE CANCER

Prostate cancer is the second most commonly diagnosed cancer in men (following skin cancer) and the second leading cause of death (following lung cancer). In 2003, approximately 220,900 men in the United States were diagnosed with prostate cancer, and about 28,900 died from the disease.[2]

Etiology and Risk Factors

The cause of prostate cancer is unknown, but it is known that two types of tumors are diagnosed in the clinical setting. A latent form can be identified in as many as 30% of men during the fifth decade of life and about 60% to 70% of men in their 80s. Clinically aggressive prostate cancer affects about one in six American men, and it demonstrates the local invasion and metastatic properties of other forms of cancer. Therefore researchers must determine the factors that cause the initiation of prostate cancer and the factors that cause it to progress to the clinically aggressive form that causes men to die of the disease without treatment. Whereas these factors are not yet known, a discussion of the risk factors associated with both forms of prostate cancer provides clues that are likely to solve this persistent mystery.

Men with a family history of prostate cancer are at high risk for developing adenocarcinomas, and 10% of all cases are believed to be inherited. For example, a focus for prostate cancer susceptibility at a young age has been located on the long arm of chromosome 1 and *PCAP* and *CAPB* genes (both components of chromosome 1) have been identified as leading to an increased risk for prostate cancer. Additional research has identified a gene on the X chromosome (*HPCX*) that appears more often in men with prostate cancer, suggesting that the familial predisposition may exhibit heterogeneity (susceptibility based on the expressions of more than one gene). Of note, genetic predisposition to breast cancer has progressed along similar lines and shared susceptibility loci on chromosome 1 suggests a possible biologic linkage to breast cancer in the women of certain families as well as prostate cancer in the men of these families.

Although 10% are thought to be inherited, the remaining 90% must be classified as sporadic. Nevertheless, it is postulated that sporadic and inherited cancers have similar etiologies from a biochemical perspective. Research into noninherited prostate cancer has led to hypotheses that these tumors may arise from damage or loss of genes that control essential cellular processes such as *replication* (cell replacement) or *apoptosis* (programmed cellular death).

In addition to increases in our understanding of possible causes of the initiation of prostate malignancies, research during the past decade has greatly increased our understanding of the processes that cause a prostate tumor to progress from a slow growing to a clinically relevant (and potentially deadly) cancer. Genetic factors associated with this progression include damage to chromosome 10q affecting the *PTEN/MMAC* suppressor gene, abnormalities of chromosome 12 resulting in loss of the tumor suppression of gene *p27*, and over- expression of gene *MYC* owing to alterations in the long arm of chromosome 8q. In addition, an abnormality of the AR locus of the X chromosome has been identified that is hypothesized to contribute to the progression of advanced stage prostate cancers from hormone-sensitive to hormone-independent tumors, an ominous event that greatly limits effective treatment options.

Prostate cancer risk rises with aging, particularly when men reach the sixth decade of life. Approximately three of four men diagnosed with prostate cancer will be aged 65 years or older. In contrast to this trend, the risk for clinically aggressive tumors appears to be greater among younger men, especially among those diagnosed during their 50s or earlier.

Race also acts as a risk factor for developing prostate cancer as well as the likelihood of experiencing a clinically aggressive tumor. For example, African-American men

COMPLEMENTARY AND ALTERNATIVE THERAPY

Selenium Supplements and Prostate Cancer Risk

A randomized trial of selenium brewers' yeast-based supplements (200 µg/day) versus a placebo failed to have an effect on the primary endpoint of the trial (recurrence of skin cancer). However, a secondary endpoint from the trial was the incidence of prostate cancer, and the results showed a 65% decrease in the risk of prostate cancer in the men taking the supplement versus the placebo.

This initial and potentially exciting finding must be weighed against other evidence from the same trial. For example, only men with baseline plasma selenium levels of less than 121.6 ng/ml benefited from the supplement. Men with higher baseline selenium levels either experienced no reduced risk or a slight increase in risk of prostate cancer and other cancers. In addition, it seems that former smokers had the most benefit from the study. This study reinforces the observation that men with initially deficient levels of plasma selenium potentially have the most to gain by taking a supplement or, ideally, by getting more selenium from food sources such as brazil nuts, fish, garlic, poultry, and mushrooms.

Reference

Duffield-Lillico, A., et al. (2002). Baseline characteristics and the effect of selenium supplementation on cancer incidence in a randomized clinical trial: A summary report of the Nutritional Prevention of Cancer Trial. *Cancer Epidemiology Biomarkers Prevention, 11*, 630-639.

COMPLEMENTARY AND ALTERNATIVE THERAPY

Zinc Supplements and Prostate Cancer

Researchers examined the relationship between supplemental zinc intake and prostate cancer risk among 46,974 U.S. men in the Health Professionals Follow-up Study. During 14 years of follow-up (1986 to 2000), a total of 2901 new cases of prostate cancer were documented, and 434 of these cases were classified as advanced prostate cancer. Supplemental zinc intake at dosages up to 100 mg/day was not associated with the risk of prostate cancer (the RDA for men is 11 mg/day). However, compared with non-users, men who took more than 100 mg/day of zinc supplements had a relative risk of 2.29 (p trend = 0.003), and men who consumed zinc supplements for 10 or more years had a relative risk of 2.37 (p trend <0.001).

Past studies of zinc suggest that it may enhance the activity of telomerase and may reduce the efficacy of bisphosphonates. Zinc may also cause immune dysfunction, impair antioxidant defense, reduce the effect of selenium, and increase IGF-I and testosterone and growth factors. A 131-item food frequency questionnaire was used in this study. Supplemental zinc provided 32% of the total zinc intake (the largest source), with beef (11%) and breakfast cereals (5%) representing other large sources of zinc.

Reference

Leitzmann, M., et al. (2003). Zinc supplement use and risk of prostate cancer. *Journal of the National Cancer Institutes, 95,* 1004-1007.

are at greatest risk for developing prostate cancer compared with any other group, and this risk incorporates a greater likelihood of having an advanced stage tumor at initial diagnosis or dying of prostate cancer. In contrast, Asian Americans have a lower risk for prostate cancer with compared with whites or blacks. This difference is greatest in Asians residing in Asia, and it diminishes when Asian men migrate to the United States, reflecting the contribution of environmental and dietary risk factors.

The greatest dietary risk factor for prostate cancer is the consumption of a diet that is high in saturated animal fats (see the Complementary and Alternative Therapy feature on Prostate Cancer and Dietary Fat Intake on the website). In contrast, consumption of green and yellow vegetables or lycopenes contained in tomatoes is associated with a reduced risk of prostate cancer, indicating a probable protective effect (see the Complementary and Alternative Therapy feature on Fruits and Vegetables and Prostate Cancer Risk on the website). Vitamin D deficiency also may increase the risk for prostate cancer, but this risk may be reduced with adequate exposure to sunlight, a critical component of vitamin D metabolism in the human. (See the Complementary and Alternative Therapy features on Selenium Supplements and Prostate Cancer Risk and on Zinc Supplements and Prostate Cancer, above.

Testosterone and DHT, essential to the growth and development of the prostate, play an important but poorly understood role in prostate cancer initiation and progression. Absence of functioning testes is associated with absence of BPH or prostate cancer and consumption of a low-fat, high-fiber diet (known to reduce circulating testosterones) diminishes prostate cancer risk. Male pattern baldness (associated with increased levels of testosterone) is also associated with an increased risk of prostate cancer.

Environmental and occupational risk factors include living in an urban area and specific occupations such as fertilizer, textile, and rubber industries and work with batteries containing cadmium.

Sexually transmitted virus-like organisms have been found in prostate cancer tissue, suggesting that viruses may act as a risk factor; however, the magnitude of this risk remains unclear. High levels of testosterone have also been linked to development of prostate cancer.

Several potential risk factors have been identified but largely disproved when further research was completed.

For example, neither BPH nor vasectomy has been associated with prostate cancer.

See the Complementary and Alternative Therapy feature on Prostate Cancer Prevention with Finasteride on the website.

Pathophysiology

More than 90% of all cancers arising from the prostate are adenocarcinomas. They typically arise from the peripheral zone of the prostate gland, in contrast to BPH that originates in the transitional zone. A tumor becomes clinically relevant when local invasion or distant metastasis interrupts the function of the urinary and other organ systems producing morbidity or death. Whereas no premalignant lesion has been definitely associated with prostate cancer, high-grade prostatic intraepithelial neoplasia (PIN) has been found to occur in the same location as adenocarcinomas.

The magnitude of local invasion or metastasis is evaluated according to a staging system. The tumor, node, metastases (TNM) (see Chapter 19) or Jewett systems (see Chapter 36) are used to stage prostate cancers. Applied to prostate cancer, stages T1 and T2 (Jewett stages A and B) tumors remained contained within the prostatic capsule and diagnosed as *localized prostate cancer*. In contrast, stage T3 and T4 (Jewett stages C and D) tumors have spread beyond the prostatic capsule and are classified as *advanced stage prostate cancers*. They are associated with metastatic spread to lymph nodes (N1) or spread to distant organs (M1).

The likelihood that an individual tumor will behave in a clinically aggressive manner is evaluated as grade. The Gleason system is typically used to grade prostate cancers. It is based on 10 possible grades according to how well-differentiated tumor cells appear on microscopic analysis. Poorly differentiated *(anaplastic)* cells are associated with a greater risk of aggressive behavior, whereas more highly differentiated cells are less aggressive. Gleason grades 5 to 7 are associated with a 40% chance of metastasis; Gleason grades 8 to 10 are associated with a 75% chance.

Clinical Manifestations

Men with localized prostate cancer typically have no clinical manifestations, and early detection relies on measurement of the serum PSA combined with DRE because these tests have about a 50% accuracy when performed in isolation. The American Cancer Society and American Urological Association recommend regular testing on all men between 50 and 70 years of age and routine testing beginning at age 40 years for African Americans or any man with one or more first-order relatives with prostate cancer. Screening may be completed annually, but more recent research has led to recommendations that men whose PSA is less than 1 should be retested every 5 years and men whose PSA is between 1 and 2 undergo annual testing. DRE and PSA measurement in men older than 70 years of age must be judged on an individual basis; it is *not* recommended in men whose life expectancy is less than 10 years.

Prostate-specific antigen is a glycoprotein produced by the prostate gland, and it is elevated in men with certain prostate conditions such as prostate cancer, BPH, or prostatitis. Normal PSA levels are less than 2.6 ng/ml.[32] When the PSA is 2.6 to 10 ng/ml, the likelihood of prostate cancer is judged as moderate, but values greater than 10 ng/ml indicate a high level of suspicion. A variety of factors other than prostate cancer may elevate the PSA. DRE elevates the PSA only slightly, and it may be measured before or after the DRE has been completed. Prostatitis sharply elevates the PSA, and a period of 6 weeks or longer should pass before PSA is measured in a man with a recent history of a prostate infection. Recent urethral instrumentation such as catheterization or cystoscopy acutely elevates the PSA, and they should not be performed immediately before PSA measurement.

Several techniques have been developed to increase the PSA test's ability to predict the presence of prostate cancer. A fractionated PSA measures free versus protein-bound PSA in the blood. Men with prostate cancer have a higher proportion of their PSA bound to protein, whereas the proportion of free PSA is higher in men with BPH. Measurements of PSA density (PSAD) are particularly useful in men whose original values fall in the moderate suspicion range (2.6 to 10 ng/ml). PSAD combines the serum PSA value and prostate volume assessed via transrectal prostatic ultrasound. Scores are calculated by dividing the PSA by the prostatic volume; men with a score above 0.15 are more likely to have cancer than men with lower values. PSA velocity (PSAV) involves the rate of change in PSA level over time. Men who have a PSAV that rises more than 0.7 ng/ml/yr or that increases 20% or more a year are considered at high risk of having prostate cancer.[32]

Digital rectal examination requires careful palpation of the prostate and seminal vesicles; it is typically performed by a physician or nurse practitioner. The man may be examined while supine, in a lithotomy position, or in stirrups based on the examiner's preference. The client is warned that the examination will cause mild discomfort and pressure in the rectum. A DRE that reveals one or more hardened nodules, asymmetry between the palpable lobes, induration or a stony gland fixed to the rectal wall is suspicious for prostate cancer.

Abnormality of the PSA or DRE indicates the need for more definitive evaluation with a transrectal ultrasound and biopsy. An isolated elevation in PSA should be confirmed several weeks later before proceeding with further testing, including prostate biopsy.[14] Preparation for the procedure includes careful explanation of the procedure. The client is counseled that the probe will produce a sensation of rectal pressure and may cause a desire to defecate. Tissue biopsy generates a sudden noise, but no sensation of a needle stick. All anticoagulant medications, including prescribed agents, over-the-counter drugs such as aspirin, or dietary supplements such as high-dose vitamin E, should be discontinued 7 days before and 1 day following TRUS with biopsy. Bowel cleansing using an enema or stimulant may be required in selected clients. Antimicrobial therapy may be given on the day of the procedure. Following ultrasound and biopsy, the client is instructed to monitor the stool for excessive bleeding.

Pathologic analyses of biopsies are used to determine the presence of a malignancy and its stage. If prostate cancer is found, additional tests are ordered to clarify the stage of the cancer. A bone scan, chest x-ray, and computed tomography (CT) or magnetic resonance imaging (MRI) of the abdomen and pelvis are completed to identify the presence of nodal or distant organ metastasis. A specific imaging scan can be used to locate metastases of prostate cancer in soft tissue. Capromab pendetide (ProstaScint) targets prostate-specific membrane antigen (PSMA), which is found in prostate cancer cells. Two sessions 4 days apart are required. The ProstaScint scan is especially useful in finding "skipped" metastases (i.e., abdominal lymph node involvement without pelvic lymph node involvement), but it is expensive.

Outcome Management
■ Nursing Management of Clients Undergoing Diagnosis

Provide Support. Men with prostate cancer and their significant others need ongoing sensitive support and accurate information to make the difficult decisions required of them. Their concerns are considerable and may include the choices of available treatments, fear of death, anxiety about residual disability and illness, feelings of loss of control, and the possible effects of the illness on people in their social network and in their marriage. After diagnosis, prostate cancer can affect their masculinity and self-esteem. Depression and fatigue are common after many treatments for prostate cancer.

Suggest Resources. Increased awareness of prostate cancer has led to the development of many resources, including books, articles, and Internet websites in the public sector. Local and national prostate cancer support groups have organized. Information is also available from the American Cancer Society (Man to Man program), the American Foundation for Urologic Disease in Baltimore (800-242-2383), and US TOO International in Hinsdale, IL (800-808-7866).

Be sure to include the client's partner or spouse in planning care at the time of diagnosis and when the client is choosing treatment as well as when he is adapting to the treatment. The partner usually takes on essential support responsibilities when the client is gathering information and coping with the disease and treatments.

■ Surgical Management of Localized Prostate Cancer

Radical Prostatectomy. Radical prostatectomy is the treatment of choice for localized prostate cancer, provided the client's health is adequate to undergo the physical stress of anesthesia and surgery, he has a life expectancy of 10 to 15 years, and he elects surgery when presented with a fair and balanced explanation of all the available treatment options. Radical surgery involves removing the entire prostate gland (rather than just enucleation), its outer capsule, the seminal vesicles, sections of the vas deferens, adjacent lymph nodes, and (in many cases) the bladder neck. Bilateral prostatic lymph node dissection (BPLND) is usually limited to clients with higher PSA values and Gleason scores. Open surgical approaches include the retropubic (see Figure 40-2, *C*) and perineal (see Figure 40-2, *D*) approaches. Radical retropubic surgery is the most commonly performed procedure; it offers several potential advantages to alternative approaches. Specifically, preservation of one or both neurovascular bundles of the prostate reduces the risk for ED and may moderate incontinence risk. In contrast, the perineal approach is associated with a reduced risk for urinary incontinence, but preservation of the neurovascular bundles cannot be achieved with this approach, and it may increase the risk for anal sphincter damage and fecal incontinence.

Laparoscopic radical prostatectomy with or without robotic assistance is gaining popularity in some institutions. Four to five small incisions are made and 5- to 10-mm trocars are placed to gain access to the prostate. Anatomic manipulations are similar to that used for traditional radical prostatectomy, and the prostate, capsule, and seminal vesicles are removed. Advantages include absence of the larger incision required for open surgery with reduced operative time and a potentially faster recovery period. Disadvantages include prolonged anesthesia time and a greater risk for positive margins compared with open surgery, indicating incomplete tumor removal.

Complications following radical prostatectomy include bleeding, infection, urinary incontinence, ED, rectal injury, and anal sphincter damage with fecal incontinence. The risk of urinary incontinence is greatest immediately following catheter removal; it will gradually subside over the first 2 postoperative years to 35% to 50%. The vast majority will have only occasional, mild UTI, but about 8% will have significant, chronic UTI requiring continuous use of containment pads or devices. The risk of ED exists for all techniques, but preservation of at least some spontaneous erectile activity may be as high as 70% when radical retropubic prostatectomy is combined with preservation of both neurovascular bundles in otherwise healthy men with good sexual function before surgery. The risk of anal sphincter damage and fecal incontinence may be higher in men undergoing radical perineal prostatectomy and the risk for rectal damage requiring temporary diversion is higher for laparoscopic procedures.

Cryosurgical Ablation. In cryosurgical ablation of the prostate, the surgeon uses guided TRUS to insert cryoprobes into desired areas of the prostate to freeze and thereby destroy the tissue. A warming tube in the urethra keeps the urethral tissue from freezing. Cryosurgery may be an option for clients with localized cancer and other serious medical conditions that preclude them as candidates for radical surgery. Complications associated with cryoablation include urinary incontinence and ED.

■ Nursing Management of the Surgical Client

Prevent Injury. The physical nursing care for the client with prostatic cancer is based on the same principle applied to all clients undergoing other major abdomino-pelvic surgery (see Chapter 16). The client will return from surgery with an indwelling catheter and a midline incision *(retropubic approach)* or U-shaped perineal incision *(perineal approach)*. Monitor urine output closely for the first several days; reddish-colored urine is anticipated during the immediate postoperative period, but a yellow hue should return by postoperative day 2. Notify the physician immediately if brisk bleeding or passage of clots occurs. If catheter blockage occurs, promptly contact the urologist but avoid irrigation that may compromise delicate anastomoses. Compression devices for the lower extremities are maintained over the first 1 to 2 postoperative days, particularly if the client has undergone perineal prostatectomy requiring placement stirrups.

Incisional pain is usually managed by nonpharmacologic interventions, oral opioid drugs, and NSAIDs. Bladder spasms are managed using the same interventions described for the surgical management of BPH. Constipation is avoided because it places potentially harmful stress against the delicate urethral anastomosis. Maintain the client on a low roughage diet, combined with regular ambulation to encourage peristalsis and stool softeners as directed. Enemas should be avoided, particularly if the client has undergone radical perineal prostatectomy.

Men are typically discharged 2 to 3 days after surgery. The indwelling catheter can be removed as early as postoperative day 3, but it is more often left in place for 2 to 3 weeks. While the catheter remains indwelling, special care must be taken to avoid traction against the urethra while the anastomotic site heals.

Provide Support. The psychosocial and emotional care of these clients differs from care of clients with BPH because issues such as cancer and sexual image must be addressed. Thoughts of postoperative self-care at home can be overwhelming. Both the client and significant other need detailed instructions, much reassurance, and resources for supplies and advice if concerns surface at home. Sildenafil (Viagra) or intraurethral alprostadil (MUSE) is given to many clients after prostatectomy to maintain blood flow to the corpora cavernosa during recovery and reduce the risk or severity of ED.

■ Medical Management of Localized Prostate Cancer

Options for localized prostate cancer include watchful waiting, external beam or interstitial radiation therapy, and hormone deprivation. Controversy exists regarding the most effective management of prostate cancer.

Watchful waiting requires DRE, serum PSA, and completion of a lower urinary tract symptom score such as the IPSS every 6 to 12 months. The physician also monitors the man's constitutional manifestations of disease progression, including unintended weight loss, hematuria, bone pain, or pathologic fracture. Watchful waiting is reserved for highly selected cases; strong indications are men aged 70 years or older with well-differentiated, small-volume tumors and a life expectancy of less than 10 years. Men over 70 years of age with low-volume, moderately differentiated tumors are strong candidates if their life expectancy is 5 years or less. Watchful waiting can be combined with dietary measures designed to slow tumor progression. Men are advised to reduce their intake of saturated fats and to increase their intake of lycopenes, selenium, and soya-containing foods. (See the Complementary and Alternative Therapy feature on Flaxseed and a Low-Fat Diet for Men with Prostate Cancer, below.)

Decrease Tumor Growth

Radiation Therapy. Two techniques are used to deliver radiation to prostate tumors. External-beam radiation irradiates the prostate and pelvic region using a ma-

COMPLEMENTARY AND ALTERNATIVE THERAPY

Flaxseed and a Low-Fat Diet for Men with Prostate Cancer

A small pilot study investigated 20 men with prostate cancer who were going to undergo a radical prostatectomy (surgical removal of the prostate). For the 3 to 4 weeks before their surgery, participants consumed 3 grounded tablespoons of flaxseed daily and followed a diet containing less than 20% of calories from fat. The participants did not experience prostate-specific antigen (PSA) decreases overall, but on average their cholesterol levels dropped by 27 points (from 207 to 180 mg/dl). Testosterone levels decreased by an average of 62 points (from 418 to 356 ng/dl). A further look at men with Gleason scores of 6 or less showed that PSA levels decreased from 8.3 to 6.7 ng/ml. In addition, pathologic markers changes suggested that this dietary change slowed the growth of their tumors.

Reference

Demark-Wahnefried, W., et al. (2001). Pilot study of dietary fat restriction and flaxseed supplementation in men with prostate cancer before surgery: Exploring the effects on hormonal levels, prostate-specific antigen, and histopathologic features. *Urology, 58,* 47-52.

chine that resembles diagnostic x-ray machines. It is delivered over multiple treatments during a period of 6 weeks or longer. Traditional radiotherapy is being replaced with newer, conformal techniques that generate three-dimensional CT images to focus the radiation and limit the exposure of adjacent structures. Conformal techniques allow the delivery of a higher radiation dose without increasing the risk of complications. Proton-beam radiotherapy combines conformal imaging and charged protons to target more specifically prostate cancer cells while limiting damage to the overlying skin or adjacent structures including the bladder and rectum.

Brachytherapy requires the implantation of radioactive iodine-125 or pallidium-103 seeds directly into the prostate. They emit highly localized radiation energy to kill localized cancer cells without excessive harm to nearby healthy cells. Proper placement of these seeds is critical, and a preprocedural map of the prostate gland, using ultrasound or CT, is obtained. A grid is then placed over the perineum and ultrasonic or CT imaging used to deliver seeds to the prostate alone. These seeds remain in the body, but their radioactivity declines over a period of months.

Hormone therapy is used in highly selected cases of localized prostate cancer. Treatment is associated with significant adverse side effects, however, and its use is limited primarily to men with advanced stage disease.

■ Medical Management of Advanced Prostate Cancer

Hormone Deprivation/Chemotherapy. Medical management involves hormonal deprivation therapy and chemotherapy (see the Integrating Pharmacology feature on Medications for Prostate Cancer, below). Hormonal deprivation therapy is designed to block androgen (testos-

INTEGRATING PHARMACOLOGY

Medications for Prostate Cancer

Hormonal deprivation therapy is the most common medical treatment for men with advanced prostate cancer. Hormonal deprivation is designed to block androgen (testosterone) production and includes estrogens, gonadotropin-releasing hormone analogs, and antiandrogens. Chemotherapy is used primarily for palliation.

Hormonal Deprivation Therapy

Luteinizing Hormone-Releasing Hormone (LHRH) agonists (also called gonadotropin-releasing hormone analogs) are used as first line therapy for advanced stage prostate cancer. These drugs act by causing an initial surge in luteinizing hormone (LH) and testosterone, rapidly followed by a decline in testosterone levels similar to those achieved by castration. The primary forms of LHRH agonists are leuprolide (Lupron) and goserelin (Zoladex). Leuprolide acetate is administered as a deep intramuscular injection every 1 to 4 months, leuprolide acetate for injectable suspension (Eligard) is administered subcutaneously every 3 to 4 months, and goserelin is administered subcutaneously every 1 to 3 months. Viadur is a newer technique for delivering leuprolide. A cylindrical device implanted in the upper arm delivers a small dose of leuprolide over a period of 12 months. Hot flashes, erectile dysfunction, loss of libido, and minor weight gain caused by water retention are common side effects.

Alternatives to LHRH agonists include oral *nonsteroidal antiandrogens* (drugs that block androgenic effects at the level of the tumor cell such as cyproterone acetate and medroxyprogesterone acetate). Examples of antiandrogens include bicalutamide (Casodex), flutamide (Eulexin), and nilutamide (Nilandron). These medications block androgens produced by the adrenal glands and are often combined with LHRH therapy called maximal an-

drogen blockade (MAB). The nonsteroidal antiandrogens are administered orally. Gynecomastia, diarrhea, and erectile dysfunction are common side effects.

The beneficial effects associated with *estrogen (diethylstilbestrol, or DES)* are not yet understood. Oral therapy is avoided because of the high risk for adverse cardiovascular side effects. Several trials throughout the world have investigated parenteral DES and found it to be beneficial while avoiding the unacceptable side effects associated with oral administration.

Intermittent hormone deprivation therapy using the MAB technique is an alternative to ongoing therapy. Potential advantages include periods of "rest" between treatments, allowing relief from adverse side effects; however, definitive studies comparing this technique to ongoing therapy are not available and initial results do not favor the efficacy of this technique as compared to ongoing hormone deprivation.

Chemotherapy

Chemotherapy is used for palliation (alleviation of manifestations) when prostate cancer is hormone-resistant or independent. Chemotherapeutic agents may be given singly or in combination, depending on protocols. Examples of agents sometimes used are cyclophosphamide (Cytoxan), fluorouracil, estramustine phosphate (Emcyt), doxorubicin (Adriamycin), mitomycin (Mutamycin), paclitaxel (Taxol), and etoposide (VP-16, Etopophos). Mitoxantrone (Novantrone) is a chemotherapeutic drug used in combination with corticosteroids to relieve pain in hormone-resistant prostate cancer. This treatment is often successful after just one dose. Zoledronic acid (Zometa) is a bisphosphonate that may be administered for prostate cancer bone metastases. It delays or reduces bone metastases by improving bone strength.[21]

terone) production and includes a selection or combination of bilateral orchiectomy, estrogens, gonadotropin-releasing hormone analogs, and antiandrogens. The greatest amount of androgen (about 90%) is produced in the testicles, and small amounts are produced in the adrenal glands (10%). (See the Complementary and Alternative Therapy features on Acupuncture for Hot Flash Reduction in Men and on Weight Lifting for Men Receiving Androgen Deprivation Therapy for Prostate Cancer, below.)

Androgen deprivation can be achieved by several techniques. *Orchiectomy* is a technically simple procedure that removes both testes. It is also irreversible, however, and associated with profound adverse psychological effects. Thus when presented with options for managing advanced prostate cancer, the vast majority of men prefer medical castration using hormonal agents or similar drugs.

■ Nursing Management of the Medical Client

Provide Education. Nursing care depends on the type of medical therapy. Explain how treatments help prostate cancer, their side effects, and expected outcomes. Repetitive explanations are often necessary because clients must absorb much information and make decisions during a period when they may be in a state of shock. Provide information in a variety of formats, and include telephone numbers to be called when the client or partner has questions.

Explain Side Effects. Educate the man undergoing external-beam radiation about the rationale for radiation treatments, the necessity for multiple treatments, and the need to strictly attend all sessions to maximize the likelihood of success. Advise clients about possible adverse side effects, including radiation-induced cystitis or proctitis. Radiation cystitis is defined as inflammation of the bladder wall in response to unavoidable irradiation needed to treat a prostate malignancy. Tell the client that he may note dysuria (discomfort with voiding), daytime voiding frequency, an increase in the number of times he awakens to void, and suprapubic discomfort. The physician may prescribe an antimuscarinic agent such as tolterodine or oxybutynin or a urinary analgesic such as phenazopyridine. Reassure the client that radiation cystitis usually subsides within 4 to 6 weeks of radiation therapy.

Inform the client that radiation proctitis, characterized by frequent defecation, bowel cramping or urgency, and the defecation of blood and mucus, may occur. Reassure the client that, like radiation cystitis, it peaks during the latter stages of treatment but usually subsides

COMPLEMENTARY AND ALTERNATIVE THERAPY

Acupuncture for Hot Flash Reduction in Men

In 1998 the National Institutes of Health (NIH) stated that acupuncture could help with chemotherapy-induced nausea and postoperative pain. Acupuncture also is being tested for other conditions. For example, there is some preliminary research that acupuncture may reduce the risk of xerostomia (dry mouth) from radiation treatment for head and neck cancer.

Another condition, hot flashes, is also receiving attention. Researchers treated just 7 men who were experiencing hot flashes after prostate cancer androgen suppression treatment. These men were treated with acupuncture for 12 weeks (30 minutes twice a week for 2 weeks, then once a week for 10 weeks). After this treatment period, there was an average reduction in hot flashes of 70%. There was still a 50% reduction in the average number of hot flashes 3 months after the acupuncture was stopped. This is only a preliminary study, and a placebo group was not included in this investigation. Health professionals should tell their clients that in many states only an M.D. or D.O. degree is required to deliver acupuncture. Therefore clients need to check for some type of training or accreditation when looking for an acupuncturist.

Reference
Frisk, J., et al. (1999). Acupuncture treatment of vasomotor symptoms in men with prostatic carcinoma: A pilot study. *Journal of Urology, 161,* 853-856.

COMPLEMENTARY AND ALTERNATIVE THERAPY

Weight Lifting for Men Receiving Androgen Deprivation Therapy for Prostate Cancer

A total of 155 men with prostate cancer who were scheduled to receive androgen deprivation therapy for at least 3 months were randomly assigned to a weight-lifting program 3 times a week for 12 weeks ($n = 82$) or to a control group ($n = 73$). Men assigned to the weight-lifting program experienced less fatigue with activities of daily living ($p = 0.002$) and had higher quality of life scores ($p = 0.001$) compared to men in the control group. Men who lifted weights had higher levels of upper body ($p = 0.009$) and lower body ($p < 0.001$) muscular fitness versus men in the control group. The 12-week weight-lifting intervention did not improve body weight, body mass index, waist circumference, or subcutaneous skinfolds. However, lifting weights should be advocated for men receiving androgen deprivation therapy because of the profound impact on fatigue and quality of life.

Reference
Data from Segal, R., et al. (2003). Resistance exercise in men receiving androgen deprivation therapy for prostate cancer. *Journal of Clinical Oncology, 21,* 1653-1659.

within 4 to 6 weeks of the end of therapy. Mild manifestations can be managed by frequent defecation and antimuscarinic medications similar to those used for acute cystitis. In addition, counsel men to avoid or reduce their intake of foods or beverages likely to irritate the bowel or bladder, including caffeine and heavily spiced or fatty foods. The man is advised to avoid any rectal biopsies owing to the risk of subsequent bleeding or fistula formation.

Advise the client that external-beam radiation therapy may irritate the perineal skin. Teach him to cleanse the perineal skin with a mild cleanser and lukewarm water, paying special attention to skin folds, followed by dusting with a very small amount of cornstarch-based or talcum-based powder. Wearing loose cotton clothing also may relieve skin irritation. Radiation treatments also produce fatigue and loss of appetite. Counsel the client and partner that consumption of as many as six small meals per day, concentrating on foods that are high in protein and carbohydrates, will reduce these manifestations. A multivitamin should be taken daily throughout radiation therapy.

Preparation for brachytherapy typically includes bowel cleansing and administration of prophylactic antibiotics. An oral bowel stimulant such as magnesium citrate may be combined with a cleansing enema to prepare the bowel. Advise the client to maintain a clear liquid diet 12 to 24 hours preceding the study as directed. Instruct the client that the procedure is likely to produce rectal pressure or mild discomfort when the ultrasound probe is placed, but pain is not associated with implantation of radioactive seeds. A catheter is left in place that may be removed on the day of the procedure. Complete a voiding trial when removing the catheter (refer to the discussion of BPH earlier in this chapter). Teach the client that seed implantation will cause inflammation of the prostate that is likely to provoke bothersome LUTS, including daytime voiding frequency, an increase in nocturia, and difficulty initiating a urinary stream. These manifestations are typically transient and subside as prostatic inflammation diminishes.

Although rectal bleeding is uncommon after brachytherapy, you should instruct the client to monitor his stool for passage of large volumes of bright red blood, and advise him about how to manage radiation cystitis and proctitis. In addition, advise the client to avoid rectal biopsies that may cause excessive bleeding or fistula formation.

Teach the client and partner the principles of radiation safety following brachytherapy in consultation with the radiation oncologist and based on institutional policies. Advise the client that his semen is likely to have a brownish color over the first 1 to 2 months following implantation, and intercourse should be avoided during this period. In addition, intercourse with the intention of bearing children is strictly contraindicated unless cleared

> **CASE STUDY** *evolve*
> ## Cancer of the Prostate at the End of Life
> Everett Larson is a 72-year-old man who has been widowed for 15 years. Mr. Larson is being visited at this time to be admitted into hospice for end-stage prostate cancer. Mr. Larson lives alone in his own home and would like to stay there indefinitely.... *Case Study continued on the website and CD-ROM with discussions, multiple-choice questions, and a nursing care plan.* *evolve*

by the urologist or radiation oncologist. Clients are also taught to refrain from having children (or adults) sit in their lap for a prolonged period of time during the first 2 months following therapy.

Provide Support. Encourage men with prostate cancer and their significant others to attend relevant support groups or to subscribe to publications by organizations mentioned earlier. The best ways for clients to control fear and to keep a positive attitude are to learn as much as they can about treatments and to meet other men with prostate cancer. A health care provider who specializes in ED can best counsel a couple about ways to achieve sexual satisfaction.

Relieve Pain. When a client has metastases, assess pain levels (see Chapter 22) as well as activities of daily living. Keeping a pain diary is useful for the client's and the provider's awareness. Men tend to be stoic about pain and may have misconceptions about taking opioids. Carefully explain that addiction and decreasing drug effectiveness are not problems when cancer pain is being treated. Better pain control helps a man stay active and in control of his life. (See the Case Study feature on Cancer of the Prostate at the End of Life, above).

PROSTATITIS

Prostatitis (inflammation of the prostate gland) is a common and often perplexing problem. Traditionally, prostatitis was classified into four categories: acute bacterial, chronic bacterial, abacterial, and prostatodynia. This system has now been replaced by the National Institutes of Health (NIH) taxonomy with the following categories: category 1, acute bacterial prostatitis; category 2, chronic bacterial prostatitis; category 3, chronic pelvic pain syndrome (includes abacterial prostatitis and prostatodynia); and category 4, asymptomatic inflammatory prostatitis.[64] Category 1 is defined as an acute bacterial infection of the prostate causing intense local inflammation and pain as well as systemic illness or sepsis. Category 2 is a localized bacterial infection of the prostate that produces moderate localized discomfort but no systemic illness. Category 3 is diagnosed when men experience chronic pelvic pain in the absence of objective evidence of bacterial infection of the prostate. The NIH defines two subtypes of category 3: category 3A is diagnosed when manifestations are associated with objective evidence of prostatic inflammation, and category 3B is diagnosed when manifestations occur in the absence of such findings. Category 4 is diagnosed when pathologic analysis of a prostate biopsy or TURP specimen reveals evidence of infection and inflammation despite absence of reported manifestations.

Prostatitis is the most common urologic disorder in men younger than 50 years of age. About two million American men seek care for manifestations of prostatitis each year.

Etiology and Risk Factors

Category 1 (acute bacterial) prostatitis is typically caused by gastrointestinal or sexually transmitted bacteria. It causes severe localized prostatic inflammation that may interfere with the client's ability to urinate. Most men also experience systemic illness that may require hospitalization in severe cases. Although most cases have no apparent causes, risk factors include a recent bout of epididymitis, unprotected penetrative anal intercourse, urethral stricture or meatal stenosis, and recent catheterization or cystoscopy.

The etiology of category 2 (chronic bacterial) prostatitis is unknown. It is uncommon and accounts for less than 10% of all men with nonacute manifestations of prostatitis. Gastrointestinal (gram-negative) organisms are the most common cause of chronic prostatitis. Possible causes of bacterial invasion in men with chronic prostatitis include poor relaxation of the pelvic floor muscles during urination, causing turbulence and movement of bacteria from urethra to prostatic ducts.

Category 3 prostatic accounts for the remaining 90% of men with nonacute manifestations. Its etiology remains unknown.

Category 4 prostatitis is a pathologic diagnosis. Whether its presence predisposes clients to prostatitis or prostate cancer is not known.

Pathophysiology

Category 1 (acute bacterial) prostatitis leads to sepsis (bacterial invasion of the bloodstream) and a systemic immunologic response. Local immunologic responses include rapid rise in immunoglobulins A (IgA) and IgG, and the PSA protein. The PSA will return to normal within 6 weeks of treatment, but IgA and IgG levels remain elevated for 6-12 months. The reasons why some clients with a bacterial infection develop systemic responses while others experience only local inflammation with mild to moderately bothersome manifestations remains unknown.

Little is known about the pathophysiologic of category 3 prostatitis. Some researchers speculate that the

pain produced by this syndrome arises from pelvic muscle myalgia rather than prostatic inflammation, whereas other research reveals indirect evidence that turbulence of urine causes reflux of urate into the prostatic ducts with subsequent inflammation. Some recent research has attempted to link category 3 prostatitis with interstitial cystitis, a chronic abacterial inflammation of the bladder predominant in women.

Clinical Manifestations

The client's manifestations depend on the category of prostatitis. The client with acute bacterial prostatitis presents with abrupt onset of urinary urgency, frequency, nocturia, and dysuria, and he may have urinary retention. Fever, chills, and malaise are present, and the client complains of low back and perineal pain. He appears quite ill and may be experiencing nausea and vomiting. The prostate is extremely tender and boggy when examined. Prostate massage (expression of prostate secretions via digital rectal examination) is avoided because it is painful to the client and may exacerbate bacteremia. Bacteriuria and pyuria will reveal infection, and a urine culture is used to guide antibiotic therapy in category 1 prostatitis.

Many clinical manifestations of categories 2 and 3 prostatitis are similar. Bothersome LUTS include frequent daytime urination, nocturia, and a seemingly paradoxic combination of urinary urgency and hesitancy when micturition is attempted. Localized pain manifestations include the perineum (area between the rectum and scrotum), testes, tip of the penis, as well as dysuria and pain during or after ejaculation.

Assessment of category 1 prostatitis relies on urinalysis and urine culture; a blood culture may also be obtained. The client is evaluated for urinary retention, and vital signs are taken to determine the severity of systemic illness.

Assessment of category 2 and 3 prostatitis relies on examination of the urine and expressed prostatic secretions. A four-glass test was traditionally used to diagnose prostatitis, but this procedure has largely been replaced with a two-specimen technique. The client is instructed to arrive at the clinic with a comfortably full bladder. He washes the glans penis and retracts the foreskin (if uncircumcised). A midstream urine specimen is collected and analyzed via dipstick, microscopy, and culture when indicated (specimen 1). Immediately following urination, the physician will perform a DRE and any urethral discharge will be collected for microscopic analysis and culture (if feasible). This second specimen is the expressed prostatic secretion (EPS).[64]

Outcome Management
■ Medical Management

Reduce Inflammation. Clients with category 1 (acute bacterial) prostatitis may be so ill that they need hospitalization and intravenous (IV) antibiotics. Practically all antibiotics diffuse into the prostate when it is acutely inflamed, and a broad-spectrum fluoroquinolone is the drug of choice. An oral antibiotic is given when feasible, but clients with severe systemic illness may require parenteral drugs initially. Transurethral instrumentation is avoided unless absolutely necessary for urinary retention. The client should have at least 4 weeks of antibiotic therapy to eradicate the infection completely and to prevent chronic prostatitis.

The choice of antibiotic for chronic bacterial prostatitis is limited to those able to penetrate the fat and cholesterol internal environment of the *nonacute* prostate. Fluoroquinolones, such as ciprofloxacin or levofloxacin, remain the drugs of choice, and trimethoprim-sulfamethoxazole (Bactrim or Septra) is an excellent alternative. Long-term therapy (usually 30 days) is necessary, particularly when trimethoprim-sulfamethoxazole is administered.

Several treatment options can be used in men with category 3 prostatitis. Alpha-adrenergic blockers may be prescribed to reduce turbulence within the prostatic urethra and relieve urinary hesitancy. NSAIDs, hot sitz baths, and regular sexual activity (ejaculation) may provide transient relief from pelvic pain. In addition, an empiric trial of a fluoroquinolone has provided relief in some clients. Pelvic-floor muscle rehabilitation, particularly focusing on muscle relaxation, may be taught to relieve myalgia. Surgery may be considered for the client with chronic bacterial prostatitis when medical therapy does not improve manifestations that affect the man's quality of life. (See the Complementary and Alternative Therapy feature on Non-Bacterial Chronic Prostatitis and Quercetin, below.)

COMPLEMENTARY AND ALTERNATIVE THERAPY

Non-Bacterial Chronic Prostatitis and Quercetin

A total of 30 men with chronic non-bacterial prostatitis who had this condition for at least 6 months (ages 26 to 72 years) were allocated to take a 500-mg supplement called quercetin (a natural anti-inflammatory) or a placebo twice daily for 1 month. Subjects receiving the supplement experienced a significant improvement in their symptoms over the placebo. Their prostatic white blood count decreased, pain decreased, quality of life improved, and their perception of their overall condition improved. A larger and longer trial is needed, but this study is important because of a lack of medicines to effectively treat this problem.

Reference
Shoskes, D., et al. (1999). Quercetin in men with category III chronic prostatitis: A preliminary prospective, double-blind, placebo-controlled trial. *Urology, 54*, 960-963.

■ Nursing Management of the Medical Client

Teach all clients with prostatitis techniques of pelvic muscle relaxation to relieve discomfort associated with pelvic muscle hypertonicity and urinary hesitancy. Constipation can be a painful problem for clients with prostatitis. It should be managed by adequate fluid intake combined with adequate of dietary fiber and exercise.

The client may be uncomfortable, frustrated, and fearful that the manifestations will never go away or may lead to something more serious than infection. He may have sexual or fertility concerns or may believe that the infection can be sexually transmitted. Clients need much reassurance and teaching. They should understand the importance of complying with the total treatment course and know the side effects of prescribed medications. Clients should also be taught that recent research suggests that increasing sexual activity or masturbation may help to decrease prostatic gland congestion.

TESTICULAR AND SCROTAL DISORDERS
TESTICULAR CANCER

Testicular cancer is the most common and serious solid tumor cancer in men between 15 and 35 years of age. It rarely occurs in men younger than age 15 or older than age 40. It is rare, with about 7600 cases diagnosed and 400 deaths in the United States in 2003.[2] In many cases it is curable, sometimes even in an advanced stage. Testicular cancer is less common in African-American and Asian men. The incidence is about the same in Hispanic men as in white men. In Israel, the rate is three times higher in Jewish men than in non-Jewish men. Testicular cancer is about twice as frequent in high socioeconomic groups.

Etiology and Risk Factors

The cause of testicular cancer is unknown. Family history, exogenous estrogen, and cryptorchidism (undescended testicles) are known risk factors. Cryptorchidism is the major risk factor. Surgery (orchiopexy) is recommended soon after birth, but it does not completely eliminate the risk of cancer.

The male offspring of women who used estrogen in the form of diethylstilbestrol (DES) during the first trimester of pregnancy (called *DES sons*) or who were exposed to estrogen-progestin combinations frequently used in diagnostic tests to confirm pregnancy are at greater risk for testicular cancer. Between 1940 and 1970, DES was given to pregnant women who had a high risk of spontaneous abortion. DES sons also have an increased risk of genitourinary abnormalities such as micropenis, meatal stenosis, varicocele, hypoplastic testicles, infertility, and abnormal semen.

Children with an undescended testicle should be closely observed. Men 15 to 45 years of age should practice monthly testicular self-examination (see Chapter 39). Men at high risk for testicular cancer should see a physician for yearly examinations. Early detection can lead to early diagnosis and cure.

Pathophysiology

Most testicular cancers (90% to 95%) are germinal cell tumors, such as seminoma (about 30% to 40% of all tumors), embryonal carcinoma (about 20%), teratocarcinoma, or choriocarcinoma. Seminomas generally carry a favorable prognosis (about a 90% 5-year survival rate) because they are usually localized, metastasize late, and are radiosensitive.

Nongerminal tumors make up the remainder of testicular tumors and are classified as either interstitial cell tumors or testicular adenomas. They arise from interstitial cells or cells that compose the fibrous and vascular networks. They are usually benign.

Metastasis occurs primarily through lymphatic spread. Drainage from the right testis is to the inter-aortocaval nodes, whereas the left drains to the preaortic nodes. Rectoperineal nodes are commonly affected. Distant metastasis occurs most commonly to the lung and rarely to the liver, viscera, bone, or brain.

Choriocarcinoma spreads via the bloodstream. Even after surgical removal, testicular cancer can occur in the other testicle. Carcinoma in situ (localized), although rare, frequently involves both testes. Rarely, testicular tumors are secondary to cancers in another primary site.

Clinical Manifestations

Most commonly, men with testicular tumors experience a painless enlargement, noted as heaviness, in the testicle (in about 75% of cases). Some men describe it as a dragging sensation. Pain is rarely felt; however, the tumor is often found after an injury because the testicle is examined as a result of the injury. A thorough description of family and birth histories and manifestations is the first step in assessment.

Assessment findings suggesting metastasis to the retroperitoneal lymph nodes include back pain, vague abdominal pain, nausea and vomiting, bowel and bladder changes, anorexia, and weight loss. If the lungs are involved, manifestations may include cough, dyspnea, and hemoptysis.

The next step is physical examination of the scrotum and testicles, in which the health care provider determines the location and size of any nodule. If there is a nodule, a light may be held against the scrotum to see whether it is transilluminated (to see whether light passes through) (see Figure 39-11). Whereas cysts and hydroceles are transilluminated, tumors and hernias are not.

Ultrasonography of the testes follows. If tumor is suspected, chest x-ray studies and CT scans are ordered to detect metastases. An IVP may be ordered to detect urinary tract involvement.

Blood tests are ordered. Alpha-fetoprotein (AFP), beta human chorionic gonadotropin (beta-HCG), and lactic acid dehydrogenase (LDH) are the tumor markers used to detect testicular cancer. Elevated AFP is not seen in clients with testicular seminomas. Beta-HCG can be elevated in either seminomas or nonseminomas and, when elevated, may cause gynecomastia in men with testicular cancer. LDH is often elevated in germinal testicular cancers because of the cancer's cell activity, and this elevation also suggests metastasis because LDH is produced in the liver, kidney, and brain.

Testicular cancer is verified by inguinal exploration. If a definite mass is not found, a frozen biopsy may be done. If there is still suspicion, a radical orchiectomy is performed. The testis, epididymis, and vas deferens are removed. The spermatic cord is ligated just inside the internal inguinal ring to prevent seeding of the cancer. Any testicular mass is considered malignant until proved otherwise.

Staging testicular tumors helps to guess at prognosis and to determine treatment options. Testicular tumors are staged as follows:
- *Stage I$_a$:* Tumor confined to testicle (T1 N0 M0)
- *Stage I:* Metastasis to para-aortic or iliac nodes (T1 N1 M0)
- *Stage II:* Tumor spread to retroperitoneal nodes but disease limited to below the diaphragm (T2-3, N2, M0)
- *Stage III:* Tumor above the diaphragm or spread to body organs (usually the lungs) (T4, N3-4, M+)

Outcome Management
■ Surgical Management

Radical orchiectomy, performed to diagnose testicular cancer, is also the primary treatment. *Retroperitoneal lymph node dissection* (RPLND) may be done when there is lymph node involvement. The primary use of this procedure is controversial in advanced-stage cancer because treatment with chemotherapy for nonseminomas is very successful. Impotence rates are high after RPLND because many of the autonomic nerves necessary for ejaculation are located in this area. RPLND is performed when testicular cancer is embryonal because this type of cancer metastasizes rapidly.

In other types of testicular cancer, surgeons who perform RPLND believe that it limits the amount of chemotherapy needed. This approach may be used as an adjunct to chemotherapy when only a partial response is achieved. A thoracoabdominal or transabdominal incision is made, and modified dissection techniques are used. The newest approach is a *laparoscopic node dissection.* A smaller incision and fewer complications (especially retrograde ejaculation) result after laparoscopic surgery.

■ Nursing Management of the Surgical Client

Clients undergoing radical orchiectomy usually require a short hospital stay and experience few complications. The scrotal area is tender and slightly swollen after surgery. Ice bags are applied to the scrotum, and a scrotal support is worn when the client is ambulating. Teach the client self-care strategies and how to monitor for the development of complications. Provide written instructions, a resource he can call if questions or concerns arise, and a follow-up appointment with the surgeon. The client needs to be aware that testicular cancer can recur in the other testicle, and he should know how to do testicular self-examination.

If the client undergoes RPLND, hospitalization is longer, depending on the approach used. Counseling about potential infertility problems and sperm banking takes place before the procedure.

Postoperatively, the client must be monitored closely for possible problems associated with major abdominal surgery. The client requires adequate pain control to comply with ambulation and vigorous coughing and deep breathing to prevent respiratory complications. Anxiety and fear about cancer, sexuality, quality of life, and life expectancy are issues that must frequently be addressed. Be sure that follow-up appointments are made with the surgeon and oncologist for further treatment if appropriate.

■ Medical Management

Medical management follows radical orchiectomy during the treatment of testicular cancer. A period of close follow-up and observation is necessary to detect recurrence and plan future care.

Destroy Cancer Cells

Radiation Therapy. Low-grade seminomas are particularly radiosensitive. The perineum and pelvis are irradiated, as are the mediastinal and supraclavicular nodes if peritoneal nodes are positive for cancer. Side effects include common complications associated with pelvic radiation: irritable bowel and bladder problems, skin reactions, fatigue, nausea, and anorexia. Radiation may also cause temporary or permanent infertility. Side effects are usually minimal because the dose and number of treatments required are low. Almost 95% of clients with low-stage seminomas survive more than 5 years.

Chemotherapy. Nonseminomatous tumors are not radiosensitive, and they and high-grade seminomas are therefore treated with chemotherapy. The major agent used is cisplatin in combination with vinblastine and bleomycin. Cisplatin in combination with other agents dramatically increases the long-term survival rate for men with testicular cancer. These agents, in combination with a variety of others, have been used to treat metastatic disease or refractory tumors with some success. (Complications of these chemotherapeutic agents are covered in Chapter 19.) Cisplatin has nephrotoxic effects, bleomycin causes pneumonitis, and vinblastine causes peripheral neuropathy.

■ Nursing Management of the Medical Client

During assessment of a man born between 1940 and 1971, ask whether his mother took any medication during pregnancy to prevent pregnancy or miscarriage. If he appears at particular risk but does not know these details, it may be necessary to obtain the mother's medical history. Information and referral are available through DES Action, Long Island Jewish-Hillside Medical Center, New Hyde Park, NY 11040.

Supportive nursing care for these young men is important during both diagnosis and treatment. Be aware of the threat to sexuality that this condition and its treatment pose to young men. Chapter 19 reviews the care of clients undergoing chemotherapy and radiation therapy.

A Testicular torsion **B** Hydrocele **C** Varicocele

FIGURE 40-4 Disturbances of the testicles.

TESTICULAR TORSION

Testicular torsion (Figure 40-4, *A*) occurs when a testicle is mobile and the spermatic cord twists, cutting off the blood supply. It is the most common testicular disorder in children. It can occur at any age but is most usual at puberty, and about 30% of cases occur in men in their 20s. Manifestations usually arise suddenly with acute scrotal swelling and severe pain as blood supply to the testicles is interrupted.

If testicular torsion is suspected, a testicular scan and Doppler ultrasonography are performed to assess the blood supply. Torsion causes a decrease (blood supply would be increased with epididymitis).

Testicular torsion is an emergency requiring immediate surgical intervention. The spermatic cord is untwisted and the testicle is immobilized by suturing it to the scrotum (orchiopexy). Without prompt surgery, the testicle may atrophy or develop an abscess. If the testicle is necrotic, it is removed. Because there is a risk that the other testicle will be susceptible to torsion, it is also affixed to the scrotum at the time of surgery.

ORCHITIS

Orchitis is a rare, acute testicular inflammation, usually caused by a viral infection. Mumps orchitis, which occurs in about 30% of men who develop mumps after puberty, is usually bilateral.

Assessment reveals edematous and extremely tender testicles, reddened scrotal skin, fever, and prostration. Treatment includes bed rest, scrotal support, local heat to the scrotum, and medications for pain reduction, fever, and infection. An acute phase may last about a week. Permanent sterility may occur if both testicles are affected, whereas decreased fertility may result if only one is affected.

EPIDIDYMITIS

Epididymitis is more common than orchitis. Infections in the urethra, prostate, or bladder can spread along the vas deferens; infections also spread through the lymphatic and vascular systems. Bladder outlet obstruction can cause reflux of infected urine. Epididymitis can occur as a complication related to urethral instrumentation, such as catheterization or instrumentation in transurethral surgeries, but its frequency has decreased since prophylactic antibiotics have been prescribed after such procedures. Sexually transmitted organisms frequently cause the condition in younger men, and urinary pathogens cause epididymitis in older men. Trauma is a noninfectious cause.

Epididymitis is almost always unilateral. Early in the disease, a client has local pain and swelling. As epididymitis progresses, the testis becomes involved (epididymo-orchitis), the entire scrotum becomes reddened and painful, and an inflammatory hydrocele can occur. After the acute phase, fibrosis and occlusion may result, with subsequent sterility. Recurrences are common when other conditions are unresolved. Treatment is the same as for orchitis.

HYDROCELE, HEMATOCELE, AND SPERMATOCELE

Hydrocele (Figure 40-4, *B*) is a painless collection of clear, yellow fluid in the scrotum caused by an opening between the peritoneum and the tunica vaginalis or by an imbalance in production and reabsorption of fluid within the tunica vaginalis. The soft intrascrotal mass is translucent to light. Often, if the hydrocele is due to a communication with the peritoneum, it decreases in size when the man lies down. If constant discomfort, embarrassment, or impaired circulation occur, aspiration or surgical drainage may be performed. Hydroceles can conceal a testicular tumor or inguinal hernia.

A hematocele is a collection of blood in the tunica vaginalis caused by trauma. Hematoceles are less likely than hydroceles to be transilluminated on light examination. They require only drainage.

A spermatocele is a cystic dilation of part of the epididymis that contains a milky fluid and dead spermatozoa. It is painless, and surgery is usually not required.

VARICOCELE

Varicocele (Figure 40-4, *C*) is a dilation and varicosity of the pampiniform plexus (the network of veins supplying the testicles) within the scrotum. They usually arise slowly. Ninety percent of varicoceles are left-sided because the left spermatic vein enters the renal vein at a 90-degree angle, causing back pressure. Pain may be relieved by masturbation or sexual intercourse. Varicoceles are found in 19% to 41% of men who are evaluated for infertility. A right-sided varicocele suggests tumor or retroperitoneal fibrosis.

On palpation, with the man standing, a varicocele feels like a mass of tortuous veins above and posterior to the testicle. When the man lies down, the mass abates. Treatment includes the use of a scrotal support. Surgery is performed if there is severe pain or if the varicocele is thought to contribute to infertility.

VASECTOMY (ELECTIVE STERILIZATION)

A vasectomy is an elective surgical procedure to ensure a permanent method of contraception. It is sometimes performed after a prostatectomy to prevent retrograde epididymitis. The surgery is usually performed in the urologist's office or in an outpatient setting with the use of local anesthesia. The procedure, performed through a

FIGURE 40-5 Vasectomy.

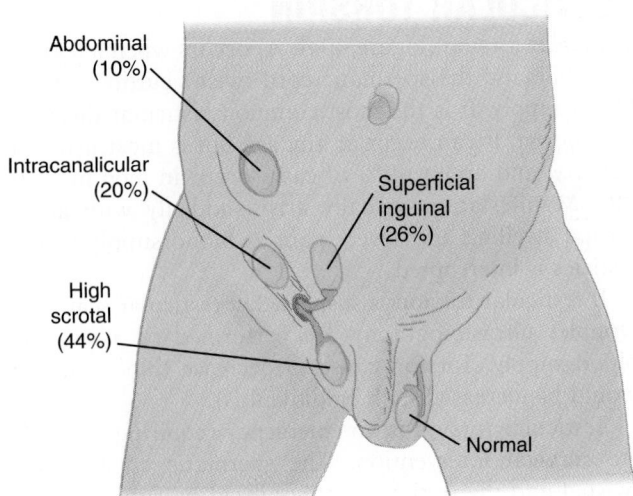

FIGURE 40-6 Undescended or mispositioned testis (cryptorchidism).

small incision in the scrotum, involves cutting out a segment of the vas deferens, ligating the ends, and tucking them into different tissue planes to prevent reanastomosis (Figure 40-5).

Slight pain, swelling, and bruising occur postoperatively, but discomfort is controlled with ice, a mild analgesic such as acetaminophen (aspirin is avoided to prevent bleeding), and rest for a few days. A scrotal support also increases client comfort. The client can resume heavy lifting and sexual intercourse about a week after surgery. The client must continue to practice other means of birth control until the follow-up semen analysis shows azoospermia (absence of sperm) because live sperm are left in the ampulla of vas deferens. Bleeding, infection, and mild chronic pain (rare) are complications that can occur after vasectomy.

The client must consider vasectomy a permanent means of contraception. Vasovasostomy, which is a surgical reversal of a vasectomy, can be done; however, it is expensive and fertility is not guaranteed.

UNDESCENDED OR MISPOSITIONED TESTICLES

The most common congenital testicular condition is malpositioned undescended testes (cryptorchidism) (Figure 40-6). Testes normally descend from the abdomen into the scrotum before birth, but sometimes they do not. One or both testicles may be arrested in the abdomen, inguinal canal (canalicular), low pelvis, or high scrotum. An ectopic testicle descends to the wrong area outside the normal path of decent (e.g., perineum). A retractile testicle descends into the scrotum but pulls back into the inguinal canal because of a hyperactive cremasteric reflex. Complete absence of a testicle may also occur.

Undescended testicles occur in about 4% of full-term male infants and are more common in premature infants. Many resolve by the first year of life. Inguinal hernias and torsion commonly occur with undescended testicles.

Cryptorchidism is associated with infertility. High body temperature, endocrine understimulation, and an abnormal epididymis that seems to accompany an undescended testicle cause changes that prevent normal fertility in the future. The incidence of testicular cancer is high in men with undescended testes if the condition is not corrected before puberty. A man with an undescended testicle has a 1 in 80 chance of testicular cancer development. Correction, however, does not guarantee prevention.

Treatment, which is surgical, is performed when the child is between 9 and 12 months old and certainly by 18 months, not only to allow time for spontaneous descent but also to decrease the risk of total infertility and testicular cancer. An inguinal incision is used so that additional repair (i.e., hernia repair or excision of connective tissue bands) or orchiectomy (should the testicle look abnormal) can be done.

Retractile testes usually descend and stay in the scrotum by puberty, but surgery is not required. HCG has sometimes been used to promote passage of the testicle into the scrotum. Luteinizing hormone-releasing hormone (LHRH) is administered as a nasal spray in Europe, but it has not been approved for use in the United States.

If the cryptorchidism is bilateral, the child should be assessed for intersexuality (an intermingling of female and male characteristics with external characteristics often contradictory to internal characteristics), especially if the condition is associated with other genital abnormalities. Continuous follow-up through the childbearing years is necessary to detect malignancy and to deal with infertility issues if they arise. Clients and their parents should learn how to do testicular self-examination.

INFERTILITY

Infertility is a situation in which regular, unprotected intercourse does not result in a pregnancy over a 12-month period. Infertility affects 20% to 35% of couples in the United States who are trying to have children, and requests for infertility services are increasing rapidly.

A male factor contributes partially or totally to the couple's inability to conceive in about 50% of the cases. It is best, however, that the two partners be treated together. Minimal fertility *(subfertility)* in one partner can be offset by strong fertility in the other. If both partners are minimally fertile, infertility is more likely. Awareness of these statistics alerts health care professionals to clients who may have concerns about infertility but who have difficulty expressing them. Male factors for infertility are discussed in this chapter.

Etiology and Risk Factors

Pretesticular (hormonal) causes involve endocrine dysfunction and account for about 3% to 25% of cases. Examples are pituitary and adrenal tumors, thyroid disorders, diabetes, and cirrhosis.

Testicular causes are most common. Varicoceles are found in 19% to 41% of infertility cases. Other testicular causes include congenital abnormalities, torsion, genitourinary infection, trauma, and exposure to substances known to interfere with spermatogenesis (sperm formation). Cryptorchidism is directly related to infertility.

Post-testicular causes include congenital blockage of the vas deferens and other malformations of structures distal to the testes. Additional causes include epididymitis, emotional factors, surgical procedures that cause retrograde ejaculation, and some medical conditions such as renal disease or paraplegia.

Infection of the prostate, epididymis, or testicle can affect fertility. The mumps virus attacks the testicle in 5% to 37% of adults who acquire the infection. Of these men, 16% to 65% have bilateral involvement. Although rare in the Western world, tuberculosis is a genital infection seen in other countries and in immigrants to the United States.

Whether testicular trauma and infertility are related is a matter of controversy. The formation of anti-sperm antibodies is one theory. Some surgical procedures cause retrograde ejaculation.

Chemicals, drugs, and other substances that affect spermatogenesis are called *gonadotoxins* (e.g., heavy use of alcohol, marijuana, and anabolic steroids). Many medications, including allopurinol, cimetidine, nitrofurantoin, sulfasalazine, and chemotherapeutic drugs, have been related to infertility. Alpha-adrenergic blockers and ganglion blockers can cause retrograde ejaculation and may thus be a secondary cause of inability to conceive. Exposure to agricultural, industrial, and warfare agents is an increasing concern. Lead, agent orange (a herbicide used as a defoliant in Vietnam), and some pesticides affect fertility. Tobacco smoke has been investigated as a cause of infertility, but a clear link has not been established; data suggest that smoking may be involved in subfertility. Radiation and hyperthermia also affect fertility.

Problems with intercourse are responsible for infertility in about 5% of couples. These include ED, premature ejaculation, unfavorable timing or frequency of intercourse, excessive masturbation, and aberrant sexual behaviors. Many water-soluble lubricants used during intercourse can be toxic to sperm.

Pathophysiology

The pathophysiologic mechanisms involved in infertility vary, and the problem is often complex. Hormonal imbalance between the hypothalamus, pituitary gland, and testicles can interfere with the production and maturation of sperm. Hypoxia of the testicle and elevated scrotal temperature cause germ cell damage. Seminal WBCs present in genitourinary infections are believed to release bioactive cytokines that affect spermatogenesis.

Some viruses and bacteria directly destroy cells or cause enough inflammation to cause tissue necrosis. Sexually transmitted diseases (STDs), particularly gonorrhea and infection with *Chlamydia trachomatis*, may account for cases of infertility because they can cause testicular atrophy, but a clear relationship has not been proved. Immune responses may prevent the formation of normal sperm. Gonadotoxins can decrease the number of sperm, decrease motility (the forward movement of sperm), or cause abnormal morphology. Congenital factors and trauma can impair patency of the ductal system that extends from the testicles through the prostate.

Clinical Manifestations

Assessment of infertility includes obtaining a detailed occupational, sexual, medical, and reproductive history and conducting a thorough physical examination. During an examination, the presence of testicles and their size, varicocele or other scrotal and penile abnormalities, and secondary sex characteristics are noted. A prostate massage and specimens of secretions may be obtained for culture to check for infection. A post-ejaculatory urine specimen may also be checked for the presence of sperm, which suggests retrograde ejaculation.

Semen analysis is performed on more than one specimen. Semen volume and viscosity, number and concentration of sperm, motility, and morphology are analyzed. The presence of white blood cells or agglutination of sperm is noted. A normal semen analysis would show the following values:

- Semen volume, 1.5 to 5 ml
- Concentration, >20 million sperm/ml
- Total sperm count, >50 to 60 million
- Motility, 60% grade 2 or higher (on a scale of 1 to 4)
- Morphology, 60% normal

Motility refers to the forward movement of sperm; *morphology* refers to sperm form and size. Normally, sperm have one head and one tail. Abnormal sperm may be immature, may have misshapen heads, or may have two tails. Some infertility specialists consider slightly lower percentages for sperm count, motility, and morphology to be adequate when evaluating semen quality. Other more specific tests may be done to evaluate semen, such as checking for viscosity, coagulation, and the presence of fructose.

Serum endocrine studies are conducted to assess testosterone, prolactin, LH, and follicle-stimulating hormone (FSH). For example, if testosterone levels are normal, nonhormonal causes are pursued. If testosterone levels and prolactin levels are low but LH levels are high, primary testicular disease may be suspected. If FSH levels are high, spermatogenesis is probably arrested. If FSH levels are normal, *azoospermia* (absence of sperm) or *oligospermia* (scarcity of sperm) is probably caused by obstruction in the post-testicular ducts, which may be corrected by microsurgery.

If anatomic abnormalities are suspected, imaging techniques such as Doppler ultrasonography, MRI, cavernosography, and color flow Doppler imaging are ordered. A testicular biopsy may be performed if sperm are absent or scarce along with normal hormone levels. Clients are carefully selected for such studies because the tests are costly and, when invasive, may cause testicular damage.

Outcome Management
■ Medical Management

Pretesticular Causes. Treatment of male infertility with pretesticular causes varies. No treatment is available for primary testicular failure or hypogonadism. Testosterone may be prescribed to correct low testosterone levels. A testosterone patch is applied directly to the scrotum (Testoderm) or to the torso or extremities (Androderm). Scrotal skin is five times more permeable, and there is concern about too much absorption and side effects. With both transdermal methods, skin irritation or contact dermatitis is experienced in about 9% of clients. Testosterone is contraindicated for men with prostate cancer or severe bladder outlet obstruction. Hyperprolactinemia may be treated by surgical removal of a pituitary tumor or by administration of bromocriptine (Parlodel).

Treatment of male sexual dysfunction is discussed under Erectile Dysfunction later in this chapter. For oligospermia caused by excessive frequency of ejaculation, recommend that the couple have intercourse only once every 36 hours during the woman's periovulatory period because it takes 24 hours for a normal sperm count to be generated after ejaculation.

Testicular Causes. Treatment of male infertility with testicular causes also varies. Instruct the client to avoid factors that depress spermatogenesis such as heat, drugs, alcohol, and marijuana. He should keep the testicles cool by avoiding hot baths and tight clothing or by using a commercially prepared, water-dampened scrotal-cooling device; keeping the testes cool appears to improve the sperm count. Advise the client to maintain good nutrition. Medications such as HCG or testosterone (Depo-Testosterone) are sometimes prescribed as hormonal treatments. Nonhormonal therapy may consist of kallikrein, steroids, indomethacin, arginine, zinc, or vitamins. Varicocele is treated surgically.

Post-Testicular Causes. Treatment of male infertility with post-testicular causes involves correcting ejaculatory abnormalities and obstruction. Ejaculatory abnormalities may be corrected by the split-ejaculate technique. The first half of the ejaculate contains more sperm than the second half. The first half may be used for artificial insemination or may be deposited in the vagina during intercourse, followed by withdrawal of the penis. Absence of ejaculation or retrograde (backward) ejaculation may be treated with drugs such as ephedrine, imipramine, or antihistamines. When the client experiences retrograde ejaculation, artificial insemination may be performed using sperm from urine obtained by centrifugation. Obstructive infertility is treated by surgery.

Appropriate antimicrobial drugs are used to treat genitourinary infections. Male infertility with immunologic causes may be treated with steroids and artificial insemination of sperm that have been washed to remove antibodies contained in the sperm.

■ Nursing Management of the Medical Client

Provide Support. The client and his partner are often highly emotional in the diagnostic phase, and your sensitivity can ease their concerns somewhat. Both may need help and support to express their feelings and concerns about infertility. Failure to conceive may make several demands on the couple, threatening their individual self-concepts, gender roles, relationship, and sexual interaction. Guilt and blame about previous sexual activity, STDs, or abortion may come between them. Some men find masturbation (necessary to obtain a semen sample) difficult for personal, cultural, or religious reasons. Many men do not know what chemicals they have been exposed to at the workplace or elsewhere. Fear and anxiety may be lessened during your assessment and teaching sessions. This provides you with the opportunity to support, respond to questions, and explain diagnostic and treatment procedures. Emphasize the need for consistent follow-up to evaluate progress.

Referral for counseling or support groups, or both, for infertile couples may be appropriate. A nationally known support group in the United States is RESOLVE (Department P, Box 474, Belmont, MA 02178).

Provide Education. Because thorough and complete fertility assessment is expensive and can be ineffective, the client needs to understand the testing and the reasons for the various examinations. Explain fully how to collect a specimen for sperm analysis so that results are accurate. Written as well as verbal instructions are important because anxiety levels may be high. The man should refrain from sexual activity for 3 days before collecting a semen sample and should take the specimen immediately (within 1 hour) to the laboratory for analysis. Masturbation is the preferred method because some semen is lost during intercourse. Condoms and lubricants may make the sperm immotile. The specimen should be kept close to the body to maintain normal temperature. Two to three interval specimens are required for evaluation because results can vary. Ensure that the client understands the medical regimen suggested and the importance of following it closely.

Prevent Infertility. If possible, it is more effective to prevent infertility than to treat it. Clients who want to conceive at present or in the future can try to prevent infertility by doing the following:

1. Avoiding gonadotoxins, as discussed earlier
2. Decreasing exposure to occupational and environmental hazards
3. Keeping the scrotum cool by avoiding excessive heat, hot baths, and tight clothing
4. Avoiding transmission of STDs by limiting the number of sexual partners and by using condoms
5. Developing effective means of stress reduction
6. Eating a well-balanced, nutritious diet

PENILE DISORDERS
PHIMOSIS

Phimosis occurs when the penile foreskin (prepuce) is constricted at the opening, making retraction difficult or impossible. The condition can be congenital or a result of inflammation, infection, or local trauma. It is not usually painful, but it can lead to obstructive uropathy if it is severe enough. Prolonged phimosis, caused by chronic inflammation and irritation, predisposes to penile cancer. Assessment reveals edema, erythema, tenderness, and purulent discharge. Intervention includes controlling infection with local treatment and broad-spectrum antimicrobial drugs.

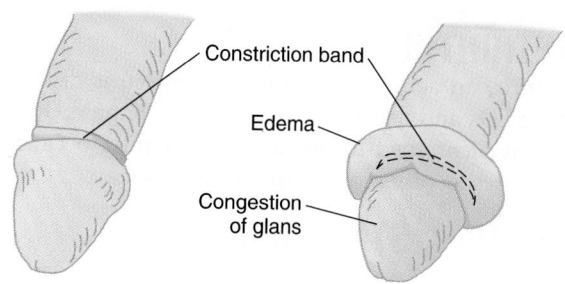

FIGURE 40-7 Paraphimosis.

Effective genital hygiene is essential to prevent acquired penile disorders. In uncircumcised males, the man cleans the penis by pulling the foreskin back gently and washing the area with a washcloth. This technique should be done daily to eliminate the normally accumulated smegma, and the foreskin should be returned to its normal position.

Routine *circumcision* (surgical removal of the foreskin) of male infants has not been considered medically necessary by the American Academy of Pediatrics and other health professionals and health organizations. Some parents have religious or cultural reasons for continuing the practice of circumcision. The operation may be indicated for clients with penile infection, phimosis, or paraphimosis. The rate of penile cancer is almost nil in circumcised men. The procedure should be done with the client under general anesthesia. Potential risks include excessive bleeding, infection, and penile trauma.

PARAPHIMOSIS

Paraphimosis (Figure 40-7) occurs when a tight foreskin, once retracted, cannot be returned to its normal position. This sometimes happens after rigorous cleaning, masturbation, sexual intercourse, catheter insertion, or cystoscopy if the foreskin is not returned to its normal position. Circulation is thus impeded, and the glans swells rapidly. It is painful and edema is common. The foreskin can be gently compressed either manually or with an elastic wrap. The client can then attempt manual reduction by gently pulling the foreskin. Surgical incision of the foreskin with local anesthesia may be necessary if the condition does not resolve.

POSTHITIS AND BALANITIS

Posthitis (foreskin inflammation) and *balanitis* (inflammation of the glans penis and the mucous membrane beneath it) are caused by irritation and invasion of microorganisms. Good hygiene and thorough drying of the penis are recommended. It is important to assess for diabetes, which predisposes the client to secondary infection. Antibiotics may help control local infection. Circumcision may be necessary.

URETHRITIS

Urethritis, an acute urethral inflammation, is discussed under STDs and urinary disorders (see Chapters 36 and 43). It is mentioned throughout this chapter because it predisposes to other genitourinary disorders.

URETHRAL STRICTURE

Urethral stricture is caused by urethral scarring or narrowing. It may be congenital or caused by untreated or severe urethritis or urethral injury (including urologic instrumentation, e.g., cystoscopy). Manifestations are caused by obstruction: small-caliber urinary stream, hyperdistended bladder, infection, fever, and dysuria. Urethral strictures are released surgically by urethral dilation or urethroplasty. See Chapter 36 for further information.

EPISPADIAS

Epispadias (Figure 40-8, *A*) is a rare congenital condition in which the urethral meatus opens dorsally on top of the penis, proximal to the glans, most commonly at the abdominal-penile junction. Surgery is required to correct urinary incontinence and to return the urethra to a normal position in the penis.

HYPOSPADIAS

Hypospadias (Figure 40-8, *B*) is a congenital condition in which the urethral meatus opens on the ventral side of the penis. Common locations include the glans penis, penile shaft, penoscrotal junction, and perineum. *Chordee* (curvature of the penis) is often associated with hypospadias. Hypospadias occurs in about two to eight per thousand live male births.

Early assessment of internal reproductive organ development is necessary to confirm the child's gender. For psychological reasons, hypospadias should be repaired before the child starts school. It is important to ask about this condition when taking the history.

PEYRONIE'S DISEASE

Fibrous plaques develop in the connective tissue in Peyronie's disease, usually near the dorsal midline of the penile shaft in middle-aged and older men. Although the etiologic mechanism is unknown, one theory is that the disease is caused by an abnormal fibrotic reaction to trauma. The disease has two phases: acute and chronic. Pain is more likely during the initial phase, and plaques begin to develop. This phase can last about 12 to 18 months. Pain usually subsides during the chronic phase, but fibrosis is increased.

Diagnosis may be made during history taking, although men usually seek a physician because of concern about penile lumps (fear of cancer), painful erection, or ED. The man may have penile curvature on erection, painful erection, and unsatisfactory vaginal penetration. Peyronie's disease is often associated with Dupuytren's contracture of the hand tendons.

Some cases improve spontaneously. Reassure the client that this is not a malignant condition and does not lead to development of cancer. If a client is not having discomfort and has soft plaques and minimal curvature, the physician may advise waiting several months before instituting therapy. Medical treatment includes vitamin E, para-aminobenzoic acid, tamoxifen, and colchicine. Intralesional injections, local radiation, and ultrasonography have also been used. Surgical correction is necessary when previous treatments have failed and the client is unable to perform sexually.

PRIAPISM

Priapism is a prolonged, persistent penile erection without sexual desire. It can last hours or even days and may be very painful. The condition is sometimes associated with leukemia or sickle cell anemia. Self-injection of medications (mainly papaverine) to treat impotence is the other common cause. It may also result from some

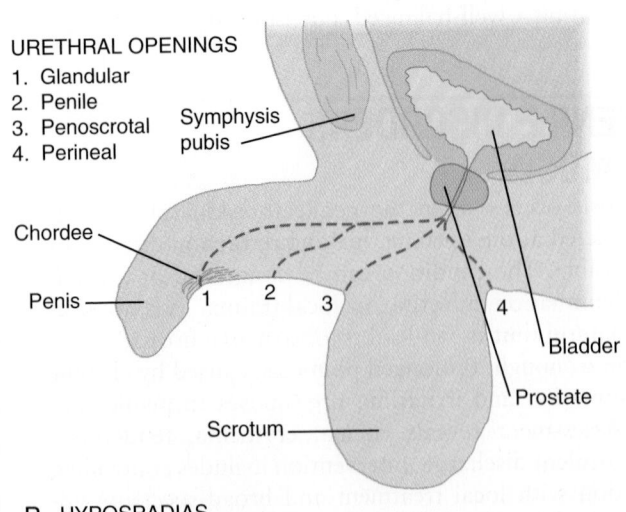

A EPISPADIAS

B HYPOSPADIAS

FIGURE 40-8 Epispadias (**A**) and hypospadias (**B**).

medications, such as anticoagulants, alcohol, phenothiazine, alpha-adrenergic blockers, and marijuana.

Two major types of priapism have been defined according to a physiology-based system. *High-flow* arterial priapism, the less common type, usually occurs after trauma and is less painful. *Low-flow* veno-occlusive priapism, the more common form, is an emergency situation and is extremely painful.

In the client with low-flow priapism, circulation to the penis is compromised, predisposing to ischemia and permanent ED. The client may also be unable to void. Treatment in most cases consists of aspiration of blood from the penis followed by serial intracavernosal injections of phenylephrine.

Low-flow priapism must be resolved within 24 hours to prevent penile ischemia, gangrene, fibrosis, and ED. If the more conservative treatments are unsuccessful, more invasive therapy is required to prevent permanent damage. Surgical treatment is designed to drain the congested blood from the corpora cavernosa.

High-flow priapism can often be treated with ice and compression. If these measures are not successful, the client may require selective embolization or ligation of the traumatized artery.

Be sensitive to the embarrassing nature of this problem. Men are often reluctant to admit that this problem has occurred and yet may be in severe pain. Be understanding, and try to make the client comfortable while decreasing the client's embarrassment about the problem.

PENILE CANCER

Penile cancer is rare. It usually affects the foreskin in older, uncircumcised men who have suffered chronic irritation and have poor hygiene practices. Associated genital cancer sometimes develops in sexual partners (e.g., cervical cancer in females). Any dry, wart-like, painless growth on the penis or foreskin that fails to respond to antibiotics should be assessed for cancer. If an early diagnosis is made, excision and circumcision may be all that is necessary.

Many men find penile problems embarrassing and consequently do not seek medical attention for months. By this time, a lesion may be ulcerated, involve the foreskin and penile shaft, and have metastasized to the inguinal nodes. Penile shaft resection or sometimes penectomy and dissection of enlarged inguinal nodes may be necessary. Dissection of the pelvic lymph nodes carries a risk of long-term lymphedema affecting one or both lower extremities.

PENILE AND SCROTAL INJURIES

Although fairly protected, the penis and scrotum can sustain various injuries. *Nonpenetrating* injuries result from sudden force, such as a straddle injury or penile fracture during intercourse. Underlying structures can be bruised or ruptured. Items placed around the penis

that strangulate may also cause significant tissue damage. *Penetrating* injuries usually involve knife or gunshot wounds but also include self-emasculation attempts and amputation. The male genitalia can also be injured by radiation, chemical or electrical burns, and avulsion (from accidents caused by working with machinery).

Hemorrhage is immediate, whether microscopic or obvious. Pain and edema accompany bleeding. Minor hemorrhage is controlled by ice packs, bed rest, analgesia, and scrotal elevation. Direct compression and pressure dressings may be needed if bleeding is worse. For penile injury, a retrograde urethrogram is obtained to rule out urethral injury. If the urethra is intact, an indwelling catheter is inserted. If bleeding from the penis is noted, urethral disruption is assumed and instrumentation is contraindicated. For scrotal injury, scrotal ultrasonography is performed.

Surgery is necessary to drain a hematoma, to debride necrotic tissue, or to repair damage, including reanastomosis if appropriate. Microsurgical techniques are used. Postoperative antibiotics are given, and catheterization continues until penile injuries are healed. Often further operations are required for repair of strictures, skin grafting, or reconstruction. If scrotal skin is avulsed, the remaining scrotal skin is usually replaced over the scrotal organs; scrotal skin regenerates. When this is not possible, surgeons may perform skin grafts and temporarily reimplant the testes into subcutaneous thigh pouches. These clients need professional approaches and much explanation and reassurance to reduce anxiety. If the client has sustained self-inflicted injuries, psychological referral is part of the care.

When the urinary tract is disrupted, urine can escape into the peritoneum, scrotum, or penile tissue, thus creating an emergency condition. Assessment reveals discoloration of tissue, shock, and fever. Emergency intervention includes alternative drainage of urine (urethral or suprapubic catheter) and drainage of the tissues with a Penrose drain.

ERECTILE DYSFUNCTION

Our understanding of ED (impotence) has expanded significantly over the last two decades, as have the options for managing this common disorder. ED is defined as an inability to achieve or maintain an erection sufficient for sexual activity. Occasional erectile failure may occur because of a variety of self-limiting factors, but consistent failure that affects 50% of attempts at sexual activity is considered clinically relevant.

Etiology and Risk Factors

Both psychological and physiologic factors typically combine to cause ED. Important psychological factors include performance anxiety, stress and fatigue, low self-esteem, depression, and changes in a relationship. After experiencing failure once, a man may be so anxious that he "fails" again and again, worsening the problem.

A variety of physiologic factors may contribute to ED. Although aging does not cause ED, multiple age-related factors increase the risk of ED. For example, an increase in local nerves (both adrenergic and cholinergic receptors) may promote penile flaccidity while reducing the penile response to nitric oxide (the primary neurotransmitter responsible for a penile erection). Diminished testosterone levels, combined with raises in estradiol and serum prolactin, may reduce libido, leading to a decline in the number of erections in older men, an increase in the time needed to achieve sexual arousal, and an increase in the interval between successful erections. Nevertheless, it must be emphasized that *none* of these changes inevitably leads to ED, and many older men enjoy successful erections and intercourse throughout their lifetimes. Other endocrine disorders associated with sexual dysfunction include hyperprolactinemia and thyroid dysfunction. Increased prolactin blocks testosterone effectiveness and decreases the desire for sexual activity; both hyperthyroidism and hypothyroidism predispose to ED.

Major medical risk factors for ED include cardiovascular disease, hypertension, diabetes mellitus, long-term cigarette smoking, renal failure, neurologic disorders affecting the spinal cord, stroke, and chronic obstructive pulmonary disease. Congenital defects affecting gonadal development and testosterone production predispose men to erectile dysfunctions, although surgical castration does *not* necessarily lead to impotence. Multiple medications may produce ED, including antihypertensives, anticholinergics, α-adrenergic agonists (decongestants), and certain antidepressants. Illicit drugs, such as cannabis, cocaine, and the hallucinogens, impair erectile function, as does alcohol.

Surgical procedures associated with a risk of ED include extensive abdominopelvic and spinal procedures. Open prostatectomy and TURP occasionally produce erectile dysfunction, but radical prostatectomy carries a high risk for impotence. Urethral stricture or injury, genital trauma, pelvic bone fracture or Peyronie's diseases (painful curvature of the penis) are also associated with ED.

Pathophysiology

A normal erection comprises two phases. When the penis is flaccid, local arterioles provide enough blood flow to meet nutritional needs of penile tissues but not enough for rigidity. A variety of sensory and psychological stimuli may trigger the release of neurotransmitters and paracrines from local nerve receptors and blood vessels producing an erection. The erection begins with relaxation of smooth muscle of local arterioles and si-

nusoids (blood filled sinuses) within the corpora cavernosa. As arterial blood fills the sinusoids, tumescence (an increase in penile length and circumference) occurs initially. When the cavernous bodies reach the limits imposed by their fibrous outer covering (the tunica albuginea), however, veins and venules within are compressed, and the erection achieves sufficient rigidity for vaginal penetration. Following a period of rigidity, the penis returns to a flaccid state. This requires increased tone in the smooth muscle of the arterioles and sinusoids of the cavernous bodies and reversal of venous compression. Although the endocrine system influences erectile function via effects on the development of secondary sex characteristics and libido, individual erections are controlled by neurovascular mechanisms. Interruption of any one of these physiologic events as a result of a physiologic disorder or psychological dysfunction leads to erectile failure and may cause ED unless it is corrected.

Clinical Manifestations

A detailed medical and sexual history is the first step in determining the cause of ED. A focused physical examination is performed to identify contributing factors such as congenital defects of the male reproductive system, neurologic deficits, or cardiovascular disease such as hypertension. Laboratory tests often include serum testosterone and LH levels as well as prolactin levels and thyroid function. A nocturnal penile tumescence study may be completed to identify the presence of nocturnal erections and their quality. Specialized tests such as color duplex Doppler ultrasonography or dynamic infusion cavernosometry are completed in highly selected cases when potentially reversible vascular problems are suspected as the principal cause of erectile dysfunction.

Outcome Management
■ Medical Management

Correct Psychological Problems. Sometimes just giving accurate information about normal sexual function, alternative sexual activity, and dispelling myths is all that is necessary for a client to deal with ED. Myths about sexual activity greatly influence outcome success. Behavioral modification techniques (the best known were developed by Masters and Johnson in the 1960s) may be used when psychogenic causes are identified as the principal cause of ED, and counseling is often invaluable as part of a multimodal management plan.

Correct Physiologic Problems. When physiologic causes are involved, several approaches may be used. Medications may be altered and recreational drugs such as cigarette smoking or alcohol consumption stopped. Medical conditions causing ED need to be treated if possible. Low serum testosterone can be augmented using a parenteral or transcutaneous delivery system, *provided* hypogonadism or deficiency or endogenous testosterone has been identified during evaluation.

Stimulate Erection

Medications. See the Integrating Pharmacology feature on Medications for Erectile Dysfunction, below. See also the Complementary and Alternative Therapy features on Korean Red Ginseng for Erectile Dysfunction and on L-Arginine and Erectile Dysfunction on p. 1048.

Vacuum Erection Devices. Vacuum erection devices are legitimate medically prescribed pumps that mechanically achieve an erection. A cylinder is placed over the penis and a pump is used to create vacuum suction, thus drawing blood into the corpora cavernosa. When an erection is achieved, a compression ring is applied to the base of the penis and the cylinder is removed for intercourse. The ring must be removed within about 30 minutes to prevent tissue damage caused by interrupted circulation. Bruising and cold penile skin and a lack of spontaneity are minor problems that may result. Priapism occurs rarely.

■ Nursing Management of the Medical Client

Provide Support. A sensitive, caring approach is vital for nurses who work with these clients because embarrassment may cause many men to avoid treatment. Just knowing that ED is common and treatment alternatives are available can be reassuring to the client. Involve the sexual partner when the client permits.

Provide Education. Teach the client about normal erectile physiology, factors that interfere, and how different approaches correct the problem. Inform the client about public or community resources. If medication is used, explain how to administer the medication and caution the client to follow directions as prescribed and not to use the medication more often then directed.

The client who must use intracorporeal injections needs to know how to draw up medication into a sy-

INTEGRATING PHARMACOLOGY
Medications for Erectile Dysfunction

A myriad of medications have become available for treatment of erectile dysfunction. Most of these medications block the action of phosphodiesterase 5 (PDE5) or dilate vessels in the corpora cavernosa.

PDE5 inhibitors include sildenafil (Viagra), vardenafil (Levitra), and tadalafil (Cialis). These drugs block the action of PDE5, a substance that promotes the metabolism of cyclic GMP and nitric oxide. Blockade of this drug prolongs and enhances the actions of these substances within the corpora cavernosa. The drugs do not generate an erection as do the injectable agents; instead, they enhance the client's ability to achieve and sustain an erection that must be stimulated by psychological, visual, tactile, and other factors. Side effects may include headache, a flushed feeling, dyspepsia, nasal congestion, and a color tinge or other mild visual disturbances. Sildenafil is *absolutely contraindicated* for any man taking nitrates in any form. Vardenafil and tadalafil are more selective to the PDE5 isoenzyme and have been proven effective for treatment of ED in men regardless of comorbid conditions such as hypertension, diabetes, or coronary artery disease. Caution must be observed when men are taking alpha-adrenergic blockers or have a peptic ulcer.

Intracavernosal vasodilating drugs such as papaverine, phentolamine, and prostaglandin E₁ (PGE₁) (Casodex) can be injected. Combinations of these drugs may be given in a single injection. Because pain, bruising, and fibrosis at the injection site and priapism are possible side effects, it is recommended that injections be given not more than two or three times per week.

Intraurethral instillation of an alprostadil (PGE₁) pellet (Muse) has been successful. This approach eliminates injection of the penis, but the technique must be accurately performed to achieve erection. This approach can be a good one for a client who is obese or has problems with dexterity or vision. The drug should not be given more than twice in a 24-hour period. Side effects are the same as described before; intraurethral pain and minor bleeding may occur. PGE₁ administration is contraindicated if penile anatomy is abnormal or the client has urethritis. A gel version and a creme version of alprostadil are in final phase 3 trials in the United States. These versions are topically applied to the head of the penis before intercourse.

Yohimbe, an alpha-adrenergic blocking agent, causes vasodilation of the corpora cavernosa and may alleviate erectile dysfunction in some cases. Side effects include fluid retention, nausea, orthostatic hypotension, and diaphoresis; studies have shown that yohimbine is often ineffective for men with moderate to severe erectile dysfunction.

Apomorphine (Uprima) is a sublingual dopaminergic agonist (not an opioid) that acts on the central nervous system and has been used effectively in Europe and Latin America since 2001. Approval by the U.S. Food and Drug Administration (FDA) is pending, and U.S. clinical trials are ongoing with apomorphine nasal spray.

Penile Prosthesis. The following are the two basic categories of penile prostheses (Figure 40-9):

1. *Inflatable* prostheses come in one-piece, two-piece, and three-piece units that are hydraulic devices. In the one-piece prosthesis, the reservoir, pump, and cylinders fit within the penis. Two-piece units have a reservoir-pump system within the scrotum. The reservoir on the three-piece devices is implanted in the abdominal cavity and the pump is implanted in the scrotum.
2. *Semirigid* prostheses can be malleable, with spring-like mechanisms that help make the penis more erect for intercourse, or mechanical, with cable strands in the device that can be bent to make the penis more erect.

Ice and penile or scrotal elevations are used postoperatively to minimize swelling. Pain should be well controlled with medication. Sexual activity can usually be resumed 6 to 8 weeks after surgery when healing is complete and pain is controlled. Infection, extrusion of the prosthesis, and mechanical failure are some of the complications after surgery.

Revascularization. Revascularization surgical procedures attempt to restore circulation to the corpora cavernosa. Although initially successful, these techniques are uncommon because they lack durability.

■ Nursing Management of the Surgical Client

Care of the client having surgery for ED is the same as that of any surgical client. Penile circulation and dressing should be observed consistently as ordered. En-

ringe, cleanse the site, inject the medication, and safely dispose of equipment. He should know that bruising might occur. Injections should be given at the 2 o'clock or 10 o'clock position, and sites should be rotated to minimize fibrotic changes. Intraurethral pellets require using the applicator correctly, careful insertion and waiting about 10 minutes for an erection to occur. Standing or walking during this time and stimulation are important.

■ Surgical Management

Surgical management of ED includes implantation of a penile prosthesis, revascularization procedures, and incision of Peyronie's plaques. Penile prostheses are most common if medical therapy is not effective and if the client is a good surgical candidate.

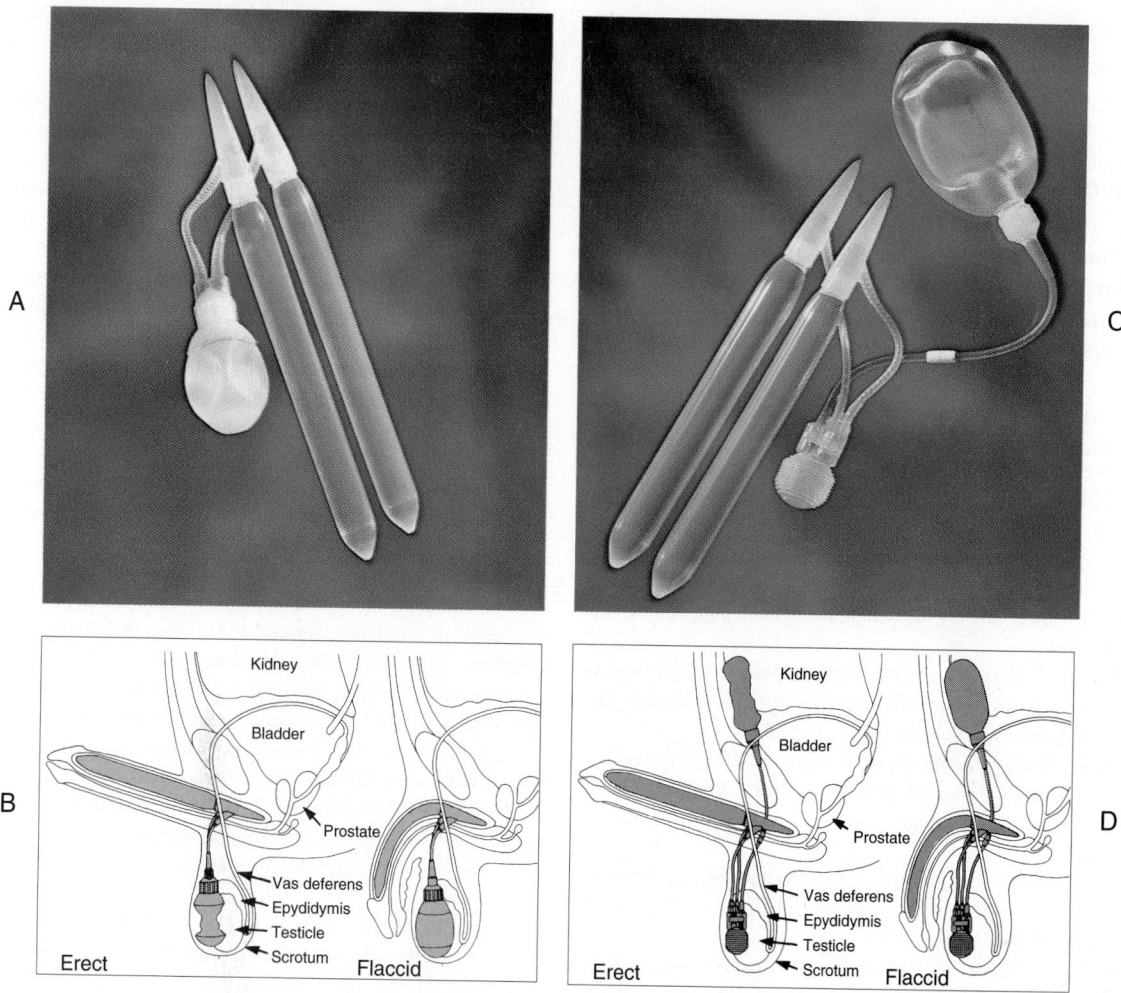

FIGURE 40-9 Penile prostheses. **A,** Mark II (two-piece inflatable penile prosthesis). **B,** Mark II prosthesis erect and flaccid. **C,** Alpha I (three-piece inflatable penile prosthesis). **D,** Alpha 1 prosthesis erect and flaccid. (Courtesy of Mentor, Santa Barbara, CA.)

courage the client to use pain medication before the pain becomes severe. All clients are given antibiotics before and after surgery. The client is taught preoperatively how to use the prosthesis and cautioned not to use it before healing has occurred. These men need a great deal of emotional support because of secrecy with friends, emotional issues with partners, and sometimes doubt about the decision to have surgery related to pain.

CONCLUSIONS

Male genital and reproductive disorders can be complex problems for both the client and the nurse. The client often finds that these disorders threaten sexuality and sexual function or normal urinary elimination. These effects may be physiologic, but complex psychosocial problems also arise.

Prostate disorders are among the most common problems experienced by men throughout their lifetime. Can-

cers of the male reproductive tract can be life threatening, but if they are detected early, they can be cured or at least controlled for long periods. Problems such as ED and infertility directly affect both partners, who experience the diagnostic and treatment phases together. The nurse acts as a caregiver, educator, support, and resource person.

THINKING CRITICALLY *evolve*

1. Your client underwent a laser-assisted TURP yesterday. Closed bladder irrigation is being used, and his urine is dark to bright red with multiple clots. He is complaining of intense cramping pain in the lower abdomen. What further assessments should you make? What could be causing the cramping pain? What nursing action should you take?

Factors to Consider. Is the dark to bright red urine output normal at this stage? What does the nature of the client's pain tell you about its likely cause?

2. A young man in his early 20s is given a diagnosis of testicular cancer, and he is very concerned about the treatment's effects on his ability to perform sexually and to father children. What issues should you discuss with him?

Factors to Consider. What impact might a bilateral orchiectomy or a radical lymph node dissection have on erectile function and fertility? What might be the effect of a unilateral orchiectomy? What options for fathering children are important to consider before the client undergoes treatment?

Discussions for these questions can be found on the website and the CD-ROM.

BIBLIOGRAPHY

 1. Albaugh, J., et al. (2002). Health care clinicians in sexual health medicine: Focus on erectile dysfunction. *Urologic Nursing, 22*(4), 217-232.

2. American Cancer Society. (2003). *Cancer facts and figures.* Atlanta: Author.

 3. Ames, C.D., & Gray, M. (2000). Voiding dysfunction after radiation to the prostate for prostate cancer. *Journal of Wound, Ostomy and Continence Nursing, 27*(3), 155-167.

4. Amling, C., Kane, C., Riffenburg, R., et al. (2001). Relationship between obesity and race in predicting adverse pathologic variables in patients undergoing radical prostatectomy. *Urology, 58*(5), 723-728.

5. Blatt, H., et al. (2001). Utilization of a self-administered questionnaire to assess rectal function following prostate brachytherapy. *Urologic Nursing, 21*(5), 356-359.

6. Bodell, A., & Shore, D. (2002). Prostate cancer screening in asymptomatic men in a community setting. *Urologic Nursing, 22*(1), 31-37.

7. Boon, T.A., Van Venrooij, G.E., & Eckhardt, M.D. (2001). Effect of diabetes mellitus on lower urinary tract symptoms and dysfunction in patients with benign prostatic hyperplasia. *Current Urology Reports, 2*(4), 297-301.

8. Broderick, G., & Lue, T. (2002). Evaluation and nonsurgical management of erectile dysfunction and priapism. In P. Walsh, et al. (Eds.) *Campbell's urology* (8th ed., pp 1619-1672). Philadelphia: W.B. Saunders.

9. Butler, L., et al. (2001). Quality of life post radical prostatectomy: A male perspective. *Urologic Nursing, 21*(4), 283-288.

10. Burnett, A.L. (1999). Neurophysiology of erectile function and dysfunction. In Hellstrom W.J.G. (Ed.). *Handbook of sexual dysfunction* (pp. 12-17). San Francisco: American Society of Andrology.

11. Colwell, J.C., & Goldberg, M. (2000). A review of radiation proctitis in the treatment of prostate cancer. *Journal of Wound, Ostomy, & Continence Nursing, 27*(3),179-187.

12. Cox, B., et al. (2002). Vasectomy and risk of prostate cancer. *Journal of the American Medical Association, 287*(23), 3110-3115.

13. de la Rosette, J.J., Alivizatos, G., & Laguna, M.P. (2001). Transurethral hot water balloon thermoablation. *Current Urology Reports, 2*(4), 302-305.

14. Eastham, J., et al. (2003). Variation of serum prostate-specific antigen levels: An evaluation of year-to-year fluctuations. *Journal of the American Medical Association, 289*(20), 2696-2700.

15. Eastham, J., & Scardino, P. (2002). Radical prostatectomy. In P. Walsh, et al. (Eds.) *Campbell's urology* (8th ed., pp. 3080-3106). Philadelphia: W.B. Saunders.

16. Eisenburger, M., & Carducci, M. (2002). Chemotherapy for hormone-resistant prostate cancer. In P. Walsh, et al. (Eds.) *Campbell's urology* (8th ed., pp. 3209-3226). Philadelphia: W.B. Saunders.

17. Fitzpatrick, J., & Mebust, W. (2002). Minimally invasive and endoscopic management of benign prostatic hyperplasia. In P. Walsh, et al. (Eds.) *Campbell's urology* (8th ed., pp. 1379-1422). Philadelphia: W.B. Saunders.

18. Floratos, D.L., de La Rosette J. (2001). Heat treatment of the prostate: Where do we stand in 2000? *Current Opinion in Urology, 11*(1), 35-41.

19. Foley, S.J., et al. (2000). A prospective stud of the natural history of hematuria associated with benign prostatic hyperplasia and the effect of finasteride. *Journal of Urology, 163*(2), 496-503.

20. Fox, S., et al. (1999). Male genitourinary cancer sexuality questionnaire. *Urologic Nursing, 19*(2), 101-107.

21. Gaines, K. (2002). Zoledronic acid (Zometa): Bisphosphonate for prostate cancer/bone metastases. *Urologic Nursing, 22*(6), 398-400.

22. Goldstein, M. (2002). Surgical management of male infertility and other scrotal disorders. In P. Walsh, et al. (Eds.) *Campbell's urology* (8th ed., pp. 1475-1530). Philadelphia: W.B. Saunders.

23. Gray, M., & Moore, K. (In press). *Urologic disorders.* St. Louis: Mosby.

24. Gray, M., & Allensworth, D. (1997). Medical management of benign prostatic hyperplasia. *Urologic Nursing, 17*(4), 137-141.

25. Gray, M. (1998). Psychometric analysis of the international prostate symptom score. *Urologic Nursing, 18,* 175-183.

26. Gray M., Petroni, G.R., & Theodorescu, D. (1999). Urinary function following radical prostatectomy: A comparison of the retropubic and perineal approaches. *Urology, 53,* 881-889.

27. Gray, M., & Allensworth, D. (1999). Electrovaporization of the prostate: Initial experiences and nursing management. *Urologic Nursing, 19*(1), 25-31.

28. Gray, M. (2001). Etiology of erectile dysfunction. *Clinician Reviews, 11* (Supplement), 9-14.

29. Gray M. (2002). Prostate cancer primer. *Urologic Nursing, 22,* 151-169.

30. Gray, M., & Brown, K.C. (2002). Genitourinary system. In J. Thompson, G. McFarland, J. Hirsh, & S. Tucker (Eds.), *Clinical Nursing* (5th ed., pp. 917-999). St. Louis: Mosby.

31. Grayhack, J.T., McVary, K.T., & Kozlowski, J.A. (2002). Benign prostatic hyperplasia. In J. Gillenwater, et al. (Eds.) *Adult and pediatric urology* (4th ed., pp. 1402-1470). Philadelphia: Lippincott Williams & Wilkins.

32. Gretzer, M., & Partin, A. (2003). *Campbell's urology updates: PSA and PSA molecular derivatives, 1*(1), 1-12.

 evolve *Did you remember to check out the bonus material on the Evolve website and the CD-ROM, including free self-assessment exercises?*

http://evolve.elsevier.com/Black/medsurg/

33. Han, M., Alfert, H., & Partin, A. (2002). Retropubic and suprapubic open prostatectomy. In P. Walsh, et al. (Eds.) *Campbell's urology* (8th ed., pp. 1423-1434). Philadelphia: W.B. Saunders.

 34. Helke, C., et al. (2001). Is transurethral vaporesection of the prostate better than standard transurethral resection? *European Urology, 39*(5), 551-557.

35. Hewitt, A. (2001). Early catheter removal following radical perineal prostatectomy: A randomized clinical trial. *Urologic Nursing, 21*(1), 37-44.

36. Incrocci, L., & Slob, A. (2002). Incidence, etiology, and therapy for erectile dysfunction after external beam radiotherapy for prostate cancer. *Urology, 60*(1), 1-7.

37. Jarow, J., et al. (2002). Male infertility evaluation guidelines. *The Journal of Urology, 167*(5), 2138-2144.

38. Jemal, A., et al. (2002). Cancer statistics, 2002. *CA Cancer Journal for Clinicians, 52*, 23-47.

39. Joseph, A. (2001). Male pelvic anatomy/post-prostatectomy incontinence. *Urologic Nursing, 21*(1), 25-29.

40. Kirby, R. (2000). The natural history of benign prostatic hyperplasia: What have we learned in the last decade? *Urology, 56*(5 suppl 1), 3-6.

41. Kirby, R.S., Kirby, M.G., & Riad, N.F. (2000). *Men's health.* Oxford, UK: Isis Medical Media.

42. Kupeli, S., et al. (1999). Combined transurethral resection and vaporization of the prostate using newly designed electrode: A promising treatment alternative for benign prostatic hyperplasia. *Journal of Endourology, 13*(3), 225-228.

43. Laumann, E., Paik, A., & Rosen, R. (1999). Sexual dysfunction in the United States: Prevalence and predictors. *Journal of the American Medical Association, 281*(6), 537-544.

44. Lepor, H., & Lowe, F. (2002). Evaluation and nonsurgical management of benign prostatic hyperplasia. In P. Walsh, et al. (Eds.) *Campbell's urology* (8th ed., pp. 1337-1378). Philadelphia: W.B. Saunders.

45. Lewis, R., & Jordon, G. (2002). Surgery for erectile dysfunction. In P. Walsh, et al. (Eds.) *Campbell's urology* (8th ed., pp. 1673-1708). Philadelphia: W.B. Saunders.

46. Lue, T. (2002). Physiology of penile erection and pathophysiology of erectile dysfunction and priapism. In P. Walsh, et al. (Eds.) *Campbell's urology* (8th ed., pp. 1591-1617). Philadelphia: W.B. Saunders.

47. Lynch, D.F., & Pettaway, C.A. (2002). Tumors of the penis. In P. Walsh, et al. (Eds.) *Campbell's urology* (8th ed., pp. 2945-2981). Philadelphia: W.B. Saunders.

48. Marks, L., et al. (2002). Herbal formulation for prostate cancer. *Urology, 60*(3), 369-377.

49. McCallum, T., Moore, K., & Griffiths, D. (2001). Urinary incontinence after radical prostatectomy: Implications and urodynamics. *Urologic Nursing, 21*(2), 113-119, 124.

50. McClain, R., & Gray, M. (2000). Prostate cancer management for nurse practitioners. *Clinical Advice for Nurse Practitioners, 3*, 37-50.

51. Middleton, L., & Lessick, M. (2003). Inherited urologic malignant disorders: Nursing implications. *Urologic Nursing, 23*(1), 15-30.

52. Moore, K., & Estey, A. (1999). The early postoperative concerns of men after radical prostatectomy. *Journal of Advanced Nursing, 29*(5), 1121-1129.

53. Moul, J., & Civitelli, K. (2001). Managing advanced prostate cancer with Viadur (leuprolide acetate implant). *Urologic Nursing, 21*(6), 385-396.

54. Moyad, M. (2003). Osteoporosis part III—not just for bone loss: Potential benefits of calcium and vitamin D for overall general health, *Urologic Nursing, 23*(1), 69-74.

55. Ng, C. (2001). Assessment and intervention knowledge of nurses in managing catheter patency in continuous bladder irrigation following TURP. *Urologic Nursing, 21*(2), 97-111.

56. Parrott, B. (2003). TUNA of the prostate in an office setting: Nursing implications. *Urologic Nursing, 23*(1), 33-40.

57. Pound, C., et al. (1999). Natural history of progression after PSA elevation following radical prostatectomy. *Journal of the American Medical Association, 281*(17), 1591-1597.

58. Quallich, S., & Ohl, D. (2002). Penile prosthesis case study. *Urologic Nursing, 22*(2), 91-95.

59. Quallich, S., & Ohl, D. (2002). Penile prosthesis: Patient teaching and perioperative care. *Urologic Nursing, 22*(2), 81-90.

60. Roehrborn, C.G., & McConnell, J.D. (2002). Etiology, pathophysiology, epidemiology and natural history of BPH. In P. Walsh, A. et al. (Eds.). *Campbell's urology* (8th ed., pp. 1297-1336). Philadelphia: W.B. Saunders.

61. Sattelle, K. (2002). Men's health in focus. *Professional Nurse, 17*(11), 633.

62. Sigman, M., & Jarow, J. (2002). Male infertility. In P. Walsh, et al. (Eds.) *Campbell's urology* (8th ed., pp. 1475-1531). Philadelphia: W.B. Saunders.

63. Shinohara, K., & Carroll, P. (2002). Cryotherapy for prostate cancer. In P. Walsh, et al. (Eds.) *Campbell's urology* (8th ed., pp. 3171-3181). Philadelphia: W.B. Saunders.

64. Shoskes, D., Katske, F., & Kim, S. (2001). Diagnosis and management of acute and chronic prostatitis. *Urologic Nursing, 21*(4), 255-264.

65. Shipley, W., et al. (1999). Radiation therapy for clinically localized prostate cancer: A multi-institutional pooled analysis. *Journal of the American Medical Association, 281*(17), 1598-1604.

66. Stamey, T., et al. (1999). Biological determinants of cancer progression in men with prostate cancer. *Journal of the American Medical Association, 281*(15), 1395-1400.

67. Townsend, C. (Ed.) (2001). *Sabiston textbook of surgery* (16th ed.). Philadelphia: W.B. Saunders.

68. Wallace, M., & Powel, L. (2002). *Prostate cancer: Nursing assessment, management and care.* New York: Springer-Verlag.

Management of Women with Reproductive Disorders

Francie Bernier

The major themes of all gynecologic disorders are sexuality and self-concept, including body image and self-esteem. Any disorder of the reproductive tract may lead to changes in sexual functioning or sexual identity. Change in sexual habits, such as abstinence from sexual activities or use of different positioning during vaginal intercourse, can be related to this diagnosis as well. The disorders and their treatments have the potential to change a woman's perceived or actual body structure, possibly leading to shame, embarrassment, and other negative emotions.

Alterations in sexuality and body image have a major effect on some women's feminine identity. Even in the 19th century, the common medical view was that the reproductive organs dominated a woman's body. Some aspects of this view, which reduces women's identity to the functioning of their body parts, persist in modern culture.

Contraception is a major health issue in various religious groups. Many religions, such as the Church of Jesus Christ of Latter-Day Saints (Mormons), the Roman Catholic Church, some Orthodox Jewish groups, and Baha'i, encourage followers to be fruitful and multiply. Sterilization and abortion are opposed by religious doctrine in many groups.

MENSTRUAL DISORDERS
CULTURAL INFLUENCES

Attitudes toward menstruation are often culturally based, and adolescent girls may be taught a variety of folk beliefs and practices at the time of puberty. Among Hispanic Americans, for example, menstruating females are not permitted to walk barefooted, wash their hair, or take showers or baths. Some Hispanic Americans believe that sour or iced foods cause menstrual blood to coagulate. Some Puerto Rican women have been taught that drinking lemon or pineapple juice will increase menstrual cramping. The nurse should be aware of these beliefs and respect cultural practices.

Some Arab women who practice Islam, such as Palestinians, Lebanese, Jordanians, and Saudi Arabians, and some African women have ethnoreligious prohibitions and duties during and after menstruation. In Islam, blood is considered to be unclean (*najis*). The blood of menstruation, as well as blood lost during childbirth, renders the woman ritually impure. In Islamic legal language, the term used for menstruation is *hayz* and the menstruating woman is called *ha'iz*. Because one must be in a pure state in order to pray, the *ha'iz* are forbidden

Nursing Outcomes Classification (NOC)
for Nursing Diagnoses—Women with Reproductive Disorders

Constipation
  Bowel Elimination
  Hydration
Risk for Dysfunctional Grieving
  Concentration
  Family Coping
  Grief Resolution

Psychosocial Adjustment: Life Change
  Role Performance
Risk for Infection
  Immune Status
  Knowledge: Infection Control
  Risk Control
  Risk Control: Sexually Transmitted
    Diseases

Risk Detection
Tissue Integrity: Skin and Mucous
  Membranes
Treatment Behavior: Illness or Injury
Wound Healing: Primary Intention
Wound Healing: Secondary Intention

to perform certain acts of worship, such as touch the Koran, enter a mosque, pray, and participate in certain feasts. During the menstrual period, sexual intercourse is forbidden for both men and women. When the menstrual flow stops, the woman performs *ghusl,* a washing ritual to purify herself.

In the Navajo culture, a ceremony called the *kinaalda* announces the achievement of menarche (beginning of menstruation). Although fertility was the goal of the ceremony in the past, the most common reason for the *kinaalda* today is educational, to equip the girl to participate in society as an adult female. Menstruating Navajo women may not look at sand painting, enter a ceremonial *hogan,* attend or lead a sing, or join in the dancing that occurs at certain ceremonies.

In various cultures, menstruating women may be subject to restrictions on work and physical activities as well as rules related to the disposal of menstrual fluid and the proper disposal of sanitary napkins. Attitudes toward intercourse during menstruation are variable. Many religions also require or encourage women to engage in certain practices during and after menstruation. It is easy to understand why reproductive disorders can have such far-reaching effects on women.

REACTIONS TO MANIFESTATIONS

Women may experience some menstrual problems during their 30 or more years of menstruating. They tend to seek professional help for obvious abnormalities, such as excessive and irregular vaginal bleeding; however, they may not bring other menstrual problems to the attention of health care providers.

Women react to menstrual problems individually. Although some promptly seek health care, others do not, for various reasons. For example, one woman may hesitate and may be unable to discuss menstruation. She may view the subject as a personal and intimate problem that should be kept private. Another woman may have low self-esteem or may have been told that problems are to be expected. Therefore she may dismiss her own complaints as unimportant or may not seek help, expecting the problems will disappear in time. Others may desire a relief of manifestations or may fear that the treatment will be worse than the problem. It is not uncommon for

menstrual problems to remain undetected unless the nurse is skillful and sensitive in assessment. The nurse may identify a menstrual problem during a discussion of contraception or other needs. Some of the most common menstrual problems are dysmenorrhea (painful menstruation), premenstrual syndrome (PMS), and abnormal uterine bleeding.

DYSMENORRHEA

Dysmenorrhea is estimated to affect 30% to 75% of women. *Primary* dysmenorrhea is believed to be caused by either a prostaglandin excess or an increased sensitivity to prostaglandins with no underlying pathologic pelvic disorders. Prostaglandins are hormone-like secretions that cause smooth muscle contraction. *Secondary* dysmenorrhea begins with an underlying disease condition.

Etiology and Risk Factors

There are no preventive measures for dysmenorrhea, which has a variety of causes. The causes can be grouped according to five factors that affect the reproductive system in various ways:
  • Elevated levels of uterine prostaglandins
  • Endocrine factors
  • Myometrial factors
  • Biochemical factors
  • Psychosocial factors

Secondary dysmenorrhea is suspected when pain is concentrated in a specific area, is unilateral, or begins after age 20 years. It may be caused by the following:
  • Pelvic inflammatory disease (PID)
  • Endometriosis
  • Adenomyosis (invasion of uterine myometrium by endometrial tissue) (see the Unit 9 Anatomy and Physiology Review)
  • Uterine prolapse
  • Uterine myomas
  • Polyps

Pathophysiology

Prostaglandin synthesis at the time of menstruation appears to produce strong myometrial contractions. The severe muscle spasms constrict blood vessels supplying the uterus, causing ischemia and pain. The excess prostaglandins in smooth muscle also help explain the presence of gastrointestinal (GI) manifestations, headache, and other manifestations.

Clinical Manifestations

Primary dysmenorrhea characteristically begins 1 to 2 months after menarche (onset of menses) in conjunction with ovulatory cycles. Generally, it increases in severity over several years with a decline when the woman reaches her mid-20s. Primary dysmenorrhea often decreases significantly after childbirth.

The discomfort of primary dysmenorrhea commonly begins 1 to 2 days before the onset of menstrual flow. The more severe discomfort is usually experienced during the first 24 hours of flow and typically subsides by the second day. More than half of the women experiencing dysmenorrhea also have systemic manifestations, such as nausea and vomiting, diarrhea, syncope, headache, and back pain.

Diagnosis is based on a thorough history, including medications used for symptomatic relief. A physical examination is performed to rule out underlying pathologic causes of dysmenorrhea.

Outcome Management
■ Medical Management

The current approach to primary dysmenorrhea emphasizes prevention and education. For women with mild manifestations who want to avoid medication, nonpharmacologic remedies might be effective. For example, biofeedback, therapeutic touch, or acupuncture might be helpful. Nutritional measures include decreasing the intake of sodium and increasing the intake of vitamin B_6, calcium, magnesium, and protein.

Administer Oral Contraceptives. If contraception as well as relief of dysmenorrhea is desired, combination oral contraceptives may relieve menstrual pain. The combination inhibits ovulation, resulting in decreased endometrial prostaglandin production and a concurrent reduction of uterine activity. For the woman with a contraceptive *intrauterine device* (IUD), removal of the IUD may lead to relief. Another form of contraception may be desired.

Promote Exercise. Exercise, such as aerobic exercise and swimming, has also been used as a remedy for dysmenorrhea. Exercise increases blood flow of beta-endorphins, the body's endogenous opiates, making them available for pain reduction. The exact mechanism responsible for pain reduction is not known.

Administer Prostaglandin Synthesis Inhibitors. *Prostaglandin synthesis inhibitors* (antiprostaglandin agents) may provide relief by decreasing prostaglandin activity, even in the presence of ovulatory cycles. Some commonly prescribed medications in this group are ibuprofen (Motrin), mefenamic acid (Ponstel), indomethacin (Indocin), and naproxen (Naprosyn). Ibuprofen (Advil) and naproxen (Aleve) are available as nonprescription drugs in lower doses, which makes them easy to obtain. Other medications—such as the COX-2 inhibitors, including celecoxib (Celebrex) and rofecoxib (Vioxx)—used for the treatment of arthritis pain have been helpful for those who suffer from dysmenorrhea. However, it frequently takes up to 2 to 3 hours for theses medications to reach a blood level to produce effective pain management.

These medications may have GI side effects. Other possible side effects are sodium and water retention, rashes, and potential allergic reactions. For maximum effectiveness, the medications should be administered either before or at the onset of menses. Sometimes a client may have to try several prostaglandin synthesis inhibitors to find the one with maximum effectiveness for her.

Treatment of secondary dysmenorrhea is directed toward the underlying cause, such as endometriosis or PID (see the discussion later in this chapter). Antiprostaglandin agents may provide some relief.

■ Nursing Management of the Medical Client

Education and supportive reassurance are important nursing interventions for clients with primary dysmenorrhea. Provide information about the mechanisms involved in dysmenorrhea and the actions and possible side effects of any prescribed medications. Assess the client's general health status. Encourage adequate nutrition, decreased caffeine intake, and appropriate rest, sleep, and exercise. Assess stress, which may increase manifestations, and explore methods of stress management.

PREMENSTRUAL SYNDROME

Premenstrual syndrome is defined as a combination of emotional and physical manifestations that occur cyclically in the female before menstruation and regress or disappear during menstruation. PMS is somatic (a physical syndrome), not psychic, in origin. It is a complex mechanism involving not only the endocrine system but the autonomic and central nervous systems as well. A predominant alteration is the retention of body fluids.

The incidence of PMS is difficult to determine because of its variable manifestations and the lack of a clear understanding about the syndrome. PMS manifestations peak in women 30 to 40 years old. Variable reports in the literature indicate that 20% to 60% of all women experience some form of PMS.

Etiology and Risk Factors

The cause of PMS is unclear. However, neuroendocrine mechanisms appear to be involved. It is not clear whether PMS is a single syndrome or a group of separate disorders. Some suggested causes of PMS are as follows:

- Estrogen-progesterone imbalance, especially in estrogen excess and a progesterone deficiency, or estrogen deficiency at time of manifestations
- Interaction among estrogen, progesterone, and aldosterone
- Excess of prolactin, hypothyroidism, or hypoglycemia
- Dietary factors, such as deficiency of vitamin B₆, magnesium, or both
- Lifestyle factors, such as increased stress and poor diet

Health promotion and health maintenance activities include good nutrition, vitamin and mineral supplements, stress management, exercise, and rest.

Clinical Manifestations

Typically, manifestations of PMS appear during the last few premenstrual days and are relieved suddenly with full menstrual flow. However, manifestations may begin with ovulation and may not be relieved until during or toward the end of menses. Characteristically, manifestations gradually worsen until menses begin.

Various manifestations are attributable to PMS, including altered emotional states, behavioral changes, somatic problems, changes in appetite, and motor effects. Different sets of manifestations are experienced by individual women. Emotional manifestations may include tension, depression, irritability, hostility, insomnia, loneliness, a tendency to cry easily, and indecision. Forgetfulness and mental confusion may occur. Psychosis and suicidal tendencies are possible and rare.

Somatic problems are headache, breast tenderness and abdominal bloating, peripheral edema, joint pain and backache, hives, constipation, and exacerbation of pre-existing conditions, such as migraine and herpes. Because PMS manifestations usually do not occur during the menstrual flow, women may not associate them with the menstrual cycle.

To date, there is no objective method of diagnosing PMS. The diagnosis is usually made by documenting the cyclic nature of the manifestations on a menstrual calendar. A diary of manifestations and menstrual periods is an essential part of the assessment when PMS is suspected. Manifestations must occur for a minimum of three menstrual cycles. The diagnosis is confirmed according to the timing of manifestations rather than on the presence of particular manifestations.

Outcome Management
■ Medical Management
Relieve Manifestations

Vitamins and Minerals. Daily intake of vitamin B₆ and elimination of caffeine have improved some premenstrual manifestations. Nonprescription over-the-counter medications include calcium, vitamins A and C,

magnesium, and trace elements. Essential fatty acid supplements are often recommended. (See the Complementary and Alternative Therapy feature on Calcium Supplements and PMS, below.)

Medications. Prescription medications commonly include oral spironolactone (Aldactone), progesterone, oral contraceptives, and anti-anxiety agent or selective serotonin re-uptake inhibitors (SSRIs) such as sertraline hydrochloride (Zoloft), paroxetine hydrochloride (Paxil), or fluoxetine hydrochloride (Prozac).

Spironolactone (Aldactone) is a synthetic steroid aldosterone antagonist that inhibits the physiologic effect of aldosterone on the distal renal tubules. It is commonly used to treat the edema associated with excessive aldosterone secretion.

Progesterone may relieve physiologic and psychological manifestations. Bromocriptine (Parlodel) reduces serum prolactin concentrations by inhibiting prolactin release from the anterior pituitary gland. It has been used successfully to reduce breast pain in some cases of PMS.

Sedatives and analgesics, including antiprostaglandin agents, are often prescribed. Antidepressants may be prescribed for severe PMS.

Nursing Management of the Medical Client

Nurses are in a key position to help women identify and cope with PMS when it is present. Clients who are in poor physical condition may be particularly susceptible to premenstrual difficulties. Thus the nursing assessment includes general lifestyle, sleep and dietary habits, and overall health maintenance.

Provide Education. Once the diagnosis of PMS is confirmed, the client needs accurate information about the

---

COMPLEMENTARY AND ALTERNATIVE THERAPY   **EB**

Calcium Supplements and PMS

One well-designed, randomized, controlled trial of calcium supplements for treating manifestations of premenstrual syndrome (PMS) found a greater than 50% reduction in the manifestation complex scores after 3 months in more than half of the participants taking 1200 mg of supplemental elemental calcium carbonate. The number needed to treat (NNT) from this study versus a placebo was 6 for a 50% reduction. This makes elemental calcium one of the more preferred agents to reduce the manifestations of PMS because it was so effective and because the adverse effects were the same as placebo.

Reference
Thys-Jacobs, S., et al. (1998). *American Journal of Obstetrics and Gynecology, 179,* 444-452.

syndrome and reassurance about the physiologic basis of the manifestations. Women often benefit from the opportunity to talk about their feelings and experiences with PMS, especially because of the confusion and misconceptions surrounding the syndrome. Instructions on how to take medications are important.

Encourage Lifestyle Modifications. Suggested dietary modifications include reducing intake of salt and refined carbohydrates. Eating small, frequent meals to stabilize blood glucose levels can decrease fatigue, irritability, and craving. A calcium intake of at least 1000 mg/day may also decrease manifestations (see the Complementary and Alternative Therapy feature on Calcium Supplements and PMS on p. 1056.) It may also be helpful to reduce alcohol and caffeine intake and to stop smoking.

Give careful attention to stress management and reduction. Weight reduction may decrease manifestations. Daily exercise (such as aerobics, jogging, or swimming) has been recommended to improve circulation, reduce stress, and promote a sense of well-being.

Improve Coping. Another major nursing responsibility is helping the client and her significant others cope with the manifestations of PMS. Keep in mind the client's particular lifestyle and preferences. For example, a reallocation of responsibilities within the family might help to reduce her stress. If the client prefers to retain her current responsibilities, explain how she might manage them in ways that minimize stress.

Support groups or educational sessions may be helpful as well. These sessions can serve as a forum for sharing information, providing mutual support, and discussing feelings. You can help form such a group if none exist in the area.

ABNORMAL UTERINE BLEEDING

Abnormal uterine bleeding encompasses a wide variety of menstrual disorders, such as lack of menstrual flow and irregular or excessive uterine bleeding. Changes in menstrual patterns can create anxiety in any woman. Associated manifestations disrupt activities of daily living. Sometimes abnormal uterine bleeding indicates an underlying pathologic disease. The term *dysfunctional uterine bleeding* refers to abnormal uterine bleeding for which no organic cause can be found through the usual assessment techniques. The presence of abnormal uterine bleeding necessitates careful assessment by a qualified health care provider.

AMENORRHEA

Amenorrhea means the absence of menses. *Primary* amenorrhea occurs if a woman has not begun to menstruate by the age of 16 years. *Secondary* amenorrhea is the absence of menses for 6 months in a woman who previously had regular cyclic bleeding or 12 months in a woman with a history of irregular bleeding.

Etiology and Risk Factors
There are many causes of amenorrhea, and they may appear alone or in combination (Figure 41-1).

Clinical Manifestations
Results of the physical examination are usually normal. Laboratory tests and, on occasion, endometrial biopsy may be used to identify and treat amenorrhea.

Outcome Management
■ Medical Management
Treatment depends on the woman's needs and the cause of the amenorrhea. Particularly important are her wishes regarding childbearing. If pregnancy is not desired at this time, progesterone may be prescribed. If pregnancy is desired, ovulation induction with clomiphene citrate (Clomid) may be undertaken.

■ Nursing Management of the Medical Client
Rule Out Pregnancy. The absence of spontaneous menstrual flow in a female older than 16 years requires careful assessment, including history and physical examination. Pregnancy also must be ruled out for any woman of childbearing age experiencing secondary amenorrhea. Ask about the presence of manifestations of pregnancy, such as breast tenderness, nausea, urinary frequency, weight gain, fatigue, and changes in food tolerance. Even if the client has been consistently using birth control, pregnancy must be considered.

Young girls may deny having had sexual intercourse (penile penetration), but may admit, on careful questioning, that they have engaged in sexual play involving ejaculation between the thighs or near the introitus (opening into the vagina). Pregnancy can result from the migration of sperm in these situations, and a pregnancy test is necessary. If the pregnancy test result is positive, an ultrasound study should be performed to determine fetal size and to confirm estimated date of confinement (EDC). Additionally, if the test result is positive, the client should be offered appropriate opportunity to discuss her wishes about continuing or terminating the pregnancy.

Provide Teaching. Teaching opportunities are an important part of nursing care. Depending on the cause of amenorrhea, the client may need help in reducing energy drain from excessive physical activity and in controlling stress. Assess her general health, and help her plan and make changes as indicated.

MENORRHAGIA
The term *menorrhagia* means excessive vaginal bleeding at normal intervals.

FIGURE 41-1 Primary and secondary causes of amenorrhea. *GnRH,* Gonadotropin-releasing hormone; *ACTH,* adrenocorticotropin-releasing hormone.

Etiology and Risk Factors

There are a number of causes of menorrhagia, including the following:

- Anovulatory menstrual cycles
- Uterine fibroids and adenomyosis
- Anatomic lesions
- Spontaneous abortion
- Inflammatory processes (e.g., endometritis and salpingitis)
- Blood dyscrasias (disordered cellular elements)
- Hypothyroidism
- Use of an IUD
- Endometrial carcinoma
- Medications (e.g., anticoagulants)

Clinical Manifestations

Assessing the amount of blood loss can be difficult. Many women are unable to give a reliable history of blood loss. Asking the client to compare the number of pads or tampons used during the abnormal period with the number used during a normal cycle is a way of de-

termining abnormality. Significant blood loss may be considered if the client is changing her pad or tampon every 1 to 2 hours. Because this information may not be adequate, a hematocrit or hemoglobin measurement may be performed to check for anemia.

Another test for significant uterine bleeding is transvaginal uterine ultrasound, which may reveal an increased thickness of the endometrium indicating abnormal tissue growth.

Outcome Management
■ Medical Management

Medical management may involve prescription of (1) estrogens and progestins, alone or in combination, (2) oral contraceptives, or (3) antifibrinolytic agents, depending on which factors are thought to be associated with the bleeding.

■ Surgical Management

An endometrial biopsy may be performed to determine the cause of uterine bleeding. A tiny amount of uterine tissue is removed and sent to the pathologist for evaluation. The specimen is analyzed for hormone effects on the tissues and for any irregular or abnormal tissue growth. Often, the tissue demonstrates abnormal tissue proliferation that responds to hormone therapy.

Outpatient endometrial ablation (removal) is used to permanently stop uterine bleeding. A laser fiber is inserted into the uterus through a hysteroscope (an endoscope used to examine the cervix and uterus), and the laser beam is directed at destroying the endometrium. The destroyed tissue is then removed by irrigation of the uterus with saline. Sterility caused by uterine scarring is a likely consequence of the procedure.

Another procedure is known as *ThermaChoice*. ThermaChoice carefully destructs the hormone-enriched endometrial lining. The procedure is not done under general anesthesia. Once the cervix is dilated, a special balloon is inserted into the uterus. The balloon is inflated with a hot liquid that causes a burn within the uterus. The balloon is removed after the procedure. Because no general anesthesia is given, the client can go home the same day.

■ Nursing Management of the Surgical Client

Other than an explanation of biopsy and the obtaining of informed consent for the procedure, no preoperative care is required before an endometrial biopsy, although emotional support is indicated. For an ablation, preoperative care includes having the client restrict food and fluid intake for anesthesia. The client is placed in the lithotomy position for this procedure.

Postoperatively, a perineal pad is in place. The pad should be checked and changed frequently. There may also be vaginal packing, which is usually removed within 24 hours.

During the first few hours, monitor vital signs and assess for excessive vaginal bleeding. Assess the client's ability to urinate. Urination may be difficult, especially if vaginal packing is exerting pressure on the urethra. Report excess bleeding, inability to void, or excessive pain. The client usually experiences only minimal uterine cramping postoperatively. Mild analgesics, such as acetaminophen and codeine (Tylenol No. 3), usually relieve any discomfort. The client should avoid aspirin for the first 24 to 48 hours to prevent excessive bleeding.

Follow-up instructions are as follows:
1. Avoid strenuous activity for about 1 week.
2. Do not douche or engage in vaginal or rectal intercourse until your physician judges that healing is complete.
3. Expect a small amount of pinkish vaginal discharge, followed by a dark red or dark brown discharge, during the healing process.
4. Subsequent menstrual periods may or may not be affected. Your next menses may not occur, may be on schedule, or may vary from the usual time.
5. Call your physician if any complications such as excessive bleeding (more than one pad per hour),

excessive pain, or temperature elevation of greater than 100° F occur.
6. Return for a follow-up appointment.

METRORRHAGIA

Metrorrhagia (vaginal bleeding between menses) may occur as spotting or outright bleeding. Possible causes include ectopic pregnancy, spotting with ovulation, cervical polyps, breakthrough bleeding with oral contraceptives, and those listed for menorrhagia.

Pregnancy, as well as the presence of malignant or nonmalignant cells or hormonal or physical abnormalities, needs to be ruled out or treated appropriately. Anemia caused by excessive blood loss should be treated. For breakthrough bleeding in conjunction with the use of oral contraceptives or *hormone replacement therapy* (HRT), assess the length of time the hormones have been given, how long the bleeding has been present, and the amount of bleeding the client is experiencing in order to suggest any change in oral contraceptive or HRT dosing.

MENOPAUSE

Physiologic menopause (cessation of menstruation) is discussed in the Unit 9 Anatomy and Physiology Review.

SURGICAL MENOPAUSE

Menopause may be induced at any age by surgical removal of the ovaries, ablation with chemicals, or pelvic irradiation. *Hysterectomy* is the removal of only the uterus, not the ovaries, and does not usually cause surgical menopause. On occasion, the surgical intervention may have menopausal manifestations. In these instances, it is possible that blood vessels supplying the ovaries have been injured. The resulting loss of blood supply causes the ovaries to atrophy. Another possible cause is the hormone imbalance produced by removal of the uterus and its loss as a hormone receptor.

PERIMENOPAUSAL CHANGES

A wide variety of physical and psychosocial manifestations have been attributed to the perimenopausal period, but the only manifestations due to menopause itself (not the associated changes that are due to aging or stressful life events) are vasomotor instability, menstrual irregularities, and vaginal changes. A positive clinical manifestation is a follicle-stimulating hormone (FSH) level greater than 40 mIU/ml, indicating the intense attempt of the pituitary gland to stimulate the ovaries to produce estrogen, with the subsequent low serum estradiol level.

Vasomotor Instability
Manifestations of vasomotor instability, such as "hot flashes," night sweats, and the occasional palpitations

and dizziness associated with menopause, appear to be caused by hormonal changes.

Hot flashes are sudden involuntary waves of heat that begin in the upper chest or neck and proceed up the face and head. These sensations last from a few seconds to an hour and are exacerbated by anything that increases heat production in the body. A hot flash may or may not be accompanied by a *hot flush,* which consists of a measurable change in skin temperature, a visible pink to bright red change in the skin, and perspiration.

A *night sweat* is a hot flash with or without a hot flush that occurs in the night, is accompanied by perspiration, which can be profuse, and is often followed by chills. Hot flashes have been described as the following:

1. *Mild hot flash.* A warm feeling, often so fleeting it is barely noticeable. It may or may not be accompanied by dampness and slight flushing.
2. *Moderate hot flash.* A warm to extremely warm feeling that lasts longer and is more noticeable than a mild hot flash. It is often accompanied by sweat and sometimes by flushing.
3. *Severe hot flash.* An intense or extremely hot feeling, usually accompanied by profuse and very uncomfortable sweating or flushing. The thermal discomfort of a severe hot flash may lead a woman to stop her activity at the time of the hot flash and to seek relief by using a fan, showering, removing or changing clothes, or lying down. Other bodily sensations associated with a severe hot flash are feelings of waves of heat, dizziness, a feeling of suffocation, inability to concentrate, and chest pain.

Generally, the manifestations of the hot flash occur about 45 seconds before the hot flush. In perimenopausal women, the reported incidence of the hot flash varies from 68% to 92%. There is a great variance in both the quantitative and qualitative aspects of women's experiences of hot flashes. Some women in other cultures do not all report experiencing hot flashes; thus the hot flash may not be a universal manifestation, or it may not be culturally acceptable for women to discuss menopausal manifestations.

Atrophic Vaginitis and Other Changes

The vaginal mucous membrane is especially responsive to low estrogen levels. When these levels remain low both during and following menopause, the vaginal walls become thinner and drier, with greater sensitivity and susceptibility to infection. These changes lead to the manifestations of atrophic vaginitis in menopausal women. Other manifestations are vaginal irritation, burning, pruritus, increased leukorrhea (vaginal discharge), bleeding, and dyspareunia (difficult or painful intercourse).

Vaginal epithelium loses its elasticity and subcutaneous fat after menopause. Pubic hair may become thinner. As the epidermal layer thins, the labia minora flatten and become flush with the labia majora. Other urogenital changes may be related to the loss of the estrogen-rich mucosal layer of the urethra and urethral atrophy associated with a higher incidence of cystitis and urethritis. In addition, these manifestations may also be confused with a urinary tract infection (UTI) or vaginitis.

The pubococcygeus muscles tend to lose their tone, and stress urinary incontinence (see Chapter 36) also may occur. In addition, manifestations of urge incontinence, such as urgency, frequency, and urine loss, may increase and may be confused with persistent UTI.

Some women experience difficulty sleeping. Others have backache, joint pain, and other manifestations of osteoporosis (a skeletal disorder characterized by the loss of bone mass and bone calcium). The calcium loss leads to an increased predisposition to bone collapse or fracture. Estrogen has been shown to inhibit bone breakdown and loss. A decrease or absence of estrogen in conjunction with other risk factors may lead to osteoporosis.

Many myths abound about the occurrence of depression at the time of menopause, but no relationship between depression and menopause has been clinically demonstrated. However, some women appear to complain of depression or emotional changes at menopause more than at any other time in their lives. A woman's experience of menopause is affected not only by hormonal changes but also by her life circumstances and relationships. Psychosocial stress at the time of menopause, however, may affect menopausal manifestations.

Outcome Management
■ Medical Management

Replace Hormones. HRT (estrogen plus progesterone) may be part of the medical management of perimenopausal, menopausal, and postmenopausal manifestations. Women must be informed of the advantages and risks of HRT so that they can make informed decisions about treatment.[60] Several studies report the benefits and risks of the long-term use of HRT (see the Evidence-Based Practice in Action feature on Hormone Replacement Therapy on p. 1061).

It is often difficult for women to decide to begin and continue HRT because of conflicting information and fears related to an increase in the incidence of breast and uterine cancer associated with the treatment. Some researchers have claimed that the risk of breast cancer actually decreases with HRT, although further study is necessary to support this claim. HRT alleviates vasomotor instability, vaginal and urinary tract atrophy, and dyspareunia. Recent findings show no benefit to HRT and incidence of dementia and cognitive impairment.[39,44] (See the Complementary and Alternative Therapy feature on Alternative Medicines for Hot Flashes on p. 1062.)

In the middle to late 1970s, evidence of an association between ERT and endometrial cancer was discovered. In subsequent years, this association has been studied ex-

E B EVIDENCE-BASED PRACTICE IN ACTION

Hormone Replacement Therapy

Over the past 30 years, researchers have questioned the use of hormone replacement therapy (HRT) for relief of menopausal manifestations and the associated long-term sequelae of estrogen deprivation in women. Women have dreaded the menopausal years as not only a sign of advancing age, but because of the unpleasant and annoying mood swings and insomnia; vasomotor manifestations such as hot flashes and headaches, and pelvic floor dysfunction such as incontinence, vaginal prolapse, and sexual dysfunction. More significant are the life-threatening conditions such as cardiovascular disease and an increased hip-fracture risk from osteoporosis associated with menopause. Because estrogen deprivation has been associated with these changes, hormone replacement has been used and advocated to decrease or eliminate the annoying manifestations and improve cardiovascular health while lessening the incidence of osteoporosis.

Estrogen and progesterone are often prescribed to women who have a uterus in place and are experiencing manifestations or conditions associated with menopause. The combined therapy of estrogen and progesterone, known as HRT, is recommended to protect the endometrium from the development of hyperplasia, a potentially precancerous condition that is the forerunner to uterine cancer. Women who do not have a uterus in place are able to take estrogen only as replacement therapy (ERT). With the elimination of vasomotor manifestations reduced pelvic floor dysfunction, and improvement in cardiovascular and osteoporosis risk, hormone replacement appeared to significantly improve the clinical manifestations while decreasing the risk of life-threatening conditions associated with menopause.

However, the Heart and Estrogen/Progestin Replacement Study (HERS), a secondary prevention trial of estrogen in postmenopausal women with heart disease, reported observational data that suggest no overall benefit to HRT with an unexpected excess of cardiovascular events.[4] Since July 2002, when the data from the Women's Health Initiative (WHI) investigation was released, health care professionals have been reluctant to prescribe estrogen with or without progesterone because the literature has revealed conflicting reports to the risks and benefits of HRT or estrogen replacement therapy (ERT).[3,8] Concerns about the associated higher incidence of breast and uterine cancer risk and an increase in cardiovascular events have been the focus of menopausal research as a result of the Women's Health Initiative investigation.[3,8] The study did not report findings on women who have undergone a hysterectomy and are taking ERT alone.[8]

Subsequent data published suggest that estrogen and progestin increased the incidence of dementia and did not prevent mild cognitive impairment in postmenopausal women.[5,6] Both ERT and HRT decrease the risk of osteoporosis and are considered preventive measures against osteoporosis but not as effective as alendronate (Fosamax) alone. Combination therapy of HRT and alendronate (Fosamax) prevented bone loss in older women better than HRT alone or alendronate alone.[2] However, alendronate was superior to HRT in preventing bone loss in these women.[2] Combination therapy with HRT and alendronate was the most effective in prevention of bone loss in older women.[2] The optimal duration of therapy for osteoporosis prevention is not known but is considered lifelong. Biphosphonate drugs that prevent or improve bone mass in those women who have osteoporosis are alendronate (Fosamax) and risedronate (Actonel). Alendronate and risedronate are only taken daily or once a week and can be given with HRT. Raloxifene (Evista), an estrogen receptor modulator, prevents osteoporosis and may provide cardioprotective effects without increasing cancer risk. The possible cardioprotective effects of ERT, HRT, and raloxifene are being investigated. Raloxifene cannot be given to women who are taking HRT and ERT.

Until recently, women who had a risk of breast cancer or a history of breast cancer, a history of deep venous thrombosis, and a history of previous uterine cancer were not candidates for HRT or ERT. However, the newer studies (HERS and WHI) have reported that the use of HRT may be related to a higher breast cancer incidence and increased cardiovascular disease risk than the previous literature previous reports.[3,8] These studies did not report the relationship of ERT to these life-threatening conditions. The arguments question the risk factors of the women taking the HRT in these studies, the type of estrogen and progestin administered, and the dosing of the drug therapy.[3,8]

Other supplements for the treatment of menopause have been under consideration. Phytoestrogens or soy based products have shown some evidence that they offer protection against a wide range of human conditions, including breast cancer, cardiovascular disease, cognitive dysfunction, osteoporosis, and menopausal manifestations. Phytoestrogens can be found in high concentrations of legumes, such as soybeans, soy products, chickpeas, red clover, sweet potatoes, carrots, garlic, and green beans. Clinical application of these products has not been fully established. However, phytoestrogens or soy may offer a safe and inexpensive alternative with relatively no side effects to current HRT and ERT therapy.[1,7]

Implications

The studies discussed have generated much controversy regarding whether women on HRT and ERT should consider stopping current replacement therapy or begin taking replacement therapy with the onset of menopause. Physicians and nurses are challenged by the concerns of women who have been taking HRT or ERT regularly. The decision by the client and health care professional to begin or to continue on HRT or ERT should be individualized based on the client's health risks and associated clinical manifestations of menopause. Therefore nurses can provide the client the opportunity to discuss and provide the necessary education regarding choices in treatment of menopausal symptom relief and menopausal disease prevention.

Continued

📖 EVIDENCE-BASED PRACTICE IN ACTION

Hormone Replacement Therapy—cont'd

References

1. Ewies, Anyman. (2002). Phytoestrogens in the management of the menopause. *Obstetrics & Gynecology Survey, 57*(5),306-311.
2. Greenspan, S., Resnick, N., & Parker, R. (2003). Combination therapy with hormone replacement and alendronate for prevention of bone loss in elderly women: A randomized controlled trial. *Journal of the American Medical Association, 289*(19), 2525-2533.
3. Grady, D., et al. (2002). Cardiovascular disease outcomes during 6.8 years of hormone therapy: Heart and estrogen/progestin replacement study follow-up (HERS II). *Journal of the American Medical Association, 288*(1), 49-57.
4. Hlatky, M.A., et al. (2002). Quality-of-life symptoms in postmenopausal women after receiving hormone therapy: results from the Heart and Estrogen/Progestin Replacement Study (HERS) trial. *Journal of the American Medical Association, 287*(5), 591-597.
5. Rapp, S., et al. (2003). Effect of estrogen plus progestin on global cognitive function in postmenopausal women. The women's health initiative memory study: A randomized controlled trial. *Journal of the American Medical Association, 289*(20), 2663-2672.
6. Shumacher, S., et al. (2003). Estrogen plus progestin and the incidence of dementia and mild cognitive impairment in postmenopausal women. The women's health initiative memory study: A randomized control trial. *Journal of the American Medical Association, 289*(20), 2651-2662.
7. Tsourounis, C. (2001). Clinical effects of phytoestrogens. *Clinical Obstetrics & Gynecology, 44* (4), 836-842.
8. Writing Group for the Women's Health Initiative Investigators. (2002). Risks and benefits of estrogen plus progestin in healthy postmenopausal women: Principal results from the Women's Health Initiative randomized controlled trial. *Journal of the American Medical Association, 288*, 321-333.

COMPLEMENTARY AND ALTERNATIVE THERAPY

Alternative Medicines for Hot Flashes

A recent analysis of 29 randomized controlled trials for hot flash reduction or menopausal manifestations was conducted. Researchers followed data on black cohosh, red clover, dong quai, evening primrose oil, ginseng, a Chinese herbal formula, soy and soy extracts, vitamin E, and wild yam cream. After analysis, researchers reported no consistent evidence that complementary therapies benefit women with menopausal manifestations; harm or adverse effects were not studied.

A further look at these data, however, shows that soy did show some benefit in 6 of the 11 randomized trials and that vitamin E demonstrated a small benefit in 1 randomized trial. In addition, flaxseed (which is high in plant estrogens) was not reviewed, and the verdict on acupuncture is not complete. Therefore other agents may show a benefit in the future, and other clinical trials are still being completed.

Reference

Kronenberg, F., & Fugh-Berman, A. (2002). Complementary and alternative medicine for menopausal symptoms: A review of randomized, controlled trials. *Annals of Internal Medicine, 137,* 805-813.

tensively. Today, estrogen is given with a progestational agent to simulate normal endometrial tissue. The progestin provides a protective effect against endometrial cancer. *Unopposed ERT* (estrogen without progestin) is no longer recommended for a woman with an intact uterus. It is generally accepted that estrogens should not be given to women with the following features:

- Known or suspected breast or uterine cancer or any estrogen-dependent cancer (or a strong family history of the same)
- Undiagnosed abnormal uterine bleeding
- Previous or present thrombophlebitis
- Acute liver disease
- Risk factors such as obesity, varicosities, hypertension, and heavy smoking, which become even more significant when they occur in combination
- Additional risk factors related to uterine fibromyomas, severe varicose veins, chronic hepatic dysfunction, and diabetes mellitus, which require thorough assessment before estrogen is prescribed

The use of ERT or HRT should be individualized according to the client's needs and wishes, risks, and individual manifestations. The risk for women with fibrocystic breast disease is unclear, but careful assessment must be made. Risks should be assessed for endometrial cancer, osteoporosis, cardiovascular disease, and breast cancer. Both ERT and HRT are effective against perimenopausal hot flashes, atrophic vaginitis, and urinary tract changes. Unless otherwise indicated, HRT or ERT may or may not be considered for lifelong replacement therapy. Dosage may decrease with the client's age. Some recent research suggests that hormone replacement therapy be taken for only 5 years.[10]

Hormone therapy is considered replacement of female hormones and should be discussed as such with the client before it is started. If a client opts for ERT or HRT, she should be monitored for the development of breast cancer or any complication with annual breast examinations and mammography. Women must receive adequate education regarding the risk factors and anticipated effects of HRT as well as signals of impending problems it may cause. See the Complementary and Alternative Therapy feature on Hormone Replacement Therapy and Obesity on the website.

Treatment regimens vary for estrogen-progesterone combinations. In some cases, estrogens may be used for 25 days each month or continually, whereas progesterones may be prescribed for 10 to 14 days a month. A low-dose continuous progesterone therapy may be given along with continuous ERT. The advantage of continuous combined therapy is the elimination of withdrawal bleeding. Bleeding usually ceases in about 4 months.

Side effects of high-dose progesterone therapy include bloating, depression, acne, breast tenderness, and premenstrual tension; however, adjusting the dose can generally lessen these effects, as with continuous therapy, or lengthening the duration of therapy. Side effects of progesterone may unfavorably alter the ratio of high-density-lipoprotein (HDL) and low-density-lipoprotein (LDL) cholesterol. Therefore unopposed estrogen has been recommended for the client whose uterus has been surgically removed.

Transdermal estrogen patches are an alternative when oral estrogens cannot be tolerated or when the hepatic effects of estrogen (increased secretion of renin substrate causing hypertension and increased clotting factors as a result of liver stimulation) are a problem.

Vaginal estrogen is indicated for any woman experiencing urogenital manifestations of menopause (e.g., atrophic vaginitis, incontinence, and vaginal dryness). Vaginal estrogen can be delivered in continuous dosing, such as in a vaginal ring that is changed every 3 months. A small amount of vaginal cream, 0.5 to 1 g, can be inserted into the vagina at bedtime, several times per week. Vagifem, a topical vaginal estrogen in pill form, is the newest topical therapy. The tablet is inserted into the vagina several times a week. Clients report that this type of topical estrogen replacement is less messy than the previously mentioned types.

■ Nursing Management of the Medical Client

Provide Education. Nurses have a unique role in providing education for women undergoing menopause and their partners or significant others. The role involves providing support, education, and assistance in moving through this normal life experience as comfortably as possible. Accurate information about menopause and what to expect can be helpful and reassuring. Provide educational information about the risks and benefits of estrogen therapy.

To help clients cope with the minor discomforts of menopause, you may recommend the following self-care advice:

1. *Relief of vaginal dryness.* Intercourse and masturbation aid circulation and keep tissues flexible; use water-soluble vaginal lubricants as often as needed. Topical estrogen cream or other vaginal estrogen preparations eliminate manifestations.
2. *Prevention of osteoporosis.* Take part in weight-bearing exercises; increase calcium intake; stop smoking; reduce alcohol and caffeine intake.
3. *Prevention of UTIs.* Increase fluid intake (six to eight glasses of water per day); attempt to void every 2 to 3 hours; maintain good perineal hygiene; wear cotton underwear.
4. *Pelvic relaxation.* Perform Kegel (pelvic floor) exercises to increase muscle tone (see later discussion and Chapter 36); lose weight if appropriate.

Remind women experiencing menopause of the value of good health habits. Balanced nutrition and adequate sleep and rest are important. Phytoestrogens (plant estrogens), found in soy products, flaxseed oil, nuts, and brown rice, have a very mild estrogenic effect that may reduce vaginal dryness. Exercising at least three to four times per week for 45 minutes improves bone and cardiovascular health.

POSTMENOPAUSAL BLEEDING

Postmenopausal bleeding (vaginal bleeding occurring after menopause) is a manifestation, not a diagnosis (Figure 41-2). Careful assessment is necessary because it may be a manifestation of many conditions of the lower reproductive tract: atrophic vaginitis, cervical polyps, uterine fibroids (leiomyoma), endometrial hyperplasia, cervical erosion, and uterine or cervical cancer.

■ PELVIC INFLAMMATORY DISEASE

The term *pelvic inflammatory disease* refers to ascending pelvic infection that involves the upper genital tract.

Etiology and Risk Factors

Chlamydia trachomatis, gonococci, staphylococci, streptococci, and other pus-producing (pyogenic) organisms commonly cause PID. A common risk factor is an untreated bacterial infection. Most of these infections are sexually transmitted. The lack of condom use increases the risk of passing the bacteria between partners.

Health promotion actions are to advise clients to avoid (1) unprotected intercourse, (2) sex with multiple partners, especially with use of an IUD, (3) IUD for birth control, and (4) douches. To maintain health, clients should seek treatment immediately when manifestations of PID appear and if a sexual partner has a sexually transmitted disease (STD).

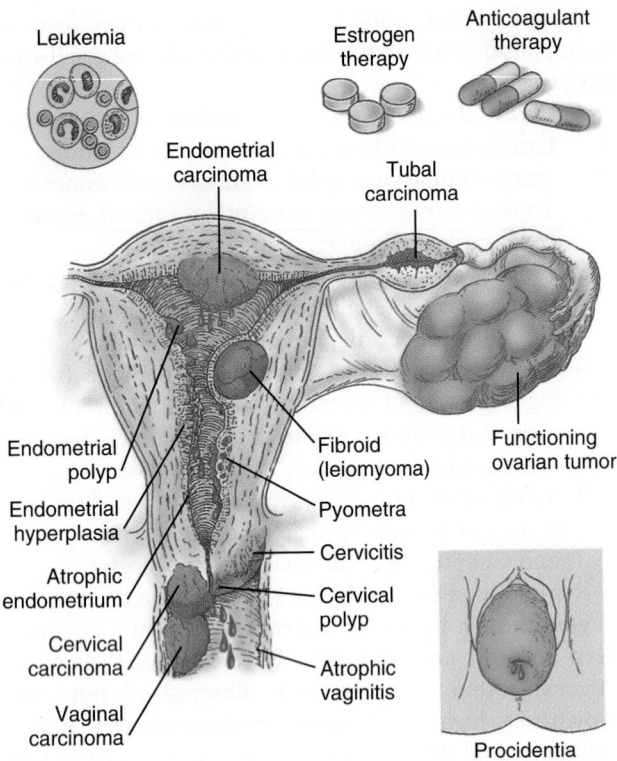

FIGURE 41-2 Causes of postmenopausal bleeding.

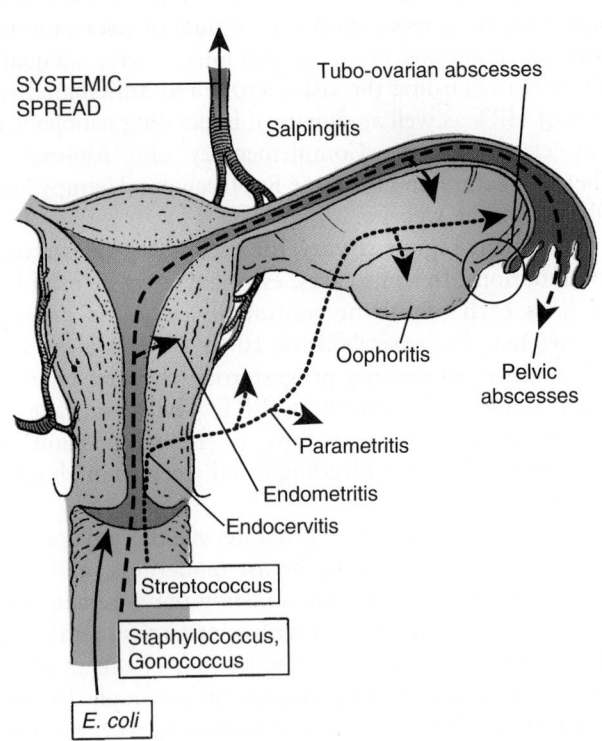

FIGURE 41-3 Routes of spread of pelvic inflammatory disease.

Health restoration activities include advising clients to complete the full course of medications used to treat a PID and to follow health promotion recommendations to prevent reinfection.

Pathophysiology

Once an infection is in the upper genital tract, the bacteria may travel along several routes (Figure 41-3). Tuberculosis (TB), a rare cause of PID, travels through the blood and affects the fallopian tubes and sometimes the ovaries, uterus, and pelvic peritoneum. The woman's excreta are contaminated until the antituberculin medications have taken effect.

C. trachomatis and gonococcal and staphylococcal organisms spread along the uterine endometrium to the fallopian tubes, where an acute *salpingitis* (inflammation of the fallopian tubes) occurs. The tubes become partially occluded and may drain pus, leukocytes, and other debris into the pelvic cavity, causing pelvic peritonitis, or the material may form a pocket around the ovary, causing a tubo-ovarian abscess.

Streptococci spread similarly, but they tend to travel via the uterine or cervical lymphatics across the parametrium to the tubes or ovaries. Pelvic cellulitis and occasional thrombophlebitis of the major pelvic veins with additional risk of the development of emboli may occur. Another route of infection is from the pelvic cavity itself. Organisms such as *Escherichia coli* may be extruded from a ruptured bowel, causing peritonitis.

Although septic shock and other complications may appear, the most common is a pelvic abscess.

More than 50% of women with a history of PID have difficulty becoming pregnant or experience an ectopic pregnancy after the infection has cleared. These problems are due to scarring by the inflammatory process and subsequent closing and scarring of the fallopian tubes.

Clinical Manifestations

PID may be "silent" (asymptomatic), especially in the early stage. Clinical manifestations of PID include malaise, fever, chills, anorexia, nausea and vomiting, aching and tachycardia. In addition, the woman usually experiences acute, sharp, severe aching pain on both sides of the abdomen or pelvis. Pain is worsened by urination or defecation and may be accompanied by a heavy, purulent, and, possibly, odorous discharge. Occasionally, vaginal bleeding occurs. The rapidity of onset of PID depends on (1) the virulence (degree of severity) of the infecting organism, (2) the status of the client's pelvic organs, and (3) the client's general health.

Other helpful clues to PID are obtained from the history. A history of acute lower genital tract infection is significant. Other data, including a thorough sexual history, are important. A history of contraceptive use is established because the presence of an IUD correlates with a higher incidence of PID.

The long-term sequelae of untreated, silent PID may be detected when attempts to achieve a pregnancy have proved unsuccessful. During a clinical evaluation of the client, routine screening tests, such as cultures, may yield positive results. The usual laboratory tests for infection, including multiple cultures, are performed. Some practitioners perform a culture of any evident drainage and obtain specimens from various sites, such as the cervix, vagina, and urethra. Additional specimens from the vagina and the adjacent structures may be obtained to evaluate for bacterial infection of the genital tract. If multiple organisms are found, several types of antibiotics may be necessary to treat the infection.

Histologic examination of endometrial biopsy specimens, colposcopy (examination with use of a large color-filtering, magnifying instrument), or ultrasonography to identify an abscess may also be used in the diagnosis of PID.

Outcome Management
■ Medical Management

Eliminate Causative Organism. Most clients with PID are treated as outpatients, receiving antibiotics appropriate to the specific organism causing the infection. They are cautioned to avoid sexual activity, douching, and other activities that might enhance the infectious process. With improvement, the client should return to the clinic in a week for reevaluation of status. Advise the client being treated at home for PID to return sooner if her condition deteriorates or if manifestations increase.

Hospitalization may be necessary for a client with PID who is acutely ill. During hospitalization, antibiotics are administered in maximal doses if the cause of PID is bacterial; PID resulting from TB is treated with antituberculosis medications. Treatment with medication is aimed at removing or destroying the causative organism.

■ Surgical Management

Some abscesses must be removed by surgical intervention. Others may rupture, causing peritonitis. The type of surgical intervention and its timing, either acute or after initial medical management, varies with the health care provider's philosophy and the presenting problem. Treatment of some women with PID includes a laparotomy. Occasionally, the uterus, ovaries, and fallopian tubes are removed if they are involved by the infection. Surgery performed during the acute phase of PID increases the woman's risk of postoperative complications. This risk must be balanced against that of continuing unsuccessful medical therapy, which often leads to chronic PID.

■ Nursing Management of the Medical-Surgical Client

Promote Drainage and Comfort. If in bed, the woman should be instructed to maintain a semi-Fowler's position to promote downward drainage. Pain management is important. Sitz baths or heat applied periodically to the lower back or abdomen may help relieve the pain.

Analgesics are also used. Document the amount, color, odor, and appearance of the vaginal discharge. It is a nursing responsibility to assist with perineal care frequently.

Provide Support. Nursing care of the woman experiencing PID is directed toward providing health information and psychosocial support to the client and her significant others. Because PID is often caused by STDs, there may be guilt feelings and emotional stress within the relationship. Usually, the woman's sexual partner requires treatment whether symptomatic or not.

Some women are infertile after PID. This loss of fertility may be difficult for the client and her significant other to accept. Plan and provide time for the expression of such feelings.

Provide Education. Education is important for the client with PID. Women with PID can benefit from factual discussion about the infection, recognizing the manifestations of recurrences, and general hygienic and sexual measures to help prevent new infections. The client should be instructed to wash the perineal area regularly with soap and water, to wipe the perineum from front to back after elimination, to change tampons and pads several times a day during menses, and to wash hands before and after changing tampons or pads.

Balanced nutrition, adequate rest, sleep, and exercise can improve general health and reduce the risk of infection. Inform clients when sexual activity can be resumed, how to ensure the safety of sexual encounters, and when other restrictions can be lifted.

CHRONIC PELVIC INFLAMMATORY DISEASE

Chronic PID can occur if the acute phase of the illness does not respond to treatment or if treatment is inadequate. Clinical manifestations of chronic PID include chronic pelvic discomfort, menstrual disturbances or dysfunctional uterine bleeding, constipation, malaise, and periodic return of acute manifestations. Sterility, one of the more serious complications, results from destruction of part of the fallopian tubes and loss of their patency (their being wide open).

Treatment of chronic PID is aimed at removing the offending organism and improving the client's general health. If treatment is unsuccessful, surgical removal of the pelvic organs may be necessary.

▋ UTERINE DISORDERS
ENDOMETRIOSIS

Endometriosis is an abnormal condition in which *endometrium,* the tissue that normally lines the uterus, is located in internal sites other than in the uterus.

Endometriosis most commonly affects women in their mid-30s. It occasionally occurs in women younger than 20 years of age. There is a familial predisposition, and the highest incidence is in white women who are nulliparous (have not given birth).

Etiology and Risk Factors

The cause of endometriosis is unknown, although a few theories have been proposed, for instance:

1. *Retrograde menstruation theory.* Menstrual secretions flow backward through the fallopian tubes and deposit particles of viable endometrial tissue outside the uterine cavity. Spread then occurs as endometrial tissue reproduces itself, a process called *metaplasia.*
2. *Vascular and lymphatic dissemination theory.* Spread (metastasis) of endometrial tissue occurs through the lymphatic and vascular systems to locations outside the uterus. This may explain some of the distant sites of metastasis, such as the lungs and kidneys.

Pathophysiology

Although the abnormally located endometrial tissue is usually confined to the pelvic cavity, it may be found in other areas. The most common sites are the ovary and the dependent portion of the pelvic peritoneum. Rarely, tissue may lie outside the pelvis, such as in surgical scars, lungs, and extremities. Possible sites are shown in Figure 41-4.

Regardless of the site, this misplaced endometrial tissue responds to hormonal stimulation and bleeds, producing a variety of manifestations. Scarring and inflammation occur at these extrauterine sites. Repeated episodes of intraperitoneal bleeding, due to hormonal stimulation of the endometrial tissue, cause adhesions. Scarring and adhesions cause the organs and peritoneal surface to become fixed to each other.

Because endometrial tissue is hormone-dependent, the tissue usually atrophies with the normal ovarian regression associated with menopause; it also regresses during pregnancy.

Infertility is a major complication of endometriosis. Usually, the infertility is due to scarring, leading to obstruction of the fallopian tubes.

Clinical Manifestations

Manifestations of endometriosis relate more to the *site* than to the *extent* of disease present. Pain is the most characteristic manifestation; however, about 25% of women with this condition are asymptomatic. Pain typically begins before the menstrual period, lasting for the duration of menstruation and sometimes for several days afterward. The intensity of pain is not correlated with the extent of endometriosis. Pain usually reaches its peak just before the onset of menstrual flow and during the first 1 or 2 days of the menstrual period. The pain may be located in several areas, making the diagnosis more difficult to confirm. Unfortunately, some health care providers may view some women with endometriosis as

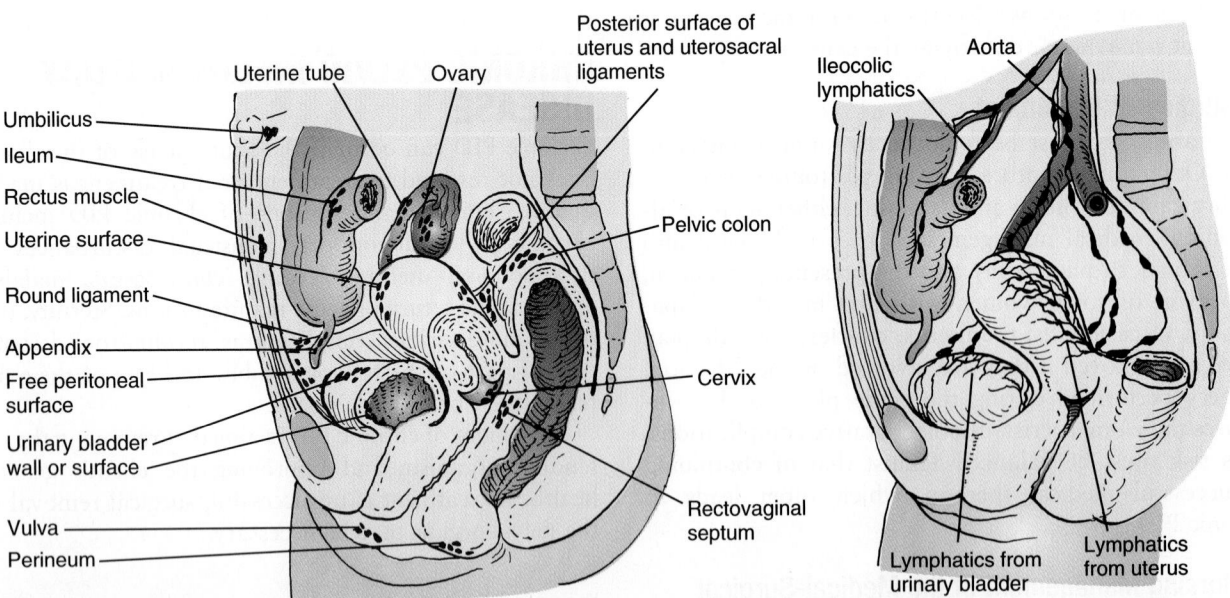

A. SITES OF ENDOMETRIOSIS

B. LYMPHATICS

FIGURE 41-4 Endometriosis. **A,** Sites of endometriosis. The locations most frequently affected are the ovaries and the dependent pelvic peritoneum. However, many other sites may be involved. **B,** Pelvic and lymph nodes are important.

having psychosomatic complaints and drug-seeking behaviors.

Other manifestations of endometriosis are dyspareunia, menstrual irregularities, and infertility in the absence of tubal obstruction. When the condition occurs inside the ovary, it can produce a "chocolate" cyst, or *endometrioma*. Severe pain is associated with the presence or rupture of this cyst. Implants of endometrium on the ureters may cause obstruction. Rectal implants may be associated with bleeding, diarrhea, or obstruction. Bowel involvement may cause painful defecation.

The diagnosis is generally made from the history, a pelvic examination, and observation of lesions either by laparoscopic examination or pelvic surgery. Direct observation of lesions is necessary for a definitive diagnosis.

Outcome Management
■ Medical Management

Appropriate treatment of endometriosis depends on the client's manifestations, age, number of children (parity), and extent of disease. When manifestations and extent of disease are mild, the client is given support, information, and coping strategies for pain management. Mild analgesics may be helpful. If manifestations become severe or the disease progresses, additional treatment is generally necessary.

Reduce Manifestations. Medication may inhibit endometriosis enough to allow pregnancy or, at least, relieve manifestations. Hormonal intervention includes inducing a *pseudopregnancy* (false pregnancy) with oral contraceptives, progesterone, or both. During the course of this treatment, progestins cause the endometrial implants to slough off. Theoretically, then, the endometrial tissue no longer functions in abnormal sites. This type of treatment is not successful in all women.

The other hormonal treatment is to induce *ovarian suppression* or *pseudomenopause* (false menopause). Danazol (Danocrine) is an antigonadotropin testosterone derivative that inhibits gonadotropin release, causing ovarian suppression and regression of endometriosis. The medication provides rapid and safe relief of manifestations. Side effects may include acne, hirsutism (excess hair), weight gain, decreased breast size, hot flashes, and vaginal dryness.

Leuprolide (Lupron), a synthetic analog of luteinizing hormone (LH), reduces endometrial pain and lesions. The client can administer it herself monthly in an intramuscular (IM) injection or daily in a subcutaneous (SC) injection. This medication also carries associated menopausal side effects.

Nafarelin (Synarel) acts as a synthetic analog of gonadotropin-releasing hormone (GnRH). Lesions are reduced because endometrial lesions are sensitive to ovarian hormones. It is administered intranasally twice a day and may create menopausal side effects.

Hormonal treatments are expensive, costing from $100 to more than $300 per month.

■ Surgical Management

Exploratory or therapeutic surgery directed at endometriosis may make pregnancy possible. Conservative surgical intervention involves restoring normal anatomy and removing or destroying endometriotic foci. A carbon dioxide laser may be used to vaporize adhesions and endometrial implants. Even if the client claims that pregnancy is not desirable at this time, conservative surgery should be considered.

More radical surgery involves removing the uterus, as many implants as possible, and, possibly, the ovaries. This procedure has wide-reaching consequences for affecting sexuality, cardiovascular health, and the risk of osteoporosis unless HRT is also given. This surgical intervention is used only when other measures have failed and the client does not wish to preserve fertility. It causes surgically induced menopause and permanent sterility.

Controversy exists about the use of HRT after such an extensive surgical procedure. The client with a history of endometriosis who undergoes surgically induced menopause may be at risk for induction of additional growth of endometrial implants if she is given some form of HRT after the procedure, particularly in the first few months postoperatively. Conservative surgery is effective for most women. More radical surgery is almost completely effective.

■ Nursing Management of the Medical-Surgical Client

Nursing care of the woman with endometriosis depends on (1) severity of manifestations, (2) extent of disease, (3) age, and (4) childbearing status. Nursing care consists of support during the diagnostic process as the client considers the various treatment options.

Nursing interventions should include discussion of information about the nature of endometriosis, its treatment, and ways to cope with the manifestations. Yoga and relaxation techniques may provide relief. If infertility is an issue, provide information and support in decision-making in this area as well.

Surgical management is similar to that discussed for abdominal hysterectomy, tubal ligation, or laparoscopy (see later discussion).

BENIGN UTERINE TUMORS (LEIOMYOMAS)

Leiomyomas are the most common tumors of the female genital tract. They occur in more than 20% to 30% of all women during the menstrual years. The incidence is two to three times greater in African-American women than in white women. Leiomyomas are more common in women approaching menopause.

Leiomyomas are known by various names related to the tissue involved such as fibroids, fibromas, fibromyomas, fibroleiomyomas, myomas, and fiber balls. Leiomyomas are composed mainly of muscle and fibrous connective tissue.

Etiology and Risk Factors

The cause of leiomyomas is unknown. Their growth seems to be related to estrogen stimulation because the fibroids often enlarge with pregnancy and shrink with menopause. A leiomyoma begins as a simple proliferation of smooth muscle cells. It has been suggested that this type of proliferation is stimulated by physical or mechanical means and may occur at points of maximal stress within the myometrium. Because there are many points of stress within the uterus resulting from contractions, fibroids are often multiple (Figure 41-5).

Pathophysiology

Leiomyomas develop from the uterine myometrium. Growth is usually associated with proliferation of the smooth muscle cells. Estrogen and other hormones influence growth of the muscle cells. Manifestations usually decrease after menopause.

Classification

Leiomyomas may be classified according to their location (those occurring in the uterine body are most common; see Figure 41-5):

1. *Intramural.* Found in the uterine wall, surrounded by myometrium. Clinical manifestations include increased uterine size, vaginal bleeding between menses, and dysmenorrhea.
2. *Submucosal.* Located directly under the endometrium, involving the endometrial cavity. May become pedunculated (grow on a stalk). Clinical manifestations include prolonged vaginal bleeding and cramps, and the tumor may be seen protruding through the cervix.
3. *Subserosal.* Found on the outer surface (under the serosa) of the uterus. Tends to become pedunculated, to wander, and to be multiple and large. Clinical manifestations include backache, constipation, and bladder problems.
4. *Wandering or parasitic.* A pedunculated leiomyoma that twists on its pedicle, breaks off, then attaches to other tissues, particularly the omentum.
5. *Intraligamentary.* Implants on the pelvic ligaments. May displace the uterus or involve the ureters.
6. *Cervical.* Occur infrequently and may obstruct the cervical canal.

Clinical Manifestations

Frequently, leiomyomas are asymptomatic. Manifestations relate to tumor size, location, and number. Additionally, abnormal bleeding, often resulting in hypermenorrhea (excessive uterine bleeding), is frequently related to the hormone dependence of the fibroid.

Manifestations vary widely and occur in about half of clients with leiomyomas. When present, manifestations often relate to the size, location, and number of leiomyomas. The onset of manifestations most commonly occurs in a client's late 40s and early 50s, just before menopause. Once menopause begins, manifestations often cease. It is rare for manifestations to begin after menopause, when leiomyomas tend to regress with decreasing estrogen stimulation. If new manifestations develop during these years, other diagnoses, such as cancer, need to be ruled out.

The most common clinical manifestation is abnormal uterine bleeding, which may be excessive in either amount or duration. Additionally, it may be accompanied by anemia, with manifestations of tiredness, weakness, and lethargy. Dysmenorrhea and a sense of pelvic pressure are often present. Urinary frequency is common when the tumor presses on the bladder. Urinary retention also may occur when bladder function is compromised by tumor size. Constipation, hydroureter (abnormal distention of ureter with urine), hydronephrosis (distention of kidney due to abnormal accumulation of urine in the kidney pelvis), abdominal pain, and dyspareunia are less common manifestations.

Occasionally, the client may have vaginal discharge, which may be foul or water-tinged and blood-tinged. Abdominal pressure occurs if the leiomyoma is large enough to cause abdominal distention. The tumor may be palpable. Also, the client may experience sterility

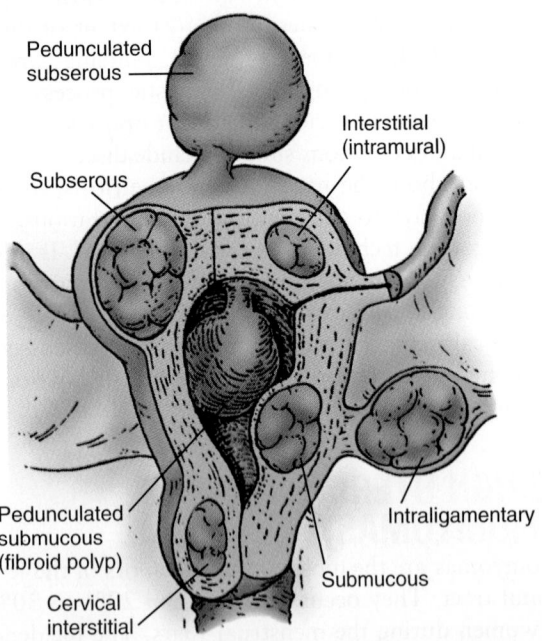

FIGURE 41-5 Sites of leiomyomas (fibroids). Uterine leiomyomas, depending on their location and size, may interfere with passage of sperm and implantation of a fertilized ovum.

or have a history of one or more spontaneous abortions.

A characteristic history, confirmed by findings of abdominal and pelvic examinations, usually establishes the diagnosis. Ultrasonography may demonstrate an abnormal uterine shape. Various disorders, such as cancer and a problem pregnancy, must be ruled out before treatment is planned.

Outcome Management
■ Medical Management

A plan of treatment for leiomyomas depends on manifestations, age of the client, location and size of the tumors, onset of complications, and client's desire to preserve fertility. Leiomyomas can be assessed every 6 months by a practitioner if the client is not pregnant; if there is no excessive bleeding or pressure on the bladder, bowel, or ureters; and if the tumor is not rapidly growing.

GnRH analogs (see Endometriosis earlier in this chapter) may be administered to reduce size and inhibit growth of tumors. Malignant degeneration is rare. A rapid increase in the size of the leiomyoma, as indicated by manifestations or detected on examination, should be thoroughly evaluated, and aggressive therapy should be considered.

■ Surgical Management

Surgical treatment may involve cutting off the blood supply to the fibroid with uterine artery embolization or *myomectomy* (removal of a tumor without removal of the uterus). Both procedures preserve the reproductive organs and reproductive capability. However, because of the increased risk that additional leiomyomas may develop later, a hysterectomy may be the preferred procedure.

Hysterectomy

 Indications. Three types of hysterectomy may be performed:

1. *Total hysterectomy*—removal of the uterus and cervix. Can be performed either abdominally or vaginally.
2. *Total hysterectomy with bilateral salpingo-oophorectomy* (TAH-BSO)—removal of uterus, cervix, fallopian tubes, and ovaries. Can be performed vaginally or abdominally.
3. *Radical hysterectomy*—same as a TAH-BSO plus removal of the lymph nodes, upper third of the vagina, and parametrium. Usually performed if a malignant tumor is found.

 Contraindications. The only contraindication to hysterectomy is any health condition that prevents surgery.

 Complications. Hemorrhage and infection are the primary complications.

 Outcomes. It is expected that the client will return home in 2 to 4 days and resume regular activities within 4 to 6 weeks, depending on the type of hysterectomy performed. Pain, abnormal bleeding, and anemia, if present, will cease. For all procedures except myomectomy, menstruation ends.

■ Nursing Management of the Surgical Client

Preoperative Care

The client seeks medical help because of some form of abnormal uterine bleeding, dyspareunia, or pelvic pain. Obtain a thorough history from the client, especially if there are complaints of irregular bleeding. It is also important to assess the client's knowledge of her condition and the surgery. Listen carefully for any questions she has about sexuality after treatment.

Reduce Pain. Before surgery is performed, the client can be taught ways to reduce pain associated with intercourse, such as assuming positions in which leiomyomas are not pressed on during intercourse and using water-soluble lubricants. Pain medications can be used for severe pain. Sometimes, sitz baths or the application of heat to the lower abdomen may be helpful.

Provide Education. The client undergoing a hysterectomy has many learning needs. Frequently, a woman undergoing gynecologic surgery needs help understanding the problem and the proposed operation. She needs to understand her options and the differences among the procedures proposed.

If a hysterectomy is planned, inform the client about the loss of fertility. If the ovaries are to be removed in conjunction with the hysterectomy, discuss surgical menopause and HRT. Some women are relieved that the operation will remove the risk of unwanted pregnancy and monthly menstrual manifestations.

Discuss how sexual intercourse may change after a hysterectomy. Although the client's ability to achieve orgasm should not change, the vagina will be shortened and there may be scar tissue.

The client whose ovaries are removed may complain of a decrease in *libido* (sexual desire). This is due to the loss of testosterone that is normally produced by the ovaries. HRT may include a small daily dose of testosterone. Tell the client that once healing has occurred, intercourse should be pain-free. Answer any questions asked, and encourage the client and her significant other to express their feelings and concerns about sexuality.

Postoperative Care
Assessment

Perform the usual postoperative assessments. Evaluation of psychological manifestations is also important.

The proximity of the bladder to the female reproductive organs increases the risk of urinary problems, which must be monitored postoperatively. A Foley catheter is usually inserted at the time of surgery to prevent bladder distention and injury during surgery; the catheter is often left in place for 24 hours postoperatively. Potential postoperative problems related to the placement of a Foley catheter are UTI and temporary urinary retention due to voiding dysfunction.

Assess GI function by listening for bowel sounds, noting distention, and determining whether the abdomen is soft or firm. Passing of flatus (bowel gas) indicates the return of GI function. After an abdominal hysterectomy, assess the abdominal incision for bleeding and intactness.

Assess vaginal bleeding. One saturated pad should be necessary in 4 hours after abdominal or vaginal hysterectomy. Excessive bleeding should be considered if one sanitary napkin is saturated in 1 hour or less.

Diagnosis, Outcomes, Interventions

Diagnosis: Risk for Dysfunctional Grieving.

Some women experience grief about their loss of the female reproductive organs, making *Risk for Dysfunctional Grieving related to loss of reproductive capacity and perceived loss of femininity* an appropriate nursing diagnosis for a client undergoing hysterectomy.

Outcomes. The client can be expected to go through a grieving process over her loss after hysterectomy and may express her feelings about the loss.

Interventions. When reproductive ability is lost, the client may undergo a grief response. It is important for the nurse to understand the grieving process and to be able to help the woman understand that this response is normal. Some women experience relief rather than grief. Support normal grieving, including temporary denial, which is a part of the grieving process. If the client continues to experience grief beyond the normal degree or time expected, she may require counseling.

Diagnosis: Risk for Infection.

During surgery for a hysterectomy, a Foley catheter is inserted, leading to the nursing diagnosis *Risk for Infection related to surgical intervention and presence of a urinary catheter.*

Outcomes. The client will remain free of infection, or will report any infection immediately for proper diagnosis and treatment.

Interventions

Prevent Urinary Infection. When a Foley catheter is in place, instruct the client to keep the urinary drainage catheter below the level of the bladder, drink at least 2 to 4 L of liquid daily, and report any urinary pain or discomfort. Check the urinary drainage system closely for leaks and kinks in the system, provide complete perineal care every shift, and report any change in color or odor of the urine. When a Foley catheter is discontinued, monitor the client for the first void. Voiding frequently in small amounts, inability to void, and bladder distention or hematuria should be reported to the physician.

Prevent Retention. Often, a suprapubic catheter is placed instead of a Foley catheter. This allows the client to clamp the catheter and attempt to void as soon as she is ambulatory. If the suprapubic area becomes distended when the catheter is clamped and the client is unable to void, the suprapubic catheter can be opened and drained. Using a suprapubic catheter avoids the need for recatheterization of a client who cannot void.

Diagnosis: Constipation.

Because of bowel manipulation during surgery, the nursing diagnosis *Constipation related to bowel manipulation during surgery* is appropriate.

Outcomes. The client will not become constipated, and bowel distention will be treated, as evidenced by return to a normal bowel pattern and absence of abdominal distention.

Interventions

Promote Peristalsis. Pain and discomfort after abdominal hysterectomy usually center on the incision and postoperative gas pains. After abdominal hysterectomy, GI functioning returns slowly. Uncomfortable gas pains are often experienced during the early postoperative period. Early, frequent ambulation helps improve GI function. If gas pains persist, a small enema may be prescribed to facilitate peristalsis and prevent constipation. Continue to encourage frequent ambulation to facilitate the return of normal GI functioning. Drinking warm fluids may encourage the return of peristalsis.

Evaluation

It is expected that the client will recover from a hysterectomy without complications. She can return to normal activities within 4 to 6 weeks without permanent problems.

■ Self-Care

The client should understand the type of surgery she has had and the follow-up needed. If she has had a myomectomy, pregnancy is still an option. She must continue to have routine gynecologic examinations and to use birth control measures until her physician judges that she can attempt a pregnancy. If she has undergone TAH-BSO, discuss menopause and HRT with her. Discharge teaching should also include the following instructions:

1. Eat a well-balanced diet, drink six to eight glasses of water daily, and get plenty of rest.
2. Avoid heavy lifting for about 6 weeks to prevent straining on the abdominal muscles and surgical sites.
3. Avoid activities that increase pelvic congestion, such as aerobic activity, horseback riding, and prolonged standing. Optimal circulation is necessary to promote healing of pelvic tissues.
4. Avoid vaginal and rectal intercourse and douching until healing is complete, usually in about 6 weeks. These activities can interfere with healing of the vaginal cuff or other healing tissues and can introduce infection.
5. Report any fresh bleeding and any abnormal vaginal discharge to the surgeon.
6. Return for follow-up care as requested by the surgeon.

ENDOMETRIAL (UTERINE) CANCER

Endometrial cancer is the most common malignancy of the female genital reproductive system. In 2003, the American Cancer Society estimated that 40,100 new cases of uterine cancer would be diagnosed in the United States. The 5-year survival rate is 96% if the cancer is discovered at an early stage.[1]

Etiology and Risk Factors

Endometrial cancer is thought to be related to overstimulation of the endometrium from excessive circulating estrogen. Common sources of excessive estrogen are successive anovulatory menstrual cycles and unopposed ERT (estrogen without progestin) in a woman who still has her uterus. Other factors are history of pelvic radiation, other reproductive cancer, family history, history of diabetes or hypertension, obesity, and hyperestrogenism (early menarche, late menopause, dysfunctional uterine bleeding, delayed onset of ovulation).

Health promotion actions include advising overweight women to lose weight and use of HRT (estrogen and progestin) or raloxifene (Evista) instead of estrogen therapy. Health maintenance actions are to advise women to have yearly pelvic examinations even after menopause, ensure that high-risk women undergo endometrial biopsy at regular intervals, and inform the client to have postmenopausal bleeding assessed.

Pathophysiology

In women with endometrial cancer, the cell type is usually adenocarcinoma, a tumor that involves the glands. This relatively slow-growing tumor metastasizes late in its course and tends to spread slowly to other organs. Most commonly, the carcinoma invades the uterus, causing uterine enlargement. The cancerous process may ex-

tend along the endometrial surface to the cervix or fallopian tubes and ovaries. It can spread to other peritoneal structures, including the lymphatics and blood vessels. It can then spread to the vagina, through the lymphatics to other areas, and, occasionally, to distant sites such as the brain and lungs.

Clinical Manifestations

Because there is no practical, accurate method of screening for endometrial cancer, the cancer is usually discovered after the first manifestations appear. The most significant manifestation is some type of abnormal uterine bleeding, especially in the postmenopausal woman. Other manifestations relate to invasion, metastasis to other organs, or both (Figure 41-6).

A diagnosis of endometrial cancer is usually established by pelvic examination and pathologic analysis of an endometrial biopsy specimen. Women at high risk may undergo endometrial biopsy at each annual or biannual pelvic examination. An endovaginal ultrasound study of the endometrium may be used to detect a thickened endometrium, or a hysteroscope (a small intrauterine instrument that visualizes uterine contents) with biopsy may be used to assist in the diagnosis.

Outcome Management
■ Surgical Management

Endometrial cancer is generally treated with surgery, radiation, or a combination. Early endometrial cancer is

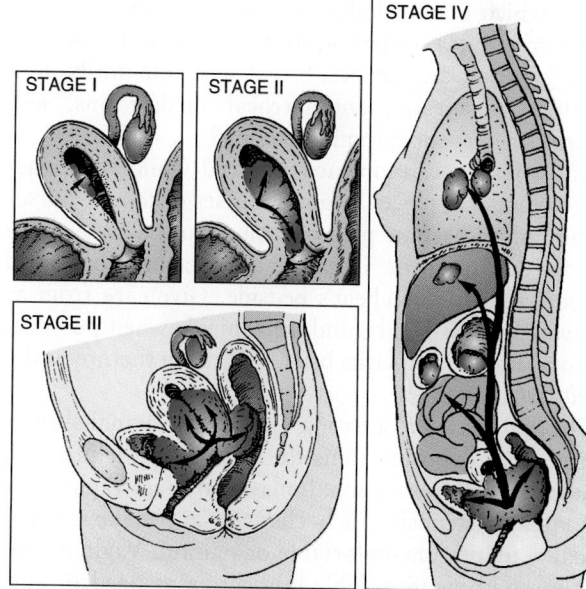

FIGURE 41-6 Staging uterine cancer. *Stage I,* The tumor is confined to the uterine corpus. *Stage II,* The cancer has also invaded the cervix. *Stage III,* The cancer has spread beyond the uterus but remains confined to the pelvis, such as in the bladder or rectum. *Stage IV,* Highest level of invasiveness because the cancer has spread beyond the pelvis, causing metastatic disease and large masses, such as in the liver or lungs.

surgically treated with a TAH-BSO. Surgery may be preceded or followed by irradiation, either external of internal. Surgical management is the same as for benign uterine tumors (leiomyomas).

■ Medical Management

External irradiation is discussed in Chapter 19. If intracavity (internal) radiation therapy (IRT) or brachytherapy is selected, an applicator is placed through the vagina into the uterus with the use of anesthesia. Correct placement is verified by x-ray study, and the client is taken to a hospital room. A radiologist places a radioactive isotope in the applicator, which remains for 1 to 3 days.

Precancerous endometrial changes may be treated with the hormone progesterone. Chemotherapy and hormonal therapy with tamoxifen (Nolvadex) are used to treat late stages of endometrial cancer.

■ Nursing Management of the Medical-Surgical Client

Nursing care of the surgical client is the same as described for the client with benign uterine tumors (leiomyomas).

While the radioactive implants are in place, the client is strictly isolated in a private room. She must remain on bed rest, with the head of the bed flat or elevated no more than 20 degrees. Movement is restricted except for deep breathing and leg exercises. A Foley catheter is inserted to prevent dislodgment of the implants, and the client is given a low-residue diet to prevent bowel movements, which may dislodge the implant. Increased fluid intake, to prevent urinary stasis, is encouraged. You may also administer antiemetics, broad-spectrum antibiotics, sedatives, analgesics, antidiarrheal medications, and heparin (to prevent thrombophlebitis).

Radiation precautions are enforced while a radioactive implant is in place. Pregnant nurses or female nurses attempting to become pregnant must not be assigned to care for such a client. Organize care so that you spend minimal time at the client's bedside. Give care from as far away as possible, behind lead shields when possible. Visitors should keep visits brief. Radiation therapy is detailed in Chapter 19.

The high dose of radiation may cause vaginal shrinkage, because exposure thins the vaginal epithelium and reduces vaginal lubrication. It may also cause vaginal adhesions and stenosis. Such changes can make vaginal sexual activities uncomfortable or painful. Vaginal penetration, with water-soluble lubrication as needed, during the course of irradiation and in subsequent months minimizes the possibility of vaginal stenosis and contracture. Depending on personal preference, vaginal penetration and dilation can be accomplished with the woman's own fingers, a vaginal dilator, or her sexual partner's fingers or penis. Vaginal dilators can be used for 10 minutes per day with water-soluble lubricants until sexual activity is resumed in 2 to 6 weeks. Support for the woman experiencing body image changes is extremely important.

CERVICAL CANCER

The incidence of invasive cervical cancer has steadily decreased over the years, whereas that of cervical carcinoma in situ (localized) has risen. The decrease is largely attributed to the prevalence of screening with the Papanicolaou test (Pap smear). About 12,200 new cases of invasive cervical cancer are expected to be diagnosed in 2003, with approximately 4100 cervical cancer deaths expected.[1] The diagnosis of noninvasive cervical cancer is expected to be 4 times greater than invasive cervical cancer. The death rate appears to decline about 2% per year.[1] The incidence in African-American and Native American women is nearly twice as high as in white women. Spanish-speaking women younger than 39 years are the least likely to have Pap smears.

Etiology and Risk Factors

The exact cause of cervical cancer is unknown, although chronic irritation is often present before diagnosis of cervical cancer. Human papillomavirus (HPV) is the leading cause of cervical cancer. There is a strong relationship between the presence of the types 16 and 18 and cervical intraepithelial neoplasia (CIN).[13,22,27] (See the Evidence-Based Practice in Action feature on Human Papillomavirus and Cervical Cancer on p. 1073.) CIN has increasingly progressed to carcinoma in situ and invasive cervical cancer. The following are other risk factors:

- Having multiple sexual partners or a partner who has had multiple sexual partners
- Early age of first intercourse
- Smoking tobacco
- Low socioeconomic status
- Untreated chronic cervicitis
- STDs
- Having a sexual partner with a history of penile or prostate cancer

Health promotion actions involve instructing clients (1) to avoid and to seek early treatment of vaginal or cervical infection, (2) to limit the number of sexual partners, and (3) to use condoms to limit the transmission of STDs and HPV. A yearly Pap smear for high-risk women is a health maintenance activity. After three or more consecutive annual examinations with normal results of Pap smears, the client with average risk may undergo Papanicolaou testing less frequently, at the discretion of the health care provider. Pap smears are important because cervical carcinoma in situ is potentially 100% curable.

Pathophysiology

Cervical dysplasia (an abnormal alteration in cell structure), the earliest premalignant change noted in cervical epithelium, is further divided into several levels:

- Mild dysplasia, or CIN 1
- Moderate dysplasia, or CIN 2

EB EVIDENCE-BASED PRACTICE IN ACTION

Human Papillomavirus and Cervical Cancer

Cervical cancer remains one of the leading causes of female cancers in the United States Since the 1960s, the survival rate has increased from 47% to 58% to 57% to 71% due to the impact of Papanicolaou (Pap) smear screening. However, despite the increase in the survival rate, the mortality rate from advanced cervical cancer is unchanged at 8% to 10%.[6] The primary goal of Pap smear testing is to prevent cervical cancer by identifying and treating abnormal cervical cells that have become or have the potential to become cervical neoplasia or cervical cancer. Up to 25% of the female population do not have annual Pap smears. Barriers to having annual Pap smears are related to low income, low education, minority status, lack of knowledge, attitudes and beliefs, low perceived cancer susceptibility, embarrassment, language and certain cultural beliefs, sexual trauma, childhood sexual abuse, sexual violence, and avoidance of coping mechanism, commonly associated with post-traumatic stress disorder.[2]

Human papillomavirus (HPV), a sexually transmitted disease (STD), has been linked to cervical cancer. It is estimated that more than 50% of sexually active men and women ages 15 to 49 years are infected with one or more of the 38 strains of HPV. Of theses 38 strains of HPV typing, only two have been linked to genital warts, whereas all others have been linked to cervical cancer. Invasive cancers of the vagina, vulva, penis, and anus have been linked with genital HPV infection, but are rare compared to the incidence of cervical cancer.[4]

Pap smears allow for early detection and treatment of HPV-associated cervical lesions, leading to a decreased cervical cancer rate and mortality in women. The best protection against the HPV infection is abstinence from sexual activity. Although condoms have been associated with a decreased incidence of STDs, evidence suggests that HPV infection may not be prevented by the use of condoms because the port of viral entry may not be protected by a condom.[4]

More than 50,000 Pap smears are performed annually in the United States. However, because of the less than optimal assurance standards in the processing and reading of the slides, results of Pap smears may carry a 25% to 50 % false-negative report rate.[3] New technologies have improved the sensitivity of the Pap test and, although they are more expensive to perform, they can be cost-effective in the early detection and prevention of cervical cancer.

Three newer techniques that are more effective than the Pap smear are the *Papnet, AutoPap,* and *ThinPrep. Papnet* combines automated microscopy and computerized analysis to reduce screening errors. *ThinPrep* is a semiautomated, liquid-based slide preparation system. A liquid-based slide preparation filters the noncellular material and deposits the cells in a thin layer on the slide.[1] These tests are more expensive to prepare and read. Therefore they may be offered every few years to those who are not at risk for cervical cancer.

Implications

The most frequently reported risk factors for cervical cancer are initiating sexual intercourse at age 15 years or younger or having more than 10 sexual partners.[5] Additional risk factors are a history of smoking and infection with human immunodeficiency virus. The best cancer prevention tool is consistent health prevention and maintenance. Therefore nurses have an important role to question clients about present and past sexual activity, including sexual abuse while taking consistent sexual histories and history of past Pap smear findings. They also must provide follow-up care when Pap smears are abnormal. Education for clients and their partners at routine medical visits as well as continuous updating of information for health care providers encourage dissemination of information about risk factors including HPV, availability of Pap smear screening, and the treatment of abnormal Pap smears.

References

1. Brown, A., & Garber A.M. (1999). Cost-effectiveness of 3 methods to enhance the sensitivity of Papanicolau Testing. *Journal of the American Medical Association, 281*(4), 347-353.
2. Farley, M., Golding, J., Minkoff, J.R. (2002). Is a history of trauma associated with a reduced likelihood of cervical cancer? *Journal for Family Practitioners, 51*(10), 827-831.
3. Mandelblatt, J., et al. (2002). Benefits and cost of using HPV testing for screen for cervical cancer. *Journal of the American Medical Association, 287*(18), 2372-2390.
4. Manhart, L., & Koutsky, L. (2002). Do condoms prevent genital HPV infection, external genital warts, or cervical neoplasia?: A meta-analysis. *Sexually Transmitted Diseases, 29*(11), 725-735.
5. Manos, M., et al. (1999). Identifying women with cervical neoplasia using human papillomavirus DNA testing for equivocal Papanicolaou results. *Journal of the American Medical Association, 281*(17), 1605-1610.
6. O'Mera, A. (2002). Changing the face of cervical cancer: ongoing efforts. *Current Opinion of Obstetrics and Gynecology, 14*(1), 1-3.

- Severe dysplasia, or CIN 3
- Carcinoma in situ

Potentially, all women with carcinoma in situ and 91% of women with nonmetastatic disease can be cured. Five to 10 years may elapse between the preinvasive and invasive stages of cervical cancer. Most cervical cancers are of the squamous cell type. Squamous cell carcinoma usually begins at the squamocolumnar junction, near the external end of the cervix. The spread of squamous cell cervical cancer occurs first by direct extension to the vaginal mucosa, the lower uterine segment, parametrium, pelvic wall, bladder, and bowel. Distant metastasis occurs mainly through lymphatic spread, with some spread occurring through the circulatory system to the liver, lungs, or bones.

On occasion, cervical adenocarcinomas occur, but they are more difficult to identify. Adenocarcinoma generally involves the endocervical glands.

Clinical Manifestations

There are no early indications of carcinoma in situ or early cervical cancer. An abnormal Pap smear result, however, indicates the need for further assessment. Newer techniques for Pap smear collection have brought about better diagnostic collection of cells. The newer Pap smear collections are called *Papnet, AutoPap,* and *Thin Pap.* These procedures have different methods of viewing the cells collected.

Abnormal Pap smear results may be followed by HPV deoxyribonucleic acid (DNA) testing to confirm malignancy or repeating of the Pap smear. Another effective diagnostic test involves swabbing the cervix with vinegar solution (acetic acid) and the use of a colposcope (a microscope with special colored lenses) that enhances and illuminates the abnormal cells on the cervix.

Assessment findings in late stages of cancer include the presence of vaginal discharge and bleeding, especially after intercourse. Metrorrhagia, postmenopausal bleeding, and *polymenorrhea* (increased frequency of menstrual bleeding) may be present. Early bleeding also may occur as spotting or contact bleeding from cervical trauma secondary to sexual intercourse or douching. This early minimal bleeding increases in amount and duration as the cancer progresses.

Vaginal discharge, which is normally watery, becomes dark and foul-smelling as the disease advances. With infection of the neoplastic area, the discharge becomes more profuse and malodorous. Concurrent bleeding makes this condition more unpleasant.

Other assessment findings that develop as the disease progresses relate to the areas involved in the malignant process. They include (1) pressure on the bowel, bladder, or both, (2) bladder irritation, (3) rectal discharge, (4) manifestations of ureteral obstruction, and (5) heavy, aching abdominal pain. Fistulae may form as the malignancy erodes through the walls of adjacent organs.

Pain is another late manifestation. It usually becomes a difficult problem with the onset of *cachexia,* or general wasting syndrome. This syndrome often accompanies the terminal stage of cervical cancer.

Pap Smear

The Pap smear is the primary diagnostic tool for cervical cancer. Further assessment of an abnormal Pap smear result typically includes repetition of cytologic and pelvic examinations. Colposcopic examination can often locate lesions for biopsy. Biopsy specimens are collected with the aid of a colposcope. After the cervix is wiped clean of any mucus or discharge, acetic acid is placed on it. The practitioner views the cervix through the colposcope, looking for abnormalities of color and cell formation. Tiny biopsy specimens are collected from any areas under suspicion. Colposcopy is an office procedure that causes mild discomfort.

Cold Conization

Occasionally, biopsy specimens may be obtained by cold conization, a procedure that may be performed when colposcopic examination is not considered adequate and a larger specimen is necessary. A cone-shaped section of the cervix is obtained with a scalpel. This procedure enables more tissue to be provided for analysis, thus increasing the chances of identifying an area of invasive carcinoma or carcinoma in situ. The procedure is particularly helpful if areas such as the endocervical glands are involved and are not readily visualized.

Sometimes analysis of the tissue removed during a cold conization demonstrates that a wide area of normal tissue surrounds an excised malignancy. When this situation occurs, conization serves not only as the diagnostic procedure but also as the only treatment needed. This procedure allows the woman to maintain reproductive capacity. Cautery (burning of abnormal cervical tissue) or *cryosurgery* (freezing of cervical tissue) may be performed instead of cold conization.

Loop Electrocautery Excision Procedure

A loop electrocautery excision procedure (LEEP) is the newest and most common procedure. A LEEP is performed to excise the cervical areas causing concern. Once the clinician has identified the lesions with colposcopy, a paracervical nerve block is administered for anesthesia, and the lesion or lesions are totally removed by a low-voltage diathermy loop (an electrical current causing burning). There is less risk with this procedure because it is performed in the ambulatory setting without general anesthesia.

Outcome Management
■ Medical Management

Irradiation is used as primary therapy for early cervical cancer. It is usually curative, but it induces menopause. Intracavity radiation is described previously (see Endometrial [Uterine] Cancer earlier in this chapter), and external irradiation is discussed in Chapter 19. In 1999, cancer experts recommended a change in the treatment of advanced surgical cancer, urging that chemotherapy be added to the standard treatment using irradiation.

Treatment of clients with cervical cancer during pregnancy varies, depending on the stage of the cancer, the duration of the pregnancy, and the client's wish to preserve fertility. A client can usually complete the pregnancy if CIN or carcinoma in situ is diagnosed. She may then be treated with cold conization or a LEEP 2 to 3 months postpartum if she desires further childbearing. If a pregnant woman has invasive cervical carcinoma, however, abortion is recommended up to 24 weeks into the pregnancy. After 24 weeks, therapy is delayed until the fetus is viable (28 to 32 weeks) and a cesarean section is performed. The client may then be treated with either hysterectomy or irradiation in the postpartum period.

■ Nursing Management of the Medical Client

Prevent Complications. For the care of a client with radiation implants, see Endometrial (Uterine) Cancer earlier; external radiation is discussed in Chapter 19.

Prevent Recurrence. All clients who have been treated conservatively for cervical cancer need information about recurrence. Encourage clients who have been treated for cervical cancer to have frequent health examinations to identify manifestations of recurrence of the cancer. Pelvic examinations and Pap smears should be scheduled every 3 months for the first 2 years, as advised by the physician.

■ Surgical Management

Treatment may range from cryosurgery, conization, laser therapy, or LEEP for localized tumors to a radical hysterectomy for invasive cancer:

1. *Cryosurgery* is the local freezing of abnormal cells and tissues with volatile gases such a nitrous oxide or carbon dioxide. Cell death results from dehydration and cell membrane destruction; dead tissue then sloughs off with a heavy discharge for 2 to 3 weeks.
2. *Conization* is the removal of a small cone of tissue with a sharp instrument (see earlier discussion).
3. *Laser therapy* or *LEEP* (see later discussion) may also be performed to remove abnormal tissue. Laser therapy causes a burn of the tissues, leading to an increase in sloughing discharge for several weeks. There may also be minimal bleeding.

A total abdominal hysterectomy can be used to treat carcinoma in situ in women who have finished childbearing or to treat invasive cancer. *Pelvic exenteration* (Figure 41-7), a radical procedure, is performed if the cancer has spread. This procedure involves removal of

A   Normal anatomy

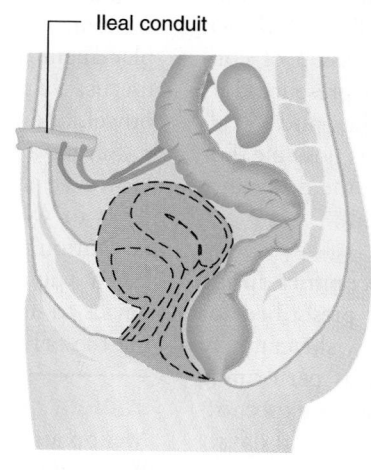

Ileal conduit

B   Anterior exenteration

FIGURE 41-7 Pelvic exenteration. **A,** Natural pelvic structures. **B,** Anterior exenteration: formation of the ileal conduit. **C,** Posterior exenteration: formation of colostomy. **D,** Total exenteration: formation of both ileal conduit and colostomy.

Colostomy

C   Posterior exenteration

Ileal conduit — — Colostomy

D   Total exenteration

all pelvic organs, including the uterus, fallopian tubes, ovaries, vagina, bladder, rectum, and colon. In addition, an ileal conduit and ileostomy may be performed if removal of the bladder or colon is indicated.

■ Nursing Management of the Surgical Client

For care of the client with a hysterectomy, see Benign Uterine Tumors (Leiomyomas). For care of the client with an ileal conduit, see Chapter 36. For care of the client with a colostomy or ileostomy, see Chapter 35.

Cryosurgery, Laser Therapy, LEEP

Explain Procedure. Nursing preparation of a client for cryosurgery, laser therapy, or a LEEP involves informing the client that a surgical incision will not be made. Explain that the procedure is performed with a vaginal speculum in place, as during a routine pelvic examination. During treatment, a few clients experience headaches, dizziness, flushing, and some cramping.

Provide Support. During the procedure, provide psychological support by (1) staying with the client, (2) informing her of what is to be done, (3) talking with her, listening to her, and facilitating her expression of concerns, (4) continuing to acknowledge her presence during the procedure rather than excluding her, and (5) allowing her to retain as much self-control as possible. For example, tell her what she can do during the procedure to help it move along quickly and smoothly.

Promote Comfort. Assess the client's discomfort during the procedure. A mild analgesic may be prescribed for pain following the procedure. Discuss how she can help manage postprocedure discomfort, such as performing slow, deep breathing. Tell the client what to expect afterward; mild cramping may continue for several days.

Encourage Perineal Hygiene. A clear, watery discharge usually occurs for up to several weeks. This is followed by a malodorous discharge containing debris from the sloughing of dead cells. If the discharge continues longer than 8 weeks, an infection is suspected.

Meticulous perineal hygiene minimizes the risk of infection and makes the client more comfortable. Healing takes about 6 weeks. The client should take showers during this time, avoiding tub and sitz baths.

Radical Hysterectomy

After a radical hysterectomy, the vagina is shortened and the trigone region of the bladder and the sigmoid colon may adhere to the vaginal apex. This may cause dyspareunia, the pain of which may be felt deep in the pelvis. Recommend that during penile penetration the client keep her thighs adducted and use her thumb and index finger at the vaginal opening to encircle the shaft of the penis, providing extra length to the vagina.

Despite vigorous treatment, some women with cervical cancer become terminally ill (see Chapter 23 for palliative care). In this situation, the goals of care change and are directed toward physiologic and psychosocial comfort. Pain reduction (see Chapter 22) may be accomplished through use of opioid analgesics. Palliative irradiation may also be used as a pain reduction measure in some cases.

■ Modifications for Older Clients

In older clients, cervical cancer may be treated with less invasive methods. The older client undergoing internal irradiation treatments should be monitored closely after treatment for development of fistulae.

UROGENITAL DISPLACEMENT AND PROLAPSE

Urogenital displacement and prolapse occur with relaxation and descent of the pelvic organs adjacent to the vagina. This is a common problem found in menopausal women. The organs that descend with urogenital displacement and then prolapse are the urethra, bladder, uterus, vaginal apex if the uterus has been removed, bowel, and rectum.

Surgery has been successful in reducing prolapse. However, some women who are poor surgical candidates or who choose not to proceed with a surgical intervention may elect a nonsurgical approach, such as using a vaginal support device known as a *pessary* (a device to hold the organs in correct position) or increasing the pelvic floor support with Kegel exercises.

Etiology and Risk Factors

Menopause causes a decrease in circulating estrogens. With a decrease of estrogen, the supporting structures of the pelvic floor lose their elasticity and ability to support, causing relaxation and prolapse of the urogenital organs.

Additional factors that put a woman at risk for development of prolapse are multiparity, childbirth trauma, chronic straining, and inability to maintain the perineal musculature. The occurrence of prolapse has decreased with improved obstetric care. Better preparation of women for labor and the rare use of forceps during delivery have helped. Help prevent prolapse by encouraging pregnant clients to seek qualified obstetric care and instructing them to perform Kegel exercises before and after delivery.

Cystocele and Urethrocele

A *cystocele* involves a descent of the urinary bladder because of weakened pelvic floor muscles; it is seen as a protrusion of the anterior part of the vaginal wall (Figure 41-8, *A* and *B*). A *urethrocele* (prolapse of the urethra) often accompanies a cystocele as the bladder descends into the vagina. Urinary difficulties caused by the cystocele and urethrocele include incontinence, urinary tract infections, and urinary retention. Additionally, the client may complain of vaginal pressure with or without pelvic discomfort.

Rectocele and Enterocele

A *rectocele* is the protrusion of the vaginal wall musculature that supports the rectum (see Figure 41-8, *C* and *D*). A rectocele can produce constipation, incomplete emptying of the rectum, fecal incontinence, and rectal or vaginal pressure. To completely empty the rectum, some women find it necessary to support the posterior wall of the vagina with a finger while having a bowel movement.

An *enterocele* is the descent of the bowel and protrusion of the upper portion of the posterior wall of the vagina. It often accompanies a rectocele and is usually without manifestations when it is seen alone.

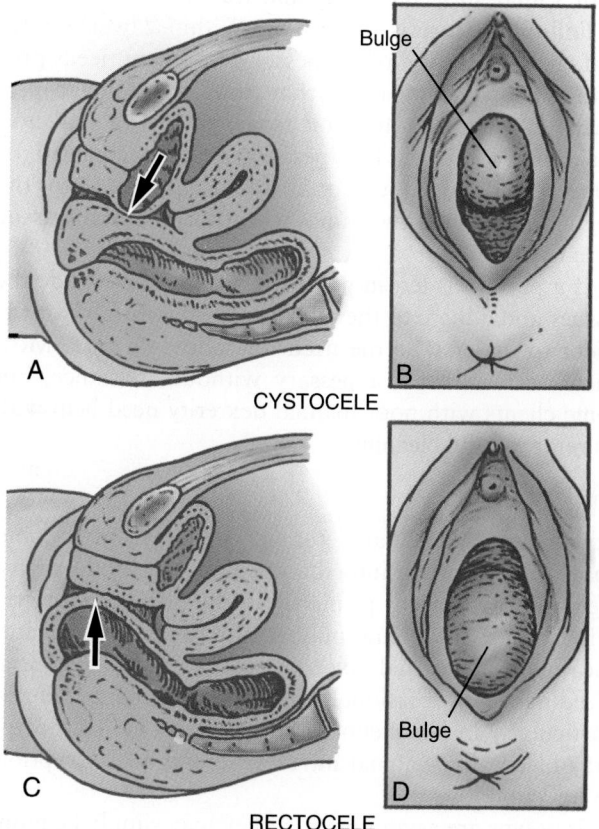

FIGURE 41-8 **A,** Cystocele. Note the bulging of the anterior vaginal wall. The urinary bladder is displaced downward. **B,** The cystocele pushes the anterior vaginal wall downward into the vagina. **C,** Rectocele. **D,** Note the bulging of the posterior vaginal wall.

Vaginal or Uterine Prolapse

Vaginal or uterine prolapse is the descent of the uterus into the vagina (Figure 41-9). The associated manifestations are increasing vaginal pressure, dyspareunia, and backache. As the prolapse descends through the vagina, there may be bleeding from irritation and ulcerations on the prolapsing cervix.

Clinical Manifestations

Manifestations of displacement and prolapse often depend on the level of descent and clinical signs. Some clients present with significant descent but have no manifestations. Clinically, prolapse should be assessed by the level of the descent. The grading scale is as follows.

- *Grade 0:* No descent
- *Grade 1:* Descent half way between the ischial spines and the hymenal ring
- *Grade 2:* Descent to the hymenal ring
- *Grade 3:* Descent halfway beyond the hymenal ring
- *Grade 4:* Descent fully outside the hymenal ring

Outcome Management
■ Surgical Management

Treatment of prolapse depends on the extent of prolapse and the client's health status. The most effective treatment is reconstructive surgery. A vaginal pessary may be used if surgery is not desired or the health status of the client is less than optimal.

The cystocele is often corrected by a procedure called an *anterior colporrhaphy;* an additional procedure called a *Burch colposuspension* may be included if a urethrocele is present (see Chapter 36). The rectocele is usually corrected with a *posterior repair.* The accompanying enterocele is often corrected at the same time by one of various enterocele reconstructive procedures. Hence, an anterior and posterior (A & P) repair involves both procedures.

A hysterectomy may be performed at the same time as the reconstructive surgery if the client does not want to preserve fertility and if the uterus has descended into the vagina. The hysterectomy is performed by way of incisions through the vaginal wall into the pelvic cavity and supportive structures. The uterus is removed from its supporting broad, round, and uterosacral ligaments. The supporting ligaments are then attached to the vaginal cuff to maintain vaginal length.

■ Nursing Management of the Surgical Client

Prevent Bladder Distention. During the operation and for at least the first 24 hours afterward, the bladder is kept decompressed. If a Foley catheter is placed, it is usually removed as soon as the client is ambulatory. When the catheter is removed, the client must be taught to keep her bladder empty by voiding every 2 hours to avoid placing pressure along the suture line. If a suprapubic

FIRST-DEGREE PROLAPSE   SECOND-DEGREE PROLAPSE   THIRD-DEGREE PROLAPSE

FIGURE 41-9 Uterine prolapse. Note the progressive prolapse of the uterus into the vagina until it is visible externally.

catheter is placed, bladder retraining is begun once the client is ambulatory.

Monitor Bleeding. Postoperatively, monitor the client closely for excessive vaginal bleeding. There is normally a small to moderate amount of frank vaginal bleeding. If heavy vaginal bleeding is accompanied by a rapidly distending, rigid abdomen, referred shoulder pain, and indications of shock, immediate surgery may be indicated. Other times of potential bleeding are the 4th, 9th, 14th, and 21st days after surgery as sutures dissolve. If vaginal packing, a drain, or both are in place, the surgeon usually removes them after 24 to 48 hours.

■ Medical Management

The vaginal pessary has been used more successfully recently as an alternative to surgery or as a comfort measure during the wait for surgery. This device holds the prolapsing vaginal organs in the correct position. Pessaries come in different sizes and styles. A well-fit pessary should be comfortable. For proper compliance, then, the client should not experience any discomfort from the pessary during activities. She should be able to void normally with the pessary in place, and she should be comfortable inserting and removing it.

■ Nursing Management of the Medical Client

Teach Pelvic Floor (Kegel) Exercises. Mild manifestations may be relieved by pelvis-strengthening Kegel exercises. These exercises may be prescribed to help a client achieve pubococcygeal muscle control. Instruct the client to practice alternately tightening and relaxing her rectal and vaginal muscles. She tightens these muscles as if she were trying to hold back a bowel movement or a stream of urine. She holds this tightened position for a few seconds and then relaxes the muscles. Over time, she should hold the contraction for a longer period. Kegel exercises can be performed frequently during the day, whenever

the client thinks of them, or for a specified number of times two or three times a day.

Teach Pessary Care. Because a pessary has the potential to irritate the vaginal mucosa, instruct the client to remove the device daily and to reinsert it after cleaning it with a mild, unscented soap and water.

Follow-up care is important. Within 2 weeks after fitting and insertion of the pessary, the client needs professional reassessment. At that time, the clinician performs a pelvic examination to assess the vaginal mucosa for irritation. The pessary may be changed or removed. Estrogen cream is often inserted into the vagina at bedtime two times a week to maintain tissue integrity.

If a pessary is left in place too long, it may erode the tissues and adhere to the mucosa. It is important for the client to understand the need for follow-up care. Most clients can care for a pessary without assistance, but some clients with poor manual dexterity need help with its removal and cleaning.

POLYPS

Polyps are pedunculated tumors arising from the mucosa and extending into the opening of a body cavity. Genital polyps occur primarily in the uterus and cervix (Figure 41-10). Uterine polyps may cause hypermenorrhea, intermenstrual bleeding, and postmenopausal bleeding. They occasionally undergo malignant changes, particularly in postmenopausal women. Cervical polyps may bleed after vaginal intercourse and are susceptible to infection.

If polyps are asymptomatic, they may simply be monitored. Because cervical polyps have a pedicle, they are easily removed by ligation. This procedure is usually performed in the physician's office. Uterine polyps are not easily removed because of their location within the uterus. Uterine polyps do not usually need to be removed

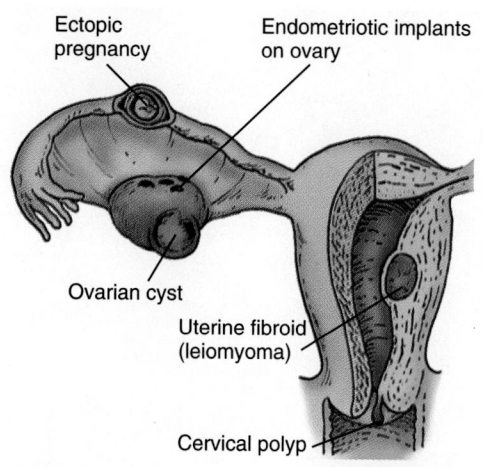

FIGURE 41-10 Common sites of common benign gynecologic lesions.

unless they become symptomatic; if they must be removed, hysteroscopy is usually performed.

OVARIAN DISORDERS
BENIGN OVARIAN TUMORS

Benign ovarian tumors are either solid or cystic. Ovarian tumors are often asymptomatic until they are large enough to cause discomfort associated with pressure; this characteristic makes their early detection difficult. Typical manifestations associated with pressure are constipation, urinary frequency, a full feeling in the abdomen, vague pelvic aching and sensations of heaviness, painful defecation, and dyspareunia. Acute pain may be experienced during menses or with rupture. With an increasing growth, the client's abdominal girth increases, and her clothes may not fit as well. Generally, the client is unable to become pregnant.

Late and rare manifestations of a benign tumor include marked abdominal distention with dyspnea, peripheral edema, and anorexia. Pelvic pain may be present as a later manifestation if the ovarian tumor is growing rapidly. If the tumor produces hormones, menstrual irregularities and masculinizing or feminizing effects may be seen.

Complications include (1) hemorrhage into a cyst, with rupture and possible infection, (2) torsion (twisting) of a cystic pedicle, and (3) malignant changes.

Treatment depends on the type of tumor. Some small cystic masses can be treated with ovarian suppression, which is usually achieved with the use of birth control pills. Placing the ovaries in a pseudopregnancy state suppresses ovarian function and, in most cases, decreases the size of ovarian cystic masses.

Tumors can be removed surgically if they are growing rapidly or disrupt the function of the pelvic organs or the ovary. Removal can be achieved through laparoscopy or with open abdominal surgery. Surgery may include removal of (1) only the tumor, (2) the tumor and the ovary or ovaries, or (3) the tumor, both ovaries and tubes, and the uterus. The type of nursing care needed depends on the extent of surgery performed.

Ovarian cysts are physiologic tumors of ovaries. They are common and may or may not have manifestations. When manifestations do occur, the woman may experience pelvic pain that is often worse on one side, pressure in the lower abdomen, backache, and menstrual irregularities.

A client with an ovarian cyst may be monitored for a month or two to determine whether the cyst might regress without intervention. If the cyst does not regress but is small, oral contraceptive therapy may provide a noninvasive therapy. Explain the treatment plan and condition to the client, and provide information about follow-up health care appointments and how to seek emergency care if needed.

A *follicular cyst* is caused by an unruptured follicle at the time of ovulation. It is often asymptomatic and frequently disappears without intervention. Sometimes, however, a cyst continues to enlarge as a result of hormone stimulation. Oral contraceptive therapy may be used if the cyst is small. Surgical intervention is required if the cyst increases in size and does not respond to medical management.

Corpus luteum cysts form when the corpus luteum fails to regress after discharging the ovum. Oral contraceptive therapy may be helpful for small cysts. However, surgical excision of the corpus luteum may be necessary. The remainder of the ovary can usually be saved.

OVARIAN CANCER

Ovarian cancer, although not the highest in incidence among reproductive tumors, is the leading cause of death from genital reproductive malignancies and accounts for about 4% of all cancer deaths in women. The death rates have risen over time, probably because of a lack of early detection methods. An estimated 25,400 new cases of ovarian cancer were expected to have been detected in the United States in 2003, with 14,300 deaths.[1] White women show higher rates of ovarian cancer than do African-American women.

Etiology and Risk Factors

The cause of ovarian cancer is unknown. Risk factors include the following:

- Age older than 40 years
- Family history of ovarian or breast cancer (mutations in *BRCA1* or *BRCA2* genes have been observed in families)[38,52]
- Family history of hereditary nonpolyposis colorectal cancer (HNPCC)
- Nulliparity

- History of infertility
- History of dysmenorrhea
- Use of ovulation-stimulating medications (a high number of ovulations increases the chances that a tumor suppressor gene called *p53* can be mutated)

Health promotion factors include telling clients that ovarian cancer may be prevented by anything that interrupts constant ovulatory cycles, such as more than one full-term pregnancy, oral contraceptive use, breastfeeding, and bilateral oophorectomy. Health maintenance activities include routine pelvic examinations, determinations of CA-125 antigen levels in high-risk women, and performance of transvaginal ultrasound combined with bimanual pelvic examination and Doppler studies for lesions in question. Prophylactic mastectomy and oophorectomy may be performed in women with *BRCA1* or *BRCA2* mutations as a way of increasing life expectancy.

Pathophysiology

Most ovarian cancers are epithelial tumors, although some are adenocarcinomas. Ovarian cancer tends to grow and spread silently until manifestations of pelvic pressure on adjacent organs or abdominal distention cause the woman to seek medical care. When these pressure-related manifestations finally appear, the malignancy has usually spread to the fallopian tubes, uterus, and ligaments. Ovarian cancer often spreads to the other ovary and associated structures (Figure 41-11). The cancer may invade bowel surfaces, the omentum, liver, and other organs. When the pelvic blood vessels become involved, distant metastasis occurs. The usual routes of spread are lymphatic spread, hematogenous spread (through blood), local extension, and peritoneal seeding.

Clinical Manifestations

Clinical manifestations of ovarian cancer include (1) abdominal distention with increasing abdominal girth, (2) urinary frequency and urgency, (3) pleural effusion, (4) malnutrition with weight loss, (5) pain from pressure caused by the growing tumor and the effects of urinary or bowel obstruction, (6) constipation, (7) ascites with dyspnea, and, ultimately, (8) general severe pain. Indications of ovarian cancer do not typically appear until the malignancy is well established, which is often not until it has spread. Unless the malignancy is diagnosed early, when it is most likely asymptomatic, most affected clients eventually have terminal cancer.

Identification of a pelvic mass by palpation is usually the first assessment finding. However, detecting such a mass may be difficult in a woman who is obese or who cannot relax during the examination. Palpation of the ovary in postmenopausal women should always be con-

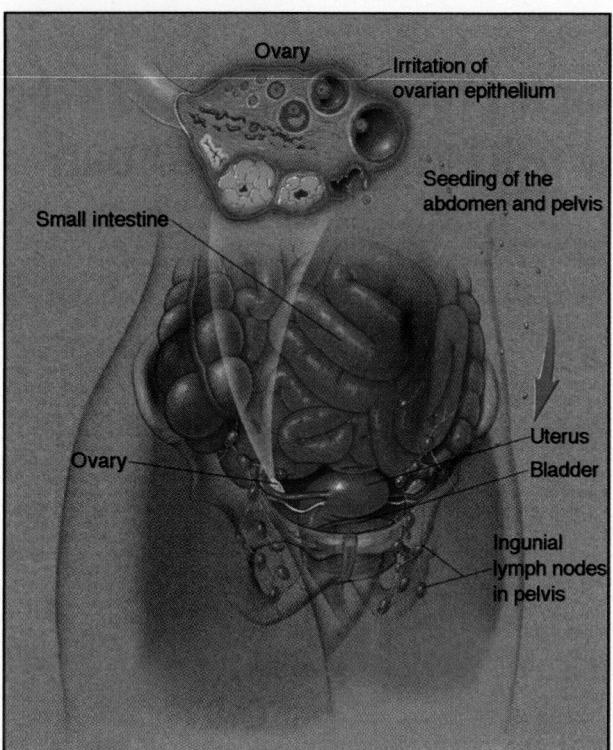

FIGURE 41-11 A, Etiology of ovarian cancer shown by irritation of the ovarian epithelium. **B,** Metastasis occurs through the lymphatic system or by direct seeding of the abdomen and pelvis. (From Shurpin, K.M. [1997]. Ovarian cancer: When to suspect this silent killer is at work. *American Journal of Nursing,* 97[4], 34-35.)

sidered an abnormal finding and should be followed up with pelvic sonogram to rule out abnormalities.

When an ovarian mass is suspected, a complete evaluation is performed. This includes an intravenous pyelogram (IVP), computed tomography (CT) scan, and, possibly, a barium enema study. Ultrasonography can determine whether the mass is solid or cystic. Generally, after the evaluation, exploratory surgery is performed to directly visualize the ovaries, obtain biopsy specimens of the adjacent structures, and perform a resection if the mass is malignant.

A serum CA-125 determination may be used as a tumor marker to track tumor growth and regression. This test should not be the only one used to determine the presence of ovarian cancer because it can give false-positive and false-negative results.

A new diagnostic blood test may soon be available that measures levels of a chemical in the body called lysophosphatidic acid (LPA), which stimulates the growth of ovarian cancer cells. Elevated levels of LPA would indicate that a woman has ovarian cancer. This test is more precise than CA-125 measurement. Further research is needed before the LPA test becomes readily available.[38,52]

Outcome Management
■ Surgical Management

The extent of an ovarian malignancy is determined by exploratory surgery. Ovarian cancer is usually treated aggressively. A young woman with a borderline malignancy may be treated conservatively with a TAH-BSO. The surgery of choice is a TAH-BSO, partial or complete omentectomy, and removal of all visible tumor. The less residual tumor left, the better the prognosis.

Some women with ovarian cancer recover following treatment. Oncologists may recommend a second-look laparotomy in women who are clinically free of disease and who have received chemotherapy for 6 to 24 months to aid in the decision whether to continue treatment. During this procedure, multiple biopsy specimens are collected and analyzed to determine the presence or absence of residual tumor.

■ Medical Management

Adjuvant therapy varies with the stage of the disease. With stage I ovarian cancer, women typically receive irradiation or chemotherapy after surgery to destroy cancer cells that may have spread into the abdominal cavity. Systemic chemotherapy may be administered (see Chapter 19). Women with stage II or higher ovarian cancers typically receive the same treatment as those with stage I disease, with the inclusion of pelvic and, possibly, abdominal radiation.

■ Nursing Management of the Medical-Surgical Client

For the nursing care of the client who has undergone TAH-BSO, see the discussion earlier in this chapter; for care of the client with cancer, see Chapter 19; for palliative care, see Chapter 23.

VAGINAL DISORDERS
VAGINAL DISCHARGE AND PRURITUS

The female reproductive tract maintains its integrity through various natural defense mechanisms. Inflammation and infection occur when organisms disrupt or overcome these natural defenses. The resulting manifestations, although usually not life-threatening, can be uncomfortable and annoying. Vaginal discharge and itching are among the most common problems women mention to health care providers.

All women have normal, nonbloody, asymptomatic vaginal discharge called *leukorrhea*. This discharge, secreted by the endocervical glands, is a clear or white exudate that keeps vaginal mucous membranes moist and clear. As this exudate passes through the vagina, it may become cloudy and acquire a slight odor as desquamated epithelial cells, leukocytes, and normal vaginal flora are added.

The amount of vaginal discharge often varies in relation to the menstrual cycle. It is greatest at ovulation and just before menses. Pregnancy, sexual stimulation, and oral contraceptives tend to increase the discharge. Changes in the amount, color, character, or odor of vaginal discharge may indicate a problem.

Some women view normal vaginal discharge and odor as offensive and go to great lengths to eliminate it. However, use of douches or vaginal deodorants may disrupt the normal vaginal bacterial flora, causing vaginal irritation and infection. The consensus in the medical literature holds that periodic douching is unnecessary. There is evidence that douching may actually be detrimental. Douching washes away protective mucus and normal bacterial flora of the vagina and may cause overgrowth of undesirable bacteria and yeast.

The most common causes of vaginal discharge and irritation are (1) vaginal infections, (2) parasites, such as pinworms, (3) STDs (see Chapter 43), and (4) mechanical or allergic irritants. An example of a mechanical irritant is a tampon left in place too long. Some forms of contraceptive creams or foams may be allergenic irritants for some clients.

Most inflammatory and infectious vaginal problems are accompanied by pathologic vaginal discharge, which may be copious, malodorous, and abnormal in color. The discharge frequently causes itching, irritation, and redness of the vulva and surrounding areas. It may be accompanied by burning and frequency of urination, anal discomfort, and pain in the lower abdominal region.

VAGINITIS

Vaginitis is inflammation of the vagina, a common problem experienced by most women at some time in their life. Causes of vaginitis include change in normal vaginal flora, change in vaginal pH, and invasion of the vagina by virulent organisms. These conditions can be caused by congestion of the pelvic organs, mechanical irritation, vaginal infection, overmedication with antibiotics, long-term steroid therapy, uncontrolled diabetes, and acquired immunodeficiency syndrome (AIDS). Candidiasis (*Candida albicans* infection) is one of the most common causes of vaginitis. Health promotion actions related to vaginitis are described in the Client Education Guide on Preventing Vaginitis on the website.

The vagina is a cavity with a normal protective population of flora, including various bacteria. The adult vagina is normally acidic because of lactic acid formed from the glycogen in desquamating vaginal epithelium. Normal vaginal function depends on a delicate balance between hormones and bacteria. Disturbance of this balance can precipitate infection.

Vaginitis is characterized by a change in vaginal discharge. It may become profuse, odorous, and purulent. The diagnosis is confirmed by a speculum examination and microscopic examination of the discharge. Specimens may be obtained for culture if manifestations indicate an STD or bacterial infection. As a result of edema and tenderness in the vagina, the examination may be painful and must be performed as gently as possible. Some bleeding may occur during and after the examination. Inform the client beforehand about the potential for pain and possible bleeding from the intrusion of the examination.

Vaginitis can be a stubborn, discouraging problem. Early, vigorous treatment may be necessary to prevent chronicity. Treatment is aimed at correcting the cause of the vaginitis. Attention must be given to the client's overall health.

TOXIC SHOCK SYNDROME

Toxic shock syndrome (TSS) is an acute condition caused by the toxin of a local infection with *Staphylococcus aureus,* which can develop into a systemic infection. It usually occurs in women who are menstruating and are using tampons or who have chronic vaginal infections.

TSS begins suddenly with a high temperature, vomiting, and severe, watery diarrhea. Within 48 hours, a characteristic rash and hypotensive shock develop. Once the diagnosis is confirmed, antistaphylococcal antibiotics and fluid replacement therapy are begun.

Advise women to change tampons several times daily or to alternate tampons with sanitary napkins and to practice good hand-washing techniques to prevent development of TSS. If a vaginal sponge or diaphragm is used for contraception, it should be removed within 24 (diaphragm) to 30 (vaginal sponge) hours after intercourse. The diaphragm should not be used during menstruation.

ATROPHIC VAGINITIS

Atrophic vaginitis occurs in postmenopausal women. Atrophic, thin, vaginal mucosa and increased watery alkaline vaginal discharge provide an environment conducive to invasion by pyogenic bacteria. Assessment findings include a discharge with or without a bloody tinge, a vaginal burning sensation, itching of the vagina and vulva, and dyspareunia. If secondary infection is present, vulvar excoriation and burning with urination often occur. Long-term use of estrogen cream is the usual medical treatment. If a secondary infection is present, therapy with an appropriate antibiotic is added.

VAGINAL FISTULAE

Vaginal fistulae are abnormal tube-like passages from the vagina to the bladder *(vesicovaginal),* rectum *(rectovaginal),* or urethra *(urethrovaginal)* (Figure 41-12). Fistula formation is an extremely distressing problem in the genitourinary tract.

Etiology and Risk Factors

Fistulae may be congenital or may result from injury or surgery. About 10% of all fistulae occur in the female reproductive area. Vaginal fistulae may occur because of the spread of a malignant lesion, after irradiation for cancer, as a result of inflammatory disease, and after a prolonged, difficult labor and traumatic delivery.

Clinical Manifestations

Urine or flatus and feces leak into the vagina. Vaginal and vulval tissues become excoriated and irritated. Chronic urinary tract infection may result. Rectovaginal

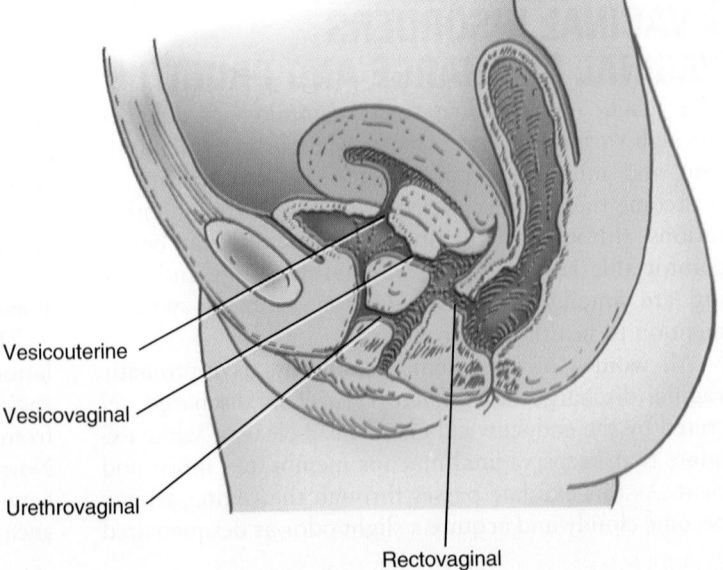

FIGURE 41-12 Locations of main types of vaginal fistulae.

Vesicouterine

Vesicovaginal

Urethrovaginal

Rectovaginal

fistulae may cause an offensive, particularly unpleasant odor. The client experiences wetness and a sensation of feeling unclean.

In addition to their unpleasant physical manifestations, vaginal fistulae produce severely distressing psychosocial problems. Clients often become social recluses. Fistulae greatly disrupt intimate relationships and social activities. Clients often do not seek professional health care until the problem becomes severe. Even then, they may be embarrassed and reluctant to discuss it.

A simple diagnostic test is the instillation of methylene blue dye into the bladder or rectum via Foley catheter and placement of a tampon in the vagina. The woman is asked to walk and perform exertional exercise for a short while. The tampon is then removed and evaluated for color and absorption. The test is considered positive if blue dye is found on the tampon. A *fistulogram* (injection of dye into the vagina) can be performed to assess the location and extent of the fistula.

Outcome Management
■ Medical-Surgical Management

The diagnosis and treatment of a vaginal fistula may be difficult. Treatment varies with the location, extent, and cause of the fistula and with the client's general health. Occasionally, a fistula heals spontaneously. Medical management is used first to treat infection because surgical management is rarely successful, especially when an infection is present. The client must be in optimal physical condition before surgery is attempted.

On occasion, a temporary colostomy may be necessary to treat a rectovaginal fistula (see Chapter 35), and a suprapubic catheter must be inserted to prevent bladder distention after a repair of a vesicovaginal fistula. Excision of either of these fistulae is difficult with a high rate of recurrence.

■ Nursing Management of the Medical-Surgical Client

An accepting attitude of health professionals to a client with a vaginal fistula is essential to help her comfortably accept and follow through with needed treatments. Help the client to minimize the manifestations and care for herself.

Prevent Infection. Some clients unadvisedly restrict their fluid intake to decrease the drainage. This action may actually increase the size of the fistula and increase the chance of infection. Make sure the woman understands the importance of increasing her fluid intake to reduce the risk of infection. Perineal hygiene measures may include cleansing the perineum every 4 hours, taking sitz baths, and changing perineal pads frequently.

If surgery is used to repair the fistula, care is directed at avoiding physical stress on the repaired area and preventing infection. A Foley or suprapubic catheter is used

after a vesicovaginal or urethrovaginal fistulectomy to drain the urinary bladder. Careful attention is necessary to keep the catheter patent and draining. Provide and encourage enough fluid intake so that internal catheter irrigation is accomplished. It is a nursing responsibility to monitor the catheter for patency. If the catheter becomes obstructed, the increased bladder pressure could adversely affect the surgical sites and cause the fistula to reopen.

Prevent Constipation. In rare instances, a client requires a colostomy following vaginal fistula repair (see Chapter 35). This procedure is usually necessary for fistulae resulting from radiation or Crohn's disease and for postoperative rectal fistulae. After corrective bowel surgery, the client's first stools may be liquid. This prevents stress on the repaired area. The stools may be maintained in a liquid state throughout the postoperative period with stool softeners and laxatives. Caution the client not to strain with a bowel movement. Enemas are avoided because of the trauma they may cause to the repaired area.

Provide Support. Surgical repair of a vaginal fistula may not be successful, even under optimal conditions. This is particularly true if a client has extensive tissue damage from tumors or irradiation. Supportive nursing care is extremely important for women experiencing this distressing disorder and for their significant others as well.

VAGINAL CANCER

Primary invasive vaginal cancer is a rare lesion, typically occurring in women older than 50 years. However, it is seen in younger women whose mothers took diethylstilbestrol (DES) during pregnancy. DES was widely prescribed in the United States from 1940 to 1970 for threatened miscarriage and other high-risk pregnancy problems. Among women who have not been exposed to DES, vaginal cancer is rare in African Americans and almost nonexistent in Jews. It was estimated that 2000 new cases of vaginal cancer would be diagnosed in the United States in 2003. Although it is rare, vaginal cancers account for about 3% of all cancers of the female reproductive system.[1]

Etiology and Risk Factors

The risk factor for vaginal (clear cell) cancer is maternal ingestion of DES. Other potential causes of vaginal cancer are (1) exposure to the drug in utero in girls and women between menarche and age 30 years (adenocarcinoma), (2) repeated pregnancies, (3) a history of STD or infection with herpes virus or HPV, (4) prior irradiation, (5) immunosuppressive therapy, and (6) significant irritation due to a poorly fitting pessary. Leukoplakia and leukorrhea are often associated with vaginal cancer.

Pathophysiology

The staging of vaginal cancer is similar to that used for other pelvic malignancies. The primary lesion and involvement of adjacent structures are considered. Primary invasive cancer tends to involve the anterior or posterior vaginal walls, or both. Complications may involve the urinary bladder or bowel, as in fistula formation.

Despite active treatment, the prognosis for vaginal cancer is generally poor. The overall cure rate reported by the American Cancer Society is about 35%. Half of women with vaginal cancer die within 18 months of diagnosis.[1] Low survival rates are due to the rarity of the cancer, which makes it difficult to identify, the typically advanced stage of the cancer when it is diagnosed, and the difficulty in treating this cancer with radiation or surgery because of the proximity of important structures.

Clinical Manifestations

Indications of vaginal cancer include foul vaginal discharge, painless vaginal bleeding, pruritus, pain (not associated with bleeding), and the presence of a vaginal mass or lesion. Urinary bladder manifestations, such as pain and frequency, may occur if a vaginal mass compresses the bladder.

EB Women exposed to DES in utero should receive careful examination of the cervix, along with cytologic examination of the cervix and any questionable area in the vagina. Colposcopy may be used to identify areas to be sampled for biopsy. During pelvic examination, Lugol's solution may be applied to any vaginal areas that appear abnormal. Lack of staining identifies suspect areas. Often, the lesions of vaginal cancer are well advanced before manifestations appear. Earlier lesions might be missed during pelvic examination.

Outcome Management
■ Medical Management

The usual treatment for vaginal cancer is either external or intravaginal radiation therapy or, less often, surgery. External radiation therapy is used for all stages of vaginal cancer. Internal radiation is generally used only in the earlier stages. The difficulty of applying radiation to the vagina without causing harm to the bladder and rectum has led some physicians to prefer surgical intervention.

■ Surgical Management

For earlier stages, radical hysterectomy, lymphadenectomy, and vaginectomy are performed. *Partial vaginectomy* refers to removal of the upper one third to one half of the vagina as part of the procedure in a radical hysterectomy. Pelvic exenteration is used in more advanced cancer if the bladder or rectum is involved; it is also indicated in a client with recurrent metastases.

■ Nursing Management of the Medical-Surgical Client

During assessment, ask young women born between 1940 and 1970 about medications their mothers may have taken during pregnancy. All those whose mothers took DES while pregnant with them should have a gynecologic examination at least twice yearly beginning at menarche, or at age 14 years, whichever comes first.

Provide Support. Vaginal surgery may be anxiety-promoting and frightening. Ostomies (see Chapters 35 and 36) also may need to be performed, adding to the client's fears and problems.

Discuss Sexuality. Sexuality is an important nursing consideration in the care of women with vaginal cancer. Postoperatively, vaginal sexual activity is not possible unless vaginal reconstruction is performed. Vaginal sex may be difficult after surgery or radiation therapy because of changes in the size and shape of the vagina. Assess the client's previous sexual history and her self-esteem to identify possible problems. Create a therapeutic environment that allows her to feel comfortable discussing sexual concerns.

Discuss the potential impact of the disease process and treatment on sexuality, as appropriate. Potential problems include fatigue, pain, dyspareunia, decreased libido, and altered body image. If a partial vaginectomy is performed, the client can probably still enjoy normal vaginal sexual activity, using large amounts of lubricant and modified positioning, because the vaginal tissue will stretch.

Promote Rest. To help the client cope with fatigue and pain, suggest that she schedule sexual activity after resting. Also, schedule pain medication so that the peak of action coincides with sexual activity. A warm bath, a back rub, alternate positioning, or relaxation techniques might also help. Advise the client to use a water-soluble lubricant during intercourse and, perhaps, a vaginal dilator at other times to prevent vaginal fibrosis and tightening.

▌VULVAR DISORDERS
VULVITIS

Vulvitis (inflammation of the vulva) is caused by direct irritation of vulvar tissues or by direct extension of irritation from the vagina to the vulva that results in itching. Risk factors associated with vulvitis include skin disorders, inflammatory problems, infection, allergies, postmenopausal atrophy and dryness, uncontrolled diabetes, pediculosis, scabies, cancer, incontinence, and poor perineal hygiene.

Medical treatment is based on the specific cause of the condition. Itching, the most common manifestation associated with vulvitis, can be severe. A local or systemic antipruritic or antihistamine agent, such as hydrocortisone cream, diphenhydramine hydrochloride (Benadryl), or hydroxyzine hydrochloride (Atarax), may be given to relieve the itching.

Teach the client the following measures to relieve itching:

1. Apply cold compresses.
2. Wear light, nonrestrictive clothing, including well-washed and well-rinsed cotton underpants. Synthetic underpants tend to keep the vulvar area warm and moist.
3. Avoid feminine hygiene sprays.
4. Apply prescribed hydrocortisone ointment or anesthetic sprays.
5. Keep the vulva clean and dry. Clean after elimination by washing the vulva with very mild soap and water; wiping with toilet tissue or a washcloth from front to back; rinsing and drying the area well; and applying cornstarch to maintain dryness.

VULVAR CANCER

Vulvar cancer is found mainly in women older than 50 years of age. It was estimated that, in 2003, approximately 4000 cases would be reported in the United States; 800 deaths from vulvar cancer were expected.[1]

Etiology and Risk Factors

Vulvar disorders (e.g., lichen sclerosus, previously called kraurosis vulvae or atrophic leukoplakia, and diabetic vulvitis) increase the risk of vulvar cancer. Contracting certain STDs, such as HPV, also increases the risk.

Pathophysiology

Vulvar cancer arises from skin, urethra, glands, or subcutaneous tissues. Approximately 90% to 95% of vulvar cancers are squamous cell carcinoma. The remaining 5% to 10% are adenocarcinoma, Paget's disease, malignant melanoma, or sarcoma.

Vulvar cancer grows slowly and remains localized for a long time. Most lesions are located in the labia, primarily the labia majora. Some are on the clitoris. Local spread may occur to the urethra, vagina, anus, and rectum. Lymphatic spread is to the inguinal, femoral, pelvic, and finally, periaortic nodes. The usual causes of death from widespread vulvar cancer are distant metastasis, urethral obstruction, infection, uremia, and hemorrhage.

The prognosis is poor with vulvar invasive lesions. Five-year survival rates for clients who have undergone vulvectomy and lymphadenectomy are approximately 30% to 55%. Recurrence as well as distant metastasis may appear in the first 2 years. In an advanced stage with node involvement, the survival rate is only 8% to 10%.

Clinical Manifestations

Lichen sclerosus is characterized by thickened gray patches of epithelium scattered over the vulva and perineum. Cracked areas in these patches provide an ideal medium for infection, which causes the tissues to ulcerate and macerate. Eventually, these areas may become malignant.

Secondary infection is characterized by a bright red, smooth, almost transparent vulvar epithelium. Lichen sclerosus is most common in postmenopausal women. With its progression, the vulvar tissues shrink and constrict the vaginal opening.

Initially, lichen sclerosus causes itching and soreness or pain but may be asymptomatic. Clinical manifestations of early vulvar cancer include pruritus, minimal vulval soreness, dyspareunia, and tissue irritation with some bleeding. The potential seriousness of these relatively mild problems may not be appreciated by women or their health care providers because the manifestations are similar to those of nonmalignant vulvar lesions. As the vulvar cancer progresses, clinical manifestations of vulvar edema and pelvic lymphadenopathy develop. Secondary infection may cause a foul-smelling discharge. Biopsy of the affected area confirms the diagnosis.

Outcome Management
■ Medical Management

When lichen sclerosus is present, a biopsy to rule out cancer is indicated. Infection is treated with an appropriate systemic or topical antibiotic, steroid creams, and hormone cream. Other manifestations are treated symptomatically.

Irradiation and chemotherapy are used less often than surgical therapy. Irradiation is not generally used because the involved tissues do not tolerate it well. Chemotherapy is typically not given unless metastasis has occurred. The agent of choice is then selected according to the extent of metastasis.

■ Nursing Management of the Medical Client

Nursing management of the client with lichen sclerosus is mainly supportive care throughout the diagnostic period. Itching can be treated symptomatically with antipruritic creams such as hydrocortisone.

■ Surgical Management

A vulvectomy is performed to remove abnormal tissue through procedures such as a skinning technique, local wide excision, or a simple or radical vulvectomy. A laser may be used in conjunction with these procedures to destroy specific abnormal tissue.

A *simple vulvectomy* involves removal of the labia majora, labia minora, and sometimes the glans clitoris. Occasionally, the perineal area is also removed, requiring plastic surgery to cover the vulvar area. However, extensive surgery is avoided if the client's condition allows a simpler procedure.

A *radical vulvectomy* (Figure 41-13) consists of excision of tissue from the anus to a few centimeters below the symphysis pubis (skin, labia majora, labia minora, and clitoris). Bilateral dissection of groin lymph nodes, such as the superficial groin and deep inguinal, femoral, iliac, hypogastric, and obturator nodes, also may be performed.

Full recovery is possible but may take 6 months or longer. Wound infections and delayed wound healing may lead to numerous problems. The long recovery and potential complications further impair the client's body image.

■ Nursing Management of the Surgical Client

Preoperative Care
For a woman experiencing vulvar surgery, psychosocial support is especially important and should begin preoperatively. Some problems you might anticipate are fear of disfigurement, grief over the loss of a body part, fear of death, and sexual concerns.

Preoperative preparation is similar to that for other gynecologic procedures. The client scheduled for a vulvectomy must understand what the surgery entails, know what preoperative procedures will be performed, and have an idea of what to expect in the postoperative period. See the Client Education Guide on Recovering *evolve* from Radical Vulvectomy on the website.

Postoperative Care
The client undergoing a radical vulvectomy is susceptible to many postoperative complications because of the ex-

tensive nature of the operation. In addition to routine postoperative care, a suction device (e.g., Hemovac), tubes, or drain must be placed in the incision to remove drainage and to reduce the risk of infection. Carefully monitor the amount of bleeding. A bed cradle is helpful in keeping bed linens away from the incision.

Prevent Thrombophlebitis. The client wears antiembolism or sequential compression stockings to prevent leg edema and thrombophlebitis, which constitutes a postoperative and a long-term problem. Keep the legs elevated as much as possible. Resuming ambulation postoperatively as early as possible helps to decrease leg edema and thrombophlebitis. The client should perform leg exercises to prevent circulatory problems. Teach the client to avoid sitting with the legs dependent, standing, and crossing the legs. A low-dose anticoagulant, such as heparin, warfarin (Coumadin), or aspirin, may be used prophylactically (as prevention) to reduce the risk of phlebitis and subsequent pulmonary embolism.

Lower extremity lymphedema can cause a change in clothing size and an upsetting change in appearance. In addition, some clients have difficulty sitting for long periods, making activities such as long automobile trips difficult.

Prevent Infection. Prevent infection in the incisional area through frequent dressing changes, perineal care or sitz baths after voiding and bowel movements, and meticulous wound care. A Foley catheter is usually in place for 7 to 14 days or until healing is adequate. If the catheter is removed, carefully monitor urination with supportive care to prevent infection and voiding dys-

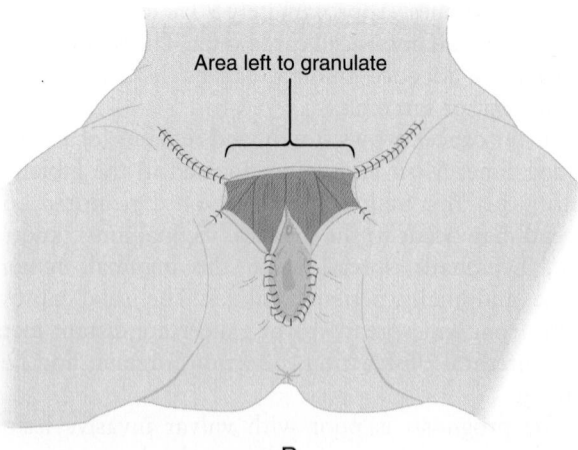

A   B

FIGURE 41-13 Radical vulvectomy. **A,** Area to be excised and line of incision *(dashed line)*. The vulvar skin, underlying subcutaneous tissue and muscles, and regional lymph nodes are excised. If the anus is involved, the incision also continues around it. Inguinal and femoral lymph nodes are resected en bloc. **B,** Completed surgery. Perineal skin is approximated to the vagina, and a large area is left open to heal gradually by filling in with granulation tissue. A simple vulvectomy (not shown) does not remove the lymph nodes. Hence the incision does not extend into the groin.

function. Additionally, it is important to monitor bowel movements. Once healing has occurred, the client may require reconstructive surgery.

Provide Support. Psychosocially, a vulvectomy may be a devastating experience for a woman because of its direct effect on the external genitalia. The surgery, especially a radical vulvectomy, may compromise the client's physical integrity and her sense of wholeness. Some important issues for a woman are fear of recurrence and metastasis, disfigurement, concern about future sexual activity, and fear of her partner's rejection.

Nursing care involves helping the woman redefine her self-image to include the physical changes of vulvectomy. Try to create an environment in which she can express her feelings. Provide opportunities for her to mourn the loss and its effect on her sexuality. Encourage her to resume her normal activities as soon as possible to reinforce her feelings of self-worth.

Stress in social relationships is common after this radical surgery. The client and her significant other may benefit from counseling aimed at developing healthy coping skills.

The effect of a vulvectomy on female sexuality has not been well described. The disfigurement secondary to the surgery can lead to body image distortion, which affects sexual functioning. Physical changes, such as removal of the clitoris, result in loss of the ability to experience orgasm. The client may experience loss of sensation within the vagina. Also, stenosis of the introitus may follow surgery, making intercourse painful or difficult; this can have a major impact on sexuality. If stenosis occurs, it can be treated with vaginal dilators. If dilation is unsuccessful, plastic surgery should be considered.

Sexual counseling should be considered for all women undergoing vulvectomy and their partners. Assist the client and her sexual partner by communicating openly with them, answering their questions, explaining structural vulvar changes, and suggesting alternative forms of sexual arousal for the client.

Promote Voiding. Some women experience unpredictable voiding difficulties following a radical vulvectomy. A client may present with complaints of incontinence, retention, or a dysfunctional voiding pattern (see Chapter 36).

BARTHOLINITIS

Inflammation of Bartholin's glands can be caused by various organisms, including gonococci, streptococci, staphylococci, and *E. coli*. The infection involves the duct of the gland, producing edema and, eventually, obstruction. Because the inflamed gland cannot drain, it swells, and an abscess forms. Cellulitis develops in the surrounding tissues, producing more pain and systemic manifestations. The abscess may rupture spontaneously or may require incision and drainage.

After the acute episode, occlusion of the duct by fibrosis and scarring causes retention of secretions and dilation of the duct. It then becomes a palpable, mobile cyst, which usually is not painful. Manifestations, which relate to the size of the cyst, include dyspareunia and pain on walking.

Systemic antibiotics specific for the causative organism are prescribed. Local heat with hot packs or sitz baths may help promote drainage. Surgery may be necessary, such as an incision and drainage or removal of the gland if cancer is suspected or for repeated infections with abscess formation.

FEMALE GENITAL MUTILATION

Female genital mutilation (FGM), often called *female circumcision*, is a medically unnecessary surgical modification of the female genitalia practiced in several African, Asian, and Middle Eastern countries. It may be seen in female immigrants from these areas. The procedure is performed on girls between ages 4 and 12 years old. Globally, FGM is estimated to affect 130 million girls and women, with approximately 2 million new FGM procedures performed yearly. About 120,000 immigrants to the United States between 1991 and 1995 originated from countries in which FGM is practiced.[31]

Of four major types, types 1 and 2 are performed in 85% of cases[31]:

- *Type 1, Sunna:* excision of the clitoral prepuce only, or *clitoridectomy* (partial or complete removal of the clitoris).
- *Type 2, Excision:* removal of prepuce and clitoris along with adjoining parts of labia minora.
- *Type 3, Infibulation:* removal of parts described in type 2 and parts of interior labia majora. The raw surfaces of the two sides of the vulva are then sutured together, obliterating the introitus. A small opening is left to allow for urine and menstrual flow.
- *Type 4, Other:* burning instead of cutting the clitoris, stretching labia minora to enhance the man's sexual pleasure, or making cuts into the vagina.

Etiology and Risk Factors

The FGM procedure originated from the belief that women are highly sexual and promiscuous. Type 3 FGM is performed to isolate women from sexual desires and temptation. Other reasons for FGM include (1) religious influences, (2) promotion of social and political cohesion, (3) distinguishing chaste from adulterous women, (4) distinguishing indigenous from non-indigenous women, and (5) economic benefits for the father. Some practitioners of FGM believe that removal of the external genitalia makes the woman cleaner and more sexually attractive. Others believe that the clitoris generates additional excitement for the male, leading to early ejaculation, so that removal of the clitoris limits sexual excitement for both genders. Still others believe that FGM after childbirth ensures fidelity in a marriage. Finally, some ethnic groups believe that the clitoris can kill a child if it touches the child's head during birth.

The decision to perform FGM is left to mothers, grandmothers, and older women. The rationale for disfavoring the practice includes marriage complications, labor complications, altered psychosexual beliefs, abandonment because of sterility, and the effects of the traumatic experience. Despite these problems, many ethnic groups, including men and women, continue to support the practice of FGM even while living in the United States.

Clinical Manifestations

Complications from FGM include the following:
- High infant mortality rate
- Hemorrhage, shock, and death during the procedure
- Keloid formation
- Chronic vaginal and pelvic infections
- Acute urinary retention
- Recurrent urinary tract infections
- Urolithiasis
- Urinary, rectal, and vaginal fistulae
- Damage to the urethra
- Prolonged labor and problems with delivery
- Psychological trauma

Clinical manifestations of these complications may lead the woman to seek health care.

Outcome Management

Management of the client with FGM is directed toward relief of clinical manifestations related to the complications. Some of these conditions are discussed earlier in this chapter and in Chapter 36. To enable childbirth, a cesarean section or *deinfibulation* (opening of the incisional area anteriorly) may be required.

When caring for a woman with FGM, remain sensitive and nonjudgmental to gain her confidence and establish a trusting, therapeutic relationship. Teach her about the complications of the procedure; this issue is extremely important if she has daughters who may be at risk for FGM. Unresolved grief and low self-esteem after the trauma of the experience or sterility caused by chronic PID may require supportive intervention or counseling.

Health care providers must act as advocates for women and girls affected by FGM by increasing professional and public awareness of the practice and its existence in the United States. Report FGM involving a girl younger than 18 years, because it is considered child abuse.

CONCLUSIONS

Female reproductive disorders can occur throughout a woman's life. These problems range from menstrual disorders to life-threatening malignancies. Nurses can provide much of the needed education to help clients become more aware of preventive measures. The physical and psychosocial care of these clients is important. The skillful and empathic nurse can assist the woman through what is often an extremely distressing diagnosis and treatment.

Nurses who need more information on reproductive issues should consult a women's health (obstetrics and gynecology) textbook. Information on contraception, tubal ligation, abortion, and other issues can be found there.

THINKING CRITICALLY *evolve*

1. The client, a 52-year-old woman, comes into the clinic stating, "I can't put up with it any longer!" Her last menstrual period was 4 months ago, and she has had severe hot flashes and night sweats for almost 6 months with no abatement. Vaginal intercourse has become so painful that she and her husband have refrained from sexual activity for 3 months. She states that the night sweats are so bad that she has had very few nights of uninterrupted sleep.
   Factors to Consider. What are your priorities for her care? What interventions might be used?

2. A 38-year-old woman enters the clinic with a complaint of acute, sharp, severe bilateral pelvic pain. She has a temperature of 102.2° F, a pulse rate of 100 beats/min, a respiratory rate of 20 breaths/min, and chills. Her cervical culture shows gonococcal infection. She uses oral contraceptives for birth control.
   Factors to Consider. Besides teaching her about antibiotic medication, what is your priority in caring for her, and what interventions are necessary?

3. The client, a 61-year-old woman, had a TAH-BSO 2 days ago for early endometrial cancer. Her Foley catheter was removed yesterday. Her temperature is 101.1° F, her pulse rate is 96 beats/min, and her respiratory rate is 16 breaths/min. Her blood pressure is 128/74 mm Hg. She complains of flank pain and urinary hesitancy. Her urine output for the past 4 hours is 120 ml, which is the total from three separate

voidings. Her urine is cloudy and has a slightly foul odor.

Factors to Consider. What is your priority, and what interventions are needed?

Discussions for these questions can be found on the website and the CD-ROM.

BIBLIOGRAPHY

1. American Cancer Society. (2003). *Cancer facts and figures.* Atlanta: Author.
2. Anonymous. (2002). Menstrual pain severely affects almost half of U.S. women. *American Journal of Operating Room Nurses, 75*(4), 788.
3. Anonymous (2002, July). Newer not necessarily better for treating dysmenorrhea. *PR Newswire, 16,* 1.
4. Brown, A.D., & Garber, A.M. (1999, January 27). Cost-effectiveness of 3 methods to enhance the sensitivity of Papanicolaou testing. *Journal of the American Medical Association, 281*(4), 347-354.
5. Byers, L., Fowler, J., & Twiggs, L. (2000). Uterus. In M. Abeloff, et al. (Eds.). *Clinical oncology* (2nd ed., pp. 1986-2015). New York: Churchill Livingstone.
6. Center for Disease Control. (2002). *DES update.* Retrieved June 16, 2003, from http://www.cdc.gov/DES/consumers/download/cdc%5Fdes%5update.pdf.
7. Clark, T., et al. (2002). Accuracy of hysteroscopy in the diagnosis of endometrial cancer and hyperplasia: A systematic quantitative review. *Journal of the American Medical Association, 288*(13), 1610-1621.
8. Compston, J., & Marsh, M. (1999). HRT and the menopause: *Current therapy.* London: Martin Dunitz.
9. Elbes, J., Farias-Eisner, R., & Berek, J. (2000). Cervix, vulva, and vagina. In M. Abeloff, et al. (Eds.). *Clinical oncology* (2nd ed., pp. 1946-1985). New York: Churchill Livingstone.
10. Grady, D., et al. (2002). Cardiovascular disease outcomes during 6.8 years of hormone therapy: Heart and estrogen/progestin replacement study follow-up (HERS II). *Journal of the American Medical Association, 288*(1), 49-57.
11. Greenspan, S., Resnick, N., & Parker, R. (2003). Combination therapy with hormone replacement and alendronate for prevention of bone loss in elderly women: A randomized controlled trial. *Journal of the American Medical Association, 289*(19), 2525-2533.
12. Harris, L. (2002). Ovarian cancer: Screening for early detection. *American Journal of Nursing, 102*(10), 46-53.
13. Hartinger, J., et al. (1999). Identifying women with cervical neoplasia: Using human papillomavirus DNA typing for equivocal Papanicolaou results. *Journal of the American Medical Association, 281*(17), 1605-1610.
14. Hlatky, M.A., et al. (2002). Quality-of-life symptoms in postmenopausal women after receiving hormone therapy: Results from the heart and estrogen/progestin replacement study (HERS) trial. *Journal of the American Medical Association, 287*(5), 591-597.
15. Howell, D. (1999). *The unofficial guide to coping with menopause.* New York: Macmillan.
16. Hulley, S., et al. (1998). Randomized trial of estrogen plus progestin for secondary prevention of coronary heart disease in postmenopausal women. *Journal of the American Medical Association, 280*(7), 605-613.
17. Jae-Hoon, K., et al. (2002). Ostepotin as a potential diagnostic biomarker for ovarian cancer. *Journal of the American Medical Association, 287*(13), 1671-1680.
18. Kellogg-Spadt, S., & Albaugh, J. (2003). Herbs, amino acids, and female libido. *Urologic Nursing, 23*(2), 160-161.
19. Kennedy, A., Sculpher, M., Coulter, A., et al. (2002). Effects of decision aids for menorrhagia on treatment choices, health outcomes, and costs: A randomized controlled trial. *Journal of the American Medical Association, 288*(21), 2701-2708.
20. Kolander, C., Ballard, D., & Chandler, C. (1999). *Contemporary women's health: Issues for today and the future.* Boston: WCB McGraw-Hill.
21. Klingman, L. (1999). Assessing the female reproductive: A guide through the gynecologic exam. *American Journal of Nursing, 99*(8), 37-44.
22. Kulasingam, S., et al. (2002). Evaluation of human papillomavirus testing in primary screening for cervical abnormalities: Comparison of sensitivity, specificity, and frequency of referral. *Journal of the American Medical Association, 288*(14), 1749-1757.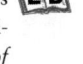
23. Lacey, J., et al. (2002). Menopausal hormone replacement therapy and risk of ovarian cancer. *Journal of the American Medical Association, 288*(3), 334-341.
24. Lightner, D. (2002). Female sexual dysfunction, *Mayo Clinic Proceedings, 77*(7), 698-702.
25. Maloney, C. (2002). Estrogen and recurrent UTIs in the postmenopausal woman. *American Journal of Nursing, 102*(8), 44-52.
26. Mandelblatt, J., et al. (2002). Benefits and costs of using HPV testing to screen cervical cancer. *Journal of the American Medical Association, 287*(18), 2372-2381.
27. Manos, M., et al. (1999). Identifying women with cervical neoplasia using human papillomavirus: DNA testing for equivocal Papanicolaou results. *Journal of the American Medical Association, 281*(17), 1605-1610.
28. Mazmanian C. (1999). Hysterectomy: Holistic care is key. *RN, 62*(6), 32-36.
29. Mills, D. (1999). *Endometriosis: A key to healing through nutrition.* Boston: Shaftesbury Dorset.
30. Moody, F. (1999). *Atlas of ambulatory surgery.* Philadelphia: W. B. Saunders.
31. Morris, R. (1999). Female genital mutilation: Perspectives, risks and complications. *Urologic Nursing, 19*(1), 13-19.
32. Morse, G. (1999) Positively reframing perceptions of menstrual cycle among women with premenstrual syndrome. *Journal of Obstetrics, Gynecology, & Neonatal Health, 28*(2), 165-174.
33. Narvane, A., et al. (2001). Serotypes of Chlamydia trachomatis and resistance for development of cervical squamous cell carcinoma. *Journal of the American Medical Association, 285*(1), 47-52.
34. Nelson, H., et al. (2002). Postmenopausal hormone replacement therapy. *Journal of the American Medical Association, 288*(7), 872-881.
35. Pasacreta, J., Jacobs, L., & Cataldo, J. (2002). Genetic testing for breast and ovarian cancer risk: The psychosocial issues. *American Journal of Nursing, 102*(12), 40-48.
36. Pearlstein, T. (2002). Selective serotonin reuptake inhibitors for premenstrual dysphoric disorder: The emerging gold standard? *Drugs, 62*(13), 1869-1885.
37. Price, S., & Wilson, L. (2003). *Pathophysiology: Clinical concepts of disease processes* (6th ed.). St. Louis: Mosby.
38. Otto, S. (2001). Gynecologic cancers. In S. Otto (Ed.). *Oncology nursing* (4th ed., pp. 248-284). St. Louis: Mosby.

39. Rapp, S., et al. (2003). Effect of estrogen plus progestin on global cognitive function in postmenopausal women. The Women's Health Initiative Memory Study: A randomized controlled trial. *Journal of the American Medical Association, 289*(20), 2663-2672.

40. Rexrode, K.M., & Mason, J.E. (2002). Postmenopausal hormone therapy and quality of life: No cause for celebration. *Journal of the American Medical Association, 287*(5), 641-642.

41. Robbins, J., & Liu, J. (2000). Alternatives to hysterectomy for the treatment of excessive uterine bleeding. *International Journal of Clinical Practice, 54*(4), 233-237.

42. Rhodes, J., et al. (1999). Hysterectomy and sexual functioning. *Journal of the American Medical Association, 282*(20), 1932-1941.

43. Sharts-Hopko, N. (2001). Hysterectomy for nonmalignant conditions. *American Journal of Nursing, 101*(9), 32-42.

44. Shumacher, S., et al. (2003). Estrogen plus progestin and the incidence of dementia and mild cognitive impairment in postmenopausal women. The women's health initiative memory study: A randomized control trial. *Journal of the American Medical Association, 289*(20), 2651-2662.

45. Solomon, D., et al. (2002). The 2001 Bethesda system: Terminology for reporting results of cervical cytology. *Journal of the American Medical Association, 287*(16), 2114-2119.

46. Sorg, D. (2001). Volvodynia: More than just pain. *American Journal of Nursing, 101*(2), 24AAA-24DDD.

47. Spies, J. (2002). Leiomyomata treated with uterine artery embolization: Factors associated with successful symptom and imaging outcome. *Journal of the American Medical Association, 287*(10), 1241.

48. Stearns, V., et al. (2003). Paroxetine controlled release in the treatment of menopausal hot flashes: A randomized controlled trial. *Journal of the American Medical Association, 289*(21), 2827-2834.

49. Stewart, F., et al. (2001). Clinical breast and pelvic examination requirements for hormonal contraception. *Journal of the American Medical Association, 285*(17), 2232-2240.

50. Stoler, M. (2002). New Bethesda terminology and evidence-based management guidelines for cervical cytology findings. *Journal of the American Medical Association, 287*(16), 2141-2142.

51. Teaffy, N. (1999). *Perimenopause: Preparing for the change: A guide to the early stages of menopause and beyond* (2nd ed.). Rocklin, CA: Prima.

52. Thigpen, J. (2000). Ovaries and fallopian tubes. In M. Abeloff, J., et al. (Eds.). *Clinical oncology* (2nd ed., pp. 2016-2040). New York: Churchill Livingstone.

53. Tiedmann, D. (2000). Ovarian cancer. *RN, 63*(10), 36-42.

54. Todd, A. (2002) An alternative to hysterectomy. *RN, 65*(3), 30-33.

55. Vleck, J., & Safranek, S. (2002). What medications are effective for treating symptoms of premenstrual syndrome (PMS)? *Journal of Family Practice, 51*(10), 894.

56. World Congress on Endometriosis. (1998). *Understanding and managing endometriosis: Advances in research and practice.* Proceedings of the Sixth World Congress on Endometriosis, June 30-July 4, 1998. Quebec City, Canada: Author.

57. Wright, T., et al. (2002). Consensus guidelines for the management of women with cervical cytological abnormalities. *Journal of the American Medical Association, 287*(16), 2120-2129.

58. Wright, T., Holinka, C., Ferenczy, et al. (2002). Estradial-induced hyperplasia in endometrial biopsies from women on hormone replacement therapy. *American Journal Surgical Pathology, 10*, 1269-1275.

59. Writing Group for the Women's Health Initiative Investigators. (2002). Risks and benefits of estrogen plus progestin in healthy postmenopausal women. Principal results from the women's health initiative: Randomized controlled trial. *Journal of the American Medical Association, 288*(3), 321-333.

60. U. S. Preventive Services Task Force. (2003). Postmenopausal hormone replacement therapy for the primary prevention of chronic conditions: Recommendations and rationale. *American Journal of Nursing, 103*(6), 83-91.

Management of Clients with Breast Disorders

Melissa Craft

---

evolve

Web Enhancements

Case Study
Breast Cancer with Mastectomy
Client Education Guide
Arm Care After Axillary Lymph Node Dissection (English Version and Spanish Translation)
Postmastectomy Exercises (Spanish Translation)
Clinical Pathway
Mastectomy

Ethical Issues in Nursing
Communication Problem or Ethical Dilemma?
Tables
TNM Staging System for Breast Cancer
Appendix C
Laboratory Values of Clinical Importance in Medical-Surgical Nursing

---

A woman who finds a breast lump or other breast problem will probably first suspect cancer, even though 8 of 10 lumps are benign. Despite many misconceptions regarding the etiology of breast cancer, public awareness about this health threat has grown dramatically. In the past, the subject was avoided, or if information was shared, it was often inaccurate. Now breast cancer is openly discussed, and information about this topic is frequently presented in mass media. With the recent media focus on breast cancer awareness and early detection, the public is becoming more aware of the roles that breast self-examination, clinical examination, and especially routine mammograms have in the early detection of a breast mass.

Nurses have a responsibility to teach the public about breast lesions and cancer, to correct misconceptions, and to provide accurate information concerning normal breasts and breast disease, detection, and treatment. Facts about the disease, treatment, and prognosis need to be shared openly with all members of society, particularly the underserved. If women understand the importance of early detection and treatment, they are more likely to have regular mammograms and less likely to delay seeking medical care when an abnormality is found. Delay in seeking medical care is often due to (1) fear that the problem is cancer and (2) lack of knowledge that breast cancer can be curable if caught early.

BREAST CANCER IN WOMEN

Breast cancer is the most common malignancy in women in the United States and is second only to lung cancer as a cause of cancer death.[18] The incidence of breast cancer in the United States has been increasing gradually for the past 30 years. In 2003, the number of new cases of breast cancer diagnosed in women in the United States was estimated at 211,300, with 40,200 deaths caused by the disease.[2] At age 85 years, a woman's risk for breast cancer is one in eight, depending on where she lives. The

---

evolve *Be sure to check out the bonus material on the Evolve website and the CD-ROM, including free self-assessment exercises.*
http://evolve.elsevier.com/Black/medsurg/

Nursing Outcomes Classification (NOC)
for Nursing Diagnoses—Clients with Breast Disorders

Deficient Knowledge
  Knowledge: Disease Process
  Knowledge: Health Resources
  Knowledge: Illness Care
  Knowledge: Medication
  Knowledge: Prescribed Activity
  Knowledge: Treatment Procedures
  Knowledge: Treatment Regimen
Disturbed Body Image
  Grief Resolution
  Psychosocial Adjustment: Life Change
  Self-Care: Activities of Daily Living
    (ADL)
  Self-Esteem
**Effective Therapeutic Regimen
Management**
  Decision Making

Family Participation in Professional
  Care
  Knowledge: Diet
  Knowledge: Disease Process
  Knowledge: Medication
  Knowledge: Treatment Procedures
  Knowledge: Treatment Regimen
  Participation: Health Care Decisions
**Imbalanced Nutrition: Less Than Body
Requirements**
  Nutritional Status: Food and Fluid In-
    take
  Nutritional Status: Nutrient Intake
Risk for Impaired Skin Integrity
  Tissue Integrity: Skin and Mucous
    Membranes
  Treatment Behavior: Illness or Injury

Wound Healing: Primary Intention or
  Secondary Intention
**Risk for Ineffective Individual Coping
and Risk for Compromised Family
Coping**
  Caregiver Emotional Support Coping
  Decision-Making
  Family Coping
  Family Normalization
  Family Participation in Professional
    Care
  Information Processing
  Role Performance
  Social Support
Risk for Injury
  Symptom Control

---

highest incidence of breast cancer occurs in the United States and Europe.

Before 1990, there was little evidence of any decrease in the United States age-standardized death rate from breast cancer. Currently, breast cancer mortality appears to be declining among all women. Between 1989 and 1995, death rates decreased by 1.6% annually for all races combined. Between 1995 and 1998, the decrease accelerated to a decline of 3.4% annually.[28] (Breast cancer in men is rare and is discussed later in this chapter.) The decrease in mortality may be ascribed to the combined benefits of early detection and better treatment.[45] There is some evidence that the death rate is higher in black women older than 75 years of age, but it remains unclear whether this is related to socioeconomic factors or basic tumor biology.[9,38] The increase in early diagnosis due to mammography and the generally increased awareness of breast cancer among women and their physicians have resulted in detection of smaller tumors, which are more likely to be localized and to be treated successfully.[18]

Probably the most important encouragement to breast cancer detection has been the discovery that screening mammography reduces breast cancer deaths by 30%.[1,49] The Breast and Cervical Cancer Mortality Act of 1990 was enacted to ensure that underinsured or uninsured women receive mammograms and appropriate treatment services.[12] In 2000, the Breast and Cervical Cancer Treatment and Prevention Act (BCCTP) was

The authors would like to thank Michelle Goodman and Stephanie Mellon-Reppen for their contribution to this chapter in the sixth edition of *Medical-Surgical Nursing*.

passed to help provide treatment to women diagnosed with breast and cervical cancer. This act made it possible for each state to enact legislation that would make women diagnosed through the services of the BCCTP eligible to receive Medicaid benefits for treatment. This underscores the need for states to act on this matching funding proposal and for the women to be screened through BCCTP-funded agencies.[12] Women need to understand the importance of mammography in detecting breast cancers while tumors are small. Likewise, they should understand that the treatment is less toxic and more effective for all modalities used when the disease is detected early, even before the tumor is palpable. With regard to surgery, less tissue is removed when the tumor is small; therefore better cosmesis is possible. With irradiation of a smaller volume of diseased tissue, cure is more likely and a lower dose is needed for radiation therapy. With adjuvant treatment, a small tumor burden means that systemic therapy may not be needed; if it is needed, then drug treatment is more successful. Smaller tumors also mean less regional node involvement and fewer complications associated with axillary node dissection.[20]

Nurses need to provide current and accurate information concerning the latest approaches to breast cancer treatment and related complications. Encouraging the client to participate in research, if appropriate, is especially important, so that critical questions regarding breast cancer therapy can be addressed. Clients and their families are required to make many difficult decisions. The nurse can be especially helpful by ensuring that the client understands treatment options and by providing clarification when appropriate.

Etiology and Risk Factors

The cause of breast cancer is not known. Many women are anxious about their risk for breast cancer, and many tend to overestimate their risk. Even though genetic, hormonal, or biochemical factors are likely to be involved, 70% of women with breast cancer have no known risk factors.

Age and Ethnicity

All women are at risk for breast cancer, and the most important single risk factor is age. Risk increases with age, although the rate of increase slows after menopause. The annual incidence of breast cancer in American women older than age 65 years is 10 times higher than that in women 30 to 35 years of age.[59] African-American women younger than 50 years have a higher age-specific incidence of breast cancer than that in Caucasian women.[38] However, between 1992 and 1998, incidence rates were relatively unchanged in women of all racial and ethnic groups.[3]

Edwards and colleagues, in their examination of the impact of race on survival in breast cancer, found that not only are African-American women less likely to be cured than their non–African-American counterparts, but they also survive for a shorter time until death from breast cancer.[18] Even when matched for tumor stage, they are more at risk for micrometastatic disease and early death. It is not clear whether these findings are related to tumor biology, host response, or variability in treatment. Psychosocial and socioeconomic factors have a major role in governing access to medical care. Uninsured clients and those insured by Medicaid present with more advanced disease, have a higher risk of death, and have lessened survival compared with privately insured clients.[9,38]

Breast cancer incidence among Hispanic women living in North America is only 40% to 50% as great as that among non-Hispanic white women. Asian women born in Asia have a very low lifetime risk of breast cancer, but their daughters born in North America have the same lifetime risk of breast cancer as for American white women.[9] However, in a recent report to the nation on cancer, Edwards writes that "rates other than for whites and blacks should be interpreted with caution because of possible misreporting and misclassification of race/ethnicity."[18]

Ovarian and Hormonal Function

Early menarche (first menses) and late menopause (cessation of menses) lead to an increased total lifetime number of ovulatory menstrual cycles and a corresponding 30% to 50% increase in breast cancer risk. The woman who experiences natural menopause before age 45 years has a risk for breast cancer that is half that of the woman whose menopause occurs after age 55 years.[1] Likewise, oophorectomy before a woman reaches menopause lowers her risk of breast cancer by approximately two thirds. Both nulliparity (no births) and age older than 30 years at first live birth are associated with a nearly doubled risk of subsequent breast cancer.[59]

The use of hormone replacement therapy (HRT) has also demonstrated a small but significant increase in risk for breast cancer in women who have used it for more than 10 years. The Women's Health Initiative (WHI) study, which includes women randomized to receive hormones or placebo, conducted by the National Heart, Lung, and Blood Institute (NHLBI), in 2002 announced that, after 5.2 years of follow-up, the data and safety monitoring board had recommended stopping the estrogen plus progestin versus placebo arm of the study because the risks exceeded the benefits.[39,63] The risks implicated in their decision were for breast cancer, coronary heart disease, and stroke. Although benefits in reduction of osteoporosis, colon cancer, and endometrial cancer were observed, these did not outweigh the risks. This excessive risk to benefit was not seen in the estrogen only arm during the 10th interim analysis in spring 2002, and this study is to continue as planned until 2005, the planned termination. Note that absolute excess risk or risk reduction of estrogen plus progestin to the individual woman is low. In a year's time, 10,000 women taking the combined therapy versus 10,000 women not taking it would have seven more coronary heart disease events, eight more strokes, eight more pulmonary embolisms, eight more invasive breast cancers, six fewer colorectal cancers, and five fewer hip fractures.[63] This study was not designed to look at the short-term risks and benefits of HRT such as hot flashes, insomnia, mood and cognitive change, and urogenital atrophy, gallbladder disease, and stroke.[37] Previous studies have indicated that using HRT for less than 5 years or short-term use is considerably less likely to increase the risk of breast cancer and the WHI study did not indicate an increased risk of breast cancer until after 3 years.[37] Therefore it is possible that, for short-term use, there may be more benefit than risk.[36,39,42] It has been recommended that combination HRT not be prescribed for long-term use.[37] The American Heart Association has recommended making HRT decisions based on noncoronary benefits and risks. The choice for each woman must be individual and frequently involves a formal risk-benefit analysis.

At present there is no convincing evidence that oral contraceptive use affects the risk of breast cancer. The question is difficult to address because the oral contraceptives in use currently are vastly different (dosages are much lower) from those used 15 and 20 years ago. Even if oral contraceptives influence the incidence of breast cancer, it would be only of historical interest because the drugs used years ago are not comparable to those used today. However, women who have a strong family history of breast cancer may have an increased risk related to earlier formulations of oral contraceptives. It is unclear what the effect may be of recent lower doses on this client population.[11,24]

Benign Breast Disease

Benign breast disease is not any more common in women with other risk factors for breast cancer. Nonproliferative lesions (e.g., cysts, duct ectasia, mild hyperplasia, and fibroadenoma) do not increase the risk of breast cancer; however, cellular atypia or atypical hyperplasia (a proliferative disease) is an example of a histologic change associated with a higher risk. Complex fibroadenomas, sclerosing adenosis, epithelial calcification, and papillary apocrine changes increase the relative risk of breast cancer two-fold to three-fold, but the exact incidence and factors that influence malignant transformation are not well determined.[1] Studies indicate that women with a family history of breast cancer and atypical hyperplasia have at least a three-fold increased risk of breast cancer.[60]

Family History

Family history is one of the known risk factors for breast cancer. Breast cancer due to the inheritance of a specific germ line mutation from either maternal or paternal relatives is rare. In fact, the breast cancer susceptibility gene BRCA1 and BRCA2 and the p53 tumor suppressor gene have been identified in fewer than 10% of all women with breast cancer. (See the Genetics Link feature on Breast Cancer Susceptibility Genes: BRCA1 and BRCA2,

below.) Certain populations have a higher incidence of BRCA mutations than the general population (e.g., native Icelanders and Ashkenazi Jews).[1] Depending on the familial context, the lifetime risk of breast cancer, ovarian cancer, or both associated with carrying a mutation ranges from 50% to 85%.[1] Families with several affected first-degree relatives and clients with early-onset disease have been found to harbor mutations at a higher frequency. Commercial testing for mutations in BRCA1 and BRCA2 as well as for less common mutations that predispose to breast cancer, such as HNPCC (hereditary nonpolyposis colon cancer) and Li-Fraumeni are available.[1] The decision to undergo genetic testing is individual and carries both benefits and limitations. Comprehensive breast cancer screening and high-risk counseling centers are ideal mechanisms for providing women with individualized evaluation, education, screening, and, when appropriate, genetic testing.[59]

In addition to hereditary breast cancer, it is estimated that approximately 15% to 20% of breast cancer cases are familial.[59] Like hereditary cancer, a clustering of two or more relatives are affected; however, the ages of onset are older and a clear inheritance pattern may not be demonstrated. Familial breast cancer is probably related to a combination of genetic and environmental factors, and studies on these families may yield discovery of additional breast cancer genes.

Environmental and Dietary Factors

An increased incidence of breast cancer has been reported in women who received mantle radiation for the treatment of Hodgkin's disease, particularly if they were younger than 20 years of age.[30,31] The latency period is

---

GENETICS LINKS

Breast Cancer Susceptibility Genes: BRCA1 and BRCA2

Description
Major cancer susceptibility genes may account for 5%-10% of breast cancer cases. Two genes (BRCA1 and BRCA2) have been identified and are thought to account for approximately 75% of all hereditary breast cancer. Other breast cancer susceptibility genes exist and contribute to a much smaller amount. Disease-causing mutations result in a predisposition to breast and ovarian cancer and other cancers, including prostate, colon, and others. Features suggestive of a BRCA1/BRCA2 family include multiple affected family members, early age of onset, and bilateral disease.

Genetics
BRCA1 and BRCA2 mutations are estimated to occur in 1 of every 300 to 800 individuals. These mutations are inherited in an autosomal dominant manner, with each offspring of an affected parent having a 50% risk of inheriting the mutation.

Diagnosis/Testing
Clinical molecular testing for BRCA1/BRCA2 is clinically available for an affected individual who is at high risk for having a BRCA1/BRCA2 mutation or for at-risk family members of an individual who has an identified mutation. Multiple molecular laboratory methods are used to identify mutations, but identification of all disease-causing mutations cannot be guaranteed.

Management
Education and counseling of affected individuals and family members is essential. Recommendations are made for cancer screening of individuals who have a BRCA1 or BRCA2 mutation. Some women choose to have prophylactic mastectomy and oophorectomy to reduce the risk of cancer.

between 10 and 25 years. The disease in this group typically presents more aggressively, with a high rate of nodal involvement and bilaterality. It is for this reason that all persons who receive mantle radiation for Hodgkin's disease, especially those treated before age 20 years, receive a regular mammography follow-up examination to detect these lesions early.[31] Sophisticated, modern radiation therapy techniques have lowered the incidence of breast cancer and other long-term complications in these clients.[31]

Alcohol intake is the best-established dietary risk factor for breast cancer in epidemiologic studies. The positive correlation of alcohol intake with breast cancer risk has been established, and it appears that moderate alcohol intake (one to two drinks per day) increases the risk of breast cancer by altering estrogen metabolism.[55] Recent studies have suggested that drinking in moderation, defined, as about one drink per day is an example of a modifiable risk factor for breast cancer.[50] Folic acid has been shown to reduce the risk of breast cancer in women who consume alcohol and continues to be studied in several trials.[64] (See the Complementary and Alternative Therapy feature on Multivitamins, Alcohol, and Breast Cancer, below.) As is commonly observed, Japanese women living in Japan have a very low incidence of breast cancer. When they move to the United States, their risk for breast cancer approximates that of native white women within one generation.

In a large study involving nearly 338,000 women, there was no apparent correlation between breast cancer risk and dietary intake of fat.[28] There is a possibility that the influence of dietary fat, obesity, and high caloric intake may impact postmenopausal breast cancer differently than premenopausal breast cancer. (See the Complementary and Alternative Therapy feature on Diet and Breast Cancer: Everything in Moderation?, below.) Identification of separate risk factors for premenopausal and postmenopausal women may determine a role for fat intake in the future.[59] Epidemiologic evidence does not support any substantial increase in breast cancer risk associated with caffeine consumption. Studies have shown that consumption of fruits and vegetables is not significantly related to a reduction in breast cancer risk.[56,59] Passive cigarette smoking has also been shown to be unrelated to breast cancer risk, but a new study suggests that active smoking may impart a small risk, especially when smoking is initiated at young ages.[19] More importantly, for nurses in particular, several recent studies have suggested that working at night may increase the relative risk of breast cancer by 60%.[15,47] The risk appeared to be related to the amount of time spent working at night. Working night shifts increased risk by about the same amount as alcohol use and delayed childbirth.[25] This could have obvious implications for nursing both individually and collectively.[33]

COMPLEMENTARY AND ALTERNATIVE THERAPY

Multivitamins, Alcohol, and Breast Cancer

The large prospective Nurses' Health Study had previously found that women taking a cheap multivitamin daily for many years could significantly reduce their risk of colon cancer or heart disease. However, researchers also looked at the impact of this supplement on breast cancer risk. A total of 88,818 women were followed for 16 years. Researchers found that taking a multivitamin with approximately 400 to 600 μg of folic acid could slightly reduce the risk of breast cancer in women who also were already drinking 1 to 2 alcoholic drinks per day. Alcohol is estrogenic and seems to reduce folic acid levels in the body. Thus there may be an added advantage for women taking multivitamins if they also drink alcohol compared to women who drink but do not take a daily multivitamin.

Reference

Hankinson, S., et al. (1999). A prospective study of folate intake and the risk of breast cancer. *Journal of the American Medical Association, 281,* 1632-1637.

COMPLEMENTARY AND ALTERNATIVE THERAPY

Diet and Breast Cancer: Everything in Moderation?

Researchers in this study were motivated by the observation that in many studies there seems to be a U-shaped association of body mass index and survival in breast cancer. In other words, moderate and healthy weight may be associated with a better survival rate as opposed to extremes in weight (too thin or too heavy). The researchers wanted to see if this relationship is true for diet. A total of 477 women with surgically resected T1 to T3, N0/1, M0 breast cancer completed a food frequency questionnaire approximately 9.3 +/− 4.6 weeks after diagnosis (reporting their intakes of food over the previous 12 months). Median follow-up of the survivors was 6.1 years.

Researchers found a nonlinear survival association for protein, oleic acid, cholesterol, polyunsaturated-saturated fat ratio, and percentage of calories from fat and percentage of calories from carbohydrates. Their data suggest that the midrange (moderation) intake of most major energy or food sources was associated with the most favorable outcomes, whereas extremes in diet were associated with less favorable outcomes. In summary, moderate diets or lifestyles that produce a normal body mass index may be associated with the best breast cancer outcomes.

Reference

Goodwin, P., et al. (2003). Diet and breast cancer: Evidence that extremes in diet are associated with poor survival. *Journal of Clinical Oncology, 21,* 2500-2507.

Nurses have a unique role in fostering health promotion and in teaching women about breast cancer as well as in identifying a woman's individual risk for breast cancer. Because most women—especially those with any family history of breast cancer—greatly overestimate their risk for breast cancer, it is helpful to instruct women about the known risk factors and, as indicated, provide support to lessen some of their fears (Table 42-1). Counseling, with appropriate referrals when required, should always accompany specific recommendations for clients with significant risks. The American Cancer Society published new screening guidelines in May 2003. These guidelines help women determine the appropriate screening for their individual risk. The new guidelines also state that women who are at increased risk for breast cancer may benefit from more frequent screenings and additional imaging modalities (e.g., ultrasound and magnetic resonance imaging [MRI]).[54a]

Health Promotion Activities

Although no known agent or practice guarantees that a woman will remain free of breast cancer, methods are under investigation that may alter the risk and therefore can be considered health promotion activities.

Chemoprevention. Chemoprevention is the use of a drug to prevent the development of a certain malignancy. Two agents have been found to decrease the risk of breast cancer: tamoxifen (Nolvadex) (see the Integrating Pharmacology feature on Medications for Breast Cancer on p. 1097) and raloxifene (Evista).

Tamoxifen is an agent commonly used in clients who have breast tumors with receptors for estrogen. Fisher and colleagues[22] looked at tamoxifen and its role in decreasing the incidence of breast cancer in high-risk clients. In this study, 13,388 high-risk women were randomized to receive either placebo or tamoxifen 20 mg/day. Tamoxifen reduced the risk of invasive breast cancer by 49% overall; however, endometrial cancer developed in twice as many women in the tamoxifen group as in the placebo group. In another study, 7705 women with osteoporosis were randomized to receive either a placebo or raloxifene.[14] Over 33 months, nearly twice as many invasive breast cancers were seen in the placebo group as in the raloxifene group.

In contrast to the tamoxifen trial, there was no increase in the incidence of endometrial cancer in women who received raloxifene. Because raloxifene has never been compared with tamoxifen as a chemopreventive agent and has not been studied in women at high risk for breast cancer, the National Surgical Adjuvant Breast Project (NSABP) is conducting a double-blind study that will compare these two drugs in 22,000 high-risk women. Tamoxifen is currently the more widely used of the two drugs; it costs approximately $100 in the United States for a 1-month supply and is covered by most insurance plans.

TABLE 42-1	*American Cancer Society Guidelines for Early Breast Cancer Detection, 2003*
Women at Average Risk	Begin mammography at age 40.
	For women in their 20s and 30s, it is recommended that clinical breast examination be part of a periodic health examination, preferably at least every 3 years. Asymptomatic women ages 40 and over should continue to receive a clinical breast examination as part of a periodic health examination, preferably annually.
	Beginning in their 20s, women should be told about the benefits and limitations of breast self-examination (BSE). The importance of prompt reporting of any new breast symptoms to a health professional should be emphasized. Women who choose to do BSE should receive instruction and have their technique reviewed on the occasion of a periodic health examination. It is acceptable for women to choose not to do BSE or to do BSE irregularly.
	Women should have an opportunity to become informed about the benefits, limitations, and potential harms associated with regular screening.
Older Women	Screening decisions in older women should be individualized by considering the potential benefits and risks of mammography in the context of current health status and estimated life expectancy. As long as a woman is in reasonably good health and would be a candidate for treatment, she should continue to be screened with mammography.
Women at Increased Risk	Women at increased risk of breast cancer might benefit from additional screening strategies beyond those offered to women of average risk, such as earlier initiation of screening, shorter screening intervals, or the addition of screening modalities other than mammography and physical examination, such as ultrasound or magnetic resonance imaging. However, the evidence currently available is insufficient to justify recommendations for any of these screening approaches.

From Smith, R. et al. (2003). American Cancer Society guidelines for breast cancer screening: Update 2003. *CA Cancer Journal for Clinicians, 53*, 141-169.

Prophylactic Mastectomy. The only other measure that may predictably prevent the occurrence of breast cancer and be considered a method of health promotion is prophylactic mastectomy. All of the breast tissue is removed in a woman who does not have evidence of breast cancer. Women who may benefit from this procedure are those who have a strong family history of breast cancer, a history of breast cancer in the other breast, a history of atypical hyperplasia on repeated surgical biopsies, or presence of a mutated *BRCA1* or *BRCA2* gene. Breast cancer incidence may be reduced as much as 90% in women who have a prophylactic mastectomy.[27] However, it is not known whether prophylactic mastectomy is superior to careful clinical and radiologic screening of high-risk women, especially with the emergence of the role of MRI in the screening of high-risk breast cancer clients.[59]

Lifestyle Changes. Women can also be encouraged to make changes in lifestyle to lower their potential risk for breast cancer. For instance, they can decrease their consumption of alcohol. Although a moderate decrease in dietary fat intake does not appear to reduce the risk of breast cancer, decreasing fat intake to 20% of dietary calories is a worthwhile goal.[1]

Exercise may have an indirect role in the prevention of breast cancer. Exercise leads to a decrease in body fat, thereby reducing the amount of free estrogen stored in body fat. Hence, it is another health promotion activity.

Health Maintenance Activities

Health maintenance involves optimal screening and early detection of breast cancer. Regardless of the method used, regular and careful physical examination is the key to identifying asymptomatic cancerous lesions. When combined with mammography, physical examination decreases mortality, especially in women older than age 50 years. According to the National Cancer Advisory Board (NCAB), a committee that advises and consults with the director of the National Cancer Institute (NCI), data presented at the Consensus Development Conference showed that regular screening mammography of average-risk women in their 40s re-

INTEGRATING PHARMACOLOGY
Medications for Breast Cancer

Many women with breast cancer receive tamoxifen as one part of their treatment. Generally it is the last modality used in their multimodality regimen. Dosing is 20 mg/day for 5 years.[1,2,7]

Tamoxifen is a drug classified as a selective estrogen receptor modulator. It works by competing for the binding site normally occupied by estrogen. By blocking the ability of estrogen to bind with estrogen receptor positive breast cancer cells, it controls and even prevents the growth of breast cancer cells.

Tamoxifen is usually well tolerated and has limited potential for drug interactions. There are side effects, however, and some may affect the breast cancer survivor's quality of life. Side effects include hot flashes, mood swings, depression, and anecdotal reports of memory changes.[5] Recent literature, however, reports a statistically insignificant relationship between tamoxifen and depression in the first breast cancer prevention trial. Day[3] and Ernst et al.[4] demonstrated a weaker association between tamoxifen and brain metabolism in older women than what was projected, thereby decreasing some concern about mentation effects of tamoxifen in older women. Other side effects include an increased risk for stroke, pulmonary emboli, cataracts, endometrial cancer, and vaginal dryness.[6] Women should be followed up by their oncologist and family practitioner and gynecologist to monitor for any negative sequelae of taking tamoxifen.

Implications
With increasing numbers of premenopausal women taking tamoxifen, it is important to recognize that amenorrhea, although likely, is not guaranteed, and that the woman could become pregnant. Tamoxifen is thought to be teratogenic, so premenopausal women should practice some form of birth control while taking it.

References
1. *Breast Cancer Facts and Figures. 2001-2002.* Atlanta, GA: American Cancer Society.
2. Breast care guidelines. (2002). National Comprehensive Cancer Network, as obtained from www.acr.org on 10/16/02.
3. Day, R., Ganz, P.A., & Constantino, J.P. (2001). Tamoxifen and depression: More evidence from the NSABP Breast Cancer Prevention (P-1) randomized study. *Journal of the National Cancer Institute, 93*(21), 615-624.
4. Ernst, T., et al. (2002). The effects of tamoxifen and estrogen on brain metabolism in elderly women. *Journal of the National Cancer Institute, 94*(8), 592-597.
5. Ganz, P.A. (2001). Impact of tamoxifen adjuvant therapy on symptoms, functioning and quality of life. *Journal of the National Cancer Institute,* Monograph #30. 130-134.
6. Makia, J. (2001). Breast cancer: Risk prevention and tamoxifen. *American Journal of Nursing, 101*(4), 26-35.
7. What you need to know about breast cancer. Retrieved 10/3/02 from http://www.cancer.gov/cancer-info.

duces deaths from breast cancer by about 17% to 24%.[8,13] On the basis of this finding, the NCAB recommended to the NCI that women between the ages of 40 and 49 years have screening mammograms every 1 to 2 years if they are at average risk for breast cancer. In November 2000, the American College of Radiology (ACR), the American Cancer Society, the American Medical Women's Association, and numerous women's groups issued a statement that supports annual screening mammography starting at age 40 years. The ACR believes that clinical trials have shown that having screening mammograms every year, compared to every 1 to 2 years, allows the detection of cancers at an earlier stage.[10] The U.S. Preventive Services Task Force (USPSTF) reaffirmed the value of mammography for women older than 40 years in January 2002. Predicted breast cancer rates increased 5.9% in 2002, which the USPSTF speculates is related to better screening as well as the aging of "baby boomers."[2]

Once a mammogram reveals an area suggestive of cancer, an ultrasound study is a useful complement to diagnostic mammography as a means for distinguishing cystic from solid masses. For women with particularly dense breasts or with implants, MRI scanning and digital mammography provide improved sensitivity. It is hoped that better mammography technology, including digitized radiography, routine use of magnified views, and greater skill in interpretation, combined with MRI and positron-emission tomography (PET) scanning, will make it possible to identify breast cancers at an earlier stage. A large prospective trial is underway to determine whether digital mammography is superior to film mammography. Digital mammography may decrease false-positive rates and possibly detect more cancers. Although it is more expensive initially, digital mammography may be more cost-effective in the long run because of easier storage and fewer false-positive results.[8,40,43]

Health care professionals and health care advocates have for many years promoted breast self-examination (BSE) as a key component of early cancer detection because most breast cancers are detected by the woman herself, usually after the mass has grown to the size of 2.5 cm or larger. The only reason the cancer is detected then is that the mass is large enough to be felt. A better goal would be to detect the cancer while it is still small, before it can be felt (Figure 42-1). The only way to do this is by regular mammography and physical examination by a trained clinician (see Chapter 39). BSE has not been proven to save lives or to increase survival. There is insufficient evidence to recommend for or against the teaching of BSE.[3] Teaching a woman to examine her breasts is an important strategy for increasing her awareness of the risk of breast cancer. See Chapter 2 and Figure 2-4 for a discussion of BSE.

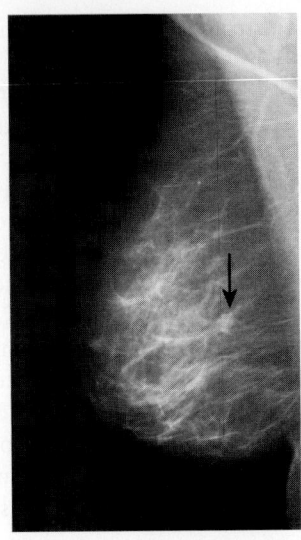

FIGURE 42-1 Screening mammogram of a 56-year-old woman with a strong family history of breast cancer, right mediolateral oblique view. The mammogram shows a small, irregular, nonpalpable mass *(arrow)*, which was highly suggestive of malignancy. Refer to Figure 39-8 for a view of a normal mammogram.

Health Restoration Activities

Arm exercises and positioning after surgery to prevent lymphedema, obtaining a prosthesis, and breast reconstruction are health restoration activities. If lymphedema develops despite exercises and positioning, referral to a physical therapist or specialized nurse for lymphedema management is recommended.

Pathophysiology

Breast cancers are malignant tumors that typically begin in the ductal-lobular epithelial cells of the breast and spread via the lymphatic system to the axillary lymph nodes. The tumor may then metastasize to distant regions of the body, including lungs, liver, bone, and brain. The finding of breast cancer in the axillary lymph nodes is an indicator of the tumor's ability for potential distant spread and is not merely contiguous growth into the adjacent region of the breast. Most primary breast cancers are adenocarcinomas located in the upper outer quadrant of the breast (Figure 42-2).

Carcinoma in Situ

Malignant-appearing cells confined to the ductal or lobular units without permeation of the basement membrane represent carcinoma in situ. *Ductal carcinoma in situ* (DCIS) is a precursor of infiltrating carcinoma. Pathologists classify DCIS as high, intermediate-grade, or low-grade according to the growth pattern of cells occupying the ducts, their nuclear features, mitotic activity, presence of necrosis, and type of microcalcifications.

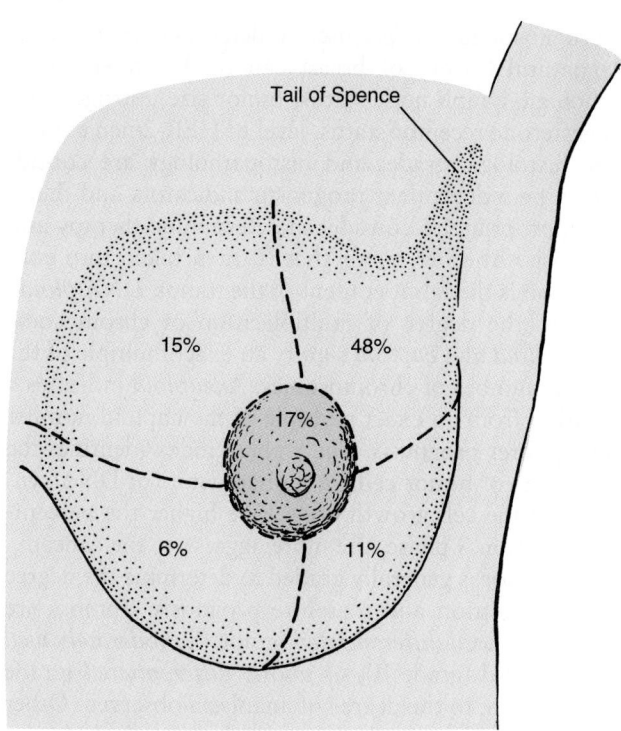

FIGURE 42-2 Frequency of occurrence of breast cancer according to location. The highest occurrence is in the upper outer quadrant and in the tail of Spence.

Low-grade DCIS tends to be the most common and is typically multifocal; high-grade DCIS is second in prevalence and tends to be architecturally contiguous and associated with prominent microcalcifications. High-grade DCIS tends to be estrogen receptor–negative, shows increased expression for human epidermal growth factor receptor (HER-2)/neu protein (c-erbB2), and has a mutated p53 tumor suppressor gene.

Ipsilateral (affecting the same side) invasive carcinoma develops within 10 years in approximately 30% of cases of DCIS. Left untreated, intraductal carcinoma transforms into invasive ductal carcinoma.

Lobular carcinoma in situ (LCIS) is characterized by a solid proliferation of atypical cells expanding lobular units. In contrast to DCIS, LCIS is usually found incidentally and is not typically associated with microcalcifications. LCIS has a lower tendency to develop into infiltrating carcinoma.

Invasive Breast Cancer

Most breast cancers (75%) are infiltrating ductal carcinomas. They typically metastasize to regional lymph nodes and beyond. Lobular carcinomas account for about 5% to 10% of cases and usually present as a generalized thickening. Tumor types that are associated with a favorable prognosis include tubular (accounting for 2% of cases), medullary (5% to 7%), and mucinous

(colloid) carcinoma (3%). These histologic types tend to have low-grade histology, positive estrogen and progesterone receptors status, diploid deoxyribonucleic acid (DNA) content, low S phase fraction (discussed later under Prognosis and Defining Extent of Disease), and no oncogenic markers. Tumors with poor clinical prognosis are those associated with high-grade histology and dermal lymphatic invasion designated as "inflammatory carcinoma." Inflammatory breast cancer is characterized by skin redness and induration. Edema and warmth are other common associated findings. Frequently, palpable axillary and supraclavicular nodes and distant metastases are involved.

Clinical Manifestations

Most breast cancers present as painless, nontender, hard, irregularly shaped, nonmobile masses. About 60% of cancers are somewhat movable, 40% have regular borders by palpation, and 40% can feel soft or cystic. Even when no mass is present, other physical findings, such as nipple discharge, induration, and dimpling, can suggest malignancy. Heat and erythema of the breast skin may be related to inflammation but may also indicate inflammatory carcinoma. Skin edema is characteristic of malignant disease. The edema is due to the invasion and obstruction of dermal lymphatics by the tumor. If a tumor is suspected on the basis of the physical findings, a diagnostic mammogram is indicated.

Radiographic Findings

Additional diagnostic films of the affected breast, as well as localized compression and magnification views, increase the specificity of identifying the abnormality. Digital mammography and computer-assisted diagnosis (CAD) may be useful to evaluate the lesion, because these tests allow more variations in exposure and show the differences in tissue contrast more clearly. CAD uses a software program to target lesions suspected to be malignant. The specificity of the image is enhanced by on-screen evaluation that allows manipulation of contrast, which improves detection.

Fine-Needle Aspiration

Fine-needle aspiration (FNA) is performed on an outpatient basis. The purpose is to determine whether a solid lump is a cyst or to confirm a clinically apparent diagnosis. If the mass turns out to be a cyst, the lump should disappear after the aspiration. If a lump is solid, a cytologic specimen may be obtained by making several passes into the lesion to retrieve small cell samples; this technique can reduce the incidence of false-negative results. If the FNA results are negative and the physician suspects cancer from the clinical findings, excisional biopsy (open) is indicated.

Stereotactic Needle-Guided Biopsy

Stereotactic needle-guided biopsy (SNB) is used mainly to target and identify nonpalpable lesions in the breast that have been detected with mammography. The basic goal is to immobilize the breast from fixed horizontal and vertical coordinates to calculate the exact position of the lesion within a three-dimensional field. SNB permits biopsy diagnosis of benign disease without the trauma or scarring of an open biopsy.

Ultrasound Core Biopsy

Ultrasound-guided breast biopsy is used when the lesion can be seen on ultrasound. It is easier for the client than a stereotactic biopsy because she can lie on her back and does not have to have her breast immobilized during the procedure. A local anesthetic is used to anesthetize the area and a biopsy is performed using a large-bore biopsy needle.

Open Biopsy

Excisional or open biopsy may be chosen when the lesion is determined to be solid and indeterminate in nature, when results of cytologic or histologic analysis are insufficient, or when the clinical or mammographic findings suggest malignancy. A wire-localized biopsy procedure similar to the stereotactic method can be used; the aim of this procedure is to assist the surgeon in locating the nonpalpable lesion for the purpose of excisional biopsy and to minimize the volume of tissue removed to avoid unnecessary deformity.

Prognosis and Defining Extent of Disease

Once a diagnosis of cancer is made, the cancer needs to be evaluated further to determine the most appropriate therapy. For example, if breast-conserving surgery (lumpectomy) is being considered, the presence of microcalcifications must be evaluated further to determine whether the disease in the breast is multifocal.

The tumor is staged according to the extent of local, regional, and distant spread. *Staging* permits an accurate definition of the extent of the disease and therefore a more accurate prognosis. The American Joint Committee on Cancer (AJCC) staging system for breast cancer is based on the tumor-node-metastasis (TNM) system, presented on the website. Prognosis for breast cancer is associated primarily with the extent of disease at detection. The tumor staging is based on (1) the size of the primary tumor; (2) whether it extends to the chest wall or skin; (3) the presence of axillary lymph nodes; (4) whether they are matted, fixed, or mobile; and (5) the presence of distant metastases (Figure 42-3). The 5-year survival rate for breast cancer based on stage of disease is presented in Table 42-2.

Prognostic factors are used to determine prognosis or the natural history of breast cancer. At present, only pathologic lymph node status, tumor size, estrogen and progesterone receptor status, level of HER-2/neu expression, histologic grade, and histopathology are considered to be independent prognostic indicators and therefore appropriate to consider in determining therapy and prognosis. Another factor that is often taken into consideration is the DNA content of the tumor. *DNA ploidy* refers to the degree of multiplication of chromosome sets. *Diploid* and *euploid* signify an exact multiple of the haploid number of chromosomes. *Aneuploid* indicates a deviation from an exact multiple of the haploid number and a poorer prognosis. The S phase index identifies the percentage of tumor cells in S phase (start of DNA synthesis) of the cell growth cycle. The higher the percentage of cells in S phase, the more aggressive the cancer.

The tumor is generally graded to determine the degree of differentiation and therefore prognosis. Tumors are classified as *well differentiated* (grade I), *moderately well differentiated* (grade II), or *poorly differentiated* (grade III) according to the degree of anaplasia observed. Other factors identified on the pathology report include nucleus size and shape, presence or absence of mitotic figures, and degree of tubule formation. Dermal lymphatic invasion and microvascular invasion may also be predictive of metastatic disease.

The 2002 National Comprehensive Cancer Network (NCCN) practice guidelines for breast cancer recommends evaluation of the level of HER-2/neu expression for all newly diagnosed clients.[10] Research has shown that the HER-2/neu expression is used in the selection of appropriate adjuvant chemotherapy and to predict the benefit of using trastuzumab in women with recurrent or metastatic cancer.[13,41,53] Steroid receptor status is an accepted predictive factor for response to endocrine therapies. If the tumor is determined to be estrogen receptor positive and progesterone receptor positive, antiestrogen therapy is an appropriate therapeutic option with or without chemotherapy. Anastrozole, a steroidal aromatase inhibitor, may provide an alternative to tamoxifen for estrogen receptor–positive postmenopausal women. Whether to use anastrozole instead of tamoxifen should be decided after individual consultation.[10]

Tumor markers are not considered useful preoperatively when adjuvant therapy for cure is planned. Tumor markers are assessed as part of the work-up of advanced disease and generally have significance only in a woman with metastatic disease. Carcinoembryonic antigen (CEA), CA-125, and CA 15-3 are substances produced by the tumor and are present in the serum of the woman with breast cancer. A tumor marker is expected to be present only in metastatic disease, in which case it is assessed on a monthly basis to monitor response to therapy. Pretreatment assessment also includes a metastatic work-up to determine extent of disease. Tests are se-

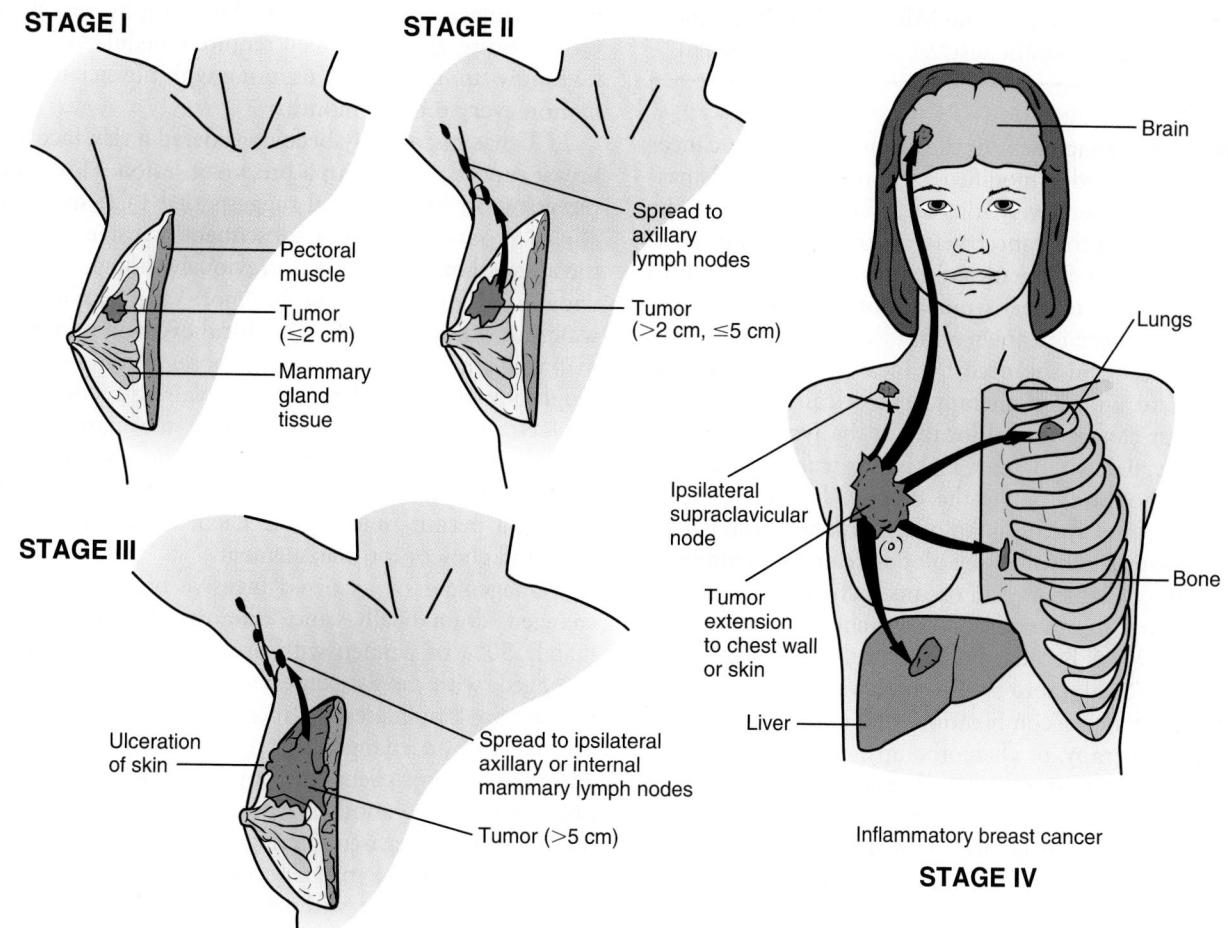

STAGE I

Pectoral muscle

Tumor (≤2 cm)

Mammary gland tissue

STAGE II

Spread to axillary lymph nodes

Tumor (>2 cm, ≤5 cm)

STAGE III

Ulceration of skin

Spread to ipsilateral axillary or internal mammary lymph nodes

Tumor (>5 cm)

Brain

Lungs

Ipsilateral supraclavicular node

Tumor extension to chest wall or skin

Bone

Liver

Inflammatory breast cancer

STAGE IV

FIGURE 42-3 Clinical staging of breast cancer. *Stage I,* Tumor 2 cm or less in diameter and confined to the breast. *Stage II,* Tumor up to 5 cm, or early metastasis to axillary lymph nodes. *Stage III,* Tumor larger than 5 cm with involvement of the ipsilateral axillary or internal mammary lymph nodes. *Stage IV,* Distant metastasis, such as to brain, bone, or liver; ipsilateral supraclavicular lymph node; skin or extension to chest wall; or inflammatory breast cancer.

lected according to the clinical presentation and the likelihood of metastatic disease. A chest x-ray film and a bone scan are possible useful baseline studies. A bone scan is usually not indicated unless the client has invasive breast cancer that is at least stage II or III. Only 30% to 60% of clients with a true-positive bone scan have increased alkaline phosphatase levels, and only 20% of clients with elevated alkaline phosphatase levels are disease-free. If the bone scan is abnormal, then radiographs of the affected sites are necessary to confirm metastatic disease and to exclude a benign etiologic mechanism.

A complete metabolic panel and physical examination detects any liver dysfunction and may identify the need for a liver scan. The liver scan is usually not done unless there is reason to suspect that the disease has spread or if the disease is at stage III. When metastatic disease is strongly suspected, an MRI study or a computed tomography (CT) scan may be ordered to further define and measure the extent of disease. A PET scan is not usually

TABLE 42-2	Five-Year Survival Rate for Breast Cancer by Stage
Stage	**5-Year Survival (% of Patients)**
0	99
I	92
IIA	82
IIB	65
IIIA	47
IIIB	44
IV	14

Data from Surveillance Epidemiology End Results (SEER), National Cancer Institute, *http://www.seer.ims.nci.nih.gov*, April 25, 2000.

indicated unless results of the MRI or CT scan are indeterminate and metastatic disease is strongly suspected.

Outcome Management

In the past, management of the client with breast cancer typically included a modified radical or a radical mastectomy. Postoperatively, the surgeon would assure the woman that all the cancer was removed and that treatment was ended. The current management approach to localized breast cancer is much more complicated, because much more is known about the systemic nature of breast cancer and the need for local control as well as appropriate adjuvant therapy. Historically, it was believed that cancer spread locally to the lymph nodes in an orderly, defined manner. If this was true, radical mastectomy should eliminate the disease. However, breast cancer does not spread in an orderly manner and cancer cells metastasize through the bloodstream and lymphatic system to other tissues and organs such as skin, regional lymph nodes, or more distant sites, including bone, lung, liver, and brain. Because breast cancer is a systemic disease, less radical, more breast-conserving surgical procedures are done in combination with radiation therapy, hormonal therapy, or chemotherapy.

Soon after a biopsy-proven diagnosis of breast cancer, the client should consult with a team of interdisciplinary consultants before deciding on the definitive approach to management of her breast cancer. Most insurance companies encourage this consultation because there are numerous approaches to the management of breast cancer and an interdisciplinary approach is not only most advantageous for the client but also most efficient and cost-effective. The interdisciplinary team generally includes a medical oncologist, a radiation oncologist, and a surgical oncologist. An oncology nurse, a nutritionist, and a psycho-oncologist are also vital members of the team, because many clients have questions concerning quality of life, how to maintain nutrition, and ways to promote communication among family members.

PRIMARY BREAST CANCER

Carcinoma in situ (meaning that the cancer has not invaded the tissue of origin) is becoming more of an issue in local control of breast cancer, owing to the success of mammography in detecting these small cancers. DCIS is generally managed by local excision with or without radiation. The risk of local recurrence following breast-sparing surgery is approximately 10% at 10 years. Whether radiation therapy is necessary for all clients is uncertain. Some clients with DCIS may be appropriately treated with excision alone. Selection criteria relate to the client's age, tumor size, grade, margin, willingness to accept potential increased risk of local recurrence, and other health problems.[10] The addition of tamoxifen as therapeutic as well as prophylactic treatment following local treatment is gaining acceptance. (See the Integrat-

ing Pharmacology feature on Medications for Breast Cancer on p. 1097.) Women require scheduled diagnostic follow-up mammograms along with physician examination every 6 to 12 months.

LCIS has historically been considered a risk factor for breast cancer rather than a precursor lesion. However, a recent report by Page et al suggests that LCIS may actually carry more risk for a subsequent invasive cancer in the affected breast than was previously thought and that wide local excision may be more appropriate than watchful waiting.[40a] Following local excision options for management range from careful observation and mammography at 6- to 12-month intervals to bilateral prophylactic mastectomy—options that for many women appear either too conservative or too extreme. The physician-nurse team needs to explain the options carefully and permit time for the client to understand her risks and choices for management.

Management of localized invasive breast cancer has changed dramatically since the mid-1980s. Approximately 30% of women with breast cancer are currently managed with breast-conserving surgery. Many more women are candidates for this procedure, but surgeons are reluctant to change, and research takes many years and thousands of clients to prove that one form of therapy is superior to another. However, several studies have indicated that breast-conserving treatments, consisting of the removal of the primary tumor by some form of lumpectomy with or without irradiation to the breast, may result in survival that is equal to that of more extensive procedures, including mastectomy and modified radical mastectomy.[1] Similarly, the addition of radiation therapy to mastectomy does not improve 10-year survival rates and is not indicated if the surgical margins are clear and if no other factors place the client at high risk for local recurrence. However, recent studies have suggested a survival advantage for women with positive axillary nodes even after mastectomy and axillary node dissection. The current NCCN guidelines call for consideration of postmastectomy irradiation in women such as these.[44]

At the time of the initial consultation, a plan of care is devised and the goal of therapy is determined. It is crucial to identify clients at substantial risk for recurrence because they do benefit from systemic therapy. Likewise, in a woman with a tumor smaller than 1 cm with no evidence of axillary node involvement, there is little justification for adjuvant chemotherapy. When the tumor is larger than 1 cm and there is evidence of axillary lymph node involvement, other parameters are assessed, such as estrogen receptor status and measures of tumor growth rate. These help determine not only the need for adjuvant chemotherapy but also whether a doxorubicin-containing regimen is appropriate. For example, tumors with a high proportion of cells in the S phase of cell division are associated with a greater risk of relapse, and chemotherapy offers a greater survival benefit. Cancers that lack either estrogen or progesterone receptors are more likely to recur than those that are estrogen receptor positive and progesterone receptor positive. Tumors with a poor nuclear grade have a higher degree of recurrence than tumors with a good nuclear grade.

Tumors that overexpress HER-2/neu protein (c-erbB2) or that have a mutated p53 gene have a poorer prognosis. Tumors that overexpress HER-2/neu protein are more likely to respond to higher doses of doxorubicin. (The presence of c-erbB2 is determined at the time of surgery and usually appears on the pathology report.) HER-2/neu status (positive or negative) is usually considered in therapeutic decisions about the use of a doxorubicin- or taxane-containing regimen.

■ Surgical Management

The extent of the surgical intervention is determined by the clinical presentation and by the possibility of resecting the tumor with clean margins. The goal is to preserve the breast, because there is no evidence that a mastectomy is more beneficial than lumpectomy plus radiation therapy. However, because of size or the multifocal or multicentric extent of disease, a mastectomy may be necessary to provide adequate tumor removal.

Breast-Preserving Procedures

Indications. Breast-preserving procedures are selected for stage I and stage II breast cancers. Such conservative surgical approaches may be appropriate, depending on the size of the primary tumor. Clients with small invasive cancers generally require a wide local excision under local or general anesthesia for partial mastectomy involving removal of the tumor plus a 1- to 2-cm margin of normal tissue (lumpectomy). A variation of the procedure is the quadrantectomy (removal of the quadrant of the breast in which the cancer is located).

Radiation therapy is begun once healing is confirmed, as long as the client is not receiving a doxorubicin- or taxane-containing regimen. If the individual is to receive either of these two chemotherapeutic agents plus radiation, then the radiation therapy commences 3 weeks after the last course of chemotherapy. If the client is to receive methotrexate (Mexate) and 5-fluorouracil (5-FU) with or without cyclophosphamide (Cytoxan), the radiotherapy may begin with the chemotherapy, may be sandwiched in after the third course and continued for 5 to 6 weeks, or may begin a few weeks after the last course of chemotherapy.

Contraindications. Breast-conserving surgery is not performed when women cannot tolerate irradiation because of prior radiation therapy to the breast or chest wall, pregnancy, or pre-existing rheumatic disorders, such as arthritis, lupus, and scleroderma. Other contraindications are extensive intraductal involvement requiring a wide incision, the presence of two cancers simultaneously in the same breast, diffuse malignant microcalcifications throughout the breast, and large, aggressive tumors. Client preference for a complete breast removal, client fear of radiation side effects, and inability to travel to and from a radiation therapy facility are additional contraindications.

Complications. Although rare, infection, cellulitis, hematoma, and, less commonly, lymphedema may occur after the surgery.

Outcomes. After breast-conserving surgery with radiation therapy or chemotherapy or both, the client will remain free of cancer and its recurrence.

Mastectomy

Indications. Mastectomy is the treatment of choice when the following apply:
- The tumor involves the nipple-areola complex
- The tumor is larger than 7 cm
- The tumor exhibits extensive intraductal disease involving multiple quadrants of the breast
- The woman cannot comply with daily radiation therapy

A *modified radical mastectomy* is an en bloc removal of the breast, axillary lymph nodes, and overlying skin, with the muscles left intact. Owing to more sophisticated diagnostic techniques that detect breast cancers of a smaller size and at an earlier stage, this procedure is done much less frequently than it was 10 years ago. In a *total* or *simple* prophylactic *mastectomy*, used most commonly to prevent cancer in high-risk women, breast tissue and some skin are removed, including the nipple and areola complex. Lymph nodes are not removed in a prophylactic mastectomy.

Contraindications. Although not contraindicated for treatment of small tumors, mastectomy is usually not used for stage I and stage II tumors unless the client prefers this approach.

Complications. Possible complications of breast surgery include lymphedema, infection, seroma, hematoma, and cellulitis. Because clients are often discharged from the hospital within a few days of surgery, they should be taught to report any unusual manifestations early. Any evidence of infection, such as fever, chills, or an area of redness or inflammation along the incision line, should be reported to the physician. Any increase in drainage, foul odor, or separation at the incision site should be reported immediately.

Outcomes. After surgery and adjuvant chemotherapy or radiation therapy, the client will remain free of cancer and its recurrence. If a cancer-free state cannot be achieved, the focus is on promoting quality of life for the client. See the Clinical Pathway on Mastectomy on the *evolve* website.

Axillary Dissection

The role of axillary dissection is in transition. In women with clinically negative node disease and a primary tumor that is 1 to 2 cm in size, a node dissection is probably not necessary.[1] The NCCN Practice Guidelines state that in clients who have particularly favorable tumors, those in whom the selection of adjuvant systemic therapy will not be altered, and older clients or those with serious comorbid conditions, axillary node dissection could be considered optional.[10] The number of positive axillary nodes may help determine the need for chemotherapy as well as whether more aggressive therapy is required. Information regarding nodal status is also valuable in determining prognosis and eligibility for research protocols and high-dose chemotherapy regimens.

Recognizing that most women with breast cancer benefit from adjuvant chemotherapy, hormonal therapy, or both, some authorities claim that it is no longer necessary to determine the status of the axillary lymph nodes in clients with breast cancer. However, the lymph node status in clients with early breast cancer remains the most powerful predictor of recurrence and survival. Furthermore, nearly one third of clients with clinically negative nodes are found to have pathologically involved nodes. Information obtained from pathologic examination of axillary lymph nodes frequently changes the adjuvant therapy plan for women with nonpalpable axillary lymph nodes.[62]

In some cases, axillary node dissection is not necessary because its findings would not affect the choice of therapy. For example, a client presenting with a large primary cancer or evidence of metastatic disease that requires extensive surgery does not need an axillary dissection, nor does a client undergoing mastectomy for a tumor greater than 5 cm or a client in whom the surgical margins are positive for residual tumor. In both of these cases, the risk of local recurrence is sufficiently high to warrant the use of postmastectomy radiotherapy to the chest wall and supraclavicular areas. Women who have four or more positive axillary lymph nodes also are at increased risk for local recurrence; chest wall and regional lymph node irradiation is recommended in this setting and has been shown to substantially reduce the risk of local recurrence.[10]

Sentinel Node Biopsy

Nodal assessment may be conducted using the sentinel node biopsy, a diagnostic test to determine the status of regional lymph nodes. The sentinel node is the first lymph node to receive lymphatic drainage from a tumor. The node can be detected by injection of a blue dye or radioactive colloid around the primary tumor, which travels to and identifies the first draining (sentinel) node. The sentinel lymph node can reveal whether there are lymphatic metastases, making extensive axillary dissection obsolete.[48]

The procedure is technically challenging but has been rapidly adopted into clinical practice because of the advantages it offers over traditional axillary node dissection.[52] Clients who have sentinel node procedures versus axillary node dissections may have less lymphedema, numbness, pain, and arm stiffness; increased arm mobility and arm strength; and better quality of life scores.[62] Specific recommendations for its use, training, and interpretation of results have been addressed recently.[48] The AJCC staging guidelines were revised in 2002 to reflect sentinel node information, and the specific use of these results to plan care is continuing to be evaluated.[51]

■ Nursing Management of the Surgical Client

Preoperative Care
Assessment

The preoperative time, before the biopsy for breast cancer and before a woman knows whether she has cancer in her breast or not, is extremely stressful, constituting a psychological emergency. To put off the biopsy for more than just a few days is often impossible for the woman once a cancer is suspected. Once the diagnosis is established, the woman can return to the routines of her life, or if the biopsy result is positive, she can begin to mobilize her resources to determine the next step. Initially, the woman may be in shock and perhaps even denial, because her decision to undergo the biopsy procedure may have been based largely on her recognition that 8 of 10 breast masses are benign. A few days are often needed for the woman to recover from the diagnosis of cancer before beginning the consultation process.

Most women do not sign consent for an immediate surgical resection or mastectomy upon evidence of a positive biopsy result. Generally, women are given ample time to evaluate the options for management once the diagnosis is confirmed. Most authorities recommend that definitive surgery be performed within 2 weeks of the biopsy, but some women need more time to sort through the copious literature before deciding on a course of treatment. Physicians are required to present the risks and benefits of each of the numerous treatment options for breast cancer and to allow the woman to choose her course of treatment. The options include (1) mastectomy alone, (2) mastectomy with immediate reconstruction, and (3) breast-preserving treatment. Because there is no absolute right answer for many women, each option must be fully considered. Every woman with breast cancer deserves time to deliberate and to participate actively in the decision-making process. Because the possibilities for treatment may be overwhelming, it is appropriate to refer the woman to a comprehensive breast center in which all disciplines are available to address her concerns regarding therapy.

The plan for treatment, which may include surgery, radiation therapy, chemotherapy, hormone therapy, or biologic immunomodulation therapy, is laid out before treatment is begun. In addition, clients should be offered a research protocol if they are eligible. Be familiar with these multimodality protocols for treating breast cancer. It is an enormous challenge to help clients understand and feel confident in their decisions regarding therapy. To be knowledgeable about the client's options for therapy, make every effort to be present for the initial discussion between the physicians and the client and family. Then clarify any misconceptions the client and family members may have, and reinforce what they have been told regarding the therapy.

Diagnosis, Outcomes, Interventions

Diagnosis: Deficient Knowledge.
The nursing diagnosis may be expressed as *Deficient Knowledge related to inexperience and new information regarding available options for treatment.*

Outcomes. The client will understand the available treatment options, as evidenced by her questions and statements concerning options and her ability to explain her choice.

Interventions

Explain Options. The woman should receive information about recommendations and treatment options before surgery or treatment is initiated. The nurse can help women understand treatment options.[1]

Initiate Teaching Plan. Because the typical hospital stay for a modified radical mastectomy or lumpectomy and axillary node dissection surgery is 1 to 3 days, preoperative teaching is done on an outpatient basis, usually in the physician's office. Give clients written instructions regarding postoperative care, including wound care and hand and arm care. Some clients may even go home the day of their surgery. There is some evidence that clients who are discharged early may not have as much anxiety and depression as clients who have longer hospital stays after surgery.[35] With appropriate support at home and visits from home care nurses, this may be an excellent option for some clients. Nursing assessment provides data about knowledge deficits for use in formulating a teaching plan. This plan includes preoperative activities, explanations of surgery, postoperative care, discharge planning, and a discussion of any limitations the woman

may have as a result of surgery. Encourage the woman to question her physicians about lymph node dissection versus lymph node sampling. Because the woman's anxiety level may be so high that she cannot remember new information, it is important to provide written as well as oral instructions. Give instructions in the presence of a family member. Because clients are discharged early postoperatively, they also need emergency phone numbers and instructions regarding whom to call if they have a question or a problem after discharge. Evaluate the client's and family members' learning, and repeat information as often as is necessary.

Diagnosis: Risk for Ineffective Individual Coping and Risk for Compromised Family Coping.
The nursing diagnosis may be expressed as *Ineffective Individual Coping and Compromised Family Coping related to diagnosis of cancer and surgical changes in breast.*

Outcomes. The client will cope with the diagnosis of cancer and surgical changes in the breast, as evidenced by her statement of acceptance and decisions about treatment. Family members will also cope effectively, as evidenced by support given to the client.

Interventions. Preoperatively or before any treatment, assess the client's and significant others' coping ability and concerns. Do not rush the assessment. Identify the coping mechanisms usually used by the client and her significant others. Are there any potentially disabling coping patterns? Use this information as the basis of support. The woman may fear pain, mutilation, death, loss of control, and the hospital environment. Use these findings to establish a plan of care to help the client use positive, growth-producing coping and to avoid disabling coping.

Evaluation

For a positive outcome, the client will be adequately prepared for surgery and its outcomes. Recovery from the surgical procedure is usually uncomplicated. Delayed grieving, even for months following mastectomy, is not uncommon, because intellectually the woman knows the surgery is necessary and because her grief is overshadowed at first by fear of dying.

Postoperative Care
Assessment

Assess the client's psychological reaction to the surgery. Also, inspect the wound and drains, assess for the presence of clinical manifestations of infection and pain, and perform routine postoperative assessments as discussed in Chapter 16.

Diagnosis, Outcomes, Interventions

Diagnosis: Disturbed Body Image.
A nursing diagnosis of *Disturbed Body Image related to impending changes in breast and sexuality* may be appropriate.

Outcomes.
The client will begin to exhibit her presurgical or baseline positive body image, as evidenced by wearing usual make-up and using her own nightgown or other feminine attire after surgery.

Interventions

Initiate Referral. Because the hospital stay is short (1 to 3 days) or that of an outpatient, there may be little opportunity for the woman to express her usual feelings regarding her femininity and the manner in which she might display a positive adaptation to her surgery. In this case, it is appropriate merely to ask the woman if she feels that she or family members might benefit from a consultation with the psycho-oncologist, social worker, or sex therapist. Ask whether she would like to talk to someone who has had a similar surgical procedure, possibly someone from the American Cancer Society's Reach for Recovery program. (See the Case Study feature on Breast Cancer with Mastectomy, below.)

Assess Coping Strategies. Women who undergo surgery for breast cancer experience a sense of loss—changes in life routines, social interactions, self-concept, and body image—and fear of death. Recovery during the postoperative period after mastectomy requires a great deal of energy. Fatigue is a persistent complaint for 6 months or more after surgery. A client's usual coping strategies may not be effective. Not everyone perceives or handles stress in the same way. Displacement, projection, denial, hope, prayer, meditation, stoicism, fatalism, and any combination of these reactions may be used as coping mechanisms. Clients who have surgically lost a breast may adapt in the same way as they would to any loss.

Encourage Self-Care Activities. Effective postoperative care is essential for successful psychosocial and physical rehabilitation. During the 1- to 3-day hospital stay, the focus of nursing care is on recovery from surgery and anesthesia as well as on discharge planning for self-care postoperative management. The client's self-image improves with self-care activities.

Explain Possible Body Image Concerns After Discharge. The full impact of losing a breast or having breast cancer may not be felt until a while after the client goes home. Many women are surprised by events such as the amount of pain and discomfort, marked fatigue, slow incision healing, and arm swelling. Ordinary motions, such as shifting to a comfortable position in bed, may be difficult and painful. As time passes, however, the woman and her significant others reorganize and restructure their lives. During this time, the woman resumes her role in society. Important changes in this role may be necessary. Individual women cope differently; feelings of sexual inadequacy, poor body image, and loss of a sense of femininity are common. Because body image is further altered by weight gain and alopecia if the woman is undergoing chemotherapy, she should be encouraged to purchase a wig and other hair coverings before hair loss. Fatigue, decreased libido, and periods of depression are common in women receiving chemotherapy and radiation therapy. Treatment for cancer may hasten menopause in perimenopausal women or bring the return of manifestations in women who are menopausal but have had to discontinue hormone replacement therapy. Hence, women want to discuss quality of life concerns such as osteoporosis, hot flashes, and mood swings, and ask about the safety of phytoestrogens. See the Evidence-Based Practice in Action feature on Menopausal Manifestations: Safety of Phytoestrogens in Breast Cancer Survivors on p. 1107.

Discuss Strategies to Improve Body Image. Gradually the woman will decide whether to conceal her incision from significant others or let it be seen. The incision may be camouflaged for a woman by an appropriately fitted brassiere or a special bathing suit or evening dress, but doubts and fears about her attractiveness may affect even the most secure woman. You can offer understanding and facilitate communication between the client and significant others. The woman may wish to talk with other breast cancer survivors who have faced similar problems due to breast cancer. Breast cancer support groups may also be beneficial, but they should be composed of women in similar stages of illness. A woman who is undergoing adjuvant therapy for curative breast cancer, for example, may be overwhelmed and fright-

---

CASE STUDY *evolve*
Breast Cancer with Mastectomy

Samantha Guern is a 33-year-old African American who presents to a free health care clinic with complaints of a painless rash on her left breast. She indicates that she does not perform breast self-examination and has not noticed any pain or tenderness in either breast. A mammogram is ordered, and Samantha is informed that a follow-up ultrasound examination and biopsy of the lump may be necessary. Samantha is tearful and asks, "How will I pay for these tests? What if you find something awful?" Consider appropriate responses that the nurse might make. . . .*Case Study continued on the website and the CD-ROM with discussions, multiple-choice questions, and a nursing care plan.* *evolve*

EVIDENCE-BASED PRACTICE IN ACTION

Menopausal Manifestations: Safety of Phytoestrogens in Breast Cancer Survivors

Many women with breast cancer are premenopausal or peri-menopausal. The treatment for cancer may hasten menopause, bringing on premature manifestations such as hot flashes, mood swings, vaginal dryness, and concerns about long-term effects of decreased estrogen such as osteoporosis. Postmenopausal women on hormone replacement therapy (HRT) may have to discontinue HRT when the diagnosis of breast cancer is made. In either case, the outcome is the same, numbers of women must deal with real or potential health and quality of life concerns.

The question of whether soy and other phytoestrogens are appropriate or even helpful for these women is frequently asked.[3] With so much contradictory information regarding hormone therapy and breast cancer risk, it is appropriate to critically analyze the data relevant to the use of phytoestrogens in breast cancer survivors.

Two studies reported no statistical difference in hot flashes between the experimental and control group.[8,10] This is consistent with the literature that indicates a strong placebo effect with any intervention for hot flashes. Long-term effects of phytoestrogens on osteoporosis, cardiovascular disease, and cognitive function have not been well established and in many cases have been contradictory.[1,2,4,5,9]

The safety of using phytoestrogens in women with breast cancer is debated. Some studies indicate isoflavones (a form of phytoestrogens found in soybeans and red clover) may actually reduce the risk of breast cancer, similar to the action of tamoxifen.[1,6] However, two other studies question this conclusion and indicate that genistein may increase cancer risk or tumor growth.[4,7]

The use of phytoestrogens in women who have had breast cancer is complicated by the uncontrolled dosing and packaging of these agents. Although there may be some benefit in taking them, there is no clear evidence that their efficacy can overcome any potential risks in breast cancer clients, particularly those with estrogen receptor–positive disease. The North American Menopause Society recommends that women whose clinicians concur with their decision to use phytoestrogens do so by incorporating whole soy foods into their diet and avoid packaged supplements that may lead to higher doses and potentially negative outcomes.[9]

References

1. Fotsis, T., et al. (1993). Genistein, a dietary-derived inhibitor of in vitro angiogenesis. *Proceedings of the National Academy of Science USA, 90,* 2690-2694.

2. Harris, P.F., et al. (2002). Prevalence and treatment of menopausal symptoms among breast cancer survivors. *Journal of Pain and Symptom Management, 23*(6), 501-509.

3. Loprinzi, C.L., Barton, D.L., & Rhodes, D. (2001). Management of hot flashes in breast-cancer survivors. *Lancet Oncology, 2*(4), 199-204.

4. McMichael-Phillips, D.F., et al. (1998). Effects of soy-protein supplementation on epithelial proliferation in the histologically normal human breast. *American Journal of Clinical Nutrition, 68*(6 suppl.), 1431S-1435S.

5. Messina, M.J., & Loprinzi, C.L. (2001). Soy for breast cancer survivors: A critical review of the literature. *Journal of Nutrition, 131*(11 suppl.), 3095S-3108S.

6. Peterson, G., Barnes, S. (1996). Genistein inhibits both estrogen and growth factor-stimulated proliferation of human breast cancer cells. *Cell Growth Differentiation, 7,* 1345-1351.

7. Petrakis, N.L., et al. (1996). Stimulatory influence of soy protein isolate on breast secretion in pre- and postmenopausal women. *Cancer Epidemiological Biomarkers Preview, 5,* 785-794.

8. Quella, S.K., et al. (2000). Evaluation of soy phytoestrogens for the treatment of hot flashes in breast cancer survivors: A North Central Cancer Treatment Group Trial. *Journal of Clinical Oncology, 18*(5), 1068-1074.

9. The role of isoflavones in menopausal health: Consensus opinion of the North American Menopause Society. (2000). *Menopause: The Journal of the North American Menopause Society, 7*(4), 215-229.

10. Van Patten, C.L., et al. (2002). Effect of soy phytoestrogens of hot flashes in postmenopausal women with breast cancer: A randomized, controlled clinical trial. *Journal of Clinical Oncology, 20*(6), 1449-1455.

ened by the discussions and concerns of women with advanced metastatic breast cancer.

Diagnosis: Risk for Impaired Skin Integrity. The nursing diagnosis may be expressed as *Risk for Impaired Skin Integrity related to surgery or radiation therapy.*

Outcomes. The client will remain free of impairment in skin integrity after surgery or radiation therapy, as evidenced by healing skin without redness, infection, hematoma formation, or breakdown.

Interventions

Provide and Explain Dressing and Drain Care. Postoperatively, a pressure dressing is usually used initially. Explain that a drain, connected to gentle suction, prevents blood or serum collection in the operative space after a modified radical mastectomy or axillary node dissection.

Instruct the woman about emptying the drain and recording the amount of drainage. Advise her to notify the physician if the drain becomes plugged or dislodged, or shows any sign of infection, or if frank bleeding develops.

When changing the dressing, gently encourage the woman to look at the incision. Seeing the incision for the first time is often difficult, but the nurse's matter-of-fact approach can help. In future dressing changes, teach methods of cleaning the incision at home and of watching for manifestations of infection.

Prevent Skin Complications Following Radiation Therapy. During radiation therapy, scaling, flaking, dryness, itching, erythema, hair loss, rash, or dry desquamation of the involved skin may occur. Careful treatment of the skin is important in minimizing the skin effects of radiation therapy. Instruct women not to wash the area with soap but to rinse it with water only. No lotion or powder is to be put on the skin that overlies the radiation port. If the area under the arm becomes reddened because of friction, moisture, or radiation damage, place soft, clean gauze pad between skinfolds to prevent skin breakdown.

Diagnosis: Risk for Injury. The nursing diagnosis may be expressed as *Risk for Injury related to increased risk of infection and lymphedema secondary to axillary node dissection.*

Outcomes. The client will not experience injury, as evidenced by absence of infection or lymphedema.

Interventions. Arm edema (e.g., lymphedema) occurs less commonly than in the past owing to the performance of less extensive mastectomy procedures and less extensive axillary dissection. Lymphedema results from insufficient transport of water and protein from the skin and subcutaneous tissue because of an inadequate development or eradication of lymphatic vessels. Lymphedema following axillary dissection has been reported in as many as 70% of cases, although probably a more accurate estimate of the average occurrence of lymphedema as a significant consequence of local therapy for breast cancer is 20% in the United States and Europe.[1] Clearly the major risk for lymphedema exists when complete axillary dissection with stripping of the axillary vein and nodal irradiation is combined with mastectomy.

Older age, obesity, and lifting of heavy objects such as grocery bags and suitcases are also thought to increase the risk of lymphedema. Arm edema, stiffness, pain, and numbness have been reported in 40% to 50% of clients approximately 1 month after beginning radiation therapy to the axilla. Lymphedema occurring years after surgery or radiation

therapy is generally the result of infection, inflammation, or recurrent tumor.

Prevent Lymphedema. In the early postoperative period, encourage arm exercises, (see the Client Education Guide on Postmastectomy Exercises on p. 1109) elevate the arm on a pillow so that the elbow is level with the heart and the hand rests just higher than the elbow. The goal is to promote lymphatic drainage and prevent infection.

Administer Antibiotics for Infection. If a woman complains of redness, swelling, and a generalized area of warmth on the affected arm with or without fever, she should be examined for possible infection in the hand or arm. If an infection is present, the woman may need to be admitted to the hospital for intravenous antibiotics to treat the infection. Such infections can occur from a slight cut on the hand, and even though they may seem innocuous, they pose a serious threat to these clients.

Minimize Lymphedema. Wearing an elastic bandage or a custom-fitted pressure-gradient elastic sleeve may be helpful in the months following surgery if lymphedema is present. Some women think that wearing a sleeve while they are on an airplane minimizes swelling due to pressure changes in the airplane, although no studies have confirmed the efficacy of this practice.

Emphasize that it is important to prevent lymphedema. Once lymphedema occurs, it is more likely to occur again and be progressive. This is because the tissue, like a balloon, is a potential space that, once expanded, will expand again to that size and beyond with little provocation.

Available treatments include application of compression garments, intermittent pneumatic compression, and massage by a trained physiotherapist. Clients can obtain more information from the National Breast Cancer Coalition, the International Society of Lymphology, and the Oncology Nursing Society.

Evaluation

The client who has undergone breast surgery for cancer will be discharged from the hospital 24 to 72 hours postoperatively. The surgical wounds may be healed within 4 weeks. Regaining complete use of the affected arm and shoulder may take as long as 6 weeks to several months, depending on the extent of the surgical procedure, rate of healing, compliance with exercises, and the degree of postoperative complications.

■ Self-Care

To promote self-care, the client needs to learn about postoperative arm exercises, postoperative care, and care of the breast prosthesis. A referral to Reach for Recovery may also be helpful.

CLIENT EDUCATION GUIDE
Postmastectomy Exercises

When to Begin	Purpose	Exercises: Perform Exercises 5-10 Times Each, Three Times a Day
Postoperative days 1-5	Prevent and/or reduce swelling	Position arm against your side in a relaxed position. Elbow should be level with your heart, with the wrist just above the elbow when resting. Rotate wrist in a circular fashion. Touch fingers to shoulder and extend arm fully.
After drains are removed	Promote muscle movement without stretching	While standing, brace yourself with your other arm and bend over slightly, allowing your affected arm to hang freely. Swing the arm in small circles and gradually increase in size. Make 10 circles—rest—repeat in the opposite direction. Swing arm forward and back as far as you can without pulling on the incision. While standing, bend over slightly and swing arms across the chest in each direction. While sitting in a chair, rest both arms at your side. Shrug both shoulders, then relax. While sitting or standing, pull shoulders back, bring the shoulder blades together.
After sutures are removed	To stretch and regain full range of motion. To gain mobility of your shoulder, you must move it in *all* directions, several times a day	While lying in bed with arm extended, raise arm over your head and extend backwards. While lying in bed, grasp a cane or short pole with both hands across your lap. Extend arms straight up and over your head and return. Repeat, rotating the cane clockwise and then counterclockwise while over your head. While standing, extend arm straight over your head and down. Extend your elbow out from your side at a 90° angle—hold it for 10 seconds—relax. Extend your arm straight out from your side even with your shoulder—extend arm straight up toward the ceiling. Stand at arm's length facing a wall. Extend arms so your fingertips touch the wall. Creep fingers up the side of the wall, stepping forward as necessary. Repeat the procedure going down the wall—keep arms extended. Stand sideways to the wall. Extend arm out so fingers touch the wall. Creep up the wall a little more each day. Use hand and arm normally.
After 6 weeks	To strengthen arm and shoulder and to regain total use of arm and shoulder	Begin water aerobics. Begin overall fitness program. Begin aerobics, Jazzercise, or other resistive exercises. Avoid using weights, as these may increase arm edema and subsequent swelling.

From Chapman, D., & Goodman, M. (1997). Breast cancer. In S. Groenwald, M. Frogge, & M. Goodman (Eds.), *Cancer nursing principles and practice* (4th ed.), pp. 916-979. Boston: Jones & Bartlett.

Teach Arm Exercises. In the early postoperative period (days 1 and 2), encourage the client to focus on the elbow, wrist, and hand of the affected side. The client performs active elbow flexion and extension, gently squeezes a soft rubber ball, and does deep breathing to facilitate lymph flow. Shoulder shrugs and active range of motion, including flexion and abduction, can be added on the second postoperative day. Encourage self-care activities (e.g., feeding, combing hair, washing face) and other activities that use the arm, with care taken not to abduct the arm or to raise the arm or elbow above shoulder height until the drains are removed.

Approximately 10 days after surgery, the client can begin active assisted range of motion exercises (see Client Education Guide on Postmastectomy Exercises on p. 1109). Tell the client to do these exercises at least twice a day as tolerated. Provide pain medication 30 minutes before exercises to permit the client to perform exercises with reduced pain. Women who do not carry out these exercises as instructed are at greater risk for lymphedema and loss of shoulder joint mobility. (Arrangements for a physical therapist to assist with range of motion and strengthening exercises may need to be made at the same time surgery is planned because of the shortened hospital stay.) Always provide written and oral instructions about arm precautions. (See the Client Education Guide feature on Arm Care After Axillary Lymph Node Dissection on the website.)

Refer to Reach for Recovery. The Reach for Recovery program of the American Cancer Society is a rehabilitation program for breast cancer survivors, specifically those who have had breast surgery. This program helps women meet common psychosocial, physical, and cosmetic needs. With authorization of the physician and the client's permission, volunteers from this program visit the hospital or the home and give the woman information and help, including the following:

1. A kit, ball, book, rope, and temporary soft cotton prosthesis for women who have had a mastectomy
2. Instruction sheet for and demonstration of postoperative axillary node dissection exercises
3. Discussion of brassiere comfort, various breast prostheses, clothing adjustments, and personal problems as appropriate

Provide Breast Prosthesis. Women who have had a mastectomy may wear a temporary lightweight prosthesis immediately after the sutures and drains are removed. This may facilitate adjustment to the loss of the breast. A soft cotton breast form may be supplied by the Reach for Recovery visitor; cotton padding inserted into a pocket sewn into a lightweight brassiere is also a good temporary substitute. A permanent prosthesis should not be purchased until the wound has healed completely because the contours of the incision site may change. Cocoa butter may be rubbed into the incision once healing has occurred to help soften the scar and prevent scar contracture.

Some women choose breast reconstruction. If a woman chooses to have a prosthesis, even temporarily while considering breast reconstruction, she should choose one that is appropriate for her. A breast prosthesis may be purchased in foundation departments in most large stores or at medical-surgical supply stores that sell durable medical equipment. Most of these stores have experienced sales associates to help women obtain the proper fit. Most private and government insurance plans pay for at least the first breast prosthesis and brassiere,

as long as a written prescription from the physician accompanies the receipt. Many plans also pay for yearly replacements.

■ Surgical Management for Breast Reconstruction

Many women have feelings of loss, depression, and alterations in body image after mastectomy. Breast reconstruction is an accepted component of the treatment plan. In the 1990s, improvements were made to surgical prostheses and surgical techniques, helping women become more confident in their choice to have reconstructive surgery and retain their self-confidence and body image, thereby enhancing their quality of life. The goal for clients having reconstructive surgery is to "feel whole again." This includes appearing "normal" in a bathing suit as well as in the nude.

The only contraindications to breast reconstruction are the client's need for chest wall irradiation and the physical inability to withstand additional surgery due to a co-morbid condition. Breast reconstruction is not contraindicated by a woman's age, her need for adjuvant chemotherapy, a poor prognosis, or even the presence of metastatic disease. The timing of the breast reconstruction may be immediate (at the time of the mastectomy) or delayed, even until years after mastectomy. When adjuvant chemotherapy is planned, the surgeon may prefer to wait until the chemotherapy is completed to begin reconstructing the breast.

Several surgical techniques can be used to reconstruct the breast mound and nipple-areola complex. The choice of technique is based upon the client's wishes, the amount of tissue available, and whether the woman has had radiation therapy in the past. The simplest method of reconstruction involves the insertion of an implant into a pocket of skin purposely left by the surgeon. This approach is best for women with small or moderate-size breasts, in whom the implant is of a size similar to the remaining breast. Other methods of reconstruction include the following.

Tissue Expanders

A tissue expander is a deflated silicone envelope that is inserted under the chest muscles and expanded slowly over 6 to 8 weeks by adding 60 to 200 ml of saline per week via a remote percutaneous injection port. When the skin overlying the breast mound is sufficiently overinflated to accommodate the implant comfortably, the expander is removed and the implant is inserted. Many times the expanded implant is expanded to become the permanent implant.

Transverse Rectus Abdominis Muscle Flap

The transverse rectus abdominis muscle (TRAM) flap procedure is commonly referred to as the "tummy tuck." A low transverse elliptical incision is made, and abdom-

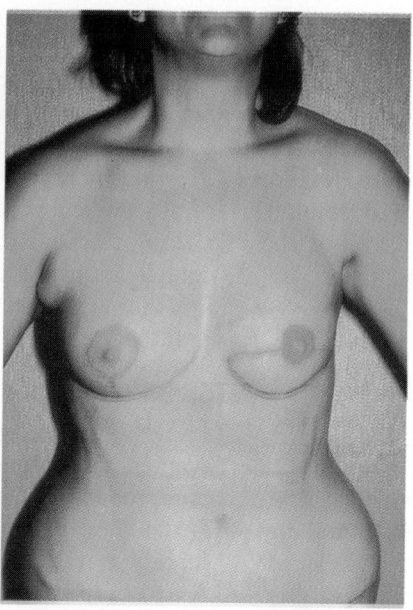

FIGURE 42-4 Breast reconstruction using transverse rectus abdominis myocutaneous flaps. **A,** Preoperative appearance. **B,** Postoperative appearance.

FIGURE 42-5 An ideal result of reconstructive surgery using a latissimus dorsi myocutaneous flap and an implant. **A,** Preoperative appearance. **B,** Postoperative appearance. A subpectoral implant is used in the right breast for symmetry.

inal muscle and fat are tunneled under the abdominal skin to the mastectomy site. Tissue viability and perfusion are retained by the superior epigastric vessel. The tissue can also be transferred as a free flap. The donor site in the abdomen is closed as for a modified abdominoplasty (Figure 42-4). Contraindications to the TRAM flap are the presence of abdominal scars and inadequate abdominal tissue.

Latissimus Dorsi Muscle Flap

The latissimus dorsi muscle, a large fan-shaped muscle beneath the scapula, is used when inadequate skin is available at the mastectomy site. It is considered an expendable muscle because alternative muscle groups are able to adduct the humerus and rotate the shoulder posteriorly. An ellipse of skin along with the latissimus

dorsi muscle is tunneled through the axilla and rotated onto the mastectomy site. The viability of the tissue is maintained through the thoracodorsal vessels (Figure 42-5).

Gluteal Muscle Free Flaps

A much less common form of breast construction involves the use of the gluteus muscle. The muscle and overlying skin are lifted from their bed and connected to the chest wall using an operating microscope.

Nipple-Areola Reconstruction

Some women elect also to have the nipple-areola reconstructed. To achieve symmetry, nipple reconstruction should be delayed for several months following breast reconstruction. During the healing process, the contour of the reconstructed breast may change as the incisions heal and edema subsides. Areola can be reconstructed with a tattoo or by nipple sharing. The dark tissue of the areola is most commonly reconstructed by tattooing. Nipple projection is constructed with a skate flap (Figure 42-6). Many years ago, the nipple was removed from the breast before amputation and stored ("banked") on the inner thigh. This procedure is no longer performed because of the risk of cancer spread.

■ Nursing Management of the Client with Breast Reconstruction

Preoperative Care
Preoperatively, the nurse reinforces the physician's instructions regarding the goals of reconstruction and any postoperative care needs. It is important that the client have realistic expectations of the outcome of the surgery. The client may be shown pictures of reconstructed breasts to familiarize her with what can be achieved. The client may express anger, disbelief, and fear related to the surgery, especially if the reconstruction is being combined with a mastectomy for a known carcinoma. Many women will at the same time express relief that the cancer surgery is being done and the cancer is being removed. Some will find comfort in discussing their feelings of disbelief at this time. Periods of depression are normal.

Encourage clients to express their feelings and fears with family members and to seek assistance from the psycho-oncology service or chaplain if appropriate. Assess risks for anesthesia-related problems and operative blood loss before surgery. Advise any client who smokes cigarettes to stop, because smoking compromises flap and skin circulation.

Postoperative Care
In addition to providing the postoperative nursing care required by any person having surgery, after reconstructive breast surgery you will assess the flap or breast area

FIGURE 42-6 Nipple-areola reconstruction.

for color, temperature, and capillary refill. If any area appears dusky and congested with blood, the flap may be suffering from venous obstruction. A flap that is pale is not receiving blood and may be experiencing arterial constriction. Whenever circulation or perfusion is in question, notify the physician immediately. The success of this surgical procedure is directly dependent on astute nursing assessment and proper physician notification of complications. Laser Doppler flow may be used to monitor skin perfusion after free flap transfer.

Inform a woman with a recent subpectoral implant that initially the implant feels very firm and is higher on the chest than a normal breast. Over time, the muscle stretches, allowing the implant to drop and soften. Women with subpectoral implants do not wear bras, because the implant needs to move into the pocket created in the chest wall. Women who undergo other types of surgery may return from the operating room wearing a bra to support the breasts. A front-closing support bra without underwires is preferred. Wearing a bra also helps some women feel more normal, encouraging a return to wellness. Psychosocial readjustment to breast reconstruction, including incorporation of the reconstructed breast into the woman's body image, usually occurs 3 to 4 months after surgery. A recent study indicated that writing letters to their new/lost breasts may facilitate the adjustment of breast cancer clients to their reconstructed breasts.[43a]

■ Medical Management
Eliminate or Prevent Spread of Cancer. After surgery or instead of surgery, it may be possible to prevent further extension of cancer or to completely eliminate the cancer cells by using radiation therapy, chemotherapy, or hormonal therapy.

Radiation Therapy. Radiation therapy is used in breast cancer treatment as follows:
- The breast and underlying chest wall are irradiated after lumpectomy or quadrantectomy as adjuvant therapy for stage I or II breast cancer.
- Women who are poor surgical candidates because of health problems such as heart disease typically receive radiation therapy to the affected breast.
- The chest wall is irradiated if it is involved or for local control after mastectomy with positive margins.
- The axilla is irradiated in women at high risk for axillary metastases who are poor surgical candidates for axillary dissection or who have gross disease that was not surgically excised.
- The supraclavicular region is irradiated if positive axillary nodes are found.
- Additional areas are irradiated for management of metastatic disease to the brain, bone, or skin.

Radiation in combination with lumpectomy or quadrantectomy is an accepted treatment for early-stage breast cancer. An axillary dissection or a sentinel node biopsy is usually done for staging purposes. Radiation therapy, when used to treat micrometastatic disease following mastectomy, successfully reduces the risk of local recurrence and therefore of distant metastases. The utility of radiation therapy following mastectomy or modified radical mastectomy comes into question when the client is also receiving adjuvant chemotherapy, tamoxifen, or both. (See the Integrating Pharmacology feature on Medications for Breast Cancer on p. 1097.) Recent studies indicate a survival advantage for radiation therapy in postmastectomy node-positive women.[10] However, the use of postoperative radiation therapy is not indicated in clients with negative axillary nodes except when there is evidence of disease at the deep margins of the tumor.

When chemotherapy is given with radiation therapy, the radiotherapy may be given concomitantly or sandwiched with the chemotherapy, or given sequentially after completion of the chemotherapy. Concomitant therapy results in a greater incidence of skin reactions than has been reported with sequential treatment. The only situation in which radiation therapy might be given before chemotherapy is in a case in which there are negative axillary nodes (and therefore low risk for distant disease) and positive surgical margins, when the risk for local recurrence is great. The real risk to women with breast cancer is systemic disease. Therefore chemotherapy is critically important to eradicate any micrometastatic disease wherever it may be, including the chest.

Radiation therapy can be administered through an external beam or via brachytherapy or iridium implants. For external beam irradiation, the radiation is administered on an outpatient basis 5 days a week for 5 to 6 weeks to the entire breast (and possibly the lymphatics),

usually with a boost to the tumor bed. The total dose of radiation is approximately 5000 rads. Regional lymph nodes may be treated if they have not been removed.

Interstitial implant therapy using iridium[192] (Ir) is an in-hospital procedure. The insertion of the iridium implant may be done using local anesthesia. Stainless steel guide needles are threaded through the tumor area at 1-cm intervals. Flexible plastic tubes are inserted in the guide needles. The guide needles are then removed, leaving the tube in place. Strands of radioactive iridium seeds are threaded through each tube (Figure 42-7). The seeds, at 1-cm intervals, form a grid with those above and below to cover the tissues evenly with radiation.

At the end of the insertion procedure, a button is attached to the end of the tubes and the ends are crimped and cut to prevent the seeds from falling out. An x-ray film confirms the location of the implant. The implant usually must remain in place for 2 or 3 days. The procedure is mildly uncomfortable. The woman is able to be up and about in her room. Radiation precautions related to time, distance, and shielding are maintained (see Chapter 19). Because of the excellent results from breast reconstruction, most women opt for complete tumor removal rather than the use of implants, which potentially leave residual disease behind. A new method of administering brachytherapy involves using a tiny bag that is inflated inside the surgical cavity. The radiation source is placed and the client is finished with her radiation in a week. Studies show that in a select group of screen-detected, node-negative women with tumors less than 1 cm, the Mammocite brachytherapy device may reduce the time, inconvenience, and toxicity associated with traditional radiotherapy.[58]

FIGURE 42-7 Radiation therapy is given via an external beam (**A**) or iridium implants (**B**).

Side effects of radiation therapy to the breast include the following:

- Temporary skin changes such as itching, dryness, tenderness, redness, swelling, and dry desquamation
- Moist desquamation, especially in skinfolds
- Fatigue
- Dry throat may occur owing to radiation scatter, especially if the supraclavicular area is irradiated
- Pneumonitis (rare), which may present as a dry cough and dyspnea, a result of inflammatory changes in the irradiated underlying lung
- Arm edema (rare), occurring more commonly with axillary irradiation
- Increased susceptibility to rib fracture in the irradiated field
- Difficulty in obtaining optimal doses of chemotherapy in women receiving chemotherapy concurrently with radiation therapy because of the effect of radiation on bone marrow

Radiation therapy can be emotionally taxing and physically fatiguing. Nursing support is needed during the 5- to 7-week treatment period. Women receiving radiation therapy have many of the same fears as those having a mastectomy: fear of death, fear of mutilation, and feelings of sexual inadequacy. These are compounded by the stress of daily treatment and the fatigue that occurs with coping with a chronic illness, often while recovering from the side effects of chemotherapy. (See the Complementary and Alternative Therapy feature on Pentoxifylline and Vitamin E for Previously Treated Breast Cancer Clients to Reduce Radiation-Induced Fibrosis, above.)

Systemic Chemotherapy

Localized Breast Cancer. Adjuvant systemic chemotherapy for early stage I and stage II breast cancer generally follows local surgical intervention and includes combinations of cyclophosphamide (Cytoxan), doxorubicin (Adriamycin), methotrexate (Mexate), 5-fluorouracil (5-FU), paclitaxel (Taxol), and docetaxel (Taxotere), with or without tamoxifen (Nolvadex or Anastrozole). Six cycles of cyclophosphamide, methotrexate, and 5-fluorouracil (CMF) and four cycles of doxorubicin and cyclophosphamide with methotrexate, 5-fluorouracil, or leucovorin (Wellcovorin) all are standard adjuvant (curative) therapy for breast cancer.

For the most part, clients are divided into three groups: those who have no involved axillary lymph nodes, those with one to three involved nodes, and those with four or more involved nodes. Adjuvant systemic therapy is usually not given to women whose tumors are 0.5 cm or less in greatest diameter and without lymph node involvement. Clients whose tumors are larger than 0.5 cm but less than 1 cm and without lymph node involvement may be divided into those with a low risk of

COMPLEMENTARY AND ALTERNATIVE THERAPY

Pentoxifylline and Vitamin E for Previously Treated Breast Cancer Clients to Reduce Radiation-Induced Fibrosis

Radiation-induced fibrosis (RIF) is not a common complication of radiation therapy, but it is a condition that needs a treatment. A total of 24 women with 29 RIF areas involving the skin and underlying tissue were involved in this clinical study. These clients were previously irradiated for breast cancer (7 +/− 4 years) and were randomly assigned to 4 groups: 800 mg/day of pentoxifylline (PTX) plus 1000 international units/day of vitamin E; PTX plus placebo; placebo plus vitamin E; and placebo alone.

The primary endpoint was the measure of relative regression in the RIF surface after 6 months of treatment. A total of 22 clients with 27 RIF areas were analyzed at 6 months. Mean RIF surface regression was significant with combined PTX and vitamin E compared to just placebo alone (60% versus 43%; $p = 0.038$). Researchers concluded that 6 months of treatment with PTX plus vitamin E (synergistic effect) can significantly reduce superficial RIF. However, a larger study is obviously needed to determine if these conclusions are accurate.

Reference
Delanian, S., et al. (2003). Randomized, placebo-controlled trial of combined pentoxifylline and tocopherol for regression of superficial radiation-induced fibrosis. *Journal of Clinical Oncology, 21,* 2545-2550.

recurrence and those who have unfavorable prognostic features that warrant consideration of adjuvant therapy. Unfavorable prognostic features include lymphatic invasion, high S phase fraction, high nuclear and histologic grades, and HER-2–positive status.

Clients with lymph node involvement or with tumors larger than 1 cm in diameter are appropriate candidates for adjuvant systemic therapy. Cytotoxic chemotherapy using CMF or a regimen of cyclophosphamide, doxorubicin, and 5-FU (CAF) or just cyclophosphamide and doxorubicin (AC) is appropriate for node-negative clients. For those clients who have positive lymph nodes, chemotherapy regimens that contain an anthracycline (doxorubicin) are preferred. The addition of paclitaxel may be superior to AC alone for node-positive women who are estrogen receptor–negative, particularly in clients who overexpress HER-2/neu.[10] For women who have receptor-positive tumors, tamoxifen therapy for 5 years is also recommended. (See the Integrating Pharmacology feature on Medications for Breast Cancer on p. 1097.) The addition of tamoxifen therapy significantly improves the 10-year survival outlook for this population.[17] The benefit of the addition of tamoxifen therapy to chemotherapy is less clear for women younger than

50 years of age with hormone receptor–positive tumors. The additive benefit of chemotherapy to tamoxifen therapy for women 50 years of age or older with hormone receptor–positive tumors may not provide a large absolute benefit. Therefore the decision to give both adjuvant treatments should be individualized, especially in those women with an already favorable prognosis or in older women with co-morbidities.[10]

The decision to use tamoxifen with or without chemotherapy in women with estrogen receptor–positive disease should be based on the absolute magnitude of risk reduction expected with the systemic therapy and the individual client's willingness to experience toxicity in order to achieve that incremental risk reduction. For women with estrogen receptor–negative disease, the choice is for adjuvant chemotherapy. A meta-analysis has shown that combination chemotherapy on the average produces an absolute improvement of 7% to 11% in 10-year survival rates for women younger than 50 years of age and of 2% to 3% for those aged 50 to 69 years.[17,57]

In some instances, the physician may recommend primary, induction, or "neoadjuvant" chemotherapy (i.e., given before surgery). Primary chemotherapy is beneficial because the physician can evaluate response to chemotherapy directly, which is impossible once the cancer is removed. Therefore the physician can know whether the choice of chemotherapy is optimal. In addition, the tumor may actually shrink so much that the disease may be "downstaged," permitting a breast-preserving procedure.

However, although preoperative chemotherapy was as effective as postoperative chemotherapy, the results have not demonstrated higher cure rates or influenced survival for stage I and II breast cancers. It does, however, offer the opportunity to observe the biologic response of the tumor to the effects of chemotherapy.[29,32,46,54] When given to clients with inflammatory breast cancer, primary chemotherapy permits shrinkage of the tumor and possible mastectomy, whereas without prior chemotherapy, it might not be possible to obtain clear surgical margins.

Advanced Localized Breast Cancer. When a client has more extensive (stage III) yet curable disease, her options and decisions for therapy are even more difficult and controversial. Women with unfavorable stage IIIA or IIIB breast cancers generally require a more aggressive management approach. Affected women typically have larger tumors (>5 cm), direct invasion of the skin of the breast or the chest wall, or fixed or matted axillary lymphadenopathy. Usually, these women undergo preoperative chemotherapy, with or without hormone therapy, followed by surgery and radiotherapy. An alternative approach involves the use of high-dose combination chemotherapy, followed by an additional combination of agents that are also active in breast cancer. The concept is to minimize the risk of drug resistance and to attempt

to kill cells before they have an opportunity to mutate to resistance. The addition of paclitaxel every 3 weeks for four cycles following the standard doxorubicin (Adriamycin) and cyclophosphamide regimen every 3 weeks for four cycles for women with node-positive breast cancer is associated with increased relapse-free survival. However, the 2002 NCCN guidelines state that mature results from this trial and others are required before definitive results can be made. Subsequent analysis of the data from the previous study showed a benefit only in women with estrogen receptor–negative disease.[10]

Other adjuvant treatments under investigation include the combination of paclitaxel and the monoclonal antibody trastuzumab (Herceptin). When these two agents are combined, there appears to be significant synergy with little increased toxicity.[34,54] The most common side effects are acute fever or chills and the potential for cardiac dysfunction. The combination of trastuzumab and anthracyclines is associated with more incidents of cardiac dysfunction; therefore combination chemotherapy with anthracyclines and trastuzumab is not recommended.[34] HER-2 is overexpressed in 25% to 30% of human breast cancers and indicates a worse prognosis in clients who have positive axillary lymph nodes. Despite the association of HER-2 overexpression with poor prognosis, a clinical response to taxanes was three times more likely to occur in HER-2–positive clients than in HER-2–negative clients.[7] Several large, randomized controlled, trials are underway evaluating the use of trastuzumab and paclitaxel as single and combined agents for adjuvant breast cancer. The results of these trials will help clinicians recommend the best treatments for individual clients.[26,54]

Dose intensification requiring the use of colony-stimulating factors or autologous hematopoietic support is not considered standard therapy in adjuvant breast cancer. Research conducted by the National Surgical Adjuvant Breast Project included two randomized trials (NSABP B22 and NSABP B25) of dose intensification, and neither one to date has demonstrated that higher doses of drug given in a compressed time period are superior to standard dosing of the same drugs (doxorubicin and cyclophosphamide).[6,21] Furthermore, the toxicity associated with dose intensification is significant. Although pilot trials of autologous bone marrow transplant procedures for women with multiple positive nodes have shown some success, more research is needed to demonstrate the efficacy of bone marrow transplantation in breast cancer.[5]

■ Nursing Management of the Medical Client Assessment

Nursing management of the woman receiving chemotherapy for breast cancer centers on her need for information and instructions regarding self-care procedures.

Because in most cases the woman undergoes breast surgery in the hospital and goes home 1 to 3 days later, there is often little time to discuss her concerns regarding chemotherapy and radiation therapy. Even though the client does not start these treatments until complete healing has taken place (usually 3 to 4 weeks after surgery), the nurse has an important role in providing the client and family members with information regarding the side effects of chemotherapy and radiation therapy. In planning care, be sure to consider the emotional, social, cognitive, spiritual, and physical impact of the diagnosis and treatment on the woman and her family.

Diagnosis, Outcomes, Interventions

Diagnosis: Effective Therapeutic Regimen Management.
The nursing diagnosis may be expressed as *Effective Therapeutic Regimen Management related to chemotherapy and radiation therapy.*

Outcomes. The client will understand the purpose and goals of chemotherapy and radiation therapy as evidenced by her statements concerning the necessity for treatment and possible side effects associated with that treatment.

Interventions

Teach About Radiation Therapy. Teaching is a major role of the nurse who is caring for clients receiving radiation therapy.

Include in the teaching plan instructions regarding skin care, sun protection, and management of fatigue. If the client is receiving chemotherapy concurrently, there is heightened risk for infection due to neutropenia. Therefore instruct clients to report any evidence of infection. Monitor blood counts on a weekly basis. Tell the client that written materials, including the booklet *Radiation Therapy and You,* are available from the NCI free of charge by calling 1-800-4-CANCER. See Chapter 19 for further information on radiation therapy.

Teach About Chemotherapy. Nurses are responsible for teaching clients about the side effects of chemotherapy. The booklet *Chemotherapy and You* (also available free of charge from the NCI) explains the purpose of chemotherapy and possible side effects. Once the regimen is selected, discuss side effects. Teach the client the names of the drugs, how the drugs are given, expected side effects and their management, preventive measures, and complications that need to be reported to the physician or nurse (e.g., infection, fever, bruising, bleeding, mouth sores).

Vary the teaching plan, depending on the drug regimen selected, because the side effects are different for each of the drugs. For example, not all chemotherapy agents cause hair loss. Women receiving methotrexate and 5-FU do not experience hair loss, whereas women receiving doxorubicin and cyclophosphamide have complete hair loss at 2 to 3 weeks after their first injection. Cyclophosphamide taken orally for 14 days and methotrexate and 5-FU given by injection twice a month cause a gradual thinning of the hair, but generally the woman can get by without a wig, especially if her hair is kept short. Methotrexate and 5-FU can cause diarrhea and stomatitis, which may interrupt therapy. Advise women taking cyclophosphamide by mouth for the 14-day regimen to drink eight glasses of water a day to prevent hemorrhagic cystitis. Paclitaxel may cause neurologic toxicity; therefore clients need to be assessed for difficulty with gait, constipation, and fine motor movements.

Diagnosis: Imbalanced Nutrition: Less Than Body Requirements.
The nursing diagnosis may be expressed as *Imbalanced Nutrition: Less Than Body Requirements related to nausea, vomiting, and stomatitis secondary to chemotherapy.*

Outcomes. The client will maintain adequate nutrition, as evidenced by absence of nausea and vomiting, control of stomatitis, intake of adequate calories, and no or minimal weight loss.

Interventions. Nausea, vomiting, anorexia, stomatitis, and taste change are common side effects of chemotherapy agents. Some drugs, specifically doxorubicin and methotrexate, cause stomatitis 4 to 5 days after the injection.

Provide Oral Hygiene. To minimize the severity of the stomatitis, the client is instructed to perform oral hygiene three to four times a day and to rinse with baking soda and water to maintain a basic environment in the oral cavity. Bacteria thrive in an acid environment. If a client experiences any mouth soreness, she should suck on ice during injection of the chemotherapy agent. This simple form of cryotherapy helps to minimize exposure of the oral cavity to the irritating effects of chemotherapy agents.

Prevent Nausea and Vomiting. Nausea and vomiting are usually preventable when antiemetic medications are taken on a schedule rather than just as needed. A combination of a dopamine antagonist, a serotonin antagonist, and a steroid is usually adequate to prevent nausea and vomiting from chemotherapy. Because chemotherapy slows colonic transit time, clients often experience epigastric distress and bloating after administration of these agents. In addition, the serotonin antagonists can be constipating. For these reasons, encourage clients to eat lightly, taking primarily liquids for the 3 days following chemotherapy. Drugs such as metoclopramide (Reglan) are useful to enhance gastric emptying and to reduce bloating. Most women who receive chemotherapy for breast cancer do not lose weight; in fact, they gain weight. Women receiving CMF therapy may gain between 15 and 25 pounds during their therapy. Counsel clients to control their weight and to watch what they are eating.

Evaluation

Many factors affect the duration of the chemotherapy regimen. The following are some considerations:
- Whether the chemotherapy is adjuvant
- Stage at which the breast cancer was diagnosed
- Co-morbidities
- Whether the disease remains stable during chemotherapy

■ Self-Care

Teach About Follow-Up Surveillance. The highest risk factor for breast cancer is a history of breast cancer. Therefore instruct clients that they require follow-up cancer surveillance for the rest of their lives. Most women are emotional and apprehensive after completing their adjuvant therapy. For the most part, they are happy to be finished but nervous that they are no longer receiving any therapy to oppose the cancer. If they are receiving tamoxifen, remind them that it is treatment for their cancer as well as a medicine to help prevent breast cancer. Women express fear that the cancer will come back. It is important to acknowledge and discuss the fact that they will worry and feel afraid, so that they can realize that such feelings are normal.

Explain that the physical examination by the physician every 3 to 4 months is designed to detect any problem early and that they should make every effort to keep their appointments. The surveillance schedule involves a physical examination every 3 to 4 months for 3 years, every 6 months for 2 years, and then once a year. A mammogram and a chest film (optional) are obtained every 12 months. Routine chemistry screening is done every year. For women on tamoxifen who still have their uterus, a pelvic examination is done every year.

Routine liver, bone, and brain scans are not indicated as surveillance tests for recurrent disease.[10] Until research determines that early institution of therapy is critical to the outcome, the goal of surveillance is to detect the disease just as the disease becomes symptomatic.[1]

Promote Acceptance of Body Image. For the woman who has had a mastectomy (a less common procedure than in the past), acceptance of the change in body image takes time. Evaluate adaptation to this loss by asking the woman how she feels about the loss and whether she thinks it would be helpful to see a social worker or psycho-oncologist to discuss strategies for coping. Adaptation and acceptance of the loss may be evident by her ability to discuss plans for a permanent prosthesis or by her questions regarding breast reconstruction. Do not insist that a woman look at her incision; she needs to wait until she is ready. A woman's reluctance to look at the incision is in no way evidence of inability to accept her loss.

Inform women of outside resources that can help them adapt to the changes imposed by the disease. For example, breast cancer support groups and other resources help the woman and her significant other learn to cope. Information about where to buy a prosthesis and a wig is helpful. Even having the telephone number and name of a person who can help with a wig or prosthesis can make a difficult time more bearable. (See the Complementary and Alternative Therapy feature on Exercise for Breast Cancer Survivors, below.)

LOCAL RECURRENCE

Nearly 80% of local recurrences appear within 5 years of mastectomy.[1] Local recurrence after mastectomy generally presents as an isolated nodule in or under the skin of the chest wall, usually near the mastectomy scar. Breast reconstruction does not interfere with early detection of a local recurrence. A complete staging work-up is conducted to define the extent of recurrence. Wide local excision and radiation therapy have been the standard form of local treatment for clients with local recurrence after mastectomy. Hormone therapy is appropriate if the tumor is estrogen receptor positive, or chemotherapy is recommended in view of the very high risk for distant metastases. The goal of therapy is control of local and distant disease.

Local recurrence after breast-preserving surgery and radiation therapy carries a better prognosis than that associated with local recurrence after mastectomy.

COMPLEMENTARY AND ALTERNATIVE THERAPY

Exercise for Breast Cancer Survivors

A total of 53 postmenopausal breast cancer survivors were randomly allocated to an exercise group ($n = 25$) or control group ($n = 28$). The exercise group trained on cycle ergometers 3 times a week for 15 weeks, and the control group did not train. Peak oxygen consumption increased significantly in the exercise group, as did overall quality of life scores compared to the control group. Thus exercise training should be advocated in postmenopausal breast cancer survivors (and possibly all survivors) because of a significant effect on cardiopulmonary function and quality of life.

Reference
Courneya, K., et al. (2003). Randomized controlled trial of exercise training in postmenopausal breast cancer survivors: Cardiopulmonary and quality of life outcomes. *Journal of Clinical Oncology, 21*, 1660-1668.

Mastectomy is the standard form of therapy for local recurrence, as long as there is no evidence of supraclavicular node involvement or distant metastases.

METASTATIC BREAST CANCER
■ Medical Management

Determine Extent of Disease. Despite adjuvant therapy, after varying periods of disease-free survival, nearly half of clients who have received treatment for apparently localized breast cancer develop metastatic disease. The majority of cases occur within 2 years of definitive surgery, but several initial breast cancer recurrences occur more than 5 years after initial therapy.[1] In general, the clinical course and presentation of metastatic disease are variable in terms of growth rate and responsiveness to systemic therapy. As a result of the heterogeneous nature of breast cancer, the disease may present as aggressive visceral disease in multiple organs, as a small skin recurrence such as in a supraclavicular lymph node, or as metastatic bone disease.

Selection of therapy depends on the extent of disease and whether any visceral organs are involved. The goal of therapy is control of disease and optimal palliation with prolongation of life and minimal disruption of the woman's lifestyle and quality of life. Life expectancy after breast cancer recurrence is variable. If disease recurs in the liver, most women die within 3 years of the recurrence. Others with disease in bone or skin may survive for many years. Women with more aggressive disease tend to be *premenopausal*, with estrogen receptor–negative, HER-2–positive disease that recurs in liver or lung. Women with less aggressive disease tend to be *postmenopausal*, with estrogen receptor–positive disease that is HER-2–negative and recurs in bone and skin.

All clients with suspected metastatic disease undergo a metastatic work-up to determine the extent of disease. Typically, a physical examination, serum chemistry profiles, a complete blood count, chest radiograph, and a bone scan are obtained initially. If the client has clinical manifestations associated with organ dysfunction, a CT scan of the area is appropriate. A CT scan or MRI study of the chest, abdomen, or pelvis may also be done if the client is being considered for a research protocol. Serum markers may be ordered and include CEA, CA-125, and CA 15-3. Serum markers that are elevated are monitored monthly to evaluate response to therapy.

Prevent Further Extension of Cancer. Once extent of disease is determined, an overall therapeutic approach is established based on the client's age, disease-free interval, hormone receptor status, and location and extent of disease. For older women with limited and non–life-threatening disease, no significant manifestations of disease, and estrogen receptor–positive tumors, hormone therapy is the initial treatment of choice. If the disease involves liver or lung or if the tumor is estrogen receptor negative, the choice of treatment is chemotherapy, with or without trastuzumab if the tumor is HER-2 positive. Radiation therapy is instituted only if the disease is symptomatic.

The basic philosophy of management for metastatic breast cancer is to use all therapies to their fullest worth, but not to the point of toxicity, when the treatment becomes worse than the disease. A treatment that creates a stable condition is still a worthwhile treatment. Treatments are not abandoned until their utility is fully spent. The emphasis is on the need for therapeutic options.

Endocrine Therapy. As stated earlier, when a woman is known to have breast cancer, her tissue sample is tested for the presence of estrogen and progesterone receptors. Estrogen and progesterone receptor assays are performed using radioimmunoassay and immunohistochemical techniques. The more strongly estrogen receptor positive the tumor, the more likely it is that the disease will respond to hormone therapies. Yet although more than 60% of human breast cancers are estrogen receptor positive, no more than two thirds of them will respond to endocrine therapy.

Hormone therapies are generally classified as *ablative* (removal of the hormone) or *additive* (addition of a hormone); both types change the hormonal environment sufficiently to affect tumor growth. The response rates for all hormonal manipulations are basically similar. Women who have a response to one hormonal intervention often have a response to a second after the first becomes ineffective.

In general, the least toxic intervention is chosen first. Once the disease is no longer controlled with a specific approach, the next least toxic agent is selected, and so forth. There is no therapeutic benefit to combining hormone therapies. It is generally accepted practice to continue each therapy for as long as it provides benefit before instituting other therapy. Even withdrawing a hormone manipulation may result in a therapeutic response.

Antiestrogens. If the woman has not previously received tamoxifen, it is typically the first hormonal agent given because of its limited toxicity. Tamoxifen works in premenopausal women, but it is more active in the absence of ovarian function and is therefore especially effective in postmenopausal women. Tamoxifen is a partial estrogen agonist that has mixed estrogenic and antiestrogenic properties; it has a favorable effect on cardiac status and opposes calcium loss as women age. Side effects include nausea, hot flashes, weight gain, menstrual irregularities, and thromboembolic events in 1% to 2% of cases. The risk of endometrial cancer is minimal (3 cases per 1000 women annually in postmenopausal women).[61]

Other antiestrogens include toremifene (Fareston), raloxifene, and long-acting ICI 182,780 (Faslodex).

Ablative Endocrine Procedures. Ablative endocrine procedures have been replaced by specific, well-tolerated hormone treatments. In premenopausal women, it is possible to administer goserelin (Zoladex), a luteinizing hormone–releasing hormone (LHRH) agonist that causes a medical oophorectomy. Injections are given every 1 to 3 months depending on the preparation. The only difference between surgical oophorectomy and medical oophorectomy is that results with surgical intervention are immediate and permanent.

For women in whom initial hormone ablation therapy fails, administration of either megestrol acetate (Megace) or an aromatase inhibitor is an option. Aromatase inhibitors prevent the peripheral conversion or aromatization of other steroids (namely, androgens to estrogen), primarily in body fat. The efficacy of aromatase inhibitors is limited to postmenopausal women. In clinical trials it appears that anastrozole (Arimidex) and letrozole (Femara) as aromatase inhibitors are associated not only with less toxicity but also with greater efficacy and even survival than have been reported for megestrol acetate.[1]

Chemotherapy. Eventually, all hormone-responsive tumors become refractory to hormone manipulation, and chemotherapy becomes the treatment of choice. The selection of combination chemotherapy again is guided by the toxicity of the regimen and the extent of disease. A doxorubicin-containing regimen is usually selected if the client has lung or liver disease, because the response is usually prompt and durable. CMF is also a good option and is somewhat less toxic. The taxanes with or without trastuzumab are excellent options, as is vinorelbine (Navelbine). All of these drugs and drug combinations are options for the woman with metastatic disease, and each offers some degree of response and tumor control.

For the most part, metastatic breast cancer is considered an incurable disease. However, long-term responses have been seen with aggressive high-dose chemotherapy regimens, including autologous stem cell transplantation. This latter procedure involves having the woman donate her own bone marrow, either through bone marrow aspiration or through peripheral stem cell apheresis. The client then is given very high-dose chemotherapy, followed by reinfusion of her own marrow or stem cells after the chemotherapy has destroyed her own marrow. Further information on bone marrow transplantation is found in Chapter 81.

Another treatment option for women with bone metastases is a bisphosphonate added to the chemotherapeutic or hormonal therapy regimen. Pamidronate (Aredia), clodronate (Ostac), and zoledronic acid (Zometa) not only reduce pain and incidence of complications but also help the bone to heal and prolong survival of the client without complications associated with bone metastases. The drugs improve bone strength and make the bone more resistant to bone metastasis.[23] Pamidronate and zoledronic acid are given intravenously over 2 hours every month. Adjuvant clodronate therapy has been shown to decrease the risk of bone metastases.[1,23]

BREAST CANCER IN MEN

Breast cancer in men is rare, with approximately 1300 new cases diagnosed and nearly 400 deaths due to breast cancer projected for 2003.[2] The average age at onset is about 60 years (10 years older than the average for women). Factors associated with an increased risk of breast cancer in men include the following:

- A first-degree male or female relative with breast cancer
- Presence of the *BRCA2* gene
- Klinefelter's syndrome
- Hepatic schistosomiasis
- Exposure to ionizing radiation
- Prolonged heat exposure

Breast cancer in men tends to be identified at a more advanced stage, possibly because of the unexpected nature of the disease and the fact that the mass is usually painless and located beneath the nipple-areola complex. Generally, the mass is detected when it becomes large, ulcerates, or becomes fixed to underlying muscle. Assessment findings indicating male breast cancer include a painless lump beneath the areola or, more often, nipple discharge, retraction, crusting, or ulceration.

Biopsy is necessary for diagnosis of male breast cancer. The most common histologic type is infiltrating ductal carcinoma. Most male breast cancers are estrogen receptor positive and respond to endocrine therapy. Staging of disease is the same as for women. Axillary dissection is done to determine nodal status and prognosis

A modified radical mastectomy is usually required to obtain clear margins. Radiation therapy may be indicated, depending on the size of the primary tumor. Chemotherapy, usually a doxorubicin-containing regimen, may be administered as adjuvant therapy and followed by radiation. Tamoxifen therapy is appropriate for adjuvant therapy. In the presence of metastatic disease, an LHRH agonist (goserelin) is appropriate hormonal manipulation and takes the place of orchiectomy. The pattern of metastasis is similar to that of female breast cancer.

BENIGN BREAST DISEASE

Most women have a profound underlying fear of breast cancer. For some women the fear is so great that they are immobilized and ignore the problem altogether. This is why some women who see a physician because of a lump, pain, or nipple discharge present with breast cancer at an advanced stage. Mastalgia, or breast pain, is frequently linked emotionally to the fear of breast cancer. Become sensitive to the emotional aspects associated with breast problems, take clients' fears seriously, provide reassurance through discussion, and perform appropriate evaluation.

The basic techniques of breast evaluation consist of the following:

- A breast-oriented medical history, including the woman's age, menstrual history, family and personal history of breast cancer, last mammogram, and current or past history of hormone therapy
- Clinical breast examination
- Mammography
- Biopsy of a persistent palpable mass

Fibrocystic Breasts

Fibrocystic breasts are the most frequently occurring pathologic problem in the female breast.[50] The exact cause is unknown, although some evidence indicates hormonal imbalance and even high caffeine consumption may be associated. The fibrocystic condition typically improves during pregnancy and lactation. It occurs during the reproductive years and may diminish with menopause.

Typical fibrocystic lesions are fluid-filled cysts that are round, well circumscribed, and movable. Depending on the amount of fluid in the cyst, the cyst may feel soft or hard. Assessment findings may include nodularity and tenderness. Pain is common, and the cysts frequently increase in size premenstrually. Cysts are generally aspirated rather than undergo surgical biopsy. If there is any question, however, a biopsy is done. A biopsy is necessary when the cyst recurs after being aspirated. A fibrocystic change in the breast is considered a risk factor for breast cancer when it is accompanied by cellular proliferation and atypia.

Hyperplasia and Atypical Hyperplasia

Ductal hyperplasia is found in 20% of all breast biopsy specimens. Atypical lobular hyperplasia is found in 1% of breast biopsy specimens. The diagnosis of hyperplasia and atypical hyperplasia can be confirmed only by pathologic examination of breast tissue from a biopsy. The presence of hyperplasia or atypical hyperplasia indicates an increased risk for breast cancer. Ductal lavage, a new technique of washing a duct out with normal saline and analyzing the cells to determine abnormalities, has been shown to be an optional diagnostic tool for women with nipple discharge. Women who are found to have atypia may receive tamoxifen to reduce the risk of breast cancer.[22] The STAR trial, a double-blind study evaluating the use of tamoxifen and raloxifene for breast cancer chemoprevention, will be benefi-

cial in determining optimal chemoprevention with minimal side effects.

Fibroadenoma

Fibroadenoma is a common breast tumor that usually occurs in young women, most frequently between ages 15 and 30 years. This tumor is generally a nontender, round, firm, or rubbery mass 1 to 3 cm in diameter. Movability of the adenoma in the breast tissue is one of its most distinctive characteristics. Fibroadenomas are readily diagnosed by imaging or biopsy.

Papilloma

Intraductal papillomas are lesions growing in the terminal portion of a duct (solitary) or throughout the duct system of a sector of breast (multiple or intraductal). Papillomas typically occur in women in their 40s. Solitary intraductal papillomas are usually not precancerous. Multiple papillomas may be indicative of an increased risk of cancer. Intraductal papilloma is usually identified as a serous, serosanguineous, or bloody discharge from the nipple. Often, no mass is palpable, although a small soft tumor in a central or periareolar portion of the breast is usually present. Examination by biopsy is necessary to determine whether the lesion is benign or malignant.

Duct Ectasia

Duct ectasia, a disease of ducts in the subareolar zone, occurs in aging breasts, usually in perimenopausal or postmenopausal women. Manifestations may include a palpable dilated duct; a thick, sticky nipple discharge; and burning pain, itching, and inflammation. There appears to be no association with cancer.

Mastodynia and Mastalgia

Mastodynia and mastalgia refer to breast pain. Breast pain is the most common breast complaint. Pain is not usually associated with breast cancer. Many women have cyclic premenstrual mastodynia. Women with cyclic premenstrual mastodynia usually have lumpy breast (nodularity) and pain for the week before menses. After any other problems have been ruled out, treatment is symptomatic. Wearing a well-fitting brassiere for support, particularly during jogging and other bouncing exercise, may be helpful. Decreasing caffeine intake may also be helpful.

Gynecomastia

Gynecomastia (hypertrophy of one or both male breasts) is common at puberty and in older men. The hormonal mechanism causing gynecomastia is not well understood, although several drugs, an increase in estrogen levels, tumors, and thyroid and hepatic problems may contribute. Usually the situation is temporary. If the gynecomastia causes severe psychosocial trauma, reduction mammoplasty can be performed, or antiestrogen (tamoxifen) or synthetic androgen (danazol [Danocrine]) medications may be administered.

MAMMAPLASTY

Mammaplasty is the surgical revision in the size or shape of the breast. It is often performed electively for cosmetic reasons to enlarge or reduce breast size.

Breast Augmentation

Clients seeking breast augmentation are often young women who have had chronic feelings of inadequacy and self-consciousness because of small or undeveloped breasts. Some clients are mature women who have postpartum breast atrophy. Current prostheses are durable, seamless, silicone rubber envelopes filled with saline. The prosthesis is inserted beneath existing breast tissue or the pectoralis muscle (called subpectoral placement) through an inframammary (under the breast), transaxillary (through the axilla), or periareolar (around the nipple) incision (Figure 42-8).

Thorough preoperative breast assessment is essential to rule out breast cancer. Mammography is generally not recommended in women younger than 35 years of age unless they have a positive family history of cancer or a suspicious lump. Surgery is performed on an outpatient basis. Nurses provide teaching and support, mostly over the telephone.

Early complications of breast augmentation include changes in breast or nipple sensation, hematoma (collection of clotted blood), infection, or leakage from the

prosthesis. The most frequent complication is capsule formation (development of fibrous sacs of scar tissue enclosing the implant), followed by contracture of the scar. These complications cause excessive breast firmness and distortion of the breast into a hard, round ball. Possible causes of capsular contracture include infection and formation of a seroma (a collection of serosanguineous fluid) or hematoma. The basic problem in these processes is that the body's defense mechanisms respond to the prosthesis as a foreign body, and scar tissue forms around the prosthesis to wall it off. Capsule formation is usually treated with open (surgical) capsulotomy. Open capsulotomy, performed under general anesthesia, involves incising the capsule.

Breast massage may be prescribed postoperatively with smooth-walled implants or after capsulotomy to reduce capsule formation. Breast massage typically begins postoperatively according to the surgeon's instructions. Teach the woman to push each breast up, to the side, and toward the middle of the chest, supporting the breast in each position for a count of 10. Discharge instructions usually include the following:

- To reduce edema, maintain a head-elevated position for a week when in bed.
- To reduce hematoma formation, get plenty of rest for a week (no excessive activity, take it easy).
- To avoid moving the pectoralis muscle and irritating the surgical site, do not raise the arms above the head for 3 weeks (e.g., while washing or brushing hair), do not play golf or tennis or swim for 6 weeks, sleep on the back and not on the stomach or sides, and be careful when closing car doors.
- Because of their anticoagulant effect, do not use aspirin or aspirin-containing compounds.
- Notify the physician if bleeding occurs or if a fever with temperature greater than 37.6° C (99.6° F) develops.

Reduction Mammaplasty

Reduction mammaplasty surgically reduces the size of large, pendulous breasts. Women usually seek such surgery to reduce the physical and psychosocial discomforts of large breasts, such as back pain, the presence of bra strap indentations in the shoulders, inability to wear normal clothing styles, intertriginous dermatitis (skin breakdown under large breasts), and distress from others' comments about breast size.

Excess breast tissue is removed through incisions under the breast (Figure 42-9). The nipple is transposed on a pedicle of tissue or grafted onto the newly formed breast. A possible complication is loss of blood supply to the nipple-areola complex. Any duskiness or pallor around the nipple-areola complex should be reported to the physician. Altered sensation and the inability to perform breast-feeding are common findings after this procedure.

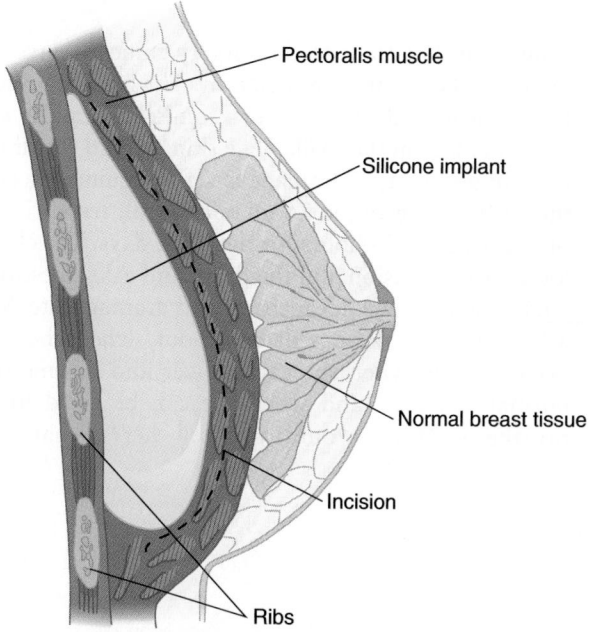

FIGURE 42-8 Augmentation mammaplasty is achieved by insertion of a saline-filled implant beneath the pectoral muscle. The incision is represented by a *dashed line.*

Pectoralis muscle

Silicone implant

Normal breast tissue

Incision

Ribs

FIGURE 42-9 Reduction mammaplasty, in which breasts are surgically reduced. Excess breast tissue is removed, and the breast is recontoured. The nipple is relocated (e.g., moved higher) on a pedicle of tissue. The pedicle supplies the nipple with blood until new blood vessels form.

Epithelium to be removed from pedicle and new areolar site

Skin incisions

Area to be resected

Areola on pedicle to be relocated as indicated

PENDULOUS BREAST BEFORE SURGERY

SAME BREAST AFTER RECONTOURING

Mastopexy

Mastopexy is the correction of mammary ptosis (drooping) to achieve an improved breast contour and position. Mastopexy may be performed with subcutaneous mastectomy or on normal breasts to improve contour. Postoperative care is similar to that with other types of breast surgery.

CONCLUSIONS

Diseases of the breast are usually benign conditions that occur throughout the life cycle. Breast cancer, however, has greatly increased in incidence over the past 30 years. The nurse has a vital role in teaching clients early detection methods so that breast cancer can be detected at a curable stage.

All diseases of the breast potentially pose problems in body image and sexuality. Even benign fibrocystic changes can cause breast tenderness and possibly interfere with sexual functioning. Breast cancer and the possibility of mastectomy as treatment can be extremely threatening to a woman's body image. The nurse can help the client cope with these potential threats and successfully adapt to any changes that occur.

THINKING CRITICALLY *evolve*

1. The pathology report of your client's breast biopsy reads: "8 mm invasive ductal carcinoma, invasive carcinoma to the margins, estrogen receptor–positive and progesterone receptor–positive." The client is considering further treatment and asks you what her options are. How would you respond?

Factors to Consider. What treatment options might the client have? What interventions might be required?

2. Your client has come to the surgery clinic 10 days after a modified radical mastectomy. The breast incision line is clean and intact. A Jackson-Pratt drain is sutured in place in the axilla. The skin around the drain is clean and intact. Drainage is serosanguineous, and the client has recorded 25 ml and 20 ml, respectively, of drainage per 24 hours for the last 2 days. The client looks at the incision and the drain and asks questions while you examine her incision and drainage site. She asks when the drain will come out, when she can drive her car, when she can shower and resume her normal activities, and when she can be fitted for a prosthesis. What would you tell her? What else

should you assess? What medical and nursing care does this client need during her appointment? What other teaching needs does she have?

Factors to Consider. Think about what structures are removed as part of the modified radical mastectomy. What are the functions of these structures? What functional limitations can be expected to affect the client's self-care needs? Consider the client's needs in this immediate postoperative period, in a few months, and over the long term.

3. Two years ago, your client's stage II cancer of the right breast was treated with a quadrantectomy (margins negative), axillary lymph node dissection (8 of 19 nodes positive), radiation therapy of the chest and axilla, and six courses of CAF (Cytoxan [cyclophosphamide], Adriamycin [doxorubicin], 5-fluorouracil) chemotherapy. Today, she presents with pain, tingling, and swelling of her right hand and arm. She states that although she noticed intermittent problems with slight swelling over the past 6 months, it has become severe over the past 2 weeks and is affecting her ability to work as a court stenographer. What further information should you assess? What are your priority interventions?

Factors to Consider. What do pain, tingling, and swelling of the hand and arm suggest in a client who has undergone lymph node dissection? Should a referral to a physical therapist for lymphedema management be made?

Discussions for these questions can be found on the website and the CD-ROM.

BIBLIOGRAPHY

1. Abeloff, M., et al. (2000). Breast. In M. Abeloff, et al. (Eds.), *Clinical oncology* (2nd ed., pp. 2051-2159). New York: Churchill Livingstone.
2. American Cancer Society. (2003). *Cancer facts and figures.* Atlanta: Author.
3. American Cancer Society. (2002). *Breast cancer facts and figures 2001-2002.* Atlanta: Author.
4. American Joint Committee. (2002). Revision of the American Joint Committee on Cancer Staging System for Breast Cancer. *Journal of Clinical Oncology, 20,* 3628-3636.
5. Anonymous. (2002). What's the verdict on mammograms? *American Journal of Nursing, 102*(5), 19.
6. Anonymous. (2002). Benefit of a high-dose epirubicin regimen in adjuvant chemotherapy for node-positive breast cancer patients with poor prognostic factors: 5-year follow-up results of French Adjuvant Study Group 05 randomized trial. *Journal of Clinical Oncology, 19*(3), 602-611
7. Baselga, J.B., et al. (1997). HER-2 overexpression and paclitaxel sensitivity in breast cancer: Therapeutic implications. *Oncology, 11*(3), 43-48.
8. Berns, E.A., Hendrick, R.E., Cutter, G.R. (2002). Performance comparison of full-field digital mammography to screen-film mammography in clinical practice. *Medical Physics, 29*(5), 830-834
9. Bradley, C.J., Given, C.W., & Roberts, C. (2002). Race, socioeconomic status, and breast cancer treatment and survival. *Journal of the National Cancer Institute, 94*(7), 490-496.
10. Breast care guidelines. (2003). National Comprehensive Cancer Network, as obtained from on http://www.nccn.org on 10/20/03.
11. Burke, W. (2000). Oral contraceptives and breast cancer: A note of caution for high-risk women. *Journal of the American Medical Association, 284*(14), 1837-1838.
12. Centers for Disease Control (2002). Breast and cervical cancer fact sheet as obtained from http://www.cdc.gov/cancer/nbccedp on 10/20/03.
13. Cooke, A.L., Stanton, P. (2001). HER-2 as a prognostic and predictive marker for breast cancer. *Annals of Oncology, 12*(suppl. 1), S23-S28.
14. Cummings, S.R., et al. (1999). The effect of raloxifene on risk of breast cancer in post menopausal women: Results from the Multiple Outcomes of Raloxifene (MORE) trial. *Journal of the American Medical Association, 281*(3), 2189-2197.
15. Davis, S., Mirick, D.K., & Stevens, R.G. (2002). Night shift work, light at night, and risk of breast cancer. *Journal of the National Cancer Institute, 93,* 1557-1562.
16. Early Breast Cancer Trialists' Collaborative Group. (1998). Tamoxifen for early breast cancer: An overview of the randomized trials. *Lancet, 351,* 1451-1467.
17. Early Breast Cancer Trialists' Collaborative Group. (1998). Polychemotherapy for early breast cancer: An overview of randomized trials. *Lancet, 352,* 930-942.
18. Edwards, B.K., et al. (2002). Annual report to the nation on the status of cancer, 1973-1999, featuring implications of age and aging on U.S. cancer burden. *Cancer, 94*(10), 2766-2791.
19. Egan, K.M. (2002). Active and passive smoking in breast cancer: Prospective results from the Nurses' Health Study. *Journal of the American Medical Association, 287*(18), 138-145.
20. Erickson, V.S., et al. (2001). Arm edema in breast cancer patients. *Journal of the National Cancer Institute, 93*(2), 96-111.
21. Fisher, B., et al. (1999). Further evaluation of intensified and increased total dose of cyclophosphamide for the treatment of primary breast cancer: Findings from National Surgical Adjuvant Breast and Bowel Project B-25. *Journal of Clinical Oncology, 17*(11), 3374-3388.
22. Fisher, B., et al. (1998). Tamoxifen for prevention of breast cancer. Report of the National Surgical Adjuvant Breast and Bowel Project: Project P-1 Study. *Journal of the National Cancer Institute, 90,* 1371-1388.
23. Gaines, K. (2002). Zoledronic acid (Zometa): Bisphosphonate for prostate cancer/bone metastases. *Urologic Nursing, 22*(6), 398-400.
24. Grabrick, D.M., et al. (2000). Oral contraceptives: Special concerns in high-risk women. *Journal of the American Medical Association, 284*(14), 1791-1797.
25. Hansen, J. (2001). Increased breast cancer risk among women who work predominantly at night. *Journal of the American Medical Association, 285*(7), 1274-1277.
26. Harris M, Smith I. (2002). The development and clinical use of trastuzumab. *Endocrine Related Cancer, 9*(2), 75-85.
27. Hartmann, L.C., et al. (1999). Efficacy of bilateral prophylactic mastectomy in women with a family history of breast cancer. *New England Journal of Medicine, 340,* 77-84
28. Howe, H.L., et al. (2001). The annual report to the nation on the status of cancer (1973-1998). Featuring cancers with recent increasing trends. *Journal of the National Cancer Institute, 93*(11), 824-842.

29. Ikeda, T., et al. (2002). The role of neoadjuvant chemotherapy for breast cancer treatment. *Breast Cancer, 9*(1), 8-14.

30. Itami, J. (2002) Hodgkin lymphoma. *Nippon Acta Radiologica, 62*(5), 215-220.

 31. Kaste, S.C., et al. (1998). Breast masses in women treated for childhood cancer: Incidence and screening guidelines. *Cancer, 82*, 784-792.

32. Lawrence, G., Crawford, J., & Sherman, F. (2002). Evaluating neoadjuvant chemotherapy in breast cancer. *Journal of Clinical Oncology, 20*(12), 2905-2906.

 33. Malone, R.E. (2002). Night shifts and breast cancer risk: Policy implications. *Journal of Emergency Nursing, 28*(2), 169-171.

 34. McKeage, K., & Perry, C.M. (2002). Trastuzumab: A review of its use in the treatment of metastatic breast cancer overexpressing HER-2. *Drugs, 62*(1), 209-213.

 35. Murphy, A., & Holcombe, C. (2001). Effects of early discharge following breast surgery. *Professional Nurse, 16*(5), 1087-1090.

36. Nelson, H.D. (2002). Assessing benefits and harms of hormone replacement therapy: Clinical applications. *Journal of the American Medical Association, 288*(7), 882-884.

 37. Nelson, H.D., et al. (2002). Postmenopausal hormone replacement therapy: Scientific review. *Journal of the American Medical Association, 288*(7), 872-881.

 38. Newman, L.A., et al. (2002). Ethnicity related differences in the survival of young breast carcinoma patients. *Cancer, 95*(1), 21-26.

 39. NIH. (2002). NHLBI stops trial of estrogen plus progestin due to increased breast cancer risk, lack of overall benefit. NIH news release. Obtained from http://www.nih.gov on 7/9/02.

40. Obenauer, S., et al. (2002). Screen film vs full-field digital mammography: Image quality, detectability and characterization of lesions. *European Radiology, 12*(7), 1697-1702.

 40a. Page, D.L., et al. (2003). Atypical lobular hyperplasia as a unilateral predictor of breast cancer risk: A retrospective cohort study. *Lancet, 361*, 125-129.

 41. Paik, S., et al. (2000). HER-2 and choice of adjuvant chemotherapy for invasive breast cancer: National Surgical Adjuvant Breast and Bowel Project Protocol B-15. *Journal of the National Cancer Institute, 92*, 1991-1998.

 42. Questions and answers on hormone replacement therapy. (2002). The American College of Obstetrics and Gynecologists. Obtained from http://www.acog.org/from-home/publications/press-releases.

43. Radiologic Society of North America. (2002). "Diagnosing" the effectiveness of digital mammography. RSNA news in *RSNA Link:* http://www.rsna.org.

 43a. Rancour, P., & Brauer, K. (2003). Use of letter writing as a means of integrating an altered body image: A case study. *Oncology Nursing Forum, 30*, 841-846.

44. Recht, A., et al. (2001). Postmastectomy radiotherapy: Clinical practice guidelines of the American Society of Clinical Oncology. *Journal of Clinical Oncology,19*, 1539-1569.

45. Ries, L.A., et al. (Eds.). (2001). *SEER Cancer Statistics Review, 1973-1998.* Bethesda, MD: National Cancer Institute.

46. Sapuner, F., & Smith, I.E. (2000). Neoadjuvant chemotherapy for breast cancer. *Annals of Medicine, 32*(1), 43-50.

47. Schernhammer, E.S., et al. (2001). Rotating night shifts and risk of breast cancer in women participating in the Nurses' Health Study. *Journal of the National Cancer Institute, 93*, 1563-1568.

48. Schwartz, G.F., Giuliano, A.E., & Veronesi, U. (2002). Proceedings of the Consensus Conference on the Role of Sentinel Lymph Node Biopsy in Carcinoma of the Breast April 19 to 22, 2001, Philadelphia, Pennsylvania. *Human Pathology, 33*(6), 579-589.

49. Screening for Breast Cancer. (2002). *Guide to clinical preventive services 3rd edition: Periodic updates.* Rockville, Md: U.S. Preventive Services Task Force.

50. Singletary, K.W., & Gapstur, S.M. (2001). Alcohol and breast cancer. Review of epidemiologic and experimental evidence and potential mechanisms. *Journal of the American Medical Association, 286*, 2143-2152.

51. Singletary, S.E., et al. (2002). Revision of the American Joint Committee on Cancer Staging System for Breast Cancer. *Journal of Clinical Oncology, 20* (17), 3628-3636.

52. Singletary, S.E. (2001). Systemic treatment following sentinel lymph node biopsy in breast cancer: Who, what and why? *Journal of the American College of Surgery, 192:* 220-230.

53. Slamon, D., et al. (1998). Addition of Herceptin to first-line chemotherapy for HER-2 overexpressing metastatic breast cancer markedly increases anticancer activity: A randomized multinational controlled phase III trial [Abstract]. *Proceedings of the American Society of Clinical Oncology, 17,* 98a.

54. Smith, I. (2001). Future direction in the adjuvant treatment of breast cancer: The role of trastuzumab. *Annals of Oncology, 12*(suppl. 1):S75-S79.

54a. Smith, R.A., et al. (2003). American Cancer Society guidelines for breast cancer screening: Update 2003. *CA Cancer Journal for Clinicians, 53,* 141-169.

55. Smith-Warner, S.A., et al. (2001). Alcohol and breast cancer in women: A pooled analysis of cohort studies. *Journal of the American Medical Association, 279,* 535-540.

56. Smith-Warner, S.A., et al. (2001). Intake of fruits and vegetables and risk of breast cancer. A pooled analysis of cohort studies. *Journal of the American Medical Association, 285*(6), 769-775.

57. Tan, A.R., & Swain, S.M. (2001). Adjuvant chemotherapy for breast cancer: An update. *Seminars in Oncology, 28*(4), 359-376.

58. Vicini, F., et al. (2002). The emerging role of brachytherapy in the management of patients with breast cancer. *Seminars in Radiation Oncology, 12*(1), 31-39.

59. Vogel, V.G. (2000). *Management of people at high risk for breast cancer.* Boston: Blackwell Scientific Publications.

60. Webb, P.M., et al. (2002). History of breast cancer, age and benign breast disease. *International Journal of Cancer, 100*(3), 375-378.

61. Wickerham, D.L., et al. (2002). Association of tamoxifen and uterine sarcoma. *Journal of Clinical Oncology, 20,* 2758-2760.

62. Wong, S.L., et al. (2002). Optimal use of sentinel lymph node biopsy versus axillary node dissection in patients with breast carcinoma. *Cancer, 95*(3), 478-486.

63. Writing Group for the Women's Health Initiative. (2002). Risks and benefits of estrogen plus progestin in healthy women. Principle results from the Women's Health Initiative Randomized Control Trial. *Journal of the American Medical Association, 288*(3), 321-333.

64. Zang, S., et al. (1999). A prospective study of folate intake and the risk of breast cancer. *Journal of the American Medical Association, 281,* 1632-1641.

Management of Clients with Sexually Transmitted Diseases

Meg Blair

SEXUALLY TRANSMITTED DISEASES: AN OVERVIEW

The term *sexually transmitted disease* (STD) refers to any infection contracted primarily through sexual activities or contact. *STD* has replaced the older term *venereal disease* (VD), which referred to diseases transmitted only by sexual intercourse. STD is also known as sexually transmitted infection (STI). More than 50 organisms are known to spread through sexual activity. The five most widely known STDs are chlamydia, gonorrhea, syphilis, genital herpes, and genital warts. Other infections are chancroid, lymphogranuloma venereum, granuloma inguinale, trichomoniasis, human immunodeficiency virus (HIV), and some enteric and ectoparasitic infections. The number of STDs is increasing as new agents are implicated in the sexual transmission of disease.

STDs share the following characteristics:
1. STDs can be transmitted by any sexual activity between opposite-sex or same-sex partners (not only vaginal-penile sex but also oral and anal sex).
2. Having one STD confers no immunity against future reinfection with that STD or with any other STD (except, possibly, for hepatitis B).
3. Sexual partners of infected clients need to be assessed for treatment (see individual diseases for specific recommendations).
4. STDs affect people from all socioeconomic classes, cultures, ethnicities, and age-groups.
5. Women bear a disproportionate number of the effects of STDs.
6. Frustration, anger, anxiety, fear, shame, and guilt are common emotions associated with an STD diagnosis.
7. STDs frequently coexist in the same client.

The last fact may be responsible for some treatment failures. Current treatment guidelines for STDs are available in the United States from the Centers for Disease Control and Prevention (CDC) in Atlanta and on the CDC website http://www.cdc.gov.

STDs are a serious public health problem. Recognized since the beginning of recorded history, these diseases are

Nursing Outcomes Classification (NOC)
for Nursing Diagnoses—Clients with Sexually Transmitted Diseases

Anxiety
  Anxiety Control
  Coping
  Impulse Control
  Social Interaction Skills
Ineffective Health Maintenance
  Health Belief: Perceived Resources

Health Promoting Behavior
Health Seeking Behavior
Knowledge: Health Behaviors
Knowledge: Health Promotion
Knowledge: Health Resources
Knowledge: Treatment Regimen
Participation: Health Care Decisions

Psychosocial Adjustment: Life Changes
Risk Detection
Self-Direction of Care
Social Support
Treatment Behavior: Illness or Injury

associated with substantial morbidity and, in some cases, mortality. The incidence of STDs continues to increase worldwide, and infections are becoming more severe. STDs also facilitate the development of HIV infection and AIDS. Thus the scope of the health problem they create is increasing rather than decreasing. It is a matter of public concern that treatments for STDs be safe, inexpensive, and effective.

Except for the common cold and influenza, STDs are the most prevalent communicable diseases in the United States, which has the highest STD rate in the industrialized world. Most sources describe STD rates as epidemic. Symptomatic STDs are diagnosed in more than 15 million people in the United States annually, not including HIV infection and AIDS, and 86% of affected people are between 15 and 29 years of age. Another 40 million people are infected with human papillomavirus (HPV), which causes genital warts. It is estimated that 50% of all Americans will have been exposed to or will contract an STD by age 30 years. Although AIDS is probably the best publicized and most dangerous, the most common STDs are chlamydial infection, gonorrhea, genital herpes, genital warts, and syphilis.

Official national incidence statistics for STDs are published by the CDC and by local health authorities, but the actual incidence is unknown. Accurate statistics are difficult to compile for a number of reasons. Statistics reflect the accuracy of case reporting, and reporting is not mandatory for all STDs. Rates for some STDs, such as genital herpes and genital warts, are based on estimates derived from local studies and physicians' reports. These estimates are thought to be low. Even rates developed from mandatory case reporting are believed to be low. There are several causes for physician and clinic underreporting.

The costs of STDs are staggering, both in medical expense and in emotional suffering. Up to $17 billion a year is spent to treat STDs and their sequelae (consequences), including at least $2 billion a year to treat subsequent infertility. These figures, like statistics, can be misleading. For instance, women, who are two times more likely to be infected with an STD than men, are less likely to receive treatment, often because the STD is asymptomatic. Also, STDs can lead to infertility. The cost of treating infertility due to STDs is an indirect cost of the STD. Many couples in lower socioeconomic classes cannot afford infertility treatments. Hence, infertility services are used most often by middle-class and upper-class couples.

Etiology and Risk Factors

STDs can be caused by bacteria, viruses, protozoa, fungi, and ectoparasites. Although younger people have the highest rates for STDs (particularly for chlamydia and gonorrhea), all age groups are at risk. Anyone who engages in intimate physical contact can contract and transmit an STD. Many health care providers do not always acknowledge that fact, especially in regard to middle- or upper-class clients. Health care providers often fail to consider that adolescents or older adults are sexually active. Research shows that health care professionals are unskilled and uncomfortable taking a client's sexual history, which can lead to underscreening.

The fetus or neonate can be infected across the placenta or during vaginal birth. Infants and children can be infected through child abuse. Children and adolescents are particularly vulnerable due to biologic variables and because they are more likely to have more frequent unprotected sex and shorter term relationships leading to multiple partners, and they face obstacles in obtaining health care services. In children, peer group pressure and the belief that they are invincible also are factors when considering the presence of STDs. Older adults can be infected or can experience residual effects from infections contracted earlier. Some manifestations of STDs can be mistaken for other age-related diseases. When a client complains of manifestations that could be an STD, then STDs should be part of the differential diagnosis.

The worldwide increase in the incidence of STDs is a result of many factors. Antibiotic-resistant strains of bacteria have become more common. For example, the incidence of gonorrhea has risen since the evolution of penicillinase-producing *Neisseria gonorrhoeae*. Some strains of gonorrhea are also resistant to quinolone antibiotics. The use of intrauterine devices (IUDs) and oral contraceptives may lower women's resistance to infection and facilitate transmission of STDs. Women may not think to use an infection barrier *in addition to* effective contraception. Sterilized women often do not use condoms. Many people have a cavalier attitude about infection and illness in general because of advances made in antimicrobial therapy, and thus do not consider STDs to be serious diseases with possible complications.

Lack of knowledge also plays a role in the incidence of STDs. Clients may find it difficult to obtain accurate information, even from health professionals. Politics and religion continue to affect the controversy over sex education in schools. Accurate information about sex and STDs is not always presented in a manner designed for young people. Information presented to children and adolescents must take into account their age, developmental level, and culture (see the Evidence-Based

Practice in Action feature on Teaching Adolescents About Sexually Transmitted Diseases—What Works?, below). Research continues on the best ways to educate individuals and encourage them to change risky behaviors.

The following are specific risk factors for acquiring STDs:

- Intravenous (IV) drug use
- Other substance abuse
- High-risk sexual activity (use of prostitutes, multiple or casual sexual partners, sex with IV drug users and infected people, unprotected sex, exchanging sex for money or drugs)
- Younger age
- Younger age at *sexarche* (the beginning of sexual activity)

EB EVIDENCE-BASED PRACTICE IN ACTION

Teaching Adolescents About Sexually Transmitted Diseases—What Works?

The goal of educating people about STDs is to convince them to change their behavior when it comes to risky sexual practices. This is difficult in all populations, but presents special challenges when working with adolescents. Besides being biologically more susceptible to STDs, many social and developmental influences create barriers to safe behavior in this age-group.[1]

Developmentally, adolescents are trying to create identities separate from their parents. This often leads to conflict as the teen seemingly rejects advice from older people. Where a parent or teacher may seem hopelessly out-of-date, a peer educator can provide a credible role model and is often preferred by teens. Teens use concrete reasoning and have a present-oriented and short-term view of events. An adolescent girl might not be able to conceptualize acquiring a disease that has no manifestations and that may affect her fertility in 10 to 15 years. A teen may say she is in a "long-term" relationship, when, in reality, the relationship may endure a matter of weeks. Some teens cannot complete a task requiring multiple steps (physically using a condom correctly). Egocentrism often leads teens to believe they can "tell" who has an STD and who is "safe."

Often sexuality messages are presented in ways that appeal to adults: scare tactics can work when the audience thinks in abstract and future-oriented terms. But to reach teens, teaching must be done in ways that appeal to them. The best programs seem to have the following concepts. Within a sound theoretical framework, the program should focus on reducing a specific risky behavior and use a variety of interactive teaching methods that help the student personalize the material. Instruction should include dealing with social pressure and opportunities to practice communication skills. Reinforcement of values and norms can be done with peer educators who "normalize" the message.[2]

A successful HIV-risk reduction program developed with teen input included colorful posters, pocket calendars for participants,

"giveaways" (snacks, condoms, bus tokens), teaching methods that were seen as fun and inventive, and small group activities. Presentations were modeled after computer games, students wrote commercials and rap songs about using condoms, and they viewed videos and played card games with messages about HIV. Students also participated in role plays that required increasingly sophisticated communication skills. The instructors were proficient in using language and references that resonated with the teens.[3]

When working with individual teens, focus on a specific behavior and present-oriented consequences. (The risk profiler at http://www.unspeakable.com is a good reference; other good websites are http://www.thebody.com/surveys/sexsurvey.html; http://www.studenthlth.pitt.edu/studenthealthed_wbpage/ sexual-health/links_for_shi/selftest.html). Help the teen formulate ways of avoiding the risk and allow him or her to practice needed skills. Use terms the teen can understand. Ask concrete but open-ended questions about behaviors that do not require the teen to formulate a judgment about behavior. Honest, respectful, caring, and forthright health care providers are valued by teens.

References

1. Holmes, K., et al. (1999). *Sexually transmitted diseases* (3rd ed.). New York: McGraw-Hill.
2. Lane, M.A., et al. (1999). Features of sexually transmitted disease services important to African American adolescents. *Archives of Pediatric and Adolescent Medicine, 153*, 829-833.
3. Morrison-Beedy, D., et al. (2002). Adolescents' input on the development of an HIV risk reduction intervention. *Journal of the Association of Nurses in AIDS Care, 13*(1), 21-27.

- Inner city residence
- Poverty
- Poor nutrition
- Poor hygiene

According to the CDC, STD prevention and health promotion should focus on five major concepts:

- Education (particularly on risky behaviors)
- Detection of active disease (including asymptomatic infections)
- Effective diagnosis and treatment
- Evaluation and treatment of sexual partners (see CDC guidelines; generally all partners in the last 60 days, or most recent)
- Pre-exposure vaccination if available

Sex education in schools, risk-reduction counseling, promotion of safer sex, and an open, accepting attitude from health professionals can increase knowledge levels. Health professionals must be comfortable asking clients about sexual activity and must provide information in a way that does not "turn off" the client or cause embarrassment. Substitute objective descriptors of activity for judgmental phrases. Instead of asking "Are you unfaithful?" rather ask "How many sexual partners have you had?" Instead of using labeling terms such as "homosexual," ask questions such as "Do you have sex with men, women, or both?" Many people who have had same-sex partners do not identify themselves as "homosexual." "Sexually active" is another phrase that should be avoided because people tend to equate that with vigorous activity or multiple partners.

Health maintenance consists of the following:

- Screening high-risk people
- Maintaining a high index of suspicion for asymptomatic infections
- Providing accurate, timely diagnosis and treatment
- Performing follow-up after treatment when indicated
- Reporting cases of STDs
- Identifying and treating sexual partners of clients with STDs

Health restoration includes measures to reverse the effects of disease, such as infertility (see Chapters 40 and 41). Although some STDs can be passed nonsexually, most are transmitted sexually because the causative organisms thrive in a warm, dark, moist environment within the body and survive only very briefly outside that environment. Therefore their transmission requires intimate contact. Prevention and control must focus on breaking the chain of sexual transmission of disease.

Pathophysiology

An STD occurs when an individual is infected by an organism through sexual contact. Some STDs remain localized; others spread and become systemic. Some STDs present as an acute episode; others are chronic illnesses. See sections on specific STDs for more detailed information.

Clinical Manifestations

Clinical manifestations vary among the STDs and depend on the organism involved and the location of the infection (local or systemic). Diseases may be grouped according to their primary manifestation (e.g., those that cause vaginal discharge). Diagnostic testing is individualized for each condition. See specific STDs for more detailed information.

Outcome Management
■ Medical Management

Medical management focuses on eradicating the offending organism, if possible, or managing a chronic condition. The Integrating Pharmacology feature on Drugs Used to Treat Common Sexually Transmitted Diseases on p. 1129 provides a concise pharmacologic overview.

■ Nursing Management of the Medical Client

Nursing outcomes are similar to medical outcomes. The following discussion of nursing care can be generalized to all STDs. Specific details are provided in the discussion of each STD.

Assessment

A thorough nursing assessment consists of (1) general health assessment and examination, (2) sexual history, preference, and practices, (3) previous history of STDs, (4) specific complaints (60% to 80% of STDs are asymptomatic), (5) genital hygienic practices (douching), (6) contraceptive history, and (7) infection barriers used. A holistic approach also assesses lifestyle, nutrition, stress, and sexuality. High-risk clients should be screened for STDs regardless of whether manifestations are present at the time of a visit to a health care provider. Never assume that a client is not sexually active and make sure that the client understands questions exactly.

Nurses need to know about the variety of sexual activities, their effect on transmission of STDs, and the common manifestations for which to assess. Separate personal views of morality from appropriate nursing activities. Judgmental attitudes may deter clients from seeking care and may interfere with therapeutic relationships. Bias and prejudice can be communicated in obvious and subtle ways that make the client feel uncomfortable, judged, and discounted. A prejudiced health professional cannot provide comprehensive care. An accepting attitude may ensure treatment and prevent disease transmission.

STDs are associated with a social stigma. Ashamed, many clients try to keep the diagnosis secret. Many relate STDs with low social status and immorality, and many have misconceptions and fears about the dangers

INTEGRATING PHARMACOLOGY

Drugs Used to Treat Common Sexually Transmitted Diseases

Antibiotics

Antibiotics are used for STDs caused by bacteria, such as chlamydia, gonorrhea, and syphilis. Antibiotic therapy eradicates manifestations, cures disease, and prevents spread of disease through antimicrobial properties. Oral antibiotics should be taken evenly throughout the day. Doxycycline may lessen contraceptive effectiveness and should not be taken with dairy products, iron, or antacids. Ceftriaxone is reconstituted with lidocaine to reduce pain at injection site. Quinolone-resistant gonorrhea occurs; see CDC guidelines.[8] Clients treated for gonorrhea need to be treated for chlamydia also and vice versa.

Penicillin is the treatment of choice for syphilis. Some oral antibiotics are effective in some stages, but they must be taken long term. Clients need support to maintain compliance with therapy. Treatment in latent syphilis is primarily directed toward preventing or slowing complications. Transmission is not affected. Antibiotic treatment of bacterial vaginosis alleviates irritating vaginal manifestations and cures disease. Clients should avoid alcohol during oral therapy and for 24 hours afterward.

Chancroid is treated with either oral azithromycin or an injection of ceftriaxone. Granuloma inguinale is treated with oral doxycycline, and another bacterial disease, bacterial vaginosis, is treated with metronidazole.

Antiviral Agents

Antiviral therapy is used for human papillomavirus (HPV) infection and for herpes. The main goal of therapy in HPV infection is to remove symptomatic warts. Each topical drug has specific directions regarding frequency of application, duration of treatment, and adjunct skin care. Topical ointments should be applied wearing a glove. Podofilox/podophyllin prevents cell division. Imiquimod is an immune-enhancer that stimulates local immune response. Cryotherapy causes cell lysis. Acid application causes protein coagulation and wart destruction. Interferons inhibit viral replication and may have an immunostimulating effect. Systemic interferons have no effect, but can be injected directly into the wart.

Antiviral therapy used in herpes offers partial control and more rapid resolution of manifestations in acute episodes and provides suppressive therapy for clients who suffer frequent recurrences. All drugs interfere with viral replication. Treatment for recurrent episodes should begin with the prodromal phase. No drug is curative. Commonly used drugs for herpes include acyclovir, famciclovir, and valacyclovir.

Antiprotozoan Therapy

Treatment for trichomoniasis with oral metronidazole relieves manifestations, cures disease, and halts transmission. Topical metronidazole does not reach therapeutic levels for treatment for this condition, so it is given orally.

Modified from the *2002 Sexually Transmitted Diseases Treatment Guidelines*[8] with further information from *Mosby's Nursing Drug Reference.*[25]

of STDs. Other problems may surface with discovery of an STD. For example, a newly infected client may be angry with the presumed responsible sexual partner or may hesitate to identify or inform the sexual partner or partners about the STD. When a marital or committed relationship is involved, questions about infidelity or infertility may arise.

Clients can seek treatment from various sources: health department STD clinics, physician offices, emergency departments, Planned Parenthood clinics, and other community-based clinics. All points of service must be prepared to deal with STDs and have staff sensitive to the needs of these clients. Strict confidentiality is essential. It is especially, but not exclusively, important to homosexual men and lesbians, who may be at risk for discrimination if their sexual orientation is disclosed.

Diagnosis, Outcomes, Interventions

Diagnosis: Ineffective Health Maintenance. The client with an STD needs to improve health behaviors, which makes *Ineffective Health Maintenance related to lack of understanding of the causes, treatments, and prevention of STDs* the priority nursing diagnosis.

Outcomes. The client will understand the cause, treatment, and prevention of specific STDs, as evidenced by client's statements, the client's avoidance of STDs, successful treatment of an STD, and, if possible, the absence of recurrence of the STD.

Interventions

Teach About STDs. Provide accurate, specific, factual information about the transmission, prevention, and treatment of STDs in terms the client can understand (see the Client Education Guide on Sexually Transmitted Diseases on the website). Clarify any misinformation the client has about STDs; for example, many people erroneously believe that oral contraceptives protect them against STDs and do not use condoms in conjunction with their contraceptives. Often women who have been surgically sterilized, who have IUDs, or who are postmenopausal (and who do not need birth control) fail to consider condom use for disease protection. Teaching methods should consider religious and cultural concerns. (See the Bridge to Home Health Care on Teaching About Sexually Transmitted Infections on the website for information on teaching clients about STDs in a sensitive manner.) Include the following topics in teaching sessions about specific STDs:

1. Name, nature, and seriousness of the condition
2. Mode of transmission
   a. Any sexual activity can spread STDs, not just intercourse.
   b. High-risk activities include sexual relations with new or multiple partners.
3. Actions the client should take to prevent the spread of infection to others
   a. Clients should always use a new latex condom for each sexual act (male and female condoms are available).
   b. Clients should finish all prescribed medications.
   c. Sexual partners should be evaluated and treated if needed.
   d. Clients should refrain from sexual relations until both partners have been treated.
   e. Clients should refrain from sexual relations if either partner has any manifestations of an STD.
4. Incubation periods
5. Manifestations of infection
6. Asymptomatic problems
7. When and how to seek treatment
   a. Be sure the client understands the difference between Papanicolaou (Pap) smears and STD examinations; both are not always done at the same time. (Most people seeking treatment or screening for STDs assume the Pap smear and testing for all diseases is being done. Explain to clients if this is not the case.)
8. Treatment methods
   a. Teach clients about medication or other treatments.
9. Follow-up care (when and how to obtain it)
10. Consequences of not completing treatment
    a. Infertility
    b. Chronic abdominal pain
    c. Higher risk of ectopic pregnancy or spontaneous abortion
11. Risks and consequences of recurrent infections, for example, STDs increase the risk of acquiring HIV infection

Teach Condom Use. Promote the use of a new condom for every act of penetrating sexual activity. The latex condom (called a *rubber* in lay terms) is the most effective mechanical barrier to STDs and its use by sexually active people who are at risk should be promoted. Sexually active men and women should learn to use condoms properly, effectively, and consistently. Condom failure is primarily due to improper or inconsistent use rather than to product defect. See the Client Education Guide on How to Use a Condom on the website for instructions on correct condom use.

There are several barriers to using condoms. Women may not believe they are empowered to make healthy choices. Condoms require male cooperation, and many women are in relationships defined by an imbalance of power in which they cannot insist on condom use. Some studies have shown that the fear of losing a sexual partner is greater for some women than the fear of contracting an STD, even AIDS. Older people may not have experience with condoms. Condoms may not be acceptable to some clients for religious, cultural, or ethnic reasons.

Use Therapeutic Communication. When caring for clients with STDs, nurses obtain privileged or private information and provide instruction about these diseases. Both activities require sensitivity and skillful interaction. The successful nurse needs to be adept in interpersonal communication. Such clients need encouragement, support, and accurate information.

Identify Resources. Nurses play a pivotal role in identifying community and national resources available to clients. Most public health agencies have STD education, prevention, and treatment programs that are open to the public. Clients can also obtain information anonymously from the National STD Hotline (1-800-227-8922) or the National HIV/AIDS Hotline (1-800-342-AIDS), or at http://www.ashastd.org.

Diagnosis: Anxiety. The client with an STD often experiences a great deal of uncertainty, which makes *Anxiety related to threat to biologic integrity and threat to self-concept* an important nursing diagnosis.

Outcomes. The client will experience a decrease in anxiety, as evidenced by verbal statements, showing acceptance of the condition, and demonstrating appropriate coping methods.

Interventions

Provide Support. STDs can threaten a client's self-concept and pose potential physical problems, such as infertility and fetal damage. The client may express guilt, apprehension, and fear of rejection. Help the client reduce anxiety by being warm and supportive, facilitating the expression of feelings, and encouraging effective coping strategies.

Help with Problem-Solving. Assist the client with learning and problem-solving once anxiety is reduced. Role-playing and practicing negotiation skills may help a woman become more assertive in being able to ensure her sexual health.

Other Diagnoses. Risk for Situational Low Self-Esteem, Acute Pain, Impaired Tissue Integrity, and Risk for Ineffective Therapeutic Regimen Management.

Evaluation

It is expected that the STD will be successfully treated and, if possible, eradicated. The client will be able to state the cause, manifestations, treatment, and prevention of STDs and will remain free of STDs.

DISEASES CHARACTERIZED BY URETHRITIS OR CERVICITIS
CHLAMYDIAL INFECTIONS

Chlamydial infection is the nation's most common bacterial STD. The number of new cases per year is estimated to be at least 4 million at a cost of $2.2 billion per year.

Etiology and Risk Factors

The causative organism, *Chlamydia trachomatis*, is a nonmotile, gram-negative bacterium. This organism is the most common cause of what was previously diagnosed as nonspecific vaginitis in women and of nongonococcal urethritis (NGU) in men.

C. trachomatis is transmitted by intimate sexual contact. Women usually acquire the infection during vaginal intercourse with an infected man, but it can also be transmitted through oral-anal contact or anal penetration. The infection does not cross the placenta, but passage through the birth canal of an infected mother can cause conjunctivitis and pneumonia in a newborn. The incubation period is 7 to 21 days.

Pathophysiology

Chlamydial infection is known as "the great sterilizer" and is considered the most important cause of pelvic inflammatory disease (PID) and tubal infertility. Undetected and untreated cases can have serious, irreversible consequences. *C. trachomatis* causes inflammation that leads to scarring and ulceration of involved tissue. In women, the infection can extend to the endometrium and salpinx (fallopian tube); the major consequence is salpingitis (inflammation of the fallopian tubes) with subsequent infertility or high risk of ectopic (tubal) pregnancy. Secondary extension to the peritoneum can cause PID (see Chapter 41). In men, the infection can cause a urethral stricture that may extend to the *epididymis*. Sterility can result from the ensuing epididymitis. A serious systemic complication more common in

men is Reiter's syndrome, which consists of urethritis, polyarthritis, and conjunctivitis.

Clinical Manifestations

Chlamydial infections primarily affect the cervix, urethra, and rectum. In most cases, the infection is asymptomatic for an extended period. In women, the primary site of infection is the endocervix. The cervix becomes edematous and produces a yellow, mucopurulent vaginal discharge. This discharge may be accompanied by spotting at menstrual midcycle or with sexual intercourse. *C. trachomatis* also causes urethritis with dysuria (painful or difficult urination) and urinary frequency in women. In 65% of women who had urinary manifestations and negative urine culture results, one study found that results of culture for *C. trachomatis* were positive. Involvement of Bartholin's duct produces a purulent discharge.

In males, the chief manifestation is urethritis with dysuria (painful and difficult urination) and clear to mucopurulent discharge. In both sexes, proctitis (rectal inflammation) and pharyngitis (inflammation of the pharynx) may develop with rectal and orogenital contact.

Because chlamydial infection may produce few or no manifestations, clients tend not to seek medical treatment and the diagnosis is difficult and often missed. Because chlamydial and gonorrheal infections often coexist, diagnostic tests and treatment are recommended for both when either condition is suspected. Presumptive treatment for chlamydial infection in clients being treated for gonorrhea is appropriate and cost-effective, particularly when testing for *C. trachomatis* is not performed.

The definitive test for the fast and accurate diagnosis of chlamydial infection has yet to be developed. The best and most sensitive diagnostic test is tissue culture of cellular material from the urethra, endocervix, or rectum. This test, however, is expensive and technically difficult.

Rapid nonculture detection tests performed on urogenital secretions are readily available, including direct fluorescent antibody (DFA) microscopy, enzyme-linked immunosorbent assay (ELISA), nucleic acid amplification tests, and monoclonal antigen-antibody tests to detect *C. trachomatis* antigens. Although less accurate than cultures, these tests are more convenient, less expensive, and quicker. The ELISA test can be used to detect *C. trachomatis* antigen in the initial 10 to 20 ml of voided urine. Some testing can be performed via a self-administered vaginal swab. Screening is recommended for all asymptomatic, high-risk clients in whom chlamydia might be present. Priority groups for testing are (1) high-risk pregnant women, (2) adolescents, and (3) women age 20 to 24 years who have new or multiple sexual partners or who do not use condoms routinely. Many sources also recommend testing any woman with a history of infertility, ectopic pregnancies, or spontaneous abortions.

Outcome Management
■ Medical Management

Eradicate Disease and Manifestations. The treatment of choice for chlamydial infection is doxycycline (Vibramycin) given orally for 7 days or one dose of azithromycin (Zithromax). To prevent complications, it is imperative that treatment be aggressive and started when the disease is suspected (before test results are back), and that the entire course of antibiotics be completed. Antibiotics are almost always effective; therefore test of cure is not necessary unless manifestations persist or recur. If testing for chlamydial infection is not available, treatment is prescribed on the basis of clinical diagnosis only or as co-treatment for gonorrhea. All sexual partners within the last 60 days should be examined and treated. When the client's last sexual contact occurred more than 60 days before diagnosis, the last partner should be treated. The CDC recommends that medications be dispensed on site and that the first dose be directly observed to improve compliance.

■ Nursing Management of the Medical Client

Eradicate Disease and Manifestations. Instruct clients about the greater risk of infection with multiple sexual partners and inform them of the serious danger of sterility, particularly for women. Stress that this infection may have a long latency period. Infected clients should scrupulously avoid all sexual activity until both partners are cured, and they should use condoms thereafter.

GONORRHEA

Gonorrhea (also known as *clap, white, drips, strain,* and *dose* in lay terms) can be divided into two categories: local and disseminated. *Local infection* can involve the mucosal surfaces of the cervix, urethra, and rectum; vestibular glands; pharynx; or conjunctiva. *Systemic infection (disseminated gonococcal infection)* involves bacteremia with polyarthritis, dermatitis, endocarditis, and meningitis. Systemic infection is more common in women.

Etiology and Risk Factors

Gonorrhea is one of the most prevalent STDs in the United States; more than 650,000 new cases are reported each year. Some studies show that gonorrhea may be grossly underreported. Teenagers and young adults are at highest risk. Most cases of gonorrhea occur in people age 15 to 29 years, with the highest rate in those age 20 to 24 years.

Pathophysiology

Gonorrhea is caused by the gram-negative diplococcus *Neisseria gonorrhoeae.* The causative organism is highly contagious, but does not survive long outside the body. Gonorrhea, therefore, is almost always transmitted by direct sexual contact. The few rare exceptions are infection in infants, who can contract gonorrhea during vaginal birth, and infection of medical personnel through broken skin. The incubation period is 3 to 8 days.

Clinical Manifestations

The endocervical canal is the primary site of gonorrheal infection in women. In most women, the urethra is also infected. Infection can also involve the vestibular glands and anus. The vagina is resistant to the infection in adulthood but not before puberty. The disease may be asymptomatic in women. There is a large *carrier population* (people who carry the organism and have no manifestations but can transmit the disease) for gonorrhea. Manifestations of gonorrhea include (1) heavy, yellow-green, purulent vaginal discharge, (2) cervical erythema, (3) a red, swollen, sore vulva, (4) abnormal menstrual bleeding, and (5) dysuria and urinary frequency.

The most common complication of gonorrhea in women is salpingitis, which can progress to PID. Both PID and salpingitis can produce infertility secondary to scarring and occlusion of the fallopian tubes. The first recognizable manifestations of gonorrhea in women may arise from PID.

Manifestations of gonorrhea are usually evident earlier in men than in women. The infection is principally one of the anterior urethra that produces a purulent discharge, dysuria, and urinary frequency. Complications include epididymitis and prostatitis, but these are not common with early and complete antibiotic therapy. In addition to the gender-specific manifestations, both men and women may have conjunctivitis or pharyngitis due to orogenital contact or proctitis from anal contact.

Disseminated infection results from gonococcal bacteremia and is often manifested by septic arthritis, skin lesions, asymmetrical arthralgias, and tenosynovitis (inflammation of the tendon and synovial membrane). Rarely, hepatic adhesions (Fitz-Hugh-Curtis syndrome), endocarditis, or meningitis occurs.

Diagnosis of gonorrhea can be made through history, physical examination, identification of the gonococcus on a smear, or culture of the exudate from infected areas. Culture with selective culture media remains the cornerstone of diagnosis.

Outcome Management
■ Medical Management

Eradicate Disease and Manifestations. All sexually active women in high-risk groups should be screened for gonorrhea on a regular basis. All clients in whom gonorrhea is detected should also be tested for chlamydial infection.

Gonorrhea is treated aggressively with antibiotics, without waiting for test results, on the basis of clinical manifestations. Before the advent of resistant organisms, penicillin was the treatment of choice. The current recommended regimen for uncomplicated gonorrhea is a single intramuscular (IM) dose of ceftriaxone (Rocephin), or a single oral dose of cefixime (Suprax), ciprofloxacin (Cipro), or ofloxacin (Floxin). Levofloxacin is also effective, but quinolone-resistant infections are increasingly common. Therefore quinolone therapy should be avoided for cases that originated in Asia or the Pacific (including Hawaii), and should probably not be used in California. A single IM injection of spectinomycin (Trobicin) can be used for clients who cannot tolerate ceftriaxone. All persons treated for gonorrhea need to be treated concurrently for chlamydial infection (see the Integrating Pharmacology feature on Drugs Used to Treat Common Sexually Transmitted Diseases on p. 1129).

For clients with disseminated gonococcal infection, the recommended regimen is administration of ceftriaxone, given IM or IV every 24 hours and continued 24 to 48 hours after improvement begins, followed by cefixime or ciprofloxacin, given orally for a full week.

After therapy for uncomplicated gonorrhea is completed, a follow-up examination and culture are not necessary because treatment failure is rare. Recurring or unresolved cases should be evaluated with a follow-up culture. Any gonococcal organisms on the second culture should be tested for antibiotic sensitivity and possible resistant organisms.

■ Nursing Management of the Medical Client

Eradicate Disease and Manifestations. Discuss the importance of identifying and treating all sexual partners, because there seems to be a reservoir population of asymptomatic men. Recurrence due to reinfection may indicate the need for improved client education and sexual partner referral. Investigation of the client's sexual contacts is essential for the prevention and control of gonorrhea. All sexual partners within the 60 days before diagnosis (or the last contact if greater than 60 days) should undergo examination, culture, and treatment. Reporting sexual contacts can be difficult and frightening for an infected client. Ask for contact information in a positive, nonthreatening way.

Warn pregnant clients of the danger of infecting their newborns during delivery. Clients receiving treatment for gonorrhea must understand the importance of taking the *complete* course of prescribed medication.

■ DISEASES CHARACTERIZED BY ULCERATIONS
SYPHILIS

Syphilis (lay terms are *bad blood, lues, pox,* and *syph*) is a systemic, highly infectious STD. It became less prevalent after the advent of penicillin, but the disease has not been eradicated. The incidence of syphilis peaked in the early 1990s and declined for a few years. In 1997, 75% of all U.S. counties reported no new cases, which has led the CDC to call for its complete eradication. However, the incidence is now increasing in many areas; this is

worrisome because syphilis is often a "herald" disease for HIV infection.

Etiology and Risk Factors

Syphilis is caused by the delicate motile (self-moving) spirochete *Treponema pallidum*. Although *T. pallidum* cannot survive long outside the body, it is highly infectious. Sexual transmission of *T. pallidum* occurs only when the mucocutaneous lesions of primary and secondary syphilis are present. Adolescents, young adults, and men who have sex with men are at greatest risk. Syphilis is a known cofactor for development of HIV infection.

Pathophysiology

T. pallidum enters the body through intact mucous membranes or abraded skin, almost exclusively by direct sexual contact. After entry, the organisms multiply locally and disseminate systemically through the bloodstream and lymphatics. The infection can also be passed transplacentally from an untreated pregnant woman to her fetus during any stage of the disease (*congenital syphilis*).

In rare instances, syphilis has been contracted through nonsexual personal contact, accidental inoculation, or blood transfusion from a syphilitic donor. Syphilis can progress to irreversible blindness, mental illness, paralysis, heart disease, and death.

Clinical Manifestations

Syphilis is characterized by well-defined sequential stages that occur over years: primary, secondary, latent (early latent and late latent), and tertiary.

Primary Stage

The principal manifestation of primary syphilis is the appearance of a genital chancre. A *chancre* is an oval ulcer with a raised firm border that does not bleed readily and is painless unless infected (Figure 43-1). The chancre develops at the site of inoculation, usually the genitalia, anus, or mouth. Most commonly, a single chancre occurs about 4 weeks after initial infection. Chancres in women often remain unnoticed. Lymphadenopathy may occur as lymph glands near the chancre become enlarged. Nodes are painless, firm, and discrete. If untreated, a chancre heals spontaneously in 4 to 6 weeks, leaving a thin, atrophic scar.

Secondary Stage

If the primary disease is untreated, secondary syphilis develops 6 to 8 weeks after infection. The following are indications of the second stage:

1. *Generalized rash.* Typically, a maculopapular and nonpruritic rash appears; the rash can be anywhere but often appears on the palms of the hands and

FIGURE 43-1 Ulcer of primary syphilis. (Courtesy of Dr. Rodney M.S. Basler.)

soles of the feet (few other diseases cause a rash in these locations); the rash is infectious.

2. *Generalized, nontender, discrete lymphadenopathy.*
3. *Mucous patches.* Gray, superficial patches occur on the mucous membranes in the mouth and may be accompanied by a sore throat.
4. *Condylomata lata.* Broad-based, flat papules usually can be easily distinguished from the typical narrow-based, pedunculated growth of condylomata acuminata (genital warts). Condylomata lata may develop in warm, moist body areas—most commonly on the labia or anus or at the corners of the mouth. They are highly contagious.
5. *General flu-like manifestations,* including nausea, anorexia, constipation, headache, muscle, joint, and bone pain, and a chronically elevated temperature.
6. *Patchy hair loss* from eyebrows and scalp (alopecia).

Secondary stage manifestations usually disappear after 2 to 6 weeks. A latency period then begins.

Latent Stage

Latent syphilis is defined as that period after infection with *T. pallidum* when a client is seroreactive (with a positive blood test) but shows no other evidence of disease. During this stage, syphilis is noninfectious except via transplacental spread or blood transfusion. Syphilis is not transmitted by sexual contact during the latent phase unless a secondary syphilitic mucocutaneous skin lesion reoccurs during early latent syphilis. Latent syphilis usually occurs 1 to 2 years after the primary lesion and can last as long as 50 years. About 66% of those infected remain in this stage without further problems.

Tertiary Stage

In 1 to 35 years after the primary infection, about 33% of clients with untreated syphilis experience devastating, irreversible complications, such as chronic bone and joint inflammation, cardiovascular problems (for example, valvular involvement, aneurysms), granulomatous lesions *(gummas)* on any part of the body, and ophthalmic, auditory, and central nervous system problems. This stage, although not infectious, may be terminal if untreated (see Chapter 74 for manifestations of neurosyphilis [syphilis affecting the central nervous system]).

Diagnosis

The diagnosis of syphilis is based on health assessment and various direct and indirect laboratory studies. A *direct test* identifies the causative organism; an *indirect test* identifies antibodies of the causative agent. *T. pallidum* cannot be grown in culture. Primary or secondary stage lesions can be scraped and the causative organism identified directly with dark-field microscopy (DFA) testing. Dark-field examination must be done by an expert, because other spirochetes closely resembling *T. pallidum* are present in oral and genital mucosa. This test confirms a diagnosis of syphilis in the primary stage (when other tests are generally negative) and the secondary stage.

Serologic tests for syphilis are indirect tests that detect antibodies. These antibodies are not present in the serum until 4 weeks *after* the appearance of the chancre. Such tests include the following:

- The Venereal Disease Research Laboratory (VDRL)
- Rapid plasma reagin (RPR), which uses an antigen to detect the antibody relatively specific for *T. pallidum*
- Fluorescent treponemal antibody absorption (FTA-ABS) tests
- *T. pallidum* particle agglutination (TP-PA)

The VDRL test for nonspecific antibodies is the most commonly used screening test. Results are negative in the early primary stage, before antibodies to *T. pallidum* are formed and are present in the circulation. Results may be falsely positive if the VDRL test is performed during the early stages of several common viral illnesses (mumps, measles, hepatitis, chickenpox, infectious mononucleosis; also presence of systemic lupus erythematosus may yield a false-positive test). Results are given as "nonreactive," "borderline," "weakly reactive," or "reactive." Reactive and weakly reactive results are considered to be positive.

The FTA-ABS serologic test is more specific because it measures antibodies specific to *T. pallidum*. It is used when the VDRL result is positive but the diagnosis of syphilis is still uncertain. The FTA-ABS test result usually becomes positive 3 to 4 weeks after infection. Once positive, FTA-ABS test results usually remain positive for the client's life, regardless of treatment or cure. Cerebrospinal fluid may be examined for characteristic findings in late neurosyphilis.

Syphilis often coexists with other infections. The CDC recommends that all clients with syphilis be counseled on the risks of HIV infection and AIDS and encouraged to undergo HIV testing, plus screening for other common STDs.

Outcome Management
■ Medical Management

Eradicate Disease and Manifestations. Parenteral penicillin remains the treatment of choice for all stages of syphilis; however, the structural changes present in late syphilis are irreversible despite successful treatment. The dosage schedule and length of therapy are determined by the stage of the disease and current guidelines for treatment. For primary, secondary, and early latent syphilis, the treatment of choice is benzathine penicillin G, given IM in one dose. Late latent syphilis (or latent of unknown duration) is treated with three weekly penicillin injections. Neurosyphilis is treated with IV aqueous crystalline penicillin G.

Use of penicillin to treat syphilis in clients with penicillin allergy is a complicated issue. Clients who are pregnant or noncompliant with therapy or who have neurosyphilis should undergo desensitization and treatment with penicillin. Desensitization guidelines are available from the CDC. For nonpregnant clients who are allergic to penicillin, doxycycline or tetracycline may be given, but they are not as effective as penicillin.

Treatment failure can occur with any given regimen. Compliance is often a problem. Clients should be reexamined clinically and evaluated with serologic testing at 6, 12, and 24 months after treatment. No definitive criteria for cure exist. With successful treatment, ideally, no evidence of disease should be present and serial serologic test values should decline.

Treating sexual partners is also a complex issue; treatment is best guided by information available from the CDC. All people who have had sexual contact with the client who has primary syphilis must be identified and evaluated. Most practitioners treat sexual contacts as if they have primary syphilis whether or not they show evidence of infection.

■ Nursing Management of the Medical Client

Eradicate Disease and Manifestations. A client with syphilis needs information and psychosocial support to deal with this complex illness. Individualize health teaching to meet the client's particular needs and psychosocial situation. A diagnosis of syphilis can be frightening and difficult to accept.

Clients with primary or secondary syphilis should abstain from sexual contact for at least 1 month after treatment. Adequate treatment should be curative, but reinfection is possible and can be detected with clinical examinations and monitoring of serologic test values. Proper follow-up, although essential, is time-consuming and difficult. Many clients do not understand the severe consequences of not obtaining adequate treatment.

GENITAL HERPES

Genital herpes is a recurrent, systemic viral infection. Although recognized for centuries, genital herpes has received renewed attention because of its epidemic incidence. Now one of the most common STDs (50 million cases in the United States), it is the most frequent cause of genital ulceration. Its peak incidence is among adolescents and young adults.

Etiology and Risk Factors

Caused by herpes simplex virus (HSV) type 2, the infection is closely related to other herpes infections, such as the classic cold sore caused by HSV type 1. HSV type 1 infection is mainly nongenital, occurring above the waist (often on the lips or nose). HSV type 2 infection occurs primarily below the waist as a sexually transmitted genital infection. It is possible for HSV type 1 to cause genital infections and for HSV type 2 to cause oral lesions (Figure 43-2).

Pathophysiology

The HSV organism is present in the exudate of the lesion. Herpes can be transmitted while a lesion is present and for 10 days after a lesion has healed. Genital herpes is usually transmitted by direct contact with the exudate during sexual activity, but transmission is possible by *fomites* (objects that can harbor pathogenic microorganisms), such as towels used by an infected person. Many cases of genital herpes are acquired from people who do not know they have an infection or who are asymptomatic at the time of sexual contact. Newborns can be infected during vaginal delivery when active genital lesions are present. Cesarean section prevents this transmission.

Clinical Manifestations

Many people with HSV type 2 infection have mild or unrecognized disease. Manifestations of genital herpes

FIGURE 43-2 Typical herpes vesicles. (Courtesy of Dr. Rodney M.S. Basler.)

usually occur 3 to 7 days after contact. Initially, a burning sensation (paresthesia) is noted at the site of inoculation. Next, numerous small vesicles with an erythematous border form painful, shallow ulcers that then crust and heal with a scar in about 2 to 4 weeks.

The major problem with HSV is recurrence. Up to 75% of clients have a recurrent infection within 1 year of the first episode. The virus is believed to lie dormant in the body, probably in nerve ganglions, until it is activated, at which point another episode of genital herpes, with characteristic lesions, occurs. Stress, infection, trauma, menses, or sexual activity may trigger recurrent episodes.

Characteristically, recurrent genital herpes causes only local manifestations. Prodromal (pre-onset) manifestations of a burning sensation may occur before the vesicles erupt. The vesicles tend to reappear at the sites of previous infection, but they can involve new sites. Manifestations are similar to, but usually less severe than, those in the primary infection. Vesicles rupture in 24 to 48 hours, and the syndrome generally lasts 7 to 10 days.

Potential complications of HSV infections include disseminated infections, meningitis, and transverse myelitis. Women are at risk for spontaneous abortion, and it has been suggested that HSV type 2 predisposes to carcinoma of the cervix.

A diagnosis of genital herpes is often made visually. The diagnosis is confirmed by a viral culture, direct immunofluorescence staining, or antigen detection testing of the vesicular exudate. A Pap smear can also be performed; the presence of multinucleated giant cells in the Pap smear, with or without inclusion bodies, is characteristic of a herpes infection.

Outcome Management
■ Medical Management

Reduce Manifestations. Genital herpes is a chronic disease without a cure. Treatment does not cure HSV infection or prevent its spread. Management focuses on preventing or lessening occurrences and giving palliative care. The recommended treatment for an acute primary infection is acyclovir (Zovirax) or famciclovir, antiviral agents, taken orally for 7 to 10 days. Episodic recurrences are treated with acyclovir, valacyclovir (Valtrex), or famciclovir (Famvir) taken for 5 days.

Clients with frequent recurrences (six or more episodes in 1 year) take daily suppressive therapy. Daily acyclovir taken for 4 months to 3 years may prevent or reduce the frequency and severity of recurrence in most people. Clients should begin oral suppressive therapy when they first recognize the prodromal sensations or first become symptomatic. The need for daily suppressive therapy should be reevaluated after 1 year. Severe disease is treated with IV acyclovir.

■ Nursing Management of the Medical Client

Prevent Reinfection. When the vesicles of herpes rupture, they release a highly contagious exudate. Clients and health care providers should wash their hands thoroughly after any contact with the herpetic lesions to avoid further spread. HSV infections of the eye are particularly serious. Infected clients should have separate towels and other personal items and avoid touching their eyes. Clients should use condoms during latent periods because the possible risk of transmission exists even when lesions are not present. Women should have annual pelvic examinations and Pap smears.

Provide Support. Coping with genital herpes may cause tremendous psychosocial stress. Although recurrence cannot always be predicted, nurses can help clients identify possible triggers. Reappearance of the disease can significantly affect sexual activity. Support groups may help clients deal with the anger, guilt, and shame that many commonly feel. Stress reduction techniques may be helpful. Sexual partners should be offered counseling, evaluation, and treatment if needed.

Reduce Pain. The pain of herpes lesions is problematic. Palliative measures include (1) keeping the involved area clean and dry, (2) wearing loose-fitting, nonsynthetic undergarments, and (3) using sitz baths, cooling applications, and analgesic medications, such as aspirin, for pain reduction.

CHANCROID

Chancroid is a highly contagious infection caused by the gram-negative bacillus *Haemophilus ducreyi*. The initial papules or pustules produce multiple painful, irregular, and deep genital ulcers, often accompanied by tender inguinal lymphadenopathy (Figure 43-3). Although chancroid is more common in the tropics, the incidence is endemic in many areas of the United States. Chancroid is **E B**

FIGURE 43-3 Chancroid lesions. (Courtesy of Dr. Rodney M.S. Basler.)

well established as a cofactor for HIV transmission. There is a high rate of HIV and syphilis infection in clients with chancroid. Clients with chancroid should also be tested for HIV infection, HSV infection, and syphilis.

Definitive diagnosis requires the culture of *H. ducreyi*. It is difficult to isolate the organism, and culture of *H. ducreyi* is not widely available. A clinical diagnosis may be made if the client has painful genital ulcers and regional lymphadenopathy (especially tender inguinal adenopathy), and does not have evidence of syphilis or genital herpes. People with whom the client has had sexual contact within 10 days before the onset of manifestations should be examined and treated. Recommended treatment is oral azithromycin or ceftriaxone given IM in a single dose; alternatively, ciprofloxacin or erythromycin may be given orally.

LYMPHOGRANULOMA VENEREUM

Lymphogranuloma venereum is a systemic infection that is rare in the United States. It is caused by certain strains of *C. trachomatis*. The primary lesion is a small, painless papule on the glans penis or the vaginal mucosa that heals spontaneously and may go unnoticed.

The most common clinical manifestations are markedly tender, enlarged, and inflamed inguinal lymph nodes *(buboes)*, which are usually unilateral and appear 2 to 6 weeks after the primary lesion. Eventually, draining ulcerations, scarring, lymphatic obstruction, and marked external genital deformity may occur. Rectal fibrosis and strictures are late sequelae.

Definitive diagnosis is made with a positive culture for *C. trachomatis*. Recommended therapy is doxycycline, given orally for 21 days. Oral erythromycin is an alternative.

GRANULOMA INGUINALE

Granuloma inguinale (donovanosis) is a chronic infection endemic in some tropical and developing areas but rare in the United States. It is caused by the small gram-negative bacillus *Calymmatobacterium granulomatis*.

Granuloma inguinale is characterized by genital and perianal papular lesions without lymphadenopathy. These become painless, gradually enlarging, ulcerating granulomatous lesions that cause tissue destruction. The lesions are highly vascular, bleed easily, and have a beefy-red appearance. Diagnosis is made by microscopic identification of Donovan's bodies (inclusion bodies of the causative organism) in a smear taken from edge scrapings of the lesion.

Treatment consists of a long course of an antibiotic such as trimethoprim-sulfamethoxazole or doxycycline. Relapses can occur despite adequate treatment. IV aminoglycosides are given for infections that do not improve with first-line antibiotics. All partners who have had sexual contact with an infected client within 60 days before diagnosis need evaluation and treatment.

INFECTION WITH HUMAN PAPILLOMAVIRUS
GENITAL WARTS (CONDYLOMATA ACUMINATA)

Etiology and Risk Factors

Genital warts are diagnosed in 5.5 million people each year. Caused by human papillomavirus (HPV), they are usually transmitted by sexual contact. Genital warts have become epidemic, in part because they are often asymptomatic and undiagnosed. Factors that may favor their development include HIV, pregnancy, smoking, drug or alcohol use, poor nutrition, and fatigue.

Pathophysiology

More than 30 types of HPV affect the genital tract. The natural history of HPV is complex and poorly understood. Infection with certain strains of HPV is strongly associated with carcinomas of the genitals, including the cervix. See the Evidence-Based Practice in Action feature on Human Papillomavirus Screening for Women with Abnormal Pap Smear Results on p. 1138.

Clinical Manifestations

Genital warts are benign growths that typically occur in multiple, painless clusters on the vulva, vagina, cervix, perineum, anorectal area, urethral meatus, or glans penis 1 to 2 months after exposure (Figure 43-4). Oral, pharyngeal, and laryngeal lesions can also occur. HPV can cause laryngeal papillomatosis in infants born to mothers with vaginal warts.

Diagnosis is typically made visually. Subclinical (asymptomatic or not visible) warts can be identified through Pap smear and colposcopy (examination of vagina and cervical tissues with a scope containing a magnifying lens) of the cervix. Acetic acid applied to tissue infected with HPV turns a characteristic whitish color. Biopsies may be performed to differentiate warts from carcinoma or condylomata lata of the secondary stage of syphilis.

Outcome Management
■ Medical Management

Remove Visible Warts. There is no cure for genital warts. A variety of chemical, mechanical, and ablative techniques are used for visible lesions, but no specific antiviral therapy for the HPV is available, and no treatment is considered optimal. Treatment varies according to the site and severity of the warts and is client preference. Treatment is more successful if the warts are small and have been present for less than a year. Treatment of subclinical cases is not recommended if the client does not also have cervical squamous cell lesions. Experts

EB EVIDENCE-BASED PRACTICE IN ACTION

Human Papillomavirus Screening for Women with Abnormal Pap Smear Results

Cervical cancer is the second most common cancer affecting women worldwide and is a significant cause of morbidity and mortality, particularly in the developing world. Rates of cervical cancer deaths have plunged in the United States due to the use of the Papanicolaou (Pap) smear, but there are still large areas where the death rate from this preventable cancer is unacceptably high. The American Cancer Society estimated 12,000 new cases in 2002 and 4800 deaths.

Although the Pap smear is recognized as an invaluable tool, there are several well-known problems with it. Many women are not routinely screened and may go years without a Pap smear. This is a particular problem for older women. Whatever the cause, more than half the women with cervical cancer have not had a Pap smear in at least 3 years, despite repeated contacts with health care providers.

Cervical cancer is a sexually transmitted disease in 90% to 100% of all cases. The link between cervical cancer and the human papillomavirus (HPV) is well established; this relationship is "stronger than that of tobacco with lung cancer."[3] Several types of HPV are strongly oncogenic; their DNA has been found in 90% to 100% of cervical cancers. New techniques allow testing of women with abnormal Pap smears for high-risk HPV DNA. The results provide useful information, particularly for women with the confusing results of ASCUS (atypical squamous cells of undetermined significance).

Only a few high-risk types of HPV exist. Women whose test results are negative for high-risk HPV can be managed with a conservative approach. Women whose test results are positive for high-risk HPV can have treatment decisions tailored to their increased risk of developing advanced lesions and cancer. HPV DNA testing has a sensitivity for detecting high-grade lesions and invasive cancers that is equal to or superior to that of Pap smears.[1]

According to the 2001 Consensus Guidelines for the Management of Women with Cervical Cytological Abnormalities, three treatment options exist for ASCUS: serial repeat testing, colposcopy, or HPV DNA testing. The preferred option is to collect the HPV DNA sample with the Pap smear and analyzing it only if the Pap result is abnormal ("reflex testing"). Women whose tests are positive for high-risk HPV should be referred for colposcopy. HPV DNA testing is also recommended for women with low-grade squamous intraepithelial lesions (LSIL) after colposcopy shows no cancer, and HPV DNA testing is in the algorithm for postmenopausal women. Two negative tests for high-risk HPV lends an almost 100% negative predictive value for invasive disease.[2,6]

Several studies have attempted a cost-benefit analysis for HPV screening. One study showed that triennial Pap/HPV screening up to age 75 years was very cost-effective, but biennial Pap/HPV screening saved the most lives. This study has the drawback of eliminating screening in an underserved group (older women). Although the rate of cervical cancer decreases after age 45 years, many older women present with more advanced lesions that progress faster than in younger women.[4]

HPV infection is relatively rare in women older than age 40 years, so a positive test for high-risk HPV DNA is clinically significant. In this age group, the combination of Pap smears with HPV testing may offer the greatest benefit. In women younger than 25 years, as many as 70% test positive for HPV and, in many, the infections regress within months. HPV DNA testing in this age group may not be as predictive of further pathology because HPV infection may be transient.[5]

Self-collected vaginal swabs for HPV DNA are being developed. One study showed the results of self-collected HPV swabs and Pap smears to be virtually identical; both methods identified an equal number of high-grade lesions and invasive cancers.[7] The greatest benefit for this technique may be in resource-poor areas of the world and among women adverse to the gynecologic examination.

References

1. ALTS Group. (2000). Human papillomavirus testing for triage of women with cytologic evidence of low-grade squamous intraepithelial lesions: Baseline data from a randomized trial. *Journal of the National Cancer Institute, 92,* 397-402.
2. American Society for Colposcopy and Cervical Pathology. (2002). Consensus guidelines for the management of women with cervical cytological abnormalities. Available at http://www.asccp.org.
3. Burk, R.D. (1999). Human papillomavirus and the risk of cervical cancer. *Hospital Practice, 34*(12), 103-111.
4. Mandelblatt, J., et al. (2002). Benefits and costs of using HPV testing to screen for cervical cancer. *Journal of the American Medical Association, 287,* 2372-2381.
5. McFadden, S., & Schumann, L. (2001). The role of human papillomavirus in screening for cervical cancer. *Journal of the American Academy of Nurse Practitioners, 13*(3), 116-125.
6. Wright, T., et al. (2002). 2001 Consensus guidelines for the management of women with cervical cytological abnormalities. *Journal of the American Medical Association, 287,* 2120-2129.
7. Wright, T.C., et al. (2000). HPV DNA testing of self-collected vaginal samples compared with cytologic screening to detect cervical cancer. *Journal of the American Medical Association, 283,* 81-86.

FIGURE 43-4 Genital warts (condylomata acuminata). (Courtesy of Dr. Rodney M.S. Basler.)

consider the "watch and wait" approach an acceptable treatment option in uncomplicated cases.

Topical Therapy. The most common pharmacologic treatment is podophyllin resin in compound tincture of benzoin or trichloroacetic acid (TCA) applied topically (by a health care professional) to the warts *only*. Treatments are repeated weekly until all the lesions have disappeared and the skin is healed. Podophyllin is contraindicated during pregnancy because of its *abortifacient* (abortion-causing) properties.

Topical podofilox and Imiquimod cream are approved for self-application by clients at home. For safe application, the client must be able to see and reach the warts easily. Podofilox is also contraindicated during pregnancy. If warts persist, other modes of therapy should be considered (see the Integrating Pharmacology feature on Drugs Used to Treat Common Sexually Transmitted Diseases on p. 1129).

Other Treatment. Warts can be treated with cryotherapy using liquid nitrogen or a cryoprobe. Carbon dioxide lasers, electrocautery, and simple surgical excision can be used on extensive warts. The antiviral drug interferon has also been used, but it is expensive and is associated with a high rate of adverse side effects.

It is not necessary to evaluate and treat sexual partners of clients with genital warts, because treatment is not effective in eradicating the disease or its spread. Female partners should be referred for a Pap smear, and all sexual partners should be offered the opportunity to be examined and tested for other STDs.

■ Nursing Management of the Medical Client

Inform clients with genital warts that no cure exists and that female clients are at increased risk for genital malignancy. HPV infections are strongly associated with cancer of the cervix and vulva in women and squamous cell carcinoma of the penis in men. All women with genital warts should receive a Pap smear and, when indicated, cervical colposcopy and biopsy. Encourage condom use. See the Evidence-Based Practice in Action feature on Human Papillomavirus Screening for Women with Abnormal Pap Smear Results on p. 1138.

DISEASES CHARACTERIZED BY VAGINAL DISCHARGE

Infections manifested by vaginal discharge include trichomoniasis and vaginitis (bacterial and yeast). Although occasionally transmitted sexually, candidiasis (vaginal yeast infection) is generally not considered an STD. Recurrent vaginal yeast infections are a common manifestation of HIV infection in women (vaginitis is discussed in Chapter 41).

TRICHOMONIASIS

Etiology and Risk Factors

Trichomoniasis is a protozoal infection causing vulvovaginitis. Although not life-threatening, the incidence is high worldwide and the disease remains a major health problem. Often asymptomatic, trichomoniasis affects 3 million people annually, and its role in PID and infertility may be greatly underestimated.

Pathophysiology

Trichomoniasis is caused by the anaerobic, flagellated, parasitic protozoan *Trichomonas vaginalis*. The organism is almost always transmitted sexually. *T. vaginalis* prefers an alkaline environment (pH 6 to 7), and alterations in the vaginal *flora* (the usual bacteria and fungi)—from douching, for instance—make a woman more susceptible to infection. Trichomoniasis can be resistant to treatment, and recurrence is common.

Clinical Manifestations

Manifestations may be minor, especially in men. In women, manifestations include a copious, malodorous, yellow-green vaginal discharge. This is irritating to the vulva and causes severe itching, burning, and excoriation and maceration of the vulvar tissues. Occasionally, the cervix is covered with punctate (point-like) hemorrhages ("strawberry cervix"). The vaginal mucosa appears reddened and slightly edematous. Some women experience dyspareunia (pain during sexual intercourse).

If trichomoniasis extends to the urethra, urinary frequency and burning with urination may occur. This is the most common manifestation in a man. Anal involvement may also occur, either asymptomatically or with a slight discharge. Bladder and anal involvement are more common when the infection becomes chronic.

The diagnosis can be made by examining a fresh, warm specimen of vaginal exudate in a saline wet mount under a microscope in which the highly motile organisms are seen. Cultures are rarely necessary. The vaginal speculum used during the examination must be inserted without lubrication to avoid destroying the organism. If possible, instruct the client not to douche before the vaginal examination.

Outcome Management
■ Medical Management

EB **Eradicate Disease and Manifestations.** The preferred treatment of trichomoniasis is a single oral dose of metronidazole (Flagyl) with simultaneous treatment of all sexual partners for a cure. Metronidazole should not be taken during the first trimester of pregnancy because it may adversely affect fetal development. *T. vaginalis* itself does not affect the fetus. Single-dose metronidazole therapy is usually curative, but recurrence is common. Instruct clients to seek prompt treatment if manifestations return. Metronidazole may be given in a 7-day regimen for recurrent infection.

■ Nursing Management of the Medical Client

Advise clients taking metronidazole not to drink alcoholic beverages, because doing so might cause nausea, vomiting, and headaches. This prohibition includes all alcohol-containing products, such as cough syrup. Emphasize the importance of good perineal hygiene. Treatment should continue through the client's menstrual period because the vagina is more alkaline during this time and a flare-up is more likely to occur. Metronidazole can be taken without regard to meals. Advise clients that urine may turn dark, reddish brown.

BACTERIAL VAGINOSIS

Bacterial vaginosis, formerly known as nonspecific or *Gardnerella* vaginitis, is a common condition in adults. It is the most common cause of vaginal discharge in women, although many clients are asymptomatic.

Etiology and Risk Factors

Bacterial vaginosis is linked to sexual activity, particularly having multiple sex partners, although not all cases are caused by sexual activity. It is often seen in women who douche, and it can occur after other genital infections and invasive gynecologic procedures.

Pathophysiology

Like the organisms responsible for vulvovaginal *Candida* (yeast) infections, the causative bacteria are found in the normal vagina. The infection is caused by the overgrowth of a number of different organisms, including *Gardnerella vaginalis* and vaginal anaerobes. Overgrowth may occur when the normal flora and pH of the vagina are altered and replaced with high numbers of anaerobic bacteria.

Clinical Manifestations

The vulvovaginitis produced by bacterial vaginosis is mild or asymptomatic. The main manifestation is a mild to moderate, malodorous vaginal discharge. The discharge is usually thin, watery, and grayish white and tends to adhere to the vaginal wall. The odor is described as "fishy" and is often more noticeable after sexual intercourse. Manifestations are almost always confined to the vulvovaginal area. Mild vaginal burning and irritation may occur, but redness and pruritus are not common.

Evaluation is mainly by physical examination of the vagina, microscopic examination of the discharge, and determination of the pH of the discharge. The diagnosis is determined by the presence of at least three of the following manifestations:

- A homogeneous gray or white discharge that adheres to the vaginal wall
- Vaginal fluid pH above 4.5 (normal pH is 4.0 to 4.5)
- Positive result of the "whiff" test—a fishy odor elicited when potassium hydroxide (KOH) is added to the vaginal fluid
- Presence of *clue cells* (desquamated vaginal epithelial cells characteristically stippled by the adherence of coccobacilli to their surfaces) on either a saline wet mount or a Gram's stain of vaginal fluid

Outcome Management
■ Medical Management

The recommended treatment of bacterial vaginosis in nonpregnant women is metronidazole (Flagyl), given orally or intravaginally for 7 days. Single-dose regimens can be used to improve compliance, but they are less effective than the 7-day regimen. Pregnant women are treated with lower doses of metronidazole to minimize exposure to the fetus. Alternative treatment includes metronidazole in a high, single dose, or clindamycin orally or intravaginally.

■ Nursing Management of the Medical Client

Bacterial vaginosis is not necessarily transmitted sexually, although its occurrence is associated with sexual activity. Treatment of male partners is recommended only with recurrent or resistant infection. Recurrence is common.

ACQUIRED IMMUNODEFICIENCY SYNDROME

AIDS is a viral STD that has reached epidemic proportions worldwide. HIV infection has had an effect on the transmission of STDs, and vice versa. People with AIDS are more susceptible to other STDs. These coexistent

STDs require more aggressive therapy and tend to recur. Conversely, people infected with an STD, especially those with genital ulcerations, are more susceptible to HIV infection. On the positive side, national campaigns to prevent and control the transmission of HIV have had a beneficial effect on the incidence of some STDs (e.g., reduced incidence of hepatitis B in the homosexual population). AIDS is discussed in Chapter 80.

VACCINE-PREVENTABLE DISEASES

Vaccines for STDs are receiving increasing attention as possible strategies for control of STDs. Currently, vaccines are available for hepatitis B and hepatitis A. Trials are under way for vaccines against other STDs. Every person seeking screening or treatment of STDs should be offered the hepatitis B vaccine, and certain high-risk groups (men who have sex with men, people who have sex with IV drugs users) should be offered the hepatitis A vaccine.

HEPATITIS

Hepatitis A is caused by a virus and is most commonly transmitted through oral-fecal contamination. The virus is also found in serum and saliva. Risk factors for hepatitis A include (1) household or sexual contact with people who have the virus, (2) homosexual activity, and (3) IV drug abuse or sexual contact with an IV drug user. Measures that are typically used to decrease the spread of other STDs do not stop the transfer of this virus.

Sexual contact is the most frequently reported mode of transmission for the hepatitis B virus (HBV) (30% to 60% of all cases), although blood-borne and perinatal transmission also occur. Clients at high risk for sexually transmitted hepatitis B are (1) heterosexuals with multiple sexual partners, (2) sexual partners of IV drug users, and (3) men who have sex with men. The incidence of sexually transmitted hepatitis B has decreased dramatically in the homosexual population, probably as a result of the modification of high-risk sexual behaviors to prevent AIDS.

Hepatitis C is associated with sexual activity (20% of cases). Sexually oriented risk factors include having multiple partners, having sex with an IV drug user, and engaging in sexual activities that cause trauma. See Chapter 49 for further discussion of hepatitis A and B.

DISEASES CAUSED BY INFESTATIONS
PEDICULOSIS PUBIS AND SCABIES

Cutaneous infestation with pubic lice (pediculosis pubis) or mites (scabies) results either from close physical contact with an infected person or from contact with contaminated objects of an infected person, such as linens and clothing. Because sexual transmission is possible,

these conditions are included in any list of STDs. For further discussion, see Chapter 51.

SEXUALLY TRANSMITTED ENTERIC INFECTIONS

Gastroenteritis caused by enteric pathogens are typically acquired from food or water contaminated with fecal matter. Since the mid-1970s, it has been recognized that these pathogens can also be transmitted by oral and anal sexual contact. Sexually transmitted enteric infections include shigellosis, salmonellosis, amebiasis, and giardiasis. Men who have sex with men are at highest risk for these infections. See Chapter 35 for discussion of gastroenteritis.

MANAGEMENT OF CLIENTS REPORTING SEXUAL ASSAULT

Victims of sexual assault need immense support from health care professionals, a discussion of which is beyond the scope of this chapter. Regarding STDs, a sexual assault victim needs an immediate physical examination, including tests for pregnancy, gonorrhea, chlamydial infection, trichomoniasis, HIV, hepatitis A and B, and syphilis. Follow-up testing should be repeated in 2 weeks; syphilis and HIV testing should also be repeated at 6, 12, and 24 months. Prophylaxis for HIV infection is described in Chapter 80.

CONCLUSIONS

STDs are more prevalent than ever before. This phenomenon is attributable to many factors. The improper and indiscriminate use of antibiotics has produced a number of resistant organisms. Sexual activity, especially among adolescents and young adults, has increased. Many STDs are asymptomatic and go undetected. Nurses are in a unique position to help clients protect, salvage, or restore their sexual health and have an ever-increasing responsibility and role in the prevention, early detection, and treatment of STDs.

THINKING CRITICALLY evolve

1. A 20-year-old unmarried man comes to a walk-in STD clinic with a purulent urethral discharge. The diagnosis is uncomplicated gonorrhea. The client has no known allergies. He is sexually active with multiple partners. He gives a temporary address. What are the priorities of care? What are the priority interventions?

Factors to Consider. What effect would the client's status as a walk-in client have on your planning? Consider the fact that gonorrhea often leads to PID in women. What effect would the temporary address have on your planning and need for identification of partners? What diseases are likely to coexist with gonorrhea?

2. Your client is a 65-year-old widowed woman who comes for treatment of acute, symptomatic genital herpes. Her male sexual contact told her when their sexual relationship began that he had a history of genital herpes but that, because he had no active lesions, there was no risk of her becoming infected. She is humiliated by having contracted herpes and tells you that she feels dirty and contaminated. She also states that she knows nothing about condoms and, furthermore, that she "wouldn't be caught dead buying them." What are the goals of her care? What interventions might be used?

Factors to Consider. How accurate is the client's knowledge about the transmission of genital herpes? What are her psychosocial needs? What obstacles to buying condoms can you identify, and how will you help this client control her sexual health?

3. A 25-year-old monogamous woman seeks outpatient treatment for the irritating, malodorous vaginal discharge of trichomoniasis. She has had trichomoniasis before, and metronidazole (Flagyl) was prescribed. What interventions should the care of this client include?

Factors to Consider. Knowing that metronidazole is usually curative, consider what might have caused this recurrence.

Discussions for these questions can be found on the website and the CD-ROM.

BIBLIOGRAPHY

1. Alter, M.J. (1999). Epidemiology of hepatitis C. *Hepatology*, 26(suppl. 1), S25-S65.
2. Anonymous. (2002). Gonorrhea rates rising among hardest-hit. *AIDS Alert*, 17(5), 63-65.
3. Anonymous. (2001). Photoclinic: Secondary syphilis. *Consultant*, 41, 628.
4. Anonymous. (2000). Photoclinic: Foresee your next patient. Lymphogranuloma venereum. *Consultant*, 40, 1905.
5. Blake, D.R., & Woods, E.R. (2001). The future is here: Noninvasive diagnosis of STDs in teens. *Contemporary OB/Gyn*, 46(3), 103-104, 106, 109.
6. **EB** Bull, S.S., et al. (2000). Acceptability and feasibility of urine screening for chlamydia and gonorrhea in community organizations: Perspectives from Denver and St. Louis. *American Journal of Public Health*, 90, 285-286.
7. **EB** Centers for Disease Control. (2002). Nonoxynol-9 spermicide contraception use—United States, 1999. *MMWR*, 51, 289-392.
8. **EB** Centers for Disease Control. (2002). Sexually transmitted diseases treatment guidelines—2002. *MMWR 51(RR06)*.
9. **EB** Centers for Disease Control. (1999). Prevention of hepatitis A through active or passive immunization: Recommendations of the Advisory Committee on Immunization Practices. *MMWR, 48(RR-12)*.
10. **EB** Cohen, F., et al. (1999). Persistent stress as a predictor of genital herpes recurrence. *Archives of Internal Medicine*, 159, 2430-2436.
11. **EB** Corey, L., et al. (1999). Recombinant glycoprotein vaccine for the prevention of genital HSV-2 infection. *Journal of the American Medical Association*, 282, 331-340.
12. **EB** Duncan, B., & Hart, G. (1999). Sexuality and health: The hidden costs of screening for *Chlamydia trachomatis*. *British Medical Journal*, 318, 931-933.
13. **EB** Duncan, B., et al. (2001). Qualitative analysis of psychosocial impact of diagnosis of *Chlamydia trachomatis*: Implications for screening. *British Medical Journal*, 322, 195-199.
14. Grigg, E. (2000). Sexually transmitted infections and older people. *Nursing Standard*, 14(39), 48-53.
15. **EB** Hicks, N.R., et al. (1999). Evidenced based case report: Chlamydia infection in general practice. *British Medical Journal*, 318, 790-792.
16. Holmes, K.K., et al. (1999). *Sexually transmitted diseases* (3rd ed.). New York: McGraw-Hill.
17. Kelley, L.S. (1999). Evaluating change in quality of life from the perspective of the person: Advanced practiced nursing and Parse's Goal of Nursing. Holistic *Nurse Practitioner*, 13(4), 61-70.
18. **EB** King, E.A., et al. (2002). Bacterial vaginosis and *Chlamydia trachomatis* among pregnant abused and nonabused Hispanic women. *Journal Obstetrics, Gynecologic, and Neonatal Nursing*, 29, 606-612.
19. Mangione-Smith, R., McGlynn, E.A., & Hiatt, L. (2002). Screening for *Chlamydia* in adolescents and young women. *Archives of Pediatric and Adolescent Medicine*, 154, 1108-1113.
20. Morse, S., Holmes, K., & Ballard, R. (2002). *Atlas of sexually transmitted diseases and AIDS* (3rd ed.). London: Mosby.
21. Pace, B. (2000). JAMA patient page: Syphilis. *Journal of the American Medical Association*, 284, 520.
22. Pagana, K.D., & Pagana, T.J. (2002). *Mosby's manual of diagnostic and laboratory tests* (2nd ed.). St. Louis: Mosby.
23. **EB** Roddy, R.E., et al. (2002). Effect of nonoxynol-9 gel on urogenital gonorrhea and chlamydial infection. *Journal of the American Medical Association*, 287, 1117-1122.
24. Saunders, C.S. (2000). Monitoring HPV infection. *Patient Care*, 34(5), 142-144, 147, 151-154.
25. Skidmore-Roth, L. (2002). *Mosby's nursing drug reference*. St. Louis: Mosby.
26. **EB** Stevens-Simon, C., et al. (2000). The prevalence of genital human papillomavirus infections in abused and nonabused preadolescent girls. *Pediatrics*, 106, 645-649.
27. **EB** Turner, C.F., et al. (2002). Untreated gonococcal and chlamydial infection in a probability sample of adults. *Journal of the American Medical Association*, 287, 726-733.
28. **EB** Vastag, B. (2002). CDC: Rates are up for gonorrhea, down for syphilis. *Journal of the American Medical Association*, 285, 155.
29. Weiner, H.R. (1999). Chlamydia infection: The hidden epidemic. *Emergency Medicine*, 31(11), 88-90, 95.
30. Williams, L.A., et al. (1999). Elimination and reintroduction of primary and secondary syphilis. *American Journal of Public Health*, 89, 1093-1097.

Unit 10

Metabolic Disorders

Anatomy and Physiology Review

The Metabolic Systems

Robert G. Carroll

Metabolism depends on the availability of fuel (glucose and fatty acids), oxygen, and the balance of *anabolic* (building) against *catabolic* (breakdown) processes. Regulation of this balance is dynamic and is one function of the endocrine and neuroendocrine systems. Metabolic processes affect all cells of the body, and whole-body metabolic regulation involves numerous endocrine structures, the liver, muscle, and fat cells.

Endocrine secretions, together with the nervous system, coordinate the balance of metabolism, reproduction, water and electrolyte balance, and nutrient absorption. Metabolism is closely regulated by thyroid hormone, with some influence exerted by cortisol and epinephrine. Growth and development are regulated by growth hormone (also called *somatotropin*), with thyroid hormone, insulin-like growth factors, and the sex hormones providing significant effects. Plasma glucose is closely regulated by insulin, with glucagon and the metabolic hormones cortisol, growth hormone, and epinephrine having a role. Endocrine agents involved in water and electrolyte balance, nutrient absorption, and reproduction are described in Units 6 and 8.

The liver and pancreas have both endocrine and exocrine roles. The exocrine secretions assist the digestion and absorption of the diet (see the Unit 6 Anatomy and Physiology Review). The endocrine role is tied closely to metabolism, particularly the regulation of plasma glucose. Plasma glucose represents the balance of glucose absorption from the diet, movement into and out of storage pools, new glucose synthesis from amino acids *(gluconeogenesis)*, and, finally, glucose consumption by the tissues. The liver plays a central role in these processes and is a good point to begin the discussion of metabolism.

STRUCTURE OF THE METABOLIC SYSTEMS

LIVER

The liver is the largest gland in the body, representing about 2.5% of body weight. It lies in the upper right quadrant of the abdomen, just below the diaphragm. The rib cage encloses the liver except for the lower margin. The lungs extend over the liver's upper portion. The lower portion of the liver provides a "roof" for the stomach and intestines. A peritoneal covering blankets most of the liver and also the adjacent gallbladder. The liver divides at the falciform ligament into two major lobes, right and left (Figure U10-1). These two lobes, in turn, divide into superior and inferior portions of the posterior, anterior, medial, and lateral segments.

Liver blood flow represents about 20% of the cardiac output, about 1 L/min. The hepatic artery supplies the liver with about one third of its blood, and the portal vein supplies the other two thirds (see Figure U10-1, *B*). The hepatic artery carries oxygenated blood; the portal vein carries deoxygenated blood. The superior and inferior mesenteric veins and the splenic vein, which receive blood from the pancreas, spleen, stomach, intestines, and gallbladder, join to form the portal vein. The portal vein carries nutrients, metabolites, and toxins from the digestive organs to the liver for processing, detoxification, or assimilation. Blood pressure in the hepatic sinuses is low; hence, any process elevating central venous pressure causes liver engorgement. Similarly, any process impeding blood flow through the liver causes engorgement of vessels draining the digestive organs. The liver is an important reservoir for blood, with contraction of the hepatic venules and veins moving about 500 ml into the circulation.

The functional unit of the liver is the *lobule,* and the *hepatocyte* is the major cell. Hepatocytes are arranged in a hub-like fashion around a central vein. One side of the polyhedral hepatocyte faces the *hepatic sinusoids* (the capillary system of the liver); another faces the bile canaliculi. As incoming blood from the portal vein and the hepatic artery enters the sinusoids and passes through the liver lobules, many substances are exchanged between the blood and the hepatocytes. Lymphatic ducts drain excess interstitial fluid. Bile is formed in the hepatocytes, is secreted into the *bile canaliculi,* and travels through bile ductules to the gallbladder. Endothelial and *Kupffer's cells* form the walls of the sinusoids.

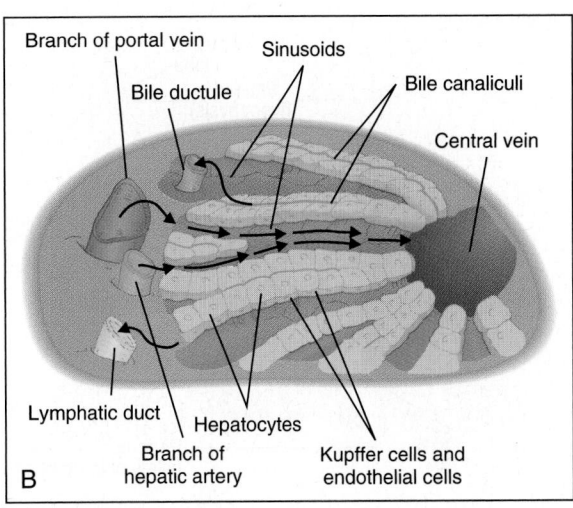

FIGURE U10-1 The liver and vascular drainage systems. Blood enters the liver from the hepatic artery, and the hepatic portal vein supplies the liver with blood from the digestive organs. *Inset,* Liver lobule. Blood from the hepatic artery and portal vein is processed by the hepatocytes as it flows through the sinusoids into the central vein. Lymphatics and bile ducts leave the liver through separate pathways.

Kupffer's cells are an important part of the mononuclear phagocyte system (formerly the reticuloendothelial system). This system is so effective that fewer than 1% of the bacteria entering the portal system from the intestine pass through the liver. After leaving the sinusoids, blood flows into the central vein, the hepatic veins, and the inferior vena cava.

ENDOCRINE SYSTEM

The endocrine glands are distributed throughout the body. *Endocrine* tissues (*endo,* "within") secrete a compound (hormone) that is carried by the blood to act on a target tissue. This is in contrast to *exocrine* (*exo,* "outside") tissues, which secrete across an epithelium, such as sweat and pancreatic peptidases (the lumen of the gastrointestinal [GI] tract is "outside" the body), and *paracrine* (*para,* around) cells, whose secretions do not need to be transported in the blood to reach their target tissue.

Hormones are generally classified on the basis of molecular structure as follows:

1. *Steroids.* Steroids are derived from cholesterol and are consequently poorly soluble in water. After secretion, steroids are transported in the blood by carrier proteins. Steroids diffuse across the cell membrane of the target tissue and bind to a cytoplasmic-binding protein. The steroid-binding protein complex enters the nucleus, where it alters deoxyribonucleic acid (DNA) transcription. There is usually a lag of minutes to hours before steroids exert their effects.

2. *Peptides.* Proteins and *polypeptides* are synthesized in the endoplasmic reticulum of the endocrine tissue and are secreted in vesicles. After transport in the blood, they bind to cell membrane receptors on the target tissues and activate either second messenger systems or ion channels. Peptide hormones such as insulin generally have rapid response times.

3. *Amino acid derivatives.* The derivatives of tyrosine include thyroid hormone and the catecholamines epinephrine, norepinephrine, and dopamine. Thyroid hormone alters DNA synthesis through a pathway similar to that for steroids, but the catecholamines bind cell membrane receptors, similar to the mechanism of peptides. Their response time is immediate.

The major endocrine organs described in this review include the pituitary, the thyroid, the parathyroid, the

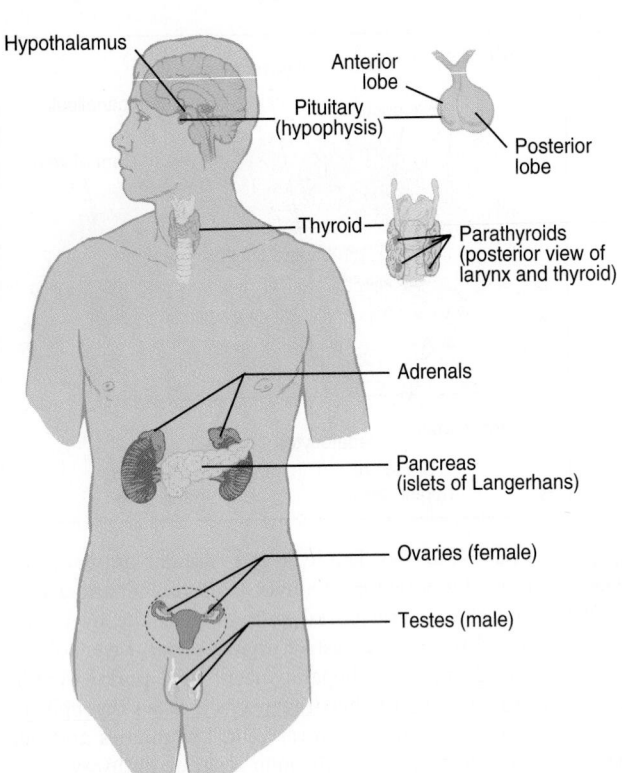

Hypothalamus

Anterior lobe

Pituitary (hypophysis)

Posterior lobe

Thyroid

Parathyroids (posterior view of larynx and thyroid)

Adrenals

Pancreas (islets of Langerhans)

Ovaries (female)

Testes (male)

FIGURE U10-2 Major organs of the endocrine system.

pancreas, the adrenal, and, to a lesser extent, the gonads (Figure U10-2). Other organs have important endocrine secretions, including the kidney (renin and erythropoietin), the heart (atrial natriuretic peptide), and the placenta of a pregnant female (human chorionic gonadotropin [HCG], estrogen, progesterone, and the growth hormone somatomammotropin). See the Anatomy and Physiology Reviews for Units 8, 9, and 12.

Hypothalamus and Pituitary Gland

The pituitary gland *(hypophysis)* is a small (1 g) extension on the dorsal surface of the hypothalamus, connected to the hypothalamus by the hypophyseal stalk (Figure U10-3). The pituitary has three histologically distinct sections, two of which secrete hormones in humans:

1. The *anterior pituitary (adenohypophysis)* is glandular tissue that contains a variety of secretory cell types.
2. The *posterior pituitary (neurohypophysis)* is neural tissue that contains glia cells and terminal axons from cells of the hypothalamus.
3. The *pars intermedia* is a vestigial remnant in humans, with little physiologic significance.

The hypothalamus lies dorsal to the pituitary gland and regulates secretion of both the anterior and the posterior pituitary hormones. The hypophyseal stalk has

two distinct pathways leading from the hypothalamus to the pituitary.

The *neural stalk* contains axons originating in the hypothalamus that terminate in the posterior pituitary. Cell bodies are in the supraoptic and paraventricular nuclei, and axons terminate in the posterior pituitary, where the synaptic terminals secrete hormones rather than make synaptic connections with another neuron.

The *hypothalamo-hypophyseal portal system* provides a vascular connection between the median eminence of the hypothalamus and the anterior pituitary. Arterial blood enters the capillaries of the hypothalamus. Blood flows through portal vessels in the hypophyseal stalk before entering a second set of capillaries (sinuses) in the anterior pituitary. Blood then exits the anterior pituitary and joins with other venous drainages. This vascular supply ensures that releasing and inhibiting hormones secreted in the median eminence of the hypothalamus remain concentrated until delivered to the target cells of the anterior pituitary.

The *anterior pituitary* is the end organ for growth hormone and prolactin secretion. The other anterior pituitary hormones act on endocrine target organs to stimulate the release of additional hormones. In the *posterior pituitary* are glia-like cells, which support and nourish the nerve endings. Oxytocin and antidiuretic hormone (ADH) are synthesized in the hypothalamus and transported to the posterior pituitary gland for secretion.

Thyroid and Parathyroid

The thyroid gland is located in the neck, just below the cricoid cartilage, and is somewhat H-shaped (Figure U10-4). The right and left lateral lobes lie on either side of the trachea. The lobes are connected by a thin mass of tissue (the *isthmus*), which stretches over the surface of the trachea. Each lobe is composed of irregularly shaped lobules, which consist of a multitude of tiny sacs (follicles) filled with a jelly-like, iodine-containing substance called *colloid* (see Figure U10-4, inset). The main component of colloid is thyroglobulin—the storage form of the hormone thyroxine. The *parathyroid glands* are four small glands near, attached to, or embedded in the thyroid gland.

Endocrine Pancreas

The pancreas (see Figure U10-2) contains islets of Langerhans, which secrete three hormones that regulate blood glucose: (1) *alpha* cells secrete *glucagons*, (2) *beta* cells secrete *insulin,* and (3) *delta* cells secrete *somatostatin,* identical to the growth hormone inhibitory hormone secreted by the hypothalamus. The close proximity of these cells within the islets allows a coordinated paracrine regulation of pancreatic secretion because insulin inhibits glucagon release and somatostatin inhibits both insulin and glucagon release.

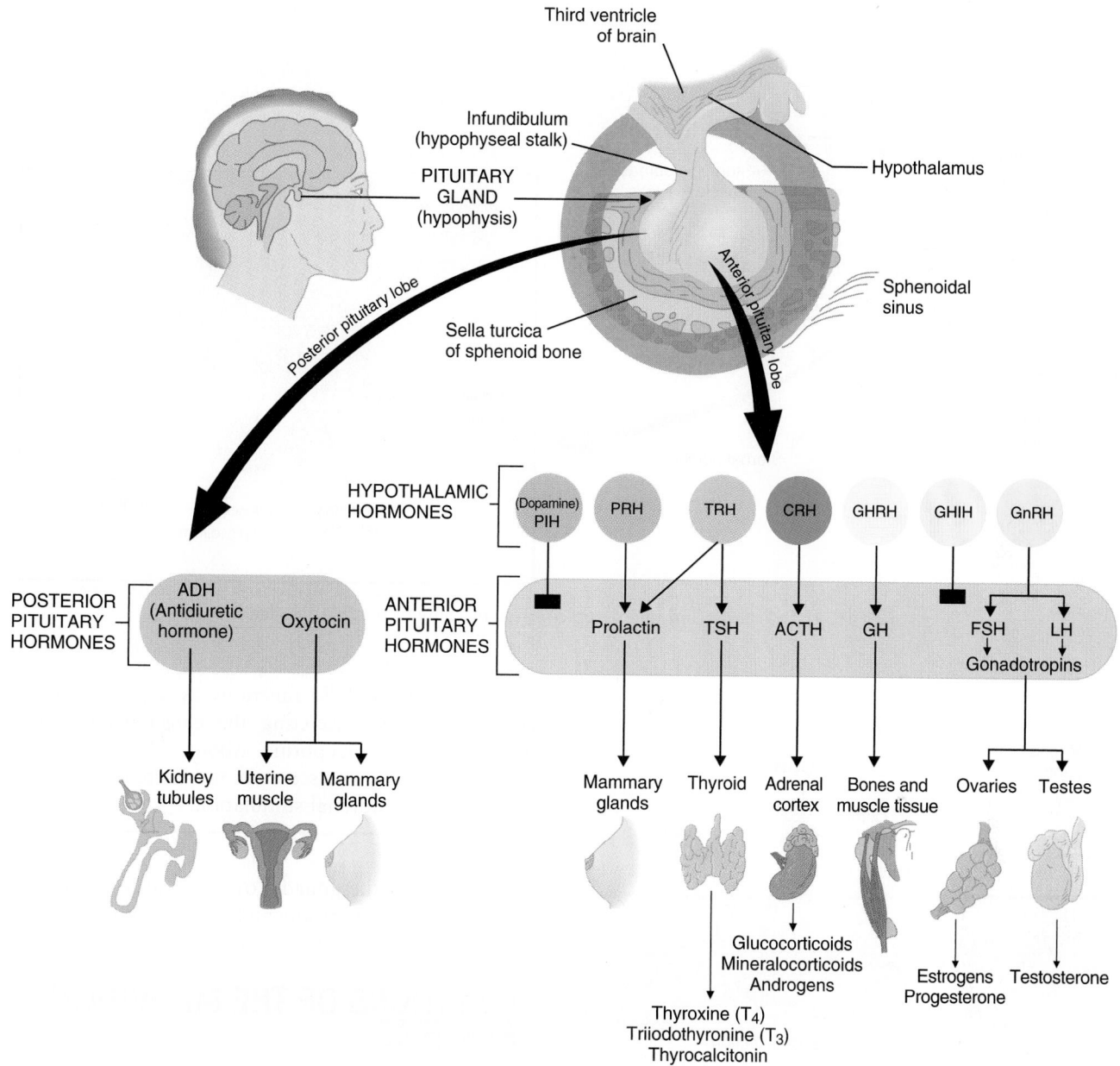

FIGURE U10-3 Hypothalamus, pituitary gland, and target tissues. The pituitary gland is suspended from the hypothalamus by the infundibular or hypophyseal stalk. Hormones released from the hypothalamus travel in a portal vascular system to the anterior pituitary gland, where they stimulate (or inhibit) the release of anterior pituitary hormones. Posterior pituitary hormones are synthesized in the hypothalamus and are released from axons in the posterior pituitary gland.

Adrenal Glands

The adrenal glands are paired endocrine organs situated at the superior poles of the kidneys. The adrenal gland is divided into an outer cortex and an inner medulla (Figure U10-5). The *cortex* has three zones. The outer *zona glomerulosa* secretes the mineralocorticoids aldosterone and corticosterone. The inner *zona fasciculata* and *zona reticularis* secrete the glucocorticoids cortisol and corti-

costerone as well as androgen sex hormones. Corticosterone and deoxycorticosterone are secreted in small amounts and exert both glucocorticoid and mineralocorticoid effects. Adrenal cortical hormones are steroids formed from a cholesterol nucleus. Deficits in synthetic enzymes often lead to overproduction of other adrenal hormones. Stimuli that enhance adrenal cortical secretions also cause hypertrophy of the appropriate cortical zones.

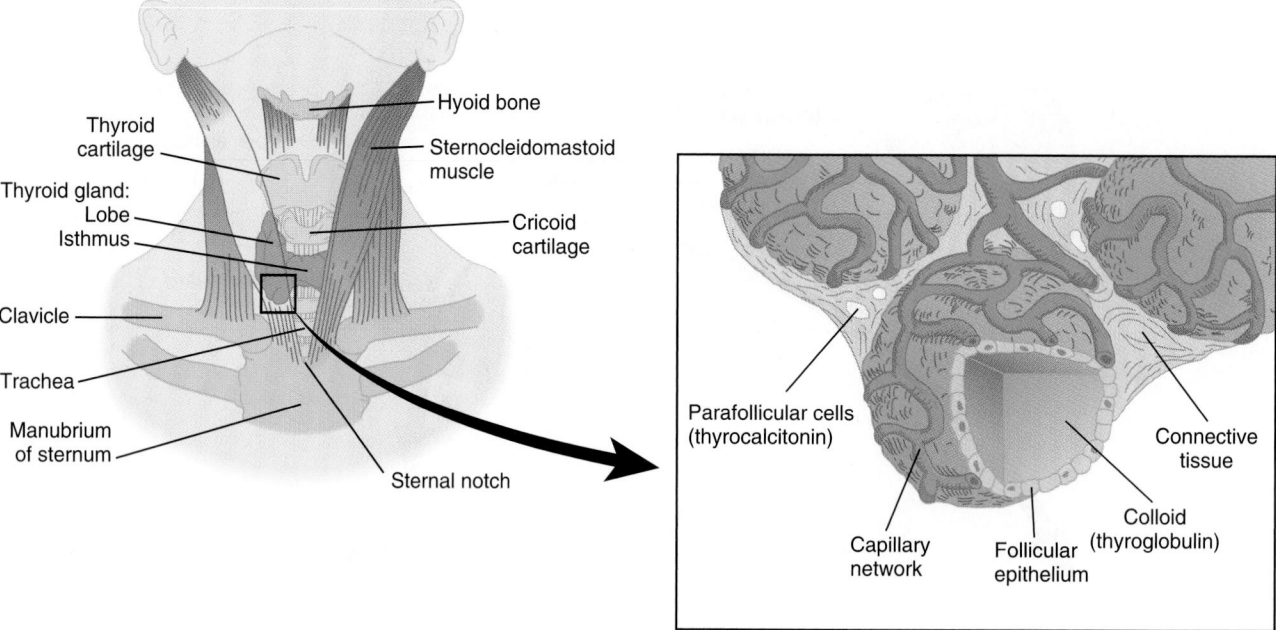

FIGURE U10-4 Gross and microscopic *(inset)* anatomy of the thyroid gland.

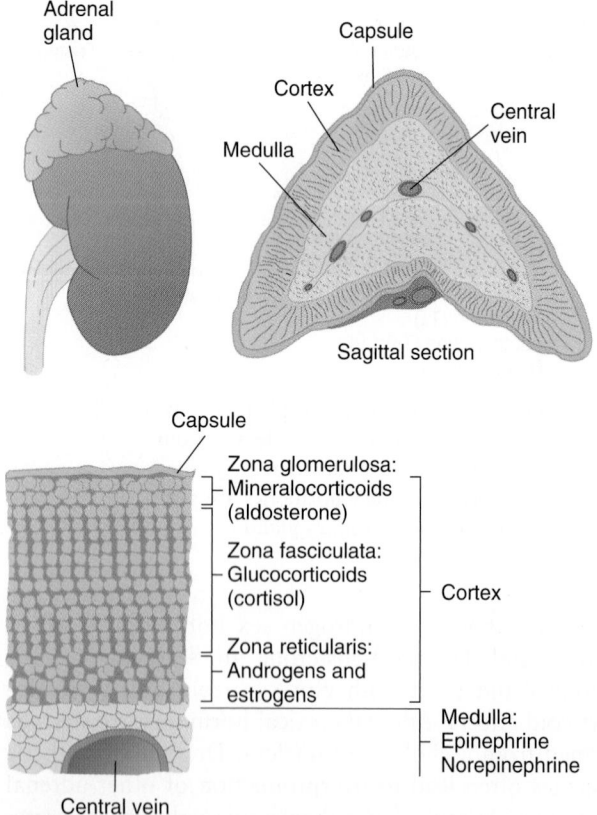

FIGURE U10-5 Gross and microscopic anatomy of the adrenal gland.

The *adrenal medulla* functions as a postganglionic sympathetic nerve, secreting the catecholamines epinephrine and norepinephrine. About 80% of the basal (resting) catecholamine secretion is epinephrine, but this ratio varies with adrenal stimulation.

Gonads
The structure of the gonads (ovaries and testes) is covered in the Unit 9 Anatomy and Physiology Review.

FUNCTIONS OF THE METABOLIC SYSTEMS
LIVER
The liver plays a central role in the regulation of metabolic substrates, glucose, and fatty acids. Additionally, hepatic synthesis provides most of the proteins circulating in the plasma.

The liver is the major storage organ for *glycogen,* a polymer of glucose. In addition to storage, the liver converts glucose to glycogen *(glycogenesis),* breaks down glycogen into glucose *(glycogenolysis),* and forms glucose from other sugars *(galactose and fructose)* or amino acids *(gluconeogenesis).* The regulation of these processes is discussed later.

The major functions of the liver in relation to fat metabolism are as follows:
- Oxidation of fatty acids for energy
- Formation of most lipoproteins

- Synthesis of cholesterol and phospholipids
- Synthesis of fat from proteins and carbohydrates

The liver provides energy from fats by splitting them into glycerol and fatty acids; when the fatty acids are oxidized, tremendous amounts of energy are released.

Most of the cholesterol synthesized in the liver is converted into bile salts; the remainder is transported in the lipoproteins throughout the body. Phospholipids are also synthesized in the liver and transported in lipoproteins. The cholesterol and phospholipids help form cell membranes and intracellular structures and are involved in cellular function.

The primary functions of the liver in relation to protein metabolism are as follows:

- Deamination of amino acids
- Formation of urea for removal of ammonia from the body
- Formation of plasma proteins
- Biotransformation of hormones, drugs, and other substances

Degradation is the process of excess amino acid catabolism. This process begins in the liver with deamination, the removal of amino groups ($-NH_2$). Ammonia (NH_3), which results from deamination, is converted into urea by the liver and is excreted by the kidneys and intestines. Ammonia can also be formed in the intestines by bacterial action. In severe liver disease or damage, ammonia that is normally converted to urea by the liver accumulates to dangerously high levels in the blood. As a result, a severe toxic state *(hepatic encephalopathy)* develops.

The liver also synthesizes plasma proteins, such as albumin, prothrombin, fibrinogen, and clotting proteins (factors V, VI, VII, IX, and X). Albumin is essential for maintaining plasma oncotic pressure; the other proteins contribute to blood clotting. Plasma oncotic pressure prevents intravascular fluid from moving out into the extravascular spaces, where it manifests as *ascites* and varying degrees of peripheral edema. Vitamin K, a fat-soluble vitamin, must be present for synthesis of several clotting proteins. Assimilation of vitamin K depends on the presence of bile in the intestine. Gamma globulins are the only plasma proteins not synthesized by the liver.

The liver primarily detoxifies and biotransforms hormones, drugs, and other chemicals. Some substances are deactivated by deamination, hydroxylation, oxidation, or reduction. Through conjugation, other substances become soluble in water, resulting in their excretion through the bile and, therefore, in feces or urine.

Clients with compromised liver function are at high risk for untoward reactions to many medications, all opiates, and many chemicals. The two major problems that result are prolonged action and increased potency of the substance.

ENDOCRINE SYSTEM

Regulation of endocrine secretions is generally by a negative feedback loop, linking the hormone to a response, to another hormone, or to glucose or some other plasma compound. Endocrine agents also have significant trophic effects on the target tissues, with high hormone levels often causing hypertrophy, and inadequate hormone levels causing atrophy, of the target tissues. Regulation of endocrine systems is often integrated with the nervous system. When the distinction between endocrine and nervous systems is blurred, the system is described as the *neuroendocrine system.*

Hypothalamus and Pituitary Gland

The hypothalamus regulates secretion of anterior and posterior pituitary hormones. Five hypothalamic-releasing hormones and two hypothalamic inhibitory hormones regulate secretion of the six anterior pituitary hormones (see Figure U10-3).

Growth Hormone (Somatotropin)

The anterior pituitary is the end organ for secretion of growth hormone, which exerts several effects:

- Stimulates growth in almost all body tissues, causing both an increase in cell size *(hypertrophy)* and an increase in cell number *(hyperplasia)*
- Diverts amino acids into protein synthesis *(anabolism)* and decreases protein breakdown *(catabolism)*
- Enhances the use of free fatty acids as metabolic substrates, which depletes body fat stores
- Increases plasma glucose levels but protects amino acid pools (discussed later)

Insulin has an important permissive, or facilitatory, role in growth hormone–mediated growth. It enhances the entry of both glucose and amino acids into cells. Growth hormone exerts some of its effects through an intermediary, the somatomedins, or insulin-like growth factors.

Growth hormone secretion is enhanced by various stressful and normal stimuli, including starvation, chronic protein deficiency, hypoglycemia, low plasma levels of free fatty acids, exercise, and the first hours of sleep. Hypothalamic secretion of growth hormone releasing and inhibitory hormones is the primary regulator of growth hormone release.

Prolactin

The hypothalamus is the end organ for prolactin secretion. Hypothalamic control of prolactin is unique in that the normal control of prolactin release is by hypothalamic prolactin inhibitory hormone. Consequently, interruption of the hypothalamo-hypophyseal portal system increases pituitary prolactin release. Prolactin-releasing hormone is important in the suckling reflex (see the Unit 9 Anatomy and Physiology Review).

Antidiuretic Hormone and Oxytocin

Nerve endings in the *posterior pituitary* secrete oxytocin and antidiuretic hormone (ADH), also known as *vasopressin*. Oxytocin, formed primarily in the paraventricular nucleus of the hypothalamus, promotes uterine contraction during parturition, causing expression of milk ("let-down") following suckling (see the Unit 9 Anatomy and Physiology Review). ADH is formed primarily in the supraoptic nucleus and is released by increases in plasma osmolarity or by low blood pressure. Stress and trauma can also promote ADH release. The mechanism of ADH control of water and electrolyte balance is discussed in the Unit 8 Anatomy and Physiology Review.

Thyroid Gland

Thyroid hormone is a conglomerate of three (T_3) or four (T_4) iodinated tyrosine residues. Triiodothyronine (T_3) and thyroxine (T_4) together are called *thyroid hormone.* Thyroid hormone is lipid soluble, and 99% of thyroid hormone in the plasma is bound to thyroid-binding globulin. Of the two thyroid hormones, T_3 has the most rapid effect on target tissues, requiring 3 days for peak effect; T_4 (the more common) requires 11 days for peak effect.

Thyroid hormone has several functions:

- It increases metabolism, enhancing carbohydrate consumption and increasing the size and density of mitochondria.
- It assists in acclimatization to cold environments by increasing metabolic rate (heat production is a byproduct of metabolism).
- It increases DNA translation and transcription.
- It increases protein synthesis but also has protein catabolic effects.
- It promotes growth and is required for normal growth in children.

Finally, thyroid hormone has a permissive effect to increase other endocrine secretions.

Thyroid hormone is formed in epithelium-lined follicles that contain the glycoprotein thyroglobulin. Thyroglobulin can contain five to six thyroid hormone molecules. Dietary iodine is required for thyroid hormone synthesis. Iodine is oxidized within the follicles and binds a tyrosine residue (T_1) of thyroglobulin. Iodinated tyrosines are coupled while still part of the thyroglobulin molecule, forming T_3 and T_4. The mature hormone is released by digestion of thyroglobulin, with recycling of unused iodine, T_1, and T_2.

Release of thyroid hormone is regulated by negative feedback by T_4 on thyroid-stimulating hormone (TSH) release at the anterior pituitary. TSH stimulates proteolysis of thyroglobulin, releasing T_3 and T_4. TSH also stimulates iodine uptake by the thyroid for new thyroid hormone synthesis, increasing the activity of thyroid gland cells and increasing thyroid hormone synthesis. TSH release is controlled by the hypothalamic tripeptide thyrotropin-releasing hormone (TRH). Cold exposure is a potent stimulus for TRH release, but the feedback loop for the effect of temperature on TRH is not yet established.

Parathyroid Glands

The endocrine secretion of the parathyroid glands is the polypeptide parathyroid hormone (PTH). A fall in serum calcium levels causes release of PTH: PTH acts on bone, the GI tract, and kidneys to increase circulating plasma calcium levels, an action coordinated with vitamin D and calcitonin (discussed later).

Endocrine Pancreas

The islets of Langerhans of the pancreas secrete three hormones that regulate blood glucose: (1) insulin, (2) glucagon, and (3) somatostatin.

Insulin

Insulin is a small protein derived successively from a pre-prohormone and a prohormone. Insulin circulates as a free hormone, has a short plasma half-life of about 6 minutes, and is cleared from the plasma primarily by the liver and kidneys. Insulin binds to receptors on the surface of target tissues and enhances glucose transport across the membrane. Insulin decreases blood glucose by enhancing uptake, use, and storage of glucose in hepatic, muscle, and adipose tissues (discussed later). Insulin enhances amino acid transport into cells; it acts synergistically with growth hormone to promote cell hypertrophy and hyperplasia.

Note that the brain is refractory to insulin and must use glucose for a metabolic substrate. Because the brain glucose transporter has a much higher glucose affinity than the insulin-sensitive transporter, only a severe decline in the blood glucose level can lead to hypoglycemic shock.

Insulin is released after ingestion and absorption of carbohydrates. The initial phase, from release of stored insulin, peaks in 5 minutes. A delayed phase, from synthesis of new insulin, persists until blood glucose returns to fasting levels. The ability of insulin to control plasma glucose levels is the basis of the glucose tolerance test (GTT). In the absence of insulin, fats are used as metabolic substrates. The incomplete oxidation of fatty acids results in the ketoacidosis that is characteristic of untreated diabetes mellitus. The lack of insulin elevates blood glucose, causing an osmotic diuresis (see the Unit 8 Anatomy and Physiology Review). Finally, the lack of insulin promotes protein catabolism and inhibits growth.

Glucagon

Glucagon is an extremely potent hormone that is released when blood glucose levels drop below 90 mg/dl. Glucagon acts on the liver to elevate plasma glucose, an action opposite that of insulin (discussed later). The second messenger for glucagon is cyclic adenosine monophosphate (cAMP); it allows excessively high glucagon levels to affect other tissues (enhancing cardiac contractility, enhancing bile secretion, and inhibiting gastric acid secretion). Protein ingestion enhances glucagon release as well as insulin release. This simultaneous secretion of insulin and glucagon allows cells to use and store glucose without severely decreasing plasma glucose levels. Glucagon is also released during exercise and helps prevent hypoglycemia despite enhanced glucose use by muscle.

Somatostatin

Somatostatin is a small polypeptide with a short (2-minute) half-life; it has many inhibitory actions. Somatostatin is released after ingestion of a meal and inhibits the release of both insulin and glucagon. The net action of somatostatin is to delay nutrient absorption by the GI tract, thus prolonging the duration of intestinal food absorption after a meal.

Adrenal Glands

Adrenal Cortex

Aldosterone. The primary mineralocorticoid secreted by the adrenal cortex is aldosterone. About 50% of aldosterone is free in the plasma; the remainder is bound. Aldosterone is degraded in the liver and is excreted in the urine and feces as a glucuronide or sulfate. Infusion of aldosterone causes a drop in plasma potassium levels by increasing renal excretion of potassium. Plasma potassium concentration is the primary regulator of aldosterone release through a negative feedback control mechanism. Angiotensin II can also promote aldosterone synthesis and release, and adrenocorticotropic hormone (ACTH) has a permissive role in aldosterone production and secretion.

Cortisol. The primary glucocorticoid secreted by the adrenal cortex is cortisol. Following secretion, 94% of cortisol is bound in the plasma to transcortin, a cortisol-binding globulin, and 6% is free. Cortisol is degraded in the liver and is excreted in the urine and feces as a glucuronide or sulfate. Cortisol is a potent metabolic regulatory hormone, increasing plasma glucose and promoting use of alternate metabolic substrates for energy (discussed later). Cortisol stimulates appetite, which leads to central deposition of fat in some central adipose tissues despite the use of fat from peripheral tissues (see the clinical description of Cush-

ing's syndrome). Cortisol's metabolic changes assist the transition to nonglucose support of metabolism in starvation.

Cortisol release is regulated by a hypothalamus-pituitary-adrenal cascade. The hypothalamus secretes corticotropin-releasing hormone (CRH), which is carried by the hypothalamo-hypophyseal portal system to the anterior pituitary gland, where it stimulates ACTH release. ACTH travels in the blood to the adrenal gland, where it promotes conversion of cholesterol to pregnenolone, the rate-limiting step in adrenal glucocorticoid and androgen secretion. Because of a common synthetic pathway, pituitary ACTH also stimulates adrenal androgen production.

The release of ACTH coincides with the release of other compounds formed from the same pre-prohormone. These include (1) melanocyte-stimulating hormone (which stimulates pigment production in epidermal cells), (2) beta-lipotropin (which may stimulate aldosterone release), and (3) the opiate beta-endorphin.

Cortisol is generally described as a stress hormone. Painful stimuli promote release of CRH from the hypothalamus. Emotional stress generated in the limbic system also promotes hypothalamic release of CRH. Cortisol has significant anti-inflammatory effects, retarding the development and enhancing the resolution of the inflammatory response. Glucocorticoid secretion exhibits a strong diurnal rhythm, which is highest in the early morning and lowest in the late evening.

Adrenal Medulla

The adrenal medulla secretes the catecholamines epinephrine and norepinephrine, whose actions mimic those of the sympathetic nervous system but have a longer duration. Epinephrine has strong beta-adrenergic effects and is a potent stimulator of heart rate and contractility. Epinephrine has strong metabolic effects and increases the metabolic rate by up to 100%. These effects include increasing metabolic substrates in the plasma by lipolysis and glycogenolysis (discussed later).

Gonads

The sex hormones have important trophic and metabolic effects. The synthetic pathways for estrogens and androgens share many common precursors with each other and with the adrenal cortical steroids. Consequently, sex hormones originate predominantly from the gonads but are secreted in lower amounts from the adrenal glands.

Androgens, primarily testosterone, have a potent anabolic action. Testosterone is controlled by the hypothalamic-pituitary axis, and gonadotropin-releasing hormone (GnRH) and luteinizing hormone (LH) act on the Leydig cells of the testes to promote testosterone synthesis and release. The reproductive significance of testosterone is discussed in the Unit 9 Anatomy and Physiology Review. A secondary effect of testosterone is to promote protein synthesis as well as the musculoskeletal growth that accompanies puberty.

In the female, LH also stimulates androgen production in the ovarian thecal cells, but the aromatase of the ovarian granulose cells converts the androgens into the estrogen estradiol. The puberty-related increase in musculoskeletal growth and onset of menstruation are results of increases in the cyclic release of estrogen and progesterone (see the Unit 9 Anatomy and Physiology Review).

METABOLIC SUBSTRATES

Plasma Glucose

Glucose is the primary metabolic substrate for the body. The plasma glucose level is normally about 100 mg/dl in both the fed and fasted states. Glucose entry into most cells is insulin dependent. The notable exception is in the brain; cerebral glucose utilization is independent of insulin and requires a plasma glucose level of only 60 mg/dl; levels below this will disrupt brain function.

Plasma glucose represents the balance between glucose absorption from the diet, movement into and out of storage pools, and utilization by the tissues. Glucose storage pools include glycogen, the glycerol component of fat, and amino acids. Although only insulin acts to de-

crease plasma glucose levels, the hormones glucagon, cortisol, growth hormone, and epinephrine all can elevate plasma glucose levels. This multiple endocrine control allows protection of one or more glucose storage pools (Figure U10-6). For example, glucagon mobilizes all storage pools, resulting in increased plasma glucose. Growth hormone prevents gluconeogenesis but increases glucose by the other mechanisms. Cortisol preserves glycogen and fat stores in the center of the body but mobilizes all other glucose pools, including gluconeogenesis. Epinephrine mobilizes fat and glycogen pools.

After a meal, excess plasma glucose is moved into storage, facilitated by insulin. During periods of fasting, glucose is moved from the storage pools, first from glycogen, then from fats, and—if the fast is sufficiently long—from the amino acid pools.

Plasma Amino Acids

Plasma amino acid levels are not controlled by a tight negative feedback mechanism. Ingestion of a protein-rich meal, however, increases both insulin and growth hormone levels. Growth hormone alone enhances cellular uptake of amino acids and preserves amino acid stores (by blocking gluconeogenesis) when insulin is not elevated. When insulin is elevated, the combined action of growth hormone and insulin greatly enhances uptake of amino acids.

FIGURE U10-6 Regulation of metabolic substrates. Cells consume glucose or fatty acids to support metabolism. Plasma glucose is regulated by multiple endocrine mechanisms, which act primarily on the movement into and out of storage pools. Glucose is stored if the plasma glucose level is above 110 mg/dl; glucose is mobilized from storage pools if the plasma glucose level is below 90 mg/dl. FFA, free fatty acid.

Plasma Free Fatty Acids

Free fatty acids are the baseline metabolic substrate and are used unless insulin shifts metabolism to glucose as a metabolic fuel. The heart in particular can oxidize free fatty acids and thus is not as dependent on glucose as a metabolic substrate as the remainder of the body is. In the American diet, food is ingested with sufficient frequency that insulin levels are high, and glucose is normally used as the metabolic fuel. When metabolized, fatty acids are incompletely oxidized, however, with ketone bodies produced as a metabolic by-product.

Plasma levels of free fatty acids are not controlled by a tight negative feedback mechanism. A drop in plasma glucose levels, however, causes the release of epinephrine, cortisol, and growth hormone, all of which promote lipolysis. This results in the movement of fatty acids from the storage pool in fat cells into the plasma pool, providing an alternative substrate for metabolism when glucose availability is limited.

Plasma Calcium

The plasma calcium level (Ca^{2+}) is tightly regulated around 9.4 mg/dl, with a normal range of 9 to 10 mg/dl. About 40% of plasma Ca^{2+} is tightly bound to plasma proteins, and an additional 10% is combined in non-ionized salts with citrate and phosphate. About 5 mg/dl (50%) of plasma Ca^{2+} is free.

More than 99% of calcium within the body is stored in bone, most of it combined with phosphate in hydroxyapatite crystals. Regulation of plasma calcium levels involves balancing dietary absorption, renal excretion, and exchange between the plasma and storage areas. PTH and vitamin D_3 are the major regulators of plasma calcium, with a minor role for the hormone calcitonin.

Infusion of PTH results in elevated plasma calcium levels and decreased plasma phosphate levels. The increase in plasma calcium occurs by enhancing dietary calcium absorption (via vitamin D_3), by decreasing renal calcium excretion, and by mobilizing calcium from the bone storage pools. Plasma calcium is the primary regulator of PTH release. PTH synthesis and release are stimulated by a drop in plasma calcium and help to regulate calcium levels during pregnancy and lactation.

Dietary absorption of calcium requires activated vitamin D. Vitamin D can be absorbed from the diet or synthesized through ultraviolet (sun) light action on 7-dehydrocholesterol. Vitamin D is then converted successively in liver and kidney to 1-25-hydroxycholecalciferol, the active form.

Calcitonin is a polypeptide secreted by the parafollicular C cells of the thyroid gland. Although infusion of calcitonin decreases the plasma calcium concentration, its role in regulating plasma calcium levels is minor.

Alterations in plasma calcium levels produce physiologic changes. Hypocalcemia increases neuronal excitability. Motor neurons exhibit spontaneous depolarizations, leading to tetanic muscular contractions. The hand is particularly susceptible, resulting in carpopedal spasm. Hypercalcemia depresses neuronal and muscle activity.

EFFECTS OF AGING

With aging, the functions of the liver, biliary system, and exocrine pancreas all begin to deteriorate. In the liver, the number and size of hepatic cells is reduced, leading to a decreased weight and mass. Fibrotic tissue also increases, leading to a decrease in protein synthesis, liver enzymes, and cholesterol synthesis. The decrease in enzyme activity diminishes the liver's ability to detoxify drugs and increases the risk of toxic levels of a variety of medications in older adults.

The pancreas is also affected by the process of aging, with calcification of the pancreatic vessels, and by changes in the size of the ducts through distention and dilation. These changes lead to decreased production of lipase, resulting in reduced fat absorption and digestion. Older people also may experience a decreased absorption of fat-soluble vitamins and an increase of fat excreted through the feces (steatorrhea).

CONCLUSIONS

Metabolic regulation is a complex body function, involving the GI tract, liver, muscle, and fat tissues. The multiple endocrine systems that regulate the availability of metabolic fuels reflect the essential role of glucose and fatty acids in survival. The process is complicated by the fact that the body must cope both with periods of excess nutrients (after a meal) and with prolonged fasting.

BIBLIOGRAPHY

1. Berne, R., and Levy, M. (1998). *Physiology* (4th ed.). St. Louis: Mosby.
2. Kierszenbaum, A.L. (2002). *Histology and cell biology: An introduction to pathology*. St. Louis, Mosby.
3. Guyton, A., and Hall, J. (2001). *Textbook of medical physiology* (10th ed.). Philadelphia: W.B. Saunders.
4. Silverthorn, D. (2001). *Human physiology* (2nd ed). Saddle River, NJ: Prentice Hall.

Chapter 44

Assessment of the Endocrine and Metabolic Systems

Dianne M. Smolen

evolve

Web Enhancements

Assessment Terms
English and Spanish
Appendix A
Religious Beliefs and Practices Affecting Health Care

http://evolve.elsevier.com/Black/medsurg/

Appendix B
A Health History Format That Integrates the Assessment of Functional Health Patterns
Appendix C
Laboratory Values of Clinical Importance in Medical-Surgical Nursing

Clients with endocrine or metabolic system disorders may have specific complaints such as nausea, diarrhea, or fatigue. These clients may also have vague, intermittent, generalized manifestations. Because of the different functions of the endocrine glands and the organs of metabolism, and because most glands and organs are relatively inaccessible, there is no single, uniform assessment for clients with endocrine or metabolic disorders. Assessment of clients with such disorders usually focuses on the manifestations of hormone excess or deficiency or metabolic dysfunction. For these reasons, it is important to assess the client's presenting clinical manifestations, health history, physical examination, diagnostic tests, and family and social history. After completing a thorough assessment, analyze the data related to the client's current situation.

HISTORY

During the health history interview, help the client sequence the recalled experiences and manifestations. Linking events and clinical manifestations aids the diagnostic process.

Biographical and Demographic Data

Note biographical and demographic data, such as the client's age, gender, ethnic background, and geographical residence. Some disorders, such as gallbladder disease, diabetes mellitus, and hepatitis, are associated with age or gender as well as where a person lives. For example, as a person ages, fewer hormones and metabolic secretions may be produced or their effect on target organs may diminish.

Current Health

Chief Complaint

Thorough investigation of the client's chief complaint is necessary for accurate assessment. Like gastrointestinal manifestations, the manifestations of endocrine and metabolic disorders may be ambiguous with a puzzling origin. Indicate the onset, duration, intensity, and characteristics of manifestations and any alterations in growth patterns, especially changes in weight, height, or hand, foot, or head size.

evolve *Be sure to check out the bonus material on the Evolve website and the CD-ROM, including free self-assessment exercises.*

http://evolve.elsevier.com/Black/medsurg/

Symptom Analysis

In this discussion, common manifestations related to the endocrine and metabolic systems are grouped by body system as follows (see Chapter 4).

Integumentary Manifestations and Changes in Appearance

- Red, noninflammatory blisters and erosions on dorsum (back) of hands? They are commonly demonstrated in clients infected with hepatitis C virus.
- Jaundiced skin? These causes include viral hepatitis, cirrhosis, and obstructive or cholestatic liver disease.
- Unexplained puncture holes? These may be the route of entry for hepatitis [type B or C] or other pathogens.
- Spider angiomas? Petechiae? Dilated abdominal veins? These may indicate hepatic cirrhosis.
- Skin lesions that do not heal? These may indicate pancreatic dysfunction (see Chapter 48).
- Hyperpigmentation or hypopigmentation? Addison's disease, caused by chronic adrenocortical insufficiency, causes excessive pigmentation of skin; areas of hypopigmentation *[vitiligo]* may indicate other endocrine disorders.
- Hard, nonpitting edema? This occurs in adult hypothyroidism *(myxedema)*.
- Delayed healing? This may indicate diabetes mellitus.
- Changes in hands, head, feet, and face? Acromegaly produces enlargement of the head, hands, and feet and coarsening of facial features. Adrenocortical hyperfunction (Cushing's syndrome) is manifested in moon facies, thin extremities, and truncal obesity.
- Growth delayed? Stunted *(dwarfism)*? Excessive *(gigantism)*? Inappropriate *(acromegaly)*? All of these may indicate a pituitary or other type of endocrine disorder.
- Changes in hair distribution, amount, or texture? Excessive hair *(hirsutism)* may indicate ovarian or adrenocortical disorders; loss of pubic and ancillary hair may indicate a pituitary problem; dry, brittle hair may indicate hypothyroidism; and soft, silky hair may indicate hyperthyroidism.

Cardiovascular Manifestations

- Nosebleeds or bruising easily? Hemorrhoids? *Ascites* (fluid accumulation in peritoneal cavity)? Edema of limbs? All may be indicative of a hepatic disorder in which fluid overload results from the liver's improper functioning and metabolism of hormones, such as aldosterone and antidiuretic hormone (ADH).
- Changes in vital signs? Hyperthyroidism may cause elevation of body temperature and pulse rate.
- Hypertension? This may be caused by an adrenal tumor (pheochromocytoma). Insufficient secretion of ADH from the pituitary gland can cause dehydration; oversecretion can cause excessive retention of body water.

- Increased heart rate and flushing? This may occur in hyperthyroidism and in pheochromocytoma.
- Kussmaul's respiration (deep, rapid breathing)? This is a direct result of diabetic ketoacidosis.

Neurologic Manifestations

- Weakness? Generalized or localized? This may indicate late manifestations of diabetes mellitus.
- Mild depression? This may be a manifestation of pancreatic cancer or an endocrine disorder.
- Changes in mental status or mood (increased irritability)? Extreme alterations in consciousness, such as coma, may occur in uncontrolled diabetes mellitus.
- Emotional lability? Alterations in consciousness? These manifestations may indicate liver or endocrine disorders.
- Drowsiness? A change in mental status and neurologic manifestations can signal the development of hepatic encephalopathy or uncontrolled diabetes mellitus.
- Pain? If radiating to the back, it can be a manifestation of a pancreatic, gallbladder, or biliary tract disorder.
- Tremors? If uncontrolled, can indicate hyperthyroidism.
- Loss of sensation, especially in hands or feet? This suggests diabetes mellitus.

Ophthalmic Manifestations

- Bulging eyes *(exophthalmos)*? This is characteristic of hyperthyroidism.
- Diminished or blurred vision? Visual problems may be caused by diabetes mellitus; visual loss may be caused by a pituitary tumor.

Gastrointestinal Manifestations

- An enlarged, red tongue *(glossitis)*? This may be present in clients with diabetes mellitus.
- Weight gain or loss or changes in appetite? This may indicate an endocrine or metabolic disorder. For example, increased eating but loss of weight may indicate hyperthyroidism; gaining weight may suggest hypothyroidism. Excessive appetite *(polyphagia)* may be indicative of diabetes mellitus.
- Excessive thirst *(polydipsia)*? This may indicate diabetes mellitus.
- Abdominal pain? Right upper quadrant discomfort suggests gallbladder or liver disorders.
- Nausea or vomiting? This occurs in 70% of clients with pancreatitis.
- Anorexia? This is especially prevalent in liver disorders.
- Fatty food intolerance? This may be indicative of pancreatic or biliary tract disease.
- Excessive eructation (belching or *aerophagia*)? This suggests gallbladder disease.
- Heartburn *(pyrosis)*? This may be a manifestation of cholecystitis or refluxed acid or bile.

- Disturbed bowel pattern, such as diarrhea (dark-colored, tarry stools)? This may be caused by hyperthyroidism or a biliary tract problem.
- Constipation? This may indicate hypothyroidism or a biliary disorder.
- Clay-colored stools or *acholic* (without bilirubin) stools? This may occur briefly in viral hepatitis; it is common in obstructive jaundice.
- Fatty, foul-smelling stools *(steatorrhea)?* This may occur with chronic pancreatitis or after gastric surgery; it is partially the result of rapid gastric emptying, which prevents adequate mixing with pancreatic and biliary secretions.

Genitourinary and Reproductive Manifestations

- Dark yellow or tea-colored urine? This indicates impaired excretion of bilirubin caused by hepatocellular disease.
- Frequent urination *(polyuria)?* This may be indicative of diabetes mellitus.
- Menstrual cycle irregularities (including amenorrhea)? Loss of libido? Loss or premature development of secondary sex characteristics? Impotence or infertility? These sexual changes are characteristics of endocrine disorders.
- Renal problems? Calcium stone formation may be caused by hyperparathyroidism (because calcium is resorbed from bone).

Other Manifestations

- Yellow sclerae? This suggests biliary obstruction.
- Fever? This may indicate an acute gallbladder, pancreas, or liver problem.
- Intolerance of alcohol or medications? Fatigue? Malaise? All occur with hepatitis or endocrine disorders.
- Dehydration? This may indicate insufficient levels of ADH.
- Bone or joint pain? Hyperparathyroidism may cause calcium to be reabsorbed from bone and contribute to bone pain, fracture, or both. Adrenal insufficiency (Cushing's syndrome) may produce a rapid breakdown of bone.
- Muscle cramps? Tetany? This may result from inadequate secretion of parathyroid hormone.

Past Health History

Childhood and Infectious Diseases

Ask the client and family members about any episodes of endocrine or metabolic disorders that the client may have experienced as a child or an adolescent. For example, did the client have any growth patterns that were different from those of other members of the family? Did these changes in body size occur after physical maturation?

Have there been any changes in head circumference or size of the hands or feet? For instance, has the client needed to buy hats, gloves, rings, or shoes in a larger size?

Ask about changes in the amount and distribution of hair, such as increased facial hair (women), decreased hair (men), or changes in pubic or axillary hair (both men and women). Has the client had any episodes of excessive thirst and urination? In addition, ask female clients about their menstrual history, pregnancies, or fertility problems.

Immunizations

Inquire about the client's immunization status. Did the client receive the routine childhood vaccinations (see Chapters 4 and 21)? Were the vaccinations given when the client was an infant or later in life? Was a tetanus shot received recently? Has the client been immunized against hepatitis A or B or ever received post-exposure immunization for hepatitis A?

Major Illnesses and Hospitalizations

Ask the client to identify any illnesses or injuries to the head or neck. Is there a history of head trauma, such as from a forceful blow? Trauma can lead to hypopituitarism. Has the client been hospitalized for surgery to the head or neck? Is there a history of surgery, chemotherapy, or radiation therapy to the head or neck? Ask about diagnosis or treatment for related disorders, such as primary brain or spinal cord tumors, metastatic tumors, meningitis, brain infarctions, diabetes mellitus, diabetes insipidus, hypertension, and goiter.

Have the client describe any past problems with jaundice, hepatitis, abdominal pain, gallbladder disease, anemia, or changes in bowel elimination, such as diarrhea, clay-colored stools, or melena. Has the client ever been hospitalized for any of these disorders or ever had surgery of the liver or gallbladder?

Have diagnostic procedures, such as a gallbladder x-ray study, liver biopsy, or ultrasound examination of the gallbladder ever been performed? Has the client ever received a transfusion of blood or blood products?

Procedures Causing Skin or Membrane Disruption

Has the client had recent blood tests, transfusions of blood products, dental procedures, ear or other body piercing, tattooing, or any intravenous injection with a potentially contaminated needle? Note such procedures in an assessment, because breaks in the skin may be the route of entry for hepatitis virus (type B or C) or other pathogens.

Medications

Ask specifically about the use of hormones and steroids, including name, dose, and duration of use. Does the client have a history of taking anabolic steroids? Ask about medications that the client is currently taking or has taken previously, including over-the-counter drugs. Many drugs and chemicals are potentially hepatotoxic, such as alcohol, gold compounds, mercury, phosphorus, anabolic steroids, acetaminophen, isoniazid, halothane, sulfonamides, arsenic, thiazide diuretics, zidovudine (azidothymidine), and anticancer drugs, such as methotrexate. Other medications to ask about are oral contraceptives, anesthetic agents, and antipsychotic agents.

Ask about the use of alternative therapies, such as herbal medicines. Herbal medicines used in the treatment of non–insulin-dependent diabetes include aloe vera juice, beans (*Phaseolus* species), bitter gourd, karela (*Momordica charantia*), black tea (*Camellia sinensis*), fenugreek (*Trigonella foenum-graecum*), gumar (*Gymnema sylvestre*), macadamia nut, and Madagascar periwinkle (*Catharanthus roseus*). Effects of these herbs include lowering of blood pressure (fenugreek), a boosting of insulin production (gurmar), and increased use of available insulin (black tea).

Kelp (*Fucus vesiculosus*) may help with weight loss in hypothyroid disorders. Milk thistle (*Silybum marianum*) is used for treatment and prophylaxis of chronic hepatotoxicity, inflammatory liver disorders, and certain types of cirrhosis. See Chapter 5 for additional information on complementary and alternative therapies.

Allergies

Ask the client about known allergies to food or medications. Specifically ask about reactions to iodine. Iodine is contained in contrast media used in some diagnostic studies of the metabolic system.

Family Health History

When assessing a client with an endocrine or metabolic disorder, inquire about the family history. A number of endocrine disorders are inherited or tend to run in families. Has any family member had problems similar to those of the client? Disorders to inquire about include growth and development problems, obesity, goiter, hypothyroidism or hyperthyroidism, hypertension, low blood pressure (hypotension), diabetes mellitus, diabetes insipidus, autoimmune diseases (Addison's disease), and problems with the adrenal glands (pheochromocytoma).

Ask the client whether any family members have had cancer (especially of the bowel, liver, or pancreas), jaundice, bleeding disorders, hepatitis, nutritional deficiencies, alcoholism, obesity, pancreatic disease, or gallbladder disease. A history of these disorders in family members increases the risk of their development in the client.

Psychosocial History

Assessment of the psychosocial history and lifestyle patterns provides data about the client's physical and psychological status. Inquire about the client's occupation, environment, and habits.

Occupation, Geographical Location, and Environment

Because *stress* can increase the severity of disorders such as diabetes mellitus, ask about the client's stress tolerance and coping patterns. Stress can be either *physiologic* (caused by illness) or *emotional*. Ask about job-related stressors, such as amount of time spent on the job both in the work setting and at home. Do strained interpersonal relationships at work contribute to increased stress levels? Does the client have opportunities to retreat from the workplace and to engage in recreational activities?

Ask about the home environment and family interpersonal relationships and obligations. What support systems are available to the client? Does the client report effective current coping strategies? If possible, ask family members to corroborate or to help identify behavior changes.

Ask about the client's occupation and work environment. Are there any factors that are known to cause liver damage? For example, heavy metals such as mercury and lead, anesthetic agents such as nitrous oxide, and chemicals such as carbon tetrachloride and certain pesticides are known hepatotoxins. Does the client engage in activities that increase the risk of exposure to substances that cause hepatitis or pancreatitis? Ask about the following:

- Any close contact with hazardous waste
- Travel in areas where hepatitis or pancreatitis is endemic
- Eating raw or steamed shellfish (oysters, clams, scallops) from polluted water
- Swimming or bathing in polluted water
- Any known contact with hepatitis-infected animals or people
- Ingestion of mushrooms that have not been purchased in a store

Exercise, Nutrition, and Habits

When assessing the client for endocrine or metabolic disorders, consider other aspects of lifestyle and coping. Ask about exercise, food intake, sleep and rest patterns, and the use of alcohol, illicit drugs, or tobacco products. Ask about usual patterns as well as any alteration in patterns. Related to food intake, investigate the following:

- Food preferences
- Daily intake of proteins, carbohydrates, fats, and sodium
- Changes in eating patterns, including onset of changes
- Meal preparation (by whom, style of preparation)
- Recent development of food intolerances

In the case of a chronic condition such as diabetes mellitus, careful control is crucial to prevent complications. Diet and physical activity are important in the management of both type 1 and type 2 diabetes (see **EB** Chapter 47). Type 2 (non–insulin-dependent) diabetes mellitus, is often prevented through diet and physical activity. According to *Healthy People 2010*, the goal of the U.S. Department of Health and Human Services is **EB** "through prevention programs, reduce the disease and economic burden of diabetes, and improve the quality of life for all persons who have or are at risk for diabetes."[12] You have an important role in helping clients adjust to chronic conditions such as diabetes mellitus or liver disease by assisting them to adopt health-seeking behaviors related to diet, exercise, and necessary medication.

Carefully explore the client's use of alcohol and other mind-altering substances. Pay attention to alcohol use patterns, because alcoholism often accompanies liver and pancreatic disease, causing fatty infiltration of the liver.

Be alert to whether the client provides confusing or conflicting data. Is the client's behavior altered in any way as the assessment proceeds? For example, does the client become angry, silent, or tearful? If significant others are present, do they corroborate the client's account? The client who does not acknowledge a substance abuse problem may not provide reliable information about usage. The client who takes illicit drugs may be unwilling to describe drug use patterns. If you suspect that the client's history is unreliable, ask significant others to provide additional information. (Chapter 26 discusses alcoholism and other drug use.)

Review of Systems

If an endocrine or metabolic disorder is suspected, a careful review of systems is important because endocrine and metabolic disorders can affect multiple systems. During this review, ask about the integumentary, cardiovascular, neurologic, gastrointestinal, and genitourinary systems, and mental status (see Chief Complaint and Symptom Analysis on pp. 1154 and 1155). Specifically, inquire about jaundice, pruritus (itching), abdominal swelling indicating edema or ascites (fluid-filled abdomen), dark-colored urine, clay-colored stools, bleeding tendencies (purpura), spider angiomas (spider nevi or telangiectasia), fatigue, excessive thirst, excessive urination, and weight loss or weight gain. Detailed questions for the review of systems may be found on the website **evolve** for this book for Chapter 4.

PHYSICAL EXAMINATION

Physical assessment of endocrine or metabolic (liver, biliary, or pancreatic) dysfunction involves careful examination of the entire body and is integrated throughout the interaction with the client. Specifically, the assessment covers general health and nutritional status along with the skin, head, neck, thorax, abdomen, upper and lower extremities, and genitalia. Examine all body systems in a systematic manner from head to toe (see Chap-

ter 4) using inspection, auscultation, percussion, and palpation.

Before the examination, ask the client to point to any painful area; examine that area last. As stated earlier, hepatic or biliary pain is often located in the right upper quadrant (Figure 44-1). Pain that is dull and difficult to localize or describe may arise from an organ (viscera). Somatic pain is sharp, piercing, and easy to localize; it arises from nerve endings in the peritoneum.

General Appearance and Nutritional Status

Begin by assessing general appearance and health status. Is the client alert and responding appropriately to questions? Observe the client's mood, level of consciousness (orientation, alertness), verbal and nonverbal behavior, memory, affect, and speech patterns. Note any anxiety or nervousness, depression, apathy, or anger.

Does the client appear acutely or chronically ill? Ask about use of alcohol and other substances. Because handwriting deteriorates with diminishing liver function, obtain a handwriting sample for subsequent comparison **EB** in case the client has progressive hepatocellular damage (see Chapter 49).

Assess nutritional status. Weigh the client and determine the amount of subcutaneous fat and muscular development. Obesity may accompany gallbladder disease. Ask whether the client has a pattern of right upper quadrant pain after eating certain high-fat foods (nuts, chocolate). Clients with a history of substance abuse or cir-

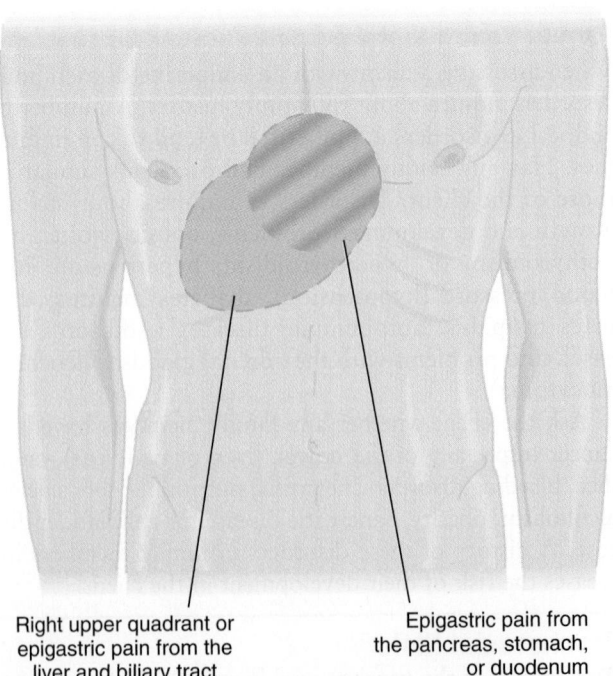

Right upper quadrant or epigastric pain from the liver and biliary tract

Epigastric pain from the pancreas, stomach, or duodenum

FIGURE 44-1 Location of abdominal pain with hepatic, biliary, or pancreatic disorders.

rhosis may be malnourished. Observe the client's state of dress, growth and development, and body size. Chapter 30 describes the assessment of nutrition.

Vital Signs

Measure and assess vital signs. Temperature is elevated in hyperthyroidism or may be low-normal or below normal in hypothyroidism. Observe respirations for altered rate and rhythm. Blood pressure alterations include hypotension, hypertension, and widening pulse pressure. Pulse rate may vary orthostatically.

Integument

Observe hair texture and distribution over body surfaces. Note brittleness or loss of hair (alopecia). Inspect the skin for color, pigmentation, striae, ecchymoses, or mottling. Palpate the skin for texture, thickness, moisture, and diaphoresis. Inspect and palpate the nails for color, texture, brittleness, presence of ridges, and peeling.

Head

Inspect the contour and shape of the head. Note symmetry and the proportion of facial features. Observe skin color for erythema or rash over the cheeks. Observe facial expression for anxiety.

Eyes

Inspect and palpate the eyebrows, noting hair distribution. Observe eye position, symmetry, shape, and eyelid lag. Note color of sclerae: Are they yellowish or white? Assess visual acuity, extraocular movements, and visual fields. Inspect for lens opacity and eye edema.

Complete ophthalmoscopic assessment includes observing the retinas. See Chapter 66 for a discussion of how to use an ophthalmoscope and Chapter 47 for a description of retinal changes associated with diabetes mellitus.

Nose

Inspect mucosa for swelling and color. Listen for noisy or labored breathing.

Mouth

Note size and shape of the jaw. Inspect the color of the oral mucosa and the condition of the client's teeth. Note malocclusion. Observe tongue size and activity for fasciculations.

Neck

Listen to the client's voice for hoarseness or huskiness. Note clarity, pitch, and volume of speech. Ask the client to swallow and observe for difficulty in swallowing or pain; repeat this maneuver with the client's neck in a hyperextended position. Inspect the neck for symmetry, alignment, thickness, or bulging over the thyroid gland, and examine the midline position of the trachea. Observe for scars related to thyroidectomy, trauma, or other neck surgery. Note presence of hyperpigmentation.

Observe for forceful pulsations over the carotid arteries. Palpate the thyroid gland unless it is noticeably enlarged; vigorous palpation can stimulate release of thyroid hormone, which increases the risk of precipitating a thyroid crisis in a client with thyroid hyperplasia. If the thyroid gland is enlarged, auscultate the lobes for bruits.

The thyroid gland may be palpated by means of an anterior or posterior approach (Figure 44-2). In both approaches, gently run a finger down the anterior part of the neck, locating the thyroid and cricoid cartilages and the isthmus of the thyroid gland. The isthmus feels soft and compressible compared with the firmer cartilage ring just superior to it. Ask the client to swallow while you palpate the isthmus. It should rise in the neck and should not be enlarged. Figure 44-2 explains the anterior and posterior approaches for palpating the lobes of the thyroid gland. The thyroid gland is normally nonpalpable. If it is palpable, note the texture of the gland because it is usually smooth and firm, without lumps, roughness, hardness, asymmetry, or tenderness (see the Physical Assessment Findings in the Healthy Adult feature on The Thyroid Gland on p. 1160).

Extremities

Examine the arms and legs for size, shape, and symmetry, and check their proportionality to the trunk. The distance from the symphysis pubis to the heel is usually about half of the body's total height. Note peripheral edema. Palpate and note peripheral pulse amplitude (see Chapter 4). Assess deep tendon reflexes and observe their relaxation time (see Chapter 69).

Upper Extremities

Ask the client to extend the hands with palms down; observe for fine tremors and for reddened palms (palmar erythema). Inspect for thenar wasting, Dupuytren's contracture, and nail clubbing (see Chapter 61). Note the size of the client's hands in proportion to the rest of the body. Assess grip strength and muscle strength of the fingers and arms (see Chapter 27).

Lower Extremities

Note the color and distribution of hair. Assess the size of the client's feet in proportion to the rest of the body. Inspect for corns and calluses. Separate the toes, and observe for deformities and skin changes, such as thickening, fissures, and nail thickening. Palpate and note pedal pulses (see Chapter 4). Assess leg muscles for weakness (see Chapter 27).

A   Posterior approach

B   Anterior approach

FIGURE 44-2 Palpation of the thyroid. **A,** Posterior approach. Stand behind the client. Ask the client to lower the chin to relax the neck muscles, and tilt the head slightly to the right. To examine the right lobe of the thyroid, use the fingers of your left hand to displace the trachea slightly to the right. This moves the thyroid laterally. You can then palpate between the trachea and the sternocleidomastoid for the right lobe with the fingers of your right hand. Ask the client to swallow while you palpate; doing so causes the gland to rise in the neck. Repeat for the left lobe by reversing your hand placement and positioning the client toward the left. Projection of the thyroid can be enhanced by having the client drink water. **B,** Anterior approach. Stand in front of the client. To palpate the thyroid gland's right lobe, flex the client's head toward the right to relax the neck muscles on that side. Use the fingers of your right hand to displace the trachea slightly to the client's right. Then ask the client to swallow while you palpate the right lobe of the thyroid with the fingers of your left hand. Repeat for the left lobe. You can also assess for thyroid enlargement by palpating deep on each side of the sternocleidomastoid muscle.

Thorax

In males, inspect for gynecomastia (breast enlargement), which can develop because of decreased metabolism of estrogen when the liver is dysfunctional. Auscultate for extra heart sounds, such as a systolic murmur (see Chapter 56).

Abdomen

Assessment of the abdomen includes inspection, auscultation, percussion, and palpation. Table 44-1 summarizes the key points of a physical examination for endocrine and metabolic disorders.

Inspection

Note areas of hyperpigmentation, such as in scars or striae. Observe the client for manifestations of pain during light palpation; examine painful areas last. Charac-

---

PHYSICAL ASSESSMENT FINDINGS IN THE HEALTHY ADULT*
The Thyroid Gland

Inspection
The thyroid gland is not normally seen on inspection.

Palpation
The gland rises and falls with swallowing. Isthmus at midline, soft. Right lobe slightly larger than the left lobe. Texture rubbery without nodules. Nontender.

Auscultation
No bruits heard over either lobe.

*Findings for the metabolic system are found in Chapter 30 as part of the abdominal assessment.

TABLE 44-1 Key Points of a Physical Examination: Endocrine and Metabolic Disorders

Steps	Normal or Common Findings	Significant or Abnormal Findings
Inspection Note:		
Color of skin	Same as or lighter than other areas	Redness, cyanosis, jaundice, lesions, ecchymosis, needle marks, or hematomas
Eyes	White sclerae	Sclerae: yellow tint
Symmetry, contour, shape of abdomen	Flat, rounded abdomen	Distended, asymmetrical, masses
Surface of abdomen	Smooth	Tight, shiny; engorged, prominent veins, spider angiomas
Rectal area	No dilated veins (hemorrhoids)	Presence of distended veins (hemorrhoids)
General nutritional state Weigh Observe for ascites	Adequate for height and build	Obesity or malnutrition
Auscultation Place stethoscope (warmed) over right upper quadrant. Listen for vascular sounds or friction rubs	No venous hums No friction rubs	Venous hum with both diastolic and systolic components
Percussion *Abdomen:* Note percussion sounds in four quadrants	Tympany over abdomen, bladder, intestines, and aorta, and dull over liver, spleen, pancreas, kidneys, and uterus	Dullness over enlarged organs; indicates need for further assessment for ascites
Liver: Span. Percuss upward from below client's umbilicus on the right midclavicular line (MCL) until dullness is heard. Mark this point. Percuss downward from lung resonance in right MCL to dullness and measure distance between two marks.	Liver span is 6-12 cm; no tenderness	Liver span is greater than 12 cm
Note if tender, soft, or firm, smooth or nodular	Slightly tender, soft, smooth surface	Nodular, more than slightly tender, hard
Spleen: Note size. Percuss downward in left posterior axillary line, beginning with lung resonance until dullness is heard	Dullness between ribs 6 and 10	Dullness extends above sixth rib or covers large area—indicates enlargement
Palpation Use palmar surface of extended fingers		
Liver: Palpate lightly on right side, and then palpate deeply	No tenderness, pain, masses	Tenderness, rigidity, nodules, enlarged
Spleen: Note: If spleen can be percussed, it is best not to palpate it. Palpate lightly on left side, distal to MCL	No tenderness, pain, masses	Tenderness, rigidity, nodules, enlarged
Adaptations for Older Adults		
Inspection Contour	Sagging and rounded because of loss of muscle tone and accumulation of fat	
Palpation Note liver span and borders	Span may be shortened, but border is more easily palpated	Right upper quadrant or epigastric pain from the liver and biliary tract Epigastric pain from pancreas, stomach, or duodenum

teristics of ascites include a distended abdomen with tight and glistening skin, bulging flanks, and prominent abdominal veins. Measure abdominal girth if ascites is present. Ascites may account for recent rapid onset of weight gain with accompanying loss of muscle mass.

Auscultation

Auscultation for possible hepatic or biliary problems is performed by gently placing a warmed stethoscope on the right upper quadrant while the client is supine. Note whether a soft hum is heard during both the systolic and diastolic components of the heartbeat. A *hum* indicates increased collateral circulation between the portal and systemic venous systems, as might occur in hepatic cirrhosis.

Listen for a *friction rub* (a grating sound heard with respiratory ventilation). A friction rub suggests inflammation of the peritoneal surface of an organ, as from a liver tumor, chlamydial or gonococcal perihepatitis, or recent liver biopsy.

If a systolic *bruit* (swishing sound indicating vascular turbulence) accompanies a hepatic friction rub, carcinoma of the liver is suspected.

Percussion

Percuss the abdomen, especially the liver and spleen. Assess liver size by percussing the span of the liver at the right midclavicular line (RMCL) and the midsternal line (MSL). Begin by percussing in the right midclavicular line either superior or inferior to the estimated borders of the liver. Superiorly, begin at the third intercostal space (ICS) over lung resonance; percuss down the thorax until the sound changes to dull. Mark this level on the skin with a pen. Inferiorly, start over a tympanic area and percuss upward until the sound changes to dull. Also mark this with the pen.

At the midsternal line, percuss upward from above the umbilicus from tympany to dull. Mark where the sound changes. Superiorly, percuss down the sternum until the percussion note changes; mark this too. Measure the distance between each set of marks.

At the right midclavicular line, the liver span ranges from 6 to 12 cm (2½ to 5 inches); at the midsternal line, it ranges from 4 to 8 cm (1½ to 3 inches). The lower border of the liver at the right midclavicular line is usually at the right costal margin, and the upper border is between the fifth and seventh intercostal spaces.

Liver size varies with body size. Measurements larger than the norms indicate liver enlargement. Ask the client to take a deep breath and hold it while you percuss the lower liver border in the right midclavicular line again. With deep inspiration, the pressure of the diaphragm causes the liver to descend lower into the abdomen. The distance of liver descent is marked and measured, and

ranges from 2 to 3 cm (~1 inch). Use the marked level of liver descent as a guide for later palpation of the liver.

Percussion may determine spleen size, particularly if the spleen is enlarged. The spleen is located by percussion as a small area of dullness just posterior to the left midaxillary line (LMAL) between the sixth and 10th ribs. It normally has a span of approximately 7 cm (2½ to 3 inches). If the spleen enlarges, the area of dullness shifts inferiorly below the 10th rib and anteriorly toward or beyond the left anterior axillary line (LAAL).

Percussion is also used to assess for ascites in the abdomen by observing for a *fluid wave*. This infrequently performed maneuver is an advanced physical assessment technique because of the potential difficulty in detecting a fluid wave. A more common method of assessment for ascites is to measure changes in abdominal girth and weight gain over time. Another advanced assessment technique to detect ascites is the *test for shifting dullness* (Figure 44-3, A-C).

The *fluid wave test* is performed while the client is supine. Two nurses participate. One nurse places the edges of the hands on the client's abdominal midline to stabilize the abdominal wall. The second nurse places one hand on one side of the client's abdomen while briskly tapping the opposite side of the abdomen with the other hand. The second nurse feels for the movement of a fluid wave against the palpating hand opposite the side percussed (see Figure 44-3, D).

Palpation

Use palpation initially to assess for muscle guarding or tenderness. Observe the client for facial grimaces, tensing, or other indications of discomfort. Next, perform deep palpation to evaluate tenderness, indicating possible inflammation. Light and deep palpation techniques are discussed in Chapter 4.

Because the peritoneum is often involved, evaluate for localized peritoneal irritation. Press the abdomen firmly at a point away from any tender area and quickly remove the examining hand. Severe pain accompanies this maneuver when inflammation is present, indicating *rebound tenderness*.

Perform *liver palpation* standing at the client's right side. Use one of two bimanual techniques:

1. *First technique.* Place your left hand under the client's right posterior thorax over the 11th and 12th ribs, and push the thorax upward. Place the right hand below the right costal margin at the previously marked level of liver descent, as determined by percussion. Point your fingers upward toward the costal margin, then gently push up and in as the client takes a deep breath using the abdominal muscles. As the client inhales, feel for the liver's edge to slip over the finger tips as it descends. If the liver's edge is felt, it should feel firm, sharp,

smooth, and regular. Palpate at several points medially and laterally to assess the edge along its inferior border.

2. *Second technique.* Place the right hand below the right costal margin as described. Superimpose the left hand on the right hand. Perform the remainder of the maneuver as described earlier.

The liver is difficult to palpate in clients who are obese or tense or who have taut abdominal muscles because they are physically fit. Abnormal findings include a hard, nodular feel to the liver and more than minimal tenderness as perceived by the client. If extreme ascites is present, the liver edge is nonpalpable.

Spleen palpation is an advanced physical assessment technique. If percussion has shown that the spleen is enlarged, the nurse does not usually palpate it because of the possibility of rupture. If no enlargement is noted on percussion, perform spleen palpation in a manner similar to that for the liver; however, perform the technique on the left side of the abdomen below the costal margin. Ask the client to turn onto the right side, allowing gravity to bring the spleen forward and down, closer to the abdominal wall. Place your left hand behind the client's left posterior rib cage, and push forward while palpating with the right hand. The spleen is normally nonpalpable. Congestion caused by portal hypertension results in enlargement of the spleen and is a common finding in cirrhosis.

Blunt (fist) percussion is used to determine organ tenderness over the liver. This maneuver is performed after all other abdominal assessment techniques are completed to avoid producing discomfort in the presence of organ tenderness. When assessing for *liver tenderness,* use *only* indirect fist percussion over the costal margin at the right midclavicular line to avoid trauma to the liver. This maneuver is also known as a *liver tap.* For comparison, perform indirect fist percussion over the left costal margin at the midclavicular line (Chapter 4 explains blunt percussion). Tell the client what is going to be done to avoid a reaction of surprise that may be misinterpreted as tenderness. Note the client's reaction to the blows.

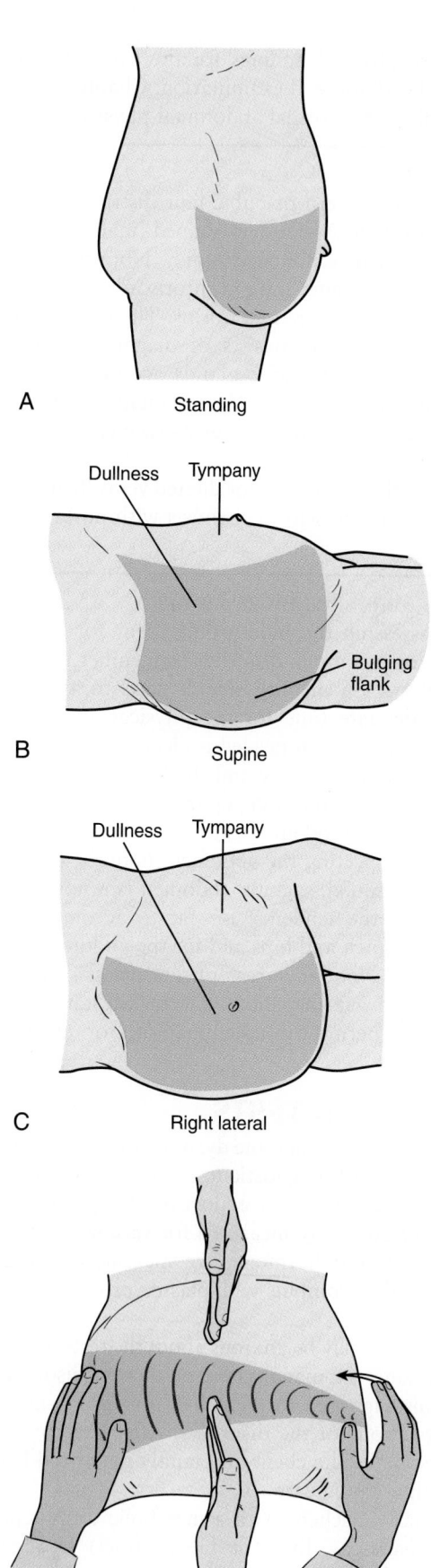

FIGURE 44-3 Testing for *shifting dullness* to assess fluid levels in ascites. Shaded areas demonstrate how fluid and percussion sound shift to the dependent side: **A,** To the lower abdomen when standing; **B,** To the flanks when supine; **C,** To the dependent side when lying on one side. **D,** Test for *fluid wave.* An assistant places the edges of his or her hands along the client's midline to stop transmission of a wave through abdominal fat. The examiner places one hand on one of the client's flanks and percusses the opposite flank sharply with the fingertips. The nonpercussing hand feels for the impulse transmitted through the fluid.

Record physical findings for the liver and spleen as part of the abdominal examination. Chapter 30 includes a recording of a normal abdominal physical assessment.

Genitalia and Rectum

Observe the pattern of pubic hair distribution, particularly in women. A diamond-shaped (male) pattern is indicative of a masculinizing tumor. Note the size of the testes in male clients and the clitoris in female clients for comparison with expected norms. The remainder of endocrine assessment consists of diagnostic studies, because the only endocrine glands accessible to physical examination are the thyroid and gonads (see Chapter 39 for further information about assessment of the reproductive system).

Inspect the rectal area for dilated veins (hemorrhoids). These may be present in cirrhosis with portal hypertension.

Modifications for Older Adults

When assessing the older adult client for possible endocrine or metabolic disorders, remember to divide the physical assessment into several parts to avoid fatigue. Allow adequate time for the physical examination so that the information needed is clearly communicated to the client. Speak clearly and distinctly when asking for specific information or giving instructions so that the request is understood and heard.

When inspecting the abdomen, note the contour and color. A rounded, sagging abdomen is a normal finding because of the tendency for fat to accumulate in the lower abdomen and hips and for the abdominal muscles to weaken. Note any areas of tenderness or discomfort because old age may blunt the manifestations of pain caused by peritoneal inflammation, for example (see Table 44-1).

DIAGNOSTIC TESTS

A client with an endocrine dysfunction may need several general types of diagnostic tests. Blood levels of various hormones specific to the endocrine glands are measured. Some hormones are measured for specific levels; others, such as thyroid hormone, are measured according to how well they combine with plasma proteins or radioactive iodine.

The client may be anxious about the tests and the possible results. In many cases, endocrine disorders have been misdiagnosed for years because of the nonspecific manifestations of the disorders. After the correct diagnosis is made, the client and family may need help coping with ongoing care.

Similarly, a client with a metabolic dysfunction (exocrine pancreas, liver, or biliary tract) frequently requires multiple diagnostic measures. No single laboratory test, radiographic study, or surgical procedure yields sufficient data to confirm a diagnosis or establish the de-

gree of malfunction. Foster a sense of self-worth and understanding in the client during repeated diagnostic procedures. Such a sense promotes cooperation and reduces the fatigue and anxiety that frequently accompany these evaluations.

In the discussion that follows, common diagnostic tests of endocrine function are identified according to specific endocrine organs: pancreas, thyroid, parathyroid, adrenal, and pituitary, after which diagnostic tests involving organs of metabolism (exocrine pancreas, liver, biliary tract, and gallbladder) are discussed. For organizational purposes, the diagnostic tests are divided into (a) laboratory studies and (b) radiographic and other diagnostic studies.

Laboratory Studies

Endocrine Function Studies

Tests of Endocrine Pancreas Function. Diagnostic assessment of pancreatic endocrine function is related to blood glucose levels. Elevated fasting blood glucose is usually the first indication of hyperglycemia. Glycosylated hemoglobin (HbA1c), or glycohemoglobin, is a measure of the average blood glucose over 3 months and can be obtained in the nonfasting state. A more detailed presentation of diagnostic tests related to diabetes appears in Chapter 47.

Tests of Thyroid Function. Several tests are available to assess thyroid function. A brief overview of the most common laboratory tests follows (Table 44-2).

Serum Thyroid-Stimulating Hormone. Measurement of the basal serum thyroid-stimulating hormone (TSH) concentration is useful in differentiating primary and secondary hypothyroidism. In primary hypothyroidism, the thyroid gland compensates for a functional abnormality that impairs the ability to synthesize hormones. This results in hypersecretion of TSH. In contrast, the serum TSH concentration is almost always low or undetectable in secondary and tertiary hypothyroidism.

Antithyroid Antibody Tests. Many thyroid disorders are presumed to have an autoimmune basis, such as Hashimoto's thyroiditis, some types of myxedema, and Graves' disease (a form of hyperthyroidism). Serologic tests may be performed to determine whether the client's blood contains antithyroid antibodies.

Serum Thyroxine and Triiodothyronine. Radioimmunoassay can be used to measure serum concentrations of thyroxine (T_4) and triiodothyronine (T_3).

T_4 is transported in the blood largely bound to thyroxine-binding globulin and is an effective indicator of thyroid function; conditions that affect thyroid-binding globulin levels alter the serum T_4 concentration. Hyperthyroidism, viral hepatitis, pregnancy, and oral contraceptives increase serum T_4; hypothyroidism, strenuous exercise, heparin, and lithium decrease serum T_4.

T_3 (like T_4) circulates in the bloodstream, attached to plasma proteins and to erythrocytes. However, T_3 binds far more readily to plasma proteins than to erythrocytes. T_3 binds to erythrocytes only when plasma protein binding sites are limited.

Analysis of T_3 and T_4 concentrations has largely replaced the older technique of estimating basal metabolic rate (BMR). BMR is calculated by measuring the amount of oxygen the body consumes when in a state of complete mental and physical relaxation.

T_3 Resin Uptake. If thyroid function is below normal or if serum protein levels are high, resin uptake of T_3 is depressed. If thyroid function is above normal or serum protein levels are low, resin uptake of T_3 is elevated. T_3 resin uptake is one test used to measure thyroid function, but it should not be the only one.

Thyrotropin-Releasing Hormone Stimulation Test. Thyrotropin-releasing hormone (TRH) is released from the hypothalamus, and it normally stimulates release of TSH from the pituitary. During the TRH stimulation test, people with thyroid disorders are given TRH intravenously. An increase in TSH levels indicates that the pituitary is functioning normally. TSH levels do not increase in the presence of hyperthyroidism or when the pituitary cells that secrete TSH are diseased.

Serum Cholesterol. The serum cholesterol level may be elevated in primary hypothyroidism, which may explain why this condition is accompanied by a marked tendency toward atherosclerosis (see Table 44-2). People with hyperthyroidism usually have a lower serum cholesterol level. Serum cholesterol is not a specific test of thyroid function, however, because its levels are influenced by many factors other than thyroid hormone levels.

Tests of Parathyroid Function. Measurement of serum calcium, phosphorus, serum alkaline phosphatase, parathyroid hormone, and osteocalcin are important to evaluate because of the relationship between the parathyroid and thyroid glands. For example, calcitonin secretion by the thyroid gland affects the plasma calcium concentration.[13] See Table 44-2 for specific information about these tests.

Tests of Adrenal Function. Adrenal function tests may be used to evaluate medullary and cortical hormones and their metabolites by assessing both serum and urine specimens. Adrenocortical hormones include cortisol (glucocorticoid), aldosterone (mineralocorticoid), and small amounts of sex hormones (androgens). Adrenal medullary hormones include epinephrine and norepinephrine (catecholamines). See Table 44-2 for specific information.

Aldosterone Levels. Plasma levels of aldosterone, angiotensin II, and renin can be measured at any time. Plasma levels of aldosterone can be increased by giving potassium, restricting sodium, or having the client assume an upright position. Plasma levels of aldosterone can be decreased by infusion of saline.

Serum Cortisol Test: Dexamethasone Suppression. Serum cortisol is measured in clients suspected to have hyperfunctioning or hypofunctioning adrenal glands. Cortisol levels usually increase and decrease during the day in a pattern called the *diurnal variation*. Cortisol levels are highest around 6 to 8 AM and gradually decrease during the day, reaching their lowest point around midnight. A cortisol suppression test involves the suppression of pituitary adrenocorticotropic hormone (ACTH) with dexamethasone. Normally after administration of dexamethasone, 24-hour levels of ketosteroid in the urine decrease by 50%. Dexamethasone can also be given at midnight and serum cortisol then assessed at 8 AM. In clients with increased adrenocortical stimulation, no decrease is seen in ketosteroid production in urine or serum levels of cortisol.

Serum Adrenocorticotropic Hormone. Serum levels of ACTH can be assessed after infusion of synthetic ACTH. Urine levels of ketosteroid would be expected to increase to 25 mg in 24 hours; plasma levels of cortisol should increase to 10 to 40 µg/dl. Urine levels of ketosteroid can be measured with 24-hour urine specimens. *Ketosteroids* are metabolites of the hormones produced by the adrenal cortex. A preservative is required for the collection bottle. If the client has an indwelling catheter, the urinary drainage bag is emptied frequently and the urine is refrigerated. Collection of 24-hour urine specimens is explained in Chapter 4.

Plasma Renin Assays. Plasma levels of renin can be used in the differential diagnosis of primary versus secondary hyperaldosteronism. Clients with primary hyperaldosteronism have too much aldosterone from an adrenal gland problem that causes decreased renin activity. Clients with secondary hyperaldosteronism have a renovascular occlusive disease or a primary renal disease that results in increased levels of plasma renin.

Urinary Catecholamines. Adrenal medullary function can be assessed through urine levels of catecholamines and their metabolites (vanillylmandelic acid). A 24-hour urine sample is collected and assayed. Adrenal medullary secretion can be suppressed by administration of ganglionic blocking agents, which normally decrease the urine levels of catecholamines. In clients with pheochro-

Text continued on p. 1176

TABLE 44-2 *Laboratory Tests for Endocrine and Metabolic Function*

Test	Normal Value*	Description
Endocrine Function Studies		
Tests of Thyroid Function		
Thyroid-stimulating hormone (TSH) assay	2-10 mU/L (SI units)	Used to differentiate primary and secondary (and tertiary) hypothyroidism. TSH increases in primary thyroid disease to increase thyroid function (T_4). Thyroid gland is unable to increase T_4 no matter how significant the stimulation because of disease of organ itself.
Antithyroglobulin antibody (thyroid autoantibody)	Titer <1:100	Measures the presence of antibodies to various thyroid gland components. They may lead to inflammation and destruction of thyroid gland.
Thyroxine index, free (FT_4)	0.8-2.4 ng/dl or 10-31 pmol/L (SI units)	Used to evaluate thyroid function.
Thyroxine (T_4)	*Adult male:* 51-154 nmol/L (SI units); *Adult female:* 64-154 nmol/L (SI units); *Adult >60 yr:* 64-142 nmol/L (SI units)	Used to assess and diagnose thyroid function, and to monitor replacement and suppressive therapy.
Triiodothyronine uptake (T_3 resin uptake)	24%-34% or 24-34 AU (arbitrary units; SI units)	Used to evaluate thyroid function. Measures T_3 that is protein bound.
Thyrotropin-releasing hormone (TRH)	Euthyroid = <10; hyperthyroid <10	Prompt increase in serum TSH level to approximately twice the baseline value in 30 minutes after an IV bolus of TRH.
Tests of Parathyroid Function		
Total serum calcium	9-10.5 mg/dl or 2.25-2.75 mmol/L	Used to evaluate parathyroid function and calcium metabolism and ionized and non-ionized calcium in serum.
Serum phosphorus	3-4.5 mg/dl or 0.97-1.45 mmol/L (SI units)	Assists in interpretation of studies investigating parathyroid and calcium abnormalities.
Serum alkaline phosphatase (ALP)	30-120 units/L or 0.5-2 μKat/L (SI units)	Used to detect and monitor diseases of the liver or bone.
Parathyroid hormone (PTH)	10-65 pg/ml or 10-65 SI units (ng/L)	Used to assist in the evaluation of hypercalcemia or hypocalcemia. It is routinely monitored in clients with chronic renal failure.
Osteocalcin	Adult >22 yr: *Male:* 5.8-14 ng/ml; *Female:* 3.1-14.4 ng/ml	Is a measure of bone turnover used to evaluate clients with diseases that affect bone mineral density and turnover.

Data from Pagana, K.D., & Pagana, T.J. (2002). *Manual of diagnostic and laboratory tests* (2nd ed.). St. Louis: Mosby.
* Normal values may differ significantly between laboratories.
† Trends in elevation are of particular importance in predicting the rapidity with which the liver is failing. If levels increase, decrease, and then increase again, liver failure may be occurring.

Procedure	Interpretation
Client may eat or drink. Obtain 5 ml venous blood	↑: Primary hypothyroidism (thyroid dysfunction) ↓: Secondary hypothyroidism (pituitary disorder); high doses of dopamine or corticosteroids
No fasting required. 3-5 ml of venous blood is obtained and sent to lab.	↑: Thyroiditis, rheumatoid arthritis, pernicious anemia, hypothyroidism, thyroid carcinoma
A venous blood sample is obtained.	↑: Hyperthyroidism ↓: Hypothyroidism
Fasting is not necessary. Instruct client to stop taking exogenous T_4 medication 1 month before testing. Venous blood specimen is collected.	↑: Hyperthyroidism, acute thyroiditis. ↓: Hypothyroidism, pituitary insufficiency, hypothalamic failure, protein malnutrition, iodine insufficiency
No fasting is required. 5-7 ml venous blood is collected.	↑: Hyperthyroidism, hypoproteinemia ↓: Hypothyroidism, hypothyroid states, hepatitis, cirrhosis
Instruct client to stop taking thyroid preparations for 3 to 4 wk before TRH test. No fasting is required. A 500-μg IV bolus of TRH is administered. Venous blood samples are obtained at intervals and TSH levels are measured.	↑: Hyperthyroidism, primary hypothyroidism (thyroid disease), secondary hypothyroidism (pituitary disease)
No fasting is required. 7 ml venous blood is collected and sent to lab.	↑: Hyperparathyroidism, metastatic tumor to bone ↓: Hypoparathyroidism, renal failure, rickets, vitamin D deficiency, osteomalacia
NPO after midnight on day of test. 5-7 ml venous blood is collected and sent to lab.	↑: Hypoparathyroidism, renal failure, hypocalcemia, bone tumors, diabetic acidosis, increased dietary or IV intake of phosphorus ↓: Hyperparathyroidism, chronic antacid ingestion, chronic alcoholism, vitamin D deficiency, and myxedema
Tell client fasting is preferred but not required. 7-10 ml venous blood sent to lab.	↑: Hyperparathyroidism, primary cirrhosis, biliary obstruction, meal high in vitamin D, healing fractures, metastatic tumor to the bone, Paget's disease, rheumatoid arthritis ↓: Hypophosphatemia, malnutrition, pernicious anemia, scurvy
Client is NPO except for water after midnight on day of test. Venous blood is collected at various intervals and sent to lab.	↑: Secondary hyperparathyroidism, non–PTH-producing tumors, congenital renal defect, hypocalcemia, chronic renal failure, malabsorption syndrome, vitamin D deficiency and rickets ↓: Hypoparathyroidism due to surgical ablation or immunoablation, hypercalcemia of malignancy, metastatic bone tumor, sarcoidosis, vitamin D intoxication
3-5 ml venous blood is collected and sent to lab.	↑: Hyperparathyroidism, osteoporosis, Paget's disease, acromegaly, hyperthyroidism ↓: Hypoparathyroidism, steroid therapy

Continued

TABLE 44-2   *Laboratory Tests for Endocrine and Metabolic Function—cont'd*

Test	Normal Value*	Description

Endocrine Function Studies—cont'd
Tests of Adrenocortical Function

Test	Normal Value*	Description
Aldosterone	**Blood:** *Supine:* 3-10 ng/dl or 0.08-0.30 nmol/L (SI units) *Upright (sitting for at least 2 hr):* Female: 5-30 ng/dl or 0.14-0.80 nmol/L (SI units) Male: 6-22 ng/dl or 0.17-0.61 nmol/L (SI units) **Urine:** 2-26 μg/24 hr or 6-72 nmol/24 hr (SI units)	Used to diagnose hyperaldosteronism. To differentiate primary aldosteronism (adrenal gland problem) from secondary aldosteronism (extra-adrenal gland problem), a plasma renin assay must be performed simultaneously. Values may be affected by diet, posture, pregnancy, and diurnal variations.
Cortisol, blood	8 AM: 5-23 μg/dl or 138-635 nmol/L (SI units) 4 PM: 3-13 μg/dl or 83-359 nmol/L (SI units)	Measure of serum cortisol. Performed on clients suspected to have hyperfunctioning or hypofunctioning of adrenal glands. Peak cortisol levels occur around 6-8 AM and lowest levels around midnight.
ACTH, serum	AM: <80 pg/ml or <18 pmol/L (SI units) PM: <50 pg/ml or <11 pmol/L (SI units)	Serum ACTH study tests anterior pituitary gland function for possible causes of either Cushing's syndrome (overproduction of cortisol) or Addison's disease (underproduction of cortisol).
ACTH stimulation	**Rapid test:** cortisol levels increase > 7 mg/dl above baseline **24-hr test:** cortisol levels >40 μg/dl **3-day test:** cortisol levels >40 μg/dl	Evaluates the ability of adrenal gland to respond to ACTH administration. Useful in evaluating the cause of adrenal insufficiency and in evaluating clients with cushingoid manifestations.
Dexamethasone suppression	**Prolonged method:** Expected values— normal *Low dose:* >50% reduction of plasma cortisol and 17-hydroxycorticosteroid (17-OCHS) levels *High dose:* >50% reduction of plasma cortisol and 17-OCHS levels **Rapid method:** *Normal:* nearly zero cortisol levels	Used for diagnosing adrenal hyperfunction (Cushing's syndrome) and distinguishing its cause. Dexamethasone suppresses ACTH secretion. Under normal circumstances, this results in reduced stimulation to adrenal glands and ultimately a decrease of 50% or more in plasma cortisol and 17-OCHS. Physical and emotional stress can alter test results as can barbiturates, estrogens, oral contraceptives, steroids, phenytoin, and tetracyclines.
Renin assay, plasma	**Upright position, sodium-restricted diet:** *Ages 20-30 yr:* 2.9-24 ng/ml/hr; *>40 yr:* 2.9-10.8 ng/ml/hr **Upright position, normal sodium diet:** *Ages 20-30 yr:* 0.1-4.3 ng/ml/hr; *>40 yr:* 0.1-3 ng/ml/hr	Measures renin, an enzyme produced by juxtaglomerular apparatus in response to decreased blood flow to kidneys. Used to evaluate hypertension. Helpful in the differential diagnosis of aldosteronism.

Data from Pagana, K.D., & Pagana, T.J. (2002). *Manual of diagnostic and laboratory tests* (2nd ed.). St. Louis: Mosby.
* Normal values may differ significantly between laboratories.
† Trends in elevation are of particular importance in predicting the rapidity with which the liver is failing. If levels increase, decrease, and then increase again, liver failure may be occurring.

Procedure	Interpretation

Blood: Client to be upright for a minimum of 2 hr before test is drawn. No fasting is necessary. Instruct client to maintain a normal sodium diet (approximately 3 g/day and avoid licorice for at least 2 wk before test. Collect and send 5-10 ml blood on ice to lab.

Urine: Explain to client how to collect a 24-hr urine sample. Note start and stop time. Keep refrigerated.

↑: Primary or secondary hyperaldosteronism, hyponatremia, hyperkalemia, laxative abuse, stress, poor perfusion states, hypovolemia or hemorrhage, pregnancy and oral contraceptives

↓: Addison's disease, steroid therapy, hypernatremia, antihypertensive therapy

Collect 7-10 ml venous blood at 8 AM and another blood sample at 4 PM.

↑: Cushing's disease, stress, syndrome, ectopic adrenocorticotropic hormone (ACTH)-producing tumors, obesity, hyperthyroidism, pregnancy

↓: Addison's disease, adrenal hyperplasia, hypopituitarism, hypothyroidism

Fasting sample. Stress may artificially increase results. Collect 20 ml heparinized venous blood in tube. Place tube in ice water and send to lab.

↑: Cushing's disease caused by bilateral adrenal hyperplasia or ectopic ACTH-producing tumors, stress, Addison's disease (primary adrenal insufficiency, surgical removal of adrenals, adrenal suppression with long-term exogenous steroid supply

↓: Secondary adrenal insufficiency (pituitary insufficiency), hypopituitarism, adrenal adenoma or carcinoma, Cushing's syndrome, exogenous steroid administration

Obtain fasting baseline blood samples for all three types of tests. Give cosyntropin IV. For rapid test: obtain plasma cortisol levels 30-60 min after drug administration. For 24-hr test, obtain cortisol levels 24 hr after drug administration. For 3-day test, obtain cortisol levels at 12, 24, 36, 48, 60, and 72 hr after start of test.

Exaggerated response: Cushing's syndrome, adrenal insufficiency. Normal or below normal response: Cushing's syndrome, adrenal insufficiency

Prolonged method: Obtain 24-hr urine sample for corticosteroids baseline and daily over 6 days. Obtain baseline plasma cortisol levels. On day 3, administer low dose of oral dexamethasone (DS). On day 5, administer high dose of oral DS. Send urine for cortisol and 17-OCHS to lab.

Rapid method: Give 1 mg dexamethasone at 11 PM to suppress ACTH formation. At 8 AM draw blood for plasma cortisol level. If no cortisol suppression occurs after administration of 1 mg of dexamethasone, administer higher dose (8 mg) to suppress ACTH production. Draw blood for cortisol level and send to lab.

Adrenal hyperfunction (Cushing's syndrome) Cushing's disease, ectopic ACTH-producing tumors, adrenal adenoma or carcinoma, bilateral adrenal hyperplasia, mental depression

Instruct client to maintain normal diet with restricted amount of sodium for 3 days before test and discontinue medications such as diuretics, steroids, antihypertensives, vasodilators, oral contraceptives for 2 to 4 wk before test. Obtain venous blood (7-12 ml) with client in upright position.

↑: Addison's disease, essential hypertension, hyperkalemia, cirrhosis, malignant hypertension, salt-losing GI disease

↓: Primary hyperaldosteronism wherein aldosterone inhibits further renin production, steroid therapy, congenital adrenal hyperplasia

Continued

TABLE 44-2	*Laboratory Tests for Endocrine and Metabolic Function—cont'd*	
Test	**Normal Value***	**Description**

Endocrine Function Studies—cont'd
Tests of Adrenocortical Function—cont'd

Cortisol, urine	<100 µg/24 hr or <276 nmol/day (SI units)	Measures urinary cortisol and is performed in clients suspected of hyperfunction or hypofunction of adrenal gland. Stress, activity, certain drugs can affect cortisol levels.
17-OCHS	*Male:* 3-10 mg/24 hr or 8.3-27.6 µmol/day (SI units) *Female:* 2-8 mg/24 hr or 5.2-22.1 µmol/day (SI units)	Urine study measures adrenocortical function by measuring cortisol metabolites (17-OCHS) in a 24-hr urine collection.
17-Ketosteroids	*Male:* 6-20 mg/24 hr or 20-70 µmol/day (SI units) *Female:* 6-17 mg/24 hr or 20-60 µmol/day (SI units)	Measures adrenal cortex function, especially related to androgenic function. Useful for evaluation and monitoring of adrenal hyperplasia and adrenal tumors.

Metabolic Function Studies
Tests of Liver, Biliary, Exocrine Pancreas Function
Tests Specific to Liver and Biliary Function

Bilirubin, serum		Used to evaluate liver function. Is part of the evaluation of adults having hemolytic anemias.
Direct (conjugated)	0.1-0.3 mg/dl or 1.7-5.1 µmol/L (SI units)	
Indirect (unconjugated)	0.2-0.8 mg/dl or 3.4-12 µmol/L (SI units)	
Total	0.3-1 mg/dl or 5.1-17 µmol/L (SI units)	
Urine bilirubin	0-0.02 mg/dl	Bilirubin is excreted into the urine and suggests disease affecting bilirubin metabolism after conjugation or defects in excretion (gallstones).
Urine urobilinogen	Random; 0.3-3.5 mg/dl; 24-hr: 0.05-2.5 mg/24 hr	Bilirubin transformed into urobilinogen by action of bacteria in the bowel. Test is rarely performed.
Fecal urobilinogen	75-275 EU/100 g	Breakdown of direct bilirubin to fecal urobilinogen occurs by action of bacteria in bowel and is excreted in stool. Test is rarely performed.
Cholesterol, serum	<200 mg/dl or <5.20 mmol/L (SI units)	Used to determine the risk for coronary heart disease and for evaluation of hyperlipidemias.

Data from Pagana, K.D., & Pagana, T.J. (2002). *Manual of diagnostic and laboratory tests* (2nd ed.). St. Louis: Mosby.
* Normal values may differ significantly between laboratories.
† Trends in elevation are of particular importance in predicting the rapidity with which the liver is failing. If levels increase, decrease, and then increase again, liver failure may be occurring.

Procedure	Interpretation
Collect 24-hr urine sample and send to lab.	↑: Cushing's disease, stress, Cushing's syndrome, ectopic ACTH-producing tumor, pregnancy, stress, hyperthyroidism, obesity ↓: Adrenal hyperplasia, Addison's disease, hypopituitarism, hypothyroidism
Withhold drugs for several days. Collect 24-hr urine sample and keep cold. Send to lab.	↑: Cushing's disease, ectopic ACTH-producing tumors, stress, Cushing's syndrome, hyperthyroidism, obesity ↓: Adrenal hyperplasia, Addison's disease, hypopituitarism, hypothyroidism
24-hr urine test; keep urine cold; may need preservative. Results may be affected by many drugs.	↑: Congenital adrenal hyperplasia, pregnancy, ACTH administration, ACTH-secreting ectopic tumors, hyperpituitarism, testosterone-secreting or androgenic-secreting tumors of the adrenal glands, ovaries, or testes, Cushing's syndrome ↓: Addison's disease, severe debilitating disease, severe stress or infection, chronic disease, hypogonadism, castration, hypopituitarism
With client NPO except for water, blood is drawn after midnight. Certain drugs may cause increased, decreased, false-positive, or false-negative results. Collect 5-7 ml blood. Protect from light and send to lab.	**Conjugated (direct):** ↑: Gallstones, extrahepatic duct obstruction, extensive liver metastasis, cholestasis from drugs **Unconjugated (indirect):** ↑: Excessive erythrocyte hemolysis: transfusion reaction, sickle cell anemia, hemolytic jaundice, hemolytic anemia, pernicious anemia, hepatitis, cirrhosis, sepsis **Total bilirubin:** measures direct and indirect levels together
10 ml urine collected and sent to lab.	↑: Gallstones, extrahepatic duct obstruction (tumor, inflammation, gallstone, scarring, surgical trauma), extensive liver metastasis, cholestasis from drugs
2- or 24-hr afternoon collection is placed in brown refrigerated bottle with sodium carbonate preservative.	↑: Erythrocyte hemolysis and certain drugs (sulfonamides) and liver, toxic or infectious hepatitis ↓: Biliary obstruction or liver damage
Entire stool specimen is sent to lab.	↑: Erythrocyte hemolysis ↓: Biliary obstruction
Client is to eat normal diet for at least 1 week before test and to fast 12-14 hr after eating a low-fat meal. Only water is permitted and no alcohol within 24 hr before the test. Collect 5-10 ml venous blood and send to lab.	↑: Familial hypercholesterolemia, familial hyperlipidemia, hypothyroidism, uncontrolled diabetes mellitus, biliary cirrhosis, pregnancy, high-cholesterol diet, nephrotic syndrome, stress ↓: Malabsorption, malnutrition, advanced cancer, chronic liver disease, hyperthyroidism, cholesterol-lowering medication, pernicious anemia, hemolytic anemia, sepsis/stress, acute myocardial infarction

Continued

TABLE 44-2 *Laboratory Tests for Endocrine and Metabolic Function—cont'd*		
Test	**Normal Value***	**Description**

Metabolic Function Studies—cont'd
Tests of Liver, Biliary, Exocrine Pancreas Function—cont'd

Liver Enzyme Tests†

Aspartate aminotransferase (AST)	0-35 units/L or 0-0.58 μKat/L (SI units)	Used in evaluation of clients with suspected coronary artery occlusive disease or suspected hepatocellular disease. Serum AST, alanine aminotransferase (ALT), and lactate dehydrogenase (LDH) released from damaged liver, heart, kidney, and muscle cells.
ALT	4-36 international units/L at 37° C or 4-36 units/L (SI units)	Used to identify hepatocellular diseases of liver. Is an accurate monitor of improvement or worsening of these diseases.
LDH and isoenzymes	*LDH:* 100-190 units/L at 37° C or 100-190 units/L (SI units) Isoenzymes: *LDH-1:* 17%-27% *LDH-2:* 27%-37% *LDH-3:* 18%-25% *LDH-4:* 3%-8% *LDH-5:* 0%-5%	An intracellular enzyme used to support the diagnosis of injury or disease involving the heart, liver, red blood cells (RBCs), kidneys, skeletal muscle, brain, and lungs. Isolated elevation of some drugs may cause increased or decreased levels.
ALP and isoenzymes	30-120 units/L or 0.5-2 μKat/L (SI units)	Used to detect and monitor diseases of the liver or bone. ALP found in liver, biliary tract epithelium, and bone.
Gamma-glutamyl transpeptidase	*Male and female >45 yr:* 8-38 units/L or 8-38 international units/L (SI units); *Female <45 yr:* 5-27 units/L or 5-27 international units/L (SI units)	A sensitive indicator of hepatobiliary disease. Also used as an indicator of heavy and chronic alcohol use
5'-Nucleotidase	0-1.6 units at 37° C or 0-1.6 units at 37° C (SI units)	Used to support diagnosis of hepatobiliary obstructive disease. 5'-Nucleotidase is an enzyme specific to liver.
Leucine aminopeptidase (LAP)	*Male:* 80-200 units/ml or 19.2-48 units/L (SI units) *Female:* 75-185 units/ml or 18-44.4 units/L (SI units)	Used to diagnose liver disorders. Aids in the differential diagnosis of clients with high levels of ALP

Protein Metabolism: Liver

Protein electrophoresis, serum		Used to diagnose, evaluate and monitor disease course in clients with impaired protein synthesis or utilization caused by chronic liver dysfunction, cancer, intestinal/renal protein-wasting states, immune disorders, impaired nutrition, and edematous states. Levels of albumin and globulin vary with condition.
Total protein	6.4-8.3 g/dl or 64-83 g/L (SI units)	
Albumin	3.5-5 g/dl or 35-50 g/L (SI units)	
Globulin	2.3-3.4 g/dl	
Alpha₁ globulin	0.1-0.3 g/dl or 1-3 g/L (SI units)	
Alpha₂ globulin	0.6-1 g/dl or 6-10 g/L (SI units)	
Beta globulin	0.7-1.1 g/dl or 7-11 g/L (SI units)	
Gamma globulin	0.5-1.7 g/dl	

Data from Pagana, K.D., & Pagana, T.J. (2002). *Manual of diagnostic and laboratory tests* (2nd ed.). St. Louis: Mosby.

* Normal values may differ significantly between laboratories.

† Trends in elevation are of particular importance in predicting the rapidity with which the liver is failing. If levels increase, decrease, and then increase again, liver failure may be occurring.

Procedure	Interpretation

Blood is drawn without special preparation. Collect venous blood daily for 3 days and then again in 1 wk.

↑: Liver diseases: hepatitis, hepatic cirrhosis, hepatic surgery; acute pancreatitis; heart diseases; skeletal muscle diseases
↓: Acute renal disease, diabetic ketoacidosis, pregnancy, chronic renal dialysis

No fasting required. Collect 7-10 ml blood and send to lab.

↑↑↑ Hepatitis, hepatic necrosis, hepatic ischemia
↑↑ Cirrhosis, cholestasis, hepatic tumor, hepatotoxic drugs, obstructive jaundice, severe burns
↑: Myositis, pancreatitis, myocardial infarction, infectious mononucleosis, shock

No fasting required. Collect 7-10 ml venous blood and send to lab.

Myocardial infarction (LDH-1, LDH-2), pulmonary disease (LDH-2, LDH-3), hepatic disease (LDH-5), RBC disease (LDH-1), skeletal muscle disease and injury (LDH-5), pancreatitis (LDH-4)

Fasting is preferred but not required except for isoenzymes. Collect 7-10 ml blood and send to lab.

↑: Primary cirrhosis, intrahepatic or extrahepatic biliary obstruction, primary or metastatic liver tumor, third trimester normal pregnancy, healing fracture, metastatic tumor to bone, hyperparathyroidism, myocardial infarction
↓: Hypophosphatemia, malnutrition, pernicious anemia, scurvy

An 8-hr fast is required. Collect 7-10 ml venous blood and send to lab.

↑: Liver diseases (hepatitis, cirrhosis, hepatic tumor or metastasis, hepatotoxic drugs, cholestasis, jaundice), pancreatic diseases, myocardial infarction, alcohol ingestion, pancreatic diseases, Epstein-Barr virus

No fasting is required. Collect 7-10 ml venous blood and send to lab.

↑: Bile duct obstruction, cholestasis, hepatitis, cirrhosis, hepatic necrosis, hepatic tumor, hepatotoxic drugs

No fasting is required. Collect 7-10 ml venous blood and send to lab.

↑: Hepatobiliary disease (hepatitis, cirrhosis, hepatic necrosis, hepatic tumor, cholestasis, gallstones)

No fasting is required. Collect 7-10 ml venous blood and send to lab.

↑: Albumin: Dehydration
↓ Albumin: Malnutrition, pregnancy, liver disease, protein-wasting enteropathies, protein-losing nephropathies, overhydration, burns, inflammatory diseases
↑: Alpha$_1$ globulin: Inflammatory diseases
↓: Alpha$_1$ globulin: Juvenile pulmonary emphysema
↑: Alpha$_2$ globulin: Nephrotic syndrome, inflammatory disease

Continued

TABLE 44-2	*Laboratory Tests for Endocrine and Metabolic Function—cont'd*	
Test	**Normal Value***	**Description**

Metabolic Function Studies—cont'd

Tests of Liver, Biliary, Exocrine Pancreas Function—cont'd

Protein Metabolism: Liver—cont'd

Protein electrophoresis, serum—cont'd

Test	Normal Value*	Description
Immunoglobulin (IG) elec- trophoresis		Used to assist in diagnosis and monitoring of therapeutic response in many disease states such as liver disorders.
IgG	565-1765 mg/dl	
IgA	85-385 mg/dl	
IgM	55-375 mg/dl	
IgD	Minimal	
IgE	Minimal	
Prealbumin	15-36 mg/dl or 150-360 mg/L (SI units)	Used to indicate liver function status as well as nutritional status.
Ammonia, plasma	80-110 μg/dl or 47-65 μmol/L (SI units)	Used to support the diagnosis of severe liver diseases and for surveillance of these diseases. Some drugs may increase or decrease blood levels.
Hemostatic Function: Liver Prothrombin time (PT)	11-12.5 seconds; 85%-100%	Used to evaluate the adequacy of the extrinsic system and common pathway in clotting mechanism. Certain drugs may increase or decrease levels.
Platelets	150,000-400,000/mm³ μL (mean = 250,000 μL) or 150-400 × 10⁹/L (SI units)	Monitors the course of disease or therapy. Most platelets exist in the bloodstream. About 25% exist in the liver and spleen.
Metabolism of Foreign Substances Bromsulphalein (BSP) excre- tion	<5% retention in 1 hr	Tests liver function.

Data from Pagana, K.D., & Pagana, T.J. (2002). *Manual of diagnostic and laboratory tests* (2nd ed.). St. Louis: Mosby.

* Normal values may differ significantly between laboratories.

† Trends in elevation are of particular importance in predicting the rapidity with which the liver is failing. If levels increase, decrease, and then increase again, liver failure may be occurring.

Procedure	Interpretation
	↓: Alpha₂ globulin: Hemolysis, Wilson's disease, hyperthyroidism, severe liver dysfunction ↑: Beta globulins: Hypercholesterolemia, iron deficiency anemia ↓: Beta globulin: Malnutrition ↑: Gamma globulin: Cirrhosis, acute and chronic infections, multiple myeloma, chronic inflammatory disease (rheumatoid arthritis, lupus) ↓ Gamma globulin: Immune disorders and deficiencies
No fasting is required. Collect 7-10 ml venous blood and send to lab. Drugs that may cause increased IG levels include isoniazid (INH), phenytoin (Dilantin), oral contraceptives, steroids, and tetanus toxoid and antitoxin.	↑: IgA: Chronic liver diseases, chronic infections ↓: IgA: Hypoproteinemia, drug immunosuppression (steroids, dextran) ↑: IgG: Chronic liver disease, autoimmune diseases, intrauterine devices, multiple myeloma ↓ IgG: Acquired immunodeficiency syndrome (AIDS), hypoproteinemia, agammaglobulinemia, drug immunosuppression, leukemia ↑: IgM: Chronic infections (hepatitis), chronic liver disorders (biliary cirrhosis), acute infections, lupus ↓: IgM: AIDS, agammaglobulinemia, hypoproteinemia, leukemia, multiple myeloma ↑: IgE: Allergy reactions (hay fever, asthma), allergic infections (parasites, aspergillosis) ↓: IgE: Agammaglobulinemia
No fasting is required. Collect venous blood and send to lab. A 24-hr urine collection may be ordered.	↑ Pregnancy, Hodgkin's disease, nephrotic syndrome ↓ Liver damage, malnutrition, burns, inflammation
No fasting is required. Collect 5-7 ml blood and send to lab.	↑: Primary hepatocellular disease, portal hypertension, severe heart failure with congestive hepatomegaly, GI bleeding and obstruction with mild liver disease, hepatic encephalopathy and hepatic coma, genetic metabolic disorder of urea cycle ↓ Essential or malignant hypertension
No fasting is required. Collect 5-7 ml venous blood and send to lab.	↑: (Prolonged PT): Liver disease (cirrhosis, hepatitis), bile duct obstruction, coumarin ingestion, salicylate intoxication, vitamin K deficiency, hereditary factor deficiency, massive blood transfusion.
No fasting is required. Collect 5-7 ml peripheral venous blood and send to lab.	↑: Malignant disorders, polycythemia vera, rheumatoid arthritis, iron-deficiency anemia ↓: Liver disease (cirrhosis, chronic active hepatitis) anemias, leukemias, hemorrhage, lupus
Blood specimen taken after fasting for 12 hr; BSP dye given, blood drawn at intervals. Dye retained with diminished hepatocellular ability to remove it from blood and excrete it.	↑: Hepatocellular disease. Test is infrequently used

Continued

TABLE 44-2	*Laboratory Tests for Endocrine and Metabolic Function—cont'd*	
Test	**Normal Value***	**Description**

Metabolic Function Studies—cont'd

Tests of Liver, Biliary, Exocrine Pancreas Function—cont'd

Antigens and Antibodies: Liver

Anti-DNA antibody	Negative: <70 international units/ml Borderline: 70-200 international units/ml Positive: >200 international units/ml	Generally used to test for systemic lupus erythematosus (SLE) but elevation occurs in chronic hepatitis.
Antimitochondrial antibody (AMA)	No AMAs at titers >1:5	Used to aid in diagnosis of primary biliary cirrhosis.
Antineutrophil cytoplasmic antibody (ANCA)	Negative normal findings	Assists in diagnosis of Wegener's granulomatosis, a regional vasculitis in kidneys, lungs and upper respiratory tract. ANCA found in clients with sclerosing cholangitis.
Antinuclear antibody (ANA and anticytoplasmic antibodies)	Negative titer (1:20)	Used to diagnose systemic lupus erythematosus (SLE) and other autoimmune diseases. Certain drugs may cause false-positive or false-negative results.
Anti-smooth muscle antibody (ASMA)	No ASMAs at titers >1:20	Aids in diagnosis of autoimmune chronic active hepatitis (CAH), which has been referred to as "lupoid" CAH.
Alpha-fetoprotein	<40 ng/ml or <40 mg/L (SI units)	Used as a tumor marker to identify cancers, such as hepatomas.

Tests Specific to Exocrine Pancreatic Function

Serum amylase with isoenzymes	60-120 Somogyi units/dl or 30-220 units/L (SI units)	Used to detect and monitor clinical course of pancreatitis. Frequently ordered when client presents with acute abdominal pain.
Serum lipase	0-160 units/L or 0-160 SI units (values are method dependent)	Used in the evaluation of pancreatic disease.
Urine amylase	Up to 5000 Somogyi units/24 hr, or 6.5-48.1 units/hr	Used to assist in making the diagnosis of pancreatitis, although other nonpancreatic diseases can cause elevated urine amylase levels. Urine amylase levels increase later than blood levels.

Data from Pagana, K.D., & Pagana, T.J. (2002). *Manual of diagnostic and laboratory tests* (2nd ed.). St. Louis: Mosby.
* Normal values may differ significantly between laboratories.
† Trends in elevation are of particular importance in predicting the rapidity with which the liver is failing. If levels increase, decrease, and then increase again, liver failure may be occurring.

mocytoma (a tumor of the adrenal medulla), ganglionic blocking agents have a negligible effect in controlling blood pressure. An older assessment test for pheochromocytoma, which involved blood pressure manipulation, is rarely performed today.

Tests of Pituitary Function

Hormone Assays. Hormonal disorders caused by malfunction of the pituitary gland can lead to a wide va-

riety of clinical manifestations, depending on which hormone is involved. Growth hormone (GH) and ADH are presented as examples of hormones secreted by the anterior (GH) and posterior (ADH) lobes of the pituitary gland. See Chapter 46 for further discussion.

Growth Hormone Levels. GH is secreted in a diurnal pattern, and its level can be assayed. In a determination of basal levels, the blood sample is usually drawn in the morning after the client has had nothing by mouth (*nil*

Procedure	Interpretation
No fasting required. Collect venous blood and send to lab.	↑: Chronic hepatitis, biliary cirrhosis, lupus, autoimmune diseases, rheumatic fever
No fasting is required. Collect 7-10 ml venous blood and send to lab.	↑: Primary biliary cirrhosis, chronic active hepatitis, lupus, syphilis, drug-induced cholestasis, autoimmune hepatitis (scleroderma, SLE), extrahepatic obstruction, acute infectious hepatitis
No fasting is required. Collect blood and send to lab.	↑: Primary sclerosing cholangitis, autoimmune hepatitis, active viral hepatitis, Crohn's disease, ulcerative colitis
No fasting is required. Collect 7-10 ml venous blood and send to lab.	↑: Cirrhosis, chronic hepatitis, SLE, rheumatoid arthritis, dermatomyositis, scleroderma, myasthenia gravis
No fasting is required. Collect 7-10 ml blood and send to lab.	↑: Mononucleosis hepatitis, primary biliary cirrhosis, viral hepatitis, malignancy
No fasting is required. Collect 7-10 ml blood and send to lab.	↑: Primary hepatocellular cancer (hepatoma), liver cell necrosis (cirrhosis, hepatitis)
No fasting is required. Collect 5-7 ml venous blood and send to lab.	↑: Acute pancreatitis, chronic relapsing pancreatitis, penetrating peptic ulcer into pancreas, GI disease, acute cholecystitis, parotiditis, ruptured ectopic pregnancy, renal failure, diabetic ketoacidosis, pulmonary infarction, after endoscopic retrograde pancreatography
NPO except for water 8-12 hr before test. Collect 5-7 ml venous blood and send to lab.	↑: Pancreatic diseases (acute, chronic, and relapsing pancreatitis, pancreatic cancer, pancreatic pseudocyst); biliary diseases (acute cholecystitis, cholangitis, extrahepatic duct obstruction); renal failure; intestinal diseases (bowel obstruction, infarction); salivary gland inflammation or tumor; peptic ulcer disease
No fasting required. Discard initial specimen and collect all urine for 24 hr. Send to lab.	↑: Acute pancreatitis, chronic relapsing pancreatitis, acute cholecystitis, parotiditis (mumps), ruptured ectopic pregnancy, diabetic ketoacidosis, post-endoscopic retrograde pancreatography

per os, NPO) for 8 to 10 hours. Usual levels for males are less than 5 ng/ml; for females, less than 10 ng/ml. GH can be stimulated by administration of (1) levodopa (500 mg, orally), (2) insulin (0.05 to 0.3 unit/kg, intravenously), or (3) bromocriptine (5 mg, orally). After the stimulus, blood is drawn at intervals for up to 120 minutes. GH levels usually peak 60 minutes after stimulation.

Dehydration Tests. ADH is synthesized by the hypothalamus and secreted by the posterior pituitary. Ab-

sence of ADH leads to diabetes insipidus. A dehydration test is used to differentiate the various types of diabetes insipidus (neurohypophyseal, neurogenic, pituitary, cranial, or central)[22] and to aid in the differential diagnosis of polyuria occurring as a result of one of the types of diabetes insipidus. Fluids are withheld long enough to result in stable hourly urinary osmolalities (4 to 18 hours). During this time, the client's vital signs, urine output, and urine specific gravity are assessed hourly. Hypovolemic shock can develop from dehydration. After the third hour of stable urinary osmolality, the client is given vasopressin as 5 units aqueous arginine vasopressin or 1 μg desmopressin by subcutaneous injection or 10 μg desmopressin by nasal spray.[22] A client without diabetes insipidus responds with decreased urine output and increased urine osmolality. A client with diabetes insipidus cannot respond and continues to produce high volumes of dilute urine (low osmolality).

Metabolic Function Studies

Tests of Liver, Biliary, Exocrine Pancreas Function. The most common laboratory tests for metabolic function (liver, biliary, and exocrine pancreas) include those used to measure levels of serum enzymes, including bilirubin, proteins, antigens, antibodies, fats, bleeding and clotting factors, and related urine and stool studies (see Table 44-2). Details on hepatitis virus infection are presented in Chapter 49.

Diagnostic Imaging and Other Studies

Endocrine Function Studies

Tests of Thyroid Structure and Function. The thyroid gland can be assessed for size, shape, position, and function by scanning, ultrasound, magnetic resonance imaging (MRI), computed tomography (CT), radionuclide imaging, fine needle aspiration, and testing the Achilles tendon reflexes (Table 44-3.)

Radioiodine Uptake. The body cannot distinguish between radiolabeled ("tagged") iodine and nonradiolabeled iodine. Consequently, the thyroid takes up radioactive iodine and processes it just as it does regular iodine. The thyroid gland selectively transports radioisotopes of iodine (^{123}I, ^{125}I, ^{131}I) and ^{99m}Tc pertechnetate, allowing thyroid imaging and quantification of radioactive tracer fractional uptake.[15] Radioiodine is excreted in the urine just as is ordinary iodine. A scintillation scanner is used to measure the amount of radioactive iodine present in the thyroid 24 hours after administration of a radioiodine isotope preparation. The laboratory may measure the client's urine output of radioactive iodine after the test.

Many factors can distort findings. Therefore before the procedure, question the client about the following, and inform the physician if the client answers "yes" to any of the following questions:

- Have you taken any iodine-containing medications within the last 30 days?
- Are you taking estrogens? (Estrogen can cause a false elevation.)
- Have you undergone x-ray studies of the gallbladder, ureters, bronchi, fallopian tubes, or heart within the last 10 years?

- Within the last 2 weeks, have you principally eaten seafood? (Seafood is so rich in iodine that ^{131}I uptake can show a falsely low reading.)

Achilles Tendon Reflexes. The Achilles tendon reflex test measures the amplitude and duration of the ankle jerk with a special instrument, which is used to tap the strong tendon at the back of the heel. Clients with hyperthyroidism may demonstrate a more rapid tendon reflex. Clients with an underactive thyroid gland or diabetes mellitus and pregnant women have slower reflexes and prolonged relaxation times. Chapter 69 covers tendon reflex testing.

Tests of Adrenal Structure and Function. The adrenal cortex can be assessed for lesions or disease by CT, MRI, adrenal venogram, and angiography. See Table 44-3.

Tests of Pituitary Structure and Function. The structure of the pituitary gland can be assessed by skull x-ray study, CT, or MRI. Tumors of the pituitary may be visualized with these studies (see Chapter 4).

Metabolic Function Studies

Liver, Gallbladder, Biliary Tract, and Pancreas

Abdominal Ultrasonography. Ultrasonographic examination provides valuable diagnostic information about liver, pancreatic, and biliary tract conditions. The technique is rapid, and little or no preparation is required. Depending on the area to be examined, the client may or may not fast before the procedure. Reassure the client that the test is painless and safe.[17] There are no specific precautions or observations after ultrasonography. See Chapter 4 for a discussion of ultrasonography.

Radiography. Many procedures used to diagnose disorders of the liver, pancreas, and biliary tract involve the use of x-rays. Plain x-ray films of the abdomen may show diaphragm elevation caused by hepatic enlargement or calcification in the abdominal organs. Upper or lower gastrointestinal series using barium contrast medium also provide important information about the accessory organs of digestion (liver, gallbladder, and pancreas). Spot x-ray films are obtained to detect pancreatic and duodenal diseases (tumor at the head of the pancreas or a stricture caused by chronic pancreatitis).

Radiologic studies with iodinated contrast media permit visualization of tubes and vessels. Before any of these procedures are performed, question the client about known hypersensitivity to iodine (see Chapter 4).

Computed Tomography. CT is used to identify and evaluate liver, biliary tract, gallbladder, and pancreatic disorders. It is useful for distinguishing cysts or tumors and differentiating obstructive from nonobstructive jaundice (Figure 44-4). The client is instructed to fast,

Text continued on p. 1184

TABLE 44-3	*Diagnostic Imaging and Other Tests for Endocrine and Metabolic Function*			
Test	**Normal Findings**	**Description**	**Procedure**	**Interpretation**

Endocrine Function Studies
Thyroid Function Studies

Test	Normal Findings	Description	Procedure	Interpretation
Thyroid scan	Normal size, shape, position, and function of thyroid gland. No areas of ↓ or ↑ uptake.	Used to visualize the thyroid gland when thyroid disease or nodule is suspected. Avoid iodine in foods, drugs, or x-ray contrast before thyroid scanning.	No fasting is required. Injection of radioactive isotope ^{131}I to identify thyroid gland. Note allergy to iodine.	Cold nodules: cancer Hot nodules: benign
Thyroid ultrasound	Normal size, shape, and position of the thyroid gland.	Indicates whether a thyroid nodule is a fluid-filled cyst or a solid tumor. Also monitors medical treatment or observation of thyroid nodule.	No fasting or sedation is required. Gel applied to neck, transducer passed over nodule, and photographs obtained of image displayed.	Test may indicate cyst, thyroid adenoma, thyroid carcinoma, goiter.
Magnetic resonance imaging	Normal size, shape, and position of gland.	Indicates presence of soft tissue lesions.	Procedure takes 30-90 minutes. Client must lie still during procedure. Cannot be done in clients with metal implants (pacemakers, infusion pumps, aneurysm clips, inner ear implants, or metal fragments in one or both eyes).	Lesion (benign or malignant) may be present.
Computed tomography	Normal size, shape, and position of gland.	Identifies location and structure of gland.	Client is NPO for 4 hr before procedure. Check client for iodine allergies. May receive contrast dye.	Lesion (benign or malignant) may be present.
Radioactive iodine uptake	None.	Used to determine the metabolic activity of the thyroid gland by measuring the absorption of ^{131}I or ^{125}I in thyroid.	Client is NPO 6-8 hr before test. Client is given PO or IV radioactive iodine. 24-hr urine collection begins after oral tracer dose is given. Uptake by the thyroid gland is measured with a scanner at 2-4 hr and 24-hour intervals.	↑: Hyperthyroidism, thyroiditis, liver cirrhosis; urine: hypothyroidism ↓: Hypothyroidism; urine: hyperthyroidism Drugs that may elevate results: barbiturates, estrogen, lithium, phenothiazines. Seafood may elevate results. Drugs that may decrease results: Lugol's solution, saturated solution of potassium iodide (SSKI), antithyroid, antihistamines.

Data from Pagana, K.D., & Pagana, T.J. (2002). *Manual of diagnostic and laboratory tests* (2nd ed.). St. Louis: Mosby; and Greenberger, N.J. & Paumgartner, G. (2001). Diseases of the gallbladder and bile ducts. In E. Baunwald, A. Fauci, D. Kaspar, et al. (Eds.). *Harrison's principles of internal medicine (15th ed, pp. 1776-1788).* New York: McGraw-Hill.

Continued

TABLE 44-3	*Diagnostic Imaging and Other Tests for Endocrine and Metabolic Function—cont'd*			
Test	**Normal Findings**	**Description**	**Procedure**	**Interpretation**

Endocrine Function Studies—cont'd
Thyroid Function Studies—cont'd

Test	Normal Findings	Description	Procedure	Interpretation
Fine needle aspiration	Normal cell configuration.	Used to provide cells for histologic studies; usually used as thyroid biopsy.	Relatively pain-free procedure. Needle used to aspirate fluid from thyroid gland.	Lesion (benign or malignant) may be present.
Achilles tendon reflexes	Normal response to tapping on the tendon.	Used to measure amplitude and duration of ankle jerk.	Tendon is struck with special instrument.	Rapid tendon reflex with hyperthyroidism. Slower tendon reflex with underactive thyroid gland or diabetes mellitus and pregnancy.

Adrenal Gland Function Studies

Test	Normal Findings	Description	Procedure	Interpretation
Computed tomography	No tumors or neoplastic disease.	Used in evaluating adrenals, guiding needles during biopsy of tumor or aspiration of fluid, and monitoring abdominal disease.	Client is NPO for 4 hr before test if contrast dye is given. Note allergy to iodine. Contrast dye may be injected and abdomen is scanned.	May depict an adenoma, cancer, pheochromocytoma, hemorrhage, myelolipoma, hyperplasia.
Magnetic resonance imaging (MRI)	No evidence of disease.	Used for evaluation or diagnosis of lesions or disease.	Procedure takes 30-90 min. Client must lie still during procedure. Test cannot be done in clients with metal implants (pacemakers, infusion pumps, aneurysm clips, inner ear implants, or metal fragments in one or both eyes).	May depict a tumor, cyst, or abscess.
Adrenal venogram	Normal adrenal veins and normal adrenal vein hormone assay.	Performed to obtain blood samples from adrenal veins and to detect adrenal disease. Adrenal disease can be localized in preparation of proposed surgical treatment.	Fasting is required. Note allergy to iodine. Contrast dye is injected to visualize adrenal veins. Blood is obtained and sent to lab for assays.	Disease is limited to one or both sides of adrenal gland: Unilateral adrenal tumor, unilateral pheochromocytoma, bilateral adrenal hyperplasia, bilateral pheochromocytoma, extra-adrenal pheochromocytoma.
Arteriography (angiography)	Normal arterial vasculature.	Used to evaluate arterial occlusive disease of adrenal organs and is helpful in evaluation of suspected neoplasms from these organs.	Client is NPO for 2-8 hr before test. Note allergy to iodine. Contrast dye is injected through catheter inserted in femoral artery; x-ray studies are obtained.	Pheochromocytoma, adrenal adenoma, adrenal carcinoma, bilateral adrenal hyperplasia.

Data from Pagana, K.D., & Pagana, T.J. (2002). *Manual of diagnostic and laboratory tests* (2nd ed.). St. Louis: Mosby; and Greenberger, N.J. & Paumgartner, G. (2001). Diseases of the gallbladder and bile ducts. In E. Baunwald, A. Fauci, D. Kaspar, et al, (Eds.). *Harrison's principles of internal medicine (15th ed, pp. 1776-1788).* New York: McGraw-Hill.

Test	Normal Findings	Description	Procedure	Interpretation
Metabolic Function Studies				
Liver, Biliary, Exocrine Pancreas Function Studies				
Tests for Liver, Gallbladder, Biliary Tract, and Pancreas				
Abdominal ultrasound	Normal liver, gallbladder, bile ducts, pancreas.	Used to visualize abdomen and organs within it.	Fasting may or may not be required. Transducer is passed over skin of organ. Test takes about 20 min.	Tumors, abscesses, cysts, gallstones in bile ducts, polyps in gallbladder, or inflammation in pancreas may be present.
Plain x-ray films	Normal size, shape, and position of organs.	May indicate a disorder of liver, gallbladder, biliary tract, or pancreas.	No fasting is required. X-ray machine is directed to organ being studied.	Tumors or diseases of organs. Hepatic enlargement or calcification in the abdominal organs.
Computed tomography (CT)	No evidence of abnormality.	Used in evaluating abdominal organs such as the liver, gallbladder, biliary tract, or pancreas and as a guide during biopsy of tumor and aspiration of fluid. With MRI, CT has replaced the liver scan in diagnosis.	Client is NPO 4 hr before test if contrast dye is given. Note allergy to iodine. Abdomen is scanned.	Liver: Tumor, abscess, bile duct dilation. Pancreas: Tumor pseudocyst, inflammation, bleeding. Gallbladder/biliary system: Gallstones, tumor, bile duct dilation.
Arteriography (angiography)	Normal arterial vasculature.	Used to evaluate arterial occlusive disease of hepatic, biliary, and pancreatic arterial vessels after administration of contrast medium. Is helpful in evaluation of suspected neoplasms arising from these organs.	Client is NPO 2-8 hr before test. Note allergy to contrast dye. Dye is injected through catheter inserted into femoral artery; x-ray films are obtained.	Abnormalities of vascular structure and function in pancreas, liver, biliary tract, and gallbladder and bleeding sites in pancreas and portal system.
Tests Specific to the Liver				
Peritoneoscopy	Normal-appearing organs.	Used to directly visualize the liver and peritoneum. Is particularly helpful in diagnosing tumors and cysts.	Client is NPO after midnight. 3-4 L of CO_2 are used to fill the peritoneal cavity to separate abdominal wall from the intra-abdominal viscera. After procedure, client may have shoulder or subcostal discomfort from pneumoperitoneum for 24 hr.	Liver tumor or cyst, abscess or infection, ascites.
Biopsy	Normal liver histology.	Used to diagnose pathologic liver conditions.	Client is NPO after midnight on day of test. After careful positioning on side, small piece of liver tissue is removed to examine under microscope. Assess client frequently for signs of hemorrhage.	Benign or malignant tumor, abscess, cyst, hepatitis.

Continued

TABLE 44-3	Diagnostic Imaging and Other Tests for Endocrine and Metabolic Function—cont'd			
Test	**Normal Findings**	**Description**	**Procedure**	**Interpretation**

Metabolic Function Studies—cont'd

Liver, Biliary, Exocrine Pancreas Function Studies—cont'd

Tests Specific to the Liver—cont'd

Test	Normal Findings	Description	Procedure	Interpretation
CT portogram	No evidence of liver abnormalities.	Provides accurate picture of liver. Is used when small tumors (usually metastases) are suspected. May be helpful to surgeon contemplating liver resection.	Client is NPO 2 to 4 hr before test. Note allergy to iodine. Contrast dye is injected through catheter positioned in splenic artery, using CT and scans.	Hepatic tumor, hepatic cyst, hepatic hemangioma.
Gallium scan	Diffuse, low level of gallium uptake, especially in the liver and spleen. No increased gallium uptake within the body.	Used where white blood cells tend to congregate; to stage gallium-avid tumors (tumors that attract high concentrations of gallium), locate areas of inflammation or infection in cases of fever of unknown origin, and monitor response to treatment of infection, inflammation, or tumor.	Give cathartic or enema. Inject gallium. Obtain total body scans at intervals.	Tumor, noninfectious inflammation (rheumatoid arthritis, sarcoidosis), infection, abscess.
Magnetic resonance imaging (MRI)	No evidence of disease.	Indications for MRI change constantly as new uses for MRI are discovered. Shows promise in evaluation of liver (and other body structures).	Client must remove all metal objects. Client must remain motionless during procedure. There are no food or fluid restrictions before test. Contrast media may be used.	Tumor.

Tests Specific to Biliary, Gallbladder, and Pancreas

Test	Normal Findings	Description	Procedure	Interpretation
Percutaneous transhepatic cholangiography	Normal gallbladder and biliary ducts.	Allows visualization of bile ducts and sometimes pancreatic ducts. Clients with jaundice can be assessed for tumors, gallstones and other diseases.	Client is NPO after midnight on day of test. Note allergy to iodine. Dye is injected into liver and x-ray films are obtained.	Tumors, strictures, or gallstones of hepatic or common bile duct; sclerosing cholangitis; biliary sclerosis; cysts of common bile duct; tumors, strictures, inflammation or cysts of pancreatic duct, anatomic biliary or pancreatic duct variations.

Data from Pagana, K.D., & Pagana, T.J. (2002). *Manual of diagnostic and laboratory tests* (2nd ed.). St. Louis: Mosby; and Greenberger, N.J. & Paumgartner, G. (2001). Diseases of the gallbladder and bile ducts. In E. Baunwald, A. Fauci, D. Kaspar, et al, (Eds.). *Harrison's principles of internal medicine* (15th ed, pp. 1776-1788). New York: McGraw-Hill.

Metabolic Function Studies—cont'd
Liver, Biliary, Exocrine Pancreas Function Studies—cont'd

Tests Specific to Biliary, Gallbladder, and Pancreas—cont'd

Test	Normal Findings	Description	Procedure	Interpretation
Endoscopic retrograde cholangio-pancreatog-raphy (ERCP)	Normal size of biliary and pancreatic ducts; no obstruction or filling defects within biliary or pancreatic ducts	Used in evaluation of jaundiced client and with unexplained upper abdominal pain or pancreatitis.	Client is NPO after midnight on day of test. Administer Versed if ordered. Fiberoptic tube is inserted into duodenum. Dye is injected and x-ray films are obtained.	Tumor, strictures, or gallstones of common bile duct; sclerosing cholangitis; biliary sclerosis; cysts of common bile duct; tumor, cysts, strictures, or inflammation of pancreatic duct; anatomic biliary or pancreatic duct variations; cancer of duodenum or ampulla.
Oral cholecysto-gram (gallbladder series)	Good visualization of gallbladder. No filling defects. No stones.	Used to evaluate the gallbladder in clients with chronic right upper quadrant abdominal pain, dyspepsia, heartburn, or fatty food intolerance.	Client eats a low-fat or fat-free meal on the evening before testing. Assess for iodine dye allergy. Administer six iopanoic acid tablets at 5-min intervals. Client is NPO except for water until after test is completed.	Stones, gallbladder polyps, chronic cholecystitis, cholesterolosis, gallbladder cancer, cystic duct obstruction.
Gallbladder nuclear scanning (cholescin-tigraphy, diisopropyl-iminodia-cetic acid [DISIDA] scanning, hepato-iminodia-cetic acid [HIDA] scanning, IDA gallbladder scanning)	Gallbladder, common bile duct, and duodenum visualization within 60 min after radionuclide injection.	Valuable in evaluating clients for suspected gallbladder disease and extrahepatic biliary obstruction. Confirms patency of (or lack of) common bile duct and cystic duct.	Fasting is preferred for at least 2 hr. IV ^{99m}Tc-labeled IDAs (DISIDA, HIDA) are administered; right upper abdomen is scanned. Serial images are obtained over 1 hr and recorded on film. Ejection fraction can be determined to evaluate emptying of the gallbladder by administering a fatty meal or cholecystokinin and then scanning the gallbladder to measure the percentage of isotope ejected.	Acute cholecystitis present when no visualization of gallbladder occurs because a gallstone is blocking the cystic duct, but the rest of the biliary tree is visualized; chronic cholecystitis; acalculous cholecystitis; cystic duct syndrome if gallbladder ejection fraction is below 35%; common bile duct obstruction secondary to gallstones, tumor, or stricture.
Magnetic resonance cholangio-pancreatog-raphy	Patent pancreatic and biliary ducts.	Used to identify pancreatic duct dilation or stricture, pancreatic duct stenosis, and pancreatic divisum. Has excellent sensitivity for bile duct dilation, biliary stricture and intraductal abnormalities. Is an alternative to ERCP when ERCP is not feasible or available.	Procedure takes 30-90 min. Client must lie still during the procedure. Test cannot be done in clients with metal implants (pacemakers, infusion pumps, aneurysm clips, inner ear implants, or metal fragments in one or both eyes).	May depict a blockage of pancreatic or biliary ducts from a stone, tumor, cyst, or abscess.

FIGURE 44-4 Computed tomographic scan of chronic pancreatitis. Pancreatic atrophy and a dilated pancreatic duct *(arrow)* are present, but there is no evidence of pancreatic calcification. (From Moss, A.A., et al. [1983]. *Computed tomography of the body.* Philadelphia: W.B. Saunders.)

except for having water, before the test. See Chapter 4 for a more detailed discussion of CT.

Angiography. Angiography allows visualization of the hepatic, biliary, and pancreatic arterial vessels after administration of contrast medium. It is used to identify abnormalities of vascular structure and function, observe masses, and note bleeding sites in the pancreas, spleen, and portal system. To inject the contrast medium, the examiner usually introduces a needle into the femoral artery. Next, the needle is exchanged for a catheter, which is then passed into the celiac artery or one of its branches (superior mesenteric or hepatic). After contrast medium injection, rapid sequence filming is done. See Chapter 4 for additional details.

Preprocedure Care

Explain the purpose of the examination to the client. The client usually takes nothing by mouth for 2 to 8 hours before the test. Ask about use of any medications that might lead to bleeding, such as anticoagulants or nonsteroidal anti-inflammatory drugs (NSAIDs). These medications should be stopped up to a week before the test. Also, ask whether the client is allergic to iodine. The contrast dye contains iodine. Bleeding or clotting tests are usually ordered before the test. Remind the client that it is necessary to lie still during the examination. Explain that there may be a sensation of pressure while the catheter is introduced. Assess the pulses distal to the insertion site for comparison with pulses afterward.

Postprocedure Care

After angiography, assess the needle insertion site for manifestations of bleeding. Clients with liver conditions often have concurrent clotting disorders, which may lead to a hematoma. Assess the pulses below the level of catheter insertion and compare with the preprocedure baseline findings.

Radionuclide Imaging. Radionuclide imaging with technetium 99m dimethylacetanilide (hepato-iminodiacetic acid [HIDA], diethyl-iminodiacetic acid [DIDA], and diisopropyl-iminodiacetic acid [DISIDA]) involves intravenous infusion of gamma-emitting isotopes. After infusion, a scintillation detector is passed over the abdomen. This procedure is used to investigate biliary obstruction and indicates whether a tumor or abscess is present in the liver, gallbladder, or pancreas. Useful isotopes include colloidal gold (^{198}Au), gallium (^{67}Ga), technetium (^{99}Tc), and selenium (^{75}Se). ^{67}Ga accumulates in inflamed tissue. ^{99}Tc is used to evaluate liver, gallbladder, and biliary tract function. ^{75}Se is useful for identifying pancreatic abnormalities.

Tests of Specific Metabolic Organ Functions
Liver

Peritoneoscopy. Insertion of a peritoneoscope through an abdominal stab wound permits direct visualization of the liver and peritoneum. Visualization of structural changes aids in the diagnosis of cirrhosis and cancer. During peritoneoscopy, the examiner may take photographs and perform a biopsy. Peritoneoscopy is relatively safe and simple.

Contraindications include infections of the abdominal cavity, clotting disorders, or intestinal obstruction. In addition, the client must be able to cooperate throughout the procedure. Obesity and ascites interfere with test results.

Preprocedure Care

Do the following to prepare a client for peritoneoscopy:
- Check that written consent has been obtained.
- Check the laboratory record to make certain the client has normal or adequate clotting factors. If not, inform the physician.
- Check the client and health care record for contraindications to preprocedural medications.
- Inquire whether the client is sensitive to local anesthetics.
- Prepare the skin, and administer preprocedural medication when appropriate.
- Instruct the client to take nothing by mouth and to empty the bowel and bladder just before the procedure begins.
- Provide adequate teaching before and during the actual procedure.

- Explain to the client that it may be difficult to breathe when air is placed in the abdominal cavity.
- Instruct the client to elevate the abdominal wall by holding the breath to protect major organs during needle insertion.

Postprocedure Care

When peritoneoscopy includes liver biopsy, bed rest for 24 hours follows the procedure (see discussion of liver biopsy in the next section). If biopsy is not performed, the client resumes activity after recovery from the effects of the medication. Complications are uncommon and are more often related to biopsy. Possible complications after peritoneoscopy are pneumothorax, subcutaneous emphysema, air embolism, bile peritonitis, perforation of a hollow organ, and shoulder or abdominal pain.

Portal Pressure Measurements. Measurements of portal pressure and flow help to (1) diagnose portal hypertension, (2) indicate the severity of portal hypertension, and (3) guide decisions about appropriate intervention, which may include surgery. Also, the indirect calculation of sinusoid pressure helps determine the location of an obstruction in the liver and thus identify the underlying disorder. Normal portal pressure is 5 to 10 mm Hg. Portal hypertension is present when the wedged venous pressure is more than 5 mm Hg higher than the inferior vena cava pressure.[6]

The following are major portal pressure measurements:
- *Wedged hepatic venous pressure.* The portal pressure is obtained indirectly by percutaneous hepatic vein catheterization. The examiner uses either an arm vein or a femoral vein.
- *Umbilical vein catheterization.* This procedure allows direct measurement of portal pressure.
- *Splenic pulp manometry.* During manometry, the examiner places a needle between two of the lower ribs and inserts a manometer into the spleen. Instruct the client to hold his or her breath during needle insertion and passage.

Preprocedure Care

Portal pressure measurements are minor surgical procedures that are performed in the operating room or a special studies laboratory. In many instances, the surgeon may concurrently inject a contrast agent. These measures require standard preoperative and postoperative care (see Chapter 16).

Postprocedure Care

Observe for bleeding or pneumothorax. Assess the incision site for hematoma formation. Other nursing care is the same as for the client after liver biopsy.

Biopsy. Biopsy is the single most valuable diagnostic study because it is often the determining factor for the final diagnosis. It involves removal of a sample of living tissue for analysis. Biopsies may be open or closed procedures.

An *open biopsy* necessitates a general anesthetic and a major abdominal incision. A client may have an open biopsy at the time of a concurrent operative procedure. An advantage of the open biopsy is that the surgeon can observe the entire liver, identify grossly altered tissue, and remove the biopsy specimen for study.

A *closed biopsy,* or percutaneous liver biopsy, is performed to aspirate a core of tissue via needle for histologic study. The biopsy is usually a "blind" procedure (Menghini's technique) performed under local anesthesia using a transpleural or subcostal approach. The primary limitation of Menghini's technique is that the surgeon cannot see where the needle is going. Needle biopsy of the liver is indicated for unexplained hepatomegaly, hepatosplenomegaly, cholestasis (stoppage of bile secretion), persistently abnormal liver function tests, or suspected primary or metastatic liver tumor.

Contraindications to percutaneous liver biopsy are severe thrombocytopenia, local infection of the lung base, prolonged prothrombin time, peritonitis, massive ascites, an uncooperative client, and extrahepatic obstructive jaundice, especially with an enlarged gallbladder. The client with cancer or amyloidosis is at increased risk for postprocedure hemorrhage. If the client is unable to remain still and cooperative during the procedure, the surgeon can accidentally puncture another organ.

Procedure

The liver biopsy procedure may be performed at the bedside, in a procedure room, or in a gastrointestinal unit using a local anesthetic. Sedation and analgesia, such as with diazepam or midazolam, may be given to help allay the client's fears and make the client more comfortable. Place the client either in the supine or left lateral position with the right arm elevated. Less frequently, you may ask the client to assume a prone position. During insertion of the needle, instruct the client to exhale and then to hold his or her breath on expiration for 5 to 10 seconds to avoid puncture of the diaphragm (Figure 44-5).

When the purpose of liver biopsy is to assess a focal lesion or abnormality, the blind procedure has definite limitations. The chance of inserting the needle into the wrong part of the liver and missing the lesion is great. With the use of concurrent ultrasonography, however, the physician can view the entire procedure and thus guide the needle. Guided biopsy allows better localization of a focal lesion or abnormality.

Fine-needle aspiration biopsy, often performed when a questionable area of the liver is localized, helps to confirm malignancy. This approach is ideal when only a few

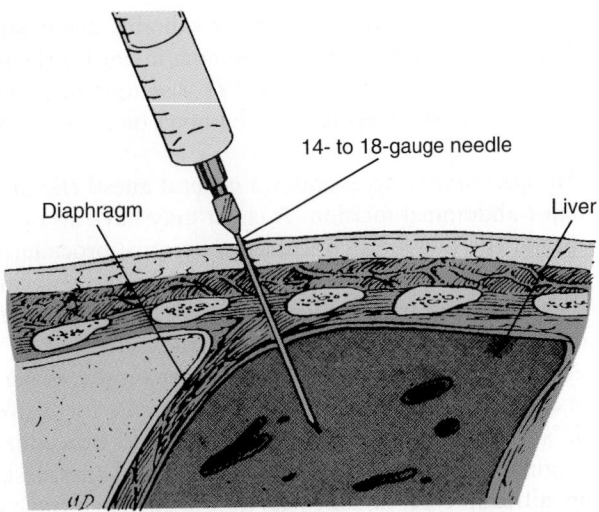

FIGURE 44-5 Percutaneous liver biopsy requires cooperation. The client must be able to lie quietly and hold his or her breath after exhaling while the biopsy needle is inserted. The insertion site is selected after careful percussion of the diaphragmatic excursion during inspiration and expiration.

cells are necessary for cytologic study. The risks of fine-needle aspiration biopsy are far less than those of a guided regular biopsy because the tissue sample is much smaller. This procedure greatly reduces risk of tumor metastasis along the needle track.

There are few contraindications to the guided regular or fine-needle aspiration biopsy procedures. Clients with impaired coagulation associated with liver disease, however, may not be appropriate candidates for the closed procedure. When biopsy is indicated for these clients, a "plugged" biopsy procedure minimizes the risk of hemorrhage. This procedure allows injection of absorbable gelatin material on withdrawal of the biopsy needle. The gelatin material applies pressure to the bleeding site and closes the potential track. The client must be able to hold his or her breath for up to 15 seconds.

Preprocedure Care

At least 2 weeks before a liver biopsy, the client must refrain from ingesting aspirin, NSAIDs, including celecoxib and rofecoxib, or anticoagulants. In addition, blood clotting tests (prothrombin time, bleeding time, partial thromboplastin time, platelet count, and hematocrit) are done beforehand.

Before the procedure is begun, the client fasts for at least 6 hours. Check the client's chart for the coagulation profile results; also check that the client has signed a consent form. Explain the procedure, including its purpose, insertion of an intravenous line during the procedure, and positioning during and after the procedure. When a client is informed about the procedure, the recovery period is smoother and less anxiety-producing

than when no information is given. Emotional support is important to decrease apprehension and to help the client feel more in control.

Postprocedure Care

After percutaneous liver biopsy, perform the following nursing assessments and interventions:

- Monitor vital signs every 15 minutes for 2 hours, every 30 minutes for 2 hours, and every 60 minutes for 4 hours.
- Assess for tachycardia and decreasing blood pressure, which may indicate hemorrhage.
- Check the puncture site by monitoring the dressing, palpating the surrounding area for crepitus, and observing for hematoma formation.
- Observe for pain in the right upper quadrant of the abdomen caused by a subcapsular accumulation of blood or bile or at the right shoulder as a result of blood on the undersurface of the diaphragm.
- Beginning 2 hours after the procedure, elevate the head of the bed 30 degrees. Two hours later, elevate it to 45 degrees. Maintain the client with bed rest for 24 hours after the procedure. Lying on the right side for the first 1 to 2 hours decreases the risk of hemorrhage and bile leakage.
- Administer postprocedure medications on an individual basis, depending on the client's physical status.
- Give vitamin K if prescribed.
- Assess respiratory status for manifestations of dyspnea.

Inherent risks of the biopsy procedure include hemorrhage and puncture of adjacent organs or structures. Hemorrhage during the first 24 hours after the procedure is the most serious complication and may result from penetration of the arterial tree or a distended vein radicle. The risk of hemorrhage increases if vascular channels are distended or if the client breathes during needle insertion into the liver. Puncture of a lung can cause pneumothorax.

A large (14- to 18-gauge) biopsy needle can penetrate a dilated intrahepatic duct if obstructive jaundice is present. Bile leakage and resultant peritonitis can develop. Bile peritonitis is treated with surgical decompression. Cross-contamination may occur after puncture of an adjacent organ. Clients with potentially effusive conditions (ascites, chronic lung disease) in addition to liver abnormality are at great risk for cross-contamination.

Other Tests. Additional tests specific to the liver include CT portogram and gallium scan (see Table 44-3).

Gallbladder, Biliary Tract, and Pancreas
Oral Cholecystography (Gallbladder Series). Cholecystography is an x-ray test for gallbladder or cystic duct disease. Oral cholecystography (OCG) has been the standard examination for gallstones for almost 50 years

but has been largely replaced by ultrasonography. Oral cholecystography is still useful for selecting clients for noninvasive treatment of gallstone disease, such as by lithotripsy or bile acid dissolution therapy. Oral cholecystography is useful in accurate identification of gallstones (90% to 95%)[10] and in assessing the patency of the cystic duct and gallbladder emptying function.

Procedure

During the test, radiography permits visualization of the gallbladder. When contraction of the gallbladder is desirable, the client consumes a high-fat meal during the procedure. After oral cholecystography, some people experience burning on urination because of the presence of the dye in the urine. Forcing fluids decreases this problem.

Poor or no visualization of the gallbladder indicates gallbladder disease, presumably because biliary obstruction prevents passage of the dye. Occasionally, stones can be visualized as shadows within the opaque medium. The test results are accurate only when gastrointestinal and liver function allows absorption and conjugation of the dye.

Preprocedure Care

The evening before the examination, the client ingests a radiopaque dye according to the fat content of the evening meal. The client who has a regular or low-fat dinner may receive ipodate sodium. After a high-fat dinner, the client must be given iopanoic acid. These dyes contain iodine. Observe the client for allergic reactions even when the health history reveals no known allergies to iodine. Possible hypersensitive reactions include nausea and vomiting, diarrhea, abdominal pain, rash, and anaphylaxis. If diarrhea develops, the radiopaque dye may not be absorbed, resulting in nonvisualization of the gallbladder.

Conjugation of the dye occurs in the liver. Be aware that these dyes are potentially toxic to the liver and kidneys, especially in clients with pre-existing hepatic or renal failure. After excretion of the opaque medium into the bile, the gallbladder concentrates the contrast medium.

Postprocedure Care

The client can eat after the examination. There is no other specific postprocedure care.

Cholangiography. Cholangiography or cholangiopancreatography allows visualization of the bile ducts. After administration of an organic iodine dye (iodipamide meglumine), x-ray filming begins. There are four types of cholangiography:

- *Intravenous cholangiography* is used for common bile duct visualization. The radiopaque dye burns intensely upon injection.
- *Percutaneous transhepatic cholangiography* involves injecting the dye directly into the ductal system through the skin via a long, slender needle.
- *Endoscopic retrograde cholangiopancreatography (ERCP).* After a local anesthetic solution is sprayed on the back of the throat, a fiberoptic endoscope is passed through the mouth to the papilla of Vater in the duodenum. The examiner passes a catheter into the common bile duct and, possibly, the pancreatic duct that allows injection of contrast material into pancreatic and biliary systems. The biliary tract and the pancreatic duct are observed for possible strictures, stones, cysts, or tumors.
- *T-tube cholangiography* involves injecting dye into a pre-existing bile drainage tube.

In all four types of cholangiography, failure of the opaque dye to pass through the bile ducts provides evidence of duct obstruction.

Preprocedure Care

Explain the procedure to the client and significant others. Check that written consent has been obtained. Ask whether the client has had a history of allergies to iodine or contrast dye. If so, inform the physician. Explain that there may be a flushing sensation when the contrast medium is injected. Food and fluids may be restricted for 8 hours.

Obtain baseline vital signs. Administer sedatives as prescribed.

Postprocedure Care

Check vital signs as ordered by the physician. A rising temperature may indicate an infection. Monitor skin color for signs of jaundice, which may indicate a disease process or the result of injury. Monitor the client for an allergic reaction for 24 hours after the procedure. Warn the client that there may be some discomfort with urination while the dye is excreted. Also, to prevent renal damage, instruct the client to drink ample amounts of fluid after administration of the dye. If the client is unable to take adequate fluids orally, intravenous hydration with or without mannitol is frequently used.

Analysis of Duodenal or Biliary Drainage. Duodenal and biliary drainage analysis assists in the diagnosis of cholelithiasis when the cholecystogram is inconclusive. Also, these procedures provide an alternative for clients allergic to iodine who cannot undergo cholecystography or cholangiography.

To prepare for the test, instruct the client to fast for 8 hours before the study. A single-lumen nasogastric tube is inserted into the stomach. The stomach contents are aspirated and the tube is slowly advanced until the aspirate changes to clear, golden, and alkaline. At this point, the tube is in the duodenum and clear golden bile ("A bile") is collected.

Next, the flow of bile into the duodenum is increased. Instillation of magnesium sulfate into the tube or intravenous administration of secretin (sometimes followed by pancreozymin) stimulates bile flow. After these bile flow stimulants are administered, it should be possible to aspirate 30 to 60 ml of concentrated bile ("B bile") from the duodenum. Bile can also be collected through an endoscope.

Collected fluid is sent to the laboratory to be analyzed for volume and bicarbonate, enzyme, and bile content. Disproportions in the bile and pancreatic juice fractions indicate obstruction in the bile or pancreatic duct. The presence of cholesterol crystals indicates lithiasis.

Other Metabolic Function Tests

Paracentesis. Paracentesis (peritoneal tap) is used to (1) extract fluid accumulations in the peritoneum (ascites), (2) relieve intra-abdominal tension, which can impair the client's respiratory status, or (3) obtain fluid for culture. After cleaning of the skin and infiltration with a local anesthetic, the physician, using sterile technique, inserts a long aspirating needle with a syringe to collect a fluid specimen. To drain ascitic fluid (if desired), the physician aseptically inserts a trocar through a small stab wound below the umbilicus. This procedure allows fluid (usually several liters) to drain slowly through a catheter into a collection bottle.

Preprocedure Care

The procedure usually takes place at the bedside. Obtain written permission before the procedure begins and explain the purpose and steps involved. Ask the client to void immediately before the procedure to decrease the risk of bladder puncture. Have the client sit upright on the edge of the bed with the feet resting on a stool and the back well supported.

Postprocedure Care

The major complication of paracentesis is *hypovolemia* and shock secondary to fluid drainage from the peritoneum, the resulting fluid shift from intravascular to interstitial space, and the sudden change in intra-abdominal pressure on the vessels. This fluid shift is exacerbated by hypoalbuminemia.

Assess vital signs and peripheral circulation every few minutes during and immediately after paracentesis. Observe for hypovolemic shock: pallor, tachycardia, decreased blood pressure, oliguria, and dyspnea.

Hepatic encephalopathy, caused by reduced tissue perfusion, is another complication resulting from drainage of ascitic fluid. Because ascitic fluid contains a high concentration of protein, the physician may pre-scribe albumin infusions for 24 hours after paracentesis to compensate for protein losses. Potassium depletion may also occur after multiple paracentesis procedures. Infection, peritonitis, and bleeding related to vessel trauma occasionally complicate paracentesis.

Carefully assess for abdominal pain after paracentesis. In addition, monitor the puncture site for persistent leakage of ascitic drainage.

CONCLUSIONS

Once you have gained a thorough knowledge of the structure and function of the endocrine and metabolic organs, you must examine the diagnostic assessment of these organs. Systematic assessment of the client with possible disorders of the endocrine and metabolic organs can lead to prompt diagnosis and treatment. You can facilitate the diagnostic process by adequately preparing the client for diagnostic procedures and by assisting with or collecting assessment data.

BIBLIOGRAPHY

1. Barkauskas, V.H. (2002). Abdomen. In V.H. Barkauskas, L.C. Baumen, & C.S. Fisher (Eds.). *Health and physical assessment* (3rd ed., pp. 384-414). St. Louis: Mosby.
2. Bickley, L.S., & Szilagyi, P.G. (2003). *Physical assessment and history taking* (8th ed.). Philadelphia: Lippincott Williams & Wilkins.
3. Conwell, D.L. (2001). Diseases of the pancreas. In T.E. Andreoli, et al. (Eds.). *Cecil essentials of medicine* (5th ed., pp. 356-363). Philadelphia: W. B. Saunders.
4. DeGroot, L.J., & Jameson, J.L. (2001). *Endocrinology* (4th ed.). Philadelphia: W. B. Saunders.
5. Ebersole, P., & Hess, P. (2001). *Geriatric nursing and healthy aging.* St. Louis: Mosby.
6. Fallon, M.B., McGuire, B.M., Abrams, G.A., & Arguedas, M.R. (2001). Disorders of the gallbladder and biliary tract. In T.E. Andreoli, et al. (Eds.). *Cecil essentials of medicine* (5th ed., pp. 398-402). Philadelphia: W.B. Saunders.
7. Friedman, L.S. (2002). Liver, biliary tract & pancreas. In L.M. Tierney, McPhee, S.J., & M.A. Papadakin (Eds.). *Current medical diagnosis and treatment 2002* (41st ed., pp. 675-720). New York: Lange Medical Books/McGraw-Hill.
8. Ganong, W.F. (2003). *Review of medical physiology* (19th ed.). Norwalk, CT: Appleton & Lange.
9. Ghany, M., & Hoglnagle, J.H. (2001). Liver and biliary tract disease. In E. Braunwald, et al. (Eds.). *Harrison's principles of internal medicine* (15th ed., pp. 1707-1711). New York: McGraw-Hill.
10. Greensberger, N.J., & Paumgartner, G. (2001). Diseases of the gallbladder and bile ducts. In E. Braunwald, et al. (Eds.). *Harrison's principles of internal medicine* (15th ed., pp. 1776-1788). New York: McGraw-Hill.
11. Guyton, A.C., & Hall, J.E. (2000). *Textbook of medical physiology* (10th ed.). Philadelphia: W. B. Saunders.
12. *Healthy people 2010: Understanding and improving health* (2000). Sudsbury, MA: Jones & Bartlett.
13. Holick, M.F., Krane, S.M., & Potts, J.T. (2001). Calcium, phosphorus, and bone metabolism: Calcium-regulating hormones. In E. Braunwald, et al. (Eds.). *Harrison's principles of internal medicine* (15th ed., pp. 2214-2227). New York: McGraw-Hill.

14. Jameson, J.L. (2001). Principles of endocrinology. In E. Braunwald, et al. (Eds.). *Harrison's principles of internal medicine* (15th ed., pp. 2019-2029). New York: McGraw-Hill.

15. Jameson, J.L., & Weetman, A.P. (2001). Diseases of the thyroid. In E. Braunwald, et al. (Eds.). *Harrison's principles of internal medicine* (15th ed., pp. 2060-2084). New York: McGraw-Hill.

16. Jarvis, C. (2000). *Physical examination and health assessment* (3rd ed.). Philadelphia: W. B. Saunders.

17. Kee, J.L. (2002). *Laboratory and diagnostic tests with nursing implications* (6th ed.). Stamford, CT: Appleton & Lange.

18. Melmed, S. (2001). Disorders of the anterior pituitary and hypothalamus. In E. Braunwald, et al. (Eds.). *Harrison's principles of internal medicine* (15th ed., pp. 2029-2052).

19. Pagana, K.D., & Pagana, T.J. (2002). *Mosby's manual of diagnostic and laboratory tests* (2nd ed.). St. Louis: Mosby.

20. Pratt, D.S., & Kaplan, M.M. (2001). Evaluation of liver function. In E. Braunwald, et al. (Eds.). *Harrison's principles of internal medicine* (15th ed., pp. 1711-1715). New York: McGraw-Hill.

21. Price, S., & Wilson, L. (Eds.). (2003). *Pathophysiology* (6th ed.). St. Louis: Mosby.

22. Robertson, G.L. (2001). Disorders of the neurohypophysis. In E. Braunwald, et al. (Eds.). *Harrison's principles of internal medicine* (15th ed., pp. 2052-2062). New York: McGraw-Hill.

23. Seidel, H.M., et al. (2003). *Mosby's guide to physical examination* (5th ed.). St. Louis: Mosby.

24. Skidmore-Roth, L. (2001). *Mosby's handbook of herbs and natural supplements.* St. Louis: Mosby.

25. Sommers, M.S., & Johnson, S.A. (2002). *Diseases and disorders: A nursing therapeutics manual* (2nd ed.). Philadelphia: F.A. Davis.

26. Swearingen, P.L. (2003). *Manual of medical-surgical nursing care* (5th ed.). St. Louis: Mosby.

27. Williams, G.H., & Dluhy, R.G. (2001). Disorders of the adrenal cortex. In E. Braunwald, et al. (Eds.). *Harrison's principles of internal medicine* (15th ed., pp. 2084-2105). New York: McGraw-Hill.

evolve Did you remember to check out the bonus material on the Evolve website and the CD-ROM, including free self-assessment exercises?
http://evolve.elsevier.com/Black/medsurg/

Management of Clients with Thyroid and Parathyroid Disorders

Anne M. Larson

evolve

Web Enhancements

Case Study
Hyperthyroidism and Postmenopausal Osteoporosis
Client Education Guide
Thyroid Supplements (English Version and Spanish Translation)

http://evolve.elsevier.com/Black/medsurg/

Appendix C
Laboratory Values of Clinical Importance in Medical-Surgical Nursing

THYROID DISORDERS

Many terms describe normal and abnormal states of thyroid function. *Euthyroidism* means that the thyroid gland is functioning normally. Like other endocrine disorders, the two primary thyroid disorders are related to increased secretion *(hyperthyroidism)* and decreased secretion *(hypothyroidism)* of the gland's hormones. Such alterations in thyroid hormone (TH) secretion result in increased or decreased rates of metabolic function, heat production, and oxygen consumption. In addition, a third disorder is related to enlargement of the thyroid gland. These enlargements are called *goiters*.

GOITER

Enlargement of the thyroid gland may be seen with both hyperthyroidism and hypothyroidism. It generally results from a lack of iodine, inflammation, or benign or malignant tumors. Enlargement may also appear in hyperthyroidism, especially Graves' disease, in which the client typically has exophthalmos as well.

Etiology and Risk Factors

The two major forms of simple goiter are endemic and sporadic.

Endemic goiter is caused principally by nutritional iodine deficiency. It tends to occur in goiter "belts," geographical areas characterized by soil and water that are deficient in iodine. Major goiter belts in the United States are the Midwest, Northwest, and Great Lakes regions. Iodine is readily available in regions with access to salt water and also through consumption of seafood. Hence goiters are less common in coastal areas.

Endemic goiter typically occurs in fall and winter months and is twice as prevalent in women as it is in men. Also, because the need for TH is particularly great during growth spurts, pregnancy, and lactation, goiter commonly develops in adolescents, pregnant women, and nursing mothers who live in iodine-deficient regions.

Sporadic goiter is not restricted to any geographical area. Major causes include the following:
- Genetic defects resulting in faulty iodine metabolism
- Ingestion of large amounts of nutritional *goitrogens* (goiter-producing agents that inhibit thyroxine [T_4] production), such as rutabagas, cabbage, soybeans, peanuts, peaches, peas, strawberries, spinach, and radishes, all of which contain goitrogenic glycosides. Ingestion of medicinal goitrogens, for example, adrenergic antagonists, glucocorticoids, dopamine,

---

evolve *Be sure to check out the bonus material on the Evolve website and the CD-ROM, including free self-assessment exercises.*
http://evolve.elsevier.com/Black/medsurg/

Nursing Outcomes Classification
for Nursing Diagnoses—Clients with Thyroid and Parathyroid Disorders

Activity Intolerance
  Activity Intolerance
  Endurance
  Energy Conservation
  Self-Care: Activities of Daily Living
Constipation
  Bowel Elimination
  Hydration
  Medication Response
  Mobility Level
Decreased Cardiac Output
  Cardiac Pump Effectiveness
  Circulation Status
  Tissue Perfusion: Peripheral
  Vital Signs Status
Hyperthermia
  Thermoregulation
  Vital Signs Status
Hypothermia
  Thermoregulation
  Vital Signs Status

Imbalanced Nutrition: Less than Body Requirements
  Nutritional Status
  Nutritional Status: Food and Fluid Intake
  Nutritional Status: Nutrient Intake
Imbalanced Nutrition: More than Body Requirements
  Nutritional Status: Food and Fluid Intake
  Nutritional Status: Nutrient Intake
  Weight Control
Impaired Social Interaction
  Role Performance
  Social Interaction Skills
  Social Involvement
Impaired Urinary Elimination
  Knowledge: Disease Process
  Symptom Control
  Symptom Severity
  Urinary Elimination

Risk for Impaired Skin Integrity
  Fluid Balance
  Immobility Consequences: Physiologic
  Nutritional Status
  Risk Control
  Risk Detection
  Thermoregulation
  Tissue Integrity: Skin and Mucous Membranes
  Tissue Perfusion: Peripheral
Risk for Injury
  Knowledge: Personal Safety
  Neurological Status
  Risk Control
  Risk Control: Visual Impairment
  Risk Detection
  Symptom Control

FIGURE 45-1 Massive thyroid enlargement caused by diffuse toxic goiter. (From Swartz, M.H. [2002]. *Textbook of physical diagnosis* [4th ed.]. Philadelphia: W.B. Saunders.)

methimazole, lithium, iodinated radiographic contrast agents, phenytoin, rifampin, carbamazepine, and propylthiouracil (PTU)

Health promotion practices include the ingestion of iodized salt and avoidance of goitrogens. Health mainte-nance or restoration interventions include teaching about the use of iodized salt.

Pathophysiology

If a person's diet lacks sufficient iodine or if production of thyroid hormones is suppressed for any other reason, the thyroid enlarges in an attempt to compensate for hormonal deficiency. Under these circumstances, goiter is essentially an adaptation to a deficiency of thyroid hormones. Enlargement of the gland also occurs in response to increased pituitary secretion of thyroid-stimulating hormone (TSH). TSH stimulates the thyroid to secrete more T_4 when blood T_4 levels are low. Eventually, the gland may become so large that it compresses structures in the neck and chest, causing respiratory problems and dysphagia.

Clinical Manifestations

Diagnosis of simple goiter is confirmed by history, clinical findings, and laboratory tests (Figure 45-1). The client is often euthyroid because the gland enlarges enough to produce normal amounts of T_4. Needle biopsy of the goiter may be indicated to rule out malignancy.

Outcome Management
■ Medical Management

When enlargement is a compensatory reaction to iodine deficiency and consequent suppression of T_4 secretion, the client can be treated with preparations of iodine and thyroid hormones. Either a strong iodine solution (Lugol's solution) or saturated solution of potassium iodide (SSKI) drops can be administered. Iodine reduces the size and vascularity of the enlarged gland. The availability of iodized salt and thyroid hormones has made replacement therapy with iodine obsolete in the United States.

The client's diet should also be higher in iodine. The client may switch to iodized salt. Dietary goitrogens (e.g., turnips, soybeans, rutabagas, and, to a lesser degree, seafood, green leafy vegetables, carrots, and peanuts) should be avoided.

Endemic goiter can be prevented altogether with the use of iodized salt. Adults require at least 50 mg of iodine per day; however, 200 to 300 mg/day is considered the minimum adequate intake needed to prevent goiter. Iodized salt, used in the United States since 1924, contains 1 part iodine to 100,000 parts of salt. Thus the average person, who ingests about 6.2 g of salt a day, is also taking 474 mg of iodine daily if the salt is iodized.

Many clients do not understand the need for iodized salt to prevent goiters. Some believe that any additive to food or water is harmful and they therefore avoid iodized salt. These two problems, along with the fact that many modern foods are processed with cheaper non-iodized salt, contribute to the potential for development of simple goiter. Nurses need to educate the public about the importance of iodized salt.

■ Surgical Management

Surgery is indicated for a goiter that is very large, does not respond to treatment, or is putting too much pressure on other structures in the neck. Surgery is discussed in detail under Hyperthyroidism.

HYPOTHYROIDISM

Hypothyroidism is a deficiency of TH resulting in slowed body metabolism, decreased heat production, and decreased oxygen consumption by the tissues. Underactivity of the thyroid gland may result from primary thyroid dysfunction, or it may be secondary to anterior pituitary dysfunction.

The frequency of hypothyroidism depends on the population being studied. The incidence of overt hypothyroidism is 1 to 2 in 1000 people in community surveys and 5 to 20 in 1000 clients seeking medical care.

Hypothyroidism affects women more than men (about 4:1). Although hypothyroidism may be congenital (cretinism) and therefore present at birth, the highest incidence is in adults between 30 and 65 years of age. About 95% of all people with hypothyroidism have the *primary* form of the disease. *Central hypothyroidism* resulting from pituitary or hypothalamic disease accounts for fewer than 10% of cases.

Some consider the term *hypothyroidism* to be synonymous with *myxedema, whereas others identify myxedema as severe hypothyroidism.* In the following discussion, *myxedema* is used to denote severe hypothy-

roidism. *Myxedema coma* is a life-threatening condition in which all body systems are severely compromised by the hypometabolic state.

Etiology and Risk Factors

Primary hypothyroidism can be caused by the following:
- Congenital defects of the thyroid (cretinism)
- Defective hormone synthesis
- Iodine deficiency (prenatal and postnatal)
- Antithyroid drugs
- Surgery or treatment with radioactive agents for hyperthyroidism
- Chronic inflammatory (autoimmune) diseases such as Hashimoto's disease, amyloidosis, and sarcoidosis

Hashimoto's disease is the most common type of autoimmune hypothyroidism. In primary hypothyroidism, TH levels are low and TSH levels are elevated, indicating that the pituitary is attempting to stimulate the secretion of thyroid hormones but the thyroid is not responding.

Secondary hypothyroidism develops when there is insufficient stimulation of a normal thyroid gland; consequently TSH levels are decreased. This condition may start as a malfunction of the pituitary or hypothalamus or it might be caused by peripheral resistance to TH. When this occurs, both TSH and TH levels are low in the serum.

Tertiary or *central hypothyroidism* can develop if the hypothalamus cannot produce thyroid-releasing hormone (TRH) and subsequently does not stimulate the pituitary to secrete TSH. It may be due to a tumor or other destructive lesion in the hypothalamic region. When this occurs, both TSH and TH levels are again low in the serum.

Subclinical hypothyroidism is defined as hypothyroidism that is diagnosed with an elevated TSH level but a normal to low-normal T_4 level. Manifestations resemble those of mild hypothyroidism with subtle cardiac defects, especially in clients with pre-existing cardiac disease. Subclinical hypothyroidism is found in 20 to 120 of 1000 persons in the community. The causes are the same as those of primary hypothyroidism. Prevalence increases with age. Low-dose levothyroxine sodium (Synthroid) is effective for the relief of manifestations and improvement in cardiac function and lipid profile.

Use of iodized salt and avoidance of goitrogens are health promotion activities. Health restoration practices involve lifelong hormone replacement.

Pathophysiology

The thyroid gland needs iodine to synthesize and secrete thyroid hormones: T_4, triiodothyronine (T_3), and thyrocalcitonin (calcitonin). Production of thyroid hormones depends on the secretion of TSH from the anterior pituitary and the ingestion of adequate protein and iodine. The hypothalamus regulates the pituitary secretion of TSH via a negative feedback system.

Decreased levels of thyroid hormones lead to overall slowing of the basal metabolic rate. This slowing of all body processes leads to *achlorhydria* (decreased secretion of hydrochloric acid in the stomach), decreased gastrointestinal tract motility, bradycardia, slowed neurologic functioning, and a decrease in heat production resulting in a decreased basal body temperature.

The most important changes caused by reduced levels of thyroid hormones are those that affect lipid metabolism. The reduction in thyroid hormones causes an increase in serum cholesterol and triglyceride levels and an increase in arteriosclerosis and coronary heart disease in clients with hypothyroidism.

Because thyroid hormones play a role in the production of red blood cells, people with hypothyroidism also show evidence of anemia, with possible vitamin B_{12} and folate deficiency.

Myxedema, a mucinous edema, is caused by accumulation of hydrophilic proteoglycans in the interstitial spaces. The cause of this problem remains unclear.

Clinical Manifestations

The manifestations of hypothyroidism depend on whether it is mild, severe (myxedema), or complicated (myxedema coma).

Mild Hypothyroidism

Clients with mild hypothyroidism (the most common form) may be asymptomatic or may experience vague manifestations so ordinary as to escape detection. For example, clients may experience sensitivity to cold, lethargy, dry skin or hair, forgetfulness, depression, and some weight gain. Constipation and fecal impaction related to slowed peristaltic action and lack of normal physical activity may be reported (Table 45-1).

As the degree of hypothyroidism worsens, the thyroid may enlarge (goiter) in an attempt to produce enough T_4. Typically, clients seek medical advice when the goiter grows large enough to distort the appearance of the neck. They may also experience respiratory distress and dysphagia if the goiter is very large.

Diagnostic tests for hypothyroidism confirm the clinical picture of hypometabolism and depressed thyroid activity. The serum TSH level is elevated in primary hypothyroidism. Radioactive iodide uptake is decreased in hypothyroidism.

Myxedema

Myxedema may develop in clients with undiagnosed or undertreated hypothyroidism who experience stress. Stressors include infection, drugs (phenothiazines, barbiturates, opioids, anesthetics), respiratory failure, heart failure, cerebral vascular accident, trauma, prolonged exposure to cold, metabolic disturbances, surgery, and seizures.

Myxedema is characterized by a dry, waxy type of swelling with abnormal deposits of mucin in the skin and other tissues. The edema is of the nonpitting type and is common in the pretibial and facial areas.

Myxedema is most commonly diagnosed in hypothyroid women in their 60s. Untreated myxedema has been associated with severe atherosclerosis and has been attributed to the increase in serum cholesterol concentrations, particularly low-density lipoproteins. TH replacement improves these changes.

Clients with myxedema may also have hypercholesterolemia, hyperlipidemia, and proteinemia as a result of T_4 changes in the synthesis, mobilization, and degradation of serum lipids. Elevated lipid levels may contribute to the later development of cardiac problems. Dilutional hyponatremia may develop as a result of the marked impairment of water excretion because of decreased delivery of sodium and volume to the distal renal tubules associated with decreased renal blood flow. Elevated creatine phosphokinase, aspartate aminotransferase, and lactate dehydrogenase may also develop secondary to altered metabolism.

Myxedema Coma

The major complication of hypothyroidism is myxedema coma, an extremely rare condition with a mortality rate approaching 100%. Myxedema coma is characterized by a drastic decrease in metabolic rate, hypoventilation leading to respiratory acidosis, hypothermia, and hypotension. Complicating conditions include hyponatremia, hypercalcemia, secondary adrenal insufficiency, hypoglycemia, and water intoxication. Myxedema coma may be brought on by stress—as from surgery or infection—or by noncompliance with thyroid treatment.

Outcome Management

Hypothyroidism is rarely a primary diagnosis. Usually, the diagnosis is made after the development of another medical problem. Clients with hypothyroidism are typically managed on an outpatient basis with TH replacement. Treatment is an ongoing, lifelong process. Clients with myxedema or myxedema coma are managed as a medical emergency.

■ Medical Management

Hypothyroidism

The desired outcomes of the medical management of hypothyroidism are to correct TH deficiency, reverse manifestations, and prevent further cardiac and arterial damage.

Correct Thyroid Hormone Deficiency. For hypothyroidism to be reversed permanently, the client must usually take TH for life. Levothyroxine sodium is the prin-

TABLE 45-1	*Manifestations of Hypothyroidism and Hyperthyroidism*	
System	**Hypothyroidism**	**Hyperthyroidism**
Cardiovascular	↓ HR + ↓ SV: ↓ CO ↓ Myocardial O$_2$ demand ↑ Peripheral vascular resistance Possible hypertension Hyperlipidemia Hypercholesterolemia Distant heart sounds	↑ HR + ↑ SV: ↑ CO ↑ O$_2$ consumption Systolic BP ↑ 10-15 mm Hg Diastolic BP ↑ 10-15 mm Hg Palpitations Rapid, bounding pulse Possible heart failure, edema
Gastrointestinal	↓ Peristalsis Anorexia Possible weight gain Constipation ↓ Protein metabolism ↑ Serum lipids Delayed glucose uptake ↓ Glucose absorption	↑ Peristalsis ↑ Appetite Weight loss Diarrhea ↑ Use of adipose and protein stores ↓ Serum lipids ↑ Gastrointestinal secretions
Musculoskeletal	Slow movements	Fatigue Muscle weakness Tremors
Integumentary	Dry, coarse, scaly skin Hair that falls out Thick, brittle nails Expressionless face Periorbital edema Thick, puffy skin: face and pretibial areas Cold intolerance	Profuse sweating Moist skin Flushed, warm skin Hair: fine, soft, straight, possible hair loss Heat intolerance
Neurologic	↓ Deep tendon reflexes Fatigue, somnolence Slow, deliberate speech Apathy, depression, paranoia Impaired short-term memory Lethargy	↑ Deep tendon reflexes Nervousness, restlessness Emotional instability: anxiety, worry, paranoia
Reproductive	Females: menorrhagia, anovulation, irregular menses, decreased libido Males: decreased libido, impotence	Females: amenorrhea, irregular menses, ↓ fertility, ↑ tendency for spontaneous abortion Males: impotence, decreased libido ↓ Sexual development prepuberty
Other	Myxedema	Exophthalmos

BP, Blood pressure; *CO,* cardiac output; *CO$_2$,* carbon dioxide; *HR,* heart rate; *O$_2$,* oxygen; *SV,* stroke volume.

cipal form of replacement therapy. Dosages vary with the client's age, the severity of the hypothyroidism, the client's general medical condition (particularly regarding cardiovascular disorders), and the client's response to medical treatment at the initiation of TH therapy. Children and older adults receive smaller doses.

Clients who respond to TH therapy receive a maintenance dose of T$_4$ daily for life. Pharmacologic goitrogens are replaced by drugs that do not interfere with TH function. The drug of choice for thyroid replacement is levothyroxine sodium, which is converted in the body to both T$_4$ and T$_3$. Desiccated thyroid and liothyronine sodium (Cytomel), once commonly used in replacement therapy, are now used infrequently because of problems with fluctuating plasma levels and side effects (see the Integrating Pharmacology feature on Medications for Thyroid Disorders on p. 1196).

Reverse Manifestations. Clients with hypothyroidism of long duration notice an improvement in manifestations

INTEGRATING PHARMACOLOGY

Medications for Thyroid Disorders

Medications used in the treatment of hyperthyroid conditions are used to reduce thyroid hormone levels. Medications used in the treatment of hypothyroid conditions are used to increase thyroid hormone levels.

Two medical treatment options exist for hyperthyroidism. First the client may be temporarily treated with anti-thyroid drugs such as propylthiouracil (PTU), which inhibits thyroid hormone synthesis. Radioactive iodine (^{131}I) offers a more permanent option because it destroys thyroid tissue. Radioactive iodine is not be given to pregnant women because it may cross fetal circulation and destroy fetal thyroid tissue.

Clients with hypothyroidism must receive lifelong thyroid hormone replacement therapy such as Synthroid (levothyroxine). Thyroid hormone levels are routinely monitored to ensure adequate dosage prescription. Thyroid hormone replacement therapy is also prescribed for clients with goiters because it promotes shrinkage of the gland.

Clients with thyrotoxicosis may receive additional drug therapy for palliative treatment. For example, beta-adrenergic blockers may be prescribed to control heart rate and tremors. Acetaminophen may be prescribed for fever.

within 2 to 3 weeks of starting medication; however, hoarseness, anemia, and changes in hair and skin may take many months to resolve.

Prevent Cardiac Complications. A client with cardiac complications starts with a small dose of TH. Large doses may precipitate heart failure or myocardial infarction by increasing body metabolism, myocardial oxygen requirements, and consequently the workload of the heart.

Myxedema Coma

The desired outcome of the medical management of myxedema coma is to reverse the condition to save the client's life. Supportive measures begin immediately and include maintaining a patent airway, giving oxygen, and replacing fluids intravenously. The client is kept warm, and vital signs are closely monitored until the client begins to recover. Vasopressors are used to maintain tissue perfusion.

Levothyroxine sodium is given intravenously with glucose and corticosteroids. When administering TH to a client with myxedema heart disease, assess the client carefully for angina, dyspnea, or orthopnea. The event that precipitated the coma (surgery, infection, noncompliance) also must be evaluated and treated.

■ Nursing Management of the Medical Client with Mild Hypothyroidism
Assessment

Carefully assess the client for manifestations of hypothyroidism. Obtain a careful history; look for evidence of decreased metabolic function, such as weight gain, excessive sleeping, and generalized fatigue. Take a thorough diet history, looking particularly at the intake of iodine. Does the client take any goitrogenic substances or reside in a goiter belt?

Ask the client about other medical conditions that might be present, such as a history of hyperthyroidism treated with surgery or radioactive iodine, both of which predispose to hypothyroidism. Does the client use any medication that might lead to hypothyroidism? Lithium, aminoglutethimide, sodium or potassium perchlorate, and cobalt can slow thyroid metabolism.

Diagnosis, Outcomes, Interventions

Diagnosis: Imbalanced Nutrition: More than Body Requirements. The slowed metabolic rate places a hypothyroid client at risk for weight gain, leading to the nursing diagnosis *Imbalanced Nutrition: More than Body Requirements related to a slowed metabolic rate resulting in weight gain.*

Outcomes. The client will return to normal weight as evidenced by loss of at least 2 pounds weekly.

Interventions. When the client begins taking thyroid medication, the activity level and decreased edema commonly result in a significant initial weight loss without any change in diet. Typically, however, appetite also increases as the medication begins to work. Therefore teach the client to maintain a low-calorie diet until weight stabilizes at the ideal body weight. The client should gain more energy as the TH level returns to normal, allowing an increase in activity to help in weight loss.

Diagnosis: Activity Intolerance. A client with hypothyroidism usually feels fatigued, which commonly leads to the nursing diagnosis *Activity Intolerance related to weakness and apathy secondary to a decreased metabolic rate and resulting in an increased heart rate and shortness of breath with activity.*

Outcomes. The client will develop increased tolerance for activity as evidenced by a return to pre-illness activity levels.

Interventions. While the client still has hypothyroidism, energy levels are decreased and the client tires easily.

Usually the result is a decreased activity level. When TH replacement begins, the client returns to a level of physical and mental activity that should gradually improve with hormone therapy.

Diagnosis: Constipation. A client with hypothyroidism has decreased gastrointestinal motility, leading to the nursing diagnosis *Constipation related to decreased peristalsis secondary to slowed metabolic rate and activity intolerance, resulting in decreased frequency of stools and painful defecation.*

Outcomes. The client will experience a return to a normal pre-illness bowel pattern as evidenced by a bowel movement at least every other day.

Interventions. Implement measures to prevent constipation and fecal impaction. As the hypothyroidism is reversed and cardiac status improves, encourage more activity. Advise the client to drink six to eight glasses of water every day and to eat foods high in fiber, such as fresh fruits, vegetables, and grains. If these measures are ineffective, a stool softener or cathartic may be indicated.

Evaluation

Once hypothyroidism has been diagnosed and replacement therapy begun, it is expected that the condition will be reversed over 3 to 12 weeks. A maintenance dosage of TH replacement is determined. If reversal of the condition does not continue, the client must be assessed for compliance with the therapeutic regimen.

■ Nursing Management of the Medical Client with Myxedema
Assessment

Observe the client for the physical manifestations of myxedema, such as periorbital and facial edema, a blank facial expression, a thick tongue, and generalized slowing of all muscle movement. The client's vital signs are also affected and must be monitored closely. The client is hypothermic. Depressed respirations precipitate respiratory acidosis. Alterations in heart rate and blood pressure follow.

Diagnosis, Outcomes, Interventions

Diagnosis: Decreased Cardiac Output. The client with myxedema is susceptible to severe arteriosclerotic heart disease and other cardiac abnormalities, leading to the nursing diagnosis *Decreased Cardiac Output related to sustained bradycardia, resulting in edema and decreased urine output.*

Outcomes. The client will maintain a normal cardiac output and will remain free of heart failure as evidenced by normal heart rate, evidence of normal perfusion, absence of edema, and urine output of at least 0.5 ml/kg/hr.

Interventions. As the client proceeds with hormone replacement therapy, the edema and puffiness start to lessen. Continue to monitor the client's intake and output, which will become more balanced. Urine output should increase significantly during thyroid therapy. Monitor the client's weight daily.

To help prevent further strain on the already overburdened heart, help the client conserve energy. For example, always help the client turn in bed. If any new cardiac manifestations occur, notify the physician immediately. Do not give TH until the physician has reappraised the client's condition.

When administering thyroid preparations, assess the client carefully for manifestations of thyrotoxicosis, such as tachycardia, increased appetite, diarrhea, sweating, agitation, tremor, palpitations, and shortness of breath. If any of these manifestations develop during thyroid therapy, notify the physician at once so that the dosage can be reduced.

Diagnosis: Hypothermia. A client with severe myxedema has a very low metabolic rate, leading to an important nursing diagnosis of *Hypothermia related to slowed metabolic rate resulting in subnormal body temperature.*

Outcomes. The client's body temperature will return to normal.

Interventions. Provide the client with a comfortable, warm environment. Remember that hypothyroidism sharply increases sensitivity to cold. If necessary, supply extra clothing and warm blankets. Encourage the client to dress warmly and to avoid extreme cold whenever possible. In cases of severe hypothermia, a warming blanket may be necessary.

Diagnosis: Risk for Injury: Myxedema Coma. A client with acute hypothyroidism is susceptible to the development of myxedema coma, leading to the nursing diagnosis *Risk for Injury: Myxedema coma related to hypersensitivity to anesthetics, sedatives, and opioids secondary to decreased metabolic rate.*

Outcomes. The client will not receive the usual doses of anesthetics, sedatives, and opioids so that development of myxedema coma will be prevented and the client will not be injured.

Interventions. The client should not receive sedatives unless it is absolutely necessary. If a sedative or opioid must be given, administer no more than one-third to one-half the usual dose. Then assess the client carefully for respiratory depression or a decreased level of consciousness.

Diagnosis: Risk for Impaired Skin Integrity. A client with myxedema is very susceptible to skin breakdown, leading to the nursing diagnosis *Risk for Impaired Skin Integrity related to edema and dryness secondary to infiltration of fluid into interstitial spaces.*

Outcomes. The client's skin will remain intact as evidenced by absence of injury and resolution of edema.

Interventions. Monitor the sacrum, coccyx, elbows, scapulae, and other pressure points for redness or tissue breakdown. Remember that edematous tissues are more susceptible to pressure ulcers. Plan a strict turning schedule for the client, and use a pressure reduction mattress.

Evaluation

It is expected that after successful treatment the client will demonstrate no evidence of heart failure, edema, or skin impairment; temperature and urine output will be normal; and no further evidence of myxedema will be seen. After the client is out of danger and alert, long-term management begins (see the following section).

■ Self-Care
Hypothyroidism is a lifelong disease that must be managed with the client's full participation. The client should understand the pharmacologic regimen, nutrition, and follow-up required to control the condition.

To promote self-care, focus your teaching on the client's need to understand the manifestations of hyperthyroidism and hypothyroidism to follow the medication regimen and diet and to seek medical attention appropriately. Evaluate the client's level of knowledge about the disorder and the importance of taking TH daily for life. Develop and implement a teaching plan based on the client's particular needs. Also provide a written list (such as the one in the Client Education Guide feature on Thyroid Supplements on the website) of the manifestations of thyroid deficiency or excess. Instruct the client about how to monitor the pulse rate. Instruct the client and his or her significant others to telephone the physician if those manifestations develop.

Monitor the client's weight weekly. Physical manifestations of hypothyroidism should decrease over 3 to 12 weeks as TH levels increase. Emphasize the need for iodized salt. Advise the client to drink sufficient fluids, increase physical activity, and eat a high-fiber diet to prevent constipation. Remind the client to have TH levels

checked routinely until they stabilize and then at regular intervals to ensure that they remain normal.

■ Modifications for Older Clients
Subclinical hypothyroidism refers to a combination of elevated TSH levels, normal T_3 and free thyroxine (FT_4) levels, and no clinical manifestations. Subclinical hypothyroidism occurs in up to 15% of postmenopausal women. The most common causes of are, in order of frequency, autoimmune thyroiditis, Hashimoto's disease, previous thyroid surgery or treatment with radioactive agents, and noncompliance with prescribed T_4 replacements.

Medical treatment is not indicated for clients who have no manifestations. Clients with generalized complaints may benefit from small doses of T_4, which indicates that their condition is symptomatic rather than subclinical. Remember that a principal hazard in giving T_4 to an older client is the development of ischemic heart disease as evidenced by angina. The response to therapy and serum levels must be observed closely. The client's pulse should be monitored daily.

The difficulty in diagnosing hypothyroidism in older adults is that the manifestations are usually vague and generic to other disease processes. Hypothyroidism must be considered in the differential diagnosis of a variety of conditions affecting older people.

HYPERTHYROIDISM
Hyperthyroidism (excessive secretion of TH) is a highly preventable endocrine disorder. Like most thyroid conditions, it is a disorder that predominantly affects women (in a female-to-male ratio of 4:1), especially women between ages 20 and 40 years.

Etiology and Risk Factors
Hyperthyroidism may be due to overfunctioning of the entire gland or, less commonly, to single or multiple functioning adenomas of thyroid cancer. Overtreatment of myxedema with TH may also result in hyperthyroidism.

The most common form of hyperthyroidism is Graves' disease (toxic, diffuse goiter), which has three principal hallmarks: hyperthyroidism, thyroid gland enlargement (goiter), and *exophthalmos* (abnormal protrusion of the eyes). Graves' disease is an autoimmune disorder mediated by immunoglobulin G (IgG) antibody that binds to and activates TSH receptors on the surface of the thyroid cells.

Other causes of hyperthyroidism include toxic nodular goiter, toxic adenoma (benign), thyroid carcinoma, subacute and chronic thyroiditis, ingestion of TH, and ingestion of amiodarone hydrochloride for atrial fibrillation. Health maintenance and restoration activities include monitoring TH levels if TH replacement is given, removal of thyroid tumors, and administration of antithyroid medications.

Pathophysiology

Graves' disease may be due to excessive stimulation of the adrenergic nervous system or excessive levels of circulating TH.

Hyperthyroidism is characterized by loss of the normal regulatory controls of TH secretion. Because the action of TH on the body is stimulatory, hypermetabolism results, with increased sympathetic nervous system activity. Excessive amounts of TH stimulate the cardiac system and increase the number of beta-adrenergic receptors, leading to tachycardia and increased cardiac output, stroke volume, adrenergic responsiveness, and peripheral blood flow. Metabolism increases greatly, leading to a negative nitrogen balance, lipid depletion, and a state of nutritional deficiency and weight loss.

Hyperthyroidism also results in altered secretion and metabolism of hypothalamic, pituitary, and gonadal hormones. If hyperthyroidism occurs before puberty, sexual development is delayed in both genders. After puberty, hyperthyroidism results in diminished libido in both men and women. Women also have menstrual irregularities and decreased fertility.

Clinical Manifestations

Because hyperthyroidism is caused by excessive secretion of TH, the clinical picture of Graves' disease is in many ways opposite to that of hypothyroidism. Assessment reveals a client who appears extremely agitated and irritable, with a hand tremor at rest. Despite a ravenous appetite, weight loss occurs as a result of the quickened metabolism. Because of the high levels of circulating TH, the client's body processes "speed up." Manifestations include loose bowel movements, heat intolerance, profuse diaphoresis (perspiration), tachycardia, and incoordination related to tremor. The skin becomes warm, smooth, and moist because of accelerated circulation to the tissues. Hair appears thin and soft.

Moreover, the client's emotions are adversely affected by the turbulent activity within the body. Moods may be cyclic, ranging from mild euphoria to extreme hyperactivity to delirium. The excessive hyperactivity in turn leads to extreme fatigue and depression, again followed by episodes of overactivity. As a result of the client's chaotic emotional state, interpersonal relationships may deteriorate, further accentuating the emotional disturbance.

Goiter, the second characteristic of Graves' disease is due to hyperplasia and hypertrophy of the thyroid cells. The gland may grow to three or four times its normal size. Cellular overgrowth results in the release of excessive amounts of TH into the blood.

Exophthalmos is the third major manifestation of Graves' disease. The cause of the ophthalmologic

changes in Graves' disease seems to be autoimmunity against retro-orbital tissues. The client who develops exophthalmos has protruding eyes and a fixed stare caused by accumulation of fluid in the fat pads and muscles that lie behind the eyeballs (Figure 45-2). Because the eyes are surrounded by unyielding bone, edema forces them forward out of their sockets, producing the typical facies of exophthalmos. In severe cases, clients may be unable to close their eyelids and must have their lids taped shut to protect the eyes. Without intervention, severe exophthalmos can progress to corneal ulceration or infection and loss of vision. In some cases, exophthalmos is not reversed by intervention and may actually worsen with radioactive iodine therapy.

The diagnosis of Graves' disease is confirmed on the basis of the client's often striking physical appearance (enlarged neck, protruding eyes, agitated expression); the manifestations of agitation, restlessness, and weight loss; and laboratory findings. Serum TH levels are usually all elevated, although they are occasionally within the normal range (so-called euthyroid Graves' disease). Serum cholesterol levels are usually depressed. See Table 44-2 for the usual laboratory findings.

Complications

The three major complications of Graves' disease are exophthalmos, heart disease, and thyroid storm (thyroid crisis, thyrotoxicosis).

Exophthalmos

Exophthalmos develops as a result of proptosis, lid retraction, muscle swelling, and tissue edema from a

FIGURE 45-2 Extreme exophthalmos in hyperthyroidism. Because the eyes are surrounded by unyielding bone, fluid accumulation in the fat pads and muscles behind the eyeballs causes protruding eyes and a fixed stare in the client with exophthalmos. Without intervention, the client with severe exophthalmos may be unable to close the eyelids and may develop corneal ulceration or infection. Eventually, this can result in total loss of vision. (From Scheie, H.G. [1977]. *Textbook of ophthalmology* [9th ed.] Philadelphia: W.B. Saunders.)

prolonged hyperthyroid condition. Manifestations may include a gritty sensation in the eye, photophobia, lacrimation, inflammatory changes, and dyslogia.

Unlike the manifestations of goiter and hyperthyroidism, exophthalmos does not necessarily regress with therapy. Diuretics may alleviate some of the periorbital edema. Glucocorticoids such as prednisone are given in large doses to reduce inflammation of the periorbital tissues. Unfortunately, steroids produce many undesirable side effects, including acute psychoses. Estrogen therapy is occasionally of value in postmenopausal women. Methylcellulose eye drops, 14% four times daily, help reduce eye irritation. Radiation therapy to the retro-orbital tissues may help in severe cases. Surgical decompression of the orbits may be performed when all other measures fail to correct exophthalmos. This procedure may save the client's vision when eye changes are severe.

A number of general nursing interventions also help to reduce eye discomfort and prevent corneal ulceration and infection. Instruct a client with exophthalmos to wear dark eyeglasses. Warn the client to avoid getting dust or dirt in the eyes. If the eyelids cannot be closed easily or at all, have the client wear a sleeping mask (available in drug stores) or lightly tape the eyes shut with nonallergic tape. Elevate the head of the bed at night, and have the client restrict salt intake to relieve edema.

Heart Disease

Heart disease poses a serious threat. Tachycardia almost always accompanies thyrotoxicosis, and atrial fibrillation may also appear. Heart failure is found among older clients with long-standing thyrotoxicosis. Propranolol is the drug of choice but is contraindicated if asthma or heart failure is a pre-existing condition. Treatment of these cardiac complications is covered in Unit 13.

Thyroid Storm (Thyrotoxicosis)

Thyroid storm (thyrotoxicosis) is a potentially fatal acute episode of thyroid overactivity characterized by high fever, severe tachycardia, delirium, dehydration, and extreme irritability. Thanks to modern intervention techniques, this once common problem seldom develops today. Factors that may precipitate a thyroid storm include undiagnosed or untreated hyperthyroidism, infection, thyroid ablation, metabolic catastrophes, surgery, trauma, labor and delivery, myocardial infarction, pulmonary embolus, medication overdose, or inadequate preparation for thyroid surgery.

A client with thyrotoxicosis may have an increase in clotting factor VIII. Despite this increase, the hyperthyroid client has increased sensitivity to coumarin derivatives because of the accelerated metabolic clearance of the vitamin K–dependent clotting factors. Thyroid storm is a clinical diagnosis; no laboratory tests differentiate hyperthyroidism from thyroid storm in general.

Outcome Management
■ Medical Management

The desired outcomes of medical management for clients with Graves' disease are to curtail the excessive secretion of TH and to prevent and treat complications. Choice of intervention is based on age, goiter size, and whether the client has other health problems. The three major forms of therapy are antithyroid medication, radioiodine therapy, and surgery.

Curtail Excessive Secretion of Thyroid Hormone

Antithyroid Medication Therapy. Antithyroid medication is recommended for clients younger than 18 years of age and for pregnant women. The major medications used to control hyperthyroidism include iodide, propylthiouracil, and methimazole (Tapazole). Adrenergic blocking agents may be administered as adjunctive therapy.

Propylthiouracil is the most commonly used antithyroid medication. It corrects hyperthyroidism by impairing TH synthesis. With the usual dosage regimen, propylthiouracil ameliorates Graves' disease within 4 to 8 weeks. Several months may pass before manifestations completely abate, however. When euthyroid, the client is given a maintenance dose of propylthiouracil, usually three times daily. Although an ideal medication in many ways, propylthiouracil causes significant side effects in about 9% of people who use it (see the Integrating Pharmacology feature on Medications for Thyroid Disorders on p. 1196).

The most serious toxic effect is agranulocytosis (see Chapter 77). A white blood cell (WBC) count should be obtained before initial administration of the medication. Instruct the client to report a sore throat, fever, or rash immediately so that further WBC tests can be performed and the client's condition can be evaluated. Less severe adverse reactions include mild allergies (rash and pruritus). Rarely does hepatitis or drug fever develop.

Methimazole blocks the action of TH in the body. Unfortunately, it produces agranulocytosis in a small percentage of people.

Iodine therapy is prescribed for two reasons: (1) to reduce the vascularity of the thyroid gland before subtotal or total thyroidectomy and (2) to treat thyroid storm. Iodine preparations act temporarily to prevent the release of TH into the circulation by increasing the amount of TH stored in the gland. The stored TH is eventually released back into the circulation, however, once again producing hyperthyroidism. For this reason, iodine preparations are usually given only for 10 to 14 days before surgery. If iodine is given for a longer period or if it is given alone (not in combination with propylthiouracil), the thyroid gland may "escape" before thyroidectomy, meaning that the iodine is no longer capable of maintaining TH storage. As a result, TH floods the circulation, and hyperthyroidism becomes more severe than before.

The iodine medication of choice is potassium iodide. Lugol's solution is also used but is more expensive than potassium iodide and tends to inactivate antithyroid preparations in the bowel.

Radioiodine Therapy. Therapy with radioactive iodine (^{131}I) is prescribed mainly for middle-aged and older clients. This intervention offers many advantages: it is economical, is simple to administer, and can be prescribed on an outpatient basis as described in the Case Study feature on Hyperthyroidism and Postmenopausal Osteoporosis, below. Radiotherapy is contraindicated for pregnant women and is rarely used for children.

The rationale behind ^{131}I therapy for Graves' disease is simple. The thyroid gland is unable to distinguish between regular iodine atoms and radioiodine atoms. Consequently, when the client receives a dose of ^{131}I, the thyroid gland picks up the radioiodine and concentrates it just as it would regular iodine. As a result, the cells that concentrate ^{131}I to make T_4 are destroyed by the local irradiation, TH secretion diminishes, and the manifestations of hyperthyroidism and goiter disappear. Because radioiodine destroys thyroid cells, however, one of the major possible complications of ^{131}I therapy is hypothyroidism. Therefore assess for manifestations of hypothyroidism after ^{131}I therapy.

The ^{131}I is dissolved in water and administered orally. The dosage is determined both by the size of the gland and by the thyroid's uptake of a tracer dose of radioiodine. After receiving the radioiodine, the client may go home unless the dosage is extremely large, in which case the client must be placed in isolation for several days to prevent radioactive contamination.

The manifestations of hyperthyroidism usually subside within 6 to 12 weeks after ^{131}I administration. Because of the delay in achieving a therapeutic response with ^{131}I, concurrent treatment with beta-adrenergic blockers may be desirable. Sometimes resistant clients require a second or, in rare instances, a third dose of radioiodine.

The client who becomes euthyroid still needs regular medical examinations because hypothyroidism may develop several years after radiotherapy. Clients who become hypothyroid require lifelong hormone replacement with thyroid preparations.

Prevent and Treat Complications

Adrenergic Blocking Agents. Adrenergic blocking agents are sometimes given as adjunctive therapy to control the activity of the sympathetic nervous system. There is now evidence that these agents are of great benefit to the "hyperthyroid heart," which has increased sensitivity to catecholamines and an increased number of beta-adrenergic receptor sites. Therefore these agents help lessen distressing manifestations such as palpitations and tachycardia. Tremor and nervousness may also be alleviated by adrenergic blocking agents. The most commonly used medication is propranolol. Treatment of Graves' hyperthyroidism may involve a long delay (i.e., weeks to months) between the start of therapy and substantial improvement or resolution of manifestations.

Dietary Therapy. The client with hyperthyroidism needs a high-calorie, high-protein diet to compensate for the hypermetabolic state. A diet of 4000 to 5000 calories with high protein levels may be necessary to prevent a negative nitrogen balance and weight loss.

Treating Thyroid Storm. Because thyroid storm is an emergency, heroic intervention is needed for control. The high fever is treated with hypothermia blankets; dehydration is reversed with the administration of intravenous fluids. Management of thyroid storm involves suppressing hormone release, inhibiting hormone synthesis, blocking conversion of T_4 to the more active T_3, inhibiting the effects of TH on body tissues, and treating the precipitating cause, if it is known.

Blockade of TH release is usually achieved by oral administration of iodides, such as potassium iodide. Sodium iodide may be given intravenously. Glucocorticoid, dexamethasone, and propylthiouracil are also commonly used oral drugs. Beta-blockers are given to decrease the effects of sympathetic nervous system stimulation and to treat tachycardia.

CASE STUDY   *evolve*

Hyperthyroidism and Postmenopausal Osteoporosis

Mrs. Gonzales is a 55-year-old Hispanic woman who presents at a free clinic for migrant farm workers. She is dressed in a lightweight sundress and sandals despite outdoor temperatures around 50° F. Mrs. Gonzales complains of pounding in her chest and shortness of breath without exertion. She relates that she has lost 20 pounds in the last 6 weeks even though she has been eating more than usual. A thyroxine (T_4) level determined at the clinic is twice the normal value. The nurse practitioner has arranged for additional outpatient diagnostic studies. . . . *Case Study continued on the website and the CD-ROM with discussions, multiple-choice questions, and a nursing care plan.* *evolve*

■ Nursing Management of the Medical Client
Assessment

Begin your assessment by obtaining a complete history. By asking questions concerning weight, appetite, activity, heat intolerance, and bowel activity, you can assess for the presence of typical manifestations of hyperthyroidism. Also ask about mood alterations. Mood swings, irritability, decreased attention span, and manic behavior may be experienced by the client with hyperthyroidism. Because the client may not be aware of some of the mood changes, consider questioning significant others about changes in the client's behavior (see the Critical Monitoring feature on Thyrotoxicosis/Thyroid Storm, below.)

Diagnosis, Outcomes, Interventions

Diagnosis: Imbalanced Nutrition: Less than Body Requirements. A client with hyperthyroidism is hypermetabolic, leading to the nursing diagnosis *Imbalanced Nutrition: Less than Body Requirements related to accelerated metabolic rate resulting in weight loss and decreased energy levels.*

Outcomes. The client's weight loss will end as evidenced by an ability to consume sufficient calories to return to ideal body weight.

Interventions. Provide the client with a well-balanced, high-calorie diet. Clients with Graves' disease are usually extremely hungry because of the increased metabolism. Six full meals a day may be needed to satisfy their appetite. Despite unusually large meals, however, clients may lose weight rapidly; they are also usually in a state of negative nitrogen balance. Therefore encourage the client to eat foods that are nutritious and contain ample amounts of protein, carbohydrates, fats, and minerals. Discourage the ingestion of foods that increase peristalsis and thus result in diarrhea, such as highly seasoned, bulky, or fibrous foods.

The client should be weighed daily, and weight losses of more than 4.4 pounds (2 kg) should be reported. If the client continues to appear malnourished despite an ample diet, supplemental vitamins, particularly vitamin B complex, may be needed.

Diagnosis: Activity Intolerance. Another nursing diagnosis related to the client's hypermetabolic state is *Activity Intolerance related to exhaustion secondary to accelerated metabolic rate resulting in inability to perform activity without shortness of breath and significant increases in heart rate.*

Outcomes. The client will engage in a normal level of activity as evidenced by ability to maintain a proper balance of rest and activity to prevent exhaustion.

Interventions. Provide the client with an environment that is restful both mentally and physically. It is a challenge to help hyperthyroid clients relax. Assign the client to a private room to promote rest and to prevent the client from disturbing others through hyperactivity and restlessness.

Diagnosis: Risk for Injury. Many ocular problems can develop in a client with hyperthyroidism. Therefore an important nursing diagnosis for this client is *Risk for Injury: Corneal ulcerations, infection, and possible blindness related to inability to close the eyelids secondary to exophthalmos.*

Outcomes. The client will not experience corneal ulceration, infection, or blindness as evidenced by the lack of further development of exophthalmos.

Interventions. Treatment should be started as soon as possible after the diagnosis is made so that exophthalmos—a potentially permanent condition—can be avoided. The client should use artificial tears and eye patches as needed to prevent irritation if exophthalmos has already developed. When treatment has begun, the exophthalmos should not increase; however, it may not diminish quickly or at all.

Diagnosis: Hyperthermia. A client with hyperthyroidism is in a hypermetabolic state, leading to the nursing diagnosis *Hyperthermia related to accelerated metabolic rate resulting in fever, diaphoresis, and reported heat intolerance.*

Outcomes. The client will not exhibit hyperthermia as evidenced by a return to normal body temperature.

CRITICAL MONITORING

Thyrotoxicosis/Thyroid Storm

These manifestations should be monitored in a client who is thought at risk for thyroid storm:

- Anxiety, short attention span, irritability
- Hyperreflexia
- Increased temperature (as high as 106° F)
- Increased pulse (as high as 200 beats/min)
- Systolic hypertension
- Dyspnea
- Augmentation of other disorders, such as atrial fibrillation, heart failure, angina pectoris (chest pain), paranoia, and anxiety

Interventions. Tell the client to stay in a cool environment. Use only a lightweight sheet for the top cover, and give the client light, loose pajamas. The client who is diaphoretic may need fresh bed sheets and clothes frequently. Encourage the client not to overexert because doing so raises the body temperature and metabolic rate.

Diagnosis: Impaired Social Interaction. A client with hyperthyroidism is hyperactive, possibly leading to the nursing diagnosis *Impaired Social Interaction related to extreme agitation, hyperactivity, and mood swings resulting in inability to relate effectively with others.*

Outcomes. The client will not suffer from impaired social interaction as evidenced by his or her ability to interact without difficulty and without agitation, hyperactivity, or mood swings.

Interventions. Explain to the client's significant others that any bizarre, difficult behavior is likely to be temporary and should improve steadily with intervention. Maintain a quiet, understanding manner when caring for a client with Graves' disease. Accept the irritation and emotional outbursts as normal expressions of the disease.

Incorporate occupational therapy into care planning. The occupational therapist may be able to provide simple activities designed to distract the client from the disorder (such as putting together a puzzle with large pieces, molding clay, or watching television). For a very restless client, discuss with the physician the need for a sedative such as diazepam (Valium) or possibly an adrenergic blocking agent.

Evaluation

The client with Graves' disease should recover from the hyperthyroidism without difficulty when the medication regimen has begun.

■ Surgical Management

Thyroidectomy
Surgery for hyperthyroidism has been performed since the early 1880s. Thyroidectomy (removal of the thyroid gland) may be total or partial. *Total* thyroidectomy is performed to remove thyroid cancer. Clients who undergo this operation must take thyroid hormones permanently. *Subtotal* thyroidectomy is performed to correct hyperthyroidism and extreme cases of simple goiter. About five sixths of the gland is removed. Because one sixth of the functioning gland is left intact, hormone replacements may not be necessary.

Indications and Contraindications. Ideally, clients selected are young and free of any condition that makes them poor operative risks (e.g., diabetes, heart disease, renal disease, drug allergies).

Preoperative preparation for a subtotal thyroidectomy is extremely important. The client must be euthyroid before the operation, if possible. Preoperative care for a client with Graves' disease includes administration of antithyroid drugs to suppress secretion of thyroid hormones and iodine preparations to reduce the size and vascularity of the organ, thereby diminishing the chance of hemorrhage (see Medical Management earlier in this chapter). The client should be adequately rested, at optimal weight, and in good health before entering the operating room. Adequate preoperative preparation may take as long as 2 to 3 months.

Postoperative orders, rationales, and associated nursing interventions after thyroidectomy are presented in Table 45-2.

Complications. Besides the usual complications of any surgery, which include hemorrhage and infection, the client after thyroidectomy is at risk for thyroid storm, tetany, respiratory obstruction, laryngeal edema, and vocal cord injury. If the client is not euthyroid, the risk of intraoperative or postoperative thyroid storm is greatly increased.

Although uncommon, respiratory obstruction may result from swelling related to the surgical site. Rarely, vocal cord paralysis may result from nerve damage. Hypoparathyroidism may result from inadvertent removal of parathyroid gland tissue. The parathyroid glands lie just behind the lobes of the thyroid and are commonly disturbed and sometimes inadvertently removed during surgery. Careful postoperative monitoring of neurologic irritability and serum calcium levels is performed for this reason.

Outcomes. Surgical treatment is effective in most people with Graves' disease. A small percentage will remain hyperthyroid, and hypothyroidism develops in some.

■ Nursing Management of the Surgical Client
Assessment

Assess the client for typical manifestations of Graves' disease. A hypermetabolic state may be obvious from apparent weight loss, and exophthalmos may be obvious as well. Also, question the client about visual difficulties, fatigue, weakness, tremors, and insomnia

Diagnosis, Outcomes, Interventions

Diagnosis: Risk for Injury: Thyroid Storm, Hypocalcemia, or Hemorrhage. The client undergoing a thyroidectomy should be euthyroid preoperatively. Thus an important nursing diagnosis is *Risk for Injury: Thyroid*

TABLE 45-2 Postoperative Orders, Rationales, and Associated Nursing Interventions After Thyroidectomy

Postoperative Order	Rationale	Associated Nursing Interventions
Take vital signs every 15 min until stable; then every hour for next 24 hr.	After thyroidectomy, hemorrhage and respiratory obstruction may develop. Elevated pulse and hypotension indicate hemorrhage and shock. Dyspnea, stridulous respirations, and retraction of neck tissues indicate respiratory obstruction.	Check dressing after checking vital signs. Observe for bleeding at front, sides, and back of neck. Examine back of neck and shoulders for bleeding because blood tends to drain posteriorly. Check dressing for tightness; uncomfortable tautness may indicate bleeding into tissues. Loosen dressing and call surgeon immediately.
Use semi-Fowler position when client is conscious, unless client is hypotensive. Support head and neck with pillows and sandbags. Ambulation on day 2 as tolerated.	Immobilization of head and neck is essential to prevent flexion and hyperextension of neck with resultant strain on suture line. Semi-Fowler position used for comfort.	Place sandbags on either side of head for immobilization and good alignment. Warn client not to extend or hyperextend neck; reassure client that sandbags will prevent moving head too much. Gently rub back of neck to relieve tension. Support client's head and neck when moving or changing position.
Give fluids by mouth as tolerated. If nausea or vomiting, notify surgeon. Start soft diet on afternoon of day 2.	Give intravenous fluids if nausea or vomiting. Otherwise, start oral fluids as soon as client is fully conscious.	Maintain intake and output record for 2-3 days. Assess for difficulty swallowing. Normally this problem lasts for only 1-2 days postoperatively. Weigh client once a full diet is started; weight lost during early postoperative period should be regained.
Give morphine sulfate or other opioid agents every 1-2 hr as needed for pain in throat area.	Meperidine and morphine sulfate are both used during early postoperative period to relieve pain and promote rest.	Do not give opioids if client has respirations below 12 breaths/min or respiratory congestion. Consult physician for further orders. Do not oversedate clients with profuse respiratory secretions; give opioids judiciously.
Cough and deep-breathe every hour. Suction mouth and trachea if necessary.	Pooling of mucous secretions in trachea, bronchi, and lungs causes respiratory obstruction with resultant atelectasis and pneumonia. Secretions must be raised to prevent respiratory complications.	Instruct client to cough and deep-breathe as taught during the preoperative period. If client cannot raise secretions, gently suction mouth and trachea.
Have tracheostomy set, endotracheal tube, laryngoscope, and oxygen on hand.	Acute respiratory obstruction due to hemorrhage, edema of glottis, laryngeal nerve damage, or tetany is an emergency. Equipment for establishing an airway and administering oxygen must be available for immediate use.	Continuously assess for manifestations of airway obstruction, such as increasing restlessness, tachycardia, apprehension, cyanosis, stridulous respiration, and retraction of neck tissues. Report any of these manifestations to the surgeon immediately.
Give continuous mist inhalation until chest is clear.	Humidification of air promotes easier breathing and helps to liquefy mucous secretions.	Keep doors closed so that moist air is retained in room.
Take temperature every 4 hr for 24 hr, then routinely.	One of the first manifestations of thyroid storm is elevated temperature.	Carefully assess for manifestations of thyroid storm: elevated temperature, extreme restlessness, agitation, and tachycardia. Report any elevation over 100° F (37.7° C) rectally or 99° F (32.2° C) orally.
Assess client for hypocalcemia and monitor calcium, magnesium, and phos-	Inadvertent removal or devascularization of the parathyroid glands can cause postoperative hypoparathyroidism.	Mild hypocalcemia can be asymptomatic. Severe hypocalcemia can produce circumoral paresthesias, positive Chvostek's on Trousseau's sign. Administer calcium supplements for hypocalcemic levels.

storm, hypocalcemia, or hemorrhage related to surgical procedure and not being in a euthyroid state.

Outcomes. Thyroid storm, hypocalcemia, or hemorrhage will be prevented or detected early, and the client will be protected from injury.

Interventions

Promote Preoperative Euthyroid State. The client must be carefully prepared for a thyroidectomy to avoid complications (e.g., thyroid storm and hemorrhage). Outcomes of successful preparation for thyroid surgery are as follows:

- The client is euthyroid before entering the operating room. Tests of thyroid function are within normal limits.
- Manifestations of thyrotoxicosis are greatly diminished or absent. The client appears rested and relaxed.
- Weight and nutritional status are normal; any weight lost earlier has been regained.
- Cardiac problems are under control, pulse rate is normal, and preoperative electrocardiograms show no dangerous dysrhythmias.

To help meet these outcomes, antithyroid drugs, iodine preparations, bed rest, a nutritious diet, and supplemental vitamins are prescribed. Cardiac monitoring is maintained. Thorough preparation may take months. When good health has been restored, however, the client can undergo surgery with confidence that the operation will be successful and the manifestations alleviated.

Provide Postoperative Care. The immediate desired outcomes of postoperative care after thyroidectomy are to maintain airway patency, minimize strain on the suture line, relieve discomfort related to the sore throat and tracheal irritation, prevent pooling of respiratory secretions, prevent or relieve complications, and monitor for decreased parathyroid function.

Monitor for Postoperative Complications. Assemble the needed equipment at the bedside before the client returns from surgery. The equipment includes a blood pressure cuff and stethoscope, additional pillows, oxygen, suction equipment, intubation supplies, and a tracheostomy set. Ampules of calcium gluconate should be on hand in the medicine room or on the emergency cart (see the Critical Monitoring feature on Intravenous Calcium Infusion, above).

As noted earlier, major complications after thyroidectomy may include the following:

- Respiratory obstruction caused by edema of the glottis, bilateral laryngeal nerve damage, or tracheal compression from hemorrhage
- Hemorrhage
- Weakness and hoarseness of the voice from trauma or damage to one laryngeal nerve

---

CRITICAL MONITORING

Intravenous Calcium Infusion

Measures for safe administration of intravenous calcium include the following:

- Dilute to reduce vein irritation and venospasm.
- Administer into a large central or deep vein.
- Confirm patency of the IV prior to administration.
- Monitor vital signs and serum calcium levels.
- Observe for hyperchloremic acidosis if calcium carbonate is administered.
- Observe for extravasation. Necrosis and sloughing may occur.
- Inject 1% procaine hydrochloride and hyaluronidase using a 25- to 27-gauge needle if extravasation occurs to reduce vasospasm

---

- Hypocalcemia and tetany from accidental removal of one or more parathyroid glands
- Thyroid storm (if the client is not euthyroid preoperatively)

Promote Voice Rest. Temporary hoarseness and voice weakness may occur if there has been unilateral injury to the recurrent laryngeal nerve during surgery. To assess the voice, ask the client's name after full recovery from the anesthesia. Have the client speak every 30 to 60 minutes thereafter, and carefully note any voice changes. If hoarseness or voice weakness is present, reassure the client that the problem will probably subside in a few days. Discourage unnecessary talking to minimize hoarseness.

Monitor and Treat Hypocalcemia. Muscle twitching and hyperirritability of the nervous system may indicate hypocalcemic tetany. Hypocalcemia can develop after thyroidectomy if the parathyroid glands are accidentally removed during surgery. Manifestations may develop 1 to 7 days after surgery. Monitor the client for Chvostek's (facial nerve irritability) and Trousseau's (carpal spasm) signs; report positive responses to the physician immediately. Also call a physician if the client develops numbness and tingling around the mouth, fingertips, or toes; muscle spasms; or twitching. Make sure calcium gluconate ampules are available at the bedside and that the client has a patent intravenous line.

Evaluation

The client should be discharged within several days of surgery without difficulty. The wound should heal within about 6 weeks without infection.

■ Self-Care

Hyperthyroidism is a chronic disease that must be managed with the client's full participation. When the immediate postoperative period and its dangers have passed, turn your attention to teaching. Several important areas should be included.

Neck Exercises. First, teach the client how to support the weight of the head and neck when sitting up in bed. Show the client how to place the hands at the back of the head when flexing the neck or moving. The client probably will be able to perform this maneuver by the first postoperative day.

Second, as the wound heals (about the 2nd to 4th postoperative day), demonstrate range-of-motion exercises to prevent contractures. With the surgeon's permission, teach the client to flex the head forward and laterally, to hyperextend the neck, and to turn the head from side to side. Have the client perform these exercises several times every day.

Medications. If a total thyroidectomy has been performed, explain self-administration of thyroid medications (see the Client Education Guide feature on Thyroid Supplements on the website and the Integrating Pharmacology feature on Medications for Thyroid Disorders on p. 1196.) Teach the client the medication regimen and the need for lifelong replacement therapy.

Follow-up Monitoring. Make an appointment for the clinic or physician's office after discharge. Serum thyroid levels must be determined to monitor treatment. Emphasize that the client who has had a thyroidectomy must see a physician at least twice yearly to avert possible complications (e.g., hypothyroidism, hypoparathyroidism, recurrent hyperthyroidism) related to hormonal replacement. TH levels must be measured at regular intervals until the replacement medication is adjusted to a maintenance dose. The client should then see the physician twice a year for examinations.

Promote Wound Healing. Teach the client how to care for the incision when it has healed by using lanolin or vitamin E cream to soften the wound and minimize the scar.

■ Modifications for Older Clients

Hyperthyroidism in older adults accounts for 10% to 15% of all thyrotoxic clients. Some clients present with typical manifestations of hyperthyroidism, especially when the diagnosis is Graves' disease. Hyperthyroidism in older people is also notorious, however, for atypical or minimal manifestations. It is often overlooked because the manifestations are not the usual ones.

Indeed, manifestations are commonly attributed to aging. Weight loss, lack of ocular findings, and normal-sized thyroid glands are commonly found on assessment. Many clients actually appear apathetic instead of hyperactive. Cardiovascular abnormalities, such as heart failure, atrial dysrhythmias (usually digoxin resistant), and various degrees of heart block may be caused by hyperthyroidism. If the cardiac condition is pre-existing, it may be exacerbated by hyperthyroidism. Relative lack of tachycardia has been documented; about 40% of older clients have heart rates under 100 beats/min.

The diagnosis of hyperthyroidism is established by appropriate laboratory tests. It is usual to find elevated T_4 and suppressed TSH levels. Hyperthyroidism in older clients is treated with radioactive iodine.

THYROIDITIS

Thyroiditis (inflammation of the thyroid gland) appears in three basic forms:
- Acute suppurative
- Subacute thyroiditis, either granulomatous (painful or de Quervain's thyroiditis) or lymphocytic (silent or painless thyroiditis)
- Chronic thyroiditis, also known as Hashimoto's disease

Etiology and Risk Factors

Acute suppurative thyroiditis is an uncommon inflammatory disease usually caused by bacterial invasion in the form of an abscess of the thyroid gland. *Streptococcus pyogenes, Staphylococcus aureus,* and *Pneumococcus pneumoniae* are the most common etiologic agents. Acute thyroiditis is more common in females. Usually, it affects women between 20 and 40 years of age, but it also occurs in children and older people. Most affected clients have a pre-existing thyroid disorder.

Subacute granulomatous thyroiditis is a self-limiting inflammatory condition. No etiologic agent has been identified, although the condition may be viral in origin and commonly follows a respiratory infection. Autoimmune abnormalities have been described. There also appears to be a genetic predisposition to the development of both subacute granulomatous and lymphocytic thyroiditis. Of people with subacute granulomatous thyroiditis, 80% are women between 40 and 50 years of age.

Chronic thyroiditis (Hashimoto's disease) is the most common form of thyroiditis. It is more prevalent in women than in men and usually occurs between 20 and 50 years of age. Hashimoto's disease is a long-term inflammatory disorder. It is most commonly caused by autoimmune destruction of the thyroid gland. Genetic predisposition also plays a role in its causation.

Pathophysiology

Acute thyroiditis is a state of acute infection and inflammation. Usually, one lobe of the thyroid is more affected than the other. Follicular destruction, cell infiltration, and colloid depletion occur. Microabscesses form.

Subacute thyroiditis has three phases:

- *Phase 1:* The condition begins with a 3- to 4-week prodromal viral illness. Fever and malaise precede the sudden onset of a tender goiter. The thyroid gland may become two to three times its normal size. Mild hyperthyroidism may be present because of sudden release of thyroid hormones into the circulation as a result of the inflammation and destruction of the thyroid gland.
- *Phase 2:* Mild hypothyroidism develops because of incomplete recovery of the injured gland and exhaustion of stored thyroid hormones. Relapse may occur. Hypothyroidism is rarely permanent.
- *Phase 3:* The recovery phase may begin 2 to 4 months after onset.

Hashimoto's disease is manifested by an enlarged thyroid gland that may produce hypothyroid manifestations if the gland is destroyed by the autoimmune system. A euthyroid state may prevail if the gland is not destroyed.

Clinical Manifestations

Manifestations of acute thyroiditis include abrupt onset of unilateral anterior neck pain with possible radiation to the ear or mandible on the affected side. Fever, diaphoresis, and other manifestations of bacterial toxicity may also be present.

Subacute granulomatous thyroiditis is usually painful, whereas subacute lymphocytic thyroiditis is usually painless. Assessment data may include characteristic anterior, unilateral neck pain that may have an abrupt onset, usually after a respiratory infection or viral episode. Radiation to the ear on the ipsilateral side may occur. Manifestations of viral infection, such as myalgia, low-grade fever, lassitude, and sore throat may occur. About 50% of clients present with thyrotoxicosis.

Subacute lymphocytic thyroiditis is characterized by occasional hyperthyroidism and a painless goiter. The goiter is firm, diffuse, and mildly enlarged.

Manifestations of chronic thyroiditis include painless, asymmetrical enlargement of the gland, which causes pressure on the surrounding structures and can lead to dysphagia and respiratory distress. Most clients are euthyroid, about 20% are hypothyroid, and fewer than 5% are hyperthyroid.

The diagnosis of thyroiditis may be confirmed by evaluation of serum T_3, FT_4, ^{131}I uptake, TSH, erythrocyte sedimentation rate, and thyroid antibodies. Clients with acute thyroiditis are typically euthyroid according to laboratory tests.

For subacute granulomatous thyroiditis, laboratory findings reveal hyperthyroidism in about 50% of clients. With subacute lymphocytic thyroiditis, laboratory diagnosis includes decreased radioactive iodine uptake, elevated T_3 and T_4, and frequently positive thyroid antibodies.

In chronic thyroiditis, immune antibodies are usually positive. Other thyroid function levels may be normal, increased, or decreased.

Outcome Management
■ Medical Management

Acute thyroiditis usually responds to parenteral antibiotic therapy. Treatment of subacute granulomatous thyroiditis is supportive. Therapy may include salicylates, nonsteroidal anti-inflammatory agents (NSAIDs), and oral glucocorticoids such as prednisone. The desired outcome of treatment in subacute lymphocytic thyroiditis is to provide relief of manifestations of hyperthyroidism with beta-adrenergic blocking agents. Antithyroid medications are not indicated.

The course of Hashimoto's disease varies. Some clients experience spontaneous remission, whereas others remain stable for years. In about one third of cases, hypothyroidism develops from gradual atrophy of the gland. Intervention is intended to reduce the size of the gland and correct any thyroid function abnormalities. Immunologic tests are not useful in monitoring these clients.

■ Surgical Management

Clients with acute thyroiditis that does not respond to medical treatment may require incision and drainage of the affected gland. Depending on the size of the thyroid area to be incised and concurrent medical problems, the procedure can be done in the physician's office or during a short stay in the hospital. A fine-needle biopsy may be performed to rule out malignancy in chronic thyroiditis.

■ Nursing Management of the Medical-Surgical Client

Nursing care of a client with thyroiditis is usually supportive until the diagnosis is made. Then, as with other thyroid disorders, care revolves around helping the client learn correct medication administration. If surgery is necessary, care is the same as discussed earlier.

Discharge teaching focuses on ensuring that the client understands the medication and how to take it. Thyroid function is monitored at regular intervals after client discharge for development of hyperthyroidism or hypothyroidism and for testing the effectiveness of medication.

THYROID CANCER

The incidence of thyroid cancer is rising. One reason may be the maturation of people who were exposed to low-dose radiation early in life. Thyroid cancer estimates for 2003 in the United States were for 22,000 new cases and about 1400 cancer deaths.[1] The ratio of females to males is about 3:1. Its incidence peaks during the 60s, but it may arise from infancy to old age. Mortality is lowest in the young if the cancer is well differentiated.

Etiology and Risk Factors

Benign adenomas are usually not dangerous, although they occasionally grow large enough to cause respiratory problems by pressing against the trachea. Malignant transformation sometimes occurs, and the benign nodules become cancerous. Also, malignant transformation of benign nodules apparently can follow prolonged stimulation of the thyroid gland by TSH. Other risk factors include genetic predisposition, a family history of thyroid cancer, and a history of radiation therapy 10 to 20 years following cancer treatment elsewhere in the body.

Pathophysiology

Papillary and follicular carcinomas are the two most frequent types of thyroid cancers. They are usually referred to as *differentiated* thyroid cancer. The papillary form accounts for about 75% of thyroid cancers, and the follicular form accounts for 15% to 20% of thyroid cancers. Both are slow-growing firm tumors that are palpable, and they may spread to regional lymph nodes in 15% (follicular) to 50% (papillary) of cases.[18]

Benign adenomas and malignant thyroid tumors constitute the third most common cause of thyroid enlargement, with hypothyroidism and hyperthyroidism being the two most common causes. Benign adenomas are usually well encapsulated and as a result do not spread into other tissues.

Clinical Manifestations

The major manifestation of thyroid cancer is the appearance of a hard, irregular, painless nodule in an enlarged thyroid gland. The nodule itself is typically solitary, rapidly enlarging, and "cold" (i.e., it does not take up radioactive iodine) in contrast to benign adenomas, which may take up radioactive iodine. The examiner can make this determination by giving a tracer dose of ^{131}I and performing a thyroid scan 24 hours later to assess ^{131}I uptake by any nodules. "Hot" nodules absorb more isotope than normal tissue and are usually benign.

If the tumor has metastasized, the lymph nodes are sometimes palpable. In long-standing cases, the client may have respiratory difficulty and dysphagia (difficulty swallowing) resulting from the enlarged thyroid pressing against neck structures. The diagnosis of thyroid cancer is confirmed by fine-needle aspiration biopsy.

Outcome Management
■ Medical Management

Without prompt, aggressive therapy, a client with thyroid cancer risks death. Chemotherapy, ^{131}I, external radiation, or TSH suppressive therapy may be used for metastasis, as discussed earlier. A client with a benign nodule is likely to undergo long-term suppression therapy with levothyroxine. The desired outcome is to suppress serum TSH without causing hypothyroidism.

EB EVIDENCE-BASED PRACTICE IN ACTION

Use of the Internet to Support People with Rare Cancers

Client education is an integral part of nursing practice. At times nurses are not aware of current trends in treatment provided outside their practice settings, or clients are dismissed before their learning needs can be met. Consumers frequently turn to the Internet to seek health-related information.[1] One study suggests that the public may not view nurses as expert health care knowledge providers.[2]

Psychosocial support was an area of need identified by one group of cancer clients. They also identified needs in the communication and information area.[3] The use of information technology to provide health-related information has been explored for a variety of health topics.[4]

Implications

Health care consumers are turning to the Internet for health-related information. Nurses are capable of providing knowledgeable health-related information. Several venues exist on the Internet to provide this information, including list servers, nursing journal sites, and general consumer health sites. Nurses must expand their thinking to encompass the necessity for monitoring health sites for current reliable information and passing this information and the availability of reliable sites on to their clients.

References
1. Clark, P., & Gomez, E. (2000). Details of demand: Consumers, cancer information, and the Internet. *Clinical Journal of Oncology Nursing, 5,* 19-24.
2. Floyd, J. (2000). The public's uses of nurses for health care advice. *Journal of Nursing Scholarship, 32,* 220.
3. Sanson-Fisher, R., Girgis, A., & Boyes, A. (2000). The unmet supportive care needs of patients with cancer. *Cancer, 88,* 226-237.
4. Schultz, P. (2002). Providing information to patients with a rare cancer: Using internet discussion forums to address the needs of patients with medullary thyroid carcinoma. *Clinical Journal of Oncology Nursing, 6*(4), 219-222.

■ Surgical Management

Treatment usually includes removal of all or part of the thyroid. Neck resection may be done for metastases to the neck. (Thyroid surgery has been covered earlier.) As with a thyroidectomy for noncancerous lesions, the major postoperative complications are respiratory distress, recurrent laryngeal damage, hemorrhage, and hypoparathyroidism.

■ Nursing Management of the Medical-Surgical Client

Nursing care of the client with thyroid cancer is similar to the care of any client undergoing a thyroidectomy. The client also needs the support and teaching that a client with cancer requires. If the client is to have chemotherapy, additional teaching is needed (see the **EB** Evidence-Based Practice in Action feature on Use of the Internet to Support People with Rare Cancers on p. 1208).

If the client has undergone a total thyroidectomy, replacement of thyroid hormones is necessary. Discharge teaching focuses on ensuring that the client understands the medication and how to take it. Home health needs reflect those of any client after thyroidectomy or receiving chemotherapy or radiation therapy. The client should be checked at regular intervals for recurrence, and thyroid function should be monitored.

■ PARATHYROID DISORDERS
HYPERPARATHYROIDISM

Hyperparathyroidism, a disorder caused by overactivity of one or more of the parathyroid glands, is classified as primary, secondary, or tertiary. It usually occurs in clients older than 60 and affects women twice as often as men. It is not related to age in clients with renal failure. The overall incidence of hyperparathyroidism is 27 per 100,000.[22]

Etiology and Risk Factors

Primary hyperparathyroidism develops when the normal regulatory relationship between serum calcium levels and parathyroid hormone (PTH) secretion is interrupted. The interruption occurs when an adenoma or hyperplasia of the gland exists without an identifying injury.

Secondary hyperparathyroidism occurs when the glands are hyperplastic because of malfunction of another organ system. It is usually the result of renal failure but may also occur with osteogenesis imperfecta, Paget's disease, multiple myeloma, or carcinoma with bone metastasis.

Tertiary hyperparathyroidism occurs when PTH production is irrepressible (autonomous) in clients with normal or low serum calcium levels.

Pathophysiology

The normal function of PTH is to increase bone resorption, thereby maintaining the proper balance of calcium and phosphorus ions in the blood (see Chapter 44). Excessive circulating PTH leads to bone damage, hypercalcemia, and kidney damage.

Primary Hyperparathyroidism

The severity of hypercalcemia reflects the quantity of hyperfunctioning parathyroid tissue. Excessive PTH stimulates transport of calcium into the blood from the intestine, kidneys, and bone. Nephrolithiasis is secondary to calcium phosphate kidney stones and deposition of calcium in the soft tissues of the kidney. Pyelonephritis may complicate the nephrolithiasis. Bone resorption related to hypercalcemia may develop.

Myopathy is a common condition characterized by neuropathic atrophy and proximal muscle weakness. Hypercalcemia can stimulate hypergastrinemia, abdominal pain, and peptic ulcer disease. Pancreatitis is also influenced by high calcium levels.

Secondary Hyperparathyroidism

Chronic renal failure and hyperphosphatemia cause secondary hyperparathyroidism. As the glomerular filtration rate (GFR) decreases in chronic renal failure, serum phosphorus levels rise, which causes the serum calcium level to fall. PTH secretion is stimulated. This increase decreases renal tubular absorption of phosphorus, causing serum phosphorus levels to return to normal. As the GFR continues to decrease, PTH is secreted in increased amounts to decrease tubular reabsorption of phosphorus and maintain serum phosphorus at or close to normal limits.

Clinical Manifestations

Some clients with hyperparathyroidism may be asymptomatic. Others have myriad manifestations arising from the skeletal disease, renal involvement, gastrointestinal tract disorders, and neurologic abnormalities, as outlined in the Critical Monitoring feature on Hyperparathyroidism and Hypoparathyroidism on p. 1210 and in Figure 45-3.

Manifestations of bone disease range from backache, joint pain, and bone pain to pathologic fractures of the spine, ribs, and long bones. In long-standing cases, assessment reveals deformity and bending of the bones. Osteitis fibrosa with superperiosteal resorption or bone cysts, arthritis, or radiologic osteoporosis may be diagnosed.

Manifestations of renal involvement include polyuria and polydipsia; the appearance of sand, gravel, or stones (calculi) in the urine; azotemia; and hypertension

FIGURE 45-3 Clinical manifestations of primary hyperparathyroidism. (Modified from Strewler, G.J., & Rosenblatt, M. [1995]. Mineral metabolism. In P. Felig, J.D. Baxter, & L.A. Frohman [Eds.], *Endocrinology and metabolism* [3rd ed., pp. 1407-1499]. New York: McGraw-Hill.)

CRITICAL MONITORING

Hyperparathyroidism and Hypoparathyroidism

These manifestations should be monitored in a client who is thought to have a diagnosis of hyperparathyroidism or hypoparathyroidism.

Hyperparathyroidism	Hypoparathyroidism
Increased bone resorption	Decreased bone resorption
Elevated serum calcium levels	Depressed serum calcium levels
Depressed serum phosphate levels	Elevated serum phosphate levels
Hypercalciuria and hyperphosphaturia	Hypocalciuria and hypophosphaturia
Decreased neuromuscular irritability	Increased neuromuscular activity, which may progress to tetany

resulting from renal damage. Without intervention, renal insufficiency may progress to fatal renal hypertension and uremia.

Hypercalcemia produces mainly gastrointestinal manifestations such as thirst, nausea, anorexia, constipation, ileus, and abdominal pain. Decreased neuromuscular ir-

ritability is also common. Often, clients have a history of peptic ulcer or gastrointestinal bleeding. Assessment may also reveal psychiatric manifestations. Listlessness, depression, and paranoia are sometimes associated with high levels of serum calcium. Finally, calcification may form in the eyes, impairing vision.

Major complications include the manifestations associated with hypercalcemia and those associated with treatment, such as dehydration, hypocalcemia, and gastrointestinal problems.

The diagnosis of hyperparathyroidism mainly rests on laboratory and x-ray findings. Serum calcium levels are elevated, serum phosphate levels are depressed, and both urine calcium and phosphorus levels are high. In addition, alkaline phosphatase is elevated in the 25% of clients who have associated bone disease (see Table 44-2). Clients with skeletal damage have the following characteristic x-ray findings: diffuse demineralization of bones, bone cysts, subperiosteal bone resorption, and loss of the lamina dura around the teeth. Ultrasonography or magnetic resonance imaging (MRI) may be used for preoperative localization of the parathyroid glands.

Outcome Management
■ Medical Management

The desired outcomes of the medical treatment of hyperparathyroidism include lowering severely elevated calcium levels and long-term management of hypercalcemia with drugs to increase bone resorption of calcium.

Lower Elevated Calcium Levels. Serum calcium levels are lowered by hydration and calciuria. Hydration can be achieved with an infusion of normal saline solution. Normal saline is the fluid of choice because it both expands the volume and acts in the kidney to inhibit the resorption of calcium. Furosemide (Lasix), a loop diuretic, may also be used to promote calciuria after rehydration has occurred. Thiazide diuretics are not used because they promote calcium retention in the kidneys. A client with hypercalcemia should have a diet low in calcium and vitamin D.

Antiresorption Agents. Drugs that inhibit bone resorption include plicamycin (Mithracin), gallium nitrate (Ganite), phosphates, and calcitonin. Plicamycin is a chemotherapeutic drug that is effective in lowering serum calcium levels. The hypocalcemic effect occurs after 24 hours and lasts about 1 to 2 weeks. The dose is about one tenth that used for cancer treatment, and the adverse effects are proportionally lower.

Gallium nitrate, a newer drug, is now being used more often because it has even fewer side effects. Glucocorticoids may be used to reduce hypercalcemia by decreasing the gastrointestinal absorption of calcium. Etidronate (Didronel) or calcitonin can be used to decrease the release of calcium by bones. (See the Integrating Pharmacology feature on Medications for Parathyroid Disorders at right.)

■ Nursing Management of the Medical Client

Assessment

There are no obvious manifestations of hyperparathyroidism and the resultant hypercalcemia. Elicit a good history from the client to determine whether any risk factors are present. The client may exhibit psychological changes, such as lethargy, drowsiness, memory loss, and emotional lability, all manifestations seen in hypercalcemia.

Diagnosis, Outcomes, Interventions

Diagnosis: Risk for Injury. The client with hyperparathyroidism is at great risk for injury, leading to the nursing diagnosis *Risk for Injury related to demineralization of bones resulting in pathologic fractures.*

Outcomes. The client will remain free from injury as evidenced by the absence of pathologic fractures or hypercalcemia.

Interventions

Prevent Fractures. Protect the client from accidents. If bone involvement exists, pathologic fractures may develop from even small bumps or minor falls. Keep the client's bed in the low position and use the side rails. If

---

INTEGRATING PHARMACOLOGY
Medications for Parathyroid Disorders

The desired outcomes of the medical treatment of hyperparathyroidism include lowering severely elevated calcium levels and long-term management of hypercalcemia with drugs to increase bone resorption of calcium.

Serum calcium levels are lowered by hydration and calciuria. Furosemide (Lasix) a loop diuretic, may be used to promote calciuria. Drugs that inhibit bone resorption include plicamycin (Mithracin), gallium nitrate (Ganite), phosphates, and calcitonin. Plicamycin is a chemotherapeutic drug that is effective in lowering serum calcium levels. The hypocalcemic effect occurs after 24 hours and lasts for about 1 to 2 weeks. Gallium nitrate may be used because it has fewer side effects.

Glucocorticoids may be used to reduce hypercalcemia by decreasing gastrointestinal absorption of calcium. In addition, Etidronate (Didronel) or calcitonin may be used to decrease the release of calcium by bones.

For clients with chronic hypoparathyroidism, the desired outcome of intervention is to restore the serum calcium level to normal concentrations. In clients with acute hypoparathyroidism, 10% calcium gluconate solution in an intravenous infusion is ordered. In chronic hypoparathyroidism, the client is given oral calcium salts (calcium gluconate, calcium lactate, or calcium carbonate) to maintain normal serum calcium levels. The client may also be given vitamin D to maintain serum calcium levels. Some clients may receive replacement of the absent hormone.

---

the client is weak or has joint or skeletal disease, help with ambulation.

Assist with Activities. If the client suffers from severe osteoporosis or pathologic fractures, some assistance may be required at home. The client may need a visiting nurse to help assess the home situation and to make recommendations about how safety might be enhanced. The home should be cleared of articles that can increase the risk of falling, such as throw rugs. The client may also need assistive devices, such as a railing in the bathroom, a bedside commode, or a walker.

Diagnosis: Impaired Urinary Elimination. The development of urinary lithiasis in clients with hyperparathyroidism may lead to the nursing diagnosis *Impaired Urinary Elimination related to renal involvement secondary to hypercalcemia and hyperphosphaturia resulting in urolithiasis, painful urination, hematuria, and spasms.*

Outcomes. The client will resume a normal urine output as evidenced by urine production of 0.5 ml/kg/hr without development of stones.

Interventions

Encourage Fluids. The client should consume at least 3000 ml of fluid each day. Dehydration is dangerous in clients with hyperparathyroidism because it increases the serum calcium level and promotes the formation of renal stones.

Prevent Urolithiasis. Cranberry juice or prune juice may help make the urine more acidic. Acidification helps to prevent renal stone formation because calcium is more soluble in acidic urine than in alkaline urine.

Strain Urine of Stones. If a kidney stone is present, strain all urine to detect gravel and stones. Save any specimens of abnormal urine for the physician to examine and for laboratory analysis. Also, observe the urine for blood and assess the client for renal colic (see Chapter 36).

Diagnosis: Imbalanced Nutrition: Less Than Body Requirements.

The client is likely to experience nutritional problems, suggesting the nursing diagnosis *Imbalanced Nutrition: Less than Body Requirements related to anorexia and nausea resulting in decreased food intake and weight loss.*

Outcomes. The client will have an adequate intake as evidenced by absence of nausea and return to or maintenance of ideal body weight.

Interventions. Encourage a low-calcium diet to correct hypercalcemia. Explain that abstaining from milk and milk products may help to alleviate some of the distressing gastrointestinal manifestations. A client who has peptic ulcers needs to take antacids or histamine receptor antagonists. Help the client create a diet that is high enough in calories without dairy products. If necessary, have the client see a dietitian to help with meal planning.

Diagnosis: Constipation.

A client with hyperparathyroidism is susceptible to bowel problems, leading to the nursing diagnosis *Constipation related to adverse effects of hypercalcemia on the gastrointestinal tract resulting in decreased frequency of stools and painful defecation.*

Outcomes. The client will maintain a normal bowel pattern as evidenced by a daily, soft, formed bowel movement.

Interventions. Work to prevent constipation and fecal impaction resulting from hypercalcemia. Help the client stay as active as the extent of bone disease allows. Increase fluid intake and the amount of fiber in the diet. The client should drink at least six to eight glasses of water a day unless contraindicated. If constipation continues despite these measures, obtain an order for a stool softener or laxative.

Evaluation

Depending on the cause of the hypercalcemia, medical management may be able to control primary hypercalcemia. If it does not, surgery may be required. If the condition is secondary to renal failure, management is more chronic.

■ Surgical Management

Parathyroidectomy

Indications. Definitive treatment of primary hyperparathyroidism is surgical removal of the gland or glands causing hypersecretion of PTH. Intra-operative, rapid parathyroid hormone assay measurement affords the ability to ensure removal of all hyperfunctioning parathyroid tissue.

Autotransplantation of the parathyroid glands is a useful modality for the management of certain forms of hyperparathyroidism and radical neck surgery. After partial parathyroidectomy, it is possible to transplant the remaining healthy parathyroid tissue to a safer location, such as the brachioradial muscle of the forearm. Reexploration of the neck in the future may cause laryngeal nerve damage and influence complications of the original surgery. Transplantation procedures take some time to come to full effect. In the meantime, the client must supplement the diet with calcium and vitamin D to prevent hypoparathyroidism and hypocalcemia.

If hyperparathyroidism is surgically treated early in its course, the chance of total recovery is good. Bone pain may disappear within 3 days after removal of parathyroid tissue, and bone lesions may heal completely. Unfortunately, serious renal disease might not be reversible by parathyroid surgery.

Complications. Complications after parathyroidectomy are similar to those following thyroidectomy and rarely occur. Hypocalcemia is a potentially life-threatening complication even if some parathyroid glands are left untouched because edema reduces their function. The client may also experience respiratory distress related to either hemorrhage or recurrent laryngeal nerve damage.

Outcomes. The cure rate for primary hyperparathyroidism after surgical removal is greater than 95%. This high success rate is directly related to the experience of the surgeon and adequate exploration of the neck.

■ Nursing Management of the Surgical Client
Assessment

The client undergoing surgery may have long-standing hyperparathyroidism and thus should be assessed for complications of the disease. Renal function should be carefully assessed preoperatively.

Diagnosis, Outcomes, Interventions

Diagnosis: Risk for Injury.
The client undergoing surgery for hyperparathyroidism is at risk for a number of complications. An important nursing diagnosis is *Risk for Injury related to preoperative drug sensitivities and postoperative complications.*

Outcomes.
The client will not suffer injury as evidenced by the absence of medication reactions preoperatively and by the absence of respiratory distress, hemorrhage, and hypocalcemia postoperatively.

Interventions

Administer Digitalis. If the client is receiving digitalis, administer this medication with extreme caution. Clients with hypercalcemia are hypersensitive to digitalis, and toxic manifestations may develop quickly.

Monitor for Postoperative Complications. During the postoperative period, new problems arise, some of which are the reverse of those found preoperatively. During the immediate postoperative period, nursing care is similar to that after thyroidectomy; that is, assess the client carefully for hemorrhage, airway obstruction, injury to the recurrent laryngeal nerve, and tetany. Also watch for manifestations of hormonal imbalance.

Mild tetany resulting from a drop in the serum calcium level is expected after removal of parathyroid tissue. Typically, the uncomfortable tingling of the hands and around the mouth that follows parathyroid resection is temporary. If it persists or is severe, however, calcium gluconate is administered intravenously.

Prevent Osteoporosis. Clients with bone disease require additional therapy after surgery. Removal of the parathyroid glands reduces bone resorption, and because bone rebuilding proceeds at a rapid rate, the client may experience the "hungry bones" syndrome. This syndrome is characterized by hypocalcemia and severe tetany resulting from the rapid utilization of calcium by the bones.

To prevent low serum calcium levels resulting from bone recalcification, instruct the client to eat foods high in calcium. Tetany is treated with injections of calcium gluconate. To maintain adequate calcium levels, the client usually takes oral calcium preparations for months until the skeletal tissues have been rebuilt. Finally, encourage ambulation as soon as possible after surgery because weight-bearing speeds the recalcification process.

Evaluation

If hypercalcemia remains unrelieved by medical management, surgery is usually therapeutic. If a partial parathyroidectomy is unsuccessful, the remaining gland may need to be transplanted to the forearm to reduce ab-sorption of the hormone. This measure usually eliminates the problem. As long as the client is closely observed in the immediate postoperative period, complications of hypocalcemia are usually controllable.

■ Modifications for Older Clients
Hyperparathyroidism in older adults is an overlooked disease. It is estimated that 1 of 1000 men and 2 of 1000 women older than 60 years of age experience hyperparathyroidism.[15] This disease often goes undiagnosed in older people because manifestations in the early stages are subtle and attributed to old age, depression, or anxiety. The manifestations intensify as the serum calcium level continues to rise and other physiologic and functional changes occur. Laboratory diagnosis is the same as for a younger client, but treatment may be complicated by medical problems and medication.

HYPOPARATHYROIDISM
Hyposecretion of the parathyroid glands produces hypoparathyroidism—the reverse of hyperparathyroidism. That is, serum calcium levels are abnormally low, serum phosphate levels are abnormally high, and pronounced neuromuscular irritability (tetany) may develop.

Hypoparathyroidism is diagnosed in women more often than men. The incidence is related to thyroid surgery. The incidence of temporary hypoparathyroidism after total thyroidectomy ranges from 6.9% to 25%. The incidence after subtotal thyroidectomy is 1.6% to 9%.[14]

Etiology and Risk Factors
The causes of hypoparathyroidism are either *iatrogenic* (treatment-induced) or *idiopathic* (without a specific cause). Iatrogenic causes include accidental removal of the parathyroid glands during thyroidectomy, infarction of the parathyroid glands because of an inadequate blood supply to the glands during surgery, and strangulation of one or more of the glands by postoperative scar tissue. Health maintenance actions include monitoring of PTH, calcium, and phosphorus levels. Calcium supplements are required for life to prevent tetany.

Idiopathic hypoparathyroidism, like Graves' disease and Hashimoto's disease, may be an autoimmune disorder with a genetic basis. It is far less common than the iatrogenic form. *Pseudohypoparathyroidism* (Albright's hereditary osteodystrophy) is an inherited form of hypoparathyroidism that involves a lack of end-organ responsiveness to PTH.

Pathophysiology
Normally PTH acts to increase bone resorption, which maintains proper serum calcium levels. The hormone also regulates phosphate clearance by the renal tubules, thereby maintaining the correct inverse balance between serum calcium and serum phosphate. Consequently, when parathyroid secretion is reduced, bone resorption slows, serum calcium levels fall, and severe neuromuscu-

lar irritability develops. Somewhat paradoxically, calcifications form in various organs, such as the eyes and basal ganglia. Also, without sufficient PTH, fewer phosphorus ions are secreted by the distal tubules of the kidney, renal excretion of phosphate falls, and serum phosphate levels rise.

The client may fully recover from the effects of hypoparathyroidism if the condition is diagnosed early, before serious complications begin. Unfortunately, cataracts and brain calcification, once formed, are irreversible.

Clinical Manifestations

The manifestations of hypoparathyroidism result mainly from low serum calcium levels. Manifestations are always more severe in clients with an elevated serum pH (alkalosis) of any cause (e.g., hyperventilation, ingestion of antacids). They worsen because, when the pH of the blood rises, the amount of ionized calcium drops, although total serum calcium remains the same. With less ionized calcium available to the body, the manifestations resulting from hypocalcemia become more severe until the alkalosis is corrected.

Acute Hypoparathyroidism

Acute hypoparathyroidism is caused by accidental damage to parathyroid tissues during thyroidectomy. It is characterized by greatly increased neuromuscular irritability, which results in tetany. Clients with tetany experience painful muscle spasms, irritability, grimacing, tingling of the fingers, laryngospasm, and dysrhythmias. Assessment also reveals Chvostek's and Trousseau's signs. In some cases, tetany is so severe that a tracheostomy is required to correct acute respiratory obstruction secondary to laryngospasm.

Chronic Hypoparathyroidism

Chronic hypoparathyroidism is usually idiopathic, resulting in lethargy; thin, patchy hair; brittle nails; dry, scaly skin; and personality changes. Ectopic or unexpected calcification may appear in the eyes and basal ganglia. Thus cataracts and permanent brain damage, accompanied by psychosis or convulsions, may develop. In addition, severe persistent hypocalcemia adversely affects the heart, causing dysrhythmias and eventual cardiac failure.

The diagnosis of hypoparathyroidism is based on the following physical examination findings related to hypocalcemia:

- Presence of Chvostek's sign (spasms of facial muscles after a tap over the facial nerve, signifying facial hyperirritability) (see Figure 14-3)
- Presence of Trousseau's sign (spasms of the wrist and hand after compression of the upper arm, as by a blood pressure cuff) (see Figure 14-3)
- Hyperactive deep tendon reflexes (DTRs)
- Circumoral paresthesia

- Numbness and tingling of fingers

The diagnosis of hypoparathyroidism also stems from the following findings:

- Laboratory findings showing low calcium, low PTH, high phosphorus, decreased urine calcium
- Radiographic studies of the skull or computed tomography (CT) of the head showing areas of calcification
- Ophthalmic examination revealing calcification of the ocular lens, which may lead to cataract formation

Complications

If treatment is not started rapidly in acute hypoparathyroidism, death can result from the respiratory obstruction secondary to tetany and laryngospasms. In chronic hypoparathyroidism, the complications are calcifications in the eye and basal ganglia; these complications can occur if treatment is delayed.

Outcome Management
■ Medical Management

Acute hypoparathyroidism (with its major manifestation of acute tetany) is a life-threatening disorder. The desired outcomes of emergency care are to elevate serum calcium levels as rapidly as possible, to prevent or treat seizures, and to control laryngeal spasm and consequent respiratory obstruction.

For clients with chronic hypoparathyroidism, the desired outcome of intervention is to restore the serum calcium level to normal concentrations. The calcium level is increased more gradually than in acute hypoparathyroidism.

Elevate Serum Calcium

Calcium Gluconate. In clients with acute hypoparathyroidism, to elevate serum calcium levels quickly, the physician prescribes 10% calcium gluconate solution in an intravenous infusion. While administering the calcium gluconate, instruct the client to inhale carbon dioxide by breathing into a paper bag. Carbon dioxide inhalation causes a mild metabolic acidosis, which elevates the amount of ionized calcium in the blood.

Oral Calcium Replacements. When the condition has stabilized and the dangers of tetany have passed, the client is given oral calcium salts to maintain normal serum calcium levels. The desired outcome of therapy for chronic hypoparathyroidism is to keep the client asymptomatic with a serum calcium level of about 8.5 to 9.2 mg/dl. The client is given oral calcium salts (calcium gluconate, calcium lactate, or calcium carbonate).

Vitamin D. The client is given vitamin D in addition to calcium supplements to maintain serum calcium levels. Commercially available forms of vitamin D include ergocalciferol (vitamin D_2) and dihydrotachysterol (Hytakerol). Although ergocalciferol is a more reliable and less expensive drug than dihydrotachysterol or dihydroxycholecalciferol, all three forms of vitamin D are effective in correcting hypocalcemia. They are available as either tablets or oily liquids. Aluminum hydroxide gel (Amphojel) is also prescribed.

Parathyroid Hormone. The ideal treatment of this PTH-deficient condition is replacement of the absent hormone. A pure form of PTH has now been synthesized and is available (see the Integrating Pharmacology feature on Medications for Parathyroid Disorders on p. 1211).

High-Calcium, Low-Phosphate Diet. A client with hypoparathyroidism should receive a diet high in calcium but low in phosphorus. Again, vitamin D is needed to maintain serum calcium levels, and clients should be encouraged to select foods or supplements enriched with vitamin D.

Address Seizures and Laryngeal Spasm. Tetany and laryngeal spasms may occur suddenly and without warning in clients at risk for acute hypoparathyroidism. Calcium gluconate should be readily available at the bedside, and in many cases an order is left to have a tracheotomy tray available at the bedside.

■ Nursing Management of the Medical Client
Assessment

Carefully assess the client at risk for acute hypoparathyroidism (e.g., the post-thyroidectomy client) for development of hypocalcemia. Question the client about any numbness or tingling around the mouth or in the fingertips or toes. Check for Chvostek's and Trousseau's signs. In addition, assess for any manifestation of respiratory distress secondary to laryngospasm.

In a client with chronic hypoparathyroidism, assess for obvious physical changes, such as dry skin and hair. Also assess for a Parkinson-like syndrome or cataracts. Assess the teeth because pits may encircle them, indicating enamel hypoplasia.

Diagnosis, Outcomes, Interventions

Diagnosis: Risk for Injury: Muscle Tetany. A client
with hypoparathyroidism is susceptible to hypocalcemia, which can lead to the nursing diagnosis *Risk for Injury: Muscle tetany related to decreased serum calcium levels.*

Outcomes. The client will remain free from injury as evidenced by a return of calcium levels to normal range, a normal respiratory rate, and blood gases within normal limits.

Interventions
Prevent Respiratory Arrest. When caring for a client with severe hypoparathyroidism, always be prepared

for laryngeal spasm and respiratory obstruction. Have an endotracheal tube, laryngoscope, and tracheostomy set available when caring for a client with acute tetany.

Monitor and Prevent Tetany. When a client is at risk for sudden hypocalcemia, as after thyroidectomy, an ampule of intravenous calcium carbonate is usually kept at the bedside for immediate use if necessary. When the intravenous tubing is removed, it is sometimes capped so that rapid venous access is available. Sometimes clients are encouraged to take in a ready source of calcium carbonate, such as Tums.

Evaluation

If the hypocalcemia is transient after a thyroidectomy, it usually resolves as edema decreases. If it is chronic, the client is usually able to manage the therapeutic regimen with minimal difficulty.

■ Self-Care
Because hypoparathyroidism can be a chronic condition, the client must be able to provide self-care. Teaching is important for the client with chronic hypoparathyroidism because this client requires lifelong medication and dietary modification.

Medications. When teaching the client about take-home medications, make sure the client knows that all forms of vitamin D, except dihydroxycholecalciferol, are slowly assimilated by the body. Therefore it may take a week or longer for the manifestations to improve.

Diet Modifications. Teach the client about a diet high in calcium but low in phosphorus. Remind the client to omit cheese and milk products, which have high phosphorus content. Explain that calcium supplements may be obtained in either tablet or solution form, depending on preference. Oral calcium administration is usually discontinued when the client responds to vitamin D preparations.

Emphasize the importance of lifelong medical care for the client with chronic hypoparathyroidism. Instruct the client to have serum calcium levels checked by a physician at least three times a year. Normal blood serum calcium levels must be maintained to prevent complications. If hypercalcemia or hypocalcemia develops, the physician will adjust the treatment regimen to correct the imbalance.

CONCLUSIONS

You must make careful assessments of clients with thyroid or parathyroid disorders. These disorders can be controlled and the manifestations reversed if they are discovered in a timely manner and prompt and proper treatment is begun. You are an important resource for these clients, who require considerable education. You are also responsible for closely monitoring any client who needs surgery for either the thyroid or parathyroid gland. The client is particularly vulnerable during this postoperative period, and high-level nursing surveillance and intervention facilitate successful recovery.

THINKING CRITICALLY *evolve*

1. A 64-year-old man comes to the clinic with a 6-month history of progressive fatigue, weakness, and dyspnea. On further questioning, you find that he has had an unintentional weight loss of 30 pounds despite an increased appetite. Your physical examination reveals an alert and oriented man who looks his stated age. He is somewhat anxious. His attention span is short, and you must repeat many questions. His heart rate is 118 beats/min; blood pressure, 154/98 mm Hg; temperature, 101° F; the skin is warm and moist; deep tendon reflexes are hyperactive. What are priorities for care?

Factors to Consider. What additional subjective and objective data should you collect to confirm a diagnosis? What medication might be started after the diagnosis is made?

2. The client is a woman with a long history of chronic renal failure. She receives dialysis three times a week. She is currently hospitalized for a complicated pneumonia. On reviewing her laboratory values, you note that her serum calcium level is 6.8 mg/dl. What are the implications for care?

Factors to Consider. What is the relationship of calcium metabolism to renal function? What are the dangers associated with this serum calcium level? What treatments should be initiated to treat this, and what should be done to prevent recurrence?

3. A middle-aged woman comes to the clinic with manifestations of weight gain, lethargy, fatigue, and severe constipation. After diagnostic evaluation, the client is given Synthroid, 0.1 mg, for hypothyroidism. What general information should you give the client about hypothyroidism? About the medication?

Factors to Consider. What should you teach about the expected therapeutic response to this medication? About side effects? How often are blood studies required for the client being treated with thyroid medications?

Discussions for these questions can be found on the website and the CD-ROM.

BIBLIOGRAPHY

1. American Cancer Society (2003). *Cancer facts & figures 2003*. Atlanta: Author.
2. Burman, K., & Wartofsky, L. (2001). Thyroid function in the intensive care setting. *Critical Care Clinics, 17*(1), 43-58.
3. Carlstedt, F., & Lind, L. (2001). Hypocalcemic syndromes. *Critical Care Clinics, 17*(1), 139-154.
4. Corbett, J.V. (2004). *Laboratory tests and diagnostic procedures* (6th ed.). Norwalk, CT: Appleton & Lange.
5. DeGroot, L., & Jameson, J. (Eds.). (2001). *Endocrinology* (4th ed.). Philadelphia: W.B. Saunders.
6. Elliott, B. (2000). Diagnosing and treating hypothyroidism. *The Nurse Practitioner, 25*(3), 92-105.
7. Facts and Comparisons Staff. (2002). *Drug facts and comparisons* (56th ed.). St. Louis: Facts & Comparisons.
8. Gahart, B., & Nazareno, A. (2003). *Intravenous medications*. St. Louis: Mosby.
9. Goldsmith, C. (1999). Hypothyroidism. Symptoms of this prevalent disorder often go unrecognized. *American Journal of Nursing, 99*(6), 42-43.
10. Holcomb, S. (2002). Thyroid disease. *Dimensions of Critical Care Nursing, 21*(4), 127-133.
11. Hueston, W. (2001). Treatment of hypothyroidism. *American Family Physician, 64*(10), 1717-1724.
12. Irvin, G., & Carneiro, D. (2000). Management changes in primary hyperparathyroidism. *Journal of the American Medical Association, 284*(8), 934-936.
13. Klein, I., & Ojamaa, K. (2001). Thyroid hormone and the cardiovascular system. *New England Journal of Medicine, 344*(7), 501-509.
14. Levine, M. (2001). Hypoparathyroidism and pseudohypoparathyroidism. In L. DeGroot & J. Jameson (Eds.), *Endocrinology* (4th ed., pp. 1133-1153). Philadelphia: W.B. Saunders.
15. Li, T. (2002). Hypothyroidism in elderly people. *Geriatric Nursing, 23*(2), 88-93.
16. Malchiodi, L. (2002). Thyroid storm. Recognizing the signs and symptoms of this life-threatening complication. *American Journal of Nursing, 102*(5), 33-35.
17. McCloskey, J., & Bulechek, G. (2000). *Nursing interventions classification (NIC)* (3rd ed.). St. Louis: Mosby.
18. Pacini, F., & DeGroot, L. (2001). Thyroid neoplasia. In L. DeGroot & J. Jameson (Eds.) *Endocrinology* (4th ed., pp 1541-1566). Philadelphia: W.B. Saunders.
19. Pagana, K., & Pagana, T. (2003). *Mosby's diagnostic and laboratory test reference* (6th ed.). St. Louis: Mosby.
20. Ringle, M. (2001). Management of hypothyroidism and hyperthyroidism in the intensive care unit. *Critical Care Clinics, 17*(1), 59-74.
21. Schultz, P. (2002). Providing information to patients with a rare cancer: Using internet discussion forums to address the needs of patients with medullary thyroid carcinoma. *Clinical Journal of Oncology Nurses, 6*(4), 219-222.
22. Silverberg, S., & Bilezikian, J. (2001). Primary hyperparathyroidism. In L. DeGroot & J. Jameson (Eds.), *Endocrinology* (4th ed., pp. 1075-1092). Philadelphia: W.B. Saunders.
23. Young, J. (1999). Action stat: Thyroid storm. *Nursing, 29*(8), 33.

evolve **Did you remember to check out the bonus material on the Evolve website and the CD-ROM, including free self-assessment exercises?**
http://evolve.elsevier.com/Black/medsurg/

Management of Clients with Adrenal and Pituitary Disorders

Anne M. Larson

evolve

Web Enhancements

http://evolve.elsevier.com/Black/medsurg/

Concept Map
Understanding Hypercortisolism (Cushing's Disease) and Its Treatment

Appendix C
Laboratory Values of Clinical Importance in Medical-Surgical Nursing

ADRENOCORTICAL DISORDERS

Glandular hypofunction and hyperfunction characterize the major disorders of the adrenal cortex. Underactivity of the adrenal cortex results in a deficiency of glucocorticoids, mineralocorticoids, and adrenal androgens. The person with adrenal hypofunction is a prime candidate for injury, deficient knowledge, and feelings of powerlessness. Overactivity of the adrenal cortex results in excessive production of glucocorticoids, mineralocorticoids, and androgens or estrogens. The person with adrenal hyperfunction needs to focus on preventing injury and infection, acquiring effective coping mechanisms, and learning about the disease process.

ADRENAL INSUFFICIENCY

Hypofunction of the adrenal cortex can originate from a disorder in the adrenal gland itself (primary adrenal insufficiency), or it may result from hypofunction of the pituitary-hypothalamic unit (secondary adrenal insufficiency).

PRIMARY ADRENAL INSUFFICIENCY

Commonly known as *Addison's disease,* primary adrenal insufficiency results from idiopathic atrophy or destruction of the adrenal glands by an autoimmune process or other disease. Thomas Addison first described this disorder in 1849.

Etiology and Risk Factors

Primary adrenal insufficiency is caused by hypofunction of the adrenal glands. It is a rare disorder, and its incidence and prevalence in the United States are unknown. An autoimmune process accounts for 75% of primary adrenal insufficiency. It is commonly seen in people with acquired immunodeficiency syndrome (AIDS). Tuberculosis is the cause in about 20% of cases of Addison's disease. Adrenal metastasis from the lung, breast, gastrointestinal tract, melanoma, or lymphoma may also cause primary adrenal insufficiency. Additional causes include bilateral adrenalectomy and hemorrhagic infarction with necrosis of the adrenal gland.

Risk factors for primary adrenal insufficiency include (1) a history of other endocrine disorders, (2) taking glucocorticoids for more than 3 weeks with sudden cessation, (3) taking glucocorticoids more than once every other day, (4) adrenalectomy, and (5) tuberculosis.

Health promotion and health maintenance activities for clients receiving glucocorticoids include instruction on the risks and benefits of this therapy and on the proper means of withdrawing glucocorticoids. Health maintenance activities for those receiving long-term steroid therapy include education about the need for supplemental steroids to prevent acute adrenal insufficiency and having parenteral steroids available for use when the client is unable to take oral steroids. Health

Nursing Outcomes Classification (NOC)
for Nursing Diagnoses—Clients with Adrenal and Pituitary Disorders

Activity Intolerance
  Activity Tolerance
  Endurance
  Energy Conservation
  Self-Care: Activities of Daily Living
    (ADL)
  Self-Care: Instrumental Activities of
    Daily Living (IADL)
Acute Pain
  Comfort Level
  Pain Control
  Pain: Disruptive Effects
  Pain Level
Deficient Knowledge
  Knowledge: Diet
  Knowledge: Disease Process
  Knowledge: Energy Conservation
  Knowledge: Health Behaviors
  Knowledge: Health Resources
  Knowledge: Illness Care
  Knowledge: Infection Control
  Knowledge: Medication
  Knowledge: Personal Safety

  Knowledge: Prescribed Activity
  Knowledge: Treatment Procedures
  Knowledge: Treatment Regimen
Disturbed Thought Processes
  Cognitive Ability
  Cognitive Orientation
  Concentration
  Decision-Making
  Distorted Thought Control
  Identity
  Information Processing
  Memory
  Neurologic Status: Consciousness
Risk for Impaired Skin Integrity
  Immobility Consequences: Physiologic
  Nutritional Status
  Risk Control
  Risk Detection
  Tissue Integrity: Skin and Mucous
    Membranes
  Tissue Perfusion: Peripheral
  Wound Healing: Primary Intention

Risk for Infection
  Immune Status
  Knowledge: Infection Control
  Nutritional Status
  Risk Control
  Risk Detection
  Tissue Integrity: Skin and Mucous
    Membranes
  Treatment Behavior: Illness or Injury
  Wound Healing: Primary Intention
Risk for Injury
  Circulation Status
  Knowledge: Personal Safety
  Neurologic Status
  Risk Control
  Risk Detection
  Safety Behavior: Fall Prevention
  Safety Behavior: Home Physical Envi-
    ronment
  Safety Behavior: Personal
  Safety Status: Physical Injury
  Symptom Control
  Vital Signs Status

restoration activities include ensuring that the client is mindful of the need for follow-up with the physician to monitor his or her steroid levels.

Pathophysiology

Autoimmunity is the most common cause of adrenal insufficiency. Lymphocytic infiltration of the adrenal cortex is the characteristic feature. Addison's disease is frequently accompanied by other immune disorders. Gradual destruction leads to chronic adrenal insufficiency. Continued loss of cortical tissue accompanies a deficiency of mineralocorticoids as well as glucocorticoids. Adrenocortical hypofunction results in decreased levels of mineralocorticoids (aldosterone), glucocorticoids (cortisol), and androgens.

Clinical Manifestations

The onset of Addison's disease is usually insidious. The client experiences mild fatigue, languor, irritability, weight loss, nausea, vomiting, and postural hypotension, usually weeks or months before the diagnosis is confirmed. As the disorder progresses, manifestations intensify. By then, the client has lost more than 90% of both adrenal cortices.

Diagnosis of Addison's disease depends primarily on blood and urine hormonal assays. Primary adrenal insufficiency is characterized by a low cortisol production rate and a high plasma adrenocorticotropic hormone (ACTH) concentration.

Other diagnostic tests may be ordered to evaluate the effects of hypofunction of the adrenals on the body: (1) serum electrolytes (especially hyponatremia and hyperkalemia in primary adrenal insufficiency and hyponatremia alone in secondary disease); (2) blood glucose; (3) complete blood count (to assess for anemia); (4) x-ray studies, computed tomography (CT); and (5) magnetic resonance imaging (MRI) of the adrenals and pituitary.

Outcome Management

Addisonian crisis is an emergent condition that requires careful monitoring in the critical care unit. Thereafter the rate of recovery is client specific. Normally, Addison's disease can be managed on an outpatient basis if the client is compliant and receives proper self-care instructions.

■ Medical Management

Addisonian Crisis

Addisonian crisis, or *acute adrenal insufficiency,* may occur when the client has been under stress without appropriate hormone replacement. Stressors include pregnancy, surgery, infection, states of dehydration or anorexia, fever, and emotional upheaval. Manifestations are related to the degree of hormone deficiency and electrolyte imbalance and include sudden penetrating pain in the back, abdomen, or legs; depressed or changed mentation; volume depletion; hypotension; loss of consciousness; and shock.

Correct Fluid and Electrolyte Imbalances. The overall desired outcome of treatment is prevention of the morbidity and mortality associated with the addisonian crisis. Untreated, addisonian crisis is fatal. The cause of the crisis must be determined and treated immediately. Hypotension and electrolyte imbalance need to be corrected quickly. Rapid rehydration is essential. An isotonic solution usually corrects the volume depletion, salt depletion, and hypotension. The client may also need oxygen, vasopressors, or volume expanders. Sodium polystyrene sulfonate (Kayexalate) may be administered orally or as an enema in combination with sorbitol. Kayexalate is a resin that releases sodium ions in exchange for potassium ions.

Correct Hypoglycemia. Hypoglycemia must be evaluated and corrected with intravenous (IV) glucose (5% dextrose [D₅] solution IV or IV glucose push bolus).

Replace Steroids. Hydrocortisone 100 mg is administered as an intravenous (IV) bolus followed by 100 mg IV every 8 hours for 24 hours. The IV hydrocortisone is tapered as the client's status dictates. Oral hydrocortisone is initiated (see the Integrating Pharmacology feature on Corticosteroids at right).

Addison's Disease

At one time Addison's disease was fatal within months. Today, with the availability of synthetic corticosteroids, clients with Addison's disease can live normal, active lives, provided they receive adequate glucocorticoid replacement. Use corticosteroids with caution. Carefully assess clients for manifestations of hypercortisolism, which can result from excessive long-term cortisol therapy. Most clients receive glucocorticoid and mineralocorticoid replacement.

Osteoporosis is a complication that may develop with excessive use of glucocorticosteroids because the protein matrix in the bones is broken down and therefore calcium cannot be retained. Closely observe clients with other medical problems that may be worsened with steroid use.

■ Nursing Management of the Medical Client

Addisonian Crisis
Assessment

Monitor the client's vital signs closely while the disease is being diagnosed. Check the pulse carefully, at least every 4 hours. Take orthostatic blood pressure (BP) readings and pulses. Report drops in BP or orthostatic changes.

INTEGRATING PHARMACOLOGY
Corticosteroids

Glucocorticoids may be prescribed for a variety of reasons and disorders because of the anti-inflammatory and immune-response suppression properties of these drugs. Glucocorticoids are categorized in three categories based on duration of action: long, intermediate, or short. Attention must also be given to the sodium-retaining capabilities of this class. For example, dexamethasone (Decadron) is a long-acting glucocorticoid that is often prescribed for head injuries because it suppresses inflammation and also has a low sodium retaining ability, which is important in averting cerebral edema.

For clients with adrenal insufficiency, steroid hormone replacement therapy is essential. Most often, short-acting glucocorticoids such as hydrocortisone (Hydrocortone) are prescribed in a divided dose regimen with two thirds of the daily dose taken in the morning and one third taken in the afternoon. This practice simulates the body's normal ebb and flow of cortisol activity. Clients must be instructed on the essential nature of this therapy and the need to comply with the drug regimen. Wearing a drug alert identification device is essential and clients must also be advised to inform all health care providers regarding their steroid dependence. Adjustments in dosages may be expected during times of stress and clients should be taught to contact their primary health care provider as needed during these situations.

Mineralocorticoids such as fludrocortisone (Florinef) are also prescribed for a variety of reasons. Primarily mineralocorticoids act to conserve sodium and therefore water, resulting in increased circulating blood volume. This makes this class of drug an ideal choice for clients with chronic syncope related to orthostatic hypotension. Clients with adrenal insufficiency typically are prescribed a single daily dose of a mineralocorticoid.

As rehydration occurs and electrolyte imbalances are corrected, assess increased physical vitality and emotional well-being. Assess bone prominences for pressure ulcers in immobilized clients. With therapy, listlessness and exhaustion should gradually disappear.

Monitor for exposure to cold and infections. Immediately inform the physician if evidence of infection develops, such as a sore throat or burning on urination. Remember, a client with Addison's disease cannot tolerate stress. Infection imposes additional stress on the body, and cortisol levels need to be higher during infectious illnesses.

Carefully assess for manifestations of sodium and potassium imbalance (see Chapter 14). Obtain daily weights for objective measurement of fluid gain or loss. If steroid replacement therapy is inadequate, sodium loss and potassium retention continue uncorrected. If the steroid dosage is too high, excessive amounts of sodium and water are retained and potassium excretion is high.

Diagnosis, Outcomes, Interventions

Diagnosis: Risk for Injury: Addisonian Crisis.
The client must be diligent in self-care, or the nursing diagnosis may be *Risk for Injury: Addisonian crisis related to adrenal insufficiency.*

Outcomes.
The client will not exhibit injury as evidenced by the absence of hypotension, shock, or other manifestations of acute adrenal insufficiency.

Interventions

Monitor for Manifestations of Crisis. Addisonian crisis usually develops over 24 to 48 hours. Closely monitor for sudden profound weakness; severe abdominal, back, and leg pain; hyperpyrexia (although this may be suppressed by steroids) followed by hypothermia; hypotension associated with high cardiac output, normal wedge pressure, and low systemic resistance; coma; renal shutdown; and death.

An adrenal crisis is a medical emergency that must be treated rapidly and vigorously. The three major desired outcomes of intervention are (1) reversal of shock, (2) restoration of blood circulation (the client usually has a deficit of at least 20% of extracellular fluid volume), and (3) replenishment with essential steroids.

Correct Fluid, Electrolyte, Steroid Imbalances. Immediately on admission, 1000 ml of normal saline with water-soluble glucocorticoid (hydrocortisone phosphate or hydrocortisone sodium succinate) added is rapidly infused. The dosage of the prescribed glucocorticoid is gradually reduced. It is administered intramuscularly (IM) or IV every 8 hours on days 1 and 2 of the crisis and gradually reduced thereafter. Hypoglycemia is controlled by a glucose infusion, either an IV bolus or IV drip as part of rehydration. Hyperkalemia is controlled or corrected with Kayexalate. The precipitating event must be corrected. Plasma, oxygen, and vasopressor medications may be indicated.

Throughout the emergency period, monitor BP, administer IV infusion and medications, monitor hourly urine output, report oliguria (a manifestation of shock), and minimize exposure to emotional and physical stress. Observe for manifestations of glucocorticoid overdose and overhydration, such as generalized edema from fluid retention, hypertension, flaccid paralysis from hypokalemia, psychosis, and loss of consciousness. Also evaluate electrolytes for hyperkalemia, hyponatremia, and hypoglycemia, and correlate these findings with the client's manifestations.

With rapid, efficient intervention, addisonian crisis usually resolves within 12 hours. The client's condition stabilizes, and the convalescent period begins. When the client can tolerate food and fluids by mouth, steroid replacement can be administered orally.

Prevent Future Crises. After the immediate crisis is over, help the client avoid further development of adrenal insufficiency. Obtain a medical identification (Medic-Alert) bracelet and an emergency kit before discharge from the hospital. Instruct the client to carry these items at all times. The client's name and diagnosis should appear on the identification bracelet, and a wallet card should state that the client receives daily hydrocortisone and that the medication must be administered by injection in an emergency.

Dexamethasone can be kept in a prepared syringe in an emergency kit with sterile alcohol wipes for cleaning the injection site. The kit should also contain written information about the client's diagnosis, prescribed drugs, dosage schedules, and emergency phone numbers, including the physician's name and phone number.

Adrenal insufficiency is a potentially life-threatening condition, but when properly recognized and treated, it has little or no effect on life span. There are no dietary or activity restrictions.

Evaluation

The outcome of treatment for addisonian crisis is easily evaluated, usually within 12 hours of treatment. By this time, the client should no longer exhibit any manifestations of addisonian crisis or death would have occurred.

■ Self-Care
Management of Addison's disease takes place in the community with regular medical follow-up of the client's status. Hence, the focus of management is on self-care. Carefully assess the client's ability to understand and perform self-care. The client needs extensive instruction in self-care activities to achieve independence. Appropriate outcomes for the client with Addison's disease are that the client's weight remains stable, vital signs and cortisol levels remain within normal limits, and the client states that fatigue has decreased.

Steroid Replacement. The client must learn how to take steroids correctly. Provide the client and his or her significant others with written instructions on self-administration of steroids. (The client and significant others should have demonstrated their ability to prepare and administer injections.) The client needs to know the following information:

- Actions of prescribed hormones (hydrocortisone, fludrocortisone)
- Importance of taking medications daily, without fail, exactly as prescribed
- Principles of self-administration of oral medications (e.g., the client must check the label on the bottle before taking the medication and documenting medications taken and their side effects)
- Manifestations of overdosage and underdosage

- Importance of hydrocortisone self-injection when unable to tolerate oral medication (because of nausea and vomiting) and during times of acute stress (motor vehicle accident, trauma) because the body is unable to provide the needed additional glucocorticoid coverage
- Need for an IM self-injection kit to be available at all times
- Need for a Medic-Alert bracelet showing the diagnosis and the need for cortisol replacement
- Need for the client to call a health care provider if questions arise after discharge from the medical center

Emphasize that the client who takes glucocorticoids must call the physician to obtain a dosage increase when experiencing stressful situations (e.g., emotional upheavals, dental extractions, minor surgery, upper respiratory infections). The general rule is to double the glucocorticoid dosage for up to 1 week, depending on manifestations, and then resume normal dosage. In addition, temporary mineralocorticoid dosage is reduced by 50% to avoid excessive salt retention and hypertension. Encourage the client to consult the physician for dose adjustment. The medication must be administered IM when nausea and vomiting prevent oral administration.

Follow-Up Monitoring. Remind clients to keep semiannual appointments with the physician, even when their health is good and self-medication is proceeding smoothly. As with diabetes mellitus, the control of Addison's disease is a lifelong responsibility.

■ Modifications for Older Clients
Adrenal diseases are uncommon in older people. The effects of normal aging on the adrenals are unclear. It appears, however, that ACTH and cortisol production remains constant throughout life. Older people may be more sensitive to the side effects of steroid therapy because these problems (e.g., osteoporosis, hypertension, diabetes) already exist.

SECONDARY ADRENAL INSUFFICIENCY
Secondary adrenal insufficiency results from dysfunction of the hypothalamic-pituitary-adrenal (HPA) axis (see the Unit 10 Anatomy and Physiology Review). The most common cause is chronic treatment with glucocorticoids for non-endocrine uses. Other causes include the following:
- Hypopituitarism resulting in decreased ACTH secretion by the pituitary gland, which causes decreased secretion of cortisol and androgens by the adrenal gland
- Pituitary tumor or infarction
- Radiation
- Suppression of hypothalamic-pituitary secretion of ACTH related to hypercortisolism caused by either

exogenous administration of corticosteroids or oversecretion of corticosteroids by an adrenal tumor (in both cases, the adrenal glands atrophy and become filled with lipids)

Secondary adrenal insufficiency is characterized by low cortisol production and low plasma ACTH. Because circulating levels of corticosteroids remain high, these clients do not experience manifestations of adrenocortical insufficiency unless steroid therapy is discontinued suddenly or the tumor is resected. If corticosteroid therapy is tapered gradually, with the dose reduced each day, adrenal gland function usually returns to normal.

Assessment reveals that clients with secondary adrenal insufficiency experience cortisol deficiency. Aldosterone continues to be secreted in sufficient amounts. Treatment involves administering glucocorticoids, as in Addison's disease. Mineralocorticoid replacement is unnecessary. Instruct the client to wear an emergency identification bracelet and to carry an emergency kit for hydrocortisone injection in case of an adrenal crisis.

ADRENOCORTICAL HYPERFUNCTION
Hyperfunction of the adrenal cortex can result in excessive production of glucocorticoids, mineralocorticoids, and androgens. Major conditions of adrenocortical hyperfunction are hypercortisolism (glucocorticoid excess) and primary aldosteronism (aldosterone excess).

HYPERCORTISOLISM
Hypercortisolism (Cushing's syndrome) was first described by Harvey Cushing in 1932. It results from overactivity of the adrenal gland, with consequent hypersecretion of glucocorticoids. Cushing's syndrome is relatively rare, and its incidence is unknown. It occurs mainly in women 20 to 40 years of age; however, it can occur up to age 60.

Etiology and Risk Factors
Iatrogenic hypercortisolism (resulting from medical interventions) accounts for most cases because of the frequent therapeutic use of high-dose glucocorticoids. Hypersecretion of cortisol can be caused by a cortisol-secreting adrenal tumor or adrenal hyperplasia, resulting from overproduction of ACTH. Adrenal tumors are responsible for about 30% of cases of Cushing's syndrome. Most (85%) are benign, but 15% are malignant. There are two sources of excessive ACTH secretion:
- Pituitary hypersecretion and pituitary tumors, which cause about 70% of cases of Cushing's syndrome. These usually benign tumors are either small basophil adenomas or large chromophobe adenomas. Pituitary hypersecretion of ACTH that results in glucocorticoid excess is called *Cushing's disease*.
- Ectopic secretion of ACTH (or *ectopic ACTH syndrome*). ACTH-secreting tumors located outside

the pituitary gland are a rare cause of Cushing's syndrome. The tumors that most frequently cause ectopic ACTH syndrome are oat cell carcinoma of the lung; pancreatic islet cell carcinoma; and carcinoid tumors of the lung, gut, thymus, and ovary.

Iatrogenic Cushing's syndrome, another form of the disorder, results from exogenous (originating outside the body, e.g., taking supplemental medication) administration of synthetic glucocorticoids in supraphysiologic amounts. Thus educating clients to avoid unnecessary use of exogenous steroids is an important health promotion activity. Health maintenance activities include (1) educating clients who are at risk for manifestations of Cushing's syndrome; (2) treating clinical manifestations of hypernatremia, hypokalemia, hyperglycemia, and hypertension; and (3) teaching clients about adrenalectomy and steroid replacement. Health restoration activities include making sure that clients understand the importance of surgery, lifelong steroid replacement, and recognizing disease complications that may have already developed (such as osteoporosis or "buffalo hump," a fat pad on the neck).

Pathophysiology

When Cushing's syndrome develops, the normal function of the glucocorticoids becomes exaggerated and the classic picture of the syndrome emerges (Figure 46-1). This exaggerated physiologic action of glucocorticoids appears as follows:

- Persistent hyperglycemia (or "steroid diabetes").
- Protein tissue wasting, which results in muscle wasting and weakness; capillary fragility, which results in ecchymosis; and osteoporosis from bone matrix wasting. Osteoporosis can become so severe that even mild trauma can cause fractures. Com-

pression fractures can develop in the osteoporotic spine, leading to kyphosis and loss of height.
- Potassium depletion, leading to hypokalemia, dysrhythmias, muscle weakness, and renal disorders.
- Sodium and water retention, which causes edema and hypertension.
- Hypertension, which eventually predisposes the client to left ventricular hypertrophy, heart failure, and stroke.
- Abnormal fat distribution (in conjunction with edema), which results in a moon-shaped face, a dorsocervical fat pad on the neck (buffalo hump), and truncal obesity with slender limbs. Also, pink and purple striae appear on the breasts, axillary areas, abdomen, and legs because of thinning of the skin. Striking changes in appearance occur after the development and cure of Cushing's syndrome. Old photographs can be useful in showing changes over time.
- Increased susceptibility to infection and lowered resistance to stress increase vulnerability to microorganisms of all types. Because of suppression of the inflammatory response, people with Cushing's syndrome show few manifestations of infection. They also demonstrate poor wound healing.
- Possible increased production of androgens can cause virilism (masculine characteristics) in women. Manifestations of virilism include acne, thinning of scalp hair, and hirsutism (excessive bodily and facial hair in a male pattern).
- Mental changes include memory loss, poor concentration and cognition, euphoria, and depression. Sometimes a condition called "steroid psychosis" develops. Depression can predispose the client to suicidal thoughts. About 80% of the clients meet the criteria for a major affective disorder: 50% with unipolar depression, 30% with bipolar illness (see the Evidence-Based Practice in Action feature on Responding to Altered Cognitive Function in Clients with Cushing's Syndrome on p. 1223 and the Concept Map on Understanding Hypercortisolism [Cushing's Disease] and Its Treatment on pp. 1224 and 1225).

FIGURE 46-1 Clinical manifestations of Cushing's syndrome.

Labels: Mood swings and personality changes "Steroid" psychosis; Thinning of scalp hair; Posterior subcapsular cataracts Increased intraocular pressure; Dorsocervical fat pad; "Moon face" Ruddy cheeks (ecchymosis) Hirsutism and acne; Hypertension; Ecchymosis; Insulin resistance; Poor wound healing Increased susceptibility to infection Capillary fragility; Protein tissue wasting, muscle weakness, thin limbs; Striae and truncal obesity; Osteoporosis Aseptic bone necrosis Pathologic fractures

Clinical Manifestations

Even for clients who have a classic cushingoid appearance, it is important to perform diagnostic studies for confirmation. Laboratory tests for Cushing's syndrome reflect hyperglycemia, fluid and electrolyte disturbances, and immunosuppressive responses that characterize excessive glucocorticoid secretion. Thus in Cushing's syndrome glucose tolerance decreases and glucosuria appears. The white blood cell count often rises above 10,000/mm³, but the total eosinophil count can drop below 50/mm³. Also, lymphocytes can fall below 20%. Both urinary 17-hydroxysteroid (17-HS) and blood cortisol levels are elevated.

EB EVIDENCE-BASED PRACTICE IN ACTION

Responding to Altered Cognitive Function in Clients with Cushing's Syndrome

Clients with Cushing's syndrome can expect lower cognitive functioning, memory problems, and depression.[1] Some of these problems improve with treatment, but residual effects may remain. There is also variation in the amount of these deficits noted across the client population afflicted with Cushing's syndrome.

Implications

Nurses must be attuned to the subtle changes that may occur as clients' disease states progress. Careful assessment is necessary to provide clients and families with adequate teaching and support. The ability of clients to perform their occupational duties may be affected and appropriate occupational therapy referrals would be imperative. Additionally, clients with depression may benefit from psychotropic drugs or psychotherapy.

References

1. Dorn, L., & Cerrone, P. (2000). Cognitive function in patients with Cushing syndrome. *Clinical Nursing Research, 9*(4), 420-441.

Normally plasma cortisol follows a diurnal pattern, increasing in the early morning (10 to 25 mg/dl), gradually falling to below 10 mg/dl in the evening, and approaching undetectable levels near midnight. Clients with Cushing's syndrome have elevated plasma cortisol levels throughout the day without diurnal variation. Urinary free cortisol (UFC) measurement is used as a screening test to identify elevated urinary excretion of free cortisol. Clients with Cushing's syndrome have UFC levels above 100 mg/day. See Table 44-2 for discussion of rapid and prolonged dexamethasone suppression tests. Suppression is interpreted as a fall in basal 17-HS of more than 50%, which is compatible with Cushing's disease and ectopic ACTH secretion.

In the plasma ACTH test, low ACTH levels point to an adrenal tumor as the cause of hypercortisolism. Overproduction of cortisol by the adrenal tumor provides negative feedback to the pituitary gland, which responds by reducing ACTH release. The high cortisol level also provides feedback to the hypothalamus, which reduces release of corticotropin-releasing hormone.

An ectopic ACTH-producing tumor usually yields a normal or elevated ACTH level. ACTH production by the tumor is independent of pituitary production of ACTH. Thus despite negative feedback to the hypothalamic-pituitary unit, ACTH levels remain high.

The inferior petrosal sinus sampling test is a radiologic test used to isolate the source of ACTH secretion (whether it is in the pituitary gland and, if so, where). The left and right petrosal sinuses carry blood from the pituitary gland to the jugular veins. Catheters are threaded into the inferior petrosal sinus via the femoral veins. With sampling of serum ACTH levels drawn from the right and left petrosal sinuses, the side of the pituitary gland producing ACTH can be identified.

If ACTH levels from the petrosal sinuses are greater than this one from a peripheral site (the arm), a pituitary tumor is identified as the source of hypercortisolism. If central ACTH levels (petrosal) and peripheral ACTH

levels (arm) are equivalent, an ectopic ACTH-secreting tumor is likely.

The development of this test has allowed neurosurgeons to perform a hemi-hypophysectomy, removing only the half of the pituitary gland that contains the microadenoma. Before the availability of this test, the entire gland usually had to be removed because of the difficulty in localizing these "invisible" tumors. An adrenal CT scan is performed to detect an adrenal mass in the right or left adrenal gland. Contrast dye is used, when possible, to enhance the clarity of the scan.

Outcome Management
■ Surgical Management

Surgical removal of even one adrenal gland requires careful inpatient monitoring because the remaining adrenal gland may have atrophied and stopped producing adrenocortical hormones. For Cushing's syndrome caused by an adrenal tumor, an adrenalectomy can be performed to remove the gland containing the tumor. In case of ectopic ACTH-secreting tumors, the tumor can be difficult to localize. If no source is found, a bilateral adrenalectomy can be performed to interrupt the production of cortisol in response to the ACTH produced by the tumor, or the client can be treated with anti-glucocorticoids while the search for the tumor continues. Laparoscopic adrenalectomy is being evaluated as an alternative to traditional adrenalectomy. Early studies indicate that it may reduce postoperative morbidity.

After successful surgical removal of the adrenals, the client receives lifelong glucocorticoid and mineralocorticoid replacement. Most physical manifestations of Cushing's syndrome resolve after bilateral adrenalectomy.

Resection of most pituitary tumors causing Cushing's disease is performed via transsphenoidal hypophysectomy (see Chapter 71). Occasionally, large or anatomically complex tumors are excised via a transfrontal approach (see later discussion of hypophysectomy). A surgical cure rate of 85% to 90% has been documented.

Understanding Hypercortisolism (Cushing's Disease) and Its Treatment

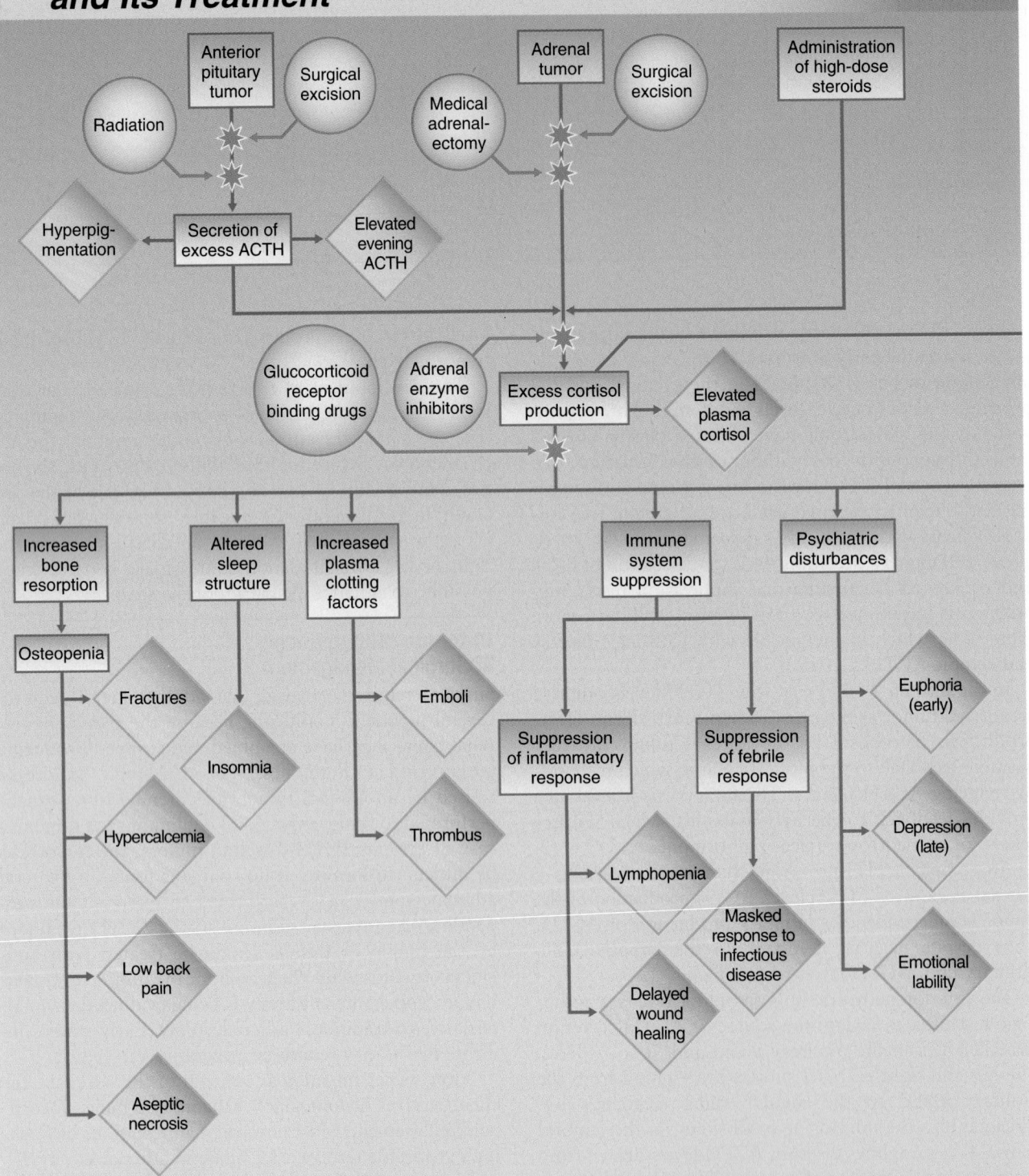

CONCEPT MAP—cont'd

evolve

Impotence ↔ Decreased libido

Hirsutism (facial hair) ↔ Oligomenorrhea

Excess androgen production → Oily facial skin

Antihypertensives

Catabolism

Muscle wasting
- Proximal muscle weakness
- Elevated serum cholesterol
- Increased appetite

Altered fat metabolism

Abnormal fat distribution
- Facial fat deposition ("moon face")
- Protruding abdomen
- Exophthalmos
- Subclavicular fat deposits ("buffalo hump")

Sympathetic nervous system stimulation

Diuretics → Moderate hypertension

Diuretics → Heart failure

Diuretics → Dependent edema

Thinning of stratum corneum

Vitamin A

Loss of subcutaneous fat

Paper-thin skin

Striae

Loss of connective tissue

No use of tape

Easy bruising

Delayed wound healing

○ Treatment   ▢ Pathology   ◇ Clinical manifestations

Because the HPA axis has been suppressed, adrenal insufficiency develops postoperatively. The axis takes 12 to 24 months to recover. Replacement steroids are indicated during this time.

■ Nursing Management of the Surgical Client

Preoperative Care
Assessment

Begin by obtaining a careful history from a client with possible Cushing's syndrome. The client may exhibit the characteristic clinical manifestations identified previously. Support the client during the diagnostic phase of care. At this point, there is often a great deal of uncertainty about the cause of the disorder. Explain to the client why these tests must be performed before treatment can be started.

During the preoperative phase, the client with Cushing's syndrome requires expert nursing assessment and care. The crucial problems of hypertension, edema, possible heart disease, diabetes mellitus, increased susceptibility to infection, decreased resistance to stress, and emotional lability (i.e., a tendency toward frequent mood changes) or instability must all be assessed and brought under control before surgery.

Diagnosis, Outcomes, Interventions

Diagnosis: Risk for Injury: Fractures, Hypertension, or Diabetes. Until the diagnosis is made and the problem treated, the client is at *Risk for Injury: Fractures, Hypertension, or Diabetes related to osteoporosis, sodium and water retention, or the presence of an insulin antagonist, respectively.*

Outcomes. Injury will not occur as evidenced by the absence of fractures. The client will not have hypertension, hyperglycemia, or diabetes.

Interventions
Prevent Injury. Protect the client from falls and accidents. Clients with Cushing's syndrome have osteoporosis and tend to develop fractures even with mild trauma. Keep the bed in its lowest position, and raise the side rails for protection. Assist clients with ambulation to avoid falls.

Monitor for Hypertension and Diabetes. Monitor vital signs at frequent intervals. Assess the client carefully for evidence of severe hypertension, such as elevated BP, headache, failing vision, irritability, and dyspnea. Check for postural hypotension (but have the client change position slowly to avoid injury from a sudden drop in BP). Obtain the client's weight daily in a consistent manner. If sodium intake is reduced, edema and weight should diminish. Obtain daily blood glucose levels via

finger stick. Positive results may indicate diabetes mellitus (steroid diabetes) caused by the insulin antagonist action of the excessive cortisol.

Diagnosis: Deficient Knowledge. A typical nursing diagnosis for the client undergoing surgery to correct adrenocortical excess is *Deficient Knowledge regarding the disease, surgery, and proper diet related to no previous instruction and new diagnosis resulting in anxiety, misinformation, and questions.*

Outcomes. The client will understand the disease, the surgery planned, and the importance of a proper diet, as evidenced by statements of understanding and choice of a proper diet.

Interventions
Explain Disease and Treatment. It is important for clients to understand their condition and the proposed treatment. Give clients an opportunity to ask questions about the treatment, and assess their understanding of it.

Provide Adequate Nutrition. Encourage a diet low in calories, carbohydrates, and sodium but with ample protein and potassium. Such a diet promotes weight loss, reduction of edema and hypertension, control of hypokalemia, and rebuilding of wasted tissue. The client with diabetes mellitus or gastric ulcers requires a special diet.

Evaluation

It is expected that clients will have minimal complications or will have had appropriate management of complications before surgery so that they can undergo the adrenalectomy successfully. The client will be able to explain the desired outcome of surgical intervention, possible complications, and related treatment. A glucocorticoid preparation will be given on the morning of surgery to prevent adrenal insufficiency during the procedure.

Postoperative Care
Assessment

Routine postoperative monitoring of the incision and special assessments for manifestations of shock, addisonian crisis, and renal shutdown are required. Assess the client's ability to perform self-care and to manage the disease for the remainder of his or her life. The client's current level of knowledge must be assessed and a teaching plan carefully developed.

Diagnosis, Outcomes, Interventions

Diagnosis: Risk for Injury. After surgery, the client may have *Risk for Injury related to complications of the surgical procedure.*

Outcomes. Injury will not occur or will be detected early as evidenced by the absence of shock, hemorrhage, infection, or addisonian crisis.

Interventions. On the morning of surgery, administer a glucocorticoid preparation IM or IV as prescribed. A water-soluble cortisol preparation (diluted in an IV infusion) may be given throughout the surgery. Cortisol protects against the development of acute adrenal insufficiency during the adrenalectomy. Even if the surgeon plans to remove only one adrenal gland, temporary glucocorticoid support may be needed until the remaining adrenal gland begins to secrete sufficient cortisol. Because of the excessive secretion of cortisol by the tumorous gland, the healthy gland can atrophy and needs time to readjust.

During the immediate postoperative phase, the major desired outcomes are prevention of shock and infection, maintenance of adequate cortisol levels, and control of pain and incisional discomfort. Observe for manifestations of shock related to hemorrhage (hypotension and a rapid, weak pulse). Document vital signs every 15 minutes. Measure urine and record hourly output, observing for oliguria, a manifestation of shock, and renal shutdown. Administer IV fluids, pressor amines, and corticosteroids as prescribed.

The manifestations of addisonian crisis resemble those of shock. Closely assess the client for this complication, and administer IV cortisol in high doses until the manifestations subside. The client will require increased amounts of steroids until the remaining adrenal gland returns to a normal level of functioning and the stress associated with the treatment subsides.

Diagnosis: Risk for Infection. The client receiving steroid replacement will be at *Risk for Infection related to lowered resistance to stress and compromised immune response.*

Outcomes. Infection will not develop or will be detected early as evidenced by the absence of leukocytosis, fever, and other manifestations of infections.

Interventions. After surgery, encourage the client to cough, turn, and deep-breathe to prevent respiratory infections. Employ meticulous sterile technique with wound care to prevent infection. Paralytic ileus is less common because the flank approach is usually used.

Protect the client from exposure to infectious organisms. Isolate the client from health care personnel and significant others who have contagious disorders. Wash your hands meticulously before contact with the client.

Because glucocorticoids suppress immune and inflammatory reactions, a client with Cushing's syndrome may have only mild manifestations of even a severe infection. The white blood cell count does not show significant elevation in immunosuppressed clients. A slight elevation

in body temperature may indicate the presence of a severe infection.

Diagnosis: Activity Intolerance. A client receiving steroids may exhibit *Activity Intolerance related to fatigue and muscle weakness from protein wasting, persistent hyperglycemia (and possible diabetes mellitus), and potassium depletion resulting in an inability to maintain a normal activity level without increased heart rate or shortness of breath.*

Outcomes. The client will be able to balance rest and activity.

Interventions. Promote mental and physical rest for the client with Cushing's syndrome. Minimize stress and confusion so that the client can achieve maximal periods of rest.

Diagnosis: Risk for Impaired Skin Integrity. A client receiving steroids is at *Risk for Impaired Skin Integrity related to tissue catabolism (thinning of skin), loss of connective tissue, and edema secondary to sodium and water retention.*

Outcomes. The client will maintain intact skin.

Interventions. Monitor the client's skin meticulously for breakdown. The client is extremely susceptible to breakdown from tissue catabolism. Avoid using tape or other irritants that may tear or excoriate the skin.

Diagnosis: Disturbed Thought Processes. The client may exhibit *Disturbed Thought Processes (memory loss, cognitive impairment, mood swings, euphoria, or depression) related to increased levels of glucocorticoids and ACTH, resulting in an inability to make decisions and remember.* (See the Evidence-Based Practice in Action feature on Responding to Altered Cognitive Function in Clients with Cushing's Syndrome on p. 1223.)

Outcomes. The client will not have memory loss, cognitive impairment, or mood swings, or these manifestations will be minimized.

Interventions. Anticipate mood swings. Clients may become easily upset by changes in their appearance caused by the disease and may also become alarmed by bizarre feelings and emotions. Reassure clients that appearance and moods should gradually return to normal after treatment unless steroid replacement is necessary. If clients need steroid therapy, some side effects will continue.

Evaluation

If the surgical management of Cushing's disease is successful, neither injury related to the surgery nor addisonian crisis will develop. If complications do occur, desired outcomes may be related to successful management of the complications, such as control of hemorrhage, prevention of shock, and control of addisonian crisis.

Appropriate outcomes also include the control of side effects of the steroid therapy. Because these cannot be completely avoided, the client's ability to control them is an appropriate area to evaluate. The client should be able to differentiate complications from the side effects of medications.

■ Medical Management

Usually, a client with primary adrenal hyperplasia is treated surgically as an inpatient. Medical management is reserved for clients with inoperable tumors or metastatic tumors that warrant palliative care (Table 46-1). The outcome, therefore, is related to achieving comfort versus cure. Medical management options include radiation therapy and administration of adrenal blocking agents or ACTH-reducing agents to decrease the effects of the adrenal hyperplasia.

Radiation Therapy. Radiation therapy can be used to treat primary pituitary tumors and other ACTH-secreting adenomas. Radiation can be applied to the pituitary gland either internally or externally. Internally, the radiation is applied through a transsphenoidal implant. Radiation must be used with care because of the proximity of the optic nerve. Radiation is not always effective in even palliative treatment of tumors and may destroy normal tissue. For ACTH-secreting adenomas, such as lung tumors, palliation is possible. Radiation therapy is commonly used concurrently with surgical or pharmacologic management to enhance its effectiveness and reduce long-term side effects.

Adrenal Blocking Agents. Medications that interfere with ACTH production or adrenal hormone synthesis are available. Mitotane (Lysodren) is a cytotoxic antihormonal agent that inhibits corticosteroid synthesis without destroying cortical cells. Aminoglutethimide (Cytadren) and trilostane (Modrastane) are other cytotoxic agents that block the synthesis of glucocorticoids and adrenal steroids.

TABLE 46-1	*Therapies for Cushing's Syndrome, Cushing's Disease, and Ectopic ACTH Syndrome*		
Condition	**Responsible Lesion**	**Therapies**	**Remarks**
Cushing's syndrome	Adrenal tumor (benign or malignant)	Adrenalectomy	Adrenalectomy for benign unilateral tumor; usually curative Bilateral adrenalectomy must be followed by lifelong administration of corticosteroids
	Adrenal carcinoma with widespread metastases	Surgery and chemotherapy (mitotane)	Chemotherapy largely unsuccessful
Cushing's disease	Pituitary tumor (or unidentified lesion) that secretes excessive amounts of ACTH	Microsurgical resection of pituitary adenoma	Pituitary surgery successful in 95% of cases
		Irradiation of pituitary gland	Irradiation successful in 75% of cases; therapeutic effects not apparent for months after initiation of therapy
		Total bilateral adrenalectomy (corrects adrenal hyperplasia caused by excessive ACTH stimulation)	Total bilateral adrenalectomy must be followed by lifelong replacement therapy with glucocorticoid and mineralocorticoid
Ectopic ACTH syndrome	Extra-adrenal malignant tumor	Surgical removal of ectopic malignant tumor; chemotherapy used to control hypercortisolism and promote remission in clients with inoperable cancer	Surgery rarely successful because metastasis usually occurs before diagnosis; chemotherapy purely palliative

ACTH, Adrenocorticotropic hormone.

ACTH-Reducing Agents. Cyproheptadine (Periactin), bromocriptine, or somatostatin is used to treat hypersecretion caused by pituitary abnormalities and resulting in increased ACTH levels. These agents appear to interfere with ACTH production, thereby reducing the effect on the adrenals.

■ Self-Care

The client with a bilateral adrenalectomy needs to learn self-care because lifelong glucocorticoid replacement is essential. If only one adrenal gland has been removed, daily cortisol replacement continues until the remaining gland functions normally (usually after 6 to 12 months). Before discharge, the client and his or her significant others need instruction on self-administration of replacement hormones (hydrocortisone). They should successfully demonstrate the injection technique before discharge. The client should also be able to repeat and comply with instructions and to remain free of addisonian crisis or adrenal insufficiency.

■ Modifications for Older Clients

Older clients may exhibit excessive manifestations of Cushing's syndrome because these clients may already have osteoporosis, hypertension, and diabetes. Older clients are also more susceptible to the side effects of steroid replacement therapy.

HYPERALDOSTERONISM

Aldosterone is the most powerful of the mineralocorticoids. Its primary role is to conserve sodium, and it also promotes potassium excretion. The incidence of primary hyperaldosteronism in the hypertensive population is unknown, affecting about 1%. It affects women twice as often as men and appears most frequently in middle-aged people.

Etiology and Risk Factors

Primary hyperaldosteronism refers to hypersecretion of aldosterone resulting from an adrenal lesion, which is usually benign. The disease, which produces secondary hypertension, hypokalemia (in most), and hypernatremia, is also known as *Conn's syndrome.*

Secondary hyperaldosteronism results from a variety of conditions that cause overproduction of aldosterone. These conditions include sodium-wasting renal disease, laxative or diuretic abuse, dehydration, cirrhosis with ascites, heart failure, and a decrease in intravascular volume. Hypertension is uncommon.

There are no particular risk factors for primary hyperaldosteronism. Risk factors for secondary hyperaldosteronism include chronic heart failure, cirrhosis with ascites, nephrotic syndrome, and hypertension caused by destructive renal artery disease. Health promotion measures, therefore, are successful treatment and control of the causative disease process. The more successfully these factors are controlled, the less secondary hyperaldosteronism is present.

Pathophysiology

Aldosterone affects tubular reabsorption of sodium and water and excretion of potassium and hydrogen ions in the renal tubular epithelial cells. These effects lead to the development of hypernatremia, hypervolemia, hypokalemia, and metabolic alkalosis. With hypervolemia and hypernatremia, BP increases, often to very high levels, and renin production is suppressed. The hypertension can lead to cerebral infarcts and renal damage.

Secondary hyperaldosteronism is a result of continuous secretion of aldosterone secondary to high levels of angiotensin II, resulting from high plasma renin activity. Decreased renal perfusion of a variety of causes is the underlying mechanism.

Clinical Manifestations

Clients with primary hyperaldosteronism may be asymptomatic, but incidental findings include hypertension, hypernatremia, and hypokalemia. Without intervention, all of the complications of chronic hypertension, such as visual disturbances, heart failure, renal damage, and stroke, may occur. Unfortunately, the renal complications resulting from long-term hypertension tend to be progressive. Therefore clients with primary hyperaldosteronism need to be identified and treated early in the course of the disease.

Hypokalemia results from excessive urinary excretion of potassium ions. This problem in turn causes muscle weakness, paralysis, or cardiac dysrhythmias because potassium loss reduces normal neuromuscular irritability. In addition, excessive potassium excretion results in polyuria. The large urine output leads to polydipsia (excessive thirst). Finally, hypokalemia leads to metabolic alkalosis because of shifting of hydrogen ions into the cells in exchange for potassium and exchange of hydrogen ions in the tubular cells for sodium ions from the tubular urine. Metabolic alkalosis causes a decrease in ionized calcium levels, which can result in tetany and respiratory suppression.

Despite sodium retention, clients with hyperaldosteronism rarely develop overt edema. Although extracellular fluid increases moderately, excessive water is normally excreted in the urine with potassium ions. Over time, the kidneys tend to adjust physiologically to excessive secretion of aldosterone, and water excretion reaches an equilibrium with sodium intake. The kidneys' eventual "escape" from the sodium-retaining and water-retaining action of aldosterone is sometimes called the *escape phenomenon.*

The diagnosis of primary hyperaldosteronism is based on low serum potassium levels, alkalosis, and elevated urinary or plasma aldosterone levels with low plasma renin levels (elevated in secondary hyperaldosteronism).

In addition, radiographic studies may reveal cardiac hypertrophy resulting from chronic hypertension. Radionuclide scanning techniques using radiolabeled iodocholesterol allow visualization of the tumors.

Outcome Management
■ Surgical Management

Surgery is the treatment of choice for the client with primary hyperaldosteronism. A unilateral or bilateral adrenalectomy must be performed. A client undergoing a unilateral adrenalectomy may need temporary replacement of glucocorticoids. A client who requires a bilateral adrenalectomy needs permanent replacement (see Addison's disease discussion). Clients usually receive glucocorticoids preoperatively to prevent adrenal hypofunction. In two thirds of cases, removal of the aldosterone-secreting tumor completely resolves the hypertension, hypokalemia, and hypernatremia. Most clients have normal BP readings by the third postoperative month.

■ Nursing Management of the Surgical Client

Help prepare the client for the diagnostic assessment so that the diagnosis of hyperaldosteronism can be achieved rapidly and the treatment performed before permanent damage occurs. Administer prescribed medications, and closely monitor the client for hypertension or renal damage. Preoperative and postoperative management is the same as that described for hypercortisolism.

Discharge planning must include client education about a low-sodium diet, medications, and manifestations of hypokalemia if the client is to be medically treated. The client should also understand the disease process and manifestations.

■ Medical Management

 A client who cannot be treated surgically may receive spironolactone (Aldactone) to increase sodium excretion and to treat the hypertension and hypokalemia. Hypertension may take 4 to 8 weeks to correct. Potassium levels should be carefully monitored for the development of hyperkalemia, especially if the client has been receiving potassium supplements or a high-potassium diet (Box 46-1). Amiloride is the drug of choice for clients who cannot tolerate spironolactone.

■ Nursing Management of the Medical Client

Assess the client's ability to manage the complex therapeutic regimen. Plan and implement a teaching program for self-care.

ADRENOMEDULLARY DISORDERS

Two important tumors occur in the adrenal medulla: *pheochromocytoma,* a tumor that causes hyperactivity of the gland, and *neuroblastoma,* a malignant tumor made up of cells resembling a neuroblast. For a complete description of neuroblastoma, an important tumor in children, consult a pediatric textbook.

> **BOX 46-1**   *Complications of Spironolactone Administration*
>
> Spironolactone is the drug of choice for primary hyperaldosteronism. It effectively lowers blood pressure and improves hypokalemia. The administration of spironolactone is complicated by the following:
> 1. Side effects such as gastrointestinal discomfort, impotence, decreased libido, gynecomastia, and menstrual irregularities.
> 2. Increase in the half-life of digoxin. The client's digoxin dosage may be reduced based on serum levels.
> 3. Concomitant therapy with salicylates. Salicylates increase renal tubular excretion of canrenone, the major active metabolite of spironolactone, thus decreasing its effectiveness.

PHEOCHROMOCYTOMA

A pheochromocytoma is a catecholamine-secreting tumor of the chromaffin cells of the sympathetic nervous system; it is usually found in the adrenal medulla. Pheochromocytomas are rare. In autopsy series, the incidence of pheochromocytoma is 0.1% in clients with diastolic hypertension. The condition is equally common in women and men. Although the disease can occur at any age, it is most common in middle age and rarely occurs after age 60 years.

Etiology and Risk Factors

The cause of pheochromocytomas is unknown. In some cases, they appear to have a familial basis. They often occur together with neuroectodermal diseases and with multiple endocrine neoplasia type IIA. There are no known risk factors for pheochromocytoma.

Pathophysiology

Usually weighing less than 200 g, a pheochromocytoma is composed of chromaffin cells, so named (Latin *affinis, affinitas,* affinity) because these cells stain brownish yellow with chromic salts. In 85% to 95% of cases, pheochromocytomas arise within the adrenal medulla. Occasionally, however, they develop from the chromaffin tissues found in the sympathetic paraganglia. Pheochromocytomas are typically benign; fewer than 10% are malignant. Because of the excessive amounts of epinephrine and norepinephrine they secrete, they can produce severe manifestations and even death (Table 46-2).

Once a pheochromocytoma is diagnosed, certain risk factors are known to influence catecholamine release. Catecholamine release occurs with various frequencies and intensities and is called a *paroxysm.* Risk factors that may stimulate a paroxysm include the following:

- Smoking
- Micturition (voiding reflex)

TABLE 46-2	*The Effects of Epinephrine and Norepinephrine*
Epinephrine	**Norepinephrine**

Cardiovascular System

Constricts superficial blood vessels; in small doses, dilates muscle, brain, and coronary vessels, thus shunting blood supply to organs; essential for "fight or flight"	Constricts blood vessels (especially peripheral), causing increased peripheral resistance
Raises blood pressure	Raises blood pressure greatly
Increases cardiac output	Decreases cardiac output because of increased peripheral resistance
Increases pulse dramatically	Increases pulse moderately
Constricts spleen, shunting stored red blood cells into general circulation	
Increases coagulability of blood	

Respiratory System

Increases rate and depth of respirations	
Dilates bronchi	

Nervous System

Stimulates central nervous system, increasing alertness and producing a feeling of fright, excitation, and impending doom	
Dilates pupils	Dilates pupils
Inhibits gastrointestinal tract	Inhibits gastrointestinal tract

Metabolism

Increases nonesterified fatty acid level of blood	Increases nonesterified fatty acid level of blood
Promotes conversion of glycogen to glucose	
Increases body metabolism	Increases body metabolism slightly

Data from DeGroot, L., & Jameson, J. (2001). *Endocrinology* (4th ed.). Philadelphia: W.B. Saunders.

- Activities that displace abdominal organs, such as bending, exercising, straining, vigorous palpation of the abdomen, and pregnancy
- Certain drugs, such as histamines, anesthetics, atropine, opiates, fentanyl, steroids, and glucagon

Without early intervention, the client is at risk for cerebral hemorrhage and cardiac failure. If a pheochromocytoma is discovered early in its development, it can usually be removed surgically.

Clinical Manifestations

A client with pheochromocytoma may show with manifestations of diabetes mellitus (elevated blood glucose and glucosuria), hypertension (elevated BP, headaches), hyperthyroidism (increased metabolic rate, diaphoresis, agitation, rapid pulse, palpitations, emotional outbursts), and psychoneurosis (emotional instability).

Hypertension is the principal manifestation of pheochromocytoma, and it can be persistent, fluctuating, intermittent, or paroxysmal (rapid onset and abrupt cessation). Typically, the client has episodes of high BP accompanied by pounding headaches. Other manifestations of sympathetic overactivity include sweating, apprehension, palpitations, nausea, and vomiting. Excessive release of catecholamines also results in excessive conversion of glycogen into glucose in the liver. Consequently, hyperglycemia and glucosuria occur during attacks. Such manifestations can develop spontaneously or may be precipitated by emotional stress, physical exertion, or change in body position.

Acute attacks may be associated with profuse diaphoresis (perspiration), dilated pupils, and cold extremities. Severe hypertension can precipitate a stroke or sudden blindness.

Because pheochromocytoma is curable, early and accurate diagnosis is essential. Current methods of diagnosis include the following:

1. *History and physical examination.* The client may describe symptomatic attacks over weeks, months, or even years. The BP may change with exertion or emotional upset. In long-standing cases, complications of intractable hypertension (such as visual disturbances), manifestations of heart disease (dyspnea, edema), and manifestations of kidney damage (albuminuria, proteinuria, and increased blood urea nitrogen) can coexist.

2. *Chemical tests* of urinary catecholamines and their metabolites (metanephrines and vanillylmandelic acid [VMA]) and of plasma catecholamine concentrations. Assays of catecholamines are performed on single-voided urine specimens, 2- to 4-hour specimens, and 24-hour urine specimens. The normal range of urinary catecholamines is up to 14 mg per 100 ml of urine, with higher levels occurring in clients with pheochromocytoma. Assays of urinary VMA levels are performed only on 24-hour urine specimens. Advise the client to avoid tea, chocolate, vanilla, and all fruits for at least 2 days before urine collection begins, and remind the client not to take any medications for 2 to 3 days before the test. Normally, the amount of VMA is less than 7 mg in 24 hours. Urinary VMA levels increase in

clients with pheochromocytoma. Plasma-free metanephrines are considered one of the best tests for excluding or confirming a pheochromocytoma.[14] Plasma catecholamine concentrations may also be determined.

3. *Direct assay* of catecholamines (epinephrine and norepinephrine) in the blood. The normal ranges of catecholamines in the blood are epinephrine, 0.02 to 0.2 mg/L, and norepinephrine, 0.1 to 0.5 mg/L.

4. *X-ray imaging.* Various radiographic techniques, such as CT and MRI, can help confirm and identify adrenomedullary tumor location.

5. *Nonspecific laboratory tests.* In the presence of pheochromocytoma, the basal metabolic rate increases, blood glucose rises to abnormal levels, and glycosuria can occur.

Outcome Management
■ Surgical Management

Adrenalectomy

Indications. The primary treatment of a pheochromocytoma is surgical removal of one or both adrenal glands, depending on whether the tumor is unilateral or bilateral. The procedure is the same as that described for Cushing's syndrome.

Contraindications. The presence of complications of pheochromocytoma may make the client a poor surgical risk. Ideally, surgery is performed before complications develop; however, high BP and vascular complications may necessitate treatment before surgery can take place. Alpha-adrenergic blocking agents, such as phentolamine (Regitine), can be used in an IV bolus or IV drip for hypertensive crisis. Oral phenoxybenzamine (Dibenzyline) is used at least 7 days preoperatively to control BP, reduce manifestations, and eliminate paroxysms before surgical removal of the affected gland.

Complications associated with pheochromocytoma that may delay surgery include hypertensive retinopathy, hypertensive nephropathy, myocarditis, increased platelet aggregation, stroke, and heart failure. Death may result from myocardial infarction, stroke, dysrhythmias, irreversible shock, renal failure, or dissecting aortic aneurysm.

Complications. The surgical procedure for pheochromocytoma is not without danger. There are two serious hazards. First, excessive discharge of pressor hormones during induction of anesthesia or manipulation of the tumor can cause extreme rises in BP and cardiac dysrhythmias. Second, after resection of the tumor, BP can fall precipitously.

Outcomes. Surgical removal of the pheochromocytoma can be curative in most cases if the growth is discovered before cardiovascular damage becomes permanent. Some clients may receive less medication at discharge after surgery. Lifelong steroid replacement must be initiated after a bilateral adrenalectomy.

■ Nursing Management of the Surgical Client

Preoperative Care
Assessment

Assess and control the client's BP preoperatively. Closely monitor the client for the development of stressful episodes before treatment has begun. Evaluate the client's neurologic status in case the client has a stroke because of the extremely elevated BP.

Diagnosis, Outcomes, Interventions

Diagnosis: Risk for Injury. The client with a pheochromocytoma is at great risk for injury preoperatively. Write the nursing diagnosis *Risk for Injury related to excessive release of epinephrine and norepinephrine preoperatively.*

Outcomes. Injury will not occur or will be detected early as evidenced by absence of hypertensive episodes and cardiovascular or cerebral damage.

Interventions. During the preoperative phase, the desired outcome of treatment is preventing attacks of acute paroxysmal hypertension, thereby lowering the risk of further damage to the cardiovascular system. Important nursing interventions include (1) promoting rest and relief from stress; (2) administering prescribed sedatives; (3) providing a diet high in vitamins, minerals, and calories; (4) prohibiting beverages containing caffeine, such as coffee, tea, and colas; and (5) monitoring vital signs. In most cases, the physician prescribes an alpha-adrenergic blocking agent, such as phenoxybenzamine.

Postoperative Care
Assessment

The first 24 to 48 hours after surgery is a critical period demanding vigilant nursing assessment. After surgery, the client should be closely monitored for adrenal insufficiency, hypotension, hemorrhage, and shock. Urine output and BP are assessed hourly.

Diagnosis, Outcomes, Interventions

Diagnosis: Risk for Injury. The client is at increased risk for such problems as hypotension postoperatively. Write the nursing diagnosis as *Risk for Injury related to postoperative hypotension, hemorrhage, and shock.*

Outcomes. Injury will not occur or will be detected early, as evidenced by a normotensive state and an absence of hemorrhage, shock, or addisonian crisis.

Interventions

Monitor and Prevent Shock. During the immediate postoperative period, observe for manifestations of shock and hemorrhage. After removal of the tumor, profound shock can develop as catecholamine levels drop. Hypotension can persist for 24 to 48 hours. Hemorrhage can occur because of the high vascularity of the adrenal glands. To prevent postoperative shock, do the following:

1. Give IV fluids as prescribed, such as blood, plasma, dextran, or glucose in water to maintain blood volume.
2. Administer IV pressors as prescribed at a rate sufficient to maintain BP within a safe range. Check BP as often as necessary to titrate the medication.
3. Carefully measure hourly urine output. If the client voids less than 0.5 ml/kg/hr, notify the physician. Oliguria can signify impending shock and consequent renal shutdown.
4. Assess the client for manifestations of hemorrhage. Check the dressing every half hour for bloody drainage. If the client is bleeding internally, an abdominal hematoma can develop, resulting in paralytic ileus or nonmechanical bowel obstruction (see Chapter 35). Manifestations of paralytic ileus include abdominal pain, distention, severe nausea, vomiting, and diminished or absent bowel sounds.
5. If cortical tissue has been resected during surgery, assess the client closely for manifestations of adrenal insufficiency (see addisonian crisis discussion). If both adrenal glands have been removed, the client must receive cortisol replacement for life.

Diagnosis: Acute Pain. Postoperatively, the client must be monitored for *Acute Pain related to surgery, headache, and other manifestations of pheochromocytoma resulting in verbal reports of pain and guarding behaviors.*

Outcomes. The client will have pain relief or reduction as evidenced by the client's statements, normotensive state, and an absence of pained expressions.

Interventions. When administering medication for incisional pain, monitor BP frequently. Although opioids, particularly meperidine, produce hypotension as a side effect, withholding pain medication can also lead to hypotension (or even hypertension) and severe pain. It is important to control the pain so that the client's level of stress decreases.

Evaluation

It is expected that the client will have no complications postoperatively or that complications that occur will be managed successfully so that the client is discharged within 4 to 5 days postoperatively. Self-care outcomes are evaluated by the client's ability to manage steroid replacement after surgery. Although side effects of steroids cannot be avoided, there are ways to minimize them, and the client's ability to control these and avoid complications can be evaluated.

■ Self-Care

After a bilateral adrenalectomy, the client must learn self-care measures. When the critical postoperative period is over, most clients experience an uneventful convalescence. A client who will be self-administering corticosteroids needs instruction concerning the administration and side effects (see Addison's disease discussion).

■ Modifications for Older Clients

Damage related to hypertensive episodes associated with the pheochromocytoma tends to affect older clients, whose cardiovascular and cerebrovascular systems may be weak and thus susceptible to damage by elevated BP.

ANTERIOR PITUITARY DISORDERS

Disorders of the pituitary gland occur most frequently in the anterior lobe. Major causes of pituitary disease include functioning tumors, nonfunctioning tumors, pituitary infarction, genetic disorders, and trauma. The three principal pathologic consequences of pituitary disorders are (1) hyperpituitarism, (2) hypopituitarism, and (3) local compression of brain tissue by expanding tumor masses.

HYPERPITUITARISM AND HYPERPROLACTINEMIA

Etiology and Risk Factors

Hyperpituitarism is defined as oversecretion of one or more of the hormones secreted by the pituitary gland. It is caused primarily by a hormone-secreting pituitary tumor, typically a benign adenoma. Syndromes associated with hyperpituitarism are Cushing's syndrome, acromegaly, amenorrhea, galactorrhea, hyperthyroidism, and, rarely, hypergonadism in the male.

Pathophysiology

Prolactin and growth hormone are the hormones most commonly overproduced by adenomas. They lead to hyperprolactinemia and acromegaly (Figure 46-2), respectively. Increased amounts of growth hormone lead to rapid growth of all body tissues. This increased growth leads to gigantism (Figure 46-3) if it occurs before closure of the epiphysis and acromegaly if it occurs after epiphyseal closure.

Clinical Manifestations

Pituitary tumors produce both systemic and local effects. Systemic effects include excessive or abnormal growth patterns related to overproduction of growth hormone, ab-

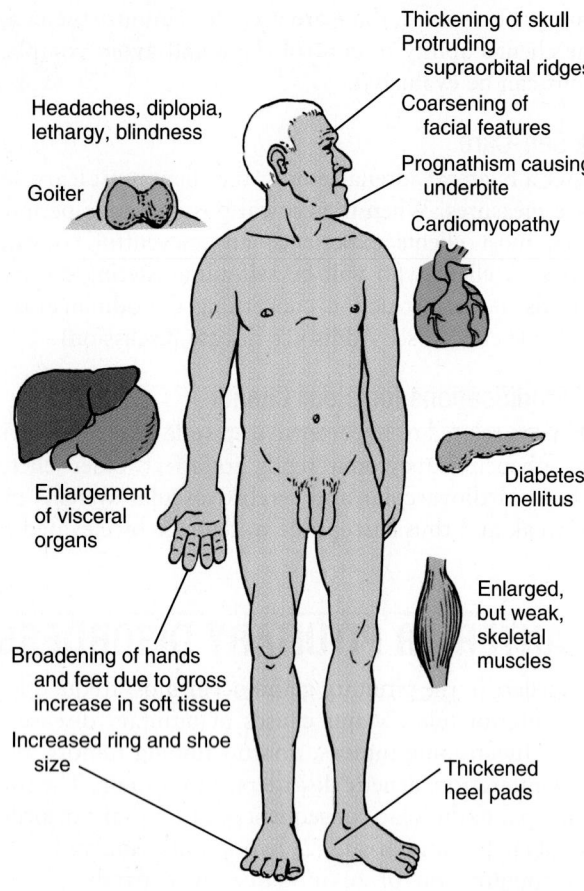

Headaches, diplopia,
lethargy, blindness

Goiter

Thickening of skull
Protruding
supraorbital ridges

Coarsening of
facial features

Prognathism causing
underbite

Cardiomyopathy

Enlargement
of visceral
organs

Diabetes
mellitus

Broadening of hands
and feet due to gross
increase in soft tissue

Enlarged,
but weak,
skeletal
muscles

Increased ring and shoe
size

Thickened
heel pads

FIGURE 46-2 Clinical manifestations of acromegaly.

normal milk secretion (galactorrhea), and overstimulation of one or more of the target glands, resulting in release of excessive thyroid, sex, or adrenocortical hormones.

Locally, pituitary tumors produce manifestations because the bony cranium that houses the tumor cannot expand to accommodate a growing mass. Local manifestations include visual field abnormalities resulting from pressure on the optic chiasm, headaches, and somnolence. See Table 46-3 for additional information related to hyperprolactinemia and acromegaly.

Outcome Management
■ Surgical Management

A client with a pituitary tumor must have the tumor resected. A variety of approaches can be used to remove a pituitary tumor. Usually, a transsphenoidal hypophysectomy is performed (see Chapter 71).

■ Nursing Management of the Surgical Client
Assessment

Most clients are frightened by the prospect of having the pituitary gland removed. Provide the client and his or her significant others with emotional support and comfort throughout the preoperative period.

The initial manifestations are vague; therefore the client may have seen many physicians and may have had multiple examinations and tests while seeking a diagnosis. The client and family may be fearful, skeptical, or relieved with the final diagnosis of pituitary tumor. Assess the client's reaction to the diagnosis, expectations for the surgery, educational needs related to the diagnosis and treatment plan, and available support network after discharge.

Physical assessment includes baseline vital signs and weight as well as neurologic assessment. The client should also have a preoperative eye examination by an ophthalmologist. These findings are essential to establish a baseline for postoperative comparison. To perform the neurologic assessment, check the following:

- Pupil equality and reactivity to light
- Handgrip for strength, equality, and ability to release on command
- Level of consciousness
- Orientation to time, place, person, and location
- Appropriate response to stimuli
- Visual acuity and visual fields

Diagnosis, Outcomes, Interventions

Diagnosis: Deficient Knowledge. Preoperatively, the client must to be taught about the surgery and its implications. A typical nursing diagnosis would be *Deficient Knowledge: Surgery and possible outcomes related to lack of instruction resulting in anxiety, misinformation, and questions.*

Outcomes. The client will understand the planned surgery and possible outcomes as evidenced by his or her statements, questions, and ability to describe the procedure and outcomes.

Interventions. Explain the surgery to the client in detail, along with potential outcomes of surgical treatment. Use drawings of the brain to explain the transsphenoidal approach. Prepare the client for the presence of an indwelling urinary catheter, IV lines, and any other lines or monitors that may be needed after surgery. Tell the client that vital signs will be monitored closely after surgery. Preoperative preparation also includes coaching the client in deep-breathing exercises and assisting in keeping records of intake and output.

Diagnosis: Risk for Injury. A typical postoperative nursing diagnosis would be *Risk for Injury related to postoperative complications.*

Outcomes. Injury will not result from surgery as evidenced by absence of addisonian crisis, balanced intake and output, no manifestations of increased intracranial pressure, normal temperature, and absence of manifestations of cerebrospinal fluid (CSF) leakage or meningitis.

FIGURE 46-3 Primary gigantism. **A,** A 22-year-old man with gigantism resulting from excess growth hormone is shown to the left of his identical twin. The increased height (**A**), enlarged hand (**B**), and enlarged foot (**C**) of the affected twin are apparent. Their height and features began to diverge at the age of approximately 13 years. (Courtesy of Robert F. Gagel, MD, and Ian McCutcheon, MD, University of Texas M.D. Anderson Cancer Center, Houston, TX.)

Interventions

Prevent Adrenal Insufficiency. Before surgery, the client usually receives an IV injection of cortisol. Glucocorticoids help the client tolerate the stress of an operation that can result in loss of adrenocortical function.

Monitor Intracranial Pressure. Treatment after transfrontal hypophysectomy resembles that for any craniotomy (see Chapter 71). Immediately after surgery, assess for cerebral edema and rising intracranial pressure (elevated BP, widened pulse pressure, low pulse rate, pupil changes, altered respiratory pattern).

Monitor for Hormonal Insufficiencies. Because the pituitary gland no longer produces tropic hormones, watch for target gland deficiencies, such as adrenal insufficiency and hypothyroidism. In addition, diabetes insipidus can occur temporarily because of antidiuretic hormone (ADH, vasopressin) deficiency, as outlined in the Critical Monitoring feature Does Your Client Have an Antidiuretic Hormone (ADH) Imbalance? on p. 1237. This deficiency is related to surgical manipulation. Maintain strict documentation of intake and output. Notify the physician if urine output is above 200 ml/hr with a specific gravity below 1.005.

Monitor for Meningitis. Assess the client carefully for meningitis, a potential complication of surgery. Report any temperature elevation, severe headache, irritability, or nuchal rigidity.

Provide Oral Hygiene. The client who has undergone transsphenoidal hypophysectomy requires frequent oral hygiene with a gauze sponge; the lips should be lubri-

TABLE 46-3	*Hyperprolactinemia and Acromegaly in Hyperpituitarism*	
	Hyperprolactinemia	**Acromegaly**
Hormone secreted	Excessive prolactin (PRL) causes prolactinoma	Excessive growth hormone (GH)
Risk factors	Hyperprolactinemia; estrogen therapy; oral contraceptive use; pregnancy may increase tumor size and dysfunction	None
Etiology	Pregnancy; hypothalamic-pituitary disorders; hypothyroidism; drug ingestion (estrogen or oral contraception)	Anterior pituitary adenoma; abnormal hypothalamic function (rare)
Pathophysiology	PRL-producing tumors deliver excess PRL systemically	GH-producing adenomas deliver excess GH systemically, leading to rapid growth in other body tissues (with exception of the CNS), causing organomegaly; increase in tumor size within confined space can result in destruction of entire pituitary and cause hypopituitarism
Clinical manifestations related to hormone oversecretion	Abnormal lactation (galactorrhea) in nonlactating breast; amenorrhea; decreased vaginal lubrication; decreased libido in men; impotence; depression; anxiety; headache; visual loss	Local overgrowth of bone: skull and mandible; soft tissue overgrowth; lethargy; weight gain; paresthesias; glucose intolerance; coarse facial features; irregular or absent menses; enlargement of hands and feet over 1-10 yr; depression; headache; visual field impairment; osteoarthritis; paresthesias; impotence
Complications related to tumor growth	Headaches; visual disturbances affecting cranial nerves III, IV, VI; hypopituitarism; infertility; decreased bone growth	Hypopituitarism; neoplasms of gastrointestinal tract; increased mortality secondary to cardiovascular atherosclerosis, cerebral atherosclerosis, congestive heart failure, respiratory disease, hypertension, diabetes mellitus
Pharmacologic intervention	Bromocriptine is treatment of choice; bromocriptine can reduce PRL levels in 90% of clients; adverse reactions may contribute to noncompliance: nausea, headaches, dizziness, nasal stuffiness, hypotension, depression	Somatostatin analog octreotide is very effective in reducing GH levels; pharmacologic treatment may cause cholelithiasis; bromocriptine is effective in 60%-80% of clients
Surgical intervention	Transsphenoidal microsurgery; complications: residual tissue may produce elevated hormone levels, visual loss, diabetes insipidus, postoperative infection	Transsphenoidal microsurgery is treatment of choice; complications: same as in hyperprolactinemia
Radiation treatment	May decrease adenoma, but local complications are common because of tissue scarring and impairment of anterior pituitary function (hypopituitarism)	Produces slower decline of GH levels, implying higher morbidity related to atherosclerotic disease, respiratory disease, hypertension, diabetes mellitus, and gastrointestinal cancer; hypopituitarism
Diagnosis	Measurement of GH, ACTH, FSH, LH, PRL, testosterone, gonadotropins; thyroid function tests (T_3, T_4, FT_4, TSH); liver function tests (LDH, CPK, AST, alkaline phosphatase); coagulation studies; kidney function tests (serum creatinine, BUN, 24-hr urine collection for protein, creatinine clearance, GFR); urinalysis; pregnancy testing; CT or MRI for pituitary adenoma localization	Radioimmunoassay or enzyme-linked immunosorbent assay for GH level; serum GH level; insulin-like growth factor; CT scan or MRI for pituitary edema localization; oral GTT may demonstrate hyperglycemia; usually, GTT suppresses normal GH release 1-2 hr after ingestion, but in acromegaly the GH level remains elevated

ACTH, Adrenocorticotropic hormone; *AST,* aspartate aminotransferase; *BUN,* blood urea nitrogen; *CNS,* central nervous system; *CPK,* Creatine phosphokinase; *CT,* computed tomography; *FSH,* follicle-stimulating hormone; *FT₄,* free thyroxine; *GFR,* glomerular filtration rate, *GH,* growth hormone; *GTT,* glucose tolerance test; *LDH,* lactate dehydrogenase; *LH,* luteinizing hormone; *MRI,* magnetic resonance imaging; *PRL,* prolactin; *TSH,* thyroid-stimulating hormone; *T₃,* triiodothyronine; *T₄,* thyroxine.

CRITICAL MONITORING

Does Your Client Have an Antidiuretic Hormone (ADH) Imbalance?

	Diabetes Insipidus	Syndrome of Inappropriate Secretion of Antidiuretic Hormone
ADH	↓	↑
Urine output	↑	↓
Urine osmolality	↓	↑
Urine specific gravity	↓	Value insignificant
Serum Na+	↑	↓
Urine Na+	↓	↑
Plasma osmolality	↑	↓
Daily weights	↓	Sudden ↑ (without edema)
Mentation changes	Related to electrolyte imbalance and hypotension	Related to degree of hyponatremia

cated with petroleum jelly. The client should not brush the teeth for 2 weeks after surgery.

Monitor for CSF Drainage. The nasal packing is usually removed in 2 to 5 days. After its removal, observe the client for rhinorrhea, which can indicate a CSF leak. Have the client report frequent postnasal drainage. Collect any serous drainage, and test it for the presence of CSF (see Chapter 69) or send it to the laboratory for analysis. It is possible for the muscle or fat graft to dislodge, causing a CSF leak. Instruct the client to avoid sneezing, coughing, and bending over from the waist to avoid disrupting the graft.

Evaluation

Appropriate outcomes after a hypophysectomy include the absence of postoperative complications and the client's ability to manage lifetime hormone replacement. If complications occur, the appropriate outcome would be that these complications are controlled without permanent problems.

■ Self-Care

After a hypophysectomy, the client must take replacement hormones for life. Instruct the client to avoid gastric irritation by taking cortisone with milk, food, or an antacid. Advise the client to notify the physician about gastritis, tarry stools, or frank blood in the stools. Some clients may also require thyroid or sex hormone replacement. In addition, some need vasopressin replacement to treat *diabetes insipidus.* As a result of deficient ADH, clients may experience polyuria (large urine output) and low urine specific gravity readings. Diabetes insipidus is usually transient after surgery but can persist, indicating the need for chronic hormone replacement.

SEXUAL DISTURBANCES

Excess secretion of gonadotropic hormones, such as luteinizing hormone (LH) and follicle-stimulating hormone (FSH), from pituitary tumors can produce sexual precocity in children. Excess prolactin secretion can cause amenorrhea or galactorrhea (excessive flow of milk) in women. Physicians consider surgical removal the treatment of choice for radiologically demonstrable tumors.

Clients with increased prolactin secretion and no radiologic or neurologic evidence of a pituitary tumor often respond to bromocriptine, an ergot-like compound. Clients with prolactinomas can be successfully treated with bromocriptine. A dopamine agonist, bromocriptine inhibits prolactin secretion. Surgery is no longer the treatment of choice in most cases.

HYPOPITUITARISM

In contrast to hyperpituitarism, hypopituitarism is a deficiency of one or more of the hormones produced by the anterior lobe of the pituitary. When both the anterior and posterior lobes fail to secrete hormones, the condition is called *panhypopituitarism.* Hypopituitarism and panhypopituitarism are rare disorders.

Etiology and Risk Factors

The nine most important causes of hypopituitarism are known as the "nine *Is*":

- Invasion (most common)—pituitary tumors, central nervous system tumors, carotid aneurysm
- Infarction—postpartum necrosis (Sheehan's syndrome), pituitary apoplexy
- Infiltration—sarcoidosis, hemochromatosis
- Injury—head trauma, child abuse
- Immunologic—lymphocytic hypophysitis
- Iatrogenic—surgery, radiation therapy
- Infectious—mycoses, tuberculosis, syphilis

- Idiopathic—familial
- Isolated—deficiency of an anterior pituitary hormone, such as growth hormone, LH, FSH, thyroid-stimulating hormone (TSH), ACTH–lipotropic pituitary hormone (ACTH-LPH), or prolactin

Clinical Manifestations

The pituitary gland has enormous functional reserve; therefore manifestations of hypopituitarism usually do not appear until 75% of the pituitary has been obliterated by tumor or thrombosis. Manifestations depend on age of onset as well as the hormones that are deficient. The onset of hypopituitarism is usually gradual. The classic course of progressive hypopituitarism is an initial loss of growth hormone and gonadotropin, followed by deficiencies of TSH, then ACTH, and finally prolactin.

Specific disorders resulting from pituitary hyposecretion include the following:

- *Short stature.* Severely stunted growth results from either a congenital lack of growth hormone or the development of a space-occupying intracranial tumor, meningitis, or brain injury during early childhood.
- *Sexual and reproductive disorders.* Deficiencies of the gonadotropins (LH and FSH) can produce sterility, diminished sex drive, and decreased secondary sex characteristics. Decreased FSH and LH lead to infertility and amenorrhea, diminished spermatogenesis, and testicular atrophy.
- *Hypothyroidism.* Because the synthesis of thyroid hormone depends on TSH, therapeutic ablation or pathologic destruction of the pituitary gland causes hypothyroidism unless the client receives thyroid hormone (see Chapter 45).
- *Secondary adrenocortical insufficiency.* Adrenal insufficiency can follow diminished synthesis of ACTH by the pituitary gland, which in turn causes diminished secretion of adrenocortical hormones by the adrenal cortex.
- *Prolactin deficiency.* This deficiency is indicated by absence of lactation in the postpartum woman.

Diagnosis of growth hormone deficiency rests on the inability of stimulating agents—such as levodopa, arginine, and insulin—to increase plasma growth hormone levels. ACTH levels can be measured to diagnose secondary adrenal insufficiency. Cortisol levels are low in both primary and secondary hypothyroidism; however, when it is a primary deficiency, ACTH levels are high. In a client with secondary hypopituitarism, ACTH levels are low. Low serum thyroid hormone levels, together with low serum TSH levels, establish the diagnosis of hypothyroidism. Sexual and reproductive disorders are diagnosed by low levels of sex steroids and low levels of plasma FSH and LH. Skull x-ray studies may reveal enlargement of the sella turcica, erosion of the sphenoid bone, or calcification of a suprasellar

mass. CT or MRI may provide an enhanced view of an x-ray finding.

Outcome Management

Treatment of hypopituitarism involves removal, if possible, of the causative factor (such as a tumor) and permanent replacement of the hormones secreted by the target organs.

■ Medical Management

Injections of human growth hormone successfully treat growth hormone deficiency. Previously, human growth hormone was scarce and available for only a few clients. Now it is produced by recombinant deoxyribonucleic acid (DNA) technology and is readily available. Medications prescribed to replace hormones include corticosteroids to correct secondary adrenocortical insufficiency, thyroid hormone to treat myxedema, and sex hormones to correct hypogonadism.

Assessment of the client with hypopituitarism focuses on target organs that depend on pituitary secretions (see specific disorders such as Addison's disease and hypothyroidism). Nursing interventions are also directed at problems resulting from deficiency at the target organ. See the appropriate secretions for specific interventions.

POSTERIOR PITUITARY (NEUROHYPOPHYSEAL) DISORDERS

Unlike the adenohypophysis, the neurohypophysis is rarely destroyed by disease. Even if the posterior lobe becomes damaged or is surgically destroyed with the anterior lobe, hormonal deficiencies usually do not develop because the hypothalamus continues to synthesize oxytocin and ADH. If the hypothalamus suffers damage, however, deficiencies of oxytocin and ADH develop even if the neurohypophysis is healthy and intact.

The major disorder of the posterior lobe is ADH deficiency, also known as *diabetes insipidus.* Excessive ADH causes a condition called the *syndrome of inappropriate antidiuretic hormone* (SIADH), which can occur with lung cancer, head injuries, cranial surgery, pituitary tumors, encephalitis, poliomyelitis, and myxedema. Table 46-4 compares diabetes insipidus and SIADH.

GONADAL DISORDERS

Testicular dysfunction can be primary, a disorder of testicular function, or secondary to a disorder of hypothalamic-pituitary function. Primary testis dysfunction can involve the seminiferous tubules (germ cells or Sertoli's cells), Leydig's cells, or both. Germ cell abnor-

TABLE 46-4	*Comparison of Diabetes Insipidus and Syndrome of Inappropriate Secretion of Antidiuretic Hormone*	
	Diabetes Insipidus (DI)	**Syndrome of Inappropriate Secretion of Antidiuretic Hormone (SIADH)**
Definition	A deficiency of antidiuretic hormone (ADH, vasopressin) results in inability to conserve water	Excessive amounts of ADH secreted from posterior pituitary and other ectopic sources
Incidence	Unknown; DI idiopathic in about 30% of all clients with DI; tumors can be related to 25% of DI cases; head injury accounts for 16%; cranial surgery for 20% of DI cases	Approximately 80% of clients with small cell carcinoma have evidence of impaired ability to excrete water secondary to ectopic production of vasopressin
Etiology	Central or neurogenic DI: CNS interruption of anatomic integrity of posterior pituitary; localized or generalized edema from head trauma, vascular lesions, centrally acting drugs, or CNS infections may also cause central DI; ADH synthesis or release is affected; may be transient or permanent Complete DI occurs when there is disruption of hypophyseal tract and a complete absence of ADH Nephrogenic DI: rare hereditary disorder; acquired structural or functional change in kidney occurs; ADH produced normally, but distal and collecting tubules cannot respond Idiopathic DI	Ectopic production of vasopressin by malignancy is most common cause (degree of vasopressin impairment is relative to extent of malignant disease); see Risk Factors below
Risk factors	Head injury, neurosurgery, hypothalamic tumors, pituitary tumors, brain infections or inflammation; drugs that inhibit vasopressin release: ethanol, glucocorticoids, adrenergic agents, phenytoin, narcotic antagonists, lithium	Vasopressin overuse (from DI); malignant conditions that may contain ectopic sources of vasopressin-like hormone: bronchogenic carcinoma; lymphoma of duodenum, brain, bladder; pancreatic cancer; prostatic cancer; increased intracranial pressure secondary to infectious processes or brain trauma; infectious processes—viral or bacterial pneumonia; drugs that may stimulate vasopressin release: vincristine, cyclophosphamide, thiazides, phenothiazines, carbamazepine, vinblastine, cisplatin, oxytocin; endocrine disorders: adrenal insufficiency, myxedema, anterior pituitary insufficiency; analgesics; vomiting
Pathophysiology: normally ADH increases kidneys' permeability to water to promote water reabsorption and decrease urinary output; ADH is normally released in response to ↑ serum osmolality and ↓ extracellular volume	With ADH deficiency: permeability of water is diminished resulting in excretion of large volumes of hypotonic fluid Three patterns may develop: (1) transient DI—abrupt onset within first few days after neurosurgery, resolves within several days; (2) permanent DI (prolonged DI)—abrupt and early onset, persists for several weeks or forever, usually occurs after damage to hypothalamus or neurohypophyseal stalk; (3) triphasic DI—immediate postinjury increase in urine volume with decrease in urine osmolality lasting 4-5 days; interphase occurs over next 5-7 days when urine volume decreases to normal and is followed by a permanent phase of polyuria	Key features of ADH excess: (1) water retention, (2) hyponatremia, (3) hypo-osmolality; a continual release of ADH causes water retention from renal tubules and collecting ducts; extracellular fluid volume increases with dilutional hyponatremia; hyponatremia suppresses renin and aldosterone secretions causing a decrease in proximal tubule reabsorption of Na^+

IM, intramuscular; *IV*, intravenous; *SC*, subcutaneous.

Continued

	TABLE 46-4	*Comparison of Diabetes Insipidus and Syndrome of Inappropriate Secretion of Antidiuretic Hormone—cont'd*

	Diabetes Insipidus (DI)	Syndrome of Inappropriate Secretion of Antidiuretic Hormone (SIADH)
Physical examination	Integumentary: dry, cool skin, dry mucous membranes Cardiovascular: tachycardia Physical manifestations related to specific electrolyte imbalance	Physical manifestations related to hyponatremia: decreased deep tendon reflexes, fatigue, headache, anorexia, nausea, decreased mental status, seizures, coma Physical manifestations related to fluid volume excess: weight gain without edema, jugular venous distention, tachycardia, tachypnea, rales
Clinical manifestations	Genitourinary: polyuria—a few liters to 18 L/day; clear urine; urinary frequency; nocturia Gastrointestinal: weight loss; polydipsia (if thirst mechanism intact) Integumentary: dry skin and mucous membranes Neurologic: mentation changes as electrolyte imbalance and hypotension worsen	Related to degree of hyponatremia: confusion, lethargy, irritability, seizures, coma Gastrointestinal: decreased motility with anorexia, nausea, vomiting; abrupt weight gain *without edema* of 5%-10%
Complications	Electrolyte imbalance; hypovolemia; hypotension; shock	Seizures; coma; permanent brain damage; disease processes already in progress may be complicated
Diagnosis	Urine: output—a few liters to 18 L/day; specific gravity 1.005; osmolality <200 mOsm/kg H_2O Plasma osmolality ↑ secondary to hypovolemia and dehydration Serum Na^+ ↑ secondary to hypovolemia and dehydration Serum osmolality >290 mOsm/kg H_2O Serum Na^+ ↓ secondary to volume depletion Water deprivation study: positive results Hypertonic saline test: positive for DI if there is little or no ↑ in plasma ADH levels	Serum Na^+ ↓; urine Na^+ ↑; blood urea nitrogen ↑; serum osmolality ↓; urine osmolality ↑; absence of hypotension, hypovolemia, or edematous states; water load test: positive for SIADH, abnormal water excretion; serum Na^+ remains ↓; serum osmolality remains ↓; urine osmolality remains ↑
Surgical management	Hypophysectomy to remove posterior pituitary tumor	None
Medical management	IV fluids; ADH replacement with DDAVP (desmopressin) IV, SC, or intranasal; nasal solution bid is drug of choice; onset of action is 1 hr, 6-24 hr duration; Pitressin tannate in oil is given IM; aqueous Pitressin is used for acute, transient form of DI	Hypertonic IV fluids to correct hyponatremia; sodium restriction; diuretics to correct low plasma osmolality; monitor urine electrolyte loss; replace electrolyte loss; demeclocycline to facilitate free water clearance; treat the underlying cause
Nursing management	1. Know which clients are at risk 2. Monitor intake and output 3. Monitor for excessive thirst or urination 4. Assess serum and urine values: ↓ specific gravity, ↓ urine osmolality, ↑ serum osmolality are early indicators of DI 5. Observe effects of DI on concurrent medical and surgical disorders 6. Client and family teaching	1. Know which clients are at risk 2. Monitor appropriate urine and serum laboratory tests 3. Assess for manifestations of hyponatremia by evaluating neurologic status 4. Monitor daily weights and intake and output 5. Observe for changes in concurrent disorders 6. Administer demeclocycline as ordered to interfere with ADH action; monitor for possible nephrotoxicity 7. Monitor for hypernatremia with fluid overcorrection 8. Client and family teaching

IM, intramuscular; *IV*, intravenous; *SC*, subcutaneous.

TABLE 46-4	*Comparison of Diabetes Insipidus and Syndrome of Inappropriate Secretion of Antidiuretic Hormone—cont'd*	
	Diabetes Insipidus (DI)	**Syndrome of Inappropriate Secretion of Antidiuretic Hormone (SIADH)**
Prognosis	Excellent if there is compliance with vasopressin therapy	Depends on cause and sodium level and serum osmolality; poor for client with bronchogenic carcinoma; seizures and coma contribute to chronic brain dysfunction

malities cause infertility by disrupting spermatogenesis. Secondary sexual development and virilization are normal because testosterone production is not interrupted. When Leydig cell function is impaired, testosterone production falls, and virilization is impaired.

Causes of primary hypogonadism include genetic defects, malnutrition, trauma, infection, renal failure, radiation, chemotherapy, and environmental toxins (such as lead or alcohol). The cause, however, is usually unknown. Klinefelter's syndrome, caused by a chromosomal anomaly with a 47,XXY chromosome constitution, is an example of a genetic disorder causing primary testicular failure.

Secondary testicular dysfunction, frequently referred to as *hypogonadotropic hypogonadism,* results from inadequate secretion of gonadotropins. This complication leads to infertility and hypoandrogenism. The extent of LH and FSH deficiency and the age of onset determine the clinical manifestations. Prepubertal hypogonadism leads to eunuchoid body proportions (resulting from deficiency in male hormones), small testes, and lack of virilization.

Causes of secondary hypogonadism include hypothalamic or pituitary tumors, trauma, degenerative lesions, and radiation. Kallmann's syndrome, which involves a deficiency of gonadotropin-releasing hormone (GRH) production by the hypothalamus, is an example of congenital secondary testicular dysfunction. People with Kallmann's syndrome do not mature normally because of gonadotropin deficiency. Midline defects, such as cleft lip or palate, color blindness, anosmia, and ataxia, are common findings.

CONCLUSIONS

Adrenal, pituitary, and gonadal disorders are not common but are extremely complex and diverse. Obtaining a thorough understanding of the adrenal, pituitary, and gonadal anatomy and physiology can help you care for clients with these disorders. Most of these conditions (such as hypopituitarism) are acute and affect many body systems, whereas others become chronic and lead to a wide variety of other problems, such as Addison's disease. Teaching is vital to the care of these clients; understand these conditions so that appropriate teaching plans can be initiated.

THINKING CRITICALLY *evolve*

1. The client is a woman with a 9-year history of Addison's disease. Normally she takes her prescribed doses of a glucocorticoid (dexamethasone [Decadron]) and a mineralocorticoid (fludrocortisone [Florinef]) without fail. She is 29 years old and is otherwise in good health. The client stayed home from work today because she began to experience nausea, vomiting, diarrhea, and fever with diaphoresis. Because of the nausea and vomiting, she did not take her medications. When her husband returned home at 5:30 PM, he found her unconscious. What events led to the client's unconsciousness? How might missing her medications have affected the client?

Factors to Consider. What acute disorder do the nausea, vomiting, diarrhea, and fever suggest? How might they affect a person with Addison's disease?

2. A 50-year-old woman has been taking glucocorticoids for 10 years for asthma. She is admitted to the hospital for sudden onset of severe low back pain. What factors may have contributed to her back pain?

Factors to Consider. What are the potential long-term effects of oral glucocorticoid therapy? What are their manifestations?

3. A 23-year-old man is admitted for a head injury related to an automobile accident. While doing your hourly checks, you note that his urine output has been 800 ml since the last check. Over the next 3 hours, the client excretes an additional 3000 ml of very clear urine. His blood pressure has dropped, and urine specific gravity is less than 1.005. What are your priorities for care?

Factors to Consider. Is the urine output within normal limits? How might his urine output be related to his head injury?

Discussions for these questions can be found on the website and the CD-ROM.

BIBLIOGRAPHY

EB
1. Carson, P. (2000). Emergency: Adrenal crisis. *American Journal of Nursing, 100*(7), 49-50.
2. Castiglione, B. (2000). Emergency: Hyperkalemia. *American Journal of Nursing, 100*(1), 55-56.
3. Coskeran, P. (1999). Management and treatment of patients with acromegaly. *Nursing Times, 95*(13), 50-52.

EB
4. Coursin, D., & Wood, K. (2002). Corticosteroid supplementation for adrenal insufficiency. *Journal of the American Medical Association, 287*(2), 236-240.
5. DeGroot, L., & Jameson, J. (Eds.) (2001). *Endocrinology* (4th ed). Philadelphia: W.B. Saunders.

EB
6. Dorn, L., & Cerrone, P. (2000). Cognitive function in patients with Cushing syndrome: A longitudinal perspective. *Clinical Nursing Research, 9*(4), 420-440.
7. Edwards, C. (2001). Primary mineralocorticoid excess syndromes. In L. DeGroot & J. Jameson (Eds.), *Endocrinology* (4th ed., pp. 1820-1844). Philadelphia: W.B. Saunders.
8. Eisenberg, A., & Redick, E. (1999). Caring for a patient after resection of pituitary adenoma. *Critical Care, 29*(12), 32cc1-2, 32cc4-6.
9. Ezzone, S. (1999). Clinical focus: SIADH. *Clinical Journal of Oncology Nursing, 3*(4), 187-188.
10. Facts and Comparisons Staff. (2002). *Drug facts and comparisons* (56th ed.). St. Louis: Facts & Comparisons.
11. Heater, D. (1999a). If ADH goes out of balance. Diabetes insipidus. *RN, 62*(7), 44-46.
12. Heater, D. (1999b). If ADH goes out of balance. SIADH. *RN, 62*(7), 47-49.
13. Jones, R., & Huether, S. (2002). Alterations of hormonal regulations. In K. McCance & S. Huether (Eds.), *Pathophysiology: The biologic basis for disease in adults and children* (4th ed., pp. 624-667). St. Louis: Mosby.
14. Lenders, J., et al. (2002). Biochemical diagnosis of pheochromocytoma. Which test is best? *Journal of the American Medical Association, 287*(11), 1427-1434.
15. Loriaux, D.L., & McDonald, W.J. (2001). Adrenal insufficiency. In L. DeGroot & J. Jameson (Eds.), *Endocrinology* (4th ed., pp. 1683-1690). Philadelphia: W.B. Saunders.
16. McCloskey, J., & Bulechek, G. (2000). *Nursing intervention classification (NIC)* (3rd ed.). St. Louis: Mosby.
17. McCowen, K., Malhotra, A., & Bistrian, B. (2001). Stress-induced hyperglycemia. *Critical Care Clinics, 17*(1), 107-124.
18. Miller, M. (2001). Syndromes of excess antidiuretic hormone release. *Critical Care Clinics, 17*(1), 11-24.
19. Molitch, M. (1999). Advances in the management of pituitary tumors. *Endocrinology and Metabolism Clinics of North America, 28*(1), 1-240.
20. Nayback, A. (2000). Hyponatremia as a consequence of acute adrenal insufficiency and hypothyroidism. *Journal of Emergency Nursing, 26*(2),130-133.
21. Nieman, L. (2001). Cushing's syndrome. In L. DeGroot, & J. Jameson (Eds.), *Endocrinology* (4th ed., pp. 1691-1715). Philadelphia: W.B. Saunders.
22. Raisbeck, E. (2002). Recognizing adrenal insufficiency. *Emergency Nurse, 10*(4), 24-26.
23. Roth, J., Koch, C., & Rother, K. (2001). Aging, endocrinology, and the elderly patient. In L. DeGroot & J. Jameson (Eds.), *Endocrinology* (4th ed., pp. 529-555). Philadelphia: W.B. Saunders.
24. Sabol, V. (2001). Addisonian crisis. *American Journal of Nursing, 101*(7), 24AAA-24DDD.
25. Sachse, D. (2001). Acromegaly. *American Journal of Nursing, 101*(11), 69-77.
26. Weinmann, M. (2001). Stress-induced hormonal alterations. *Critical Care Clinics, 17*(1), 1-10.
27. Zaloga, G., & Marik, P. (2001). Hypothalamic-pituitary-adrenal insufficiency. *Critical Care Clinics, 17*(1), 25-42.

Management of Clients with Diabetes Mellitus

James A. Fain

Diabetes mellitus is a chronic systemic disease characterized by either a deficiency of insulin or a decreased ability of the body to use insulin. Diabetes mellitus is sometimes referred to as "high sugars" by both clients and health care providers. The notion of associating sugar with diabetes is appropriate because the passage of large amounts of sugar-laden urine is characteristic of poorly controlled diabetes. However, high levels of blood glucose are only one component of the pathologic process and clinical manifestations associated with diabetes mellitus. Diabetes mellitus can be associated with serious complications, but people with diabetes can take preventive measures to reduce the likelihood of such occurrences.

In 1979, The National Diabetes Data Group[26] (NDDG) developed criteria for the classification and diagnosis of diabetes. By 1997, and again in 2003, the Expert Committee on the Diagnosis and Classification of Diabetes Mellitus[19] proposed changes to the original NDDG classification scheme. Such changes were supported by the American Diabetes Association (ADA) and the National Institute of Diabetes and Digestive and Kidney Diseases (NIDDK). Previously, diabetes was classified as either insulin-dependent diabetes mellitus (IDDM) or non–insulin-dependent diabetes mellitus (NIDDM). With the use of insulin therapy commonplace with both types of diabetes, IDDM is now referred to as type 1 diabetes, and NIDDM is referred to as type 2 diabetes. The ADA also recommended using Arabic numerals; type 1 and type 2, rather than Roman numerals in referring to the two types of diabetes.[19]

Type 1 diabetes is characterized by destruction of pancreatic beta cells, leading to absolute insulin deficiency. Type 1 diabetes affects 10% of people who have

evolve *Be sure to check out the bonus material on the Evolve website and the CD-ROM, including free self-assessment exercises.*

http://evolve.elsevier.com/Black/medsurg/

1243

Nursing Outcomes Classification (NOC)
for Nursing Diagnoses—Clients with Diabetes Mellitus

Readiness for Enhanced Therapeutic Regimen Management	Knowledge: Treatment Regimen	**Risk for Ineffective Therapeutic Regimen Management**
Health Belief: Perceived Resources	Participation: Health Care Decisions	Compliance Behavior
Health Promoting Behavior	Psychosocial Adjustment: Life Change	Knowledge: Disease Process
Health Seeking Behavior	Risk Detection	Knowledge: Treatment Regimen
Knowledge: Health Behaviors	Self-Direction of Care	Participation: Health Care Decisions
Knowledge: Health Promotion	Social Support	Treatment Behavior: Illness or Injury
Knowledge: Health Resources	Treatment Behavior: Injury or Illness	

BOX 47-1 *Types of Diabetes Mellitus and Abnormal Glucose Metabolism*

Diabetes Mellitus

1. Type 1 diabetes
2. Type 2 diabetes
3. Causes of secondary diabetes
   a. Genetic defects
   b. Diseases of the pancreas (such as pancreatitis, neoplasia, trauma/pancreatectomy)
   c. Endocrinopathies (such as acromegaly, Cushing's syndrome, pheochromocytoma, hyperthyroidism)
   d. Drug/chemical-induced (as from glucocorticoids, thyroid hormone, diazoxide, thiazides, phenytoin sodium [Dilantin], nicotinic acid)
   e. Infections (such as congenital rubella, cytomegalovirus infection)
   f. Genetic syndromes associated with diabetes (such as Down syndrome, Klinefelter's syndrome, Huntington's chorea)
4. Gestational diabetes mellitus

Pre-Diabetes Mellitus

1. Impaired glucose tolerance (IGT)
   (2-hour post-glucose load ≥140 and <200 mg/dl)
2. Impaired fasting glucose (IFG)
   (fasting blood glucose ≥110 and <126 mg/dl)

Modified from American Diabetes Association. (2003). Report of the Expert Committee on the Diagnosis and Classification of Diabetes Mellitus. *Diabetes Care, 26* (suppl. 1), S5-S20.

diabetes and is usually diagnosed before the age of 30. The most common form of diabetes; type 2, affects 90% to 95% of people who have diabetes and is usually diagnosed after age 40. Type 2 diabetes is more common among older adults and certain ethnic and racial populations.

Clients who do not have type 1 or type 2 diabetes may nevertheless be classified as having *impaired glucose tolerance (IGT)*, which is defined as a 2-hour oral glucose tolerance test (75-g glucose load) with a glucose concentration between 140 and 200 mg/dl. An *impaired fasting glucose level (IFG)* is a glucose concentration between 110 and 125 mg/dl.[19] IGT and IFG refer to a metabolic state between normal and diabetes, referred to as *prediabetes*.[1]

Diabetes may also result from other disorders or treatments. Genetic defects in the beta cells can lead to the development of diabetes. Several hormones, such as growth hormone, cortisol, glucagon, and epinephrine, can antagonize or counteract insulin. Excess amounts of these hormones (as in acromegaly, Cushing's syndrome, glucagonoma, and pheochromocytoma) cause diabetes. In addition, certain drugs (e.g., glucocorticoids and thiazides) may cause diabetes. Such types of secondary diabetes account for 1% to 2% of all diagnosed cases of diabetes.

Gestational diabetes mellitus is a diagnosis of diabetes mellitus that applies only to women in whom glucose intolerance develops or is first discovered during pregnancy. Gestational diabetes develops in 2% to 5% of all pregnant women but disappears when the pregnancy is over. It occurs more frequently in African Americans, Hispanic Americans, Native Americans, and women with a family history of diabetes; obesity is also a risk factor. See Box 47-1 for an overview of the types of diabetes mellitus.[19]

A significant public health problem, diabetes is the seventh leading cause of death in the United States. About 17 million people (6.2 % of the population) have diabetes; approximately one third of these cases are undiagnosed.[3] In addition, another 15 to 16 million people have prediabetes. Of those 17 million people with diabetes, some 3.2 million are 65 years of age or older. Diabetes imposes a heavy economic burden on the United States each year. It is estimated that more than $100 billion in direct and indirect costs (e.g., disability, work loss, and premature death) are attributed to diabetes mellitus each year.[3] The increasing burden of diabetes is alarming, but the good news is that much of the burden of this major public health problem can be prevented by early detection, improved delivery of care, and better education for diabetes self-management.

Type 1 diabetes mellitus accounts for about 10% of all known cases of diabetes mellitus in the United States. Annual incidence is 12 to 14 cases per 100,000 people younger than 20 years, with a prevalence of 1 case per 500 people younger than 16 years. It is one of the most common childhood diseases, being three to four times more common than such chronic childhood diseases as cystic fibrosis, juvenile rheumatoid arthritis, and leukemia, and 10 times more common than nephrotic syndrome or muscular dystrophy. The incidence of type 1 diabetes mellitus in males is similar to that in females, and the condition is more common in African Americans, Hispanic Americans, Asian Americans, and Native Americans than in whites.[3] Risk factors are less well defined for type 1 diabetes than for type 2 diabetes.[9]

Type 2 diabetes mellitus accounts for about 90% to 95% of all known cases of diabetes mellitus in the United States. About 8 million Americans have type 2 diabetes, with an almost equal number of cases being undiagnosed. Type 2 diabetes is present, on average, for about 6.5 years before its clinical identification and treatment. The prevalence is markedly higher in Native Americans, African Americans, and Hispanic Americans, as well as in older and obese people.[3] Diabetes is the leading cause of new blindness in adults 20 to 74 years of age and is the leading cause of end-stage renal disease, accounting for about 40% of new cases. Likewise, diabetes is responsible for more than half the number of nontraumatic amputations in the United States.[3]

Etiology and Risk Factors

Type 1 Diabetes Mellitus

Type 1 diabetes, previously called IDDM or *juvenile-onset diabetes,* is inherited as a heterogeneous, multigenic trait. Identical twins have a risk of 25% to 50% of inheriting the disease, whereas siblings have a 6% risk and offspring a 5% risk. Despite this strong familial influence, 90% of people in whom type 1 diabetes develops do not have a first-degree relative with diabetes. An association also exists between type 1 diabetes and several human leukocyte antigens (HLAs). Environmental factors such as viruses appear to trigger an autoimmune process that destroys beta cells. Islet cell antibodies (ICAs) then appear, increasing in amount over months to years as beta cells are destroyed.[27] Fasting hyperglycemia (elevated blood glucose level) occurs when 80% to 90% of beta cell mass has been destroyed.

Identification of ICAs has made it possible to detect type 1 diabetes mellitus in its preclinical stage. Autoantibodies directed against insulin are found in 20% to 60% of clients with type 1 diabetes before initiation of exogenous insulin therapy. The combination of large amounts of ICAs, presence of insulin autoantibodies, and decreased first-phase insulin secretion (representing insulin stored in beta cells) can predict the onset of type 1 diabetes mellitus within 5 years.[27]

There are no known health promotion activities to prevent type 1 diabetes mellitus; however, regular exercise and adherence to a prescribed diet may limit the development of complications. In some instances, high-risk individuals (i.e., first-degree relatives of people with type 1 diabetes) are screened, and appropriate counseling and follow-up are instituted.[9]

Health maintenance activities involve the following:
- Maintaining blood glucose at levels as normal as possible
- Preventing hypoglycemia and hyperglycemia with stress, illness, or exercise by closely monitoring blood glucose levels and taking early action; performing daily foot care
- Preventing complications of diabetes mellitus by removing or treating coexisting risk factors such as smoking, hypertension, hyperlipidemia, and use of nephrotoxic drugs

Health restoration actions include the following:
- Prompt treatment of foot abrasions or infections
- Follow-up visits to assess for complications of diabetes and to reinforce learning needs
- Yearly funduscopic examinations by an ophthalmologist with treatment as needed
- Treatment of coexisting risk factors as described previously

Type 2 Diabetes Mellitus

Type 2 diabetes mellitus, previously called NIDDM or *adult-onset diabetes,* also appears to be a heterogeneous disorder involving both genetic and environmental factors. It is not associated with HLA tissue types, and circulating ICAs are rarely present. Heredity plays a major role in the expression of type 2 diabetes. It is more common in identical twins (58% to 75% incidence) than in the general population. Obesity is a major risk factor with 85% of all people with type 2 diabetes being obese. It is unclear whether impaired tissue (liver and muscle) sensitivity to insulin or impaired insulin secretion is the primary defect in this type of diabetes.[27] In addition, the prevalence of coronary artery disease in people with type 2 diabetes is twice that in the non-diabetic population, and cardiovascular and total mortality rates are two-fold to three-fold greater than in non-diabetic people.[32] See the Evidence-Based Practice in Action feature on Can We Prevent Type 2 Diabetes? on p. 1246.

Health promotion actions for type 2 diabetes mellitus include the following:
- Eating habits based on the "Food Guide Pyramid" (as noted later)[31]
- Avoiding foods high in refined sugars and saturated fats
- Maintaining ideal body weight, starting in childhood
- Exercising regularly
- Returning to pre-pregnancy weight or ideal body weight postpartum

Health maintenance activities involve the following:

- Screening high-risk individuals (i.e., people with family history of diabetes in first or second generation; members of certain racial or ethnic backgrounds [African American, Native American, Mexican American, Asians/Pacific Islanders]; people older than age 45 years with any other risk factor; people with hypertension or hyperlipidemia; clients with previous impaired glucose tolerance; women with previous gestational diabetes mellitus or those who have had a baby weighing more than 9 pounds; and people with a history of recurrent infection, habitual physical inactivity, or polycystic ovary syndrome) by doing a fasting blood glucose level[10]
- Performing periodic assessments to determine the client's learning needs and to assess glycemic control
- Using strategies shown to reduce complications of diabetes by removing or treating coexisting risk factors such as smoking, hypertension, hyperlipidemia, and use of nephrotoxic drugs

- Performing daily foot care
- Preventing hypoglycemia or hyperglycemia by closely monitoring blood glucose levels and taking early action

Health restoration actions include the following:

- Teach diet and exercise programs to reduce obesity
- Prompt treatment of foot abrasions or infections
- Follow-up visits to assess for complications of diabetes and reinforce learning needs
- Yearly funduscopic examinations by an ophthalmologist with treatment as needed
- Treatment of previously described risk factors
- Control of angina and peripheral vascular disease

Pathophysiology

Type 1 Diabetes Mellitus

The development of type 1 diabetes mellitus can be broken down into five stages:

- *Stage 1:* genetic predisposition
- *Stage 2:* environmental trigger

EB EVIDENCE-BASED PRACTICE IN ACTION

Can We Prevent Type 2 Diabetes?

In the United States, the prevalence of diabetes among adults was 7.4% in 1995 and was expected to increase to 9% by 2025.[1] Results of several research studies over the past few years has indicated that lifestyle approaches can effectively prevent or delay the onset of type 2 diabetes.[3-6] Characteristics associated with an increased risk of type 2 diabetes include elevated fasting glucose levels (IFG) and postload oral glucose tolerance test (OGTT) concentrations, increased body mass index, central obesity, certain ethnic and racial backgrounds, family history of diabetes, and gestational diabetes.[2] Clinical trials of diabetes prevention among high-risk individuals have demonstrated the association between lifestyle interventions and decreased progression to diabetes.[3]

Implications

Knowledge of characteristics associated with an increased risk of type 2 diabetes is very useful in identifying appropriate population subgroups to target screening efforts aimed at identifying high-risk individuals and those individuals with undiagnosed diabetes. Several studies[4-5] have provided evidence that there is an association between successfully implemented lifestyle intervention (diet, physical activity, or both) and a decrease in progression to diabetes. The Diabetes Prevention Program showed reduction in incident rates of diabetes among racially and ethnically diverse group of males with IGT and a body mass index greater than 24 kg/m². The effectiveness of the lifestyle intervention group in reducing the incidence of type 2 diabetes was significantly greater than that of the medication group (metformin).[3] In addition, the UK Prospective Diabetes Study[6] estab-

lished that a reduction in blood glucose levels among individuals with type 2 diabetes can reduce rates of microvascular (and potentially macrovascular) complications. Therefore the focus of future research needs to identify the most effective lifestyle intervention in terms of clinical outcomes, time required, and cost.

References

1. American Diabetes Association. (2001). *Diabetes 2001 vital statistics.* Alexandria, VA: Author.
2. American Diabetes Association. (2003). Screening for type 2 diabetes (position statement). *Diabetes Care, 26* (suppl. 1), S21-S24.
3. Diabetes Prevention Program Research Group. (2000). Reduction in the incidence of type 2 diabetes with lifestyle intervention or metformin. *New England Journal of Medicine, 346,* 393-403.
4. Eriksson, K.F., Lindgarde, F. (1996). Poor physical fitness, and impaired early insulin response but late hyperinsulinemia, as predictors of diabetes in middle-aged Swedish men. *Diabetologia, 39,* 5473-5579.
5. Tuomilehto, J., Lindstrom, J., Eriksson, J.G. (2001). Prevention of type 2 diabetes mellitus by changes in lifestyle among subjects with impaired glucose tolerance. *New England Journal of Medicine, 344,* 1343-1350.
6. UK Prospective Diabetes Study Group. (1998). Intensive blood-glucose control with sulphonylureas or insulin compared with conventional treatment and risk of complications in patients with type 2 diabetes (UKPDS 33). *Lancet, 352,* 837-853.

- *Stage 3:* active autoimmunity
- *Stage 4:* progressive beta cell destruction
- *Stage 5:* overt diabetes mellitus

Type 1 diabetes mellitus does not develop in all people who have a genetic predisposition. Of those in whom gene markers (DR3 or DR4 HLA) indicate risk, diabetes ultimately develops in less than 1%. Environmental triggers have long been suspected in type 1 diabetes. Incidence is increased in both spring and fall, and onset is often coincidental with epidemics of various viral diseases. Active autoimmunity is directed against the beta cells of the pancreas and their products. ICAs and insulin antibodies progressively decrease the effective circulating insulin level.[27]

This slow, progressive insult to the beta cells and endogenous insulin molecules can result in an abrupt onset of diabetes. Hyperglycemia can result from acute illness or stress (see the Case Study feature on Diabetes and Pneumonia, below), which increases insulin demand beyond the reserves of the damaged beta cell mass. When the acute illness or stress resolves, the client may revert to a compensated state of variable duration in which the pancreas once again manages to produce adequate amounts of insulin. This compensated state, referred to as the *honeymoon period,* typically lasts for 3 to 12 months. The process ends when the diminishing beta cell mass cannot produce enough insulin to sustain life. The client then becomes dependent on exogenous insulin (produced outside the body) administration to survive.[27]

Type 2 Diabetes Mellitus

The pathogenesis of type 2 diabetes mellitus differs significantly from that of type 1. A limited beta cell response to hyperglycemia appears to be a major factor in its development. Beta cells chronically exposed to high

blood levels of glucose become progressively less efficient when responding to further glucose elevations. This phenomenon, termed *desensitization,* is reversible by normalizing glucose levels. The ratio of *proinsulin* (a precursor to insulin) to insulin secreted also increases.[27]

A second pathophysiologic process in type 2 diabetes mellitus is resistance to the biologic activity of insulin in both the liver and peripheral tissues. This state is known as *insulin resistance.* People with type 2 diabetes have a decreased sensitivity to glucose levels, which results in continued hepatic glucose production, even with high blood glucose levels. This is coupled with an inability of muscle and fat tissues to increase glucose uptake. The mechanism causing peripheral insulin resistance is not clear; however, it appears to occur after insulin binds to a receptor on the cell surface (Figure 47-1).

Insulin is a building (anabolic) hormone. Without insulin, three major metabolic problems occur: (1) decreased glucose utilization, (2) increased fat mobilization, and (3) increased protein utilization. (See the Concept Map feature on Understanding Diabetes Mellitus and Its Treatment on p. 1248.)

Decreased Glucose Utilization

In diabetes, cells that require insulin as a carrier for glucose can take in only about 25% of the glucose they require for fuel. Nerve tissues, erythrocytes, and the cells of the intestines, liver, and kidney tubules do not require insulin for glucose transport. However, adipose tissue along with skeletal and cardiac muscle does require insulin for glucose transport. Without adequate amounts of insulin, much of the ingested glucose cannot be used.[22]

With inadequate amounts of insulin, blood glucose levels rise. This elevation continues because the liver cannot store glucose as glycogen without sufficient insulin levels. In an attempt to restore balance and return blood glucose levels to normal, the kidney excretes the excess glucose. Glucose appears in the urine *(glucosuria).* Glu-

CASE STUDY   *evolve*
Diabetes and Pneumonia

Ms. Washington is a 44-year-old black woman who has been sick for the past week. She has been treated with erythromycin (E-Mycin) 500 mg q 6 hr and phenylpropanolamine-guaifenesin (Entex LA) q 12 hr as an outpatient after being seen in the clinic for a persistent cough, loss of voice, chest pain from coughing, fever, chills, and mild nausea without vomiting. She now reports that she has been coughing sputum that is brown to green, with small amounts of red blood present. Ms. Washington is also complaining of left shoulder pain of 3 days' duration, fatigue, sinus pressure, congestion, fullness in the ears, and postnasal drainage. She also reports frequent urination without dysuria or urgency and feeling thirsty all the time. . . . *Case Study continued on the website and the CD-ROM with discussions, multiple-choice questions, and a nursing care plan.* *evolve*

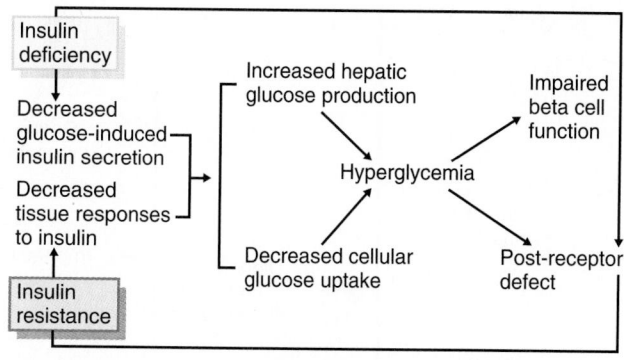

FIGURE 47-1 Relationship between insulin resistance and insulin secretion in type 2 diabetes mellitus. (Modified from American Diabetes Association [1998]. *Medical management of non-insulin dependent [type 2] diabetes* [4th ed., p. 18]. Alexandria, VA: Author.)

Understanding Diabetes Mellitus and Its Treatment

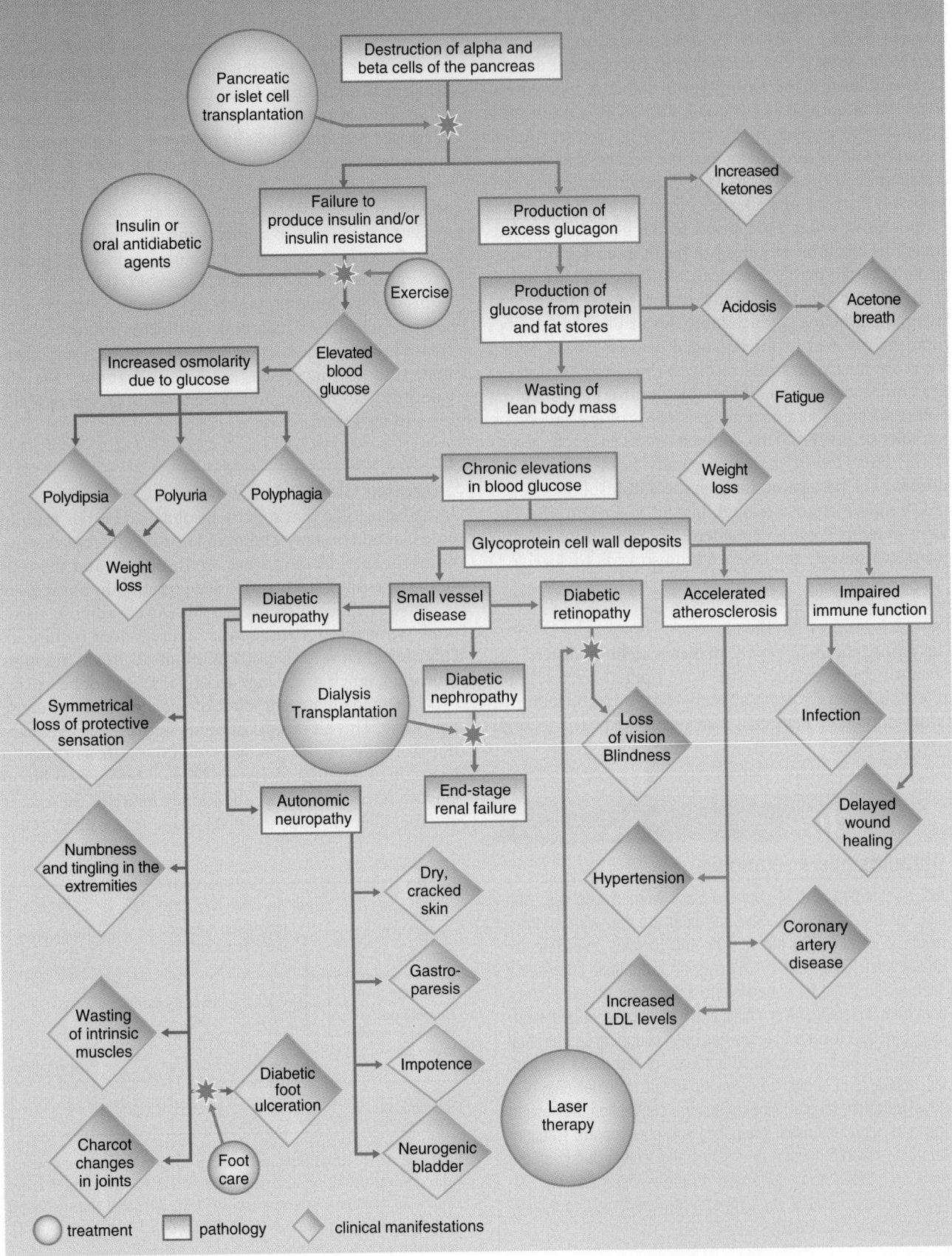

treatment — pathology — clinical manifestations

cose excreted in the urine acts as an osmotic diuretic and causes excretion of increased amounts of water, resulting in fluid volume deficit.[22,27]

Increased Fat Mobilization

In type 1 diabetes and occasionally with severe stress in type 2 diabetes, the body turns to fat stores for energy production when glucose is unavailable. Fat metabolism causes breakdown products called *ketones* to form. Ketones accumulate in the blood and are excreted through the kidneys and lungs. Ketone levels can be measured in the blood and urine; high levels can indicate uncontrolled diabetes.[22]

Ketones interfere with the body's acid-base balance by producing hydrogen ions. The pH can decrease, and metabolic acidosis (discussed later) can develop. In addition, when ketones are excreted, sodium is also eliminated, resulting in sodium depletion and further acidosis. The excretion of ketones also increases osmotic pressure, leading to increased fluid loss. Also, when fats are the primary source of energy, body lipid levels can increase to five times normal, leading to increased atherosclerosis.[22,27]

Increased Protein Utilization

Lack of insulin leads to protein wasting. In healthy people, proteins are constantly being broken down and rebuilt. In people with type 1 diabetes, without insulin to stimulate protein synthesis, the balance is altered, which leads to increased catabolism (destruction). Amino acids are converted to glucose in the liver, further elevating glucose levels. If this condition goes untreated, clients with type 1 diabetes appear emaciated. The pathophysiologic processes of diabetes continue, leading to many acute and chronic complications, as discussed later in this chapter.[22,27,32]

Clinical Manifestations

Hyperglycemia; an elevated blood glucose level, leads to common clinical manifestations associated with diabetes. In type 1 diabetes, the onset of clinical manifestations associated with hyperglycemia may be subtle with the possibility of life-threatening situations likely to happen (i.e., diabetic ketoacidosis). In contrast, type 2 diabetes may develop so gradually that some individuals may notice few or no clinical manifestations for a number of years. Clients may initially complain of numbness or tingling in their hands or feet, which is related to a long-term diabetes-related complication termed peripheral neuropathy (nerve damage in hands and feet). Other times, the diagnosis of type 2 diabetes may be made by a routine laboratory test in clients who have no clinical manifestations.

The classic clinical manifestations of diabetes are increased frequency of urination *(polyuria)*, increased thirst and fluid intake *(polydipsia)*, and, as the disease

progresses, weight loss despite increased hunger and food intake *(polyphagia)*. These clinical manifestations are caused by hyperglycemia and the accompanying spillover of excess glucose in the urine. See Tables 47-1 and 47-2 for common clinical manifestations associated with diabetes.

Diagnosis of Diabetes Mellitus

Physical examination, medical history, and laboratory tests are employed to evaluate clients with diabetes. Clinical manifestations suggest the presence of diabetes, but laboratory tests are needed to make a definitive diagnosis.

Fasting Blood Glucose

Three laboratory tests measuring blood glucose levels are used to confirm the diagnosis of diabetes. The diagnosis of diabetes is made when a client's fasting blood glucose level is greater than 126 mg/dl. Values between 110 to 126 mg/dl indicate an IFG.[19] A fasting blood glucose sample is drawn when the client has not ingested any nutrients other than water for at least 8 hours. This blood sample generally reflects glucose from hepatic production. If the client is receiving a dextrose intravenous (IV) solution, results of the test must be analyzed with that variable in mind. In clients who are known to have diabetes, food and insulin are withheld until after the specimen is obtained. The fasting blood glucose gives the best indication of overall glucose homeostasis.

Casual Blood Glucose

Clients may also be diagnosed with diabetes based on clinical manifestations and a casual (random) blood glucose level greater than 200 mg/dl.[19] A blood sample drawn without fasting for 8 hours would be considered a casual blood glucose measurement. Elevated blood glucose levels may occur after meals, after stressful events, from samples drawn from an IV site, or in cases of diabetes.

Postload Blood Glucose

A postload or postprandial (after a meal) glucose level can also be drawn and used to diagnose diabetes. Postload blood glucose samples are drawn 2 hours after a standard meal and reflect the efficiency of insulin-mediated glucose uptake by peripheral tissues. Normally, blood glucose should return to fasting levels within 2 hours. A 2-hour postload glucose level greater than 200 mg/dl during an oral glucose tolerance test (OGTT)[19] is confirmation for a diagnosis of diabetes (Box 47-2).

In older adults, postload levels are higher, typically increasing by 5 to 10 mg/dl per decade after age 50 years because of the normal decline in glucose tolerance

TABLE 47-1 Selected Clinical Manifestations of Diabetes Mellitus at Diagnosis

Clinical Manifestation	Pathophysiologic Basis	Type 1 Diabetes	Type 2 Diabetes
Cardinal manifestations			
Polyuria* (frequent urination)	Water not reabsorbed from renal tubules secondary to osmotic activity of glucose; leads to loss of water, glucose, and electrolytes	+ +	+
Polydipsia* (excessive thirst)	Dehydration secondary to polyuria causes thirst	+ +	+
Polyphagia* (excessive hunger)	Starvation secondary to tissue breakdown (catabolism) causes hunger	+ +	+
Weight loss*	Initial loss secondary to depletion of water, glycogen, and triglyceride stores; chronic loss secondary to decreased muscle mass as amino acids are diverted to form glucose and ketone bodies	+ +	−
Recurrent blurred vision	Secondary to chronic exposure of ocular lens and retina to hyperosmolar fluids	+	+ +
Pruritus, skin infections, vaginitis	Bacterial and fungal infections of the skin seem to be more common; research conflicting	+	+ +
Ketonuria	When glucose cannot be used for energy in insulin-dependent cells, fatty acids are used for energy; fatty acids are broken down into ketones in the blood and excreted by the kidneys; in type 2 diabetes, sufficient insulin is present to depress excessive use of fatty acids but not enough to permit use of glucose	+ +	−
Weakness and fatigue, dizziness	Decreased plasma volume leads to postural hypotension; potassium loss and protein catabolism contribute to weakness	+ +	+
Often asymptomatic	The body can "adapt" to a slow rise in blood glucose to a greater extent than it can to a rapid rise	−	+ +

+, Sometimes seen; + +, usually seen; −, not usually seen.
*Often referred to as *classic manifestations* of diabetes.

TABLE 47-2 Distinguishing Features of Type 1 and Type 2 Diabetes Mellitus

Feature	Type 1	Type 2
Synonyms	Insulin-dependent diabetes mellitus (IDDM), juvenile diabetes, labile or brittle diabetes	Non–insulin-dependent diabetes mellitus (NIDDM), adult or maturity-onset diabetes, mild diabetes
Age at onset	Usually occurs before age 30 yr, but may occur at any age	Usually occurs after age 30 yr, but can occur in children
Incidence	~10%	~90%
Type of onset	Usually abrupt, with rapid onset of hyperglycemia	Insidious, may be asymptomatic or mildly asymptomatic; body adapts to slow onset of hyperglycemia
Endogenous insulin production	Little or none	Below normal, normal, or above normal
Body weight at onset	Ideal body weight or thin	85% of clients are obese; may be of ideal body weight
Ketosis	Prone to ketosis, usually present at onset, often present during poor control	Resistant to ketosis, can occur with infection or stress
Manifestations	Polyuria, polydipsia, polyphagia, fatigue	Often none, may be mild manifestations of hyperglycemia
Dietary management	Essential	Essential
Exercise management	Essential	Essential
Exogenous insulin administration	Dependent on insulin for survival	20%-30% of clients may require insulin
Oral hypoglycemic agents	Not effective	Effective
Teaching needs	At diagnosis and ongoing	At diagnosis and ongoing

BOX 47-2 *Screening and Diagnosis Guidelines for Diabetes Mellitus*

Guidelines for Testing for Diabetes

Testing for diabetes should be considered in all persons at age 45. If results are normal, test should be repeated at 3-year intervals.

Testing should be considered at a younger age or performed more often for clients with the following risk factors:

- Obesity (>120% of desirable body weight or a body mass index above 25 kg/m²)
- Habitual physical inactivity
- Polycystic ovary syndrome
- Diabetes in a first-degree relative
- Racial predisposition (as in African-American, Hispanic, Native American populations)
- In women, giving birth to a baby weighing more than 9 lb or a history of gestational diabetes
- Hypertension (blood pressure >140/90 mm Hg)
- A high-density lipoprotein level <35 mg/dl or triglyceride level >250 mg/dl
- On previous testing, impaired glucose tolerance or impaired fasting glucose

Guidelines for Diagnosis of Diabetes Mellitus

Manifestations of diabetes plus casual plasma glucose concentration above 200 mg/dl (11.1 mmol/L). *Casual* is defined as any time of day without regard to time since last meal. Classic manifestations include polyuria, polydipsia, and unexplained weight loss.

OR

Fasting plasma glucose level above 126 mg/dl (7.0 mmol/L). Fasting is defined as no caloric intake for at least 8 hours.

OR

A 2-hour postload glucose level above 200 mg/dl during an oral glucose tolerance test. This test should be performed using a glucose load containing the equivalent of 75 g of anhydrous glucose dissolved in water.

Plasma Glucose Values

Fasting plasma glucose	<110 mg/dl	Normal fasting glucose
	110-126 mg/dl	Impaired fasting glucose
	>126 mg/dl	Diagnosis of diabetes
Oral glucose tolerance test, 2 hours after eating	<140 mg/dl	Normal glucose tolerance
	140-200 mg/dl	Impaired glucose intolerance
	>200 mg/dl	Diagnosis of diabetes

Modified from American Diabetes Association. (2003). Report of the Expert Committee on the Diagnosis and Classification of Diabetes Mellitus. *Diabetes Care, 26* (suppl. 1), S5-S20.

associated with aging. Smoking and drinking coffee can lead to falsely elevated values at 2 hours, whereas strenuous exercise can lead to falsely decreased values.

Glycosylated Hemoglobin

Glucose normally attaches itself to the hemoglobin molecule on a red blood cell. Once attached, it cannot dissociate. Therefore the higher the blood glucose levels, the higher the levels of glycosylated hemoglobin (HbA₁C). The term HbA₁C is referred to as an A1C.[11] The A1C is an average blood glucose level measured over the previous 3 months. It is stated as a percentage and is useful in evaluating long-term glycemic control. A1C goals must be individualized, and to avoid diabetes-related complication, the ADA recommends keeping the A1C level below 7%.[11] The ADA recommends that A1C testing be done routinely on all people with diabetes. The A1C test should be done semiannually in clients who have stable glycemic control (i.e., clients who meet target goals) and quarterly in clients who are not meeting glycemic control.[11] Conditions that increase erythrocyte turnover, such as bleeding, pregnancy, or asplenia (absence of the spleen as after splenectomy), lead to falsely low A1C concentrations. High aspirin doses, alcohol ingestion, uremia, elevated hemoglobin levels, and heparin therapy can cause falsely elevated A1C levels.

Glycosylated Albumin

Glucose also attaches to proteins, primarily albumin. The concentration of glycosylated albumin (fructosamine) represents the average blood glucose level over the previous 7 to 10 days. This measurement is useful when short-term determinations of average blood glucose are desired. The reliability and clinical applicability continue to be evaluated.

Connecting Peptide

When the proinsulin produced by pancreatic beta cells is broken apart by an enzyme, two products are formed: insulin and connecting peptide, commonly called *C-peptide*. Because C-peptide and insulin are formed in equal amounts, this test indicates the amount of endogenous insulin production. Clients with type 1 diabetes usually have no or low concentrations of C-peptide. Clients with type 2 diabetes tend to have normal or elevated levels.

Oral Glucose Tolerance Test

The OGTT is often unnecessary for the diagnosis of diabetes mellitus, especially if the client's fasting blood glucose is greater than 140 mg/dl. Bed rest, infection, trauma, medications, and stress can alter the test results. This test is not usually recommended in hospitalized clients.

The client needs a diet that offers at least 150 g of carbohydrate per day for 3 days before the test. A sample is drawn to test fasting blood glucose, and the client is given 75 g of glucose in water to drink. Blood samples are obtained at intervals afterward (e.g., at 1 and 2 hours). The client cannot consume any food or fluid other than water between the glucose load ingestion and the end of the test. Diagnosis of diabetes mellitus or impaired glucose tolerance after the glucose tolerance test is dependent on fasting and follow-up glucose levels. The oral glucose load and levels diagnostic of diabetes are different for the pregnant client undergoing testing for gestational diabetes mellitus.[19]

Ketonuria

Urine levels of ketones can be tested by clients by use of dip-strips or tablets. The presence of ketones in the urine (a condition called *ketonuria*) indicates that the body is using fat as a major source of energy, which may result in ketoacidosis. Test results are indicated by presence of color changes, indicating the presence of ketones. All clients with diabetes should test their urine for ketones during acute illness or stress, when blood glucose levels are elevated (>240 mg/dl), and when they are pregnant or have evidence of ketoacidosis (e.g., nausea, vomiting, or abdominal pain). Some ketone strips detect ketones as well as glucose. Although urine testing is important for checking ketones, urine testing for glucose is not a reliable method for monitoring.

Proteinuria

Microalbuminuria tests measure microscopic amounts of protein in the urine (proteinuria). The presence of protein (microalbuminuria) in the urine is an early manifestation of kidney disease. Testing the urine for microalbuminuria shows early nephropathy, long before it would be evident on routine urinalysis. The ADA recommends that all clients with diabetes be tested for microalbuminuria annually.[11] Some clients, however, require more frequent testing to detect progression of kidney disease related to the adverse effects of certain medications on the kidneys.

Self-Monitoring of Blood Glucose

The key to managing diabetes is to keep the blood glucose level as close to normal as possible or within a target range that is agreed upon between the client and health care provider. Self-monitoring of blood glucose (SMBG) provides immediate feedback and data on blood glucose levels. SMBG is recommended for all clients with diabetes, regardless of whether they have type 1, type 2, or gestational diabetes. SMBG is a way to know how the body responds to food, insulin, activity, and stress.[15,16]

The frequency and timing of SMBG depends on the needs and goals of each individual client. For most clients with type 1 diabetes and pregnant women taking insulin, SMBG is recommended three or more times daily. Testing should be done before each meal, before bedtime, and possibly in the middle of the night (e.g., 3:00 AM). For clients with type 2 diabetes, the frequency and timing of SMBG is mutually agreed upon by the client and health care provider. If clients with type 2 diabetes are taking oral medications, they usually do not have to monitor as often as someone with type 2 diabetes taking insulin. Extra times to SMBG should occur if the client:

- Feels ill
- Suspects hypoglycemia
- Starts taking an over-the-counter medication that affects blood glucose levels (e.g., steroid)
- Has frequent insulin reactions overnight or wakes up with high blood glucose levels
- Loses or gains weight
- Changes medication dose, eating plan, or exercise plan

Outcome Management
■ Medical Management

Medical management for clients with diabetes includes restoring and maintaining blood glucose levels to as near normal as possible by balancing diet, exercise, and the use of oral hypoglycemic agents or insulin.[4,15,16,33] In general, when diabetes is successfully managed, clients avoid the complications of hypoglycemia and hyperglycemia. However, complications may develop in some clients with diabetes despite their vigorous efforts to carefully control the disease.

Initial as well as ongoing client education is vital in helping the client manage this chronic condition. Interventions must be individualized to the client's goals, age, lifestyle, nutritional needs, maturation, activity level, occupation, type of diabetes, and ability to independently perform the skills required by the management plan. Incorporation of psychosocial aspects into the overall plan is vital.[15,16]

Regulate Blood Glucose

Promote Proper Nutrition. Dietary management is an essential component of diabetes care and management. The general goal of dietary management is to help clients with diabetes improve metabolic control by making changes in nutrition habits. Specific goals include (1) improving blood glucose and lipid levels, (2) providing consistency in day-to-day food intake (in type 1 diabetes), (3) facilitating weight management (in type 2 diabetes), and (4) providing adequate nutrition for all stages of life. (See the Complementary and Alternative Therapy feature on Lifestyle Intervention or Metformin to Prevent or Delay Type 2 Diabetes on p. 1253. Also see

COMPLEMENTARY AND ALTERNATIVE THERAPY

Lifestyle Intervention or Metformin to Prevent or Delay Type 2 Diabetes

A unique randomized, placebo-controlled trial with a mean follow-up of 2.8 years was conducted with a total of 3234 participants from 27 centers in the United States. The mean age of the participants was 51 years and 68% were women. Individuals had a body mass index (BMI) greater than or equal to 24 and a blood glucose level 5.3 to 6.9 mmol/L in the fasting state and 7.8 to 11 mmol/L 2 hours after a 75-g oral glucose load. Follow-up was 93%. Participants were allocated to an intensive program of lifestyle changes (*n* = 1079), standard lifestyle recommendations plus metformin (850 mg twice daily) for glucose control (*n* = 1073), or placebo (*n* = 1082). The intensive lifestyle change consisted of a combined intervention that would maintain a 7% or greater reduction in body weight through a low-calorie, low-fat diet and moderate physical activity. The incidence rates of diabetes were 4.8, 7.8, and 11 clients per 100 person-years for the intensive lifestyle changes, metformin, and placebo groups, respectively. Thus the lifestyle intervention reduced the risk of being diagnosed with type 2 diabetes by 50% and metformin reduced risk by 25% compared to placebo. In overweight individuals with elevated fasting and postload blood glucose concentrations, an intensive lifestyle change or metformin treatment plus standard lifestyle recommendations was more effective than standard lifestyle recommendations alone for preventing or delaying the onset of type 2 diabetes.

Reference

Diabetes Prevention Program Research Group. (2002). Reduction in the incidence of type 2 diabetes with lifestyle intervention or metformin. *New England Journal of Medicine, 346,* 393-403.

the Complementary and Alternative Therapy feature on Lifestyle Intervention to Reduce the Risk of Type 2 Diabetes on the website.)

Achieving nutrition-related goals requires a team approach that includes the client. Effective self-management requires an individualized approach, taking into account the client's personal lifestyle and diabetes management goals. A nutritional assessment is used to determine the nutrition prescription on the basis of what the client with diabetes is able and willing to do.[4] SMBG, lipid levels, blood pressure, and renal status are all essential aspects of nutrition-related management.

Promote Regular Physical Activity. A program of planned exercise is a crucial part of the treatment plan for a client with diabetes. Exercise lowers blood glucose

by increasing carbohydrate metabolism, fosters weight reduction and maintenance, increases insulin sensitivity, increases high-density lipoprotein (HDL) levels, decreases triglyceride levels, lowers blood pressure, and reduces stress and tension.[7,25]

The primary side effect of acute exercise is hypoglycemia (low glucose level). Occasionally, hyperglycemia (elevated glucose level) and ketosis can occur in clients with type 1 diabetes. Hypoglycemia is a significant risk for clients who exercise while taking insulin or oral hypoglycemics. Adjustments are sometimes needed to prevent hypoglycemia in the client taking insulin, because hepatic glucose production is blocked or partially inhibited by exogenous insulin.[25] For example, a reduction in short-acting insulin of 30% to 50% can decrease the risk of hypoglycemia. Clients who use meal planning and exercise alone to control type 2 diabetes are not at risk for hypoglycemia when exercising.

Administer Medications

Oral Antidiabetes Agents. Five chemical classes of oral antidiabetes agents are available in the United States for the management of diabetes (see the Integrating Pharmacology feature on Medications for Clients with Diabetes on p. 1254):

- Sulfonylureas (oral hypoglycemic agents)
- Meglitinides (oral hypoglycemic agents)
- Biguanides (insulin sensitizers)
- Thiazolidinediones (also insulin sensitizers)
- Alpha-glucosidase inhibitors

Pharmacologic interventions should be considered when the client cannot achieve normal or near-normal blood glucose levels with nutrition and exercise therapies.[33] Oral hypoglycemic agents are effective in people with type 2 diabetes after nutrition and exercise therapy have failed. About 35% of clients with type 2 diabetes take oral hypoglycemic agents. The client most likely to respond well to oral antidiabetes agents is one who first has diabetes after age 40 years, has had diabetes for less than 5 years, is of normal weight or obese, and either has never received insulin or has well-controlled diabetes with less than 40 units of insulin per day. Indications for these agents are (1) random blood glucose levels less than 300 mg/dl, (2) fasting blood glucose level less than 250 mg/dl, (3) and inadequate control after exercise and diet therapies.[15,33]

Insulin Therapy. Clients with type 1 diabetes do not produce enough insulin to sustain life. They depend on exogenous insulin administration on a daily basis. In contrast, clients with type 2 diabetes are not dependent on exogenous insulin for survival. They may need supplemental insulin for adequate glucose control, especially in times of stress or illness.

Insulin Sources. Insulin is obtained from a pork pancreas or made chemically by recombinant DNA technology (human insulin) with different durations of action (rapid-, short-, intermediate-, and long-acting). Most clients who require insulin therapy receive human insulin produced by recombinant deoxyribonucleic acid (DNA) technology (Table 47-3).[33] Compared with animal insulins, human insulin peaks more precisely and predictably, has a shorter duration of action, and has reduced antigenicity (ability to produce antigen response), and it does not cause lipoatrophy (loss of subcutaneous fat) or lipodystrophy (fat metabolism disturbance leading to loss of subcutaneous fat) at the injection site.

Insulin works to lower blood glucose by promoting the transport of glucose into cells, and by inhibiting the conversion of glycogen and amino acids to glucose. The type and species of the insulin used, injection technique, site of injection, level of insulin antibodies, and individual client response all can affect the onset, peak, and duration of action of insulin. Insulin injected into the abdomen is absorbed fastest, with less rapid-absorption after injection into the arm and leg, respectively. Insulin inhalers are being developed and may replace the syringes used for insulin injection. The normal secretory pattern of endogenous insulins follows a basal-level secretion, with increased production in response to an incoming carbohydrate load. In clients with type 1 diabetes, the goal is to mimic this increase with injections of exogenous insulin.

The development of rapid-acting insulin analogs was approved in 1996 to minimize the absorption limitations of regular human insulin. Rapid-acting insulin analogs, insulin lispro (Humalog), and insulin aspart (Novolog) have become the foundation in the management of clients with type 1 and type 2 diabetes. The action and potency of Humalog and Novolog are similar to those in regular human insulin. However, the onset of action begins to work about 5 minutes after they are injected; peaking in 1 hour, with a duration of action lasting about 2 to 4 hours. Both insulin analogs are approved for subcutaneous injection or with the continuous insulin infusion pump and should be taken immediately before eating. Both analogs provide many benefits in achieving glucose control and may ultimately prevent or delay diabetes-related complications. Remind clients that because insulin analogs work so quickly, hypoglycemia can develop rapidly if they do not consume adequate calories immediately after injection.[28]

Humalog and Novolog are available are premixed insulins containing both a rapid-acting and an intermediate-acting component. Humalog Mix 75/25 contains 75% insulin lispro in a crystalline protamine form (in-

INTEGRATING PHARMACOLOGY
Medications for Clients with Diabetes

Clients with type 1 diabetes must take insulin. Type 2 diabetes clients are managed with drugs in five chemical classes: alpha-glucosidase inhibitors, biguanides, meglitinides, sulfonylureas, and thiazolidinediones. The main actions of many of these drugs are either to stimulate beta cells of the pancreas to produce more insulin or to increase tissue response to insulin. Sulfonylureas and meglitinides are oral hypoglycemic agents that stimulate beta cells of the pancreas to secrete insulin. Second-generation sulfonylureas also increase tissue response to insulin (insulin sensitizer) and decrease glucose production by the liver. Biguanides increase tissue response to insulin (insulin sensitizer), decrease hepatic production of glucose, decrease absorption of glucose from the small intestine, and decrease triglyceride and low-density lipoprotein levels. Thiazolidinediones increase insulin action at receptors and postreceptors in hepatic and peripheral tissue to decrease insulin resistance and often decrease triglycerides. Alpha-glucosidase inhibitors delay the digestion of complex carbohydrates and certain sugars to blunt the peak of blood glucose and insulin levels after meals.

In addition to insulin or antidiabetic medications, many diabetic clients take an angiotensin-converting enzyme (ACE) inhibitor to decrease blood pressure and minimize nephropathic changes and take aspirin to decrease the risk of thrombus formation. Diuretics, antilipemic drugs and other antihypertensive agents may be added to prevent or treat microvascular and macrovascular complications of the diabetes.

TABLE 47-3	*Types of Human Insulin and Comparative Actions*					
Action	**Preparation**	**Appearance**	**Onset**	**Peak**	**Duration**	
Rapid-acting	Humalog (Insulin lispro)	Clear	5-10 min	1 hour	2-4 hours	
	Novolog (Insulin aspart)	Clear	5-10 min	1 hour	2-4 hours	
Short-acting	Humulin R (Regular)	Clear	0.5-2 hours	2-4 hours	4-6 hours	
	Novolin R (Regular)	Clear	0.5-2 hours	2-4 hours	4-6 hours	
Intermediate-acting	Humulin N (NPH)	Cloudy	2-4 hours	4-10 hours	10-16 hours	
	Humulin L (Lente)	Cloudy	2-4 hours	4-10 hours	10-16 hours	
	Humulin 70/30 (Premixed) (70% NPH, 30% Regular)	Cloudy	0.5-1 hour	Dual	10-16 hours	
Long-acting	Humulin U (Ultralente)	Clear	6-10 hours	None	18-20 hours	
	Lantus (Insulin glargine)	Clear	1 hour	None	24 hours	

termediate-acting) and 25% soluble (rapid-acting) insulin lispro. Novolog Mix 70/30 contains a mixture of 70% insulin aspart as the crystalline protamine form (intermediate-acting) and 30% soluble (rapid-acting) insulin aspart.[28] Administration of a mixture of insulin produces a more normal glycemia in clients than use of a single insulin. When a rapid-acting insulin is mixed with an intermediate- or long-acting insulin, the insulin should be injected within 15 minutes before a meal.[5]

Insulin Dosage. Insulin therapy should be individualized. For a client with newly diagnosed diabetes, a simple regimen with fixed doses may be used at first. The starting dose of insulin is 0.5 unit/kg/day. Two thirds of the dose is commonly given in the morning, and one third is given in the evening. The health care team works to adjust the numbers and timing of injections to smooth out normal patterns. Then the dose can be increased. Algorithms are detailed guidelines to help clients self-adjust the daily insulin dose, based on SMBG levels, food intake, exercise, and departures from normal routine (e.g., added stress or illness). These guidelines use a prospective (predictive) approach to blood glucose control.[5,33]

Insulin dosage varies greatly (Figure 47-2). In determining the dosage, the health care team must consider both the client's requirements and the client's response to the insulin. After initial stabilization, the team helps the client learn how to make adjustments in insulin doses, timing, food intake, and exercise. Unexplained fluctuations in blood glucose often occur. The team needs to help the client feel confident in his or her ability to control the diabetes.

Insulin Pump Therapy. Small portable pumps for the continuous administration of regular insulin are sometimes used (Figure 47-3). The small pump, worn externally, injects insulin subcutaneously into the abdomen through an indwelling needle site that is usually changed daily. Insulin is normally infused at a low basal rate (a rate that matches the client's basal metabolic needs), with additional infusion of larger amounts (boluses) of insulin before meals.

Insulin pumps commonly improve blood glucose control by means of continuous subcutaneous insulin infusion. However, they do not have a built-in feedback mechanism for monitoring blood glucose levels. To benefit from use of an insulin pump, the client must comply with dietary requirements and usually must deliver the correct premeal bolus of insulin. The client must also

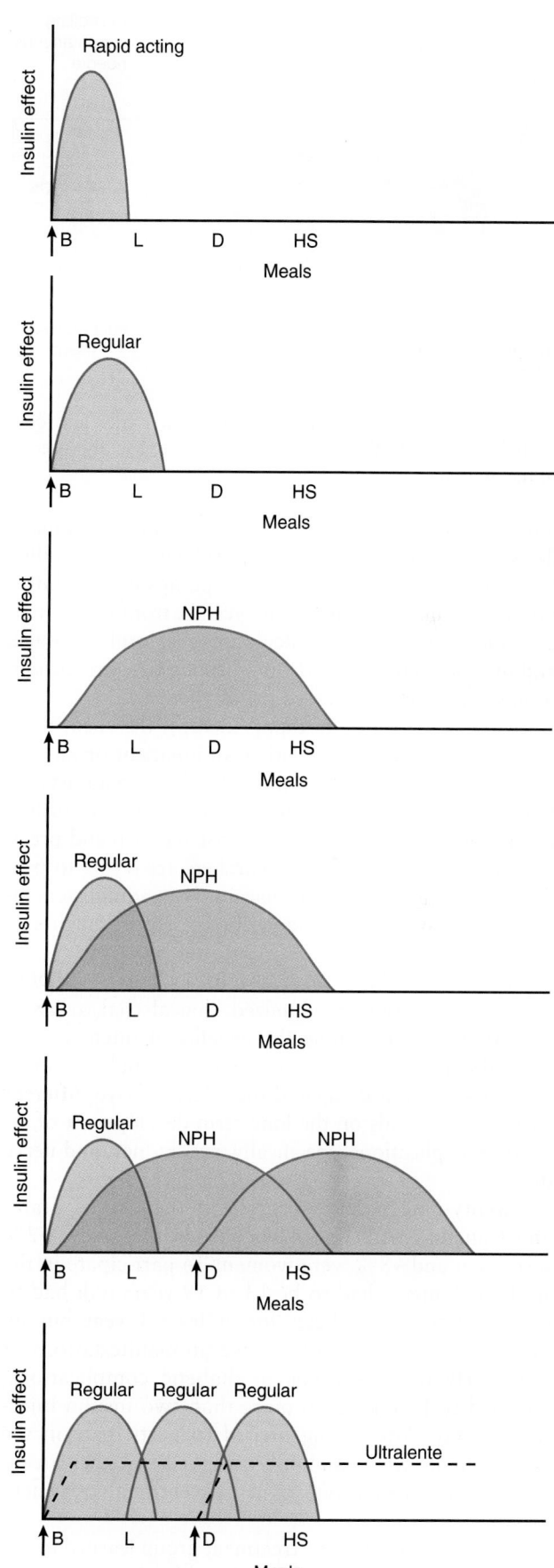

FIGURE 47-2 Insulin regimens. Only a few of a variety of possible regimens are shown here. Some clients require only one injection per day, whereas others may require split mixed doses (such as mixtures of NPH or Ultralente and regular or rapid-acting insulin) or several doses of the same type of insulin (such as NPH insulin). Insulin regimens must be individualized for each client. *B,* Breakfast; *L,* lunch; *D,* dinner; *HS,* bedtime.

Indwelling
subcutaneous
needle

Insulin
pump

Subcutaneous
tissue

FIGURE 47-3 Insulin pumps are worn externally and connected to an indwelling subcutaneous needle, usually inserted in the abdomen.

monitor blood glucose levels four times a day and make decisions about dosages by using problem-solving skills.[2] Complications from use of insulin pumps include infection at the injection site, hypoglycemia from pump malfunction or mistakes in calculating the insulin dosage, and diabetic ketoacidosis from injecting too little insulin to meet regular or increased metabolic needs.

At the start of insulin pump therapy, the client must be supervised carefully in either an inpatient or an outpatient setting. During this time, the clinician adjusts the pump for basal and bolus doses before meals, according to the client's usual diet and exercise regimen and previous insulin requirements. Researchers are trying to produce an implantable pump that not only administers insulin but also monitors blood glucose levels, much as a normal pancreas does.

Intensive Diabetes Therapy. In 1983, the NIDDK launched a 10-year, randomized clinical trial to assess the safety and determine the benefits of intensive diabetes therapy. The most comprehensive diabetes study ever conducted, it compared the effects of two different treatment methods on the long-term development of diabetes complications, specifically, eye, kidney, and nerve disease.[18]

Twenty-nine medical centers in the United States and Canada enrolled 1441 people in the study; 52% were men and 48% were women. To participate in the study, volunteers had to be 13 to 19 years old; had to have had type 1 diabetes for at least 1 year but no more than 15 years; had to have no manifestations or only early manifestations of diabetic complications; and had to be taking no more than two insulin injections a day. After being invited to participate in the study, clients were randomly assigned to either an intensive treatment group or a conventional treatment group.

Clients in the intensive treatment group learned to adjust their insulin doses to keep their blood glucose levels as close to normal as possible. Treatment included three or more insulin injections a day or the use of an insulin pump, SMBG levels four or more times a day, a special diet, an initial hospital stay, and weekly to monthly clinic visits. Clients in the conventional treatment group followed a regimen used by most people with type 1 diabetes: insulin injections once or twice a day, daily SMBG, and clinic visits every 3 months. Researchers monitored clients in both groups for manifestations of diabetic eye disease (retinopathy) as well as kidney (nephropathy) and nerve (neuropathy) disease.

Results of the trial indicated that intensive therapy delayed the onset or slowed the progression of chronic complications of diabetes by 35% to more than 70%. The risk of hypoglycemia was three times higher in the intensive treatment group than in the conventional treatment group. However, the risk of hypoglycemia was believed to be greatly outweighed by the reduction in microvascular and neurologic complications. Based on these results, it is recommended that clients with type 1 diabetes receive closely monitored intensive regimens. However, intensive therapy should be implemented with caution in clients who have repeated severe hypoglycemia or an unawareness of hypoglycemia.[18]

With the intensive therapy approach, the client must be willing to monitor blood glucose levels four to six times a day and take three to five insulin injections a day. Throughout the initiating period of intensive therapy, the clinician must assess the client's knowledge of the meal plan, monitoring techniques, management goals, and manifestations of and interventions for hyperglycemia and hypoglycemia. The client also needs to be made aware of the extra financial and emotional burdens of this approach. The family and significant others need to be involved in the teaching process. Finally, the client needs to know that neither protocol is guaranteed to prevent long-term complications.

Combination Therapy. Combination therapy is defined as the use of two or more oral antidiabetes agents or an oral agent combined with insulin. The advantage is that because the various groups of oral agents have different sites and mechanisms of action, they can complement and even augment each other.

In some clients with type 2 diabetes (mostly non-obese clients) in whom sulfonylurea agents alone failed to normalize blood glucose levels, insulin therapy has been required to achieve metabolic control very early in the course of disease. In these clients, daily insulin dosage is markedly higher than in clients with type 1 diabetes. This is attributed to insulin resistance. Because sulfonylurea agents enhance the effect of endogenous insulin by reducing insulin resistance, it has been thought that combining insulin therapy with sulfonylureas may be effective. One prescribed regimen is an injection of an intermediate-acting insulin at bedtime with daytime coverage by a sulfonylurea. This regimen is commonly called BIDS (*b*edtime *i*nsulin with *d*aytime *s*ulfonylurea).[33]

■ Nursing Management of the Medical Client

Diabetes self-management is the responsibility of clients and their families. The client with diabetes must be empowered to accept self-management and to become the focus of the team approach to treatment. Physiologic treatment of manifestations is neither the means nor the end of responsibility in dealing with a chronic disease like diabetes. Clients require consistent follow-up, updating, and reinforcement. Assessment of the client's level of acceptance of personal responsibility is necessary. This guides the practitioner to appropriate teaching and behavioral techniques to encourage a higher level of acceptance on the client's part.

Because of the multidisciplinary nature of the treatment, a team approach is recommended in managing clients with diabetes. This approach is particularly appropriate for client education when learners must acquire knowledge and skills from a variety of disciplines. Crucial members of the health care team include, whenever possible, a nurse, a dietitian, and a physician as the core members. Depending on need and availability, other members may include a psychologist, a social worker, a pharmacist, an exercise physiologist, and a podiatrist. Team meetings are planned to share information gained from individual client assessments and to develop a plan of action to respond to the client's clinical and educational priorities. The integration of various roles within the team strengthens the communication essential to client self-management.

There are two approaches to diabetes education[12-14,21]:

- The *compliance-based approach* is intended to improve client adherence to the treatment recommendations of health care professionals. It is based on the assumption that health care professionals are diabetes care experts and that, in general, clients should comply with their recommendations regarding diabetes self-management.

- In the *empowerment-based approach,* the primary purpose of diabetes education is to prepare clients to make informed decisions about their own diabetes care. This approach assumes that most clients with diabetes are responsible for making important and complex decisions.[12-14,21]

Few members of the health care team use one approach all the time to the exclusion of the other approach. Indeed, many health care professionals use some combination of the two approaches based on their own values and understanding of the purposes of education. For example, clients with newly diagnosed diabetes may wish to have the health care team make most of the decisions until they become familiar with the costs and benefits of various options in diabetes self-management.

BOX 47-3	*Education Content for Clients with Diabetes*

A. Function and structure (anatomy and physiology) of the pancreas
B. Definition of diabetes mellitus and relationship to abnormal function of pancreas
C. Manifestations of hyperglycemia
D. Methods to control hyperglycemia
  1. Diet
  2. Exercise
  3. Oral antidiabetic agents
  4. Insulin
    a. How/when/where/why to give insulin
    b. Storage/disposal of insulin and needles
E. Daily self-monitoring of blood glucose
F. Sick day rules
  1. Testing for ketones in urine
G. Complications of diabetes mellitus (definition, cause, manifestations, treatment)
  1. Acute: hypoglycemia, diabetic ketoacidosis, HHNS
  2. Chronic: microvascular and macrovascular

Survival education includes the crucial information necessary to meet the client's immediate survival needs. These vary widely from client to client. For example, insulin injection is a survival skill for a client with newly diagnosed type 1 diabetes but is unlikely to be a necessary skill in a client with newly diagnosed type 2 diabetes. Survival information varies in content, depending on the type of diabetes and age of the client but tends to focus on skills such as insulin injection, treatment of hypoglycemia, glucose self-monitoring, sick-day management, diabetic ketoacidosis, and basic dietary information. When clients are comfortable with survival skills, they can progress to more in-depth information.[15,16] Box 47-3 presents essential diabetic education content.

Assessment

Clients with diabetes must be closely assessed for level of knowledge and ability to perform self-care. The type of diabetes, clinical status of the client, and plans for treatment are also important assessments. Ask clients whether they take any vitamin, mineral, or herbal supplements to decrease blood glucose levels or for other purposes. (See the Complementary and Alternative Therapy features on Multivitamin and Mineral Supplement and the Risk of Infection in Clients with Type 2 Diabetes and on Ginseng Supplements and Blood Glucose on p. 1258.) Chromium and garlic may lower blood glucose and cholesterol levels, and magnesium may increase insulin sensitivity. Blueberries, especially European bilberries, may also decrease blood glucose levels. Niacin may impair glucose tolerance.

Multivitamin and Mineral Supplement and the Risk of Infection in Clients with Type 2 Diabetes

A randomized, double-blind, placebo-controlled trial of 130 community-dwelling adults were allocated to a multivitamin and mineral supplement or placebo daily for 1 year. More individuals taking placebo than those taking the multivitamin supplement reported an infectious illness over the year of study (73% versus 43%; $p < .001$). Infection-related absenteeism (e.g., missing work) was also higher in the placebo group (57% versus 21%; $p < .001$). The individuals with type 2 diabetes ($n = 51$) were responsible for this finding. Among diabetics receiving placebo, 93% reported an infection, whereas 17% of those receiving supplements ($p < .001$) reported an infection. A larger clinical trial is needed, but this study does initially support the use of a daily cheap multivitamin for type 2 diabetics to reduce the risk of infections (upper respiratory tract infection, lower respiratory tract infection, influenza-like syndrome, gastrointestinal infection, and urinary tract infection). Participants without diabetes ($n = 79$) did not experience any change in reported infections compared to those taking placebo in this study.

Reference

Data from Barringer, T., et al. (2003). Effect of a multivitamin and mineral supplement on infection and quality of life: A randomized, double-blind, placebo-controlled trial. *Annals of Internal Medicine, 138,* 365-371.

Ginseng Supplements and Blood Glucose

There are two common types of ginseng sold in the United States: Asian ginseng *(Panax ginseng)* and American ginseng *(Panax quinquefolius)*. A small preliminary study looked at 10 non-diabetic and 9 type 2 diabetic clients. These individuals were given a 3 g capsule of American ginseng or a placebo about 40 minutes before or while taking 25 g of glucose. In the non-diabetic clients, there was no difference between blood levels of glucose after taking the ginseng or placebo along with the sugar. However, if the ginseng was taken 40 minutes before the sugar, there was a significant reduction in glucose levels. In the type 2 diabetic clients, significant reductions in glucose levels were observed when ginseng was taken both before and at the same time the sugar was eaten. Thus ginseng may reduce large glucose increases in type 2 diabetic clients if the ginseng is taken before or during a meal. However, nondiabetic and diabetic clients should take ginseng during a meal to prevent large reductions in glucose levels. This is a small study, but it did demonstrate that American ginseng and perhaps other ginseng products may affect glucose levels, so health professionals should warn clients about the possible effect of ginseng on glucose levels.

Reference

Vuksan, V., et al. (2000). American ginseng *(Panax quinquefolius L)* reduces postprandial glycemia in nondiabetic subjects and subjects with type 2 diabetes mellitus. *Archives of Internal Medicine, 160,* 1009-1013.

Diagnosis, Outcomes, Interventions

Diagnosis: Readiness for Enhanced Therapeutic Regimen Management. The client with diabetes must be able to perform self-care to keep the condition well controlled, leading to the nursing diagnosis *Readiness for Enhanced Therapeutic Regimen Management related to lack of knowledge about diabetes mellitus, lack of knowledge about exercise regimen for diabetes management, and lack of knowledge about dietary management of diabetes mellitus and the desire to learn about effective management of diabetes mellitus.*

Outcomes. The client will relate the basic pathophysiologic mechanism of diabetes mellitus, explain the need for exercise and diet in the treatment, and list the clinical manifestations of acute and chronic complications. The client will plan an exercise program to maintain blood glucose levels at preset levels and will identify strategies to monitor for and prevent complications associated with exercise.

The client will state the relationship of dietary management to blood glucose control, and will choose foods that meet caloric needs and offer a well-balanced diet. The client will recognize the times at which it is necessary to substitute a food to maintain blood glucose control. The client will discuss with the health care team difficulties seen in compliance with plans for diet, maintain blood glucose levels within preset parameters, and maintain weight within preset parameters.

Interventions

Explain the Pathophysiology of Diabetes. You or a diabetes educator should explain to the client and family the basic pathophysiologic mechanism of diabetes and how the disorder is managed. Sometimes the information is given through classes or by videotape. The client should also receive some form of written information to reinforce the material. Also, the client should be monitored for denial or anger about the diagnosis as part of a coping response.

Plan an Exercise Program. Clients with diabetes must consult the clinician before starting an exercise program. Pre-exercise screening may include a history, physical examination, A1C, exercise stress test, foot evaluation, and laboratory determination of blood glucose level. The client with diabetes may not be able to exercise intensely to achieve a calculated heart rate because of a pre-existing cardiac condition, advanced age, or joint problems. The client should be helped to choose an exercise regimen and to set reasonable goals, because any increase in activity level is beneficial. Walking is usually well tolerated. Using a stationary bicycle or swimming is possible for clients with foot problems.

Clients with diabetes must start any new activity at a well-tolerated intensity level and duration, with gradual (over a period of weeks or months) increases in intensity and duration until preset exercise goals are reached. Exercise should include warm-up and cool-down periods before and after the activity. It is best to exercise at the same time of day, if possible. Because regular exercise is very important, have the client plan an alternative activity in case environmental or other factors make the usual exercise difficult. Unplanned exercise can be dangerous for clients taking insulin or oral hypoglycemic agents. During periods of exercise, the muscles are stimulated to take up glucose. Therefore blood glucose levels can fall abruptly.[7,25]

Prevent Complications from Exercise. Clients should make sure they are adequately hydrated before starting exercise. They should eat 15 to 30 g of carbohydrate before exercise if the blood glucose level is less than 100 mg/dl and should carry a carbohydrate snack as well as their diabetes identification. If blood glucose is 100 to 150 mg/dl, the client may exercise and have a snack later. If blood glucose is greater than 250 mg/dl and the client has not just eaten, ketone levels should be checked. Clients with this glucose level should wait to exercise, because vigorous activity can raise blood glucose levels by releasing stored glycogen. Alcohol and beta-blockers should be avoided because they may increase the risk of hypoglycemia or hyperglycemia.[7,25]

Plan Nutrition Therapy to Achieve Target Blood Glucose. A balanced nutritional plan is important for all clients, whether or not they have diabetes. Emphasize to the client and family members that they are not eating a "diabetic diet" but, rather, are following a balanced meal plan. Adherence to nutrition principles is one of the most challenging aspects of diabetes management. It requires a team effort. For an effective plan, assessment of the person's present eating patterns, knowledge of a healthy eating plan, and willingness and ability to modify patterns and nutritional needs is vital. Specific nutritional information should include the following[4]:

- Appetite
- Food allergies
- Ethnic and cultural influence on food habits
- Ability to obtain and prepare food (including financial ability)
- Community resources currently used

FIGURE 47-4 Assessment as part of the total nutritional plan for the collaborative management of diabetes. (Data from Copstead, L.C., & Banasik, J.L. [2000]. *Pathophysiology: Biological and behavioral perspectives* [2nd ed.]. Philadelphia: W.B. Saunders.)

- Amount and type of physical activity
- Chronic disease requiring dietary modification
- Gastrointestinal disease
- Vitamin, mineral, or food supplements used
- Weight patterns
- Current eating patterns
- Dietary concerns of client
- Dental and oral health
- Medications with nutritional implications

The results of this assessment form a personal profile used to arrive at individualized goals. As a member of the health care team, you must have a knowledge base of both nutritional assessment and appropriate interventions. Basic nutritional assessment includes anthropometric measures, biochemical tests, physical assessment, and dietary evaluation. No single parameter can measure the client's nutritional status or determine problems or needs. Figure 47-4 shows how assessment fits into the total nutritional plan for the collaborative management of diabetes. After the assessment, individualized goals are determined. Nutritional assessment and the client's understanding that optimal nutrition can lead to reduction of risk factors for chronic health problems and improve overall health constitute the starting point for goal selection.

For example, if the client has type 2 diabetes and is obese, emphasize that nutritional changes can help to lower blood glucose levels, decrease lipid levels, and lower blood pressure as well as help in losing weight. Weight loss also appears to increase insulin sensitivity and to normalize liver glucose production. The client should understand that dietary treatment is the best and initial treatment. If nutritional status does not improve, glucose-lowering medications, insulin, lipid-lowering agents, or antihypertensives may be required.

TABLE 47-4	*Currently Recommended Nutritional Guidelines for the Client with Diabetes Mellitus*
Calories	Sufficient to achieve and maintain reasonable weight
Protein	Adequate to ensure maintenance of body protein stores; people with diabetes have the same protein requirements as for people who do not have diabetes; in general, 10%-20% of the total daily calories should come from protein (equal to ~0.8 g/kg/day)
Fats	Less than 30% of calories should be from fat, with less than 10% of that from saturated fat sources; if individualized risk factors indicate elevated VLDL and LDL levels, total calories from saturated fat may be reduced to 7%; cholesterol intake should be limited to 300 mg/day or less
Carbohydrates	50%-60% of total calories should be from carbohydrates; simple and complex sugars do not differ appreciably in their ability to worsen hyperglycemia
Fiber	Clients with diabetes are urged to consume 20-35 g of fiber per day, which is the same as the recommendation for all Americans

LDL, Low-density lipoprotein; *VLDL,* Very-low-density lipoprotein.

A standard "diabetic diet" is no longer prescribed for all clients with diabetes; instead, many dietary options exist (Table 47-4). Basically, the client with diabetes should strive to follow the Dietary Guidelines for Americans (the "Food Guide Pyramid") issued by the U.S. Department of Agriculture (USDA) and U.S. Department of Health and Human Services (USDHHS) in 1992 for current recommended nutritional guidelines.[31]

Calories. Caloric restrictions, especially for people with lifelong obesity, may be perceived negatively. Obesity is a complex interaction between genetic and environmental factors. The most successful approach to weight reduction is unclear, but you should understand caloric restriction, regular exercise, behavior modification, and peer and professional support. Moderate caloric reduction is described as a reduction of 250 to 500 calories per day less than usual. Reduction of fat calories may be a good initial modification. Regular exercise (three to five times weekly) enhances weight loss and is a predictor of successful weight maintenance.[4]

Protein. In general, Americans with and without diabetes consume more protein than needed to meet nutritional needs. Protein should be incorporated into the diet through a variety of foods. Very-low-calorie diets are often deficient in protein and may result in accelerated protein breakdown. High protein intake increases renal workload and glomerular filtration rate. Some studies in people with diabetes indicate that lowering protein intake may delay progression of nephropathy. At present, the lower end of the recommended scale for protein intake (about 10% of daily calories) is sufficiently restricted and is recommended for clients with nephropathy. In certain cases, protein requirements vary from the adult recommended daily allowance; this is true for infants, children, adolescents, and pregnant women.[4]

Fat. The USDA national food consumption surveys reveal that most Americans eat too much fat. About 36% of calories in the average adult diet comes from fat,

with about 13% being from saturated fat. The general recommendation for Americans is to decrease total dietary fat to 30% or less of total calories, with saturated fat being decreased to less than 10%. This reduction is consistent with a diet to reduce cardiovascular disease.

Clients with type 2 diabetes often have high triglyceride levels, high low-density lipoprotein (LDL) levels, high very-low-density lipoprotein (VLDL) levels, and low high-density lipoprotein (HDL) levels. This may be the result of increased liver production of triglyceride-rich VLDLs, genetic predisposition, hyperinsulinemia, insulin resistance, or intra-abdominal fat accumulation. Limiting daily cholesterol intake to 300 mg is also recommended. All of these lipid-related dietary modifications are recommended for clients with diabetes as well as for all other Americans.[2,6,9]

The guidelines further suggest that people with elevated LDL levels should reduce their intake of saturated fat to 7% of total calories and their intake of total cholesterol to less than 300 mg/day. Whether it is better to increase fiber and carbohydrates or to replace saturated fat with unsaturated fat is still controversial.

Carbohydrates. For most of the 20th century, the most widely held belief about dietary treatment of diabetes was that sugar was to be avoided. Little or no scientific evidence supports this assumption. When fed as a single nutrient, sucrose produces a glycemic response similar to that for bread or pasta. In the United States, the average diet obtains almost half of total carbohydrate intake in the form of simple sugars. Clinical guidelines suggest that 50% to 60% of the diet should consist of carbohydrates, in either simple or complex form. An occasional high-sucrose dessert poses no problem for the client with diabetes when it is accounted for in the day's total caloric and carbohydrate plan. Because some desserts are also high in fat, however, they should be limited.[4]

Working as a team with the client and a nutritionist, make a concrete medical nutrition therapy plan. The following are some helpful questions to ask the client:

- What is your most important goal in managing your diabetes?
- What are some changes you would like to make?
- Of the changes we have talked about, what would you like to work on first?

Team members must remember their roles as providers of information and counselors. Most counseling on nutrition begins with basic overviews of nutrition, diabetes guidelines, and reading of labels. More in-depth counseling on meal planning and calorie counting, for example, can come later. Eating plans vary widely among clients. Consistency within an eating style results in lower levels of glycosylated hemoglobin than does a haphazard eating style.

Diet Management for Clients with Type 1 Diabetes. Meals should be adjusted to match insulin action. Breakfast should be eaten within 1 hour after the morning insulin dose (immediately after injection when rapid-acting insulin is used) and a carbohydrate should be eaten about 3 hours later; lunch should be eaten about 4 to 5 hours after the morning insulin dose. When multiple insulin injections are used, greater flexibility with meal timing is possible.

The following are examples of approaches used successfully to instruct clients with diabetes:

- Handouts available from government sources, such as the USDA's "Food Guide Pyramid"[31] and the USDHHS publication, which uses the four-basic-food-groups approach[30]

- Individualized menus shaped between the client and dietitian
- The exchange system, last revised in 1986, which help with uniform meal planning available from the ADA in a simple pamphlet called "Healthy Food Choices," or in an expanded version called "Exchange Lists for Meal Planning")
- Counting components of the diet, such as counting calories and grams of fat
- A point system that utilizes lists of foods with point values and a prescribed number of total points
- The total available glucose system, which looks at foods in terms of their metabolic effects (highly motivated clients who desire flexibility may like this system)

A registered dietitian who is a certified diabetes educator (CDE) should always be consulted for initial evaluation and teaching of any client with a new diagnosis of diabetes. Each client should receive an individualized meal plan based on ethnic, religious, and cultural background; eating, cooking, and work habits; and food preferences. All clients need to know the dietary basics, which include the following:

- Avoid adding sugar to foods such as coffee and cereal.
- Avoid foods that are sweetened with sugar or honey, such as jellies, jams, cakes, and ice cream.
- Check blood glucose levels regularly.
- Keep periodic appointments with health care providers for evaluation of blood glucose control.
- Be consistent about the amount, distribution, and timing of nutrients.
- Increase the amount of carbohydrate in a meal eaten before sustained exercise.
- Limit intake of saturated fat and cholesterol.

Diagnosis: Risk for Ineffective Therapeutic Regimen Management. A client with diabetes must understand and be able to self-monitor glucose levels and learn self-injection of insulin, leading to the nursing diagnosis of *Risk for Ineffective Therapeutic Regimen Management related to lack of knowledge and lack of previous experience with testing blood and urine and lack of knowledge and lack of experience with self-injection of insulin.*

Outcomes. The client will state personal goals for urine ketone and blood glucose testing parameters; demonstrate correct techniques for blood glucose testing (including timing), and demonstrate correct technique for urine ketone testing (including timing). The client will test blood glucose at regular times (including during illnesses and when traveling), and will prick the side of the finger, where nerve endings are fewer and more blood is available. The client will test urine for ketones when the glucose level is high (>240 mg/dl) or during illnesses; keep a record of all tests performed and bring this record to regular, scheduled follow-up visits; and store testing materials away from heat, light, and moisture.

The client will state that insulin lowers blood glucose, and will name the type or types of insulin prescribed and the onset, peak, and duration of each. The client will take injections at regular times, 10 to 60 minutes before meals, every day, even when ill. The client will wash hands before preparing insulin injections, demonstrate proper mixing of insulin, and withdraw prescribed dosage using sterile technique.

When taking two types of insulin, the client will withdraw the prescribed dosage of each insulin into one syringe without contaminating either bottle (regular insulin is drawn up first). A client who uses insulin glargine (Lantus) must draw up the insulin glargine in a separate syringe and not mix it with any other insulin. The client will demonstrate the correct technique of insulin injection. The client will store at least one extra bottle of insulin in the refrigerator, not use insulin past the expiration date, and will purchase insulin syringes before all of the current supply has been used.

The client will wear medical identification (MedicAlert) bracelet or necklace, or carry a diabetic identification card. The client will state manifestations, describe treatment of hypoglycemia, and will always carry something to treat hypoglycemia.

Interventions

Provide Instruction on Blood Glucose Monitoring. All clients with newly diagnosed diabetes mellitus require teaching about urine and blood glucose monitoring. All clients with diabetes may require review or update of information for self-care. Newer, more accurate blood glucose meters that are easier to use are constantly being made available. Only the basics are covered in this discussion; you must keep up-to-date on each meter's advantages and disadvantages.

Many kinds of meters are available. Each client needs to be evaluated so that the proper meter is obtained. The client's ability to calibrate the meter and to visually interpret the digital reading must be considered. Some meters can be connected to a computer, which can convert blood glucose results into bar graphs or other printouts. Glucose meters are available for the visually impaired that give audio commands for use of the device and announce the blood glucose reading.

In addition to demonstrating the techniques of blood glucose self-monitoring, discuss the normal blood glucose range, goals for good control (individualized for each client), when to test, how to record test results, and what to do for abnormal results. Consult a diabetes educator for assistance in helping the client choose an optimal meter.

Clients can use blood glucose strips if they are unable or unwilling to purchase a meter. Make sure the client is not color blind and can read the results accurately. Compare the client's results with blood glucose meter readings to check for accuracy. With some meters and strips, a 15% difference is seen between capillary blood and venous blood glucose levels. The capillary blood reading is lower. When insulin is being adjusted, make sure to account for this difference. As long as the source of blood is consistent, no adjustment is required.

Both health care agencies and clients need to verify the accuracy of their blood glucose determinations. The **EB** Joint Commission on Accreditation of Healthcare Organizations (JCAHO) and other regulating bodies dictate the procedure and frequency for quality control of meters used in health care agencies. The usefulness of many glucose meters is technique-dependent. Because treatment is based on results, correct methods of use must be ensured. Clients can perform a self-test and simultaneously send a blood specimen to the laboratory to compare results. Manufacturers of meters also provide quality-control testing solutions, which clients should be instructed to use routinely (weekly, for example). Quality control of glucose monitors is a constantly changing area; nurses and clients must keep up-to-date (see the Management and Delegation feature on Measuring and Recording Blood Glucose Levels, above).

MANAGEMENT AND DELEGATION
Measuring and Recording Blood Glucose Levels

The measurement and recording of blood glucose levels may be delegated to unlicensed assistive personnel. Delegate the data collection only to those who have demonstrated competency in performing this task. Consider the following issues:

- Initial orientation and demonstration of competence in the performance of blood glucose monitoring, including quality control and equipment management requirements.
- Instruction on the time schedule and frequency to obtain blood glucose levels.
- Proper method of recording and reporting of the blood glucose level.
- Rotation of sites from which to obtain samples in order to minimize client discomfort.

You are responsible for defining those blood glucose levels that are immediately reportable to you (e.g., levels outside the range of 70 to 180 mg/dl). Instruct assistive personnel to report any difficulty in obtaining the sample or concerns the client may raise during the process of obtaining a sample.

Verify the competency of assistive personnel in performing blood glucose level testing during orientation and annually thereafter.

Provide Instruction on Urine Testing. Urine testing for glucose is rarely done; however, urine can be tested for ketones (beta-hydroxybutyric acid, acetoacetic acid, and acetone). These substances appear in the urine of clients who are fasting, clients with poorly controlled type 1 diabetes, and clients with type 1 or type 2 diabetes who have a secondary illness. Ketones result from fat metabolism and are therefore present during fasting.[27,29] In a client with diabetes, however, the presence of ketones may indicate the serious complication of diabetic ketoacidosis (see later discussion).

Provide Instruction on Insulin Administration. When administered correctly, insulin acts as a life-saving medication for the insulin-dependent client. When administered incorrectly, it may cause complications ranging from tissue damage to lethal hypoglycemia *(insulin shock).* To administer insulin properly, the client must be familiar with insulin concentrations, syringes, storage, preparation for injection, and techniques for self-injection. See the Client Education Guide feature on Self-Injection of Insulin on p. 1263.[5] Insulin inhalers may someday replace insulin injection syringes.

Insulin Concentrations. Insulin is prescribed in units. The most commonly prescribed strength in the United

CLIENT EDUCATION GUIDE
Self-Injection of Insulin

Procedure
1. Wash hands.
2. Clean site with soap and water or 70% isopropyl alcohol (optional).
3. Store insulin vial in original carton to keep clean (or wipe top of insulin vial with 70% isopropyl alcohol).
4. Check insulin for any residue. Mix insulin by rolling the vial between your palms or by shaking the vial to resuspend all but short-acting insulins.
5. Pull air into syringe to the number of units needed.
6. Inject air into the insulin vial.
7. Invert insulin vial and draw insulin into syringe.
8. Aspirate prescribed amount of short-acting insulin into syringe first, intermediate- or long-acting insulin second.
9. Inspect syringe for air bubbles.
10. Never mix insulin glargine (Lantus) with another insulin because it has a pH of 4 and will cause precipitation when mixed with other insulins.
11. Pinch up and hold skinfold and inject at 90-degree angle.
12. If you are thin or have loose skin, inject insulin at 45-degree angle to avoid an intramuscular injection, which is absorbed faster.
13. Routine aspiration is not necessary.
14. Inject insulin.

Disposal
State laws require that needles and syringes be disposed of as a single unit in a puncture-resistant container. It is unsafe to recap, bend, or break the needle.

Syringe Reuse
The manufacturer intends that the insulin syringe and needle be disposed after one use. Research demonstrates that most people with diabetes reuse the needle and syringe until the needle becomes dull or bent or comes in contact with any surface other than skin. Most insulins have a bacteriostatic agent in them. If you reuse syringes and needles, recap the needle after each use; reusing may carry increased risk for infection, especially if you have poor personal hygiene, acute concurrent illness, or open wounds on hands. Discuss the practice of reuse with your practitioner before initiating:
- Can you safely recap the needle?
- Can you see clearly enough?
- How is your manual dexterity?
- Do you have a visible tremor?

Store syringes at room temperature. The potential benefit of using alcohol on the needle is unknown. It may remove the silicone coat on the needle and contribute to pain at the puncture site.

States is U-100. U-100 insulin contains 100 units of insulin per milliliter. It is the insulin of choice for nearly all clients. Those who require large amounts of insulin may benefit from using U-500 insulin, which contains 500 units of insulin per milliliter.[5,33]

Insulin Syringes. The most commonly used syringe can deliver a maximum of 100 units of insulin in 1 ml. However, insulin syringes are manufactured with capacities of 0.25, 0.30, 0.50, and 1 ml. For smaller prescriptions (50 units, 30 units, or less), smaller syringes are used.[7] A smaller syringe enables a more precise insulin dosage. Two lengths of needles are available: short (8 mm) and long (12.7 mm). Short needles are not recommended for obese clients because of variability of insulin absorption when injected into adipose tissue. See Figure 47-5 for examples of a 50-unit syringe, 100-unit syringe, and a syringe that has ½-unit markings.

Insulin Storage. Although manufactures recommend storing vials of insulin in the refrigerator, injecting cold insulin can sometimes make the injection more painful. When beginning use of a vial of insulin, remove it from the refrigerator. Avoid temperature extremes of less than

FIGURE 47-5 Examples of the sizes of insulin syringes that are available for precise measurement of insulin doses. **A** shows an example of a 50 unit syringe, **B** shows an example of a 100 unit syringe, and **C** shows an example of a syringe that has ½ unit markings. (Courtesy of Becton Dickinson Consumer Healthcare, Franklin Lakes, NJ.)

36° F or greater than 86° F. Vials in use may be kept at room temperature for about 1 month. A slight loss of potency may occur after 30 days at room temperature. Humalog, regular insulin cartridges, or prefilled regular insulin pens may be kept unrefrigerated for 28 days. Because of potential variations in temperature, insulin should not be left in a car or checked in airline baggage. Mark the date on the vial when it was initially opened. The client should always have a spare vial on hand.[5,33] Do not use any insulin beyond its expiration date. Inspect each vial of insulin before each use for changes (i.e., clumping, frosting, or change in clarity or color) that may affect the its potency. Visual inspection should reveal rapid and short-acting insulin as well as insulin glargine to be clear and all other insulin types to be uniformly cloudy.[5]

Insulin Preparation and Injection. Experts once thought that insulin vials should be rolled between the hands to resuspend the insulin without creating air bubbles. Now they believe that vials containing NPH and Lente suspensions should be agitated vigorously to mix the insulin to deliver consistent insulin concentrations.

To minimize the discomfort of subcutaneous insulin injection, administer the insulin at room temperature. The number of bacteria carried through a small-gauge needle is insufficient for infection to occur, and alcohol preparation is no longer considered necessary. If alcohol is used to clean the site, wait until it has evaporated completely. Have the client try to relax. Penetrate the skin quickly. Do not change the direction of the needle once it has entered the subcutaneous tissue or while it is being withdrawn.[5]

Prefilled Syringes. Prefilled syringes are chemically stable for up to 3 weeks when stored in the refrigerator. SMBG may need to be performed more frequently to check whether storage of the insulin in prefilled syringes alters its effectiveness in achieving glycemic control. Mixing regular and NPH insulins in one syringe is acceptable and convenient (insulin glargine cannot be mixed with any other insulin because it has a pH of 4.0 and will cause precipitation when mixed with other insulins). Premixed, fixed-proportion insulins are available commercially, but are not suitable when daily variations are needed in the dose or when short-acting insulin is required.[33]

Site Selection and Rotation. Certain sites are best used for insulin injection (Figure 47-6). Insulin absorption varies from site to site. To avoid possibly dramatic changes in daily insulin absorption, instruct the client to give injections in one area, about an inch apart, until the whole area has been used, before changing to another site. Tell the client to avoid sites above muscles that will be exercised heavily that day, because exercise increases the rate of absorption. The client who is taking two injections daily may use one site for the morning insulin and another site for the evening insulin. Some clinicians instruct their clients to use only the abdomen be-

FIGURE 47-6 Sites used for insulin injection. The injection site can affect the onset, peak, and duration of action of the insulin. Insulin injected into the abdomen (area I) is absorbed fastest, followed by insulin injected into the arm (area II) and the leg (area III).

cause of its more even and rapid absorption rate. Emphasize the importance of adhering to a definite injection plan for avoiding tissue damage. Rotate injection sites in one area to decrease the variability of absorption.

Techniques for Self-Injection. Most clients who take insulin learn to give themselves injections (see the Client Education Guide on Self-Injection of Insulin on p. 1263). It is primarily your responsibility to instruct clients with diabetes in the techniques for preparing and injecting insulin. The amount of teaching needed depends on the client's familiarity with insulin and the injection equipment.

Equipment that the client will purchase for home use includes insulin of the type prescribed, absorbent cotton, approved syringes with needles, and 70% ethyl or 91% isopropyl alcohol (optional). As noted, alcohol preparation of the injection site is no longer considered necessary, and cleansing of the top of the insulin vial may increase the risk of infection by transferring resident bacteria from fingers to the vial unless gloves are worn. Storing insulin in its original carton or in a container that will keep it clean may be a more practical option.

Although the prospect of daily injections for life is far from pleasant, the client's attitude toward this intervention may be largely influenced by your own attitude. A matter-of-fact approach helps the client understand and accept responsibility for self-care. Schedule a teaching session for self-injection techniques. Some clients find it difficult to inject the needle into their own skin. For these clients, you might select the site and insert the needle. Then, as the first step in self-injection, have the client push in the plunger and remove the needle. As the client gains confidence, self-injecting will be less traumatic.

Needle-Free Technology. Jet injectors, which are pen-like devices, can be used in place of insulin syringes for delivery of insulin. The needle-less devices supply sufficient force to propel a fine liquid jet of insulin through the skin and to disperse the insulin into subcutaneous tissue. Devices introduced from the 1970s through the mid-1990s were large, heavy, and expensive. Newer devices as shown in Figure 47-7 are much lighter, cheaper, and easier to clean than earlier models. The problem of safe disposal of needles is avoided with needle-less injectors.

See the Case Management feature on Diabetes on the website.

Evaluation

It is expected that clients with type 1 or type 2 diabetes will learn about the disease process and methods of control. If management is successful, complications of diabetes will be avoided as much as possible. For a client with newly diagnosed type 1 diabetes, return demonstration should be expected for all activities with increasing proficiency over time. The client should not be expected to accomplish complete self-care after a single teaching session. The amount of time required varies from client to client. Follow-up visits must be initiated to make sure that the client is following recommendations and has not experienced problems with the therapeutic regimen. Over time, periodic follow-up visits will help you monitor the client's ability to perform self-care and anticipate any potential difficulties.

■ Self-Care

Before hospital discharge, the client and family must have a basic understanding of diabetes and its management with blood glucose monitoring, insulin injections, foot care, nutrition, and exercise. Because diabetes is a chronic disorder, the client needs time to adapt to as well as to learn about the many changes that are occurring. The client should be encouraged to anticipate a usual day at work, school, or home and should be taught how and when to give insulin, how to monitor blood glucose, and what types of foods to eat.

Clients with diabetes need ongoing monitoring of their self-care ability. A1C levels are usually checked, as is the client's log of daily glucose levels and insulin. Chronic changes that result from diabetes should also be assessed on an ongoing basis, by checking the client's vision, kidney function, degree of neuropathy, blood pres-

FIGURE 47-7 A Medi-Jector VISION ® needle-less device for insulin injection. **B** shows how the jet apparatus is refilled with insulin. (Courtesy of Antares Pharma, Inc., Exton, PA.)

sure, and skin condition. If the client is older or debilitated, home nurse visits may be an excellent asset. A referral to a visiting nurse organization or home health care agency should be initiated before discharge.

■ Modifications for Older Clients

Diabetes is common among older adults and represents an important health problem for this population. Currently, 6.3 million (19%) of all people over the age of 65 years have diabetes. Many changes that occur with normal aging affect glucose levels. Blood glucose levels increase with age; fasting levels increase by about 1 mg/dl per decade and postprandial values by 6 to 13 mg/dl per decade. It is believed that peripheral receptor sites become less sensitive to insulin with time. A decline also takes place in levels of glucose-regulating hormones (glucagon and epinephrine) and in lean body mass. These changes may be accompanied by decreased physical activity and a poor diet. Older adults with diabetes mellitus are more susceptible to stroke, myocardial infarction (MI), angina, or seizures. Diminished sensations may mask the manifestations of hyperglycemia. Accompanying changes in liver and kidney function and multidrug regimens may exacerbate hypoglycemia.[20]

In general, nutritional guidelines for older clients with diabetes are no different than those for older clients without diabetes. However, older people with diabetes are at increased risk for problems that can cause functional limitations, such as the following:

- Pain
- Urinary incontinence
- Decreased vision (retinopathy, glaucoma, cataracts)
- Decreased proprioception
- Postural hypotension

Impairments in mental status, functional abilities, and sensory function may interfere with the client's ability to understand and follow the treatment plan. In the older client, the risk of acute complications from hypoglycemia may outweigh the benefits of tight glucose control. The older client may enjoy good health and do very well on an individualized treatment plan. A team approach aimed at maximizing health through optimal diet and exercise, may improve the client's quality of life, as well as achieving adequate glucose control.

■ Surgical Management
Pancreas and Pancreas-Kidney Transplantation

Indications. Some clients with type 1 diabetes receive pancreas transplants. The first pancreas transplant was completed in 1966. Eighty percent of pancreas transplantation procedures are now done concurrently with kidney transplantation. This is usually because the anti-rejection medication cyclosporine has such severe side effects, including hyperglycemia and nephrotoxicity, that adequate renal function unaffected by nephropathy must be present. The client's own pancreas is left intact (98% of its function is exocrine in nature), and the new pancreas is usually anastomosed (attached) to the iliac artery and vein, through which insulin can enter the systemic pathway. The new pancreas is placed in the lower pelvic cavity, and the duct is connected to the urinary bladder. The exocrine secretions of the new pancreas drain into the bladder and are not absorbed. The surgical procedure generally lasts from 4 to 6 hours. Pancreas-after-kidney transplants and pancreas-only transplants account for the remaining 20% of pancreas transplantation procedures.

There has been renewed interest in the surgical technique of anastomosing the transplanted pancreas to the duodenum to allow for exocrine secretions to be absorbed normally through the gastrointestinal tract. This prevents the dehydration that is common with bladder-drained pancreas transplantation. Clinical trials using the Edmonton protocol regarding transplanted pancreatic islet cells rather than transplanting the entire pancreas are being done at more than 15 sites.

Contraindications. Clients with type 1 diabetes must have well-functioning kidneys to receive only a pancreas transplant. If not, the pancreas and kidney must be transplanted simultaneously, or the pancreas must be transplanted following a successful kidney transplant. Other contraindications include problems that make the client unable to withstand the stress of surgery. Clients with type 2 diabetes do not benefit from pancreas transplantation. Type 2 diabetes results from a failure of insulin action, which cannot be improved by adding a pancreas.

Complications. Major complications of pancreas transplantation include vessel thrombosis, rejection, and infection. To help prevent thrombosis, the volume of blood flowing through the pancreas is kept at a high rate for 72 hours. Careful monitoring of laboratory values, fluid and electrolyte status, physical manifestations, and vital sign changes can alert you to possible complications. A sharp and sudden decrease in urine amylase levels, rapid increases in blood glucose, gross hematuria (blood in urine), severe pain in the iliac fossa, and tenderness in the graft area are manifestations of vessel thrombosis.

Manifestations of acute and chronic graft rejection include fever, increased serum creatinine and blood urea nitrogen (BUN) levels, weight gain, and graft tenderness. Proteinuria is a primary manifestation of chronic rejection. In addition, fever, decreased urinary amylase levels, increased serum amylase levels, hyperglycemia, and graft tenderness are manifestations of graft rejection. To prevent graft rejection, immunosuppressive therapy with monoclonal antibodies (OKT3) or polyclonal antibody preparations (cyclosporine [Sandimmune], and azathioprine [Imuran] and prednisone) is administered. See Chapter 82 for further discussion of immunosuppressive agents.

Immunosuppressive drugs may be harmful to the transplant recipient. An increase in serum creatinine levels and decreased urine output may be related to the nephrotoxic effects of cyclosporine. Decreased white blood cell counts may be associated with the myelosuppressive effects of azathioprine. Other adverse effects of immunosuppressive agents that should be monitored are discussed in Chapter 82.

Measures to prevent infection include early removal of invasive lines, adherence to sterile technique with dressing changes and catheter irrigations, pulmonary hygiene measures, and strict hand-washing practices. Antibiotics are used to treat infections.

Outcomes. It is expected that the client will recover from the pancreas or pancreas-kidney transplant surgery and will be discharged from the hospital within 7 to 10 days without the need for insulin. Within 3 to 4 months, the client resumes a normal life as long as medication and health care regimens are followed closely. Complications such as rejection and infection slow postoperative progress. The client's quality of life is improved as a result of freedom from the need for insulin and the return to a normal diet and a less restricted lifestyle. Successful transplantation is indicated by improvement in blood glucose control (levels between 60 and 110 mg/dl) and C-peptide levels.

The survival rate is 91% after transplantation. More than 65% of clients who receive transplants no longer need insulin at 1 year afterward. HLA-DR matching or mismatching affects the results. See Chapter 82 for further discussion of organ transplantation.

■ Nursing Management of the Surgical Client

Once the client has chosen transplantation as an alternative to medical care and is placed on the recipient waiting list, he or she needs to undergo an extensive physical and psychological evaluation (see Chapter 82). Nursing care focuses on assessing the client's needs for knowledge and information.

The nursing care of the client undergoing a pancreas transplantation procedure is similar to that for any client undergoing major abdominal surgery. Postoperative care is directed not only at caring for the client's postsurgical needs but also at addressing the particular needs of a client who has undergone an organ transplant. Care of the client after organ transplantation is discussed in Chapter 82; renal transplantation is discussed briefly in Chapter 38.

The major focus of care is to monitor for rejection, adverse effects of immunosuppressive agents, infection, and occlusion of vessels. Careful monitoring for changes in vital signs, laboratory values, fluid and electrolyte status, and physical manifestations is important to determine the onset of complications; thrombosis, infection, and rejection. Blood glucose levels range between 60 and 110 mg/dl, without administration of exogenous insulin. Urine amylase levels remain constant, with urine pH between 7.0 and 8.5.

Immunosuppressive therapy started before surgery must be continued on a regular schedule postoperatively to prevent rejection of the new pancreas. Nursing implications for immunosuppressive agents to prevent rejection and treat rejection are described in Chapter 82.

You are responsible not only for implementing physical care immediately after transplantation but also for addressing the psychosocial needs of the client and significant others. Keep them informed about the status of the transplanted organ. Allow them to express concerns and ask questions. See Chapter 82 for further discussion of organ transplantation.

■ Self-Care

The self-care regimen following pancreas or pancreas-kidney transplantation is complex for the client and significant others. Teach the client and significant others about long-term, ongoing care, which includes frequent follow-up to monitor the status of the new organs. Discuss self-care involved in managing medications, diet, physical activity, and manifestations of rejection and infection. Explain why continuing the present medication regimen is important and why the client should never miss a dose. Explain the manifestations of rejection and infection if the client cannot remember, needs a review, or did not receive complete information. See Chapter 82 for additional information related to transplantation.

▌ACUTE COMPLICATIONS OF DIABETES MELLITUS
HYPERGLYCEMIA AND DIABETIC KETOACIDOSIS

Hyperglycemia results when glucose cannot be transported to the cells because of a lack of insulin. Without available carbohydrates for cellular fuel, the liver converts its glycogen stores back to glucose (glycogenolysis) and increases the biosynthesis of glucose (gluconeogenesis). Unfortunately, however, these responses worsen the situation by raising the blood glucose level even higher.[27,29]

In type 1 diabetes mellitus, as the need for cellular fuel grows more critical, the body begins to draw on its fat and protein stores for energy. Excessive amounts of fatty acids are mobilized from adipose tissue cells and transported to the liver. The liver, in turn, accelerates the rate at which it produces ketone bodies (ketogenesis) for catabolism by other body tissues, particularly muscle. As fat metabolism increases, the liver may produce too many ketone bodies. Ketone bodies accumulate in the blood (ketosis) and are excreted in the urine (ketonuria). Metabolic acidosis develops from the acidic (pH-lowering) effect of the ketones acetoacetate and beta-hydroxybutyrate. This condition is called *diabetic ketoacidosis*. Severe acidosis may cause the diabetic client to lose consciousness, a condition called *diabetic coma*. Diabetic ketoacidosis always constitutes a medical emergency and requires immediate medical attention.[27,29]

Diabetic ketoacidosis is the most serious metabolic disturbance in type 1 diabetes and is a common cause of hospital admission. Diabetic ketoacidosis is identified in about 40% of clients with previously undiagnosed diabetes and is responsible for more than 160,000 hospital admissions each year. It occurs most frequently in teenagers and older adults.

Etiology and Risk Factors

Diabetic ketoacidosis is primarily a complication of type 1 diabetes mellitus, although it can also affect clients with type 2 diabetes during periods of extreme stress. A precipitating cause can be identified in 80% of clients. Common causes of diabetic ketoacidosis include the following:

- Taking too little insulin
- Skipping doses of insulin
- Inability to meet an increased need for insulin created by surgery, trauma, pregnancy, stress, puberty, or infection
- Developing insulin resistance through the presence of insulin antibodies

Pathophysiology

Diabetic ketoacidosis is marked by a relative or absolute lack of insulin. Insulin may be present, but not in suffi-

cient amounts for the increased need for glucose due to the stressors present (such as infection). When the body lacks insulin and cannot use carbohydrates for energy, it resorts to using fats and proteins. Excess production of counterregulatory hormones (glucagon, catecholamines, cortisol, and growth hormones) secondary to stress appears to play an important role in the development of diabetic ketoacidosis. These hormones antagonize the effects of insulin and foster diabetic ketoacidosis by promoting hyperglycemia, osmotic diuresis, lipolysis with secondary hyperlipidemia, and acidosis. Figure 47-8 summarizes the pathophysiologic mechanisms involved. The process of catabolizing fats for fuel gives rise to three pathologic events:

- Ketosis and acidosis
- Dehydration
- Electrolyte and acid-base imbalances

Ketosis

The metabolic effect of insufficient insulin on fat metabolism was examined previously. In diabetic ketoacidosis, buffering of acid by bicarbonate, which is excreted as carbon dioxide and water, fails to compensate for keto-

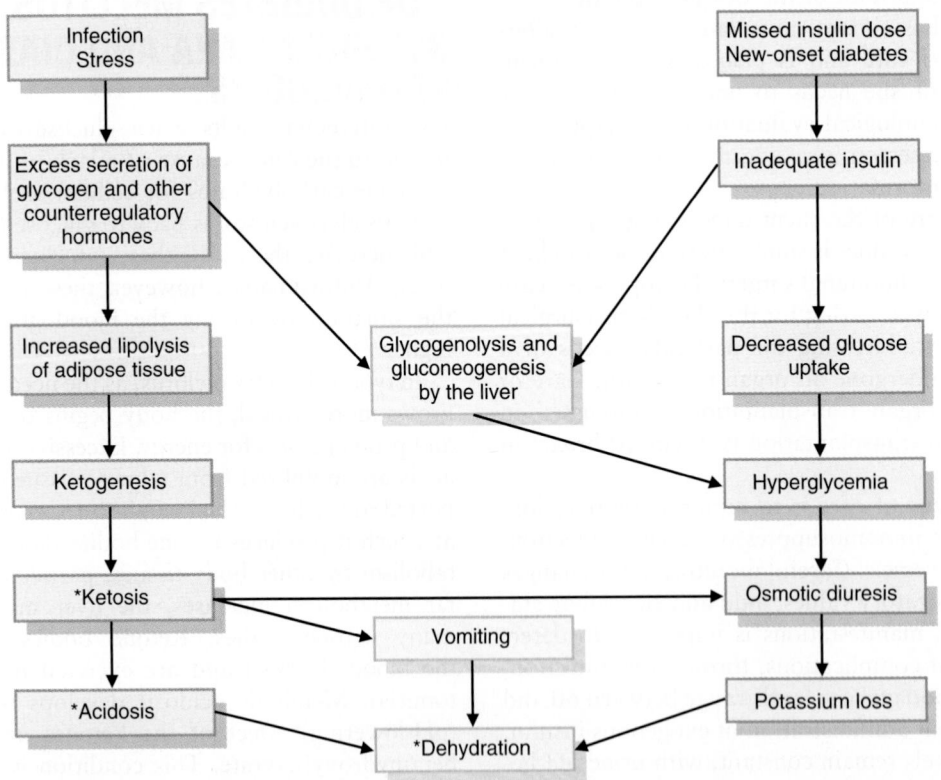

*Hallmarks of DKA

FIGURE 47-8 The pathophysiology of diabetic ketoacidosis. (Modified from White, N.H., & Henry, D.N. [1996]. Special issues in diabetes management. In D. Haire-Joshu [Ed.], *Management of diabetes mellitus: Perspectives of care across the lifespan* [2nd ed., p. 344]. St. Louis: Mosby.)

sis. Respirations increase in rate and depth (Kussmaul's respirations), and the breath has a "fruity" or acetone-like odor.

The renal system attempts to excrete enough ketone bodies to normalize pH, which leads to osmotic diuresis and hemoconcentration (excessive loss of fluid and electrolytes). Hemoconcentration impedes blood circulation and leads to tissue anoxia and lactic acid production. This increase in lactic acid further acidifies blood pH. The rising tide of ketone bodies eventually overwhelms the body's defenses against hydrogen excess. With its buffer, respiratory, and renal defense systems depleted, the body finally succumbs to its acid overload, and diabetic coma can ensue.

Dehydration

Clients with ketoacidosis lose fluids from several sources. They excrete large amounts of urine in the body's attempt to eliminate excessive glucose and ketones. Second, acidosis can cause severe nausea and vomiting, with further losses of fluid and electrolytes (notably sodium and chloride). Finally, water is lost in the breath as the body attempts to rid itself of excess acetone and carbon dioxide. Typically, clients in diabetic coma lose an amount of water equivalent to 10% of body weight, plus about 40 g of sodium. Severe dehydration resulting from these fluid losses may be followed by hypovolemic shock and lactic acidosis.

Electrolyte Imbalance

As the pH of the blood decreases (acidosis), the accumulating hydrogen moves from the extracellular fluid to the intracellular fluid. The movement of hydrogen into the cells promotes the movement of potassium out of the cells into the extracellular fluid, which results in severe intracellular potassium depletion. Initially, the intracellular potassium loss may go unrecognized because serum potassium levels are often normal or elevated. As the resulting osmotic diuresis continues, however, much potassium is excreted in the urine. If the client becomes severely dehydrated, hemoconcentration and oliguria may cause the serum potassium levels to increase even higher. In addition to potassium losses, the client in metabolic acidosis loses excessive amounts of sodium, phosphate, chloride, and bicarbonate in the urine and vomitus.

Clinical Manifestations

Common presenting manifestations of the client in diabetic ketoacidosis are listed in Box 47-4. Clinical manifestations and assessment priorities common with acute hyperglycemia are listed in Table 47-5.

> **BOX 47-4** *Common Manifestations of Diabetic Ketoacidosis*
>
> - Abdominal pain
> - Anorexia
> - Dehydration
> - Fruity odor of ketones on breath
> - Hyperpnea or Kussmaul's respirations
> - Hypotension
> - Impaired level of consciousness or coma
> - Nausea and vomiting
> - Polyuria
> - Somnolence
> - Tachycardia
> - Thirst
> - Visual disturbances
> - Warm, dry skin
> - Weakness
> - Weight loss

Outcome Management
■ Medical Management

Assessment priorities and clinical manifestations for the client with acute hyperglycemia are presented in Table 47-5. Management of diabetic ketoacidosis usually takes place in a hospital setting, with care managed by the physician, nurse, and pharmacist. Dehydration resulting in hypovolemic shock, acute tubular necrosis, and uremia are major causes of death in cases of untreated diabetic ketoacidosis. Diabetic ketoacidosis constitutes an emergency. Rapid medical care and nursing intervention are essential to correct the life-threatening abnormalities. Effective therapy is based on an understanding of metabolic changes that occur during diabetic ketoacidosis. The cornerstone of treatment is the administration of fluids, insulin, and electrolytes.

Management outcomes in diabetic ketoacidosis are rehydration, correction of electrolyte and acid-base imbalances, restoration to a state of carbohydrate catabolism from a state of fat catabolism by providing insulin, and identification and correction of those factors that precipitated the ketoacidosis. The measures to achieve these outcomes must be done with great care. Fully correcting all biochemical abnormalities may take as long as 1 week after the client is able to eat solid food. A comprehensive flow sheet should be kept to record intake and output, body weight, fluids, electrolytes, insulin, and ketones.

Rehydrate. Intravenous rehydration is required for all clients who are vomiting, are unable to drink, and have acidosis. IV infusions of isotonic or normal saline (0.9%

TABLE 47-5 *Clinical Manifestations and Priority Assessments with Acute Hyperglycemia*

Clinical Manifestations	Priority Assessments
Dehydration	Assess skin for dryness, flushed color, and "tenting."
	Assess mucous membranes for dryness.
	Monitor urine output for polyuria followed by oliguria.
	Monitor vital signs for hypotension and tachycardia.
	Monitor for fluid overload during treatment for hyperglycemia.
Electrolyte imbalances	Monitor for hyperkalemia: peaked T waves on ECG, ectopic beats, changes in heart rate, hypotension, diarrhea and hyperactive bowel sounds, muscle cramps, nausea and vomiting, hypotension.
	Monitor for hypokalemia: flattened T waves and U wave on ECG, ectopic beats, hypotension, ileus, nausea and vomiting, fatigue, lethargy, muscle weakness and cramps.
	Monitor for hyponatremia: nausea, vomiting, diarrhea, tachycardia, hypotension, lethargy, confusion, seizures, muscle weakness.
Hyperglycemia	Monitor blood glucose levels and check urine for ketones.
	Monitor for polyuria, polyphagia, and polydipsia.
	Monitor for hypoglycemia during treatment for hypoglycemia.
Hyperosmolality	Monitor serum osmolality, blood urea nitrogen, serum creatinine.
	Assess for lethargy, disorientation, and behavioral changes.
Metabolic acidosis	Monitor for hypotension, dysrrhythmias, hyperventilation, lethargy, confusion, coma, headache, acetone breath.

CRITICAL MONITORING

The Rehydration Process

- The best indication of the degree of dehydration is weight loss, which may be determined when the client's baseline weight is known; loss may be 10% of total body weight.
- Other clinical indices to monitor are tissue turgor, pulse, condition of mucous membranes, level of consciousness, thirst, hematocrit, and positional blood pressure changes (to check for orthostatic hypotension).
- For older adults and clients with heart disease, fluid replacement should be determined according to central venous pressure measurement.
- Too aggressive fluid replacement (particularly with normal saline) may induce heart failure; frequent auscultation of the lungs is vital.

BOX 47-5 *Intravenous Fluid Replacement in Diabetic Ketoacidosis**

Hour 1
Provide 15-20 ml/kg of isotonic sodium chloride (0.9%) (normal saline) or full-strength Ringer's lactate (lactated Ringer's solution).

Hour 2
Continue fluid as above at 15 ml/kg. If the client is hypernatremic, in heart failure, or is a child, consider half-strength sodium chloride (0.45% normal saline).

Hour 3
Reduce fluid intake to 7.5 ml/kg in adults. Fluid should be 0.45% normal saline.

Hour 4
Adjust fluid intake to meet clinical need. Consider urine output rate in calculation.

Modified from Bode, B. (2003). *Medical management of type 1 diabetes* (4th ed.). Alexandria, VA: American Diabetes Association.
*When blood glucose approaches 250 mg/dl, change fluid to 5% dextrose in half-strength sodium chloride (D_5 0.45% normal saline). Continue intravenous fluids until client can ingest food and drink without vomiting.

sodium chloride) are started immediately. Usually, the client receives 1000 ml of isotonic solution by the IV route during the first hour (10 to 20 ml/kg), followed by an additional 2000 to 8000 ml of solution over the next 24 hours. Clients with compromised cardiovascular function may require slower IV fluid replacement (see the Critical Monitoring feature on The Rehydration Process, above, and Box 47-5).

A nasogastric tube may be necessary if the client is comatose or is vomiting and likely to aspirate the vomitus. The client's mouth may be dry because of the nasogastric tube and the dehydration. Frequent oral care is important. Assess bowel sounds frequently for changes. Encourage the client to drink once he or she can tolerate fluids. Drinking salted broth is beneficial to replenish needed sodium. Record intake and output accurately.

Most clients require a urinary catheter. Because clients with diabetes are susceptible to infection, aseptic catheter care is essential.

Reverse Shock. If the client is in circulatory collapse, the physician may order blood, albumin, or other plasma volume expanders, such as dextran, to be administered alternately with normal saline solution. Also, the client may receive combinations of colloids and saline solution that raise serum levels of both sodium chloride and plasma protein.

Restore Potassium Balance. Because of the lowered pH in untreated ketoacidosis, potassium leaves the intracellular space, and transient hyperkalemia develops. The total body potassium level is depleted, despite a normal or elevated serum potassium level. Correct potassium replacement requires caution and timely action. Once intervention begins with fluids and insulin, dangerous hypokalemia may develop, manifested by weakness, extreme dyspnea, and even cardiac arrest. Hypokalemia occurs because potassium reenters the cells (along with glucose) after insulin administration and then is excreted in the urine with rehydration and restoration of renal function. General agreement exists on the following points of assessment and intervention:

- Frequently assess and measure urine output. Do not administer potassium to a client with low urine output; dangerous hyperkalemia may develop. Notify the physician promptly if urine output declines dramatically or is less than 0.5 ml/kg/hr.
- Assess the client continuously for evidence of hyperkalemia (bradycardia, cardiac arrest, weakness, flaccid paralysis, oliguria) or hypokalemia (weakness, flaccid paralysis, paralytic ileus, cardiac arrest). Hyperkalemia may be present during the first 4 hours of intervention. Hypokalemia usually develops 4 to 24 hours after the initial intervention.
- Replace potassium carefully following protocols (Box 47-6).
- Plan to begin potassium administration within 1 to 2 hours after starting insulin therapy and after adequate urine output is ensured.
- When the client has recovered sufficiently to resume eating and drinking, give foods and liquids that are high in potassium, such as bananas or orange juice.
- Monitor sodium chloride and phosphate levels. Sodium is replaced by normal saline. Phosphate levels can also vary to the same degree noted for potassium levels. Sometimes the physician alternates potassium chloride with potassium phosphate in the IV fluid.

Correct pH and Administer Insulin. Clients presenting in diabetic ketoacidosis usually have phosphate depletion from a combination of decreased food intake, ex-

---

> **BOX 47-6**   *Potassium Replacement in Diabetic Ketoacidosis*
>
> In clients with adequate urine output, lead II of the 12-lead electrocardiogram may be used as a guide for plasma potassium (K^+) concentration. Flattening or inversion of the T wave with U wave and prolongation of the QT interval indicate hypokalemia. Peaking of T waves, loss of P wave, and a disrupted QRS complex indicate hyperkalemia.
>
> Intravenous replacement of potassium is based on plasma K^+ concentration. If K^+ concentration is:
> - <3 mEq/L, infuse ≥0.6 mEq/kg/hr
> - 3-4 mEq/L, infuse 0.6 mEq/kg/hr
> - 4-5 mEq/L, infuse 0.2-0.4 mEq/kg/hr
> - 6 mEq/L, withhold until K^+ concentration is <6.0 mEq/L
>
> Add K^+ to replacement fluid therapy. If concentration is 20-40 mEq/L and infusion into peripheral vein causes irritation, infuse into central vein.
>
> Recheck plasma K^+ concentration every 2 hours if previous value was <4 or >6 mEq/L.

Modified from Bode, B. (2003). *Medical management of type 1 diabetes* (4th ed.). Alexandria, VA: American Diabetes Association.

---

cessive catabolism, and increased urinary excretion. As with administration of potassium, administration of insulin enhances movement of phosphate into the cells, which further reduces plasma phosphate concentration. However, administering too much phosphate can induce hypocalcemia. Calcium levels should be checked before phosphate (as potassium phosphate) is given.

Clinicians usually administer sodium bicarbonate only to clients with a blood pH of 7.1 or less. Such replacement therapy partially corrects the metabolic acidosis. As the client's condition improves, normal body mechanisms restore the blood pH to normal.

Low-dosage insulin therapy (5 to 10 units/hr) is ordered for the client in diabetic ketoacidosis. Although the blood glucose concentration is usually sharply elevated in diabetic ketoacidosis, a blood glucose level less than 300 mg/dl does not exclude the diagnosis. The client in ketoacidosis may receive an initial IV bolus of regular insulin (0.15 unit/kg) in the emergency department. Before starting an infusion of insulin, ask whether the client has already received insulin that day. Insulin should never be given subcutaneously to someone in diabetic ketoacidosis, because the subcutaneous tissues are dehydrated and poorly perfused as a result of dehydration and hypovolemic shock.[29]

Traditionally, the hyperglycemia associated with diabetic ketoacidosis is treated with an IV bolus of regular insulin. Then an insulin drip should be started. Either 0.9% (normal) saline solution or 0.45% saline may be used, depending on the degree of dehydration and concurrent medical problems. Prepare the last amount of insulin in the smallest IV bag available (e.g., 100 units of regular insulin in 100 ml of IV fluid). This gives a 1:1 ratio of regular insulin to IV fluid. Prime the IV tubing with the IV solution first, and then add the regular insulin, because insulin adheres to the IV tubing. Label the IV bag clearly with the dose and type of insulin added. The IV regular insulin must be administered meticulously by a control pump and checked frequently.

After the bolus, infuse insulin at a rate of 0.1 unit/kg/hr. If no improvement in the acidosis occurs within 2 to 4 hours, the infusion rate should be doubled. Severe insulin resistance may be precipitated by severe stress. The glucose level is normalized more quickly than pH.

Blood glucose levels need to be monitored every 30 minutes initially, preferably with a blood glucose meter. Rapid blood glucose test results allow you to adjust the insulin infusion rapidly and correctly. When the blood glucose levels approach 250 mg/dl, the insulin infusion should be reduced and 5% dextrose added to the infusion so that the blood glucose level can be maintained at about 250 mg/dl for the first 12 to 24 hours. Faster correction of hyperglycemia can lead to cerebral edema. Monitor the client's level of consciousness closely to assess for this uncommon complication. Monitor blood glucose levels every 1 to 2 hours after reaching 250 mg/dl until they are stable.[29]

As the client improves, decisions must be made about when to discontinue IV insulin and fluids and begin subcutaneous insulin administration. Normalization of the client's vital signs, correction of acidosis, and ability to take oral fluids are important considerations. Short-acting insulin is usually administered subcutaneously every 4 to 6 hours, with the first dose given 15 to 30 minutes before stopping IV insulin. The initial dose is about 0.2 unit/kg. Subsequent doses are determined by blood glucose levels.

While any metabolic abnormalities are being corrected, the cause of the client's diabetic ketoacidosis must be pursued aggressively. Cultures of urine, throat, sputum, and blood; chest x-ray films; and an electrocardiogram (ECG) may reveal the source of stress. Before discharge of the client from the hospital, the health care team reviews the situation that led to diabetic ketoacidosis and institutes teaching for risk factor reduction.

Prevent Recurrence. Primary prevention of diabetic ketoacidosis is through client education. Preventing diabetic ketoacidosis is the long-term goal of good diabetes management. Clients and their families should understand enough about ketoacidosis to avoid potential causes, to recognize its approach, to slow down or minimize its development, and to seek help fast if it begins to occur. To prevent diabetic ketoacidosis, clients with diabetes should learn to do the following:
- Take insulin in appropriate doses at appropriate times.

- Monitor blood glucose frequently, at least before each meal and at bedtime.
- Monitor urine ketone levels when blood glucose levels increase to greater than 250 mg/dl.
- Schedule regular appointments with a health care provider to review blood glucose levels, weight gains or losses, and general state of health and well-being. Recognize manifestations of infection—a major cause of diabetic ketoacidosis. The first clinical manifestations of infection (upper respiratory tract, urinary tract, or vaginal infection) should be reported immediately to the health care provider; other stressors, such as family or emotional problems, can also precipitate diabetic ketoacidosis.

The client should telephone for assistance if any of the following develop:
- Anorexia, nausea, vomiting, or diarrhea
- Ketonuria persisting for more than 8 hours
- Fever or infection
- Any manifestation of acidosis

Emphasize that the greatest weapons against diabetic ketoacidosis are regular, daily SMBG; adherence to the diabetes management program; and early recognition of and intervention in mild ketosis.

HYPERGLYCEMIC, HYPEROSMOLAR, NONKETOTIC SYNDROME

Hyperglycemic, hyperosmolar, nonketotic syndrome (HHNS) is a variant of diabetic ketoacidosis characterized by extreme hyperglycemia (600 to 2000 mg/dl), profound dehydration, mild or undetectable ketonuria, and the absence of acidosis. HHNS most commonly occurs in older clients with type 2 diabetes mellitus (Box 47-7).

Mortality with HHNS is greater than with diabetic ketoacidosis (10% to 40%), primarily because clients typically are older and commonly have significant medical problems. HHNS sometimes occurs in people with undiagnosed diabetes and in known diabetic clients after a long period of uncontrolled hyperglycemia. The precipitating factors for HHNS may be the same as those for diabetic ketoacidosis. There is almost always an identifiable precipitating factor.

The major difference between HHNS and diabetic ketoacidosis is the lack of ketonuria with HHNS. Because some residual ability to secrete insulin remains in type 2 diabetes mellitus, the mobilization of fats for energy usually does not occur. In the absence of adequate insulin, the blood becomes loaded with glucose. Glucose molecules are too large to pass into cells; therefore osmosis of water occurs from the interstitial spaces and cells to dilute the glucose in the blood. Osmotic diuresis occurs. Eventually, the cells become dehydrated.[15]

The client's fluid intake can initially balance the loss of fluid and glucose through the urine. The imbalance

BOX 47-7	*Factors Associated with Hyperglycemic, Hyperosmolar, Nonketotic Syndrome (HHNS)*

Therapeutic Agents
Glucocorticoids
Diuretics
Diphenylhydantoin
Beta-adrenergic blocking agents
L-Asparaginase
Immunosuppressive agents
Chlorpromazine
Diazoxide

Therapeutic Procedures
Peritoneal dialysis
Hemodialysis
Hyperalimentation
Surgical stress

Chronic Illness
Renal disease
Heart disease
Hypertension
Previous stroke
Alcoholism
Psychiatric diagnosis
Loss of thirst

Acute Illness
Infection
Gangrene
Urinary tract infection
Septicemia
Burns
Gastrointestinal bleeding
Myocardial infarction
Pancreatitis
Stroke

From American Diabetes Association. (1998). *Medical management of non-insulin dependent (type 2) diabetes* (4th ed.). Alexandria, VA: Author.

gradually becomes more severe as the client cannot match intake to output. In time, the client becomes obtunded and is unable to respond to thirst. At this point, the process is self-perpetuating.

The following are the four major clinical features of HHNS[15]:
- Severe hyperglycemia (600 to 2000 mg/dl)
- No or only slight ketosis
- Profound dehydration (10% to 15% loss of body water)
- Hyperosmolality (increased concentration) of plasma and elevated blood urea nitrogen

Typically, the client experiences excessive thirst, altered level of consciousness (coma or confusion), and manifestations of dehydration. The precipitating event should be determined and corrected as soon as possible, even during resuscitation. HHNS is treated with vigorous fluid replacement and administration of insulin and electrolytes. A common initial intervention is infusion of normal saline solution over a 2-hour period, followed by administration of hypotonic (0.45%) saline solution. As in diabetic ketoacidosis, potassium, sodium, chloride, and phosphates are administered intravenously.

Insulin is given via an infusion pump, but usually at lower dosages, because the client is producing some insulin. Because of severe dehydration, blood glucose levels decrease rapidly with fluid administration. Dextrose is added to the IV fluid when the blood glucose level reaches about 250 mg/dl, to prevent hypoglycemia. Because many clients who have HHNS are older and have other cardiovascular or renal disorders, fluid volume and electrolyte changes must be carefully assessed, especially if acute or chronic renal failure complicates the course.

As the population ages, an increasing number of clients will experience HHNS and you need to be alert for its manifestations. Before discharge, review the causes of HHNS with the client and family, including insulin injection (if necessary) and blood glucose testing techniques. Help the client understand how serious these acute complications are and how to prevent them in the future.

HYPOGLYCEMIA

Hypoglycemia (also known as an *insulin reaction* or hypoglycemic reaction) is a common feature of type 1 diabetes mellitus and can also be seen in clients with type 2 diabetes treated with insulin or oral agents. The precise blood glucose level at which clients have manifestations of hypoglycemia varies, but they usually do not occur until the blood glucose level is less than 50 to 60 mg/dl.

Etiology and Risk Factors
Hypoglycemic reactions may result from the following:
- An overdose of insulin or, less commonly, a sulfonylurea
- Omitting a meal or eating less food than usual
- Overexertion without additional carbohydrate compensation
- Nutritional and fluid imbalances caused by nausea and vomiting
- Alcohol intake

Inadvertent or deliberate errors in insulin dose are a frequent cause of hypoglycemia. Other changes in the schedule of meals or insulin administration, vigorous unexpected exercise, or sleeping later than usual in the morning can also cause hypoglycemia. The effects of alcohol, marijuana, or other drugs can mask a client's awareness of hypoglycemia in its earliest stages.

Hypoglycemia can also occur secondary to administration of an oral hypoglycemic agent. Most recorded cases have been in clients receiving chlorpropamide (Diabinese), which has a duration of action of 24 to 72 hours. Clients at risk for hypoglycemia while taking an oral hypoglycemic are older than age 60 years, have poor nutritional intake, use alcohol, have hepatic or renal dysfunction, and are on multi-drug regimens. Hypoglycemic reactions can be severe and prolonged.

Pathophysiology

Normally, hypoglycemia triggers counterregulatory hormones, primarily glucagon and epinephrine, to promptly increase blood glucose levels by stimulating glucose release from the liver and inhibiting insulin secretion. Under usual conditions, this leads to normoglycemia.[22]

In contrast, clients with type 1 diabetes have abnormalities in this feedback system. Typically, within the first 2 to 5 years of diabetes, the secretion of glucagon becomes deficient. Later, the secretion of epinephrine may become impaired secondary to subclinical neuropathy. The regulation of insulin absorption from subcutaneous fat also becomes impaired.

The combination of these abnormalities makes the client with type 1 diabetes susceptible to frequent development of hypoglycemia. In this respect, hypoglycemic shock is more dangerous than diabetic ketoacidosis. About 1 in 10 clients with type 1 diabetes suffer one severe reaction per year that requires emergency treatment. Untreated or prolonged hypoglycemia can cause permanent brain damage, memory loss, decreased learning ability, paralysis, and death.

Clinical Manifestations

Hypoglycemic manifestations are generally divided into two major categories (Box 47-8):

1. *Adrenergic* (autonomic) manifestations are associated with increasing epinephrine levels and are considered "mild" reactions. Cognitive deficits usually do not occur, and affected people are capable of self-treatment. Diaphoresis, although not mediated via adrenergic nerve endings, is usually grouped with the adrenergic manifestations of hypoglycemia. Adrenergic reactions usually occur during rapid decreases in blood glucose. They have been reported by clients with poorly controlled diabetes when the decrease in blood glucose level is rapid, even in the absence of hypoglycemia. These manifestations can also occur during other stressful or anxiety-provoking events. These mild reactions may produce only minimal disruptions of daily activities.[16,22]

2. *Neuroglycopenic* manifestations are associated with lack of glucose availability to the brain and resultant decrease in cognitive functioning. These reactions typically produce longer-lasting and more severe manifestations than those characteris-

---

BOX 47-8   *Manifestations of Hypoglycemia*

Adrenergic (Increased Epinephrine)

Shakiness
Irritability
Nervousness
Tachycardia, palpitations
Tremor
Hunger
Diaphoresis
Pallor
Paresthesias

Neuroglycopenic (Decreased Glucose to Brain)

Headache
Mental illness
Inability to concentrate
Slurred speech
Blurred vision
Confusion
Irrational behavior
Lethargy, severe
Loss of consciousness
Coma
Seizure
Death

---

tic of mild reactions. Common manifestations are headache, irritability, drowsiness, weakness, and tremor. The client may need assistance in treatment. Severe hypoglycemic reactions render the client unable to self-treat. The client may be awake and alert, semicomatose, or comatose.[16,22]

Hypoglycemia can occur at any time of day or night. It seems to occur most commonly during exercise, 8 to 24 hours after strenuous exercise, and in the middle of the night. Severe hypoglycemia seems to occur more often in people who have hypoglycemic unawareness, defective glucose counterregulation, and autonomic neuropathy as well as in clients receiving intensive diabetes therapy.

The period during which the client is most likely to experience an insulin reaction depends on the type of insulin given, the client's response to that type of insulin, and the timing of the insulin injection in relation to food intake. When insulin is given in the morning, short-acting preparations tend to produce reactions before lunch; intermediate-acting insulins, 2 or 3 hours before dinner; and long-acting insulins, between 2:00 AM and breakfast. NPH or Lente insulin injected before dinner (5:00 PM) can cause hypoglycemia around 2:00 AM, when the normal blood glucose level is lowest because of the decrease in metabolism, and again at around 8:00 AM, when the insulin peaks if breakfast is not eaten on time.

TABLE 47-6	*Interventions for Hypoglycemia*
Clinical Manifestations	**Interventions**
Mild Hypoglycemia Tremors Tachycardia Diaphoresis Paresthesias Excessive hunger Pallor Shakiness	10-15 g of carbohydrate, contained in the following: 4 oz orange juice 6 oz regular soda 6-8 oz 2% milk 6-8 Lifesavers candies 1 small (2-oz) tube of cake icing 4 tsp granulated sugar
Moderate Hypoglycemia Manifestations listed above plus Headache Mood swings Irritability Inability to concentrate Drowsiness Impaired judgment Slurred speech Double or blurred vision	20-30 g of carbohydrate Glucagon, 1 mg SC or IM
Severe Hypoglycemia Disorientation Seizures Unconsciousness	50% dextrose, 25 g IV Glucagon, 1 mg IM or IV

IM, Intramuscularly; *IV*, intravenously; *SC*, subcutaneously.

Outcome Management
■ Medical Management

Return Blood Glucose to Normal Levels. Management of hypoglycemia depends on the severity of the reaction (Table 47-6). To reverse mild hypoglycemia, 15 g of simple carbohydrate is given and works quickly to increase blood glucose levels. Reactions that occur during the night should be treated with a carbohydrate followed by a longer-acting mixture of carbohydrate and protein (8 ounces of milk, for example). A blood glucose test (with a glucose meter) should be performed as soon as manifestations begin. If a meter is not available, it is safer to assume and treat hypoglycemia. Blood glucose is retested in 15 to 30 minutes, and treatment is repeated if the level is not more than 100 mg/dl. Moderate reactions may need two or more treatments with 15 g of carbohydrates.

Never force an unconscious or semiconscious client to drink liquids, because fluid may be aspirated into the lungs. The unconscious client with severe hypoglycemia needs glucagon or IV glucose immediately. Family members of clients with diabetes can administer glucagon at home in the event of a serious hypoglycemic reaction. Glucagon, administered intramuscularly or subcuta-

neously in the amount of 1 mg for adults, may eliminate the need for emergency department intervention. The pharmacy dispenses glucagon in the form of a powder, with the diluent in a separate vial. Instruct family members how and when to mix and inject glucagon, and let them know that the client may experience nausea or vomiting on awakening. Even though glucagon is effective in most clients, its effect is transient and slower than that of dextrose. Hypoglycemia often recurs. Medical assistance is advisable if hypoglycemia recurs, vomiting prevents oral intake, or the client's status does not improve.

A client who experiences severe hypoglycemia in the hospital usually receives 10 to 25 g of IV glucose (as 50% or 25% dextrose) over 1 to 3 minutes. This is followed by an infusion of 5% dextrose at 5 to 10 g/hr until the client is fully recovered and able to eat.

Prevent Hypoglycemia. Because insulin reactions are common, clients with newly diagnosed diabetes must understand the following:
- Why hypoglycemia occurs
- When it is most likely to occur
- The early clinical manifestations of hypoglycemia
- The danger of severe or repeated reactions
- The importance of early intervention
- How to prevent insulin reactions

Whenever administration of insulin or an oral hypoglycemic agent begins, the client must be taught to identify clinical manifestations and to manage hypoglycemia. Once a client experiences and then fully recovers from an episode of hypoglycemia, thoroughly reassess the intervention program. In some cases, insulin reactions develop because the client carelessly prepares insulin dosages, fails to eat, or exercises excessively. Explain the dangers of repeated insulin reactions to a client who is careless in maintaining a normoglycemic balance. These dangers include loss of consciousness, trauma caused by falling after losing consciousness, injury from poor decision-making, seizures, loss of brain cells, and eventual death. Emphasize conscientious adherence to the therapeutic program.

In other cases, hypoglycemia develops because the prescribed insulin dosage is too large or the client's dietary intake is too small. Instruct the client to record the time and probable cause of any hypoglycemic episodes on the blood test record. The health care team and the client can then evaluate the record together, making appropriate changes. Teach the client with type 1 diabetes to adjust diet and insulin by monitoring results. Finally, be certain that the client with diabetes obtains a diabetic identification tag or medical identification bracelet or necklace and a diabetic identification card. Sometimes, a client who is experiencing an insulin reaction behaves as if intoxicated or mentally disturbed. By carrying proper identification, the client can avoid being arrested at a time when emergency care is desperately needed. Table 47-7 compares the data and interventions for diabetic ketoacidosis, HHNS, and hypoglycemia.

TABLE 47-7 *Acute Complications of Diabetes*

	Diabetic Ketoacidosis (DKA)	Hyperglycemic, Hyperosmolar, Nonketotic Syndrome (HHNS)	Hypoglycemia
Type of diabetes	Usually type 1; may occur in type 2	Type 2	Type 1 or type 2
Clinical manifestations	Warm/dry skin, nausea, vomiting, flushed appearance, dry mucous membranes, soft eyeballs, Kussmaul's respirations or tachypnea, abdominal pain, impaired consciousness, hypotension, tachycardia, acetone breath, acute weight loss Polyuria (early) Oliguria/anuria (late)	Same as for DKA, except Kussmaul's respirations and acetone breath usually not present Alterations in level of consciousness, severe dehydration Nausea and vomiting not present Tachypnea, shallow respirations	Mild reaction: tremors, palpitations, pallor, sweating, hunger Moderate reaction: headache, irritability, drowsiness, weakness, visual disturbances, decreased mental acuity Severe reaction: loss of consciousness, seizures
Precipitating factors	Undiagnosed diabetes Omission of insulin dose Puberty Infection Cardiovascular disorder Other physical or emotional stress, such as pregnancy or surgery Trauma	Undiagnosed diabetes Infection or other stress Medications: phenytoin sodium (Dilantin), thiazide diuretics, steroids, chlorpromazine Dialysis GI bleed Hyperalimentation, myocardial infarction Acute pancreatitis Central nervous system disorders Major burns rehydrated with high volumes of glucose	Delay or omission of meal Insulin overdosage Excessive exercise Improper timing of insulin and food
Onset of manifestations	Slow (hours to days) or quickly	Slow (hours to days)	Rapid (minutes to hours)
Laboratory findings			
Plasma glucose	300-1500 mg/dl	600-2000 mg/dl	60 mg/dl or less
Serum sodium	Normal or decreased	Normal or increased	Normal
Serum potassium	Normal or elevated at first, then decreased	Same as for DKA	Normal
Blood urea nitrogen	Elevated	Elevated	Normal
Serum ketones	Elevated	Absent	Absent
White blood cells	Elevated	Elevated	Normal or elevated
Hematocrit	Elevated	Elevated	Normal
Urine glucose	Elevated	Elevated	Absent
Urine ketones	Elevated	Absent	Absent
Arterial blood gas	Metabolic acidosis with compensatory respiratory alkalosis	Normal (metabolic acidosis of shock is profound and prolonged)	Normal or slight respiratory acidosis
pH	Less than 7.3	Usually normal or slightly decreased	Normal
Osmolality	300-350 mOsm/L	Usually over 350 mOsm/L	Normal

GI, Gastrointestinal; *IM*, intramuscularly; *IV*, intravenous; *SC*, subcutaneously; *SMBG*, self-monitored blood glucose.

TABLE 47-7	*Acute Complications of Diabetes—cont'd*		
	Diabetic Ketoacidosis (DKA)	**Hyperglycemic, Hyperosmolar, Nonketotic Syndrome (HHNS)**	**Hypoglycemia**
Acute intervention	IV regular insulin IV fluids such as normal saline or half normal saline Potassium when urine output is adequate Sodium bicarbonate, rarely Phosphate, usually Electrocardiogram Correct underlying problem	Correct underlying problem IV regular insulin IV fluids such as normal saline or half normal saline Potassium when urine output is adequate	Mild reaction: 10-15 g of simple carbohydrate Moderate reaction: one or more simple carbohydrate, glucagon may be needed, 0.5-1 mg Severe reaction: glucagon IM or SC, repeat × 1 in 10 minutes prn, may need IV glucose
Preventive measures	Prompt medical attention when necessary Plan ahead for illness care Frequent SMBG checks during illness or stressful events	Frequent SMBG checks during illness or stressful events Prompt medical attention when necessary	Sleeping late should be planned in advance; if oversleeping >45 min is planned, changes in insulin or food intake may be necessary Have short-acting carbohydrate available when exercising or reduction of insulin dose before exercise Restricting alcohol intake Double-check insulin type and dosage before administration

→ → → Wearing diabetes identification tag or bracelet. Education for self-care.→ → →

As in many chronic disorders, the client needs to develop a positive self-concept and a feeling of control. Help the client and significant others understand the complications associated with diabetes. Equally important, help the client develop and maintain self-care skills that meet emotional and social needs as well as physical ones.

OTHER HYPOGLYCEMIC DISORDERS

Other manifestations of altered counterregulatory mechanisms in type 1 diabetes mellitus are (1) hypoglycemic unawareness, (2) hypoglycemia with rebound hyperglycemia (Somogyi effect), and (3) the dawn phenomenon.

Hypoglycemic Unawareness

Hypoglycemic unawareness refers to a syndrome in which people with diabetes are unaware they are hypoglycemic and therefore do not initiate treatment. In the Diabetes Control and Complications Trial, about one third of all episodes of severe hypoglycemia seen in awake, intensively treated clients were not accompanied by manifestations of sufficient severity that clients could effectively prevent neuroglycopenia.[18] In the past, this condition was incorrectly viewed as being rare and associated only with advanced neuropathy.

Repeated episodes of hypoglycemia seem to blunt the hormonal defense mechanisms that prevent it (blunted epinephrine response) and the client's ability to perceive early manifestations. Beta-adrenergic–blocking agents (such as propranolol) can cause hypoglycemic unawareness and blunt adrenergic (epinephrine) effects in clients with diabetes, because these effects are primarily mediated by beta-adrenergic receptors. Therefore beta-blockers are contraindicated in clients with diabetes.

Clients with hypoglycemic unawareness (absence of manifestations of hypoglycemia when glucose level is less than 55 mg/dl) require consultation with an experienced physician. Increasing the frequency of SMBG levels, particularly before driving and after exercise, should be encouraged. Clients may wish to choose a slightly higher blood glucose target before meals and during the night. Self-management education and follow-up must be intensified for these clients. For clients with type 1 diabetes, maintaining good control is as much of a problem during the night as at any other time of day.

Hypoglycemia with Rebound Hyperglycemia

Hypoglycemia followed by rebound hyperglycemia, known as the *Somogyi effect* or *Somogyi phenomenon*, may complicate diabetes management. This phenomenon was implicated in the past as a common cause of fasting morning hyperglycemia. Studies have found it to be a rare occurrence. It usually results from excessive evening insulin dosing. The pathophysiology involves hypoglycemia, leading to counterregulatory hormone secretion and resultant liver production of glucose. This increase in glucose, along with insulin resistance secondary to increased hormone levels, is thought to contribute to rebound hyperglycemia.

Nocturnal rebound hyperglycemia should be investigated by SMBG levels between 2:00 and 4:00 AM and again at 7:00 AM. If early-morning levels are less than 50 to 60 mg/dl and those at 7:00 AM are greater than 180 to 200 mg/dl, rebound hyperglycemia may have occurred. Decreasing the intermediate-acting insulin dose at supper time, moving the intermediate-acting insulin dose to bedtime, or increasing the size of the bedtime snack should prevent this phenomenon.

Dawn Phenomenon

The dawn phenomenon refers to an early-morning (4 to 8 AM) increase in blood glucose level without preceding nocturnal hypoglycemia. Wearing off of insulin does not appear to be the sole cause of this phenomenon. It has been found in people with both type 1 and type 2 diabetes and probably occurs in people without diabetes. Growth hormone, increased insulin clearance, and diurnal variation in counterregulatory hormone levels seem to play a role.

The key clinical implication of the dawn phenomenon is that attempts to normalize pre-breakfast glucose levels often result in early-morning hypoglycemia. SMBG and education about bedtime snacks, manifestations of nocturnal hypoglycemia, and the importance of avoiding hypoglycemia are vital. Investigation has shown positive effects with the use of Ultralente instead of NPH insulin in the elimination of this phenomenon.

CHRONIC COMPLICATIONS OF DIABETES MELLITUS

Clients with diabetes are living longer, with an increased risk for development of chronic complications (Box 47-9). Chronic complications are the major causes of morbidity and mortality in clients with diabetes. These changes affect many body systems and can be devastating to clients and their families; they affect clients with both type 1 and type 2 diabetes. Complications are classified as one of three types[32]:

- *Macrovascular,* including coronary artery disease, cerebrovascular disease, hypertension, peripheral vascular disease, and infection
- *Microvascular,* including retinopathy and nephropathy
- *Neuropathic,* including sensorimotor and autonomic dysfunction

Sustained increases in glucose levels create an imbalance of substances used for making the matrix between cells. Enzyme systems normally convert glucose to other sugars, such as sorbitol and fructose to lower blood glu-

---

BOX 47-9 *Chronic Complications of Diabetes Mellitus*

Macrovascular Complications
- Coronary artery disease
- Cerebrovascular disease
- Hypertension
- Peripheral vascular disease
- Infection

Microvascular Complications
- Retinopathy
- Nephropathy

Neuropathic Complications
- Sensorimotor neuropathy
- Autonomic neuropathy
  - Pupillary
  - Cardiovascular
  - Gastrointestinal
  - Genitourinary

Mixed Vascular and Neuropathic Diseases
- Leg and foot ulcers

---

cose. Sorbitol, fructose, and glucose accumulate in the basement membrane of the cell and between the cells. In-tracellular accumulations of sorbitol cause intracellular edema and affect function.

The microcirculation is affected by extracellular accumulation of glucose, sorbitol, and fructose. The thick-ened basement membrane increases the distance over which nutrients and waste products must travel to and from the cell. As a result, the cells receive inadequate oxygen and nutrition and cannot rid themselves of waste. Unfortunately, the process starts as early as 2 years after the onset of diabetes.

Clinicians often see clients with diabetes in the hospital with an MI, with loss of cognitive or physical function as a result of a stroke, or with a lower limb amputation necessitated by peripheral vascular disease. Prevention of these all-too-common macrovascular health problems should be a major focus of nurses working with clients with diabetes (Table 47-8).

MACROVASCULAR COMPLICATIONS

Coronary artery disease, cerebrovascular disease, and peripheral vascular disease are more common, tend to occur at an earlier age, and are more extensive and severe in people with diabetes. Macrovascular disease (disease of large arteries) reflects atherosclerosis with deposits of lipids within the inner layer of vessel walls. The risk for development of macrovascular complications is higher in those with type 1 diabetes than with type 2 diabetes.

Clinical Manifestations	Diagnosis	Interventions
Cerebrovascular Disease		
Atherothromboembolic infarctions *(transient ischemic attacks and cerebral vascular accidents)* are more severe, have higher mortality rate, have higher recurrence rate	History Manifestations Physical examinations Computed tomography scan Magnetic resonance imaging	Same as for non-diabetics, plus improved glucose control, aspirin, dipyridamole, ticlopidine; ongoing education and support
Heart Disease (Coronary Heart Disease)		
Diabetics have a higher incidence of coronary artery changes that influence decreased oxygen and nutrients to myocardium Clients have more *angina* and higher mortality with *myocardial infarction;* manifestations are often "silent" Clients with a history of diabetes mellitus and myocardial infarction have higher incidence of *heart failure, shock,* and *dysrhythmias* *Cardiomyopathy* may occur secondary to small vessel infarctions causing myocardial fibrosis and hypertrophy Additional coronary artery disease manifestations: *Exertional weakness, peripheral edema, orthopnea, fatigue* Features such as female gender, which normally protects from premature heart disease, do not pertain to individuals with diabetes	History Manifestations Physical examination Electrocardiogram Cardiac enzymes Cardiac catheterization Stress test Autopsy	Same as for non-diabetics with cerebrovascular disease, plus improved glucose control, exercise, diet Hypertension control: Use of diuretics may worsen hyperglycemia if hypokalemia exists and may adversely affect lipid levels Beta-adrenergic blockers (may cause hypoglycemia), calcium-channel blockers, thrombolytic agents, aspirin, angioplasty, bypass surgery
Infection		
Diabetics have a higher incidence of *Pseudomonas external otitis* and *monilial skin infections;* common sites of infection in the diabetic include *urinary tract and skin*	History Manifestations Physical examination Laboratory data: serum—increased WBCs and blood glucose; urine—increased WBCs	Improved glucose control; antibiotics, antifungals as required; follow-up with laboratory data; ongoing client education
Peripheral Vascular Disease (PVD)		
The incidence of *carotid bruits, intermittent claudication, absent pedal pulses* and *ischemic gangrene* is increased in diabetes mellitus PVD and neuropathy augment the morbidity associated with trauma and infection in the lower extremity	History Manifestations Physical examinations Doppler studies Angiogram Neuropathy identification	Daily foot inspection aimed at prevention and early intervention; meticulous foot care, padded sport socks, well-fitting shoes; weight reduction; smoking cessation; safe exercise programs; ongoing education
Hypertension		
Usually asymptomatic	History Physical examinations Orthostatic blood pressures with pulse recordings Elevated blood pressure readings at 2-3 recordings Urinalysis: 24-hr urine collection for protein, creatinine clearance, and GFR Renal angiogram to evaluate for renal artery stenosis from atherosclerotic disease	Eliminate risk factors; educate client on this silent but deadly disease; diet education: low protein, low salt Pharmacologic intervention dependent on blood pressure readings: diuretics, angiotensin-converting enzyme inhibitors, calcium-channel blockers, alpha-blockers

WBC, White blood cell; *GFR,* glomerular filtration rate.

Macrovascular disease, especially coronary disease, is the most common cause of death in diabetic clients, accounting for 40% to 60% of all cases of diabetes-related macrovascular disease. The most common reason for hospitalization in diabetics is for treatment of macrovascular complications. Diabetes not only is an independent risk factor for these complications but also is a major risk factor for hypertension and hyperlipidemia. Typically, very-low-density and low-density lipoproteins are increased and high-density lipoproteins are decreased. The most characteristic lipid abnormality in diabetes is an elevated triglyceride level. Therefore the influence of diabetes in these diseases is multiplicative, not additive.

Macrovascular disease tends to occur years before the onset of clinical diabetes and to occur in people with impaired glucose tolerance at a rate similar to that in people with type 2 diabetes. This phenomenon, called *syndrome X*, further establishes the need for disease prevention and health promotion.

Health promotion activities include (1) managing obesity and maintaining ideal body weight, (2) exercising, (3) not smoking, and (4) achieving normal blood lipid levels. Health maintenance actions include (1) prompt recognition and treatment of hyperglycemia with exercise, food, and medication; (2) aggressive management of hypertension, including regular blood pressure checks; and (3) screening high-risk clients (e.g., those with a family history of diabetes). Health restoration activities involve (1) controlling angina, (2) treating peripheral vascular disease, (3) using SMBG to keep track of manifestations, (4) controlling risk factors for macrovascular disease, (5) stressing medication compliance and follow-up, and (6) working closely with the client.

Some speculate that type 2 diabetes may be one piece of a syndrome caused by insulin resistance. A well-established association has been demonstrated among hyperglycemia, hyperinsulinemia, dyslipidemia, and hypertension, which leads to coronary artery disease and stroke. The acronym CHAOS (*c*oronary artery disease, *h*ypertension, *a*dult-onset diabetes, *o*besity, and *s*tress) has been used to remind health care providers to look at the client's entire risk profile for cardiovascular disease when determining treatment for diabetes.

Successful weight reduction with a balanced diet improves lipid profiles, lessens glucose intolerance, lowers blood pressure, and eliminates obesity; otherwise, successful treatment of macrovascular disease in clients with diabetes parallels that in the non-diabetic population.[4,6,11]

CORONARY ARTERY DISEASE

Clients with diabetes are two to four times more likely than non-diabetic clients to die of coronary artery disease, and the relative risk factor for cardiovascular disease in women with type 2 diabetes is three to four times greater. Female gender does not protect the diabetic woman from premature macrovascular disease. In many clients with diabetes, macrovascular events or processes such as coronary artery disease are atypical or silent, and they often present as indigestion or unexplained heart failure, dyspnea on exertion, or epigastric pain. Coronary artery disease is common in clients younger than age 40 years if diabetes is of long duration. Clients with diabetes who have had an MI have an increased chance of complications or of having a second infarction, compared with that in non-diabetic clients who have had an MI. After an MI, diabetic clients also experience a higher incidence of heart failure, shock, and dysrhythmias. It has been suggested that insulin therapy in type 2 diabetes may actually increase the incidence of atherosclerotic disease, because such therapy often leads to weight gain and increased blood pressure.

CEREBROVASCULAR DISEASE

Prevention of cerebrovascular disease includes the same strategies as for prevention of coronary artery disease, including (1) control of hypertension, lipid levels, and obesity; (2) smoking cessation; (3) exercise; and (4) good nutritional practices.

Cerebrovascular disease, particularly atherothromboembolic infarctions manifested by transient ischemic attacks and cerebrovascular accidents (strokes), are more common and severe in diabetes. The incidence is two to three times greater in diabetic clients. The relative risk is higher in females, highest in the fifth and sixth decades of life, and much higher in clients with hypertension. In the United States, the southeastern states are often referred to as the "Stroke Belt" because of the sizable black population in that region with its increased prevalence of hypertension. Many clients presenting with stroke have undiagnosed diabetes. In clients with diabetes, strokes are more serious and carry higher recurrence and mortality rates, especially with type 2 diabetes.

It is speculated that the increased prevalence of stroke in clients with diabetes may be related to the development of diabetic nephropathy and resultant proteinuria, hypertension, and platelet adhesiveness. Clients who present with stroke and high blood glucose levels have a much poorer prognosis than that in clients with normoglycemia. Ticlopidine, a platelet aggregation inhibitor, may be more effective than aspirin in lowering the risk of stroke, especially in clients with diabetes. This drug may also cause increased cholesterol levels and neutropenia (decreased neutrophils).

HYPERTENSION

A 40% increased rate of hypertension has been noted in the diabetic population. Hypertension is a major risk factor for stroke and nephropathy. Inadequately treated hypertension augments the rate at which nephropathy develops. Individualized pharmacologic treatment for hypertension greater than 130/80 mm Hg is suggested for diabetic clients. Angiotensin-converting enzyme (ACE) inhibitors and calcium-channel blockers are the agents of choice for treatment. Beta-blockers and diuretics may increase glucose tolerance and lipid levels.

PERIPHERAL VASCULAR DISEASE

In diabetes, the incidence and prevalence of carotid bruits (abnormal sound or murmur), intermittent claudication, absent pedal (foot) pulses, and ischemic gangrene are increased. More than half of nontraumatic lower limb amputations are associated with diabetic changes such as sensory and autonomic neuropathy, peripheral vascular disease, an increased risk and rate of infection, and poor healing. This chain of events, which may lead to amputation, is illustrated in Figure 47-9.

INFECTIONS

Clients with diabetes are susceptible to infections of many types. Once infections occur, they are difficult to treat. Three factors that may contribute to the development of an infection are impaired polymorphonuclear leukocyte function, diabetic neuropathies, and vascular insufficiency. Poor glycemic control augments the importance of these factors. Infected areas heal slowly because the damaged vascular system cannot carry sufficient oxygen, white blood cells, nutrients, and antibodies to the injured site. Infections increase the need for insulin and enhance the possibility of ketoacidosis.[15,16]

Urinary tract infections are the most common type of infections affecting clients with diabetes, particularly women. One factor may be the inhibition of polymorphonuclear leukocyte activity while glucosuria is present. Glucosuria is associated with hyperglycemia. The development of a neurogenic bladder, which results in incomplete emptying and urinary retention, may also contribute to the risk of a urinary tract infection.

Diabetic foot infections are common. Their occurrence is directly related to the three factors just listed, plus hyperglycemia. Up to 40% of diabetic clients with foot infections may require amputation, and 5% to 10% will die despite amputation of the affected area. With proper education and early intervention, foot infections are usually eliminated in a timely manner. See the Care Plan feature on Foot Infections in the Client with Diabetes Mellitus on the website.[8] Effective foot care can be the initial break in the chain of events that leads to amputation (see Figure 47-9 and the Bridge to Home Health Care feature on Diabetic Foot Care on p. 1283).

MICROVASCULAR COMPLICATIONS

Microangiopathy refers to changes that occur in retinal, renal, and peripheral capillaries in diabetes. The Diabetes Control and Complications Trial has made it clear that consistent and tight glycemic control may prevent or stop microvascular changes.[18]

DIABETIC RETINOPATHY

Diabetic retinopathy is the major cause of blindness among clients with diabetes; about 80% have some form of retinopathy 15 years after diagnosis. The exact cause of retinopathy is not well understood but is probably multifactorial and associated with protein glycosylation, ischemia, and hemodynamic mechanisms. Stress from increased blood viscosity is a hemodynamic mechanism that increases permeability and decreases elasticity of capillaries.[24]

There are three types of diabetic retinopathy:
- *Nonproliferative* diabetic retinopathy is the early phase of retinopathy. It is characterized by microaneurysms (outpouching) and intraretinal "dot and blot" hemorrhages. It occurs in most clients with long-term diabetes and in many cases it does not progress or affect visual acuity.
- *Preproliferative* diabetic retinopathy involves further progression of the hemorrhages and decreasing visual acuity. It usually progresses to proliferative diabetic retinopathy.
- *Proliferative* diabetic retinopathy is the final and most vision-threatening type. The weakened and damaged vessels that have proliferated, or formed, in response to ischemia may rupture, causing retinal hemorrhage and exudates.

The retina, which is the most essential structure of the eye, has the highest rate of oxygen consumption of any tissue in the body. Consequently, if the retina is deprived of oxygen-carrying blood secondary to destruction of its capillaries, tissue anoxia (lack of oxygen) develops swiftly.[24]

Diabetic retinopathy is the leading cause of blindness in the United States among adults 20 to 74 years of age and causes from 12,000 to 24,000 new cases of blindness each year. Risk factors under investigation that may affect the development of retinopathy include chronic hyperglycemia, poor glycemic control, disease duration, hypertension, pregnancy, puberty, polyuria, and smoking (see the Client Education Guide feature on Visual Complications of Diabetes on the website).

Clinical Manifestations

Clinical manifestations of retinopathy typically do not develop until the later stages, when clients have acute vision problems. Blurred vision is a common manifestation that results from an abnormally high blood glucose level. In addition, seeing "floaters" or flashing lights may indicate hemorrhage or retinal detachment. Because of a lack of early clinical manifestations, it is important to assess the potential for visual problems in all clients with diabetes, including the date of their last dilated pupil examination.

Neuropathy and angiopathy

To break the chain:
- Teach client to always wear protective shoes, to inspect the foot daily, and to not remove corns or calluses.
- Identify clients at high risk by checking protective sensation.

Minor trauma

To break the chain:
- Recognize and treat wounds promptly.
- Assess the client's vascular status.
- Maintain good nutrition.
- Promote cessation of smoking.
- Control the client's hypertension.

Ulceration

To break the chain:
- Debride the wound.
- Administer antibiotics.
- Promote bed rest.
- Promote arterial circulation.
- Maintain good nutrition.
- Prevent edema.
- Offload the foot with splints or shoes.

Faulty healing

To break the chain:
- Obtain a CT scan to ascertain bone involvement.
- Debride the wound.
- Administer long-term antibiotic therapy.
- Maintain good nutrition.

Gangrene

Control hyperglycemia, teach self-care measures, provide psychological support.

FIGURE 47-9 Breaking the chain of events that leads to amputation in high-risk clients with diabetes mellitus. High-risk clients (those with neuropathy, vascular disease, structural deformities, abnormal gait, skin or nail deformities, or a history of previous diabetic ulcers or amputations) need frequent monitoring by the health care team. *CT,* Computed tomography. (Modified from Pecoraro, R. E., & Burgess, E. M. [1992]. Pathways to diabetic limb amputation: Basis for prevention. *Diabetes Spectrum, 5,* 329-334.)

BRIDGE TO HOME HEALTH CARE
Diabetic Foot Care

People who have diabetes often develop minor foot problems that progress to major problems, and even amputation. Many foot problems can be prevented or resolved at an early stage. The most important responsibilities of the nurse in diabetic foot care are assessment, education, and direct care measures.

The nurse who initially works with the client in the community needs to do a thorough diabetic assessment that includes evaluation of the client's knowledge, self-care ability, physical status, and needs. Physical assessment of the feet includes:
- Observation of the dermatologic condition, to detect absence of hair, diminished turgor, dry or rough skin, hyperpigmentation, fissures, calluses, ulcers, and lesions or nail problems, such as thickness or discoloration
- Evaluation of the vascular status by checking peripheral pulses, blood return after blanching, and skin temperature, consistency (to rule out edema), and color
- Examination for evidence of orthopedic problems such as hammer toes or bunions
- Evaluation of the neurologic status by testing the deep tendon reflexes and response to pain, vibration, and touch

Refer the client to a physician if anything abnormal is noted. Clients who have diabetes must receive specific education about circulation, self-inspection, protection, and daily foot care. If clients cannot safely perform the necessary tasks independently, it is imperative that other caregivers accept responsibility. Some clients need a combination of helpers including, the home health care nurse, the community health nurse at a foot care clinic, family members, and informal caregivers. Medicare reimbursement for foot care and other home health services is lim-

ited. Nurses must advocate for clients and help them obtain the most appropriate and cost-effective services.

Clients who have diabetes need to maximize the circulation of their feet. Teach them to maintain good nutrition and adequate fluid intake. Instruct them not to smoke, cross their legs, or wear restrictive clothing. Demonstrate how to do foot and ankle range-of-motion exercises by writing the alphabet with their feet. Teach them to inspect all areas of their feet daily, looking for open areas, warmth, redness, discharge, formation of calluses or corns, or anything unusual.

Encourage clients to use protective measures, such as (1) always wearing good-fitting, high-quality shoes, (2) avoiding temperature extremes, and (3) seeking immediate medical attention for any injury or problem. Teach daily care of the feet that includes washing with a mild soap; drying thoroughly, especially between the toes; moisturizing feet, except between the toes; and keeping toenails trimmed. If it is necessary to soak feet before trimming toenails, do not soak for longer than 5 to 10 minutes.

Routine foot care performed by nurses in the community may include care of the skin (washing, drying, lubricating, massaging), removal of corns and calluses (shaving to healthy skin with a file or blade), and cutting the toenails. Toenails should be cut straight across or with a slight curve following the shape of the toe and filed smooth to prevent pressure or cutting of adjacent toes.

As with any nursing procedure, appropriate infection control measures should be followed. Cleanse supplies properly, wear gloves and protective eye wear, and dispose of used blades following adequate disposal protocols for sharps.

Outcome Management

Major interventions, particularly in the early phases, include achievement of euglycemia and normalization of blood pressure. When retinopathy threatens vision, outpatient laser therapy (photocoagulation) is usually recommended. It halts or slows the decline in vision in most diabetic clients if it is used before too much damage has occurred. Although extensive photocoagulation usually diminishes peripheral vision and may decrease night vision, its success in preserving good visual acuity makes it worthwhile despite these side effects.

If the extent or location of the damage makes photocoagulation ineffective, or if the vitreous is too scarred or clouded with blood, vision may be improved with a vitrectomy, a surgical procedure that removes the vitreous and replaces it with saline solution. About 70% of

clients who have vitrectomies notice an improvement in or stabilization of their sight, and some recover enough to resume reading and driving.

NEPHROPATHY

Diabetic nephropathy is the single most common cause of end-stage renal disease (ESRD). About 35% to 45% of clients with type 1 diabetes are found to have nephropathy 15 to 20 years after diagnosis. About 20% of clients with type 2 diabetes are found to have nephropathy 5 to 10 years after diagnosis. A consequence of microangiopathy, nephropathy involves damage to and eventual obliteration of the capillaries that supply the glomeruli of the kidney. This damage leads in turn to a complex of pathologic changes and manifestations (intercapillary glomerulosclerosis, nephrosis, gross albuminuria, and hypertension). Risk factors include poor glycemic control, duration of disease, and hypertension. Some clients self-check microalbumin levels at home. This test can detect very small quantities of urinary albumin, which can indicate very early renal disease. With worsening of the nephrosis, chronic renal failure ensues. Unless the client can be maintained with hemodialysis or receives a renal transplant, uremia eventually causes death.[23]

 Clients with nephropathy monitor their blood glucose levels and blood pressure at home. ACE inhibitors can be used to decrease the microalbuminuria. Hypertension should be treated aggressively, as it can be the catalyst for the progression of nephropathy. Clients with nephropathy are taught to eat a low-protein diet and to avoid nephrotoxic drugs (e.g., gentamicin). If contrast dye is required for radiographic study, mannitol may be ordered, but the client must drink fluids after the test to clear the dye from the kidneys. Serum creatinine levels should be assessed before the administration of the contrast dye or other nephrotoxic agents.

Like diabetic retinopathy, diabetic nephropathy cannot be cured. However, prompt and adequate interventions for renal and bladder infections can prevent these causes of renal failure. Control of hypertension and tight glycemic control can contribute to a delay in the development of nephropathy or a decrease in its progression. Unsuccessfully treated nephropathy progresses to ESRD. Treatment at this point includes hemodialysis, peritoneal dialysis, or kidney transplantation.

NEUROPATHY

Neuropathy is the most common chronic complication of diabetes. Nearly 60% of diabetic clients experience it. Because nerve fibers do not have their own blood supply, they depend on the diffusion of nutrients and oxygen across the membrane. When axons and dendrites are not nourished, their transmission of impulses slows. In addition, sorbitol accumulates in nerve tissue, further diminishing both sensory and motor function. Both temporary and permanent neurologic problems may develop in clients with diabetes during the course of the illness. The neuropathy may be mild (causing minor inconveniences) or so severe that the quality of life is affected. Identified causes of diabetic neuropathy include (1) vascular insufficiency, (2) chronic elevations in blood glucose level, (3) hypertension, and (4) cigarette smoking. Clients may present with mononeuropathy or polyneuropathy and may have sensory or motor impairment, depending on which nerves are involved.[17]

A platelet-derived growth factor, becaplermin (Regranex), that stimulates the body to grow new tissue is being used to promote healing in open wounds associated with lower extremity diabetic neuropathic ulcers that extend into subcutaneous tissue or beyond. The topical agent is applied once daily, spread evenly, and covered with a saline-moistened gauze dressing. After 12 hours, the ulcer is rinsed and re-covered with saline gauze (see Chapter 20).

Mononeuropathy

Mononeuropathy, or focal neuropathy, usually involves a single nerve or group of nerves. Mononeuropathies produce sharp, stabbing pains and are usually caused by an infarction of the blood supply. The muscles innervated by nerves affected by focal neuropathies are painful and are at risk for atrophy from disuse. Treatment may include surgical decompression for compression lesions.

Polyneuropathy

Polyneuropathy, or diffuse neuropathy, involves the sensory and autonomic nerves. Sensory neuropathy is the most common type. It is commonly assessed as bilateral, symmetrical, and affecting the lower extremities. The client describes tingling, numbness, burning, and mild to total sensory loss. This complication is a major factor in injuries to the legs. Treatment includes foot care education to prevent trauma and ulcers. Painful neuropathy may be treated with tricyclic antidepressants, phenytoin, or carbamazepine. Polyneuropathy also may simply resolve spontaneously.

Autonomic Neuropathy

Autonomic neuropathy manifests itself in its effect on pupillary, cardiovascular, gastrointestinal, and genitourinary functions.

Pupillary. Autonomic neuropathy of the pupil interferes with the pupil's ability to adapt to the dark. Pupil dilation is inadequate. Clients are at risk for accidents when driving at night. The environment should be well lighted at night.

Cardiovascular. Autonomic neuropathy of the cardiovascular system is evidenced by an abnormal response to exercise. A fixed heart rate may be noted. Orthostatic hypotension may occur, which is dangerous. Resting tachycardia is another possible cardiovascular effect.

Gastrointestinal. Autonomic neuropathy commonly affects the gastrointestinal tract. The client may have dysphagia, abdominal pain, nausea, vomiting, malabsorption, postprandial hypoglycemia, diarrhea, constipation, or fetal incontinence. Gastroparesis (delayed stomach emptying) may give the client the feeling of stomach fullness. This may contribute to anorexia, decreased intake, weight loss, and labile blood glucose levels related to food malabsorption. About 20% to 30% of diabetic clients have gastroparesis, manifestations of which may be alleviated with metoclopramide (Reglan).

Genitourinary. Bladder hypotonicity, or neurogenic bladder, is a common manifestation of autonomic neuropathy. Manifestations may include straining with urination, infrequent urge to urinate with long periods of time between voiding, and a decreased urine stream. Urinary stasis may occur, leading to urinary tract infection. In the male client, autonomic neuropathy can contribute to erectile dysfunction and retrograde ejaculation. Penile injections, implantable devices, or sildenafil (Viagra) may improve function (see Chapter 40 on male reproductive problems). Women with autonomic neuropathy may experience painful intercourse, which estrogen-containing lubricants can resolve (see Chapter 41 on female reproductive problems).

■ Management of a Diabetic Client Having Surgery

Surgery is a stressful experience for anyone; for a client with diabetes, however, surgery imposes several additional stressors. Surgery interrupts the client's usual therapeutic regimen. The diet must be temporarily changed and the dosage of insulin or oral hypoglycemic agent readjusted. The stress of surgery raises blood glucose levels. The client is susceptible to infection. The surgical incision itself becomes a new potential portal of entry for pathogens. Furthermore, postoperative healing in these clients may be slower than normal.

To offset these problems, clients with diabetes require special interventions, both preoperatively and postoperatively. They may vary, depending on whether the client has type 1 or type 2 diabetes and whether the surgery is elective or performed on an emergency basis.

Preoperative Care

The goal of preoperative care for clients with diabetes is thorough regulation of blood glucose levels before surgery. Clients with type 1 diabetes need to be closely monitored for several days or even weeks before elective surgery to stabilize their condition and, thereby, to decrease surgical risk. If a client with type 1 diabetes and poor glucose control requires emergency surgery, the surgeon must choose between operating on a hypoglycemic or hyperglycemic client and postponing an emergency operation until the diabetes is controlled. In either case, the client needs constant monitoring of vital signs, frequent laboratory and bedside glucose studies, and vigilant nursing intervention.

In contrast, clients with well-controlled type 2 diabetes usually undergo surgery with only slightly more risk than that for the general population. Typically, preoperative preparation for clients with type 1 and type 2 diabetes includes the following:

- Preoperative laboratory tests, including fasting and preprandial blood glucose levels; glycosylated hemoglobin; serum electrolytes, BUN, and serum creatinine; complete blood count; ECG and cardiac enzymes; and chest radiograph

- Early-morning scheduling of surgery so that the client's diet and insulin regimen undergo as little disruption as possible

- Omission of food, water, and oral hypoglycemic agents on the morning of surgery (one long-acting hypoglycemic agent, chlorpropamide, is discontinued 1 to 2 days before surgery because of its long half-life)

- IV infusion of insulin for insulin-dependent or insulin-requiring clients, usually with glucose (5%) to prevent hypoglycemia (if the surgery is relatively minor, such as for cataract removal, the surgeon may order a 5% dextrose solution infusion and half the usual dose of intermediate-acting insulin; the anesthesiologist can monitor blood glucose levels in the operating room)

- A blood glucose determination performed and reported to the physician within 1 hour before the operation to ensure that the client (who has taken nothing by mouth since midnight) will not develop hypoglycemia during surgery

Intraoperative Care

Once the client arrives in surgery, management again depends on the severity of the diabetes and the extent of the surgery. Regular insulin, in a dose based on the client's blood glucose levels and a sliding scale or an insulin protocol, can be given by the IV route. Subcutaneous insulin should not be given intraoperatively because its absorption is affected by body temperature, circulatory blood volumes, and certain anesthetics.

Postoperative Care

After surgery, the goals of postoperative management are to stabilize the client's vital signs, correct fluid and electrolyte imbalances, reestablish control of the diabetes, prevent wound infection, and promote wound healing. The following are important postoperative interventions:

- Administer prescribed IV infusions and regular insulin until the client can take oral nourishment.

- Once the client can tolerate fluids, offer those that contain calories to prevent hypoglycemia. Once the client can eat, make food available. Discuss the client's calorie level with a dietitian to ensure that enough calories are provided for postoperative wound healing.

- Obtain a blood glucose level four to six times daily.

- Resume the client's prescribed preoperative insulin type and dosage once blood glucose control is reestablished, foods are being consumed at adequate levels, and it has been reordered by the physician.

- Observe for evidence of hypoglycemia after surgery, such as a decrease in blood pressure or an increase

CLIENT EDUCATION GUIDE
Sick Day Management for Diabetes Mellitus*

You should have an individualized plan of care prescribed by the health care team to use during illness.

Monitoring is an essential part of diabetes management, but this is even more vital during the stress of illness. Insulin requirements may be increased secondary to reduced activity and increased secretion of counterregulatory hormones. To prevent diabetic ketoacidosis, you should know the following:

Self-Monitoring of Blood Glucose. It is important to self-monitor blood glucose more frequently during illness, often every 2 to 4 hours. If pre-meal blood glucose values stay greater than 250 mg/dl, then test for urine ketones and contact your health care provider.

Ketones. Urine ketones should be monitored when you feel sick or when blood glucose is greater than 250 mg/dl. Test for ketones every 2 to 4 hours.

Insulin. Do not stop taking insulin, even if you are vomiting and unable to eat. Additional regular insulin may be required, based on self-monitored blood glucose levels.

Nutrition/Fluids. Adequate fluid intake and carbohydrates are essential during illness. Eating 10 to 15 g of carbohydrate every 1 to 2 hours and small quantities of fluid every 15 to 30 minutes is usually sufficient to prevent dehydration and ketoacidosis. Clear broth, tea, and ice chips are usually well tolerated.

Examples of foods and beverages containing about 15 g of carbohydrate are as follows:

1 regular whole Popsicle
$1/_2$ cup applesauce
$1/_2$ cup regular soft drink
$3/_4$ cup ginger ale
$1/_2$ cup orange or apple juice
1 cup Gatorade
$1/_2$ cup regular gelatin

Notify your health care provider when you have any of the following problems:

- Illness that persists more than 24 hours
- Severe abdominal pain
- Temperature greater than 100° F, oral
- Persistent diarrhea
- Vomiting with inability to take fluids for more than 4 hours
- Blood glucose levels difficult to control or moderate to high levels of ketones in urine
- Shortness of breath or chest pain
- Acute visual loss
- Other unexplained health problems

*Most applicable to clients with type 1 diabetes and those with type 2 diabetes receiving insulin therapy.

in heart rate in a client who is still unresponsive from anesthesia.

- Avoid catheterization, if possible, to prevent bladder infection.
- Change wound dressings with meticulous sterile technique to prevent wound infection.
- Assess the client's wound and incision frequently for signs of infection. Be alert for abnormal amounts of drainage or foul-smelling drainage.
- Observe for and treat manifestations of skin breakdown, especially if the client has peripheral vascular disease or neuropathy.

■ Management of a Sick Client with Diabetes

The Client Education Guide feature on Sick Day Management for Diabetes Mellitus, above, presents guidelines for the client to follow during illnesses.

CONCLUSIONS

Diabetes mellitus is a chronic disease characterized by abnormalities in carbohydrate, fat, and protein metabolism. The two major categories of diabetes mellitus are type 1 and type 2. Meal planning, exercise, and medication are the main forms of treatment. Acute complications include hyperglycemia with diabetic ketoacidosis and hypoglycemia. Chronic complications are relentlessly progressive and result from multiple changes in small and large vessels. Because diabetes is chronic, nursing management focuses on teaching the client and family how to manage the disorder on a day-to-day basis and how to assess for complications.

THINKING CRITICALLY *evolve*

1. A client with type 1 diabetes takes 14 units of regular insulin and 32 units of NPH insulin subcutaneously at 7 AM and 5 PM every day. He is now hospitalized for pneumonia and nausea. It is 9:30 AM. On entering his room, you observe the client talking to his plants. What is your priority intervention? How will his confusion be resolved?

Factors to Consider. When does regular insulin peak? What might be the underlying cause of the client's confusion? How might you confirm the presence of hypoglycemia?

2. An older woman with type 1 diabetes calls the clinic and tells the nurse that she has the flu. She tells the nurse that she usually takes Humulin N, 12 units, and Humulin R, 8 units, every morning. She has not taken her insulin this morning because of vomiting, nausea, and an inability to eat. She tells the nurse she lives alone. What telephone advice is appropriate? How often should she monitor her blood glucose levels while she is ill?

Factors to Consider. What learning needs does the client exhibit? When should the insulin be given? Is a clinic visit warranted?

3. The client is a 72-year-old woman who has a 25-year history of type 2 diabetes. She has managed her care adequately over the years; with the advent of home glucose monitoring, her blood glucose levels have been very well controlled. Her main problem is a history of significant hypertension, controlled with a daily antihypertensive. Lately, she finds that small cuts and bruises take longer than usual to heal. What are the chronic complications of diabetes mellitus? What teaching should you consider for this client?

Factors to Consider. What risks does this client face as a result of her long-term diabetic history? How would you approach teaching about complications?

Discussions for these questions can be found on the website and CD-ROM.

BIBLIOGRAPHY

 1. American College of Endocrinology. (2002). Consensus Statement on Guidelines for Diabetes. (position statement). *Endocrinology Practice, 8* (suppl. 1), 6-11.
2. American Diabetes Association. (2003). Continuous subcutaneous insulin infusion (position statement). *Diabetes Care, 26* (suppl. 1), S125.
3. American Diabetes Association. (2001). *Diabetes 2001 vital statistics.* Alexandria, VA: Author.
4. American Diabetes Association. (2003). Evidence-based nutrition principles and recommendations for the treatment and prevention of diabetes and related complications (position statement). *Diabetes Care, 26* (suppl. 1), S51-S61.
5. American Diabetes Association. (2003). Insulin administration (position statement). *Diabetes Care, 26* (suppl. 1), S121-S124.
6. American Diabetes Association. (2003). Management of dyslipidemia in adults with diabetes (position statement). *Diabetes Care, 26* (suppl. 1), S83-S86.
7. American Diabetes Association. (2003). Physical activity/exercise and diabetes mellitus (position statement). *Diabetes Care, 26* (suppl. 1), S73-S77.

8. American Diabetes Association. (2003). Preventive foot care in people with diabetes (position statement). *Diabetes Care, 26* (suppl. 1), S78-S79.
9. American Diabetes Association. (2003). Prevention of type 1 diabetes mellitus (position statement). *Diabetes Care, 26* (suppl. 1), S140.
10. American Diabetes Association. (2003). Screening for type 2 diabetes (position statement). *Diabetes Care, 26* (suppl. 1), S21-S24.
11. American Diabetes Association (2003). Standards of medical care for patients with diabetes mellitus (position statement). *Diabetes Care, 26* (suppl. 1), S33-S50.
12. Anderson, R., et al. (2003). Diabetes Empowerment Scale-Short Form (DES-SF). *Diabetes Care, 26*(5), 1641-1642.
13. Anderson, R., & Funnell, M. (2000). *The art of empowerment: Stories and strategies for diabetes educators.* Alexandria, VA: American Diabetes Association.
14. Anderson, R., et al. (1995). Patients' empowerment: Results of a randomized clinical trial. *Diabetes Care, 18*(7), 943-949.
15. Bergenstal, R., et al. (2001). Management of type 2 diabetes: A systematic approach to meeting the standards of care. In L. DeGroot & J. Jameson (Eds.), *Endocrinology* (4th ed., pp. 810-835). Philadelphia: W. B. Saunders.
16. Bode, B. (2003). *Medical management of type 1 diabetes* (4th ed.). Alexandria, VA: American Diabetes Association.
17. Boulton, A., & Malik, R. (2001). Diabetes mellitus: Neuropathy. In L. DeGroot & J. Jameson (Eds.), *Endocrinology* (4th ed., pp. 868-877). Philadelphia: W. B. Saunders.
18. Diabetes Control and Complications Trial Research Group. (1993). The effect of intensive treatment of diabetes on the development and progression of long-term complications in insulin-dependent diabetes mellitus. *New England Journal of Medicine, 329*(14), 977-998.
19. Expert Committee on the Diagnosis and Classification of Diabetes Mellitus. (2003). Report of the Expert Committee on the Diagnosis and Classification of Diabetes Mellitus. *Diabetes Care, 26* (suppl. 1), S5-S20.
20. Funnell, M.M. (1999). Care of the nursing home resident with diabetes. *Clinical Geriatric Medicine, 15,* 413-422.
21. Funnell, M.M., & Anderson, R. (2003). Patient empowerment: A look back, a look ahead. *Diabetes Educator, 29*(3), 454-458, 460.
22. Guyton, A., & Hall, J. C. D. (2000). *Textbook of medical physiology* (10th ed.). Philadelphia: W. B. Saunders.
23. Hasslacher, C. (2001). Natural course of diabetic nephropathy. In C. Hasslacher (Ed.), *Diabetic nephropathy* (pp. 19-37). New York: John Wiley & Sons.
24. Klein, R. (2001). Diabetes mellitus: Oculopathy. In L. DeGroot & J. Jameson (Eds.), *Endocrinology* (4th ed., pp. 857-867). Philadelphia: W. B. Saunders.
25. McArdle, W.D., Katch, F.I., & Katch, V.L. (2000). Essential of exercise physiology: Diabetes mellitus. Philadelphia: Lippincott Williams & Wilkins.
26. National Diabetes Data Group. (1979). Classification and diagnosis of diabetes mellitus and other categories of glucose intolerance. *Diabetes, 28,* 1039-1057.

27. Ratner, R. E. (2003). Pathophysiology of the diabetes disease state. In M.J. Franz (Ed.), *A core curriculum for diabetes education: Diabetes and complications* (5th ed., Book 1, pp. 3-18). Chicago: American Association of Diabetes Educators.

28. Rolla, A.R. (2002). Insulin analog mixes in the management of type 2 diabetes mellitus. *Practical Diabetology, 21*(4), 36-43.

29. Umpierrez, G.E., Murphy, M.B., & Kitabchi, A.E. (2002). Diabetic ketoacidosis and hyperglycemic hyperosmolar syndrome. *Diabetes Spectrum, 15*(1), 28-36.

 30. U.S. Department of Agriculture, U.S. Department of Health and Human Services. (1995). *Nutrition and your health: Dietary guidelines for Americans* (4th ed). Hyattsville, MD: USDA Human Nutrition Information Service.

31. U.S. Department of Agriculture (1992). *The food guide pyramid.* Hyattsville, MD: USDA Human Nutrition Information Service.

32. Vinicor, F. (2003). Macrovascular disease. In M.M. Funnell, et al. (Eds.), *A core curriculum for diabetes education: Diabetes and complications* (5th ed., Book 1, pp. 99-122). Chicago: American Association of Diabetes Educators.

33. White, J.R., & Campbell, R.K. (2003). Pharmacologic therapies for glucose management. In M.J. Franz (Ed), *A core curriculum for diabetes education: Diabetes management therapies* (5th ed., Book 2, pp. 95-154). Chicago: American Association of Diabetes Educators.

Management of Clients with Exocrine Pancreatic and Biliary Disorders

Dianne M. Smolen

Some disorders of the exocrine pancreas and the biliary tract are acute, and others are chronic. Manifestations are often similar to those of other conditions. The nurse plays an important role in assessing the client's manifestations and in managing the outcomes of medical and surgical treatment.

DISORDERS OF THE EXOCRINE PANCREAS

A client with a pancreatic disorder may have problems with both digestion and utilization of glucose. The relative inaccessibility of the pancreas to direct examination and the nonspecificity of manifestations associated with pancreatic disorders make the diagnosis of some conditions difficult. In addition, more than 90% of the pancreas must be damaged before fat and protein digestion problems become apparent.

ACUTE PANCREATITIS

Pancreatitis (inflammation of the pancreas) may be acute or chronic. *Acute* pancreatitis is an inflammation of the pancreas that can result in autodigestion of the pancreas by its own enzymes. Acute pancreatitis is a fairly common but a potentially lethal inflammatory process associated with edema, various amounts of autodigestion, fat necrosis, and sometimes hemorrhage.

Although the frequency is about 5000 new cases per year in the United States, with a mortality rate of about 10%, the number of clients who have recurrent acute pancreatitis or chronic pancreatitis is not known.[23]

The incidence of pancreatitis varies in different countries and depends on the cause (e.g., alcohol, gallstones, metabolic factors, drugs). In the United States, acute pancreatitis is related to alcohol consumption more commonly than to gallstones; in England, the opposite is true.

Etiology and Risk Factors

Acute pancreatitis has many causes, such as alcohol (ethanol) abuse, *cholelithiasis* (gallstones), abdominal trauma, and metabolic factors. The mechanisms by which these conditions trigger pancreatic inflammation have not been identified.

In the United States, alcohol abuse is the major cause of acute pancreatitis, with common bile duct stone disease the second most frequent occurrence. Although the exact cause is not known, acute pancreatitis is thought to result from inappropriate intrapancreatic activation of proteases, which causes autodigestion of the pancreas. Exactly how this occurs is not known. It is thought that

---

Nursing Outcomes Classification (NOC)
for Nursing Diagnoses—Clients with Exocrine Pancreatic and Biliary Disorders

Acute Pain or Chronic Pain
Comfort Level
Pain Control
Pain: Disruptive Effects
Pain Level

Anxiety
Anxiety Control
Coping
Impulse Control

Deficient Knowledge
Knowledge of: Diet
Knowledge of: Disease Process
Knowledge of: Energy Conservation
Knowledge of: Health Behaviors
Knowledge of: Health Resources
Knowledge of: Infection Control
Knowledge of: Medication
Knowledge of: Personal Safety
Knowledge of: Prescribed Activity
Knowledge of: Substance Use Control
Knowledge of: Treatment Procedure(s)
Knowledge of: Treatment Regimen

Effective Therapeutic Regimen Management
Knowledge: Treatment Regimen
Participation: Health Care Decisions
Risk Control
Symptom Control

Imbalanced Nutrition: Less Than Body Requirements
Nutritional Status
Nutritional Status: Food and Fluid Intake
Nutritional Status: Nutrient Intake

Impaired Oral Mucous Membrane
Oral Health
Tissue Integrity: Skin and Mucous Membrane

Ineffective Breathing Pattern
Respiratory Status: Airway Patency
Respiratory Status: Ventilation
Vital Signs Status

Ineffective Therapeutic Regimen Management
Decision Making
Knowledge: Disease Process
Knowledge: Treatment Regimen
Participation: Health Care Decisions
Symptom Severity
Treatment Behavior: Illness or Injury

Risk for Imbalanced Fluid Volume
Fluid Balance
Electrolyte and Acid/Base Balance
Hydration

Risk for Injury
Risk Control
Immune Status
Safety Behavior: Home Physical Environment
Safety Behavior: Personal: Safety Status: Falls Occurrence
Safety Status: Physical Injury

---

alcohol-induced pancreatitis may include a physiochemical alteration of protein that results in plugs that block the small pancreatic ductules. Biliary pancreatitis occurs when edema or an obstruction blocks the ampulla of Vater, resulting in reflux of bile into pancreatic ducts or direct injury to the acinar cells. Other causes include the following:

- Hyperlipidemia, which may occur secondary to nephritis, castration, or exogenous estrogen administration, or as hereditary hyperlipidemia
- Hypercalcemia arising as a result of hyperparathyroidism
- Familial cases with no definite mechanism defined
- Pancreatic trauma, such as penetrating or blunt external trauma, intraoperative manipulation, or ampullar manipulation and pancreatic ductal overdistention during endoscopic retrograde cholangiopancreatography (ERCP)
- Pancreatic ischemia during episodes of hypotensive shock, cardiopulmonary bypass, visceral atheroembolism, or vasculitis
- Drugs; although azathioprine and estrogens have been directly linked with the disease, many other drugs are believed to have an association (e.g., antibiotics, anticonvulsants, thiazides, sulfonamides, valproic acid, diuretics)

- Other general causes, such as pancreatic duct obstruction, obesity, duodenal obstruction, viral infection (e.g., mumps), carcinoma, scorpion venom, ERCP, peritoneal dialysis, and factors still to be determined

Avoidance of alcohol is the best way to promote health and to reduce the risk of pancreatitis. Limiting or completely stopping ingestion of alcohol may be a health promotion, health maintenance, or health restoration activity, depending on a diagnosis or potential diagnosis of pancreatitis. Recent studies found that obesity is a major risk factor for severe pancreatitis. It is thought that increased deposits of fat around the pancreas may predispose people with pancreatitis to more extensive pancreatic necrosis. Other risk factors include cholecystitis, cholelithiasis, hyperlipidemia, hypercalcemia, pancreatic tumor, pancreatic ischemia, certain medications (estrogens, azathioprine), and any condition that causes pancreatic duct obstruction. Correction of these risk factors, such as cholecystectomy for gallstones, is a health maintenance or restoration action.

Pathophysiology

The etiologic mechanism of pancreatic damage remains unclear. The pathologic changes occurring in the pancreas may be due to premature activation of proteolytic and lipolytic pancreatic enzymes. These enzymes are normally activated in the duodenum. The pancreas normally releases protease in an inactive form. Once protease is in the intestine, the action of intestinal enterokinase converts pancreatic trypsinogen (one of the proteases) into trypsin. In pancreatitis, however, activation of the proteases and lipases occurs before secretion into the intestine. When these enzymes are activated before they are secreted into the intestine, pancreatic tissue damage occurs.

Exactly how the enzymes become active in the pancreas is unknown, but they may be triggered by reflux of bile from the duodenum into the pancreatic duct or by pancreatic duct obstruction, as noted previously. The net effect of this enzymatic activation is autodigestion of the pancreas. Once pancreatic inflammation begins, a vicious circle continues the process of further tissue damage and enzyme activation. As the process becomes chronic, the pancreatic parenchyma is destroyed.

In most clients, acute pancreatitis is a mild disease; in 10% to 15% of clients, however, a severe form of illness develops that leads to a lengthy hospitalization, complications, and significant rates of morbidity and mortality. Such clients present a major medical challenge because they require an intensive care setting, hemodynamic monitoring, and frequent laboratory and radiographic evaluation.

One way to predict the severity of attack and overall prognosis on presentation is to use the predictive criteria identified in Box 48-1:

1. Clients with two or fewer prognostic manifestations, mortality is around 1%.
2. Clients with three or four manifestations have a mortality rate of about 16%.
3. Clients with five or six prognostic manifestations need intensive care, and the mortality rate reaches 40%.[7]
4. Clients with seven or more manifestations have an even higher mortality rate and truly test the limits of modern medicine.

Clinical Manifestations

Manifestations in clients with acute pancreatitis are largely the result of activation of proteases and lipases and the resulting autodigestion of the pancreas. Manifestations vary from mild, nonspecific abdominal pain to profound shock with coma and death. The predominant clinical feature is abdominal pain caused by edematous distention of the pancreatic capsule, local peritonitis resulting from enzyme release into the peritoneum, ductal spasm, or pancreatic autodigestion stimulated by increased enzyme secretion when eating.

Pain normally begins in the mid-epigastrium and achieves maximal intensity several hours later. In most clients extreme epigastric or umbilical pain radiates to the back as well as to the chest, flanks, and lower ab-

---

> **BOX 48-1** *Early Prognostic Manifestations of Acute Pancreatitis*
>
> ### Ranson/Imrie Criteria
> **At admission or diagnosis**
> Age >55 years
> Leukocytosis (white blood count) >16,000/mm³
> Hyperglycemia (blood glucose) >11 mmol/L (>200 mg/dl)
> Serum LDH >400 international units/L
> Serum AST >250 international units/L
>
> ### During Initial 48 Hours
> Fall in hematocrit by >10%
> Fluid deficit of >4000 ml
> Hypocalcemia (serum calcium <1.9 mmol/L [<8 mg/dl])
> Hypoxemia (Po_2 <60 mm Hg)
> BUN elevation to >1.8 mmol/L (>5 mg/dl) after IV fluid administration
> Hypoalbuminemia (albumin level <32 g/L [3.2 g/dl])

Data from Greenberger, N.J., & Toskes, P.P. (2001). Acute and chronic pancreatitis. In E. Braunwald et al. (Eds.), *Harrison's principles of internal medicine* (15th ed., pp. 1792-1804). New York: McGraw-Hill.
AST, Aspartate aminotransferase; *BUN,* blood urea nitrogen; *LDH,* lactic dehydrogenase; *Po_2,* partial pressure of arterial oxygen; *WBC,* white blood cells.

---

domen. In clients with alcohol-associated pancreatitis, pain often begins 12 to 48 hours after an episode of inebriation. Clients with gallstone-associated pancreatitis typically experience pain after a large meal. Nausea and vomiting are frequently present because pain stimulates the vomiting center and gastric and intestinal hypomotility.

Physical examination reveals a distressed, anxious client with abdominal distention and tenderness and fever caused by paralytic ileus of the small bowel resulting from localized peritonitis. Severe hemorrhagic pancreatitis may produce two distinctive manifestations: (1) *Turner's sign* (bluish discoloration of the left flank) and (2) *Cullen's sign* (bluish discoloration of the periumbilical area). These manifestations, which occur in fewer than 3% of cases, are the result of tissue catabolism and blood-stained retroperitoneal fluid, respectively. Jaundice, caused by common bile duct obstruction by pancreatic edema, may be present in clients with gallstone-associated pancreatitis but otherwise is uncommon in the initial phase of the disease.

Clients with severe pancreatitis may exhibit severe circulatory complications, such as hypotension; pallor; cool, clammy skin; hypovolemia; hypoperfusion; obtundation; and shock. Shock is not unusual; it may result from the following:

- Hypovolemia secondary to loss of blood and plasma proteins into the retroperitoneal space

- Increased formation and release of kinins, which cause vasodilation and increased vascular permeability
- Systemic effects of proteolytic and lipolytic enzymes released into the circulation

As many as 10% to 20% of clients have evidence of left pleural effusion or left hemidiaphragmatic elevation.

Other clinical findings include subcutaneous fat necrosis and cerebral abnormalities, such as belligerence, confusion, psychosis, and coma; these are caused by hyperosmolality, hypoperfusion and hypoxia, cerebral fat embolism, or disseminated intravascular coagulopathy. Transient hyperglycemia is found in 50% of clients, probably as a result of damage to the islet cells. All the hormonal *(endocrine)* functions of the pancreas may be disrupted from tissue damage, and diabetes may develop secondary to the disease. Hypocalcemia occurs in up to 30% of clients because calcium may be deposited in areas of necrosis and undigested intestinal fat traps calcium in feces.

Serum amylase analysis is the most widely used test for the diagnosis of pancreatitis. In most cases, hyperamylasemia is seen within 24 hours of the onset of manifestations and resolves within 7 to 14 days. Persistent hyperamylasemia may indicate the development of complications (see Chapter 44, Table 44-2).

The measurement of urinary amylase appears to be a sensitive index of pancreatitis. Some support the use of the amylase-creatinine clearance ratio in the diagnosis. Unfortunately, acute pancreatitis can occur with a normal amylase-creatinine clearance ratio.

The serum lipase value is one of the most specific indicators of acute pancreatitis because lipase is solely of pancreatic origin. The duration of hyperlipasemia often exceeds that of hyperamylasemia; however, hyperlipasemia may also be seen in perforated peptic ulcer, acute cholecystitis (inflammation of the gallbladder wall), intestinal ischemia, hereditary hyperlipidemia–associated pancreatitis, or alcohol-induced pancreatitis. Additionally, a white blood cell (WBC) count above 10,000 cells/mm³ is common; hyperglycemia, mild azotemia, abnormal liver function tests, and hypocalcemia may also be present.

Chest film findings may show left basilar atelectasis, elevated left hemidiaphragm, and left pleural effusion. Abdominal films may reveal nonspecific abnormalities, such as (1) the presence of air in the duodenal loop, indicating duodenal ileus; (2) the "sentinel loop" sign, representing a dilated proximal jejunal loop; (3) the colon "cutoff" sign, indicating distention of the transverse colon; (4) gallstones; or (5) pancreatic calcifications.

Nearly all acute pancreatitis clients have some abnormality on a computed tomography (CT) scan. Pancreatic changes include parenchymal enlargement, edema, or necrosis. A CT scan is also helpful in identifying other structural changes, such as pancreatic pseudocyst, abscess, or phlegmon. A magnetic resonance imaging (MRI) study reveals the same information as CT. Scans with radiopharmaceuticals such as technetium 99m (^{99}mTc)-labeled *N*-substituted iminodiacetic acids (HIDA, IDA, DISIDA) may be useful in acute pancreatitis to evaluate the gallbladder and biliary tree.

Although ERCP has no role in the standard diagnostic evaluation of most clients with acute pancreatitis, it has proved helpful in some clients with recurrent pancreatitis by identifying correctable abnormalities (e.g., duct abnormalities).

Pancreatitis in Clients with Acquired Immunodeficiency Syndrome

Pancreatitis has a higher incidence rate among people with acquired immunodeficiency syndrome (AIDS) because of the high incidence of infections involving the pancreas, such as cytomegalovirus, and the frequent use of certain medications administered for treatment of AIDS, such as didanosine, pentamidine, and trimethoprim-sulfamethoxazole.

Prognosis

The mortality rate for severe acute pancreatitis—more than three Ranson criteria (see Box 48-1)—is high, especially when cardiovascular, renal, or hepatic impairment is present or when pancreatic necrosis develops. Recurrences of acute pancreatitis are common in clients with alcoholic pancreatitis.

Outcome Management
■ Medical Management

Reduce Pain. Pain is usually treated with opioid analgesics, and meperidine has been the drug of choice. Morphine is contraindicated because it was once thought to cause spasm of the sphincter of Oddi, which may then potentiate ongoing pancreatic parenchymal injury. However, morphine, buprenorphine, and transdermal fentanyl have been used successfully for pain management.[11,21]

Maintain Volume Status, Electrolyte Balance, and Nutritional Status. Acute pancreatitis is commonly associated with fluid loss resulting from emesis. Fluids can accumulate in the bowel secondary to ileus or in the peripancreatic region because of edema. Management of the client involves replacing lost body fluids, correcting hypovolemia, and restoring electrolyte balance. Normally the success of fluid and electrolyte restoration is monitored by assessment of heart rate, blood pressure, and urine output. In clients with pre-existing cardiac, pulmonary, or renal disease or in those with severe pancreatitis, invasive monitoring, including urinary catheterization, central venous pressure monitoring, or monitoring cardiac output and filling via a Swan-Ganz catheter, is indicated. Clients with severe hemorrhagic pancreatitis may require transfusions of blood or clotting factors to correct coagulation problems.

Clients with acute pancreatitis commonly have a variety of electrolyte abnormalities. Clients with severe and persistent vomiting may require saline solutions containing potassium chloride. Serum calcium levels may be depressed secondary to hypoalbuminemia. Mild hyperglycemia is usually corrected with fluid volume replacement, but marked hyperglycemia or glycosuria calls for careful insulin administration.

Treatment may involve attempts to suppress pancreatic exocrine function even though they may not change the course of the disease. Therapy to decrease these enzymes may include nasogastric (NG) suction to prevent gastrin from entering the duodenum. Controlled trials, however, have indicated that NG suction may not help in treatment of mild to moderately severe acute pancreatitis. In addition, anticholinergics as well as histamine (H$_2$) blockers, protease inhibitors such as aprotinin, glucocorticoids, calcitonin, nonsteroidal anti-inflammatory drugs (NSAIDs), and glucagon have not been effective in treating pancreatitis. Pancreatitis may also be associated with nutritional problems when the client has been allowed nothing by mouth (NPO; *nil per os*), has nausea and vomiting, or has undergone NG suction. Nutritional problems are detailed later in this chapter.

Maintain Pancreatic Rest. Pancreatic rest involves withholding food and liquids by mouth initially because food ingestion increases pancreatic secretion, which may increase inflammation and pain. No food or fluids should be given orally until the client is largely free of pain and has bowel sounds. Clear liquids are then given, and gradual advancement to a regular low-fat diet is prescribed, guided by the client's tolerance and the absence of pain. Caution must be exercised, however, because premature return to oral intake has been associated with development of pancreatic abscess and reactivation of inflammation.

Clients with moderate to severe pancreatitis need to be supported nutritionally by total parenteral nutrition (TPN). Administration of a carbohydrate and amino acid solution along with lipids as a source of calories may be necessary.

Treat Complications. Complications of pancreatitis include *pancreatic* disorders (e.g., pancreatic abscess, infected necrosis), which may warrant surgery, or *nonpancreatic* disorders (e.g., colonic or bile obstruction or metabolic, renal, or pulmonary disorders). Clients with pulmonary or respiratory complications may require supportive measures, such as endotracheal intubation and positive pressure ventilation.

Other Measures. Antibiotics are not routinely administered in the treatment of acute pancreatitis of mild to moderate severity because they are without proven benefit; they are generally reserved for documented infections. Calcium gluconate must be given intravenously if

there is evidence of hypocalcemia with tetany. The role of somatostatin in severe acute pancreatitis is unknown, but octreotide and H$_2$ blocker therapy are thought to be of no benefit.

It may be necessary to perform peritoneal dialysis to rid the peritoneum of potentially toxic compounds commonly found in exudate from acute pancreatitis. Histamine, vasoactive kinins, elastase, prostaglandins, phospholipase A, trypsin, and chymotrypsin may mediate adverse systemic effects, such as hypotension, pulmonary failure, hepatic failure, and altered vascular permeability. This form of therapy is usually reserved for clients who show early clinical deterioration despite maximal intensive care support.

■ Nursing Management of the Medical Client
Assessment

Until a confirmed diagnosis is made, concentrate on preparing clients for diagnostic procedures and on assessing and treating manifestations of disease (see earlier discussion). Assess the location, severity, and character of the pain as well as the onset, duration, and precipitating or relieving factors. Evaluate the client's response to pain and the therapies used to relieve discomfort. Much of your role focuses on educating the client and his or her significant others about procedures and their rationales and monitoring of the client's pain level and respiratory status.

Diagnosis, Outcomes, Interventions

Diagnosis: Acute Pain. A common nursing diagnosis for the client with pancreatitis is *Acute Pain related to inflammation of the pancreas and surrounding tissue, biliary tract disease, obstruction of pancreatic ducts, and interruption of the blood supply.*

Outcomes. The client will demonstrate an absence of or a decrease in pain level as evidenced by verbalizing this fact and resting quietly and showing fewer expressions of pain (i.e., grimacing, guarding of the area of discomfort, crying).

Interventions

Administer Pain Medications. Administer pain medications in a timely manner. Meperidine has been the drug of choice because opioids were thought to stimulate spasm of the ducts and increase pain. With decreased use of meperidine in practice, morphine, buprenorphine, and transdermal fentanyl have been used successfully for pain management.[11,21] Other drugs are often ordered (e.g., anticholinergics, histamine-receptor antagonists) to quiet the pancreas and to decrease enzyme secretion.

Promote Pancreatic Rest. Keeping the client on NPO status (taking nothing by mouth) not only rests the gastrointestinal tract but also decreases pancreatic stimulation and pain. Allowing no oral alimentation and using an NG tube suction decrease gastrin release from the stomach and prevent gastric contents from entering the duodenum. NG suctioning, as noted earlier, while not altering the course of pancreatitis, removes hydrochloric acid (a powerful stimulant to the release of pancreatic enzymes) and helps to decrease distention, thereby promoting comfort, and should be considered elective rather than mandatory. Check the system frequently to ensure that NG suction is functioning properly.

Provide Comfort Measures. Nonpharmacologic measures are often helpful in relieving pain, relaxing the client, and enhancing the effects of opioids. Correct positioning (particularly a side-lying position with the knees curled up to the chest and a pillow pressed against the abdomen or upright in a sitting position with the trunk flexed), back rubs, relaxation techniques, and a quiet environment all help to promote comfort and rest.

Diagnosis: Risk for Imbalanced Fluid Volume.

A possible complication of acute pancreatitis is *Risk for Imbalanced Fluid Volume related to vomiting, nasogastric suctioning, NPO status, shifting of body fluids, fever, and diaphoresis.*

Outcomes. The client will remain in fluid balance, hydrated, and maintain electrolyte levels within normal limits.

Interventions. Monitor vital signs for changes in pulse and blood pressure (fluid volume changes) and respiration (acid-base imbalance). If necessary, use hemodynamic monitoring to check for changes in fluid and electrolyte status. Electrocardiographic (ECG) findings of cardiac rhythm changes may be the first indication of electrolyte imbalance.

Check laboratory values for significant changes, and observe for physical manifestations of hyperglycemia, hypocalcemia, and hypokalemia. Monitor the client's response to fluid administration and blood products by monitoring intake and output and assessing for edema, adventitious lung sounds, skin turgor, and mucous membrane alterations by. Measure abdominal girth and monitor urine output (at least 0.5 ml/kg/hr). Report significant changes promptly because these clients are at increased risk.

Diagnosis: Imbalanced Nutrition: Less Than Body Requirements.

Pancreatitis leads to many gastrointestinal manifestations, making *Imbalanced Nutrition: Less Than Body Requirements related to inability to ingest or digest food or absorb nutrients, nausea and vomiting, NPO status, and nasogastric suctioning* a common nursing diagnosis for this client.

Outcomes. The client will maintain adequate nutritional status as evidenced by maintaining normal body weight, keeping blood glucose within normal limits, and showing no evidence of muscle wasting.

Interventions. Depending on the severity of illness, these clients may be kept on NPO status for an extended time. When extended fasting is necessary, nutrition is provided through hyperalimentation and lipids (see Chapter 31). Assess the overall nutritional status of the client by checking daily weights, tissue integrity, and the presence of adequate body fat and muscle mass.

Clients with acute pancreatitis are allowed an oral diet when all abdominal pain and tenderness have resolved; however, if oral intake is resumed too soon, re-exacerbation of manifestations may occur. Therefore monitor the client's response to oral intake carefully, and begin intake slowly with liquids before the client progresses to a normal diet. As noted previously, administration of antispasmodics, anticholinergics, histamine-receptor antagonists, and antacids to reduce gastric and pancreatic secretions may provide some relief, but none of these therapies have been proven effective in shortening the duration of the disease, in reducing complications, or in reducing mortality.

If the pancreas has been severely damaged, it may be necessary to give replacement pancreatic enzymes to replace the enzyme deficit and aid digestion. Monitor the effects of these drugs. The drugs are discussed in the Integrating Pharmacology feature on Pancreatic Enzyme Replacement Therapy in Chronic Pancreatitis on p. 1300.

Diagnosis: Ineffective Breathing Pattern.

The client with acute pancreatitis has the potential for development of many problems. One appropriate nursing diagnosis is *Ineffective Breathing Pattern related to abdominal distention or ascites, pain, or respiratory complications.*

Outcomes. The client will maintain an effective breathing pattern as evidenced by a respiratory rate within normal limits, relaxed respiratory effort, absence of cyanosis, clear lungs, and a breathing pattern that supports blood gas or pulse oximetry results within normal limits.

Interventions. Assess the client's respirations for rate and effort. Your assessment should include lung auscultation for decreased lung sounds (potential for atelectasis), rales, or rhonchi (potential for pneumonia and pleural effusion), and cyanosis. Many times, these clients have been given a prescription of bed rest, which precludes the need for prophylactic nursing interventions of pulmonary hygiene (e.g., turning, coughing, deep breathing, incentive spirometry). Keeping the client comfortable with analgesics enhances full inspiration and normal breathing patterns. Positioning, such as placing the client in the semi-Fowler or a side-lying position, may facilitate normal respiration.

Diagnosis: Anxiety.
Because of the uncertainty of the disease and the possibility of recurrence, an appropriate nursing diagnosis is *Anxiety related to change in health status, change in environment, fear of pain returning, and alcohol abuse withdrawal.*

Outcomes.
The client will express and demonstrate decreasing manifestations of anxiety as evidenced by calmly discussing his or her apprehension, stating that anxiety and fear are decreasing, admitting that alcohol is a problem, seeking help with abstinence, and displaying behavior associated with relaxation (e.g., resting quietly).

Interventions.
Assess the client's level of anxiety by listening and observing. Reassure the client, and acknowledge that the unknown is frightening. Explain procedures that may cause anxiety for the client. Because clients who are in pain or who have acute anxiety may have a shortened attention span, keep instructions simple and direct. Allow significant others to remain with the client when appropriate for added reassurance and comfort.

The client must be encouraged to face the problem that alcohol is causing if it is the source of the pancreatitis. Spend time with the client to encourage him or her to talk about the problem and to explore ways to cope with the illness. Recommend groups such as Alcoholics Anonymous, and encourage the client to join such a program. Discuss supportive services available as necessary with the client and his or her significant others.

Evaluation

Within a few days of treatment, the client is expected to experience less pain and gradually resume eating and drinking. For more severe cases, the client must remain on NPO status and rest the pancreas for a much longer time. If this occurs, the client will require TPN to maintain adequate nutrition.

■ Surgical Management

Indications. Operative intervention is indicated in four specific circumstances:
- Uncertainty of diagnosis; relief of pain
- Treatment of secondary pancreatic infection: pancreatic necrosis and pancreatic abscess
- Correction of associated biliary tract disease
- Progressive clinical deterioration despite optimal supportive care

If clients with severe pancreatitis do not respond to medical management, operative intervention may be indicated to debride necrosis or, again, to exclude other possible diagnoses as causative factors.

If it is necessary to facilitate drainage of a pancreatic abscess, a laparotomy with sump drainage is usually required. It is usually necessary to resect necrotic tissue because undrained pancreatic abscesses are associated with a high mortality rate.

If the client has extensive disease of the entire gland, a subtotal pancreatectomy may be performed. The surgical procedure involves attaching a small remnant of the remaining head of the pancreas to the duodenum. A more extensive procedure, Whipple's surgical procedure (pancreaticoduodenectomy), may be necessary if the pancreatitis is confined to the head of the pancreas. In this instance, the distal third of the stomach, the duodenum, common bile duct, gallbladder, and head of the pancreas are removed.

Because it is sometimes difficult to identify acute pancreatitis, exploratory laparotomy may be indicated to eliminate processes such as perforated viscus or acute mesenteric ischemia. If uncomplicated acute pancreatitis is present, no manipulation is needed and the surgery is terminated. In presumed gallstone-associated pancreatitis, cholecystectomy and intraoperative cholangiography are favored. In clients with severe hemorrhagic pancreatitis with necrosis, debridement of necrotic tissue is performed and retroperitoneal drainage is established.

Treatment of pancreatic abscess combines antibiotic therapy and surgical drainage. Operative debridement is necessary to remove the thick, debris-filled, paste-like collections of infected necrotic material.

Contraindications. In the past, biliary tract surgery for gallstone-associated pancreatitis was deferred for up to 8 weeks; however, up to 35% (range, 11% to 48%) of clients awaiting elective surgery experienced a recurrence of pancreatitis. Today most surgeons proceed with surgery as soon as the initial manifestations of pancreatitis resolve.

Complications. Ileus, abdominal distention, and vomiting are possible postoperative complications that require NG suction if they occur. A serious complication of acute pancreatitis is adult (acute) respiratory distress syndrome (ARDS), which can occur within 3 to 7 days of the onset of pancreatitis and after the administration of large volumes of fluid and colloids given to sustain blood pressure and adequate urine output. See the Critical Monitoring feature on Manifestations of Adult (Acute) Respiratory Distress Syndrome Secondary to Acute Pancreatitis on p. 1296 for findings mandating early intervention.

Outcomes. Clients are expected to recover from the surgical procedure and not experience postoperative complications. Once bowel sounds have returned, about 3 days after surgery, the NG tube is discontinued. If tube removal is tolerated and pain is relieved, the client will

CRITICAL MONITORING

Manifestations of Adult (Acute) Respiratory Distress Syndrome Secondary to Acute Pancreatitis

- Acute respiratory distress: tachypnea, dyspnea, accessory muscle breathing, and cyanosis
- Fever and dry cough that develop over a short period
- Fine crackles heard throughout lung fields on auscultation
- Possible confusion and agitation
- Hypoxemia with partial pressure of oxygen (Po$_2$) <50 mm Hg
- Early—hypocapnia and respiratory alkalosis
- Late—hypercapnia and respiratory acidosis

begin liquids within the next 24 to 72 hours. The client is discharged once a low-fat diet is tolerated.

■ Nursing Management of the Surgical Client

Preoperative Care

Preparing a client for pancreatic surgery requires the usual preoperative care. In addition, close monitoring of WBC count, hematocrit, serum electrolytes, serum calcium, serum creatinine, urea nitrogen or blood urea nitrogen (BUN), aspartate aminotransferase (AST), lactic dehydrogenase (LDH), and arterial blood gases (ABGs) is essential. Other measures may be necessary, depending on the severity of the client's illness, such as insertion of an NG tube, continued replacement of fluids, monitoring of central venous pressure, and blood culture results.

Preoperative nursing management of the client with acute pancreatitis is similar to that described under Nursing Management of the Medical Client. Pay special attention to the nutritional status of the client as well as to the breathing pattern, fluid volume and electrolyte levels, control of pain, and possible complications as the client is prepared for surgery. The client will require preoperative teaching about the procedure and what to expect postoperatively (see Chapter 16). Encourage clients to ask questions about their condition, treatment, and progress.

Postoperative Care
Assessment

After pancreatic surgery, you should have achieved the following:
1. Have a clear idea of the surgical procedure performed, its purpose, steps, and dangers.
2. Be aware of the location and purpose of each drain inserted during surgery. If there are multiple drains,

especially external drains, assess each for proper function.
3. Continually assess tubes or drains that are in place for decompression. If a T tube or internal stent becomes nonfunctional, alert the surgeon immediately to prevent leakage at the internal insertion site. Leakage may lead to peritonitis or fistula formation. Assess for placement, location (internal or external), and proper function and patency of the drains. If the drains do not appear to be functioning, notify the physician immediately.

After pancreatic excision, it is important to know how much pancreatic tissue was removed. When there is a decrease in endocrine tissue, control of blood glucose with insulin and diet becomes necessary. Exocrine loss does not pose immediate postoperative problems but does necessitate lifelong enzyme replacement when oral ingestion is resumed. Assess the functional ability of remaining pancreatic tissue after excision of the pancreas, determining both endocrine and exocrine functioning and its long-term implications. If the client has lost all endocrine function, insulin administration will be necessary (see Chapter 47). Continue to monitor the client for manifestations of hypoglycemia and hyperglycemia.

With the loss of exocrine function, replacement of pancreatic enzyme function with medications such as pancrelipase (Pancrease) becomes necessary (see the Integrating Pharmacology feature on Pancreatic Enzyme Replacement Therapy in Chronic Pancreatitis on p. 1300). When the client begins to eat, watch for the development of diarrhea and steatorrhea (fatty stools), which indicate that insufficient pancreatic enzymes are present.

Diagnosis, Outcomes, Interventions

See the nursing diagnoses discussed under Nursing Management of the Medical Client (in the section on acute pancreatitis) relating to pain, fluid and electrolyte balance, anxiety, ineffective breathing pattern, and nutrition. All are applicable in the postoperative situation. In addition, the following nursing diagnoses are specifically related to the postoperative period.

Diagnosis: Ineffective Therapeutic Regimen Management/Effective Therapeutic Regimen Management. After pancreatectomy, the client will have many and complex learning needs, leading to the nursing diagnosis *Ineffective Therapeutic Regimen Management/Effective Therapeutic Regimen Management related to care, postoperative pain, nutritional needs, diabetic care, pancreatic enzyme replacement, or alcohol abuse and need for follow-up care.*

Outcomes. The client will understand discharge instructions, as evidenced by the ability to describe and demonstrate appropriate wound care, diet, proper diabetes care, activity and exercise level, and correct administration and side effects of the medication regimen. In addition, the client will collaborate with health providers to decide on a therapeutic regimen that is congruent with health goals and lifestyle and treatment of alcoholism if present.

Interventions. Assess the knowledge of the client and his or her significant others before providing appropriate learning guidelines preceding the client's discharge. Provide instructions for wound care. The client will require changes in diet as necessitated by diabetes. Provide guidelines for nutritional needs and an appropriate low-fat diet.

Provide the client with important information concerning diabetes, including information about hyperglycemia (polyuria, polydipsia, and polyphagia) and hypoglycemia (see Chapter 47). Explain medication (pancreatic enzymes), including action, side effects, and when to notify the physician. If the client has had surgery, routine postoperative teaching (see Chapter 16) and education about the care of drains (if still in place) will be needed.

Avoidance of alcohol is another area of postoperative education. Explain the problems that alcohol is creating and the importance of stopping drinking before irreversible damage is done.

Evaluation

If no complications arise, the client can be discharged about a week after surgery. Hence, a visiting nurse may visit the client after discharge to assess the client's ability to follow the postoperative regimen. The client will need to be seen at regular intervals to ensure compliance.

The client's ability to abstain from alcohol should be assessed carefully and further counseling provided as needed. In the short term, the client should recover from acute pancreatitis without complications. Long-term recovery, however, often depends on the client's willingness and ability to alter his or her lifestyle.

■ Self-Care

Because of the complex nature of pancreatitis and the importance of the client's understanding of how to lower the risk of recurrence, clients must become knowledgeable about the causes of the disease, treatment, possible complications, and home health care.

Before discharge home, ask the client and significant others to verbalize home health care needs related to diet; medications, including indications, dosage, frequency, and side effects; and the manifestations of recurrence.

Medications. Prepare clients for discharge by assessing their level of understanding and their learning needs.

Discuss the medication regimen with the client, including its purpose, dosage, frequency, and possible side effects. Explain that an insulin supplement may be required because of pancreatic damage. Begin your teaching as soon as possible to ensure that the client and his or her significant others are fully prepared to cope with glucose monitoring, diet, and insulin administration (see Chapter 47).

Diet Modifications. Instruct the client about dietary restrictions, such as avoiding alcohol, tea, coffee, spicy foods, and heavy meals, which stimulate pancreatic secretions and produce attacks of pancreatitis. Clients should understand the benefit of eating small, frequent meals high in protein, low in fat, and moderate to high in carbohydrate.

Teach Manifestations of Recurrence. Ensure that the client is aware of the manifestations of recurrence of pancreatitis and the importance of reporting these manifestations immediately. These manifestations include steatorrhea; severe back or epigastric pain; persistent gastritis, nausea, and vomiting; weight loss; elevated temperature; and evidence of hyperglycemia.

CHRONIC PANCREATITIS

Chronic pancreatitis is a progressive, inflammatory, destructive disease of the pancreas. The incidence in the United States is about 4 in 100,000.[24]

Pathophysiology

Chronic pancreatitis involves progressive fibrosis and degeneration of the pancreas. Characteristically, the pancreas is progressively destroyed by repeated flares of usually mild attacks of pancreatitis. After repeated attacks of acute pancreatitis, this inflammatory process results in scarring and calcification of pancreatic tissue. The damage is irreversible, affecting both endocrine and exocrine pancreatic functions.

In the United States and in other industrial countries, chronic alcoholism is the most frequent cause of chronic calcifying pancreatitis. In up to 25% of American adults, chronic pancreatitis is of unknown or idiopathic cause; it may also be hereditary. A gene for hereditary pancreatitis (cystic fibrosis transmembrane conductance regulator [*CFTR*]), transmitted as an autosomal dominant trait with variable penetrance, has been identified on chromosome 7. Protein malnutrition is a cause in other parts of the world. Other causes include untreated hyperparathyroidism, congenital anomalies, and pancreatic trauma.

Clinical Manifestations

In chronic pancreatitis, as in acute pancreatitis, pain may be continuous, intermittent, or absent with severe pain, vomiting, constipation, fever, and jaundice. The client may experience some pain relief by sitting in bed with the knees flexed and pressing a pillow to the abdomen. The client generally experiences more pain when supine. Attacks may last only a few days or as long as 2 weeks.

Because food may worsen the pain, the client usually reduces food intake, resulting in weight loss. Reduction in digestive enzyme secretion eventually causes malnutrition and contributes to the weight loss. Ultimately, because of involvement of islet tissue, hyperglycemia develops with manifestations of diabetes. Insulin-dependent diabetes mellitus occurs in up to one third of clients.

The client also suffers from (1) abdominal distention with flatus and cramps, (2) the presence of scattered calcification throughout the pancreas as noted radiographically, and (3) frequent passage of foul fatty stools (steatorrhea). Thus the clinical group of manifestations that serves as a classic presentation of chronic pancreatitis is abdominal pain, weight loss, pancreatic calcification, diabetes, and steatorrhea. Additionally, many clients present with a history of opioid analgesic abuse in an effort to control pain. Pain or digestive disturbance may motivate a person with chronic pancreatitis to seek help.

 Because clients with chronic pancreatitis have a reduced amount of functioning tissue, pancreatic enzyme analysis may be normal. Blood studies may reveal a mild leukocytosis. Glycosuria may be present. X-ray studies may show reduced bowel motility, calcifications, and adhesions. Both ultrasonography and a CT study provide useful diagnostic data. Angiography indicates vascular changes. Cholangiography and cholecystography show biliary alterations, which may be either a cause or a consequence of the pancreatic disorder.

See the Evidence-Based Practice in Action feature on Chronic Pancreatitis, Pain, Malabsorption, and Poor Nutritional Status on p. 1299.

Outcome Management
■ Medical Management

Relieve Pain. The control of pain can be a major problem and is generally the sole indication for surgical intervention. Attempts to control pain pharmacologically should begin with non-opioid analgesics and should progress to opioid analgesics, if needed. For alcohol-related pancreatitis, total abstinence from alcohol is imperative and sometimes successful in itself for pain reduction. The diet should be low in fat according to one source,[7] although another source advocates a diet moderate in fat (30%), high in protein (24%), and low in carbohydrate (40%).[9]

Steatorrhea may be treated with pancreatic supplements selected for their high lipase activity. See the Integrating Pharmacology feature on Pancreatic Enzyme Replacement Therapy in Chronic Pancreatitis on p. 1300. Concurrent administration of sodium bicarbonate H_2-receptor antagonists (e.g., ranitidine) or a proton-pump inhibitor (e.g., omeprazole) may decrease the inactivation of lipase by acid and thereby may further decrease steatorrhea.

Treatment of Endocrine Insufficiency. Exogenous insulin therapy may be necessary because of destruction of islet tissue.

Treatment of Exocrine Insufficiency. Exocrine insufficiency is treated with exogenous pancreatic enzyme therapy. See the Integrating Pharmacology feature on Pancreatic Enzyme Replacement Therapy in Chronic Pancreatitis on p. 1300. This therapy may include lipase, trypsin, or H_2-receptor antagonists.

■ Surgical Management

The four major goals of surgical intervention for chronic pancreatitis are to achieve the following:
1. Correct the primary tract disease (ampullar procedure)
2. Relieve ductal obstruction (ductal drainage procedure)
3. Alleviate pain (ablative procedure)
4. Alleviate pain (denervation procedure)

Several surgical approaches are available. The major surgical procedures are depicted in Figure 48-1.

Endoscopic or surgical drainage is indicated for pseudocysts that cause manifestations. Pancreatic ascites or pancreaticopleural fistulae resulting from a disrupted pancreatic duct can be managed by endoscopic placement of a stent across the disrupted duct. Breaking up stones (calculi) in the pancreatic duct by lithotripsy is rarely done today, but endoscopic removal of stones from the duct at ERCP or placement of a stent across pancreatic duct strictures may reduce pain. For clients with chronic pain and nondilated ducts, a percutaneous celiac plexus nerve block may be ordered, although results are often disappointing.

The prognosis for the client with chronic pancreatitis is good if acute attacks decrease in frequency. Replacement therapy for chronic fat indigestion permits a fairly normal life. If the client continues to drink alcohol, the prognosis is poor. Repeated attacks eventually cause death from shock or renal failure.

PANCREATIC PSEUDOCYSTS

Pancreatic pseudocysts are localized collections of pancreatic secretions (high concentrations of amylase, lipase, and trypsin) in a cystic structure usually adjacent to the pancreas rather than within the parenchyma. Pseudocysts account for up to 75% of all cystic lesions of the pancreas. They develop in up to 15% of clients after an attack of acute alcoholic pancreatitis, but they may be associated with acute pancreatitis of other causes, chronic pancreatitis, trauma, and pancreatic neoplasm.

EB EVIDENCE-BASED PRACTICE IN ACTION

Chronic Pancreatitis, Pain, Malabsorption, and Poor Nutritional Status

The causes of chronic pancreatitis include prolonged alcohol use, pancreatic duct obstruction, pancreas divisum, sphincter of Oddi dysfunction, hypertriglyceridemia, hyperparathyroidism, trauma, and occasionally cystic fibrosis. In about 30% of affected people, no cause is identified.[4]

Chronic pancreatitis is characterized by a gradual and irreversible loss of pancreatic tissue structure and function. There is a loss of pancreatic acinar cells and progressive scarring of pancreatic tissue that result in a decrease in enzyme output. Enzymes that are diminished include lipase, amylase, and proteases. A lack of these enzymes leads to maldigestion, malabsorption of nutrients, and eventually malnutrition if untreated. Steatorrhea, which is the passage of fat in the stool, is the primary manifestation of malabsorption. It occurs when greater than 90% of pancreatic function is lost.[1] In addition, eating induces abdominal pain, and this causes poor oral intake, weight loss, and poor nutritional status. How can these clients be managed properly to avoid weight loss, reduce their risk for nutritional deficiencies, and still be treated effectively for the pain?

According to current research, treatment for clients with chronic pancreatitis is directed toward two major problems: abdominal pain and malabsorption.[2] The pain is often severe enough to require the use of opioids, further reducing the appetite. Clients with severe and persistent pain need to avoid alcohol completely as well as large meals rich in fat. When the pain is severe enough to require opioids (and hence addiction), a number of surgical procedures may be performed to relieve that pain. Such procedures as an ERCP may provide some pain reduction. ERCP may involve sphincterotomy of the pancreatic sphincters, dilation of strictures, removal of calculi, or stenting of the pancreatic ducts. In some clients, pain reduction may come only as a result of a pancreatic resection, although these clients tend to develop pancreatic endocrine and exocrine insufficiency and must be treated with enzyme replacement therapy. Recent studies have indicated that administration of pancreatic enzymes may decrease abdominal pain in selected clients with chronic pancreatitis.[2] The clients most likely to benefit are those with mild to moderate exocrine pancreatic dysfunction.

For managing malabsorption, treatment with pancreatic enzyme replacement therapy may be helpful.[2,5] Diarrhea and steatorrhea may be improved with this treatment, although steatorrhea may not be completely corrected. Recent studies have indicated that clients with chronic pancreatitis showed evidence of better nutritional status, and fewer clients have been classified as moderate to severely malnourished based on albumin levels or percent of ideal body weight after using pancreatic enzyme supplementation.[5] Pancreatic enzyme supplementation is safe, well tolerated, and beneficial for clients with chronic pancreatitis [3]

Implications

Nurses caring for clients with chronic pancreatitis on a gastroenterology unit or in the outpatient setting should carefully monitor the client's weight, height, and serum pre-albumin and albumin levels as a part of the routine nursing assessment. These measures are effective screening methods to detect clients at risk for poor nutritional status. Documentation of the results of the assessment is also important to establish a base line of information and to monitor the client's progress. Nurses should be aware that therapy could be individualized by the physician to meet each client's nutritional needs.

References
1. Apte, M.V., Keogh, G.W., & Wilson, J.S. (1999). Chronic pancreatitis: Complications and management. *Journal of Clinical Gastroenterology, 29*(3), 225-240.
2. Greenberger, N.J., & Toskes, P. (2001). Acute and chronic pancreatitis. In E. Braunwald, et al. (Eds.), *Harrison's principles of internal medicine* (15th ed., pp. 1792-1804). New York: McGraw-Hill.
3. Pitchumoni, C.S. (1998). Chronic pancreatitis: Pathogenesis and management of pain. *Journal of Clinical Gastroenterology, 27*(2), 101-107.
4. Steer, M.L., Waxman, I., & Freedman, S. (1995). Chronic pancreatitis. *New England Journal of Medicine, 332*(22), 1482-1490.
5. Trolli, P.A., Conwell, D.L., & Zuccaro, G. (2001). Pancreatic enzyme therapy and nutritional status of outpatients with chronic pancreatitis. *Gastroenterology Nursing, 24*(2), pp. 84-87.

The most common clinical picture of a client with pancreatic pseudocyst involves abdominal pain, early satiety, nausea, and vomiting. Less common manifestations include pruritus, jaundice, sepsis, and hemorrhage. Essentially, diagnosis of pseudocyst is made through the same assessment as that used for pancreatitis.

Treatment is based on the presence or absence of manifestations, the client's age, and the size of the cyst.

Cysts smaller than 6 cm in diameter often resolve spontaneously. Clients with such cysts are followed up with frequent ultrasound studies to determine whether the cyst is decreasing in size. Clients with persistent manifestations or pseudocyst-related complications, such as infection, require operative intervention. Erosion of an inflammatory process into a blood vessel can result in a major hemorrhage into the cyst.

INTEGRATING PHARMACOLOGY

Pancreatic Enzyme Replacement Therapy in Chronic Pancreatitis

Chronic pancreatitis leads to decreased pancreatic protease secretion. Proteases break down protein into basic building blocks to be used by the body for maintenance of a healthy body. Lack of proteases leads to pancreatic stimulation causing abdominal pain. In addition, a decrease in lipase secretion results in steatorrhea (fatty stools). Proteases and lipases are necessary to help prevent maldigestion, steatorrhea, and malnutrition. In clients with chronic pancreatitis, supplementation with pancreatic enzymes provides the serine proteases and lipases necessary to correct the defects.

Pancreatic enzyme therapy is not complex and has few side effects. The effectiveness with which it works depends on factors such as enzyme formulation, dosage, frequency, and other therapies in the client's overall treatment plan. Several enzyme products are available that are enteric coated and nonenteric coated and that contain differing amounts of protease, lipase, and amylase.

Digestive enzymes such as gastric acid may alter the usual physical and chemical nature of lipase. In addition, duodenal pH can be lower than normal in chronic pancreatitis because of reduced bicarbonate secretion. Therefore acid-suppressing medications and enteric-coated enzyme preparations are often used in a client's treatment. A minimum of 30,000 international units of lipase and 10,000 international units of trypsin are needed within 4 hours postprandial to achieve adequate digestion of protein, fat, and carbohydrates.

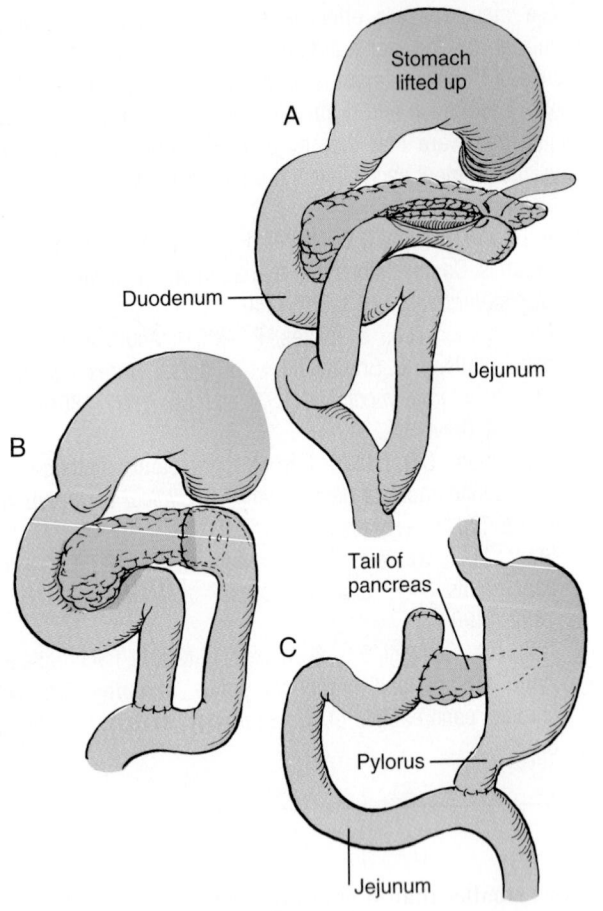

A. **Side-to-side pancreaticojejunostomy (ductal drainage)**
Indicated when gross dilation of pancreatic ducts is associated with septa and calculi. The most successful procedure, with rates of 60% to 90%.

B. **Caudal pancreaticojejunostomy (ductal drainage)**
Indicated for the uncommon cases of isolated proximal pancreatic ductal stenosis not involving the ampulla.

C. **Pancreaticoduodenal (right-sided) resection (ablative) (with preservation of pylorus) (Whipple procedure)**
Indicated when major changes are confined to head of pancreas. Preservation of pylorus avoids usual sequelae of gastric resection.

FIGURE 48-1 Surgical procedures for chronic pancreatitis and pancreatic cancer.

Surgical procedures include internal drainage of the pseudocyst (cystojejunostomy, cystogastrostomy, and cystoduodenostomy), pancreatic resection, distal pancreatectomy, and, least often, percutaneous or endoscopic drainage.

PANCREATIC CANCER

Cancer is the most common neoplasm affecting the pancreas. About 75% of cancers occur in the head, and 25% are in the body and tail of the pancreas.[7] Pancreatic cancer is the fourth most common cause of death from cancer, exceeded only by lung, colorectal, and breast (in women) or prostate (in men) cancer.[7] Of clients with pancreatic cancer, 90% die within the first year of diagnosis. Cancer of the pancreas is more common in blacks than in whites, in smokers, and in men. It appears to be linked to diabetes mellitus; the use of alcohol; a history of previous pancreatitis; smoking; ingestion of a high-fat diet; organic chemicals, such as coke, coal, gas, and benzidine; and obesity. Risk factors include age, obesity, prior abdominal radiation, and family history. Research indicates that obesity significantly increases the risk of pancreatic cancer, but physical activity appears to decrease this risk, especially among overweight people. Health promotion actions include avoidance of risk factors and pancreatitis. Health maintenance and health restoration activities are limited because of the poor prognosis associated with pancreatic cancer.

Duct cell adenocarcinoma accounts for more than 90% of cell types of malignant pancreatic exocrine tumors. Less common types of pancreatic exocrine cancer include cystadenocarcinoma and acinar cell carcinoma. Periampullary adenocarcinomas originate in the region of the ampulla of Vater. Clients typically present with jaundice, significant unexplained weight loss, and abdominal pain. Many clients are managed operatively by either resection (~30%) or palliative therapy to relieve manifestations such as jaundice.[15]

Carcinomas of the tail and body of the pancreas usually present with significant weight loss and abdominal pain. Because of their location, these tumors generally grow to a large size before manifestations occur and the diagnosis is made. Therefore the resectability rate is low (<7%), and the prognosis is poor (a 5- to 6-month mean survival). The response to chemotherapy (fluorouracil) has been disappointing.

Cystadenocarcinoma of the pancreas is seen most frequently in women 40 to 60 years of age, and it accounts for fewer than 2% of all pancreatic exocrine neoplasms. Acinar cell carcinoma of the pancreas is rare, showing no gender predominance. Surgical treatment is the same as that used for ductal adenocarcinoma.

Outcome Management
■ Medical Management

Medical treatment for pancreatic cancer includes radiation therapy (e.g., high-dose external beam, interstitial seed of iodine 125 or iridium 192, brachytherapy, and intraoperative radiation therapy) and drugs (e.g., 5-fluorouracil alone or with radiation therapy and nitrosourea, mitomycin-C, and doxorubicin). Chemotherapy has been disappointing for use in metastatic pancreatic cancer, but improved results have been reported with gemcitabine (Gemzar), which inhibits the movement of cells from the G_1 to the S phase of the cell cycle.

■ Surgical Management

Surgical treatment is Whipple's surgical procedure, when lesions are strictly limited to the head of the pancreas. The operation involves a pancreaticoduodenectomy with removal of the distal third of the stomach, pancreaticojejunostomy, gastrojejunostomy, and choledochojejunostomy (see Figure 48-1). The nursing care for these clients is similar to that for Nursing Management of the Surgical Client with acute pancreatitis.

Prognosis

Mortality rates are as high as 15% after surgical resection of pancreatic cancer. Although the potential for cure is restricted to the few who are able to undergo a complete surgical resection, the 5-year survival rate after such surgical procedures is only 10%. Nonetheless, clients who undergo resection and eventually experience recurrence of cancer survive three to four times longer than clients whose tumor is not removed.[15]

PANCREATIC TRAUMA

The pancreas is injured in fewer than 2% of persons with abdominal trauma. Two thirds of pancreatic injuries are associated with penetrating abdominal trauma, and the remainder are caused by blunt trauma. Although pancreatic trauma occurs somewhat infrequently, it is associated with high morbidity and mortality rates because of the difficulty in detecting these injuries and the likelihood of massive injury to nearby organs. Because the pancreas is retroperitoneal, clinical indicators of injury are often not obvious for several hours. Clients with penetrating abdominal trauma show manifestations of hemorrhage, progressive peritonitis, and hypovolemia.

The presentation of blunt pancreatic trauma is varied. Most people with blunt trauma have injuries to surrounding organs and vascular structures, and pancreatic trauma is discovered on treatment of these other injuries. In clients without injury to other areas, the only findings may be mild epigastric pain and tenderness; progressive deterioration yields the diagnosis of pancreatic injury. Treatment involves surgery to control hemorrhage, to debride nonviable tissue, to preserve viable tissue, and to provide drainage of pancreatic secretions.

CYSTIC FIBROSIS

Cystic fibrosis (CF) is a hereditary, chronic disease characterized by abnormal secretions of the exocrine glands. It is genetically transmitted as an autosomal recessive trait. More than 25,000 American have CF, and 850 new cases are diagnosed annually in the United States. CF is the most common fatal genetic disease of children of European-American heritage. It is diagnosed and managed in childhood, but improvements in care have allowed many clients to survive into adulthood.

Pulmonary complications are the most physically visible. Clients have obvious respiratory compromise, with frequent bronchopneumonia and chronic bronchitis. Some improvements in the management of infants and children with CF have led to a greater number of adults with CF. Typically, these adults have a small stature and appear somewhat emaciated. They are barrel-chested and have clubbed fingers. Because the digestive problems encountered with CF are generally managed with diet and oral administration of pancreatic enzymes and fat-soluble vitamins, clients are hospitalized for treatment of respiratory complications rather than for pancreatic or intestinal problems.

In addition to pulmonary problems, clients experience impaired pancreatic exocrine function because of decreased lipase released into the bowel. The result is malabsorption of lipids with blockage of the pancreatic ducts by thick mucus. Pancreatic degeneration, fibrosis, and atrophy of tissues follow, with eventual development of fatty infiltration and loss of function. The intestines have thick, viscous mucus, which may cause a thick mass within the bowel. The lack of pancreatic enzymes causes steatorrhea.

The current trend is to hospitalize the client routinely for thorough pulmonary hygiene with a full course of intravenous (IV) antibiotics, with emphasis on antifungal agents, and respiratory therapy.

Nursing management of the client with CF focuses on two major nursing diagnoses: (1) *Ineffective Airway Clearance* and (2) *Imbalanced Nutrition: Less than Body Requirements*. Interventions for clients with CF include the following:

- Prophylactic pulmonary support (expectorants, postural drainage, antibiotics)
- Administration of pancreatic enzymes
- A high-protein, high-calorie, high-salt, low-fat diet
- Replacement of fat-soluble vitamins

BILIARY TRACT DISORDERS

Disorders of the gallbladder and ducts are extremely common. In the United States alone, biliary tract disorders, specifically gallstones, account for more than 800,000 hospitalizations annually.[12] Disorders include gallstones, inflammatory conditions, infections, tumors, and congenital malformations.

The two most common conditions are gallstones and associated cholecystitis (inflammation of the gallbladder). About 98% of clients who present with symptomatic gallbladder disease have gallstones. Malignancies and congenital anomalies of the biliary tract are relatively uncommon.

Before beginning this discussion, note the list of terms (Table 48-1) used in association with these conditions.

TABLE 48-1	*Biliary Tract Terminology*
Term	**Definition**
Chole-	Pertaining to bile
Cholang-	Pertaining to bile ducts
Cholangiography	X-ray study of bile ducts
Cholangitis	Inflammation of bile duct
Cholecyst-	Pertaining to gallbladder
Cholecystectomy	Removal of gallbladder
Cholecystitis	Inflammation of gallbladder
Cholecystography	X-ray study of gallbladder
Cholecystostomy	Incision and drainage of gallbladder
Choledocho-	Pertaining to common bile duct
Choledocholithiasis	Stones in common bile duct
Choledochostomy	Exploration of common bile duct
Cholelith-	Pertaining to gallstones
Cholelithiasis	Presence of gallstones
Cholescintigraphy	Radionuclide imaging of biliary system

CHOLELITHIASIS (GALLSTONES)

About 20 million people in the United States have gallstones, and almost 475,000 cholecystectomies are performed every year. The incidence of gallstones increases with age, as do the risks associated with cholelithiasis. In the United States, more than 10% of men and 20% of women have gallstones by 65 years of age. Women account for nearly 70% of those treated for gallstones, although the mortality rate may be higher in men. Twice as many white Americans as black Americans are affected, and although gallstones are less common in blacks, cholelithiasis attributable to hemolysis occurs in more than one third of people with sickle cell anemia.

The prevalence of gallstones is much the same in Europe and Australia. Clients with diabetes mellitus, obesity, Crohn disease, and those with cirrhosis show an increased incidence.

Most of our present knowledge of cholesterol gallstones comes from the study of Pima Native American women in south-central Arizona, in whom the occurrence is 75% in those over 25 years of age. Pigment stones are dominant in Asians and in African Americans.

Etiology and Risk Factors

Gallstones are crystalline structures formed by *concretion* (hardening) or *accretion* (adherence of particles, accumulation) of normal or abnormal bile constituents. According to various theories, there are four possible explanations for stone formation.

First, bile may undergo a change in composition. Studies of subjects with cholesterol gallstones indicate that their bile is supersaturated with cholesterol but deficient in bile salts. The cholesterol saturation of bile seems to increase with age. Changes in bile composition, however, do not completely explain why gallstones form.

Second, gallbladder stasis may lead to bile stasis. Bile stasis may (1) change the composition of bile, (2) supersaturate bile with cholesterol, and (3) precipitate some bile constituents. Gallbladder stasis may result from decreased contractility and emptying of the gallbladder and spasm of the sphincter of Oddi. Circumstances in which gallbladder stasis occurs (e.g., TPN; low-fat, weight-reduction diets; spinal cord injury; pregnancy) are associated with a high rate of gallstone formation. More specifically, TPN without oral intake for longer than 1 month is associated with gallbladder sludge formation and cholelithiasis. Delayed emptying of the gallbladder may correlate with hormonal factors. In pregnant women, the female sex hormone estrogen increases, which increases dietary uptake of cholesterol and biliary cholesterol secretion. This may explain why gallstones seem to be associated with pregnancy. In addition, one of the precautions for administering estrogen substances to postmenopausal women is gallbladder disease.

Third, infection may predispose a person to stone formation. Inflammatory debris can form a *nidus* (point of origin) for stone growth. The related tissue injury may alter the composition of bile by increasing the reabsorption of bile salts and lecithin. Certain organisms may also play a part in stone formation by altering the composition of bile. For example, *Escherichia coli* increases the amount of bilirubin available for pigment stones and *Streptococcus faecalis* reduces bile salts.

Fourth, genetics and demography can affect stone formation, as shown by the higher prevalence in Pima and Chippewa Native Americans, Northern Europeans, and South Americans than in Asians.

Health promotion activities to minimize gallstone formation include maintaining a low-fat diet, maintaining ideal body weight, and limiting the number of pregnancies. Clients receiving TPN for longer than 1 month should be monitored closely as health maintenance and restoration actions. In some male clients, regular coffee consumption may help to prevent symptomatic gallstone disease.[13]

Pathophysiology

Gallstone formation involves several factors:
1. Bile must become supersaturated with cholesterol or calcium.
2. The solute must precipitate from solution as solid crystals.
3. Crystals must come together and fuse to form stones.

Gallstones are generally of three types: (1) cholesterol, (2) pigment, and (3) mixed. Because the incidence of a pure stone formation is rare, stones are generally classified by the predominant substance.

Cholesterol stones are the most common type; the incidence increases with age, and the prevalence is higher in women. Stones are usually smooth and whitish yellow to tan.

Pigment stones are present in about 30% of people with cholelithiasis in the United States. In these people, bile contains an excess of unconjugated bilirubin. Pigment stones may be black (associated with hemolysis and cirrhosis) or earthy calcium bilirubinate (associated with infection in the biliary system).

Mixed stones may be a combination of cholesterol and pigment stones or either of these with some other substance. Calcium carbonate, phosphates, bile salts, and palmitate make up the more common minor constituents.

Most gallstones are formed in the gallbladder, but they may also form in the common duct or hepatic ducts of the liver. The actual incidence is not known, however, because some stones do not cause manifestations and they pass through the ducts into the bowel unnoticed.

The pathologic findings are best interpreted from the clinical manifestations of the disease, which may be acute or chronic. Once a client becomes symptomatic, treatment and follow-up are essential to prevent progression to a more severe, sometimes fatal, complication of gallbladder disease. About one third of these complications are due to free perforation, which occurs when a gangrenous area becomes necrotic and bile breaks into the peritoneal cavity. The mortality rate is about 20% for peritonitis with systemic distribution of pepsin.

Pericholecystic abscess accounts for 50% of the complications and is the least severe, with a mortality rate of approximately 15%. Abscess formation occurs while the perforation is walled off by omentum or an adjacent organ (e.g., colon, stomach, or duodenum). Much less frequently, in about 15% of clients, a fistula occurs when the gallbladder becomes attached to a portion of the gastrointestinal tract and perforates it. The duodenum, followed by the colon, is the most common site for this event.

Occasionally, a stone is discharged into the small intestine. If the stone is large enough, it can obstruct the narrow terminal ileum, causing gallstone ileus.

Clinical Manifestations

Manifestations of biliary tract disorders are similar to those of several other conditions. Box 48-2 lists some of the more common diseases that must be differentiated from acute and chronic cholecystitis.

Fewer than half of the people with gallstones report any distress because gallstones cause no manifestations unless complications develop. The most specific and characteristic manifestation of gallstone disease is pain or biliary colic, which is caused by spasm of the biliary ducts as they try to dislodge the stones. This pain usually follows the temporary obstruction of the gallbladder

BOX 48-2 Disorders with Manifestations Similar to Those of Chronic and Acute Cholecystitis

Chronic Cholecystitis

Angina pectoris
Chronic pancreatitis
Esophagitis
Hiatal hernia
Peptic ulcer
Pyelonephritis
Spastic colitis

Acute Cholecystitis

Acute appendicitis
Acute hepatitis
Acute myocardial infarction
Acute pancreatitis
Acute pyelonephritis
Intercostal neuritis
Intestinal obstruction
Perforated ulcer
Pleurisy
Renal calculus
Right lower lobe pneumonia

outlet. Characteristically, the pain starts in the upper midline area. It may radiate around to the back and right shoulder blade, although some clients complain that it passes straight through to the back and substernal areas. The client is often restless, changing positions frequently to relieve the intensity of the pain. Pain may persist for only a few hours or several days, and the interval between attacks is variable.

If the stone is blocking the cystic duct, manifestations of acute cholecystitis (see Acute Cholecystitis) may occur. If the stone lodges in the common duct, gallstones can be complicated by *cholangitis* (inflammation of the bile duct) and pancreatitis. *Jaundice* appears only when common duct obstruction is present.

Nausea and vomiting may occur; occasionally, self-induced vomiting alleviates the manifestations. Assessment may further reveal a history of flatulence, bloating, epigastric pain, belching, intolerance for fatty foods, and vague upper abdominal sensations. Occasionally, clients who have these problems still have them after cholecystectomy.

Assessment of these clients becomes important in that manifestations of biliary colic and coronary artery disease are remarkably similar. Considering the prevalence of both these problems, accurate diagnosis is essential. Many times the diagnosis is based on the manifestations alone. Physical findings are present only during an attack

with pain, with pain being the cardinal manifestation. The right upper quadrant or epigastric area is tender to palpation with voluntary muscle guarding, but manifestations of peritonitis are absent. The gallbladder is not palpable, and the temperature is normal.

Blood test results are unremarkable. For confirmation of the presence of gallstones and acute cholecystitis, an abdominal ultrasound study is currently the test of choice. Ultrasound is very sensitive (>95%) and very specific (>95%) for gallbladder stones larger than 2 mm diameter.[7,8,12] Gallbladder nuclear scanning (cholescintigraphy, HIDA scanning, IDA scanning, or DISIDA scanning) after administration of ^{99m}Tc is also an accurate test for confirming acute cholecystitis and for viewing the gallbladder, common bile duct, and duodenum. Through the use of iminodiacetic acid analogs (IDAs) labeled with ^{99m}Tc, the biliary tract can be evaluated in a safe, accurate, and noninvasive manner. The scintillation camera emits light with each photon it receives from the gamma ray. When these light patterns are arranged in a spatial order, a realistic image of the biliary tree is apparent (see Chapter 44, Table 44-3).

In diagnosing tumors, strictures, or gallstones of the hepatic or common bile duct, the current trend is to use ERCP (see Chapter 44, Table 44-3). Magnetic resonance cholangiopancreatography (MRCP) is a newer diagnostic modality that implements MRI to evaluate the fluid-filled gallbladder and biliary and pancreatic ducts. MRCP is a noninvasive procedure that is being used with increasing frequency to diagnose gallstones (cholelithiasis) and the complications that may result.

Outcome Management
■ Medical Management

Reduce Pain. Pain may arise from contraction of the gallbladder during transient obstruction of the cystic duct by gallstones. Analgesics may be administered intramuscularly (IM) or intravenously (IV) on a schedule, with a patient-controlled analgesia (PCA) pump or as needed for pain. Antacids are given to neutralize gastric hyperacidity and to reduce associated pain, and antiemetics are given to minimize nausea and vomiting. Antibiotics are administered to reduce the likelihood of infection. Nitroglycerin may reduce biliary colic as well.

Monitor Fluid and Electrolyte Balance. During an acute attack of biliary colic, the client remains on NPO status, with IV fluids administered to maintain hydration. The client may lose fluids if an NG tube has been inserted for symptomatic relief of vomiting or if pancreatitis is a probable diagnosis.

The diet progresses according to the client's tolerance. The client is advised to avoid foods that precipitate biliary colic. Instructions may include avoiding a fatty meal or a large meal after fasting.

Nonsurgical Approaches to Eradicate Stones

Endoscopy. Retrograde endoscopy for stone removal is an important nonsurgical alternative. To remove a gallstone from the common bile duct, the physician passes an endoscope orally into the duodenum and then passes a wire snare into the common bile duct through the ampulla of Vater, securing and removing the obstructing stone (Figure 48-2). The physician may choose to enlarge the ampulla of Vater by endoscopic papillotomy to allow passage of stones. If stones remain in the common bile duct after cholecystectomy and a T tube is still in place, the physician may pass a stone-retrieving basket or other device through the T-tube tract to remove the stone.

Gallstone Dissolution (Cholesterol-Dissolving Agents).

The oral administration of agents for dissolving cholesterol gallstones, chenodeoxycholic acid (CDCA), or chenodiol, and ursodeoxycholic acid, or ursodiol (UDCA), may be used in selected clients who refuse cholecystectomy or who are not good candidates for surgery. The dose is 7 mg/kg daily of each or 8 to 13 mg/kg or ursodeoxycholic acid in divided doses daily. Both drugs act to reduce the amount of cholesterol in bile; however, each drug uses a different mechanism. The highest success rate occurs in clients with small floating, radiolucent gallstones. It is likely, however, that fewer than 10% of clients with manifestations of cholelithiasis are candidates for this type of treatment. In addition, stones tend to reoccur (30% to 50% over 3 to 5 years of follow-up), and taking medication for an indefinite time can be costly. Because of these disadvantages and the success of laparoscopic cholecystectomy, the use of oral cholesterol dissolving agents has largely been reduced to

gallstone dissolution in clients who wish to avoid or are not candidates for elective cholecystectomy.[8]

Extracorporeal Shock Wave Lithotripsy. Extracorporeal shock wave lithotripsy (ESWL) may be used as an ambulatory treatment in some cases. The client should have symptomatic cholelithiasis with fewer than four stones, each smaller than 3 cm in diameter, and no history of liver or pancreatic disease. Contraindications to the procedure are the presence of common duct stones, recent acute cholecystitis, cholangitis, and pancreatitis.

Up to 1500 shock waves are directed at the stones until they are crushed during the hour-long procedure. The minute particles are then able to travel through the biliary ductal system to be excreted via the intestine. IV conscious sedation with fentanyl citrate (Alfenta) or midazolam hydrochloride (Versed) may be used to minimize the mild discomfort that some clients experience while expelling the tiny stone fragments.

After lithotripsy, minor complications may include ecchymosis over the area of entry of the shock waves, gross or microscopic hematuria because of the proximity of the right kidney, and biliary pain when large fragments pass through the cystic duct.

Lithotripsy is used infrequently as an option for treatment in the United States today because of the emergence of laparoscopic cholecystectomy as the procedure of choice for symptomatic cholelithiasis. In addition, the procedure is less an option because about 30% of clients experience a recurrence of gallstones within 5 years of lithotripsy combined with medical litholytic therapy and because of the high cost of taking UDCA for a variable period after the procedure.[7,8]

Monitor for Complications. Monitoring for complications of gallstone disease includes observing, most commonly, for development of manifestations of biliary colic. Conditions such as bile duct obstruction, cholangitis, pancreatitis, acute calculus, and cholecystitis may occur and cause manifestations consistent with gallbladder disease and subsequent sepsis and death. People with diabetes mellitus and gallstones are more susceptible to complications of sepsis.

Because the gallbladder is left in place in all interventions except cholecystectomy, recurrence of stones is likely. Investigation continues on long-term prevention of the recurrence of gallstones.

■ Nursing Management of the Medical Client
Assessment

If the client is being admitted for evaluation and treatment of manifestations, your assessment should focus on collecting subjective and objective data and noting the client's response to medications. Assess the client's man-

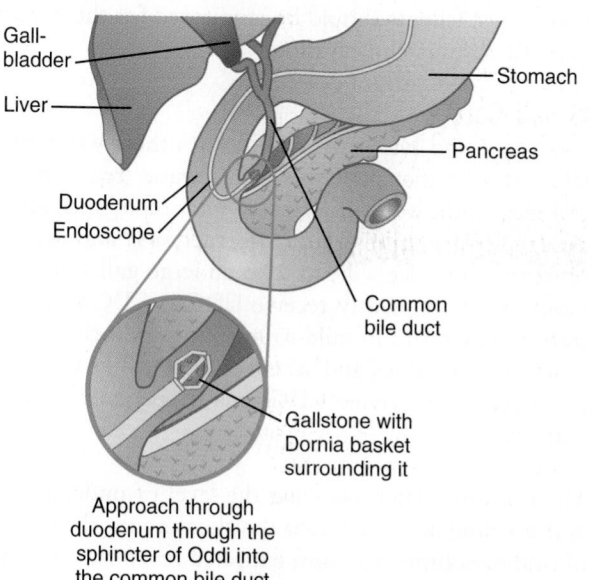

FIGURE 48-2 Retrograde cholendoscopic removal of gallstones.

ifestations carefully to help determine the diagnosis. Check vital signs at regular intervals to document inflammation associated with stones. Also assess the client's knowledge of the diagnostic process. Closely monitor the client for manifestations of obstruction from the gallstones.

Diagnosis, Outcomes, Interventions

Diagnosis: Acute Pain or Chronic Pain. Because one of the major manifestations of the disease is pain, *Acute Pain or Chronic Pain related to biliary spasms* is the major nursing diagnosis.

Outcomes. The client will demonstrate absence of or a decrease in pain as evidenced by the client's verbalizing that pain is absent or decreased and that he or she is resting quietly.

Interventions

Administer Pain Medications. Administer pain medication as ordered; document and note the client's response to the medication. Encourage the client to verbalize the effectiveness of the medication by describing whether the pain is absent or decreased.

Provide Comfort Measures. Other comforting measures may be helpful. Providing a quiet environment and using relaxation techniques, such as a back rub, or comfortable positioning may promote rest and enhance the effects of the analgesics.

Diagnosis: Risk for Imbalanced Fluid Volume. Because of the associated gastrointestinal manifestations, write the nursing diagnosis as *Risk for Imbalanced Fluid Volume related to vomiting and nasogastric suctioning.*

Outcomes. The client will maintain adequate hydration and electrolyte balance as evidenced by normal skin turgor, moist oral mucous membranes, urine output greater than 0.5 ml/kg/hr, and no manifestations of electrolyte imbalance.

Interventions

Insert a Nasogastric Tube. If the client continues vomiting, obtain an order for an NG tube with a suction attachment to relieve distention and vomiting. Suction also removes the gastric juices that stimulate cholecystokinin, which in turn causes painful contractions of the gallbladder. NG suction is usually maintained on a low intermittent setting when a single-lumen tube (e.g., Levin) is used or on a low continuous setting when a double-lumen (e.g., Salem Sump) tube is used.

Administer IV Fluids and Electrolytes. Assess and document intake, output, and electrolyte laboratory values,

communicating discrepancies to the physician. Assess the client for manifestations of dehydration, such as dry mucous membranes, poor skin turgor, and urine output less than 0.5 ml/kg/hr.

Diagnosis: Risk for Injury. The client undergoing endoscopic retrograde stone removal is assigned the nursing diagnosis *Risk for Injury related to medication during the procedure and possible introduction of bacteria into common bile duct.*

Outcomes. The client will remain free from injury and infection following endoscopic retrograde stone removal as evidenced by the airway remaining patent without aspiration and absence of manifestations of infection, such as elevated temperature.

Interventions. For the client undergoing endoscopic retrograde papillotomy or stone removal, a local anesthetic solution is sprayed on the back of the throat. This intervention facilitates the passing of the endoscope. After the endoscopic procedure, carefully check for the return of the gag reflex before allowing oral intake. If the client receives sedation, raise the side rails on the bed for protection and keep the call light within reach. Antibiotics are often administered during the procedure to minimize the risk of infection from introduction of bacteria from the intestine into the common bile duct.

Evaluation

Most clients recover from acute cholecystitis in a few days without complications. Once the biliary system is allowed to rest, inflammation decreases and recovery progresses. Clients should be monitored for the development of chronic cholecystitis.

■ Self-Care

The client and his or her significant others will need to learn about the suggested therapeutic regimen, diet changes, indications for drugs and their side effects, dosage, and administration instructions, and ways to prevent recurrence. Clients who undergo gallstone dissolution most frequently receive UDCA. CDCA administration may result in mild to moderate elevation in liver function test values and serum cholesterol levels. In addition, clients receiving CDCA may experience disabling diarrhea.

Medications. After assessing the level of understanding and learning needs, educate the client about the purpose of oral dissolution therapy, expected responses, and possible untoward reactions. Because oral dissolution medication must be taken over a long period, help the client to devise ways to remember to take the medication daily. For example, a pillbox that is divided into the days of the week clearly indicates whether the client has missed a dose.

The client who is being treated medically may be sent home with oral analgesics or other medications for comfort as well as with an oral dissolution agent. Be sure that the client and his or her significant others can relate all necessary information to the nurse before discharge.

Diet Modifications. Diet instructions may be necessary if ingestion of food precipitated the attack; that is, if a fatty food caused the biliary colic, inform the client about the need for a low-fat diet.

Prevent Recurrence. Advise the client about what to do if another attack occurs. The client has probably been encouraged by the physician to consider elective cholecystectomy or other surgical intervention before gallbladder disease progresses. Provide written material on gallbladder disease at this time to aid the client in understanding and in making decisions.

■ Surgical Management

Whether to operate on a client with asymptomatic cholelithiasis ("silent gallstones") is an area for debate. The potential for serious complications (e.g., acute cholecystitis, choledocholithiasis, sepsis) can pose a significant risk. Older people and clients with insulin-dependent diabetes have a high incidence of gallstones. Because such people are at high risk during acute biliary attacks and emergency procedures, surgeons may recommend that they undergo elective cholecystectomy to avoid later emergency surgery. Other procedures that may be performed include percutaneous cholecystolithotomy and laparoscopic cholecystectomy.

Laparoscopic Cholecystectomy

Indications. Laparoscopic cholecystectomy has become the treatment of choice for symptomatic gallbladder disease. The procedure is suitable for most clients, even those with acute cholecystitis, because there is minimal trauma to the abdominal wall. This makes it possible for clients to go home within 24 hours after the procedure and return to work within a few days instead of a few weeks, as is the case with a cholecystectomy.

With the client under general anesthesia, carbon dioxide is used to create pneumoperitoneum through a needle inserted near the umbilicus. Near the umbilicus, an endoscope is inserted through a small incision to view the gallbladder and to determine the feasibility of success associated with this procedure. Three other small incisions are created: one for grasping the gallbladder, one for suction and irrigation, and one for dissection instruments and applying clips (Figure 48-3).

Contraindications. Laparoscopic cholecystectomy is contraindicated if stones are known to exist in the common bile duct. Laparoscopic cholecystectomy does not allow exploration or removal of stones from the common duct.

Complications. Possible complications of surgery or anesthesia include damage to the biliary tract and hemorrhage. Operative cholangiography is a protective procedure for complications of cholecystectomy. Laparoscopic cholecystectomy carries a nearly twofold higher risk of major bile, vascular, or bowel complications compared with open cholecystectomy.[6] The advantages of small scars and a short hospital stay, however, have influenced surgeons to opt for this procedure more often.

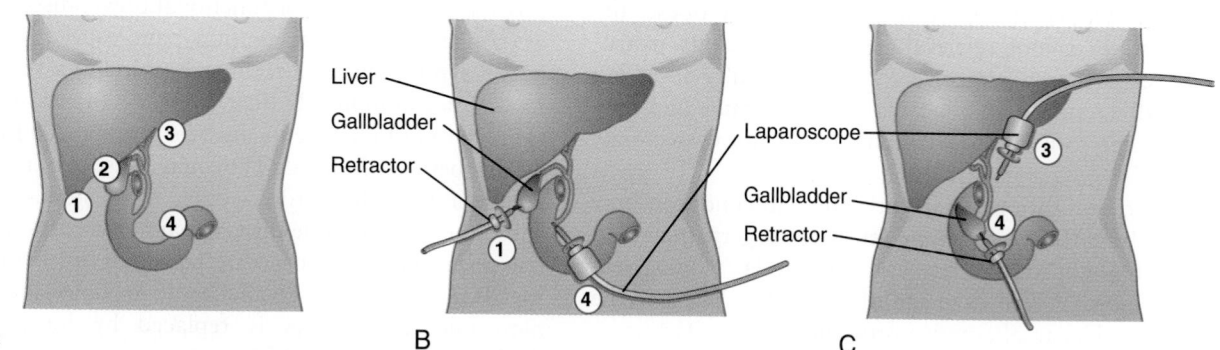

FIGURE 48-3 Laparoscopic cholecystectomy. **A,** Standard sites of four ports used in laparoscopic cholecystectomy. *1,* The lateral port is used to retract the gallbladder. *2,* The subcostal port is used to retract the gallbladder. *3,* The superior midline port is used to insert the laparoscope later in the procedure while the gallbladder is being withdrawn from the umbilical port. *4,* The umbilical port is most often used to insert the laparoscope for most of the procedure and then is used to withdraw the gallbladder after the laparoscope is moved to the superior midline port. **B,** Preparing the gallbladder for removal by ligating it from attachments (e.g., cystic duct, artery, vein). *1,* The gallbladder is retracted through the lateral port. *4,* A laparoscope is inserted through the umbilical port to visualize the gallbladder. **C,** Removal of the gallbladder. *3,* Laparoscope through the superior midline port. *4,* Removal of the gallbladder through the umbilical port.

Clients who undergo this procedure are at less risk because they are ambulatory sooner and usually require only oral analgesia. Because of the carbon dioxide pressing on the diaphragm, nausea, vomiting, and shoulder pain are more frequent if the client's head and torso are elevated too soon after surgery.

Outcomes. Most clients are discharged on the day of surgery or the day after. In most cases, they can resume normal activities and return to work after 3 to 4 days.

Cholecystectomy

Indications. A cholecystectomy consists of excising the gallbladder from the posterior liver wall and ligating the cystic duct, vein, and artery. The surgeon usually approaches the gallbladder through a right upper paramedian or upper midline incision. If necessary, the common duct may be explored through this incision. When stones are suspected in the common duct, operative cholangiography may be performed (if it has not been ordered preoperatively). The surgeon may dilate the common duct if it is not already dilated as a result of a pathologic process. Dilation facilitates stone removal. The surgeon passes a thin instrument into the duct to collect the stones, either whole or after crushing them.

After exploring the common duct, the surgeon usually inserts a T tube to ensure adequate bile drainage during duct healing *(choledochostomy)*. The T tube also provides a route for postoperative cholangiography or stone dissolution, when appropriate (Figure 48-4).

A conventional open cholecystectomy is indicated when a laparoscopic cholecystectomy does not allow for retrieval of a stone in the common bile duct and when the client's physique does not allow access to the gallbladder. Occasionally, when a client is very obese, the gallbladder is not retrievable via laparoscopic instruments. Further, a surgeon may have difficulty accessing the gallbladder in an adult with a small frame and may need to perform the conventional open cholecystectomy.

Contraindications. A client's physical condition may not be able to withstand the stress of surgery, including loss of fluid, electrolytes, and anesthesia. Cholecystotomy, incision, and drainage of the gallbladder may be performed as an alternative procedure.

Complications. After cholecystectomy, monitor the client for the usual postoperative complications, such as hemorrhage, pneumonia, thrombophlebitis, urinary retention, and ileus. The risk of bile leakage into the abdominal cavity is more applicable to surgeries involving the gallbladder. With hemorrhage and bile leakage, the client feels severe pain and tenderness in the right upper quadrant, abdominal girth increases, bile or blood may leak from the wound, blood pressure drops, and tachycardia develops.

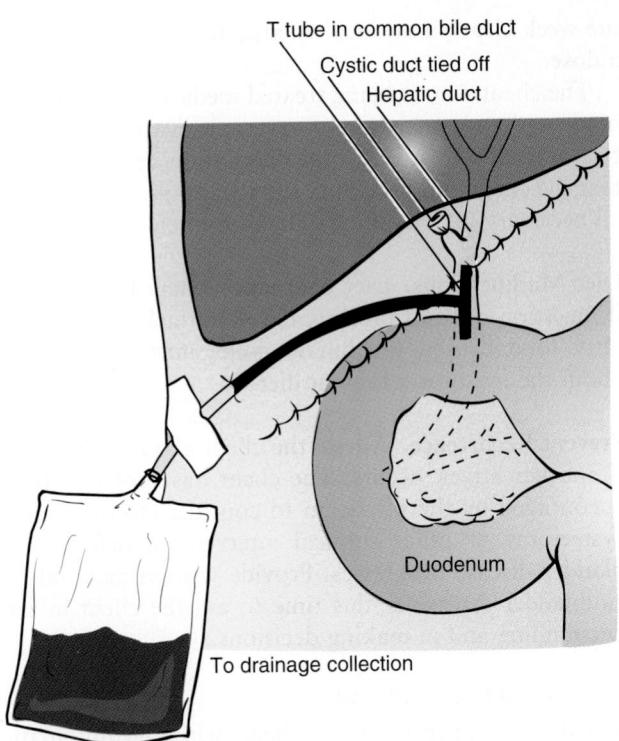

FIGURE 48-4 Placement of a T tube. The surgeon ties off the cystic duct and sutures the T tube to the common bile duct with the short arms of the T tube toward the hepatic duct and duodenum. The long arm of the T tube exits the body near the incision site. Skin suture and tape secure placement.

Outcomes. Cholecystectomy results in immediate cessation of pain in most clients and prevents development of complications such as acute cholecystitis, choledocholithiasis, and cholangitis. Persistence of manifestations after removal of the gallbladder indicates (1) a possible misdiagnosis or functional bowel disorder, such as esophagitis, peptic ulceration, pancreatitis, or irritable bowel syndrome; (2) a technical error; (3) a retained or recurrent common bile duct stone; or (4) spasm of the sphincter of Oddi. Clients must be hospitalized for about 3 days before dismissal. They may be sent home with a T tube in place for 1 to 2 weeks. When stones are present in the common bile duct, research indicates that both complications and cost can be saved if preoperative ERCP performed for suspicion of uncomplicated common bile duct stones is replaced by intraoperative cholangiography (IOC).[2]

■ Nursing Management of the Surgical Client

Preoperative Care

Preoperative care of the client facing gallbladder or biliary surgery is the same as that described in Chapter 16. In addition, preparation involves careful monitoring for early clinical findings that may indicate the onset of complications from infection or obstruction. For laparoscopic cholecystectomy, preoperative preparation involves the same measures taken for other clients going to surgery. They include (1) NPO status after midnight, (2) skin preparation (i.e., showering with antibacterial soap), (3) occasionally an enema to reduce colon mass and to reduce the chance of incontinence contaminating the operative field, and (4) sometimes an antibiotic.

Assessment

Generally, surgical management of cholelithiasis is elective and is not performed in an emergency situation unless obstruction has occurred. Consequently, although the client is typically knowledgeable about the procedure and the rationale for it, assessment of the client's knowledge of preoperative and postoperative care is needed.

Diagnosis, Outcomes, Interventions

Diagnosis: Deficient Knowledge. The preoperative client may not be completely knowledgeable about surgical procedures, particularly gallbladder surgery. The nursing diagnosis, therefore, can be *Deficient Knowledge related to gallbladder surgery and recovery.*

Outcomes. The client will indicate an understanding of the procedure, as evidenced by ability to verbalize information regarding it; will demonstrate an ability to carry out coughing, deep breathing, and leg exercises; and will have knowledge regarding the immediate postoperative course.

Interventions. Reinforce information given to the client about the surgical procedure. Determine the level of understanding and the learning needs of the client and his or her significant others. Provide material, if it is available, that can be read or viewed at the client's own pace. Give verbal instructions and a demonstration to ensure that the client can perform postoperative exercises (turning, coughing, deep breathing, and wound splinting) properly and can understand their importance.

Clients also need some knowledge of what to expect postoperatively, such as IV fluids, T-tube placement and drainage, pain control, and activity. Studies have shown that preoperative client education significantly reduces the risk for development of postoperative complications.

Diagnosis: Anxiety. Because of the surgery and associated stress, a nursing diagnosis appropriate to these clients is *Anxiety related to the procedure and outcome.*

Outcomes. The client will express and demonstrate feelings of comfort and show decreasing manifestations of anxiety as evidenced by calmly discussing his or her apprehension, affirming that anxiety is decreasing, and ventilating feelings regarding the surgical procedure and diagnosis.

Interventions. Assess the client's level of anxiety by listening and observing. Reassure the client and acknowledge that the unknown is frightening. Thoroughly explain those topics that may frighten the client, such as diagnostic or preparatory procedures. Allow significant others to stay with the client as appropriate.

Postoperative Care

Respiratory status is carefully monitored after surgery of the gallbladder or biliary tract because of the potential for development of atelectasis and pneumonia. Closely monitor drainage from all biliary tubes and drainage from the incision site, for amount, character, and color. Carefully assess cardiovascular status and manifestations of hemorrhage or shock. Hemorrhage, although rare, can occur if an inflamed gallbladder has adhered to the liver.

Analgesia for pain management is important and should be given on a regular basis to promote comfort and rest as well as to enhance the individual's ability to cough and deep breathe.

Maintain hydration and fluid balance IV until the client is no longer on NPO status and can receive fluids orally. When the client is allowed oral intake, the amount of fluid and food should be sufficient and well balanced enough to maintain renal function and body weight (minimal loss of weight). Clients are generally allowed to progress to a regular diet, with fat content included as tolerated.

Assessment

Postoperative assessment of the client is important; it includes careful monitoring of vital signs, breath and bowel sounds, and general level of responsiveness to check for complications such as hemorrhage, respiratory problems, or infection. In addition, intake is monitored to reflect renal function and output carefully measured, including wound drainage, vomiting, or nasogastric suctioning.

Assess the client's incision for redness or swelling. Monitor the level of pain as well as the location, severity, and the effectiveness of any interventions.

After a laparoscopic cholecystectomy, referred pain to the shoulder is a common postoperative pain pattern. Shoulder pain occurs because of the carbon dioxide that has not been released or absorbed by the body. Carbon dioxide causes irritation of the phrenic nerve and diaphragm and may decrease respiratory excursion.

Diagnosis, Outcomes, Interventions

Diagnosis: Risk for Injury. The postoperative client is at risk for the development of many complications leading to the nursing diagnosis *Risk for Injury related to postoperative complications of hemorrhage, infection,* *fluid and electrolyte imbalance, pulmonary changes (atelectasis, pneumonia), urinary retention, ileus, and decreased gastrointestinal motility.*

Outcomes. The client will receive appropriate assessments and interventions for early detection and prevention of injury from postoperative complications as evidenced by stable vital signs; normal pulmonary function; normal gastrointestinal function; laboratory values within normal limits; urine output of at least 0.5 ml/kg/hr; an intact incision that does not exhibit redness, odor, or purulent drainage; and no manifestations of thrombus or embolus.

Interventions

Assess Postoperatively. Take routine postoperative vital signs and assess for manifestations of shock, such as cyanosis; diaphoresis; cold, clammy skin; decreased blood pressure; and increased pulse. As vital signs are checked, check dressings and drainage tubes at the same time for unusual amounts of bleeding or drainage. If any of the aforementioned manifestations or changes occur, check vital signs frequently and notify the physician.

Prevent Pneumonia. The client should change position at least every 2 hours. While the client is awake for turning, help him or her to cough and deep breathe. Some hospitals use devices such as incentive spirometry to encourage lung expansion and spontaneous coughing. When these devices are used, it is helpful to demonstrate their use before surgery.

Auscultate the lungs for rales, rhonchi, and diminished breath sounds every 4 hours for the first 24 hours and every 8 hours thereafter. If the client had a cholecystectomy, it will be even more difficult for him or her to take deep breaths and cough because of the location of the incision. Take extra care to ensure that the client is comfortable enough to breathe normally. Many physicians and nurses believe that smaller doses of opioid given more frequently are beneficial. Splinting the incision helps as well.

Monitor Fluids and Electrolytes. Measure intake and output every 4 hours or more frequently if ordered. Assess amounts for discrepancies. Because it is not unusual for new postoperative clients to be behind on fluids for the first few hours, do not expect output to equal intake initially. Assess the client for edema along with the lung sounds every 4 hours as another assurance that the client is tolerating the fluids that are being infused.

Unless the client is otherwise compromised, such as being acutely ill at the time of surgery or having a history of other health problems (e.g., heart disease or diabetes), laboratory work probably will not be ordered until the following day. Monitor these values for indica-

tions of fluid and electrolyte imbalance (see Chapters 13 and 14).

Monitor Urine Output. Generally, the client can void within 6 hours after surgery; if not, assess the bladder for distention. The client may not to be able to void because of pain, discomfort, and position or because of an absence of feeling the need to void as a result of the effects of anesthesia and opioids. The client may need to be catheterized to empty the bladder initially.

Maintain Nasogastric Tube. Occasionally, after gallbladder surgery, the client may return with an NG tube attached to suction. Check the tube frequently to ensure that it is patent and that placement is correct for adequate drainage. A plugged or displaced tube not only causes distention, nausea, and vomiting, but it also may place undue stress on the surgical site. Auscultate bowel sounds every 4 hours to note return of normal bowel activity. Depending on the surgery, the client may or may not be allowed oral intake before bowel sounds return.

Offer oral care at least every 2 hours while the client is on NPO status. This may consist of rinsing the mouth with water, using mouthwash, swabbing with a moist swab, or assisting the client with brushing the teeth. Assess the oral mucous membranes at least every 8 hours for integrity, color, and moistness. While the client is taking nothing orally, it may be helpful to place a wet washcloth over the lips to humidify the air. Offering ice chips or sips of liquid as soon as allowed also provides much relief.

Advance Diet as Tolerated. For the more involved surgical procedure, such as a cholecystectomy, clients are usually not allowed a normal diet until they have begun to pass flatus and until bowel sounds are heard. After the client is allowed to have fluids or food, continue to assess the client for abdominal distention and normal bowel sounds to ensure that the intake is being tolerated. Because early activity also helps the return of intestinal motility, the client should be encouraged to begin progression of regular activities as soon as possible.

Prevent Infection. If the nurse is to change the dressings, the incision should be checked simultaneously for redness, swelling, drainage characteristics and amounts, and odor. If drains such as T tube are present, observe the drainage for its characteristics and amount. Check the client's temperature at least every 4 hours or more frequently if necessary. Keep the dressing and incision clean and dry because moisture enhances bacterial growth. Subjective complaints of increased pain may be the first manifestation of an infectious process taking place. For this reason, it is important to document the location, type, and amount of pain routinely so that comparison can be made and a significant change in condition can be noted immediately. Many times it is your assessment that alerts the physician and facilitates the diagnosis of infection.

Diagnosis: Acute Pain.
The client may have problems with postoperative pain. Therefore the following nursing diagnosis, *Acute Pain related to surgical procedure and incision,* is applicable.

Outcomes.
The client will feel reduction of pain, as evidenced by resting comfortably and quietly, a blood pressure and heart rate within normal limits, and the ability to tolerate postoperative exercises and activities.

Interventions.
Assess and document the level, location, and type of pain as well as the client's response to pain medication. You may need to intervene and obtain new medication orders if the ordered medication is ineffective. It may be necessary to administer medication to coincide with activity to keep the client active. Nonpharmacologic measures are also helpful. Providing a quiet environment (even limiting visitors if necessary), changing the client's position, and rubbing the client's back all are important in relaxing the client and in enhancing the effects of the pain medication. Assist the client in splinting the incision, and instruct the client on the best way to get out of bed and to lie down.

Evaluation

The client should heal without difficulty and may be discharged within about 3 to 4 days after cholecystectomy. The client will be able to resume normal activities in 4 to 6 weeks. After laparoscopic cholecystectomy, the client is usually discharged the day of or the day after surgery and can return to normal activities within 3 to 4 days.

■ Self-Care
Because the client will be faced with early discharge from the health care setting, the client should be able to verbalize and accurately demonstrate home health care needs and skills, for example, (1) identifying manifestations of infection; (2) demonstrating wound care; (3) naming medications, their purpose, side effects, and administration instructions; and (4) stating activity and dietary restrictions.

Teach the client about home health care as soon after surgery as possible to assess the client's learning potential and learning needs. Instruction should include wound care, dressing changes with a return demonstration, and assessing for manifestations of infection.

Teach Manifestations to Report. Be sure the client is knowledgeable about which manifestations should be reported to the physician and how to contact the physician. Advise the client to report fever, chills, nausea and vomiting, jaundice, dark-colored urine, pale-colored stools, and pruritus. If the client is discharged with a drain or T tube in place, he or she should know the purpose of the tube, how to secure it, how to empty it, what amounts of drainage can be expected, and abnormal characteristics of drainage.

Diet and Activity Modifications. Explain and reinforce activity and dietary restrictions thoroughly. Advise that heavy lifting (>10 pounds) or strenuous work or sports should be avoided for as long as prescribed by the physician. Instruct and question the client as to the medications he or she is being discharged with, the possible adverse effects, and the dosage and frequencies of the medications. Explain that a low-fat (to be increased gradually), a high-carbohydrate, high-protein diet is needed and that alcohol should be avoided to minimize the risk of pancreatic involvement.

■ Modifications for Older Clients
In older clients, gallstones do not necessarily cause pain, fever, or jaundice. Mental confusion, shakiness, and an elevated alkaline phosphatase may be the only manifestations of gallstones in the older population. Nonsurgical decompression techniques may be preferred in high-risk older clients.

When the older client undergoes a cholecystectomy, he or she is at greater risk for injury related to anesthesia, pain medications, and sometimes the response to the trauma of surgery. Postoperative care should be modified to prevent injury. Especially in the immediate postoperative period, the side rails should be up, the bed in low position, and the call light within easy reach.

Depending on the client's response to anesthesia and pain medication, frequent reorientation to the environment and circumstances may be necessary. In particular, be alert to the fact that older people tend to become confused after surgery, especially at night. Remind the older client how to summon help and why it is important to not get up alone. Be sure that all IV lines and drainage tubes are secure to prevent the client from inadvertently disconnecting them.

ACUTE CHOLECYSTITIS
Acute cholecystitis refers to acute inflammation of the gallbladder wall. The incidence of cholecystitis is increased in clients who are overweight, especially those with a sedentary lifestyle. Certain ethnic groups, including Chinese, Jewish, and Italians, have a higher rate of the disease.

Etiology and Risk Factors
Cholecystitis is associated with gallstones and obstruction of the cystic duct by a stone in 90% of cases.[7] Obstruction of a cystic duct by a stone is the usual cause of acute cholecystitis. In 5% to 10% of clients, however,

calculi obstructing the cystic duct are not found during surgery (*acalculous cholecystitis*, or cholecystitis without stones). In more than 50% of such cases, an underlying cause of the inflammation is not found.[8] Hepatic *Helicobacter* bacteria have been implicated in cholecystitis.

The major preventable risk factors are sedentary lifestyle and obesity. If the client increases his or her level of activity and maintains a low-fat diet, the risk of cholecystitis can be reduced. Encourage clients to engage in exercise and to follow healthy dietary habits.

Pathophysiology

Acute calculous cholecystitis, which appears to be caused by obstruction of the cystic duct, in turn causes distention of the gallbladder. Subsequently, (1) venous and lymphatic drainage is impaired, (2) proliferation of bacteria occurs, (3) localized cellular irritation or infiltration or both take place, and (4) areas of ischemia may develop. The inflamed gallbladder wall is edematous and thickened, it may have areas of gangrene, or necrosis may be present. The term *empyema* describes a gallbladder that contains pus, which is the equivalent of an intra-abdominal abscess and may be associated with severe sepsis. Recurrent episodes of acute cholecystitis cause fibrosis of the wall of the gallbladder.

Complications of untreated acute cholecystitis are usually associated with septic complications. Others are consequences of ischemia, inflammation, adhesions, and gangrene: perforation, pericholecystic abscess, and fistula.

Acalculous cholecystitis (cholecystitis without stones) is far less common than cholecystitis due to gallstones. It can be triggered by (1) multiple blood transfusions, (2) gram-negative bacterial sepsis, or (3) tissue damage after burns, trauma, or extensive surgery. Other possible contributing factors include hyperalimentation, prolonged fasting, hypotension, anesthesia, opioid analgesics, and mechanical ventilation with positive end-expiratory pressure. Clients with diabetes mellitus and systemic arteritis are also susceptible.

Clinical Manifestations

Inflammation of the gallbladder may be acute or chronic. The most common and reliable finding on physical examination is tenderness in the right upper quadrant, epigastrium, or both. Although clients with chronic and acute cholecystitis may complain of the same type of pain, the distinguishing factor is the severity and persistence of the pain. Chronic cholecystitis rarely lasts more than a few hours, whereas acute cholecystitis may last several days.

Pain in acute cholecystitis may be located in the epigastric, subscapular, or right upper quadrant regions. Sometimes the pain is referred to the right scapula. The pain usually starts suddenly, increases steadily, and reaches a peak in about 30 minutes. Abdominal examination may reveal a tender abdomen with right upper quadrant guarding. Murphy's sign may be elicited when the client is asked to take a deep breath. About 60% to 70% of clients with acute cholecystitis have experienced biliary colic episodes in the past from ductal spasm when a stone moves from the gallbladder into ducts causing waves of pain *(biliary colic)*.

In addition to pain, the following problems may be revealed in clients with acute cholecystitis:

1. Nausea and vomiting occur in about 75% of clients as a result of impulses transmitted to the vomiting center from distention of bile ducts.
2. A low-grade fever is often present from the response to inflammation, but this may be absent in older clients, immunocompromised clients, and clients receiving steroidal therapy.
3. Mild jaundice occurs in only 10% of cases.
4. Right upper quadrant tenderness, fever, and leukocytosis suggest acute cholecystitis, particularly if other assessment data support this diagnosis.

The diagnostic examination for acute cholecystitis includes the following:

1. Biliary ultrasonography is often the initial diagnostic procedure. Sonographic findings consistent with acute cholecystitis include (a) cholelithiasis, (b) focal tenderness over the gallbladder (sonographic Murphy's sign), (c) thickening of the gallbladder wall (>3 mm), and (d) distention of the gallbladder lumen (>5 cm).
2. Aminotransferase, alkaline phosphatase, and bromsulfophthalein values may be slightly abnormal. (See Chapter 44, Table 44-3 for details on each of the diagnostic tests for gallbladder and biliary disorders).
3. An abdominal x-ray study occasionally reveals the enlarged gallbladder. In 15% of cases the gallstones contain enough calcium to be visible on film.
4. CT and MRI are similar to ultrasound in visualizing gallstones but are more accurate than ultrasound in detecting acute cholecystitis complications.
5. Hepatobiliary scintigraphy (HIDA scan) (cholescintigraphy) can provide additional information (when the diagnosis is clinically obscure) by pinpointing cystic duct obstruction. Confirmation is based on nonvisualization of the gallbladder.
6. ERCP is indicated for clients with acute cholecystitis.
7. The WBC count is elevated in 85% of clients, with the exception of older clients and those receiving steroid therapy.

Outcome Management
■ Medical Management

Clients thought to have acute cholecystitis may need to be hospitalized, and initial management should include administration of antibiotics effective against organisms found in the bile in about 80% of the cases. These organisms include both gram-positive and gram-negative aerobes and anaerobes: *E. coli, Klebsiella aerogenes, S. faecalis, Clostridium welchii, Proteus* species, *Enterobacter* species, *Helicobacter* species, and anaerobic streptococci.

Antibiotics that are effective given singly include ampicillin, cephalosporins, or aminoglycosides. A combination of these drugs may be more effective in clients with diabetes mellitus or with debilitated conditions. Further medical management is the same as for symptomatic cholelithiasis (see Cholelithiasis [Gallstones]).

■ Nursing Management of the Medical Client

Assessment becomes extremely important because several other disease entities may produce the same manifestations (see Box 48-2). Collect subjective and objective data, and note the client's response to all medications.

Nursing care is the same as for the medical management of cholelithiasis except for the certainty that these clients will receive a course of antibiotics. Observe the client for the development of complications, which may include increased pain in the right upper quadrant or jaundice (from an obstruction) and decreased or absent bowel sounds (from peritonitis). For additional information on nursing management, see Nursing Management of the Medical Client under Cholelithiasis.

■ Surgical Management

Once the diagnosis of acute cholecystitis is made, the decision for early or delayed cholecystectomy depends on the risk factors. Delayed surgery is usually the correct decision for clients who have unstable angina, significant carotid artery disease, heart failure, cirrhosis, and other conditions that would increase their risk.

Cholecystectomy for the client with acute cholecystitis is more difficult than elective surgery because of the distended, inflamed gallbladder. Usually, the gallbladder must be decompressed first to allow complete visualization of all surrounding structures and to avoid injury to the extrahepatic bile ducts.

Cholecystotomy (surgical drainage of the gallbladder) is usually performed only when cholecystectomy is too dangerous, given all the risk factors. Although the procedure relieves the obstruction, the cure depends on the ability of the client's immune system to resolve the inflammatory process. Treatment of complications of cholecystotomy is usually cholecystectomy. See Nursing Management of the Surgical Client under Cholelithiasis.

ACUTE ACALCULOUS CHOLECYSTITIS

Acute acalculous cholecystitis (without stones) accounts for about 4% to 8% of all cases of acute cholecystitis. Although data are inconclusive, this condition is said to be occurring increasingly. It tends to occur after or in association with other conditions, especially major trauma, burns, or surgery. Other pre-existing conditions include the postpartum period after a prolonged childbirth, bacterial sepsis, and debilitating systemic diseases, such as cardiovascular disease, tuberculosis, and sarcoidosis. No apparent precipitating factor is present, however, in as many as 50% of the clients.

The pathologic process does not differ from that of the calculous type, although the incidence of gangrene and perforation is higher. It is debatable whether this is an inherent feature of the disease or the result of delayed diagnosis.

Recognition of the disease may be delayed when the client cannot communicate well because of concomitant disease or post-traumatic or postoperative states. The manifestations are the same as those of acute calculous cholecystitis: pain in the right upper quadrant, epigastrium, or both and vomiting. Although pain is the cardinal manifestation in the calculous type, it may be obscured or absent in acalculous cholecystitis because of opioid administration, a decreased level of consciousness, or abdominal pain from an incision or from another disease process. Significant physical findings are the same as those in acute calculous cholecystitis, and the same diagnostic procedures are used.

The standard treatment is emergency cholecystectomy because of the increased risk of gangrene and perforation.

CHRONIC CHOLECYSTITIS

Chronic cholecystitis sometimes arises as a sequela to acute cholecystitis. Typically, however, it develops independently of acute cholecystitis. In addition, it is almost always associated with gallstones. Chronic cholecystitis principally affects middle-aged and older obese women. The female-to-male ratio is 3:1.

Assessment data for chronic cholecystitis are similar to those of acute cholecystitis with certain exceptions. In chronic states, (1) the pain is less severe, (2) the temperature is not as high, and (3) the leukocyte count is lower. Vague manifestations of indigestion, epigastric pain, fat intolerance, heartburn, and flatulence accompany chronic cholecystitis. The client has usually experienced these manifestations as well as repeated attacks (mild or severe) of acute cholecystitis for a long time. Eventually, fibrous tissues begin to replace the normal muscle and mucosal tissues of the gallbladder. As a consequence, the gallbladder loses its ability to concentrate bile.

Diagnosis depends largely on ultrasonography, and other diagnostic procedures provide supplementary information. Diagnostic findings include (1) cholelithiasis, (2) gallbladder wall thickening (>3 mm), and (3) delayed visualization or nonvisualization of the gallbladder on radionuclide scanning. Scarring from chronic inflammation may partially or completely obstruct the cystic duct and thus account for this delay in visualization or nonvisualization. It may be difficult to differentiate chronic cholecystitis from other disorders. Conditions that produce manifestations similar to the manifestations of cholecystitis (acute and chronic) are listed in Box 48-2. The diagnostic process serves to rule out these conditions.

Conservative interventions include (1) a low-fat diet; (2) weight reduction; and (3) administration of anticholinergics, sedatives, and antacids. When medical intervention is ineffective, cholecystectomy may be the treatment of choice. About 90% of clients obtain relief of manifestations after cholecystectomy. Of the gallbladders removed, 95% contain stones.

CHOLEDOCHOLITHIASIS AND CHOLANGITIS

Choledocholithiasis is defined as stones in the common duct. Common bile duct calculi can arise from the gallbladder or hepatic ducts. Thus common duct stones can occur in the absence of a gallbladder and are classified as *primary. Cholangitis* is inflammation of the bile duct.

Common duct stones are found in about 15% of clients with cholelithiasis. The incidence increases with age and the frequency of gallstones in the older population may be as high as 50%.[7] Frequently, inflammation or bacteria are present, and cholangitis may develop.

Etiology and Risk Factors
The cause is essentially the same as for cholelithiasis. This condition is sometimes combined with a narrowing of the papilla, which traps stones. The risk factor for choledocholithiasis is that a small stone may pass from the gallbladder and lodge in the common bile duct.

Pathophysiology
The pathophysiology is essentially the same as for cholelithiasis. Most bile duct stones are cholesterol or mixed stones. They form in the gallbladder and move into the biliary tree through the cystic duct.

Clinical Manifestations
Common duct calculi may be asymptomatic or cause biliary colic, bile duct obstruction, cholangitis, or pancreatitis. Early manifestations of choledocholithiasis are not easily distinguished from gallbladder colic or acute cholecystitis. Pain may be mild or severe and cannot be differentiated from gallbladder pain. Jaundice is intermittent if obstruction is intermittent but may be progressive if the stone becomes impacted in the cystic duct or bile duct.

Chills and fever, frequently recurring attacks of right upper quadrant severe pain, a history of jaundice, and mild elevation of serum bilirubin are manifestations of *cholangitis.* The WBC count is normal except when cholangitis is present. It is characteristic, however, to see an elevation of serum bilirubin and alkaline phosphatase levels, which result from obstruction. The serum amylase level should always be determined to determine the presence of secondary pancreatitis.

Infrequently, manifestations of cholangitis are accompanied by shock and confusion, coma, or other central nervous system manifestations. These manifestations signal the presence of *acute toxic cholangitis,* a condition in which infected bile or pus is under pressure within the duct system. Emergency decompression of the duct system is necessary to prevent death.

To determine the diagnosis, ultrasonography, CT scan, and radionuclide imaging may be performed. Although they are not reliable for the detection of common duct stones, they can detect common duct dilation. Endoscopic retrograde cholangiography is indicated for clients with bile duct obstruction (as indicated by persistent jaundice) or bile duct dilation on ultrasonography. It allows visualization and endoscopic sphincterotomy when indicated.

Outcome Management
■ Medical Management
Medical management of pain is based on its severity and frequency and is similar to medical management described for cholelithiasis. Management of inflammation involves antibiotic therapy when cholangitis is present.

■ Surgical Management
Indications. Indications for surgical management of common duct calculi may include emergency intervention, which is rare unless severe ascending cholangitis is present. Usually, however, surgical management in some form is necessary for symptomatic choledocholithiasis.

Treatment includes hospitalization, treatment of infection, and removal of stones. The removal of stones may be accomplished surgically in clients with an intact gallbladder by cholecystectomy and choledochotomy. As many as 20% of clients undergoing cholecystectomy will prove to have common bile duct stones in addition to stones in the gallbladder. With the development and refinement of laparoscopic cholecystectomy, the management of common bile duct stones in the presence of gallstones is becoming more easily defined. To remove common bile duct stones, preoperative ERCP with endoscopic papillotomy and stone extraction followed by laparoscopic cholecystectomy is the preferred approach. Postoperative ERCP may also be done if necessary, but research indicates that when dealing with potential stones of the common bile duct, intraoperative cholangiography reduces complications and is more cost effective than performing ERCP preoperatively.

Common duct stones in a client who has previously had a cholecystectomy are best treated by endoscopic papillotomy with stone extraction is preferable to transabdominal surgery. The surgeon opens the sphincter of Oddi and allows passage of gallstones up to 1 cm. The success rate is about 90%. Extracorporeal shock wave lithotripsy is used when stones are too large to extract via the endoscopic approach. Success can be achieved in 70% to 85% of these complicated cases. Most common duct stones are found and removed at the time of cholecystectomy.

Liver function should be thoroughly evaluated preoperatively by measuring the prothrombin time. If results are abnormal, function should be restored to normal with administration of vitamin K. Antimicrobial agents (e.g., mezlocillin IV along with either metronidazole or gentamicin IV) should be given.

Another procedure, *choledochostomy,* consists of opening the common duct surgically, removing stones, and inserting a T tube for drainage. Choledochostomy may be performed in conjunction with cholecystectomy. Otherwise, cholecystectomy may be necessary at a later date.

Postoperative antibiotics are not usually given after biliary tract surgery unless specimens of the bile obtained for culture during the surgery are positive for organisms.

Contraindications. Contraindications to surgical management of choledocholithiasis include older clients and those who are poor surgical risks.

Complications. Surgical traumas or the presence of stones may result in ductal edema after choledochostomy. Inserting a T tube prevents bile from spilling into the peritoneal cavity and maintains patency of the duct (see Figure 48-4). T tubes may be attached to continuous gravity drainage or to collapsible bags in the dressing site.

Avoid tension on long tubing and obstruction by kinking. Carefully measure drainage from the T tube. The tube usually drains 300 to 500 ml in the first 24 hours. This amount decreases to less than 200 ml after 3 to 4 days. Record the volume and color of the drainage. To prevent excessive loss of bile, place the drainage bag for the T tube at the level of the abdomen rather than hanging the bag below the bed. At this height, bile flows into the bag only when pressure is high in the biliary tree.

Excessive T-tube drainage may indicate obstruction. Occasionally, it signals development of a biliary fistula. Excessive bile losses may necessitate recycling the client's bile drainage. The bile may be returned to the client through an NG tube or orally in fruit juice.

Thick bile or bile containing blood clots may prevent drainage or cause inadequate amounts of drainage from the T tube. Without intervention, bile may begin to leak from the choledochotomy site instead of through the T tube. To prevent this problem, the physician may decide to irrigate the tube with sterile saline.

On rare occasions, tube dislodgment causes failure of the T tube to drain. The tube may dislodge from the common duct when the client moves from a supine to a sitting position. This complication may result from excessive tension during T-tube insertion in surgery.

After a few days, the T tube will probably be clamped during meals to aid fat digestion.

The tube remains in place for about 10 days. A T-tube cholangiogram should be done on or about the seventh or eighth postoperative day to assess for bile duct obstruction. When the T-tube cholangiogram indicates absence of obstruction, the surgeon may decide to remove the T tube. If a retained stone is discovered during cholangiography, the client may go home with the T tube in place. The surgeon may remove the stone through the T-tube tract with a catheter later.

Outcomes. When stones are extracted, the client is likely to experience a reduction in pain and a general increase in well-being and quality of life. Encourage the client to increase his or her level of activity and maintain a low-fat diet to reduce the risk of forming additional future stones.

■ Nursing Management of the Surgical Client
Nursing management is the same as for the client with a cholecystectomy.

SCLEROSING CHOLANGITIS
Sclerosing cholangitis is an uncommon inflammatory disease of the bile ducts that causes fibrosis and thickening of their walls and multiple short, concentric strictures. The disease is progressive and gradually causes cirrhosis, portal hypertension, and death from hepatic failure. It may also predispose the client to the development of cholangiocarcinoma. Some cases are associated with inflammatory bowel disease, especially ulcerative colitis. Sclerosing cholangitis and papillary stenosis are important complications of acquired immunodeficiency syndrome (AIDS). In addition, cytomegalovirus and cryptosporidium are observed frequently in such clients, indicating that these organisms may be involved in causing primary sclerosing cholangitis.

The cause has been linked to altered immunity, toxins, and infectious agents. Clients often have the hepatocompatible antigen human leukocyte antigen-B (HLA-B), suggesting that genetic factors may play a role. The disease is most common in men 20 to 40 years of age. The male-to-female ratio is 3:2.

Usually clients present with fatigue, anorexia, weight loss, jaundice, and pruritus. They sometimes complain of vague upper abdominal pain. The diagnosis is usually made by endoscopic retrograde cholangiography, clinical findings, and liver biopsy.

Medical management consists of corticosteroids and broad-spectrum antimicrobial therapy with inconsistent, unpredictable results when cholangitis is a recurrent problem. Immunosuppressants, bile acid-binding agents, colchicine, and penicillamine have also been used with inconsistent and unpredictable results. These agents do not alter the slow, progressive course of the disease. Ursodiol, which improves primary biliary cirrhosis, is now being evaluated in the treatment of sclerosing cholangitis. Ursodiol may improve liver function test results but does not appear to alter the natural history of the disease. Cholestyramine may help control the pruritus.

The success of surgical intervention is limited by the progressive nature of the disease and the recurrent cholangitis. Surgery is generally limited to procedures to open the ducts. Cholecystectomy should not be performed unless there is definite evidence of cholecystitis or cholelithiasis. Although surgical therapy may be life saving in some circumstances, it has to be considered palliative in the overall context of the disease. The definitive management of these clients is liver transplantation, which is the procedure of choice. Survival rates with transplantation are 85% at 3 years.[7]

CARCINOMA OF THE GALLBLADDER

Although cancer of the gallbladder is the most common malignant lesion of the biliary tract, it accounts for only 5% of all cancers at autopsy. Most cancers of the gallbladder develop in conjunction with stones rather than polyps. Of all clients with this malignancy, 91% are older than 50 years of age, and the incidence in women is four times that of men; however, the incidence of bile duct cancer is predominant in men. Native Americans, Hispanics, northeastern Europeans, Israelis, and Japanese immigrants to the United States are at greatest risk for cancer of the gallbladder. At least 70% of these clients have gallstones. Adenocarcinoma accounts for 82% of all cases.

The clinical presentation differs according to stage of the disease. There is no distinct pattern because the manifestations depend on the site of the lesion, its extent, and the presence or absence of pre-existing biliary manifestations. Usually, however, the clinical manifestations are unrelenting right upper quadrant pain, weight loss, jaundice, and a palpable right upper quadrant mass.

At this point, treatment modalities and their effectiveness are widely debated. Treatment varies from radical resection, to palliative relief of duct obstruction, to chemotherapy or radiation. None of the treatments have been found to increase survival.

The prognosis for cancer of the gallbladder is poor. About 95% of clients with unresectable disease die within the first year, and fewer than 5% are alive at 5 years.[5] Trials of radiation and chemotherapy in clients with primary gallbladder cancer have been disappointing. The long-term survivors are generally those in whom the diagnosis of cancer had not been made before cholecystectomy was performed and was determined by pathologic study.

CONCLUSIONS

Biliary and exocrine pancreatic disorders are common but are extremely complex and diverse. Some of these conditions are treated without further difficulty, such as cholecystitis, whereas others can become chronic and lead to a wide variety of other problems, such as pancreatitis. Teaching is vital to the care of these clients, and the nurse must understand these conditions to initiate appropriate teaching plans.

THINKING CRITICALLY *evolve*

1. You are assigned to care for a 35-year-old writer who has been admitted with severe upper abdominal pain radiating to his back and recurrent vomiting. This is his second admission for pancreatitis. He admits to drinking 1 pint of whiskey daily on the weekends and having several drinks nightly on weekdays. His alcohol intake has been greater in the past. Laboratory data include an amylase level of 750 units/L (normal, 25 to 125 units); lipase is 5.6 units/ml (normal, 10 to 140 units); aspartate aminotransferase (AST), 150 units/L (normal, 5 to 40 units); and alanine aminotransferase (ALT), 60 units (normal, 1 to 45 units). How do you feel about caring for this client?

Factors to Consider. Are you comfortable with the client's lifestyle? Do the biochemical studies support a diagnosis of pancreatitis? What do you need to consider if he complains of pain? What should you do if you discover he is allergic to meperidine? Should a nagogastric tube be inserted?

2. A 45-year-old woman is admitted to the hospital complaining of colicky pain in the right upper abdominal quadrant. She states that the pain is worse when she eats fried foods. She also states that she has vomited on several occasions, and it seems to relieve her manifestations. What are your priorities in assessing and caring for the client?

Factors to Consider. What types of diagnostic procedures should be scheduled? Why is an accurate assessment of the clinical manifestations important? What indications warrant insertion of a nasogastric tube?

3. A 70-year-old woman comes to the emergency department with complaints of recurrent episodes of epigastric pain during the past 9 months. Chills, fever, and jaundice have occurred for the first time and have persisted for 4 days. Her white blood cell count is normal. Serum bilirubin and alkaline phosphatase values are elevated. There is no history of alcoholism, blood transfusions, or hepatitis. The client takes no medications except an occasional "Bufferin for my arthritis."

Her past medical history is unremarkable except for a cholecystectomy 10 years ago after an episode of cholecystitis. What are the priorities for care?

Factors to Consider. What are the client's clinical manifestations? Would surgical treatment alleviate the problem? What might cause stricture of the bile ducts?

Discussions for these questions can be found on the website and the CD-ROM.

BIBLIOGRAPHY

1. Ackley, B.J., & Ladwig, G.B. (2002). *Nursing diagnosis handbook.* St. Louis: Mosby.

 2. Barwood, N.T., et al. (2002). Changing methods of imaging the common bile duct in the laparoscopic cholecystectomy era in western Australia: Implications for surgical practice [Abstract]. *Journal of the American Medical Association, 287*(14), 1779.

3. Conwell, D. (2001). Diseases of the pancreas. In T.E. Andreoli, et al. (Eds.), *Cecil essentials of medicine* (5th ed., pp. 356-363). Philadelphia: W.B. Saunders.

4. Copstead, L.C., & Banasik, J.L. (2000). *Pathophysiology: Biological and behavioral perspectives* (2nd ed.). Philadelphia: W.B. Saunders.

5. Dienstag, J.L., & Isselbacher, K.J. (2001). Tumors of the liver and biliary tract. In E. Braunwald, et al. (Eds.), *Harrison's principles of internal medicine* (15th ed., pp. 588-591). New York: McGraw-Hill.

6. Fletcher, D.R., et al. (1999). Complications of cholecystectomy: Risks of the laparoscopic approach and protective effects of operative cholangiography: A population-based study [Abstract]. *Journal of the American Medical Association, 281*(22), 2072.

7. Friedman, L.S. (2002). Liver, biliary tract, and pancreas. In L.M. Tierney, S.J. McPhee, & M.A. Papadakis (Eds.), *Current medical diagnosis and treatment* (41st ed. pp. 675-720). New York: Lange Medical.

8. Greenberger, N.J., & Paumgartner, G. (2001). Diseases of the gallbladder and bile ducts. In E. Braunwald, S., et al. (Eds.), *Harrison's principles of internal medicine* (15th ed., pp. 1776-1788). New York: McGraw-Hill.

9. Greenberger, N.J., & Toskes, P.P. (2001). Acute and chronic pancreatitis. In E. Braunwald, et al. (Eds.), *Harrison's principles of internal medicine* (15th ed., pp. 1792-1804). New York: McGraw-Hill.

10. Guyton, A.C., & Hall, J.E. (2000). *Textbook of medical physiology* (10th ed.). Philadelphia: W.B. Saunders.

11. Hubbard, G., & Wolfe, K. (2003). Meperidine misuse in a patient with sphincter of Oddi dysfunction. *The Annals of Pharmacotherapy, 37*(4), 534-537.

12. Kalloo, A., & Kantsevoy, S. (2001). Gallstones and biliary diseases. In M. Borum (Ed.), *Primary Care, 28*(3), 591-606.

13. Leitzmann, M.F., et al. (1999). A prospective study of coffee consumption and the risk of symptomatic gallstone disease in men. *Journal of the American Medical Association, 281*(22), 2106-2112.

14. Malka, D., et al. (1998). Chronic obstructive pancreatitis due to a pancreatic cyst in a patient with autosomal dominant polycystic kidney disease. *Gut, 42*(1), 131-134.

15. Mayer, R.J. (2001). Pancreatic cancer. In E. Braunwald, et al. (Eds.), *Harrison's principles of internal medicine* (15th ed., pp. 591-593). New York: McGraw-Hill.

16. McCance, K.L., & Huether, S.E. (2002). *Pathophysiology: The biologic basis for disease in adults and children* (4th ed.). St. Louis: Mosby.

17. Michaud, D.S., et al. Physical activity, obesity, height, and the risk of pancreatic cancer. *Journal of the American Medical Association, 286*(8), 921-929.

18. Pagana, K.I., & Pagana, T.J. (2002). *Manual of diagnostic and laboratory tests.* St. Louis: Mosby.

19. Schlapman, N. (2001). Spotting acute pancreatitis. *RN, 64*(11), 55-59.

20. Sommers, M.S., & Johnson, S.A. (2002). *Diseases and disorders: A nursing therapeutic manual* (2nd ed.). Philadelphia: F.A. Davis.

21. Stevens, M., Esler, R., & Asher, G. (2002). Transdermal fentanyl for management of acute pancreatitis pain. *Applied Nursing Research, 15*(2), 102-110.

22. Topazian, M. (2001). Gastrointestinal endoscopy. In E. Braunwald, A.S., et al. (Eds.), *Harrison's principles of internal medicine* (15th ed., pp. 1635-1642). New York: McGraw-Hill.

23. Toskes, P.P., & Greenberger, N.J. (2001). Approach to the patient with pancreatic disease. In E. Braunwald, et al. (Eds.), *Harrison's principles of internal medicine* (15th ed., pp. 1788-1792). New York: McGraw-Hill.

24. Yeo, C.J., & Cameron, J.L. (2001). Exocrine pancreas. In C.M. Townsend, et al. (Eds.), *Sabiston textbook of surgery* (16th ed., pp. 1112-1143). Philadelphia: W.B. Saunders.

Did you remember to check out the bonus material on the Evolve website and the CD-ROM, including free self-assessment exercises?

Management of Clients with Hepatic Disorders

Dianne M. Smolen

evolve

Web Enhancements

http://evolve.elsevier.com/Black/medsurg/

Case Study
  Cirrhosis
Concept Map
  Understanding Cirrhosis and Its Treatment

Ethical Issues in Nursing
  Do Nurses Have an Obligation to Care for a Client with a
    Lifestyle Issue?
Appendix C
  Laboratory Values of Clinical Importance in Medical-Surgical
    Nursing

The liver plays a central role in many essential physiologic processes. It is the primary organ of lipid synthesis, and it detoxifies endogenous and exogenous substances such as hormones, drugs, and poisons. When the normal physiologic processes are altered, numerous hepatic and extrahepatic manifestations of liver disease appear. These manifestations offer the initial clue to liver disease, regardless of the cause.

This chapter describes the clinical features of liver diseases, their medical and surgical management, and measures the nurse can take to assist clients with such nursing diagnoses as *Impaired Skin Integrity, Excess Fluid Volume, Fatigue, and Imbalanced Nutrition: Less than Body Requirements.*

JAUNDICE

Jaundice, or icterus, is the yellow pigmentation of the sclerae, skin, and deeper tissues caused by excessive accumulation of bile pigments in the blood. It is a common manifestation of a variety of liver and biliary diseases and serves as a starting point for evaluating many of these disorders. *Bilirubin* (bile pigment), a product of red blood cell (RBC) breakdown, is deposited in the skin and excreted in the urine when present in the blood in excessive amounts *(hyperbilirubinemia).* This characteristic makes jaundice a valuable indicator of a variety of disorders involving either hemolysis or biliary obstruction. When there is an obstruction blocking the flow of bile into the intestine, jaundiced clients also may have clay-colored stools owing to lack of bilirubin and its metabolites in the intestine (see Table 49-1).

Bilirubin is formed from the breakdown of hemoglobin from RBCs by macrophages. This unconjugated bilirubin, measured as "indirect bilirubin," is not water soluble, cannot be filtered in the kidney, and thus is not excreted in the urine. Normally the unconjugated bilirubin returns to the liver via the bloodstream and is conjugated with glucuronic acid to form conjugated bilirubin (measured as "direct bilirubin"), which is water soluble. The conjugated bilirubin travels to the gallbladder and eventually to the intestines. In the bowel, bacterial action converts bilirubin to urobilinogen. A small amount of urobilinogen is absorbed into the bloodstream to be returned to the liver or excreted in the urine.

Nursing Outcomes Classification (NOC)
for Nursing Diagnoses—Clients with Hepatic Disorders

Activity Intolerance
Activity Tolerance
Endurance
Energy Conservation
Self-Care: Activities of Daily Living (ADL)

Acute Confusion
Cognitive Ability
Distorted Thought Control
Information Processing
Memory
Neurologic Status: Consciousness
Safety Behavior: Personal
Sleep

Anxiety
Anxiety Control
Aggression Control
Coping
Impulse Control

Deficient Fluid Volume
Electrolyte and Acid-Base Balance
Fluid Balance
Hydration
Nutritional Status: Food and Fluid
   Intake

Disturbed Body Image
Body Image
Distorted Thought Control
Grief Resolution
Psychosocial Adjustment: Life Change
Self-Esteem

Excess Fluid Volume
Electrolyte and Acid-Base Balance
Fluid Balance
Hydration

Fatigue
Endurance
Concentration
Energy Conservation
Nutritional Status: Energy

**Imbalanced Nutrition: Less Than Body
Requirements**
Nutritional Status
Nutritional Status: Food and Fluid
   Intake
Nutritional Status: Nutrient Intake
Weight Control

Impaired Gas Exchange
Respiratory Status: Gas Exchange
Respiratory Status: Ventilation
Electrolyte and Acid-Base Balance
Tissue Perfusion: Pulmonary
Vital Signs Status

Impaired Skin Integrity
Tissue Integrity: Skin and Mucous
   Membranes
Wound Healing: Primary Intention
Wound Healing: Secondary Intention

Ineffective Breathing Pattern
Respiratory Status: Airway Patency
Respiratory Status: Ventilation
Vital Signs Status

**Ineffective Family Therapeutic
Regimen Management**
Health Orientation
Health Promoting Behavior
Health Seeking Behavior
Knowledge: Treatment Regimen
Participation: Health Care Decisions

Treatment Behavior: Illness or Injury

Ineffective Health Maintenance
Health Beliefs: Perceived Resources
Health-Promoting Behavior
Health-Seeking Behavior

Ineffective Protection
Abuse Protection
Immune Status
Coagulation Status
Endurance

**Ineffective Therapeutic Regimen
Management**
Decision Making
Knowledge: Disease Process
Knowledge: Treatment Regimen
Participation: Health Care Decisions
Symptom Severity
Treatment Behavior: Illness or Injury

Ineffective Tissue Perfusion
Circulation Status
Cardiac Pump Effectiveness
Tissue Perfusion: Cardiac
Tissue Perfusion: Cerebral
Tissue Perfusion: Peripheral
Fluid Balance
Hydration
Urinary Elimination

Risk for Injury
Immune Status
Safety Behavior: Home Physical
   Environment
Safety Behavior: Personal
Safety Status: Falls Occurrence
Safety Status: Physical Injury

Etiology and Risk Factors

The cause of jaundice may be described according to the location of the pathologic change. It may occur because of a problem (1) outside the liver (resulting in unconjugated hyperbilirubinemia, in which the accumulated bilirubin is predominantly of the unconjugated type); or (2) in the liver or biliary tract (resulting in conjugated hyperbilirubinemia, with predominantly conjugated bilirubin). When the problem is in the liver or biliary tract, the cause may be hereditary cholestatic syndromes, hepatocellular dysfunction, or biliary obstruction.

Pathophysiology

The underlying pathophysiologic mechanism in jaundice relates to whether the jaundice results from the accumu-

lation of predominantly unconjugated or conjugated bilirubin in the serum.

Unconjugated Hyperbilirubinemia

Unconjugated hyperbilirubinemia may result from the overproduction of bilirubin as a result of hemolysis, from impaired hepatic uptake of bilirubin caused by certain drugs, or from impaired conjugation of bilirubin by glucuronide, as in Gilbert's syndrome, Crigler-Najjar syndrome, or drug reactions.

Conjugated Hyperbilirubinemia

Conjugated hyperbilirubinemia may result from the impaired excretion of bilirubin from the liver resulting from hepatocellular disease, drugs, sepsis, hereditary dis-

TABLE 49-1	*Types of Jaundice*
Types of Jaundice	**Location and Cause**
Unconjugated hyperbilirubinemia (predominant indirect-acting bilirubin)	**Increased Bilirubin Production** Hemolysis (e.g., spherocytosis, autoimmune disorders) Ineffective erythropoiesis (e.g., megaloblastic anemias, hematoma) **Decreased Hepatic Uptake** Gilbert's syndrome Drugs (e.g., rifampin, radiographic contrast agents) Neonatal **Decreased conjugation** Gilbert's syndrome Crigler-Najjar syndrome types I and II Neonatal jaundice Hepatocellular disease Drug inhibition (e.g., chloramphenicol)
Conjugated hyperbilirubinemia (predominant direct-acting bilirubin)	**Impaired Hepatic Excretion** Familial disorders (e.g., Dubin-Johnson syndrome, Rotor's syndrome, benign recurrent cholestasis, cholestasis of pregnancy) Hepatocellular disease Drug-induced cholestasis Primary biliary cirrhosis Sepsis Postoperative **Extrahepatic ("Mechanical") Biliary Obstruction** Gallstones Tumors of the head of the pancreas Tumors of bile ducts Tumors of the ampulla of Vater Biliary strictures (postcholecystectomy, primary sclerosing cholangitis) **Congenital Disorders** Biliary atresia

Data from Fallon, M.B., et al. (2001). Jaundice. In T.E. Andreoli, C.C. Carpenter, R.C. Griggs, et al. (Eds.), *Cecil essentials of medicine* (5th ed., pp. 371-375). Philadelphia: W.B. Saunders; and Friedman, L.S. (2002). Liver, biliary tract, and pancreas. In L.M. Tierney, S.J. McPhee, & M.A. Papadakis (Eds.), *Current medical diagnosis and treatment* (41st ed., pp. 675-720). New York: Lange Medical.

orders such as Dubin-Johnson syndrome, or extrahepatic biliary obstruction. The pathologic mechanism in conjugated hyperbilirubinemia varies according to the type of jaundice (mechanisms are summarized in Table 49-1). See Chapter 44, Table 44-2, for laboratory test results pertinent to liver disorders.

Hereditary Cholestatic Syndromes

Jaundice related to hereditary cholestatic syndromes or intrahepatic cholestasis (stagnation of bile in liver or bile ducts) results from faulty excretion of bilirubin conjugates, as in conditions such as Dubin-Johnson syndrome or Rotor's syndrome.

Hepatocellular Disease

Hepatocellular jaundice is due to defective uptake, conjugation, or transport of bilirubin by the liver. Liver cell

dysfunction or necrosis caused by hepatitis, for example, or defective bile transport in the bile canal and small bile duct can cause hyperbilirubinemia. Unknown channels absorb the pooled bile components into the bloodstream. Although *obstructive jaundice* usually refers to jaundice caused by an obstruction, such as a stone, hepatic cellular damage can also result in obstruction sufficient to cause jaundice.

Biliary Obstruction

Biliary obstruction, the cause of obstructive jaundice, results from impaired bilirubin transport and excretion in the biliary system. In this case, the problem arises from obstruction of an extrahepatic bile duct by gallstones.

Clinical Manifestations

Manifestations of jaundice include yellow sclerae, yellowish orange skin, clay-colored feces, tea-colored urine, *pru-*

ritus (itching), fatigue, and anorexia. Features of laboratory diagnostic tests used to identify the underlying cause and type of jaundice are found in Chapter 44, Table 44-2.

Outcome Management
■ Medical Management

Determine the Cause of Jaundice. An early goal in managing jaundice is to determine which category of disease explains the client's jaundice. The clinical evaluation is an important element in this determination and includes a carefully documented health history, physical examination, basic tests of liver function, and a complete blood count (CBC). Additional tests, such as imaging studies, serologic tests, and laboratory pathologic evaluation, may be required.

The health history should focus on specific manifestations, including the presence and character of pain, fever, or other manifestations of active inflammation and changes in appetite, weight, and bowel habits. The clinical evaluation should focus on features of the client's illness that point to hereditary cholestatic syndromes, hepatocellular disease, or biliary obstruction.

Reduce Pruritus and Maintain Skin Integrity. Pruritus, caused by an accumulation of bile salts in the skin, results from obstructed biliary excretion. Some clients experience only mild itching; others suffer such extreme itching that they tear at their skin or scratch during sleep. If skin lesions develop and become infected, antibiotics may be ordered.

Oral cholestyramine resin provides some relief by binding bile salts in the intestine so that they can be excreted. Antihistamines and phenobarbital (which enhances bile flow) may also relieve itching.

■ Nursing Management of the Medical Client
Assessment

The client should be observed closely for development of jaundice. Often the first manifestation the client notices is a change in taste, manifested as a distaste for a food or drink the client previously liked, such as coffee. Pruritus is another early manifestation of incipient jaundice. Check the sclerae daily for the development of yellow coloration.

Diagnosis, Outcomes, Interventions

Diagnosis: Impaired Skin Integrity. The most common nursing diagnosis for the client with jaundice is *Impaired Skin Integrity related to pruritus.*

Outcomes. The client's itching will be controlled as evidenced by the client's statements of relief, decreased dryness of skin, maintenance of skin and mucous membrane integrity, and a decrease in scratching.

Interventions. Administer antihistamines and phenobarbital as prescribed to relieve the itching. For clients with extreme itching, administer oral cholestyramine resin to bind with bile salts in the intestine so that they can be excreted. Suggest other interventions, including tepid water or emollient baths, avoidance of alkaline soap, and frequent application of lotions. Encourage the client to wear loose, soft clothing. Provide soft bed linens (cotton is best), and change soiled linens as soon as possible. Keep the room cool.

Diagnosis: Disturbed Body Image. Clients with jaundice often experience problems associated with the nursing diagnosis *Disturbed Body Image related to yellowing of skin and sclerae.*

Outcomes. Clients will cope with body image disturbance as evidenced by clients not isolating themselves, verbalizing and demonstrating acceptance of appearance (grooming, dress, posture, eating patterns, and self-presentation), and initiating or reestablishing support systems.

Interventions. Reassure the client that the discoloration is usually temporary. Assist the client in personal hygiene as needed, and promote activity as tolerated. Encourage clients to express their feelings about their self-image.

Diagnosis: Ineffective Health Maintenance. Clients with jaundice may lack understanding of the condition, leading to the nursing diagnosis *Ineffective Health Maintenance related to lack of knowledge of jaundice.*

Outcomes. The client will understand the cause of jaundice as evidenced by the client's statements and ability to define the illness.

Interventions. Clients often wonder why they have jaundice, how long the condition will last, and how to cope with the problem. Encourage clients with jaundice to ask questions about their health, treatment, and progress.

Evaluation

Jaundice should resolve with treatment of the underlying condition. It usually begins to disappear within 4 to 6 weeks. The return of normal stool and urine color is an indication of resolution. As the jaundice lessens, the client's appetite and body image improve and the pruritus subsides.

■ Surgical Management

Surgical exploration of the common bile duct (choledochostomy) enables the diagnostician to differentiate *choledocholithiasis* (stone in the common bile duct) from tumor. If carcinoma (usually of the head of the pancreas) is discovered during exploration, the surgeon may perform a palliative anastomosis of the gallbladder to the jejunum to bypass the common bile duct. Chapter 48 describes surgical management of the client undergoing a choledochostomy.

HEPATITIS

Simply stated, *hepatitis* is inflammation of the liver. This inflammation may be caused by viruses, toxins, or chemicals (including drugs). Jaundice usually develops, and the liver is tender. Other manifestations depend on the causative agent and the degree of organ disruption. There are several types of hepatitis, such as viral, toxic, chronic, and alcoholic.

VIRAL HEPATITIS

Viral hepatitis occurs worldwide. It is the most common blood-borne infection in the United States and many parts of the world. The most common of types of hepatitis are hepatitis A virus (HAV), hepatitis B virus (HBV), hepatitis C virus (HCV), hepatitis D virus (delta agent), and hepatitis E virus—which cause hepatitis A through E, respectively. A sixth agent, hepatitis F virus, and a seventh agent, hepatitis G, have been discovered, but they are not considered serious health threats. Agents other than hepatitis A through G that may cause viral hepatitis include rubella virus, varicella virus, retroviruses, yellow fever virus, adenoviruses, and Marburg virus. Epstein-Barr virus (which causes infectious mononucleosis), cytomegalovirus, and herpes simplex are other possible causes of viral hepatitis, especially in immunocompromised people.

Etiology, Risk Factors, and Transmission

Although the manifestations of infection are similar in hepatitis A through E plus F and G, the conditions differ related to incubation period, mode of transmission, severity, and prevention. Table 49-2 describes basic information about the various hepatitis viruses, and additional information is presented in the following paragraphs.

Hepatitis A

Hepatitis A, also known as *infectious hepatitis,* is caused by an RNA virus of the enterovirus family. Causes of epidemics include infected water, milk, and food, and especially raw shellfish from contaminated waters. People who work with animals imported from areas where hepatitis A is endemic are at increased risk, as are people who eat raw or steamed shellfish. In the general population, children under 15 years of age are at most risk.

Hepatitis A may spread to other household members before the onset of manifestations.

Hepatitis B

The major sources of HBV are carriers and clients in the acute phase of the infection. Contact with the serum of an infected person is the major mode of transmission. The virus also can be transmitted by other body fluids such as saliva and semen. HBV can survive on environmental surfaces for at least a week.

Hepatitis C

Intravenous (IV) drug use accounts for 60% of HCV transmission in the United States. The risks related to injecting (and intranasal) drug use is that shared drug paraphernalia used to prepare or inject the drug may have become contaminated with HCV. Tattooing and body-piercing tools contaminated with small amounts of blood may also contribute to HCV infection. The tattoo artist or piercer must use good health practices such as hand-washing, disposable gloves, and sterilized or disposable tattooing needles. Like hepatitis B, HCV may be spread by carriers, parenterally transmitted with risk factors similar to those for hepatitis B. See the Evidence-Based Practice in Action feature on Mass Screening for Hepatitis C: Is It Necessary? on p. 1326.

Hepatitis D

Hepatitis D is transmitted only through blood contact and is thus seen most commonly in clients exposed to blood and blood products, such as IV drug users and people with hemophilia.

Hepatitis E

The hepatitis E virus is rare in the United States. This form of hepatitis primarily affects young adults. It has a short incubation, and there is no evidence that it becomes chronic.

Hepatitis F

Hepatitis F seems to be similar to hepatitis A and E in its mode of transmission. There is no serologic test for hepatitis F, and diagnosis is by electron microscopic identification of the virus.

Hepatitis G

Hepatitis G is spread through contact with blood, blood products, and body fluids. Most clients are asympto-

TABLE 49-2	*Comparison of Seven Types of Viral Hepatitis*		
Factor	Hepatitis A (HAV)	Hepatitis B (HBV)	Hepatitis C (HCV)
Occurrence	Epidemic in areas of poor sanitation; common in fall and early winter	World-wide, especially in drug addicts, homosexuals, people exposed to blood and blood products; occurs all year	Post-transfusion, those working around blood and blood products, IV drug users; occurs all year
Incubation period	About 30 days	6 weeks to 6 months; mean 12-14 weeks	6-7 weeks
Risk factors/high-risk groups	Close personal contact or by handling feces-contaminated wastes; poor sanitation; people who work with animals from HAV endemic areas or who eat raw or steamed shellfish	Health care workers in contact with body secretions, blood, and blood products; hemodialysis and post-transfusion clients; homosexually active males and drug abusers	Similar to that for hepatitis B; also, IV drug use, intranasal cocaine use, body piercing, multiple sex partners
Transmission	Infected feces, fecal-oral route; may be airborne if copious secretions; shellfish from contaminated water; no carrier state	Most cases in United States now result from heterosexual transmission; contact with blood and body fluids; carrier state	Contact with blood and body fluids; source of infection uncertain in many clients; carrier state
Severity	Mortality low; rarely causes fulminating hepatic failure	More serious, may be fatal	Can lead to chronic hepatitis
Diagnostic tests	Anti-HAV-IgM-positive in acute hepatitis; IgG-positive after infection	HBsAg, HBV-DNA, anti-HBc-IgM, HbeAg, anti-HBsAg	Anti-HCV or anti-HDV, HCV RNA
Prophylaxis and active or passive immunity	Hygiene; immune globulin (passive), inactivated hepatitis A vaccine (active)	Hygiene, avoidance of risk factors; HBIG (passive), recombinant hepatitis B vaccine (active), hepatitis B vaccine (passive)	Hygiene anti-HCV interferon alfa-2b in combination with ribavirin (Rebetol)

Modified from Friedman, L.S. (2002). Liver, biliary tract, and pancreas. In L.M. Tierney, S.J. McPhee, & M.A. Papadakis (Eds.). *Medical diagnosis and treatment* (41st ed., pp. 675-720). New York: Lange Medical.
anti-HAV, Antibody to hepatitis A virus; *anti-HBc-IgM,* antibody to hepatitis B-IgM; *HbeAg,* hepatitis Be antigen; *anti-HCV,* antibody to hepatitis C virus; *anti-HDV,* antibody to hepatitis D virus; *anti-HEV,* antibody to hepatitis E virus; *HBsAg,* hepatitis B surface antigen; *anti-HGV,* antibody to hepatitis G virus; *HBIG,* hepatitis B immune globulin; *RNA,* ribonucleic acid; *IV,* intravenous; *anti-HBsAg,* anti-hepatitis B surface antigen; *anti-HAV-IgM,* antibody to hepatitis A virus–immune globulin M; *HDAg,* hepatitis D antigen.

matic, and chronic infection develops in 90% to 100% of infected individuals.

Prevention

To a great extent, viral hepatitis can be prevented by proper controls within the home, community, and health care facility setting. For all types of hepatitis, strict isolation of clients is not necessary, but hand-washing after bowel movements is required. Thorough hand-washing by all caregivers and attendants who come into contact with contaminated utensils, bedding, or clothing is nec-

essary. Clients with HBV and HCV should not share razors, toothbrushes, washcloths, cigarettes, or other personal items.

For the hepatitis viruses transmitted by the serum of infected people (hepatitis B, C, D, and G), medical personnel must use all necessary precautions with skin-piercing needles or instruments, for example, not recapping used needles. In addition, proper screening of blood and blood donors is essential as is sharing of accurate records between institutions (see Table 49-2).

Hepatitis D (Delta Hepatitis)	Hepatitis E (HEV)	Hepatitis F	Hepatitis G (HGV)
Hepatitis D virus causes hepatitis only in association with hepatitis B virus and only in presence of HBsAg	Parts of Asia, Africa, India, and Mexico where there is poor sanitation	Is rare and difficult to diagnose because of lack of testing methods	Associated with chronic viremia lasting 10 years; rarely causes frank hepatitis
New cases now infrequent; same as for hepatitis B	14-60 days; mean 40 days	—	—
Same as for hepatitis B	Traveling or living in areas where incidence is high	—	Health care workers in hemodialysis, IV drug users, hemodialysis clients, chronic hepatitis B or C clients
Co-infects with hepatitis B; close personal contact; carrier state	Fecal-oral route, food- or water-borne; no carrier state	—	Percutaneous
Similar to hepatitis B; more severe if occurs with chronic hepatitis B; increased risk of hepatocellular carcinoma	Illness self-limiting; mortality rate in pregnant women 10%-20%	—	Does not appear to cause liver disease
HDAg-positive (anti-HDV), HDV RNA serum	Anti-HEV	—	Anti-HGV
Hygiene; hepatitis B vaccine (active)	Hygiene, sanitation; no immunity	—	Hygiene

Hepatitis A

Household and personal contacts of clients with HAV should be given immune globulin. Administration of immune globulin (gamma globulin [Gammar]) is helpful prophylaxis both before and after exposure. Immune globulin is administered intramuscularly after exposure but not after the development of clinical manifestations. Adverse effects of intramuscular injection include pain, tenderness, and at times hematoma formation. Clients who live in or visit high-risk areas can be protected for up to 3 months by immune globulin. The earlier in the incubation period that the prophylactic immune globulin is given, the greater the protection.

Two effective inactivated hepatitis A vaccines are available and recommended for persons living in or traveling to endemic areas, clients with chronic liver disease, persons with clotting-factor disorders who are treated with concentrates, animal handlers, bisexual and homosexual men, sewage workers, illicit drug users, food handlers, and day care center caregivers. In states with a high incidence of hepatitis A, routine vaccination of all children has been recommended. For adults, either 1 ml of Havrix or Vaqta intramuscularly are recommended

EB EVIDENCE-BASED PRACTICE IN ACTION

Mass Screening for Hepatitis C: Is It Necessary?

Hepatitis C is an infection of the liver caused by the hepatitis C virus (HCV). It is the most common blood-borne infection in the United States and in many other parts of the world.[1] About 2.7 million U.S. citizens are infected according to the Centers for Disease Control and Prevention (CDC).[3] Hepatitis C–related liver disease is a leading cause of mortality and morbidity and is the most common indication for liver transplantation.

Hepatitis C is more widespread than acquired immunodeficiency syndrome (AIDS) and costs more than $600 million annually including medical treatment and work lost.[1] Many people are unaware that they are infected[4] and may even go on to develop chronic hepatitis C before they are aware of their condition. More deaths result from chronic infections and the number of clients who die from chronic hepatitis C is expected to rise as people infected 20 years ago begin to develop clinical manifestations.[5]

Given the high prevalence and potentially serious complications that develop from hepatitis C and the availability of sensitive serologic testing specific to hepatitis, mass screening for HCV may be appropriate.

Multiple factors must be considered when deciding whether HCV screening is appropriate for the entire population. These factors include the following: Only a small fraction of those infected with HCV develop progressive liver disease; the natural history of HCV infection in persons in the population whose infection will be disclosed by screening is likely to be more benign than what is described in referral clients; that is, the mortality rate corresponds to 10 hospitalizations and one death per 1000 people infected. Treatment for hepatitis C has improved a great deal, especially with the combined therapy with interferon (IFN) and ribavirin with favorable genotypes (genotypes 2 and 3) and the long-acting forms of IFN-alfa that have been developed to extend the duration of the therapeutic activity. It should be noted that for most clients with genotype 1 HCV infection, there is less than a 50% chance of cure. Also, IFN and ribavirin may cause substantial adverse effects and are expensive.[3]

Considering these factors, currently available data do not support the need for mass screening for HCV.[3,6] The current practices recommended by the National Center for Infectious Diseases include testing for people at risk for HCV infection and ensuring appropriate counseling, diagnosis, medical management and treatment; educating the public and people at risk about risk factors for HCV transmission; providing outreach and community-based programs to prevent practices that put people at risk and identifying people who need to be tested; providing surveillance to monitor acute and chronic disease trends; and evaluating the effectiveness of prevention and medical care activities.[2]

Implications

The primary goal for nurses is to help clients maintain a good quality of life with positive outcomes during the assessment, diagnostic procedures, and treatment phases of the illness. Nurses can play an integral role in supporting and comforting the client and the family during this time. Nurses are also an important part of educating the infected client and his or her family about the medication to be administered, its side effects, and changes in condition and clinical manifestations of toxicity from treatment. To prevent becoming infected with HCV themselves, family members need to learn prevention methods such as cleaning blood spills and not sharing equipment (e.g., toothbrushes, razors).

References
1. Hench, C., & Simpkins, S. (July, 2002). Hepatitis C: Risk factors, assessment and diagnosis. *Nurse Week*, 22-23.
2. Hench, C., & Simpkins, S. (August, 2002). Hepatitis C: Treatment, prevention and nursing interventions. *Nurse Week*, 17-18.
3. Kim, W.R., & Poterucha, J.J. (2001). Is it time for mass screening for hepatitis C? *The American Journal of Medicine, 111,* 667-668.
4. Lauer, G., & Walker, B.D. (2001). Hepatitis C virus infection. *New England Journal of Medicine, 345*(1), 41-53.
5. Sarbah, S.A., & Younossi, Z. (2000). Hepatitis C: An update on the silent epidemic. *Journal of Clinical Gastroenterology, 30*(2), 1-26.
6. Singer, M.E., & Younossi, Z.M. (2001). Cost effectiveness of screening for hepatitis C virus in asymptomatic, average-risk adults. *American Journal of Medicine, 111, 614-621.*

HAV vaccines, followed by a second 1-ml dose at 6 to 12 months.[8]

Hepatitis B

Until 1982 prevention of hepatitis B was based on passive immunization either with standard immunoglobulin (Ig) containing a moderate level of anti-HBs, or hepatitis B immune globulin (HBIG), containing a higher level of anti-HBs. Whereas the IG and HBIG may have reduced the frequency of clinical *illness*, it was never proved that either globulin prevented *infection*. In 1987 a genetically engineered vaccine was developed to provide active immunity. Current recommendations for immunization against HBV can be divided into those for preexposure and postexposure prophylaxis.

For preexposure prophylaxis (active immunity) against HBV in settings of frequent exposure and for those at high risk, three intramuscular injections (given in the deltoid not gluteal muscle) of HBV vaccine are recommended at 0, 1, and 6 months. Adverse reactions include headache, fever, nausea, vomiting, abdominal cramps, local soreness, redness, and swelling. Authorities strongly recommend this killed virus vaccine for all people.

Despite the availability of safe and effective vaccines, a strategy for vaccinating persons in the high-risk groups has not been successful. After introduction of the vaccines, the incidence of new hepatitis B cases continued to increase in the United States; fewer than 10% of all individuals in the high-risk group have been vaccinated. Therefore to have an impact on the incidence of HBV infection in the United States, hepatitis B vaccine is now included in the routine vaccination schedule for children (see Chapter 21). It is also recommended for adolescents and adults not previously immunized with the HBV vaccine.

For postexposure prophylaxis in persons who are not vaccinated and who sustained an exposure to HBV, a combination of hepatitis B immune globulin (HBIG) and HBV vaccine is recommended.

Hepatitis C

The transmission and prevention of HVC is similar to that of HVB. Drug therapy includes interferon (IFN) or pegylated interferon (PEG-IFN), a longer acting form of interferon than IFN (see the Integrating Pharmacology feature on Interferons at right). More commonly, a combination therapy with IFN or PEG-IFN and ribavirin (Rebetol) is administered. Interferon is given three times a week subcutaneously; oral ribavirin is given daily. For clients with HCV, genotype 1, PEG-IFN alpha combined with ribavirin in now replacing conventional IFN-alfa combined with ribavirin as the treatment of choice for chronic HCV.

Hepatitis D

Because hepatitis D must coexist with HBV, the vaccine for HBV can help to prevent hepatitis D also. The precautions that help prevent hepatitis B also are useful in preventing delta hepatitis.

Hepatitis E, F, and G

General hygiene precautions are necessary for prevention of hepatitis E. General hygiene and precautions with blood, blood products, and body fluids are necessary for prevention of hepatitis F and G. Currently no vaccines are available for hepatitis E, F, or G. Development of a vaccine for hepatitis E is in progress.

Pathophysiology

The pathophysiologic features in viral hepatitis are similar regardless of the cause. Hepatocytes undergo patho-

INTEGRATING PHARMACOLOGY

Interferons

Interferons (IFNs) are highly purified proteins and a natural product of human leukocytes within 4 to 6 hours after viral stimulation. IFNs exhibit a broad spectrum of antiviral and cytotoxic activity as well as immunomodulating properties (i.e., it favorably adjusts the immune system to combat foreign invasion of antigens and viruses better). As an immunomodulating agent, IFN enhances the phagocytic activity of macrophages and augments specific cytotoxicity of lymphocytes for target cells. IFN is species specific but not viral specific, meaning that it partially inhibits the reproduction of a virus immediately when a virus enters a cell. Thus the immune system and the IFN system of defense complement each other.

The several types of IFN include four types of alpha IFN: IFN alfa-2a, IFN alfa-2b, IFN alfa-n1, and IFN alfacon-1. The two types of beta IFN are IFN beta 1a and IFN beta 1b, but they are not used in the treatment of hepatitis. All types are produced by DNA recombinant techniques. The IFNs have been evaluated in a variety of viral infections, particularly in the treatment of chronic hepatitis B and C infections. IFN alfa-2a has been used effectively in hepatitis C and in chronic hepatitis B. IFN alfa-2b is used in chronic hepatitis B or C, IFN alfa-n1 is used in chronic hepatitis C, and IFN alfacon-1 is used in chronic hepatitis C.

The IFNs are not available for oral administration but must be given intramuscularly, subcutaneously, or intravenously. Adverse effects may differ slightly between types of IFN but primarily include flu-like manifestations: headache, fatigue, fever, chills, injection site reaction (pain, edema, hemorrhage, inflammation), pain, myalgia, arthralgia, and some central nervous systems effects such as depression and anxiety, dizziness, confusion, insomnia; respiratory effects such as cough; gastrointestinal effects such as nausea, diarrhea, and abdominal pain; and skin conditions such as rash, alopecia, pruritus, and urticaria.

Nursing implications include monitoring for and reporting any untoward clinical manifestations noted previously, withholding the IFN if manifestations of hepatitis worsen (i.e., jaundice or ascites), and monitoring laboratory tests that indicate liver, kidney, and thyroid function (e.g., serum albumin, bilirubin, alanine aminotransferase, hemoglobin and hematocrit).

logic changes induced by the body's immune response to the virus. Inflammation of the liver with areas of necrosis occurs, and the resultant damage leads to impairment of function. The degree of functional impairment depends on the amount of hepatocellular damage. The endoplasmic reticulum—responsible for protein and steroid synthesis, glucuronide conjugation, and detoxification—is the first cellular organelle (a specialized part of a cell that performs a definite function) to undergo change, and liver functions that depend on these processes are altered. Kupffer cells (fixed phagocytic cells found in sinusoids of liver) increase in both size and number. Vascular and ductular tissues undergo inflammatory changes. Healing of the damaged hepatic tissue generally occurs in 3 to 4 months.

Complications of hepatitis occur, although rarely. (See Complications of Hepatitis to follow.)

Hepatitis A

Antibodies to hepatitis A virus (anti-HAV) appear early in the course of the illness. Both immunoglobulin M (IgM) and immunoglobulin G (IgG) anti-HAV are detectable in the serum soon after the onset of illness. IgM anti-HAV titers peak during the first week of the disease and usually disappear within 3 to 6 months. Detection of IgM anti-HAV is a valid test for demonstrating acute hepatitis. IgG anti-HAV peak titers occur 1 month after onset of the disease but may stay elevated for years; this finding is therefore an indicator of past infection.

Hepatitis B

The HBV is a DNA virus that has an inner core and a surface envelope. The body forms antibodies to the viral antigens HBcAg and HBsAg. The presence of HBsAg in the blood denotes (1) a previous or resolving infection with hepatitis B; (2) a continuing, chronic infection; or (3) immunization with immunoglobulin or HBV vaccine.

Hepatitis C

The HCV is a single-stranded RNA virus with properties similar to those of the HBV and hepatitis D viruses. HCV is thought to be a pathogenic factor in conditions such as glomerulonephritis and autoimmune thyroiditis.

Hepatitis D

Hepatitis D virus is a small defective RNA virus that causes hepatitis only in HBV infection, and specifically only in the presence of HBsAg. Hepatitis D virus requires the helper function of HBV for its replication and expression. Hepatitis D virus can either infect a person simultaneously with HBV *(co-infection)* or infect a person already infected with HBV *(superinfection).*

Hepatitis E

The hepatitis E virus alters hepatocellular function in almost the same way as the other types of hepatitis viruses. It causes necrosis and liver cell damage.

Hepatitis F

The hepatitis F virus is identified by electron microscope and is difficult to diagnose as a cause of hepatitis.

Hepatitis G

Hepatitis G virus, like HCV, is a blood-borne RNA virus. Current data indicate that a large portion of clients infected with hepatitis G are also infected with HCV. Hepatitis G virus does not alter the severity of hepatitis C, nor is it associated with acute or chronic liver injury, although the latter finding requires continued study.

Clinical Manifestations

Clients with viral hepatitis all experience liver inflammation and other pathologic changes that are similar. HBV, HCV, and hepatitis D are usually the most severe, although they may be asymptomatic in some clients. The onset of manifestations ranges from abrupt to insidious according to the incubation period and the degree of infectivity.

Manifestations of viral hepatitis are systemic and vary from client to client. Manifestations that occur during the earlier (prodromal) phase may include jaundice, lethargy, irritability, myalgia, arthralgia, anorexia, nausea, vomiting, abdominal pain (caused by stretching of Glisson's capsule surrounding the liver due to inflammation), diarrhea or constipation, fever, and other flu-like manifestations. Fever is caused by the release of pyrogens in the inflammatory process. Fatigue and malaise are the result of reduced energy metabolism by the liver. Pruritus, the result of bile salt accumulation in the skin, is typically mild and transient and may be more intense at its onset and termination. Jaundice, caused by impaired excretion of conjugated bilirubin, may or may not be present; when it is, it is first seen in the sclerae of the eyes and mucous membranes.

Anicteric (without jaundice) hepatitis may or may not precede jaundice. Children with hepatitis are usually anicteric. Adults often note the appearance of darker urine (the color of tea or mahogany) and clay-colored stools a few days before clinical jaundice develops. The darker urine is from the presence of urobilinogen, which is excreted through the kidneys instead of through the bowel as normally occurs. Other manifestations often abate when jaundice appears, but they also may worsen.

If irritability and drowsiness become severe, assess for the possibility of hepatic encephalopathy. Deterioration of handwriting is an early manifestation of hepatic encephalopathy; thus at each shift ask clients to write their name and observe their writing closely for changes. *Asterixis,* an abnormal muscle tremor sometimes called "liver flap," may accompany encephalopathy. This manifestation is easily elicited by applying a blood pressure cuff on the upper arm and noting whether the tremor is **EB** present when the cuff is released. Mild depression is not uncommon because of (1) the nature of the illness (weakness, jaundice, itching, and nausea), (2) its long duration and the expense of treatment, (3) the need for confinement, and (4) forgetfulness and the inability to concentrate on completion of activities of daily living (ADLs).

Bleeding tendencies may develop either from reduced prothrombin synthesis by injured hepatic cells or from reduced absorption of the fat-soluble vitamin K as a result of reduced levels of bile in the intestines. Anemia may occur because of the decreased life span of erythrocytes (RBCs). Erythrocyte destruction results from liver enzyme alterations. A transient hyperglycemia sometimes develops, and a client with diabetes may need to increase insulin dosage at this time.

The liver is larger than normal in hepatitis and is tender to palpation. Some people with viral hepatitis have spider angiomas, palmar erythema, and gynecomastia, which disappear during the recovery period. A small percentage (5% to 15%) of clients experience splenomegaly or enlargement of the posterior cervical lymph nodes. Occasionally hepatitis B is accompanied by arthralgias, rash, vasculitis, or glomerulonephritis.

Occasionally cholestatic viral hepatitis syndrome may develop. This uncommon disease process resembles mechanical obstruction; it is difficult to differentiate cholestatic viral hepatitis from biliary tract obstruction resulting from gallstones, strictures, and tumors.

The cause and pathophysiology of this hepatitis variant are unclear. Cholestatic viral hepatitis syndrome causes jaundice, itching, and the typical flu-like and gastrointestinal problems of hepatitis, but the manifestations often last longer and are more severe. Serum bilirubin reaches levels of 10 to 15 mg/dl. Diagnostic studies reveal elevations of serum lipoproteins, globulins, cholesterol, and alkaline phosphatase. Rarely the liver progressively enlarges.

Fulminant viral hepatitis may develop. This life-threatening form resembles acute liver failure with manifestations of encephalopathy (increased excitability, insomnia, somnolence, and impaired mentation). The liver rapidly decreases in size. Other problems include gastrointestinal bleeding, disseminated intravascular coagulation (DIC), fever with leukocytosis and neutrophilia, hepatorenal problems of oliguria and azotemia, edema and ascites, hypotension, respiratory failure, hypoglycemia, bacterial infection of the respiratory or urinary tract or both, and thrombocytopenia and coagulopathy. The prognosis is poor, and death may occur before jaundice appears. Liver transplantation may be performed to save the client's life.

Presence of hepatitis B surface antigen (HBsAg) in the **EB** blood usually indicates that the person is infectious. An-

other antigen, hepatitis B early antigen (HBeAg), is often associated with progression of acute hepatitis to chronic hepatitis and indicates a highly infectious state.

Levels of serum aminotransferases first rise and then begin to fall as bilirubin starts to increase. Levels that rise, peak, drop, and then rise again indicate severe liver damage and a poor prognosis. Jaundice may not be clinically recognizable until levels are about 3 mg/dl. Bilirubin that rises above 20 mg/dl and remains elevated for a long period may indicate severe liver necrosis, which has a poor prognosis. Mild prolongation of the prothrombin time (PT) sometimes occurs. The gamma globulin fraction and alkaline phosphatase are elevated in some clients. If HBV is responsible, detection of HBsAg is possible before the level of aspartate aminotransferase (AST) (formerly serum glutamic-oxaloacetic transaminase [SGOT]) rises.

Prognosis

By 8 to 10 weeks, nearly all clients with acute viral hepatitis demonstrate normal results on liver function tests; however, the clinical course, morbidity, and mortality of viral hepatitis may vary considerably. In most cases, clients recover in 3 to 16 weeks, although results on liver function testing are abnormal for a longer time. Most clients recover completely. The mortality rate is less than 1%; this rate is reportedly higher in older people.[8]

Outcome Management
■ Medical Management

The acute manifestations of hepatitis generally subside over 2 to 3 weeks. Complete clinical and laboratory recovery occurs in hepatitis A by 9 weeks and in hepatitis B and hepatitis C by 16 weeks. Severe complications develop in fewer than 1% of clients with hepatitis. Clients who have severe nausea and vomiting and difficulty maintaining normal fluid balance need to be hospitalized if progressive deterioration occurs.

Reduce Fatigue. Rest is advisable in proportion to the severity of manifestations. Bed rest is usually not necessary but is recommended on an as-needed basis during the initial prodromal, anicteric phase of the disease, when the infection is most active and there is decreased metabolism by the liver. Return to normal activity during the convalescent period should be gradual. If pruritus disturbs rest, cholestyramine, antihistamines, emollients, and lipid creams may be prescribed.

Maintain Nutritional and Fluid Balance. No specific dietary measures are indicated, but most clients find a high calorie, low-fat, high-carbohydrate diet more easily digested and more palatable. During the most severe phase of the illness, when changes occur in the stomach or bowel, anorexia and nausea may be so extreme that oral intake of any kind is greatly reduced. In such cases, IV administration of 10% glucose is indicated. As the client's manifestations abate and appetite improves, food and fluid intake may be resumed as tolerated. All alcoholic beverages should be avoided.

Reduce Effects of Hepatitis. Few medications are available for treating viral hepatitis. Antibiotics are not prescribed. Antiemetics control nausea and vomiting, but phenothiazines should not be used because they are biotransformed in the liver and are therefore potentially toxic. Parenteral vitamin K may be given to clients with prolonged PT. Antihistamines may provide relief of pruritus but may cause sedation.

Glucocorticoids. Glucocorticoid therapy has no effect on viral hepatitis and is of no value in its treatment. Although glucocorticoids may reduce serum aminotransferase and bilirubin levels, they have no effect on liver necrosis or regeneration.

Estrogens. Estrogens can raise serum bilirubin levels. Therefore clinicians need to consider the advisability of oral contraceptive use during acute viral hepatitis.

Bile Acid Sequestrants. The administration of bile acid sequestrants cholestyramine (Questran) or colestipol (Colestid) can relieve pruritus associated with elevated levels of bile acids that may result from severe cholestatic liver disease. Both drugs bind bile acids in the gastrointestinal tract forming an insoluble complex that is excreted in the feces. The result of this action is increased clearance of cholesterol.

Immune Globulin. Immune globulin, although not used to treat viral hepatitis, does provide prophylaxis for family and friends. If given early, standard immune globulin (a preparation of proteins capable of acting as antibodies, formerly termed *immune serum globulin*) may prevent hepatitis A or mitigate the severity of manifestations. HAV does not remain in the blood long; therefore there is no healthy carrier state for HAV as there is for HBV.

Vaccines. Vaccines are available to promote immunity to HAV, HBV, and HVC. In addition to immune globulin, they may be administered prophylactically in persons exposed to infected clients.

Medications to Avoid. Clinicians administer few medications to clients with hepatitis. Medications such as chlorpromazine, aspirin, acetaminophen, and a variety of sedatives are given as infrequently as possible because of their hepatotoxic properties.

■ Nursing Management of the Medical Client

Assessment

To determine the type of hepatitis present, always begin by questioning the client about possible exposure to risk factors. Ask about common manifestations, especially jaundice, and about manifestations of disease progression, such as hepatic encephalopathy (see Hepatic Encephalopathy under Cirrhosis). Assess the results of liver function studies, and monitor them to ascertain progression of the disease. Also assess the client's and his or her family's ability to provide home and self-care. Their understanding of the disease and its implications is vital to its successful management in the home setting.

Diagnosis, Outcomes, Interventions

Diagnosis: Fatigue. The client with hepatitis has tremendous metabolic demands, leading to the nursing diagnosis *Fatigue related to decreased metabolic energy production secondary to liver dysfunction.*

Outcomes. The client will convey reduced fatigue and heightened energy as evidenced by compliance with activity restrictions and a gradual increase in activity to the pre-illness level.

Interventions. Fatigue associated with hepatitis may interfere with ADL. Most clients experience the greatest fatigue during the *anicteric phase* (before jaundice occurs) and begin to feel stronger during the icteric phase. Fatigue may persist, however, even after the jaundice clears. Clients with severe jaundice may suffer pruritus (see Jaundice for nursing interventions for *Impaired Skin Integrity related to pruritus*). During the period of severe fatigue, advise the client to rest in bed. Most clients who feel capable of being up and around can do so without harm if they rest after meals and do not engage in any activity to the point of becoming overly tired. Because prolonged bed rest itself can lead to weakness, a reasonable activity level is more conducive to recovery than enforced bed rest.

Encourage ADLs such as exercise of bathroom privileges, performance of personal hygiene measures, and self-feeding unless these activities cause excessive fatigue. Advise the client to plan rest periods while jaundice is present, especially after meals. Clients who engage in excessive activity too early in the recovery phase sometimes experience a relapse, potentially leading to liver failure.

Diagnosis: Imbalanced Nutrition: Less Than Body Requirements. For the liver to heal properly and to regenerate, nutrition is important. Clients with hepatitis often have a decreased appetite, leading to a common nursing diagnosis of *Imbalanced Nutrition: Less Than Body Requirements related to anorexia, nausea, bile stasis, and altered absorption and metabolism.*

Outcomes. The client will maintain an intake of the required calories to maintain weight as evidenced by having no weight loss and possibly having weight gain.

Interventions

Modify Diet. To help the client meet the nutritional requirements associated with hepatitis, perform the following:

1. Provide a nutritious breakfast. Because anorexia usually worsens during the day, breakfast may be the best-tolerated meal.
2. Encourage the client to avoid fatty foods, which can induce nausea.
3. Include the optimal amount of protein and carbohydrates to allow recovery of injured liver cells without overfeeding. If the client has no problem with protein metabolism, a normal intake is helpful for tissue repair. Clients with severe hepatitis who are at risk for developing hepatic encephalopathy, however, require a low-protein diet (to prevent the buildup of ammonia in the blood from incomplete clearing of protein metabolic wastes). Alterations in fat metabolism differ according to the degree of interruption of bile production and excretion.
4. Suggest multiple small meals. This approach allows the client with anorexia to ingest a diet of 2500 to 3000 calories more comfortably. Also, candy, juice, sweetened tea, and carbonated drinks can supply calories when nausea is a problem.

Avoid Alcohol. Remind the client to avoid alcohol, which is an extremely hepatotoxic agent.

Provide Vitamin Supplements. Explain that vitamin supplements are not generally necessary in uncomplicated hepatitis if the diet is adequate in nutrients. Vitamin K supplements, as ordered, may be administered if the PT is longer than normal.

Relieve Nausea and Vomiting. Clients who experience severe nausea and vomiting may obtain relief with antiemetics. Before administering these medications, review their effect on liver function. Phenothiazines such as prochlorperazine (Compazine) are usually contraindicated. If the client cannot tolerate any oral intake, provide IV nutrition.

Diagnosis: Anxiety.
Because predicting the outcome of hepatitis is difficult, the nursing diagnosis *Anxiety related to uncertainty of the effects of hepatitis* is common.

Outcomes. The client will experience a decrease in anxiety as evidenced by the ability to discuss his or her feelings about the disease.

Interventions. Encourage clients with hepatitis to express their feelings concerning the following:
- The illness
- The duration and cost of the illness
- Alterations in home life and financial status (especially for the parent of young children or for the sole family earner)
- The effect of the illness on future health problems
- The possibility of death in clients who are very ill

Suggest psychosocial and financial counseling for the client who is disturbed. Increase the client's knowledge and understanding of the illness by teaching the facts about the illness and its management. Increased knowledge can reduce anxiety.

Diagnosis: Ineffective Health Maintenance.
For the client and family members to manage hepatitis at home, the nursing diagnosis of *Ineffective Health Maintenance related to cause of disease, modes of transmission, and its course* must be addressed.

Outcomes. The client will understand the disease and its treatment as evidenced by the client's ability to state the causes of the disease and the rationales for treatment.

Interventions

Provide Client Teaching. Teaching for the client with hepatitis varies with the causative agent. Teach the client how to prevent recurrence and spread. Instruct the client to return to former activity levels slowly to avoid a relapse. Provide clear instructions concerning diet.

Administer Medications. Administer medications and provide supportive management. Discontinue any medications that may be causing inflammatory changes. Clients who cannot tolerate large doses of steroids may benefit from azathioprine and smaller steroid doses.

Promote Rest. Encourage bed rest during the active phase of the disease. The client usually remains at home to convalesce. Periods of remission may occur in which liver necrosis continues. Discuss with the client the need for help at home after discharge (such as with housework or shopping) because limits on activity will still have to be maintained. The client will need to see a physician at regular intervals after discharge to ensure that the liver is healing and no further damage has occurred.

Evaluation

Because the clinical course of acute viral hepatitis varies considerably from one client to another, the nurse must assess outcomes carefully to determine whether they have been met. Recovery without permanent liver damage is expected to occur within 1 to 4 months. Permanent damage may result if the therapeutic regimen is not followed.

■ Self-Care

Most clients recover from acute viral hepatitis, do not require hospitalization, and are appropriately managed at home. Clinical and biochemical relapses may occur before full recovery, however. In addition, complications of acute viral hepatitis may develop, necessitating careful monitoring, especially in older clients.

Avoid Hepatotoxins. There is no specific ongoing pharmacologic management of clients recovering from acute viral hepatitis. Advise the client to avoid alcohol and medications such as aspirin, acetaminophen, and sedatives because of their hepatotoxicity.

Promote Nutrition. Encourage clients to continue eating a well-balanced, nutritional diet. A low-fat, high-carbohydrate diet is generally tolerated best. A well-balanced diet promotes liver healing, leading to improved tolerance for activity.

Provide Client Teaching. One of the primary areas to cover in teaching the client and family members is how to avoid reinfection or possible spread of the infection to others. Caution the client and his or her significant others to avoid sexual activity until there is no longer a chance of disease transmission (generally after liver function tests have returned to normal) and to check with the physician before resuming sexual relations.

Promote Rest. Help the client understand the need for adequate rest so that the liver can heal on its own. The client needs to be active enough to prevent complications of immobility but not so active to risk relapse. The client is also expected to resume pre-hepatitis activities and to remain free from complications.

Prevent Infection and Reinfection. Teach the client to avoid reinfection or possible spread of the infection to other family members. You may recommend vaccination for HAV and HBV to promote health maintenance.

COMPLICATIONS OF HEPATITIS

Persons with viral hepatitis typically recover completely from the illness in 3 to 16 weeks. Clients who are otherwise healthy usually recover from hepatitis A without major sequelae. Although hepatitis A is associated with a low mortality rate, relapses weeks to months after apparent recovery may occur. Hepatitis A does not progress to chronic liver disease. Fulminant hepatitis resembling acute liver failure may occur and is primarily seen in hepatitis B and D as well as in hepatitis E and rarely in hepatitis A. Clients with hepatitis B tend to experience more complications. One in 10 persons develops chronic active hepatitis as a result of hepatitis B, of-

BOX 49-1	*Causes of Chronic Hepatitis*

Viral
Hepatitis B
Hepatitis B with superimposed hepatitis D
Hepatitis C

Drugs and Toxins
Methyldopa
Nitrofurantoin
Amiodarone
Isoniazid

Autoimmune
Presence of HLA-B8 and HLA-DR3 following hepatitis A, Epstein-Barr infection, or measles

Genetic and Metabolic Disorders
Wilson's disease
α_1–Antitrypsin deficiency
Nonalcoholic steatohepatitis

Data from Fallon, M.B., et al. (2001). Acute and chronic hepatitis. In T.E. Andreoli, et al. (Eds.).*Cecil essentials of medicine* (5th ed., p. 383). Philadelphia: W.B. Saunders.

ten leading to destruction of the liver. Cirrhosis may follow a severe case of hepatitis B or chronic active hepatitis. Primary hepatocellular carcinoma is a potential complication of chronic hepatitis. Other possible complications of hepatitis include chronic persistent hepatitis, chronic carrier state, and aplastic anemia.

Fulminant Hepatitis

Fulminant hepatitis (massive hepatic necrosis) is rare and, as noted previously, is seen primarily in hepatitis B and D as well as in hepatitis E and A. Fulminant hepatitis causes severe illness and is fatal in 1% to 2% of all cases and in up to 20% of cases occurring in pregnant women. Fulminant hepatitis involves a progression of manifestations that include jaundice, hepatic encephalopathy, and ascites. The mortality rate varies with age but approaches 90% to 100%, especially in people over 60 years of age.

Chronic Hepatitis

Chronic hepatitis exists when liver inflammation continues beyond a period of 3 to 6 months. Acute viral hepatitis in the end may lead to chronic hepatitis, with the exception of hepatitis A and E. Causes of chronic hepatitis are listed in Box 49-1.

Several categories of chronic hepatitis have been noted in the past. These categories were based on histologic criteria and included chronic persistent hepatitis (CPH), chronic lobular hepatitis (CLH), and chronic active hepatitis (CAH). CPH and CLH were thought to be milder and have a good prognosis; progression to more serious lesions was considered rare. CAH was thought to

| | **New Classification** | |
Old Classification	**Grade (Activity)**	**Stage (Fibrosis)**
Chronic persistent hepatitis	Minimal or mild	None or mild
Chronic lobular hepatitis	Mild or moderate	Mild
Chronic active hepatitis	Mild, moderate, or severe	Mild, moderate, or severe

TABLE 49-3 *Comparison of Old and New Nomenclature of Chronic Hepatitis*

Data from Dienstag, J.L., & Isselbacher, K.L. (2001). Chronic hepatitis. In E. Braunwald, et al. (Eds.), *Harrison's principles of internal medicine* (15th ed., p. 1744). New York: McGraw-Hill.

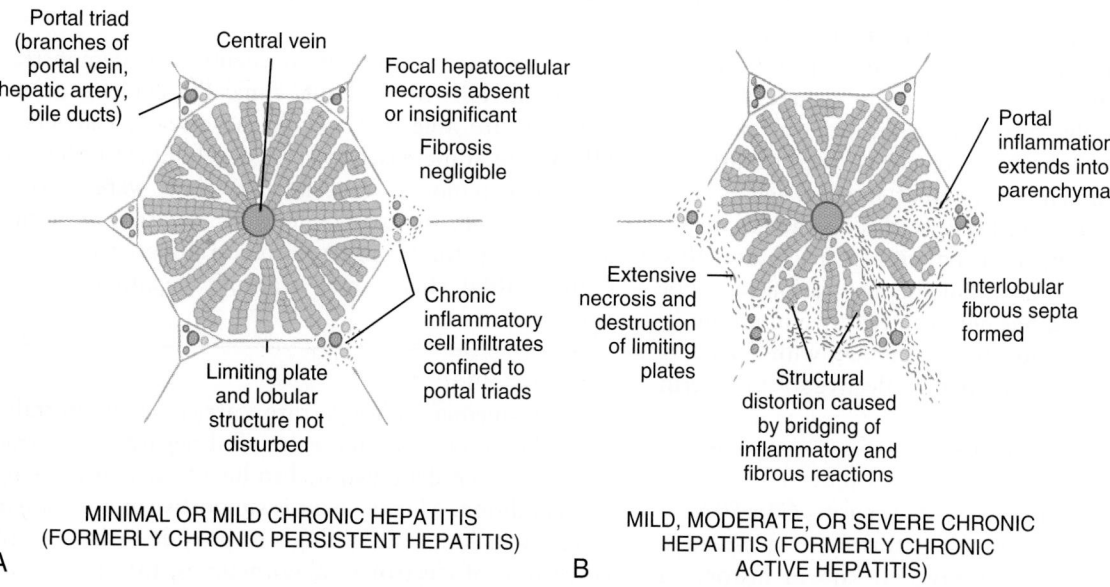

FIGURE 49-1 Comparison of structural changes with chronic hepatitis. **A,** Inflammation is confined to portal triads in minimal or mild chronic hepatitis formerly known as *chronic persistent* hepatitis. **B,** Inflammation extends into the parenchyma in mild, moderate, or severe hepatitis formerly known as *chronic active* hepatitis.

have a more serious prognosis with significant risk for progression to cirrhosis and liver failure.

More information is now available about the causes, natural history, pathogenesis, serologic features, and therapy of chronic hepatitis. The former categories have been replaced by categories based on (1) its cause or etiology; (2) its histologic activity or grade of injury as determined by the numbers and location of inflammatory cells; and (3) its degree of progression or stage as determined by degree, location, and distortion of normal architecture by fibrosis (Table 49-3).

In clients with what was formerly known as CPH, cirrhosis is absent or rare. As a general rule, clients are asymptomatic or have mild manifestations such as fatigue, anorexia, or nausea and some liver enlargement. Clients with CPH generally have an excellent prognosis. In the new nomenclature, CPH is classified by grade as *minimal* or *mild* chronic hepatitis and by stage as *absent* or *mild* fibrosis.

In clients with what was formerly known as CLH, portal inflammation with foci of necrosis and inflamma-

tion in the liver lobule occur. Progression to CAH and cirrhosis is rare. CLH corresponds in the new nomenclature to a *mild* or *moderate* grade and a stage of *absent* or *minimal fibrosis.*

Clinically CAH is characterized clinically by elevation of serum transaminase levels for more than 6 months. CAH is a progressive disorder that can lead to cirrhosis, liver failure, and death. Although some clients are asymptomatic, most clients tend to have mild to severe constitutional clinical manifestations, especially fatigue. Jaundice and hyperbilirubinemia are more common in CAH. In the new nomenclature for chronic hepatitis, what used to be CAH spans the entire spectrum of *activity grade* from *minimal,* to *mild,* to *severe chronic* hepatitis; the grade of *portal, periportal,* and *lobular* inflammation; and the *stage* of fibrosis which can be *mild, moderate,* or *severe fibrosis* as well as *cirrhosis.*

With the new classification and criteria for identification of chronic hepatitis, both serologic studies and liver biopsies are used in the diagnosis and in planning treatment (Figure 49-1). This next section addresses briefly three types of chronic hepatitis: chronic hepatitis B, chronic hepatitis C, and autoimmune hepatitis.

Chronic Hepatitis B

Chronic hepatitis B primarily affects males; nearly 400 million people worldwide and 1.25 million in the United States are affected.[9] Chronic hepatitis B follows acute HBV in about 5% of adults in the United States. Clients who are HBsAg and HBeAg positive are considered to be in a high replicative phase compared with those who are HgsAg and HBeAb positive (low replicative phase). Onset of the disease tends to be insidious. Clinical manifestations include fatigue and intermittent or persistent jaundice. Treatment of chronic HBV depends on the level of virus replication but generally includes lamivudine, 100 mg orally daily. This medication can be given instead of IFN for the treatment of chronic hepatitis B and is tolerated much better. Other antiviral agents such as adefovir dipivoxil are being studied. Strategies using multiple drugs are likely to be tried in the future. IFN may be administered also, but the medication may not be tolerated well and has not been effective in immunosuppressed persons. Short-term treatment with glucocorticoids may be helpful but are not effective for long-term therapy.

Chronic Hepatitis C

Chronic hepatitis C follows acute hepatitis C in 50% to 70% of cases. Many cases of hepatitis C are identified in asymptomatic clients who have no known history of acute hepatitis C. They discover they have chronic hepatitis C when they go to donate blood or as a result of routine laboratory screening tests. Chronic hepatitis C tends to be slowly and insidiously progressive with approximately a quarter of the cases progressing eventually to end-stage cirrhosis. Progression to cirrhosis is variable and depends on multiple factors, such as degree of liver histology, age when infected, and duration of infection. Clinical manifestations are similar to chronic hepatitis B and include fatigue. Jaundice is rare. Treatment of chronic hepatitis C is generally considered in clients under age 70 with elevated serum aminotransferase levels and more than minimal inflammation or fibrosis on liver biopsy. Standard therapy is a combination of recombinant IFN-alfa and ribavirin (see the Integrating Pharmacology feature on Interferons).[9,14,15]

Autoimmune Hepatitis

Autoimmune liver disease is generally a disease of young women and is characterized by hepatic inflammation with plasma cells and fibrosis but can occur in either gender at any age. Affected persons are often positive for human leukocyte antigen (HLA)-B8 and -DR3 and older clients, HLA-DR4. The onset is usually insidious, but about 25% of cases present as an acute attack of hepatitis or follow a viral illness such as hepatitis A, Epstein-Barr infection, or measles or exposure to a drug or toxin such as nitrofurantoin. Clinical manifestations include multiple spider nevi, acne, hirsutism, and hepatomegaly. Extrahepatic manifestations include arthritis, thyroiditis, nephritis, ulcerative colitis, and Coombs'-positive hemolytic anemia. Treatment includes prednisone with or without azathioprine. Clients who do not respond to prednisone and azathioprine may be considered for a trial medication regimen: cyclosporine, tacrolimus, or methotrexate. Liver transplantation may be required for treatment failures.[7]

Chronic Carrier State

A carrier state is possible in clients who demonstrate persistent HBsAg without clinically evident disease but who are able to transmit the disease. Carriers of HBsAg are at increased risk for development of hepatocellular carcinoma, especially if they were infected during infancy or early childhood. A carrier state may also develop for hepatitis C; blood donated by apparently healthy clients may transmit hepatitis C when transfused.

Aplastic Anemia

Aplastic anemia, although rare, carries a high mortality rate when it occurs after acute viral hepatitis. No treatment has been demonstrated to be effective in reversing this condition. Management is supportive and palliative. Therapy includes (1) IV fluids to provide hydration, (2) correction of electrolyte abnormalities, (3) medications for reduction of pain and nausea, and (4) adequate caloric intake.

TOXIC HEPATITIS

Toxins and drugs can produce a wide variety of pathologic lesions in the liver. Some agents cause toxic hepatitis, whereas others produce necrosis, cholestasis, or neoplasms. The extent and type of hepatitis produced by the toxin depend on the degree of exposure, the chemical properties of the hepatotoxin, and the genetic makeup of the individual. Most commonly, the causative agent is a toxic metabolite formed by the drug-metabolizing enzymes within the liver. Table 49-4 lists some hepatotoxic agents. Liver necrosis occurs within 2 or 3 days after acute exposure to a dose-related hepatotoxin; however, several weeks may pass before manifestations of idiosyncratic reactions appear. People experiencing either type of hepatotoxicity demonstrate abnormal results on liver function testing.

People who are repeatedly exposed to hepatotoxins in minimal amounts but over long periods may develop chronic hepatitis or cirrhosis. Clients experiencing a hypersensitivity reaction may demonstrate eosinophilia, fever, arthralgia, and sometimes *xanthomatosis* (an excessive accumulation of lipids brought about by faulty lipid metabolism).

TABLE 49-4	*Substances Known to be Hepatotoxic (Cause Alteration in Liver Morphology)*	
Principal Morphologic Change	**Class of Agent**	**Example of Substance**
Cholestasis	Anabolic steroid	Methyl testosterone
	Antithyroid	Methimazole
	Antibiotic	Erythromycin
		Nitrofurantoin
		Rifampin
		Amoxicillin-clavulinic acid
	Oral contraceptive	Norethynodrel with mestranol
	Oral hypoglycemic	Chlorpropamide
	Tranquilizer	Chlorpromazine
	Immunosuppressive	Cyclosporine
	Calcium channel blocker	Verapamil, nifedipine
Hepatitis	Oncotherapeutic	Methotrexate
	Anesthetic	Halothane
	Antihypertensive	Methyldopa, captopril
	Antibiotic	Isoniazid, rifampin
	Diuretic	Chlorothiazide
	Antidepressant	Isoniazid, amitriptyline, imipramine
	Anti-inflammatory	Ibuprofen, indomethacin
	Antifungal	Ketoconazole, fluconazole
Toxic (necrosis)	Hydrocarbon	Carbon tetrachloride
	Metal	Yellow phosphorus
	Mushroom	*Amanita phalloides*
	Analgesic	Acetaminophen

Data from Dienstag, J.L., & Isselbacher, K.J. (2001). Toxic and drug-induced hepatitis. In E. Braunwald, et al. (Eds.), *Harrison's principles of internal medicine* (15th ed., pp. 1737-1742). New York: McGraw-Hill.

Nursing intervention begins with obtaining a detailed drug history and information about past exposure and the response to a suspected agent. Ensure removal of the causative agent and adequate rest, promote alleviation of side effects (e.g., with cholestyramine for pruritus), and provide a high-calorie diet with fats and protein as tolerated. Restrict protein intake if evidence of impending hepatic encephalopathy is noted. Steroids have not proved of value in treatment of drug-induced liver disease, although they may suppress the manifestations caused by the reaction of the toxic agent.

Renal failure sometimes appears as a complication of toxic hepatitis. Assessment and interventions for renal failure are discussed in Chapter 38.

ALCOHOLIC HEPATITIS

Alcoholic hepatitis may be acute or chronic. It is caused by parenchymal necrosis resulting from heavy alcohol ingestion. Although sometimes reversible, this condition is the most frequent cause of cirrhosis. This fact is important because cirrhosis of the liver is a common cause of death among adults in the United States.

Clinical manifestations of alcoholic hepatitis usually develop after a bout of heavy drinking. Assessment reveals anorexia, nausea, abdominal pain, splenomegaly, hepatomegaly, jaundice, ascites, fever, and encephalopathy. Laboratory studies typically show anemia, leukocytosis, and an elevated serum bilirubin. Liver biopsy reveals fatty hepatic tissue. Hepatitis resulting from excessive alcohol intake carries a poor prognosis, particularly if the client continues to ingest alcohol.

Nursing interventions include providing a high-vitamin, high-carbohydrate diet and administration of folic acid and thiamine supplements and administration of parenteral fluids as ordered. Administration of liquid formulas may be useful in increasing caloric intake. Steroids sometimes have a beneficial effect, although their use remains controversial.

CIRRHOSIS

Cirrhosis of the liver is a chronic, progressive disease characterized by widespread fibrosis (scarring) and nodule formation. Cirrhosis occurs when the normal flow of blood, bile, and hepatic metabolites is altered by fibrosis and changes in the hepatocytes, bile ductules, vascular channels, and reticular cells.

TABLE 49-5	Comparison of Postnecrotic, Biliary, Cardiac, and Alcoholic Cirrhosis		
Definition	**Etiology**	**Pathology**	**Assessment Data**
Postnecrotic (Macronodular) Cirrhosis			
Most common world-wide form Massive loss of liver cells, with irregular patterns of regenerating cells	Postacute viral (types B and C) hepatitis Postintoxication with industrial chemicals Some infections and metabolic disorders	Liver small and nodular	As in alcoholic cirrhosis except less muscle wasting and more jaundice
Biliary Cirrhosis			
Bile flow decreased with concurrent cell damage to hepatocytes around bile ductules	*Primary* Chronic stasis of bile in intrahepatic ducts Cause unknown Autoimmune process implicated *Secondary* Obstruction of bile ducts outside of liver	Early-stage biopsy reveals inflammatory process with necrosis of cells and ducts Hepatocytes are lost and scar tissue remains End stage similar to postnecrotic type	Fatigue Generalized pruritus Dark urine Pale stools Jaundice Impaired bile flow Steatorrhea ↓ absorption of fat-soluble vitamins Elevated serum lipids ↑ cholesterol deposits in subcutaneous tissues Signs of portal hypertension
Cardiac Cirrhosis			
Chronic liver disease associated with severe right-sided long-term heart failure (fairly rare)	Atrioventricular valve disease Prolonged constrictive pericarditis Decompensated cor pulmonale	*Early* Dark-colored liver enlarged by blood and edema fluid *Late* Liver capsule thickens and nodular scarring occurs	Slight jaundice, enlarged liver, and ascites in person with severe cardiac impairment over 10-year span RUQ pain during acute congestion Cachexia Fluid retention Circulatory problems
Alcoholic Cirrhosis			
Alcoholic cirrhosis (Laënnec's, micronodular) Small nodules form as a result of persistence of some offending agent	Associated with alcohol abuse	Scarring and collagen tissue deposits Regenerating nodules are very small Normal lobular structure is destroyed	May produce no symptoms for long periods Onset of symptoms may be insidious or abrupt *Early:* Weakness, fatigue, weight loss *Later:* Anorexia, nausea, and vomiting Abdominal pain Ascites Menstrual irregularities Impotence Enlarged breasts in men Hematemesis Spider angiomas

Data from Chung, R.T. & Podolsky, D.T. (2001). Cirrhosis and its complications. In E. Braunwald, et al. (Eds.), *Harrison's principles of internal medicine* (15th ed., pp. 1754-1767). New York: McGraw-Hill.
AST, Aspartate aminotransferase; *IV,* intravenous; *RUQ,* right upper quadrant.

The following are the four major types of cirrhosis:
- Alcoholic (historically called *Laënnec's cirrhosis* or *micronodular* or *portal*)
- Postnecrotic (macronodular or toxin-induced)
- Biliary
- Cardiac

The types are compared in Table 49-5. The two major clinical problems in cirrhosis are (1) decreased liver function and (2) portal hypertension. The latter problem develops in severe cirrhosis.

Cirrhosis is the 10th leading cause of death in the United States, with an age-adjusted mortality rate of 9.2

Diagnosis and Prognosis	Intervention(s)
Needle biopsy of liver establishes pathologic processes Within 5 years, 75% die of complications ↑ serum aminotransferases ↑ gamma globulins	Treat complications as needed
Elevated serum bilirubin levels *Early:* 3-10 mg/100 ml *Late:* >50 mg/100 ml High elevations of alkaline phosphatase ↑ gamma globulins ↑ blood lipids Presence of lipoprotein X ↑ serum bile salts Hypoprothrombinemia ↑ antimitochondrial antibody in primary cases ↑ serum copper in primary cases	*Primary* Ursodiol Treatment is symptomatic (e.g., high-calorie diet, lower intake of fats by 30-40 g/day if problems develop) Cholestyramine for pruritus Supplement of fat-soluble vitamins *Secondary* Treatment to relieve mechanical obstruction
↑ conjugated bilirubin in serum ↑ sulfobromophthalein ↓ albumin in serum ↑ serum aminotransferases ↑ alkaline phosphatase Liver biopsy *Prognosis* Depends on course of cardiac disease	Cause of chronic heart failure is treated if possible

Liver biopsy; history of alcohol abuse; high AST; high bilirubin
  (slight); anemia
Prognosis depends on presence of complications and contin-
  ued abuse of alcohol
	Primarily supportive
	Correction of vitamin and mineral deficiencies if any (e.g., folate,
	  thiamine, pyridoxine, vitamin K, and minerals [magnesium and
	  phosphate]); treat complications as needed (e.g., ferrous sulfate
	  for anemia, IV vasopressin for esophageal varices, reduce or
	  withhold dietary protein for hepatic encephalopathy or vitamin K
	  for hemorrhagic tendency)

deaths per 100,000 population. Of those deaths, 45% were alcohol-related.[4,28] Men are more likely than women to have alcoholic (Laënnec's) cirrhosis. Worldwide, postnecrotic cirrhosis is the most common form; it is also more common in women. Mortality is higher from all types of cirrhosis in men and nonwhites.

Etiology and Risk Factors

The causes of cirrhosis have not been clearly identified, although the relationship between cirrhosis and excessive alcohol ingestion is well established. Countries with the highest incidence of cirrhosis have the greatest per

EB capita consumption of alcohol. Genetic predisposition with a familial tendency, as well as a hypersensitivity to alcohol, is seen in alcoholic cirrhosis.

The primary risk factor for cirrhosis is alcohol ingestion, especially in the absence of proper nutrition. Any client with a family history of alcoholism should avoid alcohol because of the increased risk. Hence cessation of alcohol consumption may be a health promotion, health maintenance, or health restoration activity. The amount of alcohol consumed daily appears to be a more important **EB** factor than the pattern of drinking (binge versus daily) or the type of alcoholic beverage consumed. If the client is in a poor nutritional state, the likelihood of damage is greater and the damage is more severe. Viral hepatitis is the primary risk factor for postnecrotic cirrhosis, which makes prevention of hepatitis through vaccination and good hygiene the most important health-promotion activity.

Other risk factors for cirrhosis of the liver are biliary cirrhosis with intrahepatic cholestasis or obstruction of bile ducts; use of drugs (such as acetaminophen, methotrexate, or isoniazid); hepatic congestion from severe right-sided heart failure; constrictive pericarditis; valvular disease; alpha$_1$-antitrypsin deficiency; infiltrative disease (such as amyloidosis, glycogen storage diseases, or hemochromatosis); Wilson's disease; and nutritional deficits related to jejunal bypass.

Pathophysiology

Cirrhosis is the final stage in many types of liver insults. The cirrhotic liver usually has a nodular consistency, with bands of *fibrosis* (scar tissue) and small areas of regenerating tissue. There is extensive destruction of hepatocytes. This alteration in the architecture of the liver alters flow in the vascular and lymphatic systems and bile duct channels. Periodic exacerbations are marked by bile stasis, precipitating jaundice.

Portal vein hypertension develops in severe cirrhosis. The portal vein receives blood from the intestines and spleen. Thus an increase of pressure in the portal vein causes (1) a retrograde increase in pressure resistance and enlargement of the esophageal, umbilical, and superior rectus veins, which may result in bleeding varices; (2) ascites (the result of osmotic or hydrostatic shifts leading to fluid accumulation in the peritoneum); and (3) incomplete clearing of protein metabolic wastes with a resultant increase in ammonia, thus leading to hepatic encephalopathy.

Continuation of the process as a result of unknown causes or of alcohol abuse usually results in death from hepatic encephalopathy, bacterial (gram-negative) infection, peritonitis (bacterial), hepatoma (liver tumor), or complications of portal hypertension. See the Concept Map feature on Understanding Cirrhosis and Its Treatment on pp. 1342 and 1343 for a summary of pathophysiologic changes, clinical manifestations, and treatment of cirrhosis.

Clinical Manifestations

Manifestations of cirrhosis diminish if the process is arrested at an early stage. Cirrhosis is a disease that initially progresses slowly. Thus people with cirrhosis often discover the condition incidentally when seeking health care for other problems. In the early stages of cirrhosis, findings include hepatomegaly (enlarged liver), vascular changes, and abnormal results of laboratory tests. Palpation reveals a firm (scarred), lumpy (nodular), usually enlarged liver (although the liver becomes hard and shrunken in late cirrhosis).

In advanced cirrhosis, assessment reveals the following severe complications with their physiologic bases: ascites caused by malnutrition, portal hypertension, hypoalbuminemia, and hyperaldosteronism. Gastrointestinal bleeding arises from esophageal varices (swollen veins), hypoprothrombinemia, thrombocytopenia, and portal hypertension and often results in encephalopathy. Splenomegaly (enlargement of the spleen) indicates severe portal hypertension. Anemia, leukopenia, or thrombocytopenia may result from splenomegaly. Portal hypertension may cause prominent abdominal wall veins and internal hemorrhoids. Infections may be present as a result of an enlarged, overactive spleen, causing leukopenia. In addition, the bacteria that remain in the portal venous blood bypass the liver and are not removed by Kupffer cells and hence may cause infection. Ammonia no longer removed by the liver accumulates to levels toxic to the brain, resulting in encephalopathy. Renal failure occurs with rapidly failing hepatic function. Laboratory determinations reveal impaired hepatocellular function: elevated serum levels of liver enzymes (AST, alanine aminotransferase [ALT], and lactate dehydrogenase [LDH]), hypoalbuminemia, anemia, and prolonged PT. Liver biopsy allows a definitive diagnosis and demonstrates the associated pathologic changes.

Outcome Management
■ Medical Management

Monitor for Complications. Ascites, bleeding esophageal varices, and hepatic encephalopathy are discussed in depth later in this chapter. They are the most feared complications of cirrhosis. Renal failure (hepatorenal syndrome) and infection also are deadly. Family members and the client are taught manifestations of progressive liver failure. The family members should know what manifestations they need to report to the physician and when to seek immediate assistance, such as when variceal bleeding or a decrease in the level of consciousness occurs. Clients with encephalopathy may need extensive home care.

Maximize Liver Function. Although cirrhosis is a progressive, degenerative disorder, steps are taken to minimize the risk of trauma and maximize regeneration, thereby slowing the course of the disease and prolonging life. A nutritious diet is recommended for clients with cirrhosis. The diet should be palatable, with adequate calories and protein (75 to 100 g/day) unless hepatic encephalopathy is present, in which case protein is limited. A list of foods to be included in the diet is given to the client and family. Fat intake need not be restricted. If edema or fluid retention is present, restrict sodium and fluids. If the client is receiving a thiazide diuretic, the diet should be high in potassium. The B vitamins and fat-soluble vitamins (vitamins A, D, E, and K) are commonly given to clients with alcoholic cirrhosis. Adequate rest also is important to maximize regeneration of the liver. In postnecrotic or posthepatic cirrhosis, the clinician may prescribe corticosteroids to reduce manifestations of cirrhosis and improve liver function. Other medications may be used to treat the complications.

Treat the Underlying Causes. It is important that exposure to hepatotoxins be eliminated, that use of alcohol be avoided, and that biliary obstruction be removed. Medications that should be avoided (listed in Table 49-6) are specified to the client. The client should be encouraged to seek help (e.g., from Alcoholics Anonymous [AA]) with alcohol abstinence.

Prevent Infection. Prevention of infection is accomplished by adequate rest, appropriate diet, and avoidance of hepatotoxic substances (alcoholic beverages and medications and chemicals toxic to the liver). Before the discovery of antibiotics, infection was the major cause of mortality in cirrhosis.

TABLE 49-6 Cirrhosis and Drug-Induced Liver Failure

Drugs to Restrict or Avoid	Rationale
Acetaminophen	Can cause fatal liver damage
Phenobarbital, phenytoin, chlorpromazine (Thorazine)	Stimulates liver's major drug-metabolizing system; when liver diseased or damaged, drugs may not be metabolized properly and toxicity may occur; may also cause alteration in sensory perception and thought processes related to hepatic encephalopathy
Morphine, paraldehyde, codeine	Can cause spasms and pressure in the biliary tract, thus increasing discomfort
Alcohol	Stimulates liver's major drug metabolizing system; can damage liver further

■ Nursing Management of the Medical Client

Assessment

Because the manifestations of cirrhosis are sometimes vague and nonspecific, the client may not be aware of the disease early in its course. Assess the client closely for the presence of early manifestations, such as hepatomegaly, and carefully check the laboratory data for any indication of cirrhosis. As the disease progresses, assess for manifestations of complications of cirrhosis, such as ascites, portal hypertension, or hepatic encephalopathy. These are discussed later in the chapter.

When a client with cirrhosis is hospitalized, use laboratory data and the client's physical and psychosocial assessment data to guide care planning. See the Case Study feature on Cirrhosis below for further information about these tests. Also assess the client and family members for their knowledge of the important aspects of self-care.

Diagnosis, Outcomes, Interventions

Diagnosis: Ineffective Tissue Perfusion. Because of the increased risk of bleeding in the client with cirrhosis, the nursing diagnosis *Ineffective Tissue Perfusion related to bleeding tendencies and varices that may hemorrhage* is common.

Outcomes. Hemorrhage will be prevented as evidenced by absence of bleeding, normal vital signs, and urine output of at least 0.5 ml/kg/hr.

Interventions

Monitor for Hemorrhage. Monitor the client for bleeding gums, purpura, melena, hematuria, and hematemesis. Check vital signs as ordered to assess for signs of shock.

CASE STUDY *evolve*
Cirrhosis

Mr. James is a 53-year-old man on disability from his job as a warehouse forklift driver. He became unable to work after developing idiopathic peripheral neuropathy, which resulted in frequent falls and an inability to run the controls of the forklift. He uses a cane to ambulate. Mr. James is being admitted with severe abdominal pain and coffee-grounds emesis. He reports that he had been vomiting bright red blood in the 2 days before admission. His abdomen is distended, with a measured abdominal girth of 52 inches. Mr. James also states that he has recently gained several pounds and has had shortness of breath and fatigue for the past several weeks. He reports that he smokes cigarettes but says that he does not use alcohol. . . .
Case Study continued on the website and the CD-ROM with discussions, multiple-choice questions, and a nursing care plan. *evolve*

In addition, monitor urine output. Report volume that is **EB** less than 0.5 ml/kg/hr.

Prevent Hemorrhage. Protect the client from physical injury from falls or abrasions, and give injections only when absolutely necessary, using only small-gauge **EB** needles. Be sure to apply gentle pressure after an injection, but do not rub the site because this might cause bruising.

Provide Client Teaching. Instruct the client to avoid vigorous nose-blowing and straining with bowel movements. Sometimes stool softeners are ordered to prevent straining with rupture of varices. Antidiarrheal agents may be administered to control diarrhea. If bleeding gums are noted, advise the client to use a soft tooth-brush and to refrain from flossing until the bleeding has **EB** ceased.

Diagnosis: Imbalanced Nutrition: Less Than Body Requirements.
For the liver to regenerate, the client must have adequate levels of vital nutrients; otherwise, the unmet requirements lead to the nursing diagnosis *Imbalanced Nutrition: Less Than Body Requirements related to anorexia, impaired liver function, decreased absorption of fat-soluble vitamins, and diarrhea.*

Outcomes. The client will receive adequate nutrition as evidenced by no weight loss and no manifestations of malnutrition.

Interventions
Modify Diet. The diet should provide ample protein to rebuild tissue but not enough protein to precipitate hepatic encephalopathy (75 g of high-quality protein per day). The diet should supply sufficient carbohydrates to **EB** maintain weight and to spare protein stores. A low-fat and low-sodium (200 to 1000 mg/day) diet is also suggested. Total daily calories should range between 2500 and 3000. Place the client on daily weight, intake and output, and calorie counts to assess fluid and nutritional balance.[4,28]

Closely monitor the laboratory and nutritional panels for manifestations of improvement or further deterioration. If ammonia levels rise (normal levels are 70 to 200 **EB** mg/dl in whole blood and 56 to 150 mg/dl in plasma), foods high in protein may be restricted.

If the client has ascites or edema, fluids as well as sodium should be restricted in the diet. Small, frequent meals make it easier for clients with anorexia to eat **EB** enough food. Adequate rest and a stable environmental temperature should be ensured to allow optimal use of calories. Administer prescribed medications, such as antacids, antiemetics, antidiarrheals, or cathartics to decrease gastric distress, but avoid antiemetics such as phenothiazines.

Provide Vitamin Supplements. The physician usually prescribes a maintenance multivitamin preparation or, in severe malnutrition, therapeutic levels of vitamins. Also, vitamins A, D, E, and K are supplied if fat absorption is adequate. Frequently vitamin K injections are ordered to **EB** improve blood clotting factors. The client with severe malabsorption may require IV vitamins with calcium gluconate supplementation. Encourage family or friends to provide desirable foods as permitted.

Diagnosis: Activity Intolerance.
The client with cirrhosis often experiences severe fatigue, leading to the nursing diagnosis *Activity Intolerance related to bed rest, fatigue, lack of energy, and altered respiratory function secondary to ascites.*

Outcomes. The client will maintain a balance between rest and activity as evidenced by the absence of fatigue and problems associated with immobility.

Interventions. Clinicians often prescribe rest for clients with cirrhosis, but how much rest is necessary is debated. During periods of acute malfunction, rest reduces metabolic demands on the liver and increases circulation. Long-term planning should include counseling the client to rest frequently and to avoid unnecessary fatigue.

Diagnosis: Risk for Injury.
Because the liver is in a very precarious state, intake of alcohol or other hepatotoxins should cease immediately. Otherwise the nursing diagnosis *Risk for Injury related to continued intake of hepatotoxins* becomes appropriate.

Outcomes. The client will not suffer injury from continued intake of hepatotoxins as evidenced by cessation of drinking and avoidance of medications that may cause further damage.

Interventions. Ensure that all known hepatotoxic medications (including alcohol) are removed from therapeutic regimens and that dosages of all drugs thought to be metabolized by the liver have been lowered. Avoid the administration of sedatives and opiates.

Diagnosis: Ineffective Protection.
Because of portal hypertension and decreased filtering capability of the liver, the nursing diagnosis *Ineffective Protection related to alcohol abuse and inadequate nutrition* may be appropriate.

Outcomes. The client will not experience systemic infection or spontaneous bacterial peritonitis with ascites.

Interventions. Clients with cirrhosis may experience spontaneous bacterial peritonitis with ascites; mortality is high when this occurs. Your role as nurse is to monitor for manifestations of infection and to administer antibiotics as prescribed. Antibiotics may be required to control intestinal flora that aggravate encephalopathy.

Diagnosis: Ineffective Health Maintenance.

The client with cirrhosis must become involved in self-care if the treatment is to be successful. Therefore *Ineffective Health Maintenance related to lack of knowledge of the disease and long-term treatment is an important nursing diagnosis.*

Outcomes. The client with cirrhosis will understand the disease and the implications of long-term management as evidenced by the client's statements.

Interventions. Provide the client and his or her significant others with information to manage care at home. Clients with cirrhosis will live longer if they get adequate rest, abstain from alcohol, and eat nutritious meals.

Encourage clients with a history of alcohol abuse to seek assistance from support groups such as AA to stop drinking. Even if cirrhotic changes have begun in the liver, it is vital for the client to stop drinking before irreparable damage occurs. See Chapter 26 for further information on alcoholism.

Evaluation

The outcome in cirrhosis depends on the client's ability to stop the intake of alcohol or any other substances toxic to the liver early enough to prevent irreparable liver damage. If biliary obstruction is the cause of the cirrhosis, the client must seek further medical or surgical treatment. Once extensive damage has occurred, the client will not recover and the disease will progress with manifestations of liver failure.

■ Self-Care

Clients with cirrhosis are managed at home unless they encounter complications or are in the end stage of the disease process. Hence it is important to teach them how to maintain adequate nutrition, to alternate rest and activity, and to avoid hepatotoxic substances. Refer the client to the appropriate agency or support group for assistance with alcohol cessation, such as AA, Al-Anon, or Alateen. Provide referrals to community nursing support agencies as needed. If the client is exposed to hepatotoxic agents in the workplace, suggest that the client try to change jobs. Emphasize that regular checkups and blood tests to follow the progress of the disease are needed.

COMPLICATIONS OF CIRRHOSIS

PORTAL HYPERTENSION

Portal hypertension exists when there is a persistent increase in blood pressure in the portal venous system oc-

curring as a result of increased resistance to or obstruction of blood flow through the portal venous system into the liver.

Etiology and Risk Factors

Most cases of portal hypertension in the United States are associated with cirrhosis. The portal vein is likely to be obstructed by a thrombus; a tumor is the next most common cause. Box 49-2 lists factors that may cause portal hypertension.

Pathophysiology

The normal blood flow to and from the liver depends on proper functioning of the portal vein (70% of inflow), the hepatic artery (30% of inflow), and the hepatic veins (outflow). Disease processes that damage the liver or its major vessels or alter the flow of blood through these structures are responsible for the development of portal hypertension. Portal hypertension results either from increased blood flow in the portal vein or from an increased resistance to flow within the portal venous system.

The most common cause of portal hypertension is cirrhosis. The pathophysiologic mechanism in cirrhosis is increased resistance, which is intrahepatic and primarily sinusoidal. Portal hypertension may also arise from presinusoidal obstruction, either outside the liver (as in portal vein thrombosis) or within it (as in schistosomiasis). In addition, lesions leading to portal hypertension may be postsinusoidal, either within the liver (as in veno-occlusive disease) or distal to it (as in Budd-Chiari syndrome or right-sided heart failure). Rarely portal hypertension occurs in the normal liver from markedly increased inflow beyond the capacity of the compliant portal vessels to absorb. Arterial–portal venous fistulas and massive splenomegaly resulting from infection or neoplasm are examples of causes of this type of portal

---

BOX 49-2   *Factors in the Pathogenesis of Cirrhotic Portal Hypertension*

1. *Presinusoidal obstruction*
   a. Outside liver
      (1) Portal vein thrombosis
   b. Within liver
      (1) Schistosomiasis
2. *Postsinusoidal obstruction*
   a. Distal to liver
      (1) Budd-Chiari syndrome
      (2) Right-sided heart failure
   b. Within liver
      (1) Veno-occlusive disease
3. *Increased inflow beyond vessel capacity (Sinusoidal)*
   a. Arterial-portal venous fistulas
   b. Splenomegaly

Modified from Goldman, L., Krevans, J., & Ausiello, D. (2004). *Cecil textbook of Medicine* (22nd ed.). Philadelphia: W.B. Saunders.

Understanding Cirrhosis and Its Treatment

Cessation of alcohol ingestion

Liver insult
Alcohol ingestion
Viral hepatitis
Exposure to toxins

Liver transplantation

Increased WBCs

Hepatocyte damage

Pain

Fatigue

Liver inflammation

Fever

Nausea
Vomiting

Alterations in blood and lymph flow

Anorexia

Liver necrosis

Palmar erythema

Spider angiomas

Loss of body hair

Decreased ADH and aldosterone detoxification so increased levels

Edema

Decreased androgen and estrogen detoxification so increased levels

Testicular atrophy

Gynecomastia

Menstrual changes

Decreased metabolism of protein and carbohydrate

Decreased plasma proteins

Ascites

Decreased fat metabolism

Hypoglycemia
Malnutrition

Edema

Vitamins

Decreased vitamin K absorption

Bleeding tendency

Nutrition

Bleeding precautions

Conjugated and unconjugated hyperbilirubinemia

Jaundice

Decreased bilirubin metabolism and/or Biliary tree damage or obstruction

Clay-colored stools

Decreased bile in gastrointestinal tract and Increased urobilinogen

Dark urine

Diuretics

Fluid restriction

Ascites

Edema

Esophageal varices

Liver fibrosis and scarring

Portal hypertension

Hemorrhoids

Bleeding

Portacaval shunt

Splenomegaly

Superficial abdominal varices

Bleeding

Anemia
Thrombocytopenia
Leukopenia

Delayed wound healing

Infection

Neomycin

Increased serum ammonia

Lactulose

Alterations in sleep

Foul breath

Decreased protein in diet

Liver failure

Inability to metabolize ammonia to urea

Hepatic encephalopathy

Confusion to hepatic coma

Death

Corticosteroids

Asterixis

Respiratory acidosis

○ treatment   ▭ pathology   ◇ clinical manifestations

hypertension. The degree of liver dysfunction varies with the causative process, the duration of the process, and individual client characteristics.

Normal portal venous blood pressure is 5 to 10 mm Hg. Portal hypertension exists when the pressure rises 5 mm Hg higher than the inferior vena cava pressure. Collateral vessels develop in an effort to equalize pressures between the two venous systems. The spleen and other organs that empty into the portal venous system also begin to undergo the effects of congestion. See the Concept Map feature on Understanding Cirrhosis and Its Treatment on pp. 1342 and 1343.

Clinical Manifestations

In clients with portal hypertension, assessment reveals a network of slightly tortuous epigastric vessels that branch off the area of the umbilicus and lead toward the sternum and ribs (caput medusae); an enlarged, palpable spleen; internal hemorrhoids; bruits, which may be heard over the upper abdomen; and ascites, which typically appears when there is concurrent liver disease.

Direct measurement of portal venous blood pressure is possible only during laparotomy. The diagnosis of portal hypertension often relies on indirect measurements of portal pressure—obtained at liver scanning, splenoportography, abdominal angiography, or liver biopsy—and on other laboratory data (see Chapter 44). Radiography and endoscopy procedures may be used to differentiate variceal hemorrhage from other types of gastrointestinal bleeding.

Outcome Management
■ Medical Management

One of the most serious disabling complications of portal hypertension is dilatation of the superior rectal veins, abdominal wall veins, and esophagogastric veins. With conditions such as cirrhosis, portal venous blood pressure increases, causing esophageal veins to swell and distend. These swollen, dilated veins are called *varices*. Several factors can contribute to the rupturing of varices (Figure 49-2): increased portal venous blood pressure, increased intrathoracic pressure (coughing and straining at stools), irritation by food or alcohol, and erosion by gastric juices. The veins of the stomach and esophagus are most subject to rupture; when rupture occurs, it constitutes a medical emergency.

Another mechanism that leads to hemorrhage involves the spleen. The splenic vein merges with the superior mesenteric vein to form the portal vein. When pressure increases in the portal venous system, damage to the spleen occurs. Damage to the spleen is not proportional to the increase in portal venous blood pressure. As the spleen enlarges, it destroys blood cells, especially platelets, which increases the risk of hemorrhage and anemia.

Hepatic encephalopathy is an extremely dangerous complication of portal hypertension. This problem usu-

ally arises following a period of bleeding into the gastrointestinal tract. Digestion of this blood takes place in the intestines. Because blood is a protein, this process increases ammonia in the gut and bloodstream. In turn the excessive ammonia disturbs brain function. The Critical Monitoring feature below lists assessment findings that mandate early intervention in esophageal bleeding secondary to portal hypertension. Hepatic encephalopathy is discussed later in this chapter.

Death often follows rupture of esophageal varices if the hemorrhage is not immediately controlled. To stop hemorrhage, health practitioners perform emergency measures: injection sclerotherapy, transjugular intrahepatic portosystemic shunt, administration of vasopressin, balloon tamponade, beta-adrenergic blocking agents, endoscopic electrocautery, direct ligation of the bleeding varices, transhepatic embolization of the left gastric vein, or even urgent portacaval shunt surgery. Cold saline lavage is probably ineffective but is occasionally done while the client is awaiting transport to surgery or the gastrointestinal laboratory. Fluids, especially volume expanders and blood products, are administered to maintain volume.

FIGURE 49-2 A bleeding esophageal varix. (Courtesy of Martin Sears, M.D., Internal Medicine and Diagnostic Problems, Fremont, NE.)

CRITICAL MONITORING
Esophageal Bleeding Secondary to Portal Hypertension

- Blood pressure ≤90/60 mm Hg
- Heart rate ≥100 beats/min
- Cool, clammy skin
- Distal pulses <2+ on a 0-4+ scale
- Slowed capillary refill (>2 seconds)
- Diminished orientation to person, place, and time
- Restlessness

Control Hemorrhage

Sclerotherapy. To perform sclerotherapy, the operator passes an endoscope into the esophagus and injects a sclerosing agent (e.g., morrhuate sodium) that flows into the varices. The sclerosing agent initially causes inflammation of the vein wall and then fibrosis. The operator may give repeated injections over a period of weeks until the varices are no longer prominent.

Transjugular Intrahepatic Portosystemic Shunt. For years, surgical decompression procedures were used to lower portal pressure in clients with bleeding esophageal varices. Survival rates in clients with hepatitis were not, however, improved with portal vein–systemic (portosystemic) shunt surgery. Decompression can now be accomplished without surgery through the percutaneous placement of a portosystemic shunt, called a *transjugular intrahepatic portosystemic shunt* (TIPS). In this procedure, an expandable metal stent is advanced with the aid of fluoroscopy to the hepatic veins during an angiogram and then through the liver to create a direct portacaval channel. Physiologically TIPS is similar to a side-to-side surgical shunt. Placement is successful in more than 90% of the clients, and bleeding is controlled in 90% to 95% of clients. This method offers an alternative to surgery for refractory bleeding caused by portal hypertension.

This procedure does have some difficulties, however. Stents frequently undergo stenosis or occlude over a period of months, prompting the need for another TIPS or another approach. Also, encephalopathy may develop. TIPS should be reserved for individuals who are considered poor surgical risks or who fail endoscopic or medical management.

Vasopressin. When varices rupture, IV vasopressin is routinely administered to stop variceal bleeding. Administration of vasopressin achieves temporary lowering of portal pressure. These agents reduce portal venous blood flow by constricting afferent arterioles. Direct infusion of vasopressin into the superior mesenteric artery is most effective. Serious side effects include hypothermia, myocardial and gastrointestinal tract ischemia, and acute renal failure. It is therefore contraindicated in clients with a recent myocardial infarction. Vasopressin may be given in conjunction with nitroglycerin, which is administered intravenously, sublingually, or by patch to minimize vasoconstrictive side effects. Alternatively, somatostatin is at least as effective as vasopressin. Drug therapy may stop bleeding, but it has no effect on survival.

Beta-Adrenergic Blocking Agents. The effectiveness of beta-adrenergic blocking agents (e.g., propranolol [Inderal], metoprolol [Lopressor] or nadolol [Corgard]) in the management of acute variceal bleeding is limited because they reduce the heart rate (and hence the blood pressure) and mask the early manifestations of hypoglycemia; however, studies suggest that such therapy has been effective in preventing a first episode of variceal bleeding or subsequent episodes after an initial bleed.

Balloon Tamponade. Applying pressure to ruptured varices via balloon tamponade may stop hemorrhage. For this intervention the clinician inserts a Sengstaken-Blakemore or Minnesota tube into the stomach and inflates the esophageal and gastric balloons (Figure 49-3). The pressure of the esophageal balloon against the varices may stop the bleeding. It is important to release this pressure periodically to prevent tissue necrosis. The esophageal balloon is not left inflated for more than 24 hours. Also, it is important to remove secretions and saliva that accumulate above the balloon to prevent aspiration. The Minnesota tube has an additional port for aspiration of secretions above the esophageal balloon. Ensure that the gastric balloon is inflated to prevent migration of the tube. You should also have scissors at the bedside to be able to remove the tube in an emergency. Complications of balloon tamponade may occur in 15% or more of clients and include aspiration pneumonitis as well as esophageal rupture. This intervention is performed less frequently today now that other treatment is available.

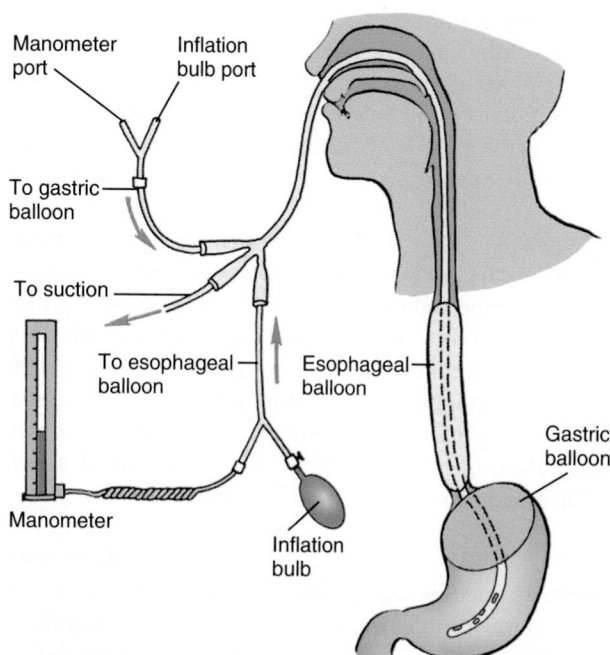

FIGURE 49-3 A Sengstaken-Blakemore tube may be used to control ruptured esophageal varices, a potential complication of portal hypertension.

■ Nursing Management of the Medical Client
Assessment

The major assessment for you to make is for the presence of hemorrhage. The other important aspect of assessment is to check for indicators of the client's clinical status after any intervention to treat the hemorrhage, such as in assessing tube function after placement of a Sengstaken-Blakemore or Minnesota tube. Monitor the client's vital signs continuously for any significant changes.

Diagnosis, Outcomes, Interventions

Diagnosis: Ineffective Tissue Perfusion. With rupture of varices, the nursing diagnosis that must be addressed immediately is *Ineffective Tissue Perfusion related to portal hypertension and rupture and hemorrhage of esophageal varices.*

Outcomes. Hemorrhage will be controlled as evidenced by the return of vital signs to normal and no further bleeding.

Interventions. The client can learn activities to help reduce the risk of rupture of esophageal varices.

Prevent Hemorrhage. The nurse should instruct the client as follows:
- Avoid straining maneuvers that increase intra-abdominal or intrathoracic pressure.
- Avoid rough foods, which may traumatize the esophagus, and spicy foods, which may irritate the esophageal mucosa.
- Develop an emergency plan in case severe esophageal varices should rupture. Include in this plan a list of all emergency telephone numbers. Discuss the plan with both the client and his or her family members.

Monitor for Hemorrhage. If hemorrhage from ruptured varices occurs, monitor blood pressure, pulse, respiration, and urine output continuously, and assist with interventions to restore circulating blood volume. Monitor vital signs closely throughout this period. This is a critical time for nursing intervention and can be a stressful time for the client, family members, and nurse. Further information on the assessment and treatment of shock and hemorrhage can be found in Chapter 83.

Diagnosis: Impaired Gas Exchange. The client with ruptured varices is susceptible to many problems. A major potential problem is addressed in the nursing diagnosis *Impaired Gas Exchange related to decreased oxygen supply secondary to aspiration pneumonitis or obstruction occurring after balloon tamponade with the Sengstaken-Blakemore tube.*

Outcomes. The client will not suffer injury related to the Sengstaken-Blakemore tube as evidenced by no respiratory distress, the absence of aspiration, and the absence of esophageal ischemia.

Interventions

Prevent Esophageal Necrosis. The pressure of the esophageal balloon on the esophagus not only stops hemorrhage but also may cause esophageal necrosis. As noted earlier, you must release the pressure on the esophagus periodically to prevent tissue damage. Consult the physician about how often to release balloon pressure because practices vary widely.

Prevent Aspiration Pneumonia. Aspiration pneumonia is another complication of balloon tamponade. The inflated balloon in the esophagus prevents saliva and secretions from reaching the stomach. Ascertain whether the tube used for tamponade has a suction port above the esophageal balloon. If not, insert a nasogastric tube to the upper balloon level or perform suctioning frequently to remove accumulating fluid.

Prevent Nares Erosion. Tubes inserted through the nose may cause erosion of the nares, especially if traction is applied to the tamponading tube (practices differ). To prevent this complication, clean and lubricate the external nares. Provide padding if necessary.

Prevent Airway Obstruction. Airway obstruction, another complication of balloon tamponade, occurs when the gastric balloon deflates or breaks and traction on the tube pulls the esophageal balloon up into the oropharynx. Keep scissors at the bedside. If this emergency arises, cut the tube and pull it out to restore airway patency. To prevent airway obstruction, label each port of the tube to prevent accidental deflation of the gastric balloon.

Diagnosis: Acute Confusion. Because of the potential buildup of ammonia, the client with bleeding varices is likely to have the nursing diagnosis *Acute Confusion related to portosystemic encephalopathy and hepatic coma occurring in conjunction with gastrointestinal bleeding and accumulation of ammonia.*

Outcomes. The client will be oriented to person, place, and time. Serum ammonia levels will not increase, and the level of consciousness will not decrease.

Interventions

Monitor Level of Consciousness. Assess the client's level of consciousness and orientation on a regular basis (after performing a baseline assessment). Ask clients to write their name each day, and assess for writing deterioration and possible rising ammonia levels. Also assess the client regularly for the development of *asterixis* (liver flap or flapping tremor). Monitor for evidence of gastrointestinal bleeding, including melena or hematemesis, because bleeding can precipitate hepatic coma. Report the bleeding promptly to the physician.

Protect from Injury. Protect the client from injury by keeping the side rails up and the bed in the lowest position. Assist the client with ambulation as needed. Use caution when administering sedatives, antihistamines, and other agents that affect the central nervous system (CNS).

Evaluation

Although the acute episode of bleeding from esophageal varices can usually be controlled, the development of varices is a clinical manifestation of deterioration of the liver and increasing portal hypertension. The client will need careful and continued follow-up to prevent recurrence or further complications.

■ Surgical Management

Endoscopic Band Ligation. In this procedure esophageal varices are ligated and strangulated with small elastic O-rings placed in the appropriate place during endoscopy. Band ligation has proved at least as effective as sclerotherapy in controlling acute variceal bleeding and preventing rebleeding. Because treatment-related complications occur less frequently with band ligation, this procedure is recommended for long-term obliteration of varices that have bled.

Portosystemic Shunt. Several surgical procedures can be used to reduce the danger of hemorrhage from varices caused by portal hypertension. These procedures involve anastomosing the high-pressure portal venous system to the low-pressure systemic venous system. This creates a portosystemic shunt.

Surgical creation of a portosystemic shunt reduces portal hypertension by sending portal venous blood directly into the inferior vena cava, bypassing the liver. Other vessels may be altered, depending on the type of shunt selected. Such a procedure lowers portal venous blood pressure, thus decreasing the risk of rupture of esophageal varices. Figure 49-4 illustrates some portosystemic (portal vein–vena cava) shunt procedures.

Overall, clients who require portosystemic shunts are poor surgical candidates because of their suboptimal nutritional status, their increased risk of infection, and their deteriorating liver function. Usually such surgery is used only as a last resort because the risk of death is high in the early operative period. The role of portosystemic shunt surgery in the management of bleeding esophageal varices after initial medical control of bleeding is uncertain.

Indications. Although surgical shunting reduces the risk of recurrent hemorrhage, the overall mortality of clients undergoing such surgery is comparable to that of clients managed medically. The similarity of outcomes is related to the increased incidence of encephalopathy in surgically managed clients when the shunted blood is not cleared of toxic substances and to the higher incidence of death from progressive liver failure with their increased longevity. For these reasons, the surgical creation of a portosystemic shunt is reserved for clients who have not responded to other treatment and who, despite periodic endoscopic sclerotherapy, continue to bleed.

Contraindications. The main contraindication to portosystemic shunt procedures is poor general health so that the client is not able to withstand the trauma, blood and fluid loss, and anesthesia of surgery.

Complications. Major complications after a shunt procedure are bacteremia and DIC, heart failure, shunt clotting, and hepatic encephalopathy. Clients must be

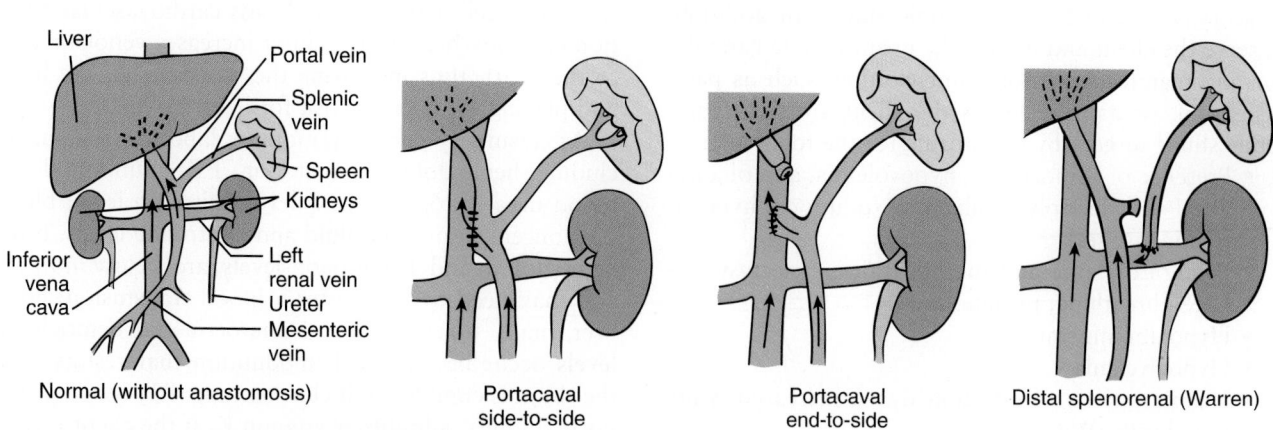

FIGURE 49-4 Some types of portacaval or portosystemic shunt procedures used to reduce portal hypertension.

monitored closely to detect the onset of these complications, and corrective measures need to be implemented quickly if they arise.

Outcomes. Clients who undergo portosystemic shunt procedures require surgery because other methods of controlling bleeding have been unsuccessful. The goal of these procedures is (1) to reduce portal venous blood flow enough to prevent variceal hemorrhage, (2) to preserve enough blood inflow to the liver to prevent hepatic encephalopathy and hepatic failure, and (3) to increase client comfort (the shunting is a palliative procedure).

■ Nursing Management of the Surgical Client

Preoperative Care

Preoperative management of the client undergoing a portosystemic shunt procedure includes an appraisal of the client's general physical condition and readiness for surgery along with assessment of the client's neurologic, respiratory, and renal systems to establish a baseline. Blood and urine may be examined for the presence of infectious organisms, and an arterial blood gas analysis may be performed to assess general respiratory function.

Blood-clotting mechanisms are analyzed as are the client's fluid and electrolyte status and levels of ammonia, protein, bilirubin, and liver enzymes. If the client has an inappropriate level of any one of these substances, measures are taken to correct the problem. If the hemoglobin and hematocrit levels are low, the client may receive a blood transfusion. The client's general nutritional status is important, and protein hydrolysates are administered by total parenteral nutrition (TPN) if indicated.

Postoperative Care
Assessment

After portosystemic shunt surgery, assess the client's respiratory, renal, and hemodynamic status. In addition, observe the client and inspect the operative site carefully for any manifestations of shunt clotting, such as pain, distention, or nausea. Assess the client after portosystemic shunt surgery by monitoring for the following:

- Presence of hemorrhage, hypovolemia, and oliguria
- Fluid and electrolyte imbalance (dilutional hyponatremia, ascites)
- Respiratory rate and rhythm (rales, atelectasis, labored breathing, pneumonia)
- Hypoalbuminemia
- Hypoglycemia
- Manifestations of infection (fever, increased white blood cells [WBCs])
- Pain levels
- Mental status (alertness)

Diagnosis, Outcomes, Interventions

Nursing diagnoses associated with care of the client after portosystemic shunt surgery include *Ineffective Tissue Perfusion, Impaired Gas Exchange,* and *Acute Confusion* (see Nursing Management of the Medical Client). In addition, *Excess Fluid Volume* is a pertinent nursing diagnosis for the client undergoing portosystemic shunt surgery.

Diagnosis: Excess Fluid Volume. The client who has undergone portosystemic shunt surgery often retains excess fluid, leading to the nursing diagnosis *Excess Fluid Volume related to retention of fluids secondary to portal hypertension, liver failure, and hemodilution of blood related to the new portosystemic shunt.*

Outcomes. A normovolemic state will be maintained as evidenced by a stable or decreasing abdominal girth and a regular respiratory rate and rhythm.

Interventions

Assess for Excess Fluid Volume. Assess the client for retention of fluid, which is likely to occur because of hemodynamic fluid shifts. Measure abdominal girth to obtain a baseline, and then recheck daily or every shift, as appropriate, to detect development of ascites. Also, monitor weight and intake and output. Output should not be less than intake. Assess for the presence of edema and document its degree, from 1+ (barely noticeable) to 4+ (deep and pitting). Be sure to check for clinical indicators of pulmonary edema, including dyspnea and orthopnea. See that appropriate pulmonary and respiratory therapy is initiated if the client has any respiratory involvement.

Monitor and Treat Postprocedure Complications. Assess the client for hepatic encephalopathy. If portal hypertension is due to liver disease, carefully monitor for postoperative hemorrhage because bleeding tendencies often arise from liver cell malfunction. Assess cardiovascular function carefully because the shunt increases venous return to the heart, thus increasing the workload of the heart and placing the client at risk for heart failure.

After surgery carefully monitor laboratory data, including hemoglobin, hematocrit, PT, ammonia level, blood urea nitrogen (BUN) level, bilirubin level, blood gas concentrations and fluid and electrolyte levels. If the hemoglobin and hematocrit levels are below normal, you may need to administer a blood transfusion; however, many times the low hematocrit and hemoglobin levels occur because of hemodilution that results after the shunt is completed. If clotting time (PT) is not within normal limits, administer vitamin K. If the client is having difficulty breathing because of ascites, it is doubly important after surgery to implement measures that improve respirations (turning, coughing, and deep-breathing; respiratory treatments; and maintaining any chest drainage system). Other areas in which you may need to intervene for clients who have undergone portosystemic shunt surgery include the following:

- Administering IV fluids plus blood or volume expanders such as dextran and maintaining line patency and prescribed flow rates
- Monitoring blood and urine values and noting any manifestations of infection (such as increased WBCs and elevated erythrocyte sedimentation rate)
- Eliminating medications that sedate, depress the CNS, or are known hepatotoxins (e.g., acetaminophen)
- Maintaining nutrition: While the client is receiving nothing by mouth, that is, is on *nil per os* (NPO) status, usually for several days postoperatively, administer TPN; when food intake begins, protein intake may be limited and increased slowly if BUN and ammonia levels and mental status remain within normal limits
- Maintaining sterile technique when changing dressing(s)
- Maintaining patency if a gastrointestinal tube is in place
- Assisting the client and his or her family to cope with postoperative discomfort and with issues pertinent to chronic liver disease and its sequelae

When emergency shunt surgery is performed, little time may be available to complete preoperative teaching of appropriate information to the client and his or her significant others. Present careful explanations postoperatively to compensate for the lack of preoperative teaching.

Evaluation

Although shunt procedures may decrease the bleeding, the long-term prognosis for the client is poor. Severe encephalopathy often develops, followed by coma and death.

Nonsurgical Alternative Procedure

Transjugular Intrahepatic Portosystemic Shunt
Transjugular intrahepatic portosystemic shunt has emerged as technique to create a portal-systemic shunt by a percutaneous approach. (See the previous section on TIPS.)

ASCITES

Etiology and Risk Factors

Ascites is the accumulation of fluid in the peritoneal cavity that results from the interaction of several pathophysiologic changes. Portal hypertension, lowered plasma colloidal osmotic pressure, and sodium retention all contribute to this condition. Disease processes that lead to these events include cirrhosis of the liver, right-sided heart failure, tuberculous peritonitis, cancer, and complications of pancreatitis.

Pathophysiology

Any process that blocks the flow of blood through the liver sinusoids to the hepatic veins and vena cava causes an increase in hydrostatic pressure in the portal venous system. Most commonly, this problem develops in cirrhosis of the liver or right-sided heart failure. As portal pressure increases, plasma leaks directly from the liver capsule and the congested portal vein into the peritoneal cavity. Congestion of lymph channels occurs, leading to the leakage of more plasma into the peritoneal cavity. Loss of plasma proteins into ascitic fluid from the portal venous system reduces oncotic pressure in the vascular compartment. Reduction in oncotic pressure limits the vascular system's ability to hold onto or collect water.

In addition, hepatocellular damage reduces the liver's ability to synthesize normal amounts of albumin. Decreased albumin synthesis leads to hypoalbuminemia, which is exacerbated by leakage of protein into the peritoneal cavity. The circulating blood volume decreases from loss of colloid osmotic pressure. The secretion of aldosterone increases to stimulate the kidneys to retain sodium and water. As a result of hepatocellular damage, the liver is unable to inactivate aldosterone. Thus sodium and water retention continue. More fluid is held, and the volume of ascitic fluid grows.

Clinical Manifestations

Ascitic fluid typically produces abdominal distention, bulging flanks, and a downward-protruding umbilicus. Although large accumulations of ascitic fluid are obvious, small or moderate amounts may be more difficult to detect. See Chapter 44 for a discussion of the assessment of a client with ascites.

Diagnostic tests to confirm the presence of ascites include paracentesis, abdominal x-ray studies, ultrasonography, and computed tomography (CT) scan. These tests may locate fluid in the peritoneal cavity. Paracentesis provides samples of fluid for analysis. Findings help determine the underlying cause of the ascites; for example, the finding of malignant cells may indicate a tumor.

Outcome Management
■ **Medical Management**
Correct Fluid and Electrolyte Imbalance. Fluid and electrolyte balance is corrected by improving renal sodium excretion and restricting sodium and water intake. This involves discontinuing medications that inhibit prostaglandin synthesis and thus impair renal sodium excretion (e.g., aspirin, ibuprofen, indomethacin).

Paracentesis. Repeated large-volume paracentesis, in combination with IV administration of albumin to maintain plasma volume, is used to manage clients with ascites resulting from cirrhosis; however, repeated removal of fluid, protein, and electrolytes from the body causes severe disturbances in homeostasis. It is becoming more common to remove the least amount of fluid, such as 100 ml, sufficient to relieve manifestations such as shortness of breath. Clients must be monitored for rupture of the umbilicus.

Albumin. The physician may prescribe IV administration of albumin to replace each liter of ascitic fluid that is removed.

Diet Modifications. The diet is low in sodium with restriction of fluids. Protein intake is moderate unless the client has manifestations of hepatic encephalopathy.

Promote Effective Breathing Pattern. Edema in the form of ascites, besides compressing the liver and thus affecting its function, may also cause shallow breathing and impaired gas exchange, resulting in respiratory compromise. When ascites is present, potassium-sparing diuretics (e.g., spironolactone) are prescribed. Oxygen may be prescribed, and arterial blood gas analysis and pulse oximetry may be ordered. Semi-Fowler or high Fowler position, as well as daily or every-shift measurement of abdominal girth, is often prescribed.

Maintain Skin Integrity. When edema is present in liver disease, the client is at increased risk for development of skin impairment and possibly infected skin lesions. If jaundice is present, tepid water or emollient baths may be ordered, along with the use of non-alkaline soaps and application of emollient lotions. If antihistamines are prescribed, observe for excessive sedation.

■ Nursing Management of the Medical Client
Assessment

Some simple assessments to perform at the bedside are the following:
- Percussion of the abdomen; if the client has ascites, the sound will be dull
- Measurement of circumference (abdominal girth)
- Assessment of the client for ascites (see Chapter 44)

Assess the amount of distress caused by the ascites. Ask whether the fluid is interfering with sleeping, eating, and breathing. Assess for the presence of a hydrothorax or misplaced point of maximal impact (PMI). See the Care Plan feature on Management of the Client with Hepatic Failure on pp. 1351 to 1354.

Diagnosis, Outcomes, Interventions

Diagnosis: Excess Fluid Volume and Deficient Fluid Volume. The client with ascites has a combination of volume problems leading to the nursing diagnoses *Excess Fluid Volume* and *Deficient Fluid Volume related to fluid shifts secondary to portal hypertension, hypoalbuminemia, and hyperaldosteronism.*

Outcomes. A normal balance of fluid between the intracellular and extracellular spaces will be maintained as evidenced by absence of hypovolemia, normal serum albumin, decreased abdominal girth, and normal blood pressure.

Interventions

Restrict Fluids. Restriction of the client's fluid intake must be strictly followed. Give medications with meals, if possible, so that mealtime fluids can be used for taking medications.

Monitor Intake and Output. Measure abdominal girth daily (sometimes twice a day), and weigh the client daily. Monitor intake and output daily. Output should be equal to or exceed intake.

Administer Albumin and Diuretics. Administer albumin and diuretics as ordered. Give the albumin first to pull fluid back into the blood vessels. Give the diuretics second to promote excretion of the extra fluid. Assess the client for electrolyte imbalance and heart failure.

Avoid Hepatotoxins. Avoid administering aspirin and nonsteroidal anti-inflammatory drugs (NSAIDs) because they inhibit prostaglandin synthesis and, as noted previously, impair sodium excretion by the kidney.

Monitor After Paracentesis. Monitor the client closely after a paracentesis procedure. Check vital signs frequently to ensure that the client has tolerated the procedure well, and check the dressing carefully to ensure that excessive amounts of fluid are not lost. Sometimes a pouch is placed to collect leaking fluid. If too much fluid is lost, the physician may suture the site closed to prevent excess loss.

Diagnosis: Ineffective Breathing Pattern. Ascites leads to many other problems. *Ineffective Breathing Pattern related to increased intra-abdominal pressure on the diaphragm* is a common nursing diagnosis in clients with ascites.

Outcomes. The client will not experience an ineffective breathing pattern as evidenced by the absence of short-

CARE PLAN

Management of the Client with Hepatic Failure

Nursing Diagnosis. Activity Intolerance related to fatigue, anemia from poor nutrition and bleeding, ascites, dyspnea from pressure of ascites on diaphragm, muscle wasting.

Outcomes. Client will feel rested with fewer complaints of fatigue and increased tolerance for activity.

Interventions	Rationales
1. Alternate rest and activity.	1. Conserves energy and reduces demands on liver.
2. Monitor hemoglobin and hematocrit.	2. Allows detection of gastrointestinal bleeding.
3. Assist with activities of daily living (ADL).	3. Conserves energy and reduces demands on the liver.
4. Administer iron supplements or blood transfusions as ordered to treat anemia.	4. Increases activity tolerance.
5. Assist with measures to decrease edema and ascites (see Fluid Volume Excess to follow).	5. Increases lung capacity.

Evaluation. Within a day after paracentesis or shunting surgery, the client will have decreased volume of ascitic fluid, tolerate activity better, perform more ADLs, and experience less dyspnea and tachycardia. If ascitic fluid reaccumulates after paracentesis, the activity intolerance will return. Continued improvement will be seen after various shunting procedures. Blood transfusions will immediately improve hemoglobin and hematocrit levels, whereas iron replacement therapy will take longer to be effective.

Nursing Diagnosis. Imbalanced Nutrition: Less than Body Requirements related to impaired utilization and storage of nutrients, increased pressure on stomach and intestines, feeling full, anorexia, nausea, loss of nutrients from vomiting.

Outcomes. Client will maintain or increase body weight to ideal weight and will consume adequate nutrients.

Interventions	Rationales
1. Weigh daily.	1. Monitors weight loss or gain.
2. Provide oral hygiene before meals.	2. Improves taste of food.
3. Administer antiemetics as ordered.	3. Relieves nausea and vomiting.
4. Provide small, frequent meals.	4. Prevents feeling of fullness and ensures adequate nutritional intake.
5. Determine food preferences and assist in selection of those that contain low or no protein and low salt, as ordered.	5. Allows preferred foods, when possible, to encourage nutrition.
6. Prevent constipation.	6. Reduces abdominal pressure.

Evaluation. With interventions, the client will maintain weight (not fluid) or begin to gain weight by consuming adequate nutrients and following diet restrictions.

Nursing Diagnosis. Ineffective Protection related to decreased filtering of bacteria by liver and impaired synthesis of clotting factors.

Outcomes. Client will remain free of infection and will have no bruising or hemorrhage.

Interventions	Rationales
1. Monitor for manifestations of hemorrhage.	1. Decreased synthesis of clotting factors can lead to hemorrhage.
2. Provide assistance with ambulation and activities of daily living.	2. Minimizes risk of trauma and injury.
3. Use small-gauge needles for injections and apply prolonged pressure after injection.	3. Minimizes risk of bleeding into tissues.
4. Recommend soft-bristle toothbrush.	4. Reduces injury to oral tissues.

Continued

CARE PLAN

Management of the Client with Hepatic Failure—cont'd

Interventions	Rationales
5. Teach to avoid vigorous blowing of nose or straining at stool.	5. Reduces risk of hemorrhage.
6. Administer vitamin K as ordered.	6. Necessary for synthesis of clotting factors.
7. Follow infection control procedures.	7. Minimizes risk of infection.
8. Monitor for manifestations of infection (temperature, leukopenia).	8. Promotes identification and treatment of infection.

Evaluation. If interventions are successful, the client will not experience hemorrhage or infection.

Nursing Diagnosis. Acute Confusion related to portal systemic encephalopathy occurring in conjunction with gastrointestinal bleeding and accumulation of ammonia in the bloodstream.

Outcomes. Client will be oriented to person, place, and time. Serum ammonia levels will not increase, and level of consciousness will not decrease.

Interventions	Rationales
1. Monitor for manifestations of encephalopathy such as disorientation, changes in handwriting or speech, or coma.	1. Liver is unable to convert ammonia to urea for excretion.
2. Encourage fluids (unless restricted).	2. Promotes excretion of ammonia and urea.
3. Give laxatives and enemas.	3. Decreases serum ammonia.
4. Provide low-protein diet.	4. Reduces generation of ammonia, which is a by-product of protein metabolism.
5. Limit activity.	5. Reduces generation of ammonia, a by-product of metabolism.
6. Treat gastrointestinal bleeding as ordered.	6. Reduces generation of ammonia, a by-product of bacterial action on blood.

Evaluation. Within 1 or 2 days of treatment, the client's serum ammonia levels will decrease and the client will become oriented to person, place, and time.

Nursing Diagnosis. Disturbed Body Image related to yellowing of skin and sclerae (jaundice), ascites, and edema.

Outcomes. Client will cope with body image disturbance, avoid isolation, and initiate or reestablish support systems.

Interventions	Rationales
1. Assess the client's response to changes in body.	1. Determines the extent of body image disturbance.
2. Promote accepting and nonjudgmental attitude.	2. Respects the client's sensitivity to body image changes.
3. Listen and encourage ventilation of feelings.	3. Helps the client feel valued.
4. Suggest clothing colors and options and makeup suggestions.	4. Enhances self-esteem.

Evaluation. Within 1 to 2 days of beginning treatment, some of the body changes will be corrected. Jaundice usually resolves in about 3 weeks. The volume of ascitic and edematous fluid can be reduced in a few days. Some degree of ascites and muscle wasting is irreversible, and the client will learn to accept the altered body image. In addition, it is expected that the client will maintain or establish new interpersonal relationships and activities.

Nursing Diagnosis. Excess Fluid Volume related to retention of fluids secondary to decreased serum albumin, increased sodium and water, portal hypertension, and possible shunting procedures causing hemodilution of blood.

Outcomes. Client will maintain a normovolemic state and adequate respirations and will have a decreased abdominal girth.

CARE PLAN

Interventions	Rationales
1. Follow sodium and fluid restrictions.	1. Helps to decrease ascites and edema.
2. Administer diuretics as ordered.	2. Promotes excretion of fluid.
3. Weigh daily.	3. Evaluates treatment measures.
4. Measure abdominal girth every day or shift.	4. Evaluates treatment measures.
5. Monitor intake and output.	5. Evaluates treatment measures.
6. Monitor electrolytes, hemoglobin, and hematocrit.	6. Diuretics may cause electrolyte imbalances; shunting may cause hemodilution.
7. Implement measures to prevent skin breakdown (see Impaired Skin Integrity to follow).	7. Edema causes skin to break down faster.
8. Administer albumin as ordered.	8. Albumin pulls fluid into blood vessels, where the action of diuretics can remove the excess fluid.
9. Assist with paracentesis procedure.	9. Paracentesis removes 1 L or more of fluid.

Evaluation. If some liver function is restored, the client will produce more albumin to promote the return of fluid into the blood vessels. Administration of albumin and diuretics will promote diuresis within hours, but repeated administration may be necessary because their effect is temporary. Paracentesis is a temporary solution; ascitic fluid will accumulate again if albumin levels remain low and portal hypertension is untreated.

Nursing Diagnosis. Ineffective Breathing Pattern related to pressure on diaphragm and reduced lung capacity secondary to ascites.

Outcomes. Client will breathe with minimal difficulty; no manifestations of hypoxia will be seen.

Interventions	Rationales
1. Place the client in the semi-Fowler or Fowler position with arms supported with pillows.	1. Relieves pressure on diaphragm.
2. Assess for manifestations such as crackles or increased respirations.	2. Identifies fluid in lungs.
3. Administer oxygen as needed.	3. Improves gas exchange.

Evaluation. Treatment of ascites will enable the client to breathe with minimal difficulty.

Nursing Diagnosis. Impaired Skin Integrity related to pruritus (itching), edema, ascites, decreased mobility.

Outcomes. Client will maintain skin integrity and obtain relief from pruritus.

Interventions	Rationales
1. Limit bathing to every 2-3 days, with sponge baths in between.	1. Keeps skin moist and minimizes itching.
2. Use warm (95-100° F) rather than hot water.	2. Cool water minimizes vasodilation and itching.
3. Avoid alkaline soaps.	3. Soaps dry skin.
4. Apply emollients (mineral oil, lanolin, baby oil).	4. Emollients reduce evaporation and keep skin moist.
5. Use cool, light cotton clothing, which promotes evaporation.	5. Minimizes irritation and itching.
6. Keep clothing and bedding dry.	6. Minimizes itching.
7. Keep the environment cool (65-70° F).	7. Minimizes vasodilation and itching.
8. Avoid activities that promote sweating.	8. Minimizes vasodilation and itching.
9. Keep nails short and smooth.	9. Prevents breaking skin integrity when scratching.
10. Administer cholestyramine as ordered.	10. Combines with bile salts and promotes intestinal elimination to decrease itching.
11. Administer diphenhydramine hydrochloride (Benadryl) at night.	11. Antihistamine that has antipruritic and sedative effect; itching is worse at night.
12. Encourage diversional activities.	12. Decreases perception of itching and improves coping.

Continued

CARE PLAN

Management of the Client with Hepatic Failure—cont'd

Interventions	Rationales
13. Encourage the client to avoid trauma.	13. May have impaired clotting activity, which will result in bruises with trauma.
14. Monitor manifestations.	14. Observes for changes that suggest improvement or worsening of condition.
15. Restrict sodium intake.	15. Prevents additional fluid retention.
16. Restrict fluids as ordered.	16. Reduces fluid retention.
17. Administer prescribed diuretics.	17. Reduces fluid retention and promotes diuresis.
18. Monitor intake and output.	18. Assesses renal function and fluid retention.
19. Weigh daily.	19. Assesses fluid retention.
20. Reposition every 2 hr.	20. Relieves pressure over bony prominences.
21. Use special mattress such as alternating air mattress or egg crate mattress.	21. Reduces the likelihood of skin breakdown.

Evaluation. After jaundice resolves in about 3 weeks, the client will have relief from pruritus, will be able to sleep without interruption, and will maintain skin integrity.

ness of breath and the presence of normal respiratory excursion.

Interventions. Position the client in the high Fowler position to facilitate breathing, and monitor his or her respiratory status for the development of atelectasis or pneumonia. Ask the client to cough, and take a deep breath hourly to maintain adequate respiratory function. The client may need to use an incentive spirometer or receive ultrasound treatments if the cough does not loosen and to bring up respiratory secretions.

Diagnosis: Impaired Skin Integrity. In clients with ascites, severe edema as well as other problems may develop, leading to the nursing diagnosis *Impaired Skin Integrity related to immobility, edema, and pressure from the abdomen.*

Outcomes. The client will maintain skin integrity.

Interventions. Turn the client frequently, providing adequate support for the distended abdomen. If the client is on bed rest, recommend a specialty mattress used to prevent skin breakdown. Inspect the client's skin carefully daily, and apply lotions and creams as necessary. Keep the skin cool, and change soiled bed linens as soon as possible.

Diagnosis: Ineffective Health Maintenance. Once the acute problems associated with ascites are controlled, the client and family members are faced with long-term control of the problem, often leading to the nursing di-

agnosis *Ineffective Health Maintenance related to lack of knowledge about ascites, treatment, and self-care.*

Outcomes. The client will understand ascites, its treatment, and self-care after discharge as evidenced by the client's statements, compliance with the treatment regimen, and abstinence from alcohol.

Interventions. Help the client to understand ascites, its treatment, and self-care needs after discharge. Discuss the causes of ascites with the client, making sure that the client understands ways to slow the recurrence. Ensure that the client understands the need for dietary modifications, fluid restrictions, and home health care measures. Help the client to understand that all intake of alcohol must stop. Refer the client to AA and other support groups for assistance with abstinence if necessary.

Evaluation

The client's ascites may be controlled to some extent, but once cirrhosis is advanced, it is difficult to control. The optimal outcome is that the client will stop drinking, thereby preventing further liver damage.

■ Surgical Management

Peritoneovenous Shunt. The client with refractory and disabling chronic ascites may obtain relief from the insertion of a peritoneovenous (LeVeen or Denver) shunt.

Indications. Insertion of a peritoneovenous shunt may be indicated for clients whose ascites is not re-

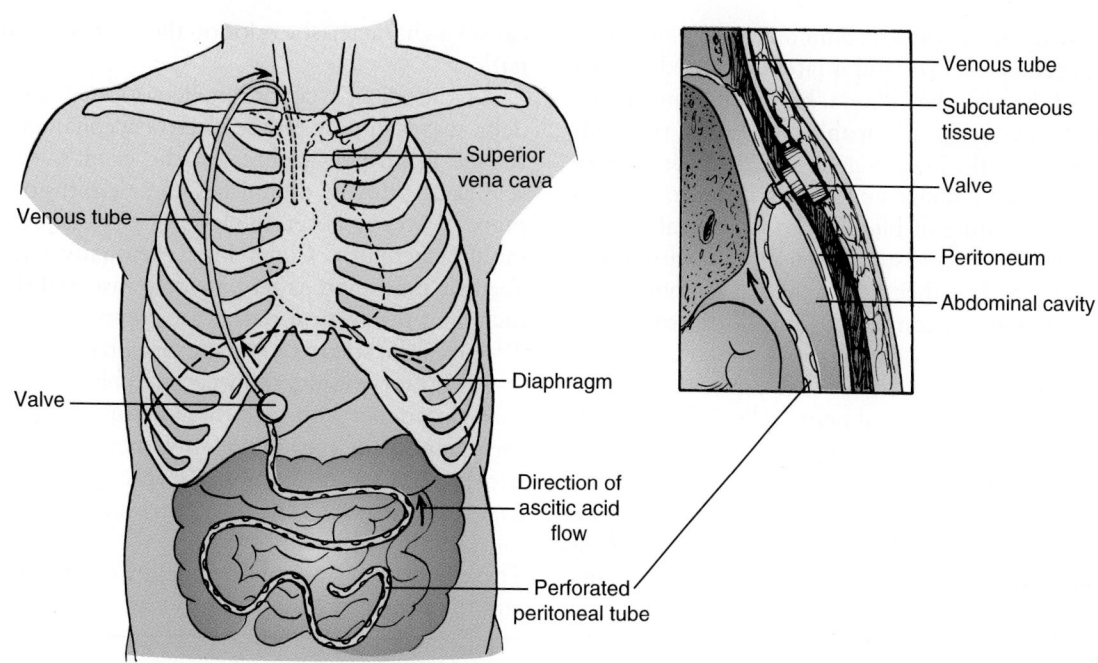

FIGURE 49-5 LeVeen peritoneovenous shunt for chronic ascites moves fluid from the peritoneal (abdominal) cavity into the superior vena cava.

sponding to medical management. As Figure 49-5 shows, a properly functioning shunt moves fluid from the peritoneal (abdominal) cavity into the superior vena cava. Resolution of ascites may be dramatic after implantation of a peritoneovenous shunt. The shunt contains a one-way valve that prevents back-flow of ascitic fluid.

Contraindications. The main contraindication to placement of a peritoneovenous shunt is that the client's state of health is too poor to withstand the trauma of surgery.

Complications. Complications of shunt implantation include infection, hemodilution, DIC, heart failure, and shunt clotting. For additional information, see the earlier discussion of surgical management of portal hypertension.

Transjugular Intrahepatic Portosystemic Shunt. The TIPS procedure is described earlier as a treatment choice for esophageal varices; however, TIPS also is useful in selected clients for the management of ascites. Even though mobilizing ascitic fluid may precipitate severe hepatic encephalopathy in some clients, TIPS remains a promising treatment for ascites.

■ Nursing Management of the Surgical Client

Preoperative and postoperative management of a client with ascites is similar to that of a client who has undergone surgery for portal hypertension and esophageal varices. See the discussion of nursing care of the client with surgical treatment of a hepatic problem.

HEPATIC ENCEPHALOPATHY

Etiology and Risk Factors

Hepatic encephalopathy constitutes a spectrum of CNS disturbances. These disturbances may appear in conjunction with severe liver injury or liver failure or after portosystemic shunt surgery. The cause of this disorder is the liver's inability to metabolize ammonia to form urea so that it can be excreted. Ammonia is a CNS depressant. Changes during the initial stages of hepatic encephalopathy include reduced mental alertness, confusion, and restlessness. Loss of consciousness, seizures, and irreversible coma occur in the terminal stage.

Pathophysiology

The specific cause of hepatic encephalopathy is unknown, but it is characterized by elevations of ammonia levels in the blood and cerebrospinal fluid (CSF). Ammonia is produced in the gastrointestinal tract when protein is broken down by bacteria, by the liver, and, in lesser amounts, by gastric juices and peripheral tissue metabolism. The kidneys are another source of ammonia in the presence of hypokalemia. More recently implicated as a cause of encephalopathy are false neurotransmitters, elevated levels of mercaptans (organic chemicals that contain the sulfhydryl radical, formed when the oxygen of an alcohol molecule is replaced by sulfur), and fatty acids.

Normally the liver converts ammonia into glutamine, which is stored in the liver and is later converted to urea and excreted through the kidneys. Blood ammonia levels rise when the liver cells are unable to perform this conversion. Failure of the liver to perform this function may be due to liver cell damage and necrosis. It also may result from the shunting of blood from the portal venous system directly into the systemic venous circulation (bypassing the liver). In either case, as blood ammonia levels rise, many unusual compounds begin to form. Some of these compounds (e.g., octopamine) apparently act as false neurotransmitters in the CNS. Ammonia also is a CNS toxin, affecting glial and nerve cells; it leads to altered CNS metabolism and function.

Any process that increases protein in the intestine, such as increased dietary protein or gastrointestinal bleeding, causes elevated blood ammonia levels and possible manifestations of hepatic encephalopathy in clients with hepatocellular failure or who have undergone portosystemic shunt surgery (Box 49-3).

Clinical Manifestations

The manifestations of hepatic encephalopathy are primarily neurologic and range from mild mental confusion to deep coma. The neurologic changes occur with cerebral accumulation of ammonia or gastrointestinal bleeding. Hepatic encephalopathy impairs memory, attention, concentration, and rate of response. Sleep pattern reversal often occurs, with the client awake at night and sleepy during the day. Handwriting and speech show significant changes as intellectual deterioration occurs. Asterixis may be present. In some clients with hepatic encephalopathy, hyperventilation with respiratory alkalosis develops because high ammonia levels stimulate the respiratory center. The presence of methylmercaptan

causes a characteristic odor on the breath called *fetor hepaticus*.

As the client's condition deteriorates, characteristic delta waves appear on the electroencephalogram (EEG). As the syndrome progresses, the client's level of consciousness slowly diminishes, and confusion becomes more severe; however, the level of CNS depression commonly fluctuates. Coma may eventually ensue, which deepens until there is no pain response and the reflexes, including the corneal reflex, are completely absent. Box 49-4 lists the stages of hepatic encephalopathy.

Laboratory results show elevated blood ammonia and CSF glutamine. Although these findings help to confirm the diagnosis of encephalopathy, they are not specific to it. Monitor serum ammonia levels, electrolytes, blood gases, and hepatic function test results (bilirubin, albumin, prothrombin, and enzymes) throughout the course. These findings help to determine the degree of imbalance and the extent of hepatic injury (see Chapter 44).

Prognosis

Although intervention usually alleviates hepatic encephalopathy, the client may die of circulatory or respi-

---

BOX 49-3 *Hepatic Encephalopathy: Causes or Precipitating Factors*

- Decrease in hepatocellular function
- Hypoxia
- Infection
- Diuretics (produce hypokalemia, alkalosis, and hypovolemia)
- Depressants: phenobarbital, narcotics, tranquilizers, and sedatives
- Gastrointestinal bleeding
- Medications containing ammonium or amino compounds
- Paracentesis
- Increased protein intake
- Constipation
- Dehydration
- Hypokalemia
- Portosystemic and portacaval shunts

BOX 49-4 *Stages of Hepatic Encephalopathy*

Stage 1
Fatigue
Restlessness
Irritability
Decreased intellectual performance
Decreased attention span
Diminished short-term memory
Personality changes
Sleep pattern reversal

Stage 2
Deterioration in handwriting
Asterixis
Drowsiness
Confusion
Lethargy
Fetor hepaticus

Stage 3
Severe confusion
Inability to follow commands
Deep somnolence, but arousable

Stage 4
Coma
Unresponsive to painful stimuli
Possible decorticate or decerebrate posturing

ratory complications, infection, or delirium and convulsions. Mortality is high among clients who progress into coma with hepatic failure. Health practitioners often use dramatic measures to reduce toxic levels of ammonia in the blood. Such measures include hemodialysis and exchange transfusions, which involve removal and replacement of about 80% of the client's blood. A liver transplant may be performed in cases of fulminant liver failure.

Outcome Management
■ Medical Management

Identify and Treat Precipitating Causes. Factors that may precipitate or severely aggravate hepatic encephalopathy in clients with severe liver disease include gastrointestinal bleeding, increased dietary protein, constipation, infection, CNS-depressant drugs (e.g., opiates, benzodiazepines), and dehydration. Gastrointestinal bleeding and increased protein intake may lead to increased bacterial formation of nitrogenous compounds that induce encephalopathy. The use of CNS-depressant drugs should be avoided in these clients.

Protein may be totally eliminated from the diet, with an intake of only fruit juices and IV fluids, although this radical restriction leads to catabolism of the client's own protein stores. The usual protein restriction is 20 to 40 g daily. The client with chronic hepatic encephalopathy may need to adjust to a long-term, low-protein diet (50 to 60 g/day), which can be difficult. Vegetable and dairy protein may be better tolerated than meats. These proteins contain fewer ammonia-forming amino acids than those in meat. A diet high in vegetables and dairy products also helps to prevent constipation, thus further reducing ammonia production.

Reduce Nitrogenous Waste (Ammonia) in Blood and Bacteria in Colon. Neomycin and lactulose are given to reduce bacteria in the intestinal tract. Because it is not absorbed into the circulation, neomycin exerts a powerful effect on the intestinal bacteria that are responsible for ammonia production. Undesirable side effects result from the depletion of intestinal flora (e.g., diarrhea, vitamin K deficiency). Also, because neomycin is nephrotoxic, its use must be avoided in clients with renal insufficiency. Lactulose, which helps decrease blood ammonia levels by reducing absorption of ammonia, is given to clients to produce two to four stools a day. Antibiotics are administered to inhibit growth of gastrointestinal bacteria, and oral magnesium sulfate or enemas are given after hemorrhage to clean out the intestines.

Maintain Fluid Volume Balance. With the accumulation of fluid in the abdominal area (ascites), bleeding, and decreased fluid intake, the client may experience a fluid volume deficit. This deficit, along with electrolyte imbalances that may occur, should be corrected. IV fluids are administered, carefully monitoring the quantity and rate of administration.

■ Nursing Management of the Medical Client
Assessment

When working with a client susceptible to hepatic encephalopathy, use interviewing and assessment techniques to evaluate psychophysiologic status. For example, has the client's normally neat handwriting become sloppy and difficult to read? Is speech slow and slurred? Observe the client for personality changes with labile feeling states, and elicit liver flap or flapping tremor (asterixis) by asking the client to dorsiflex the hand with the rest of the arm resting on the bed. (In asterixis, the hand cannot be held steady.)

The nurse who is with the client over time is often the best person to assess a change in the level of mental functioning. Early detection of a depressed or confused level of consciousness greatly improves the client's chances of recovery. To make nursing progress notes relevant, describe the client's behavior vividly and objectively, as in "States pigeons are pecking at his bedclothes," rather than offering interpretations that may have a different meaning for each reader, such as "Seems more confused." As the client progresses into coma, make ongoing neurologic checks to determine the level of consciousness. See Unit 16 for neurologic assessment of comatose clients.

Diagnosis, Outcomes, Interventions

Diagnosis: Ineffective Therapeutic Regimen Management and Ineffective Family Therapeutic Regimen Management. The client and family members are vital players in the control of encephalopathy. Thus the nursing diagnoses *Ineffective Therapeutic Regimen Management* and *Ineffective Family Therapeutic Regimen Management related to reduction in protein in the diet and long-term pharmacologic intervention with neomycin* are common with hepatic encephalopathy.

Outcomes. The client will understand and comply with the reduction of protein in the diet and long-term pharmacologic intervention with neomycin as evidenced by the client's following a low-protein diet and stating reasons why neomycin should be taken.

Interventions

Promote Low-Protein Diet. It is important that the client understand the importance of the reduced protein diet to have the motivation to remain on this diet.

Monitor for Gastrointestinal Hemorrhage. In addition to ensuring a low-protein diet, assess for manifestations of gastrointestinal bleeding, checking for bright red blood in the stool or for black, tarry stools. As previously noted, bleeding results in protein accumulation in the gastrointestinal tract, which exacerbates hepatic encephalopathy. To reverse the progression of manifestations, constipation must be prevented. Administer cathartics and enemas to hasten the exit of protein material from the intestine.

Encourage Bowel Cleansing. The client may need to learn to manage diarrhea, a possible side effect related to the laxative action of lactulose or neomycin sulfate. Intervention in severe hepatic encephalopathy commonly combines neomycin therapy with protein restriction and bowel cleansing. Administer the prescribed maintenance doses of neomycin and provide a low-protein diet for clients with chronic hepatic encephalopathy. In addition, administer oral lactulose, a combination of galactose and fructose that passes through the intestine unchanged, to decrease ammonia by trapping ammonium ions and allowing their evacuation from the bowel. As noted earlier, the appropriate lactulose dosage causes two to four soft stool evacuations daily. If severe diarrhea occurs, the dosage is reduced to prevent further electrolyte imbalance.

Diagnosis: Deficient Fluid Volume.
The client often has difficulties with fluid volume, leading to the nursing diagnosis *Deficient Fluid Volume related to bleeding, decreased intake, and ascites.*

Outcomes. The client will maintain a balanced fluid volume, as evidenced by normal blood pressure, absence of edema, absence of ascites, and balanced intake and output.

Interventions. Hypovolemia often precipitates hepatic encephalopathy by reducing hepatocellular perfusion. Fluid balance must be achieved, maintained, and monitored to prevent further hepatic injury and reduced renal perfusion. Deliver IV fluids evenly over time. Monitor vital signs frequently. If necessary, measure urine output hourly.

Electrolyte and acid-base disturbances such as hypokalemia and alkalosis may precipitate hepatic encephalopathy or may develop during its course. Laboratory tests indicate which replacement therapy is necessary.

Diagnosis: Risk for Injury.
Because of the multitude of problems faced by the client with encephalopathy, the nursing diagnosis *Risk for Injury related to loss of protective mechanisms secondary to hepatic coma* is common.

Outcomes. Injury or complications of immobility will be prevented or will be identified early as evidenced by the absence of problems related to immobility.

Interventions. Hepatic coma may create a multitude of problems for the client with encephalopathy.

Prevent Hypoxemia. Hypoxemia may precipitate hepatic encephalopathy by damaging the hepatic cell. To prevent and treat hypoxemia, attend to respiratory interventions (e.g., maintain a patent airway).

Prevent Infection. Concurrent infection, with accumulation of protein from tissue catabolism, necessitates rapid intervention. The client is particularly vulnerable to nosocomial (hospital-acquired) infections. Wash your hands thoroughly, and take other measures to prevent cross-contamination.

Prevent Ammonia Toxicity and Hypokalemia. Be alert to possible harmful accumulations of ammonia due to diuretic therapy. Hypokalemia from the use of diuretics contributes to hepatic encephalopathy by increasing ammonia production in the kidney.

Avoid Sedation. Agents with CNS-depressant effects may precipitate coma, and their use should thus be avoided. If agitation occurs in early encephalopathy, administer agents that are excreted partially through the kidney, instead of the liver (e.g., phenobarbital). *Administer phenobarbital with caution.* Know which opioids, tranquilizers, and sedatives are biotransformed by the liver; they are often contraindicated in clients with decreased hepatic function.

Prevent Complications of Immobility. The immobile client who lacks protective reflexes (blink or gag reflex) is vulnerable to numerous complications. Preventing complications requires intensive nursing intervention. Measures for intervention are discussed further in Chapter 70 on the care of the client in a coma. Prevent pneumonia and skin breakdown by turning the client frequently and promoting lung aeration.

As the body accumulates metabolic substances, physiologic disturbances develop that may produce a state of agitation. Therefore protect the client from self-injury, for example, by lowering the bed and padding the side rails. See Chapter 70 for further discussion of the comatose client and the client with neurologic disturbances.

Evaluation

The prognosis for the client with hepatic encephalopathy is poor. Generally the best outcome that can be hoped for is maintenance with slowed deterioration.

■ Self-Care
As the acute stages of cirrhosis subside, ongoing care of the client continues. If the care plan includes discharge from the hospital, provide extensive discharge teaching

for the client with cirrhosis who has experienced complications. Family members and significant others need to know how to reduce the incidence of complications from cirrhosis. Review the potential complications with the caregivers as well as how to prevent and treat them.

Medications. Review all medications along with scheduled times of administration and their intended and adverse side effects. Potential medications include lactulose, diuretics, and vitamin supplements.

Diet Modifications. Explain the importance of a well-balanced, nutritional diet to the client, with specific information about limitations on dietary protein, sodium, and water. Teach family members and significant others about the need to encourage eating and still maintain food intake within prescribed limits.

Home Modifications. Teach that the client's home may need to be altered to adjust for limitations in mobility. Safety precautions should be taken to help prevent injury to the client. The client's bedroom should be near the bathroom if the client is receiving diuretics.

Follow-Up Assessments. The client's status should be followed closely. Be sure that the client's caregivers are aware of any changes that require immediate medical attention. They should also know that diagnostic testing at regular intervals is continued to monitor the status of the liver.

FATTY LIVER (HEPATIC STENOSIS)

Lipid infiltration may lead to hepatic stenosis, or "fatty liver," one of the most common metabolic diseases of the liver. This pathologic process causes liver enlargement and increased firmness and may result in decreased function. Liver biopsy establishes the diagnosis. Laboratory studies reveal that triglyceride is the major lipid involved, but small amounts of cholesterol and phospholipid also may have infiltrated the liver.

Major causes of lipid infiltration include chronic alcoholism, protein malnutrition in early life, diabetes mellitus, obesity, Cushing's syndrome (natural or induced), jejunoileal bypass, prolonged IV hyperalimentation, chronic illnesses that involve impaired nutrition or malabsorption, some hepatotoxins (carbon tetrachloride and DDT [dichlorodiphenyltrichloroethane]), and Reye's syndrome in children.

The manifestations of fatty liver are related to the degree of fat infiltration, the amount of time fat has been accumulating, and the underlying cause. Clients with moderate to severe lipid infiltration are frequently asymptomatic; however, clients with massive infiltration experience anorexia, abdominal pain, and sometimes

jaundice. Laboratory studies demonstrate elevated serum alkaline phosphatase and bilirubin levels.

Recovery begins after the source of the problem is removed and metabolic balance and adequate nutrition are restored. Residual damage, if it occurs, usually follows persistent fatty infiltration and chronic alcoholism. Fat embolization may occur and can cause death.

Nursing intervention for clients with fatty infiltration of the liver includes the following:

- Directing attention to correction of the cause (abstinence from alcohol, control of diabetes, weight loss, or correction of the intestinal absorptive defect)
- Preparing the client for diagnostic procedures
- Giving emotional support by allowing verbalization of concerns and fears
- Giving supportive physical care including adequate nutritional intake
- Designing teaching guidelines that promote proper diet and prevent recurrence

LIVER NEOPLASMS

Tumors of the liver are either primary or metastatic. Primary liver tumors may arise from hepatocytes, connective tissue, blood vessels, or bile ducts. These tumors are either benign or malignant (Figure 49-6). Figure 49-7 presents a classification of the primary liver neoplasms. Metastatic malignant tumors arise from the gastrointestinal tract (particularly the colon), the breasts, and the lungs.

BENIGN HEPATIC TUMORS

Hepatic adenomas are benign tumors of the liver that occur most commonly in women in their 20s and 30s. Nearly 90% of cases are associated with oral contraceptive use. The fact that the tumors occur more commonly in women, especially women who take oral contraceptives, suggests a hormonal influence in their pathogenesis.

Although these tumors are classified as benign, they are nevertheless dangerous because of their vascularity. A benign adenoma may rupture, with consequent hemorrhage. Diagnosis is made by a combination of tests including sonography, CT scanning, selective hepatic arteriography, and radionuclide scanning. Liver biopsy is not warranted because the tumors are hypervascular.

Intervention for benign adenoma depends on its cause. Discontinuation of oral contraceptives or androgens, when a tumor appears to be hormone dependent, may correct the condition. Otherwise treatment may include surgical excision of the involved liver segment. If acute hemorrhage calls for surgery, the surgeon may per-

A   B

FIGURE 49-6 Benign liver tumor (**A**) and metastatic malignant liver tumor (**B**). Note the encapsulated tumor in the benign lesion and the invasiveness of malignant lesion. Satellite lesions are also present with the malignant lesion.

ORIGIN	BENIGN	MALIGNANT
Hepatocytes	Adenoma	Hepatocellular carcinoma
Connective tissue	Fibroma	Sarcoma
Blood vessels	Hemangioma	Hemangioendothelioma
Bile ducts	Cholangioma	Carcinoma

FIGURE 49-7 Classification of primary liver neoplasms.

form a hepatic lobectomy. Benign hepatic tumors are associated with an excellent prognosis if they are removed surgically before they rupture and cause death from hemorrhage.

MALIGNANT HEPATIC TUMORS
PRIMARY HEPATOCELLULAR CANCER

The rate of primary hepatocellular cancer is rising in the United States and other Western countries, presumably because of the high prevalence of hepatitis C during the last 20 to 30 years.[5,10] Other etiologic factors that may contribute to hepatoma are hepatitis B, cirrhosis, chronic liver disease, hemochromatosis, ingestion of certain mycotoxins (aflatoxins), anabolic steroid use, and long-term androgen therapy. Primary hepatocellular carcinoma is the main cause of death from cancer in many areas of the world, including sub-Saharan Africa and parts of Asia.

After the diagnosis of liver cancer and if intervention fails to terminate the neoplastic process, the client usually dies of hepatic failure within 3 to 6 months. Surgical resection of the tumor is the only method of cure and

may be attempted if the tumor is confined to one lobe. Many clients, however, do not have a resectable tumor because of underlying cirrhosis, involvement of both lobes, and distant metastases.

METASTATIC HEPATIC CANCERS

The liver is one of the common sites of metastasis for all cancers. In the United States, metastatic cancers of the liver are 20 times more common than primary liver tumors.

Etiology and Risk Factors

The liver is a common site of metastasis because of the liver's high rate of blood flow, its size, and portal venous drainage from the major abdominal organs. Tumors of the gastrointestinal tract, lung, and breast metastasize to the liver more frequently than do tumors of the prostate or thyroid.

Pathophysiology

Metastatic cancers spread to the liver in three ways: by direct extension from adjacent organs (stomach and gallbladder), via the hepatic arterial system, or via the portal venous system. Also, as a result of cell migration, the surface of the liver may become seeded with metastatic cells.

Clinical Manifestations

Clients with primary (benign and malignant) and secondary (metastatic) tumors often show similar manifestations. Early indicators of liver neoplasm are usually vague. Many clients with metastatic malignancy of the liver have the following three types of manifestations:

- Manifestations that are specific only to the primary tumor, hepatic involvement being discovered incidentally in the course of a diagnostic evaluation

- Nonspecific manifestations of anorexia, diaphoresis, fever, weight loss, and weakness
- Manifestations of active liver disease, such as abdominal pain, ascites, and hepatomegaly

Diagnostic studies and physical examination may reveal the following: elevated alkaline phosphatase, hepatomegaly, a liver mass, a friction rub or bruit over the liver, angiographic evidence of neoplasm hypoproteinemia, blood-tinged ascitic fluid, decreased liver function, and reversal of the albumin-globulin (A:G) ratio. The A:G ratio is a calculation of the distribution of two major protein fractions: albumin and globulin. The value of the A:G ratio is greater than 1, albumin divided by globulin (A:G). A high ratio is considered insignificant; however, a low ratio occurs in liver and renal diseases.

Some clients also may have metabolic derangements, such as in polycythemia, blood glucose disorders, and high levels of calcium. Other clients may present with marked leukocytosis and anemia. Jaundice occurs more often when a bile duct is the site of a primary tumor or when the tumor mass obstructs a major outflow duct. Other manifestations may be present, depending on the concurrent pathologic condition. At times the tumor process causes elevation of the diaphragm and some respiratory problems.

Although neoplasms of the liver create numerous clinical manifestations, many pathologic features may not appear until the tumors have grown quite large. Malignant tumor cells may have replaced as much as 90% of normal liver tissue before liver insufficiency becomes clinically evident.

In primary hepatocellular cancers, diagnostic tests often reveal high levels of alpha-fetoprotein (AFP). This substance is sometimes present in clients who have metastatic tumors, but levels rarely reach those found in clients with primary tumors.

A diagnosis of liver cancer is suggested by an elevated serum alkaline phosphatase level and by abnormal findings on ultrasonography, CT, liver scanning, or magnetic resonance imaging (MRI). Cytologic examination of aspirated fluid can also be used to establish the diagnosis.

Performing a liver biopsy is helpful in establishing the diagnosis. The route of access may be percutaneous, direct via laparotomy, or through a peritoneoscope. Each method has its limitations. Percutaneous procedures may cause seeding of tumor cells along the biopsy needle pathway as it is withdrawn. Laparotomy requires anesthesia, which may be too dangerous. Peritoneoscopy may be impossible if there are extensive adhesions. Because all these biopsy procedures require internal membrane puncture, be sure the client has an acceptable PT because of the risk of hemorrhage if the time is too prolonged.

Prognosis
Because hepatic tumors may be far advanced before clinical manifestations or laboratory data indicate their presence, and because severe liver disease (e.g., cirrhosis) frequently coexists, liver cancer carries a poor prognosis. In the United States, median survival from the time of diagnosis is about 6 months.

Outcome Management
■ Medical Management
Relief of Manifestations and Promotion of Palliation. As noted previously, treatment of liver cancer is aimed at relieving manifestations and supporting the client physically and emotionally. The treatment options for medical management include chemotherapy, radiation therapy, and other approaches, such as cryoablation.

Chemotherapy. Regional perfusion of the liver with infusions given directly into the hepatic artery to reduce pain or slow tumor growth may be useful and may produce fewer side effects than those incurred with systemic chemotherapy. Various chemotherapeutic agents have been used singly or in combination with other agents infused into the hepatic artery or have been given by regional infusion with other agents given systemically.

During surgery, the surgeon may implant a chemotherapy infusion pump. Such pumps, filled percutaneously, deliver medication continuously into the hepatic artery. With metastatic growths, the oncologist may prescribe systemic chemotherapy to reduce tumor size and pain.

Chemotherapeutic agents used to induce the regression of primary and metastatic tumors of the liver include 5-fluorouracil (5-FU) and doxorubicin (Adriamycin) for single-dose therapy and 5-FU with carmustine (BCNU), semustine (methyl CCNU), or streptozocin for combination therapy.

Radiation Therapy. Radiation therapy has produced disappointing results. Irradiation of liver tumors may provide temporary pain reduction but does not promote survival.

Other Approaches. Some other approaches that have been used for the treatment of primary hepatic tumor include hepatic artery embolization and chemotherapy *(chemoembolization)*, alcohol ablation via ultrasound-guided percutaneous injection, ultrasound-guided cryoablation, and gene therapy with retroviral vectors containing genes that express cytotoxic agents. Biliary drainage achieved percutaneously or through an internal stent placed surgically helps to increase the passage of bile into the duodenum, thereby decreasing jaundice and discomfort. The Food and Drug Administration (FDA) has approved a new device called *SIR-Spheres,* which consists of biocompatible microspheres containing yttrium-90 that are 20 to 40 μm in diameter. It is implanted into a hepatic tumor by injection into either the common hepatic artery or into the right or left hepatic artery using a chemotherapy catheter port.[5]

■ Nursing Management of the Medical Client

Nursing diagnoses and interventions for clients with liver neoplasms vary according to the amount of liver dysfunction and the treatment modalities. Plan to assess the client for metabolic malfunctions, pain, bleeding problems, ascites, edema, an inability to biotransform endogenous and exogenous (drug) wastes, hypoproteinemia, jaundice, and endocrine complications.

Take time to prepare the client in the diagnostic stage for the various procedures, and assess carefully for post-procedure complications. If pain is a problem, administer medication at the prescribed time and dosage. In addition, assist the client and family members to gain knowledge about the condition and to offer support necessary for them to cope with the uncertainty and fear associated with cancer. See Chapters 18 and 19 for detailed discussions of nursing care of clients with malignant tumors. See also the Care Plan feature on Management of the Client with Hepatic Failure on pp. 1351 to 1354.

■ Surgical Management

Indications. Resection is indicated for tumors that are small and confined to one liver segment or lobe. The affected segment or lobe is removed surgically. Resection is curative if the remaining unaffected liver is normal.

Liver transplantation may be considered as the therapeutic option for small unresectable tumors in a client with advanced cirrhosis; however, it may be curative in only a minority of clients. Recurrence of tumor or metastasis after transplantation has limited its usefulness.

Contraindications. The client may not be able to withstand the stress of surgery. An additional contraindication to surgery is the presence of liver disease too extensive for surgery to be beneficial.

Complications. Tumor rupture, gastrointestinal hemorrhage from varices, progressive cachexia, and hepatic failure are the primary complications of hepatic tumors. Management of the client with these complications is supportive and palliative and will vary according to the client's overall condition, degree of liver impairment, and extent of surgery.

Outcomes. Prognosis is poor. Most clients with hepatic carcinoma have a median survival time of 3 to 6 months.

■ Nursing Management of the Surgical Client

Nursing management of the client preoperatively and postoperatively includes many responsibilities. See the discussion of nursing management of the client who has undergone surgery for complications of portal hypertension, earlier in this chapter.

■ LIVER TRANSPLANTATION

■ Surgical Management

Liver transplantation is now considered a feasible form of intervention for a variety of end-stage liver diseases. The number of liver transplants has continued to grow each year. In 1999, more than 4000 people in the United States received liver transplants.[7] The demand for livers for transplantation continues to outpace availability. More than 6000 clients in the United States remain on a donor liver waiting list.

The duration of the surgical procedure is generally 8 hours but can be from 6 to 18 hours. The surgery may be *orthotopic,* involving removal of the diseased liver and insertion of the donor liver. Anastomoses of the vena cava, portal vein, hepatic artery, and bile duct are performed. In the *heterotopic* approach, the diseased liver is left in and the transplanted liver is inserted alongside it. Orthotopic surgery is by far the more common of the two. Because excessive bleeding may occur, large amounts of blood, blood products, and volume expanders are needed.

Indications. The most appropriate candidates for liver transplantation are people who, in the absence of contraindications, have severe, irreversible liver disease for which alternative medical or surgical treatments have not been successful or are not available. Ideally transplantation should be considered in clients with end-stage liver disease who are experiencing life-threatening complications of liver dysfunction, whose quality of life has increasingly deteriorated, or who are predicted to experience neurologic effects of liver damage. If the surgery is performed sufficiently early, contraindications and extrahepatic deterioration are less likely.[7]

Some of the most common conditions warranting transplantation are as follows:

- Primary and secondary biliary cirrhosis (adult)
- Hepatitis—chronic with cirrhosis, chronic viral or fulminant (usually adult)
- Primary sclerosing cholangitis (adult)
- Biliary atresia (pediatric)
- Alpha$_1$-antitrypsin deficiency (usually pediatric)
- Confined hepatic malignancy (adult or pediatric)
- Wilson's disease
- Budd-Chiari syndrome (hepatic vein thrombosis)
- Alcoholic cirrhosis

Choosing clients with alcoholic cirrhosis, chronic viral hepatitis, and primary hepatocellular malignancies as liver transplant recipients may be questionable. Clients with any one of these conditions are considered high-risk surgical candidates, but liver transplantation may be offered to carefully selected individuals. The alcoholic client, for example, must be willing to adhere to certain guidelines, such as abstinence and a substance-abuse treatment program to be eligible for the procedure. The client must be psychologically stable and have good support systems for the complex postoperative course.

Contraindications. Absolute contraindications include (1) life-threatening systemic diseases; (2) uncontrolled extrahepatic bacterial or fungal infections; (3) pre-existing advanced cardiovascular or pulmonary disease; (4) multiple uncorrectable, life-threatening congenital anomalies; (5) metastatic malignancy to the liver; (6) active alcoholism or drug abuse; (7) cholangiocarcinoma; and (8) human immunodeficiency virus (HIV) infection. See Chapter 82 for other contraindications to transplantation.

Complications. Postoperative complications can be *hepatic* or *nonhepatic*. They may include cardiovascular and pulmonary problems as well as infection, rejection, hemorrhage, atelectasis, failure of anastomosis, and acute renal failure. Rejection occurs most commonly between postoperative days 4 and 10. Manifestations of acute rejection include fever, tachycardia, right upper quadrant or flank pain, and increasing jaundice. Drugs used to stop or prevent rejection include azathioprine, cyclosporine, FK506, OKT3, and steroids such as prednisone and methylprednisolone; otherwise liver function rapidly deteriorates. Chapter 82 describes management of clients undergoing transplantation.

Outcomes. It is expected that the client will recover from the liver transplant surgery, be discharged from the hospital in 1 week, and within 3 to 4 months be able to resume a normal life as long as medication and health care regimens are followed closely. Complications such as rejection and infection will slow the progress of affected clients.

The survival rate after liver transplantation has improved steadily since 1983, about 70% in the early 1980s to 80% to 90% in the mid-1990s. The 5-year survival rate is about 60%.[7] The survival rate is higher and the quality of life better after transplantation in people who had less hepatic damage before surgery and in those who had fewer extrahepatic manifestations.

Nursing Management of the Surgical Client

Preoperative Care
Once the client has chosen transplantation as an alternative to care and is placed on the recipient waiting list,

an extensive physical and psychological evaluation is required (see Chapter 82). The client must undergo a variety of tests, including blood analysis, hepatic angiogram, abdominal CT scan, chest and hip x-ray studies, electrocardiogram (ECG), bone density studies, and nutritional assessment. The client may also have the opportunity to meet the transplant team. Matching donor and recipient organ size and blood and tissue type are important considerations in donor selection.

Focus on assessing the client's needs in relation to the amount of knowledge and information he or she has. Ascertain how the client and his or her family members are coping with the situation. In addition, the needs dictated by the extent of organ failure will guide care. The specific nursing care needs of clients during the waiting period for a liver transplant depend on the degree of end-stage liver disease.

Postoperative Care
The major focus of care is to monitor for rejection, infection, and occlusion of vessels. Immunosuppressive therapy, which is started before surgery, must be continued on a regular schedule postoperatively to prevent rejection of the new liver. The client requires constant monitoring of respiratory, cardiovascular, neurologic, and hemodynamic status. Liver function is monitored through assessment of serum transaminases (ALT, AST), bilirubin, albumin, and clotting factors. Monitor fluid and electrolyte status, blood glucose levels, and pH. Clients are always somewhat fluid overloaded from receiving extensive volumes of blood products during the long surgical procedure. This overload can lead to pulmonary edema and heart failure. Serum potassium will be decreased as a result of transplantation, and blood glucose will be increased. The serum pH will be normal to acidic.

Monitor wound drains and bile drains for patency, and note bile characteristics (amount, color, consistency). Obstruction of wound drains causes increased intra-abdominal pressure from the accumulation of ascitic fluid and blood. Obstruction of bile flow can cause damage to the liver and biliary system.

Assess the needs of family members and significant others, who may have traveled long distances from home and may be feeling powerless, stressed, and anxious. Much of the care and many of the nursing diagnoses for a client who undergoes liver transplantation are the same as for a client after any other type of surgery. See Chapter 82 for care of the client after transplantation.

■ LIVER ABSCESS

A liver *abscess* is a localized collection of pus and organisms within the parenchyma of the liver. Liver ab-

GENETICS LINKS

Hereditary Hemochromatosis

Description

An autosomal-recessive disorder of iron metabolism in which excessive iron accumulates in multiple organs such as the liver, heart, pancreas, joints, and skin. Common early clinical manifestations include abdominal pain, arthralgia, fatigue, weight loss, and lethargy. Manifestations tend to occur in men between 40 and 60 years of age and in women after menopause. Hepatic fibrosis or cirrhosis is common in untreated individuals after age 40. Other findings may include arthritis, diabetes, cardiac abnormalities, and increased skin pigmentation. Hereditary hemochromatosis (HHC) most often affects Caucasians of Northern European descent, although other ethnic groups are also affected.

Genetics

About one in nine persons in the general population is a carrier of the hemochromatosis gene. Hemochromatosis is associated mainly with mutations in a gene called *HFE,* located on chromosome 6. The two known mutations in HFE are named C282Y (the most common mutation) and H63D. Two copies of the mutant gene are necessary to cause the disorder. Offspring of carrier parents have a 25% risk of having hemochromatosis.

Diagnosis/Testing

Diagnosis of individuals with clinical manifestations is typically based on screening tests such as serum transferrin–iron saturation and serum ferritin concentration and confirmatory tests such as histologic assessment of hepatic iron stores on liver biopsy or molecular genetic testing for the C282Y and H63D mutations in the *HFE* gene.

Management

Usual therapy is removal of excess iron by phlebotomy (i.e., removal of blood). Early diagnosis and treatment to normalize serum iron levels before manifestations or organ damage develop can prevent all the potential complications of HHC. People with HHC should avoid taking iron supplements. Because HHC is common and early detection and treatment are effective, widespread screening for this disorder has been proposed and is an area of current research.

---

scess usually develops in association with one of the following three conditions:

- *Bacterial cholangitis,* which results from obstruction of the bile ducts by stone or stricture
- *Portal vein bacteremia,* which may develop following bowel inflammation or organ perforation
- *Amebiasis* (infestation with amebae from tropical or subtropical areas)

Other predisposing factors are diabetes mellitus, infected hepatic cysts, metastatic liver tumors with secondary infection, and diverticulitis.

The client commonly reports right upper quadrant pain and abdominal and right shoulder pain. Assessment may also reveal liver enlargement, tenderness, nausea, vomiting, weight loss, anorexia, fever, and diaphoresis. Sometimes a right pleural effusion develops. The liver's proximity to the base of the right lung contributes to this process.

Liver scanning is extremely valuable in diagnosis. Other useful diagnostic modalities include ultrasonography, CT, and arteriography. Laboratory data reflect slight to marked elevations of aminotransferases, alkaline phosphatase, and bilirubin. High levels indicate the presence of concurrent obstruction. Blood culture yields positive results in some cases.

Intervention in hepatic abscess consists of (1) percutaneous drainage of the abscess with antimicrobial therapy, (2) surgical drainage of large abscesses with postoperative antimicrobial therapy, or (3) antimicrobial therapy without drainage for a few months. Abscesses resulting from amebic infestation (such as by *Entamoeba histolytica*) call for treatment with metronidazole (Flagyl) or chloroquine phosphate (Aralen phosphate) instead of broad-spectrum antibiotics. Early diagnosis and therapy for uncomplicated amebic liver abscess result in mortality rate of less than 1%.

When caring for the client with liver abscess, assess vital signs regularly. High temperature and rapid pulse may indicate the presence of general sepsis, a likely complication. Encourage movement, coughing, and deep breathing to prevent or limit pulmonary complications related to hepatic abscess. Increase the client's fluid intake and provide skin care in the event of hyperpyrexia. Dispose of feces carefully, and wash your hands to prevent transmission of amebic infestations.

RARE DISORDERS

Hemochromatosis, an uncommon disorder of iron metabolism often associated with portal hypertension and hepatomegaly, and *amyloidosis,* a proteinaceous, starch-like substance that can infiltrate the liver and other organs, are two rare disorders that can occur (see the Genetic Links feature on Hereditary Hemochromatosis, above). Table 49-7 briefly describes these two disorders.

TABLE 49-7 *Rare Disorders*		
Factor	**Hemochromatosis**	**Amyloidosis**
Description/Etiology	Disorder of iron storage. Excessive amounts of iron are deposited in parenchymal cells, causing eventual damage and impaired function of organs, especially the liver, pancreas, heart, joints, and pituitary. Primary hemochromatosis is a recessive inherited metabolic defect that causes increased iron absorption from the gastrointestinal tract. Secondary hemochromatosis is caused by alcoholism, excessive intake of iron, or conditions requiring repeated blood transfusions. Common problems associated with hemochromatosis include diabetes, enlarged liver, cirrhosis, cardiac disease, increased skin pigmentation, and arthritis.	Results from deposition of insoluble proteins in extracellular spaces of organs and tissues, causing them to cease functioning; is classified according to the type of protein that forms the amyloid deposits. Primary amyloidosis (AL) is formed from the deposition of immunoglobins and causes damage to tissues of cardiac, smooth muscle, skin, kidney, and liver origin. Primary amyloidosis is often associated with multiple myeloma. Amyloidosis due to deposition of protein A (AA) occurs most often in chronic inflammations such as tuberculosis, rheumatoid arthritis, osteomyelitis, and bronchiectasis. Another type of amyloidosis is genetic and passed down through families (FAP). The tissues most affected by this type of amyloidosis include the spleen, kidney, and liver.
Diagnosis	Elevated levels of plasma iron ($>$150 mg/ml; normal is 2 to 5 g), more than 60% saturation of iron-binding protein (transferrin), manifestations of specific organ dysfunction, and liver biopsy	Liver biopsy provides best data, but there is a high incidence of postbiopsy hemorrhage or liver rupture.
Clinical manifestations	Clinical manifestations are varied and depend on the area of the body that is involved. Often arthritis prompts clients to seek medical attention.	Clinical manifestations are varied and depend on the area of the body involved.
Interventions	Phlebotomy (a surgical opening of a vein to withdraw blood) biweekly or weekly over a 1- or 2-year period (2 ml of blood = 1 mg of iron). Desferrioxamine mesylate, a chelating agent, facilitates the removal of iron from the body.	Treatment depends on the type of amyloidosis present. Genetic counseling is important for heredofamilial types, and liver transplantation has been done for FAP. In AL, stem cell transplantation and immunosuppressive drugs (melphalan) have been effective.

Data from Sipe, J.D., & Cohen, A.S. (2001). Amyloidosis. In E. Braunwald, et al. (Eds.), *Harrison's principles of internal medicine* (15th ed., pp. 1974-1979). New York: McGraw-Hill; and Powell, L.W., & Isselbacher, K.J. (2001). Hemochromatosis. In E. Braunwald, et al. (Eds.), *Harrison's principles of internal medicine* (15th ed., pp. 2257-2261). New York: McGraw-Hill.

CONGENITAL CONDITIONS

Three congenital conditions affecting the liver are Wilson's disease, Caroli's syndrome, and congenital hepatic fibrosis. Table 49-8 briefly describes these three conditions.

LIVER TRAUMA

Liver injury usually results from a penetrating injury or blunt trauma. Either can lead to laceration and hemorrhage. Penetrating injuries are usually knife or missile (gunshot) wounds. A knife wound generally is superficial and leaves a sharp clear edge, whereas missile wounds cause perforations through the liver tissue, that is, the entrance and exit points. The greater the velocity of the missile, the greater the damage. Often, a close-range missile injury is fatal because of the large amount of damage. Blunt trauma (e.g., from a steering wheel or a fall) can have various effects, ranging from small hematomas that remain under the liver capsule to large, star-like lacerations from severe impact forces.

Management of liver injuries consists of control of the hemorrhage, debridement, and drainage. Surgical resection of liver lobes may be necessary, but more often the major goal of surgical intervention is to control hemorrhage. Monitor victims of trauma carefully for falling blood pressure and tachycardia, which may indicate hemorrhage. The problem is more difficult when the liver's blood vessels or bile ducts are damaged as well. Later complications include bile peritonitis and abscess formation.

TABLE 49-8	*Congenital Conditions*		
Condition	**Description/Diagnosis**	**Symptoms**	**Intervention**
Wilson's disease	Accumulation of copper in tissues of the liver, brain, and kidney. Is usually chronic but may be acute. Acute form may be fatal. A hallmark of the disease is the presence of Kayser-Fleischer rings encircling the corneas (due to copper deposits). Copper deposits also seen in liver biopsy.	Abnormal liver function and neurologic changes. Manifests itself from early childhood to adulthood.	Penicillamine. Liver transplantation may be performed for acute disease.
Caroli's syndrome	Characterized by dilated bile ducts and cyst formations. May be localized or widespread.	Fever and bacterial cholangitis, right upper quadrant pain, and jaundice (from obstruction of biliary tract by one or more cysts or stones). Usually presents soon after birth, but may not be diagnosed until early adulthood.	Antibiotics, external biliary drainage, or liver transplantation.
Congenital hepatic fibrosis	Characterized by portal hypertension caused by portal vein fibrosis.	Upper gastrointestinal bleeding from gastric or esophageal varices.	Ranges from blood transfusions to sclerotherapy to portacaval shunting.

CONCLUSIONS

Hepatic disorders are complex and difficult for all involved. You should have a thorough understanding of the liver and its functions to care for these clients. Many hepatic disorders are the result of the client's lifestyle, further complicating an already difficult problem. The nurse must therefore consider both the physiologic and psychosocial problems associated with many hepatic disorders. Helping the client make appropriate lifestyle changes is an important nursing function.

THINKING CRITICALLY *evolve*

1. A 37-year-old man is admitted to the hospital with a 10-day history of anorexia, fatigue, malaise, low-grade fever, dark urine, and upper abdominal discomfort. There is no history of jaundice, IV drug use, or blood transfusions. He is homosexual. Alcohol intake consists of several mixed drinks nightly and wine with dinner. Findings on physical examination include temperature of 99.6° F, jaundice, blood pressure of 150/80 mm Hg, and no spider nevi. The liver measures 12 cm in the midclavicular line and is moderately tender. The spleen is not palpable. Initial laboratory data were total bilirubin, 6.8 mg/dl (normal, 0.2 to 1.2 mg/dl); alkaline phosphatase, 240 units/L (normal, 20 to 90 units/L); AST, 980 units/L (normal, 5 to 40 units/L); ALT, 1200 units/L (normal, 5 to 35

units/L). The WBC count is 5600/mm³, with a normal differential count. What are the priorities for care in this situation? What interventions might be used?

Factors to Consider. Without further data, what would appear to be the major organ systems involved? What additional information do you, as his nurse, think is necessary to obtain? If you are caring for this client and you inadvertently sustain a needle-stick from a syringe used to give an injection to this client, what action would you take?

2. A 48-year-old man arrives in the emergency department. He felt well until 2 hours ago, when he became nauseated and subsequently vomited a large amount of red blood and clots. He reports a long history of heavy alcohol use and cigarette smoking. He takes no medications. Laboratory data were hemoglobin, 9.6 g/dl; hematocrit, 28.4%; platelet count, 92,000/mm³; PT, 16.5 seconds (normal, 11 to 15); alkaline phosphatase, 120 units/L (normal, 20 to 90); AST, 265 units/L; ALT, 112 units/L. What is likely to be a major underlying cause of this client's problem? Is it reversible? Can further damage be stopped? With the client vomiting blood, what should be your priority interventions?

Factors to Consider. What gastrointestinal disorders can be manifested in people who consume large quantities of alcohol? What risks does the client face in the present situation?

3. Your client is a 68-year-old man with cirrhosis. He is admitted for treatment of ascites and acute upper right abdominal pain. His abdomen is very large, and the ascitic fluid shifts from side to side whenever he moves. Diagnostic studies reveal that the cause of the pain is cholelithiasis, and surgery is scheduled. What are the client's priority needs on admission? What complications might he face following surgery?

Factors to Consider.   What are the clinical manifestations of cirrhosis? Is the client with cirrhosis a good candidate for abdominal surgery?

Discussions for these questions can be found on the website and the CD-ROM.

BIBLIOGRAPHY

1. Ackley, B.J., & Ladwig, G.B. (2004). *Nursing diagnosis handbook* (6th ed.). St. Louis: Mosby.
2. American Cancer Society. (2003). *Cancer facts and figures.* Atlanta: Author.
3. Chene, B.L., & Decker, A.P. (2001). Battling hepatitis C. *RN, 64*(4), 54-58.
4. Chung, R.T., & Podolsky, D.K. (2001). Cirrhosis and its complications. In E. Braunwald, et al. (Eds.), *Harrison's principles of internal medicine* (15th ed., pp. 1754-1767). New York: McGraw-Hill.
5. Crawford, L. (2002). Treatment for liver tumors. *Journal of the American Medical Association, 287*(17), 2203.
6. Cummings, K.J., et al. (2001). Interferon and ribavirin vs interferon alone in the re-treatment of chronic hepatitis C previously non-responsive to interferon. *Journal of the American Medical Association, 285*(2), 193-199.
7. Dienstag, J.L. (2001). Liver transplantation. In E. Braunwald, et al. (Eds.), *Harrison's principles of internal medicine* (15th ed., pp. 1770-1776). New York: McGraw-Hill.
8. Dienstag, J.L., & Isselbacher, K.J. (2001). Acute viral hepatitis. In E. Braunwald, et al. (Eds.), *Harrison's principles of internal medicine* (15th ed., pp. 1721-1730). New York: McGraw-Hill.
9. Dienstag, J.L., & Isselbacher, K.J. (2001). Chronic hepatitis. In E. Braunwald, et al. (Eds.), *Harrison's principles of internal medicine* (15th ed., pp. 1742-1754). New York: McGraw-Hill.
10. Dienstag, J.L., & Isselbacher, K.J. (2001). Tumors of the liver and biliary tract. In E. Braunwald, et al. (Eds.), *Harrison's principles of internal medicine* (15th ed., pp. 588-591). New York: McGraw-Hill.
11. Dienstag, J.L., & Isselbacher, K.J. (2001). Toxic and drug-induced hepatitis. In E. Braunwald, et al. (Eds.), *Harrison's principles of internal medicine* (15th ed., pp. 1737-1742). New York: McGraw-Hill.
12. Dougherty, A.S., & Dreher, H.M. (2001). Hepatitis C: Current treatment strategies for an emerging epidemic. *MEDSURG Nursing, 10*(1), 9-15.
13. Fallon, M.B., et al. (2001). Jaundice. In T.E. Andreoli, et al. (Eds.), *Cecil essentials of medicine* (5th ed., pp. 371-376). Philadelphia: W.B. Saunders.
14. Fallon, M.B., et al. (2001). Acute and chronic hepatitis. In T.E. Andreoli, et al. (Eds.), *Cecil essentials of medicine* (5th ed., pp. 376-384). Philadelphia: W.B. Saunders.
15. Flamm, S. (2003). Chronic hepatitis C virus infection. *Journal of the American Medical Association, 289*(18), 2413-2417.
16. Friedman, L.S. (2002). Liver, biliary tract, and pancreas. In L.M. Tierney, S.J. McPhee, & M.A. Papadakis (Eds.), *Current medical diagnosis and treatment 2002* (41st ed., pp. 675-720). New York: Lange Medical.
17. Hench, C., & Simpkins, S. (2002, July). Hepatitis C: Risk factors, assessment and diagnosis. (Part 1 of 2). *Nurse Week*, 20-21.
18. Hench, C., & Simpkins, S. (2002, August). Hepatitis C: Treatment, prevention, and nursing interventions. (Part 2 of 2). *Nurse Week*, 17-18.
19. Kim, W.R., & Poterucha, J.J. (2001). Is it time for mass screening for hepatitis C? *American Journal of Medicine, 111*, 667-668.
20. Krumberger, J. (2002). When the liver fails. *RN, 65*(2), 26-29.
21. Lauer, G., & Walker, B.D. (2001). Hepatitis C virus infection. *New England Journal of Medicine, 345* (1), 41-53.
22. Lindseth, G. (2003). Disorders of the liver, gallbladder and pancreas. In S. Price & L. Wilson (Eds.) *Pathophysiology: Clinical concepts of disease processes* (6th ed., pp 368-401). St. Louis: Mosby.
23. Mawyer, D., & Perry, J. (2001). One nurse's fight. *RN, 64*(4), 59-60.
24. Parini, S. (2001). Hepatitis C: Speaking out about the silent epidemic. *Nursing 2001, 31*(11), 37-42.
25. Powell, L.W., & Isselbacher, K.J. (2001). Hemochromatosis. In E. Braunwald, et al. (Eds.), *Harrison's principles of internal medicine* (15th ed., pp. 2257-2261). New York: McGraw-Hill.
26. Sabiston, D.C. (2001). Liver and Surgical complications of cirrhosis and portal hypertension. In C.S. Townsend (Ed.), *Textbook of surgery: The biologic basis of modern surgical practice* (17th ed.). Philadelphia: W.B. Saunders.
27. Sip, J.D., & Cohen, A.S. (2001). Amyloidosis. In E. Braunwald, et al. (Eds.), *Harrison's principles of internal medicine* (15th ed., pp. 1974-1979). New York: McGraw-Hill.
28. Sommers, M.S., & Johnson, S.A. (2002). Cirrhosis. In M.S. Sommers & S.A. Johnson (Eds.), *Diseases and disorders: A nursing therapeutics manual* (2nd ed., pp. 253-257). Philadelphia: F.A. Davis.

Additional Online Content

The following learning tools and key reference content can be found on the Evolve website at
http://evolve.elsevier.com/Black/medsurg/

Audio Pronunciations from Dorland's Dictionary

Audio Clips, Animations, and Video Clips from Jarvis: *Health Assessment Online*

Health Assessment Images from Lemmi: *Physical Assessment Findings CD-ROM*

Fluid & Electrolyte Module

Concept Map Creator

List of Nursing Interventions Classification (NIC) Labels

List of Nursing Outcomes Classification (NOC) Labels

List of NANDA International Approved Nursing Diagnoses

APPENDIX A
Religious Beliefs and Practices Affecting Health Care

APPENDIX B
A Health History Format That Integrates the Assessment of Functional Health Patterns

APPENDIX C
Laboratory Values of Clinical Importance in Medical-Surgical Nursing

Index

b indicates numbered box material, *f* indicates illustrations, and *t* indicates tables.

I-1

Antineutrophilic cytoplasmic antibodies, normal value/significance, 2338t
Antinuclear antibody
  normal value/significance, 2338t
  in systemic lupus erythematosus, 2353t
Antinuclear antibody tests for musculoskeletal conditions, 578t
Antinuclear factor in systemic lupus erythematosus, 2352
Antioxidant vitamins for reducing cardiovascular disease, 1517
Antioxidants
  for acute respiratory distress syndrome, 1897
  mechanism of, 20
  sources of, 20
Anti-perinuclear factor in rheumatoid arthritis, 2333
Antiplatelet agents
  for angina, 1705
  for coronary heart disease, 1637
Antiretroviral agents
  classes of, 2383
  correlation to HIV life cycle, 2381f
  failure of, 2385
  for HIV infection, 2383-2387
  HIV resistance to, 2385
  initiating/maintaining, 2388-2389
  mechanism of action of, 2380
  resistance to, 2389
Antirheumatic drugs, disease-modifying, studies of, 2330, 2331
Antiseizure drugs. See Antiepileptic drugs
Antiseptic solutions for wounds, 409t
Antispasmotics
  effect on urination, 791t
  for irritable bowel syndrome, 848
  for neurogenic bladder, 904
Antithyroglobulin antibody, normal value/test description, 1166t-1167t
Antithyroid antibody tests, 1164
Antithyroid medications for Graves' disease, 1200-1201
Antivertigo agents, 1991
Antiviral agents. See also Antiretroviral agents
  for STDs, 1129
Antixoidants, appropriate use of term, 114
Antrectomy for peptic ulcer disease, 757
Anuria
  defined, 785, 942
  versus urinary retention, 893
Anus
  inspection of, 682
  palpation of, 682
  physical examination of, 780-781
  structure and function of, 774
Anxiety
  about amputation, 1523
  about anesthesia, 286
  in acute pancreatitis, 1295
  after craniotomy, 2090
  AMI-related, 1723
  with cholecystectomy, 1309
  in chronic renal failure, 967
  client, in renal trauma, 932-933
  in COPD, 1825
  in dying client, 491-492
  interventions for decreasing, 526b
  manifestations of, 525t
  mechanical ventilation-related, 1890-1891
  medications for, 492t
  pain response and, 453
  preoperative, 278
  risk for, in heart failure, 1667
  spinal fusion and, 2145
  tracheostomy-related, 1785

Anxiety (Continued)
  as universal phenomenon, 525
  in viral hepatitis, 1331
Anxiety disorders
  outcome management/interventions, 528-530
  referrals for, 529-530
Anxiolytic abuse, 549
  health consequences of, 550t-551t
Anxiolytic withdrawal, symptoms of, 544t
Anxiolytics
  in Alzheimer's disease, 2167
  effects of, 542t
Anzemet. See Dolasetron (Anzemet)
Aorta, disorders of, impotence and, 1476
Aortic aneurysm
  abdominal, resection of, acute renal failure and, 947
  dissecting
    differential assessment of, 1564t-1565t
    hypertension due to, 1495b
  palpation for, 1482, 1483f
Aortic dissection, 1532-1533
Aortic regurgitation
  clinical manifestations of, 1603-1604
  etiology/risk factors, 1603
  management of, 1604
  manifestations of, 1602-1603
  pathophysiology of, 1603
Aortic stenosis
  clinical manifestations of, 1603
  etiology/risk factors, 1603
  management of, 1604
  manifestations of, 1602
  pathophysiology of, 1603
Aortic valve disease, 1602-1604
Aortic valve stenosis/regurgitation, manifestations of, 1600t
Aortoiliac stenosis, 1511, 1511f
Aphasia
  Broca's, 1998, 2112-2113
  defined, 2112
  in epilepsy, 2075
  global, 2112
  with hemiplegia, 2113
  motor/nonfluent, 2113
  sensory/fluent, 2113
  stroke-induced, 2112-2113
  Wernicke's, 2112-2113
Apheresis for chronic myelogenous leukemia, 2406
Aphthasol. See Amlexanox (Aphthasol)
Aphthous stomatitis, 719, 719f
Aplastic anemia
  agranulocytosis and, 2301
  hereditary versus acquired, 2291-2292, 2292t
  lab findings in, 2287t
  manifestations/management of, 2291-2293
Aplastic crisis in sickle cell anemia, 2296
Apley's scratch test, purpose, techniques, findings, 573t
Apnea
  respiratory pattern in, 1751f
  sleep. See Sleep apnea
Apocrine glands
  structure and function of, 1371
  sympathetic/parasympathetic stimulation of, 2014t
Apolipoprotein E in Alzheimer's disease, 324
Apomorphine (Uprima) for erectile dysfunction, 1047
Apoptosis
  definition and role in cell death, 345, 345f
  in heart failure, 1651
  in metastasis, 344-345
Appearance, assessing, 88
Appendectomy, 813

Appendicitis, 812-814, 812f
  clinical manifestations of, 812f, 812-813
  etiology, risk factors, pathophysiology, 812
  outcome management of, 813-814
Appendicular skeleton, 558
Appetite
  changes in, assessment of, 672-673
  interventions for increasing, 696-697
  loss of. See also Anorexia nervosa
    in gastrointestinal disorders, 743
Applanation tonometry, 1912
Apraxia
  assessing, 2031
  stroke-related, 2114
Aqueous flow, promoting, in glaucoma, 1945-1946
Aqueous humor
  composition of, 1912
  normal flow of, 1944f
Arachnoid, structure and function of, 2004
Arava. See Leflunomide (Arava)
Arcus senilis, 1914
  assessing for, 1923
  in cardiovascular exam, 1571
ARDS. See Acute respiratory distress syndrome; Adult respiratory distress syndrome
Aredia. See Pamidronate (Aredia)
ARF. See Acute renal failure
L-Arginine supplements for erectile dysfunction, 1048
Argyll Robertson pupil in neurosyphilis, 2151
Arimidex. See Anastrozole (Arimidex)
Arm exercises after breast cancer surgery, 1109-1110
Arnica for skin disorders, 1378
Aromatase inhibitor in cancer treatment, 367b
Aromatherapy, 110
  description of, 116t
Arousal
  early morning, in hospital, 517
  physiology of, 438, 508-510, 509f
Arousal disorders, 514
Arrhythmias. See Dysrhythmias; specific dysrhythmias
ARS. See Artificial rectal sphincter
Art therapy, description of, 116t
Arterial baroreceptors in shock, 2448
Arterial blood gases
  analysis of, 252, 252b, 1764-1765
  in complex acid-base disorders, 257, 258
  in metabolic acidosis, 256
  in metabolic alkalosis, 255
  minimizing sampling errors in, 259, 259t
  in respiratory alkalosis, 253
Arterial blood sampling, 97
Arterial bypass surgery
  for peripheral vascular disease, 1517f, 1517-1518
  postoperative care for, 1519-1521
Arterial disorders. See also Peripheral vascular disease
  clinical manifestations of, 1476
  in lower extremities, 1477t
Arterial embolism, 1526-1527, 1527f
  versus arterial thrombosis, 1527
Arterial flow, promoting, in peripheral vascular disease, 1513, 1514
Arterial insufficiency
  manifestations of, 1476, 1477-1478
  objective/subjective data in, 1511, 1512t
Arterial occlusion
  acute, 1526-1528
  six Ps of, 1528b
Arterial oxygen, partial pressure of, in acute respiratory failure, 1877

Thyroid storm
in Graves' disease, 1200
management of, 1201
monitoring of, 1202
thyroidectomy-related, 1203, 1205
Thyroid ultrasonography, normal
findings/description, 1179t
Thyroidectomy
hypoparathyroidism after, 1213
indications/contraindications, complications,
outcomes, 1203
nursing interventions after, 1204t
for thyroid cancer, 1209
Thyroiditis
characteristics and management of, 1206-1207
chronic, 1206
Hashimoto's, 1164
subacute granulomatous, 1206-1207
subacute lymphocytic, 1207
Thyroid-releasing hormone, inadequate production
of, 1193
Thyroid-stimulating hormone
function of, 1150
increased secretion of, 1192
normal value/test description, 1166t-1167t
serum, measurement of, 1164
Thyrotoxicosis
in Graves' disease, 1200
monitoring of, 1202
palliative treatment of, 1198
Thyrotropin-releasing hormone
function of, 1150
normal value/test description, 1166t-1167t
Thyrotropin-releasing hormone stimulation test,
1165
Thyroxine, 1146
function of, 1150
normal value/test description, 1166t-1167t
serum, measurement of, 1164-1165
in subclinical hypothyroidism, 1193
Thyroxine index, normal value/test description,
1166t-1167t
TIAs. See Transient ischemic attacks
Tibial fractures, 646
Tibial nerve, assessment of, 575f
Tic, defined, 2031b
Tic douloureux, manifestations/management of,
2153-2154, 2153f
Ticlopidine for lowering stroke risk, 1280
Tidal volume, 1735, 1735f
defined, 1762t
Tilade. See Nedocromil (Tilade)
Tiludronate (Skelid) for Paget's disease, 605
Timolol maleate for glaucoma, client teaching
about, 1947t
Tinea, manifestations/management of, 1419t
Tinel's sign
in carpal tunnel syndrome, 2155, 2157f
in differential diagnosis of carpal tunnel
syndrome, 2360
Tinnitus, 1971
characteristics of, 1974
descriptors of, 1931
ginkgo biloba for, 1933
hearing loss and, 1973, 1974
in hematopoietic disorders, 2259
management of, 1975
subjective versus objective, 1974
unilateral, 1974
Tiopronin (Thiola) for preventing stone formation,
885
TIPS. See Transjugular intrahepatic portosystemic
shunt
TIPS mnemonic, 2498
Tissue donation in emergency departments,
2484

Tissue expanders for breast reconstruction, 1110
Tissue load, definition and management of,
1403-1404
Tissue perfusion
cerebral. See Cerebral perfusion
ineffective
after bypass surgery, 1521
after craniotomy, 2089
after stroke, 2123-2124
after tissue transfer, 1427
from AMI, 1719-1720
in anemia, 2284
from burn injuries, 1448-1449
in heart failure, 1666
in hepatic disorders, 1339-1340
in peripheral vascular disease, 1513-1514
in shock, 2470-2471
wound-related, 405
Tissue plasminogen activator, function of,
2244-2245
Tissues
cells of, 202
radiopaque, 98
somatic changes in, 98
TLS. See Tumor lysis syndrome
TMP-SMX. See Trimethoprim-sulfamethoxazole
(Bactrim, TMP-SMX)
TMR. See Transmyocardial revascularization
TNM staging system, 358t
Tobacco, smokeless, 337
Tobacco use. See also Nicotine; Smoking
cancer mortality due to, 335
carcinogenesis due to, 337
decline in, 335
esophageal cancer and, 737
guidelines for, 39t
oral cavity malignancies and, 722
screening/prevention measures for, 11t
surgical client's history of, 265-266
Tocopherol. See Vitamin E
Toenails
care of, 1515
ingrown, 1431
Toes
assessment of, in respiratory disorders, 1750
range of motion of, 572f
Tofranil. See Imipramine (Tofranil)
Toileting, helping clients with, 901
Tolerance
defined, 540t
drug, defined, 444b
Tolterodine (Detrol) for urge incontinence, 899
Tomography, 99-100
of musculoskeletal system, 575
Tongue, assessing, 679
Tonic seizures, 2076, 2077f
Tonic-clonic seizures, 2076
emergency management of, 2499
Tonometry, 1927-1928
Tonsillar herniation syndrome, 2193
Tonsillectomy, 1799
otalgia due to, 1981
Tonsillitis
acute, 1799-1800
chronic, 1800
Tonsilloadenectomy, 1799
Tophi, assessing, 1935
Topical anesthesia, 290, 292t, 293
action, side effects, nursing implications,
292t
Toremifene (Fareston) for preventing breast cancer
metastasis, 1119
Tositumomab (Bexxar) for cancer, 376
Total care nursing, 151
Total enteral nutrition, medical management of,
698-701

Total hip arthroplasty, 585
complications of, 586
nursing management of, 587-593
outcomes of, 586-587
Total joint arthroplasty, fat embolism syndrome
and, 629-630
Total knee arthroplasty, 593-596
continuous passive motion after, 595, 596f
contraindications to, 594
surgical technique for, 594-595
Total lung capacity
decreased, in restrictive lung disorders, 1868
defined, 1735, 1762t
Total lymphocyte count, 682-683
Total nutrient admixture, 706-707
Total parenteral nutrition
indications for, 706b
preoperative, 277
Total parenteral nutrition for inflammatory bowel
disease, 820
Touch, sense of, 1373
assessing, 2032
Tourniquet test
Brodie Trendelenburg, 1481-1482
purpose, normal values, interpretations,
2266t
Toxic dose, defined, 540t
Toxic megacolon, 817
Toxic shock syndrome, characteristics and
management of, 1082
Toxicity states, emergency management of,
2499
Toxins
bacterial, in cerebral infections, 2099-2100
chronic hepatitis due to, 1332b
hepatitis due to, 1334-1335
renal effects of, 916-917, 917b
Toxoplasma infection
of brain, 2100
opportunistic, with HIV infection, 2392
Toxoplasmosis
agent, infection site, reservoir, transmission
of, 420t
causative organism, manifestations, management
of, 2101t
Trabeculectomy for glaucoma, 1948
Trabeculoplasty, laser, for glaucoma, 1948
Trace elements in parenteral nutrition, 706
Trachea
dilation of, 1779
palpation of, 1753
physical findings in healthy adult, 1750
stenosis of, 1779
structure of, 1733
Tracheal wall, necrosis of, 1779
Tracheobronchitis, manifestations/management of,
1829-1830
Tracheoesophageal fistulas, 1779
Tracheoesophageal puncture after laryngectomy,
1793-1794, 1794f
Tracheomalacia, tracheostomy-related, 1779
Tracheostomy, 1775-1786
defined, 1775
dressings for, 1784, 1784f
healed incision after, 1794-1795, 1794f
incision for, 1776f
indications for, 1775-1776
nursing management of, 1781-1786
permanent, 1778-1779
rescue breathing and, 1781
respiratory care for, 1782
speaking valves for, 1778
Tracheostomy buttons, 1778
Tracheostomy tube cuffs
inflation/deflation of, 1777b
problems with, 1779-1780

SPECIAL FEATURES—cont'd